Basic & Clinical

Pharmacology

a LANGE medical book

Basic & Clinical
Pharmacology

sixth edition

Edited by

Bertram G. Katzung, MD, PhD
Professor of Pharmacology
Department of Pharmacology
University of California, San Francisco

APPLETON & LANGE
Norwalk, Connecticut

Notice: The authors and the publisher of this volume have taken care to
make certain that the doses of drugs and schedules of treatment are correct
and compatible with the standards generally accepted at the time of
publication. Nevertheless, as new information becomes available, changes in
treatment and in the use of drugs become necessary. The reader is advised to
carefully consult the instructions and information included in the
package insert of each drug or therapeutic agent before administration.
This advice is especially important when using new or infrequently used drugs.
The author and publisher disclaim any liability, loss, injury, or damage incurred as
a consequence, directly or indirectly, of the use and application of any of
the contents of this volume.

Prentice Hall International (UK) Limited, *London*
Prentice Hall of Australia Pty. Limited, *Sydney*
Prentice Hall Canada, Inc., *Toronto*
Prentice Hall Hispanoamericana, S.A., *Mexico*
Prentice Hall of India Private Limited, *New Delhi*
Prentice Hall of Japan, Inc., *Tokyo*
Simon & Schuster Asia Pte. Ltd., *Singapore*
Editora Prentice Hall do Brasil Ltda., *Rio de Janeiro*
Prentice Hall, Englewood Cliffs, *New Jersey*

ISBN 0–8385–0619–4
ISSN 0891–2033

Acquisitions Editor: John Dolan
Production Editor: Christine Langan
Art Coordinator: Becky Hainz-Baxter

ISBN 0-8385-0619-4

PRINTED IN THE UNITED STATES OF AMERICA

Table of Contents

Preface

This book is designed to provide a complete, authoritative, current, and readable pharmacology text for medical, pharmacy, and other health science students. It also offers special features that make it useful to house officers and practicing clinicians.

Information is organized according to the sequence used in many pharmacology courses: basic principles; autonomic drugs; cardiovascular-renal drugs; drugs with important actions on smooth muscle; central nervous system drugs; drugs used to treat inflammation, gout, and diseases of the blood; endocrine drugs; chemotherapeutic drugs; toxicology; and special topics. This sequence builds new information on information already assimilated. For example, early presentation of autonomic pharmacology allows students to integrate the physiology and neuroscience they know with the pharmacology they are learning and prepares them to understand the autonomic effects of other drugs. This is especially important for the cardiovascular and CNS groups. However, chapters can be used equally well in courses that present these topics in a different sequence.

Within each chapter, emphasis is placed on drug groups and prototypes rather than repetitive detail about individual drugs. We are pleased to see that other pharmacology textbooks are now adopting this approach. The selection and order of presentation of material are based on the accumulated experience of teaching this material to several thousand medical, pharmacy, dental, podiatry, nursing, and other health science students.

Major features that make this book especially useful to professional students include sections that specifically address the clinical choice and use of drugs in patients and the monitoring of their effects; *clinical pharmacology* is an integral part of this text. In addition, lists of the preparations available, including trade and generic names and dosage formulations, are provided at the end of each chapter for easy reference by the house officer or practitioner who is writing a chart order or prescription.

Because of the explosive increase in the number of recognized receptors, receptor nomenclature is unstable at present. In order to minimize discrepancies, we have chosen to use the receptor names given in the 1993 and 1994 issues of *Receptor Nomenclature Supplement* (special annual issues of *Trends in Pharmacological Sciences*) in most cases. Enzymes are named according to the contributor's judgment of the best current usage, usually that of *1992 Enzyme Nomenclature,* Academic Press, 1992.

Significant revisions in this edition include the following:

- Many new figures, some in color, that help to clarify important concepts in pharmacology
- Special interest sections, set off as boxed text, that provide working examples of the text material or serve to point out items of special interest
- Substantial expansion of the coverage of general concepts relating to receptors, including their molecular biology, interactions with drugs, and effector mechanisms in Chapter 2 and other chapters
- Expanded coverage of the enteric nervous system and of newly described muscarinic, norepinephrine, histamine, and serotonin receptors in appropriate chapters
- New sections on the important new fluoroquinolone antibiotics, RU 486, neurotransmitters in the enteric nervous system, current understanding of the GABA receptor, and rational prescribing and prescribing errors
- Recent changes in the clinical management of asthma, congestive heart failure, hypertension, and Alzheimer's disease
- Descriptions of important new drugs released through May 1994
- Revised bibliographies with many new references through 1993

ADDITIONAL SOURCES OF INFORMATION

Pharmacology: Examination & Board Review (Appleton & Lange) provides a succinct review of pharmacology with one of the largest available collections of sample examination questions and answers. It is especially helpful to students preparing for board-type examinations.

Drug Therapy, 2nd ed (Appleton & Lange, 1991), is a pocket-size reference to the properties, prescribing, and use of drugs on hospital wards and in outpatient practice. This clinical manual is designed for students in clinical training, house staff, and practicing physicians.

The widespread acceptance of the first five editions of *Basic & Clinical Pharmacology* over more than a decade suggests that this book fills an important need. We believe that the sixth edition will satisfy this need even more effectively. Spanish, Portuguese, Italian, and Indonesian translations are available. Translations into other languages are under way; the publisher may be contacted for additional information.

I wish to acknowledge the ongoing efforts of my contributing authors and the major contributions of the staff at Appleton & Lange and of our editor, James Ransom.

Suggestions and comments about *Basic & Clinical Pharmacology* are always welcome. They may be sent to me at the Department of Pharmacology, Box 0450, S–1210, University of California, San Francisco, CA 94143–0450.

Bertram G. Katzung, MD, PhD

San Francisco
June 1994

The Authors

David F. Altman, MD
Association of American Medical Colleges, Washington, DC.

Michael J. Aminoff, MD, FRCP
Professor of Neurology and Attending Physician, Department of Neurology, University of California, San Francisco.

Jose Alexandre M. Barbuto, MD, PhD
Visiting Scientist, Department of Medicine, University of Arizona, Arizona Cancer Center, Tucson, Arizona.

Steven L. Barriere, PharmD
Director of Professional Medical Affairs, Synergen, Inc., Boulder, Colorado.

Charles E. Becker, MD
Clinical Professor of Medicine, University of Colorado, Denver.

Leslie Z. Benet, PhD
Professor and Chairman, Department of Pharmacy, School of Pharmacy, University of California, San Francisco.

Neal L. Benowitz, MD
Professor of Medicine and Chief, Division of Clinical Pharmacology and Experimental Therapeutics, Department of Medicine, University of California, San Francisco.

Barry A. Berkowitz, PhD
President and CEO, Myco Pharmaceuticals, Inc, Cambridge, Massachusetts.

Daniel D. Bikle, MD, PhD
Professor of Medicine, Department of Medicine, and Co-director, Special Diagnostic and Treatment Unit, University of California, San Francisco, and Veterans Administration Medical Center, San Francisco.

Henry R. Bourne, MD
Professor, Departments of Pharmacology and Medicine, University of California, San Francisco.

Homer A. Boushey, MD
Professor of Medicine, Department of Medicine, University of California, San Francisco.

Alan Burkhalter, PhD
Professor of Pharmacology, Department of Pharmacology, University of California, San Francisco.

Kanu Chatterjee, MB, FRCP
Lucie Stern Professor of Cardiology and Professor of Medicine, Cardiology Division, Department of Medicine, University of California, San Francisco.

Martin S. Cohen, MD
Director of Pediatrics, Scenic General Hospital, Modesto, California.

Maria Almira Correia, PhD
Professor of Pharmacology, Department of Pharmacology, University of California, San Francisco.

Betty J. Dong, PharmD
Clinical Professor of Pharmacy and Family and Community Medicine, Schools of Pharmacology and Medicine, University of California, San Francisco.

Howard L. Fields, MD, PhD
Professor of Neurology and Physiology, Departments of Neurology and Physiology, University of California, San Francisco.

Marie L. Foegh, MD
Associate Professor, Department of Surgery, Georgetown University Medical Center, Washington.

Oscar L. Frick, MD, PhD
Professor of Pediatrics and Co-director, Allergy-Immunology Research and Training, Department of Pediatrics, University of California, San Francisco.

Alan Goldfien, MD
Professor of Medicine, Departments of Medicine, Obstetrics, Gynecology and Reproductive Sciences, and Senior Staff Member, Cardiovascular Research Institute, University of California, San Francisco.

Robert S. Goldsmith, MD, DTM&H
Professor of Tropical Medicine and Epidemiology, Department of Epidemiology and International Health, University of California, San Francisco.

Francis S. Greenspan, MD
Clinical Professor of Medicine and Radiology, Department of Medicine, and Chief, Thyroid Clinic, University of California, San Francisco.

Philip D. Hansten, PharmD
Professor of Clinical Pharmacy, Department of Pharmacy, Washington State University College of Pharmacy, Pullman, Washington.

Markus Hecker, PhD
Associate Professor of Physiology, Johann Wolfgang Goethe-University Clinic, Frankfurt am Main, Germany.

Evan M. Hersh, MD
Professor of Medicine, Department of Medicine, University of Arizona, and Chief, Hematology/Oncology, Arizona Cancer Center, Tucson, Arizona.

Brian B. Hoffman, MD
Professor of Medicine and Pharmacology, Stanford University School of Medicine, Stanford, California, and Veterans Administration Medical Center, Palo Alto, California.

Nicholas H.G. Holford, MB, ChB, MSc, MRCP(UK), FRACP
Senior Lecturer, Department of Pharmacology and Clinical Pharmacology, University of Auckland Medical School, Auckland, New Zealand.

Leo E. Hollister, MD
Professor of Psychiatry and Pharmacology, University of Texas Medical School, Houston, and Medical Director, Harris County Psychiatric Center, Houston.

Luc M. Hondeghem, MD, PhD
President and CEO, Hondeghem Pharmaceutical Consulting NV, Oostende, Belgium

Harlan E. Ives, MD, PhD
Professor of Medicine, Department of Medicine, University of California, San Francisco.

Richard A. Jacobs, MD, PhD
Associate Clinical Professor of Medicine, Department of Medicine, University of California, San Francisco.

Ernest Jawetz, MD, PhD
Professor of Microbiology and Medicine, Department of Microbiology, University of California, San Francisco.

David J. Julius, PhD
Assistant Professor of Pharmacology, Department of Pharmacology, University of California, San Francisco.

John P. Kane MD, PhD
Professor of Medicine, Department of Medicine, University of California, San Francisco.

John H. Karam, MD
Professor of Medicine, Co-director of Diabetes Clinic, and Chief of Clinical Endocrinology, University of California, San Francisco.

Bertram G. Katzung, MD, PhD
Professor of Pharmacology, Department of Pharmacology, University of California, San Francisco.

Mary Anne Koda-Kimble, PharmD
Professor of Clinical Pharmacy and Vice Chairman, Division of Clinical Pharmacy, School of Pharmacy, University of California, San Francisco.

David C. Klonoff, MD
Associate Clinical Professor of Medicine, Department of Medicine, University of California, San Francisco.

Gideon Koren, MD
Associate Professor of Pediatrics, Pharmacology, and Pharmacy, Departments of Pediatrics, Pharmacology, and Pharmacy, University of Toronto, Canada.

Nancy M. Lee, PhD
Professor of Pharmacology, Department of Pharmacology, University of Minnesota, Minneapolis.

Paul W. Lofholm, PharmD
Clinical Professor of Pharmacy, School of Pharmacy, University of California, San Francisco.

Howard I. Maibach, MD
Professor of Dermatology, Department of Dermatology, University of California, San Francisco.

Mary J. Malloy, MD
Clinical Professor of Pediatrics and Medicine, Departments of Pediatrics and Medicine, University of California, San Francisco.

Brian S. Meldrum, MB, PhD
Professor of Experimental Neurology, Department of Neurology, Institute of Psychiatry, London.

Ronald D. Miller, MD
Professor and Chairman of Anesthesia and Professor of Pharmacology, Department of Anesthesia, University of California, San Francisco.

Roger A. Nicoll, MD
Professor of Pharmacology and Physiology, Departments of Pharmacology and Physiology, University of California, San Francisco.

Kent R. Olson, MD
Associate Clinical Professor of Medicine and Adjunct Lecturer in Pharmacy, University of California, San Francisco, and Director, San Francisco Bay Area Regional Poison Control Center.

Robert A. O'Reilly, MD
Chairman, Department of Medicine, Santa Clara Valley Medical Center, Professor of Medicine, Stanford University School of Medicine, Stanford, California, and Clinical Professor of Medicine, Department of Medicine, University of California, San Francisco.

Achilles J. Pappano, PhD
Professor and Chairman, Department of Pharmacology, University of Connecticut, Farmington

William W. Parmley, MD
Professor of Medicine, Department of Medicine, Cardiology Division, University of California, San Francisco, and Chief of Cardiology, Herbert C. Moffitt Hospital, San Francisco.

Donald G. Payan, MD
Chief Science Officer, Khepri Pharmaceuticals, Inc, South San Francisco, California.

Gabriel L. Plaa, PhD
Professeur Titulaire de Pharmacologie, Département de Pharmacologie, Faculté de Médecine, Université de Montréal.

Roger J. Porter, MD
Vice President for Clinical Pharmacology, Wyeth-Ayerst Research, Philadelphia.

Peter W. Ramwell, PhD
Professor, Department of Physiology and Biophysics, Georgetown University Medical Center, Washington.

Ian A. Reid, PhD
Professor of Physiology, Department of Physiology, University of California, San Francisco.

Curt A. Ries, MD
Clinical Professor of Medicine and Hematology-Oncology, Department of Medicine, University of California, San Francisco.

James M. Roberts, MD
Professor of Obstetrics, Department of Obstetrics, Magee Women's Research Institute, Pittsburgh.

Dirk B. Robertson, MD
Associate Professor of Dermatology, Department of Dermatology, Emory University School of Medicine, Atlanta.

Sydney E. Salmon, MD
Professor of Internal Medicine and of Hematology and Oncology, University of Arizona College of Medicine, Tucson, Arizona, and Director of Arizona Cancer Center, Tucson, Arizona.

Daniel V. Santi, MD, PhD
Professor of Biochemistry and Pharmaceutical Chemistry, Departments of Biochemistry and Biophysics and Pharmaceutical Chemistry, University of California, San Francisco.

Alan C. Sartorelli, PhD
Alfred Gilman Professor of Pharmacology, and Director, Comprehensive Cancer Center, Yale University School of Medicine, New Haven.

Anthony J Trevor, PhD
Professor of Pharmacology and Toxicology, Department of Pharmacology, University of California, San Francisco.

Ching Chung Wang, PhD
Professor of Chemistry and Pharmaceutical Chemistry, Department of Pharmaceutical Chemistry, University of California, San Francisco.

David G. Warnock, MD
Professor of Medicine and Physiology, Departments of Medicine and Physiology, and Director, Division of Nephrology, University of Alabama in Birmingham, Alabama.

August M. Watanabe, MD
Professor of Medicine and Pharmacology, Indiana University School of Medicine, and Vice President, Lilly Research Laboratories, Indianapolis.

E. Leong Way, PhD
Professor Emeritus of Pharmacology, Toxicology, and Pharmaceutical Chemistry, Department of Pharmacology, University of California, San Francisco.

Walter L. Way, MD
Professor of Anesthesia and Pharmacology, Department of Anesthesia, University of California, San Francisco.

Section I.
Basic Principles

Introduction

1

Bertram G. Katzung, MD, PhD

Pharmacology can be defined as the study of substances that interact with living systems through chemical processes, especially by binding to regulatory molecules and activating or inhibiting normal body processes. These substances may be chemicals administered to achieve a beneficial therapeutic effect on some process within the patient or for their toxic effects on regulatory processes in parasites infecting the patient. Such deliberate therapeutic applications may be considered the proper role of **medical pharmacology,** which is often defined as the science of substances used to prevent, diagnose, and treat disease. **Toxicology** is that branch of pharmacology that deals with the undesirable effects of chemicals on living systems, from individual cells to complex ecosystems.

History

Prehistoric people undoubtedly recognized the beneficial or toxic effects of many plant and animal materials. The earliest written records from China and from Egypt list remedies of many types, including a few still recognized today as useful drugs. Most, however, were worthless or actually harmful. In the 2500 years or so preceding the modern era there were sporadic attempts to introduce rational methods into medicine, but none were successful owing to the dominance of systems of thought that purported to explain all of biology and disease without the need for painstaking experimentation and observation. These schools promulgated bizarre notions such as the idea that disease was caused by excesses of bile or blood in the body, that wounds could be healed by applying a salve to the weapon that caused the wound, etc.

Around the end of the 17th century, reliance on observation and experimentation began to replace theorizing in medicine as well as in the physical sciences. As the value of these methods in the study of disease became clear, physicians in Great Britain and else-

where in Europe began to apply them to the effects of traditional drugs used in their own practices. Thus, *pharmacotherapy,* the medical use of drugs, began to develop as the precursor to pharmacology. However, any understanding of the mechanisms of action of drugs was still prevented by the absence of methods for purifying active agents from the crude remedies that were available and—even more—by the lack of methods for testing hypotheses about the nature of drug actions. However, in the late 18th and early 19th centuries, François Magendie and later his student Claude Bernard began to develop the methods of experimental animal physiology and pharmacology. Advances in chemistry and the further development of physiology in the 18th and 19th centuries laid the foundation needed for understanding how drugs work at the organ and tissue levels. Paradoxically, real advances in basic pharmacology during the 19th century were accompanied by an outburst of unscientific promotion by manufacturers and marketers of worthless "patent medicines." It was not until the concepts of rational therapeutics, especially that of the controlled clinical trial, were reintroduced into medicine—about 50 years ago—that it became possible to accurately evaluate therapeutic claims.

About 50 years ago, there also began a major expansion of research efforts in all areas of biology. As new concepts and new techniques were introduced, information accumulated about drug action and the biologic substrate of that action, the receptor. During this half-century, many fundamentally new drug groups and new members of old groups have been introduced. The last 3 decades have seen an even more rapid growth of information and understanding of the molecular basis for drug action. The molecular mechanisms of action of many drugs have now been identified, and numerous receptors have been isolated, structurally characterized, and cloned. Much of that progress is summarized in this book.

The extension of scientific principles into everyday therapeutics is still going on, though the consuming public, unfortunately, is still exposed to vast amounts of inaccurate, incomplete, or unscientific information regarding the pharmacologic effects of chemicals. This has resulted in the faddish use of innumerable expensive, ineffective, and sometimes harmful remedies and the growth of a huge "alternative health care" industry. Conversely, lack of understanding of basic scientific principles in biology and statistics and the absence of critical thinking about public health issues has led to rejection of medical science by a segment of the public and a tendency to assume that all adverse drug effects are the result of malpractice.

The Nature of Drugs

In the most general sense, a drug may be defined as any substance that brings about a change in biologic function through its chemical actions. In the great majority of cases, the drug molecule interacts with a specific molecule in the biologic system that plays, as noted above, a regulatory role, ie, a **receptor** molecule. The nature of receptors is discussed more fully in Chapter 2. In a very small number of cases, drugs known as chemical antagonists may interact directly with other drugs, while a few drugs (eg, osmotic agents) interact almost exclusively with water molecules. Drugs may be synthesized within the body (eg, hormones) or may be chemicals *not* synthesized in the body, ie, xenobiotics (from Gr *xenos* "stranger"). Poisons are drugs. Toxins are usually defined as poisons of biologic origin, ie, synthesized by plants or animals, in contrast to inorganic poisons such as lead and arsenic.

In order to interact chemically with its receptor, a drug molecule must have the appropriate size, electrical charge, shape, and atomic composition. Furthermore, a drug is often administered at a location distant from its intended site of action, eg, a pill given orally to relieve a headache. Therefore, a useful drug must have the necessary properties to be transported from its site of administration to its site of action. Finally, a practical drug should be inactivated or excreted from the body at a reasonable rate so that its actions will be of appropriate duration.

A. The Physical Nature of Drugs: Drugs may be solid at room temperature (eg, aspirin, atropine), liquid (eg, nicotine, ethanol), or gaseous (eg, nitrous oxide). These factors often determine the best route of administration. For example, some liquid drugs are easily vaporized and can be inhaled in that form, eg, halothane, amyl nitrite. The common routes of administration are discussed in Chapter 3. The various classes of organic compounds—carbohydrates, proteins, lipids, and their constituents—are all represented in pharmacology. Many drugs are weak acids or bases. This fact has important implications for the way they are handled by the body, because pH differences in the various compartments of the body may alter the degree of ionization of such drugs (see below).

B. Drug Size: The molecular size of drugs in current use varies from very small (lithium ion, MW 7) to very large (eg, alteplase [t-PA], a protein of MW 59,050). However, the vast majority of drugs have molecular weights between 100 and 1000. The lower limit of this narrow range is probably set by the requirements for specificity of action. In order to have a good "fit" to only one type of receptor, a drug molecule must be sufficiently unique in shape, charge, etc, to prevent its binding to other receptors. To achieve such selective binding, it appears that a molecule should in most cases be at least 100 MW units in size. The upper limit in molecular weight is determined primarily by the requirement that drugs be able to move within the body (eg, from site of administration to site of action). Drugs much larger than MW 1000 will not diffuse readily between compartments of the body (see Permeation, below). Therefore, very large drugs (usually proteins) must be administered directly into the compartment where they have their effect. In the case of alteplase, a clot-dissolving enzyme, the drug is administered directly into the vascular compartment by intravenous infusion.

C. Drug Reactivity and Drug-Receptor Bonds: Drugs interact with receptors by means of chemical forces or bonds. These are of three major types: covalent, electrostatic, and hydrophobic. Covalent bonds are very strong and in many cases not reversible under biologic conditions. Thus, the covalent bond formed between the activated form of phenoxybenzamine and the alpha receptor for norepinephrine (which results in blockade of the receptor) is not readily broken. The blocking effect of phenoxybenzamine lasts long after the free drug has disappeared from the bloodstream and is reversed only by the synthesis of new alpha receptors, a process that takes about 48 hours. Other examples of highly reactive, covalent bond-forming drugs are the DNA-alkylating agents used in cancer chemotherapy to disrupt cell division in the neoplastic tissue.

Electrostatic bonding is much more common than covalent bonding in drug-receptor interactions. Electrostatic bonds vary from relatively strong linkages between permanently charged ionic molecules to weaker hydrogen bonds and very weak induced dipole interactions such as van der Waals forces and similar phenomena. Electrostatic bonds are weaker than covalent bonds.

Hydrophobic bonds are usually quite weak and are probably important in the interactions of highly lipid-soluble drugs with the lipids of cell membranes and perhaps in the interaction of drugs with the internal walls of receptor "pockets."

The specific nature of a particular drug-receptor bond is of less practical importance than the fact that drugs which bind through weak bonds to their receptors are generally more selective than drugs which bind through very strong bonds. This is because weak bonds require a very precise fit of the drug to its receptor if an interaction is to occur. Only a few receptor types are likely to provide such a precise fit for a particular drug structure. Thus, if we wished to design a highly selective short-acting drug for a particular receptor, we would avoid highly reactive molecules that form covalent bonds and instead choose molecules that form weaker bonds.

A few substances that are almost completely inert in the chemical sense nevertheless have significant pharmacologic effects. For example, xenon, an "inert gas," has anesthetic effects at elevated pressures.

D. Drug Shape: The shape of a drug molecule must be such as to permit binding to its receptor site. Optimally, the drug's shape is complementary to that of the receptor site in the same way that a key is complementary to a lock. Furthermore, the phenomenon of **chirality** (stereoisomerism) is so common in biology that more than half of all useful drugs are chiral molecules, ie, they exist as enantiomeric pairs. Drugs with two asymmetric centers have four diastereomers, eg, labetalol, an alpha- and beta-receptor-blocking drug. In the great majority of cases, one of these enantiomers will be much more effective than its mirror image enantiomer, reflecting a better fit to the receptor molecule. For example, the $S(+)$ enantiomer of methacholine, a parasympathomimetic drug, is over 250 times more potent than the $R(-)$ enantiomer. If one imagines the receptor site to be like a glove into which the drug molecule must fit to bring about its effect, it is clear why a "left-oriented" drug will be more effective in binding to a left-hand receptor than will its "right-oriented" enantiomer.

The more active enantiomer at one type of receptor site may not be more active at another type, eg, a receptor type that may be responsible for some unwanted effect. For example, carvedilol, a drug that interacts with adrenoceptors, has a single chiral center and thus two enantiomers (Table 1–1). One of these enantiomers, the $S(-)$ isomer, is a potent beta receptor blocker. The $R(+)$ isomer is 100-fold weaker at the beta receptor. However, the isomers are approximately equipotent as alpha receptor blockers. Ketamine is an intravenous anesthetic. The $(+)$ enantiomer is a more potent anesthetic and is less toxic than the $(-)$ enantiomer. Unfortunately, the drug is still used as the racemic mixture.

Finally, because enzymes are usually stereoselective, one drug enantiomer is often more susceptible than the other to drug-metabolizing enzymes. As a result, the duration of action of one enantiomer may be quite different from that of the other.

Unfortunately, most studies of clinical efficacy and drug elimination in humans have been carried out with racemic mixtures of drugs rather than with the separate enantiomers. At present, only about 45% of the chiral drugs used clinically are marketed as the active isomer—the rest are available only as racemic mixtures. As a result, many patients are receiving drug doses of which 50% or more is either inactive or actively toxic. However, there is increasing interest—at both the scientific and the regulatory levels—in making more chiral drugs available as their active enantiomers.

E. Rational Drug Design: Rational design of drugs implies the ability to predict the appropriate molecular structure of a drug on the basis of information about its biologic receptor. Until recently, no receptor was known in sufficient detail to permit such drug design. Instead, drugs were developed through random testing of chemicals or modification of drugs already known to have some effect (Chapter 5). However, during the past 2 decades, many receptors have been isolated and characterized. A few drugs now in use were developed through molecular design based on a knowledge of the three-dimensional structure of the receptor site. Computer programs are now available that can iteratively optimize drug structures to fit known receptors. As more becomes known about receptor structure, rational drug design will become more feasible.

Drug-Body Interactions

The interactions between a drug and the body are conveniently divided into two classes. The actions of the drug on the body are termed **pharmacodynamic** processes and are presented in greater detail in Chapter 2. These properties determine the group in which the drug is classified and often play the major role in deciding whether that group is appropriate therapy for a particular symptom or disease. The actions of the body on the drug are called **pharmacokinetic** processes and are described in Chapters 3 and 4. Pharmacokinetic processes govern the absorption, distribution, and elimination of drugs and are of great practical importance in the choice and administration of a particular drug for a particular patient, eg, one with impaired renal function. The following paragraphs provide a brief introduction to pharmacodynamics and pharmacokinetics.

Table 1–1. Dissociation constants (K_d) of the enantiomers and racemate of carvedilol. The K_d is the concentration for 50% saturation of the receptors and is inversely proportionate to the affinity of the drug for the receptors.[1]

Form of Carvedilol	Inverse of Affinity for Alpha Receptors (K_d, nmol/L)	Inverse of Affinity for Beta Receptors (K_d, nmol/L)
$R(+)$ enantiomer	14	45
$S(-)$ enantiomer	16	0.4
$R,S(+/-)$	11	0.9

[1]Data from Ruffolo RR et al: The pharmacology of carvedilol. Eur J Pharmacol 1990;38:S82.

Pharmacodynamic Principles

As noted above, most drugs must bind to a receptor to bring about an effect. However, at the molecular level, drug binding is only the first in what is often a complex sequence of steps.

A. Types of Drug-Receptor Interactions: **Agonist** drugs bind to and *activate* the receptor in some fashion, which directly or indirectly brings about the effect. Some receptors incorporate effector machinery in the same molecule, so that drug binding brings about the effect directly, eg, opening of an ion channel or activation of enzyme activity. Other receptors are linked through one or more intervening **coupling molecules** to a separate **effector molecule.** The several types of drug-receptor-effector coupling systems are discussed in Chapter 2. Pharmacologic **antagonist** drugs, by binding to a receptor, *prevent* binding by other molecules. For example, acetylcholine receptor blockers such as atropine are antagonists because they prevent access of acetylcholine and similar agonist drugs to the acetylcholine receptor. These agents reduce the effects of acetylcholine and similar drugs in the body. In contrast, drugs that prevent the binding of acetylcholine to acetylcholinesterase (cholinesterase inhibitors) slow down the normal termination of action of acetylcholine released in the body and greatly increase the action of this neurotransmitter. Thus, cholinesterase inhibitors have actions in the patient that resemble those of acetylcholine receptor agonists.

B. Duration of Drug Action: Termination of drug action at the receptor level results from one of several processes. In some cases, the effect lasts only as long as the drug occupies the receptor, so that dissociation of drug from the receptor automatically terminates the effect. In many cases, however, the action may persist after the drug has dissociated, because, for example, some coupling molecule is still present in activated form. In the case of drugs that bind covalently to the receptor, the effect may persist until the drug-receptor complex is destroyed and new receptors are synthesized, as described previously for phenoxybenzamine. Finally, some receptor-effector systems incorporate **desensitization** mechanisms for preventing excessive activation when drug molecules continue to be present for long periods. See Chapter 2 for additional details.

C. Receptors and Inert Binding Sites: To function as a receptor, an endogenous molecule must first be selective in choosing ligands (drug molecules) to bind; and second, it must change its function upon binding in such a way that the function of the biologic system (cell, tissue, etc) is altered. The first characteristic is required to avoid constant activation of the receptor by promiscuous binding of large numbers of ligands. The second characteristic is clearly necessary if the ligand is to cause a pharmacologic effect. The body contains many molecules that are capable of binding drugs, however, and not all of these endogenous molecules are regulatory molecules. Binding of a drug to a nonregulatory molecule such as plasma albumin will result in no detectable change in the function of the biologic system, so the endogenous molecule can be called an inert binding site. Such binding is not completely without significance, however, since it affects the distribution of drug within the body and will determine the amount of free drug in the circulation. Both of these factors are of pharmacokinetic importance (see below and Chapter 3).

Pharmacokinetic Principles

In practical therapeutics, a drug should be able to reach its intended site of action after administration by some convenient route. In only a few situations is it possible to directly apply a drug to its target tissue, eg, by topical application of an anti-inflammatory agent to inflamed skin or mucous membrane. In other cases, drugs may be given intravenously and circulate in the blood directly to target blood vessels in another part of the body where they bring about useful effects. Much more commonly, a drug is given into one body compartment, eg, the gut, and must move to its site of action in another compartment, eg, the brain. This requires that the drug be **absorbed** into the blood from its site of administration and **distributed** to its site of action, **permeating** through the various barriers that separate these compartments. For a drug given orally to produce an effect in the central nervous system, these barriers include the tissues that comprise the wall of the intestine, the walls of the capillaries that perfuse the gut, and the "blood-brain barrier," the walls of the capillaries that perfuse the brain. Finally, after bringing about its effect, a drug should be **eliminated** at a reasonable rate by metabolic inactivation, by excretion from the body, or by a combination of these processes.

A. Permeation: Drug permeation proceeds by four primary mechanisms. Passive diffusion in an aqueous or lipid medium is most common, but active processes play a role in the movement of some drugs, especially those whose molecules are too large to diffuse readily.

1. Aqueous diffusion–Aqueous diffusion occurs within the larger aqueous compartments of the body (interstitial space, cytosol, etc) and across epithelial membrane tight junctions and the endothelial lining of blood vessels through aqueous pores that permit the passage of molecules as large as MW 20,000–30,000.* Aqueous diffusion of drug molecules is usually driven by the concentration gradient of the permeating drug, a downhill movement described by Fick's law (see below). Drug molecules

---

*The capillaries of the brain and the testes are characterized by an absence of the pores that permit aqueous diffusion of many drug molecules into the tissue. These tissues are therefore "protected" or "sanctuary" sites from many circulating drugs.

that are bound to large plasma proteins (eg, albumin) will not permeate these aqueous pores. If the drug is charged, its flux is also influenced by electrical fields (eg, the membrane potential and—in parts of the nephron—the transtubular potential).

2. Lipid diffusion–Lipid diffusion is the most important limiting factor for drug permeation because of the large number of lipid barriers that separate the compartments of the body. Because these lipid barriers separate aqueous compartments, the lipid:aqueous partition coefficient of a drug determines how readily the molecule moves between aqueous and lipid media. In the case of weak acids and weak bases (which gain or lose electrical charge-bearing protons, depending on the pH), the ability to move from aqueous to lipid or vice versa varies with the pH of the medium, because charged molecules attract water molecules. The ratio of lipid-soluble form to aqueous-soluble form for a weak acid or weak base is expressed by the Henderson-Hasselbalch equation (see below).

3. Special carriers–Special carrier molecules exist for certain substances that are important for cell function and too large or too insoluble in lipid to diffuse passively through membranes, eg, peptides, amino acids, glucose. These carriers bring about movement by active transport or facilitated diffusion and, unlike passive diffusion, are saturable and inhibitable. Because many drugs are or resemble such naturally occurring peptides, amino acids, or sugars, they can use these carriers to cross membranes.

4. Endocytosis and exocytosis–A few substances are so large that they can enter cells only by endocytosis, the process by which the substance is engulfed by the cell membrane and carried into the cell by pinching off of the newly formed vesicle inside the membrane. The substance can then be released inside the cytosol by breakdown of the vesicle membrane. This process is responsible for the transport of iron and vitamin B_{12}, each complexed with appropriate binding proteins, across the wall of the gut into the blood. The reverse process (exocytosis) is responsible for the secretion of many substances from cells. For example, many neurotransmitter substances are stored in membrane-bound vesicles in nerve endings to protect them from metabolic destruction in the cytoplasm. Appropriate activation of the nerve ending causes fusion of the storage vesicle with the cell membrane and expulsion of its contents into the extracellular space.

B. Fick's Law of Diffusion: The passive flux of molecules down a concentration gradient is given by Fick's law:

$$\text{Flux (molecules per unit time)} =$$

$$(C_1 - C_2) \times \frac{\text{Area} \times \text{Permeability coefficient}}{\text{Thickness}}$$

where C_1 is the higher concentration, C_2 is the lower concentration, area is the area across which diffusion is occurring, permeability coefficient is a measure of the mobility of the drug molecules in the medium of the diffusion path, and thickness is the thickness (length) of the diffusion path. In the case of lipid diffusion, the lipid:aqueous partition coefficient is a major determinant of mobility of the drug, since it determines how readily the drug enters the lipid membrane from the aqueous medium.

C. Ionization of Weak Acids and Weak Bases: The electrostatic charge of an ionized molecule attracts water dipoles and results in a polar, relatively water-soluble and lipid-insoluble complex. Since lipid diffusion depends on relatively high lipid solubility, ionization of drugs may markedly reduce their ability to permeate membranes. A very large fraction of the drugs in use are weak acids or weak bases (Table 1–2). For drugs, a weak acid is best defined as a neutral molecule that can reversibly dissociate into an anion (a negatively charged molecule) and a proton (a hydrogen ion). For example, aspirin dissociates as follows:

$$C_8H_7O_2COOH \rightleftharpoons C_8H_7O_2COO^- + H^+$$

| **Neutral aspirin** | **Aspirin anion** | **Proton** |

A drug that is a weak base can be defined as a neutral molecule that can form a cation (a positively charged molecule) by combining with a proton. For example, pyrimethamine, an antimalarial drug, undergoes the following association-dissociation process:

$$C_{12}H_{11}ClN_3NH_3^+ \rightleftharpoons C_{12}H_{11}ClN_3NH_2 + H^+$$

| **Pyrimethamine cation** | **Neutral pyrimethamine** | **Proton** |

Note that the protonated form of a weak acid is the neutral, more lipid-soluble form, whereas the unprotonated form of a weak base is the neutral form. The law of mass action requires that these reactions move to the left in an acid environment (low pH, excess protons available) and to the right in a basic environment. The Henderson-Hasselbalch equation relates the ratio of protonated to unprotonated weak acid or weak base to the molecule's pK_a and the pH of the medium as follows:

$$\log \frac{\text{(Protonated)}}{\text{(Unprotonated)}} = pK_a - pH$$

This equation applies to both acidic and basic drugs. Inspection confirms that the lower the pH relative to the pK_a, the greater will be the fraction of drug in the protonated form. Because the uncharged form

Table 1–2. Ionization constants of some common drugs.

Drug	pKa[1]	Drug	pKa[1]	Drug	pKa[1]
Weak acids		**Weak bases (cont'd)**		**Weak bases (cont'd)**	
Acetaminophen	9.5	Amiloride	8.7	Methadone	8.4
Acetazolamide	7.2	Amphetamine	9.8	Methamphetamine	10.0
Ampicillin	2.5	Atropine	9.7	Methyldopa	10.6
Aspirin	3.5	Bupivacaine	8.1	Methysergide	6.6
Chlorothiazide	6.8, 9.4[2]	Chlordiazepoxide	4.6	Metoprolol	9.8
Chlorpropamide	5.0	Chloroquine	10.8, 8.4[2]	Morphine	7.9
Cromolyn	2.0	Chlorpheniramine	9.2	Nicotine	7.9, 3.1[2]
Ethacrynic acid	3.5	Chlorpromazine	9.3	Norepinephrine	8.6
Furosemide	3.9	Clonidine	8.3	Pentazocine	9.7
Ibuprofen	4.4, 5.2[2]	Cocaine	8.5	Phenylephrine	9.8
Levodopa	2.3	Codeine	8.2	Physostigmine	7.9, 1.8[2]
Methotrexate	4.8	Cyclizine	8.2	Pilocarpine	6.9, 1.4[2]
Methyldopa	2.2, 9.2[2]	Desipramine	10.2	Pindolol	8.8
Penicillamine	1.8	Diazepam	3.3	Procainamide	9.2
Pentobarbital	8.1	Dihydrocodeine	8.8	Procaine	9.0
Phenobarbital	7.4	Diphenhydramine	9.0	Promazine	9.4
Phenytoin	8.3	Diphenoxylate	7.1	Promethazine	9.1
Propylthiouracil	8.3	Ephedrine	9.6	Propranolol	9.4
Salicylic acid	3.0	Epinephrine	8.7	Pseudoephedrine	9.8
Sulfadiazine	6.5	Ergotamine	6.3	Pyrimethamine	7.0
Sulfapyridine	8.4	Fluphenazine	8.0, 3.9[2]	Quinidine	8.5, 4.4[2]
Theophylline	8.8[2]	Guanethidine	11.4, 8.3[2]	Scopolamine	8.1
Tolbutamide	5.3	Hydralazine	7.1	Strychnine	8.0, 2.3[2]
Warfarin	5.0	Imipramine	9.5	Terbutaline	10.1
Weak bases		Isoproterenol	8.6	Thioridazine	9.5
Albuterol (salbutamol)	9.3	Kanamycin	7.2	Tolazoline	10.6
Allopurinol	9.4, 12.3[2]	Lidocaine	7.9		
Alprenolol	9.6	Metaraminol	8.6		

[1]The pKa is that pH at which the concentrations of the ionized and un-ionized forms are equal.
[2] More than one ionizable group.

is the more lipid-soluble, more of a weak acid will be in the lipid-soluble form at acid pH, while more of a basic drug will be in the lipid-soluble form at alkaline pH.

The most important application of this principle is in the manipulation of drug excretion by the kidney. Almost all drugs are filtered at the glomerulus. If a drug is in a lipid-soluble form during its passage down the renal tubule, a significant fraction will be reabsorbed by simple passive diffusion. If the goal is to accelerate excretion of the drug, it is important to prevent its reabsorption from the tubule. This can often be accomplished by adjusting urine pH to make certain that most of the drug is in the ionized state, as shown in Figure 1–1. As a result of this pH partitioning effect, the drug will be "trapped" in the urine. Thus, weak acids will usually be excreted faster in alkaline urine; weak bases are usually excreted faster in acid urine. Other body fluids in which pH differences from blood pH may cause trapping or reabsorption are the contents of the stomach and small intestine; breast milk; aqueous humor; and vaginal and prostatic secretions (Table 1–3).

As suggested by Table 1–2, a large number of drugs are weak bases. Most of these bases are amine-containing molecules. The nitrogen of a neutral amine has three atoms associated with it plus a pair of unshared electrons. The three atoms may consist of one carbon and two hydrogens (a *primary* amine),

two carbons and one hydrogen (a *secondary* amine), or three carbon atoms (a *tertiary* amine). Each of these three forms may reversibly bind a proton with the unshared electrons. A fourth carbon-nitrogen bond may be formed, resulting in a *quaternary* amine. However, the quaternary amine is permanently charged and has no unshared electrons with which to reversibly bind a proton. Therefore, primary, secondary, and tertiary amines may undergo reversible protonation and vary their lipid solubility with pH, but quaternary amines are always in the poorly lipid-soluble charged form.

Primary	Secondary	Tertiary	Quaternary
H	R	R	R
R:N:	R:N:	R:N:	R:N:⁺ R
H	H	R	R

Drug Groups

To learn each pertinent fact about each of the many hundreds of drugs mentioned in this book would be an impractical goal and, fortunately, is in any case unnecessary. Almost all of the several thousand drugs currently available can be arranged in about 70 groups. Many of the drugs within each group are very similar in pharmacodynamic actions and often in their pharmacokinetic properties as well. For most groups, one or more prototype drugs can be identified that typify the most important characteristics of the group.

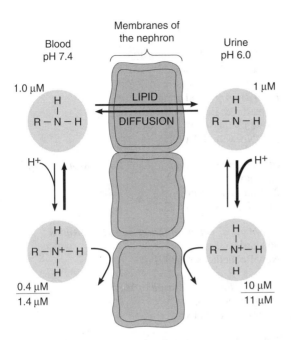

Figure 1–1. Trapping of a weak base (pyrimethamine) in the urine when the urine is more acidic than the blood. In the hypothetical case illustrated, the diffusible uncharged form of the drug has equilibrated across the membrane but the total concentration (charged plus uncharged) in the urine is almost eight times higher than in the blood.

This permits classification of other important drugs in the group as variants of the prototype, so that only the prototype must be learned in detail and, for the remaining drugs, only the differences from the prototype.

Sources of Information

Students who wish to review the field of pharmacology in preparation for an examination are referred to *Pharmacology: Examination and Board Review,* by Katzung and Trevor (Appleton & Lange, 1995). *Drug Therapy,* edited by the present author (Appleton & Lange, 1991), is intended for use by house officers and practitioners who need ready access to a compendium of available drugs and drug doses.

The references at the end of each chapter in this book were selected to provide information specific to those chapters. Three textbooks (listed alphabetically below) provide more general discussions and more extensive reference lists.

Bowman WC, Rand MJ: *Textbook of Pharmacology,* 2nd ed. Blackwell Scientific, 1980. (A large textbook with a chemical and comparative pharmacology orientation.)

Gilman AG et al (editors): *Goodman and Gilman's The Pharmacological Basis of Therapeutics,* 8th ed. Pergamon, 1990. (A large textbook with a medical orientation.)

Pratt WB, Taylor P: *Principles of Drug Action. The Basis of Therapeutics,* 3rd ed. Churchill Livingstone, 1990. (A specialized text emphasizing general principles: receptor concepts, dose-response principles, pharmacokinetics, and biochemical toxicology.)

Specific questions relating to basic or clinical research are best answered by resort to the general pharmacology and clinical specialty serials. Three periodicals can be recommended as especially useful sources of current information about drugs: *The New England Journal of Medicine,* which publishes much original drug-related research as well as frequent reviews of topics in pharmacology; *The Medical Letter on Drugs and Therapeutics,* which publishes brief critical reviews of new and old therapies, mostly pharmacologic; and *Drugs,* which publishes extensive reviews of drugs and drug groups.

Other sources of information pertinent to the USA should be mentioned as well. The "package insert" is a summary of information the manufacturer is required to place in the prescription sales package; *Physicians' Desk Reference (PDR)* is a compendium of

Body Fluid	Range of pH	Total Fluid: Blood Concentration Ratios for Sulfadiazine (acid, pK$_a$ 6.5)[1]	Total Fluid: Blood Concentration Ratios for Pyrimethamine (base, pK$_a$ 7.0)[1]
Urine	5.0–8.0	0.12–4.65	72.24–0.79
Breast milk	6.4–7.6[2]	0.2–1.77	3.56–0.89
Jejunum, ileum contents	7.5–8.0[3]	1.23–3.54	0.94–0.79
Stomach contents	1.92–2.59[2]	0.11[4]	85,993–18,386
Prostatic secretions	6.45–7.4[2]	0.21–1	3.25–1.0
Vaginal secretions	3.4–4.2[3]	0.11[4]	2,848–452

Table 1–3. Body fluids with potential for drug "trapping" through the pH-partitioning phenomenon.

[1]Body fluid protonated-to-unprotonated drug ratios were calculated using each of the pH extremes cited; a blood pH of 7.4 was used for blood drug ratio. For example, the urine:blood ratio for sulfadiazine is 0.12 at a urine pH of 5.0; this ratio is 4.65 at a urine pH of 8.0. Thus, sulfadiazine is much more effectively trapped and excreted in alkaline urine.
[2]Lentner C (editor): *Geigy Scientific Tables,* vol 1, 8th ed. Ciba Geigy, 1981.
[3]Bowman WC, Rand MJ: *Textbook of Pharmacology,* 2nd ed. Blackwell, 1980.
[4]Insignificant change in ratios over the physiologic pH range.

package inserts published annually with supplements twice a year; *Facts and Comparisons* is a more complete loose-leaf drug information service with monthly updates; the *USP DI* (vol 1, *Drug Information for the Health Care Professional*); and *AMA Drug Evaluations.* The package insert consists of a brief description of the pharmacology of the product. While this brochure contains much practical information, it is also used as a means of shifting liability for untoward drug reactions from the manufacturer onto the practitioner. Therefore, the manufacturer typically lists every toxic effect ever reported, no matter how rare. A useful and objective handbook that presents information on drug toxicity and interactions is *Drug Interactions.* Finally, the FDA has opened a computer bulletin board that carries news regarding recent drug approvals, withdrawals, warnings, etc. It can be reached using a personal computer equipped with communications software and a standard modem at 800–222–0185.

The following addresses are provided for the convenience of readers wishing to obtain any of the publications mentioned above:

AMA Drug Evaluations
535 N. Dearborn Street
Chicago, IL 60610

Drug Interactions
Lea & Febiger
600 Washington Square
Philadelphia, PA 19106

Facts and Comparisons
J.B. Lippincott Co.
111 West Port Plaza, Suite 423
St. Louis, MO 63146

Drug Therapy, 2nd edition
Appleton & Lange
25 Van Zant Street
East Norwalk, CT 06855

Pharmacology: Examination & Board Review, 3rd ed.
Appleton & Lange
25 Van Zant Street
East Norwalk, CT 06855

The Medical Letter on Drugs and Therapeutics
56 Harrison St
New Rochelle, NY 10801

The New England Journal of Medicine
10 Shattuck Street
Boston, MA 02115

Physicians' Desk Reference
Box 2017
Mahopac, NY 10541

United States Pharmacopeia Dispensing Information
12601 Twinbrook Parkway
Rockville, MD 20852

Drug Receptors & Pharmacodynamics

2

Henry R. Bourne, MD, & James M. Roberts, MD

The therapeutic and toxic effects of drugs result from their interactions with molecules in the patient. In most instances, drugs act by associating with specific macromolecules in ways that alter their biochemical or biophysical activity. This idea, now almost a century old, is embodied in the terms **receptive substance** and **receptor:** the component of a cell or organism that interacts with a drug and initiates the chain of biochemical events leading to the drug's observed effects.

Initially, the existence of receptors was inferred from observations of the chemical and physiologic specificity of drug effects. Thus, Ehrlich noted that certain synthetic organic agents had characteristic antiparasitic effects while other agents did not, though their chemical structures differed only slightly. Langley noted that curare did not prevent electrical stimulation of muscle contraction but did block contraction triggered by nicotine. From these simple beginnings, receptors have now become the central focus of investigation of drug effects and their mechanisms of action (pharmacodynamics). The receptor concept, extended to endocrinology, immunology, and molecular biology, has proved essential for explaining many aspects of biologic regulation. Drug receptors are now being isolated and characterized as macromolecules, thus opening the way to precise understanding of the molecular basis of drug action.

In addition to its usefulness for explaining biology, the receptor concept has immensely important practical consequences for the development of drugs and for making therapeutic decisions in clinical practice. These consequences—explained more fully in later sections of this chapter—form the basis for understanding the actions and clinical uses of drugs described in every chapter of this book. They may be briefly summarized as follows:

(1) Receptors largely determine the quantitative relations between dose or concentration of drug and pharmacologic effects. The receptor's affinity for binding a drug determines the concentration of drug required to form a significant number of drug-receptor complexes, and the total number of receptors often limits the maximal effect a drug may produce.

(2) Receptors are responsible for selectivity of drug action. The molecular size, shape, and electrical charge of a drug determine whether—and with what avidity–it will bind to a particular receptor among the vast array of chemically different binding sites available in a cell, animal, or patient. Accordingly, changes in the chemical structure of a drug can dramatically increase or decrease a new drug's affinities for different classes of receptors, with resulting alterations in therapeutic and toxic effects.

(3) Receptors mediate the actions of pharmacologic antagonists. Many drugs and endogenous chemical signals, such as hormones, regulate the function of receptor macromolecules as **agonists;** ie, they change the function of a macromolecule as a more or less direct result of binding to it. Pure pharmacologic **antagonists,** however, bind to receptors without directly altering the receptors' function. Thus, the effect of a pure antagonist on a cell or in a patient depends entirely upon its preventing the binding of agonist molecules and blocking their biologic actions. Some of the most useful drugs in clinical medicine are pharmacologic antagonists.

MACROMOLECULAR NATURE OF DRUG RECEPTORS

Until recently, the chemical structures and even the existence of receptors for most drugs could only be inferred from the chemical structures of the drugs themselves. Now, however, receptors for many drugs have been biochemically purified and characterized. The accompanying box describes some of the methods by which receptors are discovered and defined. Most receptors are proteins, presumably because the structures of polypeptides provide both the necessary diversity and the necessary specificity of shape and electrical charge.

The best-characterized drug receptors are **regulatory proteins,** which mediate the actions of endogenous chemical signals such as neurotransmitters, autacoids, and hormones. This class of receptors mediates the effects of many of the most useful therapeutic agents. The molecular structures and biochemical mechanisms of these regulatory receptors

HOW ARE RECEPTORS DISCOVERED?

Because today's new receptor sets the stage for tomorrow's new drug, it is important to know how new receptors are discovered. The discovery process follows a few key steps, summarized in Figure 2–1. As presented in greater detail elsewhere in this chapter, the process of defining a new receptor (stage 1 in Figure 2–1) begins by studying the relations between structures and activities of a group of drugs on some conveniently measured response. Binding of radioactive ligands defines the molar abundance and binding affinities of the putative receptor and provides an assay to aid in its biochemical purification. Analysis of the pure receptor protein tells us the number of its subunits, its size, and (sometimes) provides a clue to how it works (eg, agonist-stimulated autophosphorylation on tyrosine residues, seen with receptors for insulin and many growth factors).

These "classic" steps in receptor identification now serve as a warming-up exercise for a powerful new experimental strategy aimed at molecular cloning of the segment of DNA that encodes the receptor (stages 2–5 in Figure 2–1). The core of this strategy is the ability to identify a putative receptor DNA sequence in a representative population of cDNAs (DNA sequences complementary to the messenger RNAs expressed in an appropriate cell or tissue are obtained by means of reverse transcriptase). To do so (stage 2), investigators use biochemical and functional features of the receptor protein as handles for picking out the corresponding DNA. Thus, an antibody raised against the pure receptor protein or nucleic acid sequences based on its amino acid sequence may distinguish a bacterial colony containing putative receptor cDNA from colonies containing irrelevant cDNAs, by binding to receptor antigen expressed in the bacterium (2a) or by hybridizing to receptor DNA (2b), respectively. Alternatively, the population of cDNAs may be expressed as proteins in frog oocytes or vertebrate cells, and the putative receptor cDNA can then be detected by virtue of the protein's signaling function (2c) or its ability to bind a specific ligand (2d).

Once the putative receptor cDNA has been

identified, it is "validated" by carefully comparing the function and biochemical properties of the recombinant protein with those of the endogenous receptor that originally triggered the search (3a). The base sequence of the receptor DNA is also determined (3b), so that the amino acid sequence of the complete receptor protein can be deduced and compared with sequences of known receptors. Based on these criteria, it may then be possible to announce the identification of a new receptor (step 4).

A much greater quantity and quality of information flows from molecular cloning of the cDNA encoding a new receptor than from identifying a receptor in the "classic" way. The deduced amino acid sequence almost always resembles those of previously known receptors. Investigators can immediately place the new receptor into a specific class of known receptors, and the structural class tells us how the receptor works—whether it is a receptor tyrosine kinase, a seven-transmembrane region receptor coupled to G proteins, etc. The DNA sequence provides a probe to identify cells and tissues that express messenger RNA encoding the new receptor. Expression of the cDNA in cultured cells gives the pharmaceutical chemist an unlimited supply of recombinant receptor protein for precise biochemical analysis, tests of agonist and antagonist binding, and development of new drugs.

Finally (step 5), the receptor DNA itself provides a tool for identifying yet more receptors. Receptors within a specific class or subclass contain highly conserved regions of similar or identical amino acid (and therefore DNA) sequence. The DNA sequences corresponding to these conserved regions can be used as probes to find sequences of related but potentially novel receptors, either by DNA–DNA hybridization (2b) or as primers in a polymerase chain reaction (PCR) designed to amplify receptor DNA sequences (2e). These probes may lead to cloning DNA encoding a receptor whose ligand is unknown (an "orphan" receptor); the appropriate ligand is then sought by testing for functional and binding interactions with the recombinant receptor.

---

are described in a later section entitled Signaling Mechanisms and Drug Action.

Other classes of proteins that have been clearly identified as drug receptors include **enzymes,** which may be inhibited (or, less commonly, activated) by binding a drug (eg, dihydrofolate reductase, the receptor for the antineoplastic drug methotrexate); **transport proteins** (eg, Na^+/K^+ ATPase, the mem-

brane receptor for cardioactive digitalis glycosides); and **structural proteins** (eg, tubulin, the receptor for colchicine, an anti-inflammatory agent).

This chapter deals with three aspects of drug receptor function, presented in increasing order of complexity: (1) The first aspect is their function as determinants of the quantitative relation between the concentration of a drug and the pharmacologic re-

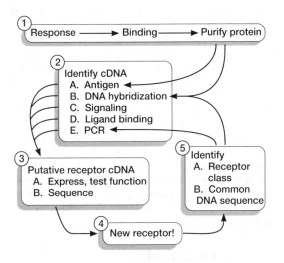

Figure 2–1. Methods used in the discovery and description of receptors. (See box: How Are Receptors Discovered?)

sponse. From this point of view, receptors are simple entities, principally characterized by their affinity for binding drug ligands and their abundance in target cells or tissues. (2) The second aspect is their function as regulatory proteins and components of chemical signaling mechanisms that provide targets for important drugs. Here receptors are considered as complex molecules whose structures and biochemical functions help to explain key features of concentration-effect relations, as well as pharmacologic selectivity. (3) The third aspect is their function as key elements of the therapeutic and toxic effects of drugs in patients. At this highest level of complexity, we discuss the crucial roles receptors play in determining selectivity of drug action, the relation between the dose of

a drug and its effects, and the therapeutic usefulness of a drug (ie, therapeutic effectiveness versus toxicity).

RELATION BETWEEN DRUG CONCENTRATION & RESPONSE

The relation between dose of a drug and the clinically observed response may be quite complex. In carefully controlled in vitro systems, however, the relation between concentration of a drug and its effect is often simple and can be described with mathematical precision. We will analyze this idealized relation first because it underlies virtually all of the more complex relations between dose and effect that occur when drugs are given to patients.

Concentration-Effect Curves & Receptor Binding of Agonists

Even in intact animals or patients, responses to low doses of a drug usually increase in direct proportion to dose. As doses increase, however, the incremental response diminishes; finally, doses may be reached at which no further increase in response can be achieved. In idealized or in vitro systems, the relation between drug concentration and effect is described by a hyperbolic curve (Figure 2–2A) according to the following equation:

$$E = \frac{E_{max} \times C}{C + EC50}$$

where E is the effect observed at concentration C, E_{max} is the maximal response that can be produced by the drug, and EC50 is the concentration of drug that produces 50% of maximal effect.

This hyperbolic relation resembles the mass action law, which predicts association between two molecules of a given affinity. This resemblance suggests

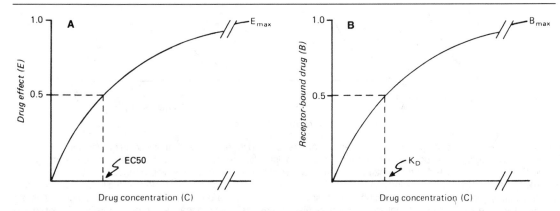

Figure 2–2. Relations between drug concentration and drug effect *(A)* or receptor-bound drug *(B)*. The drug concentrations at which effect or receptor occupancy is half-maximal are denoted EC50 and K_D, respectively.

that drug agonists act by binding to ("occupying") a distinct class of biologic molecules with a characteristic affinity for the drug receptor. With the advent of radioactive receptor ligands, including both agonists and antagonists, this occupancy assumption has been amply confirmed for a number of drug-receptor systems. In these systems, the relation between drug bound to receptors (B) and the concentration of free (unbound) drug (C) depicted in Figure 2–2B is described by an analogous equation:

$$B = \frac{B_{max} \times C}{C + K_D}$$

in which B_{max} indicates the total concentration of receptor sites (ie, sites bound to the drug at infinitely high concentrations of free drug). K_D (the equilibrium dissociation constant) indicates the concentration of free drug at which half-maximal binding is observed. This constant characterizes the receptor's affinity for binding the drug in a reciprocal fashion: If the K_D is low, binding affinity is high, and vice versa.

Note also that the EC50 and K_D may be identical but need not be, as discussed below.

Graphic representation of dose-response data is frequently improved by plotting the drug effect (ordinate) against the *logarithm* of the dose or concentration (abscissa). The effect of this purely mathematical maneuver is to transform the hyperbolic curve of Figure 2–2 into a sigmoid curve with a linear midportion (eg, Figure 2–3). This transformation makes it easier to compare different dose-response curves graphically because it expands the scale of the concentration axis at low concentrations (where the effect is changing rapidly) and compresses it at high concentrations (where the effect is changing slowly). This transformation has no special biologic or pharmacologic significance.

Receptor-Effector Coupling & Spare Receptors

When a receptor is occupied by an agonist, the resulting conformational change is only the first of many steps usually required to produce a pharma-

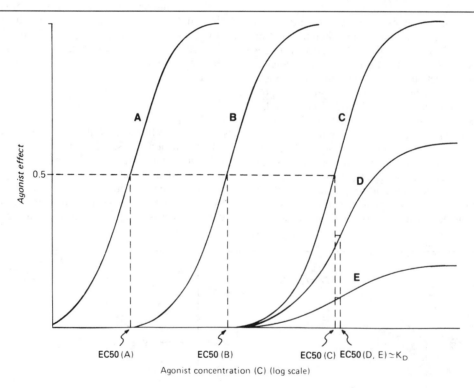

Figure 2–3. Experimental demonstration of spare receptors, using different concentrations of an irreversible antagonist. Curve *A* shows agonist response in the absence of antagonist. After treatment with a low concentration of antagonist (curve *B*), the curve is shifted to the right; maximal responsiveness is preserved, however, because the remaining available receptors are still in excess of the number required. In curve *C*, produced after treatment with a larger concentration of antagonist, the available receptors are no longer "spare"; instead, they are just sufficient to mediate an undiminished maximal response. Still higher concentrations of antagonist (curves *D* and *E*) reduce the number of available receptors to the point that maximal response is diminished. The apparent EC50 of the agonist in curves *D* and *E* may approximate the K_D that characterizes the binding affinity of the agonist for the receptor.

cologic response. The transduction process between occupancy of receptors and drug response is often termed coupling. The relative efficiency of occupancy-response coupling is partially determined by the initial conformational change in the receptor—thus, the effects of full agonists can be considered more efficiently coupled to receptor occupancy than can the effects of partial agonists, as described below. Coupling efficiency is also determined by the biochemical events that transduce receptor occupancy into cellular response.

High efficiency of receptor-effector interaction may also be envisioned as the result of spare receptors. Receptors are said to be "spare" for a given pharmacologic response when the maximal response can be elicited by an agonist at a concentration that does not result in occupancy of the full complement of available receptors. Spare receptors are not qualitatively different from nonspare receptors. They are not hidden or unavailable, and when they are occupied, they can be coupled to response. Experimentally, spare receptors may be demonstrated by using irreversible antagonists to prevent binding of agonist to a proportion of available receptors and showing that high concentrations of agonist can still produce an undiminished maximal response (Figure 2–3). Thus, a maximal inotropic response of heart muscle to catecholamines can be elicited even under conditions where 90% of the beta receptors are occupied by a quasi-irreversible antagonist. Accordingly, myocar-

dium is said to contain a large proportion of spare receptors.

How can we account for the phenomenon of spare receptors? In a few cases, the biochemical mechanism is understood, such as for drugs that act on some regulatory receptors. In this situation, the effect of receptor activation—eg, binding of GTP by an intermediate—may greatly outlast the agonist-receptor interaction (see the following section called G Proteins and Second Messengers). In such a case, the "spareness" of receptors is *temporal* in that the response initiated by an individual ligand-receptor binding event persists longer in time than the binding event itself.

In other cases, where the biochemical mechanism is not understood, we imagine that the receptors are *spare in number*. If the concentration or amount of a cellular component other than the receptor limits the coupling of receptor occupancy to response, then a maximal response can occur without occupancy of all receptors. Figure 2–4 illustrates the notion of receptors that are spare in this sense and helps to explain how the sensitivity of a cell or tissue to a particular concentration of agonist may depend not only on the affinity of the receptor for binding an agonist (characterized by the K_D) but also on the total concentration of receptors. Sensitivity may be expressed in terms of EC50, the concentration of agonist that results in half-maximal response. The K_D of the agonist-receptor interaction determines what fraction (B/B_{max}) of

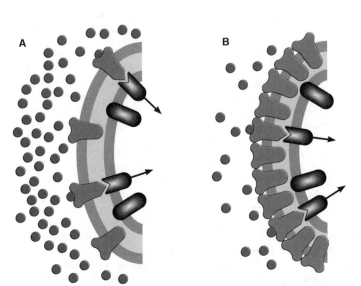

Figure 2–4. Spare receptors increase sensitivity to drug. In panel *A (left)*, the free concentration of agonist is equal to the K_D concentration; this is sufficient to bind 50% of the four receptors present, resulting in the formation of two agonist-receptor complexes. (***Note:*** When the agonist concentration is equal to the K_D, half the receptors will be occupied. Remember that $B/B_{max} = C/(C + K_D)$.) Agonist occupancy of these two receptors changes their conformation so that they bind to and activate two effector molecules, resulting in a response. Because two of four effectors are stimulated by agonist-receptor complexes, the response is 50% of maximum. In membrane *B (right)*, the receptor concentration has been increased tenfold (not all receptors are shown), and the K_D for binding of agonist to receptors remains unchanged. Now a very much smaller concentration of free agonist (= 0.05 times the K_D) suffices to occupy two receptors and consequently to activate two effector molecules. Thus, the response is 50% of maximum (just as in *A*), even though the agonist concentration is very much lower than the K_D.

total receptors will be occupied at a given free concentration (C) of agonist, regardless of the receptor concentration:

$$\frac{B}{B_{max}} = \frac{C}{C + K_D}$$

Imagine a responding cell with four receptors and four effectors (as in Figure 2–4). Here the number of effectors does not limit the maximal response, and the receptors are *not* spare in number. Consequently, an agonist present at a concentration equal to the K_D will occupy 50% of the receptors, and half of the effectors will be activated, producing a half-maximal response (ie, two receptors stimulate two effectors). Now imagine that the number of receptors increases tenfold to 40 receptors but that the total number of effectors remains constant. Now most of the receptors are spare in number. As a result, a very much lower concentration of agonist suffices to occupy two of the 40 receptors (5% of the receptors), and this same low concentration of agonist is able to elicit a half-maximal response (two of four effectors activated). Thus, it is possible to change the sensitivity of tissues with spare receptors by changing the receptor concentration. (*Note:* Changing the number of receptors does not usually change the free concentration of drug achieved by administering a given dose. This is because the concentration of receptors in a tissue is usu-. ally very small relative to effective concentrations of drugs.)

An important biologic consequence of spare receptors is that they allow agonists with low affinity for receptors to produce full responses at low concentrations, to the extent that EC50 is lower than K_D. This is important because ligands with low affinity (high K_D) dissociate rapidly from receptors, allowing rapid termination of biologic responses. High binding affinity (low K_D), on the other hand, would result in slow dissociation of agonist from receptor and correspondingly slower reversal of a biologic response.

Competitive & Irreversible Antagonists

Receptor antagonists bind to the receptor but do not activate it. The effects of these antagonists result from preventing agonists (other drugs or endogenous regulatory molecules) from binding to and activating receptors. Such antagonists are divided into two classes depending on whether or not they reversibly compete with agonists for binding to receptors. The two classes of receptor antagonism produce quite different concentration-effect and concentration-binding curves in vitro and exhibit important practical differences in therapy of disease.

In the presence of a fixed concentration of agonist, increasing concentrations of a **competitive antagonist** progressively inhibit the agonist response; high antagonist concentrations prevent response com-

pletely. Conversely, sufficiently high concentrations of agonist can completely surmount the effect of a given concentration of the antagonist, ie, the E_{max} for the agonist remains the same for any fixed concentration of antagonist (Figure 2–5A). Because the antagonism is competitive, the presence of antagonist increases the agonist concentration required for a given degree of response, and so the agonist concentration-effect curve shifts to the right.

The concentration (C′) of an agonist required to produce a given effect in the presence of a fixed concentration ([I]) of competitive antagonist is greater than the agonist concentration (C) required to produce the same effect in the absence of the antagonist. The ratio of these two agonist concentrations (the "dose ratio") is related to the dissociation constant (K_I) of the antagonist by the Schild equation:

$$\frac{C'}{C} = 1 + \frac{[I]}{K_I}$$

Pharmacologists often use this relation to determine the K_I of a competitive antagonist. Even without knowledge of the relationship between agonist occupancy of the receptor and response, the K_I can be determined simply and accurately. As shown in Figure 2–5, concentration response curves are obtained in the presence and in the absence of a fixed concentration of competitive antagonist; comparison of the agonist concentrations required to produce identical degrees of pharmacologic effect in the two situations reveals the antagonist's K_I. If C′ is twice C, for example, then [I] = K_I. K_I values derived from such experiments agree with those determined by direct measurements of binding of radiolabeled competitive antagonists to receptors.

For the clinician, this mathematical relation has two important therapeutic implications:

(1) The degree of inhibition produced by a competitive antagonist depends upon the concentration of antagonist. Thus, the extent and duration of action of such a drug will depend upon its concentration in plasma and will be critically influenced by the rate of its metabolic clearance or excretion. Different patients receiving a fixed dose of propranolol, for example, exhibit a wide range of plasma concentrations, owing to differences in clearance of the drug. As a result, the effects of a fixed dose of this competitive antagonist of norepinephrine may vary widely in patients, and the dose must be adjusted accordingly.

(2) The equation defines another important source of variability in clinical response to a competitive antagonist, ie, the concentration of agonist that is competing for binding to receptors. Here also propranolol provides a useful example: When this competitive beta-adrenoceptor antagonist is administered in doses sufficient to block the effect of basal levels of the neurotransmitter norepinephrine, resting heart rate is decreased. However, the increase in release of

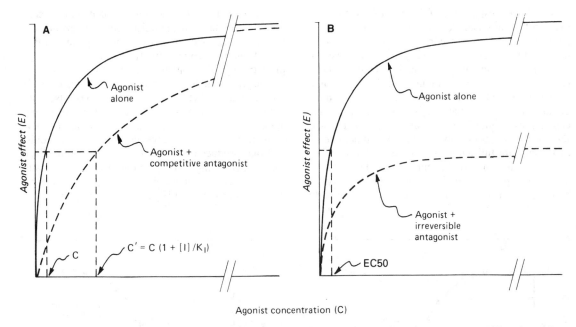

Figure 2–5. Changes in agonist concentration-effect curves produced by a competitive antagonist *(A)* or by an irreversible antagonist *(B)*. In the presence of a competitive antagonist, higher concentrations of agonist are required to produce a given effect; thus, the agonist concentration (C′) required for a given effect in the presence of concentration [I] of an antagonist is shifted to the right, as shown. High agonist concentrations can overcome inhibition by a competitive antagonist. This is not the case with an irreversible antagonist, which reduces the maximal effect the agonist can achieve, though it may not change its EC50.

norepinephrine and epinephrine that occurs with exercise, postural changes, or emotional stress may suffice to overcome competitive antagonism by propranolol and increase heart rate. Consequently, the physician who devises a dosage regimen for a competitive antagonist must always consider possible changes in endogenous agonist concentration that could influence therapeutic response.

Some receptor antagonists bind to the receptor in an **irreversible** or nearly irreversible fashion. The antagonist's affinity for the receptor may be so high that for practical purposes, the receptor is unavailable for binding of agonist. Other antagonists in this class produce irreversible effects because after binding to the receptor they form covalent bonds with it. After occupancy of a substantial proportion of receptors by such an antagonist, the number of remaining unoccupied receptors may be so low that high concentrations of agonist cannot overcome the antagonism, and a maximal agonist response cannot be obtained (Figure 2–5B). However, if spare receptors are present, a lower dose of an irreversible antagonist, however, may leave enough receptors unoccupied to allow achievement of maximum response to agonist, though a higher agonist concentration will be required (see Receptor-Effector Coupling and Spare Receptors, above).

Therapeutically, irreversible antagonists present distinctive advantages and disadvantages. Once the irreversible antagonist has occupied the receptor, it need not be present in unbound form to inhibit agonist responses. Consequently, the duration of action of such an irreversible antagonist is relatively independent of its own rate of elimination and more dependent upon the rate of turnover of receptor molecules.

Phenoxybenzamine, an irreversible alpha-adrenoceptor antagonist, is used to control the hypertension caused by catecholamines released from pheochromocytoma, a tumor of the adrenal medulla. If administration of phenoxybenzamine lowers blood pressure, blockade will be maintained even when the tumor episodically releases very large amounts of catecholamine. In this case, the ability to prevent responses to varying and high concentrations of agonist is a therapeutic advantage. If overdose occurs, however, a real problem may arise. If the alpha-adrenoceptor blockade cannot be overcome, excess effects of the drug must be antagonized "physiologically," eg, by using a pressor agent that does not act via alpha receptors.

Partial Agonists

Based on the maximal pharmacologic response that occurs when all receptors are occupied, agonists can be divided into two classes: **Partial agonists** produce a lower response, at full receptor occupancy, than do **full agonists.** As compared to full agonists, partial agonists produce concentration-effect curves that resemble curves observed with full agonists in the presence of an antagonist that irreversibly blocks receptor sites (compare Figure 2–3D and 2–6B). Nonetheless, radioligand-binding experiments have demonstrated that partial agonists may occupy all receptor sites (Figure 2–6A) at concentrations that will fail to produce a maximal response comparable to that seen with full agonists (Figure 2–4B). In addition, the failure of partial agonists to produce a "full" maximal response is not due to decreased affinity for binding to receptors. Such drugs compete, frequently

with high affinity, for the full complement of receptors. Indeed, the partial agonists' ability to occupy the total receptor population is indicated by the fact that partial agonists competitively inhibit the responses produced by full agonists (Figure 2–6C).

The precise molecular mechanism that accounts for blunted maximal responses to partial agonists is not known. It is simplest to imagine that the partial agonist produces an effect on receptors that is intermediate between the effect produced by a full agonist and that produced by a competitive antagonist. The full agonist changes receptor conformation in a way that initiates subsequent pharmacologic effects of receptor occupancy, while the "pure" competitive an-

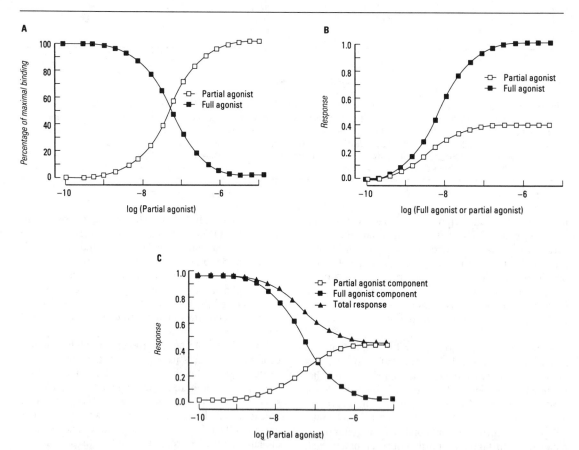

Figure 2–6. Panel A: The percentage of receptor occupancy resulting from full agonist (present at a single concentration) binding to receptors in the presence of increasing concentrations of a partial agonist. Because the full agonist (filled squares) and the partial agonist (open squares) compete to bind to the same receptor sites, when occupancy by the partial agonist increases, binding of the full agonist decreases. **Panel B:** When each of the two drugs is used alone and response is measured, occupancy of all the receptors by the partial agonist produces a lower maximal response than does similar occupancy by the full agonist. **Panel C:** Simultaneous treatment with a single concentration of full agonist and increasing concentrations of the partial agonist produces the response patterns shown in the bottom panel. The fractional response caused by a single concentration of the full agonist (filled squares) decreases as increasing concentrations of the partial agonist compete to bind to the receptor with increasing success; at the same time the portion of the response caused by the partial agonist (open squares) increases, while the total response—ie, the sum of responses to the two drugs (filled triangles)—gradually decreases, eventually reaching the value produced by partial agonist alone (compare panel B).

tagonist produces no such change in receptor conformation; in this view, the partial agonist changes receptor conformation, but not to the extent necessary to result in full activation of the occupied receptor.

To express this idea, pharmacologists refer to the **efficacy** of a drug as a way of indicating the relation between occupancy of receptor sites and the pharmacologic response. A drug may have zero efficacy (ie, may be a pure antagonist) or any degree of efficacy greater than zero. Partial agonists can be viewed as drugs with such low efficacy that even occupancy of the full complement of receptors does not result in the maximal response that can be elicited by other ("full") agonists, which have higher efficacy. The reader will see that many drugs used as competitive antagonists are in fact weak partial agonists.

Other Mechanisms of Drug Antagonism

Not all of the mechanisms of antagonism involve interactions of drugs or endogenous ligands at a single type of receptor. Indeed, **chemical antagonists** need not involve a receptor at all. Thus, one drug may antagonize the actions of a second drug by binding to and inactivating the second drug. For example, protamine, a protein that is positively charged at physiologic pH, can be used clinically to counteract the effects of heparin, an anticoagulant that is negatively charged; in this case, one drug antagonizes the other simply by binding it and making it unavailable for interactions with proteins involved in formation of a blood clot.

The clinician often uses drugs that take advantage of **physiologic antagonism** between endogenous regulatory pathways. Many physiologic functions are controlled by opposing regulatory pathways. For example, several catabolic actions of the glucocorticoid hormones lead to increased blood sugar, an effect that is physiologically opposed by insulin. Although glucocorticoids and insulin act on quite distinct receptor-effector systems, the clinician must sometimes administer insulin to oppose the hyperglycemic effects of glucocorticoid hormone, whether the latter are elevated by endogenous synthesis (eg, a tumor of the adrenal cortex) or as a result of glucocorticoid therapy.

In general, use of a drug as a physiologic antagonist produces effects that are less specific and less easy to control than are the effects of a receptor-specific antagonist. Thus, for example, to treat bradycardia caused by increased release of acetylcholine from vagus nerve endings, which may be caused by the pain of myocardial infarction, the physician could use isoproterenol, a beta-adrenoceptor agonist that increases heart rate by mimicking sympathetic stimulation of the heart. However, use of this physiologic antagonist would be less rational—and potentially more dangerous—than would use of a receptor-specific antagonist such as atropine (a competitive antagonist at the receptors at which acetylcholine slows heart rate).

SIGNALING MECHANISMS & DRUG ACTION

Until now we have considered receptor interactions and drug effects in terms of equations and concentration-effect curves. This abstract analysis explains some quantitative aspects of drug action. For a more complete explanation, we must also understand the molecular mechanisms by which a drug acts. This understanding is particularly important for drugs that mimic or block intercellular signaling by hormones and neurotransmitters.

The research of the past 10 years has revealed in considerable detail the molecular processes that transduce extracellular signals into intracellular messages that control cell function. Understanding these remarkable signaling mechanisms allows us to ask basic questions with important clinical implications: Why do some drugs produce effects that persist for minutes, hours, or even days after the drug is no longer present? How do cellular mechanisms for amplifying external chemical signals explain the phenomenon of spare receptors? Why do chemically similar drugs often exhibit extraordinary selectivity in their actions? Can the signaling mechanisms explain actions of drugs that do not interact with receptors? Do these mechanisms provide targets for developing new drugs? Our new understanding allows us not only to ask these questions but also—in many cases—to answer them.

Most transmembrane signaling is accomplished by only a few different molecular mechanisms. Each type of mechanism has been adapted, through the evolution of distinctive protein families, to transduce many different signals. These protein families include receptors on the cell surface and within the cell, as well as enzymes and other components that generate, amplify, coordinate, and terminate postreceptor signaling by chemical second messengers in the cytoplasm. This section first discusses the mechanisms for carrying chemical information across the plasma membrane, and then outlines key features of cytoplasmic second messengers.

Four basic mechanisms of transmembrane signaling are well understood (Figure 2–7). Each uses a different strategy to circumvent the barrier posed by the lipid bilayer of the plasma membrane. These strategies are (1) using a lipid-soluble ligand that crosses the membrane and acts on an intracellular receptor; (2) using a transmembrane receptor protein whose intracellular enzymatic activity is allosterically regulated by a ligand that binds to a site on the protein's extracellular domain; (3) using a ligand-gated transmembrane ion channel that can be induced to open or close by the binding of a ligand; and (4) using a transmembrane receptor protein to stimulate a GTP-binding signal transducer protein (G protein) that in turn generates an intracellular second messenger.

Of course, the signaling mechanisms for many ex-

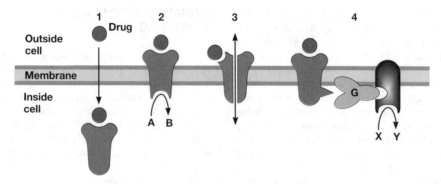

Figure 2–7. Known transmembrane signaling mechanisms: **1:** A lipid-soluble chemical signal crosses the plasma membrane and acts on an intracellular receptor (which may be an enzyme or a regulator of gene transcription); **2:** the signal binds to the extracellular domain of a transmembrane protein, thereby activating an enzymatic activity of its cytoplasmic domain; **3:** the signal binds to and directly regulates the opening of an ion channel; **4:** the signal binds to a cell-surface receptor linked to an effector enzyme by a G protein.

tracellular ligands remain unknown (eg, growth hormone, interferon, lymphokines). While the four established mechanisms do not account for all the chemical signals conveyed across cell membranes, they do transduce many of the most important signals exploited in pharmacotherapy.

Intracellular Receptors for Lipid-Soluble Agents

Several biologic signals are sufficiently lipid-soluble to cross the plasma membrane and act on intracellular receptors. One of these is a gas, nitric oxide (NO), that acts by stimulating an intracellular enzyme, guanylyl cyclase, which produces cGMP. Signaling via cGMP is described in more detail later in this chapter. Receptors for another class of ligands—including **corticosteroids, mineralocorticoids, sex steroids, vitamin D,** and **thyroid hormone**—stimulate the transcription of genes in the nucleus by binding to specific DNA sequences near the gene whose expression is to be regulated. Many of the target DNA sequences (called **response elements**) have been identified.

The detailed molecular mechanisms used by these "gene-active" receptors are well understood. Structural features common to these receptors suggest that they belong to a protein family that evolved from a common precursor. Dissection of the receptors by recombinant DNA techniques has provided insights into their molecular mechanisms. For example, removal of a carboxyl terminal segment of the glucocorticoid receptor results in a protein that binds to the DNA response element and stimulates transcription of the target gene, even in the absence of glucocorticoids. Like this experimental truncation, binding of glucocorticoid hormone to the normal receptor relieves an inhibitory constraint on the transcription-stimulating activity of the protein. Figure 2–8 schematically depicts the molecular mechanism of

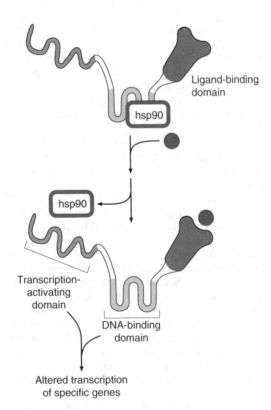

Figure 2–8. Mechanism of glucocorticoid action. The glucocorticoid receptor polypeptide is schematically depicted as a protein with three distinct domains. A heat-shock protein, **hsp90,** binds to the receptor in the absence of hormone and prevents folding into the active conformation of the receptor. Binding of a hormone ligand causes dissociation of the hsp90 stabilizer and permits conversion to the active configuration.

glucocorticoid action: In the absence of hormone, the receptor is bound to hsp90, a protein that appears to prevent normal folding of several structural domains of the receptor. Binding of hormone to the ligand-binding domain triggers release of hsp90. This allows the DNA-binding and transcription-activating domains of the receptor to fold into their functionally active conformations, so that the activated receptor can initiate transcription of target genes.

The mechanism used by hormones that act by regulating gene expression has two therapeutically important consequences: (1) All of these hormones produce their effects after a characteristic lag period of 30 minutes to several hours—the time required for the synthesis of new proteins. This means that the gene-active hormones cannot be expected to alter a pathologic state within minutes—eg, glucocorticoids will not immediately relieve the symptoms of acute bronchial asthma. (2) The effects of these agents can persist for hours or days after the agonist concentration has been reduced to zero. The persistence of effect is primarily due to the relatively slow turnover of most enzymes and proteins, which can remain active in cells for hours or days after they have been synthesized. (The persistence may also be partially due to the high affinity of receptors for the hormone, which results in slow dissociation of the hormone.) Therapeutically, it means that the beneficial (or toxic) effects of a gene-active hormone will usually decrease slowly when administration of the hormone is stopped and that there will be no simple temporal correlation between plasma concentration of the hormone and its effects.

Ligand-Regulated Transmembrane Enzymes Including Protein Tyrosine Kinases

This class of receptor molecules mediates the first steps in signaling by **insulin, epidermal growth factor (EGF), platelet-derived growth factor (PDGF), atrial natriuretic factor (ANF), transforming growth factor-beta (TGFβ)**, and several other trophic hormones. These receptors are polypeptides consisting of an extracellular hormone-binding domain and a cytoplasmic enzyme domain, which may be a protein tyrosine kinase, a serine kinase, or a guanylyl cyclase (Figure 2–9). In all these receptors, the two domains are connected by a hydrophobic segment of the polypeptide that crosses the lipid bilayer of the plasma membrane.

The tyrosine kinase signaling pathway begins with hormone binding to the receptor's extracellular domain. The resulting change in receptor conformation causes receptor molecules to bind to one another, which in turn brings together the protein tyrosine kinase domains, which become enzymatically active. Tyrosine residues in both cytoplasmic domains become phosphorylated (each is probably phosphorylated by the other). This cross-phosphorylation can intensify or prolong the duration of allosteric regulation by the hormonal ligand. For example, the tyrosine kinase activity of the autophosphorylated insulin

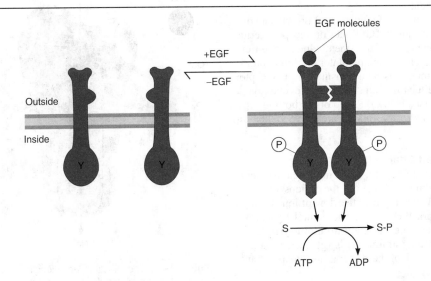

Figure 2–9. Mechanism of activation of the EGF receptor, a representative receptor tyrosine kinase. The receptor polypeptide has extracellular and cytoplasmic domains, depicted above and below the plasma membrane. Upon binding of EGF (circle), the receptor converts from its inactive monomeric state *(left)* to an active dimeric state *(right),* in which two receptor polypeptides bind noncovalently in the plane of the membrane. The cytoplasmic domains become phosphorylated *(P)* on specific tyrosine residues *(Y)* and their enzymatic activities are activated, catalyzing phosphorylation of substrate proteins *(S).*

receptor persists after insulin is removed from the binding site. Different receptors catalyze phosphorylation of tyrosine residues on different downstream signaling proteins, but only a few of these substrate proteins have been identified. Insulin, for example, uses a single class of receptors to trigger increased uptake of glucose and amino acids and to regulate metabolism of glycogen and triglycerides in the cell. Similarly, each of the growth factors initiates in its specific target cells a complex program of cellular events ranging from altered membrane transport of protons, other ions, and metabolites to characteristic changes in the expression of many genes. Some of these responses involve phosphorylation by serine and threonine kinases, while others work via transcription factors that may themselves be kinase substrates. The tyrosine kinase receptors provide attractive targets for drug development. At present, a few compounds have been found to produce effects that may be due to inhibition of tyrosine kinase activities. It is easy to imagine therapeutic uses for specific inhibitors of growth factor receptors, especially in neoplastic disorders.

The intensity and duration of action of EGF, PDGF, and other agents that act via this class of receptors are limited by receptor **down regulation.** Ligand binding induces accelerated endocytosis of receptors from the cell surface, followed by the degradation of those receptors (and their bound ligands). When this process occurs at a rate faster than de novo synthesis of receptors, the total number of cell-surface receptors is reduced (down-regulated) and the cell's responsiveness to ligand is correspondingly diminished.

A growing number of regulators of growth and differentiation, including TGFβ, act on receptor serine kinases, another class of transmembrane receptor enzymes. ANF, an important regulator of blood volume and vascular tone, acts on a transmembrane receptor whose intracellular domain, a guanylyl cyclase, generates cGMP (see below). Receptors in both groups, like the protein tyrosine kinases, are active in their dimeric forms.

Ligand-Gated Channels

Many of the most useful drugs in clinical medicine act by mimicking or blocking the actions of endogenous ligands that regulate the flow of ions through plasma membrane channels. The natural ligands include **acetylcholine, gamma-aminobutyric acid,** and the **excitatory amino acids** (glycine, aspartate, glutamate, etc). All of these agents are synaptic transmitters.

Each of these receptors transmits its signal across the plasma membrane by increasing transmembrane conductance of the relevant ion and thereby altering the electrical potential across the membrane. For example, acetylcholine causes the opening of the ion channel in the nicotinic acetylcholine receptor

(AChR), which allows Na^+ to flow down its concentration gradient into cells, producing a localized excitatory postsynaptic potential—a depolarization.

The nicotinic AChR (Figure 2–10) is one of the best characterized of all cell-surface receptors for hormones or neurotransmitters. This receptor is a pentamer made up of five polypeptide subunits (eg, two alpha chains plus one beta, one gamma, and one delta chain, all with molecular weights ranging from 43,000 to 50,000). These polypeptides, each of which crosses the lipid bilayer four times, form a cylindric structure 8 nm in diameter. When acetylcholine binds to sites on the alpha subunits, a conformational change occurs that results in the transient opening of a central aqueous channel through which sodium ions penetrate from the extracellular fluid into the cell.

The time elapsed between the binding of the agonist to a ligand-gated channel and the cellular response can often be measured in milliseconds. The rapidity of this signaling mechanism is crucially important for moment-to-moment transfer of information across synapses. It contrasts sharply with other molecular signaling mechanisms, which may require seconds, minutes, or even hours, as is the case with gene-active hormones.

G Proteins & Second Messengers

Many extracellular ligands act by increasing the intracellular concentrations of second messengers such

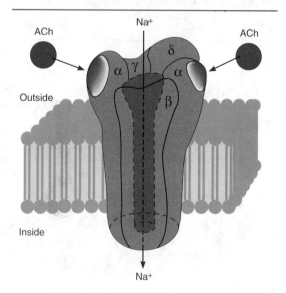

Figure 2–10. The nicotinic acetylcholine receptor, a ligand-gated ion channel. The receptor molecule is depicted as embedded in a rectangular piece of plasma membrane, with extracellular fluid above and cytoplasm below. Composed of five subunits (two α, one β, one γ, and one δ), the receptor opens a central transmembrane ion channel when acetylcholine (ACh) binds to sites on the extracellular domain of its α subunits.

as cyclic adenosine-3',5'-monophosphate (cAMP), calcium ion, or the phosphoinositides (described below). In most cases they use a transmembrane signaling system with three separate components. First, the extracellular ligand is specifically detected by a cell-surface receptor. The receptor in turn triggers the activation of a G protein located on the cytoplasmic face of the plasma membrane. The activated G protein then changes the activity of an effector element, usually an enzyme or ion channel. This element then changes the concentration of the intracellular second messenger. For cAMP, the effector enzyme is adenylyl cyclase, a transmembrane protein that converts intracellular ATP to cAMP. The corresponding G protein, called G_s, stimulates adenylyl cyclase after being activated by a host of hormones and neurotransmitters, each of which acts via a specific receptor (see Table 2–1).

G_s and other G proteins use a molecular mechanism that involves binding and hydrolysis of GTP (Figure 2–11). Significantly, this mechanism separates ligand excitation of the receptor from G protein-mediated activation of the effector, thereby allowing the transduced signal to be amplified. For example, a neurotransmitter such as norepinephrine may encounter its membrane receptor for a very short time, only a few milliseconds. When the encounter generates a GTP-bound G_s molecule, however, the duration of activation of adenylyl cyclase depends upon the longevity of GTP binding to G_s rather than upon the receptor's affinity for norepinephrine. Indeed, like other G proteins, GTP-bound G_s characteristically re-

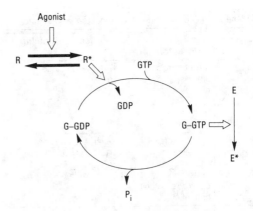

Figure 2–11. The guanine nucleotide-dependent activation-inactivation cycle of G proteins. The agonist activates the receptor *(R)*, which promotes release of GDP from the G protein *(G)*, allowing entry of GTP into the nucleotide binding site. In its GTP-bound state *(G-GTP)*, the G protein regulates activity of an effector enzyme or ion channel *(E)*. The signal is terminated by hydrolysis of GTP, followed by return of the system to the basal unstimulated state. Open arrows denote regulatory effects.

mains active for tens of seconds, which enormously amplifies the original signal. This mechanism explains how signaling by G proteins produces the phenomenon of spare receptors (described above). Even though one ligand-activated receptor molecule is required to initiate GTP binding by one G protein, the slow hydrolysis of GTP causes the active G protein to persist long after the receptor has dissociated from its agonist molecule. So at low concentrations of agonist the proportion of agonist-bound receptors may be much less than the proportion of G proteins in the active (GTP-bound) state; if the proportion of active G proteins correlates with pharmacologic response, receptors will appear to be spare—ie, a small fraction of receptors occupied by agonist at any given time will appear to produce a proportionately larger response.

The family of G proteins is quite diverse (Table 2–2); in addition to G_s, the stimulator of adenylyl cyclase, it includes other subfamilies. Members of the G_i ("i" for inhibitory) subfamily couple receptors to inhibition of adenylyl cyclase; G_i proteins also mediate receptor stimulation of the phosphoinositide second messenger system in some cells (see below) and regulation of K^+ and Ca^{2+} channels. The G_i subfamily includes two G proteins (G_{t1} and G_{t2}, also called "transducins"), that mediate phototransduction in retinal rods and cones.

Not surprisingly, receptors coupled to G proteins are structurally related to one another, comprising a family of "serpentine receptors," so called because the receptor polypeptide chain crosses the plasma membrane seven times (Figure 2–12). Receptors for adrenergic amines, serotonin, acetylcholine (muscarinic but not nicotinic), many peptide hormones,

Table 2–1. A partial list of endogenous ligands and their associated second messengers.

Ligand	Second Messenger
Adrenocorticotropic hormone	cAMP
Acetylcholine (muscarinic receptors)	Ca^{2+},phosphoinositides
Angiotensin	Ca^{2+},phosphoinositides
Catecholamines (α_1-adrenoceptors)	Ca^{2+},phosphoinositides
Catecholamines (β-adrenoceptors)	cAMP
Chorionic gonadotropin	cAMP
Follicle-stimulating hormone	cAMP
Glucagon	cAMP
Histamine (H_2 receptors)	cAMP
Luteinizing hormone	cAMP
Melanocyte-stimulating hormone	cAMP
Parathyroid hormone	cAMP
Platelet-derived growth factor	Ca^{2+},phosphoinositides
Prostacyclin, prostaglandin E_2	cAMP
Serotonin ($5-HT_4$ receptors)	cAMP
Serotonin ($5-HT_{1C}$ and $5-HT_2$ receptors)	Ca^{2+},phosphoinositides
Thyrotropin	cAMP
Thyrotropin-releasing hormone	Ca^{2+},phosphoinositides
Vasopressin (V_1 receptors)	Ca^{2+},phosphoinositides
Vasopressin (V_2 receptors)	cAMP

Table 2–2. G proteins and their receptors and effectors.

G Protein	Receptors for:	Effector/Signaling Pathway
G_s	β-Adrenergic amines, glucagon, histamine, serotonin, and many other hormones	↑Adenylyl cyclase → ↑cAMP
G_{i1}, G_{i2}, G_{i3}	$α_2$-Adrenergic amines, acetylcholine (muscarinic), opioids, serotonin, and many others	Several, including: ↓Adenylyl cyclase → ↓cAMP Open cardiac K^+ channels → ↓heart rate
G_{olf}	Odorants (olfactory epithelium)	↑Adenylyl cyclase → ↑cAMP
G_o	Neurotransmitters in brain (not yet specifically identified)	Not yet clear
G_q	Acetylcholine (eg, muscarinic), bombesin, serotonin (5-HT$_{1C}$), and many others	↑Phospholipase C → ↑IP$_3$, diacylglycerol, cytoplasmic Ca^{2+}
G_{t1}, G_{t2}	Photons (rhodopsin and color opsins in retinal rod and cone cells)	↑cGMP phosphodiesterase → ↓cGMP (phototransduction)

odorants, and even visual receptors (in retinal rod and cone cells) all belong to the serpentine family. The amino and carboxyl terminals of each of these receptors are located on the extracellular and cytoplasmic sides of the membrane, respectively. Different serpentine receptors resemble one another rather closely in amino acid sequences and in the locations of their hydrophobic transmembrane regions and hydrophilic extra- and intracellular loops, suggesting that all were derived from a common evolutionary precursor.

In parallel with these structural similarities, it appears that serpentine receptors transduce signals across the plasma membrane in essentially the same way. Often the agonist ligand—eg, a catecholamine, acetylcholine, or the photon-activated chromophore of retinal photoreceptors—is bound in a pocket enclosed by the transmembrane regions of the receptor (as in Figure 2–12). The resulting change in conformation of these regions is transmitted to cytoplasmic loops of the receptor, which in turn activate the appropriate G protein by promoting replacement of GDP by GTP, as described above. Considerable biochemical evidence indicates that the G proteins interact with amino acids in the third cytoplasmic loop of the receptor polypeptide (arrowed in Figure 2–12). The carboxyl terminal tails of these receptors, also located in the cytoplasm, can regulate the receptors' ability to interact with G proteins, as described below.

Receptor Desensitization

Receptor-mediated responses to drugs and hormonal agonists often "desensitize" with time (Figure 2–13, top). After reaching an initial high level, the response (eg, cellular cAMP accumulation, Na^+ influx, contractility, etc) gradually diminishes over seconds or minutes, even in the continued presence of the agonist. This desensitization is usually reversible. Thus, 15 minutes after removal of the agonist, a second exposure to agonist results in a response similar to the initial response. (Note that this ready reversibility distinguishes desensitization from down-regulation of the *number* of receptors, as described above for receptor tyrosine kinases.)

Although many kinds of receptors undergo desensitization, the mechanism is in most cases obscure (eg, agonist-induced desensitization of the nicotinic acetylcholine receptor). The molecular mechanism of agonist desensitization has been worked out in some detail, however, in the case of the beta adrenoceptor (Figure 2–13, bottom): Binding of agonist induces a change in conformation of the receptor's carboxyl terminal tail, making it a good substrate for phosphorylation on serine (and threonine) residues by a specific kinase, β-adrenoceptor kinase (also termed βARK). The presence of phosphoserines increases the receptor's affinity for binding a third protein, β-arrestin. Binding of β-arrestin to cytoplasmic loops of the receptor diminishes the receptor's ability to interact with G_s, thereby reducing the agonist response (ie, stimulation of adenylyl cyclase). Upon removal of agonist, however, cellular phosphatases remove phosphates from the receptor and βARK stops putting them back on, so that the receptor—and consequently the agonist response—return to normal (Figure 2–13, bottom).

Well-Established Second Messengers

A. cAMP: Acting as an intracellular second messenger, cAMP mediates such hormonal responses as the mobilization of stored energy (the breakdown of carbohydrates in liver or triglycerides in fat cells stimulated by beta-adrenomimetic catecholamines), vasopressin-mediated conservation of water by the kidney, Ca^{2+} homeostasis (regulated by parathyroid hormone), and increased rate and contraction force of the heart muscle (beta-adrenomimetic catecholamines). It also regulates the production of adrenal and sex steroids (in response to corticotropin or follicle-stimulating hormone), the relaxation of smooth muscle, and many other endocrine and neural processes.

cAMP exerts most of its effects by stimulating cAMP-dependent protein kinases (Figure 2–14). These tetrameric kinases are composed of a cAMP-binding regulatory (R) dimer and two catalytic (C) chains. When cAMP binds to the R dimer, active C chains are released, which then diffuse through the cytoplasm and nucleus, where they transfer phos-

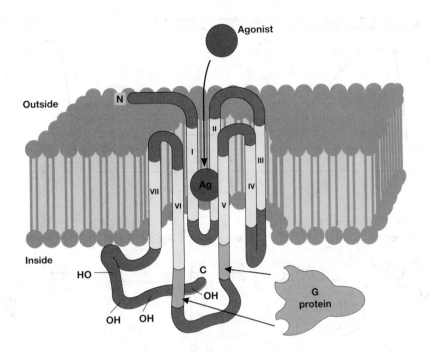

Figure 2–12. Transmembrane topology of a typical serpentine receptor. The receptor's amino *(N)* terminal is extracellular (above the plane of the membrane), and its carboxyl *(C)* terminal intracellular. The terminals are connected by a polypeptide chain that traverses the plane of the membrane seven times. The hydrophobic transmembrane segments (speckled) are designated by roman numerals *(I–VII)*. The agonist *(Ag)* approaches the receptor from the extracellular fluid and binds to a site surrounded by the transmembrane regions of the receptor protein. G proteins *(G)* interact with cytoplasmic regions of the receptor, especially with portions of the third cytoplasmic loop between transmembrane regions *V* and *VI*. The receptor's cytoplasmic terminal tail contains numerous serine and threonine residues whose hydroxyl (–OH) groups can be phosphorylated. This phosphorylation may be associated with diminished receptor-G protein interaction.

phate from ATP to appropriate substrate proteins, often enzymes.

The specificity of cAMP's regulatory effects resides in the distinct protein substrates of the kinase that are expressed in different cells. For example, liver is rich in phosphorylase kinase and glycogen synthase, enzymes whose reciprocal regulation by cAMP-dependent phosphorylation governs carbohydrate storage and release; adipocytes are rich in a lipase whose cAMP-dependent phosphorylation mediates free fatty acid release from fat cells. Similarly, phosphorylation of a kinase specific for the light chains of myosin (called myosin light chain kinase, or MLCK) is involved in relaxation of smooth muscle by beta-adrenomimetic amines. Other cell-specific responses to cAMP as a second messenger similarly depend upon the many enzymes available for regulation by phosphorylation.

When the hormonal stimulus stops, the intracellular actions of cAMP are terminated by an elaborate series of enzymes. cAMP-stimulated phosphorylation of enzyme substrates is rapidly reversed by a diverse group of specific and nonspecific phosphatases. cAMP itself is degraded to 5'-AMP by several dis-

tinct cyclic nucleotide phosphodiesterases (PDE, Figure 2–14). Competitive inhibition of cAMP degradation is one way caffeine, theophylline, and other methylxanthines produce their effects (see Chapter 19).

B. Calcium and Phosphoinositides: A second well-studied second messenger system involves hormonal stimulation of phosphoinositide hydrolysis (Figure 2–15). Some of the hormones, neurotransmitters, and growth factors that trigger this pathway (see Table 2–1) bind to receptors linked to G proteins, while others bind to tyrosine kinase receptors. In all cases, however, the crucial step is stimulation of a membrane enzyme, phospholipase C (PLC), which specifically hydrolyzes a minor phospholipid component of the plasma membrane called phosphatidyl-inositol-4,5-bisphosphate (PIP_2). PIP_2 is split into two second messengers, diacylglycerol (DAG) and inositol-1,4,5-trisphosphate (IP_3). The first of these messengers is confined to the membrane, where it activates a phospholipid- and calcium-sensitive protein kinase called protein kinase C. The other messenger, IP_3, is water-soluble and diffuses through the cytoplasm, where it triggers the release of Ca^{2+} from

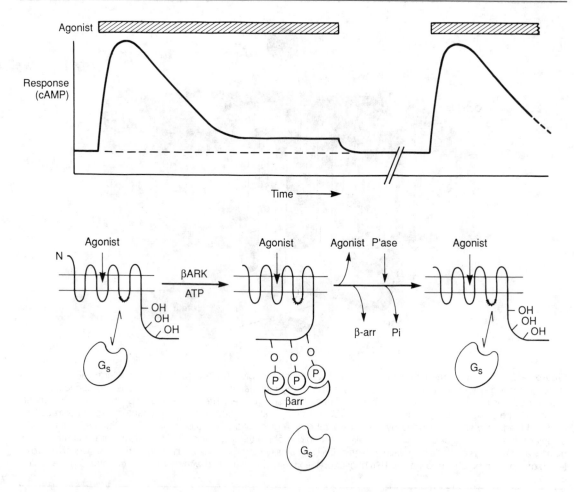

Figure 2–13. Possible mechanism for desensitization of the beta adrenoceptor. The upper part of the figure depicts the response to a β-adrenoceptor agonist (ordinate) versus time (abscissa). The break in the time axis indicates passage of time in the absence of agonist. Temporal duration of exposure to agonist is indicated by the diagonally hatched bar. The lower part of the figure schematically depicts agonist-induced phosphorylation *(P)* by β-adrenoceptor kinase (beta-adrenergic receptor kinase, βARK) of carboxyl terminal hydroxyl groups (–OH) of the beta adrenoceptor. This phosphorylation *(P)* induces binding of a protein, β-arrestin (β-arr), which prevents the receptor from interacting with G_s. Removal of agonist for a short period of time allows dissociation of β-arr, removal of phosphate *(Pi)* from the receptor by phosphatases *(P'ase),* and restoration of the receptor's normal responsiveness to agonist.

internal storage vesicles. Elevated cytoplasmic Ca^{2+} concentration promotes the binding of Ca^{2+} to the calcium-binding protein calmodulin, which regulates activities of other enzymes, including calcium-dependent protein kinases.

With its multiple second messengers and protein kinases, the phosphoinositide signaling pathway is much more complex than the cAMP pathway. For example, different cell types may contain one or more specialized calcium- and calmodulin-dependent kinases with limited substrate specificity (eg, myosin light chain kinase) in addition to a general calcium- and calmodulin-dependent kinase that can phosphorylate a wide variety of protein substrates. Also, at least nine structurally distinct types of protein kinase C have been identified.

Much of our understanding of the biologic roles of phosphoinositide second messengers comes from the use of pharmacologic agents that activate either the Ca^{2+} or the protein kinase C pathways. The concentration of cytoplasmic Ca^{2+} can be elevated by calcium ionophores, while protein kinase C is directly stimulated by binding phorbol esters or synthetic diacylglycerols. One or both of these classes of agents may reproduce the biologic response triggered by a physiologic signal using the phosphoinositide pathway.

As in the cAMP system, multiple mechanisms exist to damp or terminate signaling by this pathway. IP_3 is rapidly inactivated by dephosphorylation; diacylglycerol is either phosphorylated to yield phosphatidic acid, which is then converted back into phospholipids, or it is deacylated to yield arachidonic acid;

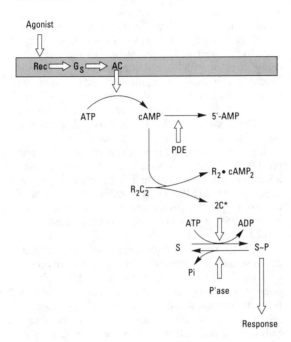

Figure 2–14. The cAMP second messenger pathway. Key proteins include hormone receptors *(Rec)*, a stimulatory G protein *(G$_s$)*, catalytic adenylyl cyclase *(AC)*, phosphodiesterases *(PDE)* that hydrolyze cAMP, cAMP-dependent kinases, with regulatory *(R)* and catalytic *(C)* subunits, protein substrates *(S)* of the kinases, and phosphatases *(P'ase)*, which remove phosphates from substrate proteins. Open arrows denote regulatory effects.

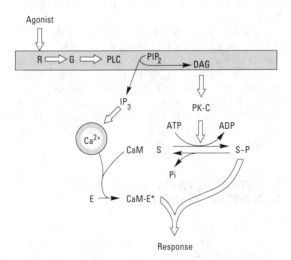

Figure 2–15. The Ca^{2+}/phosphoinositide signaling pathway. Key proteins include hormone receptors *(R)*, a G protein *(G)*, a phosphoinositide-specific phospholipase C *(PLC)*, protein kinase C *(PK-C)*, substrates of the kinase *(S)*, calmodulin *(CaM)*, and calmodulin-binding enzymes *(E)*, including kinases, phosphodiesterases, etc. (PIP$_2$, phosphatidylinositol-4,5-bisphosphate; DAG, diacylglycerol. Open arrows denote regulatory effects.)

Ca^{2+} is actively removed from the cytoplasm by Ca^{2+} pumps.

These and other nonreceptor elements of the calcium-phosphoinositide signaling pathway are now becoming targets for drug development. For example, the therapeutic effects of lithium ion, an established agent for treating manic-depressive illness, may be mediated by effects on the metabolism of phosphoinositides (see Chapter 28).

C. cGMP: Unlike cAMP, the ubiquitous and versatile carrier of diverse messages, cGMP (cyclic guanosine-3′,5′-monophosphate) has established signaling roles in only a few cell types. In intestinal mucosa and vascular smooth muscle, the cGMP-based signal transduction mechanism closely parallels the cAMP-mediated signaling mechanism. Ligands detected by cell surface receptors stimulate membrane-bound guanylyl cyclase to produce cGMP, and cGMP acts by stimulating a cGMP-dependent protein kinase. The actions of cGMP in these cells are terminated by enzymatic degradation of the cyclic nucleotide and by dephosphorylation of kinase substrates.

Increased cGMP concentration causes relaxation of vascular smooth muscle by a kinase-mediated mechanism that results in dephosphorylation of myosin light chains. In these smooth muscle cells, cGMP synthesis can be elevated by two different transmembrane signaling mechanisms, utilizing two different guanylyl cyclases. Atrial natriuretic factor (ANF), a blood-borne peptide hormone, stimulates a transmembrane receptor by binding to its extracellular (ligand binding) domain; this binding event triggers activation of the guanylyl cyclase activity that resides in the receptor's intracellular domain. The other mechanism takes advantage of the fact that cell membranes are permeable to the stimulating ligand, nitric oxide (NO, a gas). The nitric oxide is generated in vascular endothelial cells, in response to natural vasodilator agents such as acetylcholine and histamine (nitric oxide is also called endothelium-derived relaxing factor, EDRF). After entering the cell, nitric oxide binds to and activates a cytoplasmic guanylyl cyclase. A number of useful vasodilating drugs act by generating or mimicking nitric oxide (see Chapters 11 and 12).

Interplay Among Signaling Mechanisms

The calcium-phosphoinositide and cAMP signaling pathways oppose one another in some cells, and are complementary in others. For example, vasopressor agents that contract smooth muscle act by IP$_3$-mediated mobilization of Ca^{2+}, whereas agents that relax smooth muscle often act by elevation of cAMP. In contrast, cAMP and phosphoinositide second messengers act together to stimulate glucose release from the liver.

Phosphorylation: A Common Theme

Almost all second messenger signaling involves reversible phosphorylation. It plays a key role at every step, from regulation of receptors (autophosphorylation of tyrosine kinases and desensitization of receptors linked to G proteins) to kinases regulated by second messengers, and finally to substrates of these kinases that may themselves be kinases. These covalent modifications perform two principal functions in signaling, amplification and flexible regulation. In **amplification,** rather like GTP bound to a G protein, the attachment of a phosphoryl group to a serine, threonine, or tyrosine residue powerfully amplifies the initial regulatory signal by recording a molecular memory that the pathway has been activated; dephosphorylation erases the memory, taking a longer time to do so than is required for dissociation of an allosteric ligand. In **flexible regulation,** differing substrate specificities of the multiple protein kinases regulated by second messengers provide branch points in signaling pathways that may be independently regulated. In this way, cAMP, Ca^{2+}, or other second messengers can use the presence or absence of particular kinases or kinase substrates to produce quite different effects in different cell types.

RECEPTOR CLASSES & DRUG DEVELOPMENT

As we have seen, the existence of a specific drug receptor is usually inferred from studying the **structure-activity relationship** of a group of structurally similar congeners of the drug that mimic or antagonize its effects. Thus, if a series of related agonists exhibits identical relative potencies in producing two distinct effects, it is likely that the two effects are mediated by similar or identical receptor molecules. In addition, if identical receptors mediate both effects, a competitive antagonist will inhibit both responses with the same K_I; a second competitive antagonist will inhibit both responses with its own characteristic K_I. Thus, studies of the relation between structure and activity of a series of agonists and antagonists can identify a species of receptor that mediates a set of pharmacologic responses.

Exactly the same experimental procedure can show that observed effects of a drug are mediated by *different* receptors. In this case, effects mediated by different receptors may exhibit different orders of potency among agonists, and different K_I values for each competitive antagonist.

Wherever we look, more than one class of receptor seems to have evolved for every chemical signal. For example, structure-activity studies with chemical congeners of acetylcholine, histamine, and catecholamines have identified multiple receptors for each of these endogenous ligands. Ligand-binding and molecular cloning techniques continue to reveal additional receptors eg, two classes of vasopressin receptors, five molecular species of muscarinic receptors (only three of which are distinguishable by ligand-binding techniques), and multiple classes of receptors for dopamine, opioid peptides, serotonin, and others.

Why do multiple receptors for a single ligand exist? The answer is quite straightforward: Cells use more than one signaling pathway to respond to each endogenous ligand, and therefore need more than one receptor for the same ligand. Thus, acetylcholine uses a nicotinic AChR to initiate a fast excitatory postsynaptic potential (EPSP) in the postganglionic cells of autonomic ganglia and muscarinic receptors to evoke a slow EPSP, which modulates responsiveness to the fast EPSP in the same cells.

The existence of multiple receptors for each endogenous signaling ligand creates many important opportunities for drug development. Although each endogenous ligand produces multiple clinical effects, it is often therapeutically advantageous to block or mimic one set of effects without affecting the others. Subtle structural differences in the binding sites of two receptors for a ligand can make them bind congeners of the ligand with different affinities. If the affinities are sufficiently different, it may be possible to develop a drug that acts selectively, producing its effects through one receptor and not the other. Thus, β-adrenoceptor antagonists can block cardioacceleration produced by norepinephrine without preventing norepinephrine from constricting blood vessels via α_1 adrenoceptors. Clinical uses of receptor-selective drugs are described in almost every chapter of this book.

New drug development is not confined to agents that act on receptors for extracellular chemical signals. Pharmaceutical chemists are now determining whether elements of signaling pathways distal to the receptors may also serve as targets of selective and useful drugs. For example, clinically useful agents might be developed that act selectively on specific G proteins, kinases, phosphatases, or the enzymes that degrade second messengers.

RELATION BETWEEN DRUG DOSE & CLINICAL RESPONSE

We have dealt with receptors as molecules and shown how receptors can quantitatively account for the relation between dose or concentration of a drug and pharmacologic responses, at least in an idealized system. When faced with a patient who needs treatment, the physician must make a choice among a variety of possible drugs and devise a dosage regimen that is likely to produce maximal benefit and minimal toxicity. Because the patient is never an idealized system, the physician will not have precise information about the physicochemical nature of the receptors in-

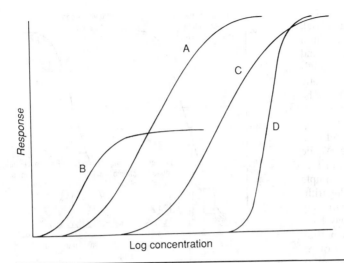

Figure 2–16. Graded dose-response curves for four drugs, illustrating different pharmacologic potencies and different maximal efficacies.

volved, the number of receptors, or their affinity for drugs. Nonetheless, in order to make rational therapeutic decisions, the physician must understand how drug-receptor interactions underlie the relations between dose and response in patients, the nature and causes of variation in pharmacologic responsiveness, and the clinical implications of selectivity of drug action.

Dose & Response in Patients

A. Graded Dose-Response Relations: To choose among drugs and to determine appropriate doses of a drug, the physician must know the relative **pharmacologic potency** and **maximal efficacy** of the drugs in relation to the desired therapeutic effect. These two important terms, often confusing to students and clinicians, can be explained by reference to Figure 2–16, which depicts graded dose-response curves that relate dose of four different drugs to the magnitude of a particular therapeutic effect, eg, lowering of blood pressure in a hypertensive patient or increasing urinary excretion of sodium in a patient with congestive heart failure.

1. Potency–Drugs A and B are said to be more potent than drugs C and D because of the relative positions of their dose-response curves along the **dose axis** of Figure 2–16. Potency refers to the concentration (EC50) or dose (ED50) of a drug required to produce 50% of that drug's maximal effect. Thus, the pharmacologic potency of drug A in Figure 2–16 is less than that of drug B, a partial agonist, because the ED50 of A is greater than the ED50 of B. Note that some doses of drug A can produce larger effects than any dose of drug B, despite the fact that we term drug B pharmacologically more potent. The reason for this is that drug A has a larger **maximal efficacy,** as described below.

Potency of a drug depends in part on the affinity (K_D) of receptors for binding the drug and in part on the efficiency with which drug-receptor interaction is coupled to response. As described above, both affinity and coupling efficiency contribute to the EC50 of a particular concentration-response relation in vitro.

For clinical use, it is helpful to distinguish between a drug's **potency** and its **efficacy.** The clinical effectiveness of a drug depends not on its potency (EC50), but on its maximal efficacy (see below) and its ability to reach the relevant receptors. This ability can depend on its route of administration, absorption, distribution through the body, and clearance from the blood or site of action. In deciding which of two drugs to administer to a patient, the physician must usually consider their relative effectiveness rather than their relative potency. However, pharmacologic potency can largely determine the administered dose of the chosen drug. In general, low potency is important only if the drug has to be administered in inconveniently large amounts.

For therapeutic purposes, the potency of a drug should be stated in dosage units, usually in terms of a particular therapeutic end point (eg, 50 mg for mild sedation, 1 μg/kg/min for an increase in heart rate of 25 beats/min). Relative potency, the ratio of equieffective doses (0.2, 10, etc), may be used in comparing one drug with another.

2. Maximal efficacy–This parameter reflects the limit of the dose-response relation on the **response axis.** Drugs A, C, and D in Figure 2–16 have equal maximal efficacy, while all have greater maximal efficacy than does drug B. The maximal efficacy (sometimes referred to simply as efficacy) of a drug is obviously crucial for making clinical decisions when a large response is needed. It may be determined by the drug's mode of interactions with receptors (as with partial agonists, described above)* or by characteristics of the receptor-effector system involved. Thus, diuretics that act on one portion of the nephron may produce much greater excretion of fluid and electrolytes than diuretics that act elsewhere. In addition, the efficacy of a drug for achieving a therapeutic end point (eg, increased cardiac contractility) may be limited by the drug's propensity to cause a toxic effect (eg, fatal cardiac arrhythmia) even if the drug could otherwise produce a greater therapeutic effect.

B. Shape of Dose-Response Curves: While the responses depicted in curves A, B, and C of Figure 2–16 approximate the shape of a simple Michaelis-Menten relation (transformed to a logarithmic plot), some clinical responses do not. Extremely steep dose-response curves (eg, curve D) may have important clinical consequences if the upper portion of the curve represents an undesirable extent of response (eg, coma caused by a sedative-hypnotic). Steep dose-response curves in patients could result from cooperative interactions of several different actions of a drug (eg, effects on brain, heart, and peripheral vessels, all contributing to lowering of blood pressure). Such steep dose-response curves could also be produced by a receptor-effector system in which most receptors must be occupied before any effect is seen.

C. Quantal Dose-Effect Curves: Despite their usefulness for characterizing the actions of drugs, graded dose-response curves of the sort described above have certain limitations in their application to clinical decision making. For example, such curves may be impossible to construct if the pharmacologic response is an either-or (quantal) event, such as prevention of convulsions, arrhythmia, or death. Furthermore, the clinical relevance of a quantitative dose-response relationship in a single patient, no matter how precisely defined, may be limited in application to other patients, owing to the great potential variability among patients in severity of disease and responsiveness to drugs.

Some of these difficulties may be avoided by determining the dose of drug required to produce a specified magnitude of effect in a large number of individual patients or experimental animals and plotting the cumulative frequency distribution of responders versus the log dose (Figure 2–17). The specified quantal effect may be chosen on the basis of clinical rele-

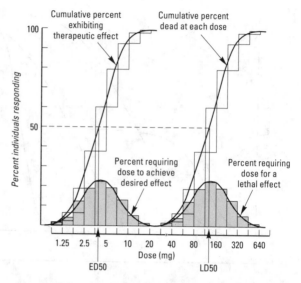

Figure 2–17. Quantal dose-effect plots. Shaded boxes (and the accompanying curves) indicate the frequency distribution of doses of drug required to produce a specified effect; ie, the percentage of animals that required a particular dose to exhibit the effect. The open boxes (and the corresponding curves) indicate the cumulative frequency distribution of responses, which are lognormally distributed.

vance (eg, relief of headache) or for preservation of safety of experimental subjects (eg, using low doses of a cardiac stimulant and specifying an increase in heart rate of 20 beats/min as the quantal effect), or it may be an inherently quantal event (eg, death of an experimental animal). For most drugs, the doses required to produce a specified quantal effect in individuals are lognormally distributed; ie, a frequency distribution of such responses plotted against the log of the dose produces a gaussian normal curve of variation (Figure 2–17). When these responses are summated, the resulting cumulative frequency distribution constitutes a quantal dose-effect curve (or dose-percent curve) of the proportion or percentage of individuals who exhibit the effect plotted as a function of log dose (Figure 2–17).

The quantal dose-effect curve is often characterized by stating the **median effective dose** (ED50), the dose at which 50% of individuals exhibit the specified quantal effect. (Note that the abbreviation ED50 has a different meaning in this context from its meaning in relation to graded dose-effect curves, described above.) Similarly, the dose required to produce a particular toxic effect in 50% of animals is called the **median toxic dose** (TD50). If the toxic effect is death of the animal, a median lethal dose (LD50) may be experimentally defined. Such values provide a convenient way of comparing the potencies of drugs in experimental and clinical settings: Thus, if the ED50s of two drugs for producing a specified

---

*Note that "maximal efficacy," used in a therapeutic context, does not have exactly the meaning the term denotes in the more specialized context of drug-receptor interactions described earlier in this chapter. In an idealized in vitro system, efficacy denotes the relative maximal efficacy of agonists and partial agonists that act via the same receptor. In therapeutics, efficacy denotes the extent or degree of an effect that can be achieved in the intact patient. Thus, therapeutic efficacy may be affected by the characteristics of a particular drug-receptor interaction, but it also depends upon a host of other factors, noted in the text.

quantal effect are 5 and 500 mg, respectively, then the first drug can be said to be 100 times more potent than the second for that particular effect. Similarly, one can obtain a valuable index of the selectivity of a drug's action by comparing its ED50s for two different quantal effects in a population (eg, cough suppression versus sedation for opiate drugs; increase in heart rate versus increased vasoconstriction for sympathomimetic amines; anti-inflammatory effects versus sodium retention for corticosteroids; etc).

Quantal dose-effect curves may also be used to generate information regarding the margin of safety to be expected from a particular drug used to produce a specified effect. One measure, which relates the dose of a drug required to produce a desired effect to that which produces an undesired effect, is the **therapeutic index.** In animal studies, the therapeutic index is usually defined as the ratio of the TD50 to the ED50 for some therapeutically relevant effect. The precision possible in animal experiments may make it useful to use such a therapeutic index to estimate the potential effectiveness of a drug in humans. Of course, the therapeutic index of a drug in humans is almost never known with real precision; instead, drug trials and accumulated clinical experience often reveal a range of usually effective doses and a different (but sometimes overlapping) range of possibly toxic doses. The clinically acceptable risk of toxicity depends critically on the severity of the disease being treated. For example, the dose range that provides relief from an ordinary headache in the great majority of patients should be very much lower than the dose range that produces serious toxicity, even if the toxicity occurs in a small minority of patients. However, for treatment of a lethal disease such as Hodgkin's lymphoma, the acceptable difference between therapeutic and toxic doses may be smaller.

Finally, note that the quantal dose-effect curve and the graded dose-response curve summarize somewhat different sets of information, although both appear sigmoid in shape on a semilogarithmic plot (compare Figures 2–16 and 2–17). Critical information required for making rational therapeutic decisions can be obtained from each type of curve: Both curves provide information regarding the **potency** and **selectivity** of drugs; the graded dose-response curve indicates the **maximal efficacy** of a drug; and the quantal dose-effect curve indicates the potential **variability** of responsiveness among individuals.

Variation in Drug Responsiveness

Individuals may vary considerably in their responsiveness to a drug; indeed, a single individual may respond differently to the same drug at different times during the course of treatment. Occasionally, individuals exhibit an unusual or **idiosyncratic** drug response, one that is infrequently observed in most patients. The idiosyncratic responses are usually caused by genetic differences in metabolism of the drug or by immunologic mechanisms, including allergic reactions.

Quantitative variations in drug response are in general more common and more clinically important: An individual patient is **hyporeactive** or **hyperreactive** to a drug in that the intensity of effect of a given dose of drug is diminished or increased in comparison to the effect seen in most individuals. (*Note:* The term **hypersensitivity** usually refers to allergic or other immunologic responses to drugs.) With some drugs, the intensity of response to a given dose may change during the course of therapy; in these cases, responsiveness usually decreases as a consequence of continued drug administration, producing a state of relative **tolerance** to the drug's effects. When responsiveness diminishes rapidly after administration of a drug, the response is said to be subject to **tachyphylaxis.**

The general clinical implications of individual variability in drug responsiveness are clear: The physician must be prepared to change either the dose of drug or the choice of drug, depending upon the response observed in the patient. Even before administering the first dose of a drug, the physician should consider factors that may help in predicting the direction and extent of possible variations in responsiveness. These include the propensity of a particular drug to produce tolerance or tachyphylaxis as well as the effects of age, sex, body size, disease state, and simultaneous administration of other drugs.

Four general mechanisms may contribute to variation in drug responsiveness among patients or within an individual patient at different times. The classification described below is necessarily artificial in that most variation in clinical responsiveness is caused by more than one mechanism. Nonetheless, the classification may be useful because certain mechanisms of variation are best dealt with according to different therapeutic strategies.

A. Alteration in Concentration of Drug That Reaches the Receptor: Patients may differ in the rate of absorption of a drug, in distributing it through body compartments, or in clearing the drug from the blood (see Chapter 3). Any of these pharmacokinetic differences may alter the concentration of drug that reaches relevant receptors and thus alter clinical response. Some differences can be predicted on the basis of age, weight, sex, disease state, or liver and kidney function of the patient, and such predictions may be used to guide quantitative decisions regarding an initial dosing regimen. Repeated measurements of drug concentrations in blood during the course of treatment are often helpful in dealing with the variability of clinical response caused by pharmacokinetic differences among individuals.

B. Variation in Concentration of an Endogenous Receptor Ligand: This mechanism contributes greatly to variability in responses to pharmacologic antagonists. Thus, propranolol, a β-adrenoceptor antagonist, will markedly slow the heart rate of a patient whose endogenous catecholamines are elevated (as in pheochromocytoma) but will not affect the resting heart rate of a well-trained marathon runner. A partial agonist may exhibit even more dramatically different responses: Saralasin, a weak partial agonist at angiotensin II receptors, lowers blood pressure in patients with hypertension caused by increased angiotensin II production and raises blood pressure in patients who produce low amounts of angiotensin.

C. Alterations in Number or Function of Receptors: Experimental studies have documented changes in drug responsiveness caused by increases or decreases in the number of receptor sites or by alterations in the efficiency of coupling of receptors to distal effector mechanisms. Although such changes have not been rigorously documented in human beings, it is likely that they account for much of the individual variability in response to some drugs, particularly those that act at receptors for hormones, biogenic amines, and neurotransmitters. In some cases, the change in receptor number is caused by other hormones; for example, thyroid hormones increase both the number of beta receptors in rat heart muscle and the cardiac sensitivity to catecholamines. Similar changes probably contribute to the tachycardia of thyrotoxicosis in patients and may account for the usefulness of propranolol, a β-adrenoceptor antagonist, in ameliorating symptoms of this disease.

In other cases, the agonist ligand itself induces a decrease in the number ("down-regulation") or coupling efficiency of its receptors. Receptor-specific desensitization mechanisms presumably act physiologically to allow cells to adapt to changes in rates of stimulation by hormones and neurotransmitters in their environment. These mechanisms (discussed above, under Signaling Mechanisms and Drug Actions) may contribute to two clinically important phenomena: first, tachyphylaxis or tolerance to the effects of some drugs (eg, biogenic amines and their congeners), and second, the "overshoot" phenomena that follow withdrawal of certain drugs. These phenomena can occur with either agonists or antagonists. An antagonist may increase the number of receptors in a critical cell or tissue by preventing down regulation caused by an endogenous agonist. When the antagonist is withdrawn, the elevated number of receptors can produce an exaggerated response to physiologic concentrations of agonist. Potentially disastrous withdrawal symptoms can result for the opposite reason when administration of an agonist drug is discontinued. In this situation the number of receptors, which has been decreased by drug-induced down regulation, is too low for endogenous agonist to produce effective stimulation. For example, the withdrawal of clonidine (a drug whose α_2-adrenoceptor agonist activity reduces blood pressure) can produce hypertensive crisis, probably because the drug downregulates α_2 adrenoceptors (see Chapter 11).

Various therapeutic strategies can be used to deal with receptor-specific changes in drug responsiveness, depending on the clinical situation. Tolerance to the action of a drug may require raising the dose or substituting a different drug. The down- (or up-) regulation of receptors may make it dangerous to discontinue certain drugs. The patient may have to be weaned slowly from the drug and watched carefully for signs of a withdrawal reaction.

D. Changes in Components of Response Distal to Receptor: Although a drug initiates its actions by binding to receptors, the response observed in a patient depends on the functional integrity of biochemical processes in the responding cell and physiologic regulation by interacting organ systems. Clinically, changes in these postreceptor processes represent the largest and most important class of mechanisms that cause variation in responsiveness to drug therapy.

Before initiating therapy with a drug, the physician should be aware of patient characteristics that may limit the clinical response. These characteristics include the age and general health of the patient and—most importantly—the severity and pathophysiologic mechanism of the disease. Once treatment is begun, the most important potential cause of failure to achieve a satisfactory response is that the diagnosis is wrong or physiologically incomplete. Thus, congestive heart failure will not respond satisfactorily to agents that increase myocardial contractility if the underlying pathologic mechanism is unrecognized stenosis of the mitral valve rather than myocardial insufficiency. Conversely, drug therapy will always be most successful when it is accurately directed at the pathophysiologic mechanism responsible for the disease.

When the diagnosis is correct and the drug is appropriate, treatment may still not produce an optimal result. An unsatisfactory therapeutic response can often be traced to compensatory mechanisms in the patient that respond to and oppose the beneficial effects of the drug. Compensatory increases in sympathetic nervous tone and fluid retention by the kidney, for example, can contribute to tolerance to antihypertensive effects of a vasodilator drug. In such cases, additional drugs may be required to achieve a useful therapeutic response.

Clinical Selectivity: Beneficial Versus Toxic Effects of Drugs

Although we classify drugs according to their principal actions, it is clear that *no drug causes only a single, specific effect.* Why is this so? It is exceedingly unlikely that any kind of drug molecule will bind to only a single type of receptor molecule, if only because the number of potential receptors in every patient is astronomically large. (Consider that the human genome encodes more than 10^5 different peptide gene products and that the chemical complexity of each of these peptides is sufficient to provide many different potential binding sites.) Even if the chemical structure of a drug allowed it to bind to only one kind of receptor, the biochemical processes controlled by such receptors would take place in multiple cell types and would be coupled to many other biochemical functions; as a result, the patient and the physician would probably perceive more than one drug effect.

Accordingly, drugs are only *selective*—rather than specific—in their actions, because they bind to one or a few types of receptor more tightly than to others and because these receptors control discrete processes that result in distinct effects. As we have seen, selectivity can be measured by comparing binding affinities of a drug to different receptors or by comparing ED50s for different effects of a drug in vivo. In drug development and in clinical medicine, selectivity is usually considered by separating effects into two categories: **beneficial** or **therapeutic effects** versus **toxic effects.** Pharmaceutical advertisements and physicians occasionally use the term **side effect,** implying that the effect in question is insignificant or occurs via a pathway that is to one side of the principal action of the drug; such implications are frequently erroneous.

It is important to recognize that the designation of a particular drug effect as either therapeutic or toxic is a value judgment and not a statement about the pharmacologic mechanism underlying the effect. As a value judgment, such a designation depends on the clinical context in which the drug is used.

It is only because of their selectivity that drugs are useful in clinical medicine. Thus, it is important, both in the management of patients and in the development and evaluation of new drugs, to analyze ways in which beneficial and toxic effects of drugs may be related, in order to increase selectivity and usefulness of drug therapy. Figure 2–18 depicts three possible relations between the therapeutic and toxic effects of a drug based on analysis of the receptor-effector mechanisms involved.

A. Beneficial and Toxic Effects Mediated by the Same Receptor-Effector Mechanism: Much of the serious drug toxicity in clinical practice represents a **direct pharmacologic extension** of the therapeutic actions of the drug. In some of these cases (bleeding caused by anticoagulant therapy; hypoglycemic coma due to insulin), toxicity may be avoided by judicious management of the dose of drug administered, guided by careful monitoring of effect (measurements of blood coagulation or serum glucose) and aided by ancillary measures (avoiding tissue trauma that may lead to hemorrhage; regulation of carbohydrate intake). In still other cases, the toxicity may be avoided by not administering the drug at all, if the therapeutic indication is weak or if other therapy is available (eg, sedative-hypnotics ordinarily should not be used to treat patients whose complaints of insomnia are due to underlying psychiatric depression).

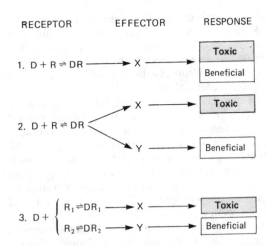

Figure 2–18. Possible relations between the therapeutic and toxic effects of a drug, based on different receptor-effector mechanisms. Therapeutic implications of these different relations are discussed in the text.

In certain situations, a drug is clearly necessary and beneficial but produces unacceptable toxicity when given in doses that produce optimal benefit. In such situations, it may be necessary to add another drug to the treatment regimen. For example, prazosin (Chapter 11) lowers blood pressure in essential hypertension by acting as an alpha₁-selective antagonist on receptors in vascular smooth muscle; as an inevitable consequence, patients will suffer from symptoms of postural hypotension if the dose of drug is large enough. (Note that postural hypotension has been called a "side effect" of prazosin, though in fact it is a direct effect, closely related to the drug's principal therapeutic action.) Appropriate management of such a problem takes advantage of the fact that blood pressure is regulated by changes in blood volume and tone of arterial smooth muscle in addition to the sympathetic nerves. Thus, concomitant administration of diuretics and vasodilators may allow the dose of prazosin to be lowered, with relief of postural hypotension and continued control of blood pressure.

B. Beneficial and Toxic Effects Mediated by Identical Receptors But in Different Tissues or by Different Effector Pathways: Examples of drugs in this category include digitalis glycosides, which may be used to augment cardiac contractility but also produce cardiac arrhythmias, gastrointestinal effects, and changes in vision (all probably mediated by inhibition of Na^+/K^+ ATPase in cell membranes); methotrexate, used to treat leukemia and other neoplastic diseases, which also kills normal cells in bone marrow and gastrointestinal mucosa (all mediated by inhibition of the enzyme dihydrofolate reductase); and congeners of glucocorticoid hormones, used to treat asthma or inflammatory disorders, which also can produce protein catabolism, psychosis, and other toxicities (all thought to be mediated by similar or identical glucocorticoid receptors). In addition to these and other well-documented examples, it is likely that adverse effects of many drugs are mediated by receptors identical to those which produce the recognized beneficial effect.

Three therapeutic strategies are used to avoid or mitigate this sort of toxicity. First, the drug should always be administered at the lowest dose that produces acceptable benefit, recognizing that complete abolition of signs or symptoms of the disease may not be achieved. Second (as described above for prazosin), adjunctive drugs that act through different receptor mechanisms and produce different toxicities may allow lowering the dose of the first drug, thus limiting its toxicity (eg, use of other immunosuppressive agents added to glucocorticoids in treating inflammatory disorders). Third, selectivity of the drug's actions may be increased by manipulating the concentrations of drug available to receptors in different parts of the body. Such "anatomic" selectivity may be achieved, for example, by aerosol administration of a glucocorticoid to the bronchi or by selective arterial infusion of an antimetabolite into an organ containing tumor cells.

C. Beneficial and Toxic Effects Mediated by Different Types of Receptors: Therapeutic advantages resulting from new chemical entities with improved receptor selectivity were mentioned earlier in this chapter and are described in detail in later chapters. Such drugs include the alpha- and beta-selective adrenoceptor agonists and antagonists, the H_1 and H_2 antihistamines, nicotinic and muscarinic blocking agents, and receptor-selective steroid hormones. All of these receptors are grouped in functional families, each responsive to a small class of endogenous agonists. The receptors and their associated therapeutic uses were discovered by analyzing effects of the physiologic chemical signals—catecholamines, histamine, acetylcholine, and corticosteroids.

A number of other drugs were discovered in a similar way, although they may not act at receptors for known hormones or neurotransmitters. These drugs were discovered by exploiting toxic effects of other agents, observed in a different clinical context. Examples include quinidine, the sulfonylureas, thiazide diuretics, tricyclic antidepressants, monoamine oxidase inhibitors, and phenothiazine antipsychotics among many others.

It is likely that some of these drugs will eventually be shown to act via receptors for endogenous agonists, as is the case with morphine, a potent analgesic agent. Morphine has been shown to act on receptors physiologically stimulated by the opioid peptides. Pharmacologists have now defined several subclasses of opioid receptors in a fashion reminiscent of earlier studies of autonomic receptors.

Thus, the propensity of drugs to bind to different classes of receptor sites is not only a potentially vexing problem in treating patients it also presents a continuing challenge to pharmacology and an opportunity for developing new and more useful drugs.

REFERENCES

Becker AB, Roth RA: Insulin receptor structure and function in normal and pathological conditions. Annu Rev Med 1990;41:99.

Bell RM, Burns DJ: Lipid activation of protein kinase C. J Biol Chem 1990;266:4661

Berridge MJ: Inositol trisphosphate and calcium signaling. Nature 1993;361:315

Bourne HR, DeFranco AL: Signal transduction and intracellular messengers. In: *Oncogenes and the Molecular Origins of Cancer.* Weinberg R (editor). Cold Spring Harbor Press, 1989.

Changeux JP: The acetylcholine receptor: Its molecular biology and biotechnological prospects. Bioessays 1989; 10:48.

Edelman AM, Blumenthal DK, Krebs EG: Protein serine/threonine kinases. Annu Rev Biochem 1987;56:567.

Freissmuth M, Casey PJ, Gilman AG: G proteins control diverse pathways of transmembrane signaling. FASEB J 1989;3:2125.

Goldstein A, Aronow L, Kalman SM: *Principles of Drug Action: The Basis of Pharmacology,* 2nd ed. Wiley, 1974.

Kenakin TP: *Pharmacologic Analysis of Drug-Receptor Interaction.* Raven Press, New York, 1987.

Kobilka B: Adrenergic receptors as models for G protein-coupled receptors. Annu Rev Neurosci 1992;15:87.

Levitski A: From epinephrine to cyclic AMP. Science 1988; 241:800.

Lowenstein CJ, Snyder SH: Nitric oxide, a novel biologic messenger. Cell 1992;70:705.

Ullrich A, Schlesinger J: Signal transduction by receptors with tyrosine kinase activity. Cell 1990;61:203.

Wong SK, Garbers DL: Receptor guanylyl cyclases. J Clin Invest 1992; 90:299.

Pharmacokinetics & Pharmacodynamics: Rational Dose Selection & the Time Course of Drug Action

3

Nicholas H.G. Holford, MB, ChB, FRACP, & Leslie Z. Benet, PhD

The goal of therapeutics is to achieve a desired beneficial effect with minimal adverse effects. When a medicine has been selected for a patient, the clinician must determine the dose that most closely achieves this goal. A rational approach to this objective combines the principles of pharmacokinetics with pharmacodynamics to clarify the dose-effect relationship (Figure 3–1). Pharmacodynamics governs the concentration-effect part of the interaction, whereas pharmacokinetics deals with the dose-concentration part (Holford, 1981). The pharmacokinetic processes of absorption, distribution, and elimination determine how rapidly and in what concentration and for how long the drug will appear at the target organ. The pharmacodynamic concepts of maximum response and sensitivity determine the magnitude of the effect at a particular concentration (see E_{max} and EC50, Chapter 2).

Figure 3–1 illustrates a fundamental hypothesis of pharmacology, namely, that a relationship exists between a beneficial or toxic effect of a drug and the concentration of the drug in a readily accessible site of the body (eg, blood). This hypothesis has been documented for many drugs, as indicated by the Effective Concentrations and Toxic Concentrations columns in Table 3–1. The apparent lack of such a relationship for some drugs does not weaken the basic hypothesis but points to the need to consider the time course of concentration at the actual site of pharmacologic effect (see below).

Knowing the relationship between drug concentrations and effects allows the clinician to take into account the various pathologic and physiologic features of a particular patient that make him or her different from the average individual in responding to a drug. The importance of pharmacokinetics and pharmacodynamics in patient care thus rests upon the improvement in therapeutic efficacy and reduction in toxicity that can be achieved by application of their principles.

PHARMACOKINETICS

The "standard" dose of a drug is based on trials in healthy volunteers and patients with average ability to absorb, distribute, and eliminate the drug (see The IND & NDA, Chapter 5). This dose will not be suitable for every patient. Several physiologic (eg, maturation of organ function in infants) and pathologic processes (eg, heart failure, renal failure) dictate dosage adjustment in individual patients. These processes modify specific pharmacokinetic parameters. The two basic parameters are **clearance,** the measure of the ability of the body to eliminate the drug; and **volume of distribution,** the measure of the apparent space in the body available to contain the drug. These parameters are illustrated schematically in Figure 3–2, where the volume of the compartments into which the drugs diffuse represents the volume of distribution and the size of the outflow "drain" in Figures 3–2B and 3–2D represents the clearance.

Volume of Distribution

Volume of distribution (V_d) relates the amount of drug in the body to the concentration of drug (C) in blood or plasma:

$$V_d = \frac{\text{Amount of drug in body}}{C} \qquad (1)$$

The volume of distribution may be defined with respect to blood, plasma, or water (unbound drug), depending on the concentration used in equation (1) ($C = C_b$, C_p, or C_u).

That the V_d calculated from equation (1) is an *apparent* volume may be appreciated by comparing the volumes of distribution of drugs such as digoxin or chloroquine (Table 3–1) with some of the physical volumes of the body (Table 3–2). V_d can vastly exceed any physical volume in the body because the V_d is the volume necessary to contain the amount of drug *homogeneously* at the concentration found in the

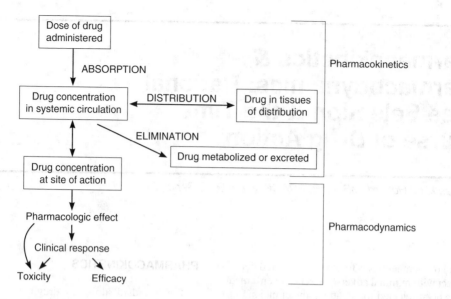

Figure 3–1. The relationship between dose and effect can be separated into pharmacokinetic (dose-concentration) and pharmacodynamic (concentration-effect) components: Concentration provides the link between pharmacokinetics and pharmacodynamics and is the focus of the target concentration approach to rational dosing. The three primary processes of pharmacokinetics are absorption, distribution, and elimination.

blood, plasma, or plasma water. Drugs with very high volumes of distribution have much higher concentrations in extravascular tissue than in the vascular compartment, ie, they are *not* homogeneously distributed. Drugs that are completely retained within the vascular compartment, on the other hand, have a minimum possible V_d equal to the blood component in which they are distributed, eg, 0.04 L/kg body weight (Table 3–2) or 2.8 L/70 kg for a drug that is restricted to the plasma compartment.

Clearance

Drug clearance principles are similar to the clearance concepts of renal physiology, in which creatinine clearance is defined as the rate of elimination of creatinine in the urine relative to its serum concentration (UV/P). At the simplest level, clearance of a drug is the ratio of the rate of elimination by all routes to the concentration of drug in a biologic fluid:

$$CL = \frac{\text{Rate of elimination}}{C} \qquad (2)$$

Clearance, like volume of distribution, may be defined with respect to blood (CL_b), plasma (CL_p), or unbound in the plasma water (CL_u), depending on the concentration measured.

It is important to note the additive character of clearance. Elimination of drug from the body may involve processes occurring in the kidney, the lung, the liver, and other organs. Dividing the rate of elimination at each organ by the concentration of drug pre-

sented to it yields the respective clearance at that organ. Added together, these separate clearances equal total systemic clearance:

$$CL_{renal} = \frac{\text{Rate of elimination}_{kidney}}{C} \qquad (3a)$$

$$CL_{liver} = \frac{\text{Rate of elimination}_{liver}}{C} \qquad (3b)$$

$$CL_{other} = \frac{\text{Rate of elimination}_{other}}{C} \qquad (3c)$$

$$CL_{systemic} = CL_{renal} + CL_{liver} + CL_{other} \qquad (3d)$$

"Other" tissues of elimination could include the lungs and additional sites of metabolism, eg, blood or muscle. The example provided in equations (3a–3d) indicates that the drug is eliminated by liver, kidney, and other tissues and that these routes of elimination account for all the pathways by which the drug leaves the body.

The two major sites of drug elimination are the kidneys and the liver. Clearance of unchanged drug in the urine represents renal clearance. Within the liver, drug elimination occurs via biotransformation of parent drug to one or more metabolites, or excretion of unchanged drug into the bile, or both. The pathways of biotransformation are discussed in Chapter 4. For most drugs, clearance is constant over the plasma or blood concentration range encountered in clinical set-

Table 3–1. Pharmacokinetic and pharmacodynamic parameters for selected drugs.

Drug	Oral Availability (F) (%)	Urinary Excretion (%)	Bound in Plasma (%)	Clearance (L/h/70 kg)[1]	Volume of Distribution (L/70 kg)	Half-Life (h)	Effective Concentrations	Toxic Concentrations
Acetaminophen	88	3	0	21	67	2	10–20 mg/L	>300 mg/L
Acyclovir	23	75	15	19.8	48	2.4	...	...
Amikacin	...	98	4	5.46	19	2.3	...	...
Amoxicillin	93	86	18	10.8	15	1.7	...	...
Amphotericin	...	4	90	1.92	53	18	...	...
Ampicillin	62	82	18	16.2	20	1.3	...	...
Aspirin	68	1	49	39	11	0.25	...	...
Atenolol	56	94	5	10.2	67	6.1	1 mg/L	...
Atropine	50	57	18	24.6	120	4.3	...	...
Captopril	65	38	30	50.4	57	2.2	50 ng/mL	...
Carbamazepine	70	1	74	5.34	98	15	6.5 mg/L	>9 mg/L
Cephalexin	90	91	14	18	18	0.9	...	...
Cephalothin	...	52	71	28.2	18	0.57	...	...
Chloramphenicol	80	25	53	10.2	66	2.7	...	...
Chlordiazepoxide	100	1	97	2.28	21	10	>0.7 mg/L	...
Chloroquine	89	61	61	45	13000	8.9	15–30 ng/mL	250 ng/mL
Chlorpropamide	90	20	96	0.126	6.8	33	...	...
Cimetidine	62	62	19	32.4	70	1.9	0.8 mg/L	...
Ciprofloxacin	60	65	40	25.2	130	4.1	...	...
Clonidine	95	62	20	12.6	150	12	0.2–2 ng/mL	...
Cyclosporine	23	1	93	24.6	85	5.6	100–400 ng/mL	>400 ng/mL
Diazepam	100	1	99	1.62	77	43	300–400 ng/mL	...
Digitoxin	90	32	97	0.234	38	6.7	>10 ng/mL	>35 ng/mL
Digoxin	70	60	25	7.8	440	39	>0.8 ng/mL	>2 ng/mL
Diltiazem	44	4	78	50.4	220	3.7	...	...
Disopyramide	83	55	2	5.04	41	6	3 mg/L	>8 mg/L
Enalapril	95	90	55	9	40	3	>0.5 ng/mL	...
Erythromycin	35	12	84	38.4	55	1.6	...	...
Ethambutol	77	79	5	36	110	3.1	...	>10 mg/L
Fluoxetine	60	3	94	40.2	2500	53	...	...
Furosemide	61	66	99	8.4	7.7	1.5	...	25 mg/L
Gentamicin	...	90	10	5.4	18	2.5	...	...
Hydralazine	40	10	87	234	105	1	100 ng/mL	...
Imipramine	40	2	90	63	1600	18	100–300 ng/mL	>1 mg/L
Indomethacin	98	15	90	8.4	18	2.4	0.3–3 mg/L	>5 mg/L
Labetalol	18	5	50	105	660	4.9	0.13 mg/L	...
Lidocaine	35	2	70	38.4	77	1.8	1.5–6 mg/L	>6 mg/L
Lithium	100	95	0	1.5	55	22	0.5–1.25 meq/L	>2 meq/L
Meperidine	52	12	58	72	310	3.2	0.4–0.7 mg/L	...
Methotrexate	70	48	34	9	39	7.2	...	10 μmol/L
Metoprolol	38	10	11	63	290	3.2	25 ng/mL	...
Metronidazole	99	10	10	5.4	52	8.5	3–6 mg/L	...
Midazolam	44	56	95	27.6	77	1.9	...	...

(continued)

Table 3–1 (cont'd). Pharmacokinetic and pharmacodynamic parameters for selected drugs.

Drug	Oral Availability (F) (%)	Urinary Excretion (%)	Bound in Plasma (%)	Clearance (L/h/70 kg)[1]	Volume of Distribution (L/70 kg)	Half-Life (h)	Effective Concentrations	Toxic Concentrations
Morphine	24	8	35	60	230	1.9	65 ng/mL	...
Nifedipine	50	0	96	29.4	55	1.8	47 ng/mL	...
Nortriptyline	51	2	92	30	1300	31	50–140 ng/mL	>500 ng/mL
Phenobarbital	100	24	51	0.258	38	4.1	10–25 mg/L	>30 mg/L
Phenytoin	90	2	89	Conc-dependent[3]	45	Conc-dependent[4]	10 mg/L	>20 mg/L
Prazosin	68	1	95	12.6	42	2.9	...	...
Procainamide	83	67	16	36	130	3	3–14 mg/L	>14 mg/L
Propranolol	26	- 1	87	50.4	270	3.9	20 ng/mL	...
Pyridostigmine	14	85	...	36	77	1.9	50–100 ng/mL	...
Quinidine	80	18	87	19.8	190	6.2	2–6 mg/L	>8 mg/L
Ranitidine	52	69	15	43.8	91	2.1	100 ng/mL	...
Rifampin	?	7	89	14.4	68	3.5	...	...
Salicyclic acid	100	15	85	0.84	12	13	150–300 mg/L	>200 mg/L
Sulfamethoxazole	100	14	62	1.32	15	10	...	...
Terbutaline	14	56	20	14.4	125	14	2.3 ng/mL	...
Tetracycline	77	58	65	7.2	105	11	...	...
Theophylline	96	18	56	2.88	35	8.1	10–20 mg/L	>20 mg/L
Tobramycin	...	90	10	4.62	18	2.2	...	...
Tocainide	89	38	10	10.8	210	14	6–15 mg/L	...
Tolbutamide	93	0	96	1.02	7	5.9	80–240 mg/L	...
Trimethoprim	100	69	44	9	130	11	...	...
Tubocurarine	...	63	50	8.1	27	2	0.6 mg/L	...
Valproic acid	100	2	93	0.462	9.1	14	30–100 mg/L	>150 mg/L
Vancomycin	...	79	30	5.88	27	5.6	...	...
Verapamil	22	3	90	63	350	4	...	...
Warfarin	93	3	99	0.192	9.8	37	...	...
Zidovudine	63	18	25	61.8	98	1.1	...	...

[1] Convert to mL/min by multiplying the number given by 16.6.
[2] Varies with concentration.
[3] Can be estimated from measured Cp using $CL = V_{max}/(K_m + Cp)$; $V_{max} = 415$ mg/d, $K_m = 5$ mg/L.
[4] Varies because of concentration-dependent clearance.

tings, ie, elimination is not saturable, and the rate of drug elimination is directly proportionate to concentration (rearranging equation [2]):

$$\text{Rate of elimination} = CL \times C \qquad (4)$$

This is sometimes referred to as "first-order" elimination. When clearance is first-order, it can be measured by calculating the area under the curve (AUC) of the time-concentration curve after a dose. Clearance is proportionate to the dose divided by AUC.

A. Capacity-Limited Elimination: For drugs that exhibit capacity-limited elimination (eg, phenytoin, ethanol), clearance will vary depending on the concentration of drug that is achieved (Table 3–1). Capacity-limited elimination is also known as saturable, dose- or concentration-dependent, nonlinear, and Michaelis-Menten elimination.

Most drug elimination pathways will become saturated if the dose is high enough. When blood flow to an organ does not limit elimination (see below), the relation between elimination rate and concentration (C) is expressed mathematically in equation (5):

$$\text{Rate of elimination} = \frac{V_{max} \times C}{K_m + C} \qquad (5)$$

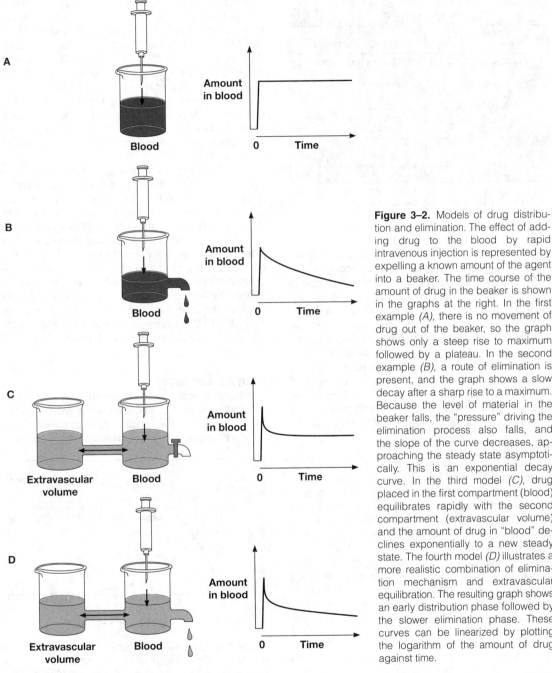

Figure 3–2. Models of drug distribution and elimination. The effect of adding drug to the blood by rapid intravenous injection is represented by expelling a known amount of the agent into a beaker. The time course of the amount of drug in the beaker is shown in the graphs at the right. In the first example *(A),* there is no movement of drug out of the beaker, so the graph shows only a steep rise to maximum followed by a plateau. In the second example *(B),* a route of elimination is present, and the graph shows a slow decay after a sharp rise to a maximum. Because the level of material in the beaker falls, the "pressure" driving the elimination process also falls, and the slope of the curve decreases, approaching the steady state asymptotically. This is an exponential decay curve. In the third model *(C),* drug placed in the first compartment (blood) equilibrates rapidly with the second compartment (extravascular volume) and the amount of drug in "blood" declines exponentially to a new steady state. The fourth model *(D)* illustrates a more realistic combination of elimination mechanism and extravascular equilibration. The resulting graph shows an early distribution phase followed by the slower elimination phase. These curves can be linearized by plotting the logarithm of the amount of drug against time.

This equation is similar to the Michaelis-Menten statement of enzyme kinetics. The maximum elimination capacity corresponds to V_{max} of the Michaelis-Menten equation, and K_m is the drug concentration at which the rate of elimination is 50% of V_{max}. It is important to note that in the nonlinear region, the increment in elimination rate becomes less as concentration increases. At concentrations that are high relative to the K_m, the elimination rate is almost independent of concentration—a state of "pseudo-zero order" elimination. If dosing rate exceeds elimination capacity, steady state cannot be achieved: The concentration will keep on rising as long as dosing continues. This pattern of capacity-limited elimination is important for three drugs in common use: ethanol, phenytoin, and aspirin. It is also the mechanism of elimina-

Table 3–2. Physical volumes (in L/kg body weight) of some body compartments into which drugs may be distributed.

Compartment and Volume	Examples of Drugs
Total body water (0.6 L/kg[1])	Small water-soluble molecules: eg, ethanol.
Extracellular water (0.2 L/kg)	Larger water-soluble molecules: eg, mannitol.
Blood (0.08 L/kg); plasma (0.04 L/kg)	Strongly plasma protein-bound molecules and very large molecules: eg, heparin.
Fat (0.2–0.35 L/kg)	Highly lipid-soluble molecules: eg, DDT.
Bone (0.07 L/kg)	Certain ions: eg, lead, fluoride.

[1]An average figure. Total body water in a young lean man might be 0.7 L/kg; in an obese woman, 0.5 L/kg.

tion for ethanol and is important when assessing the forensic significance of ethanol blood concentrations.

B. Flow-Dependent Elimination: In contrast to capacity-limited drug elimination, some drugs are cleared very readily by the organ of elimination, so that at any clinically realistic concentration of the drug, most of the drug in the blood perfusing the organ is eliminated on the first pass of the drug through it. The elimination of these drugs will thus depend primarily on the blood flow through the organ of elimination. Such drugs (listed in Table 4–6) can be called "high-extraction" drugs, since they are almost completely extracted from the blood by the organ.

Half-Life

Half-life ($t_{1/2}$) is the time required to change the amount of drug in the body by one-half during elimination (or during a constant infusion). In the simplest case—and the most useful in designing drug dosage regimens—the body may be considered as a single compartment (as illustrated in Figure 3–2B) of a size equal to the volume of distribution (V_d). While the organs of elimination can only clear drug from the blood or plasma in direct contact with the organ, this blood or plasma is in equilibrium with the total volume of distribution. Thus, the time course of drug in the body will depend on both the volume of distribution and the clearance:

$$t_{1/2} = \frac{0.7^* \times V_d}{CL} \tag{6}$$

However, many drugs will exhibit multicompartment pharmacokinetics (as illustrated in Figures 3–2C and

2D). Under these conditions, where more than one half-life term may apply to a single drug, the "true" terminal half-life as given in Table 3–1 will be greater than that calculated from equation (6). Nevertheless, half-life is a useful kinetic parameter in that it indicates the time required to attain 50% of steady state, or to decay 50% from steady-state conditions, after a change (ie, starting or stopping) in a particular rate of drug administration (the dosing regimen). Figure 3–3 shows the time course of drug accumulation during a constant-rate drug infusion and the time course of drug elimination after stopping an infusion that has reached steady state.

As an indicator of either drug elimination or distribution, half-life alone can be misleading. Disease states can affect both of the physiologically related parameters, volume of distribution, and clearance; thus, the derived parameter, $t_{1/2}$, will not necessarily reflect the expected change in drug elimination. For example, patients with chronic renal failure have a decreased renal clearance of digoxin and also a decreased volume of distribution; the increase in digoxin half-life is not as great as might be expected based on the change in renal function. The decrease in V_d is due to the decreased renal and skeletal muscle mass and consequent decreased tissue binding of digoxin.

Drug Accumulation

Whenever drug doses are repeated, the drug will accumulate in the body until dosing stops. This is because it takes an infinite time (in theory) to eliminate all of a given dose. In practical terms, this means that

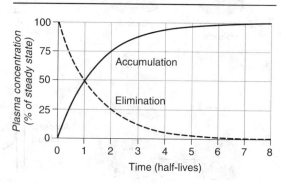

Figure 3–3. The time course of drug accumulation and elimination. *Solid line:* Plasma concentrations reflecting drug accumulation during a constant rate infusion of a drug. 50% of the steady state concentration is reached after one half-life, 75% after two half-lives, and over 90% after four half-lives. *Dashed line:* Plasma concentrations reflecting drug elimination after a constant rate infusion of a drug had reached steady state. Fifty percent of the drug is lost after one half-life, 75% after two half-lives, etc. The "rule of thumb" that 4 half-lives must elapse after starting a drug dosing regimen before full effects will be seen is based on the approach of the accumulation curve to over 90% of the final steady-state concentration.

---

*The constant 0.7 in equation (6) is an approximation to 0.693, the natural logarithm of 2. Because drug elimination can be described by an exponential process, the time taken for a twofold decrease can be shown to be proportionate to ln(2).

if the dosing interval is shorter than four half-lives, accumulation will be detectable.

Accumulation is inversely proportionate to the fraction of the dose lost in each dosing interval. The fraction lost is 1 minus the fraction remaining just before the next dose. The fraction remaining can be predicted from the dosing interval and the half-life. A convenient index of accumulation is the **accumulation factor.**

$$\text{Accumulation factor} = \frac{1}{\text{Fraction lost in one dosing interval}} \quad (7)$$

$$= \frac{1}{1 - \text{Fraction remaining}}$$

For a drug given once every half-life, the accumulation factor is 1/0.5, or 2. The accumulation factor predicts the ratio of the steady state concentration to that following the first dose. Thus, the peak concentrations after intermittent doses at steady state will be equal to the peak concentration after the first dose multiplied by the accumulation factor.

Bioavailability

Bioavailability is defined as the fraction of unchanged drug reaching the systemic circulation following administration by any route (Table 3–3). For an intravenous dose of the drug, bioavailability is equal to unity. Data on bioavailability following oral drug administration are set forth in Table 3–1 as percentages of dose available to the systemic circulation. For a drug administered orally, bioavailability may be less than 100% for two main reasons—incomplete extent of absorption and first-pass elimination.

A. Extent of Absorption: After oral administration, a drug may be incompletely absorbed, eg,

only 70% of a dose of digoxin reaches the systemic circulation. This is mainly due to lack of absorption from the gut and is in part explained by bacterial metabolism of digoxin within the intestine. Other drugs are either too hydrophilic (eg, atenolol) or too lipophilic (eg, acyclovir) to be absorbed easily, and their low bioavailability is also due to incomplete absorption. If too hydrophilic, the drug cannot cross the lipid cell membrane; if too lipophilic, the drug is not soluble enough to cross the water layer adjacent to the cell.

B. First-Pass Elimination: Following absorption across the gut wall, the portal blood delivers the drug to the liver prior to entry into the systemic circulation. A drug can be metabolized in the gut wall or even in the portal blood, but most commonly it is the liver that is responsible for metabolism before the drug reaches the systemic circulation. In addition, the liver can excrete the drug into the bile. Any of these sites can contribute to this reduction in bioavailability, and the overall process is known as first-pass loss or elimination. The effect of first-pass hepatic elimination on bioavailability is expressed as the **extraction ratio** (ER):

$$ER = \frac{CL_{liver}}{Q} \quad (8a)$$

where Q is hepatic blood flow, normally about 90 L/h in a person weighing 70 kg.

The systemic bioavailability of the drug (F) can be predicted from the extent of absorption (f) and the extraction ratio (ER):

$$F = f \times (1 - ER) \quad (8b)$$

This process is shown schematically in Figure 3–4. A drug like morphine is almost completely absorbed

Table 3–3. Routes of administration, bioavailability, and general characteristics.

Route	Bioavailability (%)	Characteristics
Intravenous	100 (by definition)	Most rapid onset
Intramuscular	≤100	Large volumes often feasible; may be painful
Subcutaneous	≤100	Smaller volumes than IM; may be painful
Oral	<100	Most convenient; first-pass effect may be significant
Rectal	<100	Less first-pass effect than oral
Inhalation	<100	Often very rapid onset
Transdermal	≤100	Usually very slow absorption; used for lack of first-pass effect; prolonged duration of action

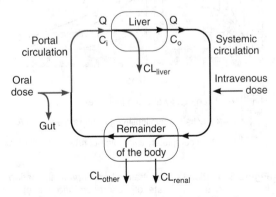

Figure 3–4. The clearance of drug by the liver is separated from the remaining systemic clearance to illustrate the effects of blood flow (Q) and extraction ratio ([C_i – C_o]/C_i) on organ clearance. The processes involved in first-pass metabolism are shown in color.

(f = 1), so that loss in the gut is negligible. However, the hepatic extraction ratio for morphine is 0.67, so (1 – ER) is 0.33. The bioavailability of morphine is therefore expected to be about 33%, which is close to the observed value (Table 3–1).

C. Rate of Absorption: In addition to the definition given above, bioavailability is sometimes used (confusingly) to indicate both the extent *and* the rate at which an administered dose reaches the general circulation.

The distinction between rate and extent of absorption is clarified in Figure 3–5. The rate of absorption is determined by the site of administration and the drug formulation. Both the rate of absorption and the extent of input can influence the clinical effectiveness of a drug. For the three different dosage forms depicted in Figure 3–5, there would be significant differences in the intensity of clinical effect. Dosage form B would require twice the dose to attain blood concentrations equivalent to those of dosage form A. Differences in rate of availability may become important for drugs given as a single dose, such as a hypnotic used to induce sleep. In this case, drug from dosage form A would reach its minimum effective concentration earlier than drug from dosage form C; concentrations from A would also reach a higher level and remain above the minimum effective concentration for a longer period. In a multiple dosing regimen, dosage forms A and C would yield the same average blood level concentrations, though dosage form A would show somewhat greater maximum and lower minimum concentrations.

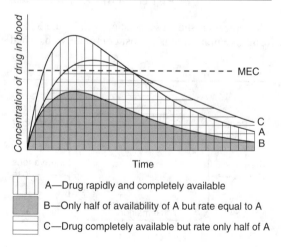

Figure 3–5. Blood concentration-time curves, illustrating how changes in the rate of absorption and extent of bioavailability can influence both the duration of action and the efficacy of the same total dose of a drug administered in three different formulations. The dashed line indicates the minimum effective concentration (MEC) of the drug in the blood.

The mechanism of drug absorption is said to be zero-order when the rate is independent of the amount of drug remaining in the gut, eg, when it is determined by the rate of gastric emptying or by a controlled-release drug formulation. In contrast, when the full dose is dissolved in gastrointestinal fluids, the rate of absorption is usually proportionate to the concentration and is said to be first-order.

Extraction Ratio & the First-Pass Effect

Disposition—systemic clearance, loss from the biologic system—is not affected by bioavailability. However, disposition can markedly affect the extent of availability because it determines the extraction ratio (equation [8a]). Of course, therapeutic blood levels may still be reached by the oral route of administration if larger doses are given. However, in this case, the levels of the drug *metabolites* will be increased significantly over those that would occur following intravenous administration. Lidocaine and verapamil are both used to treat cardiac arrhythmias and have similar bioavailability (20%), but lidocaine is never given orally because its metabolites are believed to contribute to central nervous system toxicity. Other drugs that are highly extracted by the liver include isoniazid, morphine, propranolol, verapamil, and several tricyclic antidepressants (Table 4–6).

Drugs with high extraction ratios will show marked intersubject variations in bioavailability because of differences in hepatic function and blood flow. These differences can explain the marked variation in drug concentrations that occurs among individuals given similar doses of highly extracted drugs. These considerations are also pertinent for hepatic diseases that are accompanied by significant intrahepatic or extrahepatic circulatory shunting and in the presence of surgically created anastomoses between the portal system and the systemic venous circulation. For drugs that are highly extracted by the liver, shunting of blood past hepatic sites of elimination will result in substantial increases in drug availability, whereas for drugs that are poorly extracted by the liver (for which the difference between entering and exiting drug concentration is small), shunting of blood past the liver will cause little change in availability. Drugs in Table 3–1 that are poorly extracted by the liver include chlorpropamide, diazepam, digitoxin, phenytoin, theophylline, tolbutamide, and warfarin.

Alternative Routes of Administration & the First-Pass Effect

Many routes of administration are used in clinical medicine (Table 3–3)—for convenience (eg, oral), to maximize concentration at the site of action and minimize it elsewhere (eg, topical), to prolong the duration of drug absorption (eg, transdermal), or to avoid the first-pass effect.

The hepatic first-pass effect can be avoided to a great extent by use of sublingual tablets and transdermal preparations and to a lesser extent by use of rectal suppositories. Sublingual absorption provides direct access to systemic—not portal—veins. The transdermal route offers the same advantage. Drugs absorbed from suppositories in the lower rectum enter vessels that drain into the inferior vena cava, thus bypassing the liver. However, suppositories tend to move upward in the rectum into a region where veins that lead to the liver, such as the superior hemorrhoidal vein, predominate. In addition, there are extensive anastomoses between the superior and middle hemorrhoidal veins; thus, only about 50% of a rectal dose can be assumed to bypass the liver.

Although drugs administered by inhalation bypass the hepatic first-pass effect, the lung may also serve as a site of first-pass loss by excretion and possibly metabolism for drugs administered by nongastrointestinal ("parenteral") routes. The lungs also provide a filtering function for particulate matter that may be given by intravenous injection.

THE TIME COURSE OF DRUG EFFECT

The principles of pharmacokinetics—discussed in this chapter—and those of pharmacodynamics—discussed in Chapter 2—provide a framework for understanding the time course of drug effect.

Immediate Effects

In the simplest case, drug effects are directly related to plasma concentrations, but this does not necessarily mean that effects simply parallel the time course of concentrations. Because the relationship between drug concentration and effect is not linear (recall the E_{max} model described in Chapter 2), the effect will not be always be directly proportionate to the concentration.

Consider the effect of an angiotensin-converting enzyme inhibitor, such as enalapril, on plasma angiotensin-converting enzyme (ACE). The half-life of enalapril is about 3 hours. After an oral dose of 10 mg, the peak plasma concentration at 3 hours is about 64 ng/mL. Enalapril is usually given once a day, so seven half-lives will elapse from the time of peak concentration to the end of the dosing interval. The concentration of enalapril after each half-life and the corresponding extent of ACE inhibition are shown in Figure 3–6. The extent of inhibition of ACE is calculated using the E_{max} model, where E_{max}, the maximum extent of inhibition, is 100% and the EC50 is about 1 ng/mL.

Note that plasma concentrations of enalapril change by a factor of 16 over the first 12 hours (four half-lives) after the peak, but ACE inhibition has only decreased by 20%. Because the concentrations over this time are so high in relation to the EC50, the effect

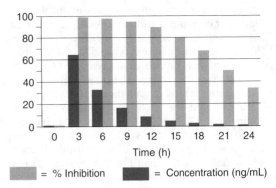

Figure 3–6. Time course of ACE inhibitor concentrations and effects. The darker bars show the plasma enalapril concentrations in nanograms per milliliter after a single oral dose. The lighter bars indicate the percentage inhibition of its target, angiotensin-converting enzyme. Note the different shapes of the concentration-time course (exponentially decreasing) and the effect-time course (linearly decreasing in its central portion).

on ACE is almost constant. After 24 hours, ACE is still 33% inhibited. This explains why a drug with a short half-life can be given once a day and still maintain its effect throughout the day. The key factor is a high initial concentration in relation to the EC50. Even though the plasma concentration at 24 hours is less than 1% of its peak, this low concentration is still half the EC50. This is very common for drugs that act on enzymes, eg, ACE inhibitors, or compete at receptors, eg, propranolol.

When concentrations are in the range between one-fourth and four times the EC50, the time course of effect is essentially a linear function of time—13% of the effect is lost every half-life over this concentration range. At concentrations below one-fourth the EC50, the effect becomes almost directly proportionate to concentration and the time course of drug effect will follow the exponential decline of concentration. It is only when the concentration is low in relation to the EC50 that the concept of a "half-life of drug effect" has any meaning.

Delayed Effects

Changes in the intensity of drug effects are often delayed in relation to changes in plasma concentration. This delay may reflect the time required for the drug to distribute from plasma to the site of action. This will be the case for almost all drugs. The delay due to distribution is a pharmacokinetic phenomenon that can account for delays of a few minutes up to a few hours. The distributional delay can account for the lag of effects after rapid intravenous injection of CNS-active agents such as thiopental.

A common reason for more delayed drug effects—especially those that take many hours or even days to occur—is the slow turnover of a physiologic substance that is involved in the expression of the drug effect. For example, warfarin works as an anticoagulant by inhibiting vitamin K epoxidase in the liver. This action of warfarin occurs rapidly, and inhibition of the enzyme is probably closely related to plasma concentrations of warfarin. The clinical effect of warfarin, eg, on the prothrombin time, reflects a decrease in the concentration of the prothrombin complex of clotting factors (Figure 33–7). Inhibition of vitamin K epoxidase decreases the synthesis of these clotting factors, but the complex has a long half-life (about 14 hours), and it is this half-life that determines how long it takes for the concentration of clotting factors to reach a new steady state and for a drug effect to become manifest reflecting the warfarin plasma concentration.

Cumulative Effects

Some drug effects are more obviously related to a cumulative action than to a rapidly reversible one. The renal toxicity of aminoglycoside antibiotics (eg, gentamicin) is greater when administered as a constant infusion as compared with intermittent dosing. It is the accumulation of aminoglycoside in the renal cortex that is thought to cause renal damage. Even though both dosing schemes produce the same average steady state concentration, the intermittent dosing scheme produces much higher peak concentrations, which saturate an uptake mechanism into the cortex; thus, total aminoglycoside accumulation is less. The difference in toxicity is a predictable consequence of the different patterns of concentration and the saturable uptake mechanism.

The effect of many drugs used to treat cancer also reflects a cumulative action, eg, the extent of binding of a drug to DNA is proportionate to drug concentration and is usually irreversible. The effect on tumor growth is therefore a consequence of cumulative exposure to the drug. Measures of cumulative exposure, such as area under the concentration time curve of the drug (AUC), have shown promise as predictors of response and—as a target AUC—provide a means to individualize treatment.

THE TARGET CONCENTRATION APPROACH TO DESIGNING A RATIONAL DOSAGE REGIMEN

A rational dosage regimen is based on the assumption that there is a *target concentration* that will produce the desired therapeutic effect. By considering the pharmacokinetic factors that determine the dose-concentration relationship, it is possible to individualize the dose regimen to achieve the target concentration. The effective concentration ranges shown in Table 3–1 are a guide to the concentrations measured when patients are being effectively treated. The initial target concentration should usually be chosen from

the lower end of this range. In some cases, the target concentration will also depend on the specific therapeutic objective—eg, the control of atrial fibrillation by digoxin often requires a target concentration of 2 ng/mL, while heart failure is usually adequately managed with a target concentration of 1 ng/mL.

Maintenance Dose

In most clinical situations, drugs are administered in such a way as to maintain a steady state of drug in the body, ie, just enough drug is given in each dose to replace the drug eliminated since the preceding dose. Thus, calculation of the appropriate maintenance dose is a primary goal. Clearance is the most important pharmacokinetic term to be considered in defining a rational steady state drug dosage regimen. At steady state (SS), the dosing rate ("rate in") must equal the rate of elimination ("rate out"). Substitution of the target concentration (TC) for concentration (C) in equation (4) predicts the maintenance dosing rate:

$$\text{Dosing rate}_{ss} = \text{Rate of elimination}_{ss}$$
$$= CL \times TC \tag{9}$$

Thus, if the desired target concentration is known, the clearance in that patient will determine the dosing rate. If the drug is given by a route that has a bioavailability less than 100%, then the dosing rate predicted by equation (9) must be modified. For oral dosing:

$$\text{Dosing rate}_{oral} = \frac{\text{Dosing rate}}{F_{oral}} \tag{10}$$

If intermittent doses are given, the maintenance dose is calculated from:

$$\text{Maintenance Dose} = \text{Dosing Rate} \times \text{Dosing Interval} \tag{11}$$

(See box: Example: Maintenance Dose Calculation.)

Note that the steady state concentration achieved by continuous infusion or the *average* concentration following intermittent dosing depends only on clearance. The volume of distribution and the half-life need not be known in order to determine the average plasma concentration expected from a given dosing rate or to predict the dosing rate for a desired target concentration. Figure 3–7 shows that at different dosing intervals, the concentration time curves will have different maximum and minimum values even though the average level will always be 10 mg/L.

Estimates of dosing rate and average steady state concentrations, which may be calculated using clearance, are independent of any specific pharmacokinetic model. In contrast, the determination of maximum and minimum steady state concentrations requires assumptions about the pharmacokinetic model. The accumulation factor (equation [7]) as-

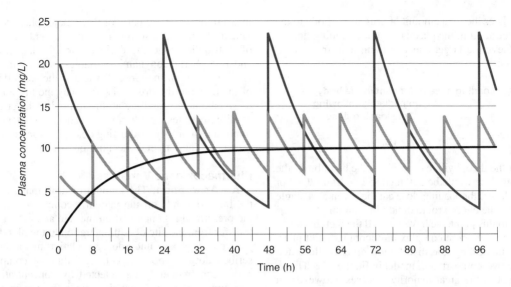

Figure 3–7. Relationship between frequency of dosing and maximum and minimum plasma concentrations when a steady-state theophylline plasma level of 10 mg/L is desired. The smoothly rising line (solid black) shows the plasma concentration achieved with an intravenous infusion of 28 mg/h. The doses for 8-hourly administration (light color) are 224 mg; for 24-hourly administration (dark color), 672 mg. In each of the three cases, the mean steady state plasma concentration is 10 mg/L.

sumes that the drug follows a one-compartment body model (Figure 3–2B), and the peak concentration prediction assumes that the absorption rate is much faster than the elimination rate. For the calculation of estimated maximum and minimum concentrations in a clinical situation, these assumptions are usually reasonable.

Loading Dose

When the time to reach steady state is appreciable, as it is for drugs with long half-lives, it may be desirable to administer a loading dose that promptly raises the concentration of drug in plasma to the target concentration. In theory, only the amount of the loading dose need be computed—not the rate of its administration—and, to a first approximation, this is so. The volume of distribution is the proportionality factor

---

EXAMPLE: MAINTENANCE DOSE CALCULATION

A target plasma theophylline concentration of 10 mg/L is desired to relieve acute bronchial asthma in a patient (Holford et al, 1993). If the patient is a nonsmoker and otherwise normal except for asthma, we may use the mean clearance given in Table 3–1, ie, 2.8 L/h/70 kg. Since the drug will be given as an intravenous infusion, F = 1.

$$\text{Dosing rate} = CL \times TC$$
$$= 2.8 \text{ L/h/70 kg} \times 10 \text{ mg/L}$$
$$= 28 \text{ mg/h/70 kg}$$

Therefore, in this patient, the proper infusion rate would be 28 mg/h/70 kg.

If the asthma attack is relieved, the clinician might want to maintain this plasma level using oral theophylline, which might be given every 12 hours using an extended release formulation to ap-

proximate a continuous intravenous infusion. According to Table 3–1, F_{oral} is 0.96. When the dosing interval is 12 hours, the size of each maintenance dose would be:

$$\text{Maintenance dose} = \frac{\text{Dosing rate}}{F} \times \text{Dosing interval}$$
$$= \frac{28 \text{ mg/h}}{0.96} \times 12 \text{ h}$$
$$= 350 \text{ mg}$$

A tablet or capsule size close to the ideal dose of 350 mg would then be prescribed at 12-hourly intervals. If an 8-hour dosing interval was used, the ideal dose would be 233 mg; and if the drug was given once a day, the dose would be 700 mg. In practice, F could be omitted from the calculation since it is so close to 1.

that relates the total amount of drug in the body to the concentration in the plasma (C_p); if a loading dose is to achieve the target concentration, then from equation (1):

$$\text{Loading dose} = \text{Amount in the body immediately following the loading dose}$$

$$= V_d \times TC \qquad (12)$$

For the theophylline example in the box above, the loading dose would be 350 mg (35 L × 10 mg/L). For most drugs, the loading dose can be given as a single dose by the chosen route of administration.

Up to this point, we have ignored the fact that some drugs follow more complex multicompartment pharmacokinetics, eg, the distribution process illustrated by the two-compartment model in Figure 3–2. This is justified in the great majority of cases. However, in some cases the distribution phase may not be ignored, particularly in connection with the calculation of loading doses. If the rate of absorption is rapid relative to distribution (this is always true for intravenous bolus administration), the concentration of drug in plasma that results from an appropriate loading dose—calculated using the apparent V_d—can initially be considerably higher than desired. Severe toxicity may occur, albeit transiently. This may be particularly important, for example, in the administration of antiarrhythmic drugs such as lidocaine, where an almost immediate toxic response may occur. Thus, while the estimation of the *amount* of a loading dose may be quite correct, the *rate of administration* can sometimes be crucial in preventing excessive drug concentrations, and slow administration of an intravenous drug (over minutes rather than seconds) is almost always prudent practice. For intravenous doses of theophylline, initial injections should be given over a 20-minute period to avoid the possibility of high plasma concentrations during the distribution phase.

When intermittent doses are given, the loading dose calculated from equation (12) will only reach the average steady state concentration and will not match the peak steady state concentration (see Figure 3–7). To match the peak steady state concentration, the loading dose can be calculated from equation (13):

$$\text{Loading Dose} = \text{Maintenance Dose} \times \text{Accumulation Factor} \qquad (13)$$

THERAPEUTIC DRUG MONITORING: RELATING PHARMACOKINETICS & PHARMACODYNAMICS

The basic principles outlined above can be applied to the interpretation of clinical drug concentration measurements on the basis of three major pharmacokinetic variables: absorption, clearance, and volume of distribution (and the derived variable, half-life); and two pharmacodynamic variables: maximum effect attainable in the target tissue and the sensitivity of the tissue to the drug. Diseases may modify all of these parameters, and the ability to predict the effect of disease states on pharmacokinetic parameters is important in properly adjusting dosage in such cases. (See box: The Target Concentration Strategy.)

Pharmacokinetic Variables

A. Absorption: The amount of drug that enters the body depends on the patient's compliance with the prescribed regimen and on the rate and extent of transfer from the site of administration to the blood.

Overdosage and underdosage relative to the prescribed dosage—both aspects of failure of compliance—can frequently be detected by concentration measurements when gross deviations from expected values are obtained. If compliance is found to be adequate, malabsorption abnormalities in the small bowel may be the cause of abnormally low concentrations. Variations in the extent of bioavailability are rarely caused by irregularities in the manufacture of the particular drug formulation. More commonly, variations in bioavailability are due to metabolism during absorption.

B. Clearance: Abnormal clearance may be anticipated when there is major impairment of the function of the kidney, liver, or heart. Creatinine clearance is a useful quantitative indicator of renal function. Conversely, drug clearance may be a useful indicator of the functional consequences of heart, kidney, or liver failure, often with greater precision than clinical findings or other laboratory tests. For example, when renal function is changing rapidly, estimation of the clearance of aminoglycoside antibiotics may be a more accurate indicator of glomerular filtration than serum creatinine.

Hepatic disease has been shown to reduce the clearance and prolong the half-life of many drugs. However, for many other drugs known to be eliminated by hepatic processes, no changes in clearance or half-life have been noted with similar hepatic disease. This reflects the fact that hepatic disease does not always affect the hepatic intrinsic clearance. At present, there is no reliable marker of hepatic drug-metabolizing function that can be used to predict changes in liver clearance in a manner analogous to the use of creatinine clearance as a marker of renal drug clearance.

C. Volume of Distribution: The apparent volume of distribution reflects a balance between binding to tissues, which decreases plasma concentration and makes the apparent volume larger, and binding to plasma proteins, which increases plasma concentration and makes the apparent volume smaller. Changes in either tissue or plasma binding can change the apparent volume of distribution determined from plasma concentration measurements. Older people have a relative decrease in skeletal muscle mass and tend to have a smaller apparent volume of distribution of digoxin. The volume of distribution may be overestimated in obese patients if based on body weight and the drug does not enter fatty tissues well, as is the case with digoxin. In contrast, theophylline has a volume of distribution (35 L) similar to that of total body water. Adipose tissue has almost as much water in it as other tissues, so that the apparent total volume of distribution of theophylline is proportionate to body weight, even in obese patients.

Abnormal accumulation of fluid—edema, ascites, pleural effusion—can markedly increase the volume of distribution of drugs such as tobramycin that are hydrophilic and—in the absence of such accumulation—have small volumes of distribution.

D. Half-Life: The differences between clearance and half-life are important in defining the underlying mechanisms for the effect of a disease state on drug disposition. For example, the half-life of diazepam increases with age. When clearance is related to age, it is found that clearance of this drug does not change with age (Klotz et al, 1975). The increasing half-life

---

THE TARGET CONCENTRATION STRATEGY

Recognition of the essential role of concentration in linking pharmacokinetics and pharmacodynamics leads naturally to the target concentration strategy. Pharmacodynamic principles can be used to predict the concentration required to achieve a particular degree of therapeutic effect. This target concentration can then be achieved by using pharmacokinetic principles to arrive at a suitable dosing regimen. The target concentration strategy is a process for optimizing the dose in an individual on the basis of a measured surrogate response such as drug concentration:

1. Choose the target concentration.
2. Predict V_d and CL based on typical population values (eg, Table 3–1) and adjustments for factors such as weight and renal function.
3. Give a loading dose or maintenance dose calculated from TC, V_d, and CL.
4. Measure the patient's response and drug concentration.
5. Revise V_d and CL based on the measured concentration.
6. Repeat steps 3–6, adjusting the maintenance dose as needed to optimize the response.

---

for diazepam actually results from changes in the volume of distribution with age; the metabolic processes responsible for eliminating the drug are fairly constant.

Pharmacodynamic Variables

A. Maximum Effect: All pharmacologic responses must have a maximum effect (E_{max}). No matter how high the drug concentration goes, a point will be reached beyond which no further increment in response is achieved.

If increasing the dose in a particular patient does not lead to a further clinical response, it is possible that the maximum effect has been reached. This can be verified by demonstrating that an increase in dose results in increased drug concentration without increased drug effect. Recognition of maximum effect is helpful in avoiding ineffectual increases of dose with the attendant risk of toxicity.

B. Sensitivity: The sensitivity of the target organ to drug concentration is reflected by the concentration required to produce 50% of maximum effect, the EC50. Failure of response due to diminished sensitivity to the drug can be detected by measuring—in a patient who is not getting better—drug concentrations that are usually associated with therapeutic response. This may be a result of abnormal physiology—eg, hyperkalemia diminishes responsiveness to digoxin—or drug antagonism—eg, calcium channel blockers impair the inotropic response to digoxin.

Increased sensitivity to a drug is usually signaled by exaggerated responses to small or moderate doses. The pharmacodynamic nature of this sensitivity can be confirmed by drug concentrations that are low in relation to the observed effect.

INTERPRETATION OF DRUG CONCENTRATION MEASUREMENTS

Clearance

Clearance is the single most important factor determining drug concentrations. The interpretation of measurements of drug concentrations depends upon a clear understanding of three factors that may influence clearance. These are the dose, the blood flow, and the intrinsic function of the liver or kidneys. Each of these factors should be considered when interpreting clearance estimated from a drug concentration measurement. It must also be recognized that changes in protein binding may lead the unwary to believe there is a change in clearance when in fact drug elimination is not altered (see box: Plasma Protein Binding: Is it Important?). Factors affecting protein binding include the following:

A. Albumin Concentration: Drugs such as phenytoin, salicylates, and disopyramide are extensively bound to plasma albumin. Albumin levels are

---

PLASMA PROTEIN BINDING: IS IT IMPORTANT?

Plasma protein binding is often mentioned as a factor playing a role in pharmacokinetics, pharmacodynamics, and drug interactions. However, there are no clinically relevant examples of changes in drug disposition or effects that can be clearly ascribed to changes in plasma protein binding. The idea that if a drug is displaced from plasma proteins it would increase the unbound drug concentration and increase the drug effect and, perhaps, produce toxicity seems a simple and obvious mechanism. Unfortunately, this simple theory, which is appropriate for a test tube, does not work in the body, which is an open system capable of eliminating unbound drug.

First, a seemingly dramatic change in the unbound fraction from 1% to 10% releases less than 5% of the total amount of drug in the body into the unbound pool because less than one-third of the drug in the body is bound to plasma proteins even in the most extreme cases, eg, warfarin. Drug displaced from plasma protein will of course distribute throughout the volume of distribution, so that a 5% increase in the amount of unbound drug in the body produces at most a 5% increase in pharmacologically active unbound drug at the site of action.

Second, when the amount of unbound drug in plasma increases, the rate of elimination will increase (if clearance is unchanged), and after four half-lives the unbound concentration will return to its previous steady state value. When drug interactions associated with protein binding displacement and clinically important effects have been studied, it has been found that the displacing drug is also an inhibitor of clearance, and it is the change in *clearance* of the unbound drug that is the relevant mechanism explaining the interaction.

---

low in many disease states, resulting in lower total drug concentrations.

B. α_1-Acid Glycoprotein Concentration: α_1-Acid glycoprotein is an important binding protein with binding sites for drugs such as quinidine, lidocaine, and propranolol. It is increased in acute inflammatory disorders and causes major changes in total plasma concentration of these drugs even though drug elimination is unchanged.

C. Capacity-Limited Protein Binding: The binding of drugs to plasma proteins is capacity-limited. Therapeutic concentrations of salicylates, disopyramide, and prednisolone show concentration-dependent protein binding. Because unbound drug concentration is determined by dosing rate and clearance—which is not altered, in the case of these low-extraction-ratio drugs, by protein binding—increases in dosing rate will cause corresponding changes in the pharmacodynamically important unbound concentration. Total drug concentration will increase less rapidly than the dosing rate would suggest as protein binding approaches saturation at higher concentrations.

Dosing History

An accurate dosing history is essential if one is to obtain maximum value from a drug concentration measurement. In fact, if the dosing history is unknown or incomplete, a drug concentration measurement loses all predictive value.

Timing of Samples for Concentration Measurement

Information about the rate and extent of drug absorption in a particular patient is rarely of great clinical importance. However, absorption usually occurs during the first 2 hours after a drug dose and varies according to food intake, posture, and activity. Therefore, it is important to avoid drawing blood until absorption is complete (about 2 hours after an oral dose). Attempts to measure peak concentrations early after oral dosing are usually unsuccessful and compromise the validity of the measurement, because one cannot be certain that absorption is complete.

Some drugs such as digoxin and lithium take several hours to distribute to tissues. Digoxin samples should be taken at least 6 hours after the last dose and lithium just before the next dose (usually 24 hours after the last dose). Aminoglycosides distribute quite rapidly, but it is still prudent to wait 1 hour after giving the dose before taking a sample.

Clearance is readily estimated from the dosing rate and mean steady state concentration. Blood samples should be appropriately timed to estimate steady state concentration. Provided steady state has been reached (at least three half-lives of constant dosing), a sample obtained near the midpoint of the dosing interval will usually be close to the mean steady state concentration.

Initial Predictions of Volume of Distribution and Clearance

A. Volume of Distribution: Volume of distribution is commonly calculated using body weight (70 kg body weight is assumed for the values in Table 3–1). If a patient is obese, drugs that do not readily penetrate fat (eg, tobramycin and digoxin) should have their volumes calculated from ideal body weight as shown below:

$$\text{Ideal body weight (kg)} = 52 + 1.9 \text{ kg/in over}$$
$$5 \text{ feet(men)} \qquad (14)$$
$$= 49 + 1.7 \text{ kg/in over } 5 \text{ feet(women)}$$

Patients with edema, ascites, or pleural effusions offer a larger volume of distribution to the aminoglycoside antibiotics (eg, tobramycin) than is predicted by body weight. In such patients, the weight should be corrected as follows: Subtract an estimate of the weight of the excess fluid accumulation. Use the resultant "normal" body weight to calculate the normal volume of distribution. Finally, this normal volume should be increased by 1 L for each estimated kilogram of excess fluid. This correction is important because of the relatively small volumes of distribution of these water-soluble drugs.

B. Clearance: Drugs cleared by the renal route often require adjustment of clearance in proportion to renal function. This can be conveniently estimated from the creatinine clearance, determined from a single blood sample (Bjornsson, 1979).*

$$\text{Creatinine clearance (L/h)} = \frac{160 - \text{Age (years)}}{22 \times \text{Serum creatinine (mg/dL)}} \times \frac{\text{weight (kg)}}{70} \tag{15}$$

(× 0.9 if female)

Note: If serum creatinine is measured in mmol/L, the 22 in the denominator should be replaced by 250.

The predicted clearance in women is 90% of the calculated value, because they have a smaller muscle mass per kilogram and it is muscle mass that determines creatinine production. Because of the difficulty of obtaining complete urine collections, creatinine clearance calculated in this way is at least as reliable as estimates based on urine collections. Ideal body weight should be used for obese patients, and correction should be made for muscle wasting in severely ill patients.

Revising Individual Estimates of Volume of Distribution & Clearance

The commonsense approach to the interpretation of drug concentrations compares predictions of pharmacokinetic parameters and expected concentrations to measured values. If measured concentrations differ by more than 20% from predicted values, revised estimates of V_d or CL for that patient should be calculated using equation (1) or equation (2). If the change calculated is more than a 100% increase or 50% decrease in either V_d or CL, the assumptions made about the timing of the sample and the dosing history should be critically examined.

For example, if a patient is taking 0.25 mg of digoxin a day, a clinician may expect the digoxin concentration to be about 1 ng/mL. This is based on typical values for bioavailability of 70% and total clearance of about 7 L/h (CL_{renal} 4 L/h, $CL_{nonrenal}$ 3 L/h). If the patient has heart failure, the nonrenal (hepatic) clearance might be halved because of hepatic congestion and hypoxia, so the expected clearance would become 5.5 L/h. The concentration is then expected to be about 1.3 ng/mL. Suppose that the concentration actually measured is 2 ng/mL. Common sense would suggest halving the daily dose to achieve a target concentration of 1 ng/mL. This approach implies a revised clearance of 3.5 L/h. The smaller clearance compared with the expected value of 5.5 L/h may reflect additional renal functional impairment due to heart failure.

This technique will often be misleading if steady state has not been reached. At least a week of regular dosing (three to four half-lives) must elapse before the implicit method will be reliable.

Failure to compare the expected concentration with the measured value in patients taking digoxin and quinidine explains why the major pharmacokinetic interaction between these two drugs went unnoticed for over 10 years, yet the doubling of steady state concentrations by the action of quinidine on digoxin clearance can be detected in almost every patient taking this drug combination.

REFERENCES

Benet LZ, Mitchell JR, Sheiner LB: Pharmacokinetics: The dynamics of drug absorption, distribution, and elimination. In: *Goodman and Gilman's The Pharmacological Basis of Therapeutics,* 8th ed. Gilman AG et al (editors). Pergamon, 1990.

Benet LZ, Williams RL: Design and optimization of dosage regimens: Pharmacokinetic data. In: *Goodman and Gilman's The Pharmacological Basis of Therapeutics,* 8th ed. Gilman AG et al (editors). Pergamon, 1990.

Bjornsson TD: Use of serum creatinine concentrations to determine renal function. Clin Pharmacokinet 1979;4:200.

Burton ME, Vasko MR, Brater DC: Comparison of drug dosing methods. Clin Pharmacokinet 1985;10:1.

Holford NHG et al: Theophylline target concentration in severe airways obstruction—10 or 20 mg/L? Clin Pharmacokinet 1993. [In press.]

Holford NHG, Sheiner LB: Understanding the dose-effect relationship. Clin Pharmacokinet 1981;6:429.

Klotz U et al: The effects of age and liver disease on the disposition and elimination of diazepam in adult man. J Clin Invest 1975;55:347.

Zito RA, Reid PR: Lidocaine kinetics predicted by indocyanine green clearance. N Engl J Med 1978;298:1160.

*A similar equation, the Cockcroft-Gault equation, is given in Chapter 62.

4

Drug Biotransformation

Maria Almira Correia, PhD

Humans are exposed daily to a wide variety of foreign compounds called **xenobiotics**—substances absorbed across the lungs or skin or, more commonly, ingested either unintentionally as compounds present in food and drink or deliberately as drugs for therapeutic or "recreational" purposes. Exposure to environmental xenobiotics may be inadvertent and accidental or—when they are present as components of air, water, and food—inescapable. Some xenobiotics are innocuous, but many can provoke biologic responses. Some of the toxic effects of these substances are discussed in Chapters 58–60. Such biologic responses often depend on conversion of the absorbed substance into an active metabolite. The discussion that follows is applicable to xenobiotics in general (including drugs) and to some extent to endogenous compounds.

WHY IS DRUG BIOTRANSFORMATION NECESSARY?

Renal excretion plays a pivotal role in terminating the biologic activity of a few drugs, particularly those that have small molecular volumes or possess polar characteristics such as functional groups fully ionized at physiologic pH. Most drugs do not possess such physicochemical properties. Pharmacologically active organic molecules tend to be lipophilic and remain unionized or only partially ionized at physiologic pH. They are often strongly bound to plasma proteins. Such substances are not readily filtered at the glomerulus. The lipophilic nature of renal tubular membranes also facilitates the reabsorption of hydrophobic compounds following their glomerular filtration. Consequently, most drugs would have a prolonged duration of action if termination of their action depended solely on renal excretion. An alternative process that may lead to the termination or alteration of biologic activity is metabolism. In general, lipophilic xenobiotics are transformed to more polar and hence more readily excretable products. The role metabolism may play in the inactivation of lipid-soluble drugs can be quite dramatic. For example, lipophilic barbiturates such as thiopental and pentobarbital would have extremely long half-lives if it were not for their metabolic conversion to more water-soluble compounds. On the other hand, lipophilic substances such as DDT that are stored in fat and protected from the major organs of drug metabolism may persist in body fat years after exposure has ceased.

Metabolic products are often less pharmacodynamically active than the parent drug and may even be inactive. However, some biotransformation products have enhanced activity or toxic properties, including mutagenicity, teratogenicity, and carcinogenicity. It is noteworthy that the synthesis of endogenous substrates such as steroid hormones, cholesterol, and bile acids involves many enzyme-catalyzed pathways associated with the metabolism of xenobiotics. The same is true of the formation and excretion of endogenous metabolic products such as bilirubin, the end catabolite of heme. Finally, drug-metabolizing enzymes have been exploited through the design of pharmacologically inactive prodrugs that are converted in vivo to pharmacologically active molecules.

THE ROLE OF BIOTRANSFORMATION IN DRUG DISPOSITION

Most metabolic biotransformations occur at some point between absorption of the drug into the general circulation and its renal elimination. A few transformations occur in the intestinal lumen or intestinal wall. In general, all of these reactions can be assigned to one of two major categories called phase I and phase II reactions (Figure 4–1).

Phase I reactions usually convert the parent drug to a more polar metabolite by introducing or unmasking a functional group (–OH, –NH$_2$, –SH). Often these metabolites are inactive, though in some instances activity is only modified.

If phase I metabolites are sufficiently polar, they may be readily excreted. However, many phase I products are not eliminated rapidly and undergo a subsequent reaction in which an endogenous substrate such as glucuronic acid, sulfuric acid, acetic

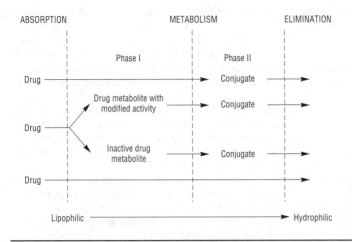

Figure 4–1. Phase I and phase II reactions in drug biodisposition. Phase II reactions may also precede phase I reactions.

acid, or an amino acid combines with the newly established functional group to form a highly polar conjugate. Such conjugation or synthetic reactions are the hallmarks of phase II metabolism. A great variety of drugs undergo these sequential biotransformation reactions, although in some instances the parent drug may already possess a functional group that may form a conjugate directly. For example, the hydrazide moiety of isoniazid is known to form an N-acetyl conjugate in a phase II reaction. This conjugate is then a substrate for a phase I type reaction, namely, hydrolysis to isonicotinic acid (Figure 4–2). Thus, phase II reactions may actually precede phase I reactions.

WHERE DO DRUG BIOTRANSFORMATIONS OCCUR?

Although every tissue has some ability to metabolize drugs, the liver is the principal organ of drug metabolism. Other tissues that display considerable activity include the gastrointestinal tract, the lungs, the skin, and the kidneys. Following oral administration, many drugs (eg, isoproterenol, meperidine, pentazocine, morphine) are absorbed intact from the small intestine and transported first via the portal system to the liver, where they undergo extensive metabolism. This process has been called a **first-pass effect.** Some orally administered drugs (eg, clonazepam, chlorpromazine) are more extensively metabolized in the intestine than in the liver. Thus, intestinal metabolism may contribute to the overall first-pass effect. First-pass effects may so greatly limit the bioavailability of orally administered drugs that alternative routes of administration must be employed to achieve therapeutically effective blood levels. The lower gut harbors intestinal microorganisms that are capable of many biotransformation reactions. In addition, drugs may be metabolized by gastric acid (eg, penicillin), digestive enzymes (eg, polypeptides such as insulin), or by enzymes in the wall of the intestine (eg, sympathomimetic catecholamines).

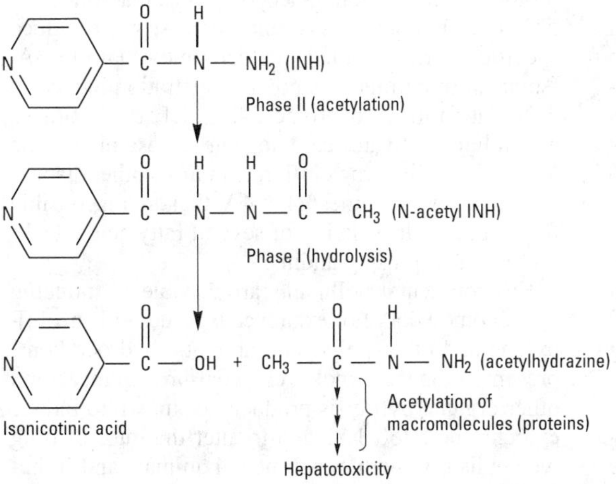

Figure 4–2. Phase II activation of isoniazid *(INH)* to a hepatotoxic metabolite.

Although drug biotransformation in vivo can occur by spontaneous, noncatalyzed chemical reactions, the vast majority are catalyzed by specific cellular enzymes. At the subcellular level, these enzymes may be located in the endoplasmic reticulum, mitochondria, cytosol, lysosomes, or even the nuclear envelope or plasma membrane.

MICROSOMAL MIXED FUNCTION OXIDASE SYSTEM

Many drug-metabolizing enzymes are located in the lipophilic membranes of the endoplasmic reticulum of the liver and other tissues. When these lamellar membranes are isolated by homogenization and fractionation of the cell, they re-form into vesicles called **microsomes.** Microsomes retain most of the morphologic and functional characteristics of the intact membranes, including the rough and smooth surface features of the rough (ribosome-studded) and smooth (no ribosomes) endoplasmic reticulum. Whereas the rough microsomes tend to be dedicated to protein synthesis, the smooth microsomes are relatively rich in enzymes responsible for oxidative drug metabolism. In particular, they contain the important class of enzymes known as the mixed function oxidases (MFO), or monooxygenases. The activity of these enzymes requires both a reducing agent (NADPH) and molecular oxygen; in a typical reaction, one molecule of oxygen is consumed (reduced) per substrate molecule, with one oxygen atom appearing in the product and the other in the form of water.

In this oxidation-reduction process, two microsomal enzymes play a key role. The first of these is a flavoprotein, NADPH-cytochrome P450 reductase. One mole of this enzyme contains 1 mol each of flavin mononucleotide (FMN) and flavin adenine dinucleotide (FAD). Because cytochrome c can serve as an electron acceptor, the enzyme is often referred to as NADPH-cytochrome c reductase. The second microsomal enzyme is a hemoprotein called cytochrome P450 that serves as the terminal oxidase. In fact, the microsomal membrane harbors multiple forms of this hemoprotein, and this multiplicity is increased by repeated administration of exogenous chemicals (see below). The name cytochrome P450 is derived from the spectral properties of this hemoprotein. In its reduced (ferrous) form, it binds carbon monoxide to give a complex that absorbs light maximally at 450 nm. The relative abundance of cytochrome P450, as compared to that of the reductase in the liver, contributes to making cytochrome P450 heme reduction a rate-limiting step in hepatic drug oxidations.

Microsomal drug oxidations require cytochrome P450, cytochrome P450 reductase, NADPH, and molecular oxygen. A simplified scheme of the oxidative cycle is presented in Figure 4–3. Briefly, oxidized (Fe^{3+}) cytochrome P450 combines with a drug substrate to form a binary complex (step ←). NADPH donates an electron to the flavoprotein reductase, which in turn reduces the oxidized cytochrome P450-drug complex (step ↑). A second electron is introduced from NADPH via the same flavoprotein reductase, which serves to reduce molecular oxygen and to form an "activated oxygen"-cytochrome P450-substrate complex (step →). This complex in turn transfers "activated" oxygen to the drug substrate to form the oxidized product (step ↓).

The potent oxidizing properties of this activated oxygen permit oxidation of a large number of substrates. Substrate specificity is very low for this enzyme complex. High solubility in lipids is the only common structural feature of the wide variety of structurally unrelated drugs and chemicals that serve as substrates in this system (Table 4–1).

Enzyme Induction

An interesting feature of some of these chemically dissimilar drug substrates is their ability, on repeated administration, to "induce" cytochrome P450 by enhancing the rate of its synthesis and/or reducing its rate of degradation. Induction results in an acceleration of metabolism and usually in a decrease in the pharmacologic action of the inducer and also of coadministered drugs. However, in the case of drugs metabolically transformed to reactive metabolites, enzyme induction may exacerbate metabolite-mediated tissue toxicity.

Various substrates appear to induce forms of cytochrome P450 having different molecular weights and exhibiting different substrate specificities and immunochemical and spectral characteristics. The two forms that have been most extensively studied are (1) cytochrome P450 2B1 (formerly P450b), which is induced by treatment with phenobarbital; and (2) cytochrome P450 1A1 (cytochrome P_1450, or P448), which is induced by polycyclic aromatic hydrocarbons (PAHs), of which 3-methylcholanthrene is a prototype. In addition, glucocorticoids, macrolide antibiotics, anticonvulsants, and some steroids induce specific forms called cytochromes P450 3A. Isoniazid or chronic ethanol administration induces a different form, cytochrome P450 2E1, that oxidizes ethanol and activates carcinogenic nitrosamines. The VLDL-lowering drug clofibrate induces other distinct isozymes, cytochromes P450 4A, that are responsible for omega-hydroxylation of several fatty acids, leukotrienes, and prostaglandins.

Environmental pollutants are capable of inducing cytochrome P450. For example, exposure to benzo[a]pyrene and other polycyclic aromatic hydrocarbons, present in tobacco smoke, charcoal-broiled meat, and other organic pyrolysis products, is known to induce cytochrome P450 1A1 and to alter the rates of drug metabolism in both experimental animals and in hu-

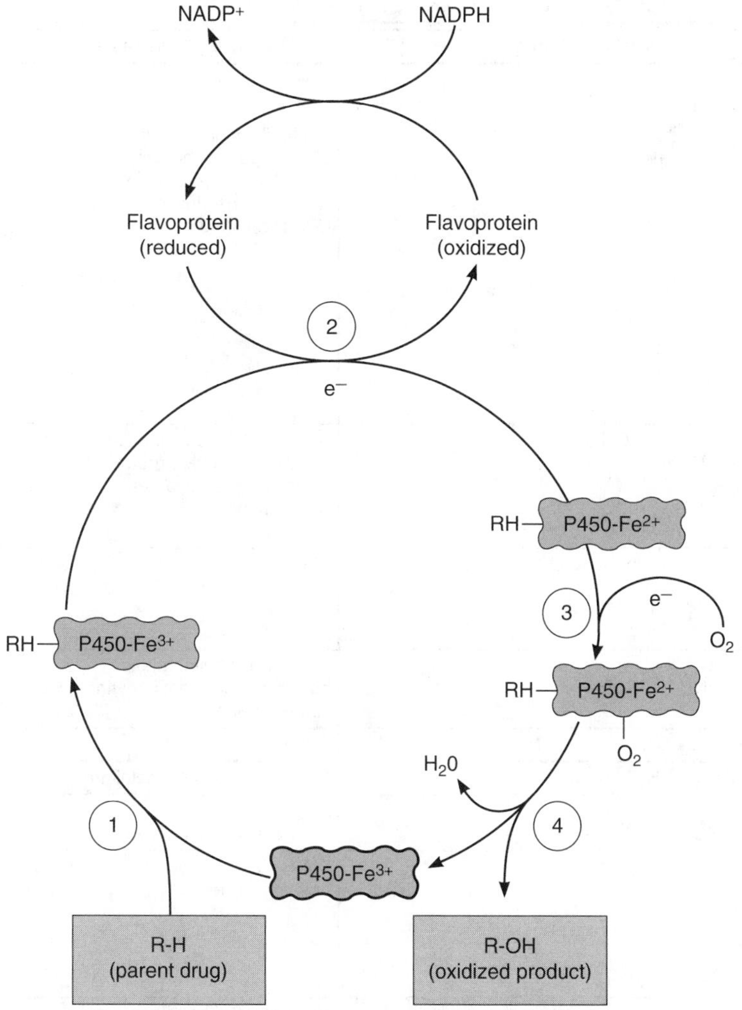

Figure 4–3. Cytochrome P450 cycle in drug oxidations. (RH, parent drug; ROH, oxidized metabolite; e^-, electron.)

mans. Other environmental chemicals known to induce specific cytochromes P450 include the polychlorinated biphenyls (PCBs), which are used widely in industry as insulating materials and plasticizers, and 2,3,7,8-tetrachlorodibenzo-*p*-dioxin (dioxin, TCDD), a trace by-product of the chemical synthesis of the defoliant 2,4,5-T (Chapter 58).

Increased synthesis of P450 requires enhanced transcription and translation. A cytoplasmic receptor for polycyclic aromatic hydrocarbons (eg, benzo[*a*]-pyrene, dioxin) has been identified, and the translocation of the inducer-receptor complex into the nucleus and subsequent activation of regulatory elements of genes have been documented. A similar receptor for the other class of inducing chemicals (eg, phenobarbital) has not yet been identified (Gonzalez, 1989).

Enzyme Inhibition

Certain drug substrates may inhibit cytochrome P450 enzyme activity. A well-known inhibitor is proadifen (SK&F 525-A). This compound binds avidly to the cytochrome molecule and thereby competitively inhibits the metabolism of potential substrates. Imidazole-containing drugs such as cimetidine and ketoconazole bind tightly to the heme-iron of cytochrome P450 and effectively reduce the metabolism of endogenous substrates (testosterone) or other coadministered drugs through competitive inhibition. However, macrolide antibiotics such as troleandomycin, erythromycin, and other erythromycin derivatives are metabolized, apparently by cytochrome P450 3A1, to metabolites that complex the cytochrome heme-iron and render it catalytically inactive. Some substrates irreversibly inhibit cytochrome P450 via covalent interaction of a metabolically generated reactive intermediate that may react with either the apoprotein or the heme moiety of the cytochrome. The antibiotic chloramphenicol is metabolized by cytochrome P450 to a species that alkylates its apocytochrome and thus also inactivates the

Table 4–1. Phase I reactions.

Reaction Class	Structural Change	Drug Substrates
Oxidations		
Cytochrome P450-dependent oxidations: Aromatic hydroxylations		Acetanilide, propranolol, phenobarbital, phenytoin, phenylbutazone, amphetamine, warfarin, 17α-ethinyl estradiol, naphthalene, benzpyrene
Aliphatic hydroxylations	$RCH_2CH_3 \rightarrow RCH_2CH_2OH$ $RCH_2CH_3 \rightarrow RCHCH_3$ $\qquad\qquad OH$	Amobarbital, pentobarbital, secobarbital, chlorpropamide, ibuprofen, meprobamate, glutethimide, phenylbutazone, digitoxin
Epoxidation	$RCH = CHR \rightarrow R - \overset{H}{\underset{\diagdown O \diagup}{C}} - \overset{H}{C} - R$	Aldrin
Oxidative dealkylation N-Dealkylation	$RNHCH_3 \rightarrow RNH_2 + CH_2O$	Morphine, ethylmorphine, benzphetamine, aminopyrine, caffeine, theophylline
O-Dealkylation	$ROCH_3 \rightarrow ROH + CH_2O$	Codeine, p-nitroanisole
S-Dealkylation	$RSCH_3 \rightarrow RSH + CH_2O$	6-Methylthiopurine, methitural
N-Oxidation Primary amines	$RNH_2 \rightarrow RNHOH$	Aniline, chlorphentermine
Secondary amines	$\begin{matrix} R_1 \\ \diagdown \\ \quad NH \\ \diagup \\ R_2 \end{matrix} \rightarrow \begin{matrix} R_1 \\ \diagdown \\ \quad N - OH \\ \diagup \\ R_2 \end{matrix}$	2-Acetylaminofluorene, acetaminophen
Tertiary amines	$\begin{matrix} R_1 \\ \diagdown \\ R_2 - N \\ \diagup \\ R_3 \end{matrix} \rightarrow \begin{matrix} R_1 \\ \diagdown \\ R_2 - N \rightarrow O \\ \diagup \\ R_3 \end{matrix}$	Nicotine, methaqualone
S-Oxidation	$\begin{matrix} R_1 \\ \diagdown \\ \quad S \\ \diagup \\ R_2 \end{matrix} \rightarrow \begin{matrix} R_1 \\ \diagdown \\ \quad S = O \\ \diagup \\ R_2 \end{matrix}$	Thioridazine, cimetidine, chlorpromazine
Deamination	$RCHCH_3 \rightarrow R - \overset{OH}{\underset{NH_2}{C}} - CH_3 \rightarrow R - \overset{}{\underset{O}{C}}CH_3 + NH_3$	Amphetamine, diazepam
Desulfuration	$\begin{matrix} R_1 \\ \diagdown \\ \quad C = S \\ \diagup \\ R_2 \end{matrix} \rightarrow \begin{matrix} R_1 \\ \diagdown \\ \quad C = O \\ \diagup \\ R_2 \end{matrix}$	Thiopental

Table 4–1. Phase I reactions.

Reaction Class	Structural Change	Drug Substrates
Cytochrome P450-dependent oxidations: (cont'd)		
	$\begin{array}{c} R_1 \\ \diagdown \\ \diagup \quad P=S \rightarrow \\ R_2 \end{array} \begin{array}{c} R_1 \\ \diagdown \\ \diagup \quad P=O \\ R_2 \end{array}$	Parathion
Dechlorination	$CCl_4 \rightarrow [CCl_3^\bullet] \rightarrow CHCl_3$	Carbon tetrachloride
Cytochrome P450-independent oxidations:		
Flavin monooxygenase (Ziegler's enzyme)	$R_3N \longrightarrow R_3N^+ \rightarrow O^- \xrightarrow{H^+} R_3N^+OH$	Chlorpromazine, amitriptyline, benzphetamine
	$\begin{array}{c} RCH_2N-CH_2R \rightarrow RCH_2-N-CH_2R \\ \quad\; H \qquad\qquad\qquad\;\; OH \\ \qquad\qquad\qquad\qquad \downarrow \\ \qquad\qquad RCH=N-CH_2R \\ \qquad\qquad\qquad\qquad O^- \end{array}$	Desipramine, nortriptyline
	$\begin{array}{c} -N \\ \diagdown \\ \diagup \quad -SH \rightarrow \\ -N \end{array} \begin{array}{c} -N \\ \diagdown \\ \diagup \quad -SOH \rightarrow \\ -N \end{array} \begin{array}{c} -N \\ \diagdown \\ \diagup \quad -SO_2H \\ -N \end{array}$	Methimazole, propylthiouracil
Amine oxidases	$RCH_2NH_2 \rightarrow RCHO + NH_3$	Phenylethylamine, epinephrine
Dehydrogenations	$RCH_2OH \rightarrow RCHO$	Ethanol
Reductions Azo reductions	$RN=NR_1 \rightarrow RNH-NHR_1 \rightarrow RNH_2 + R_1NH_2$	Prontosil, tartrazine
Nitro reductions	$RNO_2 \rightarrow RNO \rightarrow RNHOH \rightarrow RNH_2$	Nitrobenzene, chloramphenicol, clorazepam, dantrolene
Carbonyl reductions	$\begin{array}{c} RCR' \rightarrow RCHR' \\ \;\; \| \qquad\quad\; \| \\ \;\; O \qquad\quad OH \end{array}$	Metyrapone, methadone, naloxone
Hydrolyses Esters	$R_1COOR_2 \rightarrow R_1COOH + R_2OH$	Procaine, succinylcholine, aspirin, clofibrate, methylphenidate
Amides	$RCONHR_1 \rightarrow RCOOH + R_1NH_2$	Procainamide, lidocaine, indomethacin

enzyme. A growing list of inhibitors that attack the heme moiety includes the steroids ethinyl estradiol, norethindrone, and spironolactone; the anesthetic agent fluroxene; the barbiturates secobarbital and allobarbital; the analgesic sedatives allylisopropylacetylurea, diethylpentenamide, and ethchlorvynol; the solvent carbon disulfide; and propylthiouracil.

PHASE II REACTIONS

Parent drugs or their phase I metabolites that contain suitable chemical groups often undergo coupling or conjugation reactions with an endogenous substance to yield drug conjugates (Table 4–2). In general, conjugates are polar molecules that are readily excreted and often inactive. Conjugate formation in-volves high-energy intermediates and specific transfer enzymes. Such enzymes (transferases) may be located in microsomes or in the cytosol. They catalyze the coupling of an activated endogenous substance (such as the uridine 5'-diphosphate [UDP] derivative of glucuronic acid) with a drug (or endogenous compound), or of an activated drug (such as the S-CoA derivative of benzoic acid) with an endogenous substrate. Because the endogenous substrates originate in the diet, nutrition plays a critical role in the regulation of drug conjugations.

Drug conjugations were once believed to represent terminal inactivation events and as such have been viewed as "true detoxification" reactions. However, this concept must be modified, since it is now known that certain conjugation reactions (acyl glucuronidation of nonsteroidal anti-inflammatory drugs, O-sul-

Table 4–2. Phase II reactions.

Type of Conjugation	Endogenous Reactant	Transferase (Location)	Types of Substrates	Examples
Glucuronidation	UDP glucuronic acid	UDP-glucuronyl transferase (microsomes)	Phenols, alcohols, carboxylic acids, hydroxylamines, sulfonamides	Nitrophenol, morphine, acetaminophen, diazepam, N-hydroxydapsone, sulfathiazole, mepro-bamate, digitoxin, digoxin
Acetylation	Acetyl-CoA	N-Acetyl transferase (cytosol)	Amines	Sulfonamides, isoniazid, clonazepam, dapsone, mescaline
Glutathione conjugation	Glutathione	GSH-S-transferase (cytosol, microsomes)	Epoxides, arene oxides, nitro groups, hydroxylamines	Ethacrynic acid, bromobenzene
Glycine conjugation	Glycine	Acyl-CoA glycine transferase (mitochondria)	Acyl-CoA derivatives of carboxylic acids	Salicylic acid, benzoic acid, nicotinic acid, cinnamic acid, cholic acid, deoxy-cholic acid
Sulfate conjugation	Phosphoadenosyl phosphosulfate	Sulfotransferase (cytosol)	Phenols, alcohols, aromatic amines	Estrone, aniline, phenol, 3-hydroxycoumarin, acetaminophen, methyl-dopa
Methylation	S-Adenosyl-methionine	Transmethylases (cytosol)	Catecholamines, phenols, amines, histamine	Dopamine, epinephrine, pyridine, histamine, thiouracil
Water conjugation	Water	Epoxide hydrolase (microsomes)	Arene oxides, *cis*-disubstituted and monosubstituted oxiranes	Benzopyrene 7,8-epoxide, styrene 1,2-oxide, carbamazepine epoxide
		(cytosol)	Alkene oxides, fatty acid epoxides	Leukotriene A_4

fation of N-hydroxyacetylaminofluorene, and N-acetylation of isoniazid) may lead to the formation of reactive species responsible for the hepatotoxicity of the drug.

METABOLISM OF DRUGS TO TOXIC PRODUCTS

It is becoming increasingly evident that metabolism of drugs and other foreign chemicals may not always be an innocuous biochemical event leading to detoxification and elimination of the compound. Indeed, several compounds have been shown to be metabolically transformed to reactive intermediates that are toxic to various organs. Such toxic reactions may not be apparent at low levels of exposure to parent compounds when alternative detoxification mechanisms are not yet overwhelmed or compromised and the availability of endogenous detoxifying cosubstrates (glutathione, glucuronic acid, sulfate) is not limited. However, when these resources are exhausted, the toxic pathway may prevail, resulting in overt organ toxicity or carcinogenesis. The number of specific examples of such drug-induced toxicity is expanding rapidly. An example is acetaminophen (paracetamol)-induced hepatotoxicity (Figure 4–4).

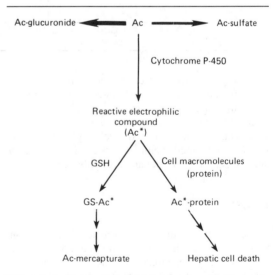

Figure 4–4. Metabolism of acetaminophen *(Ac)* to hepatotoxic metabolites. (GSH, glutathione; GS, glutathione moiety; Ac*, reactive intermediate.)

This analgesic antipyretic drug is quite safe in therapeutic doses (1.2 g/d for an adult). It normally undergoes glucuronidation and sulfation to the corresponding conjugates, which together comprise 95% of the total excreted metabolites. The alternative cytochrome P450-dependent glutathione (GSH) conjugation pathway accounts for the remaining 5%. When acetaminophen intake far exceeds therapeutic doses, the glucuronidation and sulfation pathways are saturated, and the cytochrome P450-dependent pathway becomes increasingly important. Little or no hepatotoxicity results as long as glutathione is available for conjugation. However, with time, hepatic glutathione is depleted faster than it can be regenerated, and accumulation of a reactive and toxic metabolite occurs. In the absence of intracellular nucleophiles such as glutathione, this reactive metabolite (thought to be an N-hydroxylated product or an N-acetylbenzoiminoquinone) reacts with nucleophilic groups present on cellular macromolecules such as protein, resulting in hepatotoxicity (Figure 4–4).

The chemical and toxicologic characterization of the electrophilic nature of the reactive acetaminophen metabolite has led to the development of effective antidotes—cysteamine and N-acetylcysteine. Administration of N-acetylcysteine (the safer of the two) within 8–16 hours following acetaminophen overdosage has been shown to protect victims from fulminant hepatotoxicity and death.

Similar mechanistic interpretations can be invoked to explain the nephrotoxicity of phenacetin and the hepatotoxicity of aflatoxin and of benzo[a]pyrene, a pyrolytic product of organic matter present in cigarette tar and smoke and in smoked foods.

CLINICAL RELEVANCE OF DRUG METABOLISM

The dose and the frequency of administration required to achieve effective therapeutic blood and tissue levels vary in different patients because of individual differences in drug distribution and rates of drug metabolism and elimination. These differences are determined by genetic factors and nongenetic variables such as age, sex, liver size, liver function, circadian rhythm, body temperature, and nutritional and environmental factors such as concomitant exposure to inducers or inhibitors of drug metabolism. The discussion that follows will summarize the most important variables relating to drug metabolism that are of clinical relevance.

Individual Differences

Individual differences in metabolic rate depend on the nature of the drug itself. Thus, within the same population, steady state plasma levels may reflect a 30-fold variation in the metabolism of one drug and only a twofold variation in the metabolism of another.

Genetic Factors

Genetic factors that influence enzyme levels account for some of these differences. Succinylcholine, for example, is metabolized only half as rapidly in persons with genetically determined defects in pseudocholinesterase as in persons with normally functioning pseudocholinesterase. Analogous pharmacogenetic differences are seen in the acetylation of isoniazid (Figure 4–5) and the hydroxylation of warfarin. The defect in slow acetylators (of isoniazid and similar amines) appears to be caused by the synthesis of less of the enzyme rather than of an abnormal form of it. Inherited as an autosomal recessive trait, the slow acetylator phenotype occurs in about 50% of blacks and whites in the USA, more frequently in Europeans living in high northern latitudes, and much less commonly in Asians and Inuits (Eskimos). Similarly, genetically determined defects in the oxidative metabolism of debrisoquin, phenacetin, guanoxan, sparteine, phenformin, and others have been reported (Table 4–3). The defects are apparently transmitted as autosomal recessive traits and may be expressed at any one of the multiple metabolic transformations that a chemical might undergo in vivo.

Two genetic variations of these drug metabolism polymorphisms have been particularly well investigated and so afford some insight into possible underlying mechanisms. First is the debrisoquin/sparteine oxidation type of polymorphism, which apparently occurs in 3–10% of Caucasians and is inherited as an autosomal recessive trait. In affected individuals, the cytochrome P450-dependent oxidations of debrisoquin, sparteine, phenformin, dextromethorphan, metoprolol, bufuralol, and several beta-adrenoceptor blockers and tricyclic antidepressants are impaired.

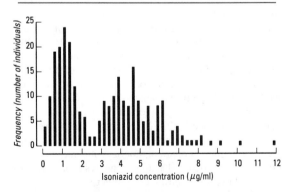

Figure 4–5. Genetic polymorphism in drug metabolism. The graph shows the distribution of plasma concentrations of isoniazid in 267 individuals 6 hours after an oral dose of 9.8 mg/kg. This distribution is clearly bimodal. Individuals with a plasma concentration greater than 2.5 mg/mL at 6 hours are considered slow acetylators. (Redrawn, with permission, from Evans DAP, Manley KA, McKusick VA: Genetic control of isoniazid metabolism in man. Br Med J 1960;2:485.)

Table 4–3. Some examples of genetic polymorphisms in drug metabolism.

Defect	Drug & Therapeutic Use	Clinical Consequences[1]
Oxidation	Bufuralol (β-adrenoceptor blocker)	Exacerbation of β-blockade, nausea
Oxidation	Debrisoquin (antihypertensive)	Orthostatic hypotension
Oxidation	Ethanol	Facial flushing, cardiovascular symptoms
N-Acetylation	Hydralazine (antihypertensive)	Lupus erythematosus-like syndrome
N-Acetylation	Isoniazid (antitubercular)	Peripheral neuropathy
Oxidation	Mephenytoin (antiepileptic)	Overdose toxicity
Oxidation	Sparteine (antiarrhythmic)	Oxytocic symptoms
Ester hydrolysis	Succinylcholine (neuromuscular blocker)	Prolonged apnea
Oxidation	Tolbutamide (hypoglycemic)	Cardiotoxicity

[1]Observed or predictable.

Findings from studies indicate that these defects in oxidative drug metabolism are probably co-inherited. The precise molecular basis for the defect appears to be faulty expression of the cytochrome P450 protein resulting in the absence of the necessary isozyme.

A second well-studied genetic drug polymorphism involves the stereoselective aromatic (4)-hydroxylation of the anticonvulsant mephenytoin. This polymorphism, which is also inherited as an autosomal recessive trait, occurs in 3–5% of Caucasians and 18–23% of Japanese populations. It is genetically independent of the debrisoquin/sparteine polymorphism. In normal "extensive metabolizers," S-mephenytoin is extensively hydroxylated at the 4 position of the phenyl ring before its glucuronidation and rapid excretion in the urine, whereas R-mephenytoin is slowly N-demethylated to nirvanol. "Poor metabolizers," however, appear to totally lack the stereospecific S-mephenytoin hydroxylase activity, so both S- and R-mephenytoin enantiomers are N-demethylated to nirvanol before excretion. The molecular basis for this defect is probably the expression of a mutant P450 isozyme that largely resembles the normal form but still exhibits sufficient structural microheterogeneity to significantly alter its substrate affinity and stereoselectivity, and consequently, its function. It is clinically important to recognize that the safety of a drug may be severely reduced in individuals who are poor metabolizers. For example, poor metabolizers of mephenytoin show signs of profound sedation and ataxia after doses of the drug that are well tolerated by normal metabolizers.

Additional genetic polymorphisms in drug metabolism that are inherited independently from those already described are being discovered. Studies of theophylline metabolism in monozygotic and dizygotic twins that included pedigree analysis of various families have revealed that a distinct polymorphism may exist for this drug and may be inherited as a recessive genetic trait. Genetic drug metabolism polymorphisms also appear to occur for aminopyrine, tolbutamide, and carbocysteine oxidations.

Although genetic polymorphisms in drug oxidations often involve specific cytochrome P450 isozymes, such genetic variations can occur at other sites. The recent descriptions of a polymorphism in the oxidation of trimethylamine, believed to be metabolized largely by the flavin monooxygenase (Ziegler's enzyme), suggest that genetic variants of other non-P450-dependent oxidative enzymes may also contribute to such polymorphisms.

Environmental Factors

Environmental factors also contribute to individual variations in drug metabolism. Cigarette smokers metabolize some drugs more rapidly than nonsmokers because of enzyme induction (see above). Industrial workers exposed to some pesticides metabolize certain drugs more rapidly than nonexposed individuals. Such differences make it difficult to determine effective and safe doses of drugs that have narrow therapeutic indices.

Age & Sex

Increased susceptibility to the pharmacologic or toxic activity of drugs has been reported in very young and old patients as compared to young adults (Chapter 62). Although this may reflect differences in absorption, distribution, and elimination, differences in drug metabolism cannot be ruled out—a possibility supported by studies in other mammalian species indicating that drugs are metabolized at reduced rates during the prepubertal period and senescence. Slower metabolism could be due to reduced activity of metabolic enzymes or reduced availability of essential endogenous cofactors. Similar trends have been observed in humans, but incontrovertible evidence is yet to be obtained.

Sex-dependent variations in drug metabolism have been well documented in rats but not in other rodents. Young adult male rats metabolize drugs much faster than mature female rats or prepubertal male rats. These differences in drug metabolism have been clearly associated with androgenic hormones. A few clinical reports suggest that similar sex-dependent differences in drug metabolism also exist in humans for ethanol, propranolol, benzodiazepines, estrogens, and salicylates.

Drug-Drug Interactions
During Metabolism

Many substrates, by virtue of their relatively high

lipophilicity, are retained not only at the active site of the enzyme but remain nonspecifically bound to the lipid membrane of the endoplasmic reticulum. In this state, they may induce microsomal enzymes; depending on the residual drug levels at the active site, they also may competitively inhibit metabolism of a simultaneously administered drug.

Enzyme-inducing drugs include various sedative-hypnotics, tranquilizers, anticonvulsants, and insecticides (see Table 4–4). Patients who routinely ingest barbiturates, other sedative-hypnotics, or tranquilizers may require considerably higher doses of warfarin or dicumarol, when being treated with this oral anticoagulant, to maintain a prolonged prothrombin time. On the other hand, discontinuance of the sedative may result in reduced metabolism of the anticoagulant and bleeding—a toxic effect of the enhanced plasma levels of the anticoagulant. Similar interactions have been observed in individuals receiving various combination drug regimens such as antipsychotics or sedatives with contraceptive agents, sedatives with anticonvulsant drugs, and even alcohol with hypoglycemic drugs (tolbutamide).

It must also be noted that an inducer may enhance not only the metabolism of other drugs but also its own metabolism. Thus, continued use of some drugs may result in a pharmacokinetic type of tolerance—progressively reduced effectiveness due to enhancement of their own metabolism.

Conversely, simultaneous administration of two or more drugs may result in impaired elimination of the more slowly metabolized drug and prolongation or potentiation of its pharmacologic effects (Table 4–5).

Table 4–4. Partial list of drugs that enhance drug metabolism in humans.

Inducer	Drug Whose Metabolism is Enhanced
Benzo[a]pyrene	Theophylline
Chlorcyclizine	Steroid hormones
Ethchlorvynol	Warfarin
Glutethimide	Antipyrine, glutethimide, warfarin
Griseofulvin	Warfarin
Phenobarbital and other barbiturates[1]	Barbiturates, chloramphenicol, chlorpromazine, cortisol, coumarin anticoagulants, desmethylimipramine, digitoxin, doxorubicin, estradiol, phenylbutazone, phenytoin, quinine, testosterone
Phenylbutazone	Aminopyrine, cortisol, digitoxin
Phenytoin	Cortisol, dexamethasone, digitoxin, theophylline
Rifampin	Coumarin anticoagulants, digitoxin, glucocorticoids, methadone, metoprolol, oral contraceptives, prednisone, propranolol, quinidine

[1]Secobarbital is an exception. See Table 4–5 and text.

Table 4–5. Partial list of drugs that inhibit drug metabolism in humans.

Inhibitor	Drug Whose Metabolism Is Inhibited
Allopurinol, chloramphenicol, isoniazid	Antipyrine, dicumarol, probenecid, tolbutamide
Cimetidine	Chlordiazepoxide, diazepam, warfarin, others
Dicumarol	Phenytoin
Diethylpentenamide	Diethylpentenamide (Novonal)
Disulfiram	Antipyrine, ethanol, phenytoin, warfarin
Ethanol	Chlordiazepoxide (?), diazepam (?), methanol
Ketoconazole	Cyclosporine, astemizole, terfenadine
Nortriptyline	Antipyrine
Oral contraceptives	Antipyrine
Phenylbutazone	Phenytoin, tolbutamide
Secobarbital	Secobarbital
Troleandomycin	Theophylline, methylprednisolone

Both competitive substrate inhibition and irreversible substrate-mediated enzyme inactivation may augment plasma drug levels and lead to toxic effects from drugs with narrow therapeutic indices. For example, it has been shown that erythromycin inhibits the metabolism of the antihistamine terfenadine and leads to the expression of adverse effects such as cardiac arrhythmias. Similarly, allopurinol both prolongs the duration and enhances the chemotherapeutic action of mercaptopurine by competitive inhibition of xanthine oxidase. Consequently, to avoid bone marrow toxicity, the dose of mercaptopurine is usually reduced in patients receiving allopurinol. Cimetidine, a drug used in the treatment of peptic ulcer, has been shown to potentiate the pharmacologic actions of anticoagulants and sedatives. The metabolism of chlordiazepoxide has been shown to be inhibited by 63% after a single dose of cimetidine; such effects are reversed within 48 hours after withdrawal of cimetidine.

Impairment of metabolism may also result if a simultaneously administered drug irreversibly inactivates a common metabolizing enzyme, as is the case with secobarbital or novonal (diethylpentenamide) overdoses. These compounds, in the course of their metabolism by cytochrome P450, inactivate the enzyme and result in impairment of their own metabolism and that of other cosubstrates.

Interactions Between Drugs & Endogenous Compounds

Various drugs require conjugation with endogenous substrates such as glutathione, glucuronic acid, and sulfate for their inactivation. Consequently, different drugs may compete for the same endogenous substrates, and the faster-reacting drug may effectively deplete endogenous substrate levels and impair the metabolism of the slower-reacting drug. If the latter has a steep dose-response curve or a narrow margin of safety, potentiation of its pharmacologic and toxic effects may result.

Diseases Affecting Drug Metabolism

Acute or chronic diseases that affect liver architecture or function markedly affect hepatic metabolism of some drugs. Such conditions include fat accumulation, alcoholic hepatitis, active or inactive alcoholic cirrhosis, hemochromatosis, chronic active hepatitis, biliary cirrhosis, and acute viral or drug hepatitis. Depending on their severity, these conditions impair hepatic drug-metabolizing enzymes, particularly microsomal oxidases, and thereby markedly affect drug elimination. For example, the half-lives of chlordiazepoxide and diazepam in patients with liver cirrhosis or acute viral hepatitis are greatly increased, with a corresponding prolongation of their effects. Consequently, these drugs may cause coma in patients with liver disease when given in ordinary doses.

Liver cancer has been reported to impair hepatic drug metabolism in humans. For example, aminopyrine metabolism is slower in patients with malignant hepatic tumors than in normal controls. These patients also exhibit markedly diminished aminopyrine clearance rates. Studies of liver biopsy specimens from patients with hepatocellular carcinoma also indicate impaired ability to oxidatively metabolize drugs in vitro. This is associated with a correspondingly reduced cytochrome P450 content.

Cardiac disease, by limiting blood flow to the liver, may impair disposition of those drugs whose metabolism is flow-limited (Table 4–6). These drugs are so readily metabolized by the liver that hepatic clearance is essentially equal to liver blood flow. Pulmonary disease may also affect drug metabolism as indicated by the impaired hydrolysis of procainamide and pro-

Table 4–6. Rapidly metabolized drugs whose hepatic clearance is blood flow-limited.

Alprenolol	Lidocaine
Amitriptyline	Meperidine
Clomethiazole	Morphine
Desipramine	Pentazocine
Imipramine	Propoxyphene
Isoniazid	Propranolol
Labetalol	Verapamil

caine in patients with chronic respiratory insufficiency and the increased half-life of antipyrine in patients with lung cancer. Impairment of enzyme activity or defective formation of enzymes associated with heavy metal poisoning or porphyria also results in reduction of hepatic drug metabolism. For example, lead poisoning has been shown to increase the half-life of antipyrine in humans.

Although the effects of endocrine dysfunction on drug metabolism have been well explored in experimental animal models, corresponding data for humans with endocrine disorders are scanty. Thyroid dysfunction has been associated with altered metabolism of some drugs and of some endogenous compounds as well. Hypothyroidism increases the half-life of antipyrine, digoxin, methimazole, and practolol, whereas hyperthyroidism has the opposite effect. A few clinical studies in diabetic patients indicate no apparent impairment of drug metabolism, as reflected by the half-lives of antipyrine, tolbutamide, and phenylbutazone. In contrast, the metabolism of several drugs is impaired in male rats treated with diabetogenic agents such as alloxan or streptozocin. These alterations are abolished by administration of insulin, which has no direct influence on hepatic drug-metabolizing enzymes. Malfunctions of the pituitary, adrenal cortex, and gonads markedly impair hepatic drug metabolism in rats. On the basis of these findings, it may be supposed that such disorders could significantly affect drug metabolism in humans. However, until sufficient evidence is obtained from clinical studies in patients, such extrapolations must be considered tentative.

REFERENCES

Correia MA, Ortiz de Montellano P: Inhibitors of cytochrome P-450 and possibilities for their therapeutic application. In: *Frontiers in Biotransformation,* vol 8. Ruckpaul K (editor). Taylor & Francis, 1993.

Dayer P et al: Contribution of the genetic status of oxidative metabolism to variability in the plasma concentrations of beta-adrenoceptor blocking agents. Eur J Clin Pharmacol 1983;24:797.

Desmond PV et al: Cimetidine impairs elimination of chlordiazepoxide (Librium) in man. Ann Intern Med 1980; 93:266.

Gilmore DA et al: Age and gender influence the stereoselective pharmacokinetics of propranolol. J Pharmacol Exp Ther 1992;261:1181.

Gonzalez F: The molecular biology of cytochrome P450s. Pharmacol Rev 1989;40:243.

Gonzalez FJ et al: Characterization of the common genetic defect in humans deficient in debrisoquin metabolism. Nature 1988;331:442.

Gonzalez FJ: Human cytochromes P450: problems and prospects. Trends Pharmacol Sci 1992;13:346.

Guengerich FP (editor): *Mammalian Cytochromes P-450:*

Structure, Mechanism and Biochemistry. Plenum Press, 1986.

Guengerich FP: Reactions and significance of cytochrome P-450 enzymes. J Biol Chem 1991:266:10019.

Jenner P, Testa B (editors): *Concepts in Drug Metabolism.* Part B of: *Drugs and the Pharmaceutical Science Series,* vol 10. Marcel Dekker, 1981.

Kroemer HK, Klotz U: Glucuronidation of drugs. A re-evaluation of the pharmacological significance of the conjugates and modulating factors. Clin Pharmacokinet 1992;23:292.

La Du BN, Mandel G, Way EL (editors): *Fundamentals of Drug Metabolism and Drug Disposition.* Williams & Wilkins, 1971.

Miller LG: Recent developments in the study of the effects of cigarette smoking on clinical pharmacokinetics and clinical pharmacodynamics. Clin Pharmacokinet 1989; 17:90.

Minchin RF, Boyd MR: Localization of metabolic activation and deactivation systems in the lung: Significance to the pulmonary toxicity of xenobiotics. Annu Rev Pharmacol Toxicol 1983;23:217.

Murray M: P450 enzymes. Inhibition mechanisms, genetic regulation, and effects of liver disease. Clin Pharmacokinet 1992;23:132.

Nelson DR et al: The P450 superfamily; update on new sequences, gene mapping, accession numbers, early trivial names of enzymes, and nomenclature. DNA Cell Biol 1993;12:1.

Ortiz de Montellano PR, Correia MA: Suicidal destruction of cytochrome P-450 during oxidative drug metabolism. Annu Rev Pharmacol Toxicol 1983;23:481.

Testa B, Jenner P (editors): *Drug Metabolism: Chemical and Biological Aspects.* Marcel Dekker, 1976.

Vessell ES: Genetic and environmental factors causing variation in drug response. Mutation Res 1991;247:241.

Waxman DJ, Azaroff L: Phenobarbital induction of cytochrome P-450 gene expression. Biochem J 1992;281: 577.

Wood AJJ, Zhou H-H: Ethnic differences in drug disposition and responsiveness. Clin Pharmacokinet 1991;20: 350.

Zanger UM et al: Absence of hepatic cytochrome P450bufI causes genetically deficient debrisoquin oxidation in man. Biochemistry 1988;27:5447.

Zhou H-H et al: Racial differences in drug response: Altered sensitivity to and clearance of propranolol in men of Chinese descent as compared with American males. N Engl J Med 1989;320:565.

5

Basic & Clinical Evaluation of New Drugs

Barry A. Berkowitz, PhD, & Bertram G. Katzung, MD, PhD

During the past 60 years, new drug developments have revolutionized the practice of medicine, converting many once fatal diseases into almost routine therapeutic exercises. One cause of this medical advance has been a fundamental improvement in the means of developing and testing new drugs. This process has been greatly accelerated by new technology, by financial motivation, and by governmental support of medical research. In most countries, the testing of drugs is now regulated by legislation and closely monitored by governmental agencies. This chapter summarizes the process by which new therapeutic agents are discovered, developed, and regulated. While the examples used reflect the USA experience, the pathway of new drug development generally is the same worldwide.

The first step in the development of a new drug is the discovery or synthesis of a potential new drug molecule (Figure 5–1). By law, the safety and efficacy of drugs must be defined before they can be marketed. In addition to in vitro studies, most of the biologic effects of the molecule must be characterized in animals before human drug trials can be started. Human testing must then go forward in three conventional phases before the drug can be considered for approval for general use. A fourth phase of data gathering follows after approval for general use.

Enormous costs, from $100 million to over $350 million, are involved in the development of a single successful new drug. These costs include the labor invested in searching for useful new molecules—5000–10,000 may be synthesized for each successful new drug introduced—and the costs of detailed basic and clinical studies and promotion of the ultimate candidate molecule. It is primarily because of the economic investment and risks involved that most new drugs are now developed in the laboratories of pharmaceutical companies. At the same time, the incentives to succeed in drug development are equally enormous. The worldwide market for ethical (prescription) pharmaceuticals in 1991 was estimated to be $141 billion.

DRUG DISCOVERY

Most new drug candidates are identified through one of three approaches: (1) chemical modification of a known molecule; (2) random screening for biologic activity of large numbers of natural products, banks of previously discovered chemical entities, or large libraries of peptides and nucleic acids; or (3) rational drug design based on an understanding of biologic mechanisms and chemical structure. The development of the thiazide diuretics from the much less useful carbonic anhydrase inhibitors (Chapter 15) is an example of the first approach. The discovery of cyclosporine, an important immunosuppressant derivative of a fungus, illustrates the second approach. An early example of the third approach was the development of H_2 histamine antagonists (Table 5–1). Based on the suspected existence of different types of histamine receptors, rational molecular modification led to the introduction of cimetidine, as described in the case study accompanying the text. Rational drug design has made major strides in the past 10 years, as illustrated by the development of angiotensin-converting enzyme inhibitors from a study of the structure-activity relationships of enzyme active site inhibitors and by the current development of hypothetical drug structures with computer assistance.

Regardless of the source of the candidate molecule, testing it involves a sequence of experimentation and characterization called **drug screening.** A variety of biologic assays at the molecular, cellular, organ, and whole animal levels are used to define the activity and selectivity of the drug. The type and number of initial screening tests depend on the pharmacologic goal. Antiinfective drugs will generally be tested first against a variety of infectious organisms, hypoglycemic drugs for their ability to lower blood sugar, etc. However, the molecule is usually studied for a broad array of actions to establish the selectivity of the drug. This has the advantage of demonstrating unsuspected toxic effects and occasionally discloses a previously unsuspected therapeutic action. The selection of molecules for further study is most efficiently conducted in animal models of human disease. Where

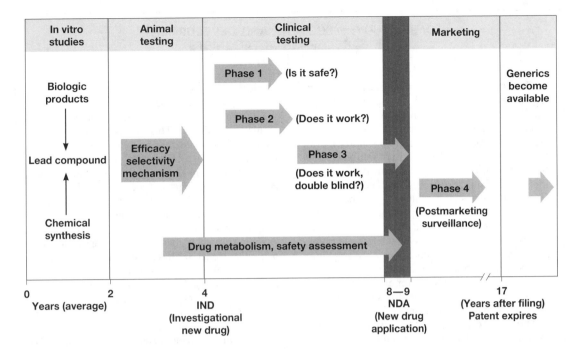

Figure 5–1. The development and testing process required to bring a drug to market in the USA. Some of the requirements may be different for drugs used in life-threatening diseases.

Table 5–1. A history of the development of H_2 receptor blockers.

Compound and Characteristics	Structure	Antagonist Activity (in vivo ID_{50}, $\mu mol/kg$)[1]
Histamine The starting point.		Agonist
N-Guanylhistamine The first lead compound. A weak partial agonist.		800
Burimamide Thiourea compound with a longer side chain. Weakly active in humans.		6.1
Metiamide Active in humans but toxic.		1.6
Cimetidine Replaces the thiourea with an N–CN substituent. Retains high potency with decreased toxicity. Launched the major series of drugs for the treatment of acid-peptic disorders.		1.4

[1]Activity in the anesthetized rate against histamine stimulation of acid secretion. The ID_{50} is the intravenous dose required to produce 50% inhibition. From Brimblecombe RW et al, 1978; and Black J, 1989.

CASE STUDY: DISCOVERY AND DEVELOPMENT
OF H$_2$-RECEPTOR ANTAGONISTS
(Table 5–1)

The idea: The H$_2$ receptor blockers are the largest-selling drug group in the world today. Their discovery began with the observations that histamine is a potent stimulant of gastric acid secretion and that the classic antihistamines (now known to be H$_1$ blockers) did not inhibit this action. To James Black, who had already developed the first useful β-adrenoceptor blockers, these observations suggested that there might be distinct subtypes of histamine receptors serving different functions and that these receptors could be stimulated or blocked in a selective manner by drugs.

The clinical need: Peptic ulcers are very common and can be treated by suppressing gastric acid secretion. The clinical need for effective acid suppression was not met by the drugs or the surgery then in use to treat ulcer disease.

The biologic hypothesis: Black's biologic hypothesis was that histamine could be selectively blocked at the receptors that mediate histamine's effects on acid secretion. Functional experimental systems existed that could be used as models and assays for effect and were capable of being measured with definite end points. It was believed that some of these experimental systems were reasonable models of human ulcer disease.

The chemical hypothesis: The chemical hypothesis was based on the fact that the then existing antihistaminic drugs were ineffective for treatment of acid-related gastrointestinal disorders and had no obvious chemical similarity to the structure of histamine. The research team reasoned that *chemical modification of histamine itself* might result in a selective antagonist for the postulated gastric histamine receptors.

Development: The chase began in 1964 when Black came to Smith Kline and French Laboratories in England. After some early difficulties had been overcome, a large number of compounds based on histamine's structure were synthesized and tested. Following adequate demonstration of the safety and efficacy of several compounds in preclinical models, testing in humans was undertaken. The first selective H$_2$ antagonist, burimamide, lacked adequate potency and clinical activity. The structure of burimamide was further altered to produce the more potent metiamide.

Clinical trials with this compound revealed good efficacy but also unexpected and serious toxicity: granulocytopenia. Further rational analysis finally yielded cimetidine. This molecule successfully completed clinical trials and was approved as the first selective H$_2$-receptor antagonist in 1974. The search had taken 12 years. In 1992, the sales of H$_2$-receptor antagonists exceeded \$4 billion.

The project at Smith Kline was carried out with considerable waxing and waning of management support. Since the statistics of drug discovery and development show that most drug candidates fail, pessimists generally have the odds in their favor. Two types of errors can be made in drug development. Drugs that lack sufficient safety and efficacy can be inappropriately supported and approved. However, it is equally possible that drugs which could prove to be safe and effective might be prematurely abandoned. In the case of the H$_2$ blockers, the project was kept alive by a few champions of the idea and eventually proved dramatically successful.

Postscript: Significant market-related factors affect decisions on drug discovery and development. The estimated market for gastric acid-related disorders during the 1960s was for annual sales of \$30 million—perhaps too small an amount to justify efforts that seemed to go on forever, with success unassured. In hindsight, that original market estimate proved to be 100-fold too low. Innovative, safe, and effective drugs can create new markets and indeed seem to increase the incidence of diagnosis of the target disease. Like H$_2$-receptor blockers, most drug classes with major sales potential (antianxiety agents, beta-blockers, converting enzyme inhibitors) of the past 2 decades created new markets that were not predicted on the basis of prospective market analysis.

At Smith Kline and other companies, even the tremendous success of a top-selling drug, while markedly strengthening the company and providing significant profits for investors and for further research and development, may not be enough to develop successor compounds or sustain sufficient growth for survival as an independent company. In 1989, Smith Kline merged with Beecham Pharmaceuticals.

good models exist (eg, hypertension), we generally have adequate drugs. Good drugs are conspicuously lacking for diseases for which models are not yet available, eg, Alzheimer's disease.

Some of the studies performed during drug screening are listed in Table 5–2 and define the **pharmacologic profile** of the drug. For example, a broad range of tests would be performed on a drug designed to act as an antagonist at vascular alpha adrenoceptors for the treatment of hypertension. At the molecular level, the compound would be screened for receptor binding affinity to cell membranes containing alpha receptors, other receptors, and binding sites on enzymes. Early studies would be done on liver cytochrome P450 to determine whether the molecule of

interest is likely to be a substrate or inhibitor of these enzymes.

Effects on cell function would be studied to determine the efficacy of the compound. Evidence would be obtained about whether the drug is an agonist, partial agonist, or antagonist at alpha receptors. Isolated tissues would be utilized to further determine the pharmacologic activity and selectivity of the new compound in comparison with reference compounds. Comparison with other drugs would also be undertaken in other vitro preparations such as gastrointestinal and bronchial smooth muscle. At each step in this pathway, the compound would have to meet specific performance criteria to be carried further.

Whole animal studies are generally necessary to

Table 5–2. Pharmacologic profile tests.

Experimental Method or Target Organ	Species/Tissue	Route of Administration	Measurement
Molecular			
Receptor binding (example: α-adrenoceptors)	Cell membrane fractions from organs or cultured cells	In vitro	Receptor affinity and selectivity.
Enzyme activity (examples: tyrosine hydroxylase, dopamine-β-hydroxylase, monoamine oxidase)	Sympathetic nerves/adrenal glands; purified enzymes	In vitro	Enzyme inhibition and selectivity.
Cytochrome P-450	Liver	In vitro	Enzyme inhibition; effects on drug metabolism.
Cellular			
Cell function	Cultured cells	In vitro	Evidence for receptor activity—agonism or antagonism (example: effects on cyclic nucleotides).
Isolated tissue	Blood vessels: arteries/veins, heart, lung, ileum (rat or guinea pig)	In vitro	Effects on vascular contraction and relaxation; selectivity for vascular receptors; effects on other smooth muscles.
Systems/disease models			
Blood pressure	Dog, cat (anesthetized)	Parenteral	Systolic-diastolic changes.
	Rat, hypertensive (conscious)	Oral	Antihypertensive effects.
Cardiac effects	Dog (conscious)	Oral	Electrocardiography.
	Dog (anesthetized)	Parenteral	Inotropic, chronotropic effects, cardiac output, total peripheral resistance.
Peripheral autonomic nervous system	Dog (anesthetized)	Parenteral	Effects on response to known drugs and electrical stimulation of central and peripheral autonomic nerves.
Respiratory effects	Dog, guinea pig	Parenteral	Effects on respiratory rate/amplitude, bronchial tone.
Diuretic activity	Dog	Oral, parenteral	Natriuresis, kaliuresis, water diuresis, renal blood flow, glomerular filtration rate.
Gastrointestinal effects	Rat	Oral	Gastrointestinal motility/secretions.
Circulating hormones, cholesterol, blood sugar	Rat, dog	Parenteral, oral	Serum concentration.
Blood coagulation	Rabbit	Oral	Coagulation time, clot retraction, prothrombin time.
Central nervous system	Mouse, rat	Parenteral, oral	Degree of sedation, muscle relaxation, locomotor activity, stimulation.

determine the effect of the drug on organ systems and disease models. Cardiovascular and renal function studies would be first performed in normal animals. For the hypothetical antihypertensive drug, animals with hypertension would then be treated to see if blood pressure was lowered and to characterize other effects of the compound. Evidence would be collected on duration of action and efficacy following oral and parenteral administration. If the agent possessed useful activity, it would be further studied for possible adverse effects on other major organ systems, including the respiratory, gastrointestinal, endocrine, and central nervous systems.

These studies might suggest the need for further chemical modification to achieve more desirable pharmacokinetic or pharmacodynamic properties. For example, oral administration studies might show that the drug was poorly absorbed or rapidly metabolized in the liver; modification to improve bioavailability might be indicated. If the drug is to be administered chronically, an assessment of tolerance development would be made. For drugs related to those known to cause physical dependency, abuse potential would also be studied. An explanation of pharmacologic mechanism would be sought.

The result of this procedure (which may have to be repeated several times with variants of the original molecules to produce a promising molecule) is a **lead compound,** ie, a leading candidate for a successful new drug. A patent application may be filed for a novel compound that is efficacious or for a previously known chemical entity that has been discovered to have a new therapeutic use.

Advances in molecular biology and biotechnology have introduced new approaches and new problems to the drug discovery and development process. New information about the structure of receptors is making possible more rational drug design. A better understanding of second messenger processes is revealing second messenger receptors as a new class of drug targets. Insertion of the genes for active peptides or proteins into bacteria, yeast, or mammalian cells makes it possible to synthesize, isolate, and purify large quantities of the desired molecule. Human insulin, human growth hormone, interferon, hepatitis vaccines, tissue plasminogen activator, erythropoietin, antihemophilic factor, and bone marrow growth factors produced by these biotechnology approaches are now available for use.

PRECLINICAL SAFETY & TOXICITY TESTING

Candidate drugs that survive the initial screening and profiling procedures must be carefully evaluated for potential risks before clinical testing is begun. Depending on the proposed use of the drug, preclinical toxicity testing includes most or all of the procedures shown in Table 5–3. While no chemical can be certified as completely "safe" (*free* of risk), since every chemical is toxic at some level of dosage, it is possi-

Table 5–3. Safety tests.

	Approach	Comment
Acute toxicity	Acute dose that is lethal in approximately 50% of animals. Determine maximum tolerated dose. Usually 2 species, 2 routes, single dose.	Compare with therapeutic dose.
Subacute toxicity	Three doses, 2 species. Up to 6 months may be necessary prior to clinical trial. The longer the duration of expected clinical use, the longer the subacute test.	Clinical chemistry, physiologic signs, autopsy studies, hematology, histology, electron microscopy studies. Identify target organs of toxicity.
Chronic toxicity	One to 2 years. Required when drug is intended to be used in humans for prolonged periods. Usually run concurrently with clinical trial.	Goals of subacute and chronic tests are to show which organs are susceptible to drug toxicity. Tests as noted above for subacute.
Effect on reproductive performance	Effects on animal mating behavior, reproduction, parturition, progeny, birth defects.	Examines fertility, teratology, perinatal and postnatal effects, lactation.
Carcinogenic potential	Two years, 2 species. Required when drug is intended to be used in humans for prolonged periods.	Hematology, histology, autopsy studies.
Mutagenic potential	Effects on genetic stability of bacteria (Ames test) or mammalian cells in culture; dominant lethal test in mice.	Increasing interest in this problem.
Investigative toxicology	Determine sequence and mechanisms of toxic action. Develop new methods for assessing toxicity.	May allow rational and earlier design of safer drugs.

ble to estimate the risk associated with exposure to the chemical under specified conditions if appropriate tests are performed.

The major kinds of information needed from the preclinical toxicity study are (1) acute toxicity—effects of large single doses up to the lethal level; (2) subacute and chronic toxicity—effects of multiple doses, which are especially important if the drug is intended for chronic use in humans; (3) effects on reproductive functions, including teratogenicity; (4) carcinogenicity; (5) mutagenicity; and (6) investigative toxicology. In addition to the studies shown in Table 5–3, several quantitative estimates are desirable. These include the "no-effect" dose—the maximum dose at which the specified toxic effect is not seen; the minimum lethal dose—the smallest dose that is observed to kill any animal; and, if necessary, the median lethal dose (LD50)—the dose that kills approximately 50% of the animals (see Chapter 2). Historically, the latter value (LD50) was determined with a high degree of precision and was used to compare toxicities of compounds relative to their therapeutic doses. It is now realized that a high degree of precision may not be necessary to compare toxicity (Malmfors, 1983). Therefore, the median lethal dose is now estimated from the smallest number of animals possible. These doses are used to calculate the initial dose to be tried in humans, usually taken as 1/100–1/10 of the no-effect dose in animals.

It is important to recognize the limitations of preclinical testing. These include the following:

(1) Toxicity testing is time-consuming and expensive. During the last decade, the total cost of preclinical pharmacology and toxicology studies was estimated to be at least $41 million per successful drug. Two to 5 years may be required to collect and analyze data.

(2) Large numbers of animals are used to obtain preclinical data. Scientists are properly concerned about this situation, and progress is being made toward reducing the numbers required while still obtaining valid data (Malmfors, 1983; Zbinden, 1981). Cell and tissue culture in vitro methods are increasingly being used, but their predictive value is still severely limited. Nevertheless, some segments of the public attempt to bring to a halt all animal testing in the unfounded belief that it has become unnecessary.

(3) Extrapolation of toxicity data from animals to humans is not completely reliable (Jelovsek, 1989; Dixon, 1980). For any given compound, the total toxicity data from all species have a very high predictive value for its toxicity in humans. However, there are limitations on the amount of information it is practical to obtain.

(4) For statistical reasons, rare adverse effects are unlikely to be detected, just as in clinical trials (see below).

EVALUATION IN HUMANS

Only about 10% of the compounds that enter clinical trials are ever approved for sale. Federal law in the USA requires that the study of new drugs in humans be conducted in accordance with stringent guidelines. Scientifically valid results are not guaranteed simply by conforming to government regulations, however, and the design and execution of a good clinical trial requires the efforts of a clinician-scientist or clinical pharmacologist, a statistician, and frequently other professionals as well. The need for careful design and execution is based upon three major factors inherent in the study of any therapeutic measure—pharmacologic or nonpharmacologic—in humans:

(1) The variable natural history of most diseases: Many diseases tend to wax and wane in severity; some disappear spontaneously with time; even malignant neoplasms may on occasion undergo spontaneous remissions. A good experimental design must take into account the natural history of the disease under study by evaluating a large enough population of subjects over a sufficient period of time. Further protection against errors of interpretation caused by fluctuations in severity of the manifestations of disease is provided by utilizing a crossover design, which consists of alternating periods of administration of test drug, placebo preparation (the control), and the standard treatment (positive control), if any, in each subject. These sequences are systematically varied, so that different subsets of patients receive each of the possible sequences of treatment. An example of such a design is shown in Table 5–4.

(2) The presence of other diseases and risk factors: Known or unknown diseases and risk factors (including life-styles of subjects) may influence the results of a clinical study. For example, some diseases alter the pharmacokinetics of drugs (Chapters 3 and 4). Concentrations of a blood component being monitored as a measure of the effect of the new agent may be influenced by other diseases or other drugs. Attempts to avoid this hazard usually involve the crossover technique (when feasible) and proper selection and assignment of patients to each of the study groups. This requires that careful medical and phar-

Table 5–4. Typical crossover design for comparing a mythical new analgesic, "Novent," with placebo and a known active drug, aspirin, in the management of chronic pain. Each therapeutic period lasts 7 days, with 1 week between treatment periods for washout of the preceding medication.

Patient Group	Medication Given		
	Week 1	Week 3	Week 5
I	Aspirin	Placebo	"Novent"
II	Placebo	"Novent"	Aspirin
III	"Novent"	Aspirin	Placebo

macologic histories (including use of recreational drugs) be obtained and that statistically valid methods of randomization be used in assigning subjects to particular study groups.

(3) Subject and observer bias: Most patients tend to respond in a positive way to any therapeutic intervention by interested, caring, and enthusiastic medical personnel. The manifestation of this phenomenon in the subject is the **placebo response** (Latin "I shall please") and may involve objective physiologic and biochemical changes as well as changes in subjective complaints associated with the disease. The placebo response is usually quantitated by administration of an inert material, with exactly the same physical appearance, odor, consistency, etc, as the active dosage form. The magnitude of the response varies considerably from patient to patient. However, the incidence of the placebo response is fairly constant, being observed in 20–40% of patients in almost all studies. Placebo "toxicity" also occurs but usually involves subjective effects: stomach upset, insomnia, sedation, etc.

Subject bias effects can be quantitated—and discounted from the response measured during active therapy—by the **single-blind design.** This involves use of a placebo or dummy medication, as described above, which is administered to the same subjects in a crossover design, if possible, or to a separate control group of subjects. Observer bias can be taken into account by disguising the identity of the medication being used—placebo or active form—from both the subjects and the personnel evaluating the subjects' responses **(double-blind design).** In this design, a third party holds the code identifying each medication packet, and the code is not broken until all of the clinical data have been collected.

The Food & Drug Administration

The Food and Drug Administration (FDA) is the administrative body that oversees the drug evaluation process in the United States and grants approval for marketing of new drug products. The FDA's authority to regulate drug marketing derives from several pieces of legislation (Table 5–5). If a drug has not been shown through adequately controlled testing to be "safe and effective" for a specific use, it cannot be marketed in interstate commerce for this use.* Unfortunately, "safe" means different things to the patient, the physician, and society. As noted above, complete absence of risk is impossible to demonstrate (and probably never occurs), but this fact is not understood by the average member of the public, who assumes that any medication sold with the approval of the FDA must indeed be free of serious, if not minor, "side effects." This confusion continues to be a major cause of litigation and dissatisfaction with medical care (Feinstein, 1988; Shulman, 1989).

The history of drug regulation reflects several medical and public health events that precipitated major shifts in public opinion. The Pure Food and Drug

---

*Although the FDA does not directly control drug commerce within states, a variety of state and federal laws control intrastate production and marketing of drugs.

Table 5–5. Major legislation pertaining to drugs in the USA.

Law	Purpose and Effect
Pure Food and Drug Act of 1906	Prohibited mislabeling and adulteration of drugs.
Opium Exclusion Act of 1909	Prohibited importation of opium.
Amendment (1912) to the Pure Food and Drug Act	Prohibited false or fraudulent advertising claims.
Harrison Narcotics Act of 1914	Established regulations for use of opium, opiates, and cocaine (marijuana added in 1937).
Food, Drug, and Cosmetic Act of 1938	Required that new drugs be safe as well as pure (but did not require proof of efficacy). Enforcement by FDA.
Durham-Humphrey Act of 1952	Vested in the FDA the power to determine which products could be sold without prescription.
Kefauver-Harris Amendments (1962) to the Food, Drug, and Cosmetic Act	Required proof of efficacy as well as safety for new drugs and for drugs released since 1938; established guidelines for reporting of information about adverse reactions, clinical testing, and advertising of new drugs.
Comprehensive Drug Abuse Prevention and Control Act (1970)	Outlined strict controls in the manufacture, distribution, and prescribing of habit-forming drugs; established programs to prevent and treat drug addiction.
Orphan Drug Amendments of 1983	Amends Food, Drug, and Cosmetic Act of 1938, providing incentives for development of drugs that treat diseases with less than 200,000 patients in USA.
Drug Price Competition and Patent Restoration Act of 1984	Abbreviated new drug applications for generic drugs. Required bioequivalence data. Patent life extended by amount of time drug delayed by FDA review process. Cannot exceed 5 extra years or extend to more than 14 years post-NDA approval.
Expedited Drug Approval (1992)	Allowed accelerated FDA approval for drugs of high medical need. Required detailed postmarketing patient surveillance.

Act of 1906 (Table 5–5) became law mostly in response to revelations of unsanitary and unethical practices in the meat-packing industry. The Federal Food, Drug, and Cosmetic Act of 1938 was largely a reaction to a series of deaths associated with the use of a preparation of sulfanilamide that was marketed before it and its vehicle were adequately tested. Thalidomide is another example of a drug that altered drug testing methods and stimulated drug-regulating legislation. This agent was introduced in Europe in 1957 and 1958 and, based on animal tests then commonly used, was promoted as a "nontoxic" hypnotic. In 1961, the first reports were published suggesting that thalidomide was responsible for a dramatic increase in the incidence of a rare birth defect called **phocomelia,** a condition involving shortening or complete absence of the limbs. Epidemiologic studies soon provided strong evidence for the association of this defect with thalidomide use by women during the first trimester of pregnancy, and the drug was withdrawn from sale worldwide. An estimated 10,000 children were born with birth defects because of maternal exposure to this one agent. The tragedy led to the requirement for more extensive testing of new drugs for teratogenic effects and played an important role in stimulating passage of the Kefauver-Harris Amendments of 1962, even though the drug was never approved for use in the USA. Unfortunately, this episode also generated widespread fear of all drugs used in pregnancy, caused much unnecessary litigation, and resulted in the withdrawal from the market of drugs that are probably not teratogenic.

Of course it is impossible, as noted above, to certify that a drug is absolutely safe, ie, free of all risk. It is possible, however, to identify most of the hazards likely to be associated with use of a new drug and to place some statistical limits on frequency of occurrence of such events in the population under study. As a result, an operational and pragmatic definition of "safety" can usually be reached that is based upon the nature and incidence of drug-associated hazards as compared to the hazard of nontherapy of the target disease.

The IND & NDA

Once a drug is judged ready to be studied in humans, a Notice of Claimed Investigational Exemption for a New Drug (IND) must be filed with the FDA (Figure 5–1). The IND includes (1) information on the composition and source of the drug, (2) manufacturing information, (3) all data from animal studies, (4) clinical plans and protocols, and (5) the names and credentials of physicians who will conduct the clinical trials.

It often requires 4–6 years of clinical testing to accumulate all required data. Testing in humans is begun after sufficient acute and subacute animal toxicity studies have been completed. Chronic safety testing in animals is usually done concurrently with clinical trials. In each of the three formal phases of clinical trials, volunteers or patients must be informed of the investigational status of the drug as well as possible risks and must be allowed to decline or to consent to participate and receive the drug. These regulations are based on the ethical principles set forth in the Declaration of Helsinki (Editor's Page, 1966). In addition to the approval of the sponsoring organization and the FDA, an interdisciplinary institutional review board at the facility where the clinical drug trial will be conducted critically reviews the plans for testing in humans.

In phase 1, the effects of the drug as a function of dosage are established in a small number of healthy volunteers. (If the drug is expected to have significant toxicity, as is usually the case in cancer and AIDS therapy, volunteer patients with the disease are used in phase 1 rather than normal volunteers.) Phase 1 trials are done to determine whether humans and animals show significantly different responses to the drug and to establish the probable limits of the safe clinical dosage range. These trials are nonblind or "open," ie, both the investigators and the subjects know what is being given. Many predictable toxicities are detected in this phase. Pharmacokinetic measurements of absorption, half-life, and metabolism are often done in phase 1. Phase 1 studies are usually performed in research centers by specially trained clinical pharmacologists.

In phase 2, the drug is studied for the first time in patients with the target disease to determine its efficacy. A small number of patients (10–200) are studied in great detail. A single-blind design is often used, with an inert placebo medication and an older active drug (positive control) in addition to the investigational agent. Phase 2 trials also are usually done in special clinical centers (eg, university hospitals). A broader range of toxicities may be detected in this phase.

In phase 3, the drug is evaluated in much larger numbers of patients—sometimes thousands—to further establish safety and efficacy. Using information gathered in phases 1 and 2, trials are designed to minimize errors caused by placebo effects, variable course of the disease, etc. Therefore, double-blind and crossover techniques (like that set out in Table 5–4) are frequently employed. Phase 3 trials are usually performed in settings similar to those anticipated for the ultimate use of the drug. Phase 3 studies can be difficult to design and execute and are usually expensive because of the large numbers of patients involved and the masses of data that must be collected and analyzed. The investigators are usually specialists in the disease being treated. Certain toxic effects—especially those caused by sensitization—may first become apparent in phase 3.

If phase 3 results are positive, application will be made for permission to market the new agent. The process of applying for marketing approval requires submission of a New Drug Application (NDA) to the FDA. The application contains, often in hundreds of volumes, full reports of all preclinical and clinical data pertaining to the drug under review. A decision on approval by the FDA may take 3 years or longer. In cases where an urgent need is perceived (eg, cancer chemotherapy), the process of preclinical and clinical testing and FDA review may be accelerated. For serious diseases, the FDA may permit extensive but controlled marketing of a new drug before phase 3 studies are completed; for life-threatening diseases, it may permit controlled marketing even before phase 2 studies are finished (Young, 1988).

Once approval to market a drug has been obtained, phase 4 begins. This constitutes monitoring the safety of the new drug under actual conditions of use in large numbers of patients. Final release of a drug for general prescription use should be accompanied by a vigilant postmarketing surveillance program. The importance of careful and complete reporting of toxicity after marketing approval by the FDA can be appreciated by noting that many important drug-induced effects have an incidence of 1:10,000 or less. Table 5–6 shows the sample size required to disclose drug-induced increases of events that occur with different frequencies in the untreated population (and some examples of such events). Because of the small numbers of subjects in phases 1–3, such low-incidence drug effects will not generally be detected before phase 4 no matter how carefully the studies are executed. Phase 4 has no fixed duration.

Table 5–6. Study size as a function of effect frequency.[1]

Number of exposed people required to detect a 2-fold increase in incidence of a rare effect with a 20% probability of missing a real effect and a 5% probability of concluding that an effect exists when one does not. One nonexposed control is required per exposed subject. If the drug increases the risk more than 2-fold, the number of subjects required is decreased.

Frequency of Effect in Nonexposed Controls	Example	Number of Exposed Subjects Required
1/100	Any congenital cardiac defect[2]	1800
1/1000	Facial clefts[3]	18,000
1/10,000	Tricuspid atresia[4]	180,000
1/100,000	Myocardial infarction[5]	1,800,000

[1]Modified and reproduced, with permission, from Finkle W: Sample size requirements for detection of drug-induced disease. Report of Joint Commission on Prescription Drug Use, Appendix V, 1980.
[2]Frequency of all forms of congenital cardiac malformations is about one in 111 live births.
[3]Frequency of facial cleft malformations is about one in 700 live births.
[4]Frequency of tricuspid valve atresia is about one in 8500 live births.
[5]Frequency of myocardial infarction in women nonsmokers 30–39 years of age is about 4 in 100,000.

The time from the filing of a patent application to approval for marketing of a new drug may be 5 years or much longer. Since the lifetime of a patent is 17 years in the USA, the owner of the patent (usually a pharmaceutical company) has exclusive rights for marketing the product for only a limited time after approval of the NDA. Because the FDA review process can be lengthy, the time consumed by the review process is sometimes added to the patent life. However, the extension (up to 5 years) cannot increase the total life of the patent to more than 14 years postNDA approval. After expiration of the patent, any company may produce and market the drug as a *generic* product without paying license fees to the original patent owner. However, a trademark (the drug's proprietary trade name) may be legally protected indefinitely. Therefore, pharmaceutical companies are strongly motivated to give their new drugs easily remembered trade names. For example, "Librium" is the trade name for the antianxiety drug "chlordiazepoxide." For the same reason, the company's advertising material will emphasize the trade name. (See section on generic prescribing in Chapter 66.)

Orphan Drugs

Drugs for rare diseases—so-called orphan drugs—can be difficult to research, develop, and market. Proof of drug safety and efficacy in small populations must be established, but doing so effectively is a complex process. For example, clinical testing of drugs in children is severely restricted, even with widely used drugs, and a number of rare diseases affect the very young. Furthermore, because basic research in the pathophysiology and mechanisms of rare diseases tends to receive little attention or funding in both academic and industrial settings, rational targets for drug action may be relatively few. In addition, the cost of developing a drug can greatly influence decisions and priorities when the target population is relatively small.

The Orphan Drug Amendments of 1983, which amended the 1938 Federal Food, Drug, and Cosmetic Act, provide incentives for the development of drugs for treatment of diseases affecting fewer than 200,000 patients in the United States. For the last 10 years, FDA has maintained an office of Orphan Product Development ([301] 443–4903) to provide special assistance to scientists with an interest in these products. Information on orphan drugs is available from a number of agencies, including The National Organization for Rare Diseases, ([800] 999–6673) and the Pharmaceutical Manufacturers Association Commission on Drugs for Rare Diseases ([202] 835–3550).

As of 1993, over 500 biologic or drug descriptions were registered with the FDA as orphan drugs, of which 189 were for products in development. The FDA has approved marketing applications for 87 orphan drugs to treat more than 74 rare diseases.

Adverse Reactions to Drugs

Severe adverse reactions to marketed drugs are uncommon, though less dangerous toxic effects, as noted elsewhere in this book, are frequent for some drug groups. Life-threatening reactions probably occur in less than 2% of patients admitted to medical wards (Adverse drug reactions, 1981). The mechanisms of these reactions fall into two main categories. Those in the first group are often extensions of known pharmacologic effects and thus are predictable. These toxicities are generally discovered by pharmacologists, toxicologists, and clinicians involved in phase 1–3 testing. Those in the second group, which may be immunologic or of unknown mechanism (Rawlins, 1981), are generally unexpected and may not be recognized until a drug has been marketed for many years. These toxicities are therefore usually discovered by clinicians. It is thus important that practitioners be aware of the various types of allergic reactions to drugs. These include IgE-mediated reactions such as anaphylaxis, urticaria, and angioedema; IgG- or IgM-mediated reactions of the lupus erythematosus type; IgG-mediated responses of the serum sickness type, which involve vasculitis; and cell-mediated allergies involved in contact dermatitis. They are discussed in Chapter 57.

Evaluating a Clinical Drug Study

The periodical literature is the chief source of clinical information about new drugs, especially those very recently released for general use. Such information may include new indications or major new toxicities and contraindications. Therefore, health practitioners should be familiar with the sources of such information (noted in Chapter 1) and should be prepared to evaluate it. Certain general principles can be applied to such evaluations and are discussed in detail in the Riegelman reference listed below. These principles are conveniently stated in the form of questions every reader should ask while examining the paper.

A. Ethical Considerations: Were appropriate ethical and procedural safeguards available to the patients? Was informed consent obtained?

B. Statement of Objectives: What were the objectives of the study? Are the goals clearly defined and stated? A poorly defined goal such as "to study the effects of minoxidil" (an antihypertensive drug) is much less likely to lead to useful results than a clearly defined objective such as, "to measure the effect of minoxidil on renal function in severely hypertensive adult males."

C. Experimental Methods: Were the experimental methods appropriate to the study goals? Does the author state the accuracy (precision) and reliability (reproducibility) of the methods? Are the methods sensitive enough so that small but biologically important changes could be detected?

D. Statistical Methods: How were the patients selected? Were there enough subjects? Are the subjects representative of the population most likely to receive the drug or of the population for which the reader would like to use the drug? If the project was a long-term or outpatient study, were any patients lost to follow-up? How was this accounted for? Were placebo and positive control treatments included? How were patients assigned to the various groups? Was a crossover design feasible, and was one used? Were patients receiving any other therapy during the trial? How was this controlled or accounted for? Were appropriate statistical tests applied?

E. Conclusions: Do the data, even if sound, justify the conclusions? Does the drug offer significant advantages of cost, efficacy, or safety over existing agents, or is it merely new? Extrapolation from the study population to other groups must be very carefully scrutinized.

A well-written report in a journal subject to peer review usually provides explicit answers to all of the above questions. Absence of clear answers to these questions justifies skepticism about the investigation and the authors' conclusions.

REFERENCES

Adverse drug reactions. (Editorial.) Br Med J 1981; 282:1819.

Beyer KH: *Discovery, Development, and Delivery of New Drugs,* SP Medical & Scientific Books, 1978.

Black J: Drugs from emasculated hormones: The principle of syntopic antagonism. Science 1989;245:486

Brimblecombe RW, et al: Characterization and development of cimetidine as histamine H_2-receptor antagonist. Gastroenterology 1978;74:339

Chappell WR, Mordenti J: Extrapolation of toxicological and pharmacological data from animals to humans. Adv Drug Res 1991;20:1.

Collins JM, Grieshaber CK, Chabner BA: Pharmacologically guided phase I clinical trials based upon preclinical drug development. J Natl Cancer Inst 1990;82:1321.

Dixon RL (editor): Extrapolation of laboratory toxicity data to man: Factors influencing the dose-toxic response relationship. (Symposium.) Fed Proc 1980;39:53.

Editor's Page: Code of ethics of the World Medical Association: Declaration of Helsinki. Clin Res 1966;14:193.

Feinstein AR: Scientific standards in epidemiologic studies of the menace of daily life. Science 1988;242:1257.

Fredd S: The FDA and the physician. Am J Gastroenterol 1988;83:1088.

Jelovsek FR, Mattison DR, Chen JJ: Prediction of risk for human developmental toxicity: How important are animal studies? Obstet Gynecol 1989;74:624.

Jick H: Drugs: Remarkably nontoxic. N Engl J Med 1974; 291:824.

Kessler DA: The regulation of investigational drugs. N Engl J Med 1989;320:281.

Laughren TP: The review of clinical safety data in a new drug application. Psychopharmacol Bull 1989;25:5.

Malmfors T, Teiling A: LD50: Its value for the pharmaceutical industry in safety evaluation of drugs. Acta Pharmacol Toxicol 1983;52(Suppl 2):229.

Mattison N, Trimble AG, Lasagna L: New drug development in the United States, 1963 through 1984. Clin Pharmacol 1988;43:290.

McKhann GM: The trials of clinical trials. Arch Neurol 1989;46:611.

Moscucci M et al: Blinding, unblinding, and the placebo effect: An analysis of patients' guesses of treatment assignment in a double-blind clinical trial. Clin Pharmacol Ther 1987;41:259.

Nolan PE Jr: Generic substitution of antiarrhythmic drugs. Am J Cardiol 1989;64:1371.

Rawlins MD: Clinical pharmacology: Adverse reactions to drugs. Br Med J 1981;282:974.

Riegelman RK: *Studying a Study and Testing a Test: How to Read the Medical Literature.* Little, Brown, 1981.

Schwartzman D: *Innovation in the Pharmaceutical Industry.* Johns Hopkins Univ Press, 1976.

Sheiner LB: The intellectual health of clinical drug evaluation. Clin Pharmacol Ther 1991;50:4.

Shulman SR: The broader message of Accutane. Am J Public Health 1989;79:1565.

Sibille M et al: Adverse events in phase one studies: A study in 430 healthy volunteers. Eur J Clin Pharmacol 1992; 42:389.

Spilker B: *Guide to Clinical Interpretation of Data.* Raven Press, 1986

Spilker B: The development of orphan drugs: An industry perspective. In: *Orphan Diseases and Orphan Drugs.* Scheinberg JH, Walshe JM (editors). Manchester Univ Press, 1986.

Venning GR: Identification of adverse reactions to new drugs. (Five parts.) Br Med J 1983;286:199, 289, 365, 458, 544.

Waller PC: Measuring the frequency of adverse drug reactions. Br J Clin Pharmacol 1992;33:249.

Young FE, Nightingale SL: FDA's newly designated treatment INDs. JAMA 1988;260:224.

Zbinden G, Flury-Reversi M: Significance of LD$_{50}$-test for the toxicological evaluation of chemical substances. Arch Toxicol 1981;47:77.

SECTION II.
Autonomic Drugs

Introduction to Autonomic Pharmacology

6

Bertram G. Katzung, MD, PhD

The motor (efferent) portion of the nervous system can be divided into two major subdivisions: the **autonomic** and the **somatic** divisions. The autonomic nervous system (ANS) is largely autonomous (independent) in that its activities are not under direct conscious control. It is concerned primarily with visceral functions—cardiac output, blood flow to various organs, digestion, etc—that are necessary for life. The somatic division is largely nonautomatic and is concerned with consciously controlled functions such as movement, respiration, and posture. Both systems have important afferent (sensory) inputs that provide sensation and modify motor output through reflex arcs of varying size and complexity.

The nervous system has several properties in common with the other major system for control of body function: the endocrine system. These include high-level integration in the brain, the ability to influence processes in distant regions of the body, and extensive use of negative feedback. Both systems use chemicals for the transmission of information. In the nervous system, chemical transmission occurs between nerve cells and between nerve cells and their effector cells. Chemical transmission takes place through the release of small amounts of transmitter substances from the nerve terminals into the synaptic cleft. The transmitter crosses the cleft by diffusion and activates or inhibits the postsynaptic cell by binding to a specialized receptor molecule.

By using drugs that mimic or block the actions of chemical transmitters, we can selectively modify many autonomic functions. These functions involve a variety of effector tissues, including cardiac muscle, smooth muscle, vascular endothelium, glands, and presynaptic nerve terminals. Autonomic drugs are useful in a large number of clinical conditions.

ANATOMY OF THE AUTONOMIC NERVOUS SYSTEM

The autonomic nervous system lends itself to division on anatomic grounds into two major portions: the **sympathetic (thoracolumbar)** division and the **parasympathetic (craniosacral)** division (Figure 6–1). Both divisions originate in nuclei within the central nervous system and give rise to preganglionic efferent fibers that exit from the brain stem or spinal cord and terminate in motor ganglia. The sympathetic preganglionic fibers leave the central nervous system through the thoracic and lumbar spinal nerves, giving rise to the alternative name "thoracolumbar system." The parasympathetic preganglionic fibers leave the central nervous system through the cranial nerves (especially the third, seventh, ninth, and tenth) and the third and fourth sacral spinal roots.

Most of the sympathetic preganglionic fibers terminate in ganglia located in the paravertebral chains that lie on either side of the spinal column. The remaining sympathetic ganglia are located in prevertebral ganglia, which lie in front of the vertebrae. From these ganglia, postganglionic sympathetic fibers run to the tissues innervated. Some preganglionic parasympathetic fibers terminate in parasympathetic ganglia located outside the organs innervated: the ciliary, pterygopalatine, submandibular, otic, and several pelvic ganglia. The majority of parasympathetic preganglionic fibers terminate on ganglion cells distributed diffusely or in networks in the walls of the innervated organs. It is important to remember that the terms sympathetic and parasympathetic are anatomic ones and do not depend on the type of transmitter chemical released from the nerve endings nor on the kind of

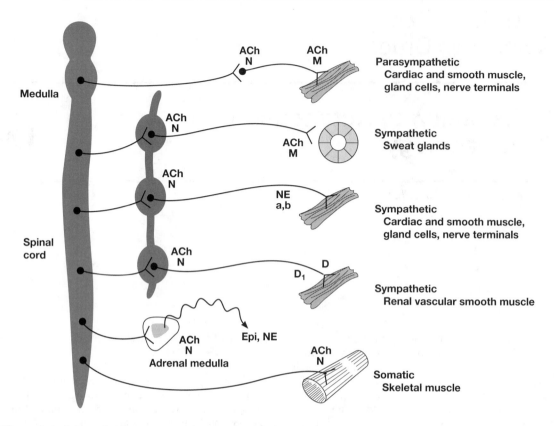

Figure 6–1. Schematic diagram comparing some anatomic and neurotransmitter features of autonomic and somatic motor nerves. Only the primary transmitter substances are shown. Parasympathetic ganglia are not shown because most are in or near the wall of the organ innervated. Note that some sympathetic postganglionic fibers release acetylcholine or dopamine rather than norepinephrine. The adrenal medulla, a modified sympathetic ganglion, receives sympathetic preganglionic fibers and releases epinephrine and norepinephrine into the blood. (ACh, acetylcholine; D, dopamine; Epi, epinephrine; NE, norepinephrine; N, nicotinic receptors; M, muscarinic receptors.)

effect—excitatory or inhibitory—evoked by nerve activity.

In addition to these clearly defined peripheral motor portions of the autonomic nervous system, there are large numbers of afferent fibers that run from the periphery to integrating centers, including the enteric plexuses in the gut, the autonomic ganglia, and the central nervous system. Many of the sensory neurons that end in the central nervous system terminate in the integrating centers of the hypothalamus and medulla and evoke reflex motor activity that is carried to the effector cells by the efferent fibers described above. There is increasing evidence that some of these sensory fibers also have important peripheral motor functions (see Nonadrenergic, Noncholinergic Systems, below).

The **enteric nervous system (ENS)** is a collection of neurons located in the wall of the gastrointestinal system (Figure 6–2). It is sometimes considered a third division of the ANS. The enteric nervous system includes the myenteric plexus (the plexus of Auerbach) and the submucous plexus (the plexus of Meissner) (see Furness, 1987). These neuronal networks receive preganglionic fibers from the parasympathetic system as well as postganglionic sympathetic axons. They also receive sensory input from within the wall of the gut. Fibers from the cell bodies in these plexuses travel to the smooth muscle of the gut to control motility. Other motor fibers go to the secretory cells. Sensory fibers transmit information from the mucosa and from stretch receptors to motor neurons in the plexuses and to postganglionic neurons in the sympathetic ganglia. The parasympathetic and sympathetic fibers that synapse on enteric plexus neurons appear to play a modulatory role, as indicated by the observation that deprivation of input from both ANS divisions does not halt activity in the plexuses nor in the smooth muscle and glands innervated by them.

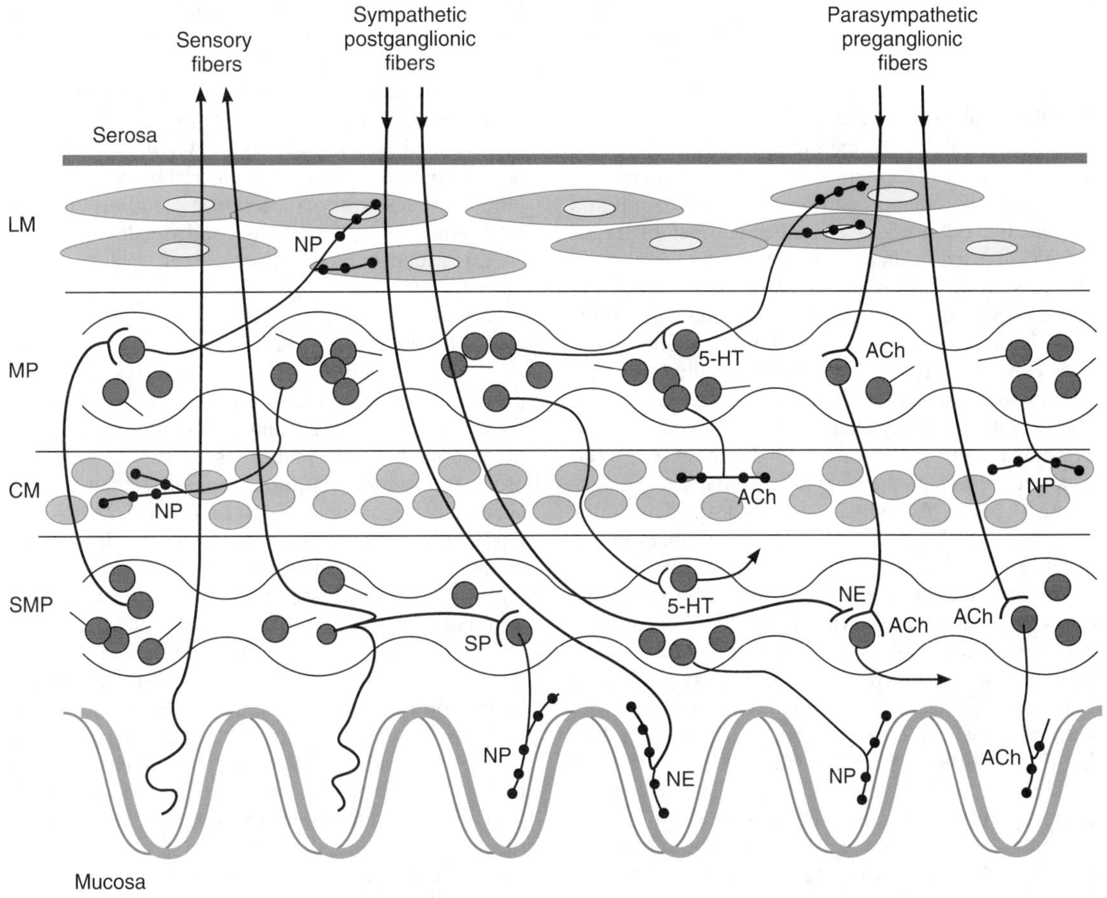

Figure 6–2. A highly simplified diagram of some of the circuitry of the enteric nervous system (ENS). The ENS receives input from both the sympathetic and the parasympathetic systems and sends afferent impulses to sympathetic ganglia and to the central nervous system. Many transmitter or neuromodulator substances have been identified in the ENS; see Table 6–1. (LM, longitudinal muscle layer; MP, myenteric plexus; CM, circular muscle layer; SMP, submucosal plexus; ACh, acetylcholine; NE, norepinephrine; NP, neuropeptides; SP, substance P; 5-HT, serotonin.)

NEUROTRANSMITTER CHEMISTRY OF THE AUTONOMIC NERVOUS SYSTEM

An important traditional classification of autonomic nerves is based on the primary transmitter molecules—acetylcholine or norepinephrine—released from their terminal boutons and varicosities. A large number of peripheral autonomic nervous system fibers synthesize and release acetylcholine; they are **cholinergic** fibers, ie, they act by releasing acetylcholine. As shown in Figure 6–1, these include all preganglionic efferent autonomic fibers and the somatic (nonautonomic) motor fibers to skeletal muscle as well. Thus, almost all efferent fibers leaving the central nervous system are cholinergic. In addition, all parasympathetic postganglionic and a few sympa-

thetic postganglionic fibers are cholinergic. Most postganglionic sympathetic fibers release norepinephrine (noradrenaline); they are **noradrenergic** (often called simply "adrenergic") fibers—ie, they act by releasing norepinephrine. These transmitter characteristics are presented schematically in Figure 6–1. As noted above, a few sympathetic fibers release acetylcholine. There is considerable evidence that dopamine is released by some peripheral sympathetic fibers. Adrenal medullary cells, which are embryologically analogous to postganglionic sympathetic neurons, release a mixture of epinephrine and norepinephrine. In recent years it has been recognized that most autonomic nerves also release several transmitter substances, or *cotransmitters*, in addition to the primary transmitter.

Four key features of neurotransmitter function represent potential targets of pharmacologic therapy: synthesis, storage, release, and termination of action. These processes are discussed in detail below.

Cholinergic Transmission

The terminals of cholinergic neurons contain large numbers of small membrane-bound vesicles concentrated near the synaptic portion of the cell membrane (Figure 6–3) as well as a smaller number of larger vesicles located farther from the synaptic membrane. Vesicles are initially synthesized in the neuron soma and transported to the terminal. They may also be recycled several times within the terminal. These vesicles contain acetylcholine in high concentration and certain other molecules (eg, peptides) that may act as cotransmitters. Acetylcholine is synthesized in the cytoplasm from acetyl-CoA and choline through the catalytic action of the enzyme choline acetyltransferase (ChAT). Acetyl-CoA is synthesized in mitochondria, which are present in large numbers in the nerve ending. Choline is transported from the extracellular fluid into the neuron terminal by a sodium-dependent membrane carrier (Figure 6–3, carrier A). This carrier can be blocked by a group of drugs called hemicholiniums. Once synthesized, acetylcholine is transported from the cytoplasm into the vesicles by an antiporter that removes protons (Figure 6–3, carrier B). This transporter can be blocked by vesamicol (Anderson, 1983). Acetylcholine synthesis is a rapid process capable of supporting a very high rate of transmitter release. Storage of acetylcholine is accomplished by the packaging of "quanta" of acetylcholine molecules (usually 1000–50,000 molecules in each vesicle).

Release of transmitter is dependent on extracellular calcium and occurs when an action potential reaches the terminal and triggers sufficient influx of calcium ions. It has recently been shown that the increased Ca^{2+} concentration "destabilizes" the storage vesicles by interacting with a special protein associated with the vesicular membrane (synaptotagmin; Brose et al, 1992). Fusion of the vesicular membranes with the terminal membrane occurs, with exocytotic expulsion of—in the case of somatic motor nerves—several hundred quanta of acetylcholine into the synaptic cleft. The amount of transmitter released by one depolarization of an autonomic postganglionic nerve terminal is probably smaller. In addition to acetylcholine, one or more cotransmitters may be released at the same time (Table 6–1). The ACh vesicle-release process is blocked by botulinum toxin through an interaction with another vesicle-associated protein, synaptobrevin (Schiavo et al, 1992).

After release from the presynaptic terminal, acetylcholine molecules may bind to and activate an acetylcholine receptor (**cholinoceptor**). Eventually (and usually very rapidly), all of the acetylcholine released will diffuse within range of an **acetylcholinesterase** (AChE) molecule. AChE very efficiently splits ace-

tylcholine into choline and acetate, neither of which has significant transmitter effect, and thereby terminates the action of the transmitter (Figure 6–3). Most cholinergic synapses are richly supplied with acetylcholinesterase; the half-life of acetylcholine in the synapse is therefore very short. Acetylcholinesterase is also found in other tissues, eg, red blood cells. (Another cholinesterase with a lower specificity for acetylcholine, butyrylcholinesterase [pseudocholinesterase], is found in blood plasma, liver, glia, and many other tissues.)

Adrenergic Transmission

Adrenergic neurons (Figure 6–4) also transport a precursor molecule into the nerve ending, then synthesize the transmitter, and finally store it in membrane-bound vesicles, but the synthesis of the adrenergic transmitters is more complex than that of acetylcholine, as indicated in Figure 6–5. In the adrenal medulla and certain areas of the brain, norepinephrine is further converted to epinephrine. Several important processes in the noradrenergic nerve terminal are potential sites of drug action. One of these, the conversion of tyrosine to dopa, is the rate-limiting step in norepinephrine synthesis. It can be inhibited by the tyrosine analogue metyrosine (Figure 6–4). A high-affinity carrier for catecholamines located in the wall of the storage vesicle can be inhibited by the reserpine alkaloids (Figure 6–4, carrier B). Depletion of transmitter stores results. Another carrier transports norepinephrine and similar molecules into the cell cytoplasm (Figure 6–4, carrier 1, commonly called uptake 1). It can be inhibited by cocaine and tricyclic antidepressant drugs, resulting in an increase of transmitter activity in the synaptic cleft.

Release of the vesicular transmitter store from noradrenergic nerve endings is similar to the calcium-dependent process described above for cholinergic terminals. In addition to the primary transmitter (norepinephrine), ATP, dopamine-β-hydroxylase, and certain peptide cotransmitters are also released into the synaptic cleft. Indirectly acting sympathomimetics—eg, tyramine and amphetamines—are capable of releasing stored transmitter from noradrenergic nerve endings. These drugs are poor agonists (some are inactive) at adrenoceptors but are taken up into noradrenergic nerve endings by uptake 1. In the nerve ending, they may displace norepinephrine from storage vesicles, inhibit monoamine oxidase, and have other effects that result in increased norepinephrine activity in the synapse. Their action does not require vesicle exocytosis and is not calcium-dependent.

Norepinephrine and epinephrine can be metabolized by several enzymes, as shown in Figure 6–6. Because of the high activity of monoamine oxidase in the mitochondria of the nerve terminal, there is a significant turnover of norepinephrine even in the resting terminal. Since the metabolic products are ex-

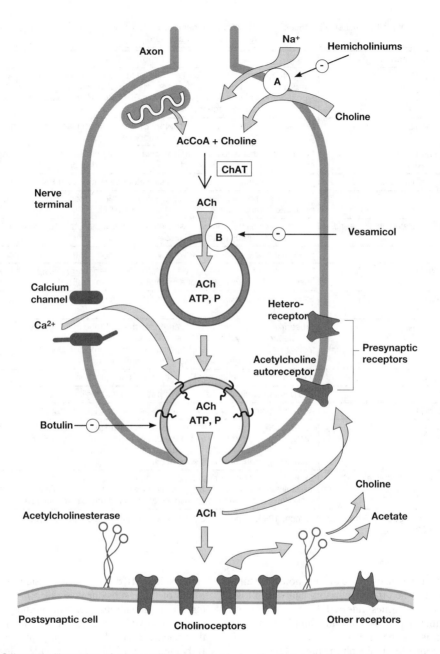

Figure 6–3. Schematic illustration of a generalized cholinergic junction (not to scale). Choline is transported into the presynaptic nerve terminal by a sodium-dependent carrier *(A)*. This transport can be inhibited by hemicholinium drugs. ACh is transported into the storage vesicle by a second carrier *(B)* that can be inhibited by vesamicol. Peptides *(P)*, ATP, and proteoglycan are also stored in the vesicle. Release of transmitter occurs when voltage-sensitive calcium channels in the terminal membrane are opened, allowing an influx of calcium. The resulting increase in intracellular calcium causes fusion of vesicles with the surface membrane and exocytotic expulsion of ACh and cotransmitters into the junctional cleft. This step is blocked by botulin. Acetylcholine's action is terminated by metabolism by the enzyme acetylcholinesterase. Receptors on the presynaptic nerve ending regulate transmitter release.

Table 6–1. Some of the transmitter substances found in autonomic nervous system (ANS), enteric nervous system (ENS), and nonadrenergic, noncholinergic neurons.[1]

Substance	Probable Roles
Acetylcholine (ACh)	The primary transmitter at ANS ganglia, at the somatic neuromuscular junction, and at parasympathetic postganglionic nerve endings. A primary excitatory transmitter to smooth muscle and secretory cells in the ENS. Probably also the major neuron-to-neuron ("ganglionic") transmitter in the ENS.
Adenosine triphosphate (ATP)	May act as a cotransmitter at inhibitory ENS neuromuscular junctions. Inhibits release of ACh and norepinephrine from ANS nerve endings.
Calcitonin gene-related peptide (CGRP)	Found with substance P in cardiovascular sensory nerve fibers. Present in some secretomotor ENS neurons and interneurons. A cardiac stimulant.
Cholecystokinin (CCK)	May act as a cotransmitter in some excitatory neuromuscular ENS neurons.
Dopamine	An important postganglionic sympathetic transmitter in renal blood vessels. Probably a modulatory transmitter in some ganglia and the ENS.
Enkephalin and related opioid peptides	Present in some secretomotor and interneurons in the ENS. Appear to inhibit ACh release and thereby inhibit peristalsis. May *stimulate* secretion.
Galanin	Present in secretomotor neurons; may play a role in appetite-satiety mechanisms.
Gamma-aminobutyric acid (GABA)	May have presynaptic effects on excitatory ENS nerve terminals. Has some relaxant effect on the gut. Probably not a major transmitter in the ENS.
Gastrin-releasing peptide (GRP)	Extremely potent excitatory transmitter to gastrin cells. Also known as mammalian bombesin.
Neuropeptide Y (NPY)	Present in some secretomotor neurons in the ENS and may inhibit secretion of water and electrolytes by the gut. Causes long-lasting vasoconstriction. It is also a cotransmitter in many parasympathetic postganglionic neurons and sympathetic postganglionic norarenergic vascular neurons.
Nitric oxide (NO)	A cotransmitter at inhibitory ENS neuromuscular junctions.
Norepinephrine (NE)	The primary transmitter at most sympathetic postganglionic nerve endings.
Serotonin (5-HT)	A cotransmitter at excitatory neuron-to-neuron junctions in the ENS.
Substance P (and related "tachykinins")	Substance P is an important sensory neuron transmitter in the ENS and elsewhere. Tachykinins appear to be excitatory cotransmitters with ACh at ENS neuromuscular junctions. Found with CGRP in cardiovascular sensory neurons. Substance P is a vasodilator (probably via release of nitric oxide).
Vasoactive intestinal peptide (VIP)	Excitatory secretomotor transmitter in the ENS; may also be an inhibitory ENS neuromuscular cotransmitter. A probable cotransmitter in many cholinergic neurons. A vasodilator (found in many perivascular neurons) and cardiac stimulant.

[1]Data from Furness et al, 1992; Llewellyn-Smith, 1989; Lundgren, Svanik, and Jivegard, 1989; Kromer, 1990; and Wharton and Gulbenkian, 1989.

creted in the urine, an estimate of catecholamine turnover can be obtained from laboratory analysis of total metabolites (sometimes referred to as "VMA and metanephrines") in a 24-hour urine sample. However, metabolism is not the primary mechanism for termination of action of norepinephrine physiologically released from noradrenergic nerves. Termination of noradrenergic transmission results from several processes, including simple diffusion away from the receptor site (with eventual metabolism in the plasma or liver) and reuptake into the nerve terminal (**uptake**1) or into perisynaptic glia or smooth muscle cells (**uptake**2) (Figure 6–4).

Cotransmitters in Cholinergic & Adrenergic Nerves

As previously noted, the vesicles of both cholinergic and adrenergic nerves contain other substances in addition to the primary transmitter. Some of the substances identified to date are listed in Table 6–1. Many of these substances are also *primary* transmitters in the nonadrenergic, noncholinergic nerves described below. Their roles in the function of nerves that release acetylcholine or norepinephrine are not fully understood. They may provide a slow, long-lasting action to supplement or modulate the more transient effects of the primary transmitter. They may also participate in feedback inhibition of the same or nearby nerve terminals.

AUTONOMIC RECEPTORS

A great deal has been learned about the chemical nature of autonomic receptors during the last decade, and this field is one of the most active research areas in pharmacology. Historically, structure-activity analyses, with careful comparisons of the potency of

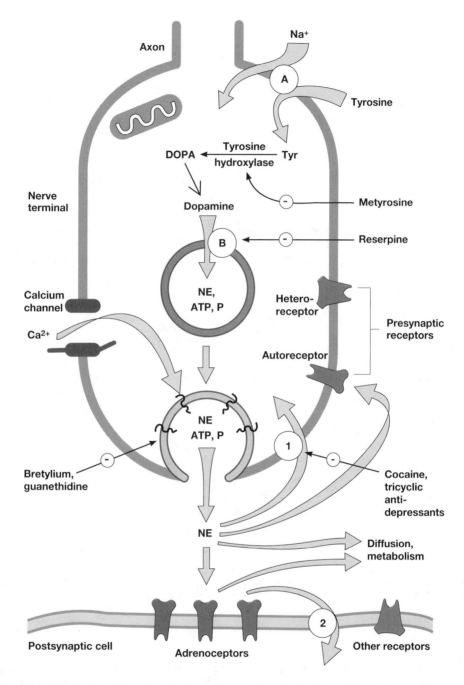

Figure 6–4. Schematic diagram of a generalized noradrenergic junction (not to scale). Tyrosine is transported into the noradrenergic ending or varicosity by a sodium-dependent carrier (A). Tyrosine is converted to dopamine (see Figure 6–5 for details), which is transported into the vesicle by a carrier (B) that can be blocked by reserpine. The same carrier transports norepinephrine (NE) and several other amines into these granules. Dopamine is converted to NE in the vesicle by dopamine-β-hydroxylase. Release of transmitter occurs when an action potential opens voltage-sensitive calcium channels and increases intracellular calcium. Fusion of vesicles with the surface membrane results in expulsion of norepinephrine, cotransmitters, and dopamine-β-hydroxylase. Release can be blocked by drugs such as guanethidine and bretylium. After release, norepinephrine diffuses out of the cleft or is transported into the cytoplasm of the varicosity (uptake 1 [1], blocked by cocaine, tricyclic antidepressants) or into the postjunctional cell (uptake 2 2). Regulatory receptors are present on the presynaptic terminal.

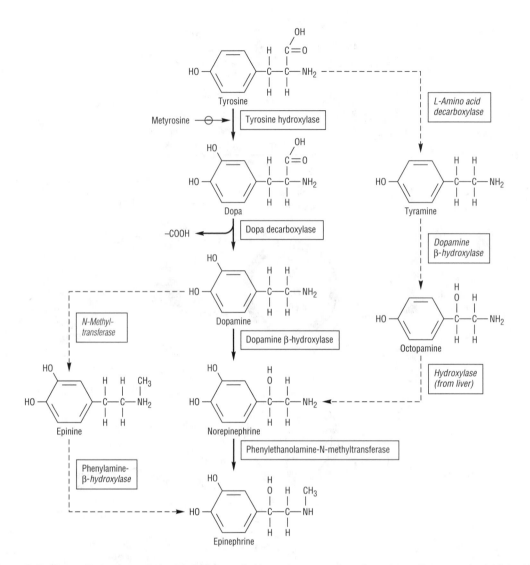

Figure 6–5. Biosynthesis of catecholamines. The rate-limiting step, conversion of tyrosine to Dopa, can be inhibited by metyrosine (alphamethyl tyrosine) The alternative pathways shown by the dashed arrows have not been found to be of physiologic significance in humans. However, tyramine and octopamine may accumulate in patients treated with monoamine oxidase inhibitors. (Reproduced, with permission, from Greenspan FS, Baxter JD (editors): *Basic & Clinical Endocrinology,* 4th ed. Appleton & Lange, 1994.)

series of autonomic analogues, led to the definition of different autonomic receptor subtypes, including muscarinic and nicotinic cholinoceptors, and alpha, beta, and dopamine adrenoceptors (Table 6–2). Molecular biology has provided a new approach by making possible the discovery and expression of genes that code for related receptors within these groups. (See Chapter 2 box: How Are Receptors Discovered?)

The primary acetylcholine receptor subtypes were named after the alkaloids originally used in their identification: muscarine and nicotine. These names are readily converted into adjectives—thus, mus-

carinic and nicotinic receptors. In the case of receptors associated with noradrenergic nerves, the coining of simple adjectives from the names of the agonists (noradrenaline, phenylephrine, isoproterenol, etc) was not practicable. Therefore, the term **adrenoceptor** is widely used to describe receptors that respond to catecholamines such as norepinephrine. By analogy, the term **cholinoceptor** denotes receptors (both muscarinic and nicotinic) that respond to acetylcholine. In North America, receptors were colloquially named after the nerves that usually innervate them; thus, **adrenergic** (or noradrenergic) **receptors** and **cholinergic receptors.** The adrenoceptors can be

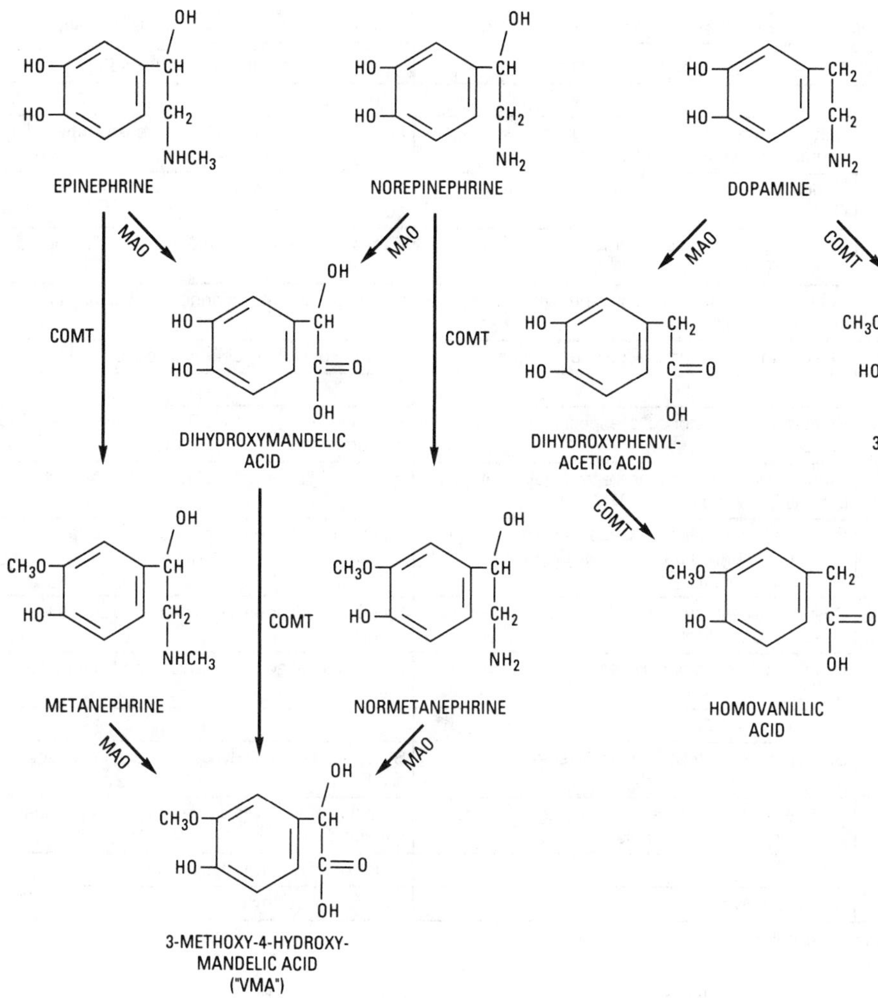

Figure 6–6. Metabolism of catecholamines by catechol-O-methyltransferase *(COMT)* and monoamine oxidase *(MAO).* (Modified and reproduced, with permission, from Greenspan FS, Baxter JD (editors): *Basic & Clinical Endocrinology,* 4th ed. Appleton & Lange, 1994.)

subdivided into alpha-adrenoceptor and beta-adrenoceptor types on the basis of both agonist and antagonist selectivity. Development of more selective blocking drugs has led to the naming of subclasses within these major types, eg, within the alpha-adrenoceptor class, α_1 and α_2 receptors differ in both agonist and antagonist selectivity. Specific examples of such selective drugs are given in the chapters that follow.

Much progress has been made in isolating and purifying receptor proteins and in many cases has permitted the determination of the peptide sequences of these proteins and their three-dimensional conformations. Independent studies based on cDNA libraries have confirmed and extended the numbers of subtypes of cholinoceptors and adrenoceptors. For example, genes have been discovered for five different muscarinic cholinoceptors (Buckley, 1989).

NONADRENERGIC, NONCHOLINERGIC NEURONS

It has been known for many years that autonomic effector tissues contain nerve fibers that do not show the histochemical characteristics of either cholinergic or adrenergic fibers. Both motor and sensory nonadrenergic, noncholinergic fibers are present. Although peptides are the most common transmitter substances found in these nerve endings, other substances, especially purines, are also present in many nerve terminals (Table 6–1). Improved immunologic assay methods now permit accurate identification and quantitation of peptides stored in and released from the fiber terminals. In addition, it has been found that capsaicin, a neurotoxin derived from chili peppers, can cause the release of transmitter from such neu-

Table 6–2. Autonomic receptor types with documented or probable effects on peripheral autonomic effector tissues.

Receptor Name	Typical Locations	Result of Ligand Binding
Cholinoceptors		
Muscarinic M_1	CNS neurons, sympathetic postganglionic neurons, some presynaptic sites.	Formation of IP_3 and DAG, increased intracellular calcium.
Muscarinic M_2	Myocardium, smooth muscle, some presynaptic sites.	Opening of potassium channels, inhibition of adenylyl cyclase.
Muscarinic M_3	Exocrine glands, vessels (smooth muscle and endothelium).	Formation of IP_3 and DAG, increased intracellular calcium.
Nicotinic N_N	Postganglionic neurons, some presynaptic chlinergic terminals.	Opening of Na^+, K^+ channels, depolarization.
Nicotinic N_M	Skeletal muscle neuromuscular endplates.	Opening of Na^+, K^+ channels, depolarization.
Adrenoceptors		
Alpha$_1$	Postsynaptic effector cells, especially smooth muscle.	Formation of IP_3 and DAG, increased intracellular calcium.
Alpha$_2$	Presynaptic adrenergic nerve terminals, platelets, lipocytes, smooth muscle.	Inhibition of adenylyl cyclase, decreased cAMP.
Beta$_1$	Postsynaptic effector cells, especially heart, lipocytes, brain, presynaptic adrenergic and cholinergic nerve terminals.	Stimulation of adenylyl cyclase, increased cAMP.
Beta$_2$	Postsynaptic effector cells, especially smooth muscle and cardiac muscle.	Stimulation of adenylyl cyclase and increased cAMP.
Beta$_3$	Postsynaptic effector cells, especially lipocytes.	Stimulation of adenylyl cyclase and increased cAMP.
Dopamine receptors		
D_1 (DA_1), D_5	Brain; effector tissues, especially smooth muscle of the renal vascular bed.	Stimulation of adenylyl cyclase and increased cAMP.
D_2(DA_2)	Brain; effector tissues especially smooth muscle; presynaptic nerve terminals.	Inhibition of adenylyl cyclase; increased potassium conductance.
D_3[1]	Brain.	Inhibition of adenylyl cyclase.
D_4[1]	Brain, cardiovascular system.	Inhibition of adenylyl cyclase.

[1]May be subtypes of the D_2 receptor.

rons and, if given in high doses, destruction of the neuron. Use of these research tools has led to the accumulation of a large amount of information, much of which is still incompletely understood.

The enteric system in the gut wall (Figure 6–2) is the most extensively studied system containing nonadrenergic, noncholinergic neurons in addition to cholinergic and adrenergic fibers. In the guinea pig small intestine, for example, these neurons respond to immunofluorescent probes for one or more of the following: calcitonin gene-related peptide, cholecystokinin, dynorphin, enkephalins, gastrin-releasing peptide, 5-hydroxytryptamine (serotonin), neuropeptide Y, somatostatin, substance P, and vasoactive intestinal peptide. Some neurons contain as many as five different possible transmitters. This system apparently "interprets" the motor outflow of the ANS and provides the necessary synchronization of impulses that, for example, ensures forward, not backward, propulsion of gut contents and relaxation of sphincters when the gut wall contracts.

The sensory fibers in the nonadrenergic, noncholinergic systems are probably better termed "sensory-efferent" or "sensory-local effector" fibers be-cause, when activated by a sensory input, they are capable of releasing transmitter peptides from the sensory ending itself, from local axon branches, and from collaterals that terminate in the autonomic ganglia. These peptides are potent agonists at many autonomic effector tissues. It is not yet known whether drugs currently in clinical use act through the modification of these sensory-efferent processes, but selective inhibitors are being actively sought.

FUNCTIONAL ORGANIZATION OF AUTONOMIC ACTIVITY

A basic understanding of the interactions of autonomic components with each other and with their effector organs is essential for an appreciation of the actions of autonomic drugs, especially because of their significant "reflex" effects.

Central Integration

At the highest level—midbrain and medulla—the two divisions of the autonomic nervous system and the endocrine system are integrated with each other, with sensory input, and with information from higher central nervous system centers. These interactions are such that early investigators called the parasympathetic system a **trophotropic** one (ie, leading to growth) and the sympathetic system an **ergotropic** one (ie, leading to energy expenditure) that was activated for "fight or flight." While such terms offer lit-

tle insight into the mechanisms involved, they do provide simple descriptions applicable to many of the actions of the systems (Table 6–3). For example, slowing of the heart and stimulation of digestive activity are typical energy-conserving "rest and digest" actions of the parasympathetic system. In contrast, cardiac stimulation, increased blood sugar, and cutane-

Table 6–3. Direct effects of autonomic nerve activity and autonomic drugs on some organ systems.

Organ	Effect of			
	Sympathetic		Parasympathetic	
	Action[1]	Receptor[2]	Action	Receptor[2]
Eye				
Iris				
Radial muscle	Contracts	α_1	...	...
Circular muscle	...	...	Contracts	M_3
Ciliary muscle	[Relaxes]	β	Contracts	M_3
Heart				
Sinoatrial node	Accelerates	β_1	Decelerates	M_2
Ectopic pacemakers	Accelerates	β_1	...	...
Contractility	Increases	β_1	Decreases (atria)	M_2
Vascular smooth muscle				
Skin, splanchnic vessels	Contracts	α	...	...
Skeletal muscle vessels	Relaxes	β_2	...	...
	[Contracts]	α	...	...
	Relaxes	M^4	...	...
Endothelium	...	...	Releases EDRF	$M_3{}^3$
Bronchiolar smooth muscle	Relaxes	β_2	Contracts	M_3
Gastrointestinal tract				
Smooth muscle				
Walls	Relaxes	$\alpha_2{}^5, \beta_2$	Contracts	M_3
Sphincters	Contracts	α_1	Relaxes	M_3
Secretion	...	...	Increases	M_3
Myenteric plexus	Inhibits	α	Activates	M_1
Genitourinary smooth muscle				
Bladder wall	Relaxes	β_2	Contracts	M_3
Sphincter	Contracts	α_1	Relaxes	M_3
Uterus, pregnant	Relaxes	β_2	...	
	Contracts	α	Contracts	M_3
Penis, seminal vesicles	Ejaculation	α	Erection	M
Skin				
Pilomotor smooth muscle	Contracts	α	...	...
Sweat glands				
Thermoregulatory	Increases	M	...	..
Apocrine (stress)	Increases	α	...	...
Metabolic functions				
Liver	Gluconeogenesis	$\alpha/\beta_2{}^6$	...	...
Liver	Glycogenolysis	α/β_2	...	...
Fat cells	Lipolysis	$\beta_3{}^7$	...	...
Kidney	Renin release	β_1	...	...
Autonomic nerve endings				
Sympathetic			Decreases NE release	M
Parasympathetic	Decreses ACh release	α		

[1]Less important actions are in brackets.
[2]Specific receptor type: α = alpha, β = beta, M = muscarinic. Muscarinic receptor subtypes are determined mostly in animal tissues.
[3]The endothelium of most blood vessels releases EDRF (endothelium-derived relaxing factor), which causes marked vasodilation, in response to muscarinic stimuli. However, unlike the receptors innervated by sympathetic cholinergic fibers in skeletal muscle blood vessels, these muscarinic receptors are not innervated and respond only to circulating muscarinic agonists.
[4]Vascular smooth muscle in skeletal muscle has sympathetic cholinergic dilator fibers.
[5]Probably through presynaptic inhibition of parasympathetic activity.
[6]Depends on species.
[7]Alpha$_2$ inhibits; β_1 and β_3 stimulate.

ous vasoconstriction are responses produced by sympathetic discharge that are suited to fighting or surviving attack.

At a more subtle level of interactions in the brain stem, medulla, and spinal cord, there are important cooperative interactions between the parasympathetic and sympathetic systems. For some organs, sensory fibers associated with the parasympathetic system exert reflex control over motor outflow in the sympathetic system. Thus, the sensory carotid sinus baroreceptor fibers in the glossopharyngeal nerve have a major influence on sympathetic outflow from the vasomotor center. This example is described in greater detail below. Similarly, parasympathetic sensory fibers in the wall of the urinary bladder significantly influence sympathetic inhibitory outflow to that organ. Within the enteric nervous system, sensory fibers from the wall of the gut synapse on both preganglionic and postganglionic motor cells that control intestinal smooth muscle and secretory cells (Figure 6–2).

Integration of Cardiovascular Function

Autonomic reflexes are particularly important in understanding cardiovascular responses to autonomic drugs. As indicated in Figure 6–7, the primary controlled variable in cardiovascular function is **mean arterial pressure.** Changes in any variable contributing to mean arterial pressure (eg, peripheral vascular resistance) will evoke powerful **homeostatic** secondary responses that tend to compensate for the directly evoked change. The homeostatic response may sometimes be sufficient to prevent any change in mean arterial pressure and to reverse the drug's effects on heart rate. A slow infusion of norepinephrine provides a useful example. This agent produces direct effects on both vascular and cardiac muscle. It is a powerful vasoconstrictor and, by increasing peripheral vascular resistance, increases mean arterial pressure. In the absence of reflex control—in a patient who has had a heart transplant, for example—the drug's effect on the heart is also stimulatory; ie, it increases heart rate and contractile force. However, in a subject with intact reflexes, the negative feedback baroreceptor response to increased mean arterial pressure causes decreased sympathetic outflow to the heart and a powerful increase in parasympathetic (vagus nerve) discharge at the cardiac pacemaker. As a

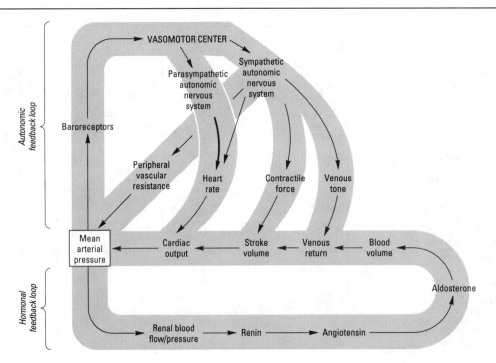

Figure 6–7. Autonomic and hormonal control of cardiovascular function. Note that two feedback loops are present: the autonomic nervous system loop and the hormonal loop. The sympathetic nervous system directly influences four major variables: peripheral vascular resistance, heart rate, force, and venous tone. It also directly modulates renin production (not shown). The parasympathetic nervous system directly influences heart rate. Angiotensin II directly increases peripheral vascular resistance (not shown). The net feedback effect of each loop is to compensate for changes in arterial blood pressure. Thus, decreased blood pressure due to blood loss would evoke increased sympathetic outflow and renin release. Conversely, elevated pressure due to the administration of a vasoconstrictor drug would cause reduced sympathetic outflow and renin release and increased parasympathetic (vagal) outflow.

Table 6–4. Autoreceptor, heteroreceptor, and modulatory effects in peripheral synapses.

Transmitter/Modulator	Receptor Type	Neuron Terminals Where Found
Inhibitory effects		
Acetylcholine	M_2	Adrenergic, enteric nervous system
Norepinephrine	Alpha$_2$	Adrenergic
Dopamine	D_2; less evidence for D_1	Adrenergic
Serotonin (5-HT)	5-HT$_1$, 5-HT$_2$, 5-HT$_3$	Cholinergic preganglionic
ATP and adenosine	P_1	Adrenergic, autonomic presynaptic, and ENS cholinergic neurons
Histamine	H_3, possibly H_2	H_3 type identified on CNS adrenergic and serotonergic neurons
Enkephalin	Delta (also mu, kappa)	Adrenergic, ENS cholinergic
Neuropeptide Y	NPY	Adrenergic, some cholinergic
Prostaglandin E_1, E_2	EP$_3$	Adrenergic
Excitatory effects		
Epinephrine	Beta$_2$	Adrenergic, somatic motor cholinergic
Acetylcholine	N_M	Somatic motor cholinergic
Angiotensin II	AII-1	Adrenergic

result, the *net* effect of ordinary pressor doses of norepinephrine is to produce a marked increase in peripheral vascular resistance, a moderate increase in mean arterial pressure, and a consistent *slowing* of heart rate. Bradycardia, the reflex compensatory response elicited by this agent, is *the exact opposite of the drug's direct action;* yet it is completely predictable if the integration of cardiovascular function by the autonomic nervous system is understood.

Presynaptic Regulation

The principle of negative feedback control is also found at the presynaptic level of autonomic function. While not yet as completely understood as the baroreceptor reflex, important presynaptic feedback inhibitory control mechanisms have been shown to exist in noradrenergic fibers. The best-documented mechanism involves an α_2 receptor located on the nerve terminals. This receptor is activated by norepinephrine and similar molecules; activation diminishes further release of norepinephrine from these nerve endings (Table 6–4). Conversely, a presynaptic beta receptor may facilitate the release of norepinephrine. Presynaptic receptors that respond to the transmitter substances released by the nerve ending have been called **autoreceptors.** Autoreceptors are usually inhibitory, but some cholinergic fibers, especially somatic motor fibers, may have excitatory autoreceptors for acetylcholine.

Control of transmitter release is not limited to

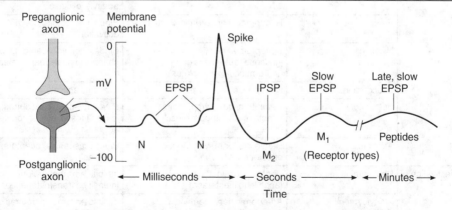

Figure 6–8. Excitatory and inhibitory postsynaptic potentials (*EPSP* and *IPSP*) in an autonomic ganglion cell. The postganglionic neuron might undergo the membrane potential changes shown schematically in the recording. The response begins with two EPSP responses to nicotinic *(N)* receptor activation, the first not achieving threshold. The action potential is followed by an IPSP, probably evoked by M_2 receptor activation (with possible participation from dopamine receptor activation). The IPSP is, in turn, followed by a slower M_1-dependent EPSP, and this is sometimes followed by a still slower peptide-induced excitatory postsynaptic potential.

modulation by the transmitter itself. Nerve terminals also carry regulatory receptors that respond to many other substances (heteroreceptors). Heteroreceptors may be activated by substances released from nerve terminals that synapse with the nerve ending. Alternatively, the ligands for these receptors may diffuse to the receptors from the blood or from nearby tissues. Some of the transmitters and receptors identified to date are listed in Table 6–4. Presynaptic regulation by a variety of endogenous chemicals probably occurs in all nerve fibers.

Postsynaptic Regulation

Postsynaptic regulation can be considered from two perspectives: modulation by the prior history of activity at the primary receptor (which may up- or down-regulate receptor number or desensitize receptors; see Chapter 2) and modulation by other temporally associated events.

The first mechanism has been well documented in several receptor-effector systems. Up- and down-regulation are known to occur in response to decreased or increased activation, respectively, of the

Table 6–5. Steps in autonomic transmission: Effects of drugs.

Process	Drug Example	Site	Action
Action potential propagation	Local anesthetics, tetrodotoxin,[1] saxitoxin[2]	Nerve axons	Block sodium channels; block conduction
Transmitter synthesis	Hemicholinium	Cholinergic nerve terminals: membrane	Blocks uptake of choline and slows synthesis
	α-Methyltyrosine (metyrosine)	Adrenergic nerve terminals and adrenal medulla: cytoplasm	Blocks synthesis
Transmitter storage	Vesamicol	Cholinergic terminals: vesicles	Prevents storage
	Reserpine	Adrenergic terminals: vesicles	Promotes depletion
Transmitter release	Many[3]	Nerve terminal membrane receptors	Modulate release
	ω-Conotoxin GVIA	Nerve terminal calcium channels	Reduces transmitter release
	Botulinus toxin	Cholinergic vesicles	Prevents release
	Latrotoxin[4]	Cholinergic and adrenergic vesicles	Causes explosive release
	Tyramine, amphetamine	Adrenergic nerve terminals	Promote transmitter release
Transmitter uptake after release	Cocaine, tricyclic antidepressants	Adrenergic nerve terminals	Inhibit uptake; increase transmitter effect on postsynaptic receptors
	6-Hydroxydopamine	Adrenergic nerve terminals	Destroys the terminals
Receptor activation/ blockade	Norepinephrine	Receptors at adrenergic junctions	Binds α receptors; causes contraction
	Phentolamine	Receptors at adrenergic junctions	Binds α receptors; prevents activation
	Isoproterenol	Receptors at adrenergic junctions	Binds β receptors; activates adenylyl cyclase
	Propranolol	Receptors at adrenergic junctions	Binds β receptors; prevents activation
	Nicotine	Receptors at nicotinic cholinergic junctions (autonomic ganglia, neuromuscular end-plates)	Binds nicotinic receptors; opens ion channel in postsynaptic membrane
	Tubocurarine	Neuromuscular end-plates	Prevents activation
	Bethanechol	Receptors, parasympathetic effector cells (smooth muscle, glands)	Binds muscarinic receptors; releases inositol trisphosphate and activates guanylyl cyclase
	Atropine	Receptors, parasympathetic effector cells	Binds muscarinic receptors; prevents activation
Enzymatic inactivation of transmitter	Neostigmine	Cholinergic synapses (acetylcholinesterase)	Inhibits enzyme; prolongs and intensifies transmitter action
	Tranylcypromine	Adrenergic nerve terminals (monoamine oxidase)	Inhibits enzyme; increases stored transmitter pool

[1]Toxin of puffer fish, California newt.
[2]Toxin of *Gonyaulax* (red tide organism).
[3]Norepinephrine, dopamine, acetylcholine, angiotensin II, various prostaglandins, etc.
[4]Black widow spider venom.

receptors. An extreme form of up-regulation occurs after denervation of some tissues, resulting in "denervation supersensitivity" of the tissue to activators of that receptor type. In skeletal muscle, for example, nicotinic receptors are normally restricted to the end-plate regions underlying somatic motor nerve terminals. Surgical denervation results in marked proliferation of nicotinic cholinoceptors over all parts of the fiber, including areas not previously associated with any motor nerve junctions. A related pharmacologic denervation supersensitivity phenomenon occurs in autonomic effector tissues after administration of drugs that deplete transmitter stores and prevent activation of the postsynaptic receptors for a sufficient period of time. For example, administration of large doses of reserpine, a norepinephrine depleter, can cause increased sensitivity of the smooth muscle and cardiac muscle effector cells served by the depleted sympathetic fibers.

The second mechanism involves modulation of the primary transmitter-receptor event by events evoked by the same or other transmitters acting on different postsynaptic receptors. Ganglionic transmission is a good example of this hierarchy (Figure 6–8). The postganglionic cells are activated (depolarized) as a result of binding of an appropriate ligand to a nicotinic (N_N) acetylcholine receptor. The resulting fast excitatory postsynaptic potential (EPSP) evokes a propagated action potential if threshold is reached. This event is often followed by a small and slowly developing but longer-lasting hyperpolarizing afterpotential—a slow inhibitory postsynaptic potential (IPSP). The hyperpolarization involves opening of potassium channels by M_2 cholinoceptors. The IPSP is followed by a small, slow excitatory postsynaptic potential apparently caused by closure of potassium channels linked to M_1 cholinoceptors. Finally, a late, very slow EPSP may be evoked by peptides released from other fibers. These slow potentials serve to modulate the responsiveness of the postsynaptic cell to subsequent primary excitatory presynaptic nerve activity. (See Chapter 20 for additional examples.)

PHARMACOLOGIC MODIFICATION OF AUTONOMIC FUNCTION

Because transmission involves different mechanisms in different segments of the autonomic nervous system, some drugs produce highly specific effects while others are much less selective in their actions. A summary of the steps in transmission of impulses, from the central nervous system to the autonomic effector cells, is presented in Table 6–5. Drugs that block action potential propagation (local anesthetics) are very nonselective in their action, since they act on a process that is common to all neurons. On the other hand, drugs that act on the biochemical processes involved in transmitter synthesis and storage are more selective, since the biochemistry of adrenergic transmission is very different from that of cholinergic transmission. Activation or blockade of effector cell receptors offers maximum flexibility and selectivity of effect: adrenoceptors are easily distinguished from

---

PHARMACOLOGY OF THE EYE

The eye is a good example of an organ with multiple ANS functions, controlled by several different autonomic receptors. As shown in Figure 6–9, the anterior chamber is the site of several tissues controlled by the ANS. These tissues include three different muscles (pupillary dilator and constrictor muscles in the iris and the ciliary muscle) and the secretory epithelium of the ciliary body.

Muscarinic cholinomimetics cause contraction of the circular pupillary constrictor muscle and of the ciliary muscle. Contraction of the pupillary constrictor muscle causes miosis, a reduction in pupil size. Miosis is usually present in patients exposed to large systemic or small topical doses of cholinomimetics, especially organophosphate cholinesterase inhibitors. Ciliary muscle contraction causes accommodation of focus for near vision. Marked contraction of the ciliary muscle, which often occurs with cholinesterase inhibitor intoxication, is called *cyclospasm*. Ciliary muscle

contraction also puts tension on the trabecular meshwork, opening its pores and facilitating outflow of the aqueous humor into the canal of Schlemm. Increased outflow reduces intraocular pressure, a very useful result in patients with glaucoma. All of these effects are prevented or reversed by muscarinic blocking drugs such as atropine.

Alpha adrenoceptors cause contraction of the radially oriented pupillary dilator muscle fibers in the iris and result in mydriasis. This occurs commonly during sympathetic discharge and when alpha agonist drugs such as phenylephrine are placed in the conjunctival sac. Beta adrenoceptors on the ciliary epithelium facilitate the secretion of aqueous humor. Blocking these receptors (with beta-blocking drugs) reduces the secretory activity and reduces intraocular pressure, providing another therapy for glaucoma.

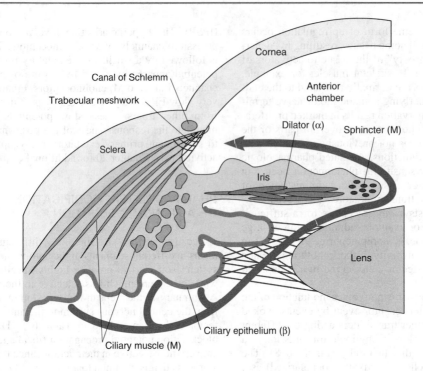

Figure 6–9. Structures of the anterior chamber of the eye. Tissues with significant autonomic functions and the associated ANS receptors are shown in this schematic diagram. Activation of the beta adrenoceptors associated with the ciliary epithelium causes increased secretion of aqueous humor (arrow). Blood vessels (not shown) in the eye are also under autonomic control and influence aqueous drainage.

cholinoceptors. Furthermore, several subgroups can be selectively activated or blocked within each major type. Some examples are given in the box: Pharmacology of the Eye.

The next four chapters provide many more examples of this useful diversity of autonomic control processes.

REFERENCES

Allen TGJ, Burnstock G: M_1 and M_2 muscarinic receptors mediate excitation and inhibition of guinea-pig intracardiac neurones in culture. J Physiol 1990;422:463.

Anderson DC, King SC, Parsons SM: Pharmacological characterization of the acetylcholine transport system in purified *Torpedo* synaptic vesicles. Mol Pharmacol 1983; 24:48.

Anderson K-E: Pharmacology of lower urinary tract smooth muscles and penile erectile tissues. Pharmacol Rev 1993; 45:253.

Bevan JA, Brayden JE: Nonadrenergic neural vasodilator mechanisms. Circ Res 1987;60:309.

Brose N et al: Synaptotagmin: A calcium sensor on the synaptic vesicle surface. Science 1992;256:1021.

Buckley NJ et al: Antagonist binding properties of five cloned muscarinic receptors expressed in CHO-K1 cells. Mol Pharmacol 1989;35:469.

Burnstock G, Hoyle CHV: *Autonomic Neuroeffector Mechanisms.* Harwood Academic Publishers, 1992.

Cassis LA, Dwoskin LP: Presynaptic modulation of transmitter release by endogenous angiotensin II in brown adipose tissue. J Neural Transm 1991;34(Suppl):129.

Duckles SP, Garcia-Villalon L: Characterization of vascular muscarinic receptors: Rabbit ear artery and bovine coronary artery. J Pharmacol Exp Ther 1990;253:608.

Eglen RM, Whiting RL: Heterogeneity of vascular muscarinic receptors. J Auton Pharmacol 1990;19:233.

Furchgott RF: Role of endothelium in responses of vascular smooth muscle to drugs. Annu Rev Pharmacol Toxicol 1984;24:175.

Furness JB et al: Roles of peptides in transmission in the enteric nervous system. Trends Neurosci 1992;15:66.

Furness JB, Costa M: *The Enteric Nervous System.* Churchill Livingstone, 1987.

Goyal RK: Muscarinic receptor subtypes. Physiology and clinical implications. N Engl J Med 1989;321:1022.

Hirning LD et al: Dominant role of N-type Ca^{2+} channels in evoked release of norepinephrine from sympathetic neurons. Science 1988;239:57.

Holzer P: Local effector functions of capsaicin-sensitive sensory nerve endings: Involvement of tachykinins, calcitonin gene-related peptide and other neuropeptides. Neuroscience 1988;24:739.

Hökfelt T et al: Coexistence of peptides with classical neurotransmitters. Experientia 1989;56(Suppl):154.

Jankovic J, Brin MF: Therapeutic uses of botulinum toxin. N Engl J Med 1991;324:1186.

Kromer W: Endogenous opioids, the enteric nervous system and gut motility. Dig Dis 1990;8:361.

Kumada M, Terui N, Kuwaki T: Arterial baroreceptor reflex: Its central and peripheral neural mechanisms. Prog Neurobiol 1990;35:331.

Langer SZ: Presynaptic regulation of monoaminergic neurons. In: *Psychopharmacology: The Third Generation of Progress.* Meltzer HY (editor). Raven Press, 1987.

Lefkowitz RJ, Hausdorff WP, Caron MG: Role of phosphorylation in desensitization of the β-adrenoceptor. Trends Pharmacol Sci 1990;11:190.

Limberger N, Späth L, Starke K: Presynaptic α_2-adrenoceptor, opioid κ-receptor and adenosine A_1-receptor interactions on noradrenalin release in rabbit brain cortex. Naunyn Schmiedebergs Arch Pharmacol 1988;338:53.

Llewellyn-Smith IJ: Neuropeptides and the microcircuitry of the enteric nervous system. Experientia 1989;56 (Suppl):247.

Lundgren O, Svanvik J, Jivegård L: Enteric nervous system. I. Physiology and pathophysiology of the intestinal tract. Dig Dis Sci 1989; 34:264.

MacDonald A et al: Contributions of α_1-adrenoceptors, α_2-adrenoceptors, and P_{2x}-purinoceptors to neurotransmission in several rabbit isolated blood vessels: Role of neuronal uptake and autofeedback. Br J Pharmacol 1992;105:347.

Maggi CA, Meli A: The sensory-efferent function of capsaicin-sensitive sensory neurons. Gen Pharmacol 1988; 19:1.

McGrath JC, Brown CM, Wilson VG: Alpha-adrenoceptors: A critical review. Med Res Rev 1989;9:407.

1994 receptor nomenclature supplement. Trends Pharmacol Sci(Suppl):1994.

Ohia SE, Jumblatt JE: Prejunctional inhibitory effects of prostanoids on sympathetic neurotransmission in the rabbit iris-ciliary body. J Pharmacol Exp Ther 1990;255:11.

Palmer RM, Ferrige AG, Moncada S: Nitric oxide release accounts for the biological activity of endothelium-derived relaxing factor. Nature 1987;327:524.

Pappano AJ, Mubagwa K: Actions of muscarinic agents and adenosine on the heart. In: *The Heart and Cardiovascular System.* Fozzard HA (editor). Raven Press, 1992.

Parsons SM et al: Transport in the cholinergic synaptic vesicle. Fed Proc 1982;41:2765.

Pfeiffer A et al: Muscarinic receptors mediating acid secretion in isolated rat parietal cells are of M_3 type. Gastroenterology 1990;98:218.

Rubanyi GM, Vanhoutte PM: Nature of endothelium-derived relaxing factor: Are there two relaxing factors? Circ Res 1987;61(Suppl 2):II–61.

Ruffolo RR Jr et al: Drug receptors and control of the cardiovascular system: Recent advances. Prog Drug Res 1991;36:117.

Schiavo G et al: Tetanus and botulinum-B neurotoxins block neurotransmitter release by proteolytic cleavage of synaptobrevin. Nature 1992;359:832.

Schwartz J-C et al: The dopamine receptor family: Molecular biology and pharmacology. Semin Neurosci 1992; 4:99.

Seeman P, Grigoriades D: Dopamine receptors in brain and periphery. Neurochem Int 1987;10:1.

Starke K, Göthert M, Kilbinger H: Modulation of neurotransmitter release by presynaptic autoreceptors. Physiol Rev 1989;69:864.

Taylor GS, Bywater RAR: Novel autonomic neurotransmitters and intestinal function. Pharmacol Ther 1989;40: 401.

Taylor SJ, Kilpatrick GJ: Characterization of histamine-H_3 receptors controlling non-adrenergic non-cholinergic contractions of the guinea-pig isolated ileum. Br J Pharmacol 1992;105:667.

Valtorta F et al: Neurotransmitter release and synaptic vesicle recycling. Neuroscience 1990;35:477.

Wagner G, Sjöstrand NO: Autonomic pharmacology and sexual function. In: *Handbook of Sexology.* Vol 6: *The Pharmacology and Endocrinology of Sexual Function.* Sitsen JMA (editor). Elsevier, 1988.

Wharton J, Gulbenkian S: Peptides in the mammalian cardiovascular system. Experientia 1989;56(Suppl):292.

7

Cholinoceptor-Activating & Cholinesterase-Inhibiting Drugs

Achilles J. Pappano, PhD, & August M. Watanabe, MD

The acetylcholine receptor stimulants and cholinesterase inhibitors together comprise a large group of drugs that mimic acetylcholine (cholinomimetic agents) (Figure 7–1). Cholinoceptor stimulants are classified pharmacologically by their *spectrum* of action depending upon the receptor type—muscarinic or nicotinic—that is activated. They are also classified by their *mechanism* of action, because some cholinomimetic drugs bind directly to (and activate) cholinoceptors while a second important group acts indirectly by inhibiting the hydrolysis of endogenous acetylcholine.

SPECTRUM OF ACTION OF CHOLINOMIMETIC DRUGS

In some of the first studies of the parasympathetic nervous system, Sir Henry Dale found that the alkaloid **muscarine** mimicked the effects of parasympathetic nerve discharge, ie, the effects were **parasympathomimetic**. Direct application of muscarine to ganglia and to autonomic effector tissues (smooth muscle, heart, exocrine glands) showed that the parasympathomimetic action of the alkaloid was mediated by receptors at the effector cells, not those in the ganglia. Therefore, by convention, the effects of acetylcholine itself and of other cholinomimetic drugs at autonomic neuroeffector junctions are referred to as parasympathomimetic effects, mediated by muscarinic receptors.

In contrast, the alkaloid **nicotine** was found to stimulate autonomic ganglia and skeletal muscle neuromuscular junctions but to have little effect on autonomic effector cells when applied in low concentrations. The ganglion and skeletal muscle receptors were therefore labeled nicotinic. When it was later demonstrated that acetylcholine is the physiologic transmitter substance at both muscarinic and nicotinic receptors, it was recognized that both receptors are subtypes of cholinoceptors.

Cholinoceptors are members of either G protein-linked (muscarinic) or ionic channel (nicotinic) families on the basis of their transmembrane signaling mechanisms. Muscarinic receptors contain seven transmembrane domains whose third cytoplasmic loop is coupled to G proteins that function as intramembrane transducers (Figure 2–12). In general, these receptors regulate the production of intracellular second messengers. Agonist selectivity is determined by the subtypes of muscarinic receptor and G protein that are present in a given cell (Table 7–1). Muscarinic receptors are located on plasma membranes of cells of organs innervated by parasympathetic nerves as well as on some tissues that are not innervated by these nerves, eg, endothelial cells (Table 7–1), and on those tissues innervated by cholinergic postganglionic sympathetic nerves.

Nicotinic receptors are part of a transmembrane polypeptide whose subunits form cation-selective ion channels (Figure 2–10). These receptors are located on plasma membranes of parasympathetic and sympathetic postganglionic cells in autonomic ganglia and also on membranes of muscles innervated by somatic motor fibers (Figure 6–1).

Because of the multiple sites of action of acetylcholine and the fact that it has both excitatory and inhibitory effects, unselective cholinoceptor stimulants in sufficient dosage can produce very diffuse and marked alterations in organ system function. Fortunately, drugs are available that have a degree of selectivity, so that desired effects can often be achieved while avoiding or minimizing adverse effects. This selectivity of action is based on several factors. Some drugs stimulate muscarinic receptors selectively, whereas others activate nicotinic receptors selectively. Some agents stimulate nicotinic receptors in ganglia preferentially and have less effect on nicotinic receptors at neuromuscular junctions. Organ selectivity can also be achieved by utilizing appropriate routes of administration ("pharmacokinetic selectivity"). For example, muscarinic stimulants can be administered topically to the external surface of the eye

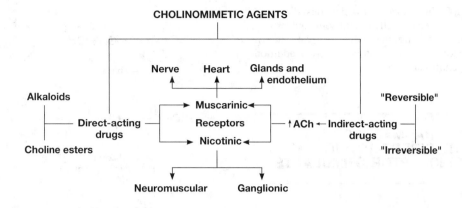

Figure 7–1. The major groups of cholinoceptor-activating drugs, receptors, and target tissues.

to modify ocular function while minimizing systemic effects.

MODE OF ACTION OF CHOLINOMIMETIC DRUGS

Cholinomimetic agents can be either direct- or indirect-acting (Figure 7–1). The direct-acting agents directly bind to and activate muscarinic or nicotinic receptors. The indirect-acting agents produce their primary effects by inhibiting the action of acetylcholinesterase, which hydrolyzes acetylcholine to

choline and acetic acid (Figure 6–3). By inhibiting acetylcholinesterase, the indirect-acting drugs increase the concentration of endogenous acetylcholine in the synaptic clefts and neuroeffector junctions, and the excess acetylcholine in turn stimulates cholinoceptors to evoke increased responses. These drugs are, in effect, *amplifiers* of endogenous acetylcholine and act primarily where acetylcholine is physiologically released.

Some cholinesterase inhibitors, even in low concentration, also inhibit butyrylcholinesterase (pseudocholinesterase), and most inhibit this enzyme when they are present in high concentrations. However, since butyrylcholinesterase is not important in the physiologic termination of action of synaptic acetylcholine, inhibition of its action plays little role in the action of indirect-acting cholinomimetic drugs. Some

Table 7–1. Subtypes and characteristics of cholinoceptors.

Receptor Type	Other Names	Location	Structural Features	Postreceptor Mechanism
M_1	M_{1a}	Nerves	7 transmembrane segments, G protein-linked	IP_3, DAG cascade
M_2	M_{2a}, cardiac M_2	Heart, nerves, smooth muscle	7 transmembrane segments, G protein-linked	Inhibition of cAMP production, activation of K channels
M_3	M_{2b} glandular M_2	Glands, smooth muscle, endothelium	7 transmembrane segments, G protein-linked	IP_3, DAG cascade
m_4[1]		?CNS	7 transmembrane segments, G protein-linked	Inhibition of cAMP production
m_5[1]		?CNS	7 transmembrane segments, G protein-linked	IP_3, DAG cascade
N_M	Muscle type, end plate receptor	Skeletal muscle neuro-muscular junction	Pentamer $(\alpha_2 \beta \delta \gamma)$[2]	Na^+, K^+ depolarizing ion channel
N_N	Neuronal type, ganglion receptor	Postganglionic cell body, dendrites	α and β subunits only as $\alpha_2 \beta_2$ or $\alpha_3 \beta_3$	Na^+, K^+ depolarizing ion channel

[1]Genes have been cloned but functional receptors have not been incontrovertibly identified.
[2]Structure in *Torpedo* electric organ and fetal muscle. In adult muscle, the γ subunit is replaced by an ε subunit. Several different α and β subunits have been identified in different mammalian tissues (Lindstrom, 1990).

cholinesterase inhibitors also have a modest direct action as well; this is especially true of some quaternary carbamates, eg, neostigmine, which activate neuromuscular nicotinic cholinoceptors directly in addition to blocking cholinesterase.

I. BASIC PHARMACOLOGY OF THE DIRECT-ACTING CHOLINOCEPTOR STIMULANTS

The direct-acting cholinomimetic drugs can be divided on the basis of chemical structure into esters of choline (including acetylcholine) and alkaloids (such as muscarine and nicotine). A few of these drugs are highly selective for the muscarinic or for the nicotinic receptor. Many have effects on both receptors; acetylcholine is typical.

Chemistry & Pharmacokinetics

A. Structure: Four important esters of choline that have been studied extensively are shown in Figure 7–2. They are permanently charged and relatively insoluble in lipids because they contain the quaternary ammonium group. Many naturally occurring and synthetic cholinomimetic drugs that are not choline esters have been identified; a few of these are shown in Figure 7–3. The muscarinic receptor is strongly stereoselective: (S)-bethanechol is almost 1000 times more potent than (R)-bethanechol.

B. Absorption, Distribution, and Metabolism: The choline esters are poorly absorbed and poorly distributed into the central nervous system because they are hydrophilic. Although they are all hydrolyzed in the gastrointestinal tract (and less active by the oral route), they differ markedly in their susceptibility to hydrolysis by cholinesterase in the body. Acetylcholine is very rapidly hydrolyzed, as described in Chapter 6; large amounts must be infused intravenously to achieve levels high enough to produce detectable effects. A large intravenous bolus injection has a brief effect, typically 5–20 seconds, whereas intramuscular and subcutaneous injections produce only local effects. Methacholine is at least three times more resistant to hydrolysis and produces systemic effects even when given subcutaneously. The carbamic acid esters, carbachol and bethanechol, are extremely resistant to hydrolysis by cholinesterase and have correspondingly longer durations of action. Presence of the β-methyl group (methacholine, bethanechol) reduces the potency of these drugs at the nicotinic receptor (Table 7–2).

The tertiary cholinomimetic alkaloids (pilocarpine, nicotine, lobeline; Figure 7–3) are well absorbed from most sites of administration. Nicotine, a liquid,

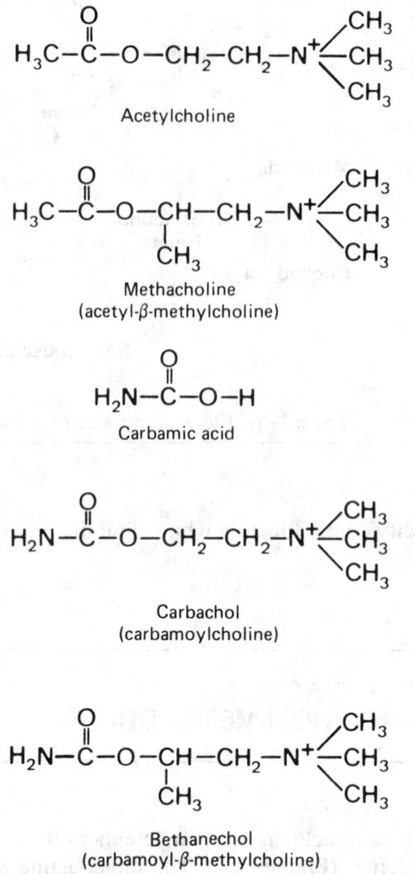

Figure 7–2. Molecular structures of four choline esters and carbamic acid. Acetylcholine and methacholine are acetic acid esters of choline and β-methylcholine, respectively. Carbachol and bethanechol are carbamic acid esters of the same alcohols.

is sufficiently lipid-soluble to be absorbed across the skin. Muscarine, a quaternary amine, is less completely absorbed from the gastrointestinal tract than the tertiary amines but is nevertheless toxic when ingested, eg, in certain mushrooms. Excretion of these amines is chiefly by the kidneys. Clearance of the tertiary amines can be accelerated by acidification of the urine. Oxotremorine is an extremely potent synthetic muscarinic agonist that has been used as a research tool. It is well distributed into the central nervous system. Lobeline is a plant derivative with lower potency than nicotine but with a similar spectrum of action. Dimethylphenylpiperazinium (DMPP) is a potent synthetic nicotinic stimulant with little access to the central nervous system. It is a research tool used for selective stimulation of ganglionic nicotinic receptors.

Pharmacodynamics

A. Mechanism of Action: Activation of the

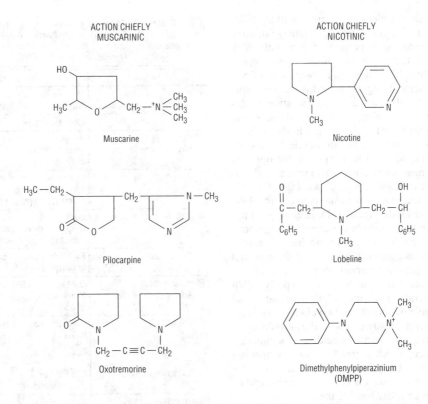

Figure 7–3. Structures of some cholinomimetic alkaloids and synthetic analogues.

parasympathetic nervous system modifies organ function by two major mechanisms. First, acetylcholine released from parasympathetic nerves can activate muscarinic receptors on effector organs to alter organ function directly. Second, acetylcholine released from parasympathetic nerves can interact with muscarinic receptors on nerve terminals to inhibit the release of their neurotransmitter. By this mechanism, acetylcholine release—and, possibly, circulating muscarinic agonists—indirectly alter organ function by modulating the effects of the parasympathetic and sympathetic nervous systems and perhaps noncholinergic, nonadrenergic systems.

The subcellular mechanism by which muscarinic stimulants alter cellular function continues to be in-

vestigated. As indicated in Chapter 6, multiple muscarinic receptor types have been cloned and several have been characterized by binding studies. Several cellular events occur when muscarinic receptors are activated, one or more of which might serve as "second messengers" for muscarinic activation. All muscarinic receptors appear to be of the "G-protein coupled" type (Chapter 2) with seven segments (Table 7–1) arranged in serpentine fashion across the membrane. An important result of muscarinic agonist binding is activation of the IP_3, DAG cascade. Some evidence implicates diacylglycerol in the opening of smooth muscle calcium channels; IP_3 evokes release of calcium from endoplasmic and sarcoplasmic reticulum. Muscarinic agonists also increase cellular concentrations of cGMP. The activation of muscarinic receptors also increases potassium flux across cell membranes. This effect is mediated by the binding of an activated G protein directly to the channel. Finally, it has been shown that activation of muscarinic receptors in some tissues (eg, heart) results in inhibition of adenylyl cyclase activity. Moreover, muscarinic agonists can attenuate the activation of adenylyl cyclase and modulate the increase in cAMP levels induced by hormones such as catecholamines. These muscarinic effects on cAMP generation are paralleled by attenuation of the physiologic response of the organ to stimulatory hormones.

Table 7–2. Properties of choline esters.

Choline Ester	Susceptibility to Cholinesterase	Muscarinic Action	Nicotinic Action
Acetylcholine chloride	++++	+++	+++
Methacholine chloride	+	++++	+
Carbachol chloride	Negligible	++	+++
Bethanechol chloride	Negligible	++	None

The mechanism of nicotinic receptor activation has been studied in great detail, taking advantage of three factors: The receptor is present in extremely high concentration in the membranes of the electric organs of electric fish; α-bungarotoxin, a component of certain snake venoms, is tightly bound to the receptors and readily labeled as a marker for isolation procedures; and activation of the receptor results in easily measured electrical and ionic changes in the cells involved. The nicotinic receptor in muscle tissues appears to be a pentamer of four types of glycoprotein subunits (one monomer occurs twice) with a total molecular weight of about 250,000 (see Figure 2–10). The nicotinic receptor in neurons consists of alpha and beta subunits only (Table 7–1). Each subunit appears to have four membrane-crossing segments. Each alpha subunit has a receptor site that, when activated by a nicotinic agonist, causes a conformational change in the protein (channel opening) that allows sodium and potassium ions to diffuse rapidly down their concentration gradients. While binding of an agonist molecule by one of the two alpha subunit receptor sites only modestly increases the probability of channel opening, simultaneous binding of agonist by both of the receptor sites greatly enhances opening probability. Thus, the primary effect of nicotinic receptor activation is depolarization of the nerve cell or neuromuscular endplate bearing the receptor.

If agonist occupancy of the nicotinic receptor is prolonged, the effector response is abolished; ie, the postganglionic neuron stops firing (ganglionic effect), and the skeletal muscle cell relaxes (neuromuscular endplate effect). Furthermore, the continued presence of the nicotinic agonist prevents electrical recovery of the postjunctional membrane. In this way, a state of "depolarizing blockade" is induced that is refractory to reversal by other agonists. As noted below, this effect can be exploited for producing muscle paralysis.

B. Organ System Effects: Most of the direct organ system effects of muscarinic cholinoceptor stimulants are readily predicted from a knowledge of the effects of parasympathetic nerve stimulation (Table 6–3) and the distribution of muscarinic receptors. Effects of a typical agent such as acetylcholine are listed in Table 7–3. The effects of nicotinic agonists are similarly predictable from a knowledge of the physiology of the autonomic ganglia and skeletal muscle motor endplate.

1. Eye–Muscarinic agonists instilled into the conjunctival sac cause contraction of the smooth muscle of the iris sphincter (resulting in miosis) and of the ciliary muscle (resulting in accommodation). As a result, the iris is pulled away from the angle of the anterior chamber, and the trabecular meshwork at the base of the ciliary muscle is opened up. Both effects facilitate the outflow of aqueous humor into the canal of Schlemm, which drains the anterior chamber.

2. Cardiovascular system–The primary car-

Table 7–3. Effects of direct-acting cholinoceptor stimulants. Only the direct effects are indicated; homeostatic responses to these direct actions may be important (see text).

Organ	Response
Eye	
Sphincter muscle of iris	Contraction (miosis).
Ciliary muscle	Contraction for near vision.
Heart	
Sinoatrial node	Decrease in rate (negative chronotropy).
Atria	Decrease in contractile strength (negative inotropy). Decrease in refractory period.
Atrioventricular node	Decrease in conduction velocity (negative dromotropy.) Increase in refractory period.
Ventricles	Small decrease in contractile strength.
Blood vessels	
Arteries	Dilatation (via EDRF) Constriction (high dose direct effect).
Veins	Dilatation (via EDRF) Constriction (high dose direct effect).
Lung	
Bronchial muscle	Contraction (bronchoconstriction).
Bronchial glands	Stimulation.
Gastrointestinal tract	
Motility	Increase.
Sphincters	Relaxation.
Secretion	Stimulation.
Urinary bladder	
Detrusor	Contraction.
Trigone and sphincter	Relaxation.
Glands	
Sweat, salivary, lacrimal, nasopharyngeal	Secretion.

diovascular effects of muscarinic agonists are reduction in peripheral vascular resistance and changes in heart rate. The direct effects listed in Table 7–3 are modified by important homeostatic reflexes, as described in Chapter 6 and depicted in Figure 6–7. Intravenous infusions of minimal effective doses of acetylcholine in humans (eg, 20–50 μg/min) cause vasodilation, resulting in a reduction in blood pressure, often accompanied by a reflex increase in heart rate. Larger doses of acetylcholine produce bradycardia and decrease conduction velocity through the atrioventricular node in addition to the hypotensive effect.

The direct cardiac actions of muscarinic stimulants include the following: (1) an increase in a potassium current ($I_{K(ACh)}$) in atrial muscle cells and in the cells of the sinoatrial and atrioventricular nodes as well; (2) a decrease in the slow inward calcium current in heart cells; and (3) a reduction in the hyperpolarization-activated current (I_f) that underlies diastolic depolarization. All of these actions contribute to the observed slowing of pacemaker rate. Effects (1) and (2) cause hyperpolarization and decreased contractility of atrial cells. As noted above, the direct slowing of sinoatrial rate and atrioventricular conduction that is produced by muscarinic agonists is often opposed by reflex sympathetic discharge, elicited by the decrease in blood pressure. The resultant interaction between sympathetic and parasympathetic effects is complex because of the previously described muscarinic modulation of sympathetic influences that occurs by inhibition of norepinephrine release and by postjunctional cellular effects. Therefore, the net effect on heart rate depends on local concentrations of the agonist in the heart and in the vessels and on the level of reflex responsiveness.

Parasympathetic innervation of the ventricles is much less extensive than that of the atria. Also, activation of muscarinic receptors in ventricles results in much less physiologic effect than that seen following activation of these receptors in atria. However, during sympathetic stimulation, the effects of muscarinic agonists on ventricular function are clearly evident because of muscarinic modulation of sympathetic effects ("accentuated antagonism"; Levy and Schwartz, 1993) as described above.

In the intact organism, muscarinic agonists produce marked vasodilation. However, in earlier studies, isolated vascular smooth muscle preparations often showed a contractile response to these agents. It is now known (Furchgott et al, 1984) that acetylcholine-induced vasodilation requires the presence of intact endothelium. Muscarinic agonists release a relaxing substance (endothelium-derived relaxing factor, or EDRF) from the endothelial cells that causes smooth muscle relaxation. Isolated vessels prepared with the endothelium preserved consistently reproduce the vasodilatory response seen in the intact organism. EDRF appears to be—at least in part—nitric oxide (NO). This substance activates guanylyl cyclase and increases cGMP in smooth muscle, resulting in relaxation (see Figure 12–2).

The cardiovascular effects of all of the choline esters are similar to those of acetylcholine, the main difference being in their potency and duration of action. Because of the resistance of methacholine, carbachol, and bethanechol to acetylcholinesterase, lower doses given intravenously are sufficient to produce effects similar to those of acetylcholine, and the duration of action of these synthetic choline esters is longer. The cardiovascular effects of most of the cholinomimetic natural alkaloids and synthetic analogues are also generally similar to those of acetylcholine.

Pilocarpine is an interesting exception to the above statement. If given intravenously (an experimental exercise), it may produce hypertension after a brief initial hypotensive response. The longer-lasting hypertensive effect can be traced to ganglionic discharge caused by activation of M_1 receptors in the postganglionic cell membrane, which close K^+ channels and elicit slow excitatory (depolarizing) postsynaptic potentials. This effect, like the hypotensive effect, can be blocked by atropine, an antimuscarinic drug.

3. Respiratory system–The smooth muscle of the bronchial tree is contracted by muscarinic stimulants. In addition, the glands of the tracheobronchial mucosa are stimulated to secrete. This combination of effects can occasionally cause symptoms, especially in individuals with asthma.

4. Gastrointestinal tract–Administration of muscarinic agonists, like stimulation of the parasympathetic nervous system, causes an increase in secretory and motor activity of the gut. The salivary and gastric glands are strongly stimulated; the pancreas and small intestinal glands less so. Peristaltic activity is increased throughout the gut, and most sphincters are relaxed. Stimulation of contraction in this organ system has been shown to involve depolarization of the smooth muscle cell membrane and increased calcium influx.

5. Genitourinary tract–Muscarinic agonists stimulate the detrusor muscle and relax the trigone and sphincter muscles of the bladder, thus promoting voiding. The human uterus is not notably sensitive to muscarinic agonists.

6. Miscellaneous secretory glands–Muscarinic agonists stimulate the secretory activity of sweat, lacrimal, and nasopharyngeal glands.

7. Central nervous system–The central nervous system contains both muscarinic and nicotinic receptors, the brain being relatively richer in muscarinic sites and the spinal cord containing a preponderance of nicotinic sites. The physiologic role of these receptors is discussed in Chapter 20. In spite of the smaller ratio of nicotinic to muscarinic receptors in the brain, nicotine and lobeline (Figure 7–3) have important effects on the brain stem and cortex. The mild alerting action of nicotine absorbed from inhaled tobacco smoke is the best-known of these effects. In larger concentrations, nicotine induces tremor, emesis, and stimulation of the respiratory center. At still higher levels, nicotine causes convulsions, which may terminate in fatal coma. The lethal effects on the central nervous system and the fact that nicotine is readily absorbed form the basis for the use of nicotine as an insecticide. Dimethylphenylpiperazinium (DMPP), a synthetic nicotinic stimulant (Figure 7–3), is relatively free of these central effects because it does not cross the blood-brain barrier.

8. Peripheral nervous system–The autonomic ganglia are important sites of nicotinic synaptic action. All of the nicotinic agents shown in Figure 7–3 are capable of causing marked activation of the nicotinic receptors, resulting in firing of action potentials in the postganglionic neurons. Nicotine itself has a somewhat greater affinity for neuronal than for skeletal muscle nicotinic receptors. The action is the same on both parasympathetic and sympathetic ganglia. The initial response therefore often resembles simultaneous discharge of both the parasympathetic and the sympathetic nervous systems. In the case of the cardiovascular system, the effects of nicotine are chiefly sympathomimetic. Dramatic hypertension is produced by parenteral injection of nicotine; sympathetic tachycardia may alternate with a vagally mediated bradycardia. In the gastrointestinal and urinary tracts, the effects are largely parasympathomimetic: nausea, vomiting, diarrhea, and voiding of urine are commonly observed. Prolonged exposure may result in depolarizing blockade.

A second class of nicotinic sites consists of chemoreceptors on sensory nerve endings—especially certain chemosensitive nerve endings in the coronary arteries and the carotid and aortic bodies. Activation of these endings elicits complex medullary responses, including respiratory alterations and vagal discharge.

9. Neuromuscular junction–The nicotinic receptors on the neuromuscular endplate apparatus are similar but not identical to the receptors in the autonomic ganglia (Table 7–1). Both types respond to acetylcholine and nicotine. (However, as discussed in Chapter 8, the receptors differ in their structural requirements for nicotinic blocking drugs.) When a nicotinic agonist is applied directly (by iontophoresis or by intra-arterial injection), an immediate depolarization of the endplate results, caused by an increase in permeability to sodium and potassium ions. Depending on the synchronization of depolarization of endplates throughout the muscle, the contractile response will vary from disorganized fasciculations of independent motor units to a strong contraction of the entire muscle. Depolarizing nicotinic agents that are not rapidly hydrolyzed (like nicotine itself) cause rapid development of depolarization blockade; transmission blockade persists even when the membrane has repolarized (discussed further in Chapters 8 and 26). In the case of skeletal muscle, this block is manifested as flaccid paralysis.

II. BASIC PHARMACOLOGY OF THE INDIRECT-ACTING CHOLINOMIMETICS

The actions of acetylcholine released from autonomic and somatic motor nerves are terminated by enzymatic destruction of the molecule. Hydrolysis is accomplished by the action of acetylcholinesterase, a protein with a molecular weight of about 320,000, which is present in high concentrations in cholinergic

synapses. The indirect-acting cholinomimetics have their primary effect at the active site of this enzyme, though some also have direct actions at nicotinic receptors. By far the most important use (in terms of amount manufactured) of these chemicals is as insecticides; a few have therapeutic applications. The chief differences between members of the group are chemical and pharmacokinetic—their pharmacodynamic properties are almost identical.

Chemistry & Pharmacokinetics

A. Structure: The commonly used cholinesterase inhibitors fall into three chemical groups: (1) simple alcohols bearing a quaternary ammonium group, eg, edrophonium; (2) carbamic acid esters of alcohols bearing quaternary or tertiary ammonium groups (carbamates, eg, neostigmine); and (3) organic derivatives of phosphoric acid (organophosphates, eg, isoflurophate). Examples of the first two groups are shown in Figure 7–4. Edrophonium, neostigmine, and ambenonium are synthetic quaternary ammonium agents used in medicine. Physostigmine (eserine) is a naturally occurring tertiary amine of greater lipid solubility that is also used in therapeutics. Carbaryl (carbaril) is typical of a large group of carbamate insecticides designed for very high lipid solubility, so that absorption into the insect and distribution to its central nervous system is very rapid.

A few of the estimated 50,000 organophosphates are shown in Figure 7–5. Many of the organophosphates (echothiophate is an exception) are highly lipid-soluble liquids. Isoflurophate (diisopropylfluorophosphate, DFP) was one of the first organophosphates synthesized and is one of the best-studied. It is still available for clinical use but has been largely superseded by drugs like echothiophate. Echothiophate, a thiocholine derivative, is of clinical interest because it retains the very long duration of action of other organophosphates but is more stable in aqueous solution. Soman is an extremely potent "nerve gas." Parathion and malathion are thiophosphate insecticides that are inactive as such; they are converted to the phosphate derivatives in animals and plants. They are somewhat more stable than compounds like isoflurophate and soman, making them more suitable for use as insecticides.

B. Absorption, Distribution, and Metabolism: Absorption of the quaternary carbamates from the conjunctiva, skin, and lungs is predictably poor, since their permanent charge renders them relatively insoluble in lipids. Similarly, much larger doses are required for oral administration than for parenteral injection. Distribution into the central nervous system is negligible. Physostigmine, in contrast, is well absorbed from all sites and can be used topically in the eye (Table 7–4). It is distributed into the central nervous system and is more toxic than the more polar quaternary carbamates. However, even the nonpolar carbamates used as insecticides are poorly absorbed

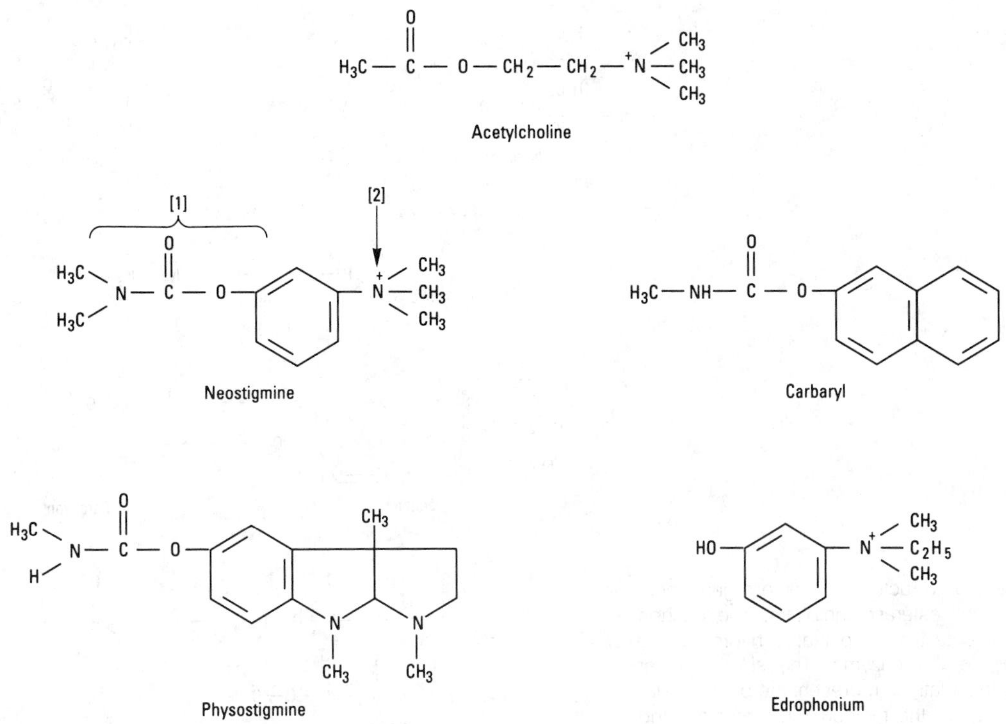

Figure 7–4. Cholinesterase inhibitors. Neostigmine exemplifies the typical compound that is an ester of carbamic acid (*[1]*) and a phenol bearing a quaternary ammonium group (*[2]*). Physostigmine, a naturally occurring carbamate, is a tertiary amine. Acetylcholine is shown in the same orientation (acid left, alcohol right) for reference. Edrophonium is not an ester but binds to the active site of the enzyme.

across the skin—the ratio of dermal:oral lethal doses for this group is much higher than the ratios for the organophosphate pesticides. The carbamates are relatively stable in aqueous solution but can be metabolized by nonspecific esterases in the body, as well as by cholinesterase. However, the duration of their effect is determined chiefly by the stability of the inhibitor-enzyme complex (see Mechanism of Action, below), not by metabolism or excretion.

The organophosphate cholinesterase inhibitors (except for echothiophate) are well absorbed from the skin, lung, gut, and conjunctiva—thereby making them dangerous to humans and highly effective as insecticides. They are relatively less stable than the carbamates when dissolved in water and thus have a limited half-life in the environment (as compared to the other major class of insecticides, the halogenated hydrocarbons, eg, DDT). Echothiophate is highly polar and more stable than most other organophosphates. It can be made up in aqueous solution for ophthalmic use and retains its activity for weeks.

The thiophosphate insecticides (parathion, malathion, and related compounds) are quite lipid-soluble and are rapidly absorbed by all routes. They must be activated in the body by conversion to the oxygen analogues (Figure 7–5), a process that occurs rapidly in both insects and vertebrates. Malathion and certain other organophosphate insecticides are also rapidly metabolized by other pathways to inactive products in birds and mammals, but not in insects; these agents are therefore considered safe enough for sale to the general public. Unfortunately, fish are not able to detoxify malathion, and significant numbers of fish have died from the heavy use of this agent on and near waterways. Parathion is not detoxified effectively in vertebrates; thus, it is considerably more dangerous than malathion to humans and livestock and is not available for general public use.

All of the organophosphates except echothiophate are fully distributed to all parts of the body, including the central nervous system. Poisoning with these agents therefore includes an important component of central nervous system toxicity.

Pharmacodynamics

A. Mechanism of Action: Acetylcholinesterase is the primary target of these drugs, but butyrylcholinesterase is also inhibited. Acetylcholinesterase is an extremely active enzyme. In the initial step, acetylcholine binds to the enzyme's active site and is hy-

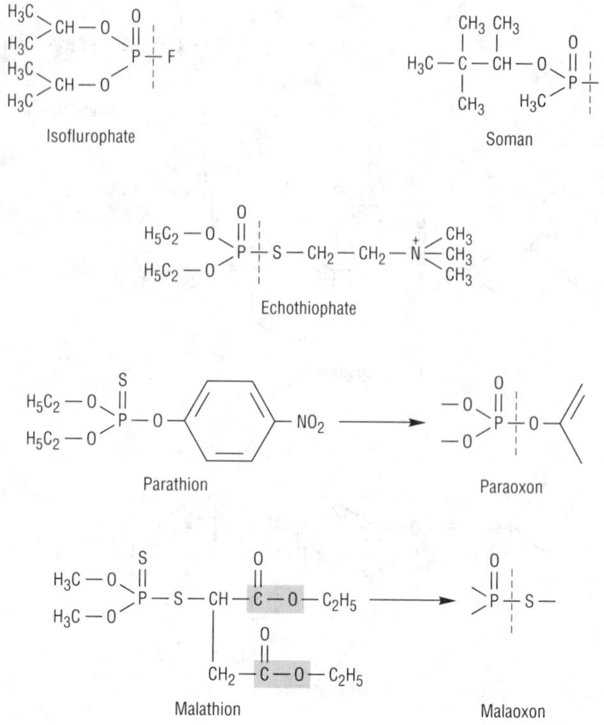

Figure 7–5. Structures of some organophosphate cholinesterase inhibitors. The dashed lines indicate the bond that is hydrolyzed in binding to the enzyme. The shaded ester bonds in malathion represent the points of detoxification of the molecule in mammals and birds.

drolyzed, yielding free choline and the *acetylated* enzyme. In the second step, the covalent acetylenzyme bond is split, with the addition of water. The entire process takes place in approximately 150 microseconds.

All of the cholinesterase inhibitors exert their effects by inhibiting acetylcholinesterase and thereby increasing the concentration of endogenous acetyl-

choline in the vicinity of cholinoceptors. However, the molecular details of their interaction with the enzyme vary according to the three chemical subgroups mentioned above.

The first group, of which edrophonium is the major example, consists of quaternary alcohols. These agents bind reversibly to the active site, thus preventing access of acetylcholine. The enzyme-inhibitor complex does not involve a covalent bond and is correspondingly short-lived (on the order of 2–10 minutes). The second group consists of carbamate esters, eg, neostigmine and physostigmine. These agents undergo a two-step hydrolysis sequence analogous to that described for acetylcholine. However, the covalent bond of the *carbamoylated* enzyme is considerably more resistant to the second (hydration) process, and this step is correspondingly prolonged (on the order of 30 minutes to 6 hours). The third group consists of the organophosphates. These agents also undergo initial binding and hydrolysis by the enzyme, resulting in a *phosphorylated* active site. The covalent phosphorus-enzyme bond is extremely stable and hydrolyzes in water at a very slow rate (hundreds of hours). After the initial binding-hydrolysis step, the phosphorylated enzyme complex may undergo a process called **aging.** This process apparently involves the breaking of one of the oxygen-phosphorus bonds of the inhibitor and results in further strength-

Table 7–4. Uses and duration of action of cholinesterase inhibitors used in therapeutics.

	Uses	Approximate Duration of Action
Alcohols		
Edrophonium	Myasthenia gravis, ileus, arrhythmias	5–15 minutes
Carbamates and related agents		
Neostigmine	Myasthenia gravis, ileus	½–2 hours
Pyridostigmine	Myasthenia gravis	3–6 hours
Physostigmine	Glaucoma	½–2 hours
Ambenonium	Myasthenia gravis	4–8 hours
Demecarium	Glaucoma	4–6 hours
Organophosphates		
Echothiophate	Glaucoma	100 hours

ening of the phosphorus-enzyme bond. The rate of aging varies with the particular organophosphate compound. If given before aging has occurred, strong nucleophiles like pralidoxime are able to split the phosphorus-enzyme bond and can be used as "cholinesterase regenerator" drugs for organophosphate insecticide poisoning (Chapter 8). Once aging has occurred, the enzyme-inhibitor complex is even more stable and is more difficult to split, even with oxime regenerator compounds.

Because of the marked differences in duration of action, the organophosphate inhibitors are sometimes referred to as "irreversible" cholinesterase inhibitors, and edrophonium and the carbamates are considered "reversible" inhibitors. In fact, the molecular mechanisms of action of the three groups do not support this simplistic description, but the terms are frequently used.

B. Organ System Effects: The most prominent pharmacologic effects of cholinesterase inhibitors are on the cardiovascular and gastrointestinal systems, the eye, and the skeletal muscle neuromuscular junction. Because the primary action is to amplify the action of endogenous acetylcholine, the effects are similar (but not always identical) to the effects of the direct-acting cholinomimetic agonists.

1. Central nervous system–In low concentrations, the lipid-soluble cholinesterase inhibitors cause diffuse activation of the EEG and a subjective alerting response. In higher concentrations, they cause generalized convulsions, which may be followed by coma and respiratory arrest.

2. Eye, respiratory tract, gastrointestinal tract, urinary tract–The effects of the cholinesterase inhibitors on these organ systems, all of which are well innervated by the parasympathetic nervous system, are qualitatively quite similar to the effects of the direct-acting cholinomimetics.

3. Cardiovascular system–The cholinesterase inhibitors can increase activation in both sympathetic and parasympathetic ganglia supplying the heart and at the acetylcholine receptors on neuroeffector cells (cardiac and vascular smooth muscles) that receive cholinergic innervation.

In the heart, the effects on the parasympathetic limb predominate. Thus, administration of cholinesterase inhibitors such as edrophonium, physostigmine, or neostigmine leads to effects on the heart that mimic the effects of vagal nerve activation. Heart rate decreases, conduction velocity through the atrioventricular junction diminishes, atrial contractility decreases, and cardiac output falls. The fall in cardiac output is attributable to bradycardia, decreased atrial contractility, and some reduction in ventricular contractility. The latter effect occurs as a result of prejunctional modulation of sympathetic activity (inhibition of norepinephrine release) as well as inhibition of postjunctional cellular sympathetic effects.

The effects of cholinesterase inhibitors on vascular smooth muscle and on blood pressure are less marked than the effects of direct-acting muscarinic agonists. This is because indirect-acting drugs can modify the tone of only those vessels that are innervated by cholinergic nerves and because the net effects on vascular tone may reflect activation of both the parasympathetic and sympathetic nervous systems. Since few vascular beds receive cholinergic innervation, the cholinomimetic effect at the smooth muscle effector tissue is minimal. Activation of sympathetic ganglia would tend to increase vascular resistance.

The *net* cardiovascular effects of moderate doses of cholinesterase inhibitors therefore consist of modest bradycardia, a fall in cardiac output, and no change or a modest fall in blood pressure. Large (toxic) doses of these drugs cause more marked bradycardia and hypotension.

4. Neuromuscular junction–The cholinesterase inhibitors have important therapeutic and toxic effects at the skeletal muscle neuromuscular junction. Low (therapeutic) concentrations moderately prolong and intensify the actions of physiologically released acetylcholine. This results in increased strength of contraction, especially in muscles weakened by curare-like neuromuscular blocking agents or by myasthenia gravis. At higher concentrations, the accumulation of acetylcholine may result in fibrillation of muscle fibers. Antidromic firing of the motor neuron may also occur, resulting in fasciculations that involve an entire motor unit. With marked inhibition of acetylcholinesterase, membrane depolarization becomes sustained and depolarizing neuromuscular blockade may ensue.

Some quaternary carbamate cholinesterase inhibitors, eg, neostigmine, have an additional *direct* nicotinic agonist effect at the neuromuscular junction. This may contribute to the effectiveness of these agents in the therapy of myasthenia.

III. CLINICAL PHARMACOLOGY OF THE CHOLINOMIMETICS

The major therapeutic uses of the cholinomimetics are for diseases of the eye (glaucoma, accommodative esotropia), the gastrointestinal and urinary tracts (postoperative atony, neurogenic bladder), the neuromuscular junction (myasthenia gravis, curare-induced neuromuscular paralysis), and the heart (certain atrial arrhythmias). Cholinesterase inhibitors are occasionally used in the treatment of atropine overdosage. **Tacrine** is a new drug with anticholinesterase and other cholinomimetic actions that is used for the treatment of Alzheimer's disease. It is discussed in Chapter 62.

Clinical Uses

A. The Eye: Glaucoma is a disease characterized by increased intraocular pressure. There are two types of acquired glaucoma: primary, which can be subdivided into angle-closure and open-angle types; and secondary, eg, caused by trauma, inflammation, or surgical procedures. Muscarinic stimulants and cholinesterase inhibitors can reduce intraocular pressure by facilitating outflow of aqueous humor and perhaps also by diminishing the rate of its secretion (see Figure 6–9). Of the direct agonists, methacholine, carbachol, and pilocarpine have been used for treatment of glaucoma. Among the cholinesterase inhibitors, physostigmine, demecarium, echothiophate, and isoflurophate have been extensively studied. Pilocarpine is by far the most commonly used.

Acute angle-closure glaucoma is a medical emergency that is usually treated initially with drugs but frequently requires surgery for permanent correction. Initial therapy often consists of a combination of a direct muscarinic agonist and a cholinesterase inhibitor (eg, pilocarpine plus physostigmine). Once the intraocular pressure is controlled and the danger of loss of vision is diminished, the patient can be prepared for corrective surgery (iridectomy). Open-angle glaucoma and some cases of secondary glaucoma are chronic diseases that are not amenable to surgical correction. Consequently, therapy is based on long-term pharmacologic management that relies greatly on the use of parasympathomimetics as well as epinephrine, the β-adrenoceptor-blocking drugs, and acetazolamide. Of the parasympathomimetics, the ones in current favor include pilocarpine (as drops, or a long-acting plastic film reservoir of drug placed in the conjunctival sac) and carbachol (drops). Longer-acting agents (demecarium, echothiophate) are reserved for cases in which control of the intraocular pressure cannot be achieved with other drugs. Other treatments for glaucoma are described in the box: Treatment of Glaucoma, Chapter 10.

Accommodative esotropia (strabismus caused by hypermetropic accommodative error) in young children is sometimes diagnosed and treated with cholinomimetic agonists. Dosage is similar to or higher than that used for glaucoma.

B. Gastrointestinal and Urinary Tracts: In clinical disorders that involve depression of smooth muscle activity *without obstruction,* cholinomimetic drugs with direct or indirect muscarinic effects may be helpful. These disorders include postoperative ileus (atony or paralysis of the stomach or bowel following surgical manipulation) and congenital megacolon. Urinary retention may occur postoperatively or postpartum or may be secondary to spinal cord injury or disease (neurogenic bladder). Cholinomimetics are also sometimes used to increase the tone of the lower esophageal sphincter in patients with reflux esophagitis. Of the choline esters, bethanechol is the most widely used for these disorders. For gastrointestinal problems, it is usually administered orally in a dose of 10–25 mg 3–4 times daily. In patients with urinary retention, bethanechol can be given subcutaneously in a dose of 5 mg and repeated in 30 minutes if necessary. Of the cholinesterase inhibitors, neostigmine is the most widely used for these applications. For paralytic ileus or atony of the urinary bladder, neostigmine can be given subcutaneously in a dose of 0.5–1 mg. If patients are able to take the drug by mouth, neostigmine can be given orally in a dose of 15 mg. In all of these situations, the clinician must be certain that there is no mechanical obstruction to outflow prior to using the cholinomimetic. Otherwise, the drug may exacerbate the problem and may even cause perforation as a result of increased pressure.

C. Neuromuscular Junction: Myasthenia gravis is a disease affecting skeletal muscle neuromuscular junctions. An autoimmune process causes production of antibodies that decrease the number of functional nicotinic receptors on the postjunctional endplates. The characteristic symptoms of weakness and fatigability that remit with rest and worsen with exercise may affect any skeletal muscle but most often involve the small muscles of the head, neck, and extremities. Frequent findings are ptosis, diplopia, difficulty in speaking and swallowing, and extremity weakness. Severe disease may affect all the muscles, including those necessary for respiration. The disease resembles the neuromuscular paralysis produced by d-tubocurarine and similar nondepolarizing neuromuscular blocking drugs (Chapter 26). Patients with myasthenia are exquisitely sensitive to the action of curariform drugs and other drugs that interfere with neuromuscular transmission, eg, aminoglycoside antibiotics.

Cholinesterase inhibitors—but not direct-acting acetylcholine receptor agonists—are extremely valuable in the therapy of myasthenia. (Some patients also respond to immunosuppressant therapy such as adrenocorticosteroids and cyclophosphamide.)

Edrophonium is sometimes used as a diagnostic test for myasthenia. A dose of 2 mg is injected intravenously after baseline measurements of muscle strength have been obtained. If no reaction occurs after 45 seconds, an additional 8 mg may be injected. Some clinicians divide the 8 mg dose into two doses of 3 and 5 mg given at 45-second intervals. If the patient has myasthenia gravis, an improvement in muscle strength that lasts about 5 minutes will usually be observed.

Edrophonium is also used to assess the adequacy of treatment with the longer-acting cholinesterase inhibitors in patients with documented myasthenia gravis. If excessive amounts of cholinesterase inhibitor have been used, patients may become paradoxically weak because of nicotinic depolarizing blockade of the motor endplate. These patients may also exhibit symptoms of excessive stimulation of muscarinic receptors (abdominal cramps, diarrhea, increased salivation, excessive bronchial secretions, miosis, bradycardia). Small doses of edrophonium (1–2 mg intravenously) will produce no relief or even worsen weakness if the patient is receiving excessive cholinesterase inhibitor therapy. On the other hand, if the patient improves with edrophonium, an increase in cholinesterase inhibitor dosage may be indicated. Clinical situations in which severe myasthenia (myasthenic crisis) must be distinguished from excessive drug therapy (cholinergic crisis) usually occur in very ill myasthenic patients and must be managed in hospital with adequate emergency and support systems (eg, mechanical ventilators) available.

Chronic long-term therapy of myasthenia gravis is usually accomplished with neostigmine, pyridostigmine, or ambenonium. The doses are titrated to optimum levels based on changes in muscle strength. These agents are relatively short-acting and therefore require frequent dosing (every 2–4 hours for neostigmine and every 3–6 hours for pyridostigmine and ambenonium; Table 7–4). Sustained-release preparations are available but should be used only at night and if needed. Longer-acting cholinesterase inhibitors such as the organophosphate agents are not used, because the dose requirement in this disease changes too rapidly to permit smooth control with long-acting drugs.

If muscarinic effects of such therapy are prominent, they can be controlled by the administration of antimuscarinic drugs such as atropine. Frequently, tolerance to the muscarinic effects of the cholinesterase inhibitors develops, so atropine treatment is not required.

Neuromuscular blockade is frequently produced as an adjunct to surgical anesthesia, using nondepolarizing neuromuscular relaxants such as curare, pancuronium, and newer agents. Following the surgical procedure, it is usually desirable to reverse this pharmacologic paralysis promptly. This can be easily accomplished with cholinesterase inhibitors; neostigmine and edrophonium are the drugs of choice. They are given intravenously or intramuscularly for prompt effect.

D. Heart: The short-acting cholinesterase inhibitor edrophonium was often used in the past for treatment of supraventricular tachyarrhythmias, particularly paroxysmal supraventricular tachycardia. By potentiating the effects of endogenous acetylcholine released from the vagus nerve endings in the atrioventricular node, atrioventricular conduction velocity was diminished, and the abnormal supraventricular tachyarrhythmia converted into normal sinus rhythm. In this application, edrophonium has been replaced by newer drugs (adenosine and calcium channel blockers).

E. Antimuscarinic Drug Intoxication: Atro-

pine intoxication is potentially lethal in children (Chapter 8) and may cause prolonged severe behavioral disturbances in adults. The tricyclic antidepressants, when taken in overdosage (often with suicidal intent), also cause severe muscarinic blockade (Chapter 29). Because the muscarinic receptor blockade produced by all these agents is competitive in nature, it can be overcome by increasing the amount of endogenous acetylcholine present at the neuroeffector junctions. Theoretically, a cholinesterase inhibitor could be used to reverse these effects. Physostigmine has been used for this application, because it enters the central nervous system and reverses the central as well as the peripheral signs of muscarinic blockade. However, as explained in the next chapter, physostigmine itself can produce dangerous central nervous system effects, and such therapy is therefore used only in patients with dangerous elevation of body temperature or very rapid supraventricular tachycardia.

Toxicity

The toxic potential of the cholinoceptor stimulants varies markedly depending on their absorption, access to the central nervous system, and metabolism.

A. Direct-Acting Muscarinic Stimulants: Drugs such as pilocarpine and the choline esters cause predictable signs of muscarinic excess when given in overdosage. These effects include nausea, vomiting, diarrhea, salivation, sweating, cutaneous vasodilation, and bronchial constriction. The effects are all blocked competitively by atropine and its congeners.

Certain mushrooms, especially those of the genus *Inocybe*, contain muscarinic alkaloids. Ingestion of these mushrooms causes typical signs of muscarinic excess within 15–30 minutes. Treatment is with atropine, 1–2 mg parenterally. (*Amanita muscaria*, the first source of muscarine, contains very low concentrations of the alkaloid.)

B. Direct-Acting Nicotinic Stimulants: Nicotine itself is the only common cause of this type of poisoning. The acute toxicity of the alkaloid is well-defined but much less important than the chronic effects associated with smoking. In addition to tobacco products, nicotine is also used in a number of insecticides.

1. Acute toxicity–The fatal dose of nicotine is approximately 40 mg, or 1 drop of the pure liquid. This is the amount of nicotine in two regular cigarettes. Fortunately, most of the nicotine in cigarettes is destroyed by burning or escapes via the "side-stream" smoke. Ingestion of nicotine insecticides and of tobacco by infants and children is usually followed by vomiting, limiting the amount of the alkaloid absorbed.

The toxic effects of a large dose of nicotine are simple extensions of the effects described previously. The most dangerous are (1) central stimulant actions, which cause convulsions and may progress to coma and respiratory arrest; (2) skeletal muscle endplate depolarization, which may lead to depolarization blockade and respiratory paralysis; and (3) hypertension and cardiac arrhythmias.

Treatment of acute nicotine poisoning is largely symptom-directed. Muscarinic excess resulting from parasympathetic ganglion stimulation can be controlled with atropine. Central stimulation is usually treated with parenteral anticonvulsants such as diazepam. Neuromuscular blockade is not responsive to pharmacologic treatment and may require mechanical respiration.

Fortunately, nicotine is metabolized and excreted relatively rapidly. Patients who survive the first 4 hours usually recover completely if hypoxia and brain damage have not occurred.

2. Chronic nicotine toxicity—The health costs of tobacco smoking to the smoker and its socioeconomic costs to the general public are still incompletely understood. However, the 1979 *Surgeon General's Report on Health Promotion and Disease Prevention* stated that "cigarette smoking is clearly the largest single preventable cause of illness and premature death in the United States." This statement was underscored by the 1983 and 1985 reports of the US Department of Health and Human Services, which estimated that up to 30% of the over 500,000 coronary heart disease deaths and 30% of the over 400,000 cancer deaths in the USA each year were attributable to smoking. Unfortunately, the fact that the most important of the tobacco-associated diseases are delayed in onset reduces the health incentive to stop smoking.

It is not known to what extent nicotine per se contributes to the well-documented adverse effects of chronic tobacco use. It appears highly probable that nicotine contributes to the increased risk of vascular disease and sudden coronary death associated with smoking. It is also probable that nicotine contributes to the high incidence of ulcer recurrences in smokers with peptic ulcer.

C. Cholinesterase Inhibitors: The acute toxic effects of the cholinesterase inhibitors, like those of the direct-acting agents, are direct extensions of their pharmacologic actions. The major source of such intoxications is pesticide use in agriculture and in the home. Approximately 100 organophosphate and 20 carbamate cholinesterase inhibitors are available in pesticides and veterinary vermifuges used in the USA.

Acute intoxication must be recognized and treated promptly in patients with heavy exposure. The dominant initial signs are those of muscarinic excess: miosis, salivation, sweating, bronchial constriction, vomiting, and diarrhea. Central nervous system involvement usually follows rapidly, accompanied by peripheral nicotinic effects, especially depolarizing neuromuscular blockade. Therapy always includes (1) maintenance of vital signs—respiration in particular may be impaired; (2) decontamination to prevent further absorption—this may require removal of all clothing and washing of the skin in cases of exposure to dusts and sprays; and (3) atropine parenterally in large doses, given as often as required to control signs of muscarinic excess. Therapy often also includes treatment with pralidoxime as described in Chapter 8.

Chronic exposure to certain organophosphate compounds, including some organophosphate cholinesterase inhibitors, causes neuropathy associated with demyelination of axons. Triorthocresylphosphate, an additive in lubricating oils, is the prototype agent of this class. The effects are not caused by cholinesterase inhibition.

PREPARATIONS AVAILABLE

Direct-Acting Cholinomimetics
 Acetylcholine (Miochol)
  Ophthalmic: 1:100 (10 mg/mL) intraocular solution
 Bethanechol (generic, Urecholine)
  Oral: 5, 10, 25, 50 mg tablets
  Parenteral: 5 mg/mL for SC injection
 Carbachol
  Ophthalmic (topical, Isopto Carbachol): 0.75, 1.5, 2.25, 3% drops
  Ophthalmic (intraocular, Miostat):0.01% solution
 Pilocarpine (generic, Isopto Carpine)
  Ophthalmic (topical): 0.25, 0.5, 1, 2, 3, 4, 6, 8, 10% solutions, 4% gel
  Ophthalmic sustained-release inserts (Ocusert Pilo-20, Ocusert Pilo-40): release 20 and 40 mcg pilocarpine/h for 1 week, respectively

Cholinesterase Inhibitors
 Ambenonium (Mytelase)
  Oral: 10 mg tablets
 Demecarium (Humorsol)
  Ophthalmic: 0.125, 0.25% drops
 Echothiophate (Phospholine)
  Ophthalmic: powder to reconstitute for 0.03, 0.06, 0.125, 0.25 % drops
 Edrophonium (generic, Tensilon)
  Parenteral: 10 mg/mL for IM or IV injection
 Isoflurophate (Floropryl)
  Ophthalmic: 0.025% ointment
 Neostigmine (generic, Prostigmin)
  Oral: 15 mg tablets
  Parenteral: 1:1000 in 10 mL; 1:2000, 1:4000 in 1 mL
 Physostigmine, eserine (generic)

Ophthalmic: 0.25% ointment; 0.25, 0.5% drops
Parenteral: 1 mg/mL for IM or slow IV injection
Pyridostigmine (Mestinon)

Oral: 60 mg tablets; 180 mg sustained-release tablets; 15 mg/mL syrup
Parenteral: 5 mg/mL for IM or slow IV injection

REFERENCES

Abou-Donia MB, Lapadula DM: Mechanisms of organophosphorus ester-induced delayed neurotoxicity: Type I and type II. Annu Rev Pharmacol 1990;30:405.

Aquilonius S-M, Hartvig P: Clinical pharmacology of cholinesterase inhibitors. Clin Pharmacokinet 1986;11:236.

Barnes PJ, Minette P, Maclagan J: Muscarinic receptor subtypes in airways. Trends Pharm Sci 1988;9:412.

Berridge MJ, Irvine RF: Inositol phosphates and cell signalling. Nature 1989;341:197.

Bognar IT, Wesner MT, Fuder H: Muscarine receptor types mediating autoinhibition of acetylcholine release and sphincter contraction in the guinea-pig iris. Naunyn Schmiedebergs Arch Pharmacol 1990;341:22.

Bonner TI et al: Identification of a family of muscarinic acetylcholine receptor genes. Science 1987;237:527.

Brown JH (editor): *The Muscarinic Receptors*. Humana Press, 1989.

Buckley NJ et al: Antagonist binding properties of five cloned muscarinic receptors expressed in CHO-K1 cells. Mol Pharmacol 1989;35:469.

Cady B: Cost of smoking. (Letter.) N Engl J Med 1983;308:1105.

Cerbai E, Klockner U, Isenberg G: The α subunit of the GTP binding protein activates muscarinic potassium channels of the atrium. Science 1988;240:1782.

Deighton NM et al: Muscarinic cholinoceptors in the human heart: Demonstration, subclassification, and distribution. Naunyn Schmiedebergs Arch Pharmacol 1990;341:14.

DiFrancesco D, Tromba C: Muscarinic control of the hyperpolarization-activated current (i_f) in rabbit sino-atrial node myocytes. J Physiol 1988;405:493.

Drachman DH: Myasthenia gravis. (Two parts.) N Engl J Med 1978;298:136, 186.

Eglen RM, Whiting RL: Heterogeneity of vascular muscarinic receptors. J Auton Pharmacol 1990;19:233.

Fielding JE: Smoking: Health effects and control. (Two parts.) N Engl J Med 1985;313:491, 555.

Freedman SB, Beer MS, Harley EA: Muscarinic M_1, M_2 receptor binding: Relationship with functional efficacy. Europ J Pharmacol 1988;156:133.

Furchgott RF et al: Endothelial cells as mediators of vasodilation of arteries. J Cardiovasc Pharmacol 1984;6:S336.

Goyal RK: Muscarinic receptor subtypes: Physiology and clinical implications. N Engl J Med 1989;321:1022.

Grana E et al: Determination of dissociation constants and relative efficacies of some potent muscarinic agonists at postjunctional muscarinic receptors. Naunyn Schmiedebergs Arch Pharmacol 1987;335:8.

Havener WH: *Ocular Pharmacology,* 5th ed. Mosby, 1983.

Hobbiger F: Pharmacology of anticholinesterase drugs. In: *Neuromuscular Junction*—Vol 42 of *Handbook of Experimental Pharmacology.* Zaimis E (editor). Springer Verlag, 1976.

Honkanen RE, Howard EF, Abdel-Latif AA: M3-muscarinic receptor subtype predominates in the bovine sphincter smooth muscle and ciliary processes. Invest Ophthalmol Vis Sci 1990;31:590.

Levy MN, Schwartz PJ (editors): *Vagal Control of the Heart.* Futura, 1993.

Lindstrom J et al: Structural and functional heterogeneity of nicotinic receptors. In: *The Biology of Nicotine Dependence.* Ciba Symposium 152. Bock G, Marsh J (editors). Wiley, 1990.

Marrion NV et al: Muscarinic suppression of the M-current in the rat sympathetic ganglion is mediated by receptors of the M_1-subtype. Br J Pharmacol 1989;98:557.

Molitor H: A comparative study of the effects of five choline compounds used in therapeutics: Acetylcholine chloride, acetyl-beta-methylcholine chloride, carbaminoyl choline, ethyl ether beta-methylcholine chloride, carbaminoyl beta-methylcholine chloride. J Pharmacol Exp Ther 1936;58:337.

Nathanson NM: Molecular properties of the muscarinic acetylcholine receptor. Annu Rev Neurosci 1987;10:195.

Noronha-Blob L et al: Muscarinic receptors: Relationships among phosphoinositide breakdown, adenylate cyclase inhibition, in vitro detrusor muscle contraction, and in vivo cystometrogram studies in guinea pig bladder. J Pharmacol Exp Therap 1989;249:843.

Pfeiffer A et al: Muscarinic receptors mediating acid secretion in isolated rat gastric mucosa cells are of M3 type. Gastroenterology 1990;98:218.

Raftery MA et al: Acetylcholine receptor: Complex of homologous subunits. Science 1980;208:1454.

Rand MJ: Neuropharmacological effects of nicotine in relation to cholinergic mechanisms. Prog Brain Res 1989;79:3.

Smoking and cardiovascular disease. MMWR Morb Mortal Wkly Rep 1984;32:677.

Watanabe AM et al: Cardiac autonomic receptors: Recent concepts from radiolabeled ligand-binding studies. Circ Res 1982;50:161.

8

Cholinoceptor-Blocking Drugs

Bertram G. Katzung, MD, PhD

Just as cholinoceptor agonists are divided into muscarinic and nicotinic subgroups on the basis of their specific receptor affinities, so the antagonists acting on these receptors fall into two major families: the **antimuscarinic** and **antinicotinic** agents. The nicotinic receptor-blocking drugs consist of ganglion-blockers and neuromuscular junction blockers. The ganglion-blocking drugs have very limited use and are discussed at the end of this chapter. The neuromuscular blockers are discussed in Chapter 26. The major emphasis in this chapter is on drugs that block muscarinic cholinoceptors.

As noted in Chapters 6 and 7, several subtypes of muscarinic receptors have been described, primarily on the basis of data from ligand-binding and cDNA-cloning experiments. A standard terminology for these subtypes is now coming into common use, and good evidence, based mostly on selective agonists and antagonists, suggests that functional differences do exist between at least three of these subtypes.

As suggested in Chapter 6, the M_1 receptor subtype appears to be located on central nervous system neurons, sympathetic postganglionic cell bodies, and many presynaptic sites. M_3 receptors are most common on effector cell membranes, especially glandular and smooth muscle cells. M_2 receptors are located in the myocardium, smooth muscle organs, and some neuronal sites.

I. BASIC PHARMACOLOGY OF THE MUSCARINIC RECEPTOR-BLOCKING DRUGS

Because the effects of parasympathetic autonomic discharge can be blocked by muscarinic antagonists, they are often called parasympatholytic drugs. However, they do not "lyse" parasympathetic nerves, and they have some effects that are not predictable from block of the parasympathetic nervous system. For these reasons, the term "antimuscarinic" is preferable.

Naturally occurring compounds with antimuscarinic effects have been known and used for millennia as medicines, poisons, and cosmetics. The prototype of these drugs is atropine. Many similar plant alkaloids are known, and hundreds of synthetic antimuscarinic compounds have been prepared.

Chemistry & Pharmacokinetics

A. Source and Chemistry: Atropine and its naturally occurring congeners are tertiary ammonium alkaloid esters of tropic acid (Figure 8–1).

Atropine (hyoscyamine) is found in the plant *Atropa belladonna,* or deadly nightshade, and in *Datura stramonium,* also known as jimsonweed (Jamestown weed) or thorn apple. **Scopolamine** (hyoscine) occurs in *Hyoscyamus niger*, or henbane. Scopolamine occurs as the $l(-)$ stereoisomer in the plant. Naturally occurring atropine is $l(-)$-hyoscyamine, but the compound readily racemizes, so the commercial material is racemic d,l-hyoscyamine. The $l(-)$ isomers of both alkaloids are at least 100 times more potent than the $d(+)$ isomers.

Semisynthetic tertiary ammonium analogues can be produced by esterifying a natural base, eg, tropine, the base in atropine, with different acids. Thus, homatropine is the mandelic acid ester of tropine. A variety of fully synthetic molecules have antimuscarinic effects.

The tertiary members of these classes (Figure 8–2) are often used for their effects in the eye or the central nervous system. Many antihistaminic (Chapter 16), antipsychotic (Chapter 28), and antidepressant (Chapter 29) drugs have similar structures and, predictably, significant antimuscarinic effects.

Quaternary ammonium antimuscarinic agents have been developed to produce more peripheral effect with reduced central nervous system effects. These drugs include both semisynthetic and synthetic molecules (Figure 8–2).

B. Absorption: The natural alkaloids and most tertiary antimuscarinic drugs are well absorbed from the gut and across the conjunctival membrane. When applied in a suitable vehicle, some, eg, scopolamine, are even absorbed across the skin (transdermal route). In contrast, only 10–30% of a dose of a quaternary

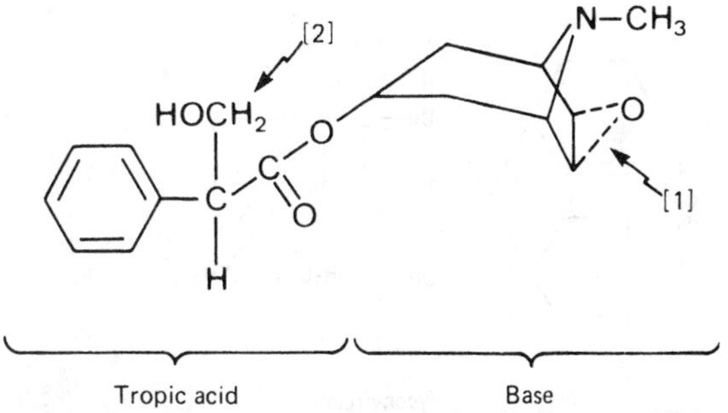

Figure 8–1. The structure of atropine (oxygen at *[1]* is missing) or scopolamine (oxygen present). In homatropine, the hydroxymethyl at *[2]* is replaced by a hydroxyl group, and the oxygen at *[1]* is absent.

antimuscarinic drug is absorbed after oral administration, reflecting the decreased lipid solubility of the charged molecule.

C. Distribution: Atropine and the other tertiary agents are widely distributed after absorption. Significant levels are achieved in the central nervous system within 30 minutes to 1 hour and may limit the dose tolerated when the drug is taken for its peripheral effects. Scopolamine is particularly rapidly and fully distributed into the central nervous system and has greater effects there than most other antimuscarinic drugs. In contrast, the quaternary derivatives are poorly taken up by the brain and therefore are relatively free—at low doses—of these central nervous system effects.

D. Metabolism and Excretion: Atropine disappears rapidly from the blood after administration, with a half-life of 2 hours. About 60% of the dose is excreted unchanged in the urine. Most of the rest appears in the urine as hydrolysis and conjugation products. The effect of the drug on parasympathetic function declines rapidly in all organs except the eye. Effects on the iris and ciliary muscle persist for 72 hours or longer.

Certain species, notably rabbits, have a specific enzyme—atropine esterase—that confers almost complete protection against the toxic effects of atropine by rapidly metabolizing the drug.

Pharmacodynamics

A. Mechanism of Action: Atropine causes reversible (surmountable) blockade of the actions of cholinomimetics at muscarinic receptors—ie, blockade by a small dose of atropine can be overcome by a larger concentration of acetylcholine or equivalent muscarinic agonist. This suggests competition for a common binding site. The result of binding to the muscarinic receptor is to prevent the actions described in Chapter 7 such as the release of IP_3 and the inhibition of adenylyl cyclase that are brought about by acetylcholine and other muscarinic agonists.

The effectiveness of antimuscarinic drugs varies with the tissue under study and with the source of agonist. The tissues most sensitive to atropine are the salivary, bronchial, and sweat glands. Secretion of acid by the gastric parietal cells is much less sensitive. Smooth muscle autonomic effectors and the heart are intermediate in responsiveness. In most tissues, antimuscarinic agents are more effective in blocking exogenously administered cholinoceptor agonists than endogenously released acetylcholine.

Atropine is highly selective for muscarinic receptors. Its potency at nicotinic receptors is much lower than at muscarinic receptors; in clinical use, actions at nonmuscarinic receptors are generally undetectable.

Atropine does not distinguish between the M_1, M_2, and M_3 subgroups of muscarinic receptors. In contrast, other antimuscarinic drugs have been found that do have moderate selectively for one or another of these subgroups (Table 8–1). Most synthetic antimuscarinic drugs are considerably less specific than atropine in interactions with nonmuscarinic receptors. For example, some quaternary ammonium antimuscarinic agents have significant ganglion-blocking actions, and others are potent histamine receptor blockers. The antimuscarinic effects of other groups, eg, antihistaminic and antidepressant drugs, have been mentioned. Their relative selectivity for muscarinic receptor subtypes has not been defined.

B. Organ System Effects:

1. Central nervous system–In the doses usually used clinically, atropine has mild stimulant effects on the central nervous system, especially the parasympathetic medullary centers, and a slower, longer-lasting sedative effect on the brain. The central vagal stimulant effect is frequently sufficient to cause bradycardia, which is later supplanted by tachycardia as the drug's antimuscarinic effects at the sinoatrial node become manifest. Scopolamine has more marked central effects, producing drowsiness when given in recommended dosages and amnesia in sensitive individuals. In toxic doses, atropine and scopolamine cause excitement, agitation, hallucinations, and coma.

The tremor of Parkinson's disease is reduced by centrally acting antimuscarinic drugs, and atropine—in the form of belladonna extract—was one of the first drugs used in the therapy of this disease. As discussed in Chapter 27, parkinsonian tremor and rigidity seem to result from a *relative* excess of cholinergic activity because of a deficiency of dopaminergic activity in the basal ganglia-striatal system. Thus, the combination of an antimuscarinic agent with a dopamine precursor drug (levodopa) may provide a more effective therapeutic approach than either drug alone.

Vestibular disturbances, especially motion sickness, appear to involve muscarinic cholinergic transmission. Scopolamine is often effective in preventing or reversing these disturbances.

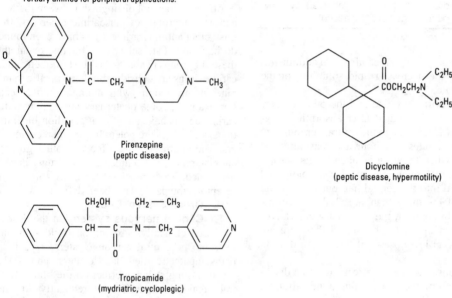

Quaternary amines for gastrointestinal applications (peptic disease, hypermotility):

Propantheline

Glycopyrrolate

Tertiary amines for peripheral applications:

Pirenzepine
(peptic disease)

Dicyclomine
(peptic disease, hypermotility)

Tropicamide
(mydriatric, cycloplegic)

Quaternary amine for use in asthma:

Ipratropium

Tertiary amine for Parkinson's disease:

Benztropine

Figure 8–2. Structures of some semisynthetic and synthetic antimuscarinic drugs.

2. Eye–The pupillary constrictor muscle (Figure 6–9) is dependent on muscarinic cholinoceptor activation. This activation is effectively blocked by topical atropine and other tertiary antimuscarinic drugs and results in unopposed sympathetic dilator activity and **mydriasis** (Figure 8–3). Dilated pupils were apparently considered cosmetically desirable during the Renaissance and account for the name belladonna (Italian, "beautiful lady") applied to the plant and its active extract because of the use of the extract as eye drops during that time.

The second important ocular effect of antimuscarinic drugs is paralysis of the ciliary muscle, or **cycloplegia.** The result of cycloplegia is loss of the ability to accommodate; the fully atropinized eye cannot focus for near vision (Figure 8–3).

Table 8–1. Muscarinic receptor subgroups and their antagonists.
(Acronyms identify selective antagonists used in research studies only.)

Property	Subgroup		
	M_1	M_2	M_3
Primary locations	Nerves	Heart, nerves, smooth muscle	Glands, smooth muscle, endothelium
Dominant effector system	↑IP$_3$, DAG	↓cAMP, ↑K channel current	↑IP$_3$, DAG
Antagonists	Pirenzepine, telenzepine dicyclomine,[2] trihexyphenidyl[3]	Gallamine,[1] methoctramine, AF-DX 116	4-DAMP, HHSD
Approximate dissociation constant[4]			
Atropine	1	1	1
Pirenzepine	10	50	200
AF-DX 116	800	100	3000
HHSD	40	200	2

[1]In clinical use as a neuromuscular blocking agent.
[2]In clinical use as an intestinal antispasmodic agent.
[3]In clinical use in the treatment of Parkinson's disease.
[4]Relative to atropine. Smaller numbers indicate higher affinity.

Key:

AF-DX 116	= 11-({2-[(Diethylamino)methyl]-1-piperidinyl}acetyl)-5,11-dihydro-6*H*-pyrido-[2,3-*b*](1,4)benzodiazepin-6-one
DAG	= Diacylglycerol
4-DAMP	= 4-Diphenylacetoxy-*N*-methylpiperidine
HHSD	= Hexahydrosiladifenidol

Both mydriasis and cycloplegia are useful in ophthalmology. They are also potentially hazardous, since acute glaucoma may be precipitated in patients with a narrow anterior chamber angle.

A third ocular effect of antimuscarinic drugs is reduction of lacrimal secretion. Patients occasionally complain of dry or "sandy" eyes when receiving large doses of antimuscarinic drugs.

3. Cardiovascular system–The atria of the heart are heavily innervated by parasympathetic (vagal) nerve fibers, and the sinoatrial node is therefore sensitive to muscarinic receptor blockade. The effect in the isolated, innervated, and spontaneously beating heart is a clear blockade of vagal slowing and a relative tachycardia. In patients, tachycardia is seen consistently when moderate to high therapeutic doses are given. However, as noted above, lower doses cause central parasympathetic *stimulation* and often result in initial bradycardia before the effects of peripheral vagal block become manifest (Figure 8–4). The same mechanisms operate in the control of atrioventricular node function; in the presence of high vagal tone, administration of atropine can significantly reduce the PR interval of the ECG by blocking muscarinic receptors in the heart. Muscarinic effects on atrial muscle are similarly blocked, but except in atrial flutter and fibrillation these effects are of no clinical significance. The ventricles, because of a lesser degree of muscarinic control, are less affected by antimuscarinic drugs at therapeutic levels. In toxic concentrations, the drugs can cause intraventricular conduction block by an unknown mechanism.

The blood vessels receive little or no direct innervation from the parasympathetic nervous system. However, as noted in Chapter 6, sympathetic cholinergic nerves cause vasodilation in the skeletal muscle vascular bed. This vasodilation can be blocked by atropine. Furthermore, almost all vessels contain uninnervated muscarinic receptors that mediate vasodilation (Chapter 7). These receptors, which are located on endothelial cells, release endothelium-derived relaxing factor (EDRF) in response to circulating direct-acting muscarinic agonists, and are readily blocked by antimuscarinic drugs. At toxic doses, and in a few patients at normal doses, antimuscarinic agents cause cutaneous vasodilation, especially in the blush area. The mechanism is unknown.

The net cardiovascular effects of atropine in patients with normal hemodynamics are not dramatic: tachycardia may occur, but there is little effect on blood pressure. However, the effects of administered direct-acting muscarinic stimulants are easily prevented.

4. Respiratory system–Both smooth muscle and secretory glands of the airway receive vagal innervation and contain muscarinic receptors. Even in normal individuals, some bronchodilation and reduction of secretion can be measured after administration of atropine. The effect is much more dramatic in patients with airway disease, although the antimus-

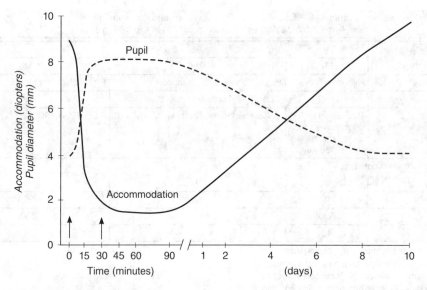

Figure 8–3. Effects of topical scopolamine drops on pupil diameter (mm) and accommodation (diopters) in the normal human eye. One drop of 0.5% solution of drug was applied at zero time, and a second drop was administered at 30 minutes *(arrows)*. The responses of 42 eyes were averaged. Note the extremely slow recovery. (Redrawn from Marron J: Cycloplegia and mydriasis by use of atropine, scopolamine, and homatropine-paredrine. Arch Ophthal 1940;23:340.)

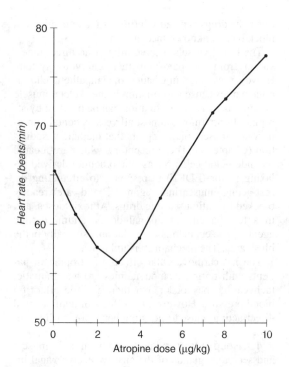

Figure 8–4. Dose-response curve for the effects of atropine on heart rate in eight healthy human subjects. Intravenous doses were given cumulatively. Lower doses slow the rate owing to stimulation of the central vagal nucleus. (Data from Porter TR et al: J Clin Invest 1990;85:1362.)

carinic drugs are not as useful as the beta-adrenoceptor stimulants in the treatment of asthma (Chapter 19). Nevertheless, the antimuscarinic agents are valuable in some patients with asthma or chronic obstructive pulmonary disease (COPD). In addition, they are frequently used prior to administration of inhalant anesthetics to reduce the accumulation of secretions in the trachea and the possibility of laryngospasm.

5. Gastrointestinal tract–Blockade of muscarinic receptors has dramatic effects on motility and some of the secretory functions of the gut. However, since local hormones and noncholinergic neurons also modulate gastrointestinal function, even complete muscarinic block cannot totally abolish activity in this organ system. As in other tissues, exogenously administered muscarinic stimulants are more effectively blocked than the effects of parasympathetic (vagal) nerve activity.

The effects of antimuscarinic drugs on salivary secretion are marked; dry mouth is a frequent symptom in patients taking antimuscarinic drugs for Parkinson's disease or peptic ulcer (Figure 8–5). Gastric secretion is blocked less effectively: the volume and amount of acid, pepsin, and mucin are all reduced, but large doses of atropine may be required. Basal secretion is blocked more effectively than that stimulated by food, nicotine, or alcohol. Pirenzepine and a more potent analogue, telenzepine, appear to reduce gastric acid secretion with fewer adverse effects than atropine and other less selective agents. This may result from a selective blockade of presynaptic excitatory muscarinic receptors on vagal nerve endings as suggested by their high ratio of M_1 to M_3 affinity (Table

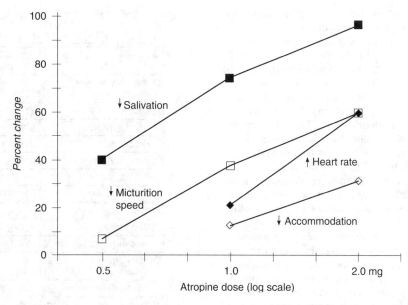

Figure 8–5. Effects of subcutaneous injection of atropine on salivation, speed of micturition (voiding), heart rate, and accommodation in normal adults. Note that salivation is the most sensitive of these variables, accommodation the least. (Data from Herxheimer A: Br J Pharmacol 1958;13:184.)

8–1), but this conclusion is not universally accepted. Pirenzepine and telenzepine are investigational in the USA. Pancreatic and intestinal secretion are little affected by atropine; these processes are primarily under hormonal rather than vagal control.

Motility of gastrointestinal smooth muscle is affected from the stomach to the colon. In general, the walls of the viscera are relaxed, and both tone and propulsive movements are diminished. Therefore, gastric emptying time is prolonged, and intestinal transit time is lengthened. Diarrhea due to overdosage with parasympathomimetic agents is readily eliminated, and even that caused by nonautonomic agents can usually be temporarily controlled. However, intestinal "paralysis" induced by antimuscarinic drugs is temporary; local mechanisms within the enteric nervous system (Chapter 6) will usually reestablish at least some peristalsis after 1–3 days of antimuscarinic drug therapy.

Several of the synthetic antimuscarinic agents are said to have "spasmolytic" activity in excess of their antimuscarinic effects. This is the result of selection of agents, through screening tests in isolated tissue, that relax the gut in the absence as well as the presence of cholinoceptor stimulants.

6. Genitourinary tract–Smooth muscle of the ureters and bladder wall is relaxed and voiding is slowed (Figure 8–5) by the antimuscarinic action of atropine and its analogues. This action is useful in the treatment of spasm induced by mild inflammatory conditions, but it also poses a hazard of precipitating urinary retention in elderly men, who may have pro-

static hypertrophy (see Clinical Pharmacology). The antimuscarinic drugs have no significant effect on the uterus.

7. Sweat glands–Thermoregulatory sweating is suppressed by atropine. The muscarinic receptors on eccrine sweat glands are innervated by sympathetic cholinergic fibers and are readily accessible to antimuscarinic drugs. In adults, body temperature is elevated by this effect only if large doses are administered, but in infants and children even ordinary doses may cause "atropine fever."

II. CLINICAL PHARMACOLOGY OF THE MUSCARINIC RECEPTOR-BLOCKING DRUGS

Therapeutic Applications

A. Central Nervous System Disorders:

1. Parkinson's disease–As described in Chapter 27, the treatment of Parkinson's disease is often an exercise in polypharmacy, since no single agent is fully effective over the (usually prolonged) course of the disease. Most of the large number of antimuscarinic drugs promoted for this application (Table 27–1) were developed before levodopa became available. Their use is accompanied by all of the adverse effects described below, but the drugs remain useful as adjunctive therapy in some patients.

2. Motion sickness–Certain vestibular disorders respond to antimuscarinic drugs (and to antihistaminic agents with antimuscarinic effects). Scopolamine is one of the oldest remedies for seasickness and is still as effective as any more recently introduced agent. It can be given by injection, by mouth, or by means of a transdermal patch. The patch formulation results in significant blood levels over 24–48 hours. Unfortunately, useful doses by any route usually cause significant sedation and dry mouth.

B. Ophthalmologic Disorders: Accurate measurement of refractive error in uncooperative patients, eg, young children, requires ciliary paralysis. In addition, ophthalmoscopic examination of the retina is greatly facilitated by mydriasis. Therefore, antimuscarinic agents, administered topically as eye drops or in ointment form, are extremely helpful in doing a complete examination. For adults and older children, the shorter-acting drugs are preferred (Table 8–2). For younger children, the greater efficacy of atropine is sometimes necessary, but the possibility of antimuscarinic poisoning is correspondingly increased. Loss of drug from the conjunctival sac via the nasolacrimal duct into the nasopharynx can be diminished by the use of the ointment form in preference to drops.

Antimuscarinic drugs should never be used for mydriasis unless cycloplegia or prolonged action is required. Alpha-adrenoceptor stimulant drugs, eg, phenylephrine, produce a short-lasting mydriasis that is usually sufficient for funduscopic examination (Chapter 9).

A second ophthalmologic use is to prevent synechia (adhesion) formation in uveitis and iritis. The longer-lasting preparations, especially homatropine, are valuable for this indication.

C. Gastrointestinal Disorders: The antimuscarinic drugs were mainly used to treat peptic ulcer until the introduction of the H_2 histamine receptor-blocking agents (see Chapter 64). Antimuscarinic agents are now rarely used for this indication, though the development of selective M_1 blockers like pirenzepine may reverse the trend. When the older agents are used for this application, quaternary antimuscarinic drugs are preferred; large doses (Table 8–3)

Table 8–3. Antimuscarinic drugs used in gastrointestinal and genitourinary conditions.

Drug	Usual Dose (mg)
Quaternary amines	
Anisotropine	50 tid
Clidinium	2.5 tid–qid
Glycopyrrolate	1 bid–tid
Hexocyclium	25 qid
Isopropamide	5 bid
Mepenzolate	25–50 qid
Methantheline	50–100 qid
Methscopolamine	2.5 qid
Oxyphenonium	5–10 qid
Propantheline	15 qid
Tertiary amines	
Atropine	0.4 tid–qid
Dicyclomine	10–20 qid
Oxybutynin	5 tid
Oxyphencyclimine	10 bid
Scopolamine	0.4 tid
Tridihexethyl	25–50 tid–qid

are required to significantly reduce gastric acid secretion. Patients who receive this treatment will have blurred vision, dry mouth, and urinary hesitancy. In the case of *gastric* peptic ulcer, antimuscarinic drugs may be contraindicated because they can slow gastric emptying and prolong the exposure of the ulcer bed to acid.

In the treatment of common traveler's diarrhea and other mild or self-limited conditions of hypermotility, the antimuscarinic agents can provide some relief. They are often combined with an opioid antidiarrheal drug, an extremely effective therapy. In this combination, however, the very low dosage of the antimuscarinic drug functions primarily to discourage abuse of the opioid agent. The classic combination of atropine with diphenoxylate, a nonanalgesic congener of meperidine, is available under many names (eg, Lomotil) in both tablet and liquid form (Chapter 64).

D. Cardiovascular Disorders: Marked vagal discharge sometimes accompanies the pain of myocardial infarction and may result in sufficient depression of sinoatrial or atrioventricular node function to impair cardiac output. Parenteral atropine or a similar antimuscarinic drug is appropriate therapy in this situation. Rare individuals without other detectable cardiac disease have hyperactive carotid sinus reflexes and may experience faintness or even syncope as a result of vagal discharge in response to pressure on the neck, eg, from a tight collar. Such individuals may benefit from the judicious use of atropine or a related antimuscarinic agent.

Table 8–2. Antimuscarinic drugs used in ophthalmology.

Drug	Duration of Mydriasis (days)	Duration of Cycloplegia (days)
Atropine	7–10	7–12
Scopolamine	3–7	3–7
Homatropine	1–3	1–3
Cyclopentolate	1	1/4–1
Tropicamide	1/4	1/4

E. Respiratory Disorders: The use of atropine became part of routine preoperative medication when anesthetics such as ether were used, because these irritant anesthetics caused a marked increase in airway secretions and were associated with frequent episodes of laryngospasm. These hazardous effects could be prevented by preanesthetic injection of atropine or scopolamine. The latter drug also produced significant amnesia for the events associated with surgery and obstetric delivery, a side effect that was considered desirable. On the other hand, urinary retention and intestinal hypomotility following surgery could be significantly exacerbated by the use of the antimuscarinic drug. With the advent of effective and nonirritant inhalational anesthetics such as halothane and enflurane, it would seem that a major reason for the routine use of antimuscarinic drugs as preanesthetic medication has been eliminated.

Inhalation of smoke from burning leaves of *Datura stramonium* has been used for centuries as a remedy for bronchial asthma. "Asthmador" cigarettes containing *D stramonium* were available without prescription for this application until recently. As described in Chapter 19, the hyperactive neural bronchoconstrictor reflex present in most individuals with asthma is mediated by the vagus, acting on muscarinic receptors on bronchial smooth muscle cells. **Ipratropium** (Figure 8–2), a synthetic analogue of atropine, is used as an inhalational drug in asthma. The aerosol route of administration provides the advantages of maximal concentration at the bronchial target tissue with reduced systemic effects. This application is discussed in greater detail in Chapter 19.

F. Cholinergic Poisoning: Severe cholinergic excess is an important medical emergency, especially in rural communities where the use of cholinesterase inhibitor insecticides is common, and in cultures where wild mushrooms are commonly eaten. The possible use of these agents as chemical warfare "nerve gases" also requires an awareness of the methods for treating acute poisoning.

1. Antimuscarinic therapy–As noted in Chapter 7, both the nicotinic and the muscarinic effects of the cholinesterase inhibitors can be life-threatening. Unfortunately, there is no effective method for directly blocking the nicotinic effects of cholinesterase inhibition, because nicotinic agonists *and* blockers when applied for prolonged periods cause blockade of transmission (Chapter 26). To reverse the muscarinic effects, a tertiary (not quaternary) amine drug must be used (preferably atropine), since the central nervous system effects as well as the peripheral effects of the organophosphate inhibitors must be treated. Large doses of atropine may be needed to combat the muscarinic effects of extremely potent agents like parathion and chemical warfare nerve gases: 1–2 mg of atropine sulfate may be given intravenously every 5–15 minutes until signs of effect (dry mouth, reversal of miosis) appear. The drug may have

to be repeated many times, since the acute effects of the anticholinesterase agent may last for 24–48 hours or longer. There is no theoretical limit to the use of atropine in this life-threatening situation, and as much as 1 gram per day may be required for as long as 1 month for full control of muscarinic excess (LeBlanc, 1986).

2. Cholinesterase regenerator compounds– A second class of compounds, capable of regenerating active enzyme from the organophosphorus-cholinesterase complex, is also available for the treatment of organophosphorus inhibitor poisoning. These **oxime** agents include **pralidoxime** (PAM), diacetylmonoxime (DAM), and others.

The oxime group (=NOH) has a very high affinity for the phosphorus atom, and these drugs are able to hydrolyze the phosphorylated enzyme if the complex has not "aged" (Chapter 7). HLö 7 is the most effective of these oximes in experimental animals (Eyer et al, 1992). Pralidoxime is the most extensively studied—in humans—of the three agents shown and the only one available for clinical use in the USA. It is most effective in regenerating the cholinesterase associated with skeletal muscle neuromuscular junctions. Because of its positive charge, it does not enter the central nervous system and is ineffective in reversing the central effects of organophosphate poisoning. Diacetylmonoxime, on the other hand, does cross the blood-brain barrier and, in experimental animals, can regenerate some of the central nervous system cholinesterase. The effect of the oximes on cholinesterase carbamoylated by the carbamate cholinesterase inhibitors is controversial.

Pralidoxime is administered by intravenous infusion, 1–2 g given over 15–30 minutes. In spite of the likelihood of aging of the phosphate-enzyme complex, recent reports suggest that administration of multiple doses of pralidoxime over several days may be useful in severe poisoning. In excessive doses, pralidoxime can induce neuromuscular weakness and

Pralidoxime

Diacetylmonoxime

HLö7

other adverse effects. Further details of treatment of anticholinesterase toxicity are given in Chapter 60.

A third approach to protection against excessive AChE inhibition lies in *pretreatment* with reversible inhibitors of the enzyme to prevent binding of the irreversible organophosphate inhibitor. This prophylaxis can be achieved with pyridostigmine or physostigmine but is reserved for situations in which possibly lethal poisoning is feared, eg, chemical warfare. An experimental cholinesterase ligand derived from hemicholinium-3 is particularly effective in animal tests (Cannon et al, 1991). Simultaneous use of atropine is required to control muscarinic excess.

Mushroom poisoning has traditionally been divided into rapid-onset and delayed-onset types. The rapid-onset type is usually apparent within 15–30 minutes following ingestion of the mushrooms. It is often characterized entirely by signs of muscarinic excess: nausea, vomiting, diarrhea, vasodilation, reflex tachycardia (occasionally bradycardia), sweating, salivation, and sometimes bronchoconstriction. Although *Amanita muscaria* contains muscarine (the alkaloid was named after the mushroom), numerous other alkaloids, including antimuscarinic agents, are found in this fungus. In fact, ingestion of *A muscaria* may produce signs of atropine poisoning, not muscarine excess. Other mushrooms, especially those of the *Inocybe* genus, cause rapid-onset poisoning of the muscarinic excess type. Parenteral atropine, 1–2 mg, is effective treatment in such intoxications.

Delayed-onset mushroom poisoning, usually caused by *Amanita phalloides, A virosa, Galerina autumnalis,* or *G marginata*, manifests its first symptoms 6–12 hours after ingestion. Although the initial symptoms usually include nausea and vomiting, the major toxicity involves hepatic and renal cellular injury by amatoxins that inhibit RNA polymerase. Atropine is of no value in this form of mushroom poisoning (see Chapter 60).

G. Other Applications: Atropine and quaternary antimuscarinic drugs have been used in the treatment of urinary urgency caused by minor inflammatory bladder disorders (Table 8–3). This approach does provide some symptomatic relief, although it is no substitute for specific antimicrobial therapy in bacterial cystitis. Oxybutynin is often used to relieve bladder spasm after urologic surgery. The antimuscarinic agents have also been used in urolithiasis to relieve the ureteral smooth muscle spasm caused by passage of the stone. However, their usefulness in this condition is debatable.

Hyperhidrosis is sometimes reduced by the antimuscarinic agents. However, relief is incomplete at best, probably because apocrine rather than eccrine glands are usually involved.

Adverse Effects

Because of the broad range of antimuscarinic ef-

fects, treatment with atropine or its congeners directed at one organ system almost always induces undesirable effects in other organ systems. Thus, mydriasis and cycloplegia are "adverse" effects when an antimuscarinic agent is being used to reduce gastrointestinal secretion or motility, even though they are "therapeutic" effects when the drug is used in ophthalmology.

At higher concentrations, atropine causes block of all parasympathetic functions; these are predictable from the organ system effects described above. However, even in gram quantities, atropine is a remarkably safe drug *in adults*. Atropine poisoning has occurred as a result of attempted suicide, but most cases are due to attempts to induce hallucinations. Poisoned individuals manifest dry mouth, mydriasis, tachycardia, hot and flushed skin, agitation, and delirium for as long as a week. Body temperature is frequently elevated. These effects are memorialized in the adage, "dry as a bone, blind as a bat, red as a beet, mad as a hatter."

Unfortunately, children, especially infants, are very sensitive to the hyperthermic effects of atropine. Although accidental administration of over 400 mg has been followed by recovery, deaths have followed doses as small as 2 mg. Therefore, atropine should be considered a highly dangerous drug when overdose occurs in infants or children.

Overdoses of atropine or its congeners are generally treated symptomatically (see Chapter 60). In the past, physostigmine or another cholinesterase inhibitor was recommended, but most poison control experts now consider physostigmine more dangerous and no more effective in most patients than symptomatic management. When physostigmine is deemed necessary, *small* doses are given *slowly* intravenously (1–4 mg in adults, 0.5–1 mg in children). Symptomatic treatment may require temperature control with cooling blankets and seizure control with diazepam.

Poisoning caused by high doses of the quaternary antimuscarinic drugs is associated with all of the peripheral signs of parasympathetic blockade but few or none of the central nervous system effects of atropine. These more polar drugs may cause significant ganglionic blockade, however, with marked orthostatic hypotension (see below). Treatment of the antimuscarinic effects, if required, can be carried out with a quaternary cholinesterase inhibitor such as neostigmine. Reversal of hypotension may require the administration of a sympathomimetic drug such as phenylephrine or methoxamine.

Contraindications

Contraindications to the use of antimuscarinic drugs are relative, not absolute. *Obvious muscarinic excess, especially that caused by cholinesterase inhibitors, can always be treated with atropine.*

Antimuscarinic drugs are contraindicated in patients with glaucoma, especially angle-closure glaucoma. Even systemic use of moderate doses may precipitate angle closure (and acute glaucoma) in patients with shallow anterior chambers.

In elderly men, atropine should always be used with caution, and should be avoided in those with a history of prostatic hypertrophy.

Because the antimuscarinic drugs slow gastric emptying, they may *increase* symptoms in patients with gastric ulcer. If a stomach ulcer is to be treated pharmacologically, H_2 histamine antagonists and other agents are preferred (see Chapter 64).

III. BASIC & CLINICAL PHARMACOLOGY OF THE GANGLION-BLOCKING DRUGS

These agents block the action of acetylcholine and similar agonists at the nicotinic receptors of both parasympathetic and sympathetic autonomic ganglia. Some members of the group also (or perhaps exclusively) block the ionic channel that is gated by the nicotinic cholinoceptor. Because of their ability to block all autonomic outflow, the ganglion-blocking drugs are still important and useful in pharmacologic and physiologic research. However, their lack of selectivity confers such a broad range of undesirable effects that they have been almost abandoned for clinical use. Their major remaining therapeutic application is for short-term blood pressure control.

Chemistry & Pharmacokinetics

All of the ganglion-blocking drugs of interest are synthetic amines. The first to be recognized as having this action was **tetraethylammonium (TEA).** Because of the very short duration of action of TEA, **hexamethonium ("C6")** was developed and was soon introduced into clinical medicine as the first effective drug for management of hypertension. As shown in Figure 8–6, there is an obvious relationship between the structures of the normal agonist acetylcholine and the nicotinic antagonists tetraethylammonium and hexamethonium. It is interesting that decamethonium, the "C10" analogue of hexamethonium, is an effective neuromuscular depolarizing blocking agent.

Because the quaternary ammonium ganglion-blocking compounds are poorly and erratically absorbed after oral administration, **mecamylamine,** a secondary ammonium compound, was developed to improve the degree and extent of absorption from the gastrointestinal tract. **Trimethaphan,** a short-acting

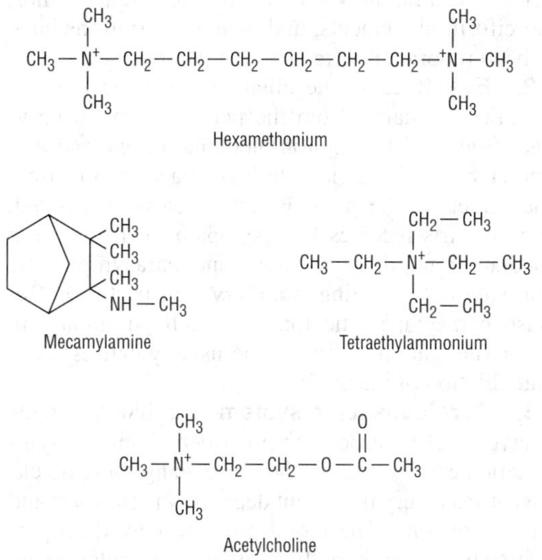

Figure 8–6. Some ganglion-blocking drugs. Acetylcholine is shown for reference. The structure of trimethaphan is shown in Chapter 11.

ganglion blocker, is inactive by the oral route and is given by intravenous infusion (Chapter 11).

Pharmacodynamics

A. Mechanism of Action: The nicotinic receptors of the ganglia, like those of the skeletal muscle neuromuscular junction, are subject to both depolarizing and nondepolarizing blockade (Chapters 7 and 27). Nicotine itself, carbamylcholine, and even acetylcholine (if given with a cholinesterase inhibitor) can produce depolarizing ganglion block.

All of the drugs presently used as ganglion blockers are classified as nondepolarizing competitive antagonists. However, evidence from many studies suggests that hexamethonium actually produces most of its blockade by occupying sites in or on the ion channel that is controlled by the acetylcholine receptor, not by occupying the cholinoceptor itself. In contrast, trimethaphan appears to block the nicotinic receptor, not the channel. According to older studies, blockade can be at least partially overcome by increasing the concentration of normal agonists, eg, acetylcholine.

As noted in Chapter 6, other receptors on the postganglionic cell modulate the ganglionic transmission process. However, their effects are not sufficient to overcome large doses of the hexamethonium-trimethaphan group.

B. Organ System Effects:

1. Central nervous system–The quaternary ammonium agents and trimethaphan are devoid of central effects because they do not cross the blood-brain barrier. Mecamylamine, however, readily enters the central nervous system. Sedation, tremor, choreiform movements, and mental aberrations have all been reported as effects of the latter drug.

2. Eye–Because the ciliary muscle receives innervation primarily from the parasympathetic nervous system, the ganglion-blocking drugs cause a predictable cycloplegia with loss of accommodation. The effect on the pupil is not so easily predicted, since the iris receives both sympathetic innervation (mediating pupillary dilation) and parasympathetic innervation (mediating pupillary constriction). Because parasympathetic tone is usually dominant in this tissue, ganglionic blockade usually causes moderate dilation of the pupil.

3. Cardiovascular system–The blood vessels receive chiefly vasoconstrictor fibers from the sympathetic nervous system; therefore, ganglionic blockade causes a very important decrease in arteriolar and venomotor tone. The blood pressure may drop precipitously, because both peripheral vascular resistance and venous return are decreased (see Figure 6–7). Hypotension is especially marked in the upright position (orthostatic or postural hypotension), because postural reflexes that normally prevent venous pooling are blocked.

Cardiac effects include diminished contractility and, because the sinoatrial node is usually dominated by the parasympathetic nervous system, a moderate tachycardia.

4. Gastrointestinal tract–Secretion is reduced, though not enough to effectively treat peptic disease. Motility is profoundly inhibited, and constipation may be marked.

5. Other systems–Genitourinary smooth muscle is partially dependent on autonomic innervation for normal function. Ganglionic blockade therefore causes hesitancy in urination and may precipitate urinary retention in men with prostatic hypertrophy. Sexual function is impaired in that both erection and ejaculation may be prevented by moderate doses.

Thermoregulatory sweating is blocked by the ganglion-blocking drugs. However, hyperthermia is not a problem except in very warm environments, because cutaneous vasodilation is usually sufficient to maintain a normal body temperature.

6. Response to autonomic drugs–Because the effector cell receptors (muscarinic, alpha, and beta) are not blocked, patients receiving ganglion-blocking drugs are fully responsive to autonomic drugs acting on the effector cell receptors. In fact, responses may be exaggerated, because homeostatic reflexes, which normally moderate autonomic responses, are absent.

Clinical Applications & Toxicity

Because of the availability of more selective autonomic blocking agents, the applications of the ganglion blockers are limited to the lowering of blood pressure. The great efficacy of trimethaphan, when aided by the orthostatic hypotensive effect of venous pooling, is valuable in the treatment of hypertensive emergencies as described in Chapter 11. Controlled hypotension can be of value in neurosurgery to reduce bleeding in the operative field. The short, controllable effect of trimethaphan lends itself to this application as well. Trimethaphan has also been used in acute pulmonary edema to reduce pulmonary vascular pressure.

The toxicity of the ganglion-blocking drugs is limited to the autonomic effects already described. For most patients, these effects are intolerable except for acute use.

PREPARATIONS AVAILABLE

Antimuscarinic Anticholinergic Drugs*
  Anisotropine (generic, Valpin)
    Oral: 50 mg tablets
  Atropine (generic)
    Oral: 0.4, 0.6 mg tablets
    Parenteral: 0.05, 0.1, 0.3, 0.4, 0.5, 0.8, 1, mg/mL for injection
    Ophthalmic (generic, Isopto Atropine): 0.5, 1, 2, 3% drops; 0.5, 1% ointments
  Belladonna alkaloids, extract or tincture (generic)
    Oral: 0.27–0.33 mg/mL liquid
  Clidinium (Quarzan)
    Oral: 2.5, 5 mg capsules

Cyclopentolate (generic, Cyclogyl, others)
  Ophthalmic: 0.5, 1, 2% drops
Dicyclomine (generic, Bentyl, others)
  Oral: 10, 20 mg capsules; 20 mg tablets; 10 mg/ 5 mL syrup
  Parenteral: 10 mg/mL for injection
Flavoxate (Urispas)
  Oral: 100 mg tablets
Glycopyrrolate (generic, Robinul)
  Oral: 1, 2 mg tablets
  Parenteral: 0.2 mg/mL for injection
Hexocyclium (Tral)
  Oral: 25 mg tablets
Homatropine (generic, Isopto Homatropine)
  Ophthalmic: 2, 5% drops

---

*Antimuscarinic drugs used in parkinsonism are listed in Chapter 27.

Isopropamide (Darbid)
 Oral: 5 mg tablets
L-Hyoscyamine (generic, Cystospaz-M, Levsinex)
 Oral: 0.125, 0.15 mg tablets; 0.375 mg timed-re-
  lease capsules; 0.125 mg/5 mL oral elixir and
  solution
 Parenteral: 0.5 mg/mL for injection
Ipratropium (Atrovent)
 Aerosol: 200 dose metered dose inhaler
Mepenzolate (Cantil)
 Oral: 25 mg tablets
Methantheline (Banthine)
 Oral: 50 mg tablets
Methscopolamine (Pamine)
 Oral: 2.5 mg tablets
Oxybutynin (generic, Ditropan)
 Oral: 5 mg tablets, 5 mg/5 mL syrup
Oxyphencyclimine (Daricon)
 Oral: 10 mg tablets
Propantheline (generic, Pro-Banthine)
 Oral: 7.5, 15 mg tablets
Scopolamine (generic)
 Oral: 0.25 mg capsules

 Parenteral: 0.3, 0.4, 0.86, 1 mg/mL for injection
 Ophthalmic (generic, Isopto Hyoscine): 0.25%
  solution
 Transdermal (Transderm-Scop): 1.5 mg patch,
  delivers 0.5 mg over 3 days
Tridihexethyl (Pathilon)
 Oral: 25 mg tablets
Tropicamide (generic, Mydriacyl Ophthalmic,
  others)
 Ophthalmic: 0.5, 1% drops

Ganglion Blockers
Mecamylamine (Inversine)
 Oral: 2.5 mg tablets
Trimethaphan camsylate (Arfonad)
 Parenteral: 500 mg/10 mL ampule

Cholinesterase Regenerator
Pralidoxime (generic, Protopam)
 Parenteral: 1 g vial with 20 mL diluent for IV ad-
  ministration; 600 mg in 2 mL autoinjector)

REFERENCES

Antimuscarinic Drugs

Amitai Y et al: Atropine poisoning in children during the Persian Gulf crisis. JAMA 1992;268:630.

Becker CE et al: Diagnosis and treatment of *Amanita phalloides*-type mushroom poisoning. West J Med 1976;125:100.

Berdie GJ et al: Angle closure glaucoma precipitated by aerosolized atropine. Arch Intern Med 1991;151:1658.

Brown JH (editor): *The Muscarinic Receptors* Humana Press, 1989.

Christofi FL, Palmer JM, Wood JD: Neuropharmacology of the muscarinic agonist telenzepine in myenteric ganglia of the guinea-pig small intestine. Eur J Pharmacol 1991;195:333.

Crowell EB, Ketchum JS: The treatment of scopolamine-induced delirium with physostigmine. Clin Pharmacol Ther 1967;8:409.

Debas HT, Mulholland MW: New horizons in the pharmacologic management of peptic ulceration. Am J Surg 1986;151:422.

Doods HN et al: Selectivity of muscarinic antagonists in radioligand and *in vivo* experiments for the putative M_1, M_2, and M_3 receptors. J Pharmacol Exp Therap 1987;242:257.

Eglen RM, Whiting RL: Muscarinic receptor subtypes: A critique of the current classification and a proposal for a working nomenclature. J Auton Pharmacol 1986;6:323.

Feldman M: Inhibition of gastric acid secretion by selective and nonselective anticholinergics. Gastroenterology 1984;86:361.

Gowdy JM: Stramonium intoxication: Review of symptomatology in 212 cases. JAMA 1972;221:585.

Higgins ST, Lamb RJ, Henningfield JE: Dose-dependent effects of atropine on behavioral and physiologic responses in humans. Pharmacol Biochem Behav 1989;34:303.

Holtmann G, Küppers U, Singer MV: Telenzepine, a new M_1-receptor antagonist, is a more potent inhibitor of pentagastrin-stimulated gastric acid output than pirenzepine in dogs. Scand J Gastroenterol 1990;25:293.

Melchiorre C et al: Antimuscarinic action of methoctramine, a new cardioselective M-2 muscarinic receptor antagonist, alone and in combination with atropine and gallamine. Europ J Pharmacol 1987;144:117.

Mikolich JR, Paulson GW, Cross CJ: Acute anticholinergic syndrome due to Jimson seed ingestion: Clinical and laboratory observation in six cases. Ann Intern Med 1975;83:321.

O'Rourke ST, Vanhoutte PM: Subtypes of muscarinic receptors on adrenergic nerves and vascular smooth muscle of the canine saphenous vein. J Pharmacol Exp Ther 1987;241:64.

Peters NL: Snipping the thread of life: Antimuscarinic side effects of medications in the elderly. Arch Intern Med 1989;149:2414.

Petrie GR, Palmer KNV: Comparison of aerosol ipratropium bromide and salbutamol in chronic bronchitis and asthma. Br Med J 1975;1:430.

Rusted JM, Warburton DM: The effects of scopolamine on working memory in healthy young volunteers. Psychopharmacology 1988;96:145.

Sigman HH, Poleski MH, Gillich A: Effects of pirenzepine on acute mucosal erosions, gastric acid, and mucosal blood flow in the spinal rat stomach. Digestion 1991;49:185.

Skorodin MS: Pharmacotherapy for asthma and chronic obstructive pulmonary disease. Current thinking, practices, and controversies. Arch Int Med 1993; 153:814.

Vybiral T et al: Effects of transdermal scopolamine on heart rate variability in normal subjects. Am J Cardiol 1990;65:604.

Wellstein A, Pitschner HF: Complex dose-response curves of atropine in man explained by different functions of M_1- and M_2-cholinoceptors. Naunyn Schmiedebergs Arch Pharmacol 1988;338:19.

Ganglion-Blocking Drugs

Fahmy NR: Nitroprusside vs. a nitroprusside-trimethaphan mixture for induced hypotension, hemodynamic effects, and cyanide release. Clin Pharmacol Ther 1985;70:264.

Gurney AM, Rang HP: The channel-blocking action of methonium compounds on rat submandibular ganglion cells. Br J Pharmacol 1984;82:623.

Mason DFJ: Ganglion-blocking drugs. In: *Physiological Pharmacology: A Comprehensive Treatise.* Vol 3. Root WS, Hoffman FG (editors). Academic Press, 1967.

Rang HP: The action of ganglionic blocking drugs on the synaptic responses of rat submandibular ganglion cells. Br J Pharmacol 1982;75:151.

Salem MR: Therapeutic uses of ganglionic blocking drugs. Int Anesthesiol Clin 1978;16:171.

Treatment of Anticholinesterase Poisoning

Cannon JG et al: Structure-activity studies on a potent antagonist to organophosphate-induced toxicity. J Med Chem 1991;34:1582.

deKort WLAM, Kiestra SH, Sangster B: The use of atropine and oximes in organophosphate intoxications: A modified approach. Clin Toxicol 1988;26:199.

DeSilva HJ, Wijewickrema R, Senanayake N: Does pralidoxime affect outcome of management in acute organophosphorus poisoning? Lancet 1992;339:1136.

Eyer P et al: HLö 7 dimethanesulfonate, a potent bispyridinium-dioxime against anticholinesterases. Arch Toxicol 1992;66:603.

Farrar HC, Wells TG, Kearns GL: Use of continuous infusion of pralidoxime for treatment of organophosphate poisoning in children. J Pediatr 1990;116:658. 199

Leadbeater L, Inns RH, Rylands JM: Treatment of poisoning by soman. Fundam Appl Toxicol 1985;5:S225.

LeBlanc FN, Benson BE, Gilg AD: A severe organophosphate poisoning requiring the use of an atropine drip. Clin Toxicol 1986;24:69.

Sharabi Y et al: Survey of symptoms following intake of pyridostigmine during the Persian Gulf war. Israel J Med Sci 1991;27:656.

Solana RP et al: Evaluation of a two-drug combination pretreatment against organophosphorus exposure. Toxicol Appl Pharmacol 1990;102:421.

Adrenoceptor-Activating & Other Sympathomimetic Drugs

9

Brian B. Hoffman, MD

The sympathetic nervous system is an important regulator of the activities of organs such as the heart and peripheral vasculature, especially in responses to stress (see Chapter 6). The ultimate effects of sympathetic stimulation are mediated by release of norepinephrine from nerve terminals that serve to activate the adrenoceptors on postsynaptic sites. Also, in response to stress, the adrenal medulla releases epinephrine, which is transported in the blood to target tissues. Drugs that mimic the actions of epinephrine or norepinephrine—**sympathomimetic drugs**—would be expected to have a wide range of effects. An understanding of the pharmacology of these agents is thus a logical extension of what we know about the physiologic role of the catecholamines.

The Mode & Spectrum of Action of Sympathomimetic Drugs

Like the cholinomimetic drugs, the sympathomimetics can be grouped by mode of action and by the spectrum of receptors that they affect. Some of these drugs (eg, norepinephrine, epinephrine) act by a *direct* mode, ie, they directly interact with and activate adrenoceptors. Others act *indirectly;* their actions are dependent on the release of endogenous catecholamines. These indirect agents may have either of two different mechanisms: (1) displacement of stored catecholamines from the adrenergic nerve ending (eg, amphetamine and tyramine) or (2) inhibition of reuptake of catecholamines already released (eg, cocaine and tricyclic antidepressants). Both types of sympathomimetics, direct and indirect, ultimately cause activation of adrenoceptors, leading to some or all of the characteristic effects of catecholamines. The selectivity of different sympathomimetics for various types of adrenoceptors is discussed below.

I. BASIC PHARMACOLOGY OF SYMPATHOMIMETIC DRUGS

IDENTIFICATION OF ADRENOCEPTORS

The effort to understand the molecular mechanisms by which catecholamines act has a long and rich history. A great conceptual debt is owed to the work done by Langley and Ehrlich 75–100 years ago in putting forth the hypothesis that drugs have their effects by interacting with specific "receptive" substances. Ahlquist, in 1948, rationalized a large body of observations by his conjecture that catecholamines acted via two principal receptors. He termed these receptors alpha and beta. Alpha receptors are those that exhibit the potency series epinephrine $\geq$ norepinephrine $>>$ isoproterenol. Beta receptors have the potency series isoproterenol $>$ epinephrine $\geq$ norepinephrine. Ahlquist's hypothesis was dramatically confirmed by the development of drugs that selectively antagonize beta receptors but not alpha receptors (see Chapter 10).

A. Beta Subtypes: Soon after the demonstration of separate alpha and beta receptors, it was found that there are at least two *subtypes* of beta receptors, designated β_1 and β_2. Beta$_1$ and β_2 receptors are operationally defined by their affinities for epinephrine and norepinephrine: β_1 receptors have approximately equal affinity for epinephrine and norepinephrine, whereas β_2 receptors have a higher affinity for epinephrine than for norepinephrine. Molecular cloning has now demonstrated the existence of a third subtype of beta receptor (β_3) and established some of the properties of each of these receptor types (Table 9–1).

B. Alpha Subtypes: Following the demonstration of the beta subtypes, it was found that there are also at least two subgroups of alpha receptors, α_1 and α_2. The subtypes of alpha receptors were originally identified with antagonist drugs that distinguished between α_1 and α_2 receptors. For example, alpha ad-

Table 9–1. Adrenoceptor types and subtypes.

Receptor	Agonist	Antagonist	Effects	Gene on Chromosome
Alpha$_1$ type	Phenylephrine, metho-xamine, cirazoline	Prazosin, corynanthine	$\uparrow$IP$_3$, DAG common to all	
Alpha$_{1A}$		WB4101, prazosin	$\uparrow$IP$_3$, DAG; $\uparrow$Ca^{2+} influx	
Alpha$_{1B}$		CEC (irreversible)	$\uparrow$IP$_3$, DAG	C5
Alpha$_{1C}$		WB4101, CEC	$\uparrow$IP$_3$, DAG	C8
Alpha$_{1D}$		WB4101	?$\uparrow$Ca^{2+} influx	C20
Alpha$_2$ type	Clonidine, BHT920	Rauwolscine, yohimbine	$\downarrow$cAMP common to all	
Alpha$_{2A}$	Oxymetazoline		$\downarrow$cAMP; $\uparrow$K$^+$ channels; $\downarrow$Ca^{2+} channels	C10
Alpha$_{2B}$		Prazosin	$\downarrow$cAMP; $\downarrow$Ca^{2+} channels	C2
Alpha$_{2C}$		Prazosin	$\downarrow$cAMP	C4
Beta type	Isoproterenol	Propranolol	$\uparrow$cAMP common to all	
Beta$_1$	Dobutamine	Betaxolol	$\uparrow$cAMP	
Beta$_2$	Procaterol, terbutaline	Butoxamine	$\uparrow$cAMP	
Beta$_3$	BRL37344		$\uparrow$cAMP	
Dopamine type	Dopamine			
D$_1$	Fenoldopam		$\uparrow$cAMP	C5
D$_2$	Bromocriptine		$\downarrow$cAMP; $\uparrow$K$^+$ channels; $\uparrow$Ca2$^+$ channels	C11
D$_4$		Clozapine	$\downarrow$cAMP	
D$_5$			$\uparrow$cAMP	C4

Key:

BRL37344	=	Sodium-4-(2-[2-hydroxy-{3-chlorophenyl}ethylamino]propyl)phenoxyacetate
BHT920	=	6-Allyl-2-amino-5,6,7,8-tetrahydro-4H-thiazolo-[4,5-d]-azepine
CEC	=	Chloroethylclonidine
DAG	=	Diacylglycerol
IP$_3$	=	Inositol trisphophate
WB4101	=	N-[2-(2,6-dimethoxyphenoxy)ethyl]-2,3-dihydro-1,4-benzodioxan-2-methanamine

renoceptors were identified in a variety of tissues by measuring the binding of radiolabeled antagonist compounds that are considered to have a high affinity for these receptors, eg, dihydroergocryptine (α_1 and α_2), prazosin (α_1), and yohimbine (α_2). These radioligands were used to measure the number of receptors in tissues and to determine the affinity (by displacement of the radiolabeled ligand) of other drugs that interact with the receptors.

The concept of subtypes *within* the α_1 group emerged out of pharmacologic experiments that indicated complex shapes of agonist dose-response curves of smooth muscle contraction in some tissues as well as differences in antagonist affinities in certain contractile responses. These experiments demonstrated the existence of two subtypes of α_1 receptor that could be distinguished on the basis of their reversible affinity for the ligand WB4101 (α_{1A}) or irreversible inactivation by chloroethylclonidine (α_{1B}; Table 9–1). The spleen and liver contain mainly α_{1B} receptors; the heart, neocortex, kidney, caudal artery, vas deferens, and hippocampus appear to have similar numbers of α_{1A} and α_{1B} receptors. Molecular cloning experiments have now confirmed the existence of multiple subtypes of alpha$_1$ receptors and established some of their properties.

The hypothesis that there are subtypes of α_2 receptors similarly emerged from pharmacologic experiments and radioligand-binding assays. Human platelets appear to contain only the α_{2A} subtype. Clinically used drugs such as prazosin, chlorpromazine, yohimbine, and oxymetazoline have different affinities for α_{2A} and α_{2B} receptors. There is additional pharmacologic evidence supporting the existence of an α_{2C} receptor. Molecular cloning has identified at least three α_2 receptors that are products of separate genes.

C. Dopamine Receptors: The endogenous catecholamine dopamine produces a variety of biologic effects that are mediated by interactions with specific dopamine receptors (Table 9–1). These receptors are distinct from alpha and beta receptors and are particularly important in the brain (see Chapters 20 and 28) and in the splanchnic and renal vasculature. As with alpha and beta adrenoceptors, there is now considerable evidence for the existence of multiple forms of dopamine receptors. Pharmacologically distinct dopamine receptor subtypes, termed D$_1$ and D$_2$, have been known for some time. More recently, molecular cloning has identified several distinct genes encoding each of these subtypes. Further complexity occurs because of the presence of introns within the coding region of the D$_2$-like receptors, which allows for alternative splicing of the exons in this major subtype. In addition, a restriction length polymorphism has been associated with a human D$_2$-like receptor (Gingrich, 1993). The terminology of the various subtypes is particularly unsettled, with the alternative series names D$_1$, D$_2$, D$_4$, D$_5$ or D$_{1A}$, D$_{2A}$,

D_{2C}, D_{1B} being used. (See 1994 Receptor Nomenclature Supplement.)

Receptor Selectivity

Examples of clinically useful sympathomimetic agonists that are relatively selective for alpha- and beta-adrenoceptor subgroups are compared with some nonselective agents in Table 9–2. Selectivity means that a drug may preferentially bind to one subgroup of receptors at concentrations too low to interact with another subgroup. For example, norepinephrine preferentially activates β_1 receptors as compared to β_2 receptors. However, selectivity is not usually absolute, and at higher concentrations related classes of receptor may also interact with the drug. As a result, the "numeric" subclassification of adrenoceptors is clinically important only for drugs that have relatively marked selectivity.

Nomenclature

The nomenclature for adrenoceptor subtypes is confusing because there is no generally agreed upon formal system; different authors may use similar names for talking about what appear to be quite different receptors. Consequently, caution is advised in reading research reports. The annual receptor nomenclature issue (1994 Receptor Nomenclature Supplement) published by the journal *Trends in Pharmacological Sciences* provides a useful introduction to current nomenclature, but it should be recognized that some of the names and descriptive data for the receptors listed are subject to rapid change.

The exact number of adrenoceptor subtypes that are actually expressed in human tissues is uncertain, but expression of subtypes has been demonstrated in tissues where the physiologic or pharmacologic importance of the subtype is not yet known. These results suggest the possibility of designing novel drugs to exploit the expression of a particular receptor subtype in a single target tissue. For example, determin-

ing which blood vessels express which subtypes of α_1 and α_2 receptors could lead to design of drugs having selectivity for certain vascular beds such as the splanchnic or coronary vessels.

MOLECULAR MECHANISMS OF SYMPATHOMIMETIC ACTION

The effects of catecholamines are mediated by cell surface receptors. As described in Chapter 2, these receptors are coupled by G proteins to the various effector proteins whose activities are regulated by those receptors. Each G protein is a heterotrimer consisting of alpha, beta, and gamma subunits. Different G proteins have distinctive alpha subunits; less variation has been found between the respective beta and gamma subunits of each of the G proteins. G proteins of particular importance for adrenoceptor function include G_s, the stimulatory G protein of adenylyl cyclase; G_i, the inhibitory G protein of adenylyl cyclase; and G_q, the protein coupling alpha receptors to phospholipase C. The activation of G protein-coupled receptors by catecholamines promotes the dissociation of GDP from the alpha subunit of the appropriate G protein. GTP then binds to this G protein, and the alpha subunit dissociates from the beta-gamma unit. The activated GTP-bound alpha subunit then regulates the activity of its effector. Some effectors of adrenoceptor-activated alpha subunits include adenylyl cyclase, cGMP phosphodiesterase, phospholipase C, and ion channels. The alpha subunit is inactivated by hydrolysis of the bound GTP to GDP and P_i, and the subsequent reassociation of the alpha subunit with the beta-gamma subunit. The beta-gamma subunit may have additional independent effects, though the physiologic significance of these effects is not yet clear.

Receptor Types

A. Alpha Receptors: The mechanism of activation of alpha receptors by catecholamines is not as well understood as that of beta receptors. The chloroethylclonidine-sensitive α_{1B} subtype has been found to stimulate the formation of inositol 1,4,5-trisphosphate, whereas the chlorethylclonidine-resistant α_{1A} subtype may or may not activate phospholipase C but may also control the gating of membrane calcium channels.

The most commonly observed effect of α_1-receptor activation is a rise in cytosolic calcium concentration. This effect does not appear to involve a change in adenylyl cyclase activity or cAMP concentration in cells except perhaps in certain regions of the brain. The mechanism that is used to produce this calcium increase is not fully defined. In certain smooth muscle cells, α_1-receptor activation leads to an influx of calcium across the membrane, probably through the opening of receptor-operated calcium channels. Al-

Table 9–2. Relative selectivity of adrenoceptor agonists.

	Relative Receptor Affinities
Alpha agonists	
Phenylephrine, methoxamine	$\alpha_1 > \alpha_2 >>>>> \beta$
Clonidine, methylnorepinephrine	$\alpha_2 > \alpha_1 >>>>> \beta$
Mixed alpha and beta agonists	
Norepinephrine	$\alpha_1 = \alpha_2;\ \beta_1 >> \beta_2$
Epinephrine	$\alpha_1 = \alpha_2;\ \beta_1 = \beta_2$
Beta agonists	
Dobutamine	$\beta_1 > \beta_2 >>>> \alpha$
Isoproterenol	$\beta_1 = \beta_2 >>>> \alpha$
Terbutaline, metaproterenol, albuterol, ritodrine	$\beta_2 >> \beta_1 >>>> \alpha$
Dopamine agonists	
Dopamine	$D_1 = D_2 >> \beta >> \alpha$

pha$_1$-receptor activation in many cells leads to the breakdown of polyphosphoinositides into inositol trisphosphate and diacylglycerol (Figure 9–1). A G protein called G$_q$ couples α_1 receptors to phospholipase C. Inositol 1,4,5-trisphosphate (IP$_3$) promotes the release of sequestered Ca^{2+} from intracellular stores, which increases the cytoplasmic concentration of free Ca^{2+} and the activation of various calcium-dependent protein kinases. Inositol 1,4,5-trisphosphate is sequentially dephosphorylated, which ultimately leads to the formation of free inositol. However, several other phosphorylated isomers of inositol may be produced and accumulate owing to the metabolism of 1,4,5-trisphosphate; the biologic significance of these other molecules is unclear. Diacylglycerol activates a protein kinase termed C kinase. The physiologic significance of C kinase is unclear; however, in some cells it promotes cell division. C kinase may also regulate long-term responses to α_1-receptor activation.

Alpha$_2$ receptors inhibit adenylyl cyclase activity and cause intracellular cAMP levels to decrease. While this effect has been well documented, it is not clear whether this action is the exclusive or major expression of α_2-receptor activation. Thus, α_2-receptor agonists cause platelet aggregation and a decrease in platelet cAMP levels, but it is not clear that aggregation is the result of the decrease in cAMP. Alpha$_2$ in-

hibition of adenylyl cyclase occurs through the mediation of the inhibitory regulatory protein, G$_i$, that couples the α_2 receptor to the inhibition of adenylyl cyclase (Figure 9–2). How the activation of G$_i$ leads to the inhibition of adenylyl cyclase is unclear. Two major possibilities are (1) that the free beta-gamma units of G$_i$ combine with the free alpha subunits of G$_s$, rendering them inactive; and (2) that the alpha subunit of G$_i$ directly inhibits adenylyl cyclase activity. Some evidence favors both of these possible mechanisms. In addition, some of the effects of α_2 adrenoceptors are independent of their ability to inhibit adenylyl cyclase; mechanisms include activation of potassium channels and closing of calcium channels.

B. Beta Receptors: The mechanism of action of beta agonists has been studied in considerable detail. Activation of all three receptor subtypes (β_1, β_2, and β_3) results in activation of adenylyl cyclase and increased conversion of ATP to cAMP (Figure 9–2). Activation of the cyclase enzyme is mediated by the stimulatory coupling protein G$_s$. cAMP is the major second messenger of β-receptor activation. For example, in the liver of many species, β-receptor activation increases cAMP synthesis, which leads to a cascade of events culminating in the activation of glycogen phosphorylase. In the heart, β-receptor activation increases the influx of calcium across the cell membrane and its sequestration inside the cell.

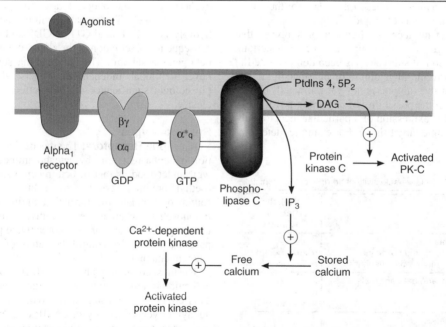

Figure 9–1. Activation of α_1 responses. Stimulation of α_1 receptors by catecholamines leads to the activation of a G$_q$ coupling protein. The α subunit of this G protein activates the effector, phospholipase C, which leads to the release of IP$_3$ (inositol 1,4,5-trisphosphate) and DAG (diacylglycerol) from phosphatidylinositol 4,5-bisphosphate *(Ptdlns 4, 5P$_2$)*. IP$_3$ stimulates the release of sequestered stores of calcium *(Ca)*, leading to an increased concentration of cytoplasmic Ca^{2+}. Ca^{2+} may then activate Ca^{2+}-dependent protein kinases, which in turn phosphorylate their substrates. DAG activates protein kinase C.

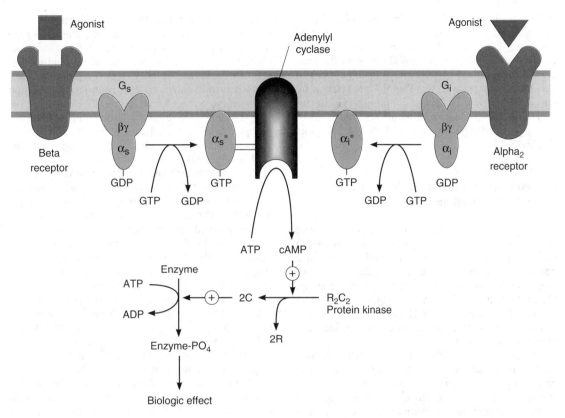

Figure 9–2. Activation and inhibition of adenylyl cyclase by agonists that bind to catecholamine receptors. Binding to beta adrenoceptors stimulates adenylyl cyclase by activating the stimulatory G protein, G_s, which leads to the dissociation of its alpha subunit charged with GTP. This α_s subunit directly activates adenylyl cyclase, resulting in an increased rate of synthesis of cAMP. Alpha$_2$ adrenoceptor ligands inhibit adenylyl cyclase by causing dissociation of the inhibitory G protein, G_i, into its subunits; ie, an α_i subunit charged with GTP and a beta-gamma unit. The mechanism by which these subunits inhibit adenylyl cyclase is uncertain. cAMP binds to the regulatory subunit *(R)* of cAMP-dependent protein kinase, leading to the liberation of active catalytic subunits *(C)* that phosphorylate specific protein substrates and modify their activity.

Beta-receptor activation also promotes the relaxation of smooth muscle. While the mechanism is uncertain, it may involve the phosphorylation of myosin light chain kinase to an inactive form (see Figure 12–1).

C. Dopamine Receptors: The D_1 receptor is typically associated with the stimulation of adenylyl cyclase (Table 9–1); for example, D_1-receptor-induced smooth muscle relaxation is presumably due to cAMP accumulation in vascular beds where dopamine is a vasodilator. D_2 receptors have been found to inhibit adenylyl cyclase activity, open potassium channels, and decrease calcium influx.

Receptor Regulation

Responses mediated by adrenoceptors are not fixed and static. The number and function of adrenoceptors on the cell surface and their responses may be regulated by catecholamines themselves, other hormones and drugs, age, and a number of disease states. These changes may modify the magnitude of a tissue's physiologic response to catecholamines. One of the best-studied examples of receptor regulation is the **desensitization** of adrenoceptors that may occur after exposure to catecholamines and other sympathomimetic drugs. After a cell or tissue has been exposed for a period of time to an agonist, that tissue often becomes less responsive to further stimulation by that agent. Other terms such as tolerance, refractoriness, and tachyphylaxis have also been used to denote desensitization. This process has considerable clinical significance because it may limit the therapeutic response to sympathomimetic agents.

The mechanisms involved in desensitization of cells to responses mediated by beta adrenoceptors have been extensively studied. There appear to be at least three distinct mechanisms. In some cells, desensitization is caused by receptor sequestration (a rapid and transient event wherein the receptors are made temporarily unavailable for activation by agonists). A second process, down-regulation (ie, disappearance of the receptors from the cell), may take place by the action of enzymes on the receptor or by decreased synthesis. Third, phosphorylation of the receptor on the cytoplasmic side by protein kinase A or β-adrenergic receptor kinase (βARK) may impair coupling of beta adrenoceptors with G_s. The phosphorylation induced by βARK may disrupt coupling to G_s, in part by facilitating association of an arrestin-like 48,000-MW protein with phosphorylated beta adrenoceptors (Figure 2–13).

CHEMISTRY & PHARMACOKINETICS OF SYMPATHOMIMETIC DRUGS

Phenylethylamine may be considered the parent compound from which sympathomimetic drugs are derived (Figure 9–3). This compound consists of a benzene ring with an ethylamine side chain. Substitutions may be made (1) on the terminal amino group, (2) on the benzene ring, and (3) on the alpha or beta carbons. Substitution by –OH groups at the 3 and 4 positions yields sympathomimetic drugs collectively known as catecholamines.

The effects of modification of phenylethylamine are to change the affinity of the drugs for alpha and beta receptors as well as to influence the intrinsic ability to activate the receptors. In addition, chemical structure determines the pharmacokinetic properties of these molecules. Sympathomimetic drugs may activate both alpha and beta receptors; however, the relative alpha-receptor versus beta-receptor activity spans the range from almost pure alpha activity (methoxamine) to almost pure beta activity (isoproterenol).

A. Substitution on the Amino Group: Increasing the size of alkyl substituents on the amino group tends to increase beta-receptor activity. For example, methyl substitution on norepinephrine, yielding epinephrine, enhances activity at β_2 receptors. Beta activity is further enhanced with isopropyl substitution at the amino nitrogen (isoproterenol). $Beta_2$-selective agonists generally require a large amino substituent group. The larger the substituent on the amino group, the lower the activity at alpha receptors; eg, isoproterenol is very weak at alpha receptors.

B. Substitution on the Benzene Ring: Maximal alpha and beta activity are found with catecholamines (drugs having –OH groups at the 3 and 4 positions). The absence of one or the other of these groups, particularly the hydroxyl at C3, without other substitutions on the ring may dramatically reduce the potency of the drugs. For example, phenylephrine (Figure 9–4) is much less potent than epinephrine; indeed, alpha activity is decreased about 100-fold and beta activity is almost negligible except at very high concentrations. However, catecholamines are subject to inactivation by catechol-O-methyltransferase (COMT), an enzyme found in gut and liver (see Chapter 6). Therefore, absence of one or both –OH groups on the phenyl ring increases the bioavailability after oral administration and prolongs the duration of action. Furthermore, absence of ring –OH groups increases the distribution of the molecule to the central nervous system. For example, ephedrine and amphetamine (Figure 9–4) are orally active, have a prolonged duration of action, and produce central nervous system effects not observed with the catecholamines.

C. Substitution on the Alpha Carbon: Substi-

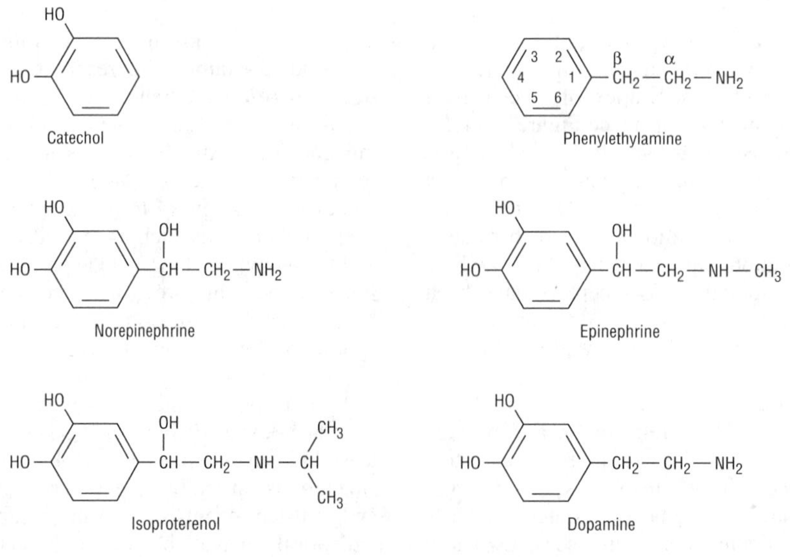

Figure 9–3. Phenylethylamine and some important catecholamines. Catechol is shown for reference.

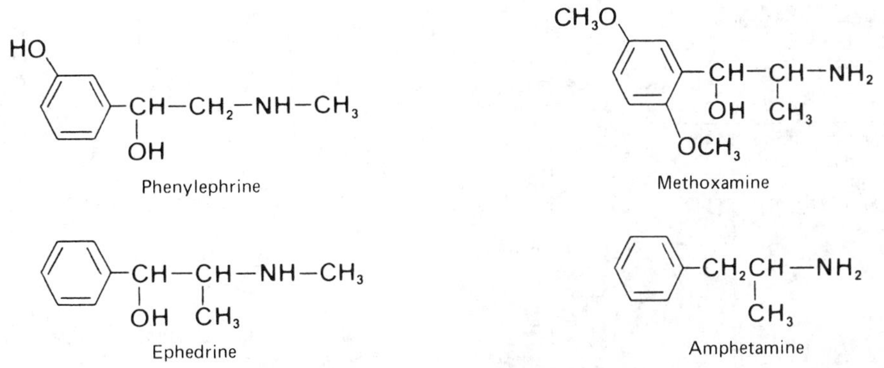

Figure 9–4. Some examples of noncatecholamine sympathomimetic drugs.

tutions at the alpha carbon block oxidation by monoamine oxidase (MAO) and prolong the action of such drugs, particularly the noncatecholamines. Ephedrine and amphetamine are examples of alpha-substituted compounds (Figure 9–4). Alpha-methyl compounds are also called phenylisopropylamines. In addition to their resistance to oxidation by MAO, phenylisopropylamines have an enhanced ability to displace catecholamines from storage sites in noradrenergic nerves. Therefore, at least a portion of their activity is dependent upon the presence of normal norepinephrine stores in the body; they are indirectly acting sympathomimetics.

D. Substitution on the Beta Carbon: Direct-acting agonists typically have a beta-hydroxyl group, though dopamine does not. In addition to activating adrenoceptors, this hydroxyl group may be important for storage of sympathomimetic amines in neural vesicles.

ORGAN SYSTEM EFFECTS OF SYMPATHOMIMETIC DRUGS

General outlines of the cellular actions of sympathomimetics are presented in Tables 6–3 and 9–3. The net effect of a given drug in the intact organism depends on its relative receptor affinity (alpha or beta), intrinsic activity, and the compensatory reflexes evoked by its direct actions.

Cardiovascular System

A. Blood Vessels: Vascular smooth muscle tone is regulated by adrenoceptors; consequently, catecholamines are important in controlling peripheral vascular resistance and venous capacitance. Alpha receptors increase arterial resistance, whereas β_2 receptors promote smooth muscle relaxation. There are major differences in receptor types in the various vascular beds (Table 9–4). The skin vessels have predominantly alpha receptors and constrict in the presence of epinephrine and norepinephrine, as do the

splanchnic vessels. Vessels in skeletal muscle may constrict or dilate depending on whether alpha or beta receptors are activated. Thus, the overall effects of a sympathomimetic drug on blood vessels depend on the relative activities of that drug at alpha and beta receptors and the anatomic sites of the vessels affected. In addition, D_1 receptors promote vasodilation of renal, splanchnic, coronary, and cerebral arteries.

Table 9–3. Distribution of adrenoceptor subtypes.

Type	Tissue	Actions
Alpha$_1$	Most vascular smooth muscle (innervated)	Contraction
	Pupillary dilator muscle	Contraction (dilates pupil)
	Pilomotor smooth muscle	Erect hair
	Rat liver	Glycogenolysis
	Heart	Increase force of contraction
Alpha$_2$	Postsynaptic CNS adrenoceptors	Propably multiple
	Platelets	Aggregation
	Adrenergic and cholinergic nerve terminals	Inhibition of transmitter release
	Some vascular smooth muscle	Contraction
	Fat cells	Inhibition of lipolysis
Beta$_1$	Heart	Increase force and rate of contraction
Beta$_2$	Respiratory, uterine, and vascular smooth muscle	Promote smooth muscle relaxation
	Skeletal muscle	Promote potassium uptake
	Human liver	Activate glycogenolysis
Beta$_3$	Fat cells	Activate lipolysis
D$_1$	Smooth muscle	Dilate renal blood vessels
D$_2$	Nerve endings	Modulate transmitter release

Table 9–4. Cardiovascular response to sympathomimetic amines.[1]

	Phenyl-ephrine	Epine-phrine	Isopro-terenol
Vascular resistance (tone)			
Cutaneous, mucous membranes (α)	↑↑	↑↑	0
Skeletal muscle (β_2, α)	↑	↓ or ↑	↓↓
Renal (α, D_1)	↑	↑	↓
Splanchnic (α)	↑↑	↓ or ↑[2]	↓
Total peripheral resistance	↑↑↑	↓ or ↑[2]	↓↓
Venous tone	↑	↑	↓
Cardiac			
Contractility (β_1)	0 or ↑	↑↑↑	↑↑↑
Heart rate (predominantly β_1)	↓↓ (vagal reflex)	↑ or ↓	↑↑↑
Stroke volume	0, ↓, ↑	↑	↑
Cardiac output	↓	↑	↑↑
Blood pressure			
Mean	↑↑	↑	↓
Diastolic	↑↑	↓ or ↑[2]	↓↓
Systolic	↑↑	↑↑	0 or ↓
Pulse pressure	0	↑↑	↑↑

[1](↑ = increase; ↓ = decrease; 0 = no change.)
[2]Small doses decrease, large doses increase.

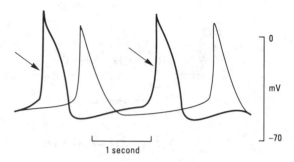

Figure 9–5. Effect of epinephrine on the transmembrane potential of a pacemaker cell in the frog heart. The arrowed trace was recorded after the addition of epinephrine. Note the increased slope of diastolic depolarization and decreased interval between action potentials. This pacemaker acceleration is typical of β_1-stimulant drugs. (Modified and reproduced, with permission, from Brown H, Giles W, Noble S: Membrane currents underlying rhythmic activity in frog sinus venosus. In: *The Sinus Node: Structure, Function, and Clinical Relevance.* Bonke FIM [editor]. Martinus Nijhoff, 1978.)

Activation of the D_1 receptors in the renal vasculature may play a major role in the natriuresis induced by pharmacologic administration of dopamine.

B. Heart: Direct effects on the heart are determined largely by β_1 receptors, though β_2 and to a lesser extent alpha receptors are also involved. Beta-receptor activation results in increased calcium influx in cardiac cells. This has both electrical (Figure 9–5) and mechanical consequences. Pacemaker activity, both normal (sinoatrial node) and abnormal (eg, Purkinje fibers), is increased (positive chronotropic effect). Conduction velocity in the atrioventricular node is increased, and the refractory period is decreased. Intrinsic contractility is increased (positive inotropic effect), and relaxation is accelerated. As a result, the twitch response of isolated cardiac muscle is increased in tension but abbreviated in duration. In the intact heart, intraventricular pressure rises and falls more rapidly, and ejection time is decreased. These direct effects are easily demonstrated in the absence of reflexes evoked by changes in blood pressure, eg, in isolated myocardial preparations and in patients with ganglionic blockade. In the presence of normal reflex activity, the direct effects on heart rate may be dominated by a reflex response to blood pressure changes.

C. Blood Pressure: The effects of sympathomimetic drugs on blood pressure can be explained on the basis of their effects on the heart, the peripheral vascular resistance, and the venous return (see Figure 6–7 and Table 9–4). A relatively pure alpha agonist such as phenylephrine increases peripheral arterial resistance and decreases venous capacitance. The enhanced arterial resistance usually

leads to a marked rise in blood pressure (Figure 9–6). In the presence of normal cardiovascular reflexes, the rise in blood pressure elicits a baroreceptor-mediated increase in vagal tone with slowing of heart rate. However, cardiac output may not diminish in proportion to this reduction in rate, since increased venous return may increase stroke volume; furthermore, direct alpha-adrenoceptor stimulation of the heart may have a modest positive inotropic action. While these are the expected effects of pure alpha agonists in normal subjects, their use in hypotensive patients usually does not lead to brisk reflex responses because in this situation blood pressure is returning to normal, not exceeding normal.

The blood pressure response to a pure beta-adrenoceptor agonist is quite different. Stimulation of beta receptors in the heart increases cardiac output. A relatively pure beta agonist such as isoproterenol also decreases peripheral resistance by dilating certain vascular beds (Table 9–4). The net effect is to maintain or slightly increase systolic pressure while permitting a fall in diastolic pressure owing to enhanced diastolic runoff (Figure 9–6). The actions of drugs with both alpha and beta effects (eg, epinephrine and norepinephrine) are discussed below.

Eye

The radial pupillary dilator muscle of the iris contains alpha receptors; activation by drugs such as phenylephrine causes mydriasis (Figure 6–9). Alpha and beta stimulants also have important effects on intraocular pressure. Present evidence suggests that alpha agonists increase the outflow of aqueous humor from the eye, while beta agonists appear to increase the production of aqueous humor. These effects are

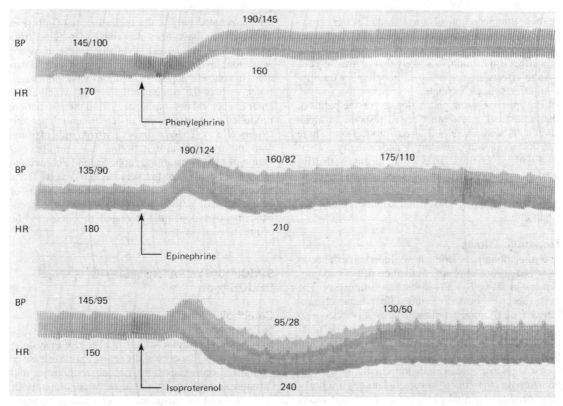

Figure 9–6. Effects of an alpha-selective (phenylephrine), beta-selective (isoproterenol), and nonselective (epinephrine) sympathomimetic, given as an intravenous bolus injection to a dog. (BP, blood pressure; HR, heart rate.) Reflexes are blunted but not eliminated in this anesthetized animal.

important in the treatment of glaucoma. Beta stimulants relax the ciliary muscle to a minor degree, causing an insignificant decrease in accommodation.

Respiratory Tract

Bronchial smooth muscle contains β_2 receptors that cause relaxation. Activation of these receptors thus results in bronchodilation (see Chapter 19 and Table 9–3). The blood vessels of the upper respiratory tract mucosa contain α_1 receptors; the decongestant action of alpha stimulants is clinically useful (see Clinical Pharmacology).

Gastrointestinal Tract

Relaxation of gastrointestinal smooth muscle can be brought about by both alpha- and beta-stimulant agents. Beta receptors appear to be located directly on the smooth muscle cells and mediate relaxation via hyperpolarization and decreased spike activity in these cells. Alpha stimulants, especially α_2-selective agonists, decrease muscle activity *indirectly* by presynaptically reducing the release of acetylcholine and possibly other stimulants within the enteric nervous system (Chapter 6). The alpha-receptor-mediated response is probably of greater pharmacologic significance than the beta-stimulant response. Alpha$_2$ re-

ceptors may also decrease salt and water flux into the lumen of the intestine.

Genitourinary Tract

The human uterus contains alpha and β_2 receptors. The fact that the beta receptors mediate relaxation can be clinically useful in pregnancy (see Clinical Pharmacology). The bladder base, urethral sphincter, and prostate contain alpha receptors that mediate contraction and therefore promote urinary continence. The specific subtype of alpha receptor involved in mediating constriction of the bladder base and prostate is uncertain and the subject of active investigation. The β_2 receptors of the bladder wall mediate relaxation. Ejaculation depends upon normal alpha-receptor (and possibly purinergic receptor) activation in the ductus deferens, seminal vesicles, and prostate. The detumescence of erectile tissue that normally follows ejaculation is also brought about by norepinephrine (and possibly neuropeptide Y) released from sympathetic nerves (deGroat, 1990). Alpha activity appears to have a similar detumescent effect on erectile tissue in female animals.

Exocrine Glands

The salivary glands contain adrenoceptors that

regulate the secretion of amylase and water. However, certain sympathomimetic drugs, eg, clonidine, produce symptoms of dry mouth. The mechanism of this effect is uncertain; it is likely that central nervous system effects are responsible, though other (peripheral) effects may contribute.

The apocrine sweat glands, located on the palms of the hands and a few other areas, respond to alpha stimulants with increased sweat production. These are the nonthermoregulatory glands usually associated with psychologic stress. (The diffusely distributed thermoregulatory eccrine sweat glands are regulated by *sympathetic cholinergic* postganglionic nerves that activate muscarinic cholinoceptors; see Chapter 6.)

Metabolic Effects

Sympathomimetic drugs have important effects on intermediary metabolism. Activation of beta adrenoceptors in fat cells leads to increased lipolysis. The beta receptors mediating this effect have characteristics of β_3 adrenoceptors. Human lipocytes also contain α_2 receptors that inhibit lipolysis by decreasing intracellular cAMP. Sympathomimetic drugs enhance glycogenolysis in the liver, which leads to increased glucose release into the circulation. In the human liver, the effects of catecholamines are probably mediated mainly by beta receptors, though alpha receptors may also play a role. Catecholamines in high concentrations may also cause metabolic acidosis. Activation of β_2 adrenoceptors by endogenous epinephrine or by sympathomimetic drugs promotes the uptake of potassium into cells, leading to a fall in extracellular potassium. This may lead to a fall in the plasma potassium concentration during stress or protect against a rise in plasma potassium during exercise. Blockade of these receptors may accentuate the rise in plasma potassium that occurs during exercise.

Effects on Endocrine & Other Function

Catecholamines are important endogenous regulators of hormone secretion from a number of glands. Insulin secretion is stimulated by beta receptors and inhibited by α_2 receptors. Similarly, renin secretion is stimulated by β_1 and inhibited by α_2 receptors; indeed, beta-receptor antagonist drugs may lower plasma renin at least in part by this mechanism. Adrenoceptors also modulate the secretion of parathyroid hormone, calcitonin, thyroxine, and gastrin; however, the physiologic significance of these control mechanisms is unclear. In high concentrations, epinephrine and related agents cause leukocytosis.

Effects on the Central Nervous System

The action of sympathomimetics on the central nervous system varies dramatically, depending on their ability to cross the blood-brain barrier. The catecholamines are almost completely excluded by this barrier, and subjective central nervous system effects are noted only at the highest rates of infusion. These effects have been described as ranging from "nervousness" to a "feeling of impending disaster," sensations that are universally regarded as undesirable. In contrast, noncatecholamines with indirect actions, such as the amphetamine agents, which easily enter the central nervous system from the circulation, produce qualitatively very different central nervous system effects. These actions vary from mild alerting, with improved attention to boring tasks; through elevation of mood, insomnia, euphoria, and anorexia; to psychotic behavior at the very highest levels. These effects are not readily assigned to either alpha- or beta-mediated actions and probably represent enhancement of dopamine-mediated processes in the central nervous system.

SPECIFIC SYMPATHOMIMETIC DRUGS

Catecholamines

Epinephrine (adrenaline) is a very potent vasoconstrictor and cardiac stimulant. The rise in systolic blood pressure that occurs after epinephrine release or administration is caused by its positive inotropic and chronotropic actions on the heart (predominantly β_1 receptors) and the vasoconstriction induced in many vascular beds (alpha receptors). Epinephrine also activates β_2 receptors in some vessels (eg, skeletal muscle blood vessels), leading to their dilation. Consequently, total peripheral resistance may actually fall, explaining the fall in diastolic pressure that is sometimes seen with epinephrine injection (Figure 9–6).

Norepinephrine (levarterenol, noradrenaline) and epinephrine have similar effects on β_1 receptors in the heart and similar potency at alpha receptors. Norepinephrine has relatively little effect on β_2 receptors. Consequently, norepinephrine increases peripheral resistance and both diastolic and systolic blood pressure. Compensatory vagal reflexes tend to overcome the direct positive chronotropic effects of norepinephrine; however, the positive inotropic effects on the heart are maintained.

Isoproterenol (isoprenaline) is an extremely potent beta-receptor agonist, having little effect on alpha receptors. The drug has positive chronotropic and inotropic actions; because isoproterenol activates beta receptors almost exclusively, it is a potent vasodilator. These actions lead to a marked increase in cardiac output associated with a fall in diastolic and mean arterial pressure and a lesser decrease or a slight increase in systolic pressure (Table 9–4 and Figure 9–6).

Dopamine, the immediate metabolic precursor of norepinephrine, activates D_1 receptors in several vascular beds, which leads to vasodilation. The effect this has on renal blood flow is of considerable clinical value. The activation of presynaptic D_2 receptors, which suppress norepinephrine release, contributes to these effects to an unknown extent. In addition, dopamine activates β_1 receptors in the heart. At low doses it has relatively little effect on overall peripheral resistance. However, at higher rates of infusion, dopamine activates vascular alpha receptors, leading to vasoconstriction. Thus, high concentrations may mimic the actions of epinephrine.

Ibopamine is an orally active butyric acid ester of methyldopamine (also called epinine). The ester linkage is hydrolyzed by nonspecific esterases in the blood to yield epinine, which has pharmacologic effects similar to those of dopamine. This compound is presently in clinical trial, and its usefulness is not yet clear.

Dobutamine is a relatively β_1-selective synthetic catecholamine. As discussed below, dobutamine also activates α_1 receptors.

Other Sympathomimetics

These agents are of interest because of pharmacokinetic features (oral activity, distribution to the central nervous system) or because of relative selectivity for specific receptor subclasses.

Phenylephrine was previously described as an example of a relatively pure alpha agonist (Table 9–2). It acts directly on the receptors. Because it is not a catechol derivative (Figure 9–4), it is not inactivated by COMT and has a much longer duration of action than the catecholamines. It is an effective mydriatic and decongestant and can be used to raise the blood pressure (Figure 9–6).

Methoxamine acts pharmacologically like phenylephrine, since it is predominantly a direct-acting alpha$_1$-receptor agonist. It may cause a prolonged increase in blood pressure due to vasoconstriction; it also causes a vagally mediated bradycardia. Methoxamine is available for parenteral use, but clinical applications are rare and limited to hypotensive states.

Ephedrine occurs in various plants and has been used in China for over 2000 years; it was introduced into Western medicine approximately 70 years ago as the first orally active sympathomimetic drug. Because it is a noncatechol phenylisopropylamine (Figure 9–4), it has high bioavailability and a long duration of action. As is the case with many other phenylisopropylamines, a significant fraction of the drug is excreted unchanged in the urine. Since it is a weak base, its excretion can be accelerated by acidification of the urine.

Ephedrine acts primarily through the release of stored catecholamines; in addition, it has some direct actions on adrenoceptors. It is nonselective and mimics epinephrine in its spectrum of effects. Because it gains access to the central nervous system, it causes a mild amphetamine-like stimulation that is not seen with the catecholamines.

Clinically, ephedrine is utilized when a prolonged duration of effect is desired, particularly after oral administration. The main applications are as a nasal decongestant and as a pressor agent.

Xylometazoline and **oxymetazoline** are direct-acting alpha agonists. These drugs have been used as topical decongestants because of their ability to promote constriction of the nasal mucosa. When taken in large doses, oxymetazoline may cause hypotension, presumably because of a central clonidine-like effect (Chapter 11). (As noted in Table 9–1, oxymetazoline has significant affinity for alpha$_{2A}$ receptors.)

Amphetamine is a phenylisopropylamine (Figure 9–4) that is important chiefly because of its use and misuse as a central nervous system stimulant (see Chapter 31). Its pharmacokinetics are similar to those of ephedrine, but amphetamine enters the central nervous system even more readily and has a much more marked stimulant effect on mood and alertness and a depressant effect on appetite. Its peripheral actions are mediated primarily through the release of catecholamines. **Methamphetamine** (N-methylamphetamine) is very similar to amphetamine with an even higher ratio of central to peripheral actions. **Phenmetrazine** (see Figure 31–1) is a variant phenylisopropylamine with amphetamine-like effects. It has been promoted as an anorexiant and is also a popular drug of abuse. **Methylphenidate** and **pemoline** are amphetamine variants whose major pharmacologic effects and abuse potential are similar to those of amphetamine. Amphetamine-like drugs appear to have efficacy in some children with attention deficit hyperactivity disorder (see Clinical Pharmacology). **Phenylpropanolamine** is an amphetamine variant with weak effects on mood that is available over the counter in numerous weight reduction medications. Though relatively safe in recommended dosage, it is associated with severe hypertension and risk of stroke or myocardial damage when taken in large doses. There is no evidence that treatment of obesity with these drugs leads to prolonged weight loss.

Receptor-Selective Sympathomimetic Drugs

Alpha$_1$-selective drugs have no special advantages over nonselective drugs. Alpha$_2$-selective agonists, on the other hand, have a paradoxical ability to *reduce* blood pressure through actions in the central nervous system even though local application may cause vasoconstriction. Such drugs (eg, clonidine, methyldopa, guanfacine, guanabenz) are useful in the treatment of hypertension and are discussed in Chapter 11.

Beta-selective agonists are very important because of the separation of β_1 and β_2 effects that has been achieved (Table 9–2). Although this separation is incomplete, it is sufficient to reduce adverse effects in several clinical applications.

Beta$_1$-selective agents include dobutamine and a partial agonist, prenalterol (Figure 9–7). Because they are less effective in activating vasodilator β_2 re-

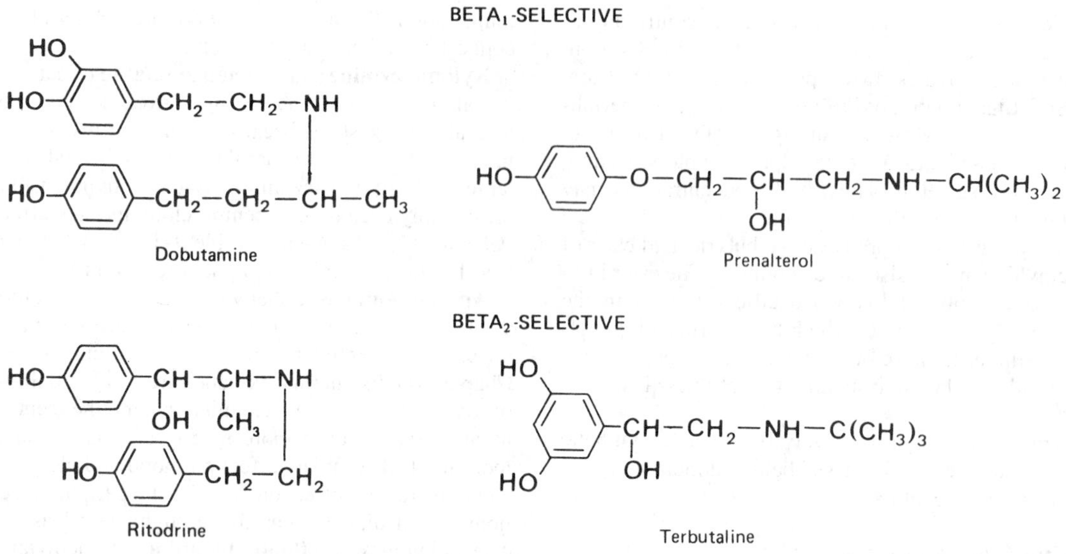

BETA₁-SELECTIVE

Dobutamine

Prenalterol

BETA₂-SELECTIVE

Ritodrine

Terbutaline

Figure 9–7. Examples of β_1- and β_2-selective agonists.

ceptors, they may increase cardiac output with less reflex tachycardia than occurs with nonselective beta agonists such as isoproterenol. Some of the important pharmacologic effects of dobutamine are critically dependent on the use of a racemic mixture. While one isomer is a good beta₁ agonist, it is likely that the other stereoisomer of dobutamine has alpha-receptor activity; this action tends to reduce vasodilation and may also contribute to the positive inotropic action caused by the isomer with predominantly beta-receptor activity. A major limitation with these drugs—as with other direct-acting sympathomimetic agents—is that tolerance to their effects may develop with prolonged use.

Beta₂-selective agents have achieved an important place in the treatment of asthma and are discussed in Chapter 19. An additional application is as uterine relaxants in premature labor (ritodrine; see below). Some examples of drugs currently in use are shown in Figures 9–7 and 19–6; many more are available or under investigation.

Special Sympathomimetics

Cocaine is a local anesthetic with a peripheral sympathomimetic action that results from inhibition of transmitter reuptake at noradrenergic synapses (see Chapter 6). It readily enters the central nervous system and produces an amphetamine-like effect that is shorter lasting and more intense. These properties and the fact that it can be smoked, "snorted," or injected for rapid onset of effect have made it a very heavily abused drug (see Chapter 31).

Tyramine (see Figure 6–5) is a normal by-product of tyrosine metabolism in the body and is also found in high concentrations in fermented foods such as cheese (Table 9–5). It is readily metabolized by MAO

and is normally inactive if ingested because of a very high first-pass effect. If administered parenterally, it has an indirect sympathomimetic action caused by the release of stored catecholamines. Thus, its spectrum of action is similar to that of norepinephrine. In pa-

Table 9–5. Foods reputed to have a high content of tyramine or other sympathomimetic agents. In a patient taking an irreversible MAO inhibitor drug, 20–50 mg of tyramine in a meal may increase the blood pressure significantly (see also Chapter 29). Note that only cheese, sausage, pickled fish, and yeast supplements contain sufficient tyramine to be consistently dangerous. This does not rule out the possibility that some preparations of other foods might contain significantly greater than average amounts of tyramine

Food	Tyramine Content of an Average Serving
Beer	(No data)
Broad beans, fava beans	Negligible (but contains dopamine)
Cheese, natural or aged	Nil to 130 mg (Cheddar, Gruyere, and Stilton especially high)
Chicken liver	Nil to 9 mg
Chocolate	Negligible (but contains phenylethylamine)
Sausage, fermented (eg, salami, pepperoni, summer sausage)	Nil to 74 mg
Smoked or pickled fish (eg, pickled herring)	Nil to 198 mg
Snails	(No data)
Wine (red)	Nil to 3 mg
Yeast (eg, dietary brewer's yeast supplements)	2–68 mg

tients treated with MAO inhibitors—particularly inhibitors of the MAO-A isoform—this effect of tyramine may be greatly intensified, leading to marked increases in blood pressure.

II. CLINICAL PHARMACOLOGY OF SYMPATHOMIMETIC DRUGS

The rationale for the use of sympathomimetic drugs in therapy rests on a knowledge of the physiologic effects of catecholamines on tissues. Selection of a particular sympathomimetic drug from the host of compounds available depends upon such factors as whether activation of alpha, β_1, or β_2 receptors is desired; the duration of action desired; and the preferred route of administration. Sympathomimetic drugs are very potent and can have profound effects on a variety of organ systems, particularly the heart and peripheral circulation. Therefore, great caution is indicated when these agents are used parenterally. In most cases, rather than using fixed doses of the drugs, careful monitoring of pharmacologic response is required to determine the appropriate dosage, especially if the drug is being infused. Generally, it is desirable to use the minimum dose required to achieve the desired response. The adverse effects of these drugs are generally understandable in terms of their known physiologic effects.

Cardiovascular Applications

A. Conditions in Which Blood Flow or Pressure Is to Be Enhanced: Hypotension may occur in a variety of settings such as decreased blood volume, cardiac arrhythmias, adverse reactions to medications such as antihypertensive drugs, and infection. If cerebral, renal, and cardiac perfusion is maintained, hypotension itself does not usually require vigorous direct treatment. Rather, placing the patient in the recumbent position and ensuring adequate fluid volume—while the primary problem is determined and treated—is usually the correct course of action. The use of sympathomimetic drugs merely to elevate a blood pressure that is not an immediate threat to the patient may increase morbidity (see Toxicity of Sympathomimetic Drugs, below). Sympathomimetic drugs may be used in a hypotensive emergency to preserve cerebral and coronary blood flow. Such situations might arise in severe hemorrhage, spinal cord injury, or overdoses of antihypertensive or central nervous system depressant medications. The treatment is usually of short duration while the appropriate intravenous fluid or blood is being administered. Direct-acting alpha agonists such as norepinephrine,

phenylephrine, or methoxamine can be utilized in this setting if vasoconstriction is desired.

Shock is a complex acute cardiovascular syndrome that results in a critical reduction in perfusion of vital tissues and a wide range of systemic effects. Shock is usually associated with hypotension, an altered mental state, oliguria, and metabolic acidosis. If untreated, shock usually progresses to a refractory deteriorating state and death. The three major mechanisms responsible for shock are hypovolemia, cardiac insufficiency, and altered vascular resistance. Volume replacement and treatment of the underlying disease are the mainstays of the treatment of shock. While sympathomimetic drugs have been used in the treatment of virtually all forms of shock, their efficacy is unclear. In most forms of shock, vasoconstriction mediated by the sympathetic nervous system is already intense. Indeed, efforts aimed at reducing rather than increasing peripheral resistance may be more fruitful if cerebral, coronary, and renal perfusion are improved. A decision to use vasoconstrictors or vasodilators is best made on the basis of information about the underlying cause, which may require invasive monitoring.

Cardiogenic shock, usually due to massive myocardial infarction, has a poor prognosis. Mechanically assisted perfusion and emergency cardiac surgery have been utilized in some settings. Optimal fluid replacement requires monitoring of pulmonary capillary wedge pressure. Positive inotropic agents such as dopamine or dobutamine may have a role in this situation. In low to moderate doses, these drugs may increase cardiac output and, compared with norepinephrine, cause relatively little peripheral vasoconstriction. Isoproterenol increases heart rate and work more than either dopamine or dobutamine. See Chapter 13 and Table 13–6 for a discussion of shock associated with myocardial infarction.

Unfortunately, the patient with shock may not respond to any of the above therapeutic maneuvers; the temptation is then great to use vasoconstrictors to maintain adequate blood pressure. While coronary perfusion may be improved, this gain may be offset by increased myocardial oxygen demands as well as more severe vasoconstriction in blood vessels to the abdominal viscera. Therefore, the goal of therapy in shock should be to optimize tissue perfusion, not blood pressure.

B. Conditions in Which Blood Flow Is to Be Reduced: Reduction of regional blood flow is desirable for achieving hemostasis in surgery, for reducing diffusion of local anesthetics away from the site of administration, and for reducing mucous membrane congestion. In each instance, alpha-receptor activation is desired, and the choice of agent depends upon the maximal efficacy required, the desired duration of action, and the route of administration.

Effective pharmacologic hemostasis, often necessary for facial, oral, and nasopharyngeal surgery, requires drugs of high efficacy that can be administered in high concentration by local application. Epinephrine is usually applied topically in nasal packs (for epistaxis) or in a gingival string (gingivectomy). **Cocaine** is still sometimes used for nasopharyngeal surgery, because it combines a hemostatic effect with local anesthesia. Occasionally, cocaine is mixed with epinephrine for maximum hemostasis and local anesthesia.

Combining alpha agonists with local anesthetics greatly prolongs the duration of infiltration nerve block; the total dose of local anesthetic (and the probability of toxicity) can therefore be reduced. **Epinephrine,** 1:200,000, is the favored agent for this application, but norepinephrine, phenylephrine, and other alpha agonists have also been used.

Mucous membrane decongestants reduce the discomfort of hay fever and, to a lesser extent, the common cold by decreasing the volume of the nasal mucosa. Unfortunately, rebound hyperemia may follow the use of these agents, and repeated topical use of high concentrations may result in ischemic changes in the mucous membrane, probably as a result of vasoconstriction of nutrient arteries. Favored short-acting topical agents include phenylephrine and phenylpropanolamine in nasal sprays and ophthalmic drops. A longer duration of action, at the cost of much lower local concentrations and greater cardiac and central nervous system effects, can be achieved by the oral administration of agents such as ephedrine or one of its isomers, pseudoephedrine. Long-acting topical decongestants include xylometazoline and oxymetazoline. All of these mucous membrane decongestants are available as over-the-counter products.

C. Cardiac Applications: Episodes of **paroxysmal atrial tachycardia** were treated in the past with alpha-agonist drugs such as phenylephrine or methoxamine. Because these drugs cause marked vasoconstriction and lead to a rise in blood pressure, a reflex vagal discharge is evoked that may convert the arrhythmia to sinus rhythm. If used for this indication, the drugs should be given by slow intravenous infusion; caution must be exercized to prevent a rise in systolic blood pressure to greater than about 160 mm Hg. While these drugs have been effective in terminating this rhythm disturbance in patients who are hypotensive, generally safer alternatives such as verapamil, adenosine, or electrical cardioversion are currently preferred (Chapter 14).

Catecholamines such as isoproterenol and epinephrine have also been utilized in the temporary emergency management of **complete heart block** and **cardiac arrest.** Epinephrine may be useful in cardiac arrest in part by redistributing blood flow during cardiopulmonary resuscitation to coronaries and to the brain. However, electronic pacemakers are both safer and more effective in heart block and should be inserted as soon as possible if there is any indication of continued high-degree block.

Congestive heart failure may respond to the positive inotropic effects of drugs such as dobutamine and prenalterol. These applications are discussed in Chapter 13. The development of tolerance or desensitization is a major limitation to the use of catecholamines in congestive heart failure.

Respiratory Applications

One of the most important uses of sympathomimetic drugs is in the therapy of bronchial asthma. This use is discussed in Chapter 19. Nonselective drugs (epinephrine), beta-selective agents (isoproterenol), and beta$_2$-selective agents (metaproterenol, terbutaline, albuterol) are all available for this indication. For most patients, the beta$_2$-selective drugs are as effective as and less toxic than the less selective agents. The intensive use of beta-adrenoceptor agonists in asthma has been associated with an increased mortality rate, though the basis for this association is uncertain.

Anaphylaxis

Anaphylactic shock and related immediate (type I) IgE-mediated reactions affect both the respiratory and the cardiovascular systems. The syndrome of bronchospasm, mucous membrane congestion, angioedema, and cardiovascular collapse usually responds rapidly to subcutaneous administration of **epinephrine,** 0.3–0.5 mg (0.3–0.5 mL of 1:1000 epinephrine solution). This drug is the agent of choice because of its great efficacy at alpha, β_1, and β_2 receptors; stimulation of all three is helpful in reversing the pathophysiologic process. Glucocorticoids and antihistamines (both H$_1$ and H$_2$ receptor antagonists) may be useful as secondary therapy in anaphylaxis; however, epinephrine is the initial treatment.

Ophthalmic Applications

Phenylephrine is an effective mydriatic agent frequently used to facilitate examination of the retina. It is also a useful decongestant for minor allergic hyperemia of the conjunctival membranes. Sympathomimetics administered as ophthalmic drops are also useful in localizing the lesion in Horner's syndrome. (See box: An Application of Basic Pharmacology to a Clinical Problem.)

Glaucoma responds to a variety of sympathomimetic and sympathoplegic drugs. (See box in Chapter 10: The Treatment of Glaucoma.) **Epinephrine** and beta-blocking agents are among the most important therapies. Used chronically, topical epinephrine (1–2% solution) lowers intraocular pressure primarily by increasing aqueous outflow. The efficacy of epinephrine may be related in part to desensitization of β-adrenoceptor-mediated responses. **Dipivefrin** is a prodrug of epinephrine formed by esterification of epinephrine with pivalic acid. The ester enjoys enhanced penetration into the anterior chamber of the eye, where it is converted back into

AN APPLICATION OF BASIC PHARMACOLOGY TO A CLINICAL PROBLEM

Horner's syndrome is a condition—usually unilateral—that results from interruption of the sympathetic nerves to the face. The effects include vasodilation, ptosis, miosis, and loss of sweating on the side affected. The syndrome can be caused by either a preganglionic or postganglionic lesion, such as a tumor. Knowledge of the location of the lesion (preganglionic or postganglionic) helps determine the optimum therapy.

An understanding of the effects of denervation on neurotransmitter metabolism permits the clinician to use drugs to localize the lesion. In most situations, a localized lesion in a nerve will cause degeneration of the distal portion of that fiber and loss of transmitter contents from the degenerated nerve ending, without affecting neurons innervated by the fiber. Therefore, a preganglionic lesion will leave the postganglionic adrenergic neuron intact, whereas a postganglionic lesion results in degeneration of the adrenergic nerve endings and loss of stored catecholamines from them. Because indirectly acting sympathomimetics require normal stores of catecholamines, such drugs can be used to test for the presence of normal adrenergic nerve endings. The iris, because it is easily visible and responsive to topical sympathomimetics, is a convenient assay tissue in the patient.

If the lesion of Horner's syndrome is postganglionic, indirectly acting sympathomimetics (eg, cocaine, hydroxyamphetamine) will not dilate the abnormally constricted pupil—because catecholamines have been lost from the nerve endings in the iris. In contrast, the pupil will dilate in response to phenylephrine, which acts directly on the alpha receptors on the smooth muscle of the iris. A patient with a preganglionic lesion, on the other hand, will show a normal response to both drugs, since the postganglionic fibers and their catecholamine stores remain intact in this situation.

epinephrine by enzymatic hydrolysis. Apraclonidine is an α_2-selective agonist that also lowers intraocular pressure and is used after laser therapy.

Genitourinary Applications

As noted above, β_2-selective agents relax the pregnant uterus. **Ritodrine, terbutaline,** and similar drugs have been used to suppress premature labor. The goal is to defer labor long enough to ensure ade-

quate maturation of the fetus. Several trials indicated that these drugs could defer delivery for days or even weeks (eg, Merkatz, 1980). However, meta-analysis of older trials and a recent randomized study suggest that beta-agonist therapy may have no significant benefit on perinatal infant mortality and may increase maternal morbidity (Canada Preterm Labor Investigators Group, 1992).

Oral sympathomimetic therapy is occasionally useful in the treatment of stress incontinence. Ephedrine or pseudoephedrine may be tried.

Central Nervous System Applications

As noted above, the amphetamine-like sympathomimetics have a mood-elevating (euphoriant) effect; this effect is the basis for the widespread abuse of this subgroup (see Chapter 31). The amphetamines also have an alerting, sleep-deferring action that is manifested by improved attention to repetitive tasks and by acceleration and desynchronization of the EEG. A therapeutic application of this effect is in the treatment of narcolepsy. The appetite-suppressing effect of these agents is easily demonstrated in experimental animals. In obese humans, an encouraging initial response may be observed, but there is no evidence that long-term improvement in weight control can be achieved with amphetamines alone. A final application of the CNS-active sympathomimetics is in the attention-deficit hyperkinetic syndrome of children, a poorly defined and overdiagnosed behavioral syndrome consisting of short attention span, hyperkinetic physical behavior, and learning problems. Some patients with this syndrome respond well to low doses of the amphetamine-like drugs.

Additional Therapeutic Uses

While the primary use of the α_2-agonist clonidine is in the treatment of hypertension (Chapter 11), the drug has been found to have efficacy in the treatment of diarrhea in diabetics with autonomic neuropathy, perhaps due to its ability to enhance salt and water absorption from the intestines. In addition, clonidine has efficacy in diminishing craving for narcotics and alcohol during withdrawal and may facilitate cessation of cigarette smoking. Clonidine has also been used to diminish menopausal hot flushes and is being used experimentally to reduce hemodynamic instability during general anesthesia.

TOXICITY OF SYMPATHOMIMETIC DRUGS

The adverse effects of adrenoceptor agonists are primarily extensions of their receptor effects in the cardiovascular and central nervous systems.

Adverse cardiovascular effects seen with pressor agents include marked elevations in blood pressure, which may cause cerebral hemorrhage or pulmonary edema. Increased cardiac work may precipitate severe angina or myocardial infarction. Beta-stimulant drugs frequently cause sinus tachycardia and may provoke serious ventricular arrhythmias. Sympathomimetic drugs may lead to myocardial damage, particularly after prolonged infusion. Special caution is indicated in elderly patients or those with hypertension or coronary artery disease.

If an adverse sympathomimetic effect requires urgent reversal, a specific adrenoceptor antagonist should be used (see Chapter 10). For example, extravasation into subcutaneous tissues of norepine-phrine being given by the intravenous route may lead to marked ischemia that can be reversed by alpha-adrenoceptor antagonists.

Central nervous system toxicity is rarely observed with catecholamines or drugs such as phenylephrine. Phenylisopropylamines commonly cause restlessness, tremor, insomnia, and anxiety. In very high doses, a paranoid state may be induced. Cocaine may precipitate convulsions, cerebral hemorrhage, arrhythmias, or myocardial infarction. The last three of these effects represent sympathomimetic toxicity. Therapy is discussed in Chapter 31.

PREPARATIONS AVAILABLE*

Amphetamine, racemic mixture (generic)
  Oral: 5, 10 mg tablets
Apraclonidine (Iopidine)
  Topical: 1% solution
Dextroamphetamine (generic, Dexedrine)
  Oral: 5, 10 mg tablets; 5 mg/5 mL elixir
  Oral sustained-release: 5, 10, 15 mg capsules
Dobutamine (Dobutrex)
  Parenteral: 250 mg/20 mL for injection
Dopamine (generic, Intropin)
  Parenteral: 40, 80, 160 mg/mL for injection; 80, 160, 320 mg/100 mL in 5% D/W for injection
Ephedrine (generic, Vatronol Nose Drops, Efedron Nasal)
  Oral: 25, 50 mg capsules; 11, 20 mg/5 mL syrups
  Parenteral: 25, 50 mg/mL for injection
  Nasal: 0.5% drops, 0.6% jelly
Epinephrine (generic, Adrenalin Chloride, others)
  Parenteral: 1:1000 (1 mg/mL), 1:10,000 (0.1 mg/mL), 1:100,000 (0.01 mg/mL) for injection
  Ophthalmic: 0.25, 0.5, 1, 2% drops
  Nasal: 0.1% drops and spray
  Aerosol for bronchospasm: 0.16, 0.2, 0.25 mg/spray (Primatene Mist, Bronkaid Mist)
Isoproterenol (generic, Isuprel)
  Oral: 10, 15 mg sublingual tablets
  Parenteral: 0.2 mg/mL for injection
Mephentermine (Wyamine Sulfate)
  Parenteral: 15, 30 mg/mL for injection
Metaraminol (generic, Aramine)
  Parenteral: 10 mg/mL for injection
Methamphetamine (generic, Desoxyn)
  Oral: 5, 10 mg tablets
  Oral sustained-release: 5, 10, 15 mg tablets
Methoxamine (Vasoxyl)
  Parenteral: 20 mg/mL for injection
Methylphenidate (generic, Ritalin-SR)
  Oral: 5, 10, 20 mg tablets
  Oral sustained-release: 20 mg tablets
Naphazoline (Privine)
  Nasal: 0.05% drops and spray
Norepinephrine (Levophed)
  Parenteral: 1 mg/mL for injection
Oxymetazoline (generic, Afrin, Neo-Synephrine 12 Hour, others)
  Nasal: 0.025, 0.05% sprays
Phenmetrazine (Preludin)
  Oral: 75 mg sustained-release tablets
Phenylephrine (generic, Neo-Synephrine)
  Parenteral: 10 mg/mL for injection
  Nasal: 0.125, 0.16, 0.25, 0.2, 0.5, 1% drops and spray; 0.5% jelly
Phenylpropanolamine (generic)
  Oral: 25, 50 mg tablets
  Oral sustained-release: 75 mg capsules
Pseudoephedrine (generic, Sudafed, others)
  Oral: 30, 60 mg tablets; 15, 30 mg/5 mL syrups; 7.5 mg/0.8 mL, 30 mg/mL drops
  Oral sustained-release: 120 mg capsules
Tetrahydrozoline (generic, Tyzine)
  Nasal: 0.05, 0.1% drops
Xylometazoline (generic, Otrivin, Neo-Synephrine Long-Acting, Chlorohist LA)
  Nasal: 0.05, 0.1% drops and spray

---

*Sympathomimetics used in the treatment of asthma are covered in Chapter 19.

REFERENCES

Barach EM et al: Epinephrine for treatment of anaphylactic shock. JAMA 1984;251:2118.

Berridge MJ: Inositol trisphosphate and diacylglycerol: Two interacting second messengers. Annu Rev Biochem 1987;56:159.

Brown CG et al: A comparison of standard dose and high dose epinephrine in cardiac arrest outside the hospital. N Engl J Med 1992;327:1051.

The Canada Preterm Labor Investigators Group: Treatment of preterm labor with the beta-adrenergic agonist ritodrine. N Engl J Med 1992;327:308.

Caron MG, Lefkowitz RJ: Catecholamine receptors: Structure, function, and regulation. Recent Prog Horm Res 1993;48:277.

Collins S, Caron MG, Lefkowitz RJ: Regulation of adrenergic receptor responsiveness through modulation of receptor gene expression. Annu Rev Physiol 1991;53:497.

Conklin BR, Bourne HR: Structural elements of G alpha subunits that interact with G beta gamma, receptors, and effectors. Cell 1993;73:631.

deGroat WC, Steers WD: Autonomic regulation of the urinary bladder and sexual organs. In: *Central Regulation of Autonomic Functions.* Loewy AD, Spyer KM (editors). Oxford, 1990.

Gingrich JA, Caron MG: Recent advances in the molecular biology of dopamine receptors. Annu Rev Neurosci 1993;16:299.

Glassman AH et al: Heavy smokers, smoking cessation, and clonidine: Results of a double-blind, randomized trial. JAMA 1988;259,2863.

Han C, Abel PW, Minneman KP: Alpha 1-adrenoceptor subtypes linked to different mechanisms for increasing intracellular Ca^{2+} in smooth muscle. Nature 1987;329:333.

Hepler JR, Gilman AG: G proteins. Trends Biochem Sci 1992;17:383.

Hurvitz LM et al: New developments in the drug treatment of glaucoma. Drugs 1991;41:514.

Kobilka B: Adrenergic receptors as models for G protein-coupled receptors. Annu Rev Neurosci 1992;15:87.

Limbird LE: Receptors linked to inhibition of adenylate cyclase: Additional signaling mechanisms. FASEB J 1988;2:2686.

Maze M, Segal IS, Bloor BC: Clonidine and other $alpha_2$ adrenergic agonists: Strategies for the rational use of these novel anesthetic agents. J Clin Anesth 1988;1:146.

Merkatz IR, Peter JB, Barden TP: Ritodrine hydrochloride: A betamimetic agent for use in preterm labor. II. Evidence of efficacy. Obstet Gynecol 1980;56:7.

Minneman KP: α_1-Adrenergic receptor subtypes, inositol phosphates, and sources of cell Ca^{2+}. Pharmacol Rev 1988;40:87.

1994 Receptor Nomenclature Supplement. Trends Pharmacol Sci, 1994.

Rasmussen H: The calcium messenger system. (Two parts.) N Engl J Med 1986;314:1094, 1164.

Ruffolo RR Jr et al: Pharmacologic and therapeutic applications of α_2-adrenoceptor subtypes. Annu Rev Pharmacol Toxicol 1993;32:243.

Ruffolo RR Jr et al: Structure and function of alpha-adrenoceptors. Pharmacol Rev 1991;43:475

Ruffolo RR Jr: Fundamentals of receptor theory: Basics for shock research. Circ Shock 1992;37:176.

Sokoloff P et al: Molecular cloning and characterization of a novel dopamine receptor (D3) as a target for neuroleptics. Nature 1990;347:146.

Spitzer WO et al: The use of β-agonists and the risk of death and near death from asthma. N Engl J Med 1992;326:501.

Tang WJ, Gilman AG: Adenylyl cyclases. Cell 1992;70:869.

10 Adrenoceptor-Blocking Drugs

Brian B. Hoffman, MD

Since catecholamines play a role in a variety of physiologic and pathophysiologic responses, drugs that block adrenoceptors have important effects, some of which are of great clinical value. These effects vary dramatically according to the drug's selectivity for alpha and beta receptors. The classification of adrenoceptors into alpha, beta, and dopamine subtypes and the effects of activating these receptors are discussed in Chapters 6 and 9. Blockade of peripheral dopamine receptors is of no recognized clinical importance at present. In contrast, blockade of central nervous system dopamine receptors is very important; drugs that act on these receptors are discussed in Chapters 20 and 28. This chapter deals with pharmacologic antagonist drugs whose major effect is to occupy either alpha or beta receptors outside the central nervous system and prevent their activation by catecholamines and related agonists.

In basic pharmacology, alpha-receptor-blocking drugs have been very useful in the experimental exploration of autonomic nervous system function; in clinical therapeutics, they have had only limited application. Although these drugs effectively block the vasoconstricting effect of catecholamines, their use in hypertension—with the exception of prazosin (and its α_1-selective analogues) and labetalol—has been of little consequence. The place of alpha-receptor antagonists in the treatment of peripheral vascular disease is uncertain. In contrast, beta-receptor-blocking drugs have been found useful in a wide variety of clinical conditions.

I. BASIC PHARMACOLOGY OF THE ALPHA-RECEPTOR-BLOCKING DRUGS

Mechanism of Action

Alpha-receptor antagonists may be reversible or irreversible in their interaction with these receptors.

Reversible antagonists may dissociate from the alpha receptor; irreversible drugs do not. Phentolamine and tolazoline are examples of reversible antagonists (Figure 10–1). Prazosin and labetalol—drugs used primarily for their antihypertensive effects—as well as several ergot derivatives (see Chapter 16) are also reversible alpha-adrenoceptor blockers. Phenoxybenzamine, an agent related to the nitrogen mustards, forms a reactive ethyleneimonium intermediate (Figure 10–1) that covalently binds to the alpha receptor, resulting in irreversible blockade. Figure 10–2 illustrates the effects of a reversible drug in comparison with those of an irreversible agent.

The duration of action of a *reversible* antagonist is largely dependent on the half-life of the drug and the rate at which it dissociates from its receptor: the shorter the half-life, the less time it takes for the effects of the drug to disappear. However, the effects of an *irreversible* antagonist may persist long after the drug has been cleared from the plasma. In the case of phenoxybenzamine, the restoration of tissue responsiveness after extensive alpha-receptor blockade is dependent on synthesis of new receptors, which may take several days.

Pharmacologic Effects

A. Cardiovascular Effects: Because arteriolar and venous tone are determined to a large extent by alpha receptors on vascular smooth muscle, alpha-receptor-blocking drugs cause a lowering of peripheral vascular resistance and blood pressure (Figure 10–3). They can prevent the pressor effects of usual doses of alpha agonists; indeed, in the case of agonists with both alpha and β_2 effects (eg, epinephrine), they convert a pressor to a depressor response (Figure 10–3). This change in response is called **epinephrine reversal.** Alpha-blockers may cause postural hypotension and reflex tachycardia. Tachycardia may be more marked with agents that block α_2 presynaptic receptors in the heart (Table 10–1), since the augmented release of norepinephrine will further stimulate beta receptors in the heart. Chronic use of alpha antagonists may result in a compensatory increase in blood volume.

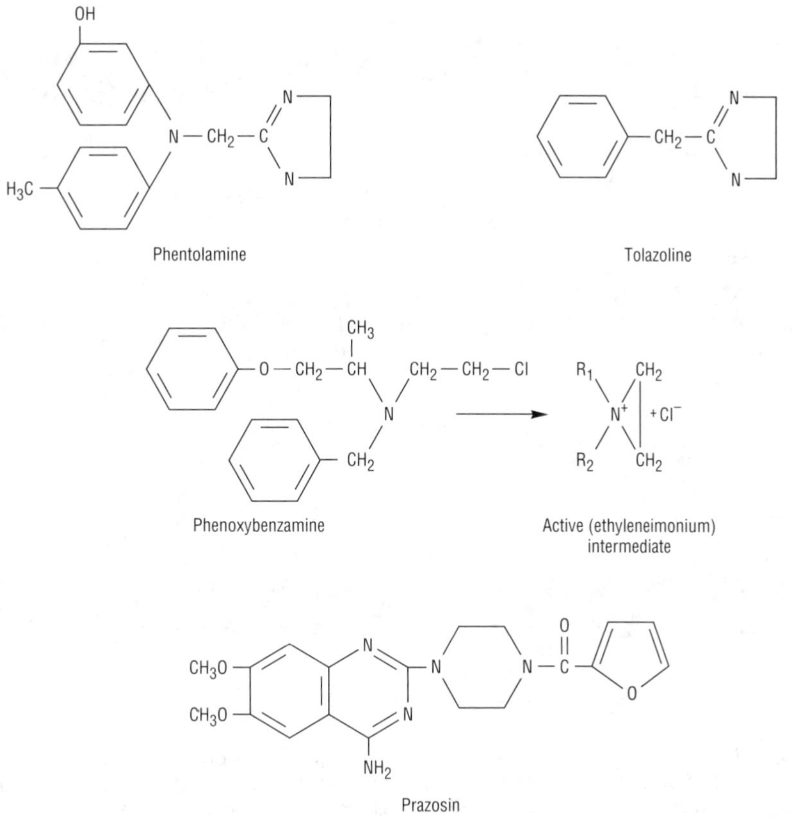

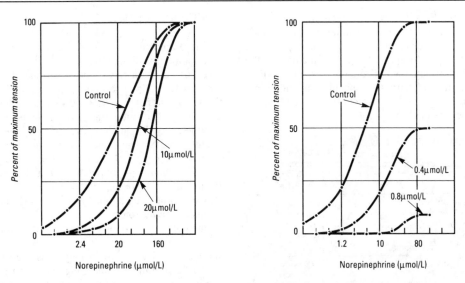

Figure 10–1. Structure of several alpha-receptor-blocking drugs.

Figure 10–2. Dose-response curves to norepinephrine in the presence of two different alpha-adrenoceptor-blocking drugs. The tension produced in isolated strips of cat spleen, a tissue rich in alpha receptors, was measured in response to graded doses of norepinephrine. **Left:** Tolazoline, a reversible blocker, shifted the curve to the right without decreasing the maximum response when present at concentrations of 10 and 20 μmol/L. **Right:** Dibenamine, an analogue of phenoxybenzamine and irreversible in its action, reduced the maximum response attainable at both concentrations tested. (Modified and reproduced, with permission, from Bickerton RK: The response of isolated strips of cat spleen to sympathomimetic drugs and their antagonists. J Pharmacol Exp Ther 1963;142:99.)

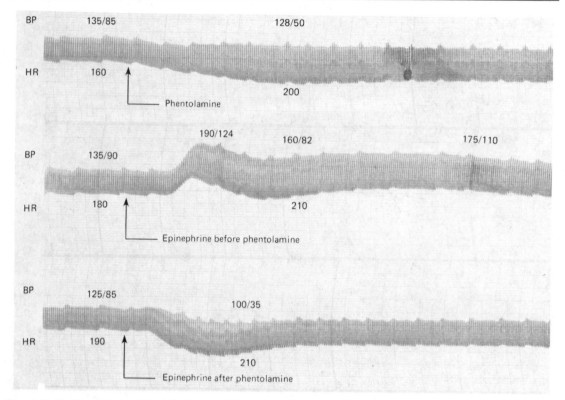

Figure 10–3. *Top:* Effects of phentolamine, an alpha-receptor-blocking drug, on blood pressure in an anesthetized dog. Epinephrine reversal is demonstrated by tracings showing the response to epinephrine before *(middle)* and after *(bottom)* phentolamine. All drugs given intravenously. (BP, blood pressure; HR, heart rate.)

B. Other Effects: Minor effects that signal the blockade of alpha receptors in other tissues include miosis, decreased adrenergic sweating, and nasal stuffiness. Alpha-receptor blockade of the base of the bladder is associated with decreased resistance to the flow of urine and retrograde ejaculation. Individual agents may have other important effects in addition to alpha blockade (see below).

Table 10–1. Relative selectivity of antagonists for adrenoceptors.

	Receptor Affinity
Alpha antagonists	
Prazosin, terazosin, doxazosin	$\alpha_1 >>>> \alpha_2$
Phenoxybenzamine	$\alpha_1 > \alpha_2$
Phentolamine	$\alpha_1 = \alpha_2$
Rauwolscine, yohimbine, tolazoline	$\alpha_2 >> \alpha_1$
Mixed antagonist	
Labetalol	$\beta_1 = \beta_2 \geq \alpha_1 > \alpha_2$
Beta antagonists	
Metoprolol, acebutolol, alprenolol, atenolol, betaxolol, celiprolol, esmolol	$\beta_1 >>> \beta_2$
Propranolol, carteolol, penbutolol, pindolol, timolol	$\beta_1 = \beta_2$
Butoxamine	$\beta_2 >>> \beta_1$

SPECIFIC AGENTS

Phentolamine, an imidazoline derivative, is a potent competitive antagonist at alpha receptors. Phentolamine causes a reduction in peripheral resistance through both alpha-receptor blockade and an additional nonadrenergic action on vascular smooth muscle. The cardiac stimulation induced by phentolamine may be reflex in part; however, a component of this stimulation is not dependent on baroreceptor activity. Alpha$_2$-receptor blockade may be involved. Phentolamine is about equally potent at α_1 and α_2 receptors. Phentolamine also inhibits responses to serotonin. Phentolamine is an agonist at muscarinic and H$_1$ and H$_2$ histamine receptors.

Phentolamine is poorly absorbed after oral administration. The principal adverse effects are related to cardiac stimulation, which may cause severe tachycardia, arrhythmias, and angina. Gastrointestinal stimulation may cause diarrhea and increased gastric acid production.

Tolazoline is similar to phentolamine. It is somewhat less potent but is better absorbed from the gastrointestinal tract. It is rapidly excreted in the urine.

Tolazoline has very limited clinical applications in peripheral vasospastic disease and in the treatment of pulmonary hypertension in newborn infants with respiratory distress syndrome. It is rarely used.

Ergot derivatives—eg, ergotamine, dihydroergotamine—cause reversible alpha-receptor blockade. However, most of the clinically significant effects of these drugs are the result of other actions; eg, ergotamine probably acts at serotonin receptors in the treatment of migraine (see Chapter 16).

Phenoxybenzamine binds covalently to alpha receptors, causing irreversible blockade of long duration (14–48 hours). It is somewhat selective for α_1 receptors but less so than prazosin (Table 10–1). The drug inhibits reuptake of released norepinephrine by presynaptic adrenergic nerve terminals. Phenoxybenzamine blocks histamine (H_1), acetylcholine, and serotonin receptors as well as alpha receptors. The role (if any) of these secondary actions in human pharmacology is not well defined.

The pharmacologic actions of phenoxybenzamine are primarily related to antagonism of alpha-receptor-mediated events. Most importantly, phenoxybenzamine blocks catecholamine-induced vasoconstriction. While phenoxybenzamine causes relatively little fall in blood pressure in supine individuals, it will reduce blood pressure when sympathetic tone is high, eg, as a result of upright posture or because of reduced blood volume. Cardiac output may be increased because of reflex effects and because of some blockade of presynaptic α_2 receptors in cardiac sympathetic nerves.

Phenoxybenzamine is absorbed after oral administration, though bioavailability is low. The drug is usually given orally, starting with low doses of 10–20 mg/d and progressively increasing the dose until the desired effect is achieved. Less than 100 mg/d is usually sufficient to achieve adequate alpha-receptor blockade.

The adverse effects of phenoxybenzamine derive from its alpha-receptor-blocking action; the most important are postural hypotension and tachycardia. Nasal stuffiness and inhibition of ejaculation also occur. Since phenoxybenzamine enters the central nervous system, it may cause less specific effects, including fatigue, sedation, and nausea. Since phenoxybenzamine is an alkylating agent, it may have other adverse effects that have not yet been characterized. Phenoxybenzamine causes tumors in animals, but the clinical implications of this observation are unknown.

Prazosin is effective in the management of hypertension (see Chapter 11). It was originally thought to be a direct-acting vasodilator, but it is now clear that the major pharmacologic action of prazosin is that of an extremely potent alpha-receptor antagonist. It is highly selective for α_1 receptors, having relatively low affinity for α_2 receptors. This may partially explain the relative absence of tachycardia seen with prazosin as compared to that seen with phentolamine and phenoxybenzamine. Prazosin leads to relaxation of both arterial and venous smooth muscle.

Prazosin is extensively metabolized in humans; because of metabolic degradation by the liver, only about 50% of the drug is available after oral administration. The half-life is normally about 3 hours.

Terazosin is another reversible α_1-selective antagonist that is effective in hypertension (see Chapter 11); it has also been approved for use in men with urinary symptoms due to prostatic hypertrophy. Terazosin has high bioavailability yet is extensively metabolized in the liver, with only a small fraction of parent drug excreted in the urine. The half-life of terazosin is about 9–12 hours. **Doxazosin** is the third α_1-selective antagonist approved for use in hypertension. It has moderate bioavailability and is extensively metabolized, with very little parent drug excreted in urine or feces. Doxazosin has active metabolites, though their contribution to the drug's effects is probably small. The parent compound has a half-life of about 22 hours.

OTHER ALPHA-ADRENOCEPTOR ANTAGONISTS

Indoramin is another α_1-selective antagonist that also has efficacy as an antihypertensive. **Urapidil** is a newer α_1 antagonist (its primary effect) that also has weak α_2-agonist and 5-HT_{1A}-agonist actions and weak antagonist action at β_1 receptors. It is used in Europe as an antihypertensive agent. **Labetalol** has both α_1-selective and beta-blocking effects; it is discussed below. Neuroleptic drugs such as chlorpromazine and haloperidol are potent alpha-receptor and dopamine-receptor antagonists. Although these drugs are not used clinically to block alpha receptors, this action may contribute to their adverse effects (eg, hypotension).

Yohimbine is an α_2-selective agent. It has no established clinical role. Theoretically, it could be useful in autonomic insufficiency by promoting neurotransmitter release through blockade of presynaptic α_2 receptors. Yohimbine may improve symptoms in some patients with painful diabetic neuropathies. It has been suggested that yohimbine improves sexual function; however, evidence for this effect in humans is limited.

It is somewhat surprising that α_2 antagonists have so little clinical usefulness. There is experimental interest in the development of highly selective antagonists to inhibit smooth muscle contraction in Raynaud's phenomenon, and for use in type II diabetes (α_2 receptors inhibit insulin secretion), and in psychiatric depression (Ruffolo et al, 1993). It is not known to what extent the recognition of multiple subtypes of α_2 receptors will lead to development of clinically useful subtype-selective new drugs.

II. CLINICAL PHARMACOLOGY OF THE ALPHA-RECEPTOR-BLOCKING DRUGS

Pheochromocytoma

The major clinical use of both phenoxybenzamine and phentolamine is in the management of pheochromocytoma. Pheochromocytoma is a tumor usually found in the adrenal medulla that releases a mixture of epinephrine and norepinephrine. Patients have many signs of catecholamine excess, including hypertension, tachycardia, and arrhythmias.

The diagnosis of pheochromocytoma is usually made on the basis of chemical assay of circulating catecholamines and urinary excretion of catecholamine metabolites, especially 3-hydroxy-4-methoxymandelic acid, metanephrine, and normetanephrine. Infusion of phentolamine has been advocated as a diagnostic test when pheochromocytoma is suspected, since patients with this tumor often manifest a greater-than-average drop in blood pressure in response to alpha-blocking drugs. However, measurement of circulating catecholamines and urinary catecholamines and their metabolites is a more reliable and safer diagnostic approach. Injection of a bolus dose of phentolamine may lead to a dangerous fall in blood pressure in a patient with a pheochromocytoma. Provocative testing for pheochromocytoma by infusion of drugs such as histamine may cause dangerous blood pressure elevation if performed improperly. Unavoidable release of stored catecholamines sometimes occurs during operative manipulation of pheochromocytoma; the resulting hypertension may be controlled with phentolamine or nitroprusside. Nitroprusside has many advantages, particularly since its effects can be more readily titrated and it has a shorter duration of action.

Alpha-receptor antagonists are most useful in the preoperative management of patients with pheochromocytoma (Figure 10–4). Administration of phenoxybenzamine in the preoperative period will prevent precipitation of acute hypertensive episodes during studies undertaken to localize the tumor and will tend to reverse chronic changes resulting from excessive catecholamine secretion such as plasma volume contraction, if present. Furthermore, the patient's operative course may be simplified. Oral doses of 10–20 mg/d may be increased at intervals of several days until hypertension is controlled. Some physicians treat patients with pheochromocytoma with phenoxybenzamine for 1–3 weeks before surgery, whereas others prefer to operate sooner. Phenoxybenzamine may be very useful in the chronic treatment of inoperable or metastatic pheochromocytoma. Although there is less experience with alternative

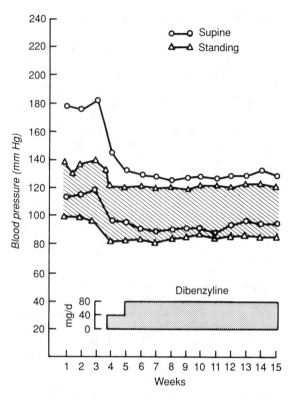

Figure 10–4. Effects of phenoxybenzamine *(Dibenzyline)* on blood pressure in a patient with pheochromocytoma. Dosage of the drug was begun in the third week as shown by the shaded bar. Supine systolic and diastolic pressures are indicated by the circles, the standing pressures by triangles and the hatched area. Note that the alpha-blocking drug dramatically reduced blood pressure. The reduction in orthostatic hypotension, which was marked *before* treatment is probably due to normalization of blood volume, a variable that is sometimes markedly reduced in patients with long-standing pheochromocytoma-induced hypertension. (Redrawn and reproduced, with permission, from Engelman E, Sjoerdsma A: Chronic medical therapy for pheochromocytoma. Ann Intern Med 1961;61:229.)

drugs, hypertension in patients with pheochromocytoma may also respond to reversible α_1-selective antagonists or to conventional calcium antagonists.

Beta-blocking drugs may be required after alpha-receptor blockade has been instituted to reverse the cardiac effects of excessive catecholamines. Beta antagonists should not be employed prior to establishing effective alpha-receptor blockade, since unopposed beta-receptor blockade could theoretically cause blood pressure elevation from increased vasoconstriction.

Pheochromocytoma is rarely treated with **metyrosine,** the α-methyl analogue of tyrosine (α-methyltyrosine). This agent is a competitive inhibitor of tyrosine hydroxylase and, in oral doses of 1–4 g/d, interferes with synthesis of dopamine (see Figure 6–5), thereby decreasing the amounts of norepinephrine and epinephrine secreted by the tumor. Metyrosine has no alpha-blocking effects but may act synergistically with phenoxybenzamine in the treatment of pheochromocytoma.

Hypertensive Emergencies

The alpha-adrenoceptor-blocking drugs have limited application in the management of hypertensive emergencies, though labetalol has been increasingly used. In theory, alpha-adrenoceptor antagonists are most useful when increased blood pressure reflects excess circulating concentrations of alpha agonists. In this circumstance, which may result from pheochromocytoma, overdosage of sympathomimetic drugs, or clonidine withdrawal, phentolamine can be used to control high blood pressure. However, other drugs are generally preferable (see Chapter 11), since considerable experience is necessary to use phentolamine safely in these settings.

Chronic Hypertension

Members of the prazosin family of α_1-selective antagonists are efficacious drugs in the treatment of mild to moderate systemic hypertension. They are generally well tolerated by most patients. Their major adverse effect is postural hypotension, which may be severe after the first dose (see Chapter 11). Nonselective alpha antagonists are not used in ordinary hypertension.

Peripheral Vascular Disease

Although alpha-receptor-blocking drugs have been tried in the treatment of peripheral vascular occlusive disease, there is no evidence that the effects are significant when morphologic changes limit flow in the vessels. Occasionally, individuals with Raynaud's phenomenon and other conditions involving excessive reversible vasospasm in the peripheral circulation do benefit from phentolamine, tolazoline, or phenoxybenzamine, though calcium channel blockers may be preferable for many patients.

Local Vasoconstrictor Excess

Phentolamine is also useful to reverse the intense local vasoconstriction caused by inadvertent infiltration of alpha agonists (eg, norepinephrine) into subcutaneous tissue during intravenous administration. The alpha antagonist is administered by local infiltration into the ischemic tissue.

Urinary Obstruction

While the primary therapy for prostatic hypertrophy is surgery, alpha-receptor blockade with phenoxybenzamine has been found to be helpful in selected patients with urinary obstruction who are poor operative risks. The mechanism of action presumably involves partial reversal of smooth muscle contraction in the enlarged prostate or in the bladder base. In addition, phenoxybenzamine may be useful in relieving bladder neck hypertonus in patients with spinal cord injury. However, the long-term safety of phenoxybenzamine has not been established. Low doses of α_1-selective antagonists are useful for some patients with obstructive symptoms. Indeed, in terms of safety, these drugs are probably preferable to phenoxybenzamine, and terazosin is approved for this indication.

Male Sexual Dysfunction

A combination of the alpha-adrenoceptor antagonist phentolamine with the nonspecific vasodilator papaverine, when injected directly into the penis, may cause erections in men with sexual dysfunction. The long-term efficacy of this form of therapy is not known; there is a risk of fibrotic reactions with long-term administration. Systemic absorption may lead to orthostatic hypotension; priapism may require direct treatment with an alpha-adrenoceptor agonist such as phenylephrine. Drugs such as PGE_1 and nitric oxide donors are being evaluated as alternative therapy for erectile dysfunction.

III. BASIC PHARMACOLOGY OF THE BETA-RECEPTOR-BLOCKING DRUGS

Drugs in this category share the common feature of antagonizing the effects of catecholamines at beta adrenoceptors. Beta-blocking drugs occupy beta receptors and competitively reduce receptor occupancy by catecholamines and other beta agonists. (A few members of this group, used only for experimental purposes, bind irreversibly to beta receptors.) Most beta-blocking drugs in clinical use are pure antagonists; ie, the occupancy of a beta receptor by such a drug causes no activation of the receptor. However, a few beta-receptor-blocking drugs are partial agonists; ie, they cause partial activation of the receptor, albeit less than that caused by the full agonists epinephrine and isoproterenol. Another major difference among the many beta-receptor-blocking drugs concerns their relative affinities for β_1 and β_2 receptors (Table 10–1). Some of these antagonists have a higher affinity for β_1 than for β_2 receptors, and this selectivity may have important clinical implications. Other major differences among beta antagonists relate to their pharmacokinetic characteristics and local anesthetic membrane-stabilizing effects.

Chemically, the beta-receptor-antagonist drugs (Figure 10–5) resemble isoproterenol (see Figure 9–3), a potent beta-receptor agonist.

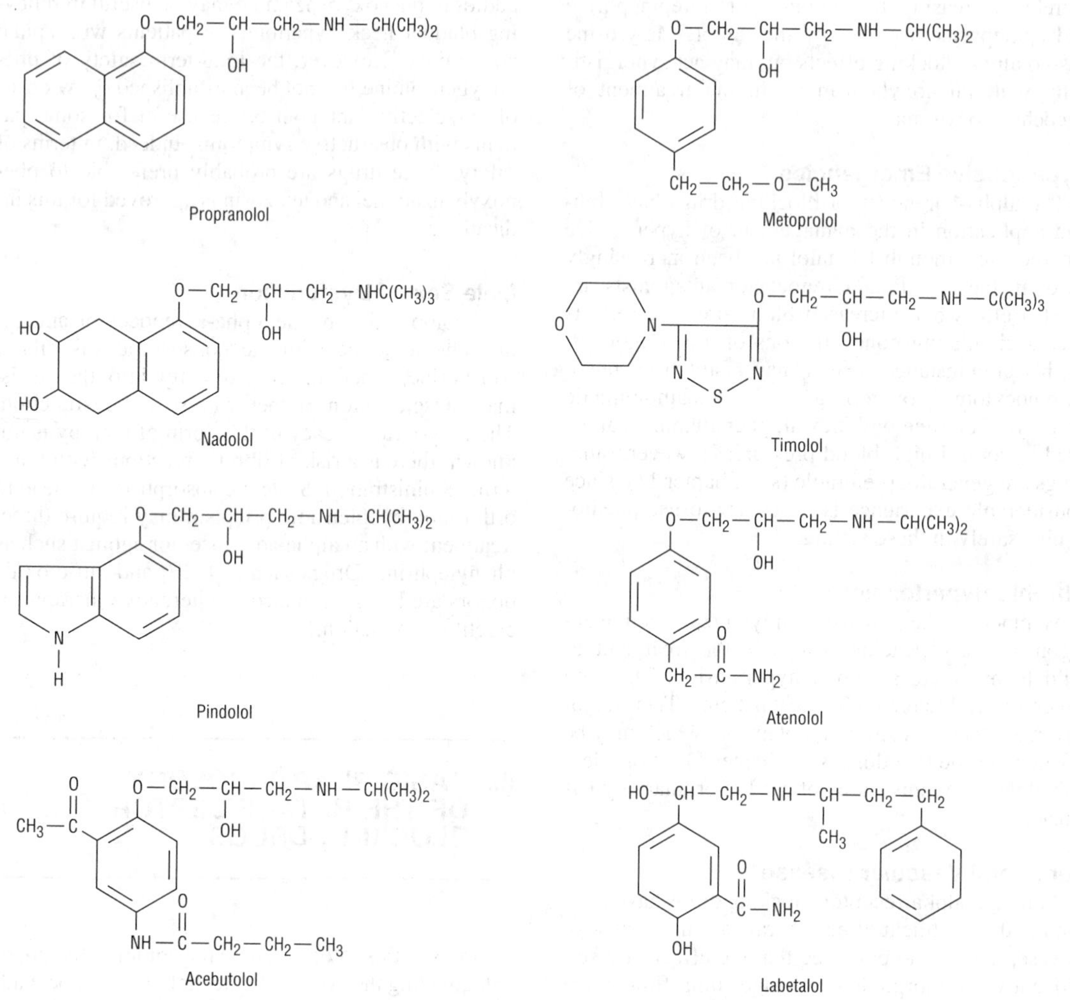

Propranolol

Metoprolol

Nadolol

Timolol

Pindolol

Atenolol

Acebutolol

Labetalol

Figure 10–5. Structures of some beta-receptor antagonists.

Pharmacokinetic Properties of the Beta-Receptor Antagonists

A. Absorption: Most of the drugs in this class are well absorbed after oral administration; peak concentrations occur 1–3 hours after ingestion. Sustained-release preparations of propranolol and metoprolol are available.

B. Bioavailability: Propranolol undergoes extensive hepatic (first-pass) metabolism; its bioavailability is relatively low (Table 10–2). The proportion of drug reaching the systemic circulation increases as the dose is increased, suggesting that hepatic extraction mechanisms may become saturated. A major consequence of the low bioavailability of propranolol is that oral administration of the drug leads to much lower drug concentrations than are achieved after intravenous injection of the same dose. Because the first-pass effect varies among individuals, there is great individual variability in the plasma concentra-

tions achieved after oral propranolol. Bioavailability is limited to varying degrees for most beta antagonists with the exception of betaxolol, pindolol, penbutolol, and sotalol.

C. Distribution and Clearance: The beta antagonists are rapidly distributed and have large volumes of distribution. Propranolol and penbutolol are quite lipophilic and readily cross the blood-brain barrier (Table 10–2). Most beta antagonists have half-lives in the range of 2–5 hours. A major exception is esmolol, which is rapidly hydrolyzed and has a half-life of approximately 10 minutes. Propranolol and metoprolol are extensively metabolized in the liver, with little unchanged drug appearing in the urine. Atenolol, celiprolol, and pindolol are less completely metabolized. Nadolol is excreted unchanged in the urine and has the longest half-life of any available beta antagonist (up to 24 hours). The half-life of nadolol is prolonged in renal failure. The elimination

	Selectivity	Partial Agonist Activity	Local Anesthetic Action	Lipid Solubility	Elimination Half-Life	Approximate Bioavailability
Acebutolol	β_1	Yes	Yes	Low	3–4 hours	50
Atenolol	β_1	No	No	Low	6–9 hours	40
Betaxolol	β_1	No	Slight	Low	14–22 hours	90
Bisoprolol	β_1	No	No	Low	9–12 hours	80
Carteolol	None	Yes	No	Low	6 hours	85
Celiprolol	β_1	Yes[1]	No	...	4–5 hours	70
Esmolol	β_1	No	No	Low	10 minutes	...
Labetalol[2]	None	Yes[1]	Yes	Moderate	5 hours	30
Metoprolol	β_1	No	Yes	Moderate	3–4 hours	50
Nadolol	None	No	No	Low	14–24 hours	33
Penbutolol	None	Yes	No	High	5 hours	>90
Pindolol	None	Yes	Yes	Moderate	3–4 hours	90
Propranolol	None	No	Yes	High	3½–6 hours	30[3]
Sotalol	None	No	No	Low	12 hours	90
Timolol	None	No	No	Moderate	4–5 hours	50

Table 10–2. Properties of several beta-receptor-blocking drugs.

[1]Partial agonist effects at β_2 receptors.
[2]Labetalol also causes α_1-selective blockade.
[3]Bioavailability is dose-dependent.

of drugs such as propranolol may be prolonged in the presence of liver disease, diminished hepatic blood flow, or hepatic enzyme inhibition. It is notable that the clinical effects of these drugs are often prolonged well beyond the time predicted from half-life data.

Pharmacodynamics of the Beta-Receptor-Antagonist Drugs

Most of the effects of these drugs are due to occupancy and blockade of beta receptors. However, some actions may be due to other effects, including partial agonist activity at beta receptors and local anesthetic action—which differ among the beta-blockers (Table 10–2).

A. Effects on the Cardiovascular System: Beta-blocking drugs given chronically *lower* blood pressure in patients with hypertension. The factors involved may include effects on the heart and blood vessels, the renin-angiotensin system, and perhaps the central nervous system. Beta-adrenoceptor-blocking drugs are of major clinical importance in the treatment of hypertension (see Chapter 11). In conventional doses, these drugs do not usually cause hypotension in healthy individuals with normal blood pressure.

Beta-receptor antagonists have prominent effects on the heart (Figure 10–6). The negative inotropic and chronotropic effects are predictable from the role of adrenoceptors in regulating these functions. Slowed atrioventricular conduction with an increased PR interval is a related result of adrenoceptor blockade in the atrioventricular node. These effects may be

clinically valuable in some patients but are potentially hazardous in others. In the vascular system, beta-receptor blockade opposes β_2-mediated vasodilation. This may result initially in a rise in peripheral resistance from unopposed alpha-receptor-mediated effects. Beta-blocking drugs antagonize the release of renin caused by the sympathetic nervous system. As noted in Chapter 11, the relation between the effects on renin release and those on blood pressure is still being debated.

B. Effects on the Respiratory Tract: Blockade of the β_2 receptors in bronchial smooth muscle may lead to an increase in airway resistance, particularly in patients with asthma. Beta$_1$-receptor antagonists such as metoprolol or atenolol may have some advantage over nonselective beta antagonists when blockade of β_1 receptors in the heart is desired and β_2-receptor blockade is undesirable. However, no currently available β_1-selective antagonist is sufficiently specific to *completely* avoid interactions with β_2-adrenoceptors. Consequently, these drugs should generally be avoided in patients with asthma.

C. Effects on the Eye: Several beta-blocking agents reduce intraocular pressure, especially in glaucomatous eyes. The mechanism usually reported is decreased aqueous humor production. (See Clinical Pharmacology and box: The Treatment of Glaucoma.)

D. Metabolic and Endocrine Effects: Beta antagonists such as propranolol inhibit sympathetic nervous system stimulation of lipolysis. The effects on carbohydrate metabolism are less clear, though

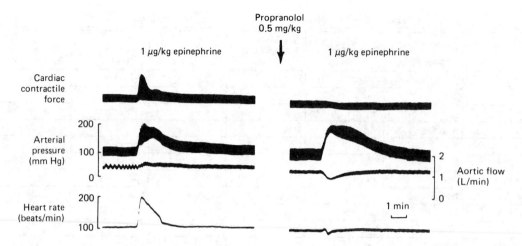

Figure 10–6. The effect in an anesthetized dog of the injection of epinephrine before and after propranolol. In the presence of a beta-receptor-blocking agent, epinephrine no longer augments the force of contraction (measured by a strain gauge attached to the ventricular wall) nor increases cardiac rate. Blood pressure is still elevated by epinephrine because vasoconstriction is not blocked. (Reproduced, with permission, from Shanks RG: The pharmacology of beta sympathetic blockade. Am J Cardiol 1966;18:312.)

glycogenolysis in the liver is at least partially inhibited after beta blockade. However, glucagon is the primary hormone employed to combat hypoglycemia. It is unclear to what extent beta antagonists impair recovery from hypoglycemia, but they should be used with caution in insulin-dependent diabetic patients. This may be particularly important in diabetic patients with inadequate glucagon reserve or in pancreatectomized patients. The chronic use of beta-adrenoceptor antagonists has been associated with increased plasma concentrations of VLDL and decreased concentrations of HDL cholesterol. Both of these changes are potentially unfavorable in terms of risk of cardiovascular disease. Although LDL concentrations generally do not change, there is a variable decline in the HDL cholesterol/LDL cholesterol ratio that may increase the risk of coronary artery disease. These changes tend to occur with both selective and nonselective beta-blockers, though they are less likely to occur with beta-blockers possessing intrinsic sympathomimetic activity (partial agonists). Interestingly, the use of *alpha*-adrenoceptor antagonists such as prazosin has been found to be associated with either no changes in plasma lipids or increased concentrations of HDL, which could be a favorable alteration. The mechanism by which alpha- and beta-receptor antagonists cause these changes is not understood.

E. Effects Not Related to Beta Blockade: Partial beta-agonist activity was significant in the first beta-blocking drug synthesized, dichloroisoproterenol. It has been suggested that retention of some intrinsic sympathomimetic activity is desirable to prevent untoward effects such as precipitation of asthma. Pindolol and other partial agonists are noted in Table 10–2. It is not yet clear to what extent partial

agonism is clinically valuable. However, these drugs may be useful in patients who develop symptomatic bradycardia or asthma with nonselective beta-adrenoceptor antagonists. Furthermore, the possibly smaller adverse effects of partial agonist drugs on plasma lipids warrant continuing study.

Local anesthetic action, also known as "membrane-stabilizing" action, is a prominent effect of several beta-blockers (Table 10–2). This action is the result of typical local anesthetic blockade of sodium channels and can be demonstrated in neurons, heart muscle, and skeletal muscle membrane. However, it is unlikely that this effect is important after systemic administration, since the concentration usually achieved by that route is too low for the anesthetic effects to be evident. Sotalol is a nonselective beta-receptor antagonist that lacks local anesthetic action but has marked class III antiarrhythmic effects, reflecting potassium channel blockade (see Chapter 14).

SPECIFIC AGENTS
(See Table 10–2.)

Propranolol is the prototype beta-blocking drug. It has low and dose-dependent bioavailability, the result of extensive first-pass metabolism in the liver. A long-acting form of propranolol is available; prolonged absorption of the drug may occur over a 24-hour period. The drug has negligible effects at alpha and muscarinic receptors; however it is moderately effective as a central serotonin receptor blocker. It has no detectable partial agonist action at beta receptors.

Metoprolol, atenolol, and other drugs (see Table 10–2) are members of the β_1-selective group. These agents may be safer in patients who experience bronchoconstrictive responses to propranolol. However, since their β_1 selectivity is rather modest, they should be used with great caution, if at all, in patients with a history of bronchospasm. Beta$_1$-selective antagonists may be preferable in patients with diabetes or peripheral vascular disease when therapy with a beta-blocker is required.

Nadolol is noteworthy for its very long duration of action; its spectrum of action is similar to that of timolol.

Timolol is a nonselective agent with no local anesthetic activity. It has excellent ocular hypotensive effects.

Pindolol, acebutolol, carteolol, celiprolol, and **penbutolol** are of interest because they have partial beta-agonist activity. They are effective in the major cardiovascular applications of the beta-blocking group (hypertension and angina). Although these partial agonists may be less likely to cause bradycardia and abnormalities in plasma lipids than are antagonists, the overall clinical significance of intrinsic sympathomimetic activity remains uncertain.

Celiprolol is a new β_1-selective antagonist like pindolol with a modest capacity to activate β_2 receptors. The drug is efficacious in hypertension and in treating angina. There is limited evidence suggesting that celiprolol may have less adverse bronchoconstrictor effects in asthma and may even promote bronchodilation (van Zyl et al, 1989). If absence of unfavorable effects in asthmatics is confirmed in longer and more extensive clinical trials, celiprolol would have significant advantages for some patients requiring a beta-receptor antagonist (see Clinical Pharmacology, Hypertension, below).

Labetalol is a reversible adrenoceptor antagonist available as a racemic mixture of two pairs of chiral isomers (the molecule has two centers of asymmetry). The SS and RS isomers are inactive, SR is a potent alpha-blocker, and the RR isomer is a potent beta-blocker. Labetalol's affinity for alpha receptors is less than that of phentolamine, but labetalol is α_1-selective. Its beta-blocking potency is somewhat lower than that of propranolol. Hypotension induced by labetalol is accompanied by less tachycardia than occurs with phentolamine and similar alpha-blockers.

Esmolol is an ultra-short-acting β_1-selective adrenoceptor antagonist. The structure of esmolol contains an ester linkage; esterases in red blood cells rapidly metabolize esmolol to a metabolite that has a low affinity for beta receptors. Consequently, esmolol has a short half-life, about 10 minutes. Therefore, during continuous infusions of esmolol, steady state concentrations are achieved quickly, and the therapeutic actions of the drug are terminated rapidly when its infusion is discontinued. Esmolol is potentially much safer to use than longer-acting antagonists in critically ill patients who require a beta-adrenoceptor antagonist. Esmolol may be useful in controlling supra-

ventricular arrhythmias, perioperative hypertension, and myocardial ischemia in acutely ill patients.

Butoxamine is selective for β_2 receptors. Selective β_2-blocking drugs have not been actively sought because there is no obvious clinical application for them.

IV. CLINICAL PHARMACOLOGY OF THE BETA-RECEPTOR-BLOCKING DRUGS

Hypertension

Many of the beta-adrenoceptor-blocking drugs have proved to be effective and well tolerated in hypertension. While many hypertensive patients will respond to a beta-blocker used alone, the drug is most often used with either a diuretic or a vasodilator. In spite of the short half-life of many beta antagonists, these drugs may be administered once or twice daily and still have an adequate therapeutic effect. Labetalol, a competitive alpha and beta antagonist, is effective in hypertension, though its ultimate role is yet to be determined. Use of these agents is discussed in detail in Chapter 11.

Considerable attention has been paid during the last decade to claims that partial agonists (eg, pindolol) have increased safety in patients with airway disease. In theory, there is much to recommend this idea, since the partial agonist beta-blockers are better agonists at β_2 than at β_1 receptors. This should result in useful bronchodilation and even added hypotensive action from the smooth muscle-relaxing action of β_2 agonism while the β_1 antagonist action reduces blood pressure. Unfortunately, there is little evidence of practical clinical differences to support this hypothesis at present. One potential advantage of partial agonist beta-blockers that has not yet been disproved is a relative lack of deleterious effect on plasma lipids (Fitzgerald, 1993).

Ischemic Heart Disease

Beta-adrenoceptor blockers reduce the frequency of anginal episodes and improve exercise tolerance in many patients with angina (see Chapter 12). These actions relate to the blockade of cardiac beta receptors, resulting in decreased cardiac work and reduction in oxygen demand. Slowing and regularization of the heart rate may contribute to clinical benefits (Figure 10–7). Large-scale prospective studies indicate that the long-term use of timolol, propranolol, oxprenolol, or metoprolol in patients who have had a myocardial infarction prolongs survival (Figure 10–8). Studies in experimental animals suggest that use of beta-receptor antagonists during the acute

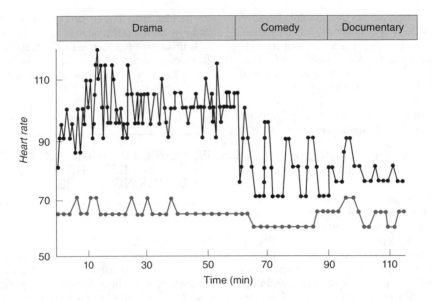

Figure 10–7. Heart rate in a patient with ischemic heart disease measured by telemetry while watching television. Measurements were begun 1 hour after receiving placebo (solid circles, black) or 40 mg of oxprenolol (color), a nonselective beta-antagonist with partial agonist activity. Not only was the heart rate decreased by the drug under the conditions of this experiment; it also varied much less in response to stimuli. (Modified and reproduced, with permission, from Taylor SH: Oxprenolol in clinical practice. Am J Cardiol 1983;52:34D.)

phase of a myocardial infarction may limit infarct size. However, this use is still controversial.

Cardiac Arrhythmias

Beta antagonists are effective in the treatment of both supraventricular and ventricular arrhythmias

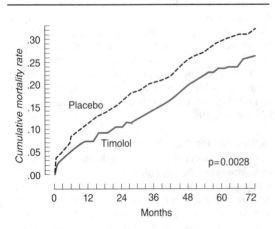

Figure 10–8. Effects of beta-blocker therapy on life-table cumulated rates of mortality from all causes over 6 years among 1884 patients surviving myocardial infarctions. Patients were randomly assigned to treatment with placebo (dashed line) or timolol (color). (Reproduced, with permission, from Pederson TR: Six-year follow-up of the Norwegian multicenter study on timolol after acute myocardial infarction. N Engl J Med 1985;313:1055.)

(see Chapter 14). In cases of sinus tachycardia and supraventricular ectopic beats, treatment should not be limited to the use of a beta antagonist; attention should be given to the underlying disease. By increasing the atrioventricular nodal refractory period, beta antagonists will slow ventricular response rates in atrial flutter and fibrillation. These drugs can also reduce ventricular ectopic beats, particularly if the ectopic activity has been precipitated by catecholamines. Sotalol has additional antiarrhythmic effects in addition to its beta-blocking action; these are discussed in Chapter 14.

Other Cardiovascular Disorders

Beta-receptor antagonists have been found to increase stroke volume in some patients with obstructive cardiomyopathy. This beneficial effect is thought to result from the slowing of ventricular ejection and decreased outflow resistance. Beta antagonists are useful in dissecting aortic aneurysm to decrease the rate of development of systolic pressure. Recent experimental evidence suggests that—paradoxically—beta antagonists may be effective in treating congestive heart failure in certain carefully selected patients, though this possibility requires more extensive studies. However, these drugs are generally contraindicated in patients with congestive heart failure who depend on sympathetic drive to maintain cardiac output.

Glaucoma
(See box: Treatment of Glaucoma)

Systemic administration of beta-blocking drugs for other indications was found serendipitously to reduce intraocular pressure in patients with glaucoma. Subsequently, it was found that topical administration also reduces intraocular pressure. The mechanism appears to involve reduced production of aqueous humor by the ciliary body, which is physiologically activated by cAMP. Timolol has been favored for local use in the eye because it lacks local anesthetic properties and is a pure antagonist. Timolol appears to have an efficacy comparable to that of epinephrine or pilocarpine in open-angle glaucoma. While the maximal daily dose applied locally (1 mg) is small compared with the systemic doses commonly used in the treatment of hypertension or angina (10–60 mg), sufficient timolol may be absorbed from the eye to cause serious adverse effects on the heart and airways in susceptible individuals. Topical timolol may interact with orally administered verapamil.

Betaxolol, carteolol, levobunolol, and metipranolol are newer beta-receptor antagonists approved for the treatment of glaucoma. Betaxolol has the potential advantage of being β_1-selective; to what extent this potential advantage might diminish systemic adverse effects remains to be determined. The drug apparently has caused worsening of pulmonary symptoms in some patients.

Hyperthyroidism

Excessive catecholamine action is an important aspect of the pathophysiology of hyperthyroidism, especially in relation to the heart (see Chapter 37). The beta antagonists have salutary effects in this condition. The beneficial effects presumably relate to blockade of adrenoceptors and perhaps to the inhibition of peripheral conversion of thyroxine to triiodothyronine. The latter action may vary from one beta antagonist to another. Propranolol is particularly efficacious in thyroid storm; it has been used cautiously in patients with this condition to control supraventricular tachycardias that often precipitate congestive heart failure.

Neurologic Diseases

Several studies suggest a beneficial effect of propranolol in reducing the frequency and intensity of migraine headache. The mechanism is not known. Since sympathetic activity may enhance skeletal muscle tremor, it is not surprising that beta antagonists have been found to reduce certain tremors (see Chapter 27). The somatic manifestations of anxiety may respond dramatically to low doses of propranolol, particularly when taken prophylactically. Propranolol is also of benefit in treating alcohol withdrawal. Beta-receptor antagonists have been found to diminish portal vein pressure in patients with cirrhosis. There is evidence that both propranolol and

---

THE TREATMENT OF GLAUCOMA

Glaucoma is a major cause of blindness in the aging population and of great pharmacologic interest because the chronic form often responds to drug therapy. The primary manifestation is increased intraocular pressure not initially associated with symptoms. Without treatment, increased intraocular pressure results in damage to the retina and optic nerve, with restriction of visual fields and, eventually, blindness. Intraocular pressure is easily measured as part of the routine ophthalmologic examination.

Two major types of glaucoma are recognized: open-angle and closed-angle (or narrow-angle). The closed-angle form is associated with a shallow anterior chamber, in which a dilated iris can occlude the outflow drainage pathway at the angle between the cornea and the ciliary body (Figure 6–9). This form is associated with acute and painful increases of pressure, which must be controlled on an emergency basis with drugs or prevented by surgical removal of part of the iris (iridectomy). The open-angle form of glaucoma is a chronic condition, and treatment is largely pharmacologic.

Because intraocular pressure is a function of the balance between fluid input and drainage out of the globe, the strategies for the treatment of closed-angle glaucoma fall into two classes: reduction of aqueous humor secretion and enhancement of aqueous outflow. Four general groups of drugs—cholinomimetics, alpha agonists, beta-blockers, and diuretics—have been found to be useful in reducing intraocular pressure and can be related to these strategies as shown in Table 10–3.

Of the four drug groups listed in Table 10–3, the beta-blockers are by far the most popular. This popularity results from convenience (once- or twice-daily dosing) and relative lack of adverse effects (except in patients with asthma or cardiac pacemaker or conduction pathway disease). Other drugs that have been reported to reduce intraocular pressure include alpha$_1$ antagonists, prostaglandin E_2, and marijuana. The use of drugs in acute closed-angle glaucoma is limited to cholinomimetics and osmotic agents preceding surgery. The onset of action of the other agents is too slow in this situation.

Table 10–3. Drugs used in glaucoma.

	Mechanism	Methods of Administration
Cholinomimetics Pilocarpine, carbachol, physostigmine, echothiophate	Ciliary muscle contraction, opening of trabecular meshwork; increased outflow	Topical drops or gel; plastic film slow-release insert
Alpha agonists Unselective Epinephrine, dipivefrin	Increased outflow	Topical drops
Alpha$_2$-selective Apraclonidine	Decreased aqueous secretion	Topical following ocular laser surgery
Beta-blockers Timolol, betaxolol, carteolol, levobunolol, metipranolol	Decreased aqueous secretion from the ciliary epithelium	Topical drops
Diuretics Acetazolamide	Decreased secretion due to lack of HCO_3^-	Oral; topically active carbonic anhydrase inhibitors in clinical trials
Ethacrynic acid (investigational)	Decreased secretion	Intraocular injection at long intervals, eg, annually

nadolol decrease the incidence of the first episode of bleeding from esophageal varices and decrease the mortality rate associated with bleeding in patients with cirrhosis (Poynard et al, 1991).

CHOICE OF A BETA-BLOCKING DRUG

Propranolol is the standard against which newer beta antagonists developed for systemic use should be compared. In many years of very wide use, it has been found to be a safe and effective drug for many indications. Since it is possible that some actions of a beta-receptor antagonist may relate to some other effect of the drug, these drugs should not be considered interchangeable for all applications. For example, only beta-antagonists known to be effective in hyperthyroidism or in prophylactic therapy after myocardial infarction should be used for those indications. It is possible that the beneficial effects of one drug in these settings might not be shared by another drug in the same class. The possible advantages and disadvantages of beta-blockers that are partial agonists have not been clearly defined in clinical settings.

CLINICAL TOXICITY OF THE BETA-RECEPTOR-ANTAGONIST DRUGS

A variety of minor toxic effects have been reported for propranolol. Rash, fever, and other manifestations of drug allergy are rare. Central nervous system effects include sedation, sleep disturbances, and depression. Rarely, psychotic reactions may occur. Discontinuing the use of beta-blockers in any patient who develops a depression should be seriously considered if clinically feasible. It has been claimed that beta-receptor antagonist drugs with low lipid solubil-

ity will be associated with a lower incidence of central nervous system adverse effects than compounds with higher lipid solubility (Table 10–2). Further studies designed to compare the central nervous system adverse effects of various drugs are required before specific recommendations can be made, though it seems reasonable to try nadolol or atenolol in a patient who experiences unpleasant central nervous system effects with other beta-blockers. Experience with the newer members of this group is too limited to permit comparison of the incidence of toxic effects.

The major adverse effects of beta-receptor antagonist drugs relate to the predictable consequences of beta blockade. Beta$_2$-receptor blockade associated with the use of nonselective agents commonly causes worsening of preexisting asthma and other forms of airway obstruction without having these consequences in normal individuals. Indeed, relatively trivial asthma may become severe after beta blockade. While β_1-selective drugs may have less effect on airways than nonselective beta antagonists, they must be used very cautiously, if at all, in patients with reactive airways. While β_1-selective antagonists are generally well tolerated in patients with mild to moderate peripheral vascular disease, caution is required in patients with severe peripheral vascular disease or vasospastic disorders.

Beta-receptor blockade depresses myocardial contractility and excitability. In patients with abnormal myocardial function, cardiac output may be dependent on sympathetic drive. If this stimulus is removed by beta blockade, cardiac decompensation may ensue. Great caution must be exercised in using beta-receptor antagonists in patients with myocardial infarction or compensated congestive heart failure. An adverse cardiac effect of a beta antagonist may be overcome directly with isoproterenol or with glucagon (glucagon stimulates the heart via glucagon receptors, which are not blocked by beta antagonists), but neither of these methods is without hazard. A very small dose of a beta antagonist (eg, 10 mg of propranolol) may provoke severe cardiac failure in a susceptible individual. Beta-blockers may interact with the calcium antagonist verapamil; severe hypotension, bradycardia, congestive heart failure, and cardiac conduction abnormalities have all been described. These adverse effects may also arise in susceptible patients taking a topical (ophthalmic) beta-blocker and oral verapamil.

There are hazards of abruptly discontinuing beta-antagonist therapy after chronic use. Evidence suggests that patients with ischemic heart disease may be at increased risk if beta blockade is suddenly interrupted. The mechanism of this effect is uncertain but might involve "up-regulation" of the number of beta receptors. Until better evidence is available regarding the magnitude of the risk, prudence dictates the gradual tapering rather than abrupt cessation of dosage when these drugs are discontinued.

The incidence of hypoglycemic episodes in diabetics that are exacerbated by beta-blocking agents is unknown. Nevertheless, it is inadvisable to use beta antagonists in insulin-dependent diabetic patients who are subject to frequent hypoglycemic reactions if alternative therapies are available. $Beta_1$-selective antagonists offer some advantage in these patients, since the rate of recovery from hypoglycemia may be faster compared with diabetics receiving nonselective beta-adrenoceptor antagonists.

Beta blockade may mask clinical signs of developing hyperthyroidism. With the growing number of patients taking beta antagonists for prolonged periods, this effect may become increasingly important.

PREPARATIONS AVAILABLE

Alpha-Blockers
Doxazosin (Cardura)
Oral: 1, 2, 4, 8 mg tablets
Phenoxybenzamine (Dibenzyline)
Oral: 10 mg capsules
Phentolamine (Regitine)
Parenteral: 5 mg/mL for injection
Prazosin (generic, Minipress)
Oral: 1, 2, 5 mg capsules
Terazosin (Hytrin)
Oral: 1, 2, 5, 10 mg tablets
Tolazoline (Priscoline)
Parenteral: 25 mg/mL for injection

Beta-Blockers
Acebutolol (Sectral)
Oral: 200, 400 mg capsules
Atenolol (Tenormin)
Oral: 25, 50, 100 mg tablets
Parenteral: 0.5 mg/mL for IV injection
Betaxolol
Oral: 10, 20 mg tablets (Kerlone)
Ophthalmic: 0.25% drops (Betoptic)
Bisoprolol (Zebeta)
Oral: 5, 10 mg tablets
Carteolol
Oral: 2.5, 5 mg tablets (Cartrol)
Ophthalmic: 1% drops (Ocupress)
Esmolol (Brevibloc)
Parenteral: 10 mg/mL for IV injection; 250 mg/mL for IV infusion
Labetalol (Normodyne, Trandate)
Oral: 100, 200, 300 mg tablets
Parenteral: 5 mg/mL for injection
Levobunolol (Betagan Liquifilm)
Ophthalmic: 0.5% drops
Metipranolol (Optipranolol)
Ophthalmic: 0.3% drops
Metoprolol (Lopressor, Toprol)
Oral: 50, 100 mg tablets
Oral sustained-release: 50, 100, 200 mg tablets
Parenteral: 1 mg/mL for injection
Nadolol (Corgard)
Oral: 20, 40, 80, 120, 160 mg tablets
Penbutolol (Levatol)
Oral: 20 mg tablets
Pindolol (Visken)
Oral: 5, 10 mg tablets
Propranolol (generic, Inderal)
Oral: 10, 20, 40, 60, 80, 90 mg tablets; 4, 8, 80 mg/mL solutions
Oral sustained release: 60, 80, 120, 160 mg capsules
Parenteral: 1 mg/mL for injection
Sotalol (Betapace)
Oral: 80, 160, 240 mg tablets
Timolol
Oral: 5, 10, 20 mg tablets (Blocadren)
Ophthalmic: 0.25, 0.5% drops (Timoptic)

Synthesis Inhibitor
Metyrosine (Demser)
Oral: 250 mg capsules

REFERENCES

Aellig WH: Clinical pharmacologic investigations of the partial agonist activity of beta-adrenoceptor antagonists. Hosp Formul 1985;20:475.

Andersson K-E: Current concepts in the treatment of disorders of micturition. Drugs 1988;35:477.

Ariëns EJ: Chirality in bioactive agents and its pitfalls. Trends Pharmacol Sci 1986;7:200.

Babamoto K, Hirokawa WT. Doxazosin: A new alpha$_1$-adrenergic antagonist. Clin Pharm 1992;11:415.

Benfield P, Sorkin EM: Esmolol: A preliminary review of its pharmacodynamic and pharmacokinetic properties, and therapeutic efficacy. Drugs 1987;33:392.

Benfield P, Clissold SP, Brogden RN: Metoprolol. Drugs 1986;31:376.

Beta blockers and lipophilicity. (Editorial.) Lancet 1987; 1:900.

Brantigan CO, Brantigan TA, Joseph N: Effect of beta blockade and beta stimulation on stage fright. Am J Med 1982;72:88.

Breslin D et al: Medical management of benign prostatic hyperplasia: A canine model comparing the in vivo efficacy of alpha-1 adrenergic antagonists in the prostate. J Urol 1993;149:395.

Cubeddu LX: New alpha$_1$-adrenergic receptor antagonists for the treatment of hypertension: Role of vascular alpha receptors in the control of peripheral resistance. Am Heart J 1988;116:133.

Feely J, Peden N: Use of beta adrenoceptor-blocking drugs in hyperthyroidism. Drugs 1984;27:425.

Fitzgerald JD: Do partial agonist beta-blockers have improved clinical utility? Cardiovasc Drugs Ther 1993; 7:303.

Frishman WH, Charlap S: Alpha adrenergic blockers. Med Clin North Am 1988;72:427.

Frishman WH, Lazar EJ, Gorodokin G: Pharmacokinetic optimisation of therapy with beta-adrenergic blocking agents. Clin Pharmacokinet 1991;20:311.

Frishman WH: Beta-adrenergic blockers as cardioprotective agents. Am J Cardiol 1992;70:21.

Gengo FM, Huntoon L, McHugh WB: Lipid-soluble and water-soluble beta blockers: Comparison of the central nervous system depressant effect. Arch Intern Med 1987;147:39.

Gold EH et al: Synthesis and comparison of some cardiovascular properties of the stereoisomers of labetalol. J Med Chem 1982;25: 1363.

Goldberg MR, Robertson D: Yohimbine: A pharmacological probe of the alpha$_2$ adrenoreceptor. Pharmacol Rev 1983;35:143.

Hjalmarson A et al: The Göteborg metoprolol trial: Effects on mortality and morbidity in acute myocardial infarction. Circulation 1983;67(Suppl 1):I–26.

Kirby RS et al: Prazosin in the treatment of prostatic obstruction: A placebo-controlled study. Br J Urol 1987; 60:136.

Lader M: Beta-adrenoceptor antagonists in neuropsychiatry: An update. J Clin Psychiatry 1988;49:213.

Leren P: Comparison of effects on lipid metabolism of antihypertensive drugs with alpha- and beta-adrenergic antagonist properties. Am J Med 1987;82(Suppl 1A):31.

Lesar TS: Comparison of ophthalmic beta-blocking agents. Clin Pharm 1987;6:451.

Limbird LE: The Alpha-2 Adrenergic Receptors. Humana Press, 1988.

Miller NE: Effects of adrenoceptor-blocking drugs on plasma lipoprotein concentrations. Am J Cardiol 1987; 60:17E.

Milne RJ, Buckley MM. Celiprolol. Drugs 1991;41:941.

Nickerson M: The pharmacology of adrenergic blockade. Pharmacol Rev 1949;1:27.

Poynard T et al: Beta-adrenergic-antagonist drugs in the prevention of gastrointestinal bleeding in patients with cirrhosis and esophageal varices: An analysis of data and prognostic factors in 589 patients from four randomized clinical trials. N Engl J Med 1991;324:1532.

Rangno RE, Nattel S, Lutterodt A: Prevention of propranolol withdrawal mechanism by prolonged small dose propranolol schedule. Am J Cardiol 1982;49:828.

Rangno RE, Langlois S: Comparison of withdrawal phenomena after propranolol, metoprolol, and pindolol. Am Heart J 1982;104:473.

Reid D et al: Double-blind trial of yohimbine in treatment of psychogenic impotence. Lancet 1987;2:421.

Riddell JG, Harron DW, Shanks RG: Clinical pharmacokinetics of beta-adrenoceptor antagonists: An update. Clin Pharmacokinet 1987;12:305.

Ruffolo RR Jr et al: Pharmacologic and therapeutic applications of alpha$_2$-adrenoceptor subtypes. Annu Rev Pharmacol Toxicol 1993;32:243.

Ruffolo RR Jr: The Alpha-1 Adrenergic Receptors. Humana Press, 1987.

Sidi AA: Vasoactive intracavernous pharmacotherapy. Urol Clin North Am 1988;15:95.

Singh BN, Thoden WR, Ward A: Acebutolol: A review of its pharmacological properties and therapeutic efficacy in hypertension, angina pectoris and arrhythmia. Drugs 1985;29:531.

Taylor SH: Intrinsic sympathomimetic activity: Clinical fact or fiction? Am J Cardiol 1983;52:16D.

Titmarsh S, Monk JP: Terazosin: A review of its pharmacodynamic and pharmacokinetic properties, and therapeutic efficacy in essential hypertension. Drugs 1987; 33:461.

van Zyl AI et al: Comparison of respiratory effects of two cardioselective beta-blockers, celiprolol and atenolol, in asthmatics with mild to moderate hypertension. Chest 1989;95:209.

Wilde MI, Fitton A, Sorkin EM: Terazosin. A review of its pharmacodynamic and pharmacokinetic properties, and therapeutic potential in benign prostatic hyperplasia. Drugs Aging, 1993;3:258.

Zentgraf M, Baccouche M, Jüneman KP: Diagnosis and therapy of erectile dysfunction using papaverine and phentolamine. Urol Int 1988; 43:65.

Section III.
Cardiovascular-Renal Drugs

Antihypertensive Agents

11

Neal L. Benowitz, MD

By some estimates, the arterial blood pressure of 15% of American adults is elevated to a degree that requires medical treatment. The prevalence varies with age, race, education, and many other variables. Sustained arterial hypertension damages blood vessels in kidney, heart, and brain and leads to an increased incidence of renal failure, coronary disease, and stroke. Effective pharmacologic lowering of blood pressure has been shown to prevent damage to blood vessels and to substantially reduce morbidity and mortality rates. Many effective drugs are available. Knowledge of their antihypertensive mechanisms and sites of action allows accurate prediction of efficacy and toxicity. As a result, rational use of these agents, alone or in combination, can lower blood pressure with minimal risk of toxicity in most patients.

HYPERTENSION & REGULATION OF BLOOD PRESSURE

Diagnosis

The diagnosis of hypertension is based on repeated, reproducible measurements of elevated blood pressure. The diagnosis serves primarily as a prediction of consequences for the patient; it seldom includes a statement about the cause of hypertension.

Epidemiologic studies indicate that the risks of damage to kidney, heart, and brain are directly related to the extent of blood pressure elevation. Even mild hypertension (blood pressure ≥ 140/90 mm Hg) in young or middle-aged adults increases the risk of eventual end organ damage. The risks—and therefore the urgency of instituting therapy—increase in pro-

portion to the magnitude of blood pressure elevation. The risk of end organ damage at any level of blood pressure or age is greater in black people and relatively less in premenopausal women than in men. Other positive risk factors include smoking, hyperlipidemia, diabetes, manifestations of end organ damage at the time of diagnosis, and a family history of cardiovascular disease.

It should be noted that the diagnosis of hypertension depends on measurement of blood pressure and not upon symptoms reported by the patient. In fact, hypertension is usually asymptomatic until overt end organ damage is imminent or has already occurred.

Etiology of Hypertension

A specific cause of hypertension can be established in only 10–15% of patients. It is important to consider specific causes in each case, however, because some of them are amenable to definitive surgical treatment: renal artery constriction, coarctation of the aorta, pheochromocytoma, Cushing's disease, and primary aldosteronism.

Patients in whom no specific cause of hypertension can be found are said to have **essential hypertension.**[*] In most cases, elevated blood pressure is associated with an overall increase in resistance to flow of blood through arterioles, while cardiac output is usually normal. Meticulous investigation of autonomic nervous system function, baroreceptor reflexes, the renin-angiotensin-aldosterone system, and the kidney has failed to identify a primary abnormality as the cause of increased peripheral vascular resistance in essential hypertension.

Elevated blood pressure is usually caused by a combination of several abnormalities (multifactorial).

---

[*]The adjective originally was intended to convey the now abandoned idea that blood pressure elevation was essential for adequate perfusion of diseased tissues.

Epidemiologic evidence points to genetic inheritance, psychologic stress, and environmental and dietary factors (increased salt and perhaps decreased calcium intake) as perhaps contributing to the development of hypertension. Increase in blood pressure with aging does not occur in populations with low daily sodium intake. Patients with labile hypertension appear more likely than normal controls to have blood pressure elevations after salt loading.

Normal Regulation of Blood Pressure

According to the hydraulic equation, arterial blood pressure (BP) is directly proportionate to the product of the blood flow (cardiac output, CO) and the resistance to passage of blood through precapillary arterioles (peripheral vascular resistance, PVR):

$$BP = CO \times PVR$$

Physiologically, in both normal and hypertensive individuals, blood pressure is maintained by moment-to-moment regulation of cardiac output and peripheral vascular resistance, exerted at three anatomic sites (Figure 11–1): arterioles, postcapillary venules (capacitance vessels), and heart. A fourth anatomic control site, the kidney, contributes to maintenance of blood pressure by regulating the volume of intravascular fluid. Baroreflexes, mediated by sympathetic nerves, act in combination with humoral mechanisms, including the renin-angiotensin-aldosterone system, to coordinate function at these four control sites and to maintain normal blood pressure.

Blood pressure in a hypertensive patient is controlled by the same mechanisms that are operative in normotensive subjects. Regulation of blood pressure in hypertensives differs from normal in that the baroreceptors and the renal blood volume-pressure control systems appear to be "set" at a higher level of blood pressure. All antihypertensive drugs act by interfering with these normal mechanisms, which are reviewed below.

A. Postural Baroreflex: (Figure 11–2.) Baroreflexes are responsible for rapid, moment-to-moment adjustments in blood pressure, such as in transition from a reclining to an upright posture. Central sympathetic neurons arising from the vasomotor area of the medulla are tonically active. Carotid baroreceptors are stimulated by the stretch of the vessel walls brought about by the internal pressure (blood pressure). Baroreceptor activation inhibits central sympathetic discharge. Conversely, reduction in stretch results in a reduction in baroreceptor activity. Thus, in the case of a transition to upright posture, baroreceptors sense the reduction in pressure that results from pooling of blood in the veins below the level of the heart as reduced wall stretch, and sympathetic discharge is disinhibited. The reflex increase in sympathetic outflow acts through nerve endings to increase peripheral vascular resistance (constriction of arterioles) and cardiac output (direct stimulation of the heart and constriction of capacitance vessels, which increases venous return to the heart), thereby restoring normal blood pressure. The same baroreflex acts in response to any event that lowers arterial pressure, including a primary reduction in peripheral vascular resistance (eg, caused by a vasodilating agent) or a reduction in intravascular volume (eg, due to hemorrhage or to loss of salt and water via the kidney).

B. Renal Response to Decreased Blood Pressure: Via control of blood volume, the kidney is primarily responsible for long-term blood pressure control. A reduction in renal perfusion pressure causes intrarenal redistribution of blood flow and increased reabsorption of salt and water. In addition, decreased pressure in renal arterioles as well as sympathetic neural activity (via beta adrenoceptors) stimulates production of renin, which increases production of angiotensin II (see Figure 11–1 and Chapter 17). Angiotensin II causes (1) direct constriction of resistance vessels and (2) stimulation of aldosterone synthesis in the adrenal cortex, which increases renal sodium absorption and intravascular blood volume.

Therapeutic Implications

Because antihypertensive therapy is not usually directed at a specific cause, it necessarily depends upon interfering with normal physiologic mechanisms that regulate blood pressure. Antihypertensive therapy is administered to an asymptomatic patient, for whom it provides no direct relief from discomfort; instead, the benefit of lowering blood pressure lies in preventing disease and death at some future time. The natural human tendency to weigh present inconvenience and discomfort more heavily than future benefit means that a major problem—perhaps *the* major problem—

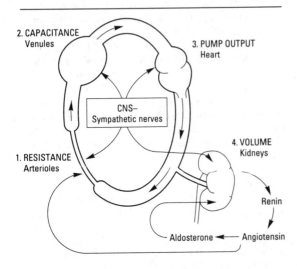

Figure 11–1. Anatomic sites of blood pressure control.

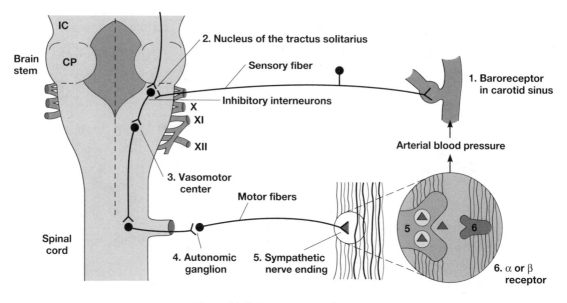

Figure 11–2. Baroreceptor reflex arc.

in antihypertensive therapy is that of providing consistent, effective drug therapy over many years in a regimen the patient will adhere to ("patient compliance").

It is essential to balance the risks of toxicity from drug treatment against the risks of not treating, which are proportionate to the extent of blood pressure elevation before treatment and vary according to the characteristics of individual patients. Accordingly, no single mode of treatment will be suitable for more than a small proportion of hypertensive patients.

I. BASIC PHARMACOLOGY OF ANTIHYPERTENSIVE AGENTS

All antihypertensive agents act at one or more of the four anatomic control sites depicted in Figure 11–1 and produce their effects by interfering with normal mechanisms of blood pressure regulation. A useful classification of these agents categorizes them according to the principal regulatory site or mechanism on which they act (Figure 11–3). Because of their common mechanisms of action, drugs within each category tend to produce a similar spectrum of toxicities. The categories include the following:

(1) Diuretics, which lower blood pressure by depleting the body of sodium and reducing blood volume and perhaps by other mechanisms.

(2) Sympathoplegic agents, which lower blood pressure by reducing peripheral vascular resistance, inhibiting cardiac function, and increasing venous pooling in capacitance vessels. (The latter two effects reduce cardiac output.) These agents are further subdivided according to their putative sites of action in the sympathetic reflex arc (see below).

(3) Direct vasodilators, which reduce pressure by relaxing vascular smooth muscle, thus dilating resistance vessels and—to varying degrees—increasing capacitance as well.

(4) Agents that block production or action of angiotensin and thereby reduce peripheral vascular resistance and (potentially) blood volume.

The fact that these drug groups act by different mechanisms permits the combination of drugs from two or more groups with increased efficacy and, in some cases, decreased toxicity. (See box: Monotherapy Versus Polypharmacy in Hypertension.)

DRUGS THAT ALTER SODIUM & WATER BALANCE

Dietary sodium restriction has been known for many years to decrease blood pressure in hypertensive patients. With the advent of diuretics, sodium restriction was thought to be less important. However, there is now general agreement that dietary control of blood pressure is a relatively nontoxic therapeutic measure and may even be preventive. Several studies

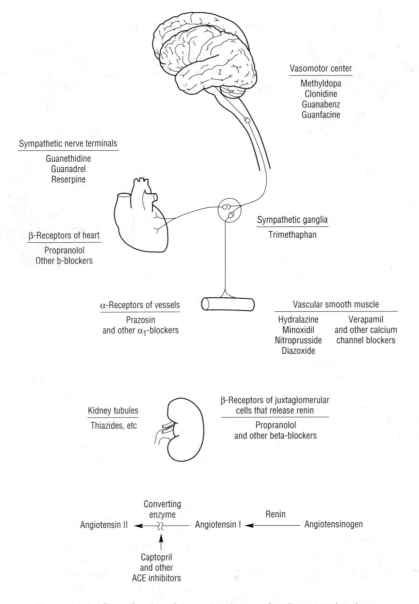

Figure 11–3. Sites of action of the major classes of antihypertensive drugs.

have shown that even modest dietary sodium restriction lowers blood pressure (though to varying extents) in many hypertensive individuals.

Mechanisms of Action & Hemodynamic Effects of Diuretics

Diuretics lower blood pressure primarily by depleting body sodium stores. Initially, diuretics reduce blood pressure by reducing blood volume and cardiac output; peripheral vascular resistance may increase. After 6–8 weeks, cardiac output returns toward normal while peripheral vascular resistance declines. Sodium is believed to contribute to vascular resistance by increasing vessel stiffness and neural reactivity, possibly related to increased sodium-calcium exchange with a resultant increase in intracellular calcium. These effects are reversed by diuretics or sodium restriction.

Some diuretics have direct vasodilating effects in addition to their diuretic action. Indapamide is a nonthiazide sulfonamide diuretic with both diuretic and vasodilator activity. As a consequence of vasodilation, cardiac output remains unchanged or increases slightly. Amiloride inhibits smooth muscle responses to contractile stimuli, probably through effects on transmembrane and intracellular calcium movement that are independent of its action on sodium excretion.

Diuretics are effective in lowering blood pressure by 10–15 mm Hg in most patients, and diuretics alone often provide adequate treatment for mild or moderate essential hypertension. In more severe hypertension, diuretics are used in combination with sympathoplegic and vasodilator drugs to control the tendency toward sodium retention caused by these agents. Vascular responsiveness—ie, the ability to either constrict or dilate—is diminished by sympathoplegic and vasodilator drugs, so that the vasculature behaves like an inflexible tube. As a consequence, blood pressure becomes exquisitely sensitive to blood volume. Thus, in severe hypertension, when multiple drugs are used, blood pressure may be well controlled when blood volume is 95% of normal but much too high when blood volume is 105% of normal.

Selection of Diuretics

The sites of action within the kidney and the pharmacokinetics of various diuretic drugs are discussed in Chapter 15. Thiazide diuretics are appropriate for most patients with mild or moderate hypertension and normal renal and cardiac function. More powerful diuretics (eg, those acting on the loop of Henle) are necessary in severe hypertension, when multiple drugs with sodium-retaining properties are used; in renal insufficiency, when glomerular filtration rate is less than 30 or 40 mL/min; and in cardiac failure or cirrhosis, where sodium retention is marked.

Potassium-sparing diuretics are useful both to avoid excessive potassium depletion, particularly in patients taking digitalis, and to enhance the natriuretic effects of other diuretics.

Dosing Considerations

Although the pharmacokinetics and pharmacodynamics of the various diuretics differ, their common therapeutic end point in treating hypertension is daily natriuresis. However, it must be recognized that in steady-state conditions (as in long-term management of hypertension), daily sodium excretion is equal to dietary sodium intake. Diuretics are necessary to oppose the tendency toward sodium retention in a relatively sodium-depleted patient. Although thiazide diuretics are more natriuretic at higher doses (up to 100–200 mg of hydrochlorothiazide), when used as a single agent, lower doses (25–50 mg) exert as much antihypertensive effect as do higher doses. Thus, a threshold amount of body sodium depletion may be sufficient for antihypertensive efficacy. In contrast to thiazides, the blood pressure response to loop diuretics continues to increase at doses many times greater than the usual therapeutic dose.

Toxicity of Diuretics

In the treatment of hypertension, the most common adverse effect of diuretics (except for potassium-sparing diuretics) is potassium depletion. Although mild degrees of hypokalemia are tolerated well by many patients, hypokalemia may be hazardous in persons taking digitalis, those who have chronic arrhythmias, or those with acute myocardial infarction. Potassium loss is coupled to reabsorption of sodium, and restriction of dietary sodium intake will therefore minimize potassium loss. Diuretics may also cause magnesium depletion, impair glucose tolerance, and increase serum lipid and uric acid concentrations. The possibility of an increased risk of coronary artery disease associated with the metabolic effects of diuretics is still under study. However, it has been found that the use of low doses minimizes these adverse metabolic effects without impairing the antihypertensive action.

DRUGS THAT ALTER SYMPATHETIC NERVOUS SYSTEM FUNCTION

In patients with moderate to severe hypertension, most effective drug regimens include an agent that inhibits function of the sympathetic nervous system. Drugs in this group are classified according to the site at which they impair the sympathetic reflex arc (Figure 11–2). This neuroanatomic classification explains prominent differences in cardiovascular effects of drugs and allows the clinician to predict interactions of these drugs with one another and with other drugs.

Most importantly, the subclasses of drugs exhibit different patterns of potential toxicity. Drugs that lower blood pressure by actions on the central nervous system tend to cause sedation and mental depression and may produce disturbances of sleep, including nightmares. Drugs that act by inhibiting transmission through autonomic ganglia produce toxicity from inhibition of parasympathetic regulation, in addition to profound sympathetic blockade. Drugs that act chiefly by reducing release of norepinephrine from sympathetic nerve endings cause effects that are similar to those of surgical sympathectomy, including inhibition of ejaculation, and hypotension that is increased by upright posture and after exercise. Drugs that block postsynaptic adrenoceptors produce a more selective spectrum of effects depending on the class of receptor to which they bind.

A few of the drugs to be discussed appear to act at more than one anatomic site, although each probably works by a single biochemical mechanism. No clinically useful drug acts primarily on baroreceptors. The **veratrum alkaloids** lower blood pressure by increasing sensitivity of baroreceptors, but they are of only academic interest because they produce erratic therapeutic effects and cause unacceptable toxicity in patients.

Finally, we should note that *all* of the agents that lower blood pressure by altering sympathetic function can elicit compensatory effects through mechanisms that are not dependent on adrenergic nerves. Thus, the antihypertensive effect of any of these agents used alone may be limited by retention of sodium and expansion of blood volume. For these reasons, sympathoplegic antihypertensive drugs are most effective when used concomitantly with a diuretic.

CENTRALLY ACTING SYMPATHOPLEGIC DRUGS

Mechanisms & Sites of Action

Methyldopa and clonidine reduce sympathetic outflow from vasopressor centers in the brain stem but allow these centers to retain or even increase their sensitivity to baroreceptor control. Accordingly, the antihypertensive and toxic actions of these drugs are generally less dependent on posture than are the effects of drugs such as guanethidine that act directly on peripheral sympathetic neurons.

Methyldopa (L-α-methyl-3,4-dihydroxyphenylalanine) is an analogue of L-dopa and is converted to α-methyldopamine and α-methylnorepinephrine; this pathway directly parallels the synthesis of norepinephrine from dopa illustrated in Figure 6–5. Alpha-methylnorepinephrine is stored in adrenergic nerve granules, where it stoichiometrically replaces norepinephrine, and is released by nerve stimulation to interact with postsynaptic adrenoceptors. However, this replacement of norepinephrine by a false transmitter in peripheral neurons is *not* responsible for methyldopa's antihypertensive effect, because the α-methylnorepinephrine released is an effective agonist at the alpha adrenoceptors that mediate peripheral sympathetic constriction of arterioles and venules. Direct electrical stimulation of sympathetic nerves in methyldopa-treated animals produces sympathetic responses similar to those observed in untreated animals.

Indeed, methyldopa's antihypertensive action appears to be due to stimulation of central alpha adrenoceptors by α-methylnorepinephrine or α-methyldopamine, based on the following evidence: (1) Much lower doses of methyldopa are required to lower blood pressure in animals when the drug is administered centrally by cerebral intraventricular injection rather than intravenously. (2) Alpha-receptor antagonists, especially α_2-selective antagonists, administered centrally, block the antihypertensive effect of methyldopa, whether the latter is given centrally or intravenously. (3) Potent inhibitors of dopa decar-

boxylase, administered centrally, block methyldopa's antihypertensive effect, thus showing that metabolism of the parent drug is necessary for its action.

The antihypertensive action of **clonidine,** a 2-imidazoline derivative, was discovered in the course of testing the drug for use as a topically applied nasal decongestant. After intravenous injection, clonidine produces a brief rise in blood pressure followed by more prolonged hypotension. The pressor response is due to direct stimulation of alpha adrenoceptors in arterioles. The drug is classified as a partial agonist at alpha receptors because it also inhibits pressor effects of other alpha agonists.

Considerable evidence indicates that the hypotensive effect of clonidine is exerted at alpha adrenoceptors in the medulla of the brain. In animals, the hypotensive effect of clonidine is prevented by central administration of alpha antagonists. Clonidine reduces sympathetic and increases parasympathetic tone, resulting in blood pressure lowering and bradycardia. The reduction in pressure is accompanied by a decrease in circulating catecholamine levels. These observations suggest that clonidine sensitizes brain stem pressor centers to inhibition by baroreflexes.

Thus, studies of clonidine and methyldopa suggest that normal regulation of blood pressure involves central adrenergic neurons that modulate baroreceptor reflexes. Both drugs bind more tightly to α_2 than to α_1 adrenoceptors. As noted in Chapter 6, α_2 receptors are located on presynaptic adrenergic neurons as well as some postsynaptic sites. It is possible that clonidine and α-methylnorepinephrine act in the brain to reduce norepinephrine release onto relevant receptor sites. Alternatively, these drugs may act on postsynaptic α_2 adrenoceptors to inhibit activity of appropriate neurons. Finally, clonidine also binds to nonadrenoceptor sites, the putative **imidazoline receptor,** which may also mediate antihypertensive effects. A number of newer agents are under study—eg, rilmenidine, moxonidine—that have much higher affinity for the I_1 imidazoline receptor than for alpha receptors and are effective antihypertensive drugs in animals and humans (Ernsberger, 1993; McKaigue, 1992).

Methyldopa and clonidine produce slightly different hemodynamic effects: clonidine lowers heart rate and cardiac output more than does methyldopa. This difference suggests that these two drugs do not have identical sites of action. They may act primarily on different populations of neurons in vasomotor centers of the brain stem.

Guanabenz and **guanfacine** are newer centrally active antihypertensive drugs that share the central alpha-adrenoceptor-stimulating effects of clonidine. They do not appear to offer any advantages over clonidine.

METHYLDOPA

Methyldopa is useful in the treatment of mild to moderately severe hypertension. It lowers blood pressure chiefly by reducing peripheral vascular resistance, with a variable reduction in heart rate and cardiac output.

Most cardiovascular reflexes remain intact after administration of methyldopa, and blood pressure reduction is not markedly dependent upon maintenance of upright posture. Postural (orthostatic) hypotension sometimes occurs, particularly in volume-depleted patients. One potential advantage of methyldopa is that it causes reduction in renal vascular resistance.

Pharmacokinetics & Dosage

Owing to extensive first-pass metabolism (primarily O-sulfate conjugation by the gastrointestinal mucosa), the bioavailability of methyldopa is low, averaging 25%, and varies among individuals. About two-thirds of the drug that reaches the systemic circulation is cleared by renal excretion, with a terminal elimination half-life of 2 hours. Impaired renal function results in reduced drug clearance.

Methyldopa enters the brain via a pump that actively transports aromatic amino acids. An oral dose of methyldopa produces its maximal antihypertensive effect in 4–6 hours, and the effect can persist for up to 24 hours. Because the effect depends upon accumulation of a metabolite, α-methylnorepinephrine, the action persists after the parent drug has disappeared from the circulation.

The maximal efficacy of methyldopa in lowering blood pressure is limited. In most patients, a dose of 2 g or less will produce maximal reduction in hypertension; if this result is not satisfactory, higher doses will usually not result in greater effects. The usual therapeutic dose is about 1–2 g/d orally in divided doses. In many patients, once-daily therapy is effective.

Toxicity

Most of the undesirable effects of methyldopa are referable to the central nervous system. Of these, the most frequent is overt sedation, particularly at the onset of treatment. With long-term therapy, patients may complain of persistent mental lassitude and impaired mental concentration. Nightmares, mental depression, vertigo, and extrapyramidal signs may occur but are relatively infrequent. Lactation, associated with increased prolactin secretion, can occur both in men and in women treated with methyldopa. This toxicity is probably mediated by an inhibiting action on dopaminergic mechanisms in the hypothalamus.

Other important adverse effects of methyldopa are development of a positive Coombs test (occurring in 10–20% of patients undergoing therapy for longer than 12 months), which sometimes makes crossmatching blood for transfusion difficult and rarely is associated with hemolytic anemia, as well as hepatitis and drug fever. Discontinuation of the drug usually results in prompt reversal of these abnormalities.

CLONIDINE

Hemodynamic studies indicate that blood pressure lowering by clonidine results from reduction of cardiac output due to decreased heart rate and relaxation of capacitance vessels, with a reduction in peripheral vascular resistance, particularly when patients are upright (when sympathetic tone is normally increased).

Reduction in arterial blood pressure by clonidine is accompanied by decreased renal vascular resistance and maintenance of renal blood flow. As with methyldopa, clonidine reduces blood pressure in the supine position and only rarely causes postural hypotension. Pressor effects of clonidine are not observed after ingestion of therapeutic doses of clonidine, but severe hypertension can complicate overdosage.

Clonidine

Pharmacokinetics & Dosage

In healthy individuals, the bioavailability of clonidine averages 75% and the half-life is 8–12 hours. About half of the drug is eliminated unchanged in the urine, suggesting that lower than usual doses may be effective in patients with renal insufficiency.

Clonidine is lipid-soluble and rapidly enters the brain from the circulation. Because of its relatively short half-life and the fact that its antihypertensive effect is directly related to blood concentration, clonidine must be given twice a day to maintain smooth blood pressure control. Therapeutic doses are commonly between 0.2 and 1.2 mg/d. However, as is not the case with methyldopa, the dose-response curve of clonidine is such that increasing doses are more effective (but also more toxic). The maximal recommended dose is 1.2 mg/d.

A transdermal preparation of clonidine that reduces blood pressure for 7 days after a single application is also available. This preparation appears to produce less sedation than clonidine tablets but is commonly associated with local skin reactions.

Toxicity

Dry mouth and sedation are frequent and may be severe. Both effects are centrally mediated and dose-dependent and coincide temporally with the drug's antihypertensive effect.

The drug should not be given to patients who are at

risk of mental depression and should be withdrawn if depression occurs during therapy. Concomitant treatment with tricyclic antidepressants may block the antihypertensive effect of clonidine. The interaction is believed to be due to alpha-adrenoceptor-blocking actions of the tricyclics.

Withdrawal of clonidine after protracted use, particularly with high doses (greater than 1 mg/d), can result in life-threatening hypertensive crisis mediated by increased sympathetic nervous activity. Patients exhibit nervousness, tachycardia, headache, and sweating after omitting one or two doses of the drug. Although the incidence of severe hypertensive crisis is unknown, it is high enough to require that all patients who take clonidine be carefully warned of the possibility. If the drug must be stopped, this should be done gradually while other antihypertensive agents are being substituted. Treatment of the hypertensive crisis consists of reinstitution of clonidine therapy or administration of alpha- and beta-adrenoceptor-blocking agents.

Other Uses of Clonidine

Clonidine is claimed to have several effects in the central nervous system that are useful apart from the therapy of hypertension. These include analgesic effects, especially when administered intrathecally (Filos et al, 1992) and amelioration of symptoms in patients withdrawing from tobacco or opioid use (Täschner, 1986). The latter action probably reflects the ability of clonidine to reduce the sympathetic outflow that ordinarily increases markedly during opioid withdrawal.

GANGLION-BLOCKING AGENTS

Historically, drugs that block stimulation of postganglionic autonomic neurons by acetylcholine were among the first agents used in the treatment of hypertension. Most such drugs are no longer available clinically because of intolerable toxicities related to their primary action (see below). Only one drug in this class (trimethaphan) is still used to treat hypertension.

Ganglion blockers competitively block nicotinic cholinoceptors on postganglionic neurons in both sympathetic and parasympathetic ganglia. In addition, these drugs may directly block the nicotinic acetylcholine channel, in the same fashion as neuromuscular nicotinic blockers (see Figure 26–5).

TRIMETHAPHAN

Trimethaphan camsylate is administered intravenously to take advantage of its rapid action in treating hypertensive crisis and to induce controlled hypotension for neurosurgery. The dependence of ganglionic

blockade on blood level and the short half-life of the drug allow precise titration of blood pressure while other drugs are taking effect.

Trimethaphan

The antihypertensive effect of trimethaphan is to a large extent dependent upon pooling of blood in capacitance vessels. Patients must be tilted head up (usually with blocks under the head of the bed) for effective blood pressure lowering. Conversely, excessive hypotension can be rapidly treated by reverse tilting.

The adverse effects of ganglion blockers are direct extensions of their pharmacologic effects. These effects include both sympathoplegia (excessive orthostatic hypotension and sexual dysfunction) and parasympathoplegia (constipation, urinary retention, precipitation of glaucoma, blurred vision, dry mouth, etc). These severe toxicities are the major reason for the abandonment of ganglion blockers for outpatient therapy of hypertension.

ADRENERGIC NEURON-BLOCKING AGENTS

These drugs lower blood pressure by preventing normal physiologic release of norepinephrine from postganglionic sympathetic neurons.

GUANETHIDINE

In high enough doses, guanethidine can produce profound sympathoplegia. The resulting high maximal efficacy of this agent made it the mainstay of outpatient therapy of severe hypertension for many years. For the same reason, guanethidine can produce all of the toxicities expected from "pharmacologic sympathectomy," including marked postural hypotension, diarrhea, and impaired ejaculation. Because of these adverse effects, guanethidine is now rarely used.

The structure of guanethidine includes a highly basic nitrogen that makes the drug too polar to enter the central nervous system. As a result, this drug has none of the central effects seen with many of the other antihypertensive agents described in this chapter.

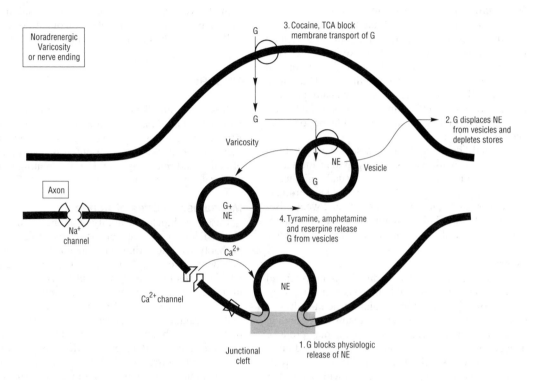

Figure 11–4. Guanethidine actions and drug interactions involving the adrenergic neuron. (G, guanethidine; NE, nor-epinephrine; TCA, tricyclic antidepressants.)

Guanethidine

Guanadrel is a guanethidine-like drug that is also available in the USA. **Bethanidine** and **debrisoquin,** antihypertensive agents not available for clinical use in the USA, are similar to guanethidine in mechanism of antihypertensive action.

Mechanism & Sites of Action

Guanethidine inhibits the release of norepinephrine from sympathetic nerve endings (Figure 11–4). This effect is probably responsible for most of the sympathoplegia that occurs in patients. Guanethidine is transported across the sympathetic nerve membrane by the same mechanism that transports norepinephrine itself (uptake 1), and uptake is essential for the drug's action. Once guanethidine has entered the nerve, it is concentrated in transmitter vesicles, where it replaces norepinephrine. Because it replaces norepinephrine, the drug causes a gradual depletion of norepinephrine stores in the nerve ending.

Inhibition of norepinephrine release is probably caused by guanethidine's local anesthetic properties on sympathetic nerve terminals. Although the drug does not impair axonal conduction in sympathetic fibers, local blockade of membrane electrical activity may occur in nerve endings, because the nerve endings specifically take up and concentrate the drug.

Because neuronal uptake is necessary for the hypotensive activity of guanethidine, drugs that block the catecholamine uptake process or displace amines from the nerve terminal (see Chapter 6) block its effects. These include cocaine, amphetamine, tricyclic antidepressants, phenothiazines, and phenoxybenzamine.

Guanethidine increases sensitivity to the hypertensive effects of exogenously administered sympathomimetic amines. This results from inhibition of neuronal uptake of such amines and, after long-term therapy with guanethidine, supersensitivity of effector smooth muscle cells, in a fashion analogous to the process that follows surgical sympathectomy (see Chapter 6).

The hypotensive action of guanethidine early in the course of therapy is associated with reduced cardiac output, due to bradycardia and relaxation of capacitance vessels, without consistent change in peripheral vascular resistance. With chronic therapy, peripheral vascular resistance decreases. Sodium and water retention may be marked during guanethidine therapy.

Pharmacokinetics & Dosage

The bioavailability of guanethidine is variable (3–50%). It is 50% cleared by the kidney. Retention of drug in nerve endings and uptake into other sites account for the very large volume of distribution and long half-life (5 days) of guanethidine. Thus, with constant daily dosing, the onset of sympathoplegia is gradual (maximal effect in 1–2 weeks), and sympathoplegia persists for a comparable period after cessation of therapy.

The daily dose required for a satisfactory antihypertensive response varies greatly among individual patients. For this reason, therapy is usually initiated at a low dose, eg, 10 mg/d. The dose should not ordinarily be increased at intervals shorter than 2 weeks. Because of the drug's long duration of action, maintenance doses need not be taken more than once a day.

Toxicity

Therapeutic use of guanethidine is often associated with symptomatic postural hypotension and hypotension following exercise, particularly when the drug is given in high doses. Injudicious treatment (excessive doses or too rapid escalation in dosage) may produce dangerously decreased blood flow to heart and brain or even overt shock. Guanethidine-induced sympathoplegia in men may be associated with delayed or retrograde ejaculation. Guanethidine commonly causes diarrhea, which results from increased gastrointestinal motility due to unopposed parasympathetic dominance in controlling the activity of intestinal smooth muscle.

Interactions with other drugs may complicate guanethidine therapy. Sympathomimetic agents such as phenylpropanolamine, at doses available in over-the-counter cold preparations, can produce hypertension in patients taking guanethidine. Similarly, guanethidine can produce hypertensive crisis by releasing catecholamines in patients with pheochromocytoma. When tricyclic antidepressants are administered to patients taking guanethidine, the drug's antihypertensive effect is attenuated, and severe hypertension may follow. A physician who is ignorant of this interaction may raise the dose of guanethidine; if the tricyclic antidepressant is then stopped, the patient may suffer severe hypotension or cardiovascular collapse from the unopposed action of guanethidine.

RESERPINE

Reserpine, an alkaloid extracted from the roots of an Indian plant, *Rauwolfia serpentina,* was one of the first effective drugs used on a large scale in the treatment of hypertension. At present, it is considered an effective and relatively safe drug for treating mild to moderate hypertension.

Mechanism & Sites of Action

Reserpine blocks the ability of aminergic transmitter vesicles to take up and store biogenic amines, probably by interfering with an uptake mechanism that depends on Mg^{2+} and ATP (Figure 6–4, carrier *B*). This effect occurs throughout the body, resulting in depletion of norepinephrine, dopamine, and serotonin in both central and peripheral neurons. Chromaffin granules of the adrenal medulla are also depleted of catecholamines, although to a lesser extent than are neurons. Reserpine's effects on adrenergic vesicles appear irreversible; trace amounts of the drug remain bound to vesicular membranes for many days. Although sufficiently high doses of reserpine in animals can reduce catecholamine stores to zero, lower doses cause inhibition of neurotransmission that is roughly proportionate to the degree of amine depletion.

Depletion of peripheral amines probably accounts for much of the beneficial antihypertensive effect of reserpine, but a central component cannot be ruled out. The effects of low but clinically effective doses resemble those of centrally acting agents (eg, methyldopa) in that sympathetic reflexes remain largely intact, blood pressure is reduced in supine as well as in standing patients, and postural hypotension is mild. Reserpine readily enters the brain, and depletion of cerebral amine stores causes sedation, mental depression, and parkinsonism symptoms.

At lower doses used for treatment of mild hyper-

Reserpine

tension, reserpine lowers blood pressure by a combination of decreased cardiac output and decreased peripheral vascular resistance.

Pharmacokinetics & Dosage

Absorption, clearance, and metabolism have not been well defined. The drug disappears rapidly from the circulation, but its effects persist much longer, owing to irreversible inactivation of catecholamine storage granules, as described above.

The usual daily dose is less than 1 mg (typically, 0.25 mg), administered orally as a single dose. Although reserpine is available in injectable form, parenteral administration is rarely indicated.

Toxicity

At the low doses usually administered, reserpine produces little postural hypotension. Most of the unwanted effects of reserpine result from actions on the brain or gastrointestinal tract.

High doses of reserpine characteristically produce sedation, lassitude, nightmares, and severe mental depression; occasionally, these occur even in patients receiving low doses (0.25 mg/d). Much less frequently, ordinary low doses of reserpine produce extrapyramidal effects resembling Parkinson's disease, probably as a result of dopamine depletion in the corpus striatum. Although these central effects are uncommon, it should be stressed that they may occur at any time, even after months of uneventful treatment. Patients with a history of mental depression should not receive reserpine, and the drug should be stopped if depression appears.

Reserpine rather often produces mild diarrhea and gastrointestinal cramps and increases gastric acid secretion. The drug should probably not be given to patients with a history of peptic ulcer.

PARGYLINE

Although pargyline and other inhibitors of monoamine oxidase lower blood pressure, they have no place in the modern treatment of hypertension. Pargyline is thought to lower blood pressure by increasing the concentration of an ineffective false transmitter in peripheral adrenergic nerve endings. Pargyline inhibits monoamine oxidase in gastrointestinal mucosa and the liver and thus allows unimpeded access of dietary tyramine to the systemic circulation. Tyramine is taken up into nerve endings and converted to octopamine (Figure 6–5), which partially replaces norepinephrine in catecholamine storage granules. Because octopamine is ineffective as a pressor agonist at postsynaptic alpha receptors, sympatholegia results even though total stores of norepinephrine may be increased.

ADRENOCEPTOR ANTAGONISTS

The pharmacology of drugs that antagonize catecholamines at alpha and beta adrenoceptors is presented in Chapter 10. Here we will concentrate on two prototypical drugs, propranolol and prazosin, primarily in relation to their use in treatment of hypertension. Other adrenoceptor antagonists will be considered only briefly.

PROPRANOLOL

Propranolol, a beta-adrenoceptor-blocking agent, is very useful for lowering blood pressure in mild to moderate hypertension. In severe hypertension, propranolol is especially useful in preventing the reflex tachycardia that often results from treatment with direct vasodilators.

Mechanism & Sites of Action

Propranolol antagonizes catecholamines at both β_1 and β_2 adrenoceptors. Both its efficacy in treating hypertension as well as most of its toxic effects result from beta blockade. When propranolol is first administered to a hypertensive patient, blood pressure decreases primarily as a result of a decrease in cardiac output associated with bradycardia. With continued treatment, however, cardiac output returns toward normal while blood pressure remains low, owing to reduction of peripheral vascular resistance.

Beta blockade in both brain and kidney has been proposed as contributing to the antihypertensive effect observed with beta-receptor blockers. In spite of conflicting evidence (Pearson, 1989), the brain appears unlikely to be the primary site of the hypotensive action of these drugs, because some beta-blockers that do not readily cross the blood-brain barrier (eg, nadolol, described below) are nonetheless effective antihypertensive agents.

Propranolol inhibits the stimulation of renin production by catecholamines (mediated by β_1 receptors). It is likely that propranolol's effect is due in part to depression of the renin-angiotensin-aldosterone system (Man in't Veld, 1983). Although most effective in patients with high plasma renin activity, propranolol also reduces blood pressure in hypertensive patients with normal or even low renin activity.

In mild to moderate hypertension, propranolol produces a significant reduction in blood pressure without prominent postural hypotension.

Pharmacokinetics & Dosage

As described in Chapter 10, effective oral doses of propranolol are greater than effective intravenous doses, owing to first-pass hepatic inactivation. The prominent first-pass effect partially accounts for the variability in doses required for clinically useful effects. The half-life is 3–6 hours.

Treatment of hypertension is usually started with 80 mg/d in divided doses. Effective antihypertensive dosage ranges from 80 to 480 mg/d. Resting bradycardia and a reduction in the heart rate during exercise are indicators of propranolol's beta-blocking effect. Measures of these responses may be used as guides in regulating dosage. Propranolol can be administered once or twice daily.

Toxicity

The principal toxicities of propranolol result from blockade of cardiac, vascular, or bronchial beta receptors and are described in more detail in Chapter 10. The most important of these predictable extensions of the beta-blocking action occur in patients with reduced myocardial reserve, asthma, peripheral vascular insufficiency, and diabetes.

When propranolol is discontinued after prolonged regular use, some patients experience a withdrawal syndrome, manifested by nervousness, tachycardia, increased intensity of angina, or increase of blood pressure. Myocardial infarction has been reported in a few patients. Although the incidence of these complications is probably low, propranolol should not be discontinued abruptly. The withdrawal syndrome may involve "up-regulation" or supersensitivity of beta adrenoceptors.

Propranolol also produces a low incidence of effects not clearly attributable to beta blockade, including diarrhea, constipation, nausea, and vomiting. Not infrequently, patients receiving propranolol complain of central nervous system effects reminiscent of those caused by methyldopa and clonidine, including nightmares, lassitude, mental depression, and insomnia.

Finally, propranolol may increase plasma triglycerides and decrease HDL-cholesterol, which theoretically could contribute to atherogenesis.

OTHER BETA-ADRENOCEPTOR-BLOCKING AGENTS

Of the large number of beta-blockers tested, most have been shown to be effective in lowering blood pressure. The pharmacologic properties of several of these agents differ from those of propranolol in ways that may confer therapeutic benefits in certain clinical situations.

1. METOPROLOL

Metoprolol is approximately equipotent to propranolol in inhibiting stimulation of β_1 adrenoceptors such as those in the heart but 50- to 100-fold less potent than propranolol in blocking β_2 receptors. Although metoprolol is in other respects very similar to propranolol, its relative cardioselectivity may be advantageous in treating hypertensive patients who also

suffer from asthma, diabetes, or peripheral vascular disease. Studies of small numbers of asthmatic patients have shown that metoprolol causes less bronchial constriction than propranolol at doses that produce equal inhibition of β_1-adrenoceptor responses. The cardioselectivity is not complete, however, and asthmatic symptoms have been exacerbated by metoprolol. Usual antihypertensive doses of metoprolol range from 100 to 450 mg/d.

2. NADOLOL, CARTEOLOL, ATENOLOL, & BETAXOLOL

Nadolol and carteolol, nonselective beta-receptor antagonists, and atenolol, a β_1-selective blocker, are not appreciably metabolized and are excreted to a considerable extent in the urine. Betaxolol is a β_1-selective blocker that is primarily metabolized in the liver but has a long half-life. These drugs can be administered once daily because of their relatively long half-lives in plasma. Nadolol is usually begun at a dosage of 40 mg/d, atenolol at a dosage of 50 mg/d, carteolol at a dosage of 2.5 mg/d, and betaxolol at a dosage of 10 mg/d. Increases in dosage to obtain a satisfactory therapeutic effect should take place no oftener than every 4 or 5 days. Patients with reduced renal function should receive correspondingly reduced doses of nadolol, carteolol, and atenolol. It is claimed that atenolol produces fewer central nervous system-related effects than other more lipid-soluble beta antagonists.

3. PINDOLOL, ACEBUTOLOL, & PENBUTOLOL

Pindolol, acebutolol, and penbutolol are partial agonists, ie, beta-blockers with intrinsic sympathomimetic activity. They lower blood pressure by decreasing vascular resistance and appear to depress cardiac output or heart rate less than other beta-blockers, perhaps because of significantly greater agonist than antagonist effects at β_2 receptors (Aellig, 1987). This may be particularly beneficial for patients with cardiac failure, bradyarrhythmias, or peripheral vascular disease. Daily doses of pindolol start at 10 mg; of acebutolol, at 400 mg; and of penbutolol, at 20 mg.

4. LABETALOL

Labetalol is given clinically as a racemic mixture of four isomeric compounds (it has two centers of asymmetry). Two of these isomers (the SS and RS isomers) are inactive, a third (SR) is a potent alpha-blocker, and the last (RR) is a potent beta-blocker. The beta-blocking isomer is thought to have selective β_2 agonist and nonselective beta antagonist action.

Labetalol has predominantly beta-blocking action, with a 3:1 ratio of beta:alpha antagonism after oral dosing. Blood pressure is lowered by reduction of systemic vascular resistance without significant alteration in heart rate or cardiac output. Because of its combined alpha- and beta-blocking activity, labetalol is useful in treating the hypertension of pheochromocytoma and hypertensive emergencies. Oral daily doses of labetalol range from 200 to 2400 mg/d. Labetalol is given as repeated intravenous bolus injections of 20–80 mg to treat hypertensive emergencies.

PRAZOSIN & OTHER α_1-BLOCKERS

Mechanism & Sites of Action

Prazosin, terazosin, and doxazosin produce most of their antihypertensive effect by blocking α_1 receptors in arterioles and venules. Selectivity for α_1 receptors may explain why these agents produce less reflex tachycardia than do nonselective alpha antagonists such as phentolamine. This receptor selectivity allows norepinephrine to exert unopposed negative feedback (mediated by presynaptic α_2 receptors) on its own release (see Chapter 6); in contrast, phentolamine blocks both pre- and postsynaptic alpha receptors, with the result that reflex stimulation of sympathetic neurons produces greater release of transmitter onto beta receptors and correspondingly greater cardioacceleration.

Alpha-blockers reduce arterial pressure by dilating both resistance and capacitance vessels. As expected, blood pressure is reduced more in the upright than in the supine position. Retention of salt and fluid occurs when these drugs are administered without a diuretic. The drugs are more effective when used in combination with other agents, such as propranolol and a diuretic, than when used alone.

Pharmacokinetics & Dosage

Prazosin is well absorbed but undergoes substantial first-pass metabolism in the liver. It is eliminated almost entirely by metabolism, with a plasma half-life of 3–4 hours, although the duration of the antihypertensive effect is longer. Plasma concentrations are increased in patients with congestive heart failure, owing primarily to reduced first-pass metabolism. Terazosin is also extensively metabolized but undergoes very little first-pass metabolism and has a half-life of 12 hours. Doxazosin has an intermediate bioavailability and a half-life of 22 hours.

Treatment with prazosin should be initiated with a low dose (1 mg 3 times daily) to prevent postural hypotension and syncope. Doses may be increased to 20 or 30 mg/d. Terazosin can often be given once daily, with doses of 5–20 mg/d. Doxazosin is usually given once daily starting at 1 mg/d and progressing to 4 mg/d or more as needed. Although long-term treatment with these alpha-blockers causes relatively little postural hypotension, a number of patients develop a precipitous drop in standing blood pressure shortly after the first dose is absorbed. For this reason, the first dose should be small and should be administered at bedtime. While the mechanism of this first-dose phenomenon is not clear, it occurs more commonly in patients who are salt- and volume-depleted.

Aside from the first-dose phenomenon, the reported toxicities of the α_1 blockers are relatively infrequent and mild. These include dizziness, palpitations, headache, and lassitude. Some patients develop a positive test for antinuclear factor in serum while on prazosin therapy, but this has not been associated with rheumatic symptoms. Unlike diuretics and beta-blockers, the α_1-blockers do not adversely and may even beneficially affect plasma lipid profiles.

OTHER ALPHA-ADRENOCEPTOR-BLOCKING AGENTS

Investigational α_1-selective blockers include pinacidil, urapidil, and cromakalim. The nonselective agents, **phentolamine** and **phenoxybenzamine,** are useful in diagnosis and treatment of pheochromocytoma and in other clinical situations associated with exaggerated release of catecholamines (eg, phentolamine may be combined with propranolol to treat the clonidine withdrawal syndrome, described above). Their pharmacology is described in Chapter 10.

VASODILATORS

Mechanism & Sites of Action

Within this class of drugs are the oral vasodilators, hydralazine and minoxidil, which are used for long-term outpatient therapy of hypertension; the parenteral vasodilators, nitroprusside and diazoxide, which are used to treat hypertensive emergencies; and the calcium channel blockers, which are used in both circumstances.

All of the vasodilators useful in hypertension relax smooth muscle of arterioles, thereby decreasing systemic vascular resistance. Sodium nitroprusside also relaxes veins. Decreased arterial resistance and decreased mean arterial blood pressure elicit compensatory responses, mediated by baroreceptors and the sympathetic nervous system (Figure 11–5), as well as renin, angiotensin, and aldosterone. These compensating responses oppose the antihypertensive effect of the vasodilator. Because sympathetic reflexes are intact, vasodilator therapy does not cause orthostatic hypotension or sexual dysfunction.

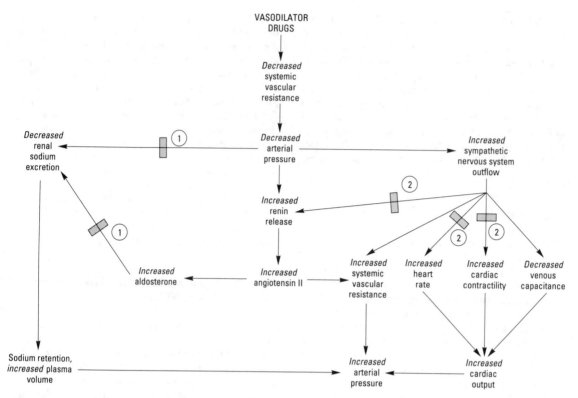

Figure 11–5. Compensatory responses to vasodilators; basis for combination therapy with beta-blockers and diuretics. ℵ Effect blocked by diuretics. ℑ Effect blocked by beta-blockers.

Vasodilators work best in combination with other antihypertensive drugs that oppose the compensatory cardiovascular responses (Figure 11–5). (See box: Monotherapy Versus Polypharmacy in Hypertension.)

HYDRALAZINE

Hydralazine, a hydrazine derivative, dilates arterioles but not veins. It has been available for many years, though it was initially thought not to be particularly effective because tachyphylaxis to hypertensive effects developed rapidly. Now the benefits of combination therapy are recognized, and hydralazine may be used more effectively, particularly in severe hypertension.

Hydralazine

Pharmacokinetics, Metabolism, & Dosage

Hydralazine is well absorbed and rapidly metabolized by the liver during the first pass, so that bioavailability is low (averaging 25%) and variable among individuals. It is metabolized in part by acetylation at a rate that appears to be bimodally distributed in the population (see Chapter 4). As a consequence, rapid acetylators have greater first-pass metabolism, lower bioavailability, and less antihypertensive benefit from a given dose than do slow acetylators. The half-life of hydralazine ranges from 2 to 4 hours, but vascular effects appear to persist longer than do blood concentrations—an observation that is consistent with experimental evidence of avid binding to vascular tissue.

Usual dosage ranges from 40 to 200 mg/d. The higher dosage was selected as the dose at which there is a small possibility of developing the lupus erythematosus-like syndrome described in the next section. However, higher dosages result in greater vasodilation and may be used if necessary. Dosing 2 or 3 times daily provides smooth control of blood pressure.

Toxicity

The most common adverse effects of hydralazine are headache, nausea, anorexia, palpitations, sweating, and flushing. In patients with ischemic heart disease, reflex tachycardia and sympathetic stimulation may provoke angina or ischemic arrhythmias. With dosages of 400 mg/d or more, there is a 10–20% incidence—chiefly in persons who slowly acetylate the drug—of a syndrome characterized by arthralgia, myalgia, skin rashes, and fever that resembles lupus erythematosus. The syndrome is not associated with renal damage and is reversed by discontinuance of hydralazine. Peripheral neuropathy and drug fever are other serious but uncommon adverse effects.

MINOXIDIL

Minoxidil is a very efficacious orally active vasodilator. The effect appears to result from the opening of potassium channels in smooth muscle membranes by minoxidil sulfate, the active metabolite. This action stabilizes the membrane at its resting potential and makes contraction less likely. Like hydralazine, minoxidil dilates arterioles but not veins. Because of its greater potential antihypertensive effect, minoxidil should replace hydralazine when maximal doses of the latter are not effective or in patients with renal failure and severe hypertension, who do not respond well to hydralazine.

Minoxidil

Pharmacokinetics, Metabolism, & Dosage

Minoxidil is well absorbed from the gastrointestinal tract and is metabolized, primarily by conjugation, in the liver. Minoxidil is not protein-bound. Its half-life averages 4 hours, but its hypotensive effect after a single dose may persist for over 24 hours, probably reflecting the persistence of its active metabolite, minoxidil sulfate.

Minoxidil is available for hypertension only as an oral preparation. Generally, patients are started on 5 or 10 mg/d in two doses, and the daily dosage is then gradually increased to 40 mg/d. Higher dosages—up to 80 mg/d—have been used in treating severe hypertension.

Even more than with hydralazine, the use of minoxidil is associated with reflex sympathetic stimulation and sodium and fluid retention. Minoxidil must be used in combination with a beta-blocker and a loop diuretic.

Toxicity

Tachycardia, palpitations, angina, and edema are observed when doses of beta-blockers and diuretics are inadequate. Headache, sweating, and hypertrichosis, which is particularly bothersome in women, are relatively common. Minoxidil illustrates how one person's toxicity may become another person's therapy. Topical minoxidil is now used as a stimulant to hair growth for correction of baldness.

SODIUM NITROPRUSSIDE

Sodium nitroprusside is a powerful parenterally administered vasodilator that is used in treating hypertensive emergencies as well as severe cardiac failure. Nitroprusside dilates both arterial and venous vessels, resulting in reduced peripheral vascular resistance and venous return. The action occurs as a result of activation of guanylyl cyclase, either via release of nitric oxide or by direct stimulation of the enzyme. The result is increased intracellular cGMP, which relaxes vascular smooth muscle.

In the absence of cardiac failure, blood pressure decreases, owing to decreased vascular resistance, while cardiac output does not change or decreases slightly. In patients with cardiac failure and low cardiac output, output increases owing to afterload reduction.

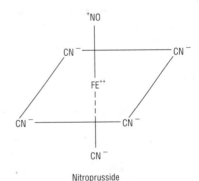

Nitroprusside

Pharmacokinetics, Metabolism, & Dosage

Nitroprusside is a complex of iron, cyanide groups, and a nitroso moiety. It is rapidly metabolized by uptake into red blood cells with liberation of cyanide. Cyanide in turn is metabolized by the mitochondrial enzyme rhodanase, in the presence of a sulfur donor, to thiocyanate. Thiocyanate is distributed in extracellular fluid and slowly eliminated by the kidney.

Nitroprusside rapidly lowers blood pressure, and its effects disappear within 1–10 minutes after discontinuation. The drug is given by intravenous infusion. Sodium nitroprusside in aqueous solution is sensitive to light and must therefore be made up fresh before each administration and covered with opaque foil. Infusion solutions should be changed after several hours. Dosage typically begins at 0.5 µg/kg/min and may be increased up to 10 µg/kg/min as necessary to control blood pressure. Higher rates of infusion, if continued for more than an hour, may result in toxicity. Because of its efficacy and rapid onset of effect, the drug should be administered by infusion pump and arterial blood pressure continuously monitored via intra-arterial recording.

Toxicity

The most serious toxicity is related to accumulation of cyanide; metabolic acidosis, arrhythmias, excessive hypotension, and death have resulted. In a few cases, toxicity after relatively low doses of nitroprusside suggested a defect in cyanide metabolism. Administration of sodium thiosulfate as a sulfur donor facilitates metabolism of cyanide. Hydroxocobalamin combines with cyanide to form the nontoxic cyanocobalamin. Both have been advocated for prophylaxis or treatment of cyanide poisoning during nitroprusside infusion. Thiocyanate may accumulate over the course of prolonged administration, usually a week or more, particularly in patients with renal insufficiency who do not excrete thiocyanate at a normal rate. Thiocyanate toxicity is manifested as weakness, disorientation, psychosis, muscle spasms, and convulsions, and the diagnosis is confirmed by finding serum concentrations greater than 10 mg/dL. Rarely, delayed hypothyroidism occurs, owing to thiocyanate inhibition of iodide uptake by the thyroid. Methemoglobinemia during infusion of nitroprusside has also been reported.

DIAZOXIDE

Diazoxide is an effective and relatively long-acting parenterally administered arteriolar dilator that is used to treat hypertensive emergencies. Injection of diazoxide results in a rapid fall in systemic vascular resistance and mean arterial blood pressure associated with substantial tachycardia and increase in cardiac output. Studies of its mechanism suggest that it prevents vascular smooth muscle contraction by opening potassium channels and stabilizing the membrane potential at the resting level.

Diazoxide

Pharmacokinetics & Dosage

Diazoxide is similar chemically to the thiazide diuretics but has no diuretic activity. It is bound extensively to serum albumin and to vascular tissue. Diazoxide is in part metabolized and in part excreted unchanged; its metabolic pathways are not well characterized. Its half-life is approximately 24 hours, but the relationship between blood concentration and hypotensive action is not well established. The blood pressure-lowering effect after a rapid injection is established within 5 minutes and lasts for 4–12 hours. It was initially thought that rapid injection was mandatory to saturate plasma protein binding so that free drug could reach vascular tissue, but this idea is no longer generally accepted. Blood pressure is in fact lowered by constant infusion, although the extent of lowering for a given total dose is greater after rapid administration.

When diazoxide was first marketed, a dose of 300 mg by rapid injection was recommended. It appears, however, that excessive hypotension can be avoided by beginning with smaller doses (75–100 mg). If necessary, doses of 150 mg may be repeated every 5 minutes until blood pressure is lowered satisfactorily. Nearly all patients respond to a maximum of three or four doses. Because of reduced protein binding, hypotension occurs after smaller doses in persons with chronic renal failure, and smaller doses should be administered to these patients. The hypotensive effects of diazoxide are also greater if patients are pretreated with beta-blockers to prevent the reflex tachycardia and associated increase in cardiac output.

Toxicity

The most significant toxicity from diazoxide has been excessive hypotension, resulting from the recommendation to use a fixed dose of 300 mg in all patients. Such hypotension has resulted in stroke and myocardial infarction. The reflex sympathetic response can provoke angina, electrocardiographic evidence of ischemia, and cardiac failure in patients with ischemic heart disease, and diazoxide should be avoided in this situation.

Diazoxide inhibits insulin release from the pancreas (probably by opening potassium channels in the beta cell membrane) and is used to treat hypoglycemia secondary to insulinoma. Occasionally, hyperglycemia complicates diazoxide use, particularly in persons with renal insufficiency.

In contrast to the thiazide diuretics, diazoxide causes renal salt and water *retention*. However, because the drug is used for short periods only, this is rarely a problem.

CALCIUM CHANNEL BLOCKERS

In addition to their antianginal (Chapter 12) and antiarrhythmic effects (Chapter 14), calcium channel blockers also dilate peripheral arterioles and reduce blood pressure. The mechanism of action in hypertension (and, in part, in angina) is inhibition of calcium influx into arterial smooth muscle cells.

Verapamil, diltiazem, and the **dihydropyridine** family **(amlodipine, felodipine, isradipine, nicardipine, and nifedipine)** are all equally effective in lowering blood pressure, and various formulations are currently approved for this use in the USA. Several others are under study. Hemodynamic differences among calcium channel blockers may influence the choice of a particular agent. Nifedipine and the other dihydropyridine agents are more selective as vasodilators and have less cardiac depressant effect than verapamil and diltiazem. Reflex sympathetic activation with slight tachycardia maintains or increases cardiac output in most patients given dihydropyridines. Verapamil has the greatest effect on the heart and may decrease heart rate and cardiac output. Diltiazem has intermediate actions. The pharmacology and toxicity of these drugs is discussed in more detail in Chapter 12. Doses of calcium channel blockers used in treating hypertension are similar to those used in treating angina or coronary spasm. Nifedipine has gained some popularity in emergency treatment of severe hypertension.

INHIBITORS OF ANGIOTENSIN

Although the causative roles of renin, angiotensin, and aldosterone in essential hypertension are still controversial, there do appear to be differences in the activity of this system among individuals. When controlled for daily sodium intake (assessed as 24-hour urinary sodium excretion) and serum potassium concentration, approximately 20% of patients with essential hypertension have inappropriately low and 20% have inappropriately high plasma renin activity. Blood pressure of patients with high-renin hypertension responds well to beta-adrenoceptor blockers, which lower plasma renin activity, and to angiotensin inhibitors—supporting a role for excess renin and angiotensin in this population.

Mechanism & Sites of Action

Renin release from the kidney cortex is stimulated by reduced renal arterial pressure, sympathetic neural stimulation, and reduced sodium delivery or increased sodium concentration at the distal renal tubule. Renin acts upon renin substrate, an α_2-globulin, to split off the inactive decapeptide angiotensin I. Angiotensin I is then converted, primarily in the lung, to the arterial vasoconstrictor octapeptide angiotensin II (Figure 11–6), which is in turn converted in the adrenal gland to angiotensin III. Angiotensin II has vasoconstrictor and sodium-retaining activity. Angiotensin II and III both stimulate aldosterone release. Angiotensin may contribute to maintaining high vascular resistance in hypertensive states associated with high plasma renin activity, such as renal arterial stenosis, some types of intrinsic renal disease, and malignant hypertension, as well as in essential hypertension after treatment with sodium restriction, diuretics, or vasodilators.

New evidence suggests that a parallel system for angiotensin generation exists in several other tissues (eg, heart) and may be responsible for trophic changes such as cardiac hypertrophy. The converting enzyme involved in tissue angiotensin II synthesis is also inhibited by the ACE inhibitors.

Renin and angiotensin II receptor antagonists that are not peptides—and therefore are orally active—are under study (see Chapter 17). Saralasin (see below) was withdrawn from regular clinical use. The drugs currently available act on the enzyme that converts angiotensin I to angiotensin II.

SARALASIN

Saralasin (1-sar-8-ala-angiotensin II) is an analogue and competitive inhibitor of angiotensin II at its receptors (Figure 11–6). Saralasin blocks the pressor and aldosterone-releasing effects of infused angiotensin II and lowers blood pressure in high-renin states such as renal artery stenosis. Saralasin also has weak agonist activity, however, so that rapid injection or administration to persons without high circulating angiotensin II may increase rather than decrease blood pressure. This partial agonist drug has proved to be a valuable research tool in determining the role of angiotensin II in hypertension.

ANGIOTENSIN-CONVERTING ENZYME (ACE) INHIBITORS

Captopril (Figure 17–2) and other drugs in this class inhibit the converting enzyme peptidyl dipeptidase that hydrolyzes angiotensin I to angiotensin II and (under the name plasma kininase) inactivates bradykinin, a potent vasodilator. Unlike saralasin, captopril has no pressor activity. Thus, the hypotensive activity of captopril probably results from an inhibitory action on the renin-angiotensin system and a

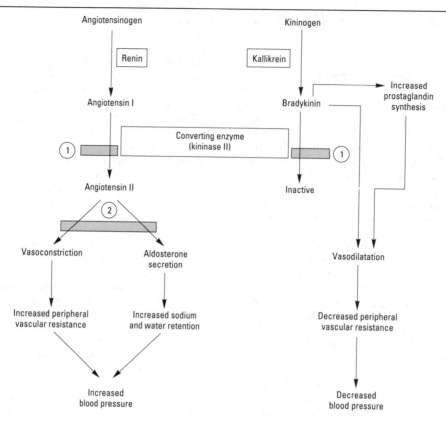

Figure 11–6. Sites of action of captopril and saralasin. א Site of captopril blockade. ℥ Site of saralasin blockade.

stimulating action on the kallikrein-kinin system (Figure 11–6).

Enalapril (Figure 17–2) is a prodrug that is converted by deesterification to a converting enzyme inhibitor, enalaprilat, with effects similar to those of captopril. Enalaprilat itself is available only for intravenous use, primarily for hypertensive emergencies. **Lisinopril** is a lysine derivative of enalaprilat. **Benazepril, fosinopril, quinapril,** and **ramipril** are recently introduced long-acting members of the class. All are prodrugs, like enalapril, and are converted to the active agents by hydrolysis, primarily in the liver.

Angiotensin II inhibitors lower blood pressure principally by decreasing peripheral vascular resistance. Cardiac output and heart rate are not significantly changed. Unlike direct vasodilators, these agents do not result in reflex sympathetic activation and can be used safely in persons with ischemic heart disease. The absence of reflex tachycardia may be due to downward resetting of the baroreceptors or to enhanced parasympathetic activity.

Although converting enzyme inhibitors are most effective in conditions associated with high plasma renin activity, there is no good correlation among subjects between plasma renin activity and antihypertensive response. Accordingly, renin measurement is unnecessary.

ACE inhibitors appear to have a particularly useful role in diabetic patients, diminishing proteinuria and stabilizing renal function (even in the absence of lowering of blood pressure). These benefits probably result from improved intrarenal hemodynamics, with decreased glomerular efferent arteriolar resistance and a resulting reduction of intraglomerular capillary pressure. ACE inhibitors have also proved to be extremely useful in the treatment of congestive heart failure. This application is discussed in Chapter 13.

Pharmacokinetics & Dosage

Captopril is rapidly absorbed, with a bioavailability of about 70% after fasting. Bioavailability is decreased by 30–40% if the drug is taken with food; however, the antihypertensive action of captopril is unaffected. It is metabolized chiefly to disulfide conjugates with other sulfhydryl-containing molecules. Less than half of an oral dose of captopril is excreted unchanged in the urine. Captopril is distributed to most body tissues, with the notable exception of the central nervous system. The half-life of captopril is less than 3 hours. Blood levels correlate poorly with clinical response.

Captopril is initially administered in doses of 25 mg 2 or 3 times each day, 1–2 hours before meals. Maximal blood pressure response is seen 2–4 hours after the dose. At 1- to 2-week intervals, doses can be increased until blood pressure is controlled.

Peak concentrations of enalaprilat occur 3–4 hours after dosing with enalapril. The half-life of enalaprilat is about 11 hours. Typical doses of enalapril are 10–20 mg once or twice daily.

Lisinopril is slowly absorbed, with peak blood levels at about 7 hours after a dose. It has a half-life of 12 hours. Doses of 10–80 mg once daily are effective in most patients.

All of the ACE inhibitors except fosinopril are eliminated primarily by the kidneys; doses of these drugs should be reduced in patients with renal insufficiency.

Toxicity

Severe hypotension can occur after initial doses of any ACE inhibitor in patients who are hypovolemic due to diuretics, salt restriction, or gastrointestinal fluid loss. Other adverse effects common to all ACE inhibitors include acute renal failure (particularly in patients with bilateral renal artery stenosis or stenosis of the renal artery of a solitary kidney), hyperkalemia, angioedema, and dry cough, sometimes accompanied by wheezing.

The use of ACE inhibitors is contraindicated during the second and third trimesters of pregnancy because of the risk of fetal hypotension, anuria, and renal failure, sometimes associated with fetal malformations or death. Captopril, particularly when given in high doses to patients with renal insufficiency, may cause neutropenia or proteinuria. Minor toxic effects seen more typically include altered sense of taste, allergic skin rashes, and drug fever, which may occur in as many as 10% of patients. The incidence of these adverse effects may be lower with enalapril and lisinopril.

Important drug interactions include those with potassium supplements or potassium-sparing diuretics, which can result in hyperkalemia. Nonsteroidal anti-inflammatory drugs may impair the hypotensive effects of ACE inhibitors by blocking bradykinin-mediated vasodilation, which is at least in part, prostaglandin mediated.

II. CLINICAL PHARMACOLOGY OF ANTIHYPERTENSIVE AGENTS

Hypertension presents a unique problem in therapeutics. It is usually a lifelong disease that causes few symptoms until the advanced stage. For effective treatment, medicines that are expensive and often produce adverse effects must be consumed daily. Thus, the physician must establish with certainty that hypertension is persistent and requires treatment and must exclude secondary causes of hypertension that might be treated by definitive surgical procedures. Persistence of hypertension, particularly in persons with mild elevation of blood pressure, should be established by finding an elevated blood pressure on at least three different office visits. Ambulatory blood pressure monitoring may be the best predictor of risk and therefore of need for therapy in mild hypertension. Recent evidence indicates that isolated systolic hypertension and hypertension in the elderly also benefit from therapy.

Once the presence of hypertension is established, the question of whether or not to treat and which drugs to use must be considered. The level of blood pressure, the age and sex of the patient, the severity of organ damage (if any) due to high blood pressure, and the presence of cardiovascular risk factors must all be considered.

Once the decision is made to treat, a therapeutic regimen must be developed and the patient must be educated about the nature of hypertension and the importance of treatment. Selection of drugs is dictated by the level of blood pressure, the presence and severity of end-organ damage, and the presence of other diseases. Severe high blood pressure with life-threatening complications requires more rapid treatment with more efficacious drugs. Most patients with essential hypertension, however, have had elevated blood pressure for months or years, and therapy is best initiated in a gradual fashion.

Successful treatment of hypertension requires that dietary instructions be followed and medications be taken as directed. Education about the natural history of hypertension and the importance of treatment as well as potential side effects of drugs is essential. Follow-up visits should be frequent enough to convince the patient that the physician thinks the illness is serious. With each follow-up visit, the importance of treatment should be reinforced and questions, particularly concerning dosing or side effects of medication, encouraged. Other factors that may improve compliance are simplifying dosing regimens and having the patient monitor blood pressure at home.

OUTPATIENT THERAPY OF HYPERTENSION

The initial step in treating hypertension may be nonpharmacologic. As discussed previously, sodium restriction may be effective treatment for as many as half of patients with mild hypertension. The average American diet contains about 200 meq of sodium per day. A reasonable dietary goal in treating hypertension is 70–100 meq of sodium per day, which can be achieved by not salting food during or after cooking and by avoiding processed foods that contain large amounts of sodium. Compliance with sodium restriction can be assessed by measuring 24-hour urinary excretion of sodium, which approximates sodium intake, before and after dietary instruction.

Weight reduction even without sodium restriction has been shown to normalize blood pressure in up to 75% of overweight patients with mild to moderate hypertension. Regular exercise has been shown in some but not all studies to lower blood pressure in hypertensive patients.

For pharmacologic management of mild hypertension, blood pressure can be normalized in most patients with a single drug. Such "monotherapy" is also sufficient for some patients with moderate hypertension. Thiazide diuretics or beta-blockers are most commonly used for initial drug therapy in such patients. Results from several large clinical trials suggest that these drugs reduce the morbidity and mortality associated with untreated hypertension. There has been concern that diuretics and beta-blockers, by adversely affecting the serum lipid profile or impairing glucose tolerance, may add to the risk of coronary disease, thereby offsetting the benefit of blood pressure reduction. Alternative choices for initial monotherapy include ACE inhibitors, calcium channel blockers, selective α_1 blockers (eg, prazosin), α,β blockers (labetalol), and central sympathoplegic

agents (eg, clonidine), though none of these have yet been shown to affect long-term outcome. The presence of concomitant disease should influence selection of antihypertensive drugs because two diseases may benefit from a single drug. For example, beta-blockers or calcium channel blockers are particularly useful in patients who also have angina, diuretics or ACE inhibitors in patients who also have congestive heart failure. Race and age also affect drug selection: blacks respond well to diuretics and calcium channel blockers and less well to beta-blockers and ACE inhibitors; older patients respond well to diuretics and beta-blockers.

If a single drug does not adequately control blood pressure, drugs with different sites of action can be combined to effectively lower blood pressure while minimizing toxicity ("stepped care"). If a diuretic is not used initially, it is often selected as the second drug. If three drugs are required, combining a diuretic, a sympathoplegic agent or an ACE inhibitor, and a direct vasodilator (eg, hydralazine or a calcium channel blocker) is often effective.

Assessment of blood pressure during office visits should include measurement of recumbent, sitting, and standing pressures. An attempt should be made to normalize blood pressure (mean blood pressure ≤ 100

MONOTHERAPY VERSUS POLYPHARMACY IN HYPERTENSION

Monotherapy of hypertension (treatment with a single drug) has become more popular since the introduction of ACE inhibitors and α_1-selective alpha-blockers because compliance is likely to be better and because in some cases adverse effects are fewer. However, moderate to severe hypertension is still commonly treated by a combination of two or more drugs, each acting by a different mechanism (polypharmacy). The rationale for polypharmacy is that each of the drugs acts on one of a set of interacting, mutually compensatory regulatory mechanisms for maintaining blood pressure (Figures 6–7 and 11–1).

For example, because an adequate dose of hydralazine causes a significant decrease in peripheral vascular resistance, there will initially be a drop in mean arterial blood pressure, evoking a strong response in the form of compensatory tachycardia and salt and water retention. The result is an increase in cardiac output that is capable of almost completely reversing the effect of hydralazine. The addition of a sympathoplegic drug (eg, propranolol) prevents the tachycardia; addition of a diuretic (eg, hydrochlorothiazide) prevents the salt and water retention. In effect, all three drugs increase the sensitivity of the cardio-

vascular system to each other's actions. Thus, partial impairment of one regulatory mechanism (sympathetic discharge to the heart) increases the antihypertensive effect of impairing regulation by another mechanism (peripheral vascular resistance). Finally, in some circumstances, a normal compensatory response accounts for the toxicity of an antihypertensive agent, and the toxic effect can be prevented by administering a second type of drug. In the case of hydralazine, compensatory tachycardia and increased cardiac output may precipitate angina in patients with coronary atherosclerosis. Addition of the beta-blocker and diuretic can prevent this toxicity in many patients.

In practice, when hypertension does not respond adequately to a regimen of one drug, a second drug from a different class with a different mechanism of action and different pattern of toxicity is added. If the response is still inadequate and compliance is known to be good, a third drug may be added. The drugs least likely to be successful as monotherapy are hydralazine and minoxidil. It is not completely clear why other drugs such as α_1-blockers and calcium channel blockers cause less marked compensatory responses for the same amount of blood pressure lowering.

mm Hg) in the posture or activity level that is customary for the patient. The extent of orthostatic hypotension and inhibition of reflex or exercise tachycardia are useful indicators of the effectiveness of or compliance with sympathoplegic therapy. In addition to noncompliance with medication, causes of failure to respond to drug therapy include excessive sodium intake and inadequate diuretic therapy with excessive blood volume (this can be measured directly), and drugs such as antidepressants and over-the-counter sympathomimetics and oral contraceptives that can interfere with actions of some antihypertensive drugs or directly raise blood pressure.

MANAGEMENT OF HYPERTENSIVE EMERGENCIES

Despite the large number of patients with chronic hypertension, hypertensive emergencies are relatively rare. Marked or sudden elevation of blood pressure may be a serious threat to life, however, and prompt reduction of blood pressure is indicated. Most commonly, hypertensive emergencies occur in patients whose hypertension is severe and poorly controlled and in those who suddenly discontinue antihypertensive medications.

Clinical Presentation & Pathophysiology

Hypertensive emergencies include hypertension associated with vascular damage (termed malignant hypertension) and hypertension associated with hemodynamic complications such as cardiac failure, stroke, or dissecting aneurysm. The underlying pathologic process in malignant hypertension is a progressive arteriopathy with inflammation and necrosis of arterioles. Vascular lesions occur in the kidney, which releases renin, which in turn stimulates production of angiotensin and aldosterone, which further increases blood pressure.

Hypertensive encephalopathy is a classic feature of malignant hypertension. Its clinical presentation consists of severe headache, mental confusion, and apprehension. Blurred vision, nausea and vomiting, and focal neurologic deficits are common. If untreated, the syndrome may progress over a period of 12–48 hours to convulsions, stupor, coma, and even death.

Treatment of Hypertensive Emergencies

The general management of hypertensive emergencies requires monitoring the patient in an intensive care unit with continuous recording of arterial blood pressure. Rapid treatment is essential, though excessively rapid lowering of blood pressure should be avoided since it can result in stroke or myocardial infarction. Fluid intake and output must be monitored carefully and body weight measured daily as an indicator of total body fluid volume during the course of therapy.

Parenteral antihypertensive medications are used to lower blood pressure rapidly (within a few hours); as soon as reasonable blood pressure control is achieved, oral antihypertensive therapy should be substituted, because this allows smoother long-term management of hypertension. The drugs most commonly used to treat hypertensive emergencies are the vasodilators sodium nitroprusside and diazoxide. Other parenteral drugs that may be effective include nitroglycerin, labetalol, trimethaphan, calcium channel blockers, hydralazine, reserpine, and methyldopa. Nonparenteral therapy with oral nifedipine, captopril, prazosin, or clonidine has also been shown to be useful in the therapy of severe hypertension.

Most patients with severe hypertension have a normal or contracted blood volume, although some, eg, those with renal failure, may be hypervolemic. Diuretics are administered to prevent the volume expansion that typically occurs during administration of powerful vasodilators. Because it is likely that the patient will have compromised renal function, a drug that works in the presence of renal insufficiency, such as furosemide, should be selected.

Dialysis may be a necessary alternative to the loop diuretics, particularly in patients with oliguric renal failure. Dialysis can remove excess fluid, correct electrolyte disturbances, and control symptoms of uremia. Uremic symptoms may be confusing in evaluating patients with hypertensive encephalopathy.

PREPARATIONS AVAILABLE

Beta-Adrenoceptor Blockers
  Acebutolol (Sectral)
    Oral: 200, 400 mg capsules
  Atenolol (generic, Tenormin)
    Oral: 25, 50, 100 mg tablets
    Parenteral: 0.5 mg/mL for injection
  Betaxolol (Kerlone)

    Oral: 10, 20 mg tablets
  Bisoprolol (Zebeta)
    Oral: 5, 10 mg tablets
  Carteolol (Cartrol)
    Oral: 2.5, 5 mg tablets
  Labetalol (Normodyne, Trandate)
    Oral: 100, 200, 300 mg tablets

Parenteral: 5 mg/mL for injection
Metoprolol (Lopressor)
Oral: 50, 100 mg tablets
Oral extended release (Toprol-XL): 50, 100, 200 mg tablets
Parenteral: 1 mg/mL for injection
Nadolol (Corgard)
Oral: 20, 40, 80, 120, 160 mg tablets
Penbutolol (Levatol)
Oral: 20 mg tablets
Pindolol (generic, Visken)
Oral: 5, 10 mg tablets
Propranolol (generic, Inderal)
Oral: 10, 20, 40, 60, 80, 90 mg tablets; Intensol, 80 mg/mL solution
Oral sustained-release (Inderal LA): 60, 80, 120, 160 mg capsules
Parenteral: 1 mg/mL for injection
Timolol (generic, Blocadren)
Oral: 5, 10, 20 mg tablets

Centrally Acting Sympathoplegic Drugs
Clonidine (generic, Catapres)
Oral: 0.1, 0.2, 0.3 mg tablets
Transdermal (Catapres-TTS): patches that release 0.1, 0.2, 0.3 mg/24 hr
Guanabenz (Wytensin)
Oral: 4, 8 mg tablets
Guanfacine (Tenex)
Oral: 1 mg tablets
Methyldopa (generic, Aldomet)
Oral: 125, 250, 500 mg tablets; 250 mg/5 mL suspension
Parenteral: 250 mg/5 mL for injection

Postganglionic Sympathetic Nerve Terminal Blockers
Guanadrel (Hylorel)
Oral: 10, 25 mg tablets
Guanethidine (generic, Ismelin Sulfate)
Oral: 10, 25 mg tablets
Reserpine (generic, Serpasil)
Oral: 0.1, 0.25, 1 mg tablets

Alpha$_1$-Selective Adrenoceptor Blockers
Doxazosin (Cardura)
Oral 1, 2, 4, 8 mg tablets
Prazosin (Minipress)
Oral: 1, 2, 5 mg capsules
Terazosin (Hytrin)
Oral: 1, 2, 5, 10 mg tablets

Ganglionic Blocking Agents
Mecamylamine (Inversine)
Oral: 2.5 mg tablets
Trimethaphan (Arfonad)
Parenteral: 500 mg/10 mL amp

Vasodilators Used in Hypertension
Diazoxide (generic, Hyperstat IV)

Parenteral: 15 mg/mL, 300 mg/20 mL amp
Hydralazine (generic, Apresoline)
Oral: 10, 25, 50, 100 mg tablets
Parenteral: 20 mg/mL for injection
Minoxidil (generic, Loniten)
Oral: 2.5, 10 mg tablets
Nitroprusside (generic, Nipride)
Parenteral: 50 mg/vial

Calcium Channel Blockers
Amlodipine (Norvasc)
Oral 2.5, 5, 10 mg tablets
Diltiazem (generic, Cardizem)
Oral: 30, 60, 90, 120 mg tablets (unlabeled in hypertension)
Oral sustained-release (Cardizem SR, Dilacor XL): 60, 90, 120, 180, 300 mg capsules
Parenteral: 5 mg/mL for injection
Felodipine (Plendil)
Oral extended release: 5, 10 mg tablets
Isradipine (DynaCirc)
Oral: 2.5, 5 mg capsules
Nicardipine (Cardene)
Oral: 20, 30 mg capsules
Oral sustained release (Cardene SR): 30, 45, 60 mg capsules
Nifedipine (generic, Adalat, Procardia)
Oral: 10, 20 mg capsules (unlabeled in hypertension)
Oral extended-release (Adalat CC, Procardia-XL): 30, 60, 90 mg tablets
Verapamil (generic, Calan, Isoptin)
Oral: 40, 80, 120 mg tablets
Oral sustained-release (generic, Calan SR, Verelan): 120, 180, 240 mg tablets; 120, 180, 240 mg capsules
Parenteral: 5 mg/2 mL for injection

Angiotensin-Converting Enzyme Inhibitors
Benazepril (Lotensin)
Oral: 5, 10, 20, 40, mg tablets
Captopril (Capoten)
Oral: 12.5, 25, 50, 100 mg tablets
Enalapril (Vasotec)
Oral: 2.5, 5, 10, 20 mg tablets
Parenteral (Enalaprilat): 1.25 mg/mL for injection
Fosinopril (Monopril)
Oral: 10, 20 mg tablets
Lisinopril (Prinivil, Zestril)
Oral: 5, 10, 20, 40 mg tablets
Quinapril (Accupril)
Oral: 5, 10, 20, 40 mg tablets
Perindopril (Aceon)
Oral: 2, 4, 8 mg tablets
Ramipril (Altace)
Oral: 1.25, 2.5, 5, 10 mg capsules

REFERENCES

Aellig WH, Clark BJ: Is the ISA of pindolol β_2-adrenoceptor selective? Br J Clin Pharmacol 1987;24:21S.

Atlas D, Diamant S, Zonnenschein R: Is the imidazoline site a unique receptor? A correlation with clonidine-displacing substance activity. Am J Hypertens 1992;5:83S.

Bauer JH, Reams GP: The role of calcium-entry blockers in hypertensive emergencies. Circulation 1987;75 (Suppl 6);V–174.

Bielen EC et al: Comparison of the effects of isradipine and lisinopril on left ventricular structure and function in essential hypertension. Am J Cardiol 1992;69:1200.

Calhoun DA, Oparil S: Treatment of hypertensive crisis. N Engl J Med 1990;323:1177.

Cohn JN, Burke LP: Nitroprusside. Ann Intern Med 1979; 91:752.

Croog SH et al: The effects of antihypertensive therapy on the quality of life. N Engl J Med 1986;314:1657.

Dahlof B et al: Morbidity and mortality in the Swedish trial in old patients with hypertension (STOP-Hypertension). Lancet 1991;338:1281.

Edelson JT et al: Long-term cost-effectiveness of various initial monotherapies for mild to moderate hypertension. JAMA 1990;263:407.

Ernsberger P et al: Moxonidine, a centrally acting antihypertensive agent, is a selective ligand for I_1-imidazoline sites. J Pharmacol Exp Ther 1993;264:172.

Filos KS et al: Intrathecal clonidine as a sole analgesic for pain relief after cesarean section. Anesthesiology 1992; 77:267.

Fletcher AE, Bulpitt CJ: How far should blood pressure be lowered?: N Engl J Med 1992;326:251.

Frohlich ED: Methyldopa: Mechanisms and treatment 25 years later. Arch Intern Med 1980;140:954.

Gifford RW Jr et al: Office evaluation of hypertension. Hypertension 1989;13:283.

Gifford RW Jr: An algorithm for the management of resistant hypertension. Hypertension 1988;11(Suppl 2):II–101.

Gifford RW Jr: Management of hypertensive crises. JAMA 1991;266:829.

Hanssens M et al: Fetal and neonatal effects of treatment with angiotensin-converting-enzyme inhibitors in pregnancy. Obstet Gynecol 1991;78:128.

Hartford M et al: Cardiovascular and renal effects of long-term antihypertensive treatment. JAMA 1988;259:2553.

Helgeland A: Treatment of mild hypertension: A five year controlled drug trial: The Oslo study. Am J Med 1980; 69:725.

Hypertension Detection and Follow-Up Program Cooperative Group: Five-year findings of the Hypertension Detection and Follow-Up Program. 1. Reduction in mortality of persons with high blood pressure, including mild hypertension. JAMA 1979;242:2562.

Hypertension Detection and Follow-Up Program Cooperative Group: Persistence of reduction in blood pressure and mortality of participants in the hypertension detection and follow-up program. JAMA 1988;259:2113.

Hypertension Detection and Follow-Up Program Cooperative Group: The effect of treatment on mortality in "mild" hypertension. N Engl J Med 1982;307:976.

Joint National Committee on Detection, Evaluation, and Treatment of High Blood Pressure: The fifth report of the Joint National Committee on Detection, Evaluation, and Treatment of High Blood Pressure (JNC V). Arch Intern Med 1993;153:154.

Joint National Committee on Detection, Evaluation, and Treatment of High Blood Pressure: Nonpharmacological approaches to the control of high blood pressure. Hypertension 1986;8:444.

Kaplan NM: Calcium entry blockers and future prospects. JAMA 1989;262:817.

Kaplan NM: Maximally reducing cardiovascular risk in the treatment of hypertension. Ann Intern Med 1988;109:36.

Kaplan NM: The appropriate goals of antihypertensive therapy: Neither too much nor too little. Ann Intern Med 1992;116:686.

Khoury AF, Kaplan NM: Alpha-blocker therapy of hypertension: An unfulfilled promise. JAMA 1991;266:394

Lam YWF, Shepherd MM: Drug interactions in hypertensive patients: Pharmacokinetic, pharmacodynamic and genetic considerations. Clin Pharmacokinet 1990;18: 295.

Langford HG et al: Dietary therapy slows the return of hypertension after stopping prolonged medication. JAMA 1985;253:657.

Law MR, Frost CD, Wald NJ: Analysis of data from trials of salt reduction. Br Med J 1991;302:819.

Leren P et al: Effect of propranolol and prazosin on blood lipids: The Oslo study. Lancet 1980;2:4.

Linas SL, Nies AS: Minoxidil. Ann Intern Med 1981;94:61.

Linas SL: The role of potassium in the pathogenesis and treatment of hypertension. Kidney Int 1991;39:771.

Lowenstein J: Clonidine. Ann Intern Med 1980;92:74.

Luke RG: Essential hypertension: A renal disease? A review and update of the evidence. Hypertension 1993; 21:380.

Maheswaran R et al: High blood pressure due to alcohol: A rapidly reversible effect. Hypertension 1991;17:787.

Makino N et al: Effect of angiotensin converting enzyme inhibitor on regression in cardiac hypertrophy. Mol Cell Biochem 1993;119:23.

Man in't Veld AJ, Schalekamp MADH: Effects of 10 different β-adrenoceptor antagonists on hemodynamics, plasma renin activity, and plasma norepinephrine in hypertension: The key role of vascular resistance changes in relation to partial agonist activity. J Cardiovasc Pharmacol 1983;5:S30.

Martin JE, Dubbert PM, Cushman WC: Controlled trial of aerobic exercise in hypertension. Circulation 1990;81: 1560.

Materson BJ et al: Single-drug therapy for hypertension in men: A comparison of six antihypertensive agents with placebo. N Engl J Med 1993;328:914.

McKaigue JP, Harron DWG: The effects of rilmenidine on tests of autonomic function in humans. Clin Pharmacol Ther 1992;52:511.

Michelson EL, Frishman WH: Labetalol: An alpha- and beta-adrenoceptor blocking drug. Ann Intern Med 1983; 99:553.

Mogensen CE: Angiotensin converting enzyme inhibitors and diabetic nephropathy: their effects on proteinuria may be independent of their effects on blood pressure. Br Med J 1992;304:327.

Moser M: Calcium entry blockers for systemic hypertension. Am J Cardiol 1987;59:115A.

Multiple Risk Factor Intervention Trial Research Group: Multiple risk factor intervention trial. JAMA 1982;248:1465.

Murphy MB et al: Glucose intolerance in hypertensive patients treated with diuretics: A fourteen-year follow-up. Lancet 1982;2:1293.

National High Blood Pressure Education Program Working Group on High Blood Pressure in Pregnancy: Working Group report on high blood pressure in pregnancy. Am J Obstet Gynecol 1990;163:1689.

National High Blood Pressure Education Program Working Group: Working Group report on hypertension and chronic renal failure. Arch Intern Med 1991;151:1280.

Pearson AA et al: A stereoselective central hypotensive action of atenolol. J Pharmacol Exp Therap 1989; 250:759.

Pollare T, Lithell H, Berne C: A comparison of hydrochlorothiazide and captopril on glucose and lipid metabolism in patients with hypertension. N Engl J Med 1989;321:868.

Report by the Management Committee: The Australian therapeutic trial in mild hypertension. Lancet 1980;1:1261.

Sanguinetti MC: Modulation of potassium channels by antiarrhythmic and antihypertensive drugs. Hypertension 1992;19:228.

Setaro JF, Black HR: Refractory hypertension. N Engl J Med 1992;327:543.

SHEP Cooperative Research Group: Implications of the Systolic Hypertension in the Elderly Program. Hypertension 1993;21:335.

SHEP Cooperative Research Group: Prevention of stroke by antihypertensive drug treatment in older persons with isolated systolic hypertension. JAMA 1991;265:3255.

Stamler J et al: INTERSALT study findings: Public health and medical care implications. Hypertension 1989;14:570.

Täschner K-L: A controlled comparison of clonidine and doxepin in the treatment of the opiate withdrawal syndrome. Pharmacopsychiatry 1986;19:91.

Task Force on Blood Pressure Control in Children: Report of the Second Task Force on Blood Pressure Control in Children–1987. Pediatrics 1987;79:1.

Toto RD et al: Reversible renal insufficiency due to angiotensin converting enzyme inhibitors in hypertensive nephrosclerosis. Ann Intern Med 1991;115:513.

Treatment of Mild Hypertension Research Group: The Treatment of Mild Hypertension Study: A randomized, placebo-controlled trial of a nutritional-hygienic regimen along with various drug monotherapies. Arch Intern Med 1991;151:1413.

van den Meiracker AH et al: Hemodynamic and hormonal adaptation to beta-adrenoceptor blockade: A 24-hour study of acebutolol, atenolol, pindolol, and propranolol in hypertensive patients. Circulation 1988;78:957.

Veterans Administration Cooperative Study Group on Antihypertensive Agents: Effects of treatment on morbidity in hypertension: 1. Results in patients with diastolic blood pressure averaging 115 through 129 mm Hg. JAMA 1967;202:1028.

Veterans Administration Cooperative Study Group on Antihypertensive Agents: Effects of treatment on morbidity in hypertension: 2. Results in patients with diastolic blood pressure averaging 90 through 114 mm Hg. JAMA 1970;213:1143.

Weber MA et al: Characterization of antihypertensive therapy by whole-day blood pressure monitoring. JAMA 1988;259:3281.

Weber MA: Clinical pharmacology of centrally acting antihypertensive agents. J Clin Pharmacol 1989;29:598.

Weber MA: Hypertension: Steps forward and steps backward–The Joint National Committee Fifth Report. Arch Intern Med 1993;153:149.

Weinberger MH et al: Dietary sodium restriction as adjunctive treatment of hypertension. JAMA 1988;259:2561.

Weinberger MH: Antihypertensive therapy and lipids: Paradoxical influences on cardiovascular disease risks. Am J Med 1986;80(Suppl 2A):64.

Weinberger MH: Optimizing cardiovascular risk reduction during antihypertensive therapy. Hypertension 1990;16:201.

Williams GH: Converting enzyme inhibitors in the treatment of hypertension. N Engl J Med 1988;319:1517.

Woosley RL, Nies AS: Guanethidine. N Engl J Med 1976;295:1053.

Working Group on Ambulatory Blood Pressure Monitoring, National High Blood Pressure Education Program Coordinating Committee: National High Blood Pressure Education Program Working Group Report on ambulatory blood pressure monitoring. Arch Intern Med 1990;150:2270.

Working Group on Hypertension in Diabetes: National High Blood Pressure Education Program. Statement on hypertension in diabetes mellitus: Final report. Arch Intern Med 1987;147:830.

Working Group on Management of Patients With Hypertension and High Blood Cholesterol: National Education Programs Working Group report on the management of patients with hypertension and high blood cholesterol. Ann Intern Med 1991;114:224.

World Health Organization: The 1986 guidelines for the treatment of mild hypertension. Hypertension 1986;8:957.

World Hypertension League: Physical exercise in the management of hypertension: A consensus statement by the World Hypertension League. J Hypertens 1991;9:283.

Vasodilators & the Treatment of Angina Pectoris

12

Bertram G. Katzung, MD, PhD, & Kanu Chatterjee, MB, FRCP

Angina pectoris is the most common condition involving tissue ischemia in which vasodilator drugs are used. Angina (pain) is caused by the accumulation of metabolites in striated muscle; angina pectoris is the severe chest pain that occurs when coronary blood flow is inadequate to supply the oxygen required by the heart. The organic nitrates, eg, **nitroglycerin,** are the mainstay of therapy in angina. Another group of vasodilators, the calcium channel blockers, is also important, especially for prophylaxis, and the beta-blockers, which are *not* vasodilators, are also useful in prophylaxis.

Ischemic heart disease is the most common serious health problem in many Western societies. By far the most frequent cause of angina is atheromatous obstruction of the large coronary vessels (**atherosclerotic** or **classic angina**). However, transient spasm of localized portions of these vessels, which is usually associated with underlying atheromas, can also cause significant myocardial ischemia and pain (**variant** or **vasospastic angina**).

The primary cause of angina pectoris is an imbalance between the oxygen requirement of the heart and the oxygen supplied to it via the coronary vessels. In classic angina, the imbalance occurs when the myocardial oxygen requirement increases, as during exercise, and coronary blood flow does not increase proportionately. The resulting ischemia usually leads to pain. Classic angina is therefore "angina of effort." (In some individuals, the ischemia may not always be accompanied by pain, resulting in "silent" or "ambulatory" ischemia.) In variant angina, oxygen delivery decreases as a result of reversible coronary vasospasm (usually superimposed on chronic obstruction).

In theory, the imbalance between oxygen delivery and myocardial oxygen demand can be corrected by **increasing delivery** (by increasing coronary flow) or **decreasing oxygen demand** (by decreasing cardiac work). Both measures are used in clinical practice. In atherosclerotic angina, reduction of demand is the easier of these goals to achieve by pharmacologic means. Traditional medical therapy achieves this goal through the use of organic nitrates—potent vasodilators—and several other classes of drugs, which decrease cardiac work. Increased delivery via increased coronary flow is difficult to achieve by pharmacologic means when flow is limited by fixed atheromatous plaques. In this situation, invasive measures (coronary bypass grafts or angioplasty) may be needed if reduction of oxygen demand does not control symptoms. In variant angina, on the other hand, spasm of coronary vessels can be reversed by nitrates or calcium channel blockers. It should be emphasized that not all vasodilators are effective in angina and, conversely, that some agents useful in angina (eg, beta-blockers) are not vasodilators.

When there is a change in the character, frequency, duration, and precipitating factors in patients with stable angina and when there are episodes of angina at rest, **unstable angina** is said to be present. This condition is caused by episodes of increased epicardial coronary artery tone or small platelet clots occurring in the vicinity of an atherosclerotic plaque. In most cases, formation of labile thrombi at the site of a fissured plaque is the mechanism for reduction in flow. It signals the imminent occurrence of a myocardial infarction and requires vigorous therapy.

History

Angina pectoris was first described as a distinct clinical entity by William Heberden in the latter half of the 18th century. In the second half of the 19th century, it was found that amyl nitrite could provide transient relief. However, it was not until the introduction of nitroglycerin in 1879 that effective relief of acute episodes of angina became possible. Subsequently, many other vasodilators (eg, theophylline, papaverine) were introduced for the treatment of angina. However, when careful double-blind clinical trials were done, these nonnitrate agents were found to be no better than placebo. In fact, several of the classic studies of the placebo effect were carried out in patients with angina. With the introduction of beta-adrenoceptor-blocking drugs, useful prophylactic therapy of angina became possible. More recently, the calcium channel blockers have been shown to be useful for prevention of anginal attacks, especially in variant angina.

PATHOPHYSIOLOGY OF ANGINA

Determinants of Myocardial Oxygen Demand

The major and minor determinants of myocardial oxygen requirement are set forth in Table 12–1. Unlike skeletal muscle, human cardiac muscle cannot develop an appreciable oxygen debt during stress and repay it later. As a consequence of its continuous activity, the heart's oxygen needs are relatively high, and it extracts approximately 75% of the available oxygen even under conditions of no stress. The myocardial oxygen requirement increases when there is an increase in heart rate, contractility, arterial pressure, or ventricular volume. These hemodynamic alterations frequently occur during physical exercise and sympathetic discharge, which often precipitate angina in patients with obstructive coronary artery disease. The relative contributions of basal metabolism and activation of contraction to the overall myocardial oxygen consumption appear to be small, but under pathologic conditions these apparently minor determinants of myocardial oxygen consumption may become relevant.

It is not possible to measure all of the determinants listed in Table 12–1 in the clinical setting. Therefore, indirect measures are often used to assess changes in myocardial oxygen demand and consumption. One commonly used index is the "double product" (heart rate × systolic blood pressure), a measure closely related to the tension-time index. The tension-time index is a more invasive measure of myocardial oxygen demand.

Determinants of Coronary Blood Flow & Myocardial Oxygen Supply

Oxygen supply is a function of myocardial oxygen delivery and extraction. Since myocardial oxygen extraction is nearly maximal at rest, there is little reserve to meet increased demands; furthermore, the oxygen content of the blood cannot be significantly increased under normal atmospheric conditions. Thus, increased myocardial demands for oxygen in the nor-

mal heart are met by augmenting coronary blood flow.

Coronary blood flow is directly related to the perfusion pressure (aortic diastolic pressure) and the duration of diastole. Because coronary flow drops to negligible values during systole, the duration of diastole becomes a limiting factor for myocardial perfusion during tachycardia. Coronary blood flow is inversely proportionate to coronary vascular bed resistance. Resistance is determined by intrinsic factors, including metabolic products and autonomic activity; by various pharmacologic agents; and by the extravascular mechanical compression of the coronary arteries. The site of autoregulation appears to be the arteriolar resistance vessels. Damage to the endothelium of coronary vessels has been shown to alter their ability to dilate in response to normal stimuli.

I. BASIC PHARMACOLOGY OF DRUGS USED TO TREAT ANGINA

Drug Action in Angina

All three of the drug groups useful in angina *decrease myocardial oxygen requirement* by decreasing peripheral vascular resistance, by decreasing cardiac output, or in both ways. In some patients, a redistribution of coronary flow may increase oxygen delivery to ischemic tissue. In variant angina, the nitrates and the calcium channel blockers may also *increase myocardial oxygen delivery* by reversing coronary arterial spasm. The mechanisms of vascular smooth muscle contraction and relaxation and the site of action of the calcium channel blockers are shown in Figure 12–1. The site of action of the nitrates (and of nitric oxide released from endothelial cells by neurohumoral agents) is shown in Figure 12–2.

NITRATES & NITRITES

Chemistry

These agents are simple nitric and nitrous acid esters of polyalcohols (Figure 12–3). They vary from extremely volatile liquids (amyl nitrite) through moderately volatile liquids (nitroglycerin) to solids (isosorbide dinitrate). Nitroglycerin may be considered the prototype of the group. Although it is used in the manufacture of dynamite, the formulations of nitroglycerin used in medicine are not explosive. The conventional sublingual tablet form of nitroglycerin may lose potency when stored as a result of volatilization and adsorption to plastic surfaces. Therefore, it should be kept in tightly closed glass containers. It is not sensitive to light.

Table 12–1. Determinants of myocardial oxygen consumption.

Major	Minor
Wall stress	
Intraventricular pressure	Activation energy
Ventricular radius (volume)	Resting metabolism
Wall thickness	
Heart rate	
Contractility	

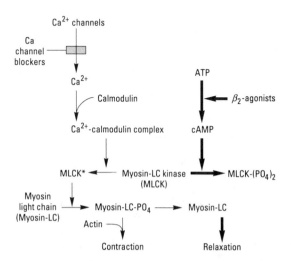

Figure 12–1. Control of smooth muscle contraction and site of action of calcium channel blocking drugs. Contraction is triggered by influx of calcium (which can be blocked by calcium channel blockers) through transmembrane calcium channels. The calcium combines with calmodulin to form a complex that converts the enzyme myosin light chain kinase to its active form *(MLCK*)*. The latter phosphorylates the myosin light chains, thereby initiating the interaction of myosin with actin. Beta$_2$ agonists (and other substances that increase cAMP) may cause relaxation in smooth muscle by accelerating the inactivation of MLCK (heavy arrows) and by facilitating the expulsion of calcium from the cell (not shown).

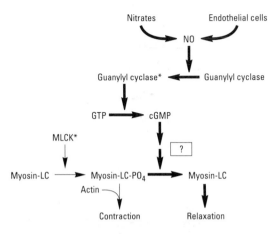

Figure 12–2. Mechanism of action of nitrates, nitrites, and other substances that increase the concentration of nitric oxide (NO) in smooth muscle cells. Steps leading to relaxation are shown with heavy arrows. (MLCK*, activated myosin light chain kinase [see Figure 12–1]; guanylyl cyclase*, activated guanylyl cyclase; ?, unknown intermediate steps.)

Structure-activity studies indicate that all therapeutically active agents in this group are capable of releasing nitric oxide (NO) in vascular smooth muscle target tissues (Harrison and Bates, 1993). Unfortunately, they all are capable of inducing cross-tolerance when given in large doses. Therefore, pharmacokinetic factors govern the choice of agent and mode of therapy when using the nitrates.

Pharmacokinetics

The use of organic nitrates is strongly influenced by the existence of a high-capacity hepatic organic nitrate reductase that removes nitrate groups in a stepwise fashion from the parent molecule and ultimately inactivates the drug. Therefore, bioavailability of the traditional oral organic nitrates (nitroglycerin and isosorbide dinitrate) is very low (typically < 10–20%). The sublingual route, which avoids the first-pass effect, is therefore preferred for achieving a therapeutic blood level rapidly. Nitroglycerin and isosorbide dinitrate are both absorbed efficiently by this route and reach therapeutic blood levels within a few minutes. However, the total dose administered by this route must be limited to avoid excessive effects; therefore, the total duration of effect is brief (15–30 minutes). When much longer duration of action is needed, oral preparations can be given that contain an amount of drug sufficient to result in sustained systemic blood levels of drug or active metabolites. Other routes of administration available for nitroglycerin include transdermal and buccal absorption from slow-release preparations; these are described below.

Amyl nitrite and related nitrites are highly volatile liquids. Amyl nitrite is available in fragile glass ampules packaged in a protective cloth covering. The ampule can be crushed with the fingers, resulting in rapid release of inhalable vapors through the cloth covering. The inhalation route provides for very rapid absorption and, like the sublingual route, avoids the hepatic first-pass effect.

Once absorbed, the unchanged nitrate compounds have half-lives of only 2–8 minutes. The partially denitrated metabolites have much longer half-lives (up to 3 hours). Of the nitroglycerin metabolites (two dinitroglycerins and two mononitro forms), the dinitro derivatives have significant vasodilator efficacy; they probably provide most of the therapeutic effect of orally administered nitroglycerin. The 5-mononitrate metabolite of isosorbide dinitrate is an active metabolite of the latter drug and is available for clinical use as isosorbide mononitrate. It has a bioavailability of 100%.

Excretion, primarily in the form of glucuronide derivatives of the denitrated metabolites, is largely by way of the kidney.

Pharmacodynamics

Nitroglycerin and its analogues are unusually selective drugs: in therapeutic doses, their action is largely on smooth muscle cells. Another action of clinical significance is on platelet aggregation.

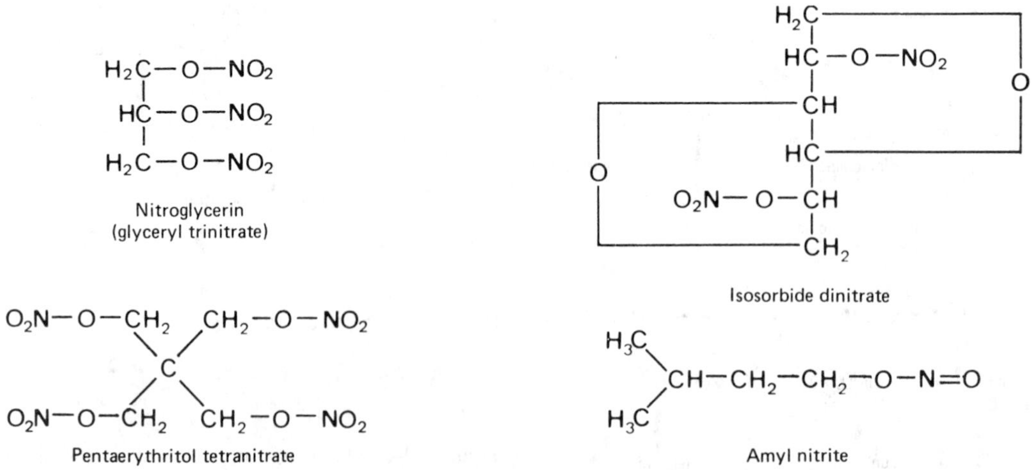

H₂C—O—NO₂
HC—O—NO₂
H₂C—O—NO₂

Nitroglycerin
(glyceryl trinitrate)

O₂N—O—CH₂   CH₂—O—NO₂
                C
O₂N—O—CH₂   CH₂—O—NO₂

Pentaerythritol tetranitrate

Isosorbide dinitrate

Amyl nitrite

Figure 12–3. Chemical structures of three nitrates and amyl nitrite.

A. Mechanism of Action in Smooth Muscle: Nitroglycerin appears to be denitrated, releasing free nitrite ion, in the smooth muscle cell as it is in other tissues, by glutathione S-transferase. A different unknown enzymatic reaction releases nitric oxide (NO) from the parent drug molecule (Harrison and Bates, 1993). Nitric oxide is a much more potent vasodilator than nitrite, which itself can release nitric oxide. As shown in Figure 12–2, nitric oxide causes activation of guanylyl cyclase and an increase in cGMP, which are the first steps toward smooth muscle relaxation. The production of prostaglandin E or prostacyclin (PGI_2) may also be involved. There is no evidence that autonomic receptors are involved in the primary nitrate response (though autonomic *reflex* responses are evoked when hypotensive doses are given). As described below, tolerance is an important consideration in the use of nitrates. While tolerance may be caused in part by a decrease in tissue sulfhydryl groups, it can be only partially prevented or reversed with a sulfhydryl-regenerating agent. The site of this cellular tolerance may be in the unknown reaction responsible for the release of nitric oxide from the nitrate, since other agents that cause vasodilation via release of nitric oxide from *endogenous* substrates, eg, acetylcholine, do not show cross tolerance with the nitrates. (See box: Coronary Steal Phenomenon.)

Nicorandil, an investigational nitrate agent, appears to combine the activity of NO release with potassium channel-opening action, thus providing an additional mechanism for causing vasodilation. See Chapter 11 for a discussion of potassium channel opening as a mechanism of vasodilation.

B. Organ System Effects: Nitroglycerin relaxes all types of smooth muscle irrespective of the cause of the preexisting muscle tone (Figure 12–4). It has practically no direct effect on cardiac or skeletal muscle.

1. Vascular smooth muscle–All segments of the vascular system from large arteries through large veins relax in response to nitroglycerin. Veins respond at the lowest concentrations, arteries at slightly higher ones. Arterioles and precapillary sphincters are dilated less than the large arteries and the veins, partly because of reflex responses (Bassenge, 1986, 1992) and partly because different vessels vary in their ability to release nitric oxide (see box). The primary direct result of an effective blood concentration is marked relaxation of the large veins with increased venous capacitance and decreased ventricular preload. Pulmonary vascular pressures and heart size are significantly reduced. In the absence of heart failure, cardiac output is reduced. Because venous capacitance is increased, orthostatic hypotension may be marked and syncope can result. Dilation of some large arteries (including the aorta) may be significant because of their large compliance. Temporal artery pulsations and a throbbing headache associated with meningeal artery pulsations are frequent effects of nitroglycerin and amyl nitrite. In the presence of heart failure, preload is usually abnormally high; the nitrates and other vasodilators, by reducing preload, may have a beneficial effect on cardiac output in this condition (see Chapter 13). However, in patients with chronic left ventricular heart failure, afterload reduction—by enhancing arterial compliance and ventriculo-aortic coupling—may also be an important mechanism for improved ventricular function.

The indirect effects of nitroglycerin consist of those reflexes evoked by baroreceptors and hormonal mechanisms responding to decreased arterial pressure (see Figure 6–7). The primary mechanism of this reflex is sympathetic discharge; this consistently results in tachycardia and increased cardiac contractility. In the case of very rapidly acting agents (eg, inhaled amyl nitrite), arterial dilation may be so marked as to cause a reflex venoconstriction.

In the isolated coronary-perfused heart (Langen-

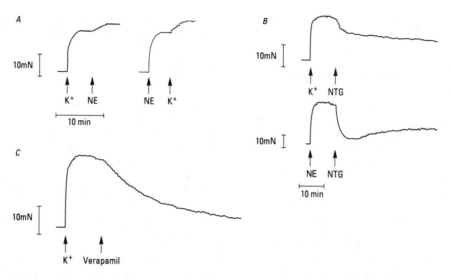

Figure 12–4. Effects of vasodilators on contractions of human vein segments studied in vitro. ***Panel A*** shows contractions induced by two vasoconstrictor agents, norepinephrine *(NE)* and potassium *(K⁺)*. ***Panel B*** shows the relaxation induced by nitroglycerin *(NTG)*, 4 μmol/L. The relaxation is prompt. ***Panel C*** shows the relaxation induced by verapamil, 2.2 μmol/L. The relaxation is slower but more sustained. (Modified and reproduced, with permission, from Mikkelsen E, Andersson KE, Bengtsson B: Effects of verapamil and nitroglycerin on contractile responses to potassium and noradrenaline in isolated human peripheral veins. Acta Pharmacol Toxicol 1978;42:14.)

CORONARY STEAL PHENOMENON

The development of useful vasodilators for management of angina has been marked by frustrating episodes when pharmacologists found that new drugs that were extremely effective vasodilators in normal animals were ineffective or even caused increased anginal symptoms in patients. It is now clear that potent arteriolar dilators (eg, hydralazine, dipyridamole) are generally ineffective in angina and may reduce perfusion of ischemic areas. In fact, dipyridamole is often used in imaging studies of the coronary circulation to demonstrate regions of poor perfusion. On the other hand, drugs that are more effective dilators of veins and large arteries and relatively ineffective dilators of resistance vessels (eg, nitrates) are very useful in angina. The reason for this apparent anomaly has been called the "coronary steal phenomenon."

Coronary steal occurs when two branches from a main coronary vessel have differing degrees of obstruction. For example, one branch may be relatively normal and capable of dilating and constricting in response to changes in oxygen demand, while the other branch is significantly obstructed and has significant arteriolar dilation—beyond the obstruction—even when cardiac oxygen demand is low, because of the accumulation of metabolites in the ischemic tissue. Perfusion in

the obstructed region may be adequate at rest, because perfusion pressure is well maintained in the main coronary artery. (Recall that perfusion in a regional vascular bed is directly proportionate to perfusion pressure in the large supply vessels and inversely proportionate to the resistance to flow in the arterioles.) If a powerful arteriolar dilator drug is administered, the arterioles in the unobstructed vessel will be forced to dilate, reducing the resistance in this area and greatly increasing flow through the already adequately perfused tissue. As a result of the reduction in resistance in the normal branch, perfusion pressure in the main coronary will diminish, flow through the obstructed branch will *decrease,* and angina may worsen.

It has been suggested that the lesser potency of the nitrates in dilating arterioles is the result of a reduced ability of these vessels to release nitric oxide from the parent nitrate molecule. There is some evidence that supplementation with thiol-containing compounds such as cysteine can increase the ability of arterioles to release nitric oxide from nitroglycerin (Harrison and Bates, 1993). If this is true, administration of acetylcysteine to prevent tolerance might cause nitroglycerin to produce effects like those of the *ineffective* arteriolar vasodilators!

dorff preparation) and in normal subjects without coronary disease, nitroglycerin can induce a significant, if transient, increase in total coronary blood flow. In contrast, there is no evidence that total coronary flow is increased in patients with angina due to atherosclerotic obstructive coronary artery disease. While some studies suggest that *redistribution* of coronary flow from normal to ischemic regions may play a role, most evidence suggests that relief of effort angina by nitroglycerin is the result of decreased myocardial oxygen requirement secondary to decreased preload and arterial pressure (see Clinical Pharmacology).

2. Other smooth muscle organs–Relaxation of smooth muscle of the bronchi, gastrointestinal tract (including biliary system), and genitourinary tract has been demonstrated experimentally. Because of their brief duration, these actions of the nitrates are rarely of any clinical value. During recent years, the use of amyl nitrite and isobutyl nitrite as purported recreational (sex-enhancing) drugs has become popular with some segments of the population. Isobutyl nitrite is not licensed or advertised as a drug but is sold over the counter under such names as Rush, Bolt, Locker Room, and Dr. Bananas.

3. Action on platelets–Nitric oxide released from nitroglycerin stimulates guanylyl cyclase in platelets as in smooth muscle. The increase in cGMP that results is responsible for a decrease in platelet aggregation (Karlberg, 1992). It is probable that this action plays a role in the observed reduction by intravenous nitroglycerin of infarct size and mortality following myocardial infarction.

4. Other effects–*Nitrite* ion reacts with hemoglobin (which contains ferrous iron) to produce **methemoglobin** (which contains ferric iron). Because methemoglobin has a very low affinity for oxygen, large doses of nitrites can result in pseudocyanosis, tissue hypoxia, and death. The plasma level of *nitrite* resulting from even large doses of organic and inorganic *nitrates* is too low to cause significant methemoglobinemia in adults. However, sodium nitrite is used as a curing agent for meats. In nursing infants, the intestinal flora is capable of converting significant amounts of inorganic nitrate, eg, from well water, to nitrite ion. Thus, inadvertent exposure to large amounts of nitrite ion can occur and may produce serious toxicity. One therapeutic application of this otherwise toxic effect of nitrite has been discovered. **Cyanide poisoning** results from complexing of cytochrome iron by the CN^- ion. Methemoglobin iron has a very high affinity for CN^-; thus, administration of sodium nitrite ($NaNO_2$) soon after cyanide exposure will regenerate active cytochrome. The cyanmethemoglobin produced can be further detoxified by the intravenous administration of sodium thiosulfate ($Na_2S_2O_3$); this results in formation of thiocyanate ion (SCN^-), a less toxic ion that is readily

excreted. Methemoglobinemia, if excessive, can be treated by giving methylene blue intravenously.

Toxicity & Tolerance

A. Acute Adverse Effects: The major acute toxicity of organic nitrates is a direct extension of therapeutic vasodilation: orthostatic hypotension, tachycardia, and throbbing headache. Glaucoma, once thought to be a contraindication, does not worsen, and nitrates can be used safely in the presence of increased intraocular pressure. Nitrates are contraindicated, however, if intracranial pressure is elevated.

B. Tolerance: With continuous exposure to nitrates, isolated smooth muscle may develop complete tolerance (tachyphylaxis), and the intact human becomes progressively more tolerant when long-acting preparations (oral, transdermal) or continuous intravenous infusions are used without interruption for more than a few hours (Steering Committee, 1991).

Continuous exposure to high levels of nitrates can occur in the chemical industry, especially where explosives are manufactured. When contamination of the workplace with volatile organic nitrate compounds is severe, workers find that upon starting their work week, they suffer headache and transient dizziness ("Monday disease"). After a day or so, these symptoms disappear owing to the development of tolerance. Over the weekend, when exposure to the chemicals is reduced, tolerance disappears, so symptoms recur each Monday. A more serious hazard of industrial exposure is the development of dependence. This may affect workers after months or years of exposure and manifests itself as variant angina occurring after 1–2 days away from the source of nitrates. In the most seriously affected individuals, coronary vasospasm may cause myocardial infarction. There is no evidence that physical dependence develops as a result of the therapeutic use of short-acting nitrates for angina, even in large doses.

The mechanisms by which tolerance develops are not completely understood. As noted above, cellular tolerance appears to play a role in that activation of guanylyl cyclase in cellular homogenates is decreased by preincubation with organic nitrates. Partial reversal of this loss of responsiveness by thiol-containing compounds (eg, acetylcysteine) and the absence of cross tolerance to other nitric oxide-dependent vasodilators (acetylcholine, nicorandil) suggests that diminished release of nitric oxide may be partly responsible for tolerance to nitroglycerin. Systemic compensation also plays a role in tolerance in the intact human. Initially, significant sympathetic discharge occurs; this increases vascular tone. After one or more days of therapy with long-acting nitrates, retention of salt and water may reverse the favorable hemodynamic changes normally caused by nitroglycerin (Parker, 1993).

C. Carcinogenicity of Nitrate and Nitrate Derivatives: Nitrosamines are small molecules with the structure R_2–N–NO formed from the combination of nitrates and nitrites with amines. Some nitrosamines are powerful carcinogens in animals, apparently through conversion to very reactive derivatives. While there is no direct proof that these agents cause cancer in humans, there is a strong epidemiologic correlation between the incidence of esophageal and gastric carcinoma and the nitrate content of food in different cultures. Nitrosamines are also found in tobacco and in cigarette smoke. There is no evidence that the small doses of nitrates used in the treatment of angina result in significant body levels of nitrosamines.

Mechanisms of Clinical Effect

The beneficial and deleterious effects of nitrate-induced vasodilation are summarized in Table 12–2.

A. Nitrate Effects in Angina of Effort: Decreased venous return to the heart and the resulting reduction of intracardiac volume are the principal hemodynamic effects. Arterial pressure decreases. Decreased intraventricular pressure and left ventricular volume are associated with decreased wall tension (Laplace relation) and decreased myocardial oxygen requirement. In rare instances, a paradoxical increase in myocardial oxygen demand may occur as a result of excessive reflex tachycardia and increased contractility.

Intracoronary, intravenous, and sublingual nitrate administration consistently increases the caliber of the epicardial coronary arteries. Coronary arteriolar resistance tends to decrease, though to a lesser extent. However, nitrates administered by the usual systemic routes also consistently *decrease* overall coronary blood flow and myocardial oxygen consumption. Intracoronary injection of small doses of nitroglycerin, which increases total coronary blood flow but does not produce systemic hemodynamic effects, does not relieve pacing-induced angina. Yet systemic administration of nitroglycerin, which decreases arterial pressure and left ventricular volume, does relieve angina despite decreased coronary blood flow. These findings indicate that the relief of effort angina with nitrates is due primarily to decreased myocardial oxygen demand, not to increased coronary blood flow.

B. Nitrate Effects in Variant Angina: Nitrates benefit patients with variant angina by relaxing the smooth muscle of the epicardial coronary arteries and relieving coronary artery spasm. Although intracoronary nitroglycerin injection appears to be the most effective method for relieving coronary artery spasm, this method of administration has little clinical relevance, and other routes of administration are also effective.

C. Nitrate Effects in Unstable Angina: Nitrates are also useful in the treatment of unstable angina, but the precise mechanism for their beneficial effects is not clear. Because both increased coronary vascular tone and increased myocardial oxygen demand can precipitate rest angina in these patients, nitrates may exert their beneficial effects both by dilating the epicardial coronary arteries and by simultaneously reducing myocardial oxygen demand.

The major mechanism for prolonged episodes of rest angina is now known to be recurrent thrombotic occlusion (presumably initiated by platelet aggregation) at the site of atherosclerotic plaques. As noted above, nitroglycerin decreases platelet aggregation, and this effect may be of importance in unstable angina.

Clinical Use of Nitrates

Some of the forms of nitroglycerin and its congeners are listed in Table 12–3. Because of its rapid onset of action (1–3 minutes), sublingual nitroglycerin is the most frequently used agent for the immediate treatment of angina. Because its duration of action is short (not exceeding 20–30 minutes), it is not suitable for maintenance therapy. The onset of action of intravenous nitroglycerin is also rapid (minutes), but its hemodynamic effects are quickly reversed by stopping its infusion. Clinical application of intravenous nitroglycerin, therefore, is restricted to the treatment of severe, recurrent rest angina. Slowly absorbed preparations of nitroglycerin include a buccal form, an oral preparation, and several transdermal forms. These formulations have been shown to provide blood concentrations for long periods, but, as noted above, doing so leads to the development of tolerance.

The hemodynamic effects of sublingual or chewable isosorbide dinitrate, pentaerythritol tetranitrate, and erythrityl tetranitrate are similar to those of nitroglycerin. The recommended dosage schedules for commonly used long-acting nitrate preparations, along with their duration of action, are listed in Table

Table 12–2. Beneficial and deleterious effects of nitrates in the treatment of angina.

	Result
Potential beneficial effects	
Decreased ventricular volume	Decreased myocardial oxygen requirement.
Decreased arterial pressure	
Decreased ejection time	
Vasodilation of epicardial coronary arteries	Relief of coronary artery spasm.
Increased collateral flow	Improved perfusion to ischemic myocardium.
Decreased left ventricular diastolic pressure	Improved subendocardial perfusion.
Potential deleterious effects	
Reflex tachycardia	Increased myocardial oxygen requirement.
Reflex increase in contractility	
Decreased diastolic perfusion time due to tachycardia	Decreased myocardial perfusion.

Table 12–3. Nitrate and nitrite drugs used in the treatment of angina.

Drug	Dose	Duration of Action
"Short-acting"		
Nitroglycerin, sublingual	0.15–1.2 mg	10–30 minutes
Isosorbide, sublingual	2.5–5 mg	10–60 minutes
Amyl nitrite, inhalant	0.18–0.3 mL	3–5 minutes
"Long-acting"		
Nitroglycerin, oral sustained-action	6.3–13 mg per 6–8 hours	6–8 hours
Nitroglycerin, 2% ointment	1–1½ inches per 4 hours	3–6 hours
Nitroglycerin, slow-release, buccal	1–2 mg per 4 hours	3–6 hours
Nitroglycerin, slow-release, transdermal	10–25 mg per 24 hours (one patch per day)	8–10 hours
Isosorbide dinitrate, sublingual	2.5–10 mg per 2 hours	1½–2 hours
Isosorbide dinitrate, oral	10–60 mg per 4–6 hours	4–6 hours
Isosorbide dinitrate, chewable	5–10 mg per 2–4 hours	2–3 hours
Isosorbide mononitrate	20 mg per 12 hours	6–10 hours
Pentaerythritol tetranitrate	40 mg per 6–8 hours	6–8 hours
Erythrityl tetranitrate	10–40 mg per 6–8 hours	6–8 hours

12–3. Although transdermal administration may provide blood levels of nitroglycerin for 24 hours or longer, the full hemodynamic effects usually do not persist for more than 8–10 hours. The clinical efficacy of slow-release forms of nitroglycerin in maintenance therapy of angina is thus limited by the development of significant tolerance. It has been suggested that a nitrate-free period of at least 8 hours between doses should be observed to reduce or prevent tolerance.

CALCIUM CHANNEL-BLOCKING DRUGS

Chemistry

Verapamil, the first clinically useful member of this group, was the result of attempts to synthesize more active analogues of papaverine, a vasodilator alkaloid found in the opium poppy. Since then, dozens of agents of varying structure have been found to have the same fundamental pharmacologic action. Four chemically dissimilar calcium channel blockers are shown in Figure 12–5. Nifedipine is the prototype of the dihydropyridine family of calcium channel blockers; dozens of molecules in this family have been investigated, and six are currently approved in the USA for angina and other indications. Nifedipine is the most extensively studied of this group, but the properties of the other dihydropyridines can be assumed to be similar to it unless otherwise noted.

Pharmacokinetics
(Table 12–4)

The calcium channel blockers are orally active agents. They are characterized by high first-pass effect, high plasma protein binding, and extensive metabolism.

Pharmacodynamics

A. Mechanism of Action: Current evidence suggests the existence of three types of voltage-dependent calcium channels (in addition to receptor-operated [eg, by α_1 receptors] calcium channels). Voltage-dependent calcium channels are categorized as L-type, T-type, or N-type, depending on whether they are characteristically large in conductance, transient in duration of opening, or neuronal in distribution. A fourth type, the P-type, may exist in other tissues. The L-type calcium channel is the dominant type in cardiac and smooth muscle and is known to contain several drug receptors. It has been demonstrated that nifedipine and other dihydropyridines bind to one site, while verapamil and diltiazem appear to bind to closely related but not identical receptors in another region. Binding of a drug to the verapamil or diltiazem receptors also affects dihydropyridine binding. These receptor regions are stereoselective, since marked differences in both stereoisomer-binding affinity and pharmacologic potency are observed for enantiomers of verapamil, diltiazem, and optically active nifedipine congeners.

Blockade by these drugs resembles that of sodium channel blockade by local anesthetics: the drugs act from the inner side of the membrane and bind more effectively to channels in depolarized membranes. Binding of the drug appears to convert the mode of operation of the channel from one in which openings occur consistently after depolarization to one in which such openings are rare. The result is a marked decrease in transmembrane calcium current (Figure 12–1) associated in smooth muscle with a long-lasting relaxation (Figure 12–4) and in cardiac muscle with a reduction in contractility throughout the heart and decreases in sinus node pacemaker rate and in atrioventricular node conduction velocity.* Smooth muscle responses to calcium influx through *receptor-operated* calcium channels are also reduced by these drugs but not as markedly. The block is partially reversed by elevating the concentration of calcium,

---

*At very low doses and under certain circumstances, some dihydropyridines *increase* calcium influx. Some special dihydropyridines, eg, Bay K 8644, appear to increase calcium influx over most of their dose range.

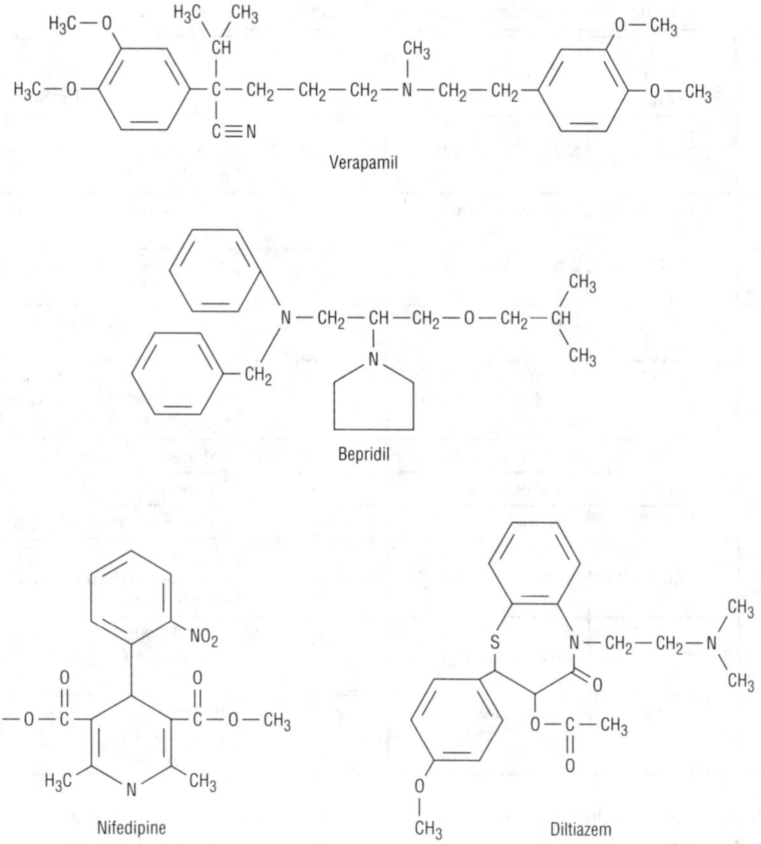

Figure 12–5. Chemical structures of several calcium channel-blocking drugs.

though the levels of calcium required are not easily attainable. Block can also be partially reversed by the use of drugs that increase the transmembrane flux of calcium, such as sympathomimetics.

T- and N-type calcium channels are less sensitive to blockade by calcium channel blockers. Therefore, tissues in which these channel types play a major role—neurons and most secretory glands—are much less affected by these drugs than are cardiac and smooth muscle.

B. Organ System Effects:

1. Smooth muscle–Most types of smooth muscle are dependent on transmembrane calcium influx for normal resting tone and contractile responses. These cells are relaxed by the calcium channel blockers (Figure 12–4). Vascular smooth muscle appears to be the most sensitive, but similar relaxation can be shown for bronchiolar, gastrointestinal, and uterine smooth muscle. In the vascular system, arterioles appear to be more sensitive than veins; orthostatic hypotension is not a common adverse effect. Blood pressure can be reduced, especially with nifedipine. Women may be more sensitive than men to the hypotensive action of diltiazem. The reduction in peripheral vascular resistance is one mechanism by which these agents may benefit the patient with angina of effort. Reduction of coronary arterial tone has been demonstrated in patients with variant angina.

Important differences in "vascular selectivity" exist among the calcium channel blockers. In general, the dihydropyridines have a greater ratio of vascular smooth muscle effects relative to cardiac effects than do bepridil, diltiazem, and verapamil (Table 12–5). Furthermore, the dihydropyridines may differ in their potency in different vascular beds. For example, nimodipine is claimed to be particularly selective for cerebral blood vessels.

2. Cardiac muscle–Cardiac muscle is highly dependent upon calcium influx for normal function. Impulse generation in the sinoatrial node and conduction in the atrioventricular node—so-called "slow response," or calcium-dependent, action potentials—may be reduced or blocked by all of the calcium channel blockers. Excitation-contraction coupling in all cardiac cells requires calcium influx, so these drugs reduce cardiac contractility and cardiac output in a dose-dependent fashion. This reduction in mechanical function is another mechanism by which the cal-

Table 12–4. Pharmacokinetics of some calcium channel blocking drugs.

Drug	Oral Bioavailability	Onset of Action (route)	Plasma Half-Life (hours)	Disposition
Dihydropyridines				
Amlodipine	65–90%	No data available	30–50	>90% bound to plasma proteins; extensively metabolized.
Felodipine	15–20%	2–5 hours (oral)	11–16	>99% bound to plasma proteins; extensively metabolized.
Isradipine	15–25%	2 hours (oral)	8	95% bound to plasma protein; extensively metabolized.
Nicardipine	35%	20 minutes (oral)	2–4	95% bound; extensively metabolized in the liver.
Nifedipine	45–70%	<1 minute (IV); 5–20 minutes (sublingual or oral)	4	About 90% bound to plasma protein; metabolized to an acid lactate. 80% of the drug and metabolites excreted in urine.
Nimodipine	13%	No data available	1–2	Extensively metabolized.
Nisoldipine	<10%	No data available	2–6	Extensively metabolized.
Nitrendipine	10–30%	4 hours (oral)	5–12	98% bound; extensively metabolized.
Miscellaneous				
Bepridil	60%	60 minutes (oral)	24–40	>99% bound to plasma proteins; extensively metabolized.
Diltiazem	40–65%	<3 minutes (IV), >30 minutes (oral)	3–4	70–80% bound to plasma protein; extensively deacylated. Drug and metabolites excreted in feces.
Verapamil	20–35%	<1½ minutes (IV), 30 minutes (oral)	6	About 90% bound to plasma protein. 70% eliminated by kidney; 15% by gastrointestinal tract.

cium channel blockers may reduce the oxygen requirement in patients with angina.

An additional benefit of calcium influx inhibition has been demonstrated in experimental myocardial infarction. Because ischemia causes membrane depolarization, calcium influx in ischemic cells is increased. Elevated intracellular calcium accelerates the activity of several ATP-consuming enzymes, which further depletes already marginal cellular energy stores, making the heart even more susceptible to ischemic damage. The calcium channel blockers have been demonstrated to protect against the damaging effects of calcium by reducing the incidence of arrhythmias and the ultimate size of developing infarctions in experimental animals.

Important differences between the available calcium channel blockers arise from the details of their interactions with cardiac ion channels and, as noted above, differences in their relative smooth muscle versus cardiac effects. Cardiac *sodium* channels are blocked by bepridil but somewhat less effectively than are calcium channels. Sodium channel block is modest with verapamil and still less marked with diltiazem. It is negligible with nifedipine and other dihydropyridines. Verapamil and diltiazem interact kinetically with the calcium channel receptor in a different manner than the dihydropyridines; they block tachycardias in calcium-dependent cells, eg, the atrioventricular node, more selectively than do the dihydropyridines. (See Chapter 14 for additional details.) On the other hand, the dihydropyridines appear to block smooth muscle calcium channels at concentrations below those required for significant cardiac effects; they are therefore less depressant on the heart than verapamil or diltiazem. Bepridil also has a significant potassium channel blocking effect in the heart. This results in prolongation of cardiac repolarization (see Chapter 14) and a distinct risk of induction of arrhythmias.

3. Skeletal muscle–Skeletal muscle is not depressed by the calcium channel blockers because it utilizes intracellular pools of calcium to support excitation-contraction coupling and does not require as much transmembrane calcium influx.

4. Cerebral vasospasm and infarct following subarachnoid hemorrhage–Nimodipine, a member of the dihydropyridine group of calcium channel blockers, has a high affinity for cerebral blood vessels and appears to reduce morbidity following a subarachnoid hemorrhage—morbidity that is probably caused by vasospasm evoked by the extravasation of blood into the tissue. Nimodipine is therefore labeled for use in patients who have had a subarachnoid hemorrhage. Some evidence suggests that calcium channel blockers may also reduce cerebral damage following thromboembolic stroke. It is not clear whether the benefits observed in this situation, if real, result from cerebral vasodilation or from reduced oxygen demand by neurons.

5. Other effects–Calcium channel blockers

Table 12–5. Vascular selectivity and clinical uses of some calcium channel blocking drugs.

Drug	Vascular Selectivity[1]	Indications[2]	Usual Dose	Toxicity
Dihydropyridines				
Amlodipine	++	Angina, hypertension	5–10 mg once daily	Headache, edema.
Felodipine	5.4	Hypertension	5–10 mg once daily	Dizziness, headache.
Isradipine	7.4	Hypertension	2.5–10 mg every 12 hours	Headache, fatigue.
Nicardipine	17.0	Angina, hypertension	20–40 mg every 8 hours orally	Edema, dizziness, headache, flushing.
Nifedipine	3.1	Angina, (hypertension, migraine, cardiomyopathy, Raynaud's phenomenon)	3–10 µg/kg IV; 20–40 mg every 8 hours orally	Hypotension, dizziness, flushing, nausea, constipation, dependent edema.
Nimodipine	++	Subarachnoid hemorrhage, (migraine)	60 mg every 4 hours orally	Headache, diarrhea.
Nisoldipine	++	Investigational for angina, hypertension	20–40 mg once daily	Probably similar to nifedipine.
Nitrendipine	14.4	Investigational for angina, hypertension	20 mg once or twice daily	Probably similar to nifedipine.
Miscellaneous				
Bepridil	—	Angina	200–400 mg orally once a day	Arrhythmias, dizziness, nausea.
Diltiazem	0.3	Angina, hypertension, (Raynaud's phenomenon)	75–150 µg/kg IV; 30–80 mg every 6 hours orally	Hypotension, dizziness, flushing, bradycardia.
Verapamil	1.3	Angina, hypertension, arrhythmias, (migraine, cardiomyopathy)	75–150 µg/kg IV; 80–160 mg every 8 hours orally	Hypotension, myocardial depression, heart failure, dependent edema.

[1]Numeric data (Spedding, 1990) give the ratio of vascular potency to cardiac potency; higher numbers mean greater vascular, less cardiac potency. Plus and minus signs reflect estimated ratio of vascular to cardiac potency: − = myocardial depression greater than vasodilation; ++ = significant degree of vasodilation greater than myocardial depression.
[2]Unlabeled indications are in parentheses.

minimally interfere with stimulus-secretion coupling in glands and nerve endings because of differences between calcium channels in different tissues, as noted above. Verapamil has been shown to inhibit insulin release in humans, but the dosages required are greater than those used in management of angina.

A significant body of evidence suggests that the calcium channel blockers may interfere with platelet aggregation in vitro and prevent or attenuate the development of atheromatous lesions in animals. Clinical studies have not yet firmly established their role in human blood clotting and atherosclerosis.

Verapamil has been shown to block the P170 glycoprotein responsible for the transport of many foreign drugs out of cancer (and other) cells; other calcium channel blockers appear to have a similar effect. Unlike calcium channel blockade, this action is not stereospecific. Increased expression of the P170 multidrug transporter protein is associated with the development of resistance to chemotherapy in cancer cells. Verapamil has been shown to partially reverse the resistance of cancer cells to many chemotherapeutic drugs in vitro. Early clinical results suggest similar effects in patients (see Chapter 56).

Toxicity

The most important toxic effects reported for the calcium channel blockers are direct extensions of their therapeutic action. Excessive inhibition of calcium influx can cause serious cardiac depression, including cardiac arrest, bradycardia, atrioventricular block, and congestive heart failure. These effects have been rare in clinical use. Bepridil consistently prolongs the cardiac action potential and in susceptible patients may cause a dangerous *torsade de pointes* arrhythmia. It is contraindicated in patients with a history of serious arrhythmias or prolonged QT syndrome. Patients receiving beta-adrenoceptor-blocking drugs are more sensitive to the cardiodepressant effects of calcium channel blockers. Minor toxicity (not usually requiring discontinuance of therapy) includes flushing, edema, dizziness, gingival hyperplasia, nausea, and constipation (Table 12–5).

Mechanisms of Clinical Effects

As mentioned previously, calcium channel blockers decrease myocardial contractile force, which in turn reduces myocardial oxygen requirements. Inhibition of calcium entry into arterial smooth muscle is associated with decreased arteriolar tone and systemic vascular resistance, resulting in decreased arterial and intraventricular pressure. Some of these drugs (eg, verapamil) also block alpha adrenoceptors, which may contribute to peripheral vasodilation. As a result of all of these effects, left ventricular wall stress declines, which reduces myocardial oxygen requirements. Decreased heart rate with the use of verapamil, diltiazem, or bepridil causes a further decrease in myocardial oxygen demand. Calcium channel-blocking agents also relieve and prevent focal coronary artery spasm—the primary mechanism of variant angina. Use of these agents has thus emerged as the most effective treatment for this form of angina pectoris.

As noted above, the calcium channel-blocking agents differ in their clinical cardiovascular effects. Sinoatrial and atrioventricular nodal tissues, which are mainly composed of slow response cells, are affected markedly by verapamil, moderately by diltiazem, and much less by nifedipine. Thus, verapamil and diltiazem decrease atrioventricular nodal conduction and are effective in the management of supraventricular reentry tachycardia and in decreasing ventricular responses in atrial fibrillation or flutter. Nifedipine does not affect atrioventricular conduction. Nonspecific sympathetic antagonism is most marked with diltiazem and much less with verapamil. Nifedipine does not appear to have this effect. Thus, significant reflex tachycardia in response to hypotension occurs most frequently with nifedipine and less so with verapamil. These differences in pharmacologic effects should be considered in selecting calcium channel-blocking agents for the management of angina.

Clinical Uses of Calcium Channel-Blocking Drugs

In addition to angina, calcium channel blockers have well-documented efficacy in hypertension (see Chapter 11) and supraventricular tachyarrhythmias (see Chapter 14). They also show promise in a wide variety of other conditions, including hypertrophic cardiomyopathy, migraine, Raynaud's phenomenon, postinfarct tissue preservation, and atherosclerosis (Scriabine, 1987; O'Rourke, 1987; Taira, 1987; Weinstein, 1989).

Approved and unlabeled indications and dosages for these drugs are set forth in Table 12–5. The choice of a particular calcium channel-blocking agent should be made with knowledge of its specific potential adverse effects as well as its pharmacologic properties. Nifedipine does not decrease atrioventricular conduction and therefore can be used more safely in the presence of atrioventricular conduction abnormalities. A combination of verapamil or diltiazem with beta-blockers may produce atrioventricular block and depression of ventricular function. In the presence of overt heart failure, all calcium channel blockers can cause further worsening of heart failure as a result of their negative inotropic effect. Controlled studies have reported a higher mortality rate in patients with congestive failure when treated with calcium channel blockers; they are therefore contraindicated in the

vasodilator treatment of heart failure. In the presence of relatively low blood pressure, nifedipine can cause further deleterious lowering of blood pressure. Verapamil and diltiazem appear to produce less hypotension and may be better tolerated in these circumstances. In patients with a history of atrial tachycardia, flutter, and fibrillation, verapamil and diltiazem provide a distinct advantage because of their antiarrhythmic effects. In the digitalized patient, verapamil should be used with caution, because it may increase digoxin blood levels through a pharmacokinetic interaction. Although increases in digoxin blood level have also been demonstrated with diltiazem and nifedipine, such interactions are less consistent than with verapamil.

BETA-ADRENOCEPTOR-BLOCKING DRUGS

Although they are not vasodilators, beta-blocking drugs (see Chapter 10) are extremely useful in the management of angina pectoris. The beneficial effects of beta-blocking agents are related primarily to their hemodynamic effects—decreased heart rate, blood pressure, and contractility—which decrease myocardial oxygen requirements at rest and during exercise. Lower heart rate is also associated with an increase in diastolic perfusion time that may increase myocardial perfusion. It has been suggested that the beta-blocking agents can cause a favorable redistribution of coronary blood flow to the ischemic myocardium based on differential effects on the coronary vascular resistance in the relatively ischemic and nonischemic myocardial segments. However, reduction of heart rate and blood pressure and consequently decreased myocardial oxygen consumption appear to be the most important mechanisms for relief of angina and improved exercise tolerance. Beta-blockers may also be valuable in treating silent or ambulatory ischemia. Because this condition causes no pain, it is usually detected by the appearance of typical electrocardiographic signs of ischemia. As shown in Figure 12–6, the total amount of "ischemic time" is reduced by chronic therapy with a beta-blocker. This improvement may account, in part, for the reduction in reinfarction and mortality in patients who are placed on beta-blocker therapy after a myocardial infarct.

Undesirable effects of beta-blocking agents include an increase in end-diastolic volume that accompanies slowing of the heart rate and an increase in ejection time. Increased myocardial oxygen requirements associated with increased left ventricular diastolic volume partially offset the beneficial effects of beta-blocking agents. These potentially deleterious effects of beta-blocking agents can be balanced by the concomitant use of nitrates as described below.

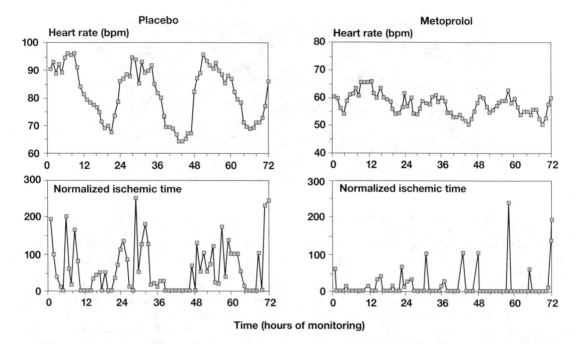

Figure 12–6. Effects of metoprolol on the heart rate and normalized ischemic time (measured by ambulatory electro-cardiographic monitoring) in nine men with severe coronary artery disease. The drug reduced the mean heart rate, magnitude of diurnal heart rate changes, and the total time during which the ECG showed evidence of ischemia. (Reproduced, with permission, from Lambert CR et al: Influence of beta-adrenergic blockade defined by time series analysis on circadian variation of heart rate and ambulatory myocardial ischemia. Am J Cardiol 1989;64:835.)

II. CLINICAL PHARMACOLOGY OF DRUGS USED TO TREAT ANGINA

Principles of Therapy of Angina

In addition to modification of the risk factors for coronary atherosclerosis (smoking, hypertension, hyperlipidemia), the treatment of angina and other manifestations of myocardial ischemia is based on reduction of myocardial oxygen demand and increase of coronary blood flow to the potentially ischemic myocardium to restore the balance between myocardial oxygen supply and demand.

Angina of Effort

Many studies have demonstrated that nitrates, calcium channel blockers, and beta-blockers increase time to onset of angina and ST depression during treadmill tests in patients with angina of effort (Figure 12–7). The double product remains consistently lower during exercise. However, although exercise tolerance increases, there is usually no change in the angina threshold, ie, the rate-pressure product at which symptoms occur.

For maintenance therapy of chronic stable angina,

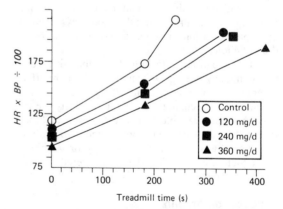

Figure 12–7. Effects of diltiazem on the "double product" in a group of 20 patients with angina of effort. In a double-blind study using a standard protocol, patients were tested on a treadmill during treatment with placebo and three doses of the drug. Heart rate *(HR)* and systolic blood pressure *(BP)* were recorded at 180 seconds of exercise (midpoints of lines) and at the time of onset of anginal symptoms (rightmost points). Note that the drug treatment decreased the double product at all times during exercise and prolonged the time to appearance of symptoms. (Data from Lindenberg BS et al: Efficacy and safety of incremental doses of diltiazem for the treatment of angina. J Am Coll Cardiol 1983;2:1129. Used with permission of the American College of Cardiology.)

Table 12–6. Effects of nitrates alone and with beta-blockers or calcium channel blockers in angina pectoris. Undesirable effects are shown in *italics*.

	Nitrates Alone	β-Blockers or Calcium Channel Blockers	Combined Nitrates With β-Blockers or Calcium Channel Blockers
Heart rate	*Reflex increase*	Decrease[1]	Decrease
Arterial pressure	Decrease	Decrease	Decrease
End-diastolic volume	Decrease	*Increase*	None or decrease
Contractility	*Reflex increase*	Decrease[1]	None
Ejection time	Decrease	*Increase*	None

[1]Nifedipine may cause a reflex *increase* in heart rate and cardiac contractility.

long-acting nitrates, calcium channel-blocking agents, or beta-blockers may be chosen; the best choice of drug will depend on the individual patient's response. In hypertensive patients, monotherapy with either calcium channel blockers or beta-blockers may be adequate. In normotensive patients, long-acting nitrates may be suitable. The combination of a beta-blocker with a calcium channel blocker (eg, propranolol with nifedipine) or two different calcium channel blockers (eg, nifedipine and verapamil) has been shown to be more effective than individual drugs used alone. If response to a single drug is inadequate, a drug from a different class should be added to maximize the beneficial reduction of cardiac work while minimizing undesirable effects (Table 12–6). Some patients may require therapy with all three drug groups.

For patients with persistent hypertension, sinus bradycardia, or atrioventricular node dysfunction, nifedipine or a longer-acting dihydropyridine is the drug of choice.

In the case of beta-blocking drugs, there is no evidence that any one agent is significantly more effective or better tolerated than the others.

Surgical revascularization and angioplasty are the only methods available that restore coronary blood flow and increase oxygen supply to the myocardium. Patients refractory to medical therapy or unable to adapt their life-style should be considered for this mode of therapy.

Vasospastic Angina

Nitrates and the calcium channel blockers are considerably more effective than the beta-adrenoceptor-blocking drugs in relieving and preventing ischemic episodes in patients with variant angina. In approximately 70% of patients treated with nitrates plus calcium channel blockers, angina attacks are completely abolished; in another 20%, marked reduction of frequency of anginal episodes is observed. Prevention of coronary artery spasm (in the presence or absence of fixed atherosclerotic coronary artery lesions) is the principal mechanism for this beneficial response. All presently available calcium channel blockers appear to be equally effective, and the choice of a particular drug should depend on the patient, as indicated above. Surgical revascularization and angioplasty are not indicated in patients with variant angina.

Unstable Angina

In patients with unstable angina with recurrent ischemic episodes at rest, recurrent thrombotic occlusions of the offending coronary artery occur as the result of fissuring of atherosclerotic plaques and platelet aggregation. In such patients, the addition of nifedipine to beta-blocker and nitrate therapy can decrease the frequency of rest angina, the incidence of myocardial infarction, and the necessity for emergency myocardial revascularization. However, nifedipine alone is not more effective than nitrates or beta-blockers in decreasing the frequency of rest angina (Kar et al, 1992). In contrast, verapamil has been found more effective than propranolol in controlling unstable angina. Aspirin has been shown to reduce the incidence of cardiac events in such patients. Intravenous heparin or thrombolytic agents may also be indicated in some patients.

PREPARATIONS AVAILABLE

Nitrates & Nitrites
Amyl nitrite (generic, Aspirols, Vaporole)
 Inhalant: 0.3 mL capsules
Erythrityl tetranitrate (Cardilate)
 Oral: 5, 10 mg tablets and sublingual tablets

Isosorbide dinitrate (generic, Isordil, Sorbitrate)
 Oral: 5, 10, 20, 30, 40, mg tablets; 5, 10 mg chewable tablets
 Oral sustained-release (generic, Sorbitrate SA, Iso-Bid): 40 mg tablets and capsules

Sublingual: 2.5, 5, 10 mg sublingual tablets

Isosorbide mononitrate (Ismo)

Oral: 20 mg tablets

Nitroglycerin

Sublingual: 0.15, 0.3, 0.4, 0.6 mg tablets; 0.4 mg/metered dose aerosol

Oral sustained-release (generic, Nitrong): 2.6, 6.5, 9 mg tablets; 2.5, 6.5, 9, 13 mg capsules

Buccal (Nitrogard): 1, 2, 3 mg buccal tablets

Parenteral (Nitro-Bid IV, Tridil): 0.5, 5 mg/mL for IV administration

Transdermal patches (Minitran, Nitro-Dur, Transderm-Nitro): to release 2.5, 5, 7.5, 10, 15 mg/24 hours

Topical ointment (generic, Nitrol): 20 mg/mL ointment (1 inch, or 25 mm, of ointment contains about 15 mg nitroglycerin)

Pentaerythritol tetranitrate (generic, P.E.T.N., Peritrate, others)

Oral: 10, 20, 40, 80 mg tablets; 30, 45, 80 mg sustained-release capsules; 80 mg sustained-release tablets

Calcium Channel Blockers

Amlodipine (Norvasc)

Oral: 2.5, 5, 10 mg tablets

Bepridil (Vascor)

Oral: 200, 300, 400 mg tablets

Diltiazem (Cardizem)

Oral: 30, 60, 90, 120 mg tablets

Oral sustained-release (Cardizem SR, Dilacor XL): 60, 90, 120, 180, 240, 300 mg capsules

Parenteral: 5 mg/mL for injection

Felodipine (Plendil)

Oral extended-release: 5, 10 mg tablets

Isradipine (DynaCirc)

Oral: 2.5, 5 mg capsules

Nicardipine (Cardene)

Oral: 20, 30 mg capsules

Oral sustained-release (Cardene SR): 30, 45, 60 mg capsules)

Nifedipine (Adalat, Procardia)

Oral: 10, 20 mg capsules

Oral sustained-release (Procardia XL): 30, 60, 90 mg tablets

Nimodipine (Nimotop)

Oral: 30 mg capsules. (Labeled for use in subarachnoid hemorrhage, not angina.)

Verapamil (generic, Calan, Isoptin)

Oral: 40, 80, 120 mg tablets

Oral sustained-release: 120, 180, 240 mg tablets; 120, 180, 240 mg capsules. (Only approved for hypertension: Calan SR, Isoptin SR, Verelan.)

Parenteral: 5 mg/2 mL for injection

Beta-Blockers Labeled for Use in Angina

Atenolol (Tenormin)

Oral: 50, 100 mg tablets

Metoprolol (Lopressor)

Oral: 50, 100 mg tablets

Propranolol (generic, Inderal)

Oral: 10, 20, 40, 60, 80, 90 mg tablets; solution, 4 and 8 mg/mL; solution, concentrated, 80 mg/mL

Oral sustained-release (Inderal LA): 80, 120, 160 mg capsules;

Nadolol (Corgard)

Oral: 20, 40, 80, 120, 160 mg tablets

REFERENCES

Abernethy DR: The pharmacokinetic profile of amlodipine. Am Heart J 1989;118:1100.

Abrams J: A reappraisal of nitrate therapy. JAMA 1988;259:396.

Allen GS et al: Cerebral arterial spasm: A controlled trial of nimodipine in patients with subarachnoid hemorrhage. N Engl J Med 1983;308:619.

Andersson K-E, Vinge E: β-Adrenoceptor blockers and calcium antagonists in the prophylaxis and treatment of migraine. Drugs 1990;39:355.

Bassenge E, Stewart DJ: Effects of nitrates in various vascular sections and regions. Z Kardiol 1986;75(Suppl 3):1.

Bassenge E, Zanzinger J: Nitrates in different vascular beds, nitrate tolerance, and interactions with endothelial function. Am J Cardiol 1992;70 (Suppl B):23B.

Beller GA: Calcium antagonists in the treatment of Prinzmetal's angina and unstable angina pectoris. Circulation 1989;80 (Suppl IV):IV–78.

Bright GE: The effects of nitroglycerin on those engaged in its manufacture. JAMA 1914;62:201.

Carmichael P, Lieben J: Sudden death in explosives workers. Arch Environ Health 1963;7:50.

Chatterjee K: Ischemic heart disease. In: *Internal Medicine.* Stein JH (editor). Little, Brown, 1990.

Chobanian A: Effects of calcium channel antagonists and other antihypertensive drugs on atherogenesis. J Hypertens 1987;5(Suppl 4):S43.

Coffman JD: Raynaud's phenomenon. An update. Hypertension 1991;17:593.

Cohn PF: Total ischemic burden: Definition, mechanisms, and therapeutic implications. Am J Med 1986;81(Suppl 4A):2.

Danish Study Group on Verapamil in Myocardial Infarction: Effect of verapamil on mortality and major events after acute myocardial infarction (The Danish Verapamil Infarction Trial II—DAVIT II). Am J Cardiol 1990;66:779.

Dickson RB, Gottesmann MM: Understanding of the molecular basis of drug resistance in cancer reveals new targets for chemotherapy. Trends Pharmacol Sci 1990;11:305.

Freedman DD, Waters DD: "Second generation" dihydropyridine calcium antagonists. Greater vascular selectivity and some unique applications. Drugs 1987;34:578.

Fuster V et al: The pathogenesis of coronary artery disease and the acute coronary syndromes. (Two parts.) N Engl J Med 1992;326:242, 310.

Ganz W, Marcus HS: Failure of intracoronary nitroglycerin to alleviate pacing-induced angina. Circulation 1972; 46:880.

Godfraind T, Miller R, Wibo M: Calcium antagonism and calcium entry blockade. Pharmacol Rev 1986;38:321.

Harrison DG, Bates JN: The nitrovasodilators. New ideas about old drugs. Circulation 1993;87:1461.

Hartman PE: Review: Putative mutagens and carcinogens in foods. 1. Nitrate/nitrite ingestion and gastric cancer mortality. Environ Mutagen 1983;5:111.

Higginbotham MB et al: Comparison of nifedipine alone with propranolol alone for stable angina pectoris including hemodynamics at rest and during exercise. Am J Cardiol 1986;57:1022.

Ignarro LJ et al: Mechanism of vascular smooth muscle relaxation by organic nitrates, nitrites, nitroprusside, and nitric oxide: Evidence for the involvement of S-nitrosothiols as active intermediates. J Pharmacol Exp Ther 1981;218:739.

Jackson CL, Bush RC, Bowyer DE: Mechanism of antiatherogenic action of calcium antagonists. Atherosclerosis 1989;80:17.

Jugdutt BI, Warnica JW: Intravenous nitroglycerin therapy to limit myocardial infarct size, expansion, and complications. Circulation 1988;78:906.

Kar S, Waikada Y, Nordlander R: The high-risk unstable angina patient. An approach to treatment. Drugs 1992; 43:837.

Karlberg K-E et al: Dose-dependent effect of intravenous nitroglycerin on platelet aggregation, and correlation with plasma glyceryl dinitrate concentration in healthy men. Am J Cardiol 1992;69:802.

Kawanishi DT et al: Response of angina and ischemia to long-term treatment in patients with chronic stable angina: A double blind randomized individualized dosing trial of nifedipine, propranolol, and their combination. J Am Coll Cardiol 1992;19:409.

Kokubun S et al: Studies on Ca channels in intact cardiac cells: Voltage-dependent effects and cooperative interactions of dihydropyridine enantiomers. Mol Pharmacol 1987;30:571.

Kukovetz WR, Holzmann S: Mechanisms of nitrate-induced vasodilation and tolerance. Eur J Clin Pharm 1990;38 (Suppl 1):S–9.

Lambert CR et al: Influence of beta-adrenergic blockade defined by time series analysis on circadian variation of heart rate and ambulatory myocardial ischemia. Am J Cardiol 1989;64:835.

Lindenberg BS et al: Efficacy and safety of incremental doses of diltiazem for the treatment of stable angina pectoris. J Am Coll Cardiol 1983;2:1129.

McDonald KM et al: Long-term oral nitrate therapy prevents chronic ventricular remodeling in the dog. J Am Coll Cardiol 1993;21:514.

Moncada S, Palmer RMJ, Higgs EA: Nitric oxide: Physiology, pathophysiology, and pharmacology. Pharmacol Rev 1991;43:109.

Multicenter Diltiazem Postinfarction Trial Research Group: The effect of diltiazem on mortality and reinfarction after myocardial infarction. N Engl J Med 1988;319:385.

Nesto RW et al: Comparison of nifedipine and isosorbide dinitrate when added to maximal propranolol therapy in stable angina pectoris. Am J Cardiol 1987;60:256.

O'Rourke RA (editor): Calcium-entry blockade: Basic concepts and clinical implications. (Symposium.) Circulation 1987;75(Suppl 6, Part 2):V–1.

Packer M et al: Prevention and reversal of nitrate tolerance in patients with congestive heart failure. N Engl J Med 1987;317:799.

Packer M: Combined beta-adrenergic and calcium-entry blockade in angina pectoris. N Engl J Med 1989; 320:709.

Parker JD, Parker JO: Effect of therapy with an angiotensin-converting enzyme inhibitor on hemodynamic and counter-regulatory responses during continuous therapy with nitroglycerin. J Am Coll Cardiol 1993;21:1445.

Parker JO et al: Effect of intervals between doses on the development of tolerance to isosorbide dinitrate. N Engl J Med 1987;316:1440.

Prida XE et al: Comparison of selective (β_1) and nonselective (β_1 and β_2) beta-adrenergic blockade on systemic and coronary hemodynamic findings in angina pectoris. Am J Cardiol 1987;60:244.

Rankin JS et al: Clinical characteristics and current management of medically refractory unstable angina. Ann Surg 1984;200:457.

Rapoport RM et al: Effects of glyceryl trinitrate on endothelium-dependent and -independent relaxation and cyclic GMP levels in rat aorta and human coronary artery. J Cardiovasc Pharmacol 1987;10:82.

Robinson BF: Relation of heart rate and systolic blood pressure to the onset of pain in angina pectoris. Circulation 1967;35:1073.

Roth A et al: Early tolerance to hemodynamic effects of high-dose transdermal nitroglycerin in responders with severe chronic heart failure. J Am Coll Cardiol 1987; 9:858.

Rouleau JL et al: Mechanism of relief of pacing-induced angina with oral verapamil: Reduced oxygen demand. Circulation 1983;67:94.

Scriabine A: Current and future indications for Ca^{2+} antagonists. Ration Drug Ther 1987;21:1.

Spedding M et al: Factors modifying the tissue selectivity of calcium-antagonists. J Neural Transm 1990;31(Suppl):5.

Steering Committee, Transdermal Nitroglycerin Cooperative Study: Acute and chronic antianginal efficacy of continuous twenty-four hour application of transdermal nitroglycerin. Am J Cardiol 1991;68:1263.

Strauss WE, Parisi AF: Combined use of calcium-channel and beta-adrenergic blockers for the treatment of chronic stable angina: Rationale, efficacy, and adverse effects. Ann Intern Med 19 1988;109:570.

Taira N: Differences in cardiovascular profile among calcium antagonists. Am J Cardiol 1987;59:24B.

Taira N: Nicorandil as a hybrid between nitrates and potassium channel activators. Am J Cardiol 1989;63 (Suppl J):18–J.

Thadani U et al: Double-blind, dose-response, placebo-controlled multicenter study of nisoldipine. A new second-generation calcium channel blocker in angina pectoris. Circulation 1991;84:2398.

Thadani U, Bittar N: Effects of 8:00 A.M. and 2:00 P.M.

doses of isosorbide-5-mononitrate during twice-daily therapy in stable angina pectoris. Am J Cardiol 1992; 70:286.

Trost BN, Weidmann P: Effects of calcium antagonists on glucose homeostasis and serum lipids in non-diabetic and diabetic subjects: A review. J Hypertens 1987; 5(Suppl 4):S81.

Tsien RW et al: Multiple types of neuronal calcium channels and their selective modulation. Trends Neurosci 1988;11:431.

Vaghy PL, Williams JS, Schwartz A: Receptor pharmacol-ogy of calcium entry blocking agents. Am J Cardiol 1987;59 (Suppl A):9–A.

Waldman SA, Murad F: Cyclic GMP synthesis and function. Pharmacol Rev 1987;39:163.

Weiner, DA: Calcium channel blockers. Med Clin North Am 1988;72:83.

Weinstein DB, Heider JG: Antiatherogenic properties of calcium antagonists. State of the art. Am J Med 1989; 86 (Suppl 4A):27.

Wong MCW, Haley EC Jr: Calcium antagonists: Stroke therapy coming of age. Stroke 1990;21:494.

13

Cardiac Glycosides & Other Drugs Used in Congestive Heart Failure

Bertram G. Katzung, MD, PhD, & William W. Parmley, MD

Congestive heart failure occurs when the cardiac output is inadequate to provide the oxygen needed by the body. Although it is believed that the primary defect in heart failure resides in the excitation-contraction coupling machinery of the heart, the clinical condition also involves many other processes and organs, including the baroreceptor reflex, the sympathetic nervous system, the kidneys, the renin-angiotensin-aldosterone system, and vasopressin.

The cardiac glycosides (**digitalis derivatives and similar agents**) comprise a group of steroid compounds that can increase cardiac output and alter the electrical functions of the heart. They also have effects on smooth muscle and other tissues. The principal therapeutic effect in congestive heart failure is an increase in cardiac contractility (a positive inotropic action), which corrects the imbalance associated with failure. Nevertheless, there is some doubt regarding the long-term efficacy of cardiac glycosides in some patients with heart failure. There is general agreement that the commonly used glycosides have a narrow margin of safety and that less toxic compounds with positive inotropic actions are needed. Several agents are candidates for this role in acute failure, including **phosphodiesterase inhibitors** and certain **beta-adrenoceptor stimulants.**

Although traditional therapy of congestive failure has placed most emphasis on correcting the failure of cardiac contractility and reversing the retention of salt and water, clinical research has shown that in some types of congestive failure, unloading the stressed myocardium—by reduction of vascular tone—gives effective relief. Thus, certain vasodilators have been used with considerable success. Such agents include **nitroprusside, hydralazine, nitroglycerin, captopril, enalapril, lisinopril,** and **other angiotensin-converting enzyme inhibitors.**

Control of Cardiac Contractility

The vigor of contraction of heart muscle is determined by several processes that lead to the movement of actin and myosin filaments in the cardiac sarcomere (Figure 13–1). Ultimately, contraction results from the interaction of calcium (during systole) with the actin-troponin-tropomyosin system, thereby releasing the actin-myosin interaction. This "activator" calcium is released from the sarcoplasmic reticulum (SR). The amount released depends upon the amount stored in the SR and upon the amount of "trigger" calcium that enters the cell through calcium channels during the plateau of the action potential. Each of these processes could, in theory, be a target of drug therapy, but only a few have proved useful thus far.

A. Sensitivity of the Contractile Proteins to Calcium: The determinants of calcium sensitivity, ie, the curve relating the shortening of cardiac myofibrils to the cytoplasmic calcium concentration, are poorly understood, but several types of drugs can be shown to affect it in vitro. For example, certain phosphodiesterase inhibitors (theophylline, etc) and some newer agents (Solaro, 1993) appear to shift this curve to lower calcium concentrations.

B. The Amount of Calcium Released From the Sarcoplasmic Reticulum: A sudden small rise in free cytoplasmic calcium, brought about by the opening of voltage-gated calcium channels in the cell membrane, triggers the opening of specialized calcium channels in the membrane of the SR and the rapid release of a large amount of the ion into the cytoplasm in the vicinity of the actin-troponin-tropomyosin complex. The amount released is proportionate to the amount stored in the SR and the amount of trigger calcium that enters the cell through the cell membrane channels. Ryanodine is a potent *negative* inotropic agent that interferes with the release of calcium through the SR channels. No drugs are available that have been shown to increase the release of calcium through these channels.

C. The Amount of Calcium Stored in the Sarcoplasmic Reticulum: The SR membrane contains a very efficient calcium uptake transporter, which maintains free cytoplasmic calcium at very low levels during diastole by pumping calcium into the membrane-limited tubules of the SR. The amount of calcium sequestered in the SR is thus determined, in part, by the amount accessible to this transporter. This in turn is dependent on the balance of calcium influx (primarily through the voltage-gated membrane cal-

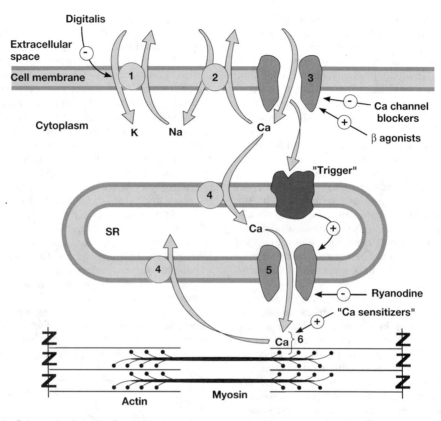

Figure 13–1. Schematic diagram of a cardiac muscle sarcomere, with sites of action of several drugs that alter contractility (numbered structures). Site *1* is Na⁺/K⁺ ATPase, the sodium pump. Site *2* is the sodium/calcium exchanger. Site *3* is the voltage-gated calcium channel. Site *4* is a calcium transporter that pumps calcium into the sarcoplasmic reticulum (SR). Site *5* is a calcium channel in the membrane of the SR that is triggered to release stored calcium by activation of the SR "trigger." Site *6* is the actin-troponin-tropomyosin complex at which activator calcium brings about the contractile interaction of actin and myosin.

cium channels) and calcium efflux, the amount removed from the cell (primarily via the sodium-calcium exchanger, a transporter in the cell membrane).

D. The Amount of Trigger Calcium: The amount of trigger calcium that enters the cell depends upon the availability of calcium channels and the duration of their opening. As described in Chapters 6 and 9, the sympathomimetics cause an increase in calcium influx through an action on these channels. Conversely, the calcium channel blockers (Chapter 12) reduce this influx and depress contractility.

E. Activity of the Sodium-Calcium Exchanger: This antiporter uses the sodium gradient to move calcium against its concentration gradient from the cytoplasm to the extracellular space. Extracellular concentrations of these ions are much less labile than intracellular concentrations under physiologic conditions. The sodium-calcium exchanger's ability to carry out this transport is thus dependent primarily on the intracellular concentrations of both ions, especially sodium.

F. Intracellular Sodium Concentration and

Activity of Na⁺/K⁺ ATPase: Na⁺/K⁺ ATPase, by removing intracellular sodium, is the major determinant of sodium concentration in the cell. The sodium influx through voltage-gated channels, which occurs as a normal part of almost all cardiac action potentials, is another determinant. As described below, Na⁺/K⁺ ATPase appears to be the primary target of cardiac glycosides. Several experimental drugs markedly increase sodium influx during action potentials by interfering with sodium channel inactivation (Hoey et al, 1993). They have been shown to have dramatic positive inotropic effects in vitro, but their role in clinical therapy has yet to be defined.

PATHOPHYSIOLOGY OF HEART FAILURE

Congestive heart failure is a syndrome with multiple causes that may involve the right ventricle, the left ventricle, or both. Cardiac output in congestive heart failure is usually below the normal range. An intrinsic biochemical defect results in decreased cardiac contractility, which is usually responsive to positive inotropic drugs. This is typical of chronic failure resulting from coronary artery disease or hypertension or acute failure resulting from myocardial infarction. Rarely, "high-output" failure may occur. In this condition, the demands of the body are so great that even increased cardiac output is insufficient. High-output failure can result from hyperthyroidism, beriberi, anemia, and arteriovenous shunts. This form of failure responds poorly to positive inotropic agents.

The primary signs and symptoms of all types of congestive heart failure include tachycardia, decreased exercise tolerance and shortness of breath, peripheral and pulmonary edema, and cardiomegaly. Decreased exercise tolerance with rapid muscular fatigue is the major direct consequence of diminished cardiac output. The other manifestations result from the attempts by the body to compensate for the intrinsic cardiac defect.

Neurohumoral reflex (extrinsic) compensation involves two major mechanisms, as described in Chapter 6 and displayed in Figure 6–7. These are the sympathetic nervous system and the renin-angiotensin-aldosterone hormonal response. The baroreceptor reflex appears to be "reset," with a lower sensitivity to arterial pressure, in patients with heart failure. As a result, baroreceptor sensory input to the vasomotor center is reduced even at normal pressures; sympathetic outflow is increased; and parasympathetic outflow is decreased (Ferguson, 1992). Increased sympathetic outflow causes tachycardia, increased cardiac contractility, and increased vascular tone. Increased arterial tone results in increased afterload and decreased ejection fraction, cardiac output, and renal perfusion. Elevation of venous tone results in increased ventricular filling pressure, dilation of the heart, and increased fiber stretch. Increased aldosterone secretion results in sodium and water retention with increased blood volume and, ultimately, edema. Other hormones may also be released.

The most important intrinsic compensatory mechanism is myocardial hypertrophy. This increase in muscle mass helps to maintain cardiac performance in the face of adverse effects such as pressure or volume overload, loss of functional tissue (myocardial infarction), or decrease in cardiac contractility. However, after an initial beneficial effect, hypertrophy can lead to ischemic changes, impairment of diastolic filling, and alterations in ventricular geometry.

Pathophysiology of Cardiac Performance

Cardiac performance is a function of four primary factors.

A. Preload: The effect of altered preload (atrial pressure) on cardiovascular performance is of considerable importance. When some measure of left ventricular performance such as stroke volume or stroke work is plotted as a function of left ventricular filling pressure, the resulting curve is termed the **left ventricular function curve** (Figure 13–2). The ascending limb (< 15 mm Hg filling pressure) represents the classic Frank-Starling relation. Beyond approximately 15 mm Hg, there is a plateau of performance. Preloads greater than 20–25 mm Hg result in pulmonary congestion. As noted above, preload is usually increased in heart failure because of increased blood volume and venous tone. Reduction of high filling pressure is the goal of salt restriction and diuretic therapy in congestive heart failure. Venodilator drugs (eg, nitroglycerin) also reduce preload by redistributing blood away from the chest into peripheral veins.

B. Afterload: Afterload is the resistance against which the heart must pump blood and is represented by aortic impedance and systemic vascular resistance. Systemic vascular resistance is frequently increased in patients with congestive heart failure. As cardiac output falls in chronic failure, there is a reflex increase in systemic vascular resistance, mediated in part by increased sympathetic outflow and circulating catecholamines and in part by activation of the renin-angiotensin system. However, elevated vascular resistance may further reduce cardiac output by

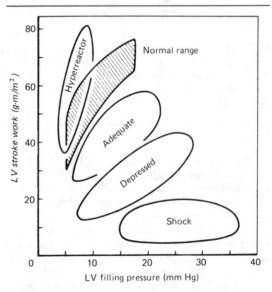

Figure 13–2. Relation of left ventricular performance to filling pressure in patients with acute myocardial infarction. The cross-hatched area is the range for normal, healthy individuals. Following infarction, there is a wide range of performance characteristics. In some patients, performance is in the normal or hypernormal range (hyperreactor). As the size of the infarct increases, however, function is shifted down and to the right. Similar depression is observed in patients with chronic congestive heart failure. (Reproduced with permission, from Swan HJC, Parmley WW: Congestive heart failure. In: *Pathologic Physiology.* Sodeman WA Jr, Sodeman TM [editors]. Saunders, 1979.)

increasing resistance to ejection. This sets the stage for the use of drugs that reduce arteriolar tone in congestive heart failure.

C. Contractility: In patients with chronic low-output failure, the primary defect appears to be a reduction in the intrinsic contractility of the myocardium. As contractility decreases, there is a reduction in the velocity of muscle shortening and the rate of intraventricular pressure development (dP/dt). This results in the reduction in pump performance of the heart that accompanies heart failure, eg, after acute myocardial infarction (Figure 13–2). However, the heart is still capable of an increase in contractility in response to inotropic drugs.

D. Heart Rate: The heart rate is a major determinant of cardiac output. As the intrinsic function of the heart decreases in failure and stroke volume diminishes, an increase in heart rate—through sympathetic activation of beta adrenoceptors—is the first compensatory mechanism that comes into play to maintain cardiac output.

I. BASIC PHARMACOLOGY OF DRUGS USED IN CONGESTIVE HEART FAILURE

DIGITALIS

Medicinal plants containing cardiac glycosides were known to the ancient Egyptians 3000 years ago, but these agents were used erratically and with variable success until the 18th century, when William Withering, an English physician and botanist, published a monograph describing the clinical effects of an extract of the foxglove plant (*Digitalis purpurea,* a major source of these agents). His book, *An Account of the Foxglove and Some of Its Medical Uses: With Practical Remarks on Dropsy and Other Diseases,* published in 1785, described in detail the indications for the use of cardiac glycosides and offered cautionary remarks about their toxicity.

Chemistry

All of the commonly used cardiac glycosides, or cardenolides—of which **digoxin** (Figure 13–3) may be considered the prototype—combine a steroid nucleus with an unsaturated five-membered lactone ring at the 17 position and a series of sugars linked to carbon 3 of the nucleus. Because they lack an easily ionizable group, their solubility is not pH-dependent.

Sources of these drugs include white and purple foxglove (*Digitalis lanata* and *D purpurea*), Mediterranean sea onion (squill), *Strophanthus gratus*, oleander, lily of the valley, milkweed, and numerous other tropical and temperate zone plants. Certain toads have skin glands capable of elaborating **bufadienolides,** which differ from the cardenolides only in having a six-membered (rather than a five-membered) lactone ring at the 17 position.

Structure-activity studies indicate that the lactone ring and the steroid nucleus are essential for activity. The other substituents—especially the sugar molecules in the 3 position—influence pharmacokinetic variables, including absorption, half-life, and metabolism. There is no clinical evidence that any of the natural cardenolides differs from the others in therapeutic index or maximal efficacy.

Pharmacokinetics

A. Absorption and Distribution: Cardenolides have both lipophilic (steroid nucleus) and hydrophilic (lactone ring, hydroxyl, sugar) groups. The balance of these two factors has an important effect on absorption, distribution, metabolism, and excretion, as shown by comparison of three representative agents:

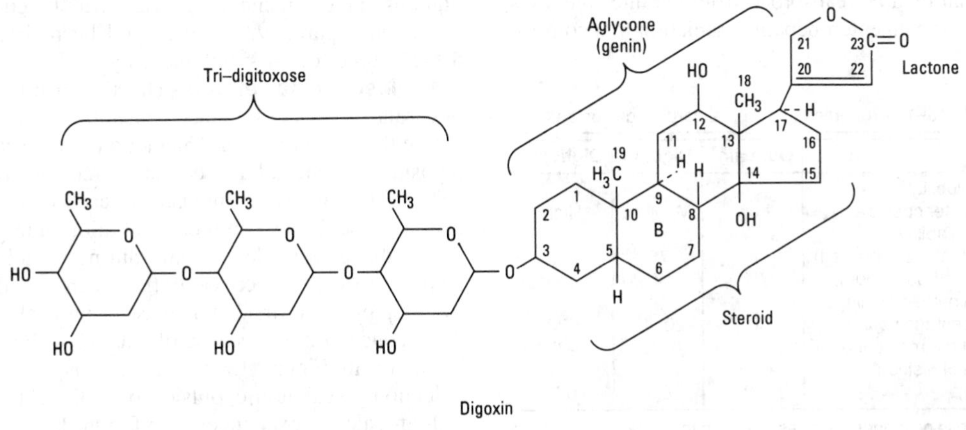

Figure 13–3. Structure of digoxin, a typical cardiac glycoside.

digoxin, digitoxin, and **ouabain** (Table 13–1). Of these three, digoxin is by far the most widely used preparation.

As noted in the table, digoxin is fairly well absorbed after oral administration. However, about 10% of individuals harbor enteric bacteria that inactivate digoxin in the gut, greatly reducing bioavailability and requiring higher than average maintenance dosage. Treatment of such patients with antibiotics can result in a sudden increase in bioavailability and digitalis toxicity. Because the safety margin of cardiac glycosides is very narrow, even minor variations in bioavailability could cause serious toxicity or loss of effect. In fact, product formulation (factors in manufacture of the tablets) can modify the bioavailability of digoxin. As a result, digoxin preparations must pass dissolution tests before they can be marketed in the USA. Digitoxin, because it is well absorbed under almost all circumstances, is not subject to this restriction. Beta-methyldigoxin, a semisynthetic derivative of digoxin often used outside the USA, is almost completely absorbed from the gut and is metabolized to digoxin in the body. Deslanoside (see Preparations Available) is also very similar to digoxin (it contains one extra sugar group).

Once absorbed into the blood, all cardiac glycosides are widely distributed to tissues, including the central nervous system. Their volumes of distribution differ, however, depending on their tendency to bind to plasma proteins. The highest tissue concentrations—for digoxin, 10–50 times higher than in plasma—are found in heart, kidney, and liver.

B. Metabolism and Excretion: Digoxin is not extensively metabolized in humans but is largely excreted unchanged by the kidneys. Its total clearance correlates closely with creatinine clearance and is significantly slowed in patients with renal disease. Equations and nomograms are available for adjusting digoxin dosage.

Digitoxin is metabolized in the liver and excreted into the gut via the bile. Cardioactive metabolites (which include digoxin) as well as unchanged digitoxin can then be reabsorbed from the intestine, thus establishing an enterohepatic circulation that contrib-

utes to the very long half-life of this agent. Renal impairment does not significantly prolong the half-life of digitoxin, so this drug may occasionally be useful in patients with erratic or rapidly failing renal function. On the other hand, a variety of hepatic enzyme-inducing drugs (see Chapter 4) can reduce the blood level of digitoxin by accelerating its metabolism.

Ouabain must be given parenterally and was therefore used only for acute therapy and rarely for more than a few doses. It is metabolized very little and excreted primarily by the kidney.

Pharmacodynamics

Digitalis has multiple direct and indirect cardiovascular effects, with both therapeutic and toxic (arrhythmogenic) consequences. In addition, it has undesirable effects on the central nervous system and gut. A small direct renal (diuretic) effect has been demonstrated.

At the molecular level, all therapeutically useful cardiac glycosides inhibit **Na^+/K^+ ATPase,** the membrane-bound transporter often called the "sodium pump." Several different forms of this enzyme have been identified, and it appears that different isoforms have differing affinities for cardiac glycosides. Very low concentrations of these drugs have occasionally been reported to *stimulate* the enzyme. In contrast, inhibition over most of the dose range has been extensively documented in all tissues studied. It is probable that this action is largely responsible for the therapeutic effect (positive inotropy) in the heart. Since the sodium pump is necessary for maintenance of normal resting potential in most excitable cells, it is likely that a portion of the toxicity of digitalis is also caused by this enzyme-inhibiting action. Other molecular-level effects of digitalis have been studied in the heart and are discussed below. The fact that the receptor for cardiac glycosides exists on the sodium pump has prompted investigators to propose that an endogenous "digitalis-like" agent must exist. (See box: Endogenous Cardiac Glycosides.)

A. Cardiac Effects: For clarity, the effects of digitalis on mechanical and electrical function are discussed separately, but it should be realized that these changes occur simultaneously.

1. Mechanical effects–The therapeutic action of cardiac glycosides on mechanical function is to increase the intensity of the interaction of the actin and myosin filaments of the cardiac sarcomere (Figure 13–1). This increased intensity is caused by an increase in the free calcium concentration in the vicinity of the contractile proteins during systole. The increase in calcium concentration is the result of a two-step process: first, an increase of intracellular sodium concentration because of Na^+/K^+ ATPase inhibition (*1* in Figure 13–1); and second, a relative reduction of calcium expulsion from the cell by the sodium-calcium exchanger (*2* in Figure 13–1) caused by the increase in intracellular sodium. Two other

Table 13–1. Properties of 3 typical cardiac glycosides.

	Ouabain[1]	Digoxin	Digitoxin
Lipid solubility (oil/water coefficient)	Low	Medium	High
Oral availability (percentage absorbed)	0	75	>90
Half-life in body (hours)	21	40	168
Plasma protein binding (percentage bound)	0	20–40	>90
Percentage metabolized	0	<20	>80
Volume of distribution (L/kg)	18	6.3	0.6

[1]Ouabain is no longer in use as a drug in the USA, but see box: Endogenous Cardiac Glycosides.

ENDOGENOUS CARDIAC GLYCOSIDES

Do all receptors on regulatory enzymes and transporters have endogenous ligands as well as an affinity for the exogenous chemicals we use as drugs? Some biologists would answer this question affirmatively, reasoning that these regulators of important processes themselves require endogenous regulators. Others argue that proteins have sufficient complexity of structure so that there is a great likelihood they will bind some completely foreign ligand molecules. Furthermore, if the binding occurs in a critical region of the protein, it is highly probable that some alteration of function of that enzyme or transporter will result, thereby causing a pharmacologic response.

The receptor for the cardiac glycosides is a case in point. The very high affinity of the Na^+/K^+ ATPase for cardiac glycosides suggests that there might be an endogenous ligand of similar structure. Like the adrenocortical hormones, the cardiac glycosides have a steroid nucleus, but the stereochemistry of the rings is quite different from that of typical cholesterol derivatives. While many plants synthesize these glycosides, in the animal kingdom only a few amphibians (poisonous toads) had been thought to have this capability.

A significant new body of evidence (reviewed by Blaustein, 1993) based on extremely sensitive immunochemical techniques now suggests that ouabain is synthesized by the adrenal and perhaps by the brain in humans and other mammals. It is claimed that ouabain is released as an endocrine and paracrine agent under certain circumstances, such as high salt intake and heart failure. It has been postulated for almost 20 years that some forms of hypertension are caused by vasoconstriction evoked by an endogenous inhibitor of the sodium pump. Elevated endogenous ouabain secretion evoked by high salt intake would provide an important link in this hypothesis. In congestive heart failure, plasma ouabain levels are said to be positively correlated with the severity of failure.

There are chemical and physiologic reasons to question these proposals (Kelly, 1992). Even if the controversial evidence is replicated, much remains to be explained about the role of endogenous ouabain. From the observation that serum ouabain is increased in patients with heart failure, we can probably conclude that failure—at least in some patients—is not caused by primary ouabain deficiency. If ouabain is indeed synthesized in the patient with heart failure, does the continued progression of the disease to the point of requiring exogenous glycoside therapy represent an inadequate endogenous supply, development of tolerance, or some other alteration?

In the meantime, it appears that one more receptor may have a surprising endogenous ligand, and if this is the case, convergent evolution in plants, toads, and mammals may have been demonstrated.

mechanisms have been proposed that may complement this well-documented action: facilitation of calcium entry through the voltage-gated calcium channels of the membrane (*3* in Figure 13–1); and an independent effect on sarcoplasmic reticulum that results in increased release of calcium from this intracellular storage site (*5* in Figure 13–1).

The net result of the action of therapeutic concentrations of a cardiac glycoside is a distinctive increase in cardiac contractility (Figure 13–4, bottom trace). In isolated myocardial preparations, the rate of development of tension and of relaxation are both increased, with little or no change in time to peak tension. The duration of the contractile response is neither shortened (as in the case of beta-adrenoceptor stimulation) nor prolonged (as in the case of methylxanthines such as theophylline). These effects occur in both normal and failing myocardium, but in the intact animal or patient the responses are modified by cardiovascular reflexes and the pathophysiology of congestive heart failure.

2. Electrical effects–The effects of digitalis on the electrical properties of the heart in the intact organism are a mixture of direct and autonomic actions. Direct actions on the membranes of cardiac cells follow a well-defined progression: an early, brief prolongation of the action potential, followed by a protracted period of shortening (especially the plateau phase). This decrease in action potential duration is probably the result of increased potassium conductance that is caused by increased intracellular calcium. (See Chapter 14 for a discussion of the effects of ionic conductances on the action potential.) All of these effects can be observed in the absence of overt toxicity. Shortening of the action potential contributes to the shortening of atrial and ventricular refractoriness (Table 13–2).

With more toxic concentrations, resting membrane potential is reduced (made less negative) as a result of inhibition of the sodium pump and reduced intracellular potassium. As toxicity progresses, oscillatory depolarizing afterpotentials appear following normally evoked action potentials (Figure 13–4, panel B). The afterpotentials (also known as "delayed afterdepolarizations") are associated with overloading of the intracellular calcium stores and oscillations in the free in-

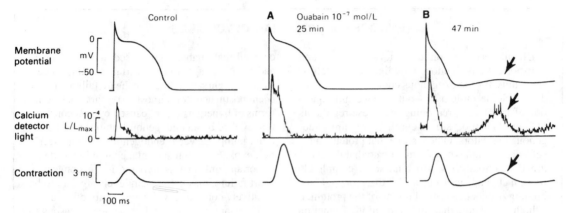

Figure 13–4. Effects of a cardiac glycoside, ouabain, on isolated cardiac tissue. The top tracing shows action potentials evoked during the control period, early in the "therapeutic" phase, and later, when toxicity is present. The middle tracing shows the light emitted by the calcium-detecting protein aequorin (relative to the maximum possible, L/L_{max}) and is roughly proportionate to the free intracellular calcium concentration. The bottom tracing records the tension elicited by the action potentials. The early phase of ouabain action *(A)* shows a slight shortening of action potential and a marked increase in free intracellular calcium concentration and contractile tension. The toxic phase *(B)* is associated with depolarization of the resting potential, a marked shortening of the action potential, and the appearance of an oscillatory depolarization, calcium increment, and contraction *(arrows)*. (Unpublished data kindly provided by P Hess and H Gil Wier.)

tracellular calcium ion concentration. When below threshold, these afterpotentials may interfere with normal conduction because of the further reduction of resting potential. Eventually, an afterpotential may reach threshold, eliciting an action potential (premature ventricular depolarization or "ectopic beat") that is coupled to the preceding normal one. If afterpotentials in the Purkinje conducting system regularly reach threshold in this way, bigeminy will be recorded on the ECG (Figure 13–5). With further toxic deterioration, each afterpotential-evoked action potential will itself elicit a suprathreshold afterpotential, and a self-sustaining arrhythmia (ventricular tachycardia) will be established. If allowed to progress, such a tachycardia may deteriorate into ventricular fibrillation.

Autonomic actions of cardiac glycosides on the heart involve both the parasympathetic and the sympathetic systems and occur throughout the therapeutic and toxic dose ranges. In the lower portion of the dose range, cardioselective **parasympathomimetic** effects predominate. In fact, these atropine-blockable effects are responsible for a significant portion of the early electrical effects of digitalis (Table 13–2). This action involves sensitization of the baroreceptors, central vagal stimulation, and facilitation of muscarinic transmission at the cardiac muscle cell. Because cholinergic innervation is much richer in the atria, these actions affect atrial and atrioventricular nodal function more than Purkinje or ventricular function. Some of the cholinomimetic effects are useful in the treatment of certain arrhythmias. At toxic levels, sympathetic outflow is increased by digitalis. This effect is not essential for typical cardenolide toxicity but sensitizes the myocardium and exaggerates all the toxic effects of the drug.

Table 13–2. Major actions of digitalis on cardiac electrical functions. (PANS = parasympathetic actions; Direct = direct membrane actions.)

	Tissue		
Variable	**Atrial Muscle**	**AV Node**	**Purkinje System, Ventricles**
Effective refractory period	↓ (PANS)	↑ (PANS)	↓ (Direct)
Conduction velocity	↑ (PANS)	↓ (PANS)	Negligible
Automaticity	↑ (Direct)	↑ (Direct)	↑ (Direct)
Electrocardiogram Before arrhythmias	Negligible	↑ PR interval	↓QT interval; T wave inversion; ST segment depression
Arrhythmias	Atrial tachycardia, atrial fibrillation	AV nodal tachycardia, AV blockade	Premature ventricular contractions, bigeminy, ventricular tachycardia, ventricular fibrillation

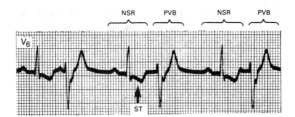

Figure 13–5. ECG record showing digitalis-induced bigeminy. The complexes marked NSR are normal sinus rhythm beats; an inverted T wave and depressed ST segment are present. The complexes marked PVB are premature ventricular beats and are the electrocardiographic manifestations of depolarizations evoked by delayed oscillatory afterpotentials as shown in Figure 13–4. (Modified and reproduced, with permission, from Goldman MJ: *Principles of Clinical Electrocardiography*, 12th ed. Lange, 1986.)

The most common cardiac manifestations of glycoside toxicity include atrioventricular junctional rhythm, premature ventricular depolarizations, bigeminal rhythm, and second-degree atrioventricular blockade. However, it is claimed that digitalis can cause virtually every variety of arrhythmia. The membrane cardiotoxicity of digitalis was described above as involving resting depolarization (due to sodium pump inhibition) and oscillatory afterdepolarizations (caused by overload of intracellular calcium). Resting depolarization may be responsible for a portion of the conduction abnormalities such as atrioventricular block. Afterdepolarizations are probably responsible for most glycoside arrhythmias involving abnormal automaticity, including premature ventricular depolarizations, bigeminy, and ventricular tachycardia.

B. Effects on Other Organs: Cardiac glycosides affect all excitable tissues, including smooth muscle and the central nervous system. The mechanism of these effects has not been fully explored but probably involves the inhibition of Na^+/K^+ ATPase in these tissues. The depolarization resulting from depression of the sodium pump would be expected to increase spontaneous activity both in neurons and in smooth muscle cells. In addition, an increase in intracellular calcium could predictably increase smooth muscle tone. This may occur when an intravenous dose of digoxin is given rapidly. However, it should be remembered that in most cases of congestive heart failure successfully treated with digitalis, a *decrease* in vascular tone is the net effect, resulting from a beneficial reduction of sympathetic tone (see below).

The gastrointestinal tract is the most common site of digitalis toxicity outside the heart. These actions include anorexia, nausea, vomiting, and diarrhea. This toxicity may be partially caused by direct effects on the gastrointestinal tract but is also the result of central nervous system actions, including chemoreceptor trigger zone stimulation.

Central nervous system effects commonly include vagal and chemoreceptor zone stimulation, as noted above. Much less often, disorientation and hallucinations—especially in the elderly—and visual disturbances are noted. The latter effect may include aberrations of color perception. Agitation and even convulsions are occasionally reported in patients taking digitalis.

Gynecomastia is a rare effect reported in men taking digitalis; it is not certain whether this effect represents a peripheral estrogenic action of these steroid drugs or a manifestation of hypothalamic stimulation.

ATPase-dependent transport processes such as production of aqueous humor and cerebrospinal fluid, as well as sodium reabsorption in the kidney, can be shown experimentally to be inhibited by cardenolides. These effects are of no clinical significance.

C. Interactions With Potassium, Calcium, and Magnesium: The concentrations of potassium and calcium in the extracellular compartment (usually measured as serum K^+ and Ca^{2+}) have important effects on sensitivity to digitalis. Potassium and digitalis interact in two ways. First, they inhibit each other's binding to Na^+/K^+ ATPase; therefore, hyperkalemia reduces the enzyme-inhibiting actions of cardiac glycosides, whereas hypokalemia facilitates these actions. Second, abnormal cardiac automaticity is inhibited by hyperkalemia (see Chapter 14); thus, moderately increased extracellular K^+ reduces the effects of digitalis, especially the toxic effects. Calcium ion facilitates the toxic actions of cardiac glycosides by accelerating the overloading of intracellular calcium stores that appears to be responsible for digitalis-induced abnormal automaticity. Hypercalcemia therefore increases the risk of a digitalis-induced arrhythmia. The effects of magnesium ion appear to be directly opposite to those of calcium. Hypomagnesemia is therefore a risk factor for arrhythmias. These interactions mandate careful evaluation of serum electrolytes in patients with digitalis-induced arrhythmias.

OTHER POSITIVE INOTROPIC DRUGS USED IN HEART FAILURE

Drugs that inhibit **phosphodiesterases,** the family of enzymes that inactivate cAMP and cGMP, have long been used in therapy of heart failure. Although they have positive inotropic effects, most of their benefits appear to derive from vasodilation, as discussed below. Aminophylline, a traditional methylxanthine compound with some phosphodiesterase-inhibiting effects, was often used in the treatment of acute pulmonary edema. It is of no value in the treatment of chronic congestive heart failure and is rarely used for acute therapy now. Newer phosphodiesterase inhibitors have been intensively studied for several decades with mixed results. The bipyridines amrinone and milrinone are the most successful of these agents found to date, but their utility is quite limited. Flosequinan, a fluoroquinolone derivative with mixed positive inotropic and vasodilating actions, was a recent addition to these candidate digitalis substitutes, but it was withdrawn because of toxicity. Clinical trials have suggested that vesnarinone, a drug with an unknown mechanism of action, may significantly lower the risk of death in patients with heart failure. (See box: Flosequinan and Vesnarinone.) A group of beta-adrenoceptor stimulants have also been used as digitalis substitutes.

BIPYRIDINES

Amrinone and **milrinone** are bipyridine compounds that can be given orally or parenterally but are only available in parenteral forms. They have elimination half-lives of 2–3 hours, with 10–40% being excreted in the urine.

Pharmacodynamics

The bipyridines increase myocardial contractility without inhibiting Na^+/K^+ ATPase or activating adrenoceptors. They appear to increase inward calcium flux in the heart during the action potential and alter the intracellular movements of calcium by influencing the sarcoplasmic reticulum. They also have a significant vasodilating effect that undoubtedly contributes to their therapeutic benefits in heart failure. Biochemical studies suggest that most of their action results from inhibition of phosphodiesterase, an action similar to that of the methylxanthines. These drugs and several investigational phosphodiesterase inhibitors appear to be relatively selective for phosphodiesterase isozyme III, a form found in cardiac and smooth muscle. Inhibition of this isozyme results in an increase in cAMP and the increase in contractility and vasodilation noted above.

When given to patients in acute heart failure, the bipyridines increase cardiac output and reduce pulmonary capillary wedge pressure and peripheral vascular resistance. There is little change in the heart rate or arterial pressure. Although the acute effects are clearly beneficial, their toxicity prevents their long-term use.

The toxicity of amrinone includes a relatively high incidence of nausea and vomiting; thrombocytopenia and liver enzyme changes have been reported in a smaller but significant number of patients. This agent is used only for short-term parenteral treatment. It may be less likely to cause cardiac arrhythmias than is digitalis. Milrinone appears less likely to cause bone marrow and liver toxicity than amrinone, but it does

cause arrhythmias. In a placebo-controlled trial in patients with severe congestive heart failure, oral milrinone increased mortality (Packer et al, 1991). Therefore, like amrinone, it is now used only intravenously and only for acute heart failure.

BETA-ADRENOCEPTOR STIMULANTS

The general pharmacology of these agents is discussed in Chapter 9. The search for positive inotropic drugs with less arrhythmogenic potential than digitalis and less tendency to increase heart rate than isoproterenol has led to the development of β_1-selective agents. At the same time, the successful use of vasodilators in congestive heart failure has resulted in an interest in selective β_2 agents for this condition.

The selective β_1 agonist that has been most widely used in patients with heart failure is **dobutamine.** This drug produces an increase in cardiac output together with a decrease in ventricular filling pressure. Some tachycardia and an increase in myocardial oxygen consumption have been reported. Thus, although dobutamine clearly increases cardiac contractility, it is unclear what net benefit it may have in patients with ischemic heart disease. The potential for producing angina or arrhythmias in such patients must be considered, as well as the tachyphylaxis that accompanies the use of any beta stimulant. Intermittent dobutamine infusion may benefit some patients with chronic heart failure.

A variety of other agents with effects at beta and dopamine adrenoceptors have been studied. Most of these, like dopamine and dobutamine, are not active orally, so they are reserved for management of acute failure or failure refractory to oral agents.

DRUGS WITHOUT POSITIVE INOTROPIC EFFECTS USED IN HEART FAILURE

The drugs most commonly used in chronic heart failure are diuretics, cardiac glycosides, and angiotensin-converting enzyme inhibitors. In acute failure, diuretics and vasodilators play important roles. Thus, drugs without positive inotropic actions on the heart play a major role in therapy.

Diuretics

The diuretics are discussed in detail in Chapter 15. Their mechanism of action in heart failure is to reduce salt and water retention, thereby reducing ventricular preload. The reduction in venous pressure has two useful effects: reduction of signs and symptoms

FLOSEQUINAN & VESNARINONE

The difficulty of developing effective new drugs for congestive heart failure is well illustrated by two newer agents.

Flosequinan is an orally active fluoroquinolone compound with a long duration of action. It has definite vasodilating effects and, probably, a positive inotropic action as well. Although it resembles the bipyridines in many respects, its mechanism of action is unknown. It is a very weak and nonselective phosphodiesterase inhibitor. It does not appear to sensitize cardiac myofibrils to calcium, and it alters neither Na^+/K^+ ATPase activity nor cAMP concentrations. The drug appeared quite promising in its initial clinical trials and was approved by the FDA for marketing in the USA. It was recommended that dosage be started at 50 mg daily, gradually increasing to a maximum of 100 mg daily. After the drug was released, an ongoing study found that mortality was increased at the 100 mg/d dosage, so a warning was published to avoid the highest dose except in patients who were unresponsive to other drugs and lower doses. Sales of the drug, even for use at lower doses, immediately declined so precipitously its manufacturer withdrew it from the market.

Vesnarinone is an orally active quinolinone agent that has been shown to have several effects on isolated cardiac muscle, including inhibition of phosphodiesterase, increase in calcium current, and prolongation of the action potential duration. Each of these effects could, in theory, produce a significant inotropic effect (see Control of Cardiac Contractility, above), and phosphodiesterase inhibition may also cause vasodilation with useful unloading of the overworked ventricles. Several clinical trials with this agent (eg, Feldman et al, 1993) have suggested that it may significantly decrease morbidity and mortality for at least 25 weeks. The latter study also showed, however, that the therapeutic margin of safety is narrow, with 60 mg daily causing a *decrease* in mortality and 120 mg daily causing a significant *increase* in deaths. It is uncertain that any of the proposed mechanisms of therapeutic effect are produced at the lower dose. If the clinical benefits can be reproduced in larger trials, it may be necessary to look for a previously unknown mechanism of benefit in heart failure.

These studies reinforce the facts that once congestive failure has occurred, the heart is extremely vulnerable to excessive stimulation, and that drugs that produce clinically useful increases in cardiac contractility are operating near the absolute limits of clinical safety. Positive inotropic drugs appear to be especially hazardous. Neither flosequinan nor vesnarinone is available for general clinical use in the USA at present.

(edema) and reduction of cardiac size, which leads to improved efficiency of pump function.

Angiotensin-Converting Enzyme Inhibitors

The ACE inhibitors are introduced in Chapter 11 and discussed again in Chapter 17. These versatile drugs reduce angiotensin II levels, which reduces peripheral resistance and thereby reduces afterload; they also reduce salt and water retention (by reducing aldosterone secretion) and in that way reduce preload. The reduction in tissue angiotensin levels also appears to reduce sympathetic activity, probably through diminution of angiotensin's presynaptic effects on norepinephrine release.

Vasodilators

The vasodilators are effective in heart failure because they provide a reduction in preload (through venodilation), or reduction in afterload (through arteriolar dilation), or both.

The clinical application of these agents in heart failure is described below.

II. CLINICAL PHARMACOLOGY OF DRUGS USED IN CONGESTIVE HEART FAILURE

DIGITALIS IN CONGESTIVE HEART FAILURE

Because it has a moderate but persistent positive inotropic effect, digitalis can, in theory, reverse the signs and symptoms of congestive heart failure. In an appropriate patient, digitalis increases stroke work and cardiac output. The increased output (and possibly a direct action resetting the sensitivity of the baroreceptors) eliminates the stimuli evoking increased sympathetic outflow, and both heart rate and vascular tone diminish. With decreased end-diastolic fiber tension (the result of increased systolic ejection and decreased filling pressure), heart size and oxygen demand decrease. Finally, increased renal blood flow improves glomerular filtration and reduces aldosterone-driven sodium reabsorption. Thus, edema fluid can be excreted, further reducing ventricular preload and the danger of pulmonary edema.

Administration & Dosage

Chronic treatment with digitalis agents requires careful attention to pharmacokinetics because of their long half-lives (Table 13–3). According to the rules set forth in Chapter 3, it will take three to four half-lives to approach steady-state total body load when given at a constant dosing rate, ie, approximately 1 week for digoxin and 1 month for digitoxin. Since it is very important not to exceed the therapeutic range of plasma digitalis concentration, such a slow approach to "digitalization" is the safest dosing technique. If a more rapid effect is required, digitalization can be achieved quickly with a large loading dose (divided into three or four portions and given over 24–36 hours) followed by maintenance doses. Typical doses used in adults are given in Table 13–3. It is essential that the patient be examined before each dose when using the rapid (three-dose) method of digitalization. Sensitive plasma digoxin assays are available at most medical centers and should be used when patient response is not as predicted from the dosing schedule.

Interactions

Important drug interactions must be considered in patients taking cardiac glycosides. All such patients are at risk of developing serious cardiac arrhythmias if hypokalemia develops, as in diuretic therapy or diarrhea. Furthermore, patients taking digoxin are at risk if given quinidine, which displaces digoxin from tissue binding sites and depresses renal digoxin clearance. The plasma level of the glycoside may double within a few days after beginning quinidine therapy, and toxic effects may become manifest. A similar interaction with other drugs, including nonsteroidal anti-inflammatory agents and calcium channel-block-

ing agents, has been reported, but clinically significant effects have not been demonstrated in humans. Quinidine does not alter volume of distribution or protein binding of digitoxin. However, it may prolong the half-life of this glycoside. As noted above, antibiotics that alter gastrointestinal flora may increase digoxin bioavailability in about 10% of patients. Finally, agents that release catecholamines may sensitize the myocardium to digitalis-induced arrhythmias.

Reduced responsiveness to cardiac glycosides may be due to intractably severe disease or patient noncompliance. In patients concurrently taking cholestyramine (see Chapter 34), digitalis absorption is reduced. The digitalis dose required for therapeutic effect must usually be increased in hyperthyroid patients because of reduction in elimination half-life.

Other Clinical Uses of Digitalis

Digitalis is useful in the management of atrial arrhythmias because of its cardioselective parasympathomimetic effects. In atrial flutter, the depressant effect of the drug on atrioventricular conduction will help control an excessively high ventricular rate. The effects of the drug on the atrial musculature may convert flutter to fibrillation, with a further decrease in ventricular rate. In atrial fibrillation, the same "vagomimetic" action helps control ventricular rate, thereby improving ventricular filling and increasing cardiac output. Digitalis has also been used in the control of paroxysmal atrial and atrioventricular nodal tachycardia. Oral or, if necessary, cautious intravenous administration of digoxin may abruptly terminate such attacks, probably as the result of its vagomimetic action. The availability of calcium channel blockers and adenosine has reduced the popularity of digoxin in this application.

Although it has been recommended in the past, digitalis is not the drug of choice in the therapy of arrhythmias associated with Wolff-Parkinson-White syndrome, because it increases the probability of conduction of arrhythmic atrial impulses through the alternative rapidly conducting atrioventricular pathway. It is explicitly contraindicated in patients with Wolff-Parkinson-White syndrome and atrial fibrillation (see Chapter 14).

Toxicity

In spite of its recognized hazards, digitalis is still a widely overused drug. In a large multicenter study, 17–27% of patients admitted for all medical conditions were taking digitalis on admission, and 5–25% of the identified group showed evidence of toxicity requiring at least temporary cessation of digitalis therapy.

Therapy of digitalis toxicity manifested as visual changes or gastrointestinal disturbances generally requires no more than reducing the dose of the drug. If cardiac arrhythmia is present and can definitely be ascribed to digitalis, more vigorous therapy may be nec-

Table 13–3. Clinical use of cardiac glycosides. (These values are appropriate for adults with normal renal and hepatic function.)

	Digoxin	Digitoxin
Half-life	40 hours	168 hours
Therapeutic plasma concentration	0.5–2 ng/mL	10–25 ng/mL
Toxic plasma concentration	>2 ng/mL	>35 ng/mL
Daily dose (slow loading or maintenance)	0.125–0.5 mg	0.05–0.2 mg
Rapid digitalizing dose	0.5–0.75 mg every 8 hours for 3 doses	0.2–0.4 mg every 12 hours for 3 doses

essary. Serum digitalis and potassium levels and the ECG should always be monitored during therapy of significant digitalis toxicity. Electrolyte status should be corrected if abnormal (see above). For patients who do not respond promptly (within one to two half-lives), calcium and magnesium as well as potassium levels should be checked. For occasional premature ventricular depolarizations or brief runs of bigeminy, oral potassium supplementation and withdrawal of the glycoside may be sufficient. If the arrhythmia is more serious, parenteral potassium and antiarrhythmic drugs may be required. Of the available antiarrhythmic agents, lidocaine, phenytoin, and propranolol are favored.

In very severe digitalis intoxication (which usually involves suicidal overdose), serum potassium will already be elevated at the time of diagnosis (because of potassium loss from the intracellular compartment). Furthermore, antiarrhythmic agents administered in this setting may lead to cardiac arrest. Such patients are best treated with "Fab fragments" of digitalis antibodies. These antibodies are produced in sheep, and although they are raised to digoxin they also recognize digitoxin. They are extremely useful in reversing severe intoxication with either of these digitalis glycosides.

Digitalis-induced arrhythmias are frequently made worse by cardioversion; this therapy should be reserved for ventricular fibrillation if the arrhythmia is glycoside-induced.

MANAGEMENT OF CHRONIC HEART FAILURE

The major steps in the management of patients with chronic heart failure are outlined in Table 13–4. Reduction of cardiac work is a traditional form of therapy that is extremely helpful in most cases. It can be accomplished by reducing activity levels, weight reduction, and—especially important—control of hypertension. Sodium restriction is the next important step. Despite the availability of efficacious diuretics, one should advise patients about the necessity for salt restriction and encourage them to avoid excess salt through dietary restraint.

If edema is present, a diuretic is usually required. It is reasonable to start with a thiazide diuretic, switching to more powerful agents as required. Furosemide, bumetanide, ethacrynic acid, and metolazone are very efficacious diuretics that should be reserved for patients with resistant edema. Sodium loss causes secondary loss of potassium, which is particularly hazardous if the patient is to be given digitalis. Therefore, serum electrolytes should be checked periodically in patients so treated. Hypokalemia can be treated with potassium supplementation or through the addition of a potassium-sparing diuretic (see Chapter 15).

When a positive inotropic drug is to be used in chronic heart failure, a cardiac glycoside is the usual choice. It should be emphasized again that digitalis is a potentially toxic agent, and only about 50% of patients with normal sinus rhythm (usually those with documented *systolic* dysfunction) will have documentable relief of congestive failure. Better results are obtained in patients with atrial fibrillation. If the decision is made to use a cardiac glycoside, digoxin is the one chosen in the great majority of cases. When symptoms are mild, slow digitalization (Table 13–3) is safest and just as effective as the rapid method. If symptoms are moderately severe, the rapid oral method may be used, but the patient should be examined before each dose with particular attention to the cardiac rhythm. An ECG should be recorded if there is any doubt about the nature of the pretherapy rhythm or changes during digitalization. Intravenous digitalization is rarely required in chronic heart failure; it should be used only in hospitalized patients with careful monitoring.

Determining the optimal level of digitalis effect may be difficult. In patients with atrial fibrillation, reduction of ventricular rate is the best measure of glycoside effect. In patients in normal sinus rhythm, symptomatic improvement and reductions in heart size, heart rate during exercise, venous pressure, or edema may signify optimum drug levels in the myocardium. Unfortunately, toxic effects may occur before the therapeutic end point is detected. If slow digitalization is being employed, simple omission of one dose and halving the maintenance dose will often bring the patient to the narrow range between suboptimal and toxic concentrations. Measurement of plasma digitalis levels is useful in patients who appear unusually resistant or sensitive; these assays are widely available for digoxin.

Vasodilator drugs are very useful agents in chronic congestive heart failure. A useful classification divides the drugs into selective arteriolar dilators, venous dilators, and drugs with nonselective vasodilatory effects (Table 13–5). The choice of agent should be based on the patient's signs and symptoms and hemodynamic measurements. Thus, in patients with

---

Table 13–4. Steps in the treatment of chronic heart failure.

1. Reduce workload of the heart.
    a. Limit activity level.
    b. Reduce weight.
    c. Control hypertension.
2. Restrict sodium.
3. Restrict water (rarely required).
4. Give diuretics.
5. Give digitalis.[1]
6. Give vasodilators.
7. Give newer inotropic drugs.

[1]Some clinicians use angiotensin-converting enzyme inhibitors before digitalis.

Table 13–5. Vasodilators for use in congestive heart failure.

Arteriolar Dilators	Combined Arteriolar and Venous Dilators	Venous Dilators
Hydralazine Minoxidil	Captopril Enalapril Lisinopril	Nitrates

high filling pressures in whom the principal symptom is dyspnea, the venous dilators will be most helpful in reducing filling pressures and the symptoms of pulmonary congestion. In patients in whom fatigue due to low left ventricular output is a primary symptom, an arteriolar dilator may be helpful in increasing forward cardiac output. In most patients with severe chronic failure that responds poorly to other therapy, the problem usually involves both elevated filling pressures and reduced cardiac output. In these circumstances, dilation of both arterioles and veins is required. In the V-HEFT trial, combined therapy with hydralazine (arteriolar dilation) and isosorbide dinitrate (venous dilation) prolonged life more than placebo in patients already receiving digitalis and diuretics (Cohn et al, 1986).

In a study comparing digoxin and captopril as first-line therapy for chronic heart failure, both agents produced similar effects (Captopril-Digoxin Multicenter Research Group, 1988). Several large studies have compared enalapril with placebo or with other vasodilators (CONSENSUS, 1987; SOLVD Investigators, 1991; Cohn et al, 1991). These studies suggest that angiotensin-converting enzyme inhibitors are superior to both placebo and other vasodilators and must be considered as first-line agents, together with diuretics and digitalis, for the treatment of chronic congestive heart failure. However, patients who are stable while receiving diuretics, digoxin, and angiotensin-converting enzyme inhibitors may deteriorate if digoxin is withdrawn, suggesting that the angiotensin-converting enzyme inhibitors cannot completely replace digitalis in these individuals (Packer et al, 1993).

Two recent studies suggest that angiotensin-converting enzyme inhibitors are also valuable in asymptomatic patients with ventricular dysfunction (Pfeffer et al, 1992; SOLVD Investigators, 1992). By reducing preload and afterload, these drugs appear to slow the rate of ventricular dilation and thus delay the onset of clinical congestive heart failure. Angiotensin-converting enzyme inhibitors thus are beneficial in all subsets of patients, from those who are asymptomatic to those in severe chronic failure.

MANAGEMENT OF ACUTE HEART FAILURE

Acute heart failure occurs frequently in patients with chronic failure. Such episodes are usually associated with increased exertion, emotion, salt in the diet, noncompliance with medical therapy, or increased metabolic demand occasioned by fever, anemia, etc. A particularly common and important cause of acute failure—with or without chronic failure—is acute myocardial infarction. Many of the signs and symptoms of acute and chronic failure are identical, but their therapies diverge because of the need for more rapid response and the relatively greater frequency and severity of pulmonary vascular congestion in the acute form.

Because of the need for rapid recognition and evaluation of changing hemodynamic status, it is much more important to obtain quantitative measurements in acute failure than in chronic failure. These measurements should include left ventricular filling pressure (pulmonary wedge pressure) and cardiac output in addition to heart rate and blood pressure. The stroke work index (approximately stroke volume index times arterial pressure) is a useful derived variable that estimates the external work performed by the left ventricle.

Measurements of stroke work index and pulmonary capillary wedge pressure from a large group of patients with acute myocardial infarction are illustrated in Figure 13–2. When filling pressure is greater than 15 mm Hg and stroke work index is less than 20 g-m/m^2, the mortality rate is high. Intermediate levels of these two variables imply a much better prognosis. It is apparent, therefore, that the effects of myocardial infarction on ventricular function are not uniform and that there can be no single standard therapy for the management of congestive failure in this condition.

Subsets of Patients Following Myocardial Infarction

Patients with acute congestive failure following myocardial infarction can be usefully characterized on the basis of three hemodynamic measurements: arterial pressure, left ventricular filling pressure, and cardiac index. One such classification is illustrated in Table 13–6.

(1) Hypovolemia: Subset 1 includes patients who are relatively hypovolemic following myocardial infarction as a result of diuretics or inadequate fluid intake. The primary hemodynamic abnormality is a low left ventricular filling pressure, which can be corrected by giving fluids. With an increase of filling pressure up to the optimal range of 15 mm Hg (Figure 13–6), hypotension often disappears and cardiac output increases.

(2) Pulmonary congestion: The second subset—patients with severe pulmonary congestion and dyspnea—is a very large one and is also repre-

Table 13–6. Therapeutic classification of subsets in acute myocardial infarction.[1]

Subset	Systolic Arterial Pressure (mm Hg)	Left Ventricular Filling Pressure (mm Hg)	Cardiac Index (L/min/m²)	Therapy
1. Hypovolemia	<100	<10	<2.5	Volume replacement.
2. Pulmonary congestion	100–150	>20	>2.5	Diuretics.
3. Peripheral vasodilation	<100	10–20	>2.5	None, or vasoactive drugs.
4. Power failure	<100	>20	<2.5	Vasodilators, inotropic drugs.
5. Severe shock	< 90	>20	<2.0	Vasoactive drugs, inotropic drugs, vasodilators, circulatory assist.
6. Right ventricular infarct	<100	RVFP>10 LVFP<15	<2.5	Provide volume replacement for LVFP, inotropic drugs. Avoid diuretics.
7. Mitral regurgitation, ventricular septal defect	<100	>20	<2.5	Vasodilators, inotropic drugs, circulatory assist, surgery.

[1]The numerical values are intended to serve as general guidelines and not as absolute cutoff points. Arterial pressures apply to patients who were previously normotensive and should be adjusted upward for patients who were previously hypertensive. (RVFP and LVFP = right and left ventricular filling pressure.)

sentative of other causes of acute heart failure. Diuretics are helpful in such patients because they reduce intravascular volume. In addition, when given intravenously, powerful diuretics such as furosemide produce an immediate increase in compliance of systemic veins. This leads to peripheral pooling of blood, which reduces central blood volume and de-

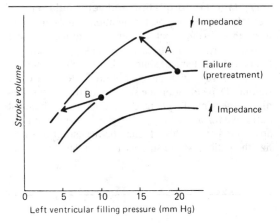

Figure 13–6. Effects of vasodilator therapy on left ventricular function. The dose is chosen to reduce filling pressure by 5 mm Hg. With the administration of a combined arteriolar dilator and venous dilator such as nitroprusside, function is shifted to a higher curve, reflecting the decreased impedance to ventricular ejection. However, the effect on stroke volume will depend on the initial filling pressure. A patient in heart failure with an initial filling pressure of 20 mm Hg will experience an increase in stroke volume along line A, up and to the left. If the patient was initially at a filling pressure of 10 mm Hg, nitroprusside would still shift performance to the upper curve, but this would result in a decrease of performance, along line B. (Reproduced, with permission, from Chatterjee K, Parmley WW: The role of vasodilator therapy in heart failure. Prog Cardiovasc Dis 1977;19:305.)

creases right and left ventricular filling pressures. Morphine sulfate also is clinically effective in the management of acute pulmonary edema. Apart from its ability to relieve the pain of infarction, the mechanisms by which it reduces pulmonary congestion are uncertain. If bronchospasm is a prominent component of the pulmonary signs, aminophylline may also be helpful, since it combines bronchodilator, vasodilator, and positive inotropic actions (see Chapter 19).

(3) Peripheral vasodilation: The third subset of patients are hypotensive and yet have warm extremities because of peripheral vasodilation. These patients may not need any therapy, since pulmonary wedge pressure is usually normal and cardiac output satisfactory. If blood pressure is extremely low, however, a vasoactive drug such as dopamine should be considered to maintain arterial perfusion pressure at the desired level.

(4) "Power failure": The fourth subset represents those patients who have a reduction in arterial pressure, though not to shock levels, together with an elevation of left ventricular filling pressure and a reduction of cardiac index. The goal of therapy in these patients is to increase cardiac output and reduce ventricular filling pressure without a further decrease in arterial pressure. Diuretics or nitrates are helpful in lowering filling pressures but will not increase cardiac output. A combined venous and arteriolar dilator such as nitroprusside is extremely beneficial in such patients. Its venodilating effects reduce right and left atrial pressures by redistributing more blood into the periphery. Its arteriolar dilating properties increase forward cardiac output by reducing systemic vascular resistance. The main limiting factor in the use of nitroprusside is the reduction in arterial pressure. If the dose is titrated carefully, however, this reduction in blood pressure may be minimized. A good rule of thumb is to consider giving nitroprusside if the systolic pressure is 90 mm Hg or higher. The effects of nitroprusside depend on the level of left ventricular filling pressure. This is illustrated diagrammatically in Figure 13–6. The middle curve in the figure represents a patient with moderately severe heart failure. If the patient has a high left ventricular filling pressure (20 mm Hg), the administration of sodium nitroprusside will shift ventricular function up and to the left, as illustrated by line *A*. If, however, the patient has been given large doses of diuretics and filling pressure has thereby been reduced to 10 mm Hg, nitroprusside will produce a different result. Although the patient moves to the upper curve with nitroprusside (line *B*), there is a reduction of stroke volume because the heart is on the steep ascending limb of the curve. This will worsen hypotension and tachycardia. If the patient is now volume-loaded to the optimal filling pressure of 15 mm Hg, the beneficial effect of nitroprusside will become evident. This example illustrates the importance of filling pressure: pulmonary wedge pressure should be maintained at about 15 mm Hg by either diuresis or volume administration, as required.

(5) Severe shock: Subset 5 represents a group of patients with cardiogenic shock following myocardial infarction. These patients have very low arterial pressures, very high filling pressures, and low cardiac indices. Although diuretics may be helpful in lowering the elevated filling pressures, they will not increase cardiac output. Furthermore, the use of vasodilators in these patients is difficult, since the accompanying hypotension may be severe and may impair perfusion of vital organs. Since the mortality rate under these circumstances is high, it is often difficult to know whether any therapy is beneficial. Nevertheless, certain approaches may be helpful. If the arterial pressure is extremely low, it is useful to consider use of a catecholamine such as dopamine. By titrating the dose of this drug, one can produce an increase in arterial pressure that is adequate for peripheral tissue perfusion. At this point, one can cautiously add nitroprusside to lower pulmonary wedge pressure. The combined effects of these two agents on the heart tend to be additive, since they work through different mechanisms. Dopamine directly increases cardiac contractility, while nitroprusside produces venous and arteriolar dilation. The addition of inotropic agents such as amrinone or dobutamine may also be useful. This therapy should be combined with an attempt to optimize left ventricular filling pressure. These patients are also candidates for circulatory assist measures (intra-aortic balloon) and consideration of cardiac catheterization and possible revascularization.

(6) Right ventricular infarction: Group 6 comprises a subset of patients who have an inferior myocardial infarction that predominantly involves the right ventricle. Their hypotension is due to the fact that the right ventricle is unable to deliver sufficient blood to the left side of the heart to optimize left ventricular filling pressure and cardiac output. Therefore, the primary therapeutic goal is to optimize left ventricular filling pressure. This may require volume infusion despite elevated central venous pressure. One should avoid using diuretics, since reduction of volume may lead to further reduction of filling pressure with associated hypotension and tachycardia. Inotropic agents may be useful.

(7) Mitral regurgitation and ventricular septal defect: A seventh subset is mentioned for completeness, though these patients are also found in other subsets, particularly those with shock. These are patients with mechanical abnormalities such as acute severe mitral regurgitation or a ruptured interventricular septum. Depending on the severity of the defect, cardiac surgery must be considered urgently as the most definitive form of therapy. However, vasodilator therapy such as nitroprusside may be necessary to stabilize the patient before surgery is possible.

PREPARATIONS AVAILABLE
(Diuretics: See Chapter 15.)

Digitalis
  Deslanoside (Cedilanid-D)
    Parenteral: 0.2 mg/mL for injection
  Digitoxin (generic, Crystodigin)
    Oral: 0.05, 0.1, 0.15, 0.2 mg tablets
  Digoxin (generic, Lanoxicaps, Lanoxin)
    Oral: 0.125, 0.25, 0.5 mg tablets; 0.05, 0.1, 0.2 mg capsules; 0.05 mg/mL elixir
    Parenteral: 0.1, 0.25 mg/mL for injection

Digitalis Antibody
  Digoxin immune fab (ovine) (Digibind)
    Parenteral: 40 mg per vial with 75 mg sorbitol lyophilized powder to reconstitute for IV injection. Each vial will bind approximately 0.6 mg digoxin or digitoxin.

Sympathomimetics Most Commonly Used in Congestive Heart Failure
  Dobutamine (Dobutrex)
    Parenteral: 250 mg/20 mL for IV infusion
  Dopamine (generic, Intropin, Dopastat)
    Parenteral: 40, 80, 160, mg/mL for IV injection; 80, 160, 320 mg/dL for IV infusion

Angiotensin-Converting Enzyme Inhibitors Labeled for Use in Congestive Heart Failure

Captopril (Capoten)
Oral: 12.5, 25, 50, 100 mg tablets
Enalapril (Vasotec)
Oral: 2.5, 5, 10, 20 mg tablets
Lisinopril (Prinivil, Zestril)
Oral: 5, 10, 20, 40 mg tablets

Other Drugs Labeled Only For Use in Congestive Heart Failure

Amrinone (Inocor)
Parenteral: 5 mg/mL for IV infusion
Milrinone
Parenteral: 5 mg/mL for IV infusion

REFERENCES

Basic Pharmacology

Blaustein MP: Physiological effects of endogenous ouabain: Control of intracellular Ca^{2+} stores and cell responsiveness. Am J Physiol 1993;264:C1367.

Doherty JE: Clinical use of digitalis glycosides. Cardiology 1985;72:225.

Hickey AR et al: Digoxin immune Fab therapy in the management of digitalis intoxication: Safety and efficacy results of an observational surveillance study. J Am Coll Cardiol 1991;17:590.

Hoey A et al: Inotropic actions of BDF 9148 and DPI 201-106 and their enantiomers in guinea-pig, rat and human atria. Eur J Pharmacol 1993;231:477.

Katz AM: Effects of digitalis on cell biochemistry: Sodium pump inhibition. J Am Coll Cardiol 1985;5(Suppl A):16A.

Kelly RA, Smith TW: Is ouabain the endogenous digitalis? (Editorial comment.) Circulation 1992;86:694.

Kelly RA, Smith TW: Recognition and management of digitalis toxicity. Am J Cardiol 1992;69:108G.

Lee JA, Allen DG: EMD 53998 sensitizes the contractile proteins to calcium in intact ferret ventricular muscle. Circ Res 1991;69:927.

LeGrand B, et al: Stimulatory effect of ouabain on T- and L-type calcium currents in guinea pig cardiac myocytes. Am J Physiol 1990;258:H1620.

Lindenbaum J et al: Inactivation of digoxin by the gut flora: Reversal by antibiotic therapy. N Engl J Med 1981;305:789.

Perrault CL et al: Differential inotropic effects of flosequinan in ventricular muscle from normal ferrets versus patients with end-stage heart failure. Br J Pharmacol 1992;106:511.

Rodin SM, Johnson BF: Pharmacokinetic interactions with digoxin. Clin Pharmacokinet 1988;15:227.

Smith TW: Digitalis: Mechanisms of action and clinical use. N Engl J Med 1988;318:358.

Solaro RJ et al: Stereoselective actions of thiadiazinones on canine cardiac myocytes and myofilaments. Circ Res 1993;73:481.

Sonnenblick EH (editor): A symposium: The role of phosphodiesterase III inhibitors in contemporary cardiovascular medicine. Am J Cardiol 1989;63(2). (Entire issue).

Sweadner KJ: Multiple digitalis receptors. A molecular perspective. Trends Cardiovasc Med 1993;3:2.

Vemuri R, Longoni S, Philipson KD: Ouabain treatment of cardiac cells induces enhanced Na^+-Ca^{2+} exchange activity. Am J Physiol 1989;256:C1273.

Wenger TL et al: Treatment of 63 severely digitalis-toxic

patients with digoxin-specific antibody fragments. J Am Coll Cardiol 1985;5(Suppl A):118A.

Pathophysiology of Heart Failure

Braunwald E: Pathophysiology of heart failure. In: *Heart Disease,* 3rd ed. Braunwald E (editor). Saunders, 1987.

Ferguson DW: Digitalis and neurohormonal abnormalities in heart failure and implications for therapy. Am J Cardiol 1992;69:24G.

Francis GS, Cohn JN: Heart failure: Mechanisms of cardiac and vascular dysfunction and the rationale for pharmacologic intervention. FASEB J 1990;4:3068.

Goto A, Yamada K, Sugimoto T: Endogenous digitalis: Reality or myth? Life Sci 1991;48:2109.

Grossmann W: Diastolic dysfunction and congestive heart failure. Circulation 1990;81(Suppl III):III-1.

Parmley WW: Pathophysiology and therapy of congestive heart failure. J Am Coll Cardiol 1989;13:771.

Rahimtoola SH: The pharmacologic treatment of chronic congestive heart failure. Circulation 1989;80:693.

Swan HJ, Parmley WW: Congestive heart failure. In: *Pathologic Physiology,* 7th ed. Sodeman WA Jr, Sodeman TM (editors). Saunders, 1985.

van Zwieten PA: Compensatory mechanisms associated with congestive heart failure as targets for drug treatment. Prog Pharmacol Clinical Pharmacol 1990;7:49.

Acute Myocardial Infarction

Califf RM, Bengtson JR: Cardiogenic shock. N Engl J Med 1994;330:1724.

Parmley W, Chatterjee K: Evaluation of cardiac function in the coronary care unit. In: *Acute Myocardial Infarction.* Donoso E, Lipski J (editors). Stratton Intercontinental, 1978.

Pasternak RC, Braunwald E, Sobel BE: Acute myocardial infarction. In: *Heart Disease,* 3rd ed. Braunwald E (editor). Saunders, 1987.

Shah PK, Swan HJC: Complications of acute myocardial infarction. In: *Cardiology.* Parmley WW, Chatterjee K (editors). Lippincott, 1988.

Verma SP et al: Modulation of inotropic therapy by venodilation in acute heart failure: A randomised comparison of four inotropic agents, alone and combined with isosorbide dinitrate. J Cardiovasc Pharmacol 1992;19:24.

Chronic Heart Failure

Brodde O-E: β_1- and β_2-adrenoceptors in the human heart: Properties, function, and alterations in chronic heart failure. Pharmacol Rev 1991;43:203.

Captopril-Digoxin Multicenter Research Group: Comparative effects of therapy with captopril and digoxin of patients with mild to moderate heart failure. JAMA 1988;259:539.

Cavero PG et al: Flosequinan, a new vasodilator: Systemic and coronary hemodynamics and neuroendocrine effects in congestive heart failure. J Am Coll Cardiol 1992;20:1542.

Chatterjee K: Digitalis, catecholamines, and other positive inotropic agents. In: *Cardiology*. Parmley WW, Chatterjee K (editors). Lippincott, 1988.

Cheitlin MD: Digitalis: Is it useful in congestive heart failure in patients in normal sinus rhythm? Cardiology 1987;74:376.

Cohn JN et al: A comparison of enalapril with hydralazine-isosorbide dinitrate in the treatment of chronic congestive heart failure. N Engl J Med 1991;325:303.

Cohn JN et al: Effect of vasodilator therapy on mortality in chronic congestive heart failure. N Engl J Med 1986; 314:1547.

CONSENSUS Trial Study Group: Effects of enalapril on mortality in severe congestive heart failure. N Engl J Med 1987;316:1429.

DiBianco R et al: A comparison of oral milrinone, digoxin, and their combination in the treatment of patients with chronic heart failure. N Engl J Med 1989;320:677.

Fonarow GC et al: Effect of direct vasodilation with hydralazine versus angiotensin-converting enzyme inhibition with captopril on mortality in advanced heart failure: The Hy-C Trial. J Am Coll Cardiol 1992;19:842.

Francis GS, McDonald KM, Cohn JN: Neurohumoral activation in preclinical heart failure: Remodeling and the potential for intervention. Circulation 1993;87(Suppl IV):IV–90.

Hall D, Zeitler H, Rudolph W: Counteraction of the vasodilator effects of enalapril by aspirin in severe heart failure. J Am Coll Cardiol 1992;20:1549.

Hood WB Jr: Controlled and uncontrolled studies of phosphodiesterase inhibitors in contemporary cardiovascular medicine. Am J Cardiol 1989;63:46A.

Horn PT, Murphy MB: New dopamine receptor agonists in heart failure and hypertension: Implications for therapy. Drugs 1990;40:487.

Konstam MA et al: Effects of the angiotensin converting enzyme inhibitor enalapril on the long-term progression of left ventricular dysfunction in patients with heart failure. Circulation 1992;86:431.

Packer M et al, for the PROMISE Study Research Group: Effect of milrinone on mortality in severe chronic heart failure. N Engl J Med 1991;325:1468.

Packer M et al: Withdrawal of digoxin from patients with chronic heart failure treated with angiotensin-converting-enzyme inhibitors. N Engl J Med 1993;329:1.

Papadakis MA, Massie BM: Appropriateness of digoxin use in medical outpatients. Am J Med 1988;85:365.

Parmley WW: Principles in the management of congestive heart failure. In: *Cardiology*. Parmley WW, Chatterjee K (editors). Lippincott, 1988.

Pfeffer MA et al, on behalf of the SAVE investigators: Effect of captopril on mortality and morbidity in patients with left ventricular dysfunction after myocardial infarction. N Engl J Med 1992;327:669.

Smith TW, Braunwald E: The management of heart failure. In: *Heart Disease,* 3rd ed. Braunwald E (editor). Saunders, 1987.

The SOLVD Investigators: Effect of enalapril on survival in patients with reduced left ventricular ejection fractions and congestive heart failure. N Engl J Med 1991;325: 293.

The SOLVD Investigators: Effect of enalapril on mortality and the development of heart failure in asymptomatic patients with reduced left ventricular ejection fractions. N Engl J Med 1992;327:685.

Agents Used in Cardiac Arrhythmias

14

Luc M. Hondeghem, MD, PhD, & Dan M. Roden, MD

Cardiac arrhythmias are a frequent problem in clinical practice, occurring in up to 25% of patients treated with digitalis, 50% of anesthetized patients, and over 80% of patients with acute myocardial infarction. Arrhythmias may require treatment because too rapid, too slow, or asynchronous contractions reduce cardiac output. Some arrhythmias can precipitate more serious or even lethal rhythm disturbances—eg, early premature ventricular depolarizations can precipitate ventricular fibrillation. In such patients, antiarrhythmic drugs may be lifesaving. On the other hand, the hazards of antiarrhythmic therapy—and in particular the fact that they can (paradoxically) *precipitate* lethal arrhythmias in some patients–has led to a reevaluation of their relative risks and benefits. In general, treatment of asymptomatic or minimally symptomatic arrhythmias should be avoided for this reason.

Arrhythmias can be treated with the drugs discussed in this chapter and with nonpharmacologic therapies such as pacemakers, cardioversion, catheter ablation, and surgery. This chapter describes the pharmacology of agents that suppress arrhythmias by a direct action on the cardiac cell membrane. Other modes of therapy are discussed briefly.

ELECTROPHYSIOLOGY OF NORMAL CARDIAC RHYTHM

The electrical impulse that triggers a normal cardiac contraction originates at regular intervals in the sinoatrial node (Figure 14–1), usually at a frequency of 60–100 beats per minute. This impulse spreads rapidly through the atria and enters the atrioventricular node, which is normally the only conduction pathway between the atria and ventricles. Conduction through the atrioventricular node is slow, requiring about 0.15 s. (This delay provides time for atrial contraction to propel blood into the ventricles.) The impulse then propagates over the His-Purkinje system and invades all parts of the ventricles. Ventricular activation is complete in less than 0.1 s; therefore, contraction of all of the ventricular muscle is synchronous and hemodynamically effective.

Arrhythmias consist of cardiac depolarizations that deviate from the above description in one or more aspects—ie, there is an abnormality in the site of origin of the impulse, its rate or regularity, or its conduction.

Ionic Basis of Membrane Electrical Activity

The transmembrane potential of cardiac cells is determined by the concentrations of several ions—chiefly sodium (Na^+), potassium (K^+), and calcium (Ca^{2+})—on either side of the membrane and the permeability of the membrane to each ion. Ion channels are the major routes by which ions diffuse through the membrane. These channels are relatively ion-specific, and the flux of ions through them is thought to be controlled by "gates" (probably flexible peptide chains or energy barriers). Each type of channel has its own type of gate (sodium, calcium, and some potassium channels are each thought to have two kinds of gates), and each kind of gate is opened and closed by specific transmembrane conditions (voltage, ionic, or metabolic).

For example, evidence suggests that sodium channels have four activation gates and one inactivation gate located between activation gates three and four. These gates open and close in response to voltage changes (see below). In most cells, resting transmembrane potential is negative. Therefore, Na^+, which is more abundant outside cells (140 mmol/L) than inside (10 mmol/L), will rapidly enter cells because of its electrical and concentration gradient if the membrane is Na^+-permeable. At rest, most cells are not significantly permeable to sodium, but at the start of each action potential, they become quite permeable (see below). Similarly, calcium enters and potassium leaves the cell with each action potential. Therefore, the cell must have a mechanism to maintain stable transmembrane ionic conditions by establishing and maintaining ion gradients. The most important of these active mechanisms is the sodium pump, Na^+/K^+ ATPase, described in Chapter 13. This pump and other active ion carriers contribute indirectly to the transmembrane potential by maintaining the gradients necessary for diffusion through channels. In ad-

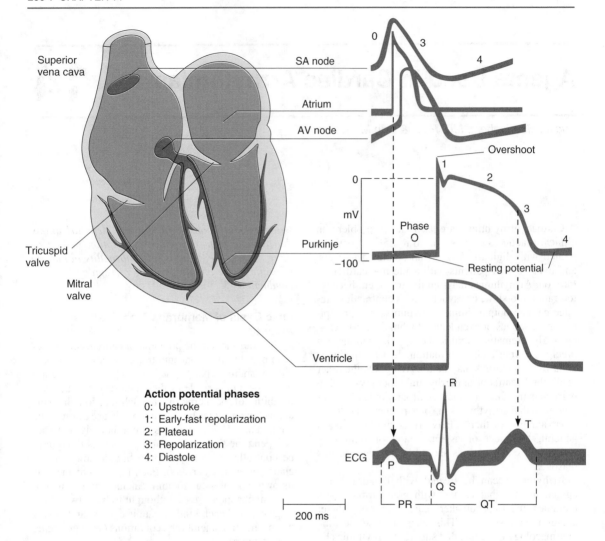

Figure 14–1. Schematic representation of the heart and normal cardiac electrical activity (intracellular recordings from areas indicated and ECG). SA node, AV node, and Purkinje cells display pacemaker activity (phase 4 depolarization). The ECG is the body surface manifestation of the depolarization and repolarization waves of the heart. The P wave is generated by atrial depolarization, the QRS by ventricular muscle depolarization, and the T wave by ventricular repolarization. Thus the PR interval is a measure of conduction time from atrium to ventricle, and the QRS duration indicates the time required for all of the ventricular cells to be activated (ie, the intraventricular conduction time). The QT interval reflects the duration of the ventricular action potential.

dition, some pumps and exchangers produce net current flow (eg, by exchanging three Na^+ for two K^+ ions) and hence are termed "electrogenic."

At any given time, the electrical potential across the cell membrane is a reflection of all the processes just described. However, under certain conditions, a useful simplification can be applied to predict the transmembrane potential. These conditions require that the cell membrane be highly permeable to one ion (eg, potassium in most cells at rest) and relatively impermeable to all others. When this is the case, the transmembrane potential, E_m, approaches the ionic equilibrium potential, E_{ion}. The equilibrium potential

is given by the **Nernst equation,** which for sodium and potassium is (at body temperature):

$$E_{ion} = 61 \times \log\left(\frac{C_e}{C_i}\right)$$

where C_e and C_i are the extracellular and intracellular concentrations, respectively, multiplied by their activity coefficients. The conditions required for application of the Nernst equation are approximated at the peak of the overshoot and during rest in most nonpacemaker cardiac cells. If the permeability is significant for both potassium and sodium, the Nernst equation is not a good predictor of membrane potential, but the **Goldman-Hodgkin-Katz (GHK) equation** may be used.

$$E_{mem} = 61 \times \log \left(\frac{P_K \times K_e + P_{Na} \times Na_e}{P_K \times K_i + P_{Na} \times Na_i} \right)$$

The Cell Membrane During Diastole

During diastole, the membrane of nonpacemaker cells is much more permeable to potassium than to other ions, so the membrane potential approaches the potassium equilibrium (Nernst) potential. For typical values of K_e (4 mmol/L) and K_i (150 mmol/L), the potassium equilibrium potential, E_K, is –96 mV. (See box: Effects of Potassium.)

In pacemaker cells (whether normal or ectopic), spontaneous depolarization (the pacemaker potential) occurs during diastole (phase 4, Figure 14–1). This depolarization results from a gradual increase of de-

polarizing current, caused by increasing permeability to sodium or calcium, and a decrease in repolarizing potassium current, caused by a decrease in potassium permeability. The effect of changing extracellular potassium is more complex in a pacemaker cell than it is in a nonpacemaker cell because the effect on permeability to potassium is much more important in a pacemaker, see box. In a pacemaker—especially an ectopic one—the end result of an increase in extracellular potassium will usually be to slow or stop the pacemaker. Conversely, hypokalemia will often facilitate ectopic pacemakers.

The Active Cell Membrane

In normal atrial, Purkinje, and ventricular cells, the action potential upstroke (phase 0) is dependent on sodium current. Depolarization to the threshold voltage results in opening of the activation (m) gates of sodium channels (Figure 14–2, middle panel). If the inactivation (h) gates of these channels have not al-

---

EFFECTS OF POTASSIUM

Just as drugs may act on two or more receptors, potassium affects two different membrane properties. As suggested in the text, the potassium concentration gradient (outside versus inside concentrations) determines the *potassium equilibrium potential* (E_K) as given by the Nernst equation. This is true of all cells and of artificial systems containing semipermeable membranes as well. Therefore, an increase in extracellular potassium concentration will reduce (make less negative) the potassium equilibrium potential, E_K. A second important effect of potassium is the ability of the extracellular potassium concentration to alter the membrane permeability to potassium. The consequences of the resulting changes in P_K are best appreciated by examining the resting potential (E_{mem}) predicted by the Goldman-Hodgkin-Katz equation. As the equation indicates, it is the *ratio of potassium permeability to sodium permeability* that determines how the concentration gradients for these two ions will influence the membrane potential. Anything that increases the potassium permeability will increase the influence of the potassium gradient and force the membrane potential closer to E_K. Since experimental evidence shows that an increase in extracellular potassium concentration increases P_K, it is not surprising that hyperkalemia will shift the membrane potential closer to E_K.

If we combine these two effects of potassium, we find that hyperkalemia will depolarize E_K and simultaneously shift E_{mem} closer to E_K. In a nonpacemaker cell, P_K is very high (during diastole) even at low and normal extracellular potassium

concentrations and E_{mem} lies relatively close to E_K at all times. On the other hand, in pacemaker cells, P_K is relatively low at normal potassium concentrations, and an increase in P_K, caused by hyperkalemia, can shift E_{mem} significantly closer to E_K. The following table shows some hypothetical examples of these effects, with Na_e, Na_i, and P_{Na} taken as 140, 10, and 1, respectively, in each condition.

Extracellular K (K_e)	K_i	P_K	E_K	E_{mem}
Nonpacemaker cell				
Low: 2.5	150	75	–108	–94
Normal: 4.0	150	100	–96	–88
High: 10.0	150	300	–72	–71
Pacemaker cell				
Low: 2.5	150	15	–108	–67
Normal: 4.0	150	20	–96	–69
High: 10.0	150	60	–72	–66

Note that in the nonpacemaker cell, both the potassium equilibrium potential (E_K) and the resting potential (E_{mem}) become significantly less negative as potassium increases. The pacemaker cell shows the same alterations in E_K, but E_{mem} is changed much less because the changes in potassium permeability are more important than changes in K_e in this cell type and have the opposite effect on resting potential. The result of increasing extracellular potassium will be to stabilize the membrane potential closer to the potassium equilibrium potential.

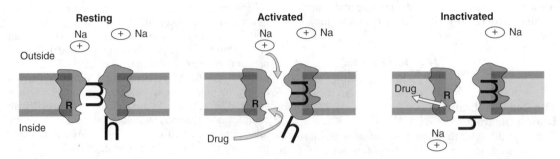

Figure 14–2. Schematic diagram of a cardiac sodium channel. The channel (color) is a protein that spans the lipid bilayer membrane. The shapes shown for the channel and its gates are purely symbolic. In the resting, fully polarized membrane *(left),* the *h* gate is open and the *m* gate is closed, preventing any movement of sodium through the channel. With an appropriate activating stimulus, the *m* gate opens, allowing a rapid influx of sodium ions *(middle).* About a millisecond later, the *h* gate closes, inactivating the channel and shutting off the sodium current *(right).* Additional stimuli applied to the inactivated channel cannot open it (the *h* gate is closed); therefore it is "unavailable." The area denoted *R* in the channel is a putative local anesthetic receptor. In the rested state, most antiarrhythmic agents have a low affinity for the receptor. When the channel is activated, drugs can access the receptor via the aqueous pathway from the inside of the cell *(arrow, middle panel).* When the channel is inactivated, the drug may be able to reach the receptor from the membrane phase *(arrow, right panel)* if it is sufficiently soluble in the membrane lipid. Most antiarrhythmic drugs are weak bases that exist partly in the neutral (lipid-soluble) and partly in the charged (water-soluble) forms, depending on the pH, and can therefore access the putative binding site via either route.

ready closed, the channels are now open or activated, and sodium permeability is markedly increased, greatly exceeding the permeability for any other ion. Extracellular sodium therefore diffuses down its electrochemical gradient into the cell, and the membrane potential very rapidly approaches the sodium equilibrium potential, E_{Na} (about +70 mV when Na_e = 140 mmol/L and Na_i = 10 mmol/L). This intense sodium current is very brief, because opening of the *m* gates upon depolarization is promptly followed by closure of the *h* gates or inactivation of the sodium channels (Figure 14–2, right panel).

Most calcium channels become activated and inactivated in what appears to be the same way as sodium channels, but in the case of the most common type of cardiac calcium channel (the "L" type), the transitions occur more slowly and at more positive potentials. The action potential plateau (phases 1 and 2) reflects the turning off of most of the sodium current, the waxing and waning of calcium current, and the slow development of a repolarizing potassium current.

Final repolarization (phase 3) of the action potential results from completion of sodium and calcium channel inactivation and the growth of potassium permeability, so that the membrane potential once again approaches the potassium equilibrium potential. These processes are diagrammed in Figure 14–3.

The Effect of Resting Potential on Action Potentials

A key factor in the pathophysiology of arrhythmias and the actions of antiarrhythmic drugs is the relationship between the resting potential of a cell and the action potentials that can be evoked in it (Figure 14–4, left panel). Because the inactivation gates of sodium channels in the resting membrane close over the potential range –75 to –55 mV, fewer sodium channels are "available" for diffusion of sodium ions when an action potential is evoked from a resting potential of –60 mV than when it is evoked from a resting potential of –80 mV. Important consequences of the reduction in peak sodium permeability include reduced upstroke velocity (called V_{max}, for maximum rate of change of membrane voltage), reduced action potential amplitude, reduced excitability, and reduced conduction velocity.

During the plateau of the action potential, most sodium channels are inactivated. Upon repolarization, recovery from inactivation takes place (in the terminology of Figure 14–2, the *h* gates reopen), making the channels again available for excitation. Another important effect of less negative resting potential is prolongation of this recovery time, as shown in Figure 14–4 (right panel). The prolongation of recovery time is reflected in an increase in the effective refractory period, ie, the time from the start of an action potential to the time when a second action potential can be evoked and propagated.

Reduction (depolarization) of the resting potential,[*] whether brought about by hyperkalemia, sodium

---

[*]The steady reduction in resting potential referred to in this section should not be confused with the abrupt depolarization involved in a normal stimulus. A brief depolarizing stimulus, whether caused by a propagating action potential or by an external electrode arrangement, causes the opening of large numbers of activation gates before a significant number of inactivation gates can close.

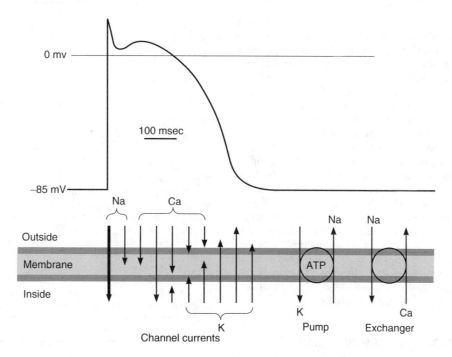

Figure 14–3. Schematic diagram of the ionic permeability changes and transport processes that occur during an action potential and the diastolic period following it. The size and weight of the arrows indicate approximate magnitudes of the ionic channel currents.

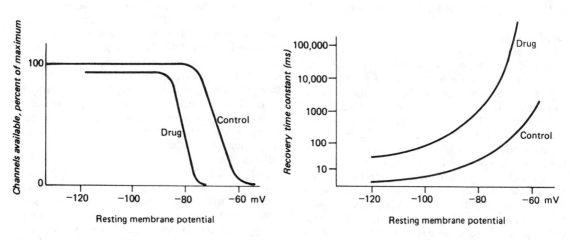

Figure 14–4. Dependence of sodium channel function on the membrane potential preceding the stimulus. As shown in the graph at **left,** the fraction of sodium channels available for opening in response to a stimulus is determined by the membrane potential immediately preceding the stimulus. The decrease in the fraction available when the resting potential is depolarized in the absence of a drug (control curve) results from the closure of h gates in the channels. The curve labeled **Drug** illustrates the effect of a typical "local anesthetic" antiarrhythmic drug. Most sodium channels are inactivated during the plateau of the action potential. The time constant for recovery from inactivation after repolarization also depends on the resting potential. The graph at **right** shows that in the absence of drug, recovery occurs in less than 10 ms at normal resting potentials (–85 to –95 mV). Depolarized cells recover more slowly (note logarithmic scale). In the presence of a sodium channel-blocking drug, the time constant of recovery is increased, but the increase is far greater at depolarized potentials than at more negative ones.

pump blockade, or ischemic cell damage, results in depressed sodium currents during the upstrokes of action potentials. Depolarization of the resting potential to levels positive to –55 mV abolishes sodium currents, since all sodium channels are inactivated. However, such severely depolarized cells have been found to support special action potentials under circumstances that increase calcium permeability or decrease potassium permeability. These "slow responses"—slow upstroke velocity and slow conduction—depend on a calcium inward current and constitute the normal electrical activity in the sinoatrial and atrioventricular nodes, since these tissues have a normal resting potential in the range of –50 to –70 mV. Slow responses may also be important for certain arrhythmias. Modern techniques of molecular biology and electrophysiology can identify multiple subtypes of calcium and potassium channels. One way in which such subtypes may differ is in sensitivity to drug therapy, so drugs targeting specific channel subtypes may be developed in the future.

MECHANISMS OF ARRHYTHMIAS

Many factors can precipitate or exacerbate arrhythmias: ischemia, hypoxia, acidosis or alkalosis, electrolyte abnormalities, excessive catecholamine exposure, autonomic influences, drug toxicity (eg, digitalis or antiarrhythmic drugs), overstretching of cardiac fibers, and the presence of scarred or otherwise diseased tissue. However, all arrhythmias result from (1) disturbances in impulse formation, (2) disturbances in impulse conduction, or (3) both.

Disturbances of Impulse Formation

The interval between depolarizations of a pacemaker cell is the sum of the duration of the action potential and the duration of the diastolic interval. Shortening of either duration results in an increase in pacemaker rate. The more important of the two, diastolic interval, is determined by three factors: maximum diastolic potential, slope of phase 4 depolarization, and threshold potential (Figure 14–5). Thus, vagal discharge slows normal pacemaker rate by making the maximum diastolic potential more negative and reducing the phase 4 slope; beta receptor-blocking drugs also reduce phase 4 slope. Acceleration of pacemaker discharge is often brought about by increased phase 4 depolarization slope, caused by hypokalemia, beta adrenoceptor stimulation, fiber stretch, acidosis, and partial depolarization by currents of injury.

Latent pacemakers (cells that show slow phase 4 depolarization even under normal conditions, eg, some Purkinje fibers) are particularly prone to acceleration by the above mechanisms. However, all cardiac cells, including normally quiescent atrial and

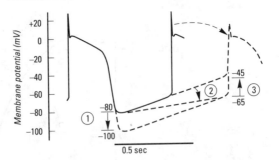

Figure 14–5. Determinants of pacemaker rate. Transmembrane potential in a Purkinje fiber pacemaker cell is shown. The rate of a pacemaker can be slowed by four mechanisms. *1,* more negative maximum diastolic potential, shown as a change from –80 to –100 mV; *2,* reduction of the slope of diastolic depolarization; *3,* more positive threshold potential, shown as a change from –65 to –45 mV; and *4* (not shown because not a common mechanism), prolongation of the action potential duration. Note that each of the changes shown results in a prolongation of the interval between the first action potential and the second from the short interval (solid line) to a longer one (dashed line).

ventricular cells, may show repetitive pacemaker activity when depolarized under appropriate conditions, especially if hypokalemia is also present.

Afterdepolarizations (Figure 14–6) are depolarizations that interrupt phase 3 (early afterdepolarizations, or EADs) or phase 4 (delayed afterdepolarizations, or DADs). Delayed afterdepolarizations, discussed in Chapter 13, often occur when intracellular calcium is increased. They are exacerbated by fast heart rates and are thought to be responsible for some arrhythmias related to digitalis excess, to catecholamines, and to myocardial ischemia. EADs, on the other hand, are exacerbated at slow heart rates and thought to be responsible for long QT-related arrhythmias. These can occur on the basis of poorly understood congenital factors and are also an increasingly recognized complication of treatment with some antiarrhythmic (and other) drugs that interfere with repolarization.

All pacemakers, normal and abnormal, are dependent upon phase 4 diastolic depolarization. Hyperkalemia, as described above, will *stabilize* the membrane potential and thus will reduce the rate of firing.[*] In hypokalemia, the membrane is less permeable to potassium and consequently more easily displaced from the potassium equilibrium potential (see box, page 207), ie, spontaneous firing is facilitated.

---

[*]Even though potassium depolarizes the membrane and depolarization can promote pacemaker activity, the effect of membrane *stabilization* is more important than that of the *depolarization,* so that increased potassium normally reduces pacemaker rate.

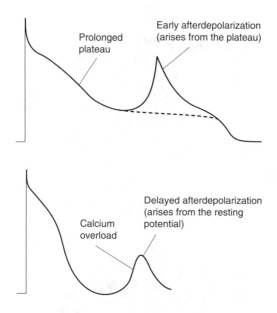

Figure 14–6. Two forms of abnormal activity, early (top) and delayed afterdepolarizations (bottom). In both cases abnormal depolarizations arise during or after a normally evoked action potential. They are therefore often referred to as "triggered" automaticity, ie, they require a normal action potential for their initiation.

Disturbances of Impulse Conduction

Severely depressed conduction may result in simple block, eg, atrioventricular nodal block or bundle branch block. Because parasympathetic control of atrioventricular conduction is significant, partial atrioventricular block is sometimes relieved by atropine. A more common but subtle abnormality of conduction is **reentry** (also known as "circus movement"), in which one impulse reenters and excites areas of the heart more than once (Figure 14–7). The path of the reentering impulse may be confined to very small areas, eg, within or near the atrioventricular node, or it may involve large portions of the atrial or ventricular walls. Furthermore, the circulating impulse often gives off "daughter impulses" that can spread to the rest of the heart. Depending on how many round trips of the pathway the impulse makes before dying out, the arrhythmia may be manifest as one or a few extra beats or as a sustained tachycardia.

In order for reentry to occur, three conditions must coexist, as indicated in Figure 14–7: (1) There must be an obstacle (anatomic or physiologic) to homogeneous conduction, thus establishing a circuit around which the reentrant wavefront can propagate; (2) there must be unidirectional block at some point in the circuit, ie, conduction must die out in one direction but continue in the opposite direction (as shown in Figure 14–7, the impulse can gradually decrease or

"decrement" as it invades progressively more depolarized tissue until it finally blocks); and (3) conduction time around the circuit must be long enough so that the impulse does not enter refractory tissue as it travels around the obstacle, ie, the conduction time must exceed the effective refractory period. Thus, reentry depends upon conduction that has been depressed by some critical amount, usually as a result of injury or ischemia. If conduction velocity is too *slow,* bidirectional block rather than unidirectional block occurs; if the reentering impulse is too weak, conduction may fail, or the impulse may arrive so late that it collides with the next regular impulse. On the other hand, if conduction is too *rapid,* bidirectional conduction rather than unidirectional block will occur. Even in the presence of unidirectional block, if the impulse travels around the obstacle too rapidly, it will reach tissue that is still refractory.

Slowing of conduction may be due to depression of sodium current, depression of calcium current (the latter especially in the atrioventricular node), or both. Drugs that abolish reentry work either by further slowing depressed conduction (by blocking the sodium or calcium current) or, less commonly, by accelerating it (by increasing the sodium or calcium current).

Lengthening (or shortening) of the refractory period may also make reentry less likely. The longer the refractory period in tissue near the site of block, the greater the chance that the tissue will still be refractory when reentry is attempted. (Alternatively, the shorter the refractory period in the depressed region, the less likely it is that unidirectional block will occur.)

I. BASIC PHARMACOLOGY OF THE ANTIARRHYTHMIC AGENTS

Mechanisms of Action

Arrhythmias are caused by abnormal pacemaker activity or abnormal impulse propagation. Thus, the aim of therapy of the arrhythmias is to reduce ectopic pacemaker activity and modify conduction or refractoriness in reentrant circuits to disable circus movement. The major mechanisms currently available for accomplishing these goals are (1) sodium channel blockade, (2) blockade of sympathetic autonomic effects in the heart, (3) prolongation of the effective refractory period, and (4) calcium channel blockade.

Antiarrhythmic drugs decrease the automaticity of ectopic pacemakers more than that of the sinoatrial node. They also reduce conduction and excitability and increase the refractory period to a greater extent in depolarized tissue than in normally polarized tis-

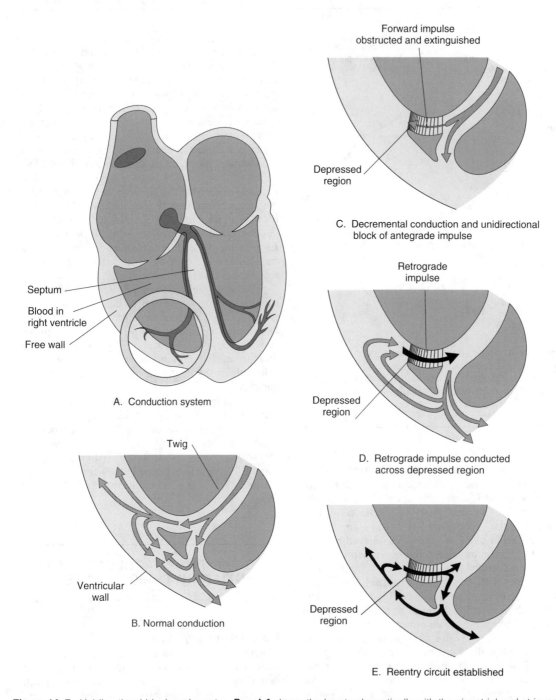

Septum

Blood in
right ventricle

Free wall

A. Conduction system

Twig

Ventricular
wall

B. Normal conduction

Forward impulse
obstructed and extinguished

Depressed
region

C. Decremental conduction and unidirectional
block of antegrade impulse

Retrograde
impulse

Depressed
region

D. Retrograde impulse conducted
across depressed region

Depressed
region

E. Reentry circuit established

Figure 14–7. Unidirectional block and reentry. **Panel A** shows the heart schematically with the sinoatrial and atrioventricular nodes and the conducting system in color. A small bifurcating twig of the Purkinje system is circled where it enters the ventricular wall. **Panel B** shows the normal passage and fate of an impulse that is conducted down the twig. It splits into two impulses at the bifurcation, and these collide (and extinguish each other) after exciting the ventricular muscle. **Panels C–E** show the sequence of events when the normal impulse finds an area of unidirectional block (blocked depressed region) in one of the branches. As shown by the path of the impulse in the depressed region **(panel C),** this weak stimulus is unable to conduct through or to "jump over" the area of block. In contrast, the wave in the undepressed branch is able to excite the entire ventricular wall **(panel D).** Because the ventricular wall constitutes a large mass of cells, the strong ventricular depolarization is able to jump the depressed region and results in a retrograde impulse (shown by the black arrow, **panels D** and **E**). The retrograde impulse may be propagated if the impulse finds excitable tissue, ie, the refractory period is shorter than the conduction time. This impulse will then reexcite tissue it had previously passed through, and a reentry arrhythmia will be established in the circuit indicated by the black arrows in panel **E.**

sue. This is accomplished chiefly by selectively blocking the sodium or calcium channels of depolarized cells (Figure 14–8). Therapeutically useful channel-blocking drugs have a high affinity for activated channels (ie, during phase 0) or inactivated channels (ie, during phase 2) but very low affinity for rested channels. Therefore, these drugs block electrical activity when there is a fast tachycardia (many channel activations and inactivations per unit time) or when there is significant loss of resting potential (many inactivated channels during rest). Their action is often described as "use-dependent" or "state-dependent," ie, channels that are being used frequently, or in an inactivated state, are more susceptible to block. Channels in normal cells that become blocked by a drug during normal activation-inactivation cycles will rapidly lose the drug from the receptors during the resting portion of the cycle (Figure 14–8). Channels in myocardium that is chronically depolarized (ie, has a resting potential more positive than –75 mV) will recover from block very slowly if at all (see also right panel, Figure 14–4).

In cells with abnormal automaticity, most of these drugs reduce the phase 4 slope (Figure 14–5) by blocking either sodium or calcium channels and thereby reducing the ratio of sodium (or calcium) permeability to potassium permeability. As a result, the membrane potential during phase 4 stabilizes closer to the potassium equilibrium potential. In addition, some agents may increase the threshold (make it more positive). Beta adrenoceptor-blocking drugs indirectly reduce the phase 4 slope by blocking the positive chronotropic action of norepinephrine in the heart.

In reentrant arrhythmias, which depend upon critically depressed conduction, most antiarrhythmic agents slow conduction further by one or both of two mechanisms: (1) steady-state reduction in the number of available unblocked channels, which reduces the excitatory currents to a level below that required for propagation (Figure 14–4, left); and (2) prolongation of recovery time of the channels still able to reach the rested and available state, which increases the effective refractory period (Figure 14–4, right).[*] As a result, early extrasystoles are unable to propagate at all; later impulses propagate more slowly and are subject to bidirectional conduction block.

Several agents prolong the duration of the cardiac action potential, perhaps through a reduction of outward repolarizing currents (eg, blockade of potassium channels) or an augmentation of inward currents (eg, activation of sodium or calcium channels during phase 2). Such prolongation is usually directly reflected in an increase in the effective refractory period, with the same beneficial results described above. These effects are also dependent upon cycle length. Unfortunately, the prolongation is commonly very small or absent at short cycle lengths, when the drug effect is most needed, and most marked following a long cycle length—ie, this effect exhibits *reverse use dependence*. Following a long compensatory pause, the prolongation can be excessive and lead to repolarization disturbances, early afterdepolarizations, and a morphologically distinctive ventricular tachycardia called torsade de pointes. "Normal" use-dependent prolongation of action potential duration would be preferable: There would be little effect at normal heart rate, but during a period of tachycardia the action potential duration would be prolonged with each beat until the refractory period became too long to allow continuation of the tachycardia. (For more details, see sections on quinidine, sotalol, and amiodarone, below.)

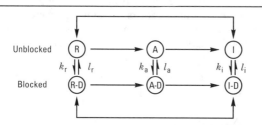

Figure 14–8. Diagram of a mechanism for the selective depressant action of antiarrhythmic drugs on sodium channels. The upper portion of the figure shows the population of channels moving through a cycle of activity during an action potential in the absence of drugs: R (rested) → A (activated) → I (inactivated). Recovery takes place via the I → R pathway. Antiarrhythmic agents that act by blocking sodium channels can bind to their receptors in the channels, as shown by the vertical arrows, to form drug-channel complexes, indicated as R-D, A-D, and I-D. Affinity of the drugs for the receptor varies with the state of the channel, as indicated by the separate rate constants (k and l) for the R → R-D, A → A-D, and I → I-D steps. The data available for a variety of sodium channel blockers indicate that the affinity of the drugs for the active and inactivated channel receptor is much higher than the affinity for the rested channel. Furthermore, recovery from the I-D state to the R-D state is much slower than from I to R. As a result, rapid activity (more activations and inactivations) and depolarization of the resting potential (more channels in the I state) will favor blockade of the channels and selectively suppress arrhythmic cells.

---

[*]In one special case, reentry may result from latent pacemaker activity, especially in Purkinje fibers. Because phase 4 depolarization in latent pacemakers results in a less negative take-off potential for any subsequent action potential, the availability of sodium channels for the upstroke of that action potential may be reduced. As illustrated by the relationship in Figure 14–4, this reduction in channel availability is very steep in the potential range of –70 to –60 mV, and conduction velocity will be similarly reduced. This reduction may be sufficient to cause unidirectional conduction block and reentry. Because they reduce phase 4 depolarization in latent pacemaker cells, antiarrhythmic drugs can therefore (at least theoretically) increase conduction velocity in latent pacemaker cells.

By these mechanisms, antiarrhythmic drugs can suppress ectopic automaticity and abnormal conduction occurring in depolarized cells—rendering them electrically silent—while minimally affecting the electrical activity in normally polarized parts of the heart. However, as dosage is increased, these agents also depress conduction in normal tissue, eventually resulting in *drug-induced* arrhythmias. Furthermore, a drug concentration that is therapeutic (antiarrhythmic) under the initial circumstances of treatment may become "proarrhythmic" (arrhythmogenic) during fast heart rates (more development of block), acidosis (slower recovery from block for most drugs), or hyperkalemia.

As noted above, extracellular potassium markedly affects the resting transmembrane potential in nonpacemaker cells. Therefore, hyperkalemia, by depolarizing the membrane and inactivating more channels, increases the depressant effects of sodium channel-blocking antiarrhythmic drugs. When antiarrhythmic drug toxicity occurs, reduction of extracellular potassium levels (eg, by elevation of serum pH) may reverse the toxicity by hyperpolarizing the myocardium. This approach should only be considered if serum potassium is normal or high, since hypokalemia may also cause arrhythmias.

II. SPECIFIC ANTIARRHYTHMIC AGENTS

The antiarrhythmic agents have traditionally been divided into four distinct classes on the basis of their dominant mechanism of action. Class I consists of the sodium channel blockers, all of which behave like local anesthetics. (In fact, the most popular parenteral antiarrhythmic drug, lidocaine, is also the most popular local anesthetic.) This is the largest group of antiarrhythmic drugs. Class I agents are frequently subdivided according to their effects on action potential duration: Class IA lengthens the duration, IB shortens it, and IC has no effect or may minimally increase action potential duration. As a group, IB agents interact (bind and unbind) rapidly with sodium channels, IC interact slowly, and IA are intermediate. Drugs that reduce adrenergic activity in the heart constitute class II. Class III is composed of drugs that prolong the effective refractory period by some mechanism other than (or in addition to) blockade of sodium channels. Class IV consists of calcium channel blockers. A fifth (unnamed) class includes adenosine, potassium, and magnesium. It is important to recognize that this classification ignores many differences among co-classified drugs and overlapping properties of drugs assigned to different groups. Thus, certain *actions* of

the drugs can be conveniently separated (block of sodium channels, prolongation of action potential duration, etc), but classifying drug action does not mean that drugs from the same class will produce the same overall effects. This is because a given drug with (for example) class I effects may also have significant class III effects, while a different drug with class I action may also have class IV effects.

In recognition of the inadequacies of the traditional classification, a new approach to classification that recognizes the multiplicity of actions of most of the drugs and the variable mechanisms of arrhythmogenesis has recently been proposed (Task Force, 1991). However, this system is not yet widely used.

SODIUM CHANNEL-BLOCKING DRUGS (CLASS I)

QUINIDINE
(Class IA)

Although quinine was used sporadically as an antiarrhythmic drug during the 18th and 19th centuries, it was not until the early years of the 20th century that quinidine, the diastereomer of quinine, came into wide use. Quinidine is among the most commonly used oral antiarrhythmic agents in the USA.

Quinidine

Cardiac Effects

Quinidine depresses pacemaker rate (especially that of ectopic pacemakers) and depresses conduction and excitability (especially in depolarized tissue) (Table 14–1). To a large extent, these actions result from quinidine's ability to bind to and block activated sodium channels, though the drug also blocks inactivated sodium channels. Recovery from block is slower and less complete in depolarized than in fully polarized tissue. Thus, quinidine lengthens the refractory period and depresses excitability and conduction in depolarized tissue more than in normal tissue.

Quinidine also lengthens the action potential duration, which is reflected in the ECG as a lengthening of the QT interval. Block of potassium channels with a reduction in repolarizing outward current is responsible for this effect (Balser et al, 1991, Snyders et al, 1992). (It should be noted that any lengthening of the action potential duration reduces the time spent at more negative diastolic membrane potentials and therefore enhances the sodium channel-blocking efficacy of quinidine.) Lengthening of the action potential duration and effective refractory period reduces the maximum reentry frequency and can slow tachycardias. This class III effect may be less marked at fast heart rates (when it is more useful) and—in some situations—excessive at slow heart rates. In experimental preparations, excessive prolongation can induce early afterdepolarizations (EADs), described previously. In patients, action potential prolongation and EADs cause torsade de pointes. This tachycardia is associated with a striking prolongation of the QT interval and appears to be the cause of quinidine syncope (see below). Plasma concentrations of quinidine are often normal in patients with this toxic effect.

Extracardiac Effects

Quinidine possesses alpha adrenoceptor-blocking properties that can cause vasodilation and a reflex increase in sinoatrial nodal rate. These effects are most prominent after intravenous administration (see below).

Toxicity

A. Cardiac: Quinidine has antimuscarinic actions in the heart that inhibit vagal effects. This can overcome some of its direct membrane effect and lead to increased sinus rate and increased atrioventricular conduction. In atrial fibrillation, the antimuscarinic action on the AV node may result in an excessively high ventricular rate. With atrial flutter, the AV coupling ratio decreases from 4:1 or more down to 1:1. However, this can be prevented by prior administration of a drug that slows atrioventricular conduction, eg, verapamil, a beta-blocker, or digitalis.

A small percentage (1–5%) of patients given quinidine develop a syndrome called "quinidine syncope," characterized by recurrent light-headedness and episodes of fainting. The symptoms are a result of drug-induced torsade de pointes, which usually terminates spontaneously but may recur frequently or become sustained. (Torsade de pointes and syncope occur with many drugs that prolong the action potential.)

In patients with sick sinus syndrome, quinidine may depress the pacemaker activity of the sinoatrial node. In toxic concentrations, this drug can depress cardiac electrical activity in any part of the heart to the point of precipitating arrhythmias or asystole. These toxic effects are more likely to occur when the serum concentrations exceed 5 µg/mL and in the presence of high serum potassium levels (> 5 mmol/L). Widening of the QRS duration by 30% by

quinidine administration is usually considered premonitory of serious toxicity. Toxic concentrations may depress contractility and lower blood pressure.

B. Extracardiac: The most common adverse effects are gastrointestinal: diarrhea, nausea, and vomiting. These may occur in one-third to one-half of patients. The drug can also cause cinchonism (headache, dizziness, tinnitus). Rarely, quinidine can cause rashes, angioneurotic edema, fever, hepatitis, and thrombocytopenia. Quinidine increases digoxin plasma levels and may precipitate digitalis toxicity in patients taking digoxin or digitoxin (see Chapter 13).

Pharmacokinetics & Dosage

Quinidine is usually administered orally and is rapidly absorbed from the gastrointestinal tract. It is 80% bound to plasma proteins. Quinidine is metabolized in the liver, but 20% is excreted unchanged in the urine. Its half-life is about 6 hours (Table 14–2) and may be longer in patients with congestive heart failure or hepatic or renal disease. Urinary excretion is enhanced in acid urine. It is usually administered orally as the sulfate, gluconate, or polygalacturonate salt. The usual dose of 0.2–0.6 g of quinidine sulfate is given 2–4 times daily. The therapeutic concentration in plasma is 3–5 µg/mL.

Parenteral administration of quinidine is occasionally necessary. Quinidine is absorbed after intramuscular injection of the sulfate in oil or the aqueous gluconate preparation. Quinidine can be given intravenously if proper precautions are observed. The intravenous dose should not exceed 10 mg/kg of quinidine gluconate and should not be given at a rate exceeding 0.5 mg/kg/min. Intravenous administration of quinidine is usually associated with a decline in blood pressure as a result of its peripheral vasodilating action. Thus, when intravenous quinidine is used, blood pressure should be carefully monitored and supported when necessary with intravenous fluids.

Therapeutic Use

Quinidine is used in nearly every form of arrhythmia: premature atrial contractions, paroxysmal atrial fibrillation and flutter, intra-atrial and atrioventricular nodal reentrant arrhythmias, Wolff-Parkinson-White tachycardias, premature ventricular contractions, and ventricular tachycardias. It has also been combined with mexiletine to enhance efficacy and reduce side effects. (Quinidine is also used for the intravenous treatment of malaria.)

PROCAINAMIDE
(Class IA)

Cardiac Effects

The electrophysiologic effects of procainamide are similar to those of quinidine. The drug may be somewhat less effective in suppressing abnormal ectopic

Table 14–1. Membrane actions of antiarrhythmic drugs.

Drug	Block of Sodium Channels		Refractory Period		Calcium Channel Blockade	Effect on Pacemaker Activity	Sympatholytic Action
	Normal Cells	Depolarized Cells	Normal Cells	Depolarized Cells			
Adenosine (Adenocard)	0	0	0	0	0	0	+
Amiodarone (Cordarone)	+	+++	↑↑	↑↑↑	+	↓↓	+
Bretylium (Bretylol)	0	0	↑↑↑	↑↑↑	0	↑↓[1]	++
Disopyramide (Norpace)	+	+++	↑	↑↑	+	↓↓	0
Esmolol (Brevibloc)	0	+	0	NA[2]	0	↓↓	+++
Flecainide (Tambocor)	+	+++	0	↑	0	↓↓	0
Imipramine (investigational)	+	++	↑	↑↑	0	↓↓	0
Lidocaine (Xylocaine)	0	+++	↓	↑↑	0	↓↓	0
Mexiletine (Mexitil)	0	+++	0	↑↑	0	↓↓	0
Moricizine (Ethmozine)	+	++	↓	↓	0	↓↓	0
Phenytoin (Dilantin)	0	+	↓	↑	+	↓	+
Procainamide (Pronestyl, others)	+	+++	↑	↑↑↑	0	↓	+
Propafenone (Rythmol)	+	++	↑	↑↑	+	↓↓	+
Propranolol (Inderal)	0	+	↓	↑↑	0	↓↓	+++
Quinidine (many trade names)	+	++	↑	↑↑	0	↓↓	+
Sotalol (Betapace)	0	0	↑↑	↑↑↑	0	↓↓	++
Tocainide (Tonocard)	0	+++	0	↑↑	0	↓↓	0
Verapamil (Calan, Isoptin)	0	+	0	↑	+++	↓↓	+

[1]Bretylium may transiently increase pacemaker rate by causing catecholamine release.
[2]Data not available.

pacemaker activity but more effective in blocking sodium channels in depolarized cells.

Perhaps the most important difference between quinidine and procainamide is the less prominent antimuscarinic action of procainamide. Therefore, the directly depressant actions of procainamide on sinoatrial and atrioventricular nodes are not as effectively counterbalanced by drug-induced vagal block as in the case of quinidine.

Procainamide

Extracardiac Effects

Procainamide has ganglion-blocking properties. This action reduces peripheral vascular resistance and can cause hypotension, particularly with intravenous use. However, in therapeutic concentrations, its peripheral vascular effects are less prominent than those of quinidine. Hypotension is usually seen only during excessively rapid procainamide infusion.

Toxicity

A. Cardiac: Procainamide's cardiotoxic effects are similar to those of quinidine. Antimuscarinic and direct depressant effects may occur. New arrhythmias may be precipitated.

B. Extracardiac: The most troublesome adverse effect of procainamide is a syndrome resembling lupus erythematosus and usually consisting of arthralgia and arthritis. In some patients, pleuritis, pericarditis, or parenchymal pulmonary disease also occurs. Renal lupus is rarely induced by procainamide. During long-term therapy, serologic abnormalities (eg, increased antinuclear antibody titer) occur in nearly all patients, and in the absence of symptoms these are not an indication to stop drug therapy. Approximately one-third of patients receiving long-term procainamide therapy develop lupus-related symptoms.

Other adverse effects include nausea and diarrhea (about 10% of cases), rash, fever, hepatitis (< 5%), and agranulocytosis (< 0.2%).

Pharmacokinetics & Dosage

Procainamide can be administered safely by the intravenous and intramuscular routes and is well absorbed orally, with 75% systemic bioavailability. The major metabolite is N-acetylprocainamide ("NAPA,"

Table 14–2. Clinical pharmacologic properties of antiarrythmic drugs.

Drug	Effect on SA Nodal Rate	Effect on AV Nodal Refractory Period	PR Interval	QRS Duration	QT Interval	Usefulness in Arrhythmias		Half-life
						Supra-ventricular	Ventricular	
Adenosine (Adenocard)	Little	↑↑↑	↑↑↑	0	0	++++	?	<10 sec
Amiodarone (Cordarone)	↓↓[1]	↑↑	↑↑	↑	↑↑↑↑	+++	+++	(weeks)
Bretylium (Bretylol)	↑↓[2]	↑↓[2]	0	0	0	0	+	4 h
Disopyramide (Norpace)	↑↓[1,3]	↑↓[3]	↑↓[3]	↑↑	↑↑	+	+++	6–8 h
Esmolol (Brevibloc)	↓↓	↑↑	↑↑	0	0	+	+	10 min
Flecainide (Tambocor)	None	↑	↑	↑↑↑	0	+[4]	++++	20 h
Imipramine (investigational)	↑[1,3]	↑	↑	↑	↑	+	+++	12 h
Lidocaine (Xylocaine)	None[1]	None	0	0	0	None[6]	+++	1 h
Mexiletine (Mexitil)	None[1]	None	0	0	0	None[5]	+++	12 h
Moricizine (Ethmozine)	None	None	↑	↑↑	0	None	+++	2–6 h[5]
Phenytoin (Dilantin)	None	None	0	↑	0	None[6]	+	24 h
Procainamide (Pronestyl, others)	↓[1]	↑↓[3]	↑↓[3]	↑↑	↑↑	+	+++	3–4 h
Propafenone (Rhythmol)	0	↑	↑	↑↑↑	0	+	+++	7 h
Propranolol (Inderal)	↓↓	↑↑	↑↑	0	0	+	+	8 h
Quinidine (many trade names)	↑↓[1,3]	↑↓[3]	↑↓[3]	↑↑	↑↑	+	+++	6 h
Sotalol (Betapace)	↓↓	↑↑	↑↑	0	↑↑↑	+++	+++	7 h
Tocainide (Tonocard)	None[1]	None	0	0	0	None[6]	+++	12 h
Verapamil (Calan, Isoptin)	↑↓	↑↑	↑↑	0	0	+++	+	7 h

[1]May suppress diseased sinus nodes.
[2]Initial stimulation by release of endogenous norepinephrine followed by depression.
[3]Anticholinergic effect and direct depressant action.
[4]Especially in Wolff-Parkinson-White syndrome.
[5]Half-life of active metabolites much longer.
[6]May be effective in atrial arrhythmias caused by digitalis.

acecainide), which is a weak sodium channel blocker and has class III activity. Excessive accumulation of NAPA has been implicated in torsade de pointes during procainamide therapy. Some individuals rapidly acetylate procainamide and develop high levels of N-acetylprocainamide. The lupus syndrome appears to be less common in these patients.

Procainamide's half-life is only 3–4 hours, which necessitates frequent dosing. Both procainamide and N-acetylprocainamide are eliminated chiefly by the kidneys. Thus, dosage must be reduced in patients with renal failure. The reduced volume of distribution and renal clearance associated with congestive heart failure also require reduction in dosage. The half-life of N-acetylprocainamide is considerably longer than that of procainamide, and it therefore accumulates more slowly. Thus, it is important to measure plasma levels of both procainamide and N-acetylprocainamide, especially in patients with circulatory or renal impairment.

If rapid effect is needed, an intravenous loading dose of up to 12 mg/kg can be given safely at a rate of 0.3 mg/kg/min or less rapidly. This dose is followed by a maintenance dose of 2–5 mg/min, with careful monitoring of plasma levels. The risk of gastrointestinal or cardiac toxicity rises at plasma concentrations greater than 8 μg/mL or NAPA concentrations greater than 20 μg/mL.

Oral procainamide is frequently used improperly. If around-the-clock antiarrhythmic activity is required, a sustained-release preparation must be administered every 6 hours in most cases. In order to control ventricular arrhythmias, a total dose of 2–5 g/d is usually required. In an occasional patient who accumulates high levels of N-acetylprocainamide and in whom that compound is active, less frequent dosing may be possible. This is also possible in renal disease, where procainamide elimination is also slowed.

Therapeutic Use

Like quinidine, procainamide is effective against most atrial and ventricular arrhythmias. However, many clinicians attempt to avoid long-term therapy because of the frequent dosing requirement and the common occurrence of lupus-related effects. Procainamide is the drug of second choice (after lidocaine) in most coronary care units for the treatment of sustained ventricular arrhythmias associated with acute myocardial infarction.

DISOPYRAMIDE
(Class IA)

Disopyramide phosphate is closely related to isopropamide, an agent long used for its antimuscarinic properties.

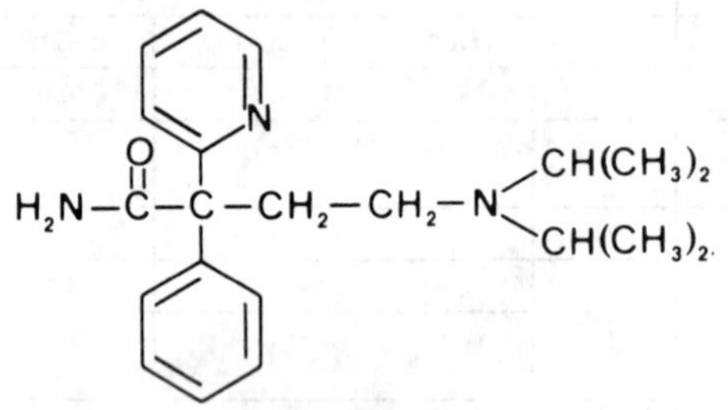

Disopyramide

Cardiac Effects
The effects of disopyramide are very similar to those of quinidine. Its cardiac antimuscarinic effects are even more marked than those of quinidine. Therefore, a drug that slows atrioventricular conduction should be administered with disopyramide in the treatment of atrial flutter or fibrillation.

Toxicity
A. Cardiac: Toxic concentrations of disopyramide can precipitate all of the electrophysiologic disturbances described under quinidine. In addition, disopyramide's negative inotropic actions are frequently troublesome in patients with preexisting left ventricular dysfunction. Moreover, in rare instances, it may produce heart failure in subjects without prior myocardial dysfunction. Because of this effect, disopyramide is not used as a first-line antiarrhythmic agent in the USA. It must be used with great caution in patients with congestive heart failure.

B. Extracardiac: Disopyramide's atropine-like activity accounts for most of its symptomatic adverse effects: urinary retention (most often, but not exclusively, in male patients with prostatic hypertrophy), dry mouth, blurred vision, constipation, and worsening of preexisting glaucoma. These effects may require discontinuance of the drug.

Pharmacokinetics & Dosage
In the USA, disopyramide is only available for oral use. Bioavailability is about 50%. The drug is exten-

sively protein-bound, but binding sites become saturated with increasing dosage, which results in a nonlinear rise in free (active) drug levels. As a result, measurements of total plasma concentration may be misleading. The drug is excreted by the kidneys and has a half-life of approximately 6–8 hours. The usual oral dose of disopyramide is 150 mg 3 times a day, but as much as 1 g/d may be required. In patients with renal impairment, this schedule must be reduced. Because of the danger of precipitating congestive heart failure, the use of loading doses is not recommended.

Therapeutic Use
Although disopyramide has been shown to be effective in a variety of supraventricular arrhythmias, in the USA it is approved only for the treatment of ventricular arrhythmias. It is most commonly used when quinidine and procainamide have been poorly tolerated or ineffective.

IMIPRAMINE
(Class IA)

Imipramine is a tricyclic antidepressant agent that also has antiarrhythmic activity. Its electrophysiologic actions and clinical spectrum of activity are similar to those of quinidine. Like disopyramide, it also has strong antimuscarinic effects. Its elimination half-life is about 12 hours. The usual daily dose is 200 mg/d in two doses. The initial dose should be smaller, because the drug's most prominent adverse effect (sedation) is lessened by slowly increasing the dose. Imipramine is marketed as an antidepressant, and its use as an antiarrhythmic agent has not been approved by the FDA.

AMIODARONE
(Classes I, II, III, & IV)

Amiodarone has been widely used as an antiarrhythmic and antianginal agent in Europe and South America. In the USA, it is only approved for use in arrhythmias. It is very effective against a wide variety of arrhythmias, but its prominent adverse effects and unusual pharmacokinetic properties have limited its use in the USA.

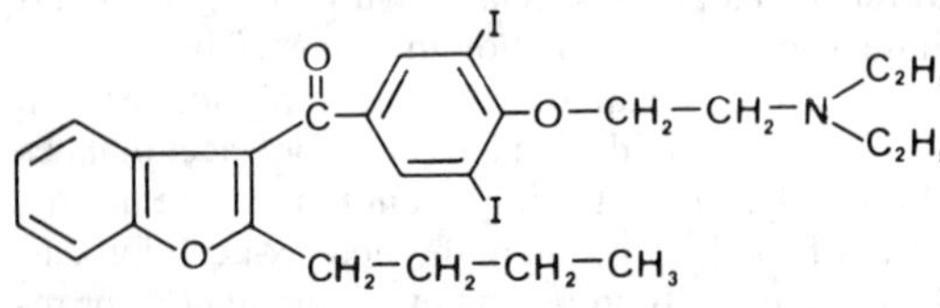

Amiodarone

Cardiac Effects

Amiodarone has a broad spectrum of actions on the heart. It is a very effective blocker of sodium channels, but unlike quinidine it has a low affinity for activated channels, combining instead almost exclusively with channels in the inactivated state. Thus, the sodium-blocking action of amiodarone is most pronounced in tissues that have long action potentials, frequent action potentials, or less negative diastolic potentials. In therapeutic concentrations, amiodarone also markedly lengthens action potential duration, probably by blocking potassium channels. Amiodarone sustains its lengthening of action potential duration quite well at fast heart rates. This is probably an important reason for its efficacy against tachycardias. Furthermore, torsade de pointes is very unusual. Amiodarone is a weak calcium channel blocker as well as a noncompetitive inhibitor of beta adrenoceptors. The drug has also been shown to be a powerful inhibitor of abnormal automaticity.

Amiodarone slows the sinus rate and atrioventricular conduction, markedly prolongs the QT interval, and prolongs QRS duration. It increases atrial, atrioventricular nodal, and ventricular refractory periods. Induction of new ventricular arrhythmias or worsening of preexisting ones occurs rarely during therapy with amiodarone. In patients with Wolff-Parkinson- White syndrome, the drug delays conduction, prolongs the effective refractory period, and may totally abolish transmission through the accessory pathways.

Amiodarone also has antianginal effects. This may result from its noncompetitive alpha and beta adrenoceptor-blocking properties as well as from its apparent ability to block calcium influx in coronary arterial smooth muscle.

Extracardiac Effects

Amiodarone causes peripheral vascular dilation, presumably through its alpha adrenoceptor-blocking and calcium channel-inhibiting effects. In some patients, this may be beneficial; rarely, it may require discontinuation of the drug.

Toxicity

A. Cardiac: In patients with sinus or atrioventricular nodal disease, amiodarone may produce symptomatic bradycardia or heart block. It may also precipitate heart failure in susceptible patients.

B. Extracardiac: Amiodarone causes a remarkable variety of extracardiac adverse effects, including potentially fatal pulmonary fibrosis. The number of amiodarone's toxic effects increases with the cumulative dose and limits the utility of this drug in long-term therapy.

Amiodarone is concentrated in tissue and can be found in virtually every organ. The most readily detected deposits are those in the cornea, which appear as yellowish-brown microcrystals in a few weeks after initiation of therapy. These corneal deposits rarely cause visual symptoms except for occasional halos in the peripheral visual fields, most prominent at night. Only infrequently does reduction of visual acuity occur, requiring discontinuation or reduction of amiodarone dosage. Skin deposits result in photodermatitis in about 25% of patients, and these patients must avoid exposure to the sun. In less than 5% of patients, a grayish-blue skin discoloration develops.

Adverse neurologic effects are common and include paresthesias, tremor, ataxia, and headaches.

Thyroid dysfunction—both hypo- and hyperthyroidism—occurs in about 5% of patients. Thyroid function should be assessed prior to and throughout the duration of amiodarone therapy.

Amiodarone may affect the gastrointestinal tract (eg, constipation, 20%), liver (eg, hepatocellular necrosis), or lung (eg, inflammation and fibrosis). Pulmonary fibrosis has been reported in 5–15% of patients; in a fraction of these, it may be fatal.

Drug interactions are very common. Amiodarone reduces clearance of warfarin, theophylline, quinidine, procainamide, flecainide, and other drugs. Although amiodarone is a highly effective antiarrhythmic agent, these adverse reactions have limited its clinical use in the USA.

Pharmacokinetics & Dosage

Amiodarone has an extremely long half-life (13–103 days). The effective plasma concentration is approximately 1–2 µg/mL, while the cardiac tissue concentration is about 30 times higher. Even with large loading doses, 15–30 days are required to load the body stores with sufficient amiodarone to estimate the drug's efficacy. Loading doses of 0.8–1.2 g daily for about 2 weeks are used, after which the patient is maintained on 0.2–1 g daily. Because of the drug's long half-life, once-daily dosage is adequate. If toxicity occurs, it persists long after drug administration is discontinued.

Therapeutic Use

Amiodarone is very effective against both supraventricular and ventricular arrhythmias. In general, relatively low dosages (200–400 mg/d) can be used against paroxysmal atrial fibrillation. Amiodarone appears to be quite effective against supraventricular arrhythmias in children, in whom it appears to be relatively safe. However, long-term experience is not yet available. Several large-scale clinical trials are under way to test amiodarone's safety and efficacy in patients with advanced heart disease.

LIDOCAINE
(Class IB)

Lidocaine is the antiarrhythmic drug most commonly used by the intravenous route. It has a low incidence of toxicity and a high degree of effectiveness in arrhythmias associated with acute myocardial infarction.

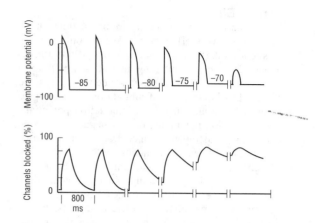

Lidocaine

Figure 14–9. Effect of membrane potential on the blocking and unblocking of sodium channels by lidocaine. **Upper trace:** action potentials in a ventricular muscle cell; **lower trace:** percentage of channels blocked by the drug. As the membrane depolarizes through –80, –75, –70 and –65 mV, an 800 ms time segment is shown. Extra passage of time is indicated by breaks in the traces. **Left side:** at the normal resting potential of –85 mV, the drug combines with open (activated) and inactivated channels during each action potential, but block is rapidly reversed during diastole because the affinity of the drug for its receptor is so low when the channel recovers to the resting state at –85 mV. **Middle:** metabolic injury has occurred, eg, ischemia due to coronary occlusion, that causes gradual depolarization over time. With subsequent action potentials arising from more depolarized potentials, the fraction of channels blocked increases because more channels remain in the inactivated state at less negative potentials (Figure 14–4, **left**), and the time constant for unblocking during diastole rapidly increases at less negative resting potentials (Figure 14–4, **right**). Because of marked drug binding, conduction block and loss of excitability in this tissue result, ie, the "sick" (depolarized) tissue is selectively suppressed.

Cardiac Effects

Lidocaine is a potent suppressor of abnormal cardiac activity, and it appears to act exclusively on the sodium channel. Its interaction with this channel differs substantially from that of quinidine. Whereas quinidine mostly blocks sodium channels in the activated state, lidocaine rapidly blocks both activated and inactivated sodium channels (Figure 14–9). As a result, a large fraction (> 50%) of the unblocked sodium channels become blocked during each action potential in Purkinje fibers and ventricular cells, which have long plateaus (and correspondingly long periods of inactivation). During diastole, most of the sodium channels in normally polarized cells rapidly become drug-free. Since lidocaine may shorten the action potential duration, diastole may be prolonged, thereby extending the time available for recovery. As a result, lidocaine has few electrophysiologic effects in *normal* cardiac tissue. In contrast, depolarized (inactivated) sodium channels remain largely blocked during diastole, and more may become blocked. Thus, lidocaine suppresses the electrical activity of the depolarized, arrhythmogenic tissues while minimally interfering with the electrical activity of normal tissues. These factors appear to be responsible for the fact that lidocaine is a very effective agent for suppressing arrhythmias associated with depolarization (eg, ischemia, digitalis toxicity), but it is relatively ineffective against arrhythmias occurring in normally polarized tissues (eg, atrial flutter and fibrillation).

Toxicity

A. Cardiac: Lidocaine is the least cardiotoxic of the currently used antiarrhythmic drugs. The drug exacerbates ventricular arrhythmias in fewer than 10% of patients (a good record). However, in about 1% of patients with acute myocardial infarction, lidocaine precipitates sinoatrial nodal standstill or worsens impaired conduction.

In large doses, especially in patients with preexisting heart failure, lidocaine may cause hypotension—partly by depressing myocardial contractility.

B. Extracardiac: Lidocaine's most common adverse effects—like those of other local anesthetics—are neurologic: paresthesias, tremor, nausea of central origin, light-headedness, hearing disturbances, slurred speech, and convulsions. Convulsions occur mostly in elderly or otherwise vulnerable patients and are dose-related, usually short-lived, and respond to intravenous diazepam. In general, if plasma levels above 9 μg/mL are avoided, lidocaine is well tolerated.

Pharmacokinetics & Dosage

Because of its very extensive first-pass hepatic metabolism, only 3% of orally administered lidocaine appears in the plasma. Thus, lidocaine must be given parenterally. Lidocaine has a half-life of about 2 hours. In adults, a loading dose of 150–200 mg administered over about 15 minutes should be followed by a maintenance infusion of 2–4 mg/min to achieve a therapeutic plasma level of 2–6 μg/mL. Determination of lidocaine plasma levels is of great value in adjusting the infusion rate. Occasional patients with myocardial infarction require (and tolerate) higher concentrations. This may be due to increased plasma _____ eactant protein _____ drug available

_____ failure, lido- _____ al body clear- _____ since these ef- _____ lf-life may not _____ rom clearance _____ isease, plasma _____ volume of dis- _____ ation half-life _____ fold or more. _____ ime to steady _____ ations may be _____ tients and pa- _____ ay be required _____ decrease liver _____ reduce lido- _____ of toxicity un- _____ infusions last- _____ ls and plasma _____ o major effect

_____ uppression of _____ after cardio- _____ that lidocaine _____ icular fibrilla- _____ nyocardial in- _____ er, whether li- _____ stered to all _____ ome analyses _____ of lidocaine _____ ossibly by in-

_____ entricular ar- _____ with Wolff- _____ toxicity.

_____ ners of lido- _____ atic metabo- _____ he oral route. _____ thmic actions _____ similar to those of lidocaine. They are useful in the treatment of ventricular arrhythmias. The therapeutic half-life of both drugs is between 8 and 20 hours, and they are administered 2 or 3 times a day. The usual daily dose of mexiletine is 600–1200 mg/d; of tocainide, 800–2400 mg/d. Both drugs cause dose-

related adverse effects that are seen frequently at therapeutic dosage. These are predominantly neurologic, including tremor, blurred vision, and lethargy. Nausea is also a common effect. Rash, fever, and agranulocytosis occur in about 0.5% of patients receiving tocainide.

Mexiletine has also shown significant efficacy in relieving chronic pain, especially pain due to diabetic neuropathy and nerve injury (Chabal et al, 1992). The usual dose is 450–750 mg/d orally. This application is unlabeled.

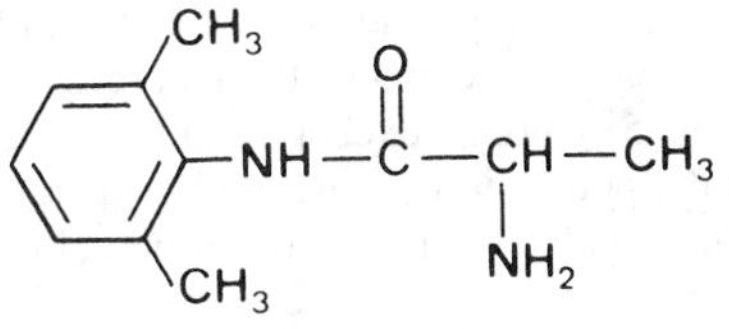

Tocainide

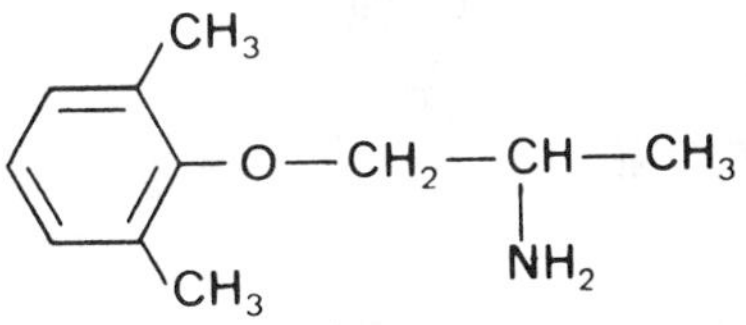

Mexiletine

PHENYTOIN
(Class IB)

Phenytoin is an anticonvulsant agent with antiarrhythmic properties (Chapter 23). Because of its limited efficacy, it should be considered a second-line drug in treatment of arrhythmias. It suppresses ectopic pacemaker activity, blocks the sodium current, and may interfere with the calcium current. It appears especially effective against digitalis-induced arrhythmias.

FLECAINIDE
(Class IC)

Flecainide is a potent sodium channel blocker used primarily for therapy of ventricular arrhythmias. It is also a potent blocker of some potassium channels, which may contribute to its efficacy in some atrial arrhythmias. It has no antimuscarinic effects. It is very effective in suppressing premature ventricular contractions. However, it may cause severe exacerbation of arrhythmia even when normal doses are administered to patients with preexisting ventricular tachyarrhythmias and those with a previous myocardial infarction and ventricular ectopy. (See box: Cardiac Arrhythmia Suppression Trial, page 226.) As a result, flecainide is currently reserved for patients with severe ventricular tachyarrhythmias, in whom the risk:benefit ratio is more favorable. Flecainide is also useful in patients with supraventricular arrhythmias, who are less prone to proarrhythmic toxicity. The drug is well absorbed and has a half-life of approximately 20 hours. Elimination is by the kidney. The usual dose of flecainide is 100–200 mg twice a day.

PROPAFENONE
(Class IC)

Propafenone has some structural similarities to propranolol and possesses weak beta-blocking activity. Its spectrum of action is very similar to that of quinidine. Its potency as a sodium channel blocker is similar to that of flecainide. Its average elimination half-life is $5\frac{1}{2}$ hours except in poor metabolizers (10% of the population), in whom it is as much as 17 hours. The usual daily dosage of propafenone is 450–900 mg in three doses. The drug is widely used in Europe. The most common adverse effects are a metallic taste and constipation.

MORICIZINE
(Class IC)

Moricizine is an antiarrhythmic phenothiazine derivative that is used for treatment of ventricular arrhythmias. It is a relatively potent sodium channel blocker that does not prolong action potential duration. It has the properties of a IC drug.

Moricizine produces multiple metabolites in humans, some of which are probably active and have long half-lives. Its most common adverse effects are dizziness and nausea. Like other potent sodium channel blockers, it can exacerbate arrhythmias.

The usual dosage of moricizine is 200–300 mg by mouth 3 times a day.

BETA ADRENOCEPTOR-BLOCKING DRUGS (CLASS II)

Cardiac Effects

Propranolol and similar drugs have antiarrhythmic properties by virtue of their beta receptor-blocking action and direct membrane effects. As described in Chapter 10, some of these drugs have selectivity for cardiac β_1 receptors; some have intrinsic sympathomimetic activity; some have marked direct membrane effects; and some prolong the cardiac action potential. The relative contributions of the beta-blocking and direct membrane effects to the antiarrhythmic effects of these drugs are not fully known. Although beta-blockers are fairly well tolerated, their efficacy for suppression of ventricular ectopic depolarizations is lower than that of sodium channel blockers. However, there is good evidence that these agents can prevent recurrent infarction and sudden death in patients recovering from acute myocardial infarction (Chapter 10).

Esmolol is a short-acting beta-blocker used primarily as an antiarrhythmic drug for intraoperative and other acute arrhythmias. See Chapter 10 for more information. Sotalol is a nonselective beta-blocking drug that prolongs the action potential (class III action).

DRUGS THAT PROLONG EFFECTIVE REFRACTORY PERIOD BY PROLONGING ACTION POTENTIAL (CLASS III)

These drugs prolong action potentials, usually by blocking potassium channels in cardiac muscle. At present, the most important agents in this category are those with additional effects that place them in one of the other subgroups. Quinidine and especially amiodarone effectively prolong action potential duration. However, as noted above, their actions on sodium channels also contribute to the measured increase in effective refractory period. Bretylium and sotalol also prolong action potential duration and refractory period and are discussed below. As noted above, action potential prolongation by these drugs exhibits "reverse" use dependence, which can contribute to torsade de pointes. Amiodarone may be an exception. A large number of newer drugs with class III actions are in clinical trials at present (see, for example, Wong et al, 1992). It is hoped that they will be less arrhythmogenic than the class I agents. There is also some evidence that several class III agents have positive rather than negative inotropic actions on the heart.

BRETYLIUM

Bretylium was first introduced as an antihypertensive agent. It interferes with the neuronal release of catecholamines but also has direct antiarrhythmic properties.

Bretylium

Cardiac Effects

Bretylium lengthens the ventricular (but not the atrial) action potential duration and effective refractory period. This effect is most pronounced in ischemic cells, which have shortened action potential durations. Thus, bretylium may reverse the shortening of action potential duration caused by ischemia. Experimentally, it has been shown that bretylium markedly increases the strength of electrical stimulation needed to induce ventricular fibrillation (ventricular fibrillation threshold) and delays the onset of fibrillation after acute coronary ligation. This antifibrillatory action appears to be independent of its sympatholytic properties.

Since bretylium causes an initial release of catecholamines, it has some positive inotropic actions when first administered. This action may also *precipitate* ventricular arrhythmias and must be watched for at the onset of therapy with the drug.

Extracardiac Effects

These are predictable from the drug's sympatholegic actions. The major adverse effect is postural hypotension. This effect can be almost totally prevented by concomitant administration of a tricyclic antidepressant agent such as protriptyline. Nausea and vomiting may occur after the intravenous administration of a bolus of bretylium.

Pharmacokinetics & Dosage

Bretylium is available only for intravenous use in the USA. In adults, an intravenous bolus of bretylium tosylate, 5 mg/kg, is administered over a 10-minute period. This dosage may be repeated after 30 minutes. Maintenance therapy is achieved by a similar bolus every 4–6 hours or by a constant infusion of 0.5–2 mg/min.

Therapeutic Use

Bretylium is usually used in an emergency setting, often during attempted resuscitation from ventricular fibrillation when lidocaine and cardioversion have failed. Only rarely does bretylium suppress premature ventricular contractions.

SOTALOL

Sotalol is a nonselective beta-blocker that also prolongs action potential duration and is an effective antiarrhythmic agent. Its D-isomer, which is currently investigational, has no beta-blocking properties but retains the effect upon repolarization. Sotalol can be used in both supraventricular and ventricular arrhythmias. The usual effective dose is 4–6 mg/kg/d given in two or three divided doses. Its major toxicities are associated with beta blockade (see Chapter 10) and with prolongation of repolarization, including torsade de pointes. Unlike quinidine, sotalol is more likely to cause torsade de pointes at higher dosages and plasma concentrations.

Sotalol

CALCIUM CHANNEL-BLOCKING DRUGS (CLASS IV)

These drugs, of which verapamil is the prototype, were first introduced as antianginal agents and are discussed in greater detail in Chapter 12. Verapamil, diltiazem, and bepridil also have antiarrhythmic effects. Nifedipine and other dihydropyridine calcium channel blocking drugs have little antiarrhythmic activity.

VERAPAMIL

Cardiac Effects

Verapamil blocks both activated and inactivated calcium channels. Thus, its effect is more marked in tissues that fire frequently, those that are less completely polarized at rest, and those in which activation depends exclusively on the calcium current, such as the sinoatrial and atrioventricular nodes. It is therefore not surprising that verapamil has marked effects on these tissues. Atrioventricular nodal conduction and effective refractory period are invariably prolonged by therapeutic concentrations. Verapamil usually slows the sinoatrial node by its direct action, but its hypotensive action may occasionally result in a small reflex increase of sinoatrial nodal rate.

Verapamil can suppress both early and delayed afterdepolarizations and may antagonize slow responses arising in severely depolarized tissue.

Extracardiac Effects

Verapamil causes peripheral vasodilation, which may be beneficial in hypertension and peripheral vasospastic disorders. Its effects upon smooth muscle produce a number of extracardiac effects (see Chapter 12).

Toxicity

A. Cardiac: Verapamil's cardiotoxic effects are dose-related and usually avoidable. A common error has been to administer intravenous verapamil to a patient with ventricular tachycardia misdiagnosed as supraventricular tachycardia. In this setting, hypotension and ventricular fibrillation can occur. Verapamil's negative inotropic effects may limit its clinical usefulness in damaged hearts (see Chapter 12). Verapamil can lead to atrioventricular block when used in large doses or in patients with partial atrioventricular block. This block can be treated with atropine, beta receptor stimulants, or calcium. In patients with sinus node disease, verapamil can precipitate sinus arrest.

B. Extracardiac: Minor adverse effects include constipation, lassitude, nervousness, and peripheral edema.

Pharmacokinetics & Dosage

The half-life of verapamil is approximately 7 hours. It is extensively metabolized by the liver; after oral administration, its bioavailability is only about 20%. Therefore, verapamil must be administered with caution in patients with hepatic dysfunction. Much smaller doses are required when the drug is administered intravenously.

In adult patients without heart failure or sinoatrial or atrioventricular nodal disease, parenteral treatment of supraventricular tachycardia consists of an initial bolus of 5 mg administered over 2–5 minutes, followed a few minutes later by a second 5 mg bolus if needed. Thereafter, doses of 5–10 mg can be administered every 4–6 hours, or a constant infusion of 0.4 μg/kg/min may be used.

Effective oral dosage ranges from 120 to 600 mg daily, divided into three or four doses.

Therapeutic Use

Reentrant supraventricular tachycardia is the major indication for verapamil, and the drug is preferred over older treatments (propranolol, digoxin, edrophonium, vasoconstrictor agents, and cardioversion). Verapamil can also reduce the ventricular rate in atrial fibrillation and flutter. It may convert atrial flutter and fibrillation to sinus rhythm. Verapamil is very rarely useful in ventricular arrhythmias.

DILTIAZEM & BEPRIDIL

These agents appear to be similar in efficacy to verapamil in the management of supraventricular arrhythmias, including rate control in atrial fibrillation. Bepridil also has action potential and QT-prolonging actions that may make it more useful in some ventricular arrhythmias but also create the risk of torsade de pointes.

MISCELLANEOUS ANTIARRHYTHMIC AGENTS

Certain agents used for the treatment of arrhythmias do not fit the conventional class I–IV organization. These include digitalis (already discussed, Chapter 13), adenosine, magnesium, and potassium.

ADENOSINE

Mechanism & Clinical Use

Adenosine is a nucleoside that occurs naturally throughout the body. Its half-life in the blood is estimated to be less than 10 seconds. Its mechanism of action involves enhanced potassium conductance and inhibition of cAMP-induced calcium influx. The results of these actions are marked hyperpolarization and suppression of calcium-dependent action potentials. When given as a bolus dose, adenosine directly inhibits atrioventricular nodal conduction and increases the atrioventricular nodal refractory period but has only mild effects on sinoatrial nodal function. Adenosine is currently the drug of choice for prompt management of paroxysmal supraventricular tachycardia because of its high efficacy (90–95%) and very short duration of action. It is usually given in a bolus dose of 6 mg followed, if necessary, by a dose of 12 mg. The drug may also be effective in rare patients with ventricular tachycardia. It is less effective in the presence of adenosine receptor blockers such as theophylline or caffeine.

Toxicity

Adenosine causes flushing in about 20% of patients and shortness of breath or chest burning (perhaps related to bronchospasm) in over 10%. Induction of high-grade atrioventricular block may occur but is very brief. Less common toxicities include headache, hypotension, nausea, and paresthesias.

MAGNESIUM

Originally used for patients with digitalis-induced arrhythmias who were hypomagnesemic, magnesium infusion has been found to have antiarrhythmic effects in some patients with normal serum magnesium levels. The mechanisms of these effects are not known, but magnesium is recognized to influence Na^+/K^+ ATPase, sodium channels, certain potassium channels, and calcium channels. Magnesium therapy appears to be indicated in patients with digitalis-induced arrhythmias if hypomagnesemia is present; it is also indicated in some patients with torsade de pointes and in some with acute myocardial infarction even if serum magnesium is normal. The full details of the action and indications of magnesium as an antiarrhythmic drug await further investigation.

POTASSIUM

The significance of the potassium ion concentrations inside and outside the cardiac cell membrane has been discussed earlier in this chapter. Its effects can be summarized as (1) a resting potential depolarizing action and (2) a membrane potential stabilizing action, caused by increased potassium permeability. Hypokalemia results in an increased risk of early and delayed afterdepolarizations, and ectopic pacemaker activity, especially in the presence of digitalis; hyperkalemia is characterized by depression of ectopic pacemakers (severe hyperkalemia is required to suppress the sinoatrial node) and slowing of conduction. Because both insufficient and excess potassium are potentially arrhythmogenic, potassium therapy is directed toward *normalizing* potassium gradients and pools in the body.

III. PRINCIPLES IN THE CLINICAL USE OF ANTIARRHYTHMIC AGENTS

The likelihood that therapy with any drug will be effective depends in part on the relationship between drug doses required to produce a desired therapeutic effect and drug doses associated with toxicity. This margin between efficacy and toxicity is particularly narrow for antiarrhythmic drugs. Therefore, individuals prescribing antiarrhythmic drugs must be thoroughly familiar with the indications, contraindications, risks, and clinical pharmacologic characteristics of each compound they use.

Pretreatment Evaluation

Several important determinations must be made prior to initiation of any antiarrhythmic therapy:

(1) Any factor that might precipitate arrhythmias must be eliminated. These include not only abnormalities of internal homeostasis, such as hypoxia or electrolyte abnormalities (especially hypokalemia or hypomagnesemia), but also drug therapy. Drugs that can precipitate arrhythmias include digitalis, all antiarrhythmic drugs, and many compounds generally not thought to have primary cardiovascular actions. For example, high doses of erythromycin, pentamidine, tricyclic antidepressants, antipsychotics (notably thioridazine), and the "nonsedating" antihista-

mines terfenadine and astemizole have all been associated with the torsade de pointes syndrome described above. Other important reversible causes of arrhythmias include underlying disease states. For example, antiarrhythmic drug therapy for atrial fibrillation is not likely to be effective in hyperthyroidism; rather, the underlying pathophysiology should be addressed with antithyroid maneuvers. Most patients who have arrhythmias have some form of underlying cardiac disease. It is important to separate this abnormal substrate from triggering factors, such as myocardial ischemia or acute cardiac dilation, which may be treatable and reversible.

(2) A firm arrhythmia diagnosis should be established. For example, the misuse of verapamil in patients with ventricular tachycardia mistakenly diagnosed as supraventricular tachycardia can lead to catastrophic hypotension and cardiac arrest. As increasingly sophisticated methods to characterize underlying arrhythmia mechanisms become available and are validated, it may be possible to direct certain drugs toward specific arrhythmia mechanisms.

(3) It is important to establish a reliable baseline upon which to judge the efficacy of any subsequent antiarrhythmic intervention. A number of methods are now available for such baseline quantitation. These include prolonged ambulatory monitoring, electrophysiologic studies that reproduce a target arrhythmia, reproduction of a target arrhythmia by treadmill exercise, or the use of transtelephonic monitoring for recording of sporadic but symptomatic arrhythmias. Whatever the baseline modality chosen, the prescriber should also recognize the phenomenon of "ascertainment" bias: Arrhythmia frequency may fluctuate over months, and patients are most likely to present to a physician when they are symptomatic. Therefore, even a completely ineffective drug intervention may appear to have antiarrhythmic properties.

(4) The mere identification of an abnormality of cardiac rhythm does not necessarily require that the arrhythmia be treated. An excellent justification for conservative treatment was provided by the Cardiac Arrhythmia Suppression Trial (CAST) (see box).

Benefits & Risks

The benefits of antiarrhythmic therapy are actually relatively difficult to establish. Two types of benefits can be envisioned: reduction of arrhythmia-related symptoms, such as palpitations, syncope, or cardiac arrest; or reduction in long-term mortality in asymptomatic patients. Among drugs discussed here, only beta-blockers have been definitely associated with reduction of mortality in relatively asymptomatic patients, and the mechanism underlying this effect is not established (see Chapter 10).

Antiarrhythmic therapy carries with it a number of risks. In some cases, the risk of an adverse reaction is clearly related to high dosages or plasma concentra-

THE CARDIAC ARRHYTHMIA SUPPRESSION TRIAL

Premature ventricular contractions (PVCs) are commonly recorded in patients convalescing from myocardial infarction. Since such arrhythmias have been associated with an increased risk of sudden cardiac death, it had been the empiric practice of many physicians to treat PVCs, even if asymptomatic, in such patients. In CAST (Cardiac Arrhythmia Suppression Trial [CAST] Investigators, 1989; Echt et al, 1991), an attempt was made to document the efficacy of such therapy in a controlled clinical trial. The effects of several antiarrhythmic drugs on arrhythmia frequency were first evaluated in an open-label fashion. Then, patients in whom antiarrhythmic therapy suppressed PVCs were randomly assigned, in a double-blind fashion, to continue that therapy or its corresponding placebo.

The results showed that mortality among patients treated with the drugs flecainide and encainide was *increased* more than twofold compared to those treated with placebo. The mechanism underlying this effect is not known, though an interaction among conduction depression by sodium channel block and chronic or acute myocardial ischemia seems likely. Whatever the mechanism, the important lesson reinforced by CAST was that the decision to initiate any form of drug therapy should be predicated on the knowledge (or at least a reasonable assumption) that any risk is outweighed by real or potential benefit.

tions. Examples include lidocaine-induced tremor or quinidine-induced cinchonism. In other cases, adverse reactions are unrelated to high plasma concentrations (eg, procainamide- or tocainide-induced agranulocytosis). For many serious adverse reactions to antiarrhythmic drugs, the *combination* of drug therapy and the underlying heart disease appears important. For example, patients with advanced conduction system disease are at increased risk for complete heart block during treatment with drugs such as quinidine or flecainide, whereas this risk is very small in patients without conduction system disease. Similarly, the development of congestive heart failure is more common during drug treatment in patients with underlying left ventricular dysfunction. Beta-blockers, verapamil, disopyramide, and flecainide are particularly prone to produce heart failure in this setting.

Several specific syndromes of arrhythmia provocation by antiarrhythmic drugs have also been identified, each with its underlying pathophysiologic mechanism and risk factors. Drugs such as quinidine or sotalol, which act—at least in part—by prolonging cardiac action potentials can result in marked QT prolongation and the distinctive polymorphic ventricular torsade de pointes. Treatment of torsade de pointes requires recognition of the arrhythmia, withdrawal of any offending agent, correction of hypokalemia, and treatment with maneuvers to increase heart rate (pacing or isoproterenol); intravenous magnesium also appears effective, even in patients with normal magnesium levels. Drugs that markedly slow conduction, such as flecainide, or high concentrations of quinidine, can result in an increased frequency of reentrant arrhythmias, notably reentrant ventricular tachycardia in patients with prior myocardial infarction in whom a potential reentrant circuit may be present. Treatment here consists of recognition, withdrawal of the offending agent, and intravenous sodium. Some patients with this form of arrhythmia aggravation cannot be resuscitated, and deaths have been reported. Thus, the prescriber is faced with the paradox that the patient most likely to benefit from antiarrhythmic therapy, such as one with advanced coronary artery disease, conduction system disease, left ventricular dysfunction, and recurrent ventricular tachycardia, is exactly that patient who is at greatest risk for adverse reactions to antiarrhythmic drugs.

In practice, the choice of drug therapies is frequently dictated not so much by expected efficacy but by toxicity profiles. The presence of certain disease states may lead the prescribing clinician away from drugs with certain toxicities and toward other drugs. In addition to left ventricular dysfunction and underlying conduction system disturbances mentioned above, noncardiovascular diseases may also influence the choice of drug therapy. For example, prostatism is a relative contraindication to disopyramide, since the drug commonly causes urinary retention even in normal individuals. It may be difficult in patients with chronic arthritis to detect the development of the procainamide-induced lupus syndrome, and this drug is therefore relatively contraindicated as well. Similarly, it may be difficult to detect amiodarone-induced pulmonary injury in patients with advanced lung disease, so the drug is relatively contraindicated. Moreover, some data suggest that such patients may actually be at increased risk for amiodarone-induced pulmonary injury.

Conduct of Antiarrhythmic Therapy

Once a decision has been made to initiate drug therapy, the next step is to decide whether the arrhythmia is immediately life-threatening. If it is, then the use of loading doses is appropriate. If it is not, loading doses may expose patients to a greater risk of toxicity, do not shorten the time required to achieve steady state, and do not alter the ultimate steady state achieved. Therefore, unless the clinical situation demands it, loading doses should be avoided.

Drug therapy can be considered effective when the target arrhythmia is suppressed (according to the measure used to quantify at baseline) and toxicities are absent. Conversely, drug therapy should not be considered ineffective unless toxicities occur at a time when arrhythmias are not suppressed. Occasionally, arrhythmias may recur at a time when plasma drug concentrations are relatively high but toxicities have not recurred. Under these conditions, the prescriber must decide whether a judicious increase in dose might suppress the arrhythmia and still leave the patient free of toxicity.

Monitoring plasma drug concentrations can be a useful adjunct to managing antiarrhythmic therapy. Widely quoted therapeutic ranges are actually derived from two concentration-response curves. The lower limit of the therapeutic range is defined as a concentration below which clinically important drug actions do not usually occur. The upper limit of the therapeutic range is a concentration beyond which additional drug efficacy is unlikely or toxicities become increasingly frequent. For a specific patient, drug efficacy or adverse effects may occur below the usual lower limit of the therapeutic range; conversely, occasional patients can be effectively treated at plasma concentrations above the upper limit and without adverse effects. Thus, the use of a concentration monitoring strategy mandates that the prescriber be aware of the potential toxicity associated with high concentrations. Plasma drug concentrations are also important in establishing compliance during long-term therapy as well as in detecting drug interactions that may result in very high concentrations at low drug dosages or very low concentrations at high dosages. For some drugs, active metabolites (which may exert pharmacologic actions similar to or different from the parent drug) contribute to a variable extent to drug actions in patients. The presence of such active drug metabolites makes interpretation of data obtained during plasma concentration monitoring particularly difficult and, in some cases, makes routine plasma concentration drug monitoring impractical.

PREPARATIONS AVAILABLE

Sodium Channel Blockers (Class I)
  Amiodarone (Cordarone)
    Oral: 200 mg tablets
  Disopyramide (generic, Norpace)
    Oral: 100, 150 mg capsules;
    Oral controlled-release (generic, Norpace CR): 100, 150 capsules
  Flecainide (Tambocor)
    Oral: 50, 100, 150 mg tablets
  Lidocaine (generic, Xylocaine)
    Parenteral: 100 mg/mL for IM injection; 10, 20 mg/mL for IV injection; 40, 100, 200 mg/mL for IV admixtures; premixed IV (5% D/W) solution
  Mexiletine (Mexitil)
    Oral: 150, 200, 250 mg capsules
  Moricizine (Ethmozine)
    Oral: 200, 250, 300 mg tablets
  Procainamide (generic, Pronestyl, others)
    Oral: 250, 375, 500 mg tablets and capsules
    Oral sustained-release (Procan-SR): 250, 500, 750, 1000 mg tablets
    Parenteral: 100, 500 mg/mL for injection
  Propafenone (Rythmol)
    Oral: 150, 300 mg tablets
  Quinidine sulfate [83% quinidine base] (generic)
    Oral: 200, 300 mg tablets; 300 mg capsules
    Oral sustained-release (Quinidex Extentabs): 300 mg tablets
  Quinidine gluconate [62% quinidine base] (generic)

    Oral sustained-release (Duraquin): 324, 330 mg tablets
    Parenteral: 80 mg/mL for injection
  Quinidine polygalacturonate [60% quinidine base] (Cardioquin)
    Oral: 275 mg tablets
  Tocainide (Tonocard)
    Oral: 400, 600 mg tablets

Beta-Blockers Labeled for Use as Antiarrhythmics (Class II)
  Acebutolol (Sectral)
    Oral: 200, 400 mg capsules
  Esmolol (Brevibloc)
    Parenteral: 10 mg/mL, 250 mg/mL for IV injection
  Propranolol (generic, Inderal)
    Oral: 10, 20, 40, 60, 80, 90 mg tablets; 4 mg/mL, 8 mg/mL solutions; Intensol, 80 mg/mL
    Oral sustained-release: 80, 120, 160 mg capsules
    Parenteral: 1 mg/mL for injection

Potassium Channel Blockers (Class III)
  Amiodarone: see Class I agents
  Bretylium (generic, Bretylol)
    Parenteral: 50 mg/mL for injection
  Sotalol (Betapace)
    Oral: 80, 160, 240 mg capsules

Calcium Channel Blockers (Class IV)
  Verapamil (generic, Calan, Isoptin)
    Oral: 40, 80, 120 mg tablets;

Oral sustained-release (Calan SR, Isoptin SR): 120, 180, 240 mg tablets and capsules

Parenteral: 5 mg/2 mL for injection

Diltiazem (generic, Cardizem; *not labeled for use in arrhythmias*)

Oral: 30, 60, 90, 120 mg tablets

Oral sustained-release: 60, 90, 120, 180, 240, 300 mg capsules

Parenteral: 5 mg/mL for intravenous injection

Bepridil (generic, Vascor; *not labeled for use in arrhythmias*)

Oral: 200, 300, 400 mg tablets

Miscellaneous

Adenosine (Adenocard)

Parenteral: 6 mg/ 2 mL for injection

Magnesium chloride

Parenteral: 1 g/20 min; repeat once if necessary

REFERENCES

Akhtar M et al: CAST and beyond: Implications of the cardiac arrhythmia suppression trial. Circulation 1990; 81:1123.

Akhtar M, Tchou P, Jazayeri M: Use of calcium entry blockers in the treatment of cardiac arrhythmias. Circulation 1989;80 (Suppl IV):IV–31.

Balser JR et al: Suppression of time-dependent outward current in guinea pig ventricular myocytes: Actions of quinidine and amiodarone. Circ Res 1991;69:519.

Belardinelli L, Pelleg A: Cardiac electrophysiology and pharmacology of adenosine. J Cardiovasc Electrophysiol 1990;1:327.

Cardiac Arrhythmia Suppression Trial (CAST) Investigators: Preliminary report: effect of encainide and flecainide on mortality in a randomized trial of arrhythmia suppression after myocardial infarction. N Engl J Med 1989;321:406.

Chabal C et al: The use of oral mexiletine for the treatment of pain after peripheral nerve injury. Anesthesiology 1992;76:513.

Coplen SE et al: Efficacy and safety of quinidine therapy for maintenance of sinus rhythm after cardioversion. Circulation 1990;82:1106.

Costard-Jaeckle A, BingLiem L, Franz MR: Frequency-dependent effect of quinidine, mexiletine, and their combination on postrepolarization refractoriness in vivo. J Cardiovasc Pharmacol 1989;14:810.

DiMarco JP et al: Adenosine for paroxysmal supraventricular tachycardia: Dose ranging and comparison with verapamil. Ann Intern Med 1990;113:104.

Drugs for cardiac arrhythmias. Med Lett Drugs Ther 1989; 31:35.

Echt DS et al for the CAST Investigators: Mortality and morbidity in patients receiving encainide, flecainide, or placebo. N Eng J Med 1991;324:781.

Fitton A, Buckley MT: Moricizine: A review of its pharmacological properties, and therapeutic efficacy in cardiac arrhythmias. Drugs 1990;40:138.

Funck-Brentano C et al: Propafenone. N Engl J Med 1990; 322:518.

Giardina EG, Wechsler ME: Low dose quinidine-mexiletine combination therapy versus quinidine monotherapy for treatment of ventricular arrhythmias. J Am Coll Cardiol 1990;15:1138.

Greene HL: The efficacy of amiodarone in the treatment of ventricular tachycardia or ventricular fibrillation. Prog Cardiovasc Dis 1989;31:319

Hondeghem LM: Molecular interactions of antiarrhythmic agents with their receptor sites. In: *Cardiac Electro-physiology: From Cell to Bedside.* Zipes DP, Jalife J (editors). Saunders, 1990.

Hondeghem LM, Katzung BG: Antiarrhythmic agents: Modulated receptor mechanism of action of sodium and calcium channel-blocking drugs. Annu Rev Pharmacol Toxicol 1984;24:387.

Hondeghem LM: Ideal Antiarrhythmic Agents: Chemical Defibrillators. J Cardiovasc Elec 1991;2:169

Katz AM: Cardiac ion channels. N Engl J Med 1993;328: 1244

Kopelman HA, Horowitz LN: Efficacy and toxicity of amiodarone for the treatment of supraventricular arrhythmias. Prog Cardiovasc Dis 1989;31:355.

Kudenchuk PJ et al: Spontaneous sustained ventricular tachyarrhythmias during treatment with type IA antiarrhythmic agents. Am J Cardiol 1990;65:446.

Latini R, Maggioni AP, Cavalli A: Therapeutic drug monitoring of antiarrhythmic drugs: Rationale and current status. Clin Pharmacokinet 1990;18:91.

Lerman BB, Belardinelli L: Cardiac electrophysiology of adenosine: Basic and clinical concepts. Circulation 1991; 83:1499.

Lesko LJ: Pharmacokinetic drug interactions with amiodarone. Clin Pharmacokinet 1989;17:130.

Levine JH, Morganroth J, Kadish AH: Mechanisms and risk factors for proarrhythmia with type Ia compared with Ic antiarrhythmic drug therapy. Circulation 1989;80:1063.

Mason JW: Amiodarone. N Engl J Med 1987;316:455.

Mason JW: A comparison of seven antiarrhythmic drugs in patients with ventricular tachyarrhythmias. N Engl J Med 1993;329:452.

Mason JW, Hondeghem LM, Katzung BG: Block of inactivated sodium channels and of depolarization-induced automaticity in guinea pig papillary muscles by amiodarone. Circ Res 1984;55:278.

Mason JW, Winkle RA: Accuracy of the ventricular tachycardia-induction study for predicting long-term efficacy and inefficacy of antiarrhythmic drugs. N Engl J Med 1980;303:1073.

Messerli FH (editor): Section 12, Part 2: Specific antiarrhythmic drugs. In: *Cardiovascular Drug Therapy.* Saunders, 1990.

Mitchell LB, Schroeder JS, Mason JW: Comparative clinical electrophysiologic effects of diltiazem, verapamil and nifedipine: A review. Am J Cardiol 1982;49:629.

Myers M et al: Benefits and risks of long-term amiodarone therapy for sustained ventricular tachycardia/fibrillation: Minimum of three-year follow-up in 145 patients. Am Heart J 1990;119:8.

Roden DM, Woosley RL: Flecainide. N Engl J Med 1986;315:361.

Roden DM et al: Clinical features and basic mechanisms of quinidine-induced arrhythmias. J Am Coll Cardiol 1986; 8:73A.

Singh BN, Nademanee K: Sotalol: A beta blocker with unique antiarrhythmic properties. Am Heart J 1987;114: 121.

Snyders D et al: Time-, state-, and voltage-dependent block by quinidine of a cloned human cardiac potassium channel. Mol Pharmacol 1992;41:322.

Stanton MS et al: Arrhythmogenic effects of antiarrhythmic drugs: A study of 506 patients treated for ventricular tachycardia or fibrillation. J Am Coll Cardiol 1989; 14:209.

Stracke H et al: Mexiletine in the treatment of diabetic neuropathy. Diabetes Care 1992;15:1550.

Task Force of the Working Group on Arrhythmias of the European Society of Cardiology: The Sicilian gambit: A new approach to the classification of antiarrhythmic drugs based on their actions on arrhythmogenic mechanisms. Circulation 1991;84:1831.

Tzivoni D et al: Treatment of torsades de pointes with magnesium sulfate. Circulation 1988;77:392.

vanWijk LM et al: Flecainide: Long-term effects in patients with sustained ventricular tachycardia or ventricular fibrillation. J Cardiovasc Pharmacol 1990;15:884.

Wong W et al: Pharmacology of the class III antiarrhythmic agent sematilide in patients with arrhythmias. Am J Cardiol 1992;69:206.

Woods KL et al: Intravenous magnesium sulphate in suspected acute myocardial infarction: Results of the second Leicester Intravenous Magnesium Intervention Trial (LIMIT-2). Lancet 1992;339:1553.

15   Diuretic Agents

Harlan E. Ives, MD, PhD, & David G. Warnock, MD

Abnormalities in fluid volume and electrolyte composition are common and important clinical problems that can become life-threatening. Drugs that block the transport functions of the renal tubules are now widely used in the treatment of these disorders.

Although various agents that increase urine flow have been described since antiquity, it was not until 1957, with the synthesis of chlorothiazide, that a practical and powerful diuretic agent became available for widespread use. Thus, the science of diuretics is relatively new. Technically, the term "diuresis" signifies an increase in urine volume, while "natriuresis" denotes an increase in renal sodium excretion. Because the important natriuretic drugs almost always also increase water excretion, they are usually called diuretics, and the increase in sodium excretion is assumed.

Many diuretic agents (loop diuretics, thiazides, amiloride, and triamterene) exert their effects on specific membrane transport proteins at the luminal surface of renal tubular epithelial cells. Others exert osmotic effects that prevent water reabsorption in the water-permeable segments of the nephron (mannitol), inhibit enzymes (acetazolamide), or interfere with hormone receptors in renal epithelial cells (spironolactone).

For the most part, each diuretic agent acts upon a single anatomic segment of the nephron (Figure 15–1). Because these segments have distinctive transport functions, the actions of each diuretic agent can be best understood in relation to its site of action in the nephron and the normal physiology of that segment. Therefore, the first section of this chapter is devoted to a review of those features of renal tubule physiology that are relevant to diuretic action. The second section is devoted to the basic pharmacology of diuretics, and the third section discusses the clinical applications of these drugs.

RENAL TUBULE TRANSPORT MECHANISMS

PROXIMAL TUBULE

Sodium bicarbonate, sodium chloride, glucose, amino acids, and other organic solutes are preferentially reabsorbed via specific transport systems in the early proximal tubule. Water is reabsorbed passively so as to maintain constant osmolality of proximal tubular fluid. As tubule fluid is processed along the length of the proximal tubule, the luminal concentrations of the solutes decrease relative to the concentration of inulin, an experimental marker that is neither secreted nor absorbed by renal tubules (Figure 15–2). The inulin concentration itself rises owing to water reabsorption by the proximal tubule. Approximately 85% of the filtered sodium bicarbonate, 40% of the sodium chloride, 60% of the water, and virtually all of the filtered organic solutes are reabsorbed in the proximal tubule.

Of the various solutes reabsorbed in the proximal tubule, the most relevant to diuretic action are sodium bicarbonate and sodium chloride. Of the currently available diuretic agents, only one (acetazolamide) acts predominantly in the proximal tubule, and that agent blocks only sodium bicarbonate reabsorption. However, proximal tubule sodium chloride reabsorption is of great theoretical interest. In view of the large quantity of sodium chloride absorbed at this site, a drug that specifically blocked proximal tubule sodium chloride transport might be a particularly powerful diuretic agent.

Sodium bicarbonate reabsorption by the proximal tubule is initiated by the action of a Na^+/H^+ exchanger located in the apical (luminal) membrane of the proximal tubule epithelial cell (Figure 15–3). This transport system allows sodium to enter the cell from the tubular lumen in one-for-one exchange with a proton from inside the cell. As in all portions of the nephron, Na^+/K^+ ATPase in the basolateral membrane pumps

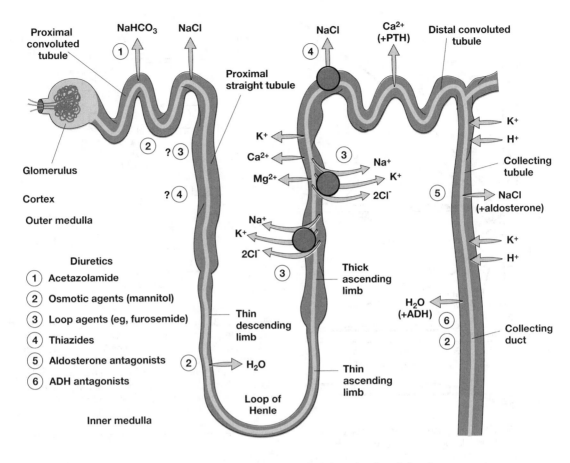

Figure 15–1. Tubule transport systems and sites of action of diuretics.

the reabsorbed Na^+ out of the cells into the interstitium and keeps the intracellular concentration of sodium low. Protons secreted into the lumen combine with bicarbonate to form carbonic acid, H_2CO_3. Carbonic acid, like bicarbonate, is not directly transported by proximal tubule cells. Instead, carbonic acid is dehydrated to CO_2 and H_2O, which readily move across the membranes. This dehydration reaction requires enzymatic catalysis, which is provided by carbonic anhydrase. Carbon dioxide produced by dehydration of carbonic acid enters the proximal tubule cell by simple diffusion and is then rehydrated back to carbonic acid. After dissociation, the H^+ is again available for transport by the Na^+/H^+ exchanger, and the bicarbonate is transported across the basolateral membrane and into the blood by a specific transporter (Figure 15–3). Thus, bicarbonate reabsorption by the proximal tubule is critically dependent upon carbonic anhydrase activity. Carbonic anhydrase is inhibited by an important diuretic: acetazolamide.

In the late proximal tubule, as bicarbonate and organic solutes have been largely removed from the tubular fluid, the residual luminal fluid closely resembles a simple NaCl solution. Under these conditions, Na^+ reabsorption continues, but the proton secreted by the Na^+/H^+ exchanger is no longer titrated by bicarbonate. This causes luminal pH to fall, activating a still poorly defined Cl^-/base exchanger (Figure 15–3). The net effect of parallel Na^+/H^+ exchange and Cl^-/base exchange is NaCl reabsorption. As yet, there are no diuretic agents that are known to act on this process. Thus, diuretic action in the proximal tubule is currently limited to inhibition of sodium bicarbonate reabsorption by carbonic anhydrase inhibitors.

Because of the high water permeability of the proximal tubule, the luminal fluid osmolality and sodium concentration remain relatively constant along the length of the proximal tubule (Figure 15–2). Thus, water is reabsorbed in direct proportion to salt reabsorption in this segment. An experimental impermeant solute like inulin will therefore rise in concentration as water is reabsorbed (Figure 15–2). If large amounts of impermeant solutes, eg, glucose or mannitol are present in the tubular fluid, water reabsorption would cause the concentration of these solutes to

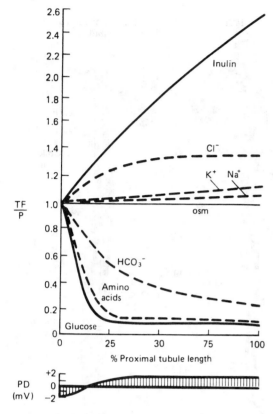

Figure 15–2. Reabsorption of various solutes in the proximal tubule in relation to tubule length. (TF/P, tubular fluid to plasma concentration ratio; PD, potential difference across the tubule.) (Reproduced, with permission, from Ganong WF: *Review of Medical Physiology*, 15th ed. Lange, 1991.)

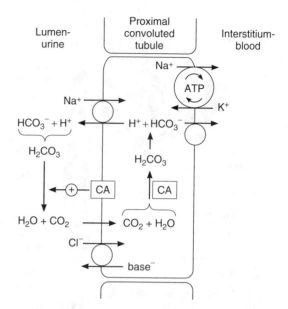

Figure 15–3. Apical membrane Na^+/H^+ exchanger and bicarbonate reabsorption in the proximal convoluted tubule cell. Na^+/K^+ ATPase is present in the basolateral membrane to maintain intracellular sodium and potassium levels within the normal range. Because of rapid equilibration, concentrations of the solutes shown are approximately equal in the interstitial fluid and the blood. Carbonic anhydrase (CA) is found in other locations in addition to the brush border.

rise to the point where osmolality of the tubular fluid is increased and further water reabsorption is blocked. This is the mechanism by which osmotic diuretics act (see below).

Organic acid secretory systems are located in the middle third of the proximal tubule (S_2 segment). These systems secrete a variety of organic acids (uric acid, *p*-aminohippuric acid, diuretics, antibiotics, etc) into the luminal fluid from the blood. Organic base secretory systems (creatinine, procainamide, choline, etc) are localized in the early (S_1) and middle (S_2) segments of the proximal tubule. These systems are important determinants in delivery of diuretics to their active sites at the luminal aspects of tubule segments along the entire nephron. In addition, these sites account for several interactions between diuretics and uric acid or other exogenous organic compounds (eg, interactions between diuretics and probenecid).

LOOP OF HENLE

The thin limb of Henle's loop does not participate in active salt reabsorption, but it does contribute to water reabsorption. Water is extracted from the thin descending limb of the loop of Henle by osmotic forces generated in the hypertonic medullary interstitium. As in the proximal tubule, impermeant solutes like mannitol or glucose in the lumen will oppose water extraction and increase the delivery of water to more distal sites.

The thick ascending limb of the loop of Henle actively reabsorbs NaCl from the lumen (about 35% of the filtered sodium), but unlike the proximal tubule and thin limb, it is extremely impermeable to water. Salt reabsorption in the thick ascending limb therefore dilutes the tubular fluid, leading to its designation as a "diluting segment." Medullary portions of the thick ascending limb contribute to medullary hypertonicity and thereby also play an important role in concentration of urine.

The NaCl transport system in the luminal membrane of the thick ascending limb is a $Na^+/K^+/2Cl^-$ cotransporter (Figure 15–4). This transporter is selectively blocked by diuretic agents known as "loop" diuretics (see below). Although the $Na^+/K^+/2Cl^-$ transporter is itself electrically neutral (two cations and two anions are cotransported), the action of the transporter leads to excess K^+ accumulation within the cell since the Na+/K+ ATPase is also pumping

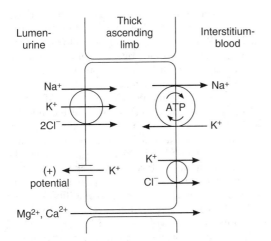

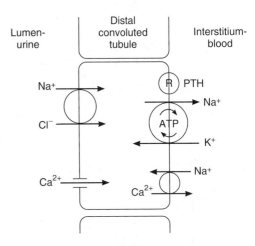

Figure 15–4. Ion transport pathways across the luminal and basolateral membranes of the thick ascending limb cell. The lumen positive electrical potential created by K^+ back diffusion drives divalent cation reabsorption via the paracellular pathway.

Figure 15–5. Ion transport pathways across the luminal and basolateral membranes of the distal convoluted tubule cell. As in all tubular cells, Na^+/K^+ ATPase is present in the basolateral membrane. (R, PTH receptor.)

potassium into the cell (from the basolateral side). This results in back diffusion of K^+ into the tubular lumen, which leads to the development of a lumen-positive electrical potential. This electrical potential provides the driving force for reabsorption of the divalent cations—Mg^{2+} and Ca^{2+}—via the paracellular pathway (between the cells). Thus, inhibition of salt transport in the thick ascending limb by loop diuretics causes an increase in urinary excretion of these divalent cations in addition to NaCl.

DISTAL CONVOLUTED TUBULE

Less NaCl is reabsorbed in the distal convoluted tubule (only about 10% of the filtered NaCl) than in the thick ascending limb. Like the thick ascending limb, this segment is relatively impermeable to water, and the NaCl reabsorption therefore dilutes the tubular fluid. The mechanism of NaCl transport in the distal convoluted tubule is electrically neutral Na^+ and Cl^- cotransport (Figure 15–5), which is pharmacologically distinct from the $Na^+/K^+/2Cl^-$ cotransporter in the thick ascending limb. The NaCl transporter is blocked by diuretics of the thiazide class. Because K^+ does not recycle across the apical membrane of the distal convoluted tubule as it does in the loop of Henle, there is no lumen-positive potential in this segment, and Ca^{2+} and Mg^{2+} are not driven out of the tubular lumen by electrical forces.

However, Ca^{2+} is actively reabsorbed by the distal convoluted tubule epithelial cell via an apical Ca^{2+} channel and basolateral Na^+/Ca^{2+} exchanger (Figure 15–5). This process is regulated by parathyroid hormone. As will be seen below, the differences in the

mechanism of Ca^{2+} transport in the distal convoluted tubule and in the loop of Henle have important implications for the effects of various diuretics on Ca^{2+} transport.

COLLECTING TUBULE

The collecting tubule is responsible for only 2–5% of NaCl reabsorption by the kidney. Despite this seemingly small contribution, the collecting tubule plays a vital role in renal physiology and in diuretic action. As the final site of NaCl reabsorption, the collecting tubule is responsible for determining the final Na^+ concentration of the urine. Furthermore, the collecting tubule (and the late distal tubule) is the site at which mineralocorticoids exert a significant influence, and this segment therefore plays an important role in volume regulation. Lastly, the collecting tubule is the major site of potassium secretion by the kidney and is thus the site at which virtually all diuretic-induced changes in potassium metabolism occur.

The mechanism of NaCl reabsorption in the collecting tubule is distinct from the mechanisms described for the other tubule segments. The **principal cells** are the major sites of Na^+, K^+, and H_2O transport (Figure 15–6), and the **intercalated cells** are the primary sites of proton secretion. Unlike the epithelial cells in the earlier nephron segments, the apical membrane of the collecting tubule principal cells does not contain cotransport systems for Na^+ and other ions. Rather, these membranes exhibit separate ion channels for Na^+ and K^+. Since these channels exclude anions, transport of Na^+ or K^+ leads to a net movement of charge across the membrane. Because the

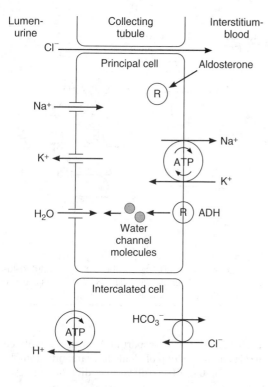

Figure 15–6. Ion and H$_2$O transport pathways across the luminal and basolateral membranes of collecting tubule and collecting duct cells. Inward diffusion of Na$^+$ leaves a lumen-negative potential, which drives reabsorption of Cl$^-$ and efflux of K$^+$. (R, aldosterone or ADH receptor.)

driving force for Na$^+$ entry into the principal cell greatly exceeds that for K$^+$ exit, Na$^+$ reabsorption predominates, and a significant (10–50 mV) lumen-negative electrical potential develops. Na$^+$ that enters the principal cell by this mechanism channel is then transported into the blood via the basolateral Na$^+$/K$^+$ ATPase as in the other nephron segments (Figure 15–6). The lumen-negative electrical potential drives the transport of Cl$^-$ back to the blood via the paracellular pathway and also drives K$^+$ out of the cell through the apical membrane K$^+$ channel. Thus, there is an important relation between Na$^+$ delivery to the collecting tubule and the resulting secretion of K$^+$. Diuretics that act upstream of the collecting tubule will increase Na$^+$ delivery to this site and will enhance K$^+$ secretion. Furthermore, if the Na$^+$ is delivered with an anion such as bicarbonate, which cannot be reabsorbed as readily as Cl$^-$, the lumen-negative potential is increased, and K$^+$ secretion will be even further enhanced. This is the basis for most diuretic-induced K$^+$ wasting, especially when concomitant volume depletion has caused enhanced aldosterone secretion.

Reabsorption of Na$^+$ and its coupled secretion of K$^+$ is regulated by aldosterone. This steroid hormone,

through its actions on gene transcription, increases the activity of both apical membrane channels and the basolateral Na$^+$/K$^+$ ATPase. This leads to an increase in the transepithelial electrical potential, and a dramatic increase in both Na$^+$ reabsorption and K$^+$ secretion (see box, opposite page, and Figure 15–7).

In the absence of antidiuretic hormone (ADH), the collecting tubule (and duct) is impermeable to water, and dilute urine is produced. However, this is the only site in the nephron at which membrane water permeability can be regulated. ADH causes intracellular vesicles containing preformed water channels to fuse with the apical membranes of the principal cells and thus increases the membrane permeability to water (Figure 15–6). ADH secretion is regulated by serum osmolality and by volume status. Thus, practical ADH antagonists would theoretically be very useful drugs for inducing water diuresis. Such agents are not yet available for clinical application.

I. BASIC PHARMACOLOGY OF DIURETIC AGENTS

CARBONIC ANHYDRASE INHIBITORS

Carbonic anhydrase is present in many nephron sites, including the luminal and basolateral membranes, the cytoplasm of the epithelial cells, and the red blood cells in the renal circulation. However, the predominant location of this enzyme is the luminal membrane of the proximal tubule (Figure 15–3), where it catalyzes the dehydration of H$_2$CO$_3$, a critical step in the proximal reabsorption of bicarbonate. Inhibitors of carbonic anhydrase thus block sodium bicarbonate reabsorption, causing sodium bicarbonate diuresis and a reduction in total body bicarbonate stores.

The carbonic anhydrase inhibitors were the forerunners of modern diuretics (see box on page 236). They are unsubstituted sulfonamide derivatives and were developed when it was noted that bacteriostatic sulfonamides caused an alkaline diuresis and hyperchloremic metabolic acidosis. With the development of newer agents, the carbonic anhydrase inhibitors are now rarely used, but there are still several specific applications that will be discussed below.

Chemistry
The structure of acetazolamide is shown in the box on page 236. The –SO$_2$NH$_2$ (sulfonamide) group is essential for activity. Alkyl substitutions at this point completely block the effects on carbonic anhydrase activity.

ELECTRICAL POTENTIAL & POTASSIUM SECRETION

The ability of mineralocorticoids to enhance K^+ secretion via their effect on electrical potential is demonstrated by the experiment shown in Figure 15–7. In adrenalectomized (ADX) rabbits, transepithelial electrical potential (left) is small (5–6 mV) and is not affected by amiloride, a diuretic agent that blocks the apical Na^+ channel (see text). K^+ secretion (right) under these conditions is very low. On the other hand, in animals treated with desoxycorticosterone acetate (DOCA), a mineralocorticoid like aldosterone, the electrical potential falls to –20 mV and K^+ secretion is enhanced sevenfold. The effects of DOCA on electrical potential and K^+ secretion are both completely reversed by blockade of the Na^+ channel with amiloride.

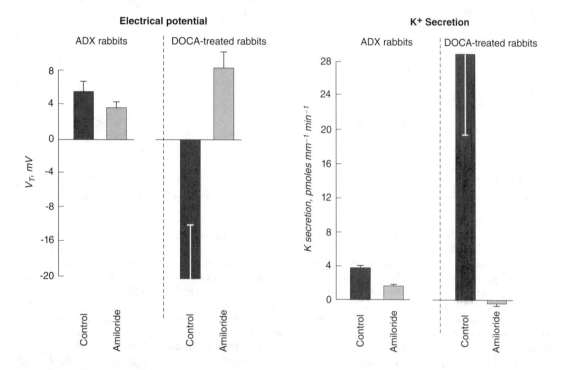

Figure 15–7. Electrical potential and potassium secretion. In adrenalectomized (ADX) rabbits, collecting tubule transepithelial voltage (left, solid bar) is positive and K^+ secretion (right, solid bar) is negligible. When rabbits are treated with a mineralocorticoid (DOCA-treated), voltage changes to –20 mV and K^+ secretion is increased more than sevenfold. The effects of DOCA are completely reversed by amiloride (shaded bars). ADX, adrenalectomized; DOCA, desoxycorticosterone acetate. (Modified and reproduced, with permission, from Wingo CS: Cortical collecting tubule potassium secretion: Effect of amiloride, ouabain, and luminal sodium concentration. Kidney Int 1985;27:886.)

Pharmacokinetics

All of the carbonic anhydrase inhibitors are well absorbed after oral administration. An increase in urine pH from the bicarbonate diuresis is apparent within 30 minutes, maximal at 2 hours, and persists for 12 hours after a single dose. Excretion of the drug is by tubular secretion in the S_2 segment of the proximal tubule, and dosing must for that reason be reduced in renal insufficiency.

Pharmacodynamics

Inhibition of carbonic anhydrase activity profoundly depresses bicarbonate reabsorption in the proximal tubule. At its maximal safely administered dosage, 85% of the bicarbonate reabsorptive capacity of the superficial proximal tubule is inhibited by acetazolamide, with an apparent IC_{50} (concentration for 50% inhibition) of 4 μmol/L. However, some bicarbonate can still be absorbed at other nephron sites by carbonic anhydrase-independent mechanisms. The overall effect of maximal acetazolamide administra-

DEVELOPMENT OF MODERN DIURETICS

Development of the thiazides and other modern diuretics began when a perceptive physician noticed that patients receiving sulfanilamide, an early antimicrobial drug, developed metabolic acidosis and a very alkaline urine. Careful study revealed that the drug was causing sodium bicarbonate diuresis. The realization that this could be a useful diuretic effect led first to the development of acetazolamide and then, by the steps shown below, to the thiazides.

The arrows in the figure indicate historical steps, not chemical reactions. When dichlorphenamide was synthesized as a competitor to acetazolamide, it was found to cause an increased ratio of sodium chloride excretion relative to sodium bicarbonate excretion—a desirable change indicating an action different from (or in addition to) carbonic anhydrase inhibition. Further molecular manipulation led to disulfamoylchloraniline, a weak diuretic but one that was cyclized to chlorothiazide, the first thiazide. This molecule has little effect on carbonic anhydrase and selectively inhibits NaCl reabsorption in the distal tubule. The loop diuretics were subsequently derived from the thiazides.

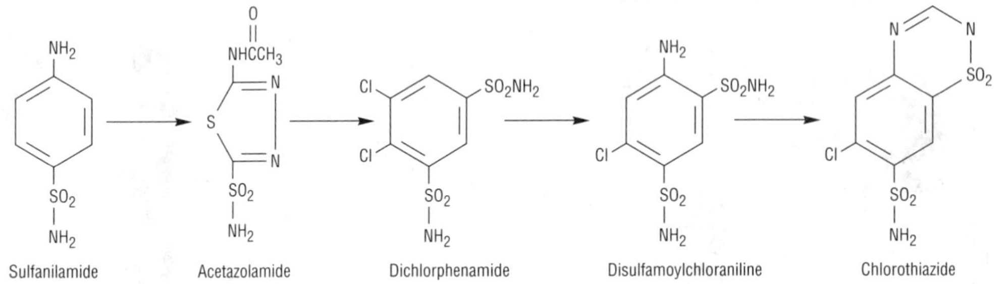

Sulfanilamide — Acetazolamide — Dichlorphenamide — Disulfamoylchloraniline — Chlorothiazide

tion is about 45% inhibition of whole kidney bicarbonate reabsorption. Nevertheless, carbonic anhydrase inhibition causes significant bicarbonate losses, resulting in hyperchloremic metabolic acidosis. Because of the toxicity of this acidosis and the fact that HCO_3^- depletion leads to enhanced NaCl reabsorption by the remaining tubule segments in the nephron, the diuretic effectiveness of acetazolamide decreases significantly with use over several days.

The major clinical applications of acetazolamide involve carbonic anhydrase-dependent bicarbonate transport at sites other than the kidney. The ciliary body of the eye secretes bicarbonate into the aqueous humor by a process similar to the reabsorption of bicarbonate from proximal tubular fluid. The only difference is that the process is reversed—bicarbonate is removed from the blood by the ciliary body and returned to the blood in the proximal tubule. Likewise, formation of cerebrospinal fluid by the choroid plexus involves bicarbonate secretion into the cerebrospinal fluid. Although these processes are in the opposite direction from that in the proximal tubule, they are equally well inhibited by carbonic anhydrase inhibitors, which in both cases dramatically alter the pH and quantity of fluid produced.

Clinical Indications & Dosage
(See Table 15–1)

A. Glaucoma: Inhibition of carbonic anhydrase decreases the rate of aqueous humor formation, thus causing a decrease in intraocular pressure. This effect is of value in both the acute and chronic management of several forms of glaucoma, making it the most common indication for use of carbonic anhydrase inhibitors. Topically active carbonic anhydrase inhibitors for use in glaucoma have been under development for some time but are not yet available.

B. Urinary Alkalinization: Uric acid and cystine are relatively insoluble in acidic urine, and enhanced renal excretion can be achieved by increasing urinary pH with carbonic anhydrase inhibitors. Similarly, renal excretion of weak acids (eg, aspirin) is enhanced by acetazolamide. In the absence of continuous bicarbonate administration, these effects of acetazolamide are of relatively short duration and are only useful in the initiation of a response. Prolonged therapy requires concomitant bicarbonate administration.

C. Metabolic Alkalosis: In most cases, maintenance of metabolic alkalosis is a consequence of decreased total body K^+ and intravascular volume, or of

Table 15–1. Carbonic anhydrase inhibitors used in treatment of glaucoma.	
	Usual Oral Dose (1–4 Times Daily)
Acetazolamide	250 mg
Dichlorphenamide	50 mg

high levels of mineralocorticoids. It is therefore treated by correction of these underlying conditions and not with acetazolamide. However, when the alkalosis is due to excessive use of diuretics in patients with severe heart failure, saline administration may be contraindicated because of elevated cardiac filling pressures. In these cases, acetazolamide can be useful in correcting the alkalosis as well as producing a small additional diuresis for the correction of heart failure. Acetazolamide has also been used to rapidly correct the metabolic alkalosis that may develop in the setting of respiratory acidosis.

D. Acute Mountain Sickness: Weakness, dizziness, insomnia, headache, and nausea can occur in mountain travelers who rapidly ascend above 3000 m. The symptoms are usually mild and last for a few days. In more serious cases, rapidly progressing pulmonary or cerebral edema can be life-threatening. By decreasing cerebrospinal fluid formation and by decreasing the pH of the cerebrospinal fluid and brain, acetazolamide can enhance performance status and diminish symptoms of mountain sickness. Prophylaxis can be achieved by starting oral acetazolamide 24 hours before the ascent. One study (Zell, 1988) recommended against routine prophylaxis for recreational hikers because the symptoms are usually mild.

E. Other Uses: Carbonic anhydrase inhibitors have been used as adjuvants for the treatment of epilepsy, in some forms of hypokalemic periodic paralysis, and to increase urinary phosphate excretion during severe hyperphosphatemia.

Toxicity

A. Hyperchloremic Metabolic Acidosis: Acidosis predictably results from chronic reduction of body bicarbonate stores by carbonic anhydrase inhibitors. Bicarbonate wasting limits the diuretic efficacy of these drugs to 2 or 3 days.

B. Renal Stones: Phosphaturia and hypercalciuria occur during the bicarbonaturic response to carbonic anhydrase inhibition. Renal excretion of solubilizing factors (eg, citrate) may also decline with chronic use. Calcium salts are relatively insoluble at alkaline pH, which means that the potential for renal stone formation from these salts is enhanced.

C. Renal Potassium Wasting: Potassium wasting can occur because $NaHCO_3$ presented to the collecting tubule causes an increase in the lumen-negative electrical potential in that segment and enhances K^+ excretion. This effect can be prevented by simultaneous administration of KCl.

D. Other Toxicities: Drowsiness and paresthesias are common following large doses. These agents accumulate in patients with renal failure, and central nervous system toxicity can be marked in this setting. Hypersensitivity reactions (fever, rashes, bone marrow suppression, interstitial nephritis) can also occur.

Contraindications

Carbonic anhydrase inhibitors should be avoided in hepatic cirrhosis. Alkalinization of the urine will decrease urinary trapping—and thus excretion—of NH_4^+ and may contribute to the development of hepatic encephalopathy.

LOOP DIURETICS

Loop diuretics selectively inhibit NaCl reabsorption in the thick ascending limb of the loop of Henle. Owing to the large NaCl absorptive capacity of this segment and the fact that diuresis is not limited by development of acidosis, as it is with the carbonic anhydrase inhibitors, these drugs are the most efficacious diuretic agents available.

Chemistry

The two prototypical drugs of this group are furosemide and ethacrynic acid. The structures of several loop diuretics are shown in Figure 15–8. Like the carbonic anhydrase inhibitors, furosemide and bumetanide are sulfonamide derivatives. These agents have a carboxyl group with a sulfamoyl moiety in the meta position (carbon number 5). A halide or phenoxy substitution is present at carbon 4, and a substituted amino group is present at carbon 2 or 3. Torsemide, a newer loop diuretic, is another sulfonamide derivative.

Ethacrynic acid—not a sulfonamide derivative—is chemically distinct from furosemide. It is a phenoxyacetic acid derivative containing an adjacent ketone and methylene group (Figure 15–8). The methylene group (shaded) forms an adduct with the free sulfhydryl group of cysteine. The cysteine adduct appears to be the active form of the drug.

Organic mercurial diuretics inhibit salt transport in the thick ascending limb. They are no longer used because of their high toxicity and are of only historical interest.

Pharmacokinetics

The loop agents are rapidly absorbed. They are eliminated by renal secretion as well as by glomerular filtration. Diuretic response is extremely rapid following intravenous injection. The duration of effect is usually 2–3 hours. Half-life is dependent on renal function. Since furosemide acts on the luminal side of the tubule, the diuretic response correlates positively with its excretion in the urine. Defects in the secretory component of its clearance may result from simultaneous administration of agents such as indomethacin and probenecid, which inhibit weak acid secretion in the proximal tubule. Metabolites of ethacrynic acid and furosemide have been identified, but it is not known if they have any diuretic activity. Torsemide has a somewhat longer half-life and duration of action than furosemide or bumetanide. It has at least one ac-

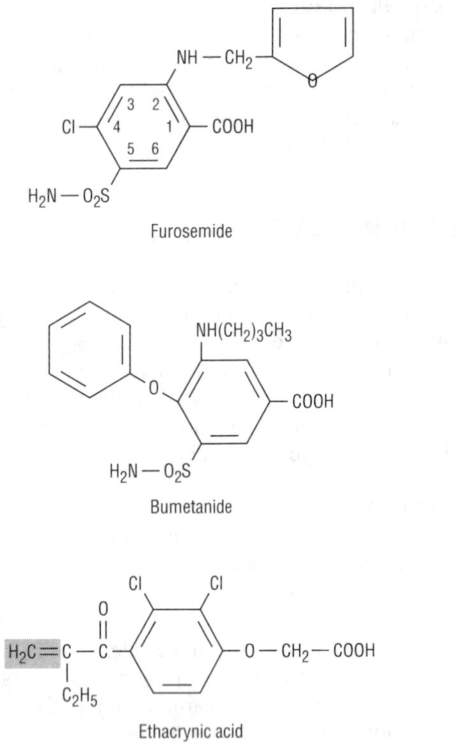

Furosemide

Bumetanide

Ethacrynic acid

Figure 15–8. Loop diuretics. The shaded methylene group on ethacrynic acid is reactive and may combine with free sulfhydryl groups.

tive metabolite with a considerably longer half-life than that of the parent compound.

Pharmacodynamics

These drugs inhibit the coupled $Na^+/K^+/2Cl^-$ transport system in the luminal membrane of the thick ascending limb of Henle's loop. By inhibiting this transporter, the loop diuretics reduce the reabsorption of NaCl and also diminish the normal lumen-positive potential that derives from K^+ recycling (Figure 15–4). This electrical potential normally drives divalent cation reabsorption in the loop. Loop diuretics, by abolishing the lumen-positive potential, cause an increase in Mg^{2+} and Ca^{2+} excretion. Prolonged use can cause significant hypomagnesemia in some patients. Since Ca^+ is actively reabsorbed in the distal convoluted tubule, loop diuretics do not generally cause hypocalcemia. However, in disorders that cause hypercalcemia, Ca^{2+} excretion can be greatly enhanced by combining loop agents with saline infusions. This effect is of great value in the acute management of hypercalcemia.

In addition to their diuretic activity, loop agents appear to have direct effects on blood flow through several vascular beds. The mechanisms for this action are not well defined. Furosemide increases renal blood

flow and causes redistribution of blood flow within the renal cortex. Furosemide and ethacrynic acid have also been shown to relieve pulmonary congestion and reduce left ventricular filling pressures in congestive heart failure before a measurable increase in urinary output occurs, and in anephric patients.

Clinical Indications & Dosage (Table 15–2)

The most important indications for the use of the loop diuretics include acute pulmonary edema, other edematous conditions, and acute hypercalcemia. The use of these drugs in these conditions is discussed below in the section on clinical pharmacology. Other indications for which the loop diuretics are useful include the following.

A. Hyperkalemia: In mild hyperkalemia—or after acute management of severe hyperkalemia—loop diuretics can significantly enhance urinary excretion of K^+ as a means of reducing total body K^+ stores. This response is enhanced by simultaneous NaCl and water administration.

B. Acute Renal Failure: Loop agents can increase the rate of urine flow and enhance K^+ excretion in acute renal failure. These drugs may convert oliguric renal failure to nonoliguric failure, which facilitates management of the patient. However, they do not seem to shorten the duration of renal failure. If a large pigment load has precipitated acute renal failure or threatens to do so, loop agents may help flush out intratubular casts and ameliorate intratubular obstruction. On the other hand, loop agents can theoretically worsen cast formation in myeloma and light chain nephropathy.

C. Anion Overdose: Bromide, fluoride, and iodide are all reabsorbed in the thick ascending limb; loop diuretics are therefore useful in treating toxic ingestions of these ions. Saline solution must be administered to replace urinary losses of Na^+ and to provide Cl^-, so as to avoid extracellular fluid volume depletion.

Toxicity

A. Hypokalemic Metabolic Alkalosis: Loop diuretics increase delivery of salt and water to the collecting duct and thus enhance the renal secretion of K^+ and H^+, causing hypokalemic metabolic alkalosis. This toxicity is a function of the magnitude of the diu-

Table 15–2. Loop diuretics: Dosages[1].	
Drug	**Daily Oral Dose**
Bumetanide	0.5–2 mg
Ethacrynic acid	50–200 mg
Furosemide	20–80 mg
Torsemide	2.5–20 mg

[1]As single dose or in two divided doses

retic effect and can be reversed by K^+ replacement and correction of hypovolemia.

B. Ototoxicity: The loop diuretics can cause dose-related hearing loss that is usually reversible. It is most common in patients who have diminished renal function or who are also receiving other ototoxic agents such as aminoglycoside antibiotics.

C. Hyperuricemia: Loop diuretics can cause hyperuricemia and precipitate attacks of gout. This is caused by hypovolemia-associated enhancement of uric acid reabsorption in the proximal tubule. It may be avoided by using lower doses of the diuretic.

D. Hypomagnesemia: Magnesium depletion is a predictable consequence of the chronic use of loop agents and occurs most often in patients with dietary deficiency of magnesium. It can be readily reversed by administration of oral magnesium preparations.

E. Allergic Reactions: Skin rash, eosinophilia, and, less often, interstitial nephritis are occasional side effects of furosemide therapy. These usually resolve rapidly after drug withdrawal. Allergic reactions are probably related to the sulfonamide moiety; they are much less common with ethacrynic acid.

F. Other Toxicities: Even more than other diuretics, loop agents can cause severe dehydration. Hyponatremia is less common than with the thiazides (see below) because loop agents diminish maximal concentrating ability. Nevertheless, patients who increase water intake in response to hypovolemia-induced thirst can become severely hyponatremic with loop agents. Loop agents are known for their calciuric effect, but hypercalcemia can occur, generally in patients who become severely dehydrated and who have another, previously occult, cause for hypercalcemia, such as an oat cell carcinoma of the lung.

Contraindications

Furosemide and bumetanide may demonstrate cross-reactivity in patients who are sensitive to other sulfonamides. Overzealous use of any diuretic is dangerous in hepatic cirrhosis, borderline renal failure, or congestive heart failure (see below).

THIAZIDES

The thiazide diuretics emerged during efforts to synthesize more potent carbonic anhydrase inhibitors (see box: Development of Modern Diuretics). It subsequently became clear that the thiazides inhibit NaCl transport independently of their effect on carbonic anhydrase activity and that they act on salt transport in the distal convoluted tubule. Some members of this group retain significant carbonic anhydrase inhibitory activity, but this effect is not related to the primary mode of action.

Chemistry

The drugs in this group are formally called benzothiadiazides, usually shortened to thiazides. The nature of the heterocyclic rings and the substitutions on these rings may vary among the congeners, but all of them retain, in common with the carbonic anhydrase inhibitors, an unsubstituted sulfonamide group (Figure 15–9).

Pharmacokinetics

All of the thiazides are absorbed when given orally, but there are differences in their metabolism. Chlorothiazide, the parent of the group, is less lipid-soluble and must be given in relatively large doses. Chlorthalidone is slowly absorbed and has a longer duration of action. Although indapamide is excreted primarily by the biliary system, enough of the active form is cleared by the kidney to exert its diuretic effect in the distal convoluted tubule.

All of the thiazides are secreted by the organic acid secretory system and compete to some extent with the secretion of uric acid by that system. As a result, the uric acid secretory rate may be reduced, with a concomitant elevation in serum uric acid level. In the steady state, uric acid production and therefore renal excretion are not affected by the thiazides.

Pharmacodynamics

Thiazides inhibit NaCl reabsorption from the luminal side of epithelial cells in the distal convoluted tubule. There may also be a small effect on NaCl reabsorption in the late proximal tubule, but this is not observed in the usual clinical setting.

Relatively little is known about the NaCl transport system that is inhibited by thiazides. As described above (under Distal Convoluted Tubule), the mode of transport appears to be an electrically neutral NaCl cotransporter that is distinct from the transporter in the loop of Henle. There is also an active reabsorptive process for Ca^{2+} in the distal convoluted tubule, which is modulated by parathyroid hormone (PTH) (Figure 15–5). In contrast to the situation in the loop of Henle, where loop diuretics inhibit Ca^{2+} reabsorption, thiazides actually enhance Ca^{2+} reabsorption in the distal convoluted tubule. The mechanism for this enhancement is not known, but it has been postulated to result from a lowering of cell Na^+ upon blockade of Na^+ entry by thiazides. The lower cell Na^+ might then enhance Na^+/Ca^{2+} exchange in the basolateral membrane (Figure 15–5), increasing overall reabsorption of Ca^{2+}. While thiazides rarely cause hypercalcemia as the result of this enhanced reabsorption, they can unmask hypercalcemia due to other causes (eg, hyperparathyroidism, carcinoma, sarcoidosis). Thiazides have proved useful in the treatment of kidney stones caused by hypercalciuria.

Clinical Indications & Dosage
(See Table 15–3)

The major indications for thiazide diuretics are (1) hypertension, (2) congestive heart failure, (3) neph-

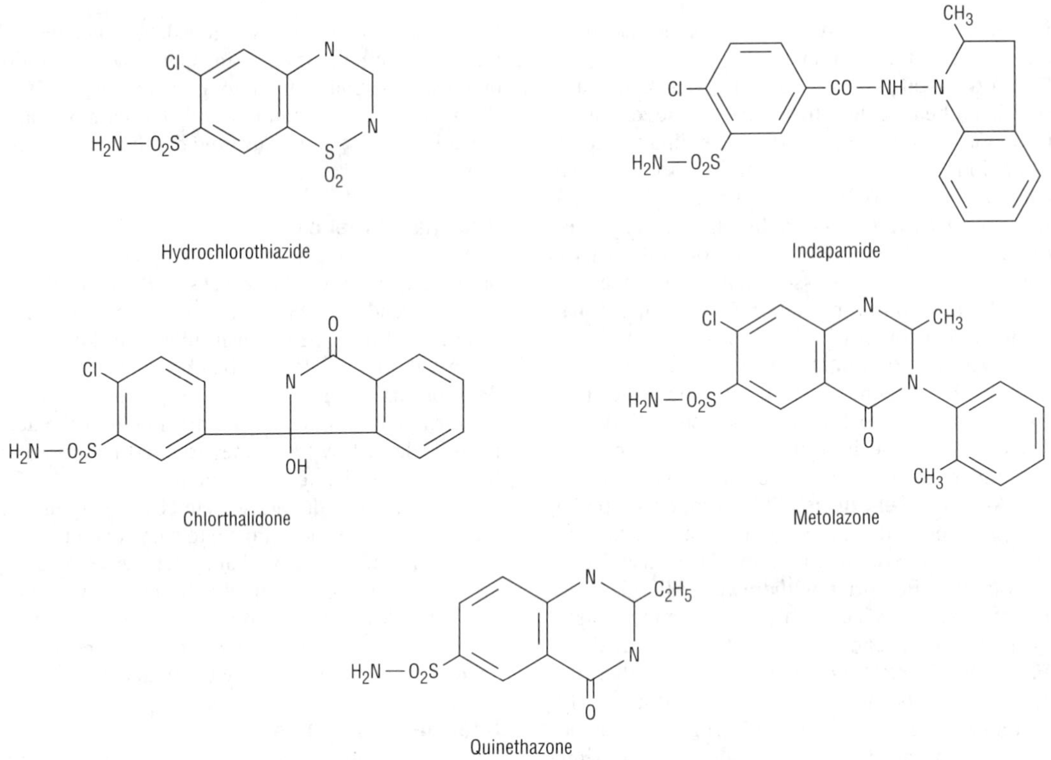

Figure 15–9. Hydrochlorothiazide and related agents.

rolithiasis due to idiopathic hypercalciuria, and (4) nephrogenic diabetes insipidus. Use of the thiazides in each of these conditions is described below in the section on clinical pharmacology.

Toxicity

A. Hypokalemic Metabolic Alkalosis and Hyperuricemia: These toxicities are similar to those observed with loop diuretics (see above).

B. Impaired Carbohydrate Tolerance: Hyperglycemia may occur in patients who are overtly dia-

betic or who have even mildly abnormal glucose tolerance tests. The effect is due both to impaired pancreatic release of insulin and to diminished tissue utilization of glucose. Hyperglycemia may be partially reversible with correction of hypokalemia.

C. Hyperlipidemia: Thiazides cause a 5–15% increase in serum cholesterol and increased low-density lipoproteins (LDL). These levels may come down toward baseline after prolonged use.

D. Hyponatremia: Hyponatremia is an important adverse effect of thiazide diuretics and can on rare occasions be life-threatening. It is due to a combination of hypovolemia-induced elevation of ADH, reduction in the diluting capacity of the kidney, and increased thirst. It can be prevented by reducing the dose of the drug or limiting water intake.

E. Allergic Reactions: The thiazides are sulfonamides and share cross-reactivity with other members of this chemical group. Photosensitivity or generalized dermatitis occurs rarely. Serious allergic reactions are extremely rare but do include hemolytic anemia, thrombocytopenia, and acute necrotizing pancreatitis.

F. Other Toxicities: Weakness, fatigability, and paresthesias may be similar to those of carbonic anhydrase inhibitors. Impotence has been reported but is probably related to volume depletion.

Table 15–3. Thiazides and related diuretics: Dosages.

	Daily Oral Dose	Frequency of Dosage
Bendroflumethiazide	2.5–10 mg	As single dose
Benzthiazide	25–100 mg	In 2 divided doses
Chlorothiazide	0.5–1 g	In 2 divided doses
Chlorthalidone[1]	50–100 mg	As single dose
Hydrochlorothiazide	25–100 mg	As single dose
Hydroflumethiazide	25–100 mg	In 2 divided doses
Indapamide[1]	2.5–10 mg	As single dose
Methyclothiazide	2.5–10 mg	As single dose
Metolazone[1]	2.5–10 mg	As single dose
Polythiazide	1–4 mg	As single dose
Quinethazone[1]	50–100 mg	As single dose
Trichlormethiazide	2–8 mg	As single dose

[1]Not a thiazide but a sulfonamide qualitatively similar to the thiazides.

Contraindications

Overzealous use of any diuretic is dangerous in hepatic cirrhosis, borderline renal failure, or congestive heart failure (see below).

POTASSIUM-SPARING DIURETICS

The members of this group antagonize the effects of aldosterone at the cortical collecting tubule and late distal tubule. Inhibition may occur by direct pharmacologic antagonism of mineralocorticoid receptors (**spironolactone**) or by inhibition of Na^+ transport through ion channels in the luminal membrane (**triamterene, amiloride**). Lesser potassium-sparing effects are occasionally seen with drugs that suppress renin or angiotensin II generation (nonsteroidal anti-inflammatory agents, beta-blockers, converting enzyme inhibitors).

Chemistry & Pharmacokinetics

Spironolactone is a synthetic steroid that acts as a competitive antagonist to aldosterone. Its onset and duration of action are therefore determined by the kinetics of aldosterone response in the target tissue. Substantial inactivation of spironolactone occurs in the liver. The overall result is a rather slow onset of action, requiring several days before full therapeutic effect is achieved.

Triamterene is metabolized in the liver, but renal excretion is a major route of elimination for the active form and the metabolites. Very little is known about the diuretic effects of the metabolites. Amiloride is excreted unchanged in the urine. Because triamterene is extensively metabolized, it has a shorter half-life and must be given more frequently than amiloride. The structures of spironolactone, triamterene, and amiloride are shown in Figure 15–10.

Pharmacodynamics

The potassium-sparing diuretics reduce Na^+ absorption in the collecting tubules and ducts. Na^+ absorption (and K^+ secretion) at this site is regulated by aldosterone. At any given rate of Na^+ delivery, the rate of distal K^+ secretion is positively correlated with the aldosterone level. As described above, aldosterone enhances K^+ secretion by increasing Na^+/K^+ ATPase activity and Na^+ and K^+ channel activities. Na^+ absorption in the collecting tubule generates a lumen-negative electrical potential, which enhances K^+ secretion. Aldosterone antagonists interfere with this process. Similar effects are observed with respect to H^+ handling by the collecting tubule, in part explaining the metabolic acidosis seen with aldosterone antagonists.

Spironolactone is a synthetic steroid that binds to cytoplasmic mineralocorticoid receptors and prevents translocation of the receptor complex to the nucleus in the target cell. Its structure is shown in Figure 15–

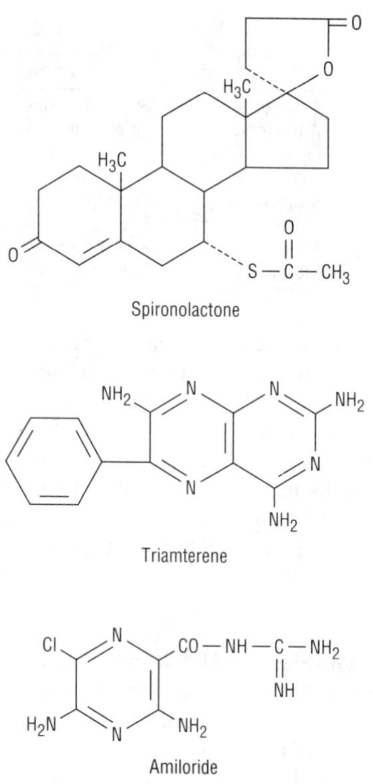

Figure 15–10. Aldosterone antagonists.

10. The drug may also reduce the intracellular formation of active metabolites of aldosterone by inhibition of 5α-reductase activity. Triamterene and amiloride do not block the aldosterone receptor but instead directly interfere with Na^+ entry through the sodium-selective ion channels in the apical membrane of the collecting tubule. Since K^+ secretion is coupled with Na^+ entry in this segment, these agents are also effective K^+-sparing diuretics.

Other Potassium-Sparing Agents

Converting enzyme inhibitors are discussed in Chapters 11 and 17. Although not used therapeutically as potassium-sparing diuretics, these agents do antagonize the effects of aldosterone by interfering with its secretion and are often associated with hyperkalemia.

Clinical Indications & Dosage
(See Table 15–4)

These agents are most useful in states of mineralocorticoid excess, due either to primary hypersecretion (Conn's syndrome, ectopic ACTH production) or to secondary aldosteronism. Secondary aldosteronism results from congestive heart failure, hepatic cirrhosis, nephrotic syndrome, and other conditions associated with renal salt retention and diminished effective intravascular volume. Use of other diuretics, like

Table 15–4. Potassium-sparing diuretics and combination preparations.

Trade Name	Potassium-Sparing Agent	Hydrochlorothiazide	Frequency of Dosage
Aldactazide	Spironolactone 25 mg	25 mg	1–4 times daily
Aldactone	Spironolactone 25 mg	. . .	1–4 times daily
Dyazide	Triamterene 50 mg	25 mg	1–4 times daily
Dyrenium	Triamterene 100 mg	. . .	1–3 times daily
Maxzide	Triamterene 75 mg	50 mg	Once daily
Maxzide-25 mg	Triamterene 37.5 mg	25 mg	Once daily
Midamor	Amiloride 5 mg	. . .	Once daily
Moduretic	Amiloride 5 mg	50 mg	Once or twice daily

thiazides or loop agents, can cause or exacerbate volume contraction and thus intensify secondary aldosteronism. In the setting of enhanced mineralocorticoid secretion and continuing delivery of Na^+ to distal nephron sites, renal K^+ wasting occurs. This is due to K^+ secretion by the collecting tubule. K^+-sparing diuretics of either type are used in this setting to blunt the K^+ secretory response and prevent depletion of the intracellular K^+ stores.

Toxicity

A. Hyperkalemia: Unlike other diuretics, these agents can cause mild, moderate, or even life-threatening hyperkalemia. The risk of this complication is greatly increased in the presence of renal disease or of other drugs that reduce renin (beta-blockers, NSAIDs) or angiotensin II (ACE inhibitors). Since most other diuretic agents lead to K^+ losses, hyperkalemia is more common when aldosterone antagonists are used as the sole diuretic agent, especially in patients with renal insufficiency. With fixed-dosage combinations of potassium-sparing and thiazide diuretics, there may be a fairly even balance, so that both the hypokalemia and the metabolic alkalosis due to the thiazide are ameliorated by the aldosterone antagonist. However, owing to variations in the bioavailability of the components of some of the fixed-dosage forms, the thiazide-associated adverse effects may predominate (eg, metabolic alkalosis, hyponatremia). For these reasons, it is generally preferable to adjust the doses of the two drugs separately.

B. Hyperchloremic Metabolic Acidosis: By inhibiting H^+ secretion in parallel with K^+ secretion, the potassium-sparing diuretics can cause acidosis similar to that seen with type IV renal tubular acidosis.

C. Gynecomastia: Synthetic steroids may cause endocrine abnormalities by effects on other steroid receptors. Gynecomastia and other adverse effects (impotence, benign prostatic hypertrophy) have been reported with spironolactone.

D. Acute Renal Failure: The combination of triamterene with indomethacin has been reported to cause acute renal failure. This has not yet been reported with other potassium-sparing agents.

E. Kidney Stones: Triamterene is poorly soluble and may precipitate in the urine, causing kidney stones.

Contraindications

These agents can cause severe, even fatal hyperkalemia in susceptible patients. Oral K^+ administration should be discontinued if aldosterone antagonists are administered. Patients with chronic renal insufficiency are especially vulnerable and should rarely be treated with aldosterone antagonists. Concomitant use of other agents that blunt the renin-angiotensin system (beta-blockers or ACE inhibitors) increases the likelihood of hyperkalemia. Patients with liver disease may have impaired metabolism of triamterene and spironolactone, and dosing must be carefully adjusted.

AGENTS THAT ENHANCE WATER EXCRETION

OSMOTIC DIURETICS

The proximal tubule and descending limb of Henle's loop are freely permeable to water. An osmotic agent that is not transported causes water to be retained in these segments and promotes a water diuresis. One such agent, mannitol, is used mainly to reduce increased intracranial pressure, but it is occasionally used to promote prompt removal of renal toxins, which may be required in acute hemolysis or after use of radiocontrast agents.

Pharmacokinetics

Mannitol is not metabolized and is handled primarily by glomerular filtration, without any important tubular reabsorption or secretion. By definition, osmotic diuretics are poorly absorbed, which means that they must be given parenterally. Mannitol is excreted by glomerular filtration within 30–60 minutes. If administered orally, mannitol causes osmotic diarrhea. This effect can be used to potentiate the effects of potassium-binding resins or eliminate toxic substances from the gastrointestinal tract in conjunction with activated charcoal (see Chapter 60).

Pharmacodynamics

Osmotic diuretics limit water reabsorption primarily in those segments of the nephron that are freely permeable to water: the proximal tubule and the descending limb of the loop of Henle. The presence of a nonreabsorbable solute such as mannitol prevents the normal absorption of water by interposing a countervailing osmotic force. As a result, urine volume increases in conjunction with mannitol excretion. The concomitant increase in urine flow rates decreases the contact time between fluid and the tubular epithelium, thus reducing Na^+ reabsorption. However, the resulting natriuresis is of lesser magnitude than the water diuresis, leading eventually to hypernatremia.

Clinical Indications & Dosage

A. To Increase Urine Volume: Osmotic diuretics are used to increase water excretion in preference to sodium excretion. This effect can be useful when renal hemodynamics are compromised or when avid Na^+ retention limits the response to conventional agents. It can be used to maintain urine volume and to prevent anuria that might otherwise result from presentation of large pigment loads to the kidney (eg, hemolysis or rhabdomyolysis). Some oliguric patients do not respond to an osmotic diuretic. Therefore, a test dose of mannitol (12.5 g intravenously) should be given prior to starting a continuous infusion. Mannitol should not be continued unless there is an increase in urine flow rate to more than 50 mL/h during the 3 hours following the test dose. If there is a response, mannitol administration (12.5–25 g) can be repeated in 1–2 hours to maintain urine flow rate greater than 100 mL/h. Prolonged use of mannitol is not advised.

B. Reduction of Intracranial and Intraocular Pressure: Osmotic diuretics reduce total body water more than total body cation content and thus reduce intracellular volume. This effect is used to reduce intracranial pressure in neurologic conditions and to reduce intraocular pressure before ophthalmologic procedures. A dose of 1–2 g/kg mannitol is administered intravenously. Intracranial pressure, which must be monitored, should fall in 60–90 minutes.

Toxicity

A. Extracellular Volume Expansion: Mannitol is rapidly distributed in the extracellular compartment and extracts water from the intracellular compartment. Initially, this leads to expansion of the extracellular fluid volume and hyponatremia. This effect can complicate congestive heart failure and may produce florid pulmonary edema. Headache, nausea, and vomiting are commonly observed in patients treated with osmotic diuretics.

B. Dehydration and Hypernatremia: Excessive use of mannitol without adequate water replacement can ultimately lead to severe dehydration, free water losses, and hypernatremia. This complication can be avoided by careful attention to serum ion composition and fluid balance.

ADH ANTAGONISTS

A variety of medical conditions, eg, tumors that secrete ADH-like peptides, cause water retention as the result of ADH excess. Unfortunately, specific ADH antagonists are still available only for investigational purposes. Two nonselective agents, Li^+ and demeclocycline, are of limited use in a few specific situations.

Pharmacokinetics

ADH antagonists currently available include Li^+ salts and tetracycline derivatives (demeclocycline). Both are orally active. Lithium is reabsorbed to some extent in the proximal tubule and thereafter is neither secreted nor absorbed. Demeclocycline is metabolized in the liver.

Pharmacodynamics

ADH antagonists inhibit the effects of ADH at the collecting tubule. While the mechanisms by which Li^+ and demeclocycline exert this action have never been conclusively demonstrated, it appears that both agents act to reduce the formation of cAMP in response to ADH and also to interfere with the actions of cAMP in the collecting tubule cells.

Clinical Indications & Dosage

A. Syndrome of Inappropriate ADH Secretion (SIADH): ADH antagonists are clinically used to manage SIADH when water restriction has failed to correct the abnormality. This generally occurs in the outpatient setting, where water restriction cannot be enforced, or in the hospital when large quantities of intravenous fluid are administered with drugs. Lithium carbonate has been used to treat this syndrome, but the response is unpredictable. Serum levels of Li^+ must be monitored closely, as serum concentrations greater than 1 mmol/L are toxic. Demeclocycline, in dosages of 600–1200 mg/d, yields a more predictable result and is less toxic. Appropriate plasma levels (2 μg/mL) can be approximated by using standard determinations of plasma tetracyclines.

B. Other Causes of Elevated ADH: ADH is also elevated in response to diminished effective circulating blood volume. When treatment by volume replacement is not possible, as in heart failure or liver disease, hyponatremia may result. As for SIADH, water restriction is the treatment of choice, but if it is not successful, demeclocycline may be considered.

Toxicity

A. Nephrogenic Diabetes Insipidus: If serum Na^+ is not monitored closely, SIADH can be replaced with nephrogenic diabetes insipidus, and severe hypernatremia can result. If Li^+ is being used primarily for an affective disorder, nephrogenic diabetes insipidus can be treated with a thiazide diuretic or amiloride (see below).

B. Renal Failure: Both Li^+ and demeclocycline

have been reported to cause acute renal failure. Long-term Li^+ therapy also causes chronic interstitial nephritis.

C. Other: Adverse effects associated with Li^+ therapy include tremulousness, mental obtundation, cardiotoxicity, thyroid dysfunction, and leukocytosis (see Chapter 28). Demeclocycline should be avoided in patients with liver disease (see Chapter 44).

DIURETIC COMBINATIONS

LOOP AGENTS & THIAZIDES

Some patients are refractory to the usual doses of loop agents or become refractory after an initial response. Since these agents have a short half-life, refractoriness may be due to an excessively long interval between doses. Renal Na^+ retention is enhanced during the time period when the drug is no longer active. After the dosing interval for loop agents is minimized or the dose is maximized, the use of two drugs acting at different nephron sites may exhibit synergy. Loop agents and thiazides in combination will often produce diuresis when neither agent acting alone is even minimally effective. There are several reasons for this phenomenon. First, salt and water reabsorption in either the thick ascending limb or the distal convoluted tubule can increase when the other is blocked. Inhibition of both will therefore produce more than an additive diuretic response. Secondly, thiazide diuretics may produce a mild natriuresis in the proximal tubule which is usually masked by increased reabsorption in the thick ascending limb. The combination of loop diuretics and thiazides will therefore blunt Na^+ reabsorption, at least to some extent, from all three segments.

Metolazone is the usual choice of thiazide-like drug in patients refractory to loop agents alone. It has been reported that metolazone may be more effective than other thiazides in renal failure, but this point is controversial, and it is likely that other members of the thiazide group are as effective as metolazone. Moreover, metolazone is available only in an oral preparation, while chlorothiazide can be given parenterally.

The combination of loop diuretics and thiazides can mobilize large amounts of fluid, even in patients who have been refractory to single agents. Therefore, close hemodynamic monitoring of these patients is essential. Routine outpatient use cannot be recommended. Furthermore, potassium wasting is extremely common and may require parenteral K^+ administration with careful monitoring of the fluid and electrolyte status.

POTASSIUM-SPARING DIURETICS & LOOP AGENTS OR THIAZIDES

Many patients who are placed on loop diuretics or thiazides develop hypokalemia at some point in their therapy. This can often be managed with dietary salt restriction, which will limit sodium delivery to the collecting tubule. When hypokalemia cannot be managed in this way, or with KCl supplements, the addition of a potassium-sparing diuretic can significantly lower potassium excretion. While this approach is generally safe, it should probably be avoided in patients with renal insufficiency, who can develop life-threatening hyperkalemia in response to potassium-sparing diuretics.

II. CLINICAL PHARMACOLOGY OF DIURETIC AGENTS

This section discusses the clinical use of diuretic agents in edematous and nonedematous states. The effects of these agents on urinary electrolyte excretion are shown in Table 15–5.

EDEMATOUS STATES

The most common reason for diuretic use is for reduction of peripheral or pulmonary edema that has accumulated as a result of diseases of the heart, kidney, or vasculature, or abnormalities in the blood oncotic pressure. Salt and water retention with edema formation often occurs when diminished blood delivery to the kidney is sensed as insufficient "effective" arterial blood volume. Judicious use of diuretics can mobilize interstitial edema fluid without significant reductions in plasma volume. However, excessive diuretic therapy in this setting may lead to further

Table 15–5. Changes in urinary electrolyte patterns in response to diuretic drugs. + = increase, − = decrease.

Agent	Urinary Electrolyte Patterns		
	NaCl	NaHCO$_3$	K$^+$
Carbonic anhydrase inhibitors	+	+++	+
Loop agents	++++	−	+
Thiazides	++	±	+
Loop agents plus thiazides	+++++	+	++
K$^+$-sparing agents	+	−	−

compromise of the effective arterial blood volume with reduction in perfusion of vital organs. Therefore, the use of diuretics to mobilize edema requires careful monitoring of the patient's hemodynamic status and an understanding of the pathophysiology of the underlying condition.

CONGESTIVE HEART FAILURE

When cardiac function is decreased by disease, the resultant changes in blood pressure and blood flow to the kidney are sensed as hypovolemia and thus induce renal retention of salt and water. This physiologic response initially expands the intravascular volume and venous return to the heart and may partially restore the cardiac output towards normal.

If the underlying disease causes cardiac function to deteriorate despite expansion of plasma volume, the kidney continues to retain salt and water, which then leaks from the vasculature and becomes interstitial or pulmonary edema. At this point, diuretic use becomes necessary to reduce the accumulation of edema, particularly that which is in the lungs. Reduction of pulmonary vascular congestion with diuretics may actually improve oxygenation and thereby improve myocardial function. Edema associated with congestive heart failure is generally managed with loop diuretics. In some instances, salt and water retention may become so severe that a combination of thiazides and loop diuretics is necessary.

In treating the heart failure patient with diuretics, it must always be remembered that cardiac output in these patients is being maintained in part by high filling pressures and that excessive use of diuretics may diminish venous return and thereby impair cardiac output. This issue is especially critical in right ventricular failure. Systemic rather than pulmonary vascular congestion is the hallmark of this disorder. Diuretic-induced volume contraction will predictably reduce venous return and can severely compromise cardiac output if left ventricular filling pressure is reduced below 15 mm Hg.

Diuretic-induced metabolic alkalosis is another adverse effect that may further compromise cardiac function. While this effect is generally treated with replacement of potassium and restoration of intravascular volume with saline, severe heart failure may preclude the use of saline even in patients who have received too much diuretic. In these cases, adjunctive use of acetazolamide can help correct the alkalosis.

Another serious toxicity of diuretic use, particularly in the cardiac patient, is hypokalemia. Hypokalemia can exacerbate underlying cardiac arrhythmias and contribute to digitalis toxicity. This can often be avoided by having the patient reduce sodium intake, thus decreasing sodium delivery to the K^+-secreting collecting tubule. Patients who are noncompliant with a low Na^+ diet must take oral KCl supplements or a K^+-sparing diuretic or must stop using the thiazide diuretic.

Finally, it should be kept in mind that diuretics can never correct the underlying cardiac disease. Drugs that improve myocardial contractility or reduce peripheral vascular resistance are more direct approaches to the basic problem. Diuretics are at best adjunctive therapy.

KIDNEY DISEASE

A variety of renal diseases may interfere with the kidney's normally critical role in volume homeostasis. Although kidney disease will occasionally cause salt wasting, most kidney diseases cause retention of salt and water. When loss of renal function is severe, diuretic agents are of little benefit, because there is insufficient glomerular filtration to sustain a natriuretic response. However, a large number of patients with milder degrees of renal insufficiency can be treated with diuretics when they retain sodium.

Many primary and secondary glomerular diseases, such as those associated with diabetes mellitus, systemic lupus erythematosus, and other disorders involving vascular damage exhibit primary retention of salt and water by the kidney. The cause of this sodium retention is not precisely known, but it probably involves disordered regulation of the renal microcirculation and tubular function through release of vasoconstrictors, prostaglandins, cytokines, and other inflammatory mediators. When these patients develop edema or hypertension, diuretic therapy can be very effective. If heart failure is present simultaneously, the caveats mentioned above should apply.

Certain forms of renal disease, particularly diabetic nephropathy, are frequently associated with development of hyperkalemia at a relatively early stage in the progression of chronic renal failure. In these cases, a thiazide or loop diuretic will enhance K^+ secretion by increasing delivery of salt to the K^+-secreting collecting tubule.

Patients with renal diseases leading to the nephrotic syndrome often present complex problems in volume management. It was taught traditionally that these patients have reduced plasma volume in conjunction with reduced plasma oncotic pressures. This explanation is probably correct in many patients with "minimal change" nephropathy. In these patients, diuretic use may cause further reductions in plasma volume that can impair glomerular filtration rate and may lead to orthostatic hypotension. However, most other causes of nephrotic syndrome are associated with an unexplained primary retention of salt and water by the kidney, leading to expanded plasma volume and hypertension despite the low plasma oncotic pressure. In these cases, diuretic therapy may be beneficial in controlling the volume-dependent component of hypertension and reducing the contribution hypertension may make to the underlying renal disease.

In choosing a diuretic for the patient with kidney disease, a number of important limitations must be kept in mind. Acetazolamide and K^+-sparing diuretics must usually be avoided because of their tendency to exacerbate acidosis and hyperkalemia, respectively. Thiazide diuretics are generally ineffective when GFR falls below 30 mL/min. Thus, loop diuretics are often the best choice in treating edema associated with kidney failure. Lastly, overzealous use of diuretics will cause renal function to decline in all patients, but in those with underlying renal disease, the consequences are all the more serious.

HEPATIC CIRRHOSIS

Liver disease is often associated with edema and with ascites in conjunction with elevated portal hydrostatic pressures and reduced plasma oncotic pressures. The mechanisms for this sodium retention are complex. They probably involve a combination of factors, including diminished renal perfusion resulting from systemic vascular alterations, diminished plasma volume as the result of ascites formation, and diminished oncotic pressure from hypoalbuminemia. In addition, there may be primary sodium retention by the kidney. Plasma aldosterone levels are usually high in response to the reduction in effective circulating volume.

When ascites and edema become severe, diuretic therapy can be useful in initiating and maintaining diuresis. Cirrhotic patients are often resistant to loop diuretics, in part because of an unexplained decrease in secretion of the drug into the tubular fluid and in part because of high aldosterone levels leading to enhanced collecting duct salt reabsorption. On the other hand, cirrhotic edema is unusual in its high degree of responsiveness to spironolactone. The combination of loop diuretics and spironolactone may be useful in some patients. However, even more than in heart failure, overly aggressive use of diuretics in this setting can be disastrous. Vigorous diuretic therapy can cause marked depletion of intravascular volume, hypokalemia, and metabolic alkalosis. Hepatorenal syndrome and hepatic encephalopathy are the unfortunate consequences of overzealous diuretic use in the cirrhotic patient.

IDIOPATHIC EDEMA

This syndrome, which occurs almost exclusively in women, consists of fluctuating salt retention and edema. Despite intensive study, the pathophysiology of this disorder remains obscure. Some studies suggest that intermittent diuretic use may actually contribute to the syndrome. Therefore, idiopathic edema should be managed with mild salt restriction alone if possible.

NONEDEMATOUS STATES

HYPERTENSION

It has long been known that the diuretic and mild vasodilator actions of the thiazides are useful in the treatment of virtually all patients with essential hypertension and may be sufficient therapy in nearly two-thirds. Moderate restriction of dietary Na^+ intake (60–100 meq/d) has been shown to potentiate the effects of diuretics in essential hypertension and to lessen renal K^+ wasting.

Until recently, a thiazide diuretic was usually the first drug to be tried in treating patients with mild essential hypertension. With increasing recognition of the adverse effects of thiazides (see above) and the development of newer antihypertensives (see Chapter 11), the use of thiazides as first-line treatment has declined somewhat. Diuretics still play an important role in patients who require multiple drugs to control blood pressure. Diuretics enhance the efficacy of many agents, particularly the angiotensin-converting enzyme inhibitors. Patients being treated with powerful vasodilators such as hydralazine or minoxidil usually require diuretics simultaneously, because the vasodilators generally cause significant volume retention and edema.

Despite their adverse effects, diuretics are likely to continue as important tools in the management of hypertension. This is particularly true in light of their low cost and effectiveness.

NEPHROLITHIASIS

Approximately two-thirds of all renal stones contain calcium phosphate or calcium oxalate. Many patients with such stones exhibit a renal "leak" of calcium that causes hypercalciuria. This can be treated with thiazide diuretics, which enhance calcium reabsorption in the distal convoluted tubule and thus reduce the urinary calcium concentration. Salt intake must be reduced in this setting, as excess dietary NaCl will overwhelm the hypocalciuric effect of thiazides. Calcium stones may also be caused by increased intestinal absorption of calcium, or they may be idiopathic. In these situations, thiazides are also effective, but should be used as adjunctive therapy with decreased calcium intake and other measures.

HYPERCALCEMIA

Hypercalcemia can be a medical emergency. Since the loop of Henle is an important site of calcium reabsorption, loop diuretics can be quite effective in promoting calcium diuresis. However, loop diuretics alone can cause marked volume contraction. If this occurs, loop diuretics are ineffective (and potentially counterproductive) because calcium reabsorption in the proximal tubule is enhanced. Thus, saline must be administered simultaneously with loop diuretics if an effective calcium diuresis is to be achieved. The usual approach is to infuse normal saline and give furosemide (80–120 mg) intravenously. Once the diuresis begins, the rate of saline infusion can be matched with the urine flow rate to avoid volume depletion. Potassium may be added to the saline infusion as needed.

DIABETES INSIPIDUS

Thiazide diuretics can reduce polyuria and polydipsia in patients who are not responsive to ADH.

The beneficial effect is mediated through plasma volume reduction, with an attendant fall in glomerular filtration rate, enhanced proximal reabsorption of NaCl and water, and decreased delivery of fluid to the diluting segments. Thus, the maximum volume of dilute urine that can be produced is lowered. This seemingly paradoxical effect of thiazides can significantly reduce urine flow in the polyuric patient. Dietary sodium restriction can potentiate the beneficial effects of thiazides on urine volume in this setting. Lithium, used in the treatment of manic-depressive disorder, is a common cause of drug-induced diabetes insipidus, and thiazide diuretics have been found to be helpful in treating it. Serum Li^+ levels must be carefully monitored in this situation, since diuretics may *reduce* renal clearance of Li^+ and raise Li^+ levels into the toxic range (Chapter 28). Lithium polyuria can also be partially reversed by amiloride, which appears to block lithium entry into collecting duct cells, much as it blocks Na^+ entry.

PREPARATIONS AVAILABLE

Acetazolamide (generic, Diamox)
Oral: 125, 250 mg tablets
Oral sustained-release: 500 mg capsules
Parenteral: 500 mg powder for injection
Amiloride (generic, Midamor)
Oral: 5 mg tablets
Bendroflumethiazide (Naturetin)
Oral: 5, 10 mg tablets
Benzthiazide (Exna)
Oral: 50 mg tablets
Bumetanide (Bumex)
Oral: 0.5, 1, 2 mg tablets
Parenteral: 0.5 mg/2 mL ampule for IV or IM injection
Chlorothiazide (generic, Diuril, others)
Oral: 250, 500 mg tablets; 250 mg/5 mL suspension
Parenteral: 500 mg powder to reconstitute for injection
Chlorthalidone (generic, Hygroton, others)
Oral: 15, 25, 50, 100 mg tablets
Demeclocycline (Declomycin)
Oral: 150 mg tablets and capsules; 300 mg tablets
Dichlorphenamide (Daranide)
Oral: 50 mg tablets
Ethacrynic acid (Edecrin)
Oral: 25, 50 mg tablets
Parenteral: 50 mg powder to reconstitute for IV injection

Furosemide (generic, Lasix, others)
Oral: 20, 40, 80 mg tablets; 8, 10 mg/mL solutions
Parenteral: 10 mg/mL for IM or IV injection
Hydrochlorothiazide (generic, Esidrix, HydroDIURIL, others)
Oral: 25, 50, 100 mg tablets; 10, 100 mg/mL solution
Hydroflumethiazide (generic, Diucardin, Saluron)
Oral: 50 mg tablets
Indapamide (Lozol)
Oral: 1.25, 2.5 mg tablets
Mannitol (generic, Osmitrol)
Parenteral: 5, 10, 15, 20, 25% for injection
Methyclothiazide (generic, Enduron, others)
Oral: 2.5, 5 mg tablets
Metolazone (Mykrox, Zaroxolyn) (**Note:** Bioavailability of Mykrox is greater than that of Zaroxolyn.)
Oral: 0.5 (Mykrox); 2.5, 5, 10 mg (Zaroxolyn) tablets
Polythiazide (Renese)
Oral: 1, 2, 4 mg tablets
Quinethazone (Hydromox)
Oral: 50 mg tablets
Spironolactone (generic, Aldactone)
Oral: 25, 50, 100 mg tablets
Torsemide (Demadex)
Oral: 5, 10, 20, 100 mg tablets

Parenteral: 10 mg/mL for injection
Triamterene (Dyrenium)
Oral: 50, 100 mg tablets

Trichlormethiazide (generic, Naqua)
Oral: 2, 4 mg tablets

REFERENCES

General

Brenner BM, Rector FC Jr (editors): *The Kidney,* 4th ed. Saunders, 1990.

Rose BD: Diuretics. Kidney Int 1991;39:336.

Warnock DG, Eveloff J: NaCl entry mechanisms in the luminal membrane of the renal tubule. Am J Physiol 1982;242:561.

Specific Agents

Ashraf N, Locksley R, Arieff AI: Thiazide-induced hyponatremia associated with death or neurologic damage in outpatients. Am J Med 1981;70:1163.

Barr WH et al: Comparison of bioavailability, pharmacokinetics, and pharmacodynamics of torasemide in young and elderly healthy volunteers. Prog Pharm Clinical Pharmacol 1990;8:1.

Battle DC et al: Amelioration of polyuria by amiloride in patients receiving long-term lithium therapy. N Engl J Med 1985;312:408.

Bear R et al: Effect of metabolic alkalosis on respiratory function in patients with chronic obstructive lung disease. Can Med Assoc J 1977;22:900.

Block WD, Shiner PT, Roman J: Severe electrolyte disturbances associated with metolazone and furosemide. South Med J 1978;71:380.

Boyer TD, Warnock DG: Use of diuretics in the treatment of cirrhotic ascites. (Editorial.) Gastroenterology 1983;84:1051.

Brown CB et al: High dose frusemide in acute renal failure: A controlled trial. Clin Nephrol 1981;15:90.

de Carvalho JG et al: Hemodynamic correlates of prolonged thiazide therapy: Comparison of responders and nonresponders. Clin Pharmacol Ther 1977;22:875.

De Marchi S, Ceddhin E: Severe metabolic acidosis and disturbances of calcium metabolism induced by acetazolamide in patients on haemodialysis. Clin Sci 1990;78:295.

DeTroyer A: Demeclocycline: Treatment for syndrome of inappropriate antidiuretic hormone secretion. JAMA 1977;237:2723.

Ellison DH et al. Adaptation of the distal convoluted tubule of the rat: Structural and functional effects of dietary salt intake and chronic diuretic infusion. J Clin Invest 1989;83:113.

Epstein M et al: Potentiation of furosemide by metolazone in refractory edema. Curr Ther Res 1977;21:656.

Giebisch G et al: Renal and extrarenal sites of action of diuretics. Cardiovasc Drugs Therap 1993;7:11.

Goldberg H et al: Mechanism of Li inhibition of vasopressin-sensitive adenylate cyclase in cultured renal epithelial cells. Am J Physiol 1988;255:F995.

Greene MK et al: Acetazolamide in prevention of acute mountain sickness: A double-blind controlled crossover study. Br Med J 1981;283:811.

Holland OB, Nixon JV, Kuhnert L: Diuretic-induced ventricular ectopic activity. Am J Med 1981;70:762.

Hollifield JW, Slaton PE: Thiazide diuretics, hypokalemia, and cardiac arrhythmias. Acta Med Scand 1981;647(Suppl):67.

Horisberger J-D, Giebisch G: Potassium-sparing diuretics. Renal Physiol 1987;10:198.

Hulter HN et al: Pathophysiology of chronic renal tubular acidosis induced by administration of amiloride. J Lab Clin Med 1980;95:637.

Indapamide: A new indoline diuretic agent. (Symposium.) Am Heart J 1983;106:183.

Koechel DA: Ethacrynic acid and related diuretics: Relationship of structure to beneficial and detrimental actions. Annu Rev Pharmacol Toxicol 1981;21:265.

Levy ST, Forrest JM, Heninger GR: Lithium-induced diabetes insipidus: Manic symptoms, brain and electrolyte correlates, and chlorothiazide treatment. Am J Psychiatry 1973;130:1014.

Links TP et al: Improvement of muscle strength in familial hypokalaemic periodic paralysis with acetazolamide. J Neurol Neurosurg Psychiatry 1988;51:1142.

Loon NR et al: Mechanism of impaired natriuretic response to furosemide during prolonged therapy. Kidney Int 1989;36:682.

McVeigh G et al: The case for low dose diuretics in hypertension: Comparison of low and conventional doses of cyclopenthiazide. Br Med J 1988;297:95.

Multicenter Diuretic Cooperative Study Group: Multiclinic comparison of amiloride, hydrochlorothiazide, and hydrochlorothiazide plus amiloride in essential hypertension. Arch Intern Med 1981;141:482.

Nakahama H et al: Pharmacokinetic and pharmacodynamic interactions between furosemide and hydrochlorothiazide in nephrotic patients. Nephron 1988;49:223.

Pollare T et al: A comparison of the effects of hydrochlorothiazide and captopril on glucose and lipid metabolism in patients with hypertension. N Engl J Med 1989;321:868.

Preisig P et al: Role of the Na^+/H^+ antiporter in rat proximal tubule bicarbonate absorption. J Clin Invest 1987;80:970.

Preisig PA, Rector FC Jr: Role of the Na^+/H^+ antiporter in rat proximal tubule NaCl absorption. Am J Physiol 1988;255:F461.

Ram CVS, Garrett B, Kaplan NM: Moderate sodium restriction and various diuretics in the treatment of hypertension: Effects of potassium wastage and blood pressure control. Arch Intern Med 1981;141:1015.

Shimuzu T et al: Effects of PTH, calcitonin, and cAMP on calcium transport in rabbit distal nephron. Am J Physiol 1990;259:F408.

Stanton BA: Cellular actions of thiazide diuretics in the distal tubule. J Am Soc Nephrol 1990;1:832.

Stokes JB: Electroneutral NaCl transport in the distal tubule. Kidney Int 1989;36:427.

Tan SY et al: Indomethacin-induced prostaglandin inhibition with hyperkalemia: A reversible cause of hyporeninemic hypoaldosteronism. Ann Intern Med 1979;90:783.

Townsend RR, Holland B: Combination of converting enzyme inhibitor with diuretic for the treatment of hypertension. Arch Intern Med 1990;150:1175.

Van Brummelen P, Woerlee M, Schalekamp MA: Long-term versus short-term effects of hydrochlorothiazide on renal haemodynamics in essential hypertension. Clin Sci 1979;56:463.

Warren SE, Blantz RC: Mannitol. Arch Intern Med 1981;141:493.

Weinberg MS et al: Anuric renal failure precipitated by indomethacin and triamterene. Nephron 1985;40:216.

Wingo CS: Cortical collecting tubule potassium secretion: Effect of amiloride, ouabain, and luminal sodium concentration. Kidney Int 1985;27:886

Wollam GL et al: Diuretic potency of combined hydrochlorothiazide and furosemide therapy in patients with azotemia. Am J Med 1982;72:929.

Zell SC, Goodman PH: Acetazolamide and dexamethasone in the prevention of acute mountain sickness. West J Med 1988;148:541.

Section IV
Drugs with Important Actions on Smooth Muscle

Histamine, Serotonin, & the Ergot Alkaloids

16

Alan Burkhalter, PhD, David Julius, PhD, & Oscar L. Frick, MD, PhD

Histamine and serotonin (5-hydroxytryptamine) are biologically active amines that are found in many tissues, have complex physiologic and pathologic effects, and are often released locally. Together with endogenous polypeptides (Chapter 17) and prostaglandins and leukotrienes (Chapter 18), they are sometimes called *autacoids* (Gk "self-remedy") or *local hormones* in recognition of these properties.

The roles of histamine and serotonin in normal physiology are not completely understood, and these compounds have no clinical application in the treatment of disease. However, compounds that selectively antagonize the actions of these amines or selectively activate certain receptor subtypes are of considerable clinical usefulness. This chapter therefore emphasizes the basic pharmacology of the agonist amines and the clinical pharmacology of the more selective agonist and antagonist drugs. The ergot alkaloids, compounds with partial agonist activity at serotonin and several other receptors, are discussed at the end of the chapter.

HISTAMINE

Histamine was synthesized in 1907 and later isolated from mammalian tissues. Early hypotheses concerning the possible physiologic roles of tissue histamine were based on similarities between histamine's actions and the symptoms of anaphylactic shock and tissue injury. Marked species variation has been observed, but in humans histamine is an important mediator of immediate allergic and inflammatory reactions; has an important role in gastric acid secretion; and functions as a neurotransmitter and neuromodulator.

I. BASIC PHARMACOLOGY OF HISTAMINE

Chemistry & Pharmacokinetics

Histamine is 2-(4-imidazoyl)ethylamine. It occurs in plants as well as in animal tissues and is a component of some venoms and stinging secretions.

Histamine

Histamine is formed by decarboxylation of the amino acid L-histidine, a reaction catalyzed in mammalian tissues by the enzyme histidine decarboxylase (E.C.4.1.1.22). Pyridoxal phosphate is required as cofactor. Once formed, histamine is either stored or rapidly inactivated. The major inactivation pathway involves, first, conversion to methylhistamine, catalyzed by imidazole-N-methyltransferase, and then oxidation to methylimidazoleacetic acid, catalyzed by diamine oxidase. A second important pathway of metabolism involves direct conversion of histamine to imidazoleacetic acid by diamine oxidase. Very little histamine is excreted unchanged. Certain tumors (systemic mastocytosis, urticaria pigmentosa, gastric carcinoid, and occasionally myelogenous leukemia) are associated with increased numbers of mast cells or basophils and with increased excretion of histamine and its metabolites.

Although histamine is found in most tissues, it is very unevenly distributed. Most tissue histamine exists in bound form in granules in mast cells or basophils; the histamine content of many tissues is directly related to their mast cell content. The bound form of histamine is biologically inactive, but many stimuli, as noted below, can trigger the release of mast cell histamine, allowing the free amine to exert its actions on surrounding tissues.

Mast cells are especially rich at sites of potential tissue injury—nose, mouth, and feet; internal body surfaces; and blood vessels, particularly at pressure points and bifurcations. Mast cells in different tissues also differ. Some mast cells found in the gastrointestinal mucosa are similar to those found in connective tissue, but others exhibit different properties. Such mucosal or atypical mast cells contain—in addition to histamine—chondroitin sulfate instead of heparin sulfate in the storage granules and exhibit different sensitivities to chemicals that cause histamine release.

Non-mast cell histamine is found in several tissues, including the brain, where it functions as a neurotransmitter. Cell bodies of histaminergic neurons are found in the tuberomamillary nucleus of the posterior hypothalamus with widespread projections to other sites. Endogenous neurotransmitter histamine may play a role in many brain functions such as neuroendocrine control, cardiovascular regulation, thermoregulation, and arousal.

Storage & Release of Histamine

In human mast cells and basophils, storage granules contain histamine complexed with the sulfated polysaccharide, heparin or chondroitin sulfate, and an acidic protein. The bound form of histamine can be released through several mechanisms.

A. Immunologic Release: The important pathophysiologic mechanism of mast cell and basophil histamine release is immunologic. These cells, if sensitized by IgE antibodies attached to their surface membranes, degranulate when exposed to the appropriate antigen (see Figure 57–7). This type of release also requires energy and calcium. Degranulation leads to the simultaneous release of histamine, ATP, and other mediators that are stored together in secretory granules. Some of these compounds, most notably ATP, serve to further potentiate mast cell degranulation via a paracrine or autocrine mechanism. Degranulated mast cells will reaccumulate histamine over a period of days to weeks. Histamine released by this mechanism is a mediator in immediate (type I) allergic reactions. Substances released during IgG- or IgM-mediated immune reactions that activate the complement cascade also release histamine from mast cells and basophils.

By a negative feedback control mechanism mediated by H_2 receptors, histamine appears to modulate its own release and that of other mediators from sensitized mast cells in some tissues. In humans, mast cells in skin and basophils show this negative feedback mechanism; lung mast cells do not. Thus, histamine may act to limit the intensity of the allergic reaction in the skin and blood.

Endogenous histamine may also have a modulating role in a variety of inflammatory and immune responses. Histamine probably plays a part in acute inflammatory responses. Upon injury to a tissue, released histamine causes local vasodilation and leakage of plasma containing mediators of acute inflammation (complement, C-reactive protein), antibodies, and inflammatory cells (neutrophils, eosinophils, basophils, monocytes, and lymphocytes). Histamine inhibits the release of lysosome contents and several T and B lymphocyte functions. Most of these actions are mediated by H_2 receptors acting through increased intracellular cAMP. Release of peptides from nerves in response to inflammation is also probably modulated by histamine, in this case acting through presynaptic H_3 receptors.

B. Chemical and Mechanical Release: Certain amines, including drugs such as morphine and tubocurarine, can displace histamine from the heparin-protein complex within cells. This type of release does not require energy and is not associated with mast cell injury or degranulation. Loss of granules from the mast cell will also release histamine, since sodium ions in the extracellular fluid rapidly displace the amine from the complex. Chemical and mechanical mast cell injury causes degranulation and histamine release. Compound 48/80, an experimental diamine polymer, specifically releases histamine from tissue mast cells by an exocytotic degranulation process requiring energy and calcium.

Pharmacodynamics

A. Mechanism of Action: Histamine exerts its biologic actions by combining with specific cellular receptors located on the surface membrane. The three different histamine receptors thus far characterized are designated H_1, H_2, and H_3 and are described in Table 16–1. All three receptor subtypes belong to the large superfamily of receptors having seven membrane-spanning regions and intracellular association with G proteins. The structures of the H_1 and H_2 receptors have been determined. In the brain, H_1 and H_2 receptors are located on postsynaptic membranes, while H_3 receptors are predominantly presynaptic. Activation of these presynaptic receptors is associated with a reduction of transmitter release, including histamine itself, norepinephrine, serotonin, and acetylcholine. Activation of H_1 receptors, which are present in endothelial and smooth muscle cells, usually elicits an increase in phosphoinositol hydrolysis and an increase in intracellular calcium. Activation of H_2 receptors, present in gastric mucosa, cardiac muscle cells, and some immune cells, increases intracellular cAMP. Activation of H_3 receptors, which are found in several areas of the central nervous system, decreases histamine release from histaminergic neurons, possibly mediated by a decrease in calcium influx.

B. Tissue and Organ System Effects of Histamine: Histamine exerts powerful effects on smooth

Table 16–1. Histamine receptor subtypes.

Receptor Subtype	Distribution	Postreceptor Mechanism	Partially Selective Agonists	Partially Selective Antagonists
H_1	Smooth muscle, endothelium, brain	↑IP_3, DAG	2-(m-fluorophenyl)-histamine[1]	Mepyramine, triprolidine
H_2	Gastric mucosa, cardiac muscle, mast cells, brain	↑cAMP	Dimaprit, impromidine	Ranitidine, tiotidine
H_3	Presynaptic: brain, myenteric plexus, other neurons	G protein-coupled	R-α-Methylhistamine, imetit	Thioperamide, iodophenpropit, impromidine

[1]Partial agonist.

and cardiac muscle, on certain endothelial and nerve cells, and on the secretory cells of the stomach. However, sensitivity to histamine varies greatly among species. Humans, guinea pigs, dogs, and cats are quite sensitive, while mice and rats are much less so.

1. Cardiovascular system–In humans, injection or infusion of histamine causes a decrease in systolic and diastolic blood pressure and an increase in heart rate (Figure 16–1). The acute blood pressure changes are caused by the direct vasodilator action of histamine on arterioles and precapillary sphincters; the increase in heart rate involves both stimulatory actions of histamine on the heart and a reflex tachycardia. Flushing, a sense of warmth, and headache may also occur during histamine administration, consistent with the vasodilation. Histamine-induced vasodilation is mediated, at least in part, by release of endothelium-derived relaxing factor (EDRF; see Chapter 6). Studies with histamine receptor antago-

nists show that both H_1 and H_2 receptors are involved in these cardiovascular responses to high doses, since a combination of H_1 and H_2 receptor-blocking agents is more effective in preventing the actions of histamine than either blocking agent alone (Figure 16–1). However, in humans, the cardiovascular effects of small doses of histamine can usually be antagonized by H_1 receptor antagonists alone.

Edema results from the action of histamine on H_1 receptors in the vessels of the microcirculation, especially the postcapillary vessels. The effect is associated with an increase in permeability of the vessel wall that has been ascribed to the separation of the endothelial cells, thus permitting the transudation of fluid and molecules as large as small proteins into the perivascular tissue. This effect is responsible for the urticaria (hives) that signals the release of histamine in the skin. New studies of endothelial cells suggest that actin and myosin within these *nonmuscle* cells

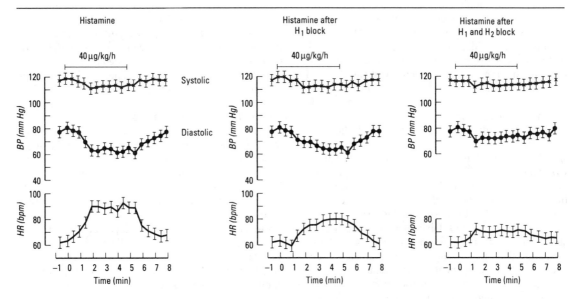

Figure 16–1. Effects of histamine and histamine antagonists on blood pressure and heart rate in humans. Histamine was infused at 40 μg/kg/h for 5 minutes as shown at the top of each panel. The H_1 antagonist was chlorpheniramine (10 mg intravenously). The H_2 antagonist was cimetidine (2 mg intravenously). (Modified and reproduced, with permission, from Torsoli A, Lucchelli PE, Brimblecombe RW [editors]: *H*-Antagonists: H_2-Receptor Antagonists in Peptic Ulcer Disease and Progress in Histamine Research. Excerpta Medica, 1980.)

contract in response to calcium influx evoked by drugs such as histamine. This contraction results in separation of the endothelial cells and increased permeability (Curry, 1992).

Direct cardiac effects of histamine include both increased contractility and increased pacemaker rate. These effects are mediated chiefly by H_2 receptors. In human atrial muscle, histamine can also decrease contractility; this effect is mediated by H_1 receptors. The physiologic significance of these cardiac actions is not clear. These cardiovascular effects may also be produced by the release of endogenous histamine from mast cells. Many of the cardiovascular signs and symptoms of anaphylaxis are due to released histamine, though other mediators are also involved.

2. Gastrointestinal tract smooth muscle– Histamine causes contraction of intestinal smooth muscle, and histamine-induced contraction of guinea pig ileum is a standard bioassay for histamine. The human gut is not as sensitive as that of the guinea pig, but large doses of histamine may cause diarrhea, partly as a result of this effect. This action of histamine is mediated by H_1 receptors.

3. Bronchiolar smooth muscle–In both humans and guinea pigs, histamine causes bronchoconstriction mediated by H_1 receptors. In the guinea pig, this effect is the cause of death from histamine toxicity, but in normal humans, bronchoconstriction following the usual doses of histamine is not marked. However, patients with asthma are very sensitive to histamine. The bronchoconstriction induced in these patients probably represents a hyperactive neural response, since such patients also respond excessively to many other stimuli, and the response to histamine can be blocked by autonomic blocking drugs such as ganglionic blocking agents as well as by H_1 receptor antagonists (see Chapter 19). Provocative tests using increasing doses of inhaled histamine are of diagnostic value for bronchial hyperreactivity in patients with suspected asthma or cystic fibrosis. Such individuals may be 100- to 1000-fold more sensitive to histamine than are normal subjects.

4. Other smooth muscle organs–In humans, histamine generally has insignificant effects on the smooth muscle of the eye and genitourinary tract. However, pregnant women who have anaphylaxis may abort as a result of histamine-induced contractions, and in some species the sensitivity of the uterus is sufficient to form the basis for a bioassay.

5. Nerve endings–Histamine is a powerful stimulant of sensory nerve endings, especially those mediating pain and itching. This H_1-mediated effect is an important component of the urticarial response and reactions to insect and nettle stings. Some evidence suggests that local high concentrations can also depolarize efferent (axonal) nerve endings (see ¶ 7, below).

6. Secretory tissue–Histamine has long been recognized as a powerful stimulant of gastric acid secretion and, to a lesser extent, of gastric pepsin and intrinsic factor production. The effect is caused by activation of H_2 receptors on gastric parietal cells (Sewing, 1986) or nearby tissue cells (Mezey, 1992) and is associated with increased adenylyl cyclase activity, cAMP concentration, and intracellular Ca^{2+} concentration. Other stimulants of gastric acid secretion such as acetylcholine and gastrin do not increase cAMP even though their maximal effects on acid output can be reduced—but not abolished—by H_2 receptor antagonists. Histamine also stimulates secretion in the small and large intestine.

Histamine has insignificant effects on the activity of other glandular tissue at ordinary concentrations. Very high concentrations can cause adrenal medullary discharge.

7. The "triple response"–Intradermal injection of histamine causes a characteristic wheal-and-flare response that was first described over 60 years ago. The effect involves three separate cell types: smooth muscle in the microcirculation, capillary or venular endothelium, and sensory nerve endings. At the site of injection, a reddening appears owing to dilation of small vessels, followed soon by an edematous wheal at the injection site and a red irregular flare surrounding the wheal. The flare is said to be caused by an axon reflex. As noted above, histamine stimulates nerve endings; the resulting impulses are thought to travel through other branches of the same axon, causing vasodilation through the release of a vasodilatory neuromediator. The sensation of itch may also accompany the appearance of these effects. The wheal is due to local edema.

Similar local effects may be produced by injecting histamine liberators (compound 48/80, morphine, etc) intradermally or by applying the appropriate antigens to the skin of a sensitized person. Although most of these local effects can be blocked by prior administration of an H_1 receptor-blocking agent, H_2 receptors may also be involved.

Other Histamine Agonists

Small substitutions on the imidazole ring of histamine significantly modify the selectivity of the compounds for the histamine receptor subtypes. For example, 2-methylhistamine is relatively more selective for H_1 receptors, while 4-methylhistamine is a relatively specific H_2 agonist. **Betazole**—a drug that was used in testing gastric acid-secreting ability—and **impromidine** are agonists at H_2 receptors and antagonists at H_3 receptors. R-α-Methylhistamine is a potent and selective H_3 receptor agonist that crosses the blood-brain barrier. It is also a potent inhibitor of histamine synthesis and release.

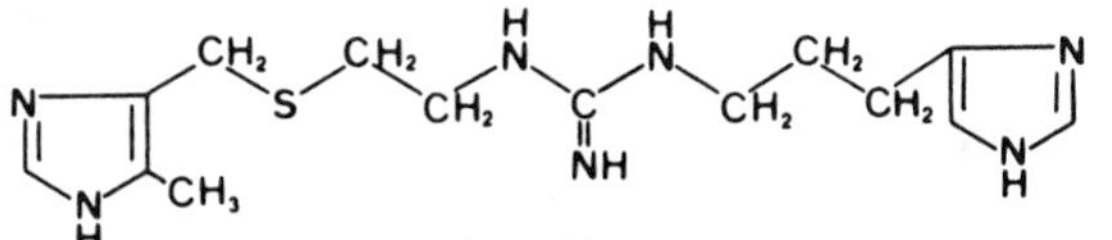

Impromidine

II. CLINICAL PHARMACOLOGY OF HISTAMINE

Clinical Uses

A. Testing Gastric Acid Secretion: Histamine was used in the past as a diagnostic agent in testing for gastric acid secreting ability. However, pentagastrin is currently used for this purpose with a much lower incidence of adverse effects.

B. Diagnosis of Pheochromocytoma: Histamine can cause release of catecholamines from adrenal medullary cells. Although this effect is not prominent in normal humans, massive release can occur in patients with pheochromocytoma. This hazardous provocative test is now obsolete, since chemical assays are available for determination of the catecholamines and their metabolites in patients suspected of having this tumor.

C. Pulmonary Function Testing: In pulmonary testing laboratories, histamine aerosol (in addition to other agents) is sometimes used as a provocative test of bronchial hyperreactivity.

Toxicity & Contraindications

Adverse effects following administration of histamine, like those of histamine release, are dose-related. Flushing, hypotension, tachycardia, headache, wheals, bronchoconstriction, and gastrointestinal upset are noted. These effects are also observed after the ingestion of spoiled fish (scombroid fish poisoning), and there is evidence that histamine produced by bacterial action in the flesh of the fish is the major causative agent.

Histamine should not be given to asthmatics (except as part of a carefully monitored test of pulmonary function) or to patients with active ulcer disease or gastrointestinal bleeding.

HISTAMINE ANTAGONISTS

The effects of histamine released in the body can be reduced in several ways. **Physiologic antagonists,** especially epinephrine, have smooth muscle actions opposite to those of histamine, but they act at differ-

ent receptors. This is important clinically because injection of epinephrine can be lifesaving in systemic anaphylaxis and in other conditions in which massive release of histamine—and other mediators—occurs.

Release inhibitors reduce the degranulation of mast cells that results from immunologic triggering by antigen-IgE interaction. Cromolyn and nedocromil appear to have this effect (see Chapter 19) and are used in the treatment of asthma, though the molecular mechanism underlying their action is presently unknown. Beta$_2$-adrenoceptor agonists also appear capable of reducing histamine release.

Histamine **receptor antagonists** represent a third approach to the reduction of histamine-mediated responses. For over 45 years, compounds have been available that competitively antagonize many of the actions of histamine on smooth muscle. However, not until the H$_2$ receptor antagonist burimamide was described in 1972 was it possible to antagonize the gastric acid-stimulating activity of histamine. The development of selective H$_2$ receptor antagonists has led not only to more precise definition of histamine's actions in terms of receptors involved but also to more effective therapy for peptic ulcer. Selective H$_3$ antagonists are not yet available for clinical use. However, a potent and selective H$_3$ receptor antagonist, thioperamide, has been introduced that competes for the binding of radiolabeled R-α-methylhistamine to this site at nanomolar concentration. Like R-α-methylhistamine, thioperamide crosses the blood-brain barrier. The availability of this agonist and antagonist will help to define the physiologic role of H$_3$ receptors.

H$_1$-RECEPTOR ANTAGONISTS

Compounds that competitively block histamine at H$_1$ receptors have been used clinically for many years, and 18 H$_1$ antagonists are currently marketed in the USA. Several are available without prescription, both alone and in combination formulations such as "cold pills" and sleep aids (see Chapter 65).

I. BASIC PHARMACOLOGY OF H$_1$-RECEPTOR ANTAGONISTS

Chemistry & Pharmacokinetics

Older H$_1$ antagonists are stable lipid-soluble amines with the general structure illustrated in Figure 16–2. There are several chemical subgroups, and the structures of compounds representing different subgroups are shown in the figure. Doses of some of these drugs are given in Table 16–2.

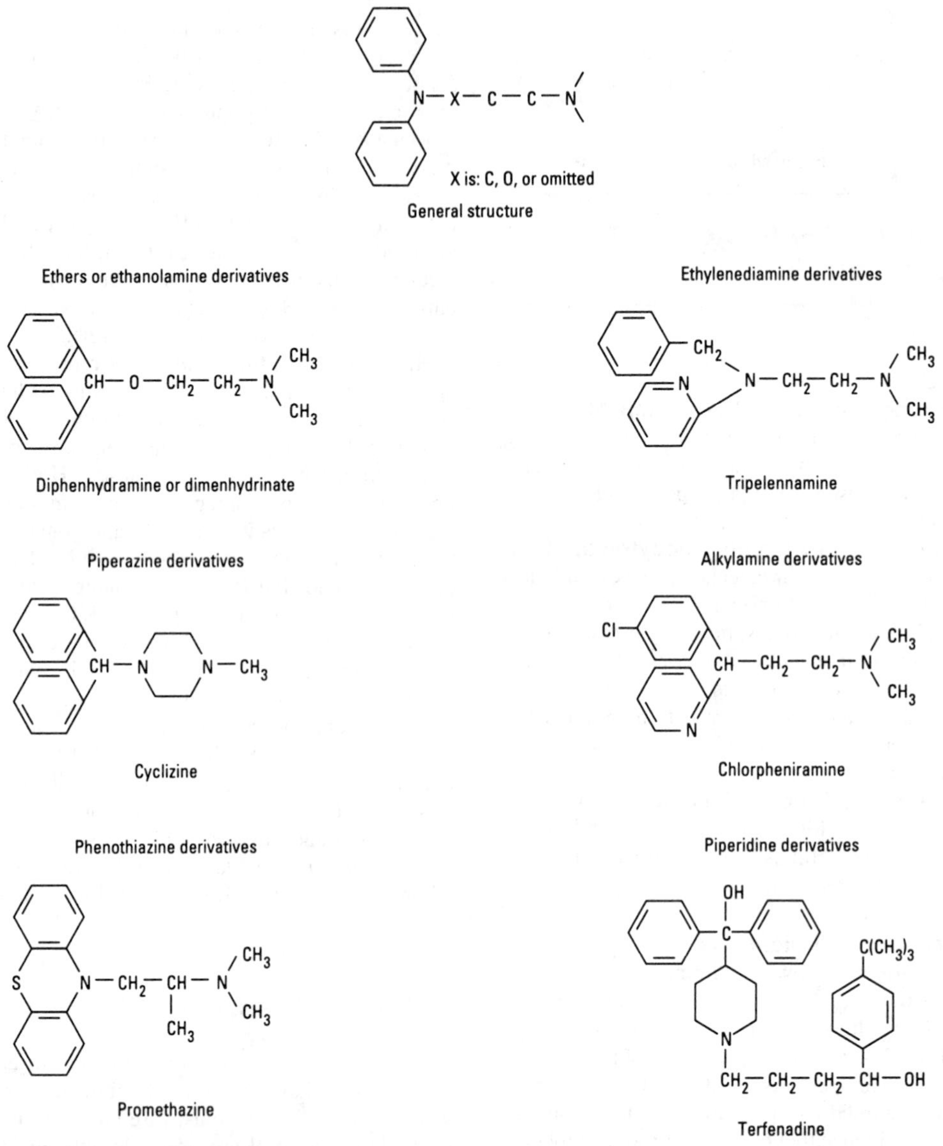

Figure 16–2. General structure of H_1 antagonist drugs and examples of the major subgroups.

Most of these agents are similar with respect to absorption and distribution. They are rapidly absorbed following oral administration, with peak blood concentrations occurring in 1–2 hours. They are widely distributed throughout the body and, except for the newer agents (terfenadine, loratadine, astemizole, and mequitazine), enter the central nervous system readily. They are extensively metabolized, primarily by microsomal systems in the liver. Most of the drugs have an effective duration of action of 4–6 hours following a single dose, but meclizine and the newer H_1-blockers are longer-acting, with a duration of action of 12–24 hours. The newer agents also are considerably less lipid-soluble and enter the central nervous system with difficulty or not at all. Both terfenadine and astemizole have active metabolites.

Pharmacodynamics

A. Histamine Receptor Blockade: H_1-receptor antagonists block the actions of histamine by reversible competitive antagonism at the H_1 receptor. They have negligible potency at the H_2 receptor and little at the H_3 receptor. For example, histamine-induced contraction of bronchiolar or gastrointestinal smooth muscle can be completely blocked by these agents, but the effects of histamine on the cardiovascular system are only partly blocked because of H_2 receptor-mediated actions (Figure 16–1). H_2 receptor-

Table 16–2. Some H_1 antihistaminic drugs in clinical use.

Drugs	Usual Adult Dose	Comments
Ethanolamines Carbinoxamine (Clistin)	4–8 mg	Slight to moderate sedation.
Dimenhydrinate (8-chlorotheophylline salt of diphenhydramine) (Dramamine, etc)	50 mg	Marked sedation; anti-motion sickness activity.
Diphenhydramine (Benadryl, etc)	25–50 mg	Marked sedation; anti-motion sickness activity.
Doxylamine (Decapryn)	1.25–25 mg	Marked sedation; now available only in OTC "sleep aids."
Ethylenediamines Antazoline	1–2 drops	Component of ophthalmic solutions.
Pyrilamine (Neo-Antergan)	25–50 mg	Moderate sedation; component of OTC "sleep aids."
Tripelennamine (PBZ)	25–50 mg	Moderate sedation.
Piperazine derivatives Cyclizine (Marezine)	25–50 mg	Slight sedation; anti-motion sickness activity.
Meclizine (Bonine, etc)	25–50 mg	Slight sedation; anti-motion sickness activity.
Alkylamines Brompheniramine (Dimetane, etc)	4–8 mg	Slight sedation.
Chlorpheniramine (Chlor-Trimeton, etc)	4–8 mg	Slight sedation; common component of OTC "cold" medication.
Dexchlorpheniramine (Polaramine)	2–4 mg	Slight sedation; active isomer of chlorpheniramine.
Phenothiazine derivatives Promethazine (Phenergan, etc)	10–25 mg	Marked sedation; antiemetic and antimuscarinic activity.
Piperidines Astemizole (Hismanal)	10 mg	Lower incidence of sedation.
Terfenadine (Seldane)	60 mg	Lower incidence of sedation.
Miscellaneous Cyproheptadine (Periactin, etc)	4 mg	Moderate sedation; also has antiserotonin activity.
Loratadine (Claritin)	10 mg	Longer action, little sedation.

mediated actions such as increase in gastric acid secretion and inhibition of histamine release from mast cells are unaffected.

B. Actions Not Caused by Histamine Receptor Blockade: The H_1-receptor antagonists have many actions not ascribable to blockade of the actions of histamine. The large number of these actions probably results from the similarity of the general structure (Figure 16–2) to the structure of drugs that have effects at muscarinic cholinoceptor, alpha-adrenoceptor, serotonin, and local anesthetic receptor sites. Some of these actions are of therapeutic value and some are undesirable.

1. Sedation–A common effect of H_1 antagonists is sedation, but the intensity of this effect varies among chemical subgroups (Table 16–2) and among patients as well. The effect is sufficiently prominent with some agents to make them useful as "sleep aids" (see Chapter 65) and unsuitable for daytime use. The effect resembles that of some antimuscarinic drugs and is considered very unlike the disinhibited sedation produced by sedative-hypnotic drugs. At ordinary dosages, children occasionally (and adults

rarely) manifest excitation rather than sedation. At very high toxic dose levels, marked stimulation, agitation, and even convulsions may precede coma. Newer H_1 antagonists are claimed to have little or no sedative action. Terfenadine (or its metabolite) is highly selective for H_1 receptors and crosses the blood-brain barrier with difficulty. Astemizole is also highly selective for H_1 receptors and is claimed to be free of sedative and autonomic blocking effects. Loratadine and cetirizine are also claimed to have few central nervous system or autonomic effects.

2. Antinausea and antiemetic actions–Several H_1 antagonists have significant activity in preventing motion sickness (Table 16–2). They are less effective against an episode of motion sickness already present. Certain H_1 antagonists, notably doxylamine (in Bendectin), were used widely in the past in the treatment of nausea and vomiting of pregnancy (see below).

3. Antiparkinsonism effects–Perhaps because of their anticholinergic effects (cf benztropine; see Chapter 27), some of the H_1 antagonists have significant acute suppressant effects on the parkinsonism symptoms associated with certain antipsychotic drugs.

4. Anticholinoceptor actions–Many of the H_1 antagonists, especially those of the ethanolamine and ethylenediamine subgroups, have significant atropine-like effects on peripheral muscarinic receptors. This action may be responsible for some of the (uncertain) benefits reported for nonallergic rhinorrhea but may also cause urinary retention and blurred vision.

5. Adrenoceptor-blocking actions–Alpha receptor-blocking effects can be demonstrated for many H_1 antagonists, especially those in the phenothiazine subgroup. This action may cause orthostatic hypotension in susceptible individuals. Beta-receptor blockade is not observed.

6. Serotonin-blocking action–Strong blocking effects at serotonin receptors have been demonstrated for some H_1 antagonists, notably cyproheptadine. This drug is promoted as an antiserotonin agent and is discussed with that drug group. Nevertheless, it has a chemical structure that resembles the phenothiazine antihistamines and is a potent H_1 blocking agent.

7. Local anesthesia–Most of the H_1 antagonists are effective local anesthetics. They block sodium channels in excitable membranes in the same fashion as procaine and lidocaine. Diphenhydramine and promethazine are actually more potent as local anesthetics than is procaine. They are occasionally used to produce local anesthesia in patients allergic to the conventional local anesthetic drugs.

II. CLINICAL PHARMACOLOGY OF H_1 RECEPTOR ANTAGONISTS

Clinical Uses

A. Allergic Reactions: The H_1 antihistaminic agents are often the first drugs used to prevent or treat the symptoms of allergic reactions. In allergic rhinitis and urticaria, in which histamine is the primary mediator, the H_1 antagonists are the drugs of choice and are often quite effective. However, in bronchial asthma, which involves several mediators, the H_1 antagonists are largely ineffective.

Angioedema may be precipitated by histamine release but appears to be maintained by bradykinins that are not affected by antihistaminic agents. For atopic dermatitis, antihistaminic drugs such as diphenhydramine are used mostly for their sedative side effects and for some control of the itching.

The H_1 antihistamines used for treating allergic conditions such as hay fever are usually selected with the goal of minimizing sedative effects; in the USA, the drugs in widest use are the alkylamines and the newer piperidines. However, the sedative effect and the therapeutic efficacy of different agents vary widely among individuals, so it is common practice to give a patient samples from each major group to determine which is the most effective with the least adverse effects in that particular individual. In addition, the clinical effectiveness of one group may diminish with continued use, and switching to another group may restore drug effectiveness for as yet unexplained reasons.

The newer H_1 blockers with lowered sedative action (terfenadine, loratadine, astemizole, and mequitazine) are used mainly for the treatment of allergic rhinitis and chronic urticaria. Several double-blind comparisons with older agents (such as chlorpheniramine) indicated about equal therapeutic efficacy. However, sedation and interference with safe operation of machinery, which occur in about 50% of subjects taking conventional antihistamines, occurred in only about 7% of subjects taking terfenadine or astemizole. The newer drugs are much more expensive.

B. Motion Sickness and Vestibular Disturbances: Scopolamine and certain H_1 antagonists are the most effective agents available for the prevention of motion sickness. The antihistaminic drugs with the greatest effectiveness in this application are diphenhydramine and promethazine. The piperazines (cyclizine and meclizine) also have significant activity in preventing motion sickness and are less sedative in most patients. Dosage is the same as that recommended for allergic disorders (Table 16–2). Both scopolamine and the H_1 antagonists are more effective in preventing motion sickness when combined with ephedrine or amphetamine.

It has been claimed that the antihistaminic agents effective in prophylaxis of motion sickness are also useful in Meniere's syndrome, but efficacy in the latter application is not well established.

C. Nausea and Vomiting of Pregnancy: Several H_1 antagonist drugs have been studied for possible use in treating "morning sickness." The piperazine derivatives were withdrawn from such use when it was demonstrated that they have teratogenic effects in rodents. Doxylamine, an ethanolamine H_1 antagonist, was promoted for this application as a component of Bendectin, a prescription medication that also contained pyridoxine. The question of fetal malformations resulting from this use of Bendectin is discussed below.

Toxicity

The wide spectrum of adverse effects of the H_1 antihistamines is described above. Several of these effects (sedation, antimuscarinic action) have been used for therapeutic purposes, especially in OTC remedies (see Chapter 65). Nevertheless, these two effects constitute the most common undesirable actions when these drugs are used to block histamine receptors. Appropriate selection of drugs with a lower incidence of these effects (Table 16–2) and trial of several drugs by the patient are the most effective methods for minimizing both toxicities.

Less common toxic effects of systemic use include excitation and convulsions in children, postural hypotension, and allergic responses. Drug allergy is relatively common, especially after topical use of H_1 antagonists. The effects of severe systemic overdosage of the older agents resemble those of atropine overdosage and are treated in the same way (see Chapters 8 and 60). Overdosage of the newer H_1-blockers, especially astemizole, may induce cardiac arrhythmias (Wiley, 1992; Saviuc, 1993), and the same effect may be caused by interaction with enzyme inhibitors (see Drug Interactions, below).

Possible teratogenic effects of doxylamine were widely publicized in the lay press after 1978 as a result of case reports of fetal malformation associated with maternal ingestion of Bendectin. However, several large prospective studies involving over 60,000 pregnancies, of which more than 3000 involved maternal Bendectin ingestion, disclosed no increase in the incidence of birth defects. In contrast, a few case-control studies of infants with malformations suggested a weak correlation between Bendectin use and certain abnormalities. Because of the continuing controversy, adverse publicity, and lawsuits, the manufacturer of Bendectin withdrew the product from the market. Our inability to define the existence and extent of risk in this situation illustrates the difficulties involved in detecting small changes in the incidence of rare pathologic events (see Chapter 5).

Drug Interactions

Significant cardiac toxicity, including QT prolongation and potentially lethal ventricular arrhythmias, has occurred in patients taking a combination of either terfenadine or astemizole and ketoconazole, itraconazole, or erythromycin. The latter three drugs inhibit the metabolism of many drugs and probably cause significant increases in blood concentrations of the antihistamines. The seriousness of this interaction is such that terfenadine and astemizole are contraindicated in patients taking ketoconazole, itraconazole, or erythromycin and in patients with liver disease. The interaction has not yet been reported in patients taking loratadine.

For those H_1 antagonists that cause significant sedation, addition of other drugs that cause central nervous system depression produces additive effects and is contraindicated while driving or operating machinery.

H_2-RECEPTOR ANTAGONISTS
(Table 16–3)

The development of H_2-receptor antagonists was described in Chapter 5 (see box: Discovery and Development of H_2-Receptor Antagonists). This development led to renewed interest in possible physiologic roles for histamine and to a classification of effects of both agonists and antagonists based upon histamine receptor subtypes. The frequency of peptic ulcer disease and related gastrointestinal complaints created great interest in the therapeutic potential of H_2-receptor antagonists. Because of the ability of this class of drugs to reduce gastric acid secretion, they are now among the most frequently prescribed drugs in the USA.

I. BASIC PHARMACOLOGY OF H_2-RECEPTOR ANTAGONISTS

Chemistry & Pharmacokinetics

The first two H_2 receptor antagonists discovered, burimamide and metiamide, are imidazole compounds with long side chains containing a thiourea group. Because of their toxic effects, these agents are no longer used. Four H_2 antagonists are currently available in the USA: cimetidine, ranitidine, famotidine, and nizatidine. Their structures and some of their pharmacokinetic properties are set out in Table 16–3.

Pharmacodynamics

A. Mechanisms of Action: Presently available H_2-receptor antagonists reversibly compete with histamine at H_2-receptor sites. This action is quite selective in that the H_2 antagonists do not affect H_1 receptor-mediated actions.

B. Organ System Effects:

1. Acid secretion and gastric motility–The most important action of H_2 receptor antagonists is to reduce the secretion of gastric acid (Figure 16–3). These drugs block the acid secretion stimulated by histamine, gastrin, cholinomimetic drugs, and vagal stimulation. The volume of gastric secretion and the concentration of pepsin are also reduced. While the ability of H_2 receptor antagonists to inhibit all phases of acid secretion has been interpreted as implicating histamine as a final common mediator of acid secretion, a more plausible hypothesis suggests that the full expression of stimuli such as gastrin and parasympathetic impulses requires the participation of histamine in some manner. See Chapter 64 for further details.

Cimetidine, ranitidine, and famotidine have little effect on gastric smooth muscle function and on lower esophageal sphincter pressure. Other gastrointestinal secretions are not significantly reduced. While there are marked potency differences among

Table 16–3. H_2 receptor-blocking drugs.

Drug	Bioavailability (Oral)	V_d	$t_{1/2\beta}$	Elimination
Cimetidine	30–80%	0.8–1.2 L/kg	1.5–2.3 hr, increased in severe renal failure	Mostly renal. Major metabolite, S-oxide.
Ranitidine	30–88%	1.2–1.9 L/kg	1.6–2.4 hr, increased in severe renal failure	Mostly renal. Small amounts of S-oxide, N-oxide, and N-desmethyl metabolites.
Famotidine	37–45%	1.1–1.4 L/kg	2.5–4 hr, increased in severe renal failure	Mostly renal. Major metabolite, S-oxide.
Nizatidine	75–100%	1.2–1.6 L/kg	1.1–1.6 hr, increased in severe renal failure	Mostly renal. Small amounts of S-oxide, N-oxide, N-desmethyl metabolites.

efficacious than the others in reducing acid secretion. Nizatidine stimulates contractile activity in the stomach, leading to decreased emptying time. This effect may be related to the ability of nizatidine to inhibit acetylcholinesterase.

2. Other effects related to H_2-receptor blockade–In doses that suppress gastric acid secretion, cimetidine and ranitidine have little effect on the heart or blood pressure. Early reports that famotidine reduces cardiac output have not been confirmed in more recent studies. Nizatidine has been reported to reduce heart rate and cardiac output in healthy subjects. These observations are consistent with the idea that endogenous histamine has a negligible role in the normal regulation of cardiovascular function. As shown in Figure 16–1, cimetidine is effective in reducing some of the actions of administered histamine on the heart and vessels.

It has been predicted that H_2 receptor antagonists may enhance certain immune responses by blocking histamine's ability to decrease mediator release from mast cells and basophils; experimentally, increases in delayed hypersensitivity reactions can be shown in some patients receiving cimetidine. However, there is no evidence that clinical hypersensitivity reactions are increased in such patients.

3. Effects not related to H_2-receptor blockade–Cimetidine and, to a much lesser extent, ranitidine can inhibit the cytochrome P450 oxidative drug-metabolizing system. Famotidine and nizatidine do not inhibit the P450 system. Ranitidine has been shown to inhibit the glucuronidation of acetaminophen in animals. Both cimetidine and ranitidine can inhibit the renal clearance of basic drugs that are secreted by the renal tubule. Cimetidine binds to androgen receptors and causes antiandrogen effects. Ranitidine, famotidine, and nizatidine do not bind to androgen receptors.

II. CLINICAL PHARMACOLOGY OF H_2-RECEPTOR ANTAGONISTS

Clinical Uses

A. Peptic Duodenal Ulcer: An estimated 10%

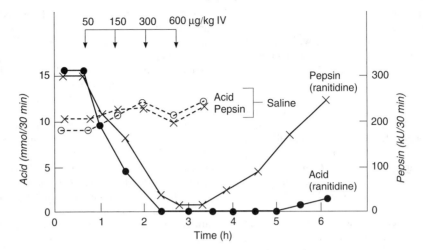

Figure 16–3. Effects of ranitidine on hypersecretion of pepsin and acid secretion in a patient. Gastric contents were collected by gastric tube for two 6-hour periods. Pepsin is quantitated as thousands of units and acid as millimoles per 30 minutes. During the first period, intravenous saline (placebo) injections were made at 40-minute intervals. During the second period, increasing intravenous ranitidine doses were given at 40-minute intervals as shown by the arrows. Ranitidine had a marked and long-lasting effect on acid secretion and a shorter but significant effect on pepsin production. (Modified and reproduced, with permission, from Danilewith M et al: Ranitidine suppression of gastric hypersecretion resistant to cimetidine. N Engl J Med 1982;306:20.)

of adults in the western world will suffer an episode of peptic ulcer disease during their lifetime. Although the mortality rate of this condition is low, the recurrence rate is high and the socioeconomic cost is great. Because it was known that "no acid = no ulcer," medical therapy—before the era of H_2-blockers—focused on reducing acidity with antimuscarinic drugs and antacids. However, antimuscarinic drugs must be used in high doses that cause significant adverse effects. Antacids relieve symptoms and, in high doses, can promote healing. However, frequent doses are required, and patient compliance is poor except during the acute symptomatic phase of the disease. The effectiveness of H_2-receptor antagonists in reducing gastric acidity coupled with their low toxicity represents a significant advance in the treatment of this disease. Results of many clinical trials show that these drugs effectively control symptoms during acute episodes and promote healing of duodenal ulcers. Prophylactic use at reduced dosage helps to prevent recurrence in many patients. Omeprazole, a very efficacious blocker of gastric acid secretion (by proton pump blockade), and sucralfate, a drug that promotes healing by coating the ulcer bed, are also available. Surgery for peptic ulcer has markedly declined as a result of drug therapy since the introduction of H_2 blockers. See Chapter 64 for further details.

For short-term management of active duodenal ulcer, once-daily doses of an H_2-blocker given at bedtime appear to be effective. Healing is promoted by cimetidine 800 mg, ranitidine 300 mg, famotidine 40 mg, or nizatidine 300 mg given once daily for up to 8 weeks. Because these drugs are eliminated by the kid-

ney, doses may be reduced in patients with poor renal function. Maintenance therapy for patients with a healed duodenal ulcer can also be accomplished by once-daily doses; cimetidine 400 mg, ranitidine 150 mg, famotidine 20 mg, or nizatidine 150 mg is effective in reducing recurrence. Most patients respond adequately, but some may become refractory to these agents for unknown reasons. These drugs are usually administered orally; cimetidine, ranitidine, and famotidine are also available for intravenous use. Hypotension and cardiac arrhythmias have been reported (rarely) following intravenous administration.

B. Gastric Ulcer: For patients with active benign gastric ulcers, administration of H_2-receptor antagonists relieves symptoms and promotes healing. Dosages are the same as for duodenal disease.

C. Erosive Esophagitis (Gastroesophageal Reflux Disorder): Erosive esophagitis often requires more frequent dosing than peptic ulcer. All four of the H_2 blockers are approved for this indication in the same or slightly higher total daily dosage, but divided into at least two daily doses.

D. Hypersecretory Conditions: Zollinger-Ellison syndrome is a usually fatal disorder in which hypersecretion of acid is caused by a gastrin-secreting tumor. Systemic mastocytosis and multiple endocrine adenomas often result in hypersecretion. In many patients, H_2 receptor-blocking drugs effectively control symptoms related to excess acid secretion. The drugs can be used before surgery or as primary treatment when surgery is not indicated. The dosages of H_2 antagonists required to reduce secretion and control symptoms are usually much larger than in ulcer patients. Multiple daily doses adjusted for each patient are usually required.

E. Other Conditions: In patients with hiatal hernia, stress-induced ulcers, and iatrogenic ulcers, the benefit of these drugs is not clearly documented.

Toxicity

H_2-blocking drugs are well tolerated, and adverse effects are reported in only 1–2% of cases. The most commonly reported effects are diarrhea, dizziness, somnolence, headache, and rash. Others include constipation, vomiting, and arthralgia. Cimetidine is associated with the most adverse effects, while nizatidine seems to produce the fewest. Other less common but more serious effects are discussed below.

A. Central Nervous System Dysfunction: Slurred speech, delirium, and confusional states are most common in elderly patients. These effects are most often associated with cimetidine, rare for ranitidine, and of unknown prevalence for famotidine and nizatidine.

B. Endocrine Effects: Cimetidine binds to androgen receptors, and antiandrogenic effects such as gynecomastia (in men) and galactorrhea (in women) have been reported. In addition, a reduction in sperm count and reversible impotence have been reported in male patients receiving high doses for hypersecretory states such as Zollinger-Ellison syndrome. These effects are rarely observed with therapy that continues for no longer than 8 weeks. Ranitidine, famotidine, and nizatidine appear to be free of endocrine effects.

C. Blood Dyscrasias: Cimetidine therapy has been associated with granulocytopenia, thrombocytopenia, neutropenia, and even aplastic anemia in a very few instances. There are also rare reports of similar effects associated with ranitidine. There is less information about these effects for famotidine or nizatidine.

D. Liver Toxicity: Reversible cholestatic effects have been reported for cimetidine. Reversible hepatitis, with or without jaundice, has been reported for ranitidine. Reversible abnormalities in liver enzyme tests have been reported for famotidine and nizatidine.

E. Pregnancy and Nursing Mothers: Animal studies have not shown any harmful effects on the fetus when H_2-blockers are administered to pregnant women. However, they cross the placenta, so these drugs should be given in this context only when absolutely necessary. All four agents are secreted into breast milk and therefore may affect the nursing infant.

Drug Interactions

Cimetidine inhibits the cytochrome P450-catalyzed oxidative drug metabolism pathway. The drug also reduces hepatic blood flow, which may further reduce clearance of other drugs. Co-administration of cimetidine with any of the following drugs may result in increased pharmacologic effects or toxicity: warfarin, phenytoin, propranolol, metoprolol, labetalol, quinidine, caffeine, lidocaine, theophylline, alprazolam, diazepam, flurazepam, triazolam, chlordiazepoxide, carbamazepine, ethanol, tricyclic antidepressants, metronidazole, calcium channel blockers, and sulfonylureas. Dosage adjustments may be necessary, especially in patients with reduced kidney function. Ranitidine in ordinary therapeutic doses does not appear to inhibit the oxidative metabolism of other drugs, but it may increase the bioavailability of ethanol by more than 40% in normal individuals. In animal studies, ranitidine has been shown to inhibit the glucuronidation of acetaminophen. Clinically significant drug interactions have not been reported for famotidine and nizatidine; however, experience with these agents is limited.

SEROTONIN (5-HYDROXYTRYPTAMINE)

Before the identification of 5-hydroxytryptamine (5-HT), it was known that when blood is allowed to clot, a vasoconstrictor substance is released from the clot; this substance was called serotonin. Independent studies established the existence of a smooth muscle stimulant in intestinal mucosa; this was called enteramine. The synthesis of 5-hydroxytryptamine in 1951 permitted the identification of serotonin and enteramine as the same metabolite of 5-hydroxytryptophan.

Serotonin is known to play a role in several diseases and is probably involved in many more. One of the more dramatic of these conditions is called **"serotonin syndrome"** and is evoked by an interaction between serotonergic agents, especially 5-HT reuptake blockers, and MAO inhibitors. This condition is described in Chapter 29. Serotonin is also one of the mediators of the signs and symptoms of carcinoid syndrome, an unusual manifestation of carcinoid tumor, a neoplasm of enterochromaffin cells. In patients whose tumor is not operable, serotonin antagonists may constitute the best treatment.

I. BASIC PHARMACOLOGY OF SEROTONIN

Chemistry & Pharmacokinetics

Like histamine, serotonin is widely distributed in

nature, being found in plant and animal tissues, venoms, and stings. It is an indoleethylamine formed in biologic systems from the amino acid L-tryptophan by hydroxylation of the indole ring followed by the decarboxylation of the amino acid. Hydroxylation at C5 is the rate-limiting step and can be blocked by *p*-chlorophenylalanine (PCPA, fenclonine) and by *p*-chloroamphetamine. These agents have been used experimentally to reduce serotonin synthesis in carcinoid syndrome.

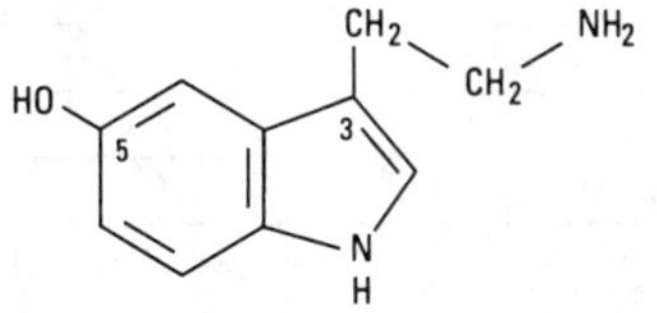

Serotonin

After synthesis, the free amine is stored or is rapidly inactivated, usually by oxidation catalyzed by the enzyme monoamine oxidase. In the pineal gland, serotonin serves as a precursor of melatonin, a melanocyte-stimulating hormone. In mammals (including humans), over 90% of the serotonin in the body is found in enterochromaffin cells in the gastrointestinal tract. In the blood, serotonin is found in platelets, which are able to concentrate the amine by means of an active carrier mechanism similar to that in the vesicles of noradrenergic and serotonergic nerve endings. Serotonin is also found in the raphe nuclei of the brain stem, which contain cell bodies of tryptaminergic (serotonergic) neurons that synthesize, store, and release serotonin as a transmitter. Brain serotonergic neurons are involved in various functions such as mood, sleep, temperature regulation, the perception of pain, and the regulation of blood pressure (see Chapter 20). Serotonin may also be involved in conditions such as depression, anxiety, and migraine. Serotonergic neurons are also found in the enteric nervous system of the gastrointestinal tract and around blood vessels. In rodents (but not in humans), serotonin is found in mast cells.

The function of serotonin in enterochromaffin cells is not clear. These cells synthesize serotonin, store the amine in a complex with ATP and with other substances in granules, and can release serotonin in response to mechanical and neuronal stimuli. Some of the released serotonin is taken up and stored in platelets.

Stored serotonin can be depleted by reserpine in much the same manner as this drug depletes catecholamines from vesicles in adrenergic nerves (see Chapter 6).

Serotonin is metabolized by monoamine oxidase, and the intermediate product, 5-hydroxyindoleacetaldehyde, is further oxidized by aldehyde dehydrogenase. When the latter enzyme is saturated, eg, by large amounts of acetaldehyde from ethanol metabolism, a significant fraction of the 5-hydroxyindoleacetaldehyde may be *reduced* in the liver to the alcohol 5-hydroxytryptophol. In humans consuming a normal diet, the excretion of 5-hydroxyindoleacetic acid (5-HIAA) is a measure of serotonin synthesis. Therefore, the 24-hour excretion of 5-HIAA can be used as a diagnostic test for tumors that synthesize excessive quantities of serotonin, especially carcinoid tumor. A few foods (eg, bananas) contain large amounts of serotonin or its precursors and must be prohibited during such diagnostic tests.

Pharmacodynamics

A. Mechanisms of Action: Serotonin exerts many actions and, like histamine, has many species differences, making generalizations difficult. The actions of serotonin are mediated through a variety of cell membrane receptors. The serotonin receptors that have been characterized thus far are described in Table 16–4. Seven major 5-HT-receptor subtypes have been identified, including both G protein-coupled receptors and a ligand-gated ion channel. Among these receptor subtypes, several lack any recognized physiologic function. Discovery of these functions awaits the development of subtype-selective drugs or the use of genetic methods to mutate or delete genes encoding these receptors from the mouse genome.

B. Tissue and Organ System Effects:

1. Cardiovascular system–Serotonin directly causes the contraction of smooth muscle. In humans, serotonin is a powerful vasoconstrictor except in skeletal muscle and heart, where it dilates blood vessels. At least part of this 5-HT-induced vasodilation requires the presence of vascular endothelial cells. When the endothelium is damaged, coronary vessels constrict (Golino, 1991). Serotonin can also elicit reflex bradycardia by activation of chemoreceptor nerve endings. A triphasic blood pressure response is often seen following injection of serotonin. Initially, there is a decrease in heart rate, cardiac output, and blood pressure caused by the chemoreceptor response. Following this decrease, blood pressure increases as a result of vasoconstriction. The third phase is again a decrease in blood pressure attributed to vasodilation in vessels supplying skeletal muscle. Pulmonary and renal vessels seem especially sensitive to the vasoconstrictor action of serotonin.

Serotonin also constricts veins, and venoconstriction with a resulting increased capillary filling appears responsible for the flush that is observed following serotonin administration. Serotonin has small direct positive chronotropic and inotropic effects on the heart that are probably of no clinical significance. However, prolonged elevation of the blood level of serotonin (which occurs in carcinoid syndrome) is associated with pathologic alterations in the endocardium (subendocardial fibroplasia) that may result in valvular or electrical malfunction.

Serotonin causes blood platelets to aggregate by activating surface 5-HT$_2$ receptors. This response, in

Table 16–4. Serotonin receptor subtypes.

Receptor Subtype	Distribution	Postreceptor Mechanism	Partially Selective Agonists	Partially Selective Antagonists
5-HT$_{1A}$	Raphe nuclei, hippocampus	↓ cAMP, K$^+$ channels	8-OH-DPAT	
5-HT$_{1B}$	Substantia nigra, globus pallidus, basal ganglia	↓ cAMP	CP 93129	
5-HT$_{1C}$	Choroid, hippocampus, substantia nigra	↑ IP$_3$		
5-HT$_{1Da,b}$	Brain	↓ cAMP	Sumatriptan	
5-HT$_{1E}$	Cortex, putamen	↓ cAMP		
5-HT$_{1F}$	Cortex, hippocampus	↓ cAMP		
5-HT$_{2A}$	Platelets, smooth muscle, cerebral cortex	↑ IP$_3$	α-Methyl-5-HT	Ritanserin
5-HT$_{2F}$	Stomach fundus	↑ IP$_3$		
5-HT$_3$	Area postrema, sensory and enteric nerves	Receptor is a Na$^+$/K$^+$ ion channel	2-Methyl-5-HT, metachlorophenyl-biguanide	Tropisetron, ondansetron, granisetron
5-HT$_4$	CNS and myenteric neurons, smooth muscle	↑ cAMP	5-Methoxytryptamine, renzapride, metoclopramide	See Bockaert, 1992, reference.
5-HT$_{5a,b}$	Brain	Unknown		
5-HT$_{6,7}$	Brain	↑ cAMP		Clozapine (5-HT$_7$)

Key: 8-OH-DPAT = 8-Hydroxy-2-(di-*n*-propylamine)tetralin
CP 93129= 5-Hydroxy-3(4-1,2,5,6-tetrahydropyridyl)-4-azaindole

contrast to aggregation induced during clot formation, is not accompanied by the release of serotonin stored in the platelets. The physiologic role of this effect is unclear.

2. Gastrointestinal tract–Serotonin causes contraction of gastrointestinal smooth muscle, increasing tone and facilitating peristalsis. This action is caused by the direct action of serotonin on smooth muscle receptors plus a stimulating action on ganglion cells located in the enteric nervous system (Chapter 6). Serotonin has little effect on secretions, and what effects it has are generally inhibitory. It has been proposed that serotonin plays an important physiologic role as a local hormone controlling gastrointestinal motility. However, large doses of antagonists of serotonin are not associated with severe constipation. On the other hand, overproduction of serotonin (and other substances) in carcinoid tumor is associated with severe diarrhea.

3. Respiration–Serotonin has a small direct stimulant effect on bronchiolar smooth muscle in normal humans. In patients with carcinoid syndrome, episodes of bronchoconstriction occur in response to elevated levels of the amine. Serotonin may also cause hyperventilation as a result of the chemoreceptor reflex or bronchial sensory nerve ending stimulation.

4. Nervous system–Like histamine, serotonin is a potent stimulant of pain and itch sensory nerve endings and is responsible for some of the symptoms caused by insect and plant stings. In addition, serotonin is a powerful activator of chemosensitive endings located in the coronary vascular bed. Activation of 5-HT$_3$ receptors on these afferent vagal nerve endings is associated with the chemoreceptor reflex (also known as the Bezold-Jarisch reflex). The reflex response consists of marked bradycardia and hypotension. The bradycardia is mediated by vagal outflow to the heart and can be blocked by atropine. The hypotension is a consequence of the decrease in cardiac output that results from bradycardia.

A variety of other agents can activate the chemoreceptor reflex. These include nicotinic cholinoceptor agonists and some cardiac glycosides, eg, ouabain.

Serotonin is present in a variety of sites in the brain. Its role as a neurotransmitter and its relation to the actions of drugs acting in the central nervous system are discussed in Chapters 20 and 29.

II. CLINICAL PHARMACOLOGY OF SEROTONIN

SEROTONIN AGONISTS

Serotonin has no clinical applications as a drug. **Buspirone,** a 5-HT$_{1a}$ agonist, has received wide attention for its utility as an effective nonbenzodiazepine anxiolytic (see Chapter 21). **Sumatriptan,** a new serotonin analogue, is a 5-HT$_{1d}$ agonist. It has been shown to be effective in the treatment of acute migraine and cluster headache attacks, strengthening the association of serotonin abnormalities with these headache syndromes (Moskowitz, 1993).

Sumatriptan

Following the subcutaneous administration of 6 mg of sumatriptan succinate, 70% of patients suffering migraine attacks will experience relief of symptoms. This degree of efficacy appears to be greater than that of other drug treatments. Most adverse effects are mild and include altered sensations (tingling, warmth, etc), dizziness, muscle weakness, neck pain, and injection site reactions. Chest discomfort occurs in 5% of patients, and chest pain has been reported. Sumatriptan is contraindicated in patients with ischemic coronary artery disease and in patients with Prinzmetal's angina. Other disadvantages of this drug include the fact that its half-life is less than 2 hours, so that its effect is often shorter than the duration of the headache. As a result several doses may be required during a prolonged migraine attack, though the drug is approved for only two doses per 24 hours. In addition, the drug is extremely expensive at present.

In addition to agonists and antagonists, compounds such as fluoxetine, which modulate serotonergic transmission by blocking reuptake of the transmitter, are among the most widely prescribed drugs for the management of depression and other behavioral disorders. These drugs are discussed in Chapter 29.

SEROTONIN ANTAGONISTS

The actions of serotonin, like those of histamine, can be antagonized in several different ways. Such antagonism is clearly desirable in those rare patients who have carcinoid tumor and may also be valuable in certain other conditions.

As noted above, serotonin synthesis can be inhibited by *p*-chlorophenylalanine and *p*-chloroamphetamine. However, these agents are too toxic for general use. Storage of serotonin can be inhibited by the use of reserpine, but the sympatholytic effects of this drug (see Chapter 11) and the high levels of circulating serotonin that result from release prevent its use in carcinoid. Therefore, receptor blockade is the major approach to therapeutic limitation of serotonin effects.

SEROTONIN RECEPTOR ANTAGONISTS

Cyproheptadine and a number of experimental drugs have been identified as competitive serotonin receptor-blocking agents. In addition, the ergot alkaloids discussed in the last portion of the chapter are partial agonists at serotonin receptors.

Cyproheptadine resembles the phenothiazine antihistaminic agents in chemical structure and has potent H$_1$ receptor-blocking actions. The actions of cyproheptadine are predictable from its H$_1$ histamine and serotonin receptor affinities. It prevents the smooth muscle effects of both amines but has no effect on the gastric secretion stimulated by histamine. It also has significant antimuscarinic effects and causes sedation.

The major clinical applications of cyproheptadine are in the treatment of the smooth muscle manifestations of carcinoid tumor and in the postgastrectomy dumping syndrome. The usual dosage in adults is 12–16 mg/d in three or four divided doses. It is also the preferred drug in cold-induced urticaria.

Ketanserin is an agent that blocks 5-HT$_{1c}$ and 5-HT$_2$ receptors and has little or no reported antagonist activity at other 5-HT or H$_1$ receptors. This drug also blocks vascular α_1 adrenoceptors. The drug blocks 5-HT$_2$ receptors on platelets and antagonizes platelet aggregation promoted by serotonin. Interest in this compound is generated by observations that it lowers blood pressure both in hypertensive animals and in hypertensive human patients. However, the exact mechanisms involved in this hypotensive action are not clear and may involve both α_1 adrenoceptors and 5-HT$_2$ receptors. Available in Europe for the treatment of hypertension and vasospastic conditions, it has not been approved in the USA.

Ritanserin, another 5-HT$_2$ antagonist, has little or no alpha-blocking action. It has been reported to alter bleeding time and to reduce thromboxane formation, presumably by altering platelet function.

Ondansetron, a 5-HT$_3$ antagonist, is approved for use in the prevention of nausea and vomiting associated with cancer chemotherapy. It is effective at a dose level of 0.1–0.2 mg/kg intravenously. The drug is also being evaluated for treatment of postsurgical nausea and vomiting, anxiety, and psychoses. Granisetron, a drug with similar properties, has recently been approved. Other congeners are in clinical trials.

Considering the diverse effects attributed to serotonin and the heterogeneous nature of 5-HT receptors, other selective 5-HT antagonists may prove to be useful clinically.

THE ERGOT ALKALOIDS

Bertram G. Katzung, MD, PhD

Ergot alkaloids are produced by *Claviceps purpurea,* a fungus that infects grain—especially rye—under damp growing or storage conditions. This fungus synthesizes histamine, acetylcholine, tyramine, and other biologically active products in addition to a score or more of unique ergot alkaloids. These alkaloids affect alpha adrenoceptors, dopamine receptors, 5-HT receptors, and perhaps other receptor types.

The accidental ingestion of ergot alkaloids in contaminated grain can be traced back more than 2000 years from descriptions of epidemics of ergot poisoning (ergotism). The most dramatic effects of poisoning are dementia with florid hallucinations; prolonged vasospasm, which may result in gangrene; and stimulation of uterine smooth muscle, which in pregnancy may result in abortion. The severity of each effect varies among reported epidemics and may represent a different mix of individual alkaloids in different crops of the fungus. In medieval times, ergot poisoning was called St. Anthony's fire after the saint whose help was sought in relieving the burning pain of vasospastic ischemia. Identifiable epidemics have occurred sporadically up to modern times (see box: Ergot Poisoning: Not Just An Ancient Disease) and mandate continuous surveillance of all grains used for food. Poisoning of grazing animals is common in many areas because the same and related fungi may grow on pasture grasses (Porter, 1992).

In addition to the effects noted above, the ergot alkaloids produce a variety of other central nervous system and peripheral effects. Detailed structure-activity analysis and appropriate semisynthetic modifications have yielded a large number of agents with documented or potential clinical value.

I. BASIC PHARMACOLOGY OF ERGOT ALKALOIDS

Chemistry & Pharmacokinetics

Two major families of compounds that incorporate the tetracyclic **ergoline** nucleus may be identified; the amine alkaloids and the peptide alkaloids (Table 16–5). Drugs of therapeutic and toxicologic importance are found in both groups.

The ergot alkaloids are variably absorbed from the gastrointestinal tract. The oral dose of ergotamine is about ten times larger than the intramuscular dose, but the speed of absorption and peak blood levels after oral administration can be improved by administration with caffeine (see below). The amine alkaloids are also absorbed from the rectum and the buccal cavity and after administration by aerosol inhaler. Absorption after intramuscular injection is slow but usually reliable. Bromocriptine is well absorbed from the gastrointestinal tract.

The ergot alkaloids are extensively metabolized in the body. The primary metabolites are hydroxylated in the A ring, and peptide alkaloids are also modified in the peptide moiety. Most of the excretory products of methysergide are demethylated at the N1 position.

Pharmacodynamics

A. Mechanism of Action: As suggested above, the ergot alkaloids act on several types of receptors. Their effects include agonist, partial agonist, and antagonist actions at alpha adrenoceptors and serotonin receptors and agonist action at central nervous system dopamine receptors (Table 16–6). In addition, as yet undefined receptors may be activated. Furthermore, some members of the ergot family have a high affinity for presynaptic receptors, while others are more selective for postjunctional receptors. There is a powerful stimulant effect on the uterus that seems to be most closely associated with agonist (or partial agonist) effects at 5-HT$_2$ receptors. Structural variations increase the selectivity of certain members of the family for specific receptor types.

B. Organ System Effects:

1. Central nervous system–As indicated by traditional descriptions of ergotism, certain of the naturally occurring alkaloids are powerful hallucinogens. Lysergic acid diethylamide (LSD, "acid") is the ergot compound that most clearly demonstrates this action. The drug has been used in the laboratory as a potent peripheral 5-HT$_2$ antagonist, but current evidence suggests that its behavioral effects are mediated by agonist effects at prejunctional (Sadzot, 1989) or postjunctional (Buckholtz, 1990) 5-HT$_2$ receptors in the central nervous system. In spite of extensive research, no clinical value has been discovered for

Table 16–5. Major ergoline derivatives (ergot alkaloids).

Amine alkaloids	Peptide alkaloids

	R_1	R_8		R_2	R_2'	R_5'
6-Methylergoline	–H	–H	Ergotamine*	–H	–CH$_3$	–CH$_2$– (phenyl)
Lysergic acid	–H	–COOH				
Lysergic acid diethylamide (LSD)	–H	$-\overset{\text{O}}{\overset{\|}{C}}-N(CH_2-CH_3)_2$	a-Ergocryptine	–H	–CH(CH$_3$)$_2$	–CH$_2$–CH(CH$_3$)$_2$
			Bromocriptine	–Br	–CH(CH$_3$)$_2$	–CH$_2$–CH(CH$_3$)$_2$
Ergonovine (ergometrine)	–H	$-\overset{\text{O}}{\overset{\|}{C}}-NHCHCH_3$ with CH_2OH				
Methysergide	–CH$_3$	$-\overset{\text{O}}{\overset{\|}{C}}-NH-CH-CH_2-CH_3$ with CH$_2$OH				

*Dihydroergtotamine lacks the double bond between carbons 9 and 10.

LSD's dramatic effects. Abuse of this drug was widespread for several decades and is discussed in Chapter 31.

Dopamine receptors in the central nervous system play important roles in extrapyramidal motor control and the regulation of prolactin release. The actions of bromocriptine on the extrapyramidal system are discussed in Chapter 27. Of all the currently available ergot derivatives, bromocriptine has the highest selectivity for the pituitary dopamine receptors. Bromocriptine directly suppresses prolactin secretion from pituitary cells by activating regulatory dopamine receptors (Chapter 36). It competes for binding to these sites with dopamine itself and with other dopamine agonists such as apomorphine.

2. Vascular smooth muscle–The action of ergot alkaloids on vascular smooth muscle is drug-, species-, and vessel-dependent, so few generalizations are possible. Ergotamine and related compounds constrict most human blood vessels in a predictable, prolonged, and potent manner (Figure 16–4). This response is partially blocked by conventional alpha-blocking agents. However, ergotamine's effect is also associated with "epinephrine reversal" (see Chapter 10) and with *blockade* of the response to other alpha agonists. This dual action represents par-

Table 16–6. Effects of ergot alkaloids at several receptors.[1]

Ergot Alkaloid	Alpha-Adrenoceptor	Dopamine Receptor	Serotonin Receptor (5-HT$_2$)	Uterine Smooth Muscle Stimulation
Bromocriptine	–	+++	–	0
Ergonovine	+	+	–(PA)	+++
Ergotamine	– –(PA)	0	+(PA)	+++
Lysergic acid diethylamide (LSD)	0	+++	– –	+
Methysergide	+/0	+/0	– – –(PA)	+/0

[1]Agonist effects are indicated by +, antagonist by –, no effect by 0. Relative affinity for the receptor is indicated by the number of + or – signs. PA means partial agonist (both agonist and antagonist effects can be detected).

ERGOT POISONING: NOT JUST AN ANCIENT DISEASE

As noted in the text, epidemics of ergotism, or poisoning by ergot-contaminated grain, are known to have occurred sporadically in ancient times and through the Middle Ages. It is easy to imagine the social chaos that might occur if fiery pain, gangrene, hallucinations, convulsions, and abortions appeared simultaneously throughout a community in which all or most of the people believed in witchcraft, demonic possession, and the visitation of supernatural punishments upon humans for their misdeeds. Such beliefs are uncommon in most cultures today. However, ergotism has not disappeared in modern times. A most convincing demonstration of ergotism occurred in the small French village of Pont-Saint-Esprit in 1951. It was described in the British Medical Journal in 1951 (Gabbai, 1951) and in a later book-length narrative account (Fuller, 1968). Several hundred individuals suffered symptoms of hallucinations, convulsions, and ischemia—and several died—after eating bread made from contaminated flour. Similar events have occurred even more recently when poverty, famine, or incompetence resulted in the consumption of contaminated grain.

Iatrogenic ergot toxicity caused by excessive use of medical ergot preparations is still frequently reported. The following case history is typical (Andersen et al, 1977).

A 58-year-old woman with a history of moderate ergotamine use for migraine was admitted to the hospital after 3 days of increasing symptoms of ischemia in the legs (pain, tenderness, cyanosis, and low skin temperature). No pulses could be palpated below the femoral vessels. The initial aortogram is shown in Figure 16–5 (left). An epidural local anesthetic was administered to block sympathetic vasoconstrictor impulses to the vessels in the pelvis and legs, but no improvement was observed. After 3 hours, an infusion of nitroprusside was started. The temperature of the skin of the large toe rose rapidly from 22 °C to 31 °C. Cyanosis disappeared, and popliteal and tibial pulses became palpable. An attempt to discontinue the nitroprusside infusion after 11 hours was followed by immediate vasoconstriction and cyanosis in the legs, so nitroprusside was restarted and continued for another 25 hours with good maintenance of circulation. Thirty-six hours after the start of the infusion, nitroprusside was discontinued with no signs of recurrent vasoconstriction. A repeat aortogram 1 week after the event appeared normal (Figure 16–5 [right]).

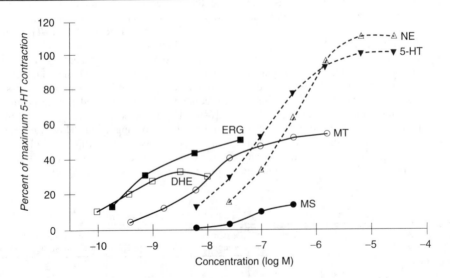

Figure 16–4. Effects of ergot derivatives on contraction of isolated segments of human basilar artery strips removed at surgery. All of the ergot derivatives are partial agonists, and all are more potent than the full agonists, norepinephrine and serotonin. (NE, norepinephrine; 5-HT, serotonin; ERG, ergotamine; MT, methylergometrine; DHE, dihydroergotamine; MS, methysergide.) (Modified and reproduced, with permission, from Müller-Schweinitzer E in: *5-Hydroxytryptamine Mechanisms in Primary Headaches.* Oleson J, Saxena PR [editors]. Raven Press, 1992.)

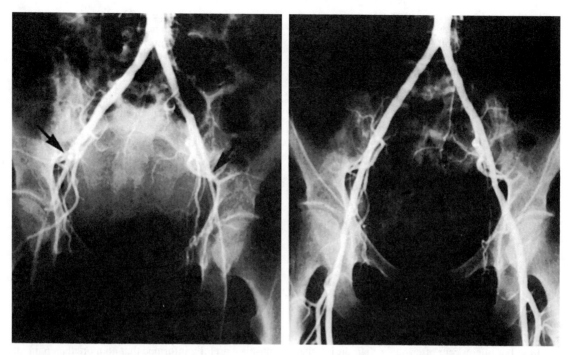

Figure 16–5. Vasospasm induced by ergotamine. Aortic angiograms taken at the time of maximum vasospasm (left panel) and 1 week after (right panel) infusion of nitroprusside. The major vessels distal to the common iliac arteries *(arrows)* are thread-like and occluded in the left panel; in the right panel, normal flow has been restored. (Modified and reproduced, with permission, from Andersen PK et al: Sodium nitroprusside and epidural blockade in the treatment of ergotism. N Engl J Med 1977;296:1271.)

tial agonist action (Table 16–5). Because ergotamine dissociates very slowly from the alpha receptor, it produces very long-lasting agonist and antagonist effects at this receptor. There is little or no effect at beta adrenoceptors.

While much of the vasoconstriction elicited by ergot alkaloids can be ascribed to partial agonist effects at alpha adrenoceptors, some may be the result of effects at 5-HT receptors. Ergotamine, ergonovine, and methysergide all have partial agonist effects at 5-HT$_2$ vascular receptors. Furthermore, different vascular beds have different sensitivities, and it is claimed that cerebral vessels, especially cerebral arteriovenous anastomotic vessels, are most sensitive to drugs such as ergotamine, dihydroergotamine, and sumatriptan (den Boer 1992). The remarkably specific antimigraine action of the ergot derivatives is thought to be related to their actions on neuronal or vascular serotonin receptors. Ergotamine, ergonovine, and methysergide are the ergot drugs most widely used for the treatment of migraine.

After overdosage with ergotamine and similar agents, vasospasm is severe and prolonged (see Toxicity, below). This vasospasm is not reversed by alpha antagonists, serotonin antagonists, or combinations of both.

Ergotamine is typical of the ergot alkaloids with a strong vasoconstrictor spectrum of action. The hydrogenation of ergot alkaloids at the 9 and 10 positions (Table 16–5) yields dihydro derivatives that have much lower direct smooth muscle and serotonin effects and more selective alpha receptor-blocking actions.

3. Uterine smooth muscle–The stimulant action of ergot alkaloids on the uterus, as on vascular smooth muscle, appears to combine alpha agonist, serotonin, and other effects. Furthermore, the sensitivity of the uterus to the stimulant effects of ergot changes dramatically during pregnancy, perhaps because of increasing dominance of alpha$_1$ receptors as pregnancy progresses. As a result, the uterus at term is more sensitive than earlier in pregnancy and far more sensitive than the nonpregnant organ.

In very small doses, ergot preparations can evoke rhythmic contraction and relaxation of the uterus. At higher concentrations, these drugs induce powerful and prolonged contracture. Ergonovine is more selective than other ergot alkaloids in affecting the uterus and is the agent of choice in obstetric applications of these drugs.

4. Other smooth muscle organs–In most patients, the ergot alkaloids have no significant effect on bronchiolar smooth muscle. The gastrointestinal tract, on the other hand, varies dramatically in sensitivity among patients. Nausea, vomiting, and diarrhea may be induced by low doses in some patients but only by high doses in others. The effect is consistent with action on the central nervous system emetic center and on gastrointestinal serotonin receptors.

II. CLINICAL PHARMACOLOGY OF ERGOT ALKALOIDS

Clinical Uses

A. Migraine: Migraine headache in its classic form is characterized by a brief "aura" that may involve visual scotomas or even hemianopia and speech abnormalities, followed by a severe throbbing unilateral headache that lasts for a few hours to 1–2 days. The disease is familial in 60–80% of patients, more common in women, and usually has its onset in early adolescence through young adulthood, waning with advancing years. Attacks are frequently precipitated by stress but often occur after rather than during the stressful episode. They vary in frequency from one attack a year to two or more a week. Excellent written descriptions by patients are available (eg, Creditor, 1982).

Although the symptom pattern varies among patients, the severity of migraine headache justifies vigorous therapy in the great majority of cases.

The pathophysiology of migraine clearly includes some vasomotor mechanism, because the onset of headache is associated with a marked increase in amplitude of temporal artery pulsations, and relief of pain by administration of ergotamine is accompanied by diminution of arterial pulsations. On the other hand, these vasomotor changes may be the result of more basic processes underlying migraine, since a number of drugs with very different vascular actions are effective in migraine. For example, even though many vasoconstrictors are able to reduce or abort a migraine attack, drug-induced dilation of the cranial vessels does not provoke a typical migraine attack. Histologic study of cranial vessels from migraine patients shows that migraine attacks are associated with a sterile neurogenic perivascular edema and inflammation. Since these tissues are well supplied with sensory nerves, such pathologic changes could indeed be associated with prolonged headache. Finally, it is claimed that many of the drugs known to be effective in clinical migraine (ergot, nonsteroidal antiinflammatory agents) are capable of preventing or reducing the perivascular tissue inflammation (Moskowitz, 1989; Buzzi, 1990).

Evidence suggests that the onset of a migrainous aura is associated with an abnormal release of serotonin from platelets, while the throbbing headache is associated with decrease of platelet and serum serotonin below normal concentrations. Other evidence implicating serotonin in migraine includes the facts that numerous serotonergic nerve fiber endings are found in and around meningeal blood vessels and that many of the drugs useful in migraine directly or indirectly influence serotonergic nerve transmission. Other chemical triggers (which may operate through serotonin) include falling levels of estrogen in women whose headache is linked to the menstrual cycle and elevated levels of prostaglandin E_1.

The efficacy of ergot derivatives in the therapy of migraine is so specific as to constitute a diagnostic test. Traditional therapy (**ergotamine**) is most effective when given during the prodrome of an attack and becomes progressively less effective if delayed. Ergotamine tartrate is available for oral, sublingual, rectal suppository, and inhaler use. It is often combined with caffeine (100 mg caffeine for each 1 mg ergotamine tartrate) to facilitate absorption of the ergot alkaloid.

The vasoconstriction induced by ergotamine is long-lasting and cumulative when the drug is taken repeatedly, as in a severe attack. Therefore, patients must be carefully informed that no more than 6 mg of the oral preparation may be taken for each attack and no more than 10 mg per week. For very severe attacks, ergotamine tartrate, 0.25–0.5 mg, may be given intravenously or intramuscularly. **Dihydroergotamine,** 0.5–1 mg intravenously, is favored by some clinicians for treatment of intractable migraine. Intranasal or oral dihydroergotamine, currently investigational, may also be effective.

Because of the cumulative toxicity of ergotamine, safer agents useful for the prophylaxis of migraine have been sought. **Ergonovine,** 0.2–0.4 mg 3 times daily, has been used. **Methysergide,** a derivative of the amine subgroup (Table 16–5), has been shown to be effective in this application in about 60% of patients. Unfortunately, significant toxicity (discussed below) occurs in almost 40% of patients. As suggested in Table 16–6, there is some evidence of a difference in the agonist:antagonist ratios of methysergide and ergotamine when assayed on serotonin receptors. Regardless of the cause, methysergide is relatively *ineffective* in treatment of impending or active episodes of migraine. The dosage of methysergide maleate for prophylaxis of migraine is 4–8 mg/d.

Although relatively free of the rapidly cumulative vasospastic toxicity of ergotamine, chronic use of methysergide may induce retroperitoneal fibroplasia and subendocardial fibrosis, possibly through its vascular effects. Therefore, it is important that patients taking methysergide have drug holidays of 3–4 weeks every 6 months (see Toxicity).

Propranolol and **amitriptyline** have also been found to be effective for the prophylaxis of migraine in some patients. Like methysergide, they are of no value in the treatment of acute migraine. **Flunarizine,**

an investigational calcium channel blocker, has been reported in preliminary trials to effectively reduce the severity of the acute attack and prevent recurrences.

Sumatriptan, discussed on page 265, appears to be an effective alternative to ergotamine for the treatment of acute migraine attacks. It is not currently available for oral or chronic use.

B. Hyperprolactinemia: Increased serum levels of the anterior pituitary hormone prolactin are associated with secreting tumors of the gland and also with the use of centrally acting dopamine antagonists, especially the antipsychotic drugs. Because of negative feedback effects, hyperprolactinemia is associated with amenorrhea and infertility in women as well as galactorrhea in both sexes.

Bromocriptine mesylate is extremely effective in reducing the high levels of prolactin that result from pituitary tumors and has even been associated with regression of the tumor in some cases. The usual dosage of bromocriptine is 2.5 mg 2 or 3 times daily. Bromocriptine has also been used in the same dosage to suppress physiologic lactation. A few cases of serious postpartum cardiovascular toxicity have been reported in association with the latter use of bromocriptine (Ruch, 1989).

C. Postpartum Hemorrhage: The uterus at term is extremely sensitive to the stimulant action of ergot, and even moderate doses produce a prolonged and powerful spasm of the muscle quite unlike natural labor. This was not appreciated when the drugs were introduced into obstetrics in the 18th century. Their use at that time to accelerate delivery caused a dramatic *increase* in fetal and maternal mortality rates. Therefore, ergot derivatives are useful only for control of late uterine bleeding and should never be given before delivery. Ergonovine maleate, 0.2 mg usually given intramuscularly, is effective within 1–5 minutes and is less toxic than other ergot derivatives for this application. It is given at the time of delivery of the placenta or immediately afterward if bleeding is significant.

D. Diagnosis of Variant Angina: Ergonovine produces prompt vasoconstriction in the coronary vessels subject to spastic responses (Prinzmetal's or variant angina; see Chapter 12). Therefore, this ergot derivative may be administered by intravenous infusion during coronary angiography to diagnose variant angina.

E. Senile Cerebral Insufficiency: Dihydroergotoxine, a mixture of dihydro-α-ergocryptine and three similar dihydrogenated peptide ergot alkaloids (ergoloid mesylates), has been promoted for many years for the relief of senility and more recently for the treatment of Alzheimer's dementia. There is no evidence of significant benefit.

Toxicity & Contraindications

The most common toxic effects of the ergot derivatives are gastrointestinal disturbances, including diarrhea and nausea and vomiting. Activation of the medullary vomiting center and of the gastrointestinal serotonin receptors is involved. Since migraine attacks are often associated with these symptoms before therapy is begun, these adverse effects are rarely contraindications to the use of ergot. However, in prophylactic management with methysergide, nausea, vomiting, and diarrhea are important factors limiting use of the drug.

A more dangerous toxic effect of overdosage with agents like ergotamine and ergonovine is prolonged vasospasm. As described above, this sign of vascular smooth muscle stimulation may result in gangrene and require amputation. Most cases involve the circulation to the arms and legs. However, bowel infarction resulting from mesenteric artery vasospasm has also been reported. Peripheral vascular vasospasm caused by ergot is refractory to most vasodilators, but infusions of large doses of nitroprusside (Dierckx, 1986) or nitroglycerin (Tfelt-Hansen, 1982), have been successful in some cases. (See box: Ergot Poisoning: Not Just an Ancient Disease.)

Chronic therapy with methysergide is associated with development of fibroplastic changes in the retroperitoneal space, the pleural cavity, and the endocardial tissue of the heart. These changes occur insidiously over months and may present as hydronephrosis (from obstruction of the ureters) or a cardiac murmur (from distortion of the valves of the heart). In some cases, valve damage may require surgical replacement (Redfield, 1992). Fortunately, in most patients, signs of toxicity regress when administration of the drug is halted. However, the potential for injury is such that all patients taking methysergide should have periodic drug holidays and should be carefully studied if signs or symptoms of fibroplasia occur.

Other toxic effects of the ergot alkaloids include drowsiness and, in the case of methysergide, occasional instances of central stimulation and hallucinations. In fact, methysergide has been used as a substitute for LSD by members of the "drug culture."

Contraindications to the use of ergot derivatives consist of the obstructive vascular diseases and collagen diseases.

There is no evidence that ordinary use of ergotamine or methysergide for migraine is hazardous in pregnancy. However, most clinicians counsel restraint in the use of these agents by pregnant patients.

PREPARATIONS AVAILABLE

Antihistamines (H₁ Blockers)

Astemizole (Hismanal)
Oral: 10 mg tablets
Azatadine (Optimine)
Oral: 1 mg tablets
Brompheniramine (generic, Dimetane, Bromphen, others)
Oral: 4, 8, 12 mg tablets; 2 mg/5 mL elixir
Oral sustained-release: 8, 12 mg tablets
Parenteral: 10 mg/mL for injection
Buclizine (Bucladin-S Softabs)
Oral: 50 mg tablets
Carbinoxamine (Clistin)
Oral: 4 mg tablets
Cetirizine (Reactine)
Oral: Data not yet available.
Chlorpheniramine (generic, Chlor-Trimeton, Teldrin, others)
Oral: 2 mg chewable tablets;, 4, 12 mg tablets; 2 mg/5 mL syrup
Oral sustained-release: 8, 12 mg tablets and capsules
Parenteral: 10, 100 mg/mL for injection
Clemastine (Tavist)
Oral: 1.34, 2.68 mg tablets; 0.67 mg/5 mL syrup
Cyclizine (Marezine)
Oral: 50 mg tablets
Parenteral: 50 mg/mL for injection
Cyproheptadine (generic, Periactin)
Oral: 4 mg tablets; 2 mg/5 mL syrup
Dexchlorpheniramine (generic, Polamine, others)
Oral: 2 mg tablets; 2 mg/5 mL syrup
Oral sustained release: 4, 6 mg tablets
Dimenhydrinate* (generic, Dramamine)
Oral: 50 mg tablets and capsules; 50 mg chewable tablets; 12.5 mg/4 mL; 15.62 mg/5 mL
Diphenhydramine (generic, Benadryl)
Oral: 25, 50 mg capsules; 25, 50 mg tablets; 12.5 mg/5 mL elixir and syrup
Parenteral: 10, 50 mg/mL for injection
Hydroxyzine (generic, Atarax, Vistaril)
Oral: 10, 25, 50, 100 mg tablets; 25, 50, 100 mg capsules; 10 mg/5 mL syrup; 25 mg/5 mL suspension
Parenteral: 25, 50 mg/mL for injection
Loratidine (Claritin)
Oral: 10 mg tablets
Meclizine (generic, Antivert, others)
Oral: 12.5, 25, 50 mg tablets; 25 mg capsules; 25 mg chewable tablets
Methdilazine (Tacaryl)
Oral: 4 mg chewable tablets; 8 mg tablets; 4 mg/5 mL syrup

Phenindamine (Nolahist)
Oral: 25 mg tablets
Promethazine (generic, Phenergan, others)
Oral: 12.5, 25, 50 mg tablets; 6.25, 25 mg/5 mL syrups
Parenteral: 25 mg/mL for injection; 50 mg/mL for IM injection
Rectal: 12.5, 25, 50 mg suppositories
Pyrilamine (generic)
Oral: 25 mg tablets
Terfenadine (Seldane)
Oral: 60 mg tablets
Trimeprazine (Temaril)
Oral: 2.5 mg tablets; 2.5 mg/5 mL syrup
Oral sustained-release: 5 mg capsules
Tripelennamine (generic, Pelamine, PBZ)
Oral: 25, 50 mg tablets; 37.5 mg/5 mL elixir
Oral sustained-release: 100 mg tablets
Triprolidine (generic, Actidil, Myidil)
Oral: 2.5 mg tablets; 1.25 mg/5 mL syrup

H₂ Blockers

Cimetidine (Tagamet)
Oral: 200, 300, 400, 800 mg tablets; 300 mg/5 mL liquid
Parenteral: 300 mg/2 mL, 300 mg/50 mL for injection
Famotidine (Pepcid)
Oral: 20, 40 mg tablets; powder to reconstitute for 40 mg/5 mL suspension
Parenteral: 10 mg/mL for injection
Nizatidine (Axid)
Oral: 150, 300 mg tablets
Ranitidine (Zantac)
Oral: 150, 300 mg tablets; 15 mg/mL syrup
Parenteral: 0.5, 25 mg/mL for injection

5-HT Agonists

Sumatriptan (Imitrex)
Parenteral: 6 mg/0.5 mL in *SELFdose* autoinjection units for subcutaneous injection.

5-HT Antagonists

Granisetron (Kytril)
Parenteral: 1 mg/mL for IV administration
Ondansetron (Zofran)
Oral: 4, 8 mg tablets
Parenteral: 2 mg/mL for IV administration

Ergot Alkaloids

Dihydroergotamine (D.H.E. 45)
Parenteral: 1 mg/mL for injection
Ergonovine (generic, Ergotrate maleate)
Oral: 0.2 mg tablets
Parenteral: 0.2 mg/mL for injection
Ergotamine [mixtures] (generic, Cafergot, others)
Oral: 1 mg ergotamine/100 mg caffeine tablets

---

*Dimenhydrinate is the chlorotheophylline salt of diphenhydramine.

Rectal: 2 mg ergotamine/100 mg caffeine suppositories
Ergotamine tartrate (Ergomar, Ergostat, others)
Sublingual: 2 mg sublingual tablets; 9 mg/mL metered-dose aerosol, 0.36 mg/dose

Methylergonovine (Methergine)
Oral: 0.2 mg tablets
Parenteral: 0.2 mg/mL for injection
Methysergide (Sansert)
Oral: 2 mg tablets

REFERENCES

Histamine

Black JW et al: Definition and antagonism of histamine H_2 receptors. Nature 1972;236:385.

Bochner BS, Lichtenstein LM: Anaphylaxis. N Engl J Med 1991;324:1785.

Curry FE: Modulation of venular microvessel permeability by calcium influx into endothelial cells. FASEB J 1992;6:2456.

DiPadova C et al: Effects of ranitidine on blood alcohol levels after ethanol ingestion: Comparison with other H_2-receptor antagonists. JAMA 1992;267:83.

Feldman M, Burton ME: Drug therapy: Histamine$_2$ receptor antagonists: Standard therapy for acid-peptic disease. (Two parts.) N Engl J Med 1990;323:1672,1749.

Guo ZG et al: Inotropic effects of histamine in human myocardium: Differentiation between positive and negative components. J Cardiovasc Pharmacol 1984;6:1210.

Haaksma EEJ, Leurs R, Timmerman H: Histamine receptors: Subclasses and specific ligands. Pharmacol Ther 1990;47:73.

Hill SJ: Distribution, properties, and functional characteristics of three classes of histamine receptors. Pharmacol Rev 1990;42:45.

Hinrichsen H, Halabi A, Kirsh W: Hemodynamic effect of H_2 receptor antagonists. Eur J Clin Invest 1992;22:9.

Hinrichsen H et al: Dose-dependent heart rate reducing effect of nizatidine, a histamine H_2-receptor antagonist. Br J Clin Pharmacol 1993:35:461.

Holmes LB: Teratogen update: Bendectin. Teratology 1983;27:277.

Honig PK et al: Terfenadine-ketoconazole interaction. Pharmacokinetic and electrocardiographic consequences. JAMA 1993;269:1513.

Howard JM et al: Famotidine, a new, potent, long-acting H_2 receptor antagonist: Comparison with cimetidine and ranitidine in the treatment of Zollinger-Ellison syndrome. Gastroenterology 1985;88:1026.

Lin JH: Pharmacokinetic and pharmacodynamic properties of histamine H_2-receptor antagonists. Relationship between intrinsic potency and effective plasma concentrations. Clin Pharmacokinet 1991;20:218.

MacGlashan DW et al: Comparative studies of human basophils and mast cells. Fed Proc 1983;42:2504.

Mezey E, Palkovits M: Localization of targets for anti-ulcer drugs in cells of the immune system. Science 1992;258:1662.

Morrow JD et al: Evidence that histamine is the causative toxin of scombroid fish poisoning. N Engl J Med 1991;324:716.

Naclerio RM: Allergic rhinitis. N Engl J Med 1991;325:860.

Nicholson AN: Antihistamines and sedation. Lancet 1983;2:211.

Pelikan Z, Knottnerus I: Inhibition of the late asthmatic response by nedocromil sodium administered more than two hours after allergen challenge. J Allergy Clin Immunol 1993;92:19.

Pollard H et al: A detailed autoradiographic mapping of histamine H_3 receptors in rat brain areas. Neuroscience 1993;52:169.

Porro GB, Keohane PP (editors): Nizatidine in peptic ulcer disease. (Symposium.) Scand J Gastroenterol 1987;22(Suppl 136):1.

Rangachari PK: Histamine: mercurial messenger in the gut. (Editorial.) Am J Physiol 1992;262(1 Part 1):G1.

Rocklin RE, Beer DJ: Histamine and immune modulation. Adv Intern Med 1983;28:225.

Saviuc P, Danel V, Dixmerias F: Prolonged QT interval and torsade de pointes following astemizole overdose. Clin Toxicol 1993;31:121.

Schwartz J-C et al: Histaminergic transmission in the mammalian brain. Physiol Rev 1991;71:1.

Sewing K-F, Hannemann H: Interaction of ranitidine and famotidine with guinea pig-isolated parietal cells. Pharmacology 1986;33:274.

Texter EC, Miyoshi A, Okabe H (editors): Famotidine: Further developments in H_2 receptor antagonist therapy. (Symposium.) Scand J Gastroenterol 1987;22(Suppl 134):U1.

Torsoli A, Lucchelli PE, Brimblecombe RW (editors): H_2 Antagonists: H_2 Receptor Antagonists in Peptic Ulcer Disease and Progress in Histamine Research. (Symposium.) International Congress Series 521. Excerpta Medica, 1980.

Ueki S et al: Gastroprokinetic activity of nizatidine, a new H_2-receptor antagonist, and its possible mechanism of action in dogs and rats. J Pharmacol Exper Ther 1993;264:152.

Wiley JF II et al: Cardiotoxic effects of astemizole overdose in children. J Pediatr 1992;120:799.

Serotonin

Bateman DN: Sumatriptan. Lancet 1993;341:221.

Bockaert J et al: The 5-HT$_4$ receptor: A place in the sun. Trends Pharmacol Sci 1992;13:141.

Buckholtz NS et al: Lysergic acid diethylamide (LSD) selectively downregulates serotonin$_2$ receptors in rat brain. Neuropsychopharmacology 1990;3:137.

Cohen ML et al: Role of 5-HT$_2$ receptors in serotonin-induced contractions of nonvascular smooth muscle. J Pharmacol Exp Ther 1985;232:770.

Cunningham D et al: Prevention of emesis in patients receiving cytotoxic drugs by GR38032F, a selective 5-HT$_3$ receptor antagonist. Lancet 1987;1:1461.

de Chaffoy de Courcelles D, Leysen JE, de Clerck F: The signal transducing system coupled to serotonin-S$_2$ receptors. Experientia 1988;44:131.

Derkach V, Surprenant A, North RA: 5-HT$_3$ receptors are membrane ion channels. Nature 1989;339:706.

Glennon RA: Serotonin receptors: Clinical implications. Neurosci Biobehav Rev 1990;14:35.

Golino P et al: Divergent effects of serotonin on coronary-artery dimensions and blood flow in patients with coronary atherosclerosis and control patients. N Engl J Med 1991;324:641.

Hesketh PJ, Gandara DR: Serotonin antagonists: A new class of antiemetic agents. J Natl Cancer Inst 1991; 83:613.

Houston DS, Vanhoutte PM: Comparison of serotonergic receptor subtypes on the smooth muscle and endothelium of the canine coronary artery. J Pharmacol Exp Ther 1988;244:1.

Humphrey PP et al: Serotonin and migraine. Ann NY Acad Sci 1990;600:587.

Julius D: Molecular biology of serotonin receptors. Annu Rev Neurosci 1991;14:335.

Kenny GNC et al: Efficacy of orally administered ondansetron in the prevention of postoperative nausea and vomiting: A dose ranging study. Br J Anaesth 1992; 68:466.

Maricq AV et al: Primary structure and functional expression of the 5-HT$_3$ receptor, a serotonin-gated ion channel. Science 1991;254:432.

Matthes H et al: Mouse 5-hydroxytryptamine$_{5A}$ and 5-hydroxytryptamine$_{5B}$ receptors define a new family of serotonin receptors: Cloning, functional expression, and chromosomal localization. Mol Pharmacol 1993;43:313.

Peroutka SJ: 5-Hydroxytryptamine-receptor subtypes. Annu Rev Neurosci 1988;11:45.

Pettersson A et al: Treatment of arterial hypertension with ketanserin in mono- and combination therapy. Clin Pharmacol Ther 1985;38:188.

Schmidt AW, Peroutka SJ: 5-Hydroxytryptamine receptor "families." FASEB J 1989;3:2242.

Sternbach H: The serotonin syndrome. Am J Psychiatry 1991;148:705.

Tecott LH, Julius D: A new wave of serotonin receptors. Curr Opin Neurobiol 1993;3:310.

The Subcutaneous Sumatriptan International Study Group: Treatment of migraine attacks with sumatriptan. N Engl J Med 1991;325:322.

Vanhoutte PM (editor): *Serotonin and the Cardiovascular System.* Raven Press, 1985.

Wagner B et al: Effect of ritanserin, a 5-hydroxytryptamine antagonist, on platelet function and thrombin generation at the site of plug formation in vivo. Clin Pharmacol Therap 1990;48:419.

Ergot Alkaloids: Historical

Fuller JG: *The Day of St. Anthony's Fire.* Macmillan, 1968; Signet, 1969.

Gabbai Dr, Lisbonne Dr, Pourquier Dr: Ergot poisoning at Pont St. Esprit. Br Med J (Sept 15) 1951;650.

King B: Outbreak of ergotism in Wollo, Ethiopia. (Letter.) Lancet 1971;1:1411.

Ergot Alkaloids: Basic Pharmacology

Berde B: Ergot compounds: A synopsis. Adv Biochem Psychopharmacol 1980;23:3.

Bredberg U et al: Pharmacokinetics of methysergide and its metabolite methylergometrine in man. Eur J Clin Pharmacol 1986;30:75.

Kalkman HO et al: Involvement of α_1 and α_2 adrenoceptors in the vasoconstriction caused by ergometrine. Eur J Pharmacol 1982;78:107.

MacLennan SJ, Martin GR: Actions of non-peptide ergot alkaloids at 5-HT$_1$-like and 5-HT$_2$ receptors mediating vascular smooth muscle contraction. Naunyn Schmiedebergs Arch Pharmacol 1990;342:120.

Müller-Schweinitzer E: Responsiveness of isolated canine cerebral and peripheral arteries to ergotamine. Naunyn Schmiedebergs Arch Pharmacol 1976;292: 113.

Müller-Schweinitzer E, Weidman H: Basic pharmacological properties. In: *Ergot Alkaloids and Related Compounds*—Vol 49 of *Handbook of Experimental Pharmacology.* Berde B, Schild HO (editors). Springer Verlag, 1978.

Sadzot B et al: Hallucinogenic drug interactions at human brain 5-HT$_2$ receptors: implications for treating LSD-induced hallucinogenesis. Psychopharmacology 1989;98:495.

Saxena PR, Ferrari MD: 5-HT$_1$-like receptor agonists and the pathophysiology of migraine. Trends Pharmacol Sci 1989;10:200.

Ergot Alkaloids: Clinical Pharmacology

Andersen PK et al: Sodium nitroprusside and epidural blockade in the treatment of ergotism. N Engl J Med 1977;296:1271.

Buzzi MG, Moskowitz MA: The antimigraine drug, sumatriptan (GR43175) selectively blocks neurogenic plasma extravasation from blood vessels in dura mater. Br J Pharmacol 1990;99:202.

Creditor MC: Occasional notes: Me and migraine. N Engl J Med 1982;307:1029.

den Boer MO, Somers JAE, Saxena PR: Lack of effect of the antimigraine drugs, sumatriptan, ergotamine, and dihydroergotamine on arteriovenous shunting in the dura mater of the pig. Br J Pharmacol 1992;107:577.

Dierckx RA et al: Intraarterial sodium nitroprusside infusion in the treatment of severe ergotism. Clin Neuropharmacol 1986;9:542.

Ferrari MD et al: Serotonin metabolism in migraine. Neurology 1989;39:1239.

Lewis PJ et al: Rapid reversal of ergotamine-induced vasospasm. Can J Neurol Sci 1986;13:72.

Malaquin F et al: Pleural and retroperitoneal fibrosis from dihydroergotamine. (Letter.) N Engl J Med 1989;321:1760.

Moskowitz MA et al: Pain mechanisms underlying vascular headaches. Rev Neurol 1989;145:181.

Moskowitz MA, Macfarlane R: Neurovascular and molecular mechanisms in migraine headaches. Cerebrovasc Brain Metab Rev 1993;5:159.

Olesen J, Saxena PR (editors): *5-Hydroxytryptamine Mechanisms in Primary Headaches.* Raven Press, 1992.

Nappi G, Micieli G: Sumatriptan in the treatment of migraine attacks. Curr Therap Res 1993;53:599.

Porter JK, Thompson FN Jr: Effects of fescue toxicosis

on reproduction in livestock. J Animal Sci 1992;
70:1594.

Raskin NH: Acute and prophylactic treatment of migraine: Practical approaches and pharmacologic rationale. Neurology 1993;43(Suppl 3):S39.

Redfield MM et al: Valve disease associated with ergot alkaloid use: Echocardiographic and pathologic correlations. Ann Intern Med 1992;117:50.

Ruch A, Duhring JL: Postpartum myocardial infarction in a patient receiving bromocriptine. Obstet Gynecol 1989;74:448.

Saxena PR, Villalon CM: Cardiovascular effects of serotonin agonists and antagonists. J Cardiovasc Pharmacol 1990;15(Suppl 7):S17.

Tfelt-Hansen P: Nitroglycerin for ergotism: Experimental studies in vitro and in migraine patients and treatment of an overt case. Eur J Clin Pharmacol 1982; 22:105.

Thorner MO et al: Hyperprolactinemia: Current concepts of management including medical therapy with bromocriptine. Adv Biochem Psychopharmacol 1980; 23:165.

Titeler M, Lyon RA, Glennon RA: Radioligand binding evidence implicates the brain 5-HT$_2$ receptor as a site of action for LSD and phenylisopropylamine hallucinogens. Psychopharmacology 1988;94:213.

Welch KMA: Drug therapy of migraine. N Engl J Med 1993;329:1476.

17

Vasoactive Peptides

Ian A. Reid, PhD

Peptides are used by most tissues for cell-to-cell communication. As noted in Chapters 6 and 20, they play important roles in the autonomic and central nervous systems. Some of the peptides found in the autonomic and central nervous systems—and a number of other peptides—exert important direct effects on vascular and other smooth muscles. These peptides include both vasoconstrictors (angiotensin II, vasopressin, endothelin, and neuropeptide Y) and vasodilators (bradykinin and other kinins, atrial natriuretic peptide, vasoactive intestinal peptide, substance P, neurotensin, and calcitonin gene-related peptide). This chapter focuses on the smooth muscle actions of the peptides.

ANGIOTENSIN

BIOSYNTHESIS OF ANGIOTENSIN

The pathway for the formation and metabolism of angiotensin II is summarized in Figure 17–1. The principal steps include enzymatic cleavage of angiotensin I from angiotensinogen by renin, conversion of angiotensin I to angiotensin II by converting enzyme, and degradation of angiotensin II by several peptidases.

Renin & Factors Controlling Renin Secretion

Renin is an aspartyl protease that specifically catalyzes the hydrolytic release of the decapeptide angiotensin I from angiotensinogen. It is synthesized as a preprohormone that is processed to prorenin, which is inactive, and then to active renin, a glycoprotein consisting of 340 amino acids.

Most (probably all) of the renin in the circulation originates in the kidneys. Enzymes with renin-like activity are present in several extrarenal tissues, including blood vessels, uterus, salivary glands, and adrenal cortex, but no physiologic role for these enzymes has been established. Within the kidney, renin is synthesized and stored in a specialized area of the nephron, the juxtaglomerular apparatus, which is composed of the afferent and efferent arterioles and the macula densa. The afferent arteriole and, to a lesser extent, the efferent arteriole contain specialized granular cells called juxtaglomerular cells that are the site of synthesis, storage, and release of renin. The macula densa is a specialized tubular segment closely associated with the vascular components of the juxtaglomerular apparatus. The vascular and tubular components of the juxtaglomerular apparatus, including the juxtaglomerular cells, are innervated by adrenergic neurons.

The rate at which renin is secreted by the kidney is the primary determinant of activity of the renin-angiotensin system. Renin secretion is controlled by a variety of factors, including a renal vascular receptor, the macula densa, the sympathetic nervous system, and angiotensin II.

A. Renal Vascular Receptor: The renal vascular receptor functions as a stretch receptor, decreased stretch leading to increased renin release and vice versa. The receptor is apparently located in the afferent arteriole, and it is possible that the juxtaglomerular cells themselves are sensitive to changes in stretch.

B. Macula Densa: The macula densa contains a different type of receptor, apparently sensitive to changes in the rate of delivery of sodium or chloride to the distal tubule. Decreases in distal delivery result in stimulation of renin secretion and vice versa. Recent evidence indicates that these changes are mediated by way of a luminal $Na^+/K^+/2Cl^-$ cotransporter sensitive to changes in luminal Cl^- concentration (Lorenz et al, 1991).

C. Sympathetic Nervous System: The sympathetic innervation of the juxtaglomerular apparatus plays an important role in the control of renin secretion. Maneuvers that increase renal neural activity cause stimulation of renin secretion, while renal denervation results in suppression of renin secretion. Norepinephrine stimulates renin secretion by a direct action on the juxtaglomerular cells. This effect is mediated by beta adrenoceptors and involves the activa-

276

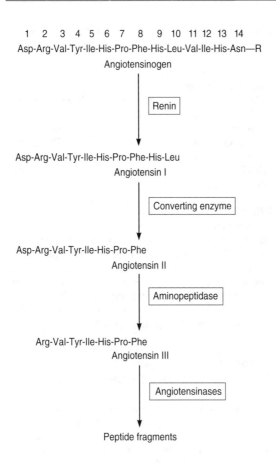

1 2 3 4 5 6 7 8 9 10 11 12 13 14
Asp-Arg-Val-Tyr-Ile-His-Pro-Phe-His-Leu-Val-Ile-His-Asn—R

Angiotensinogen

Renin

Asp-Arg-Val-Tyr-Ile-His-Pro-Phe-His-Leu

Angiotensin I

Converting enzyme

Asp-Arg-Val-Tyr-Ile-His-Pro-Phe

Angiotensin II

Aminopeptidase

Arg-Val-Tyr-Ile-His-Pro-Phe

Angiotensin III

Angiotensinases

Peptide fragments

Figure 17–1. Chemistry of the renin-angiotensin system. The amino acid sequence of the amino terminal of human angiotensinogen is shown. R denotes the remainder of the protein molecule.

tion of adenylyl cyclase and the formation of cAMP. In humans, these beta receptors are of the β_1 subtype. In some situations, norepinephrine stimulates renin secretion indirectly by way of alpha receptors. This stimulation apparently results from constriction of the afferent arteriole, with resultant activation of the renal vascular receptor and decreased delivery of sodium chloride to the macula densa. In other situations, alpha-adrenoceptor stimulation may inhibit renin secretion.

The rate of renin secretion is also influenced by circulating epinephrine and norepinephrine. These catecholamines may act via the same mechanisms as the norepinephrine released locally from the renal sympathetic nerves. However, there is evidence that a major component of the renin secretory response to circulating catecholamines is mediated by way of *extrarenal* beta receptors. The location of these receptors and the pathway by which they influence renin secretion remain to be determined.

D. Angiotensin: Angiotensin II inhibits renin secretion. The inhibition of renin secretion, which results from a direct action of the peptide on the juxtaglomerular cells, forms the basis of a short-loop negative feedback mechanism controlling renin secretion. Interruption of this feedback with antagonists of the renin-angiotensin system (see below) results in stimulation of renin secretion.

E. Pharmacologic Alteration of Renin Release: The release of renin is altered by a wide variety of pharmacologic agents. Renin release is stimulated by vasodilators (hydralazine, minoxidil, nitroprusside), beta-adrenergic agonists (isoproterenol), alpha-adrenergic antagonists, and most diuretics and anesthetics. This stimulation can be accounted for by the control mechanisms just described. Drugs that inhibit renin release are discussed below in the section on antagonists of the renin-angiotensin system.

Angiotensinogen

Angiotensinogen is the circulating protein substrate from which renin cleaves angiotensin I. Angiotensinogen in the circulation originates in the liver. Human angiotensinogen is a glycoprotein with a molecular weight of approximately 57,000. The 14 amino acids at the amino terminal of the molecule are shown in Figure 17–1. In humans, the concentration of angiotensinogen in the circulation is less than the K_m (concentration for 50% of maximum reaction rate) for the renin-angiotensinogen reaction and is therefore an important determinant of the rate of formation of angiotensin.

The production of angiotensinogen is increased by corticosteroids, estrogens, thyroid hormones, and angiotensin II. Plasma angiotensinogen concentration increases in patients with Cushing's syndrome and in patients being treated with glucocorticoids. It is also elevated during pregnancy and in women taking estrogen-containing oral contraceptives.

Angiotensin I

Although angiotensin I contains the peptide sequences necessary for all of the actions of the renin-angiotensin system, it has little or no biologic activity. Instead, it must be converted to angiotensin II by converting enzyme (Figure 17–1). Angiotensin I may also be acted on by plasma or tissue aminopeptidases to form [des-Asp[1]]angiotensin I; this in turn is converted to [des-Asp[1]]angiotensin II (commonly known as angiotensin III) by converting enzyme.

Converting Enzyme (Peptidyl Dipeptidase, PDP, Kininase II)

Converting enzyme is a dipeptidyl carboxypeptidase that catalyzes the cleavage of dipeptides from the carboxyl terminal of certain peptides. Its most important substrates are angiotensin I, which it converts to angiotensin II; and bradykinin, which it inactivates (see below). It also cleaves enkephalins and substance P, but the physiologic significance of these effects has not been established. The action of converting enzyme is restricted by a penultimate prolyl residue, and angiotensin II is therefore not hydrolyzed by converting enzyme. Converting enzyme is distributed widely in the body. In most tissues, converting enzyme is located on the luminal surface of vascular endothelial cells and is thus in close contact with the circulation.

ACTIONS OF ANGIOTENSIN II

Angiotensin II exerts important actions at several sites in the body, including vascular smooth muscle, adrenal cortex, kidney, and brain. Through these actions, the renin-angiotensin system plays a key role in the regulation of fluid and electrolyte balance and arterial blood pressure. Overactivity of the renin-angiotensin system can result in hypertension and disorders of fluid and electrolyte homeostasis.

Effects on Blood Pressure

Angiotensin II is a very potent pressor agent—on a molar basis, approximately 40 times more potent than norepinephrine. The pressor response to intravenous angiotensin II is rapid in onset (10–15 seconds) and sustained during long-term infusions of the peptide. A large component of the pressor response to intravenous angiotensin II is due to direct contraction of vascular—especially arteriolar—smooth muscle. In addition, however, angiotensin II can also increase blood pressure through actions on the brain and autonomic nervous system. The pressor response to angiotensin is usually accompanied by little or no reflex bradycardia. This is apparently because angiotensin acts on the brain to reset the baroreceptor reflex control of heart rate to a higher pressure (Reid, 1992).

Angiotensin II also interacts with the peripheral autonomic nervous system. It stimulates autonomic ganglia, increases the release of epinephrine and norepinephrine from the adrenal medulla, and—what is most important—facilitates sympathetic transmission by an action at adrenergic nerve terminals. The latter effect results from both increased release and reduced reuptake of norepinephrine. Angiotensin II also has a less important direct positive inotropic action on the heart.

Effects on the Adrenal Cortex

Angiotensin II acts directly on the zona glomerulosa of the adrenal cortex to stimulate aldosterone biosynthesis and secretion. In higher doses, angiotensin II also stimulates glucocorticoid secretion.

Effects on the Kidney

Angiotensin II acts directly on the kidney to cause renal vasoconstriction, increase proximal tubular sodium reabsorption, and, as mentioned above, inhibit the secretion of renin.

Effects on the Central Nervous System

In addition to its central effects on blood pressure, angiotensin II also acts on the central nervous system to stimulate drinking (dipsogenic effect) and increase the secretion of vasopressin and ACTH. The physiologic significance of the effects of angiotensin II on drinking and pituitary hormone secretion is not known.

Effects on Cell Growth

Angiotensin II is mitogenic for vascular and cardiac muscle cells and may contribute to the development of cardiovascular hypertrophy (Schelling, 1991). Considerable evidence now indicates that angiotensin-converting enzyme inhibitors will slow or prevent morphologic changes following myocardial infarction that would otherwise lead to congestive heart failure (Konstam et al, 1992).

ANGIOTENSIN RECEPTORS & MECHANISM OF ACTION

Angiotensin II receptors are present in a wide variety of tissues, including vascular smooth muscle, adrenal cortex, kidney, uterus, and brain. Like the receptors for other polypeptide hormones, angiotensin II receptors are located on the plasma membrane of target cells, and this permits rapid onset of the various actions of angiotensin II.

Two distinct subtypes of angiotensin II receptors termed AT_1 and AT_2 (Bumpus et al, 1991) have recently been identified on the basis of their differential affinity for peptide (CGP 42112A) and nonpeptide (losartan [DuP 753], PD 123177) antagonists (see below), and their sensitivity to sulfhydryl-reducing agents. AT_1 receptors have a high affinity for losartan and a low affinity for PD 123177 and CGP 42112A, while AT_2 receptors have a high affinity for PD 123177 and CGP 42112A and a low affinity for losartan. Angiotensin II and saralasin bind equally to both subtypes. Binding of angiotensin II to AT_1 but not AT_2 receptors is reduced by sulfhydryl-reducing agents such as dithiothreitol. The relative proportion of the two subtypes varies from tissue to tissue: AT_1 receptors predominate in vascular smooth muscle.

Most of the known actions of angiotensin II are mediated by the AT_1 receptor subtype. This receptor belongs to the G protein-coupled receptor superfamily. Binding of angiotensin II to AT_1 receptors in vascular smooth muscle results in the phospholipase C-mediated generation of inositol trisphosphate (IP_3) and diacylglycerol (DAG). IP_3 mobilizes calcium from endoplasmic reticulum, and DAG activates protein kinase C, and these two events result in smooth muscle contraction. In other tissues, AT_1 receptors are coupled to different signal transduction mechanisms, including inhibition of adenylyl cyclase. The function and signal transduction pathways for AT_2 receptors have not been identified.

METABOLISM OF ANGIOTENSIN II

Angiotensin II is removed rapidly from the circulation, with a half-life of 15–60 seconds. It is metabolized during passage through most vascular beds (a notable exception being the lung) by a variety of peptidases collectively referred to as angiotensinases. Most of the metabolites of angiotensin II are biologically inactive, but the initial product of aminopeptidase action—[des-Asp^1]angiotensin II—retains considerable biologic activity.

ANTAGONISTS OF THE RENIN-ANGIOTENSIN SYSTEM

A wide variety of agents are now available that block the formation or actions of angiotensin II. These drugs may block renin secretion, the enzymatic action of renin, the conversion of angiotensin I to angiotensin II, or angiotensin II receptors.

Drugs That Block Renin Secretion

Several drugs that interfere with the sympathetic nervous system inhibit the secretion of renin. Examples are clonidine, propranolol, and methyldopa. Clonidine inhibits renin secretion by causing a centrally mediated reduction in neural activity to the kidney, and it may also exert a direct intrarenal action. The mechanism by which methyldopa inhibits renin secretion has not been established, but it may be similar to the central action of clonidine. Propranolol and other beta-adrenoceptor-blocking drugs act by blocking the intrarenal and extrarenal beta receptors involved in the neural control of renin secretion.

Renin Inhibitors

The action of renin can be blocked by pepstatin, a pentapeptide that also inhibits the action of other proteases such as pepsin and cathepsin D. The use of pepstatin in vivo is restricted by its low solubility, but a more soluble form, N-acetylpepstatin, has been synthesized. Competitive inhibitors of renin based on the amino acid sequence around the cleavage site of angiotensinogen have been synthesized. The problem with most of these is low solubility. However, one of these peptides, Pro-His-Pro-Phe-His-Phe-Phe-Val-Tyr-Lys, is reasonably soluble and is an effective inhibitor of renin in vivo. Recently, orally active renin inhibitors have been developed. Some of these are potent, have a high specificity for renin, and lower blood pressure in hypertensive patients. Nevertheless, further improvement of the oral bioavailability and efficacy of these inhibitors is required.

Converting Enzyme Inhibitors

A nonapeptide inhibitor of converting enzyme was originally isolated from the venom of the South American pit viper, *Bothrops jararaca.* The synthetic form of this peptide, **teprotide,** is a highly effective inhibitor of converting enzyme. However, it is active only when administered intravenously. An important class of orally active angiotensin-converting enzyme (ACE) inhibitors, directed against the active site of ACE, is now extensively used. **Captopril** and **enalapril** are typical (Figure 17–2). Many potent new ACE inhibitors have been synthesized (Salvetti, 1990). It should be noted that ACE inhibitors not only block the conversion of angiotensin I to angiotensin II but also inhibit the degradation of other substances, including bradykinin, substance P, and enkephalins. This latter effect may contribute to the antihypertensive action of ACE inhibitors and may be responsible for side effects, including cough and angioedema. As noted in Chapters 11 and 13, extensive studies document the value of the ACE inhibitors in hypertension and congestive heart failure. Recent evidence suggests that these drugs may also protect against renal vascular injury in diabetes and other conditions (Björck et al, 1992).

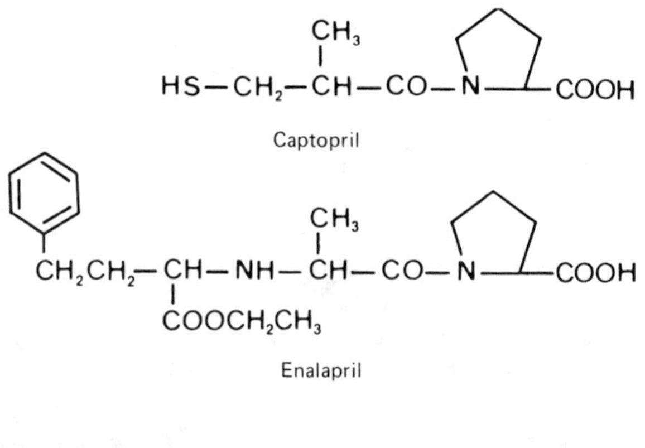

Figure 17–2. Two orally active converting enzyme inhibitors: captopril and enalapril. Enalapril is a prodrug ethyl ester that is hydrolyzed in the body.

Angiotensin Antagonists

Substitution of aliphatic residues such as glycine, alanine, leucine, isoleucine, or threonine for the phenylalanine in position 8 of angiotensin II results in the formation of potent antagonists of the action of angiotensin II. Substitution of sarcosine (N-methyl-glycine) for the amino terminal aspartic acid prolongs the half-life of the peptides and thus enhances their potency. The best-known of these antagonists is [Sar^1,Val^5,Ala^8]angiotensin-(1–8)octapeptide, or **saralasin.**

Asp-Arg-Val-Tyr-Ile-His-Pro-Phe
Angiotensin II

Sar-Arg-Val-Tyr-Val-His-Pro-Ala
Saralasin

Saralasin exhibits some agonist activity and may elicit pressor responses, particularly when circulating angiotensin II levels are low. Saralasin must be administered intravenously, and this severely restricts its use as an antihypertensive agent. However, it has been used for the detection of renin-dependent hypertension and other hyperreninemic states. In general, angiotensin analogues are less effective in lowering blood pressure than are angiotensin-converting enzyme inhibitors. This difference reflects both the partial agonist activity of angiotensin analogues and the bradykinin-potentiating action of ACE inhibitors.

Recently, a new class of nonpeptide angiotensin II antagonists has been developed. One of these, DuP 753 (losartan), is a potent and specific competitive antagonist at angiotensin AT$_1$ receptors (Figure 17–3). Losartan is orally active and does not exhibit agonist activity. It lowers blood pressure in patients with essential hypertension and is being evaluated for use in the treatment of hypertension and congestive heart failure. AT$_2$ receptor antagonists, including PD 123177 (Figure 17–3), are also available but have no clinical use at this time.

KININS

BIOSYNTHESIS OF KININS

Kinins are a group of potent vasodilator peptides. They are formed enzymatically by the action of enzymes known as kallikreins or kininogenases acting on protein substrates called kininogens. From the biochemical point of view, the kallikrein-kinin system has several features in common with the renin-angiotensin system.

Kallikreins

Kallikreins are present in plasma and in several tissues, including the kidneys, pancreas, intestine, sweat glands, and salivary glands. Kallikreins are serine proteases with active sites and catalytic properties very similar to those of enzymes such as trypsin, chymotrypsin, elastase, thrombin, plasmin, and other serine proteases. They are glycoproteins. Tissue kallikreins have molecular weights between 25,000 and 40,000; plasma kallikrein has a molecular weight of approximately 100,000.

Plasma kallikrein circulates in the blood as a precursor, prekallikrein, which is produced by the liver. Plasma kallikrein can be activated by trypsin, Hageman factor, and possibly kallikrein itself. Some glandular kallikreins exist as prekallikreins; others are

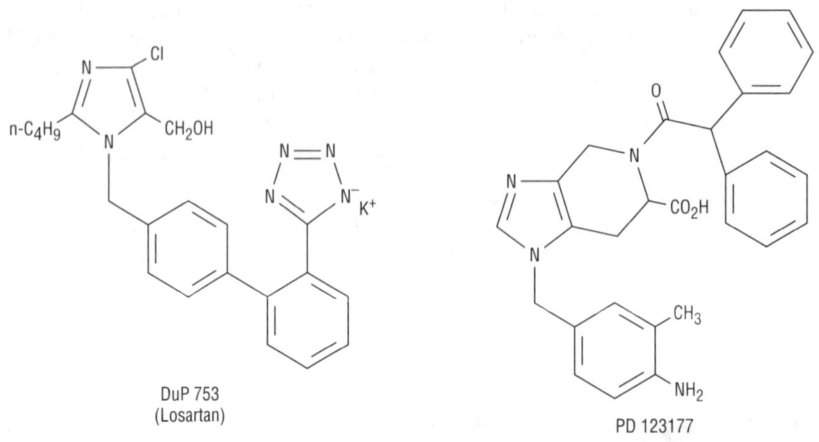

DuP 753
(Losartan)

PD 123177

Figure 17–3. Structures of the angiotensin AT$_1$-receptor antagonist DuP 753 (losartan) and the AT$_2$ antagonist PD 123177.

present in active forms. In general, the biochemical properties of glandular kallikreins are quite different from those of plasma kallikreins. It has been shown that kallikreins can convert prorenin to active renin, but the physiologic significance of this action has not been established.

Kininogens

Kininogens—the precursors of kinins—are present in plasma, lymph, and interstitial fluid. At least two kininogens are present in plasma: a low-molecular-weight form (LMW kininogen) and a high-molecular-weight form (HMW kininogen). Both are acidic glycoproteins consisting of a single polypeptide chain. About 15–20% of the total plasma kininogen is in the HMW form. It is thought that LMW kininogen crosses capillary walls and serves as the substrate for tissue kallikreins, while HMW kininogen is confined to the bloodstream and serves as the substrate for plasma kallikrein.

FORMATION OF KININS IN PLASMA & TISSUES

The pathway for the formation and metabolism of kinins is shown in Figure 17–4. Three kinins have been identified in mammals: bradykinin, lysylbradykinin (also known as kallidin), and methionyllysylbradykinin. They have the following structures:

Arg-Pro-Pro-Gly-Phe-Ser-Pro-Phe-Arg
 1   2   3   4   5   6   7   8   9
Bradykinin

Lys-Arg-Pro-Pro-Gly-Phe-Ser-Pro-Phe-Arg
Lysylbradykinin (kallidin; Lys-bradykinin)

Met-Lys-Arg-Pro-Pro-Gly-Phe-Ser-Pro-Phe-Arg
Methionyllysylbradykinin (Met-Lys-bradykinin)

Note that each kinin contains bradykinin in its structure. Each kinin is formed from a kininogen by the action of a different enzyme. Bradykinin is released by plasma kallikrein, lysylbradykinin by glandular kallikrein, and methionyllysylbradykinin by pepsin and pepsin-like enzymes. The preferred substrate for plasma kallikrein is HMW kininogen, and the preferred substrate for tissue kallikrein is LMW kininogen. Some lysylbradykinin is converted to bradykinin by an aminopeptidase. The three kinins have been found in plasma, but bradykinin is the predominant type. All three kinins are also present in urine. Lysylbradykinin is the major urinary kinin and is probably formed by the action of renal kallikrein. Bradykinin is generated from lysylbradykinin by a renal aminopeptidase. Methionyllysylbradykinin occurs in acidified urine: acid activates uropepsinogen, which then catalyzes the release of methionyllysylbradykinin from urinary kininogens.

ACTIONS OF KININS

Effects on the Cardiovascular System

Kinins produce marked vasodilation in several vascular beds, including the heart, kidney, intestine, skeletal muscle, and liver. In this respect, kinins are approximately ten times more potent than histamine. The vasodilation may result from a direct inhibitory effect of kinins on arteriolar smooth muscle or may be mediated by the release of endothelium-derived relaxing factor (EDRF, nitric oxide) or vasodilator prostaglandins such as PGE_2 and PGI_2. In contrast, the predominant effect of kinins on veins is contraction; again, this may result from direct stimulation of venous smooth muscle or from the release of venoconstrictor prostaglandins such as $PGF_{2\alpha}$. Kinins also produce contraction of most visceral smooth muscle.

When injected intravenously, kinins produce a rapid fall in blood pressure that is due to their vasodilator actions. The hypotensive response to bradykinin is of very brief duration. Intravenous infusions of the peptide fail to produce a sustained decrease in blood pressure; prolonged hypotension can only be produced by progressively increasing the rate of infusion. The rapid reversibility of the hypotensive response to kinins is due primarily to reflex increases in heart rate, cardiac output, and myocardial contractility. In some species, bradykinin produces a biphasic change in blood pressure—an initial hypotensive response followed by an increase above the preinjection level. The increase in blood pressure may be due to a reflex activation of the sympathetic nervous system, though it is worth noting that under some condi-

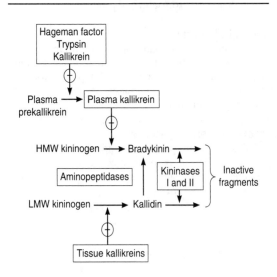

Figure 17–4. The kallikrein-kinin system. Kininase II is identical to converting enzyme peptidyl dipeptidase.

tions, bradykinin can directly release catecholamines from the adrenal medulla and stimulate sympathetic ganglia. Bradykinin also increases blood pressure when injected into the central nervous system, but the physiologic significance of this effect is not clear, since it is unlikely that kinins cross the blood-brain barrier. Kinins have no consistent effect on sympathetic or parasympathetic nerve endings.

The arteriolar dilation produced by kinins causes an increase in pressure and flow in the capillary bed, thus favoring efflux of fluid from blood to tissues. This effect may be facilitated by increased capillary permeability resulting from contraction of endothelial cells and widening of intercellular junctions, and by increased venous pressure secondary to constriction of veins. As a result of these changes, water and solutes pass from the blood to the extracellular fluid, lymph flow increases, and edema may result.

Effects on Endocrine & Exocrine Glands

As noted earlier, prekallikreins and kallikreins are present in several glands, including the pancreas, kidney, intestine, salivary glands, and sweat glands, and can be released into the secretory fluids of these glands. The function of the enzymes in these tissues is not known. The enzymes (or active kinins) may diffuse from the organs to the blood and act as local modulators of blood flow. Since kinins have such marked effects on smooth muscle, they may also modulate the tone of salivary and pancreatic ducts and help to regulate gastrointestinal motility. Kinins also influence the transepithelial transport of water, electrolytes, glucose, and amino acids and may regulate the transport of these substances in the gastrointestinal tract and kidney. Finally, kallikreins may play a role in the physiologic activation of various prohormones, including proinsulin and prorenin.

Role in Inflammation

Kinins play an important role in the inflammatory process. Kallikreins and kinins can produce all the symptoms of inflammation, and the production of kinins is increased in inflammatory lesions produced by a variety of methods.

Effects on Sensory Nerves

Kinins are potent pain-producing substances when applied to a blister base or injected intradermally. They elicit pain by stimulating nociceptive afferents in the skin and viscera.

KININ RECEPTORS & MECHANISMS OF ACTION

The biologic actions of kinins are mediated by specific receptors located on the membranes of the target tissues. Two types of kinin receptors, termed B_1 and B_2, have been identified. (Note that B here stands for bradykinin, not for beta adrenoceptor.) Bioassay studies of B_1-receptor systems indicate that Lys-bradykinin and Met-Lys-bradykinin are approximately 10 and 76 times (respectively) more potent than bradykinin. The octapeptide [des-Arg^9] bradykinin is ten times more potent, while the heptapeptide [des-Phe^8-des-Arg^9]bradykinin is inactive. Bradykinin displays the highest affinity in most B_2-receptor systems, followed by Lys-bradykinin and then by Met-Lys-bradykinin. One exception is the B_2 receptor that mediates contraction of venous smooth muscle; this appears to be most sensitive to Lys-bradykinin.

Most actions of bradykinin and kallidin are mediated by B_2 receptors, which apparently belong to the G protein-coupled family of receptors. Receptor binding sets in motion multiple signal transduction events, including calcium mobilization, chloride transport, formation of nitric oxide, and activation of phospholipase C, phospholipase A_2, and adenylyl cyclase.

METABOLISM OF KININS

Kinins are metabolized rapidly (half-life < 15 seconds) by nonspecific exo- or endopeptidases, commonly referred to as kininases. Two plasma kininases have been well characterized. **Kininase I,** apparently synthesized in the liver, is a carboxypeptidase that releases the carboxyl terminal arginine residue. **Kininase II** is present in plasma and vascular endothelial cells throughout the body. It is identical to angiotensin-converting enzyme (peptidyl dipeptidase), discussed above. Kininase II inactivates kinins by cleaving the carboxyl terminal dipeptide phenylalanyl-arginine. Like angiotensin I, bradykinin is almost completely hydrolyzed during a single passage through the pulmonary vascular bed.

DRUGS AFFECTING THE KALLIKREIN-KININ SYSTEM

Drugs that modify the activity of the kallikrein-kinin system are now available, though none is in wide clinical use. Kinin synthesis can be inhibited with the kallikrein inhibitor **aprotinin.** Competitive antagonists of B_1 and B_2 receptors are available. An example of a B_1-receptor antagonist is [Leu^8-des-Arg^9]bradykinin. B_2 receptors are blocked by [Thi^{5,8},D-Phe^7]bradykinin, which also blocks B_1 receptors to some degree. A recently developed antagonist of B_2 receptors, DArg[Hyp^3, Thi^5, $DTic^7$, Oic^8] bradykinin (Hoe 140), specifically and potently inhibits a wide variety of responses to bradykinin. Actions of kinins mediated by prostaglandin generation can be blocked nonspecifically by inhibitors of prostaglandin synthesis. Finally, the actions of kinins can be enhanced by angiotensin-converting enzyme inhibitors, which block the degradation of these peptides. However, it is difficult to determine if the effects of these agents result from accumulation of kinins or from reduced angiotensin II formation.

VASOPRESSIN

Vasopressin (antidiuretic hormone, ADH) plays an important role in the long-term control of blood pressure through its action on the kidney to increase water reabsorption. This and other aspects of the physiology of vasopressin are discussed in Chapters 15 and 36 and will not be reviewed here.

There is now considerable evidence that vasopressin also plays an important role in the short-term regulation of arterial pressure by its vasoconstrictor action. The peptide increases total peripheral resistance when infused in doses less than those required to produce maximum urine concentration. Such doses do not normally increase arterial pressure, because the vasopressor activity of the peptide is effectively buffered by a reflex decrease in cardiac output. When the influence of this reflex is removed, eg, in shock, pressor sensitivity to vasopressin is greatly increased. Pressor sensitivity to vasopressin is also enhanced in patients with idiopathic orthostatic hypotension. Higher doses of vasopressin increase blood pressure even when baroreceptor reflexes are intact. These doses are generally higher than those required to produce maximum urine concentration; however, pressor responses can be elicited when plasma vasopressin concentration is increased to levels reached during nonhypotensive hemorrhage.

VASOPRESSIN RECEPTORS & ANTAGONISTS

The actions of vasopressin are mediated by activation of specific membrane receptors. Two subtypes of vasopressin receptors have been identified: V_1 receptors that mediate the vasoconstrictor action of the peptide and V_2 receptors that mediate the antidiuretic action. V_1 effects are mediated by activation of phospholipase C, formation of inositol trisphosphate, and increased intracellular calcium concentration. V_2 effects are mediated by activation of adenylyl cyclase.

Vasopressin-like peptides selective for either vasoconstrictor or antidiuretic activity have been synthesized. The most specific V_1 vasoconstrictor agonist synthesized to date is [Phe^2, Ile^3, Orn^8]vasotocin. Selective V_2 antidiuretic analogues include 1-deamino[D-Arg^8]arginine vasopressin (dDAVP) and 1-deamino[Val^4,D-Arg^8]arginine vasopressin (dVDAVP). Specific antagonists of the vasoconstrictor action of vasopressin are also now available. One of the most potent V_1 antagonists is [1-(β-mercapto-β,β-cyclopentamethylenepropionic acid)-2-(O-methyl)tyrosine] arginine vasopressin. This compound also has antioxytocic activity but does not antagonize the antidiuretic action of vasopressin. It does not interfere with the actions of other pressor agents such as angiotensin and norepinephrine. Recently, an orally active competitive vasopressin V_1-receptor antagonist was described (Yamamura et al, 1991). Antagonists of the antidiuretic action of vasopressin are also available.

The vasopressor antagonists have been particularly useful for investigating the role of endogenous vasopressin in cardiovascular regulation. The antagonists have no cardiovascular effects when administered to animals in which circulating vasopressin levels are within or below the normal range. However, when they are administered to water-deprived rats or dogs in which circulating vasopressin levels are elevated, prompt decreases in arterial pressure or total peripheral resistance occur. Vasopressin blockade also decreases blood pressure in adrenal-insufficient animals and impairs blood pressure regulation during hemorrhage. Taken together, these and other observations demonstrate that, through its vasoconstrictor action, vasopressin plays an important role in cardiovascular regulation.

There is also some evidence that vasopressin plays a role in experimental hypertension in animals and may be involved in some forms of human hypertension. Vasopressin antagonists of the type described above will be of value in the investigation of this important question.

ATRIAL NATRIURETIC PEPTIDE

The atria of mammals contain peptides with potent natriuretic activity, variously referred to as atrial natriuretic peptides (ANP), cardionatrins, atriopeptins, and auriculins. They are derived from the carboxyl terminal end of a common precursor termed preproANP which, in humans, is a 151-amino-acid peptide. ANP is synthesized primarily in cardiac atriocytes, but small amounts are synthesized in ventriculocytes. It is also synthesized by neurons in the central and peripheral nervous systems and in the lungs. ANP circulates as a 28-amino-acid peptide with a single disulfide bridge that forms a 17-residue ring. Other peptides closely related to ANP have been identified. These include BNP, which, like ANP, is synthesized primarily in the heart; and CNP, which is synthesized primarily in the brain. The structures of the three peptides are similar (Figure 17–5), but there are differences in their biologic effects.

In healthy humans, plasma ANP concentration, as measured by radioimmunoassay, ranges from 15 to 60 pg/mL. Several factors increase the release of ANP from the heart, but the most important one appears to be atrial distention. How distention increases ANP release is not known, but cardiac innervation is not required. ANP release is also increased by volume expansion, changing from the standing to the supine position, and exercise. In each case, the increase in ANP release is probably due to increased atrial stretch, but the cellular mechanisms that link ANP release to atrial stretch have not been elucidated. ANP release can also be increased by α-adrenoceptor agonists, glucocorticoids, endothelin (see below), and vasopressin. Finally, plasma ANP concentration in-creases in various pathologic states, including congestive heart failure, primary aldosteronism, chronic renal failure, and inappropriate ADH secretion syndrome.

Administration of ANP produces prompt and marked increases in sodium excretion and urine flow. Glomerular filtration rate increases, with little or no change in renal blood flow, so that the filtration fraction increases. The ANP-induced natriuresis is apparently due to both the increase in glomerular filtration rate and a decrease in proximal tubular sodium reabsorption. ANP also inhibits the secretion of renin, aldosterone, and vasopressin; these changes may also increase sodium and water excretion. Finally, ANP decreases arterial blood pressure. This hypotensive action is due to vasodilation, which results from stimulated particulate guanylyl cyclase activity, increased cGMP levels, and decreased cytosolic free calcium concentration. ANP also antagonizes the vasoconstrictor action of angiotensin II and other vasoconstrictors, and this action may also contribute to the hypotensive action of the peptide. Three types of receptors for ANP, termed ANP_A, ANP_B, and ANP_C, have been identified. ANP_A and ANP_B recep-

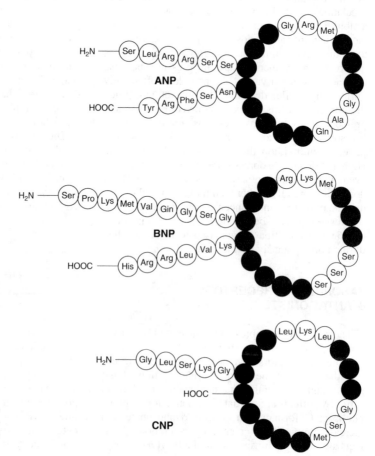

Figure 17–5. Structures of the atrial natriuretic peptides ANP, BNP and CNP. Sequences *common* to the peptides are indicated in black.

tors are linked to guanylyl cyclase; the ANP_C receptor is thought to function in the clearance of ANP.

ANP is cleared by almost all tissues and has a short half-life in the circulation (3–5 minutes). Much of this clearance involves receptor-mediated endocytosis by ANP_C receptors, which are distributed widely in the body. ANP is also degraded by the neutral endopeptidase NEP 24.11, which also metabolizes other vasoactive peptides, and by other enzymes.

There is evidence that ANP participates in the physiologic regulation of sodium excretion. For example, the natriuretic response to volume expansion is reduced, at least in some species, by ANP antibodies or by partial removal of the source of circulating ANP by atrial appendectomy. Nevertheless, additional investigation is required to fully define the physiologic significance of this peptide. Because of its ability to reduce blood volume and arterial pressure, both ANP and inhibitors of NEP 24.11, the neutral endopeptidase that metabolizes it, are being evaluated for the treatment of congestive heart failure, hypertension, renal failure, and states of fluid overload.

ENDOTHELIN

The endothelium is the source of a variety of substances with vasodilator and vasoconstrictor activity. One of these is a potent vasoconstrictor peptide called endothelin that was first isolated from cultured aortic endothelial cells.

Endothelin is a 21-amino-acid peptide containing two disulfide bridges. Three different isoforms have been identified: the originally described endothelin (ET-1) and two similar peptides, ET-2 and ET-3. Their structures are shown in Figure 17–6. Endothelin is widely distributed in the body, with high concentrations in the lung, kidney, heart, hypothalamus, and spleen. It is present in the blood but in low concentration; it probably acts locally in a paracrine or autocrine fashion rather than as a circulating hormone.

Endothelin produces a dose-dependent vasoconstriction in most vascular beds. In human mesenteric arteries, it is approximately 100 times more potent than norepinephrine. Intravenous administration of endothelin causes a transient decrease in arterial blood pressure followed by a prolonged increase. Endothelin also contracts nonvascular smooth muscle, including tracheal, uterine, and intestinal muscle. Other actions of endothelin include a positive inotropic effect, stimulation of atrial natriuretic hormone release, and proliferation of smooth muscle and other cells.

Endothelin receptors are present in many tissues and organs, including the blood vessel wall, cardiac muscle, central nervous system, lung, kidney, adrenal, spleen, and intestine. Two receptor subtypes, termed ET_A and ET_B, have been identified and sequenced. ET_A receptors have a high affinity for ET-1 and a low affinity for ET-3 and are located on smooth muscle cells, where they mediate vasoconstriction. ET_B receptors have approximately equal affinities for ET-1 and ET-3 and are located on vascular endothelial cells, where they mediate release of EDRF and prostanoids. Both receptor subtypes belong to the family of G protein-coupled receptors. Binding of en-

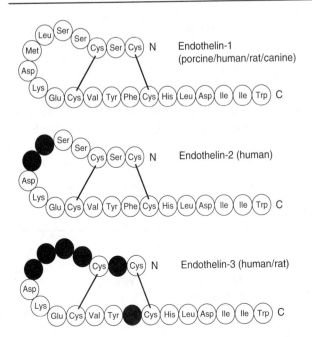

Figure 17–6. Structures of the endothelin peptides endothelin-1, endothelin-2, and endothelin-3. Sequences *different* in the three peptides are shown in black.

dothelin to its receptors results in an increase in intracellular calcium concentration. This increase results from influx of calcium into the cell via calcium channels and from stimulation of phospholipase C, formation of inositol trisphosphate, and release of calcium from the endoplasmic reticulum.

Endothelin may play an important role in cardiovascular regulation. It may also participate in hypertension and other cardiovascular diseases, but its precise role remains to be determined. Endothelin antagonists have recently been discovered and have potential for the treatment of hypertension and vascular disease.

VASOACTIVE INTESTINAL PEPTIDE

Vasoactive intestinal peptide (VIP) is a 28-amino-acid peptide closely related structurally to secretin and glucagon. Its structure is shown below.

His-Ser-Asp-Ala-Val-Phe-Thr-Asp-Asn-Tyr-Thr-Arg-Leu-Arg-Lys-Gln-Met-Ala-Val-Lys-Lys-Tyr-Leu-Asn-Ser-Ile-Leu-Asn-NH₂

Vasoactive intestinal peptide (VIP)

VIP was originally extracted from porcine lung and was subsequently purified from porcine duodenum. It is now known that VIP is widely distributed in the central and peripheral nervous systems of humans and several animal species. It is also present in the circulation, but most evidence suggests that VIP functions as a neurotransmitter or neuromodulator rather than as a classic hormone.

VIP produces marked vasodilation in most vascular beds, including the splanchnic, pulmonary, coronary, renal, and cerebral vessels. The vasodilator action of VIP is independent of norepinephrine, acetylcholine, serotonin, and histamine receptors and apparently results from a direct action of the peptide on vascular smooth muscle. As a result of this action, arterial pressure falls and cardiac output increases. The mechanism of the vasodilator action of VIP is not fully understood. However, it has been suggested that VIP binds to specific receptors in the blood vessels and stimulates cAMP production. This effect could be produced by VIP released from the nonadrenergic, noncholinergic VIP-containing nerve fibers that are associated with blood vessels or by VIP in the circulation.

In addition to dilating blood vessels, VIP relaxes tracheobronchial and gastrointestinal smooth muscle, stimulates intestinal water and electrolyte secretion, promotes hepatic glycogenolysis, causes neuronal excitation, and stimulates the release of several hormones including growth hormone, prolactin, and renin. The physiologic significance of these actions remains to be defined.

SUBSTANCE P

Substance P is an undecapeptide of the tachykinin family. It has the following structure:

Arg-Pro-Lys-Pro-Gln-Gln-Phe-Phe-Gly-Leu-Met
Substance P

Substance P is present in the central nervous system, where it is a neurotransmitter (Chapter 20); and in the gastrointestinal tract, where it may play a role as a transmitter in the enteric nervous system and as a local hormone (Chapter 6).

Substance P is a potent vasodilator and produces a marked hypotensive action in humans and in several animal species. The vasodilation apparently results from a direct inhibitory effect of the peptide on arteriolar smooth muscle. This action is mediated via specific receptors that differ from those mediating the actions of other vasodilators. In contrast to its effects on arteriolar smooth muscle, substance P stimulates contraction of venous, intestinal, and bronchial smooth muscle. It also causes secretion in the salivary glands, diuresis and natriuresis in the kidneys, and a variety of effects in the central and peripheral nervous systems. These diverse effects may result from the activation of more than one receptor type.

The amino terminal region of substance P is not essential for activity, and several carboxyl terminal fragments of the peptide, including the octa (4–11), hepta (5–11), and hexa (6–11) fragments, are also active. Indeed, depending on the preparation being studied, these peptides may be as potent as the intact undecapeptide or even more so. Analogues of substance P that are antagonists in vivo and in vitro have been synthesized.

NEUROTENSIN

Neurotensin is a tridecapeptide that was first isolated from the central nervous system but subsequently was found to be present in the gastrointestinal tract and in the circulation. It has the following structure:

Glu-Leu-Tyr-Glu-Asn-Lys-Pro-Arg-Arg-Pro-Tyr-Ile-Leu
Neurotensin

When administered into the peripheral circulation, neurotensin produces a variety of effects, including vasodilation, hypotension, increased vascular permeability, increased secretion of several anterior pituitary hormones, hyperglycemia, inhibition of gastric acid and pepsin secretion, and inhibition of gastric motility. Following administration into the cerebrospinal fluid, it produces hypothermia and analgesia. Structure-activity studies indicate that the five or six amino acid residues at the carboxyl terminal of the molecule are required for biologic activity. At present, the physiologic significance of the actions of neurotensin is not known.

CALCITONIN GENE-RELATED PEPTIDE

Calcitonin gene-related peptide (CGRP) is one of three products of the calcitonin gene. CGRP consists of 37 amino acids and displays approximately 30% structural homology with salmon calcitonin.

Like calcitonin, CGRP is present in large quantities in the C cells of the thyroid gland. It is also distributed widely in the central and peripheral nervous systems, in the cardiovascular system, the gastrointestinal tract, and the urogenital system. CGRP is found with substance P (see above) in some of these regions and with acetylcholine in others.

When CGRP is injected into the central nervous system, it produces a variety of effects, including suppression of feeding, and hypertension. The peptide also produces several effects when injected into the systemic circulation, including hypotension and tachycardia. The hypotensive action of CGRP results from the potent vasodilator action of the peptide; indeed, CGRP is the most potent vasodilator yet discovered.

NEUROPEPTIDE Y

Neuropeptide Y is a 36-amino-acid peptide that was first isolated from porcine brain. Its structure is closely related to that of pancreatic polypeptide. Neuropeptide Y is present in high concentrations in the brain and peripheral nervous system and is one of the most abundant neuropeptides. In the sympathetic nervous system, neuropeptide Y is frequently localized in noradrenergic neurons and apparently functions both as a vasoconstrictor and as a cotransmitter with norepinephrine.

Neuropeptide Y produces a variety of central nervous system effects including increased feeding, hypotension, hypothermia, and respiratory depression. Peripheral effects include vasoconstriction of cerebral blood vessels, positive chronotropic and inotropic actions on the heart, and hypertension. These effects result from prejunctional actions, including inhibition of transmitter release from sympathetic and parasympathetic nerves, and from postjunctional actions, including direct vasoconstriction, potentiation of the action of vasoconstrictors, and inhibition of the action of vasodilators. These actions are apparently mediated by multiple receptor subtypes, including postjunctional Y_1 receptors and prejunctional Y_2 receptors. The vasoconstrictor action of neuropeptide Y can be antagonized by the inositol derivative D-myo-inositol-1,2,6-trisphosphate.

PREPARATIONS AVAILABLE

Angiotensin converting enzyme inhibitors: See Chapter 11.

Vasopressin: See Chapter 15.

REFERENCES

General

Hedner T et al: Peptides as targets for antihypertensive drug development. J Hypertens 1992;10:S121.

Iverson LL: Nonopioid neuropeptides in mammalian CNS. Annu Rev Pharmacol Toxicol 1983;23:1.

Angiotensin

Bernstein KE, Alexander RW: Counterpoint: molecular analysis of the angiotensin II receptor. Endocr Rev 1992;13:381.

Björck S et al: Renal protective effect of enalapril in diabetic nephropathy. Br Med J 1992;304:339.

Bumpus FM et al: Nomenclature for angiotensin receptors. Hypertension 1991;17:720.

Carini DJ et al: Nonpeptide angiotensin II receptor antagonists: the discovery of a series of N-(biphenylylmethyl)imidazoles as potent, orally active antihypertensives. J Med Chem 1991;34:2525.

Corvol P et al: Human renin inhibitor peptides. Hypertension 1990;16:1.

Costerousse O et al: The angiotensin I converting enzyme (kininase II): Molecular organization and regulation of its expression in humans. J Cardiovasc Pharmacol 1992;20:S10.

Duc LNC, Brunner HR: Trandolapril in hypertension: Overview of a new angiotensin-converting enzyme inhibitor. Am J Cardiol 1992;70:27D.

Goldberg MR et al: Effects of losartan on blood pressure, plasma renin activity, and angiotensin II in volunteers. Hypertension 1993;21:704.

Greenlee WJ: Renin inhibitors. Med Res Rev 1990; 10:173.

Griendling KK, Murphy TJ, Alexander RW: Molecular biology of the renin-angiotensin system. Circulation 1993;87:1816.

Kleinert HD: Renin inhibitors: Discovery and development. An overview and perspective. Am J Hypertens 1989;2:800.

Kleinert HD, Baker WR, Stein HH: Renin inhibitors. Adv Pharmacol 1991;22:207

Keeton TK, Campbell WB: The pharmacologic alteration of renin release. Pharmacol Rev 1980;32:81.

Konstam MA et al: Effects of the angiotensin converting enzyme inhibitor enalapril on the long-term progression of left ventricular dysfunction in patients with heart failure. Circulation 1992;86:431.

Lorenz JN et al: Renin release from isolated juxtaglomerular apparatus depends on macula densa chloride transport. Am J Physiol 1991;260:F486.

Luther RR, Glassman HN, Boger RS: Renin inhibitors in hypertension. Clin Nephrol 1991;36:181.

Page IH, Bumpus FM (editors): Angiotensin. Springer Verlag, 1974.

Peach MJ: Renin-angiotensin system: Biochemistry and mechanisms of action. Physiol Rev 1977;57:313.

Reid IA: Actions of angiotensin II on the brain: Mechanisms and physiologic role. Am J Physiol 1984; 246:F533.

Reid IA: Interactions between ANG II, sympathetic nervous system, and baroreceptor reflexes in regulation of blood pressure. Am J Physiol 1992;262:E763.

Reid IA, Morris BJ, Ganong WF: The renin-angiotensin system. Annu Rev Physiol 1978;40:377.

Salvetti A: Newer ACE inhibitors: A look at the future. Drugs 1990;40:800.

Schelling P, Fischer H, Ganten D: Angiotensin and cell growth: A link to cardiovascular hypertrophy? J Hypertens 1991;9:3.

Smith JB: Angiotensin-receptor signaling in cultured vascular smooth muscle cells. Am J Physiol 1986; 250:F759.

Soffer RL (editor): Biochemical Regulation of Blood Pressure. Wiley, 1981.

Timmermans PBMWM et al: Angiotensin II receptors and angiotensin II receptor antagonists. Pharmacol Rev 1993;45:205.

Unger T et al: Tissue renin-angiotensin systems: fact or fiction? J Cardiovasc Pharmacol 1991;18(Suppl 2): S20.

Wyvratt MJ, Patchett AA: Recent developments in the design of angiotensin-converting enzyme inhibitors. Med Res Rev 1985;5:483.

Kinins

Bathon JM, Proud D: Bradykinin antagonists. Ann Rev Pharmacol Toxicol 1991;31:129.

Bhoola KD, Figueroa CD, Worthy K: Bioregulation of kinins: kallikreins, kininogens, and kininases. Pharmacol Rev 1992;44:1.

Dray A, Perkins M: Bradykinin and inflammatory pain. Trends Neurosci 1993;16:99.

Regoli D et al: The actions of kinin antagonists on B_1 and B_2 receptor systems. Eur J Pharmacol 1986; 123:61.

Schachter M: Kallikreins (kininogenases): A group of serine proteases with bioregulatory actions. Pharmacol Rev 1980;31:1.

Steranka LR, Farmer SG, Burch RM: Antagonists of B_2 bradykinin receptors. FASEB J 1989;3:2019.

Vavrek RJ, Stewart JM: Competitive antagonists of bradykinin. Peptides 1985;6:161.

Vasopressin

Laszlo FA, Laszlo F, De Wied D: Pharmacology and clinical perspectives of vasopressin antagonists. Pharmacol Rev 1991;43:73.

Manning M, Sawyer WH: Design, synthesis, and some uses of receptor specific agonists and antagonists of vasopressin and oxytocin. J Recept Res 1993;13:195.

Möhring J et al: Greatly enhanced pressor response to antidiuretic hormone in patients with impaired cardiovascular reflexes due to idiopathic orthostatic hypotension. J Cardiovasc Pharmacol 1980;2:367.

Montani J-P et al: Hemodynamic effects of exogenous and endogenous vasopressin at low plasma concentrations in conscious dogs. Circ Res 1980;47:346.

Reid IA, Schwartz J: Role of vasopressin in the control of blood pressure. In: Frontiers in Neuroendocrinology, vol 8. Martini L, Ganong WF (editors). Raven Press, 1984.

Sawyer WH, Grzonka Z, Manning M: Neurohypophysial peptides: Design of tissue-specific agonists and antagonists. Mol Cell Endocrinol 1981;22:117.

Thibonnier M: Signal transduction of V_1-vascular vasopressin receptors. Regul Pept 1992;38:1.

Vasopressin and cardiovascular regulation. (Symposium.) Fed Proc 1984;43:78.

Yamamura Y et al: OPC-21268, an orally effective, nonpeptide vasopressin V1 receptor antagonist. Science 1991;252:572.

Atrial Natriuretic Peptide

Awazu M, Ichikawa I: Biological significance of atrial natriuretic peptide in the kidney. Nephron 1993;63:1.

Cantin M, Genest J: The heart and the atrial natriuretic factor. Endocr Rev 1985;6:107.

Goetz KL: Physiology and pathophysiology of atrial peptides. Am J Physiol 1988;254:E1.

Maack T et al: Atrial natriuretic factor: Structure and functional properties. Kidney Int 1985;27:607.

Nakao K et al: Molecular biology and biochemistry of the natriuretic peptide system. I: Natriuretic peptides. J Hypertens 1992;10:907.

Nakao K et al: Molecular biology and biochemistry of the natriuretic peptide system. II: Natriuretic peptide receptors. J Hypertens 1992;10:1111.

Needleman P et al: The biochemical pharmacology of atrial peptides. Annu Rev Pharmacol Toxicol 1989; 29:23.

Ruskoaho H: Atrial natriuretic peptide: Synthesis, release, and metabolism. Pharmacol Rev 1992;44:479.

Tan ACITL et al: Atrial natriuretic peptide. An overview of clinical pharmacology and pharmacokinetics. Clin Pharmacokinet 1993;24:28.

Wilkins MR, Unwin RJ, Kenny AJ: Endopeptidase 24.11 and its inhibitors: Potential therapeutic agents for edematous disorders and hypertension. Kidney Int 1993;43:273.

Endothelin

Clavell A et al: Physiologic significance of endothelin: Its role in congestive heart failure. Circulation 1993; 87(Suppl V):V–45.

Haynes WG, Webb DJ: The endothelin family of peptides: Local hormones with diverse roles in health and disease? Clin Sci 1993;84:485.

Highsmith RF, Blackburn K, Schmidt DJ: Endothelin and calcium dynamics in vascular smooth muscle. Annu Rev Physiol 1992;54:257.

Lovenberg W, Miller RC: Endothelin: A review of its effects and possible mechanisms of action. Neurochem Res 1990;15:407.

Masaki T, Yanagisawa M: Physiology and pharmacology of endothelins. Med Res Rev 1992;12:391.

Miller RC, Pelton JT, Huggins JP: Endothelins: From receptors to medicine. Trends Pharmacol Sci 1993; 14:54.

Miyauchi T et al: Involvement of endothelin in the regulation of human vascular tonus: Potent vasoconstrictor effect and existence in endothelial cells. Circulation 1990;81:1874.

Rubanyi GM, Parker-Botelho LH: Endothelins. FASEB J 1991,5:2713.

Simonson MS: Endothelins: Multifunctional renal peptides. Physiol Rev 1993;73:375.

Thomas CP, Simonson MS, Dunn MJ: Endothelin: Receptors and transmembrane signals. NIPS 1992;7: 207.

Whittle BJR, Moncada S: The endothelin explosion: A pathophysiological reality or a biological curiosity? Circulation 1990;81:202.

Vasoactive Intestinal Peptide

Said SI (editor): *Vasoactive Intestinal Peptide.* Raven Press, 1982.

Substance P

Caranikas S et al: Antagonists of substance P. Eur J Pharmacol 1982;77:205.

Couture R, Regoli D: Smooth muscle pharmacology of substance P. Pharmacology 1982;24:1.

Maggio JE: Tachykinins. Ann Rev Neurosci 1988;11:13.

Nakanishi S: Substance P precursor and kininogen: Their structures, gene organizations, and regulation. Physiol Rev 1987;67:1117.

Regoli D, Escher E, Mizrahi J: Substance P: Structure-activity studies and the development of antagonists. Pharmacology 1984;28:301.

Neurotensin

Nemeroff CB, Prange AJ (editors): Neurotensin: A brain and gastrointestinal peptide. Ann NY Acad Sci 1982; 400:1.

Calcitonin Gene-Related Peptide

Goodman EC, Iversen LL: Calcitonin gene-related peptide: Novel neuropeptide. Life Sci 1986;38:2169.

Zaidi M, Breimer LH, MacIntyre I: Biology of peptides from the calcitonin genes. Q J Exp Physiol 1987; 72:371.

Neuropeptide Y

Gray TS, Morley JE: Neuropeptide Y: Anatomical distribution and possible function in mammalian nervous system. Life Sci 1986;38:389.

Sundler F et al: Neuropeptide Y in the peripheral adrenergic and enteric nervous systems. Int Rev Cytol 1986;102:243.

Walker P et al: The role of neuropeptide Y in cardiovascular regulation. Trends Pharmacol Sci 1991;12:111.

18

The Eicosanoids: Prostaglandins, Thromboxanes, Leukotrienes, & Related Compounds

Markus Hecker, PhD, Marie L. Foegh, MD, DSc, & Peter W. Ramwell, PhD

Prostaglandins (PGs) and related fatty acid derivatives of arachidonic acid are among the most potent naturally occurring autacoids and are now recognized as critically important cell regulatory substances. This is reflected in the vast literature on eicosanoids, the large number of clinical pharmacologic studies, and the increasing number of compounds entering the market. In spite of this activity, the physiologic role of the eicosanoids is still not fully defined.

EICOSANOID SYNTHESIS

Arachidonic Acid Synthesis, Reacylation, & Release

The prostaglandins and several other biologically active lipid and peptidolipid acids are formed from the same precursor through interrelated enzymatic pathways. These other lipids are nearly all carboxylic acids and include the **thromboxanes (TXs),** the **hydroperoxyeicosatetraenoic acids (HPETEs)** and **hydroxyeicosatetraenoic acids (HETEs),** the **leukotrienes (LTs),** and the more recently discovered **lipoxins (LXs)** and **epoxyeicosatetraenoic acids (EETEs).** The general term eicosanoids (Gk *eicosa* = "twenty") is used to refer to these compounds because they can all be derived from polyunsaturated fatty acids with 18-, 20-, and 22-carbon skeletons.

Among these fatty acids, arachidonic acid is the most important precursor for the biosynthesis of eicosanoids in humans. Two 18-carbon fatty acids (linoleic and α-linolenic acid) and the 20-carbon arachidonic acid are the only fatty acids known to be essential for the complete nutrition of many species of animals, including humans. Arachidonic acid is formed from linoleic acid in most mammals by desaturation and chain elongation to dihomo-γ-linolenic acid and subsequent desaturation. However, linoleic and linolenic acids are not synthesized in humans, so they must be supplied in the diet. Oils from cold-water fish supply the highly polyunsaturated fatty acids eicosapentaenoic acid and docosahexaenoic acid.

ACRONYMS USED IN THIS CHAPTER

ACTH	Adrenocorticotropic hormone
ADH	Antidiuretic hormone
EDRF	Endothelium-derived relaxing factor
EETE	Epoxyeicosatetraenoic (acid)
FSH	Follicle-stimulating hormone
HETE	Hydroxyeicosatetraenoic (acid)
HHT	Hydroxyheptadecatrienoic (acid)
HPETE	Hydroperoxyeicosatetraenoic (acid)
LH	Luteinizing hormone
LHRH	Luteinizing hormone-releasing hormone
LT	Leukotriene
LX	Lipoxin
NSAID	Nonsteroidal anti-inflammatory drugs
PAF	Platelet-activating factor
PG	Prostaglandin
PMN	Polymorphonuclear neutrophil
PTH	Parathyroid hormone
SRS-A	Slow-reacting substance of anaphylaxis
TSH	Thyroid-stimulating hormone
TX	Thromboxane

This information about the essential fatty acids is the basis for many human nutrition studies involving dietary lipids.

Eicosanoids are not stored in the cell, and their biosynthesis is limited by the availability of free precursor fatty acid. Arachidonic acid is released from membrane lipids and other lipid esters by phospholipases that are activated by both specific and nonspecific stimuli. In response to these stimuli—which vary from cell to cell—phospholipase A_2 or a combination of phospholipase C and diglyceride lipase cleaves esterified arachidonic acid from the 2 position of specific glycerophospholipids that make up part of the lipid bilayer of the cell membrane (Figure 18–1).

The amount of intracellular free arachidonic acid is partially controlled by the reincorporation of arachidonate into cellular lipids. This reacylation is regulated by two enzymes: arachidonyl-CoA synthase, which forms the activated coenzyme A fatty acid ester; and arachidonyl-CoA transferase, which adds the CoA ester to the 2-carbon of a lysophospholipid. Further transformations in the phospholipid pools may produce 1-alkyl-2-acetyl-lysophosphatidylcholine, or **platelet-activating factor (PAF),** a potent pathophysiologic mediator of asthma and shock (Figure 18–2). The inhibition of any of these enzymes leads to increased intracellular levels of free arachidonic acid.

Free arachidonic acid is metabolized mainly by two divergent enzymatic pathways that are variably distributed among different cells; prostaglandins and thromboxanes are formed by the cyclooxygenase pathway, and LTs and H(P)ETEs are produced via the lipoxygenase pathway. Not all cells make all of these products. For example, the vascular endothelium synthesizes primarily PGE_2 and PGI_2, while platelets synthesize thromboxane and 12-HETE (see below).

Prostaglandins: History & Nomenclature

Goldblatt and von Euler independently discovered a vasoactive fatty acid in human seminal fluid that decreased rabbit blood pressure. Von Euler named this active principle prostaglandin because he assumed it originated in the prostate gland (it is now known to originate in the seminal vesicles). He suggested that prostaglandin played a role in sperm transport. In 1962, Bergstrom established the structure of the first two prostaglandins and named them prostaglandin E and prostaglandin F (PGE and PGF) because of their respective partitions into ether and phosphate buffer (*fosfat* in Swedish).

Today the nomenclature of prostaglandins describes ten specific molecular groups, designated by the letters A through J, that are characterized by variations in the functional groups attached to positions 9 and 11 of the cyclopentane ring. Arachidonic acid, dihomo-γ-linolenic acid, and eicosapentaenoic acid can be used for prostaglandin biosynthesis. Therefore, each group consists of three series designated by the subscript numbers 1, 2, and 3. These numbers denote the saturation status of the aliphatic side chains; the only exception is prostacyclin (PGI_2). For PGF, the additional subscript alpha or beta signifies the spatial configuration of the carbon 9 hydroxyl group.

Prostaglandin Biosynthesis

The first two reactions in prostaglandin biosynthe-

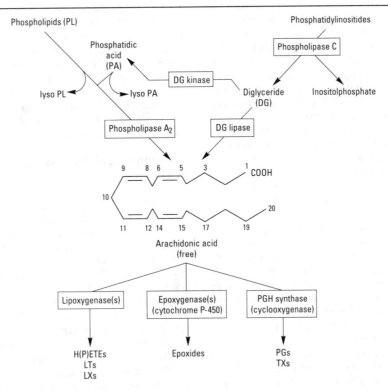

Figure 18–1. Pathways of arachidonic acid release and metabolism.

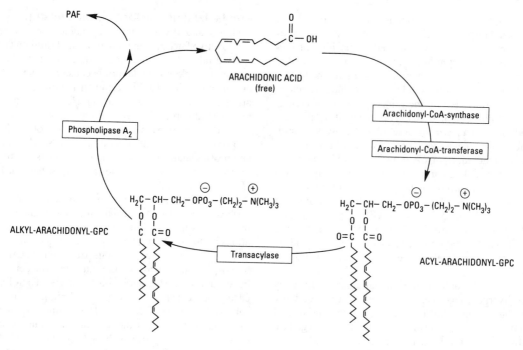

Figure 18–2. Reacylation of arachidonic acid into cellular phospholipids. (CoA, coenzyme A; GPC, glycerophosphatidylcholine; PAF, platelet-activating factor.)

sis from the polyenoic fatty acid precursors (Figure 18–3) are catalyzed by prostaglandin endoperoxide synthase. This membrane-bound hemoprotein, which exists in most animals, is distributed throughout the body (but not in erythrocytes and lymphocytes). The synthesis of prostaglandins from arachidonic acid begins with the oxygenation and cyclization of a pentane ring (the cyclooxygenase step), leading to an unstable C15-hydroperoxy-C9, C11-endoperoxide (PGG_2). The peroxidase reaction catalyzed by the same enzyme then reduces the C15-hydroperoxy group to a hydroxyl group, forming the endoperoxide PGH_2 (Figure 18–3). The cyclooxygenase reaction is inhibited by nonsteroidal anti-inflammatory drugs (NSAIDs) such as aspirin and indomethacin. There are two cyclooxygenases (Cox): Cox I and Cox II. These isoenzymes have 60% homology and are pharmacologically different. For example, aspirin and indomethacin are far more potent in inhibiting Cox I than Cox II, whereas flurbiprofen is only moderately more active in inhibiting Cox I than Cox II. Aspirin acetylates at serine 529 (Cox I) and serine 516 (Cox II), preventing prostaglandin and TXA_2 synthesis. Large amounts of 15-HETE result from acetylation of Cox II but not from acetylation of Cox I. In the body Cox I is the predominant form.

The endoperoxides provide intermediate substrates for the tissue-specific synthesis of a variety of biologically active prostaglandins. Depending on the tissue, PGH_2 is converted to PGD_2 by prostaglandin D

synthase, a cytosolic enzyme, whereas PGE_2 is formed by prostaglandin E synthase, a membrane-bound enzyme. Both enzymes require reduced glutathione as cofactor. No enzyme has been isolated that reduces PGH_2 to $PGF_{2\alpha}$ (dashed arrow in Figure 18–3). However, PGE_2 can be converted to $PGF_{2\alpha}$ by two other enzymes, prostaglandin E 9-ketoreductase and 15-hydroxyprostaglandin dehydrogenase. The presence of the enzymes, not their regulation, seems to determine which endoperoxide product predominates in a specific tissue.

Biosynthesis of Prostacyclin & Thromboxane

Aggregating platelets (thrombocytes) release thromboxane A_2 (TXA_2), which is derived from the same precursor (PGH_2) as the prostaglandins but differs in that it contains an oxan:oxetane ring. The oxetane ring of TXA_2 spontaneously hydrolyzes ($t_{1/2} = 30$ s) to the biologically inactive hemiacetal thromboxane B_2 (TXB_2). Unlike TXB_2, TXA_2 contracts smooth muscle and induces platelet aggregation at low nanomolar concentrations. TXA_2 formation is catalyzed by a cytochrome P450-like heme-thiolate protein (thromboxane synthase) that is mainly present in platelets and macrophages. Besides TXA_2, equimolar amounts of hydroxyheptadecatrienoic acid (HHT) and malondialdehyde are formed. Their biologic functions, however, are unknown.

In contrast to TXA_2, prostacyclin (PGI_2) is mainly

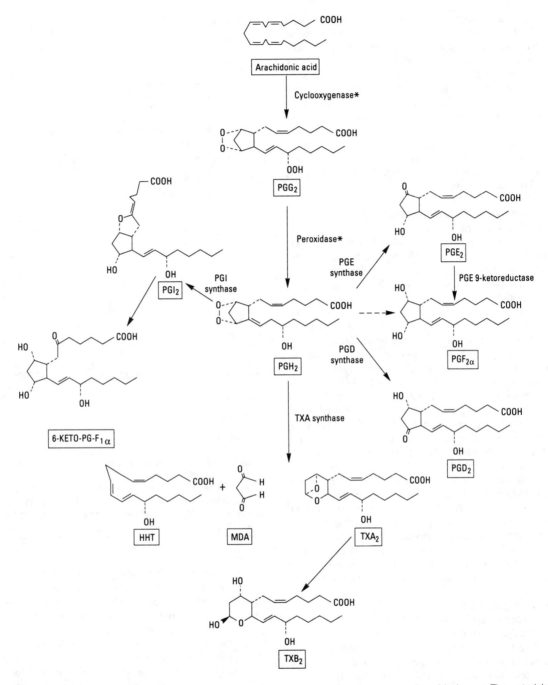

Figure 18–3. Prostaglandin and thromboxane biosynthesis. Compound names are enclosed in boxes. The asterisks indicate that both cyclooxygenase and peroxidase steps are catalyzed by the single enzyme prostaglandin endoperoxide (PGH) synthase.

produced by vascular endothelial and smooth muscle cells and strongly inhibits platelet aggregation and relaxes smooth muscle. It is synthesized by a membrane-bound cytochrome P450-like enzyme, prostacyclin synthase. PGI_2 hydrolyzes spontaneously ($t_{1/2}$ about 3 minutes) to the biologically inactive 6-keto-$PGF_{1\alpha}$. Thus, TXA_2 and PGI_2 are formed from the same precursor by two very similar but tissue-specific enzymes. This relationship corresponds well to their opposite—even antagonistic—biologic properties. Both these compounds are rapidly hydrolyzed to inactive products that can be measured easily, eg, by radioimmunoassay.

Metabolism of Arachidonic Acid by Cytochrome P450

In addition to being metabolized by the cyclooxygenase or lipoxygenase pathway (see below), arachidonic acid is also oxygenated by microsomal cytochrome P450 monooxygenases. Experimentally, the products of these reactions affect vascular tone, ion transport, cellular growth, signal transduction, hormonal responses, hemostasis, and hematopoiesis. This enzyme system oxidizes arachidonic acid to 19-hydroxy- and 19-oxoeicosatetraenoic acid (by omega-1 oxidation) and to 20-hydroxyeicosatetraenoic and eicosatetraen-1,20-dioic acids (by omega-oxidation). Other arachidonic acid metabolites are produced by hepatic and renal microsomal cytochrome P450 enzymes, including a series of epoxides (5,6-oxido-, 8,9-oxido-, 11,12-oxido-, and 14,15-oxidoeicosatetraenoic acid) that can be further converted to diols. The 11,12 oxido- product is a powerful vasodilator and causes neovascularization. Some of these arachidonic acid metabolites exhibit their biologic activity only after transcellular metabolism. In addition, both types of oxidations can occur together to yield trihydroxyarachidonic acid derivatives (lipoxins; see below). These and other closely related compounds are being investigated for their biologic activity on vascular smooth muscle and transporting epithelia.

Lipoxygenases, Hydroperoxyeicosatetraenoic Acids, & Lipoxins

The third major pathway of arachidonic acid oxygenation is by lipoxygenases, which incorporate one oxygen molecule into polyunsaturated fatty acids (Figure 18–4). The regional specificity of these lipoxygenases is designated by the position of the carbon bearing the hydroperoxy group in the product. In humans, arachidonic acid is primarily converted into 5-HPETE, 12-HPETE, and 15-HPETE. These unstable peroxides then yield their corresponding hydroxy derivatives (HETEs). There are also two forms of 12-HETE (R and S configurations) that are present in platelets and leukocytes, respectively.

The enzymes 5-lipoxygenase and 12-lipoxygenase are widely distributed in mammalian tissues and

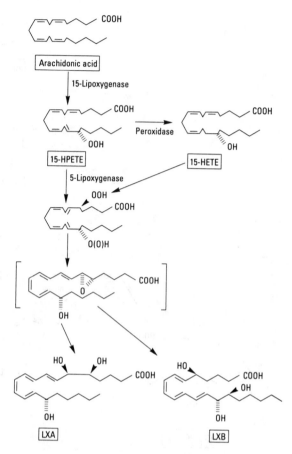

Figure 18–4. Proposed pathway of lipoxin biosynthesis. Compound names are enclosed in boxes. Both 15-HPETE and 15-HETE are substrates for polymorphonuclear leukocyte 5-lipoxygenase, which induces either LXA or LXB synthesis by oxidation at C5 and subsequent epoxide formation.

blood cells and are identical except for two amino acids that are responsible for positioning the substrate. Significant 15-lipoxygenase activity seems to be present only in eosinophils. In contrast to cyclooxygenase, lipoxygenases also occur in plants such as potatoes and soybeans. This finding may indicate that the lipoxygenase pathways of polyenoic fatty acid oxygenation are phylogenetically older. Both 5- and 15-lipoxygenase contribute to the formation of various trihydroxyeicosatetraenoic acids, including the lipoxins LXA and LXB (Figure 18–4).

Leukotriene Biosynthesis

Leukotrienes (LTs) are potent biologically active compounds that are synthesized by the 5-lipoxygenase in neutrophils, monocytes, macrophages, mast cells, and keratinocytes and also in lung, spleen, brain, and heart (Figure 18–5). Before their structure was known, they were recognized in perfusates of

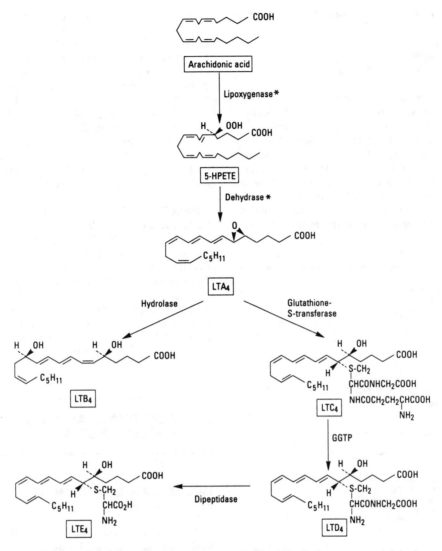

Figure 18–5. Leukotriene biosynthesis. The asterisks indicate that both the lipoxygenase and dehydrase reactions are driven by the single enzyme 5-lipoxygenase. (GGTP, γ-glutamyltranspeptidase.)

lung as the **slow-reacting substance of anaphylaxis (SRS-A)** that is released after immunologic challenge. SRS-A is a mixture of the peptidoleukotrienes LTC_4, LTD_4, and LTE_4. The name leukotriene reflects their discovery in leukocytes and the conjugated triene structure that produces their characteristic ultraviolet absorption spectrum. The subscript denotes the number of double bonds present. Leukotriene synthesis occurs only via the 5-lipoxygenase pathway, where the intermediate 5-HPETE is reduced by a dehydrase to LTA_4. In human leukocytes, a single enzyme is responsible for both the formation of 5-HPETE and its subsequent transformation to LTA_4. This product is either hydrolyzed to LTB_4 or its isomers or converted into LTC_4 by the addition of the peptide glutathione by a specific glutathione S-transferase. Removal of the glutamic acid by γ-glutamyltranspeptidase leads to the formation of LTD_4. Removal of the glycine residue by a dipeptidase yields LTE_4. The 5-lipoxygenase of human neutrophils is stimulated by calcium ions, which may translocate the enzyme from the cytosol to the membrane. This mechanism suggests a means for regulating neutrophils and so controlling their role in inflammation. Currently, the regulation of cyclooxygenase and lipoxygenases by cytokines, growth factors, and oncogenes is of considerable interest.

EICOSANOID METABOLISM

Identification of stable products of eicosanoid metabolism in plasma is important for investigational purposes. These products can be measured by radioimmunoassay or enzyme-linked immunosorbent assay (ELISA).

The Prostaglandin 15-Hydroxydehydrogenase Pathway

Prostaglandins are rapidly catabolized in the body. About 97% of an intravenous dose of PGE_2 is eliminated from the plasma within 90 seconds. Prostaglandin degradation enzymes are widely distributed in the body, with highest activities in lung, kidney, spleen, adipose tissue, and intestine. In particular, the pulmonary vascular bed is highly efficient at inactivating circulating prostaglandins (Figure 18–6). The hydroxyl group on C15, which is essential for the biologic activity of all prostaglandins, is oxidized to the corresponding ketone by the enzyme prostaglandin 15-hydroxydehydrogenase (PGDH). The 15-keto compound is reduced to the 13,14-dihydro derivative by prostaglandin 13-reductase. These first two reactions occur within a few minutes, whereas the second phase of prostaglandin catabolism entails the slower beta- and omega-oxidation of the side chains. The second phase produces polar dicarboxylic acids that are freely excreted in the urine. Another pathway forms the corresponding 13,14-dihydro derivatives by a specific oxidoreductase. The major metabolites of TXB_2 in plasma and urine are 11-dehydro-TXB_2 and 2,3-dinor-TXB_2, respectively.

Catabolism of Prostaglandins by Cytochrome P450

Cytochrome P450 monooxygenases from the liver and kidney catalyze omega-oxidation and omega-1 oxidation of some prostaglandins, including PGE_2. The significance of this pathway in relation to the dehydrogenase pathway is currently unknown. In human polymorphonuclear leukocytes, LTB_4 is further metabolized to its 20-hydroxylation product 20-hydroxy-LTB_4 and the dicarboxylic acid (20-carboxy LTB_4) by a cytochrome P450 enzyme.

I. BASIC PHARMACOLOGY OF EICOSANOIDS

MECHANISMS OF ACTION OF EICOSANOIDS

The eicosanoids are short-lived, highly potent local mediators that produce an astonishing array of biologic effects by binding to specific cell surface receptors. Several of these receptors have been isolated and solubilized. All appear to be G protein-linked (see Chapter 2). However, their pharmacologic specificity is not determined by a particular intracellular effector or second messenger system but by the distribution and number of receptors on different cell types.

For example, PGI_2 inhibits platelet aggregation by binding to receptors that specifically activate adenylyl cyclase. This leads to increased intracellular cAMP levels, which in turn activate specific protein kinases. These kinases phosphorylate internal calcium pump proteins, an action that decreases free intracellular calcium concentration. PGD_2 also inhibits platelet aggregation by activating adenylyl cyclase, but it interacts with receptors different from those used by PGI_2. In contrast, binding of TXA_2 to specific platelet receptors activates phosphatidylinositol metabolism, leading to the formation of **inositol-1,4,5-trisphosphate (IP$_3$),** another second messenger. IP_3

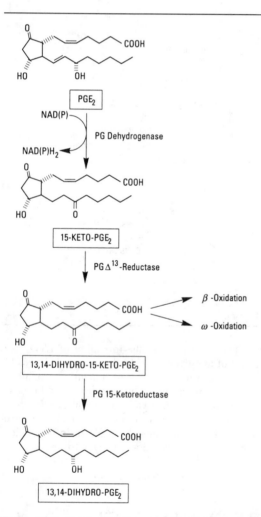

Figure 18–6. Catabolism of prostanoids. The figure illustrates the enzymatic degradation of PGE_2. PGD_2, $PGF_{2\alpha}$, 6-keto-$PGF_{1\alpha}$, and HHT can also undergo this type of metabolism, whereas TXB_2 is converted into its 2,3-dinor derivative by beta-oxidation.

causes mobilization of intracellular calcium and platelet aggregation. LTB_4 causes activation, degranulation, and superoxide anion generation in polymorphonuclear leukocytes by the secondary formation of IP_3.

Thus, the contractile effects of eicosanoids on smooth muscle may be mediated by the release of calcium, while their relaxation effects may be mediated by the generation of cAMP. The effects of eicosanoids on many body systems, including the immune system, can be similarly explained (see below). Many of the eicosanoids' contractile effects on smooth muscle can be antagonized by lowering extracellular calcium concentration or by using calcium channel-blocking drugs.

Effects of Prostaglandins & Thromboxanes

The prostaglandins and thromboxanes have major effects on smooth muscle and platelets. Other important targets include the central nervous system, autonomic postganglionic nerve terminals, sensory nerve endings, endocrine organs, and adipose tissue.

A. Smooth Muscle:

1. Vascular–Human arteriolar smooth muscle is relaxed by PGE_2 and PGI_2. These and other prostaglandins promote vasodilation by activating adenylyl cyclase. However, TXA_2 and $PGF_{2\alpha}$ act mostly as vasoconstrictors, especially on veins. Prostacyclin—which is mainly synthesized by the endothelium—originally appeared to be a circulating hormone. However, little if any PGI_2 escapes immediate degradation. In the microcirculation, PGE_2 is also an important endothelial product. Texhe potent vasodilator endothelium-derived relaxing factor (EDRF)—which is identical with nitric oxide or a closely related molecule—is released from the endothelium along with PGE_2 and PGI_2. The action of EDRF is mediated by the soluble enzyme guanylyl cyclase in vascular smooth muscle (see Figure 12–2); its effect is not blocked by NSAIDs. Thus, the regulation of the microcirculation is not dependent solely on the endothelial synthesis of prostaglandins.

2. Gastrointestinal tract–The effects of prostaglandins and thromboxanes on gastrointestinal smooth muscle vary. Longitudinal muscle is contracted by PGE_2 and $PGF_{2\alpha}$, while circular muscle is contracted by PGI_2 and $PGF_{2\alpha}$ and relaxed by PGE_2. Administration of either PGE_2 or $PGF_{2\alpha}$ results in colicky cramps (see Clinical Pharmacology of Eicosanoids, below).

3. Airways–Respiratory smooth muscle is relaxed by PGE_1, PGE_2, and PGI_2 and contracted by TXA_2 and $PGF_{2\alpha}$.

B. Platelets: As noted above, platelet aggregation can be greatly affected by eicosanoids. PGE_1 and especially PGI_2 effectively inhibit aggregation, while TXA_2 strongly facilitates aggregation.

C. Reproductive Organs:

1. Female reproductive organs–The effects of prostaglandins on the uterus are of great clinical importance. They are discussed below (see Clinical Pharmacology of Eicosanoids).

2. Male reproductive organs–The role of prostaglandins in semen is still conjectural. The major source of these prostaglandins is the seminal vesicle; the prostate and the testes synthesize only small amounts. Semen from fertile men contains about 400 μg/mL of PGE and PGF and their 19-hydroxy metabolites. There is about 20 times more PGE than PGF in fertile semen, though this ratio varies greatly among individuals. However, within individuals, this ratio remains fairly constant as long as the sperm characteristics are unchanged. The factors that regulate the concentration of prostaglandins in human seminal plasma are not known in detail, but testosterone does promote prostaglandin production. Thromboxane and leukotrienes have not been found in seminal plasma. Men with a low seminal concentration of prostaglandins are relatively infertile. Large oral doses of aspirin reduce the prostaglandin content of seminal plasma.

D. Central and Peripheral Nervous Systems:

1. Fever–PGE_1 and PGE_2 increase body temperature, especially when administered into the cerebral ventricles. Pyrogens release interleukin-1, which in turn promotes the synthesis and release of PGE_2. This synthesis is blocked by aspirin and other antipyretic compounds.

2. Sleep–When infused into the cerebral ventricles, PGD_2 induces natural sleep (as determined by electroencephalographic analysis) in a number of species, including primates.

3. Neurotransmission–PGE compounds inhibit the release of norepinephrine from sympathetic presynaptic nerve endings. Moreover, NSAIDs increase norepinephrine release, suggesting that the prostaglandins play a physiologic role in this process. Thus, vasoconstriction observed after treatment with cyclooxygenase inhibitors may be due to increased release of norepinephrine as well as inhibition of the endothelial synthesis of vasodilators (PGE_2 and PGI_2).

E. Neuroendocrinology: Both in vitro and in vivo tests have shown that some of the eicosanoids affect the secretion of neurohormones. PGE compounds promote the release of growth hormone, prolactin, thyroid-stimulating hormone (TSH), adrenocorticotropic hormone (ACTH), follicle-stimulating hormone (FSH), and luteinizing hormone (LH). However, pharmacologic effects reflecting significant release of these hormones have not yet been reported in patients receiving PGE compounds. LTC_4 and LTD_4 also stimulate LH and luteinizing hormone-releasing hormone (LHRH) secretion (see below).

Effects of Lipoxygenase- & Cytochrome P450- Derived Metabolites

Recent data indicate that 12-HPETE acts as a neurotransmitter in *Aplysia* neurons. In addition, several reports state that very high dilutions of LTC_4 specifically increase LH and LHRH release from isolated rat anterior pituitary cells. Taken together, these data indicate that products of the lipoxygenase pathway could function as neurotransmitters. Arachidonic acid epoxides also increase the release of LH from pituitary cells. However, these epoxides are far less potent than LTC_4.

The biologic functions of the various forms of hydroxy and hydroperoxy eicosaenoic acids are largely unknown, but their pharmacologic potency is impressive. For example, 12(S)-HETE stimulates the migration of aortic smooth muscle cells at concentrations as low as 1 fmol/L. This effect may be useful in promoting myointimal thickening after endothelium damage such as that caused by angioplasty. Its stereoisomer, 12(R)-HETE, is a potent inhibitor of the Na^+/K^+ ATPase in the cornea. LTB_4 is one of the most potent chemoattractants for neutrophils. It induces augmented adherence, degranulation, and oxygen radical formation in these cells. The peptidoleukotrienes, particularly LTC_4 and LTD_4, are potent bronchoconstrictors and cause increased microvascular permeability, plasma exudation, and mucus secretion—ie, they possess the properties of SRS-A. Moreover, they reduce myocardial contractility and coronary blood flow, leading to cardiac depression. Other factors (eg, PAF) are released in anaphylaxis and are discussed below. The leukotrienes have been implicated in the pathogenesis of inflammation, especially in chronic diseases.

Both LXA and LXB inhibit natural killer cell cytotoxicity, and LXA seems to exert effects similar to those of LTB_4 on neutrophils or LTC_4 on the vasculature. Thus, the multiple interactions of lipoxygenases generate compounds that can regulate specific cellular responses important in inflammation and immunity. Other cytochrome P450-derived metabolites affect nephron transport functions either directly or via metabolism to active compounds.

INHIBITION OF EICOSANOID SYNTHESIS

Corticosteroids block all the known pathways of eicosanoid synthesis, possibly by stimulating the synthesis of several inhibitory proteins collectively called lipocortins. Lipocortins inhibit phospholipase A_2 activity, probably by interfering with phospholipid binding and thus preventing the release of arachidonic acid. The nonsteroidal anti-inflammatory drugs (eg, aspirin, indomethacin, ibuprofen) block both prostaglandin and thromboxane formation by inhibiting cyclooxygenase activity. For example, aspirin is a long-lasting inhibitor of platelet cyclooxygenase and, therefore, TXA_2 biosynthesis, because it irreversibly acetylates the enzyme. Platelet cyclooxygenase cannot be restored via protein biosynthesis because platelets lack a nucleus.

The development of selective thromboxane synthase inhibitors and TXA_2 receptor antagonists has required considerable effort. The resulting compounds are quite useful for characterizing TXA_2-related effects in vitro and in vivo. They are being tested in the treatment of pulmonary hypertension and preeclampsia. Selective inhibitors of the lipoxygenase pathway are still investigational. With a few exceptions, NSAIDs do not inhibit lipoxygenase activity at concentrations that markedly inhibit cyclooxygenase activity. In fact, by preventing arachidonic acid conversion via the cyclooxygenase pathway, NSAIDs may cause more substrate to be metabolized through the lipoxygenase pathways, leading to an increased formation of (for example) the inflammatory leukotrienes. Even among the cyclooxygenase-dependent pathways, inhibiting the synthesis of one derivative may increase the synthesis of an enzymatically related product. Therefore, researchers are attempting to develop drugs that inhibit both cyclooxygenase and lipoxygenase.

II. CLINICAL PHARMACOLOGY OF EICOSANOIDS

Several approaches have been used in the clinical application of eicosanoids. First, stable, long-acting analogues of PGE_1 and PGE_2 have been developed that increase intracellular cAMP and so can be regarded as "cytoprotective" under some circumstances. Other related compounds, including prostacyclin analogues, have been approved for clinical use overseas and are being introduced in the USA. Second, enzyme inhibitors and receptor antagonists have been developed for interdiction and decreased expression of the "pathologic" eicosanoids such as the thromboxanes and leukotrienes. Third, knowledge of eicosanoid synthesis and metabolism has led to the development of new nonsteroidal anti-inflammatory drugs that inhibit cyclooxygenase with improved pharmacokinetic and pharmacodynamic characteristics. One objective, as described earlier, is to develop dual inhibitors that block both the cyclooxygenase and lipoxygenase pathways. Another goal is to decrease gastrointestinal and renal toxicity. Finally, dietary manipulation—to change the polyunsaturated fatty acid precursors in the cell membrane phospholipids and so change eicosanoid synthesis—is under active investigation.

Female Reproductive System

The physiologic role of prostaglandins in reproduction has been intensively studied since the discovery of prostaglandins in the seminal plasma of primates and sheep. It has been suggested that the prostaglandins in seminal plasma facilitate blastocyst implantation or egg transport and that uterine secretion of prostaglandins causes luteolysis. The latter theory is not true in humans but appears to be true in cattle and pigs. This finding has led to the marketing of veterinary preparations of $PGF_{2\alpha}$ and its analogues for synchronizing the ovulation of female animals.

A. Abortion: PGE_2 and $PGF_{2\alpha}$ are well known for their oxytocic action. The ability of the E and F prostaglandins and their analogues to terminate pregnancy at any stage by promoting uterine contractions has been adapted to routine clinical use. Many studies worldwide have established that prostaglandin administration efficiently terminates pregnancy. The drugs are used for first- and second-trimester abortion and priming or ripening of the cervix before abortion. These prostaglandins appear to soften the cervix by increasing proteoglycan and changing the biophysical properties of collagen.

Early studies found that intravenously administered PGE_2 and $PGF_{2\alpha}$ produced abortion in about 80% of cases. The success rate was dependent on dose, duration of infusion, and parity of the woman. Dose-limiting adverse effects included vomiting, diarrhea, hyperthermia, and bronchoconstriction.

At the present time intra-amniotic, intramuscular, or intravaginal administration is more common. Intra-amniotic administration of $PGF_{2\alpha}$ has close to a 100% success rate with fewer and less severe adverse effects than intravenous administration. The drug previously available for this route of administration, dinoprost tromethamine (a derivative of $PGF_{2\alpha}$), was recently withdrawn from the United States market. Where still available, this drug is used to induce second-trimester abortions and is usually administered as a single 40 mg intra-amniotic injection. The abortion is normally completed within 20 hours. The most serious adverse effects of this route of administration involve cardiovascular collapse. Most of the reported cases have been diagnosed as anaphylactic shock, but others may have been due to the drug's escaping into the circulation and causing severe pulmonary hypertension. In pregnant anesthetized women, 300 μg of $PGF_{2\alpha}$/min intravenously increases pulmonary resistance by 100% and increases the work of the right side of the heart threefold. Thus, only minimal amounts of the 40 mg intra-amniotic dose need to reach the circulation to cause cardiovascular effects. This problem may be avoided by instilling the drug under ultrasonic guidance.

Intramuscular injection can also be used to induce abortion. The drug used is carboprost tromethamine (15-methyl-$PGF_{2\alpha}$); the carbon 15 methyl group prolongs the duration of action. Unlike the one-time intrauterine instillation of dinoprost, carboprost is given repeatedly up to the total dose of 2.6 mg normally required to cause abortion.

Dinoprostone, a synthetic PGE_2 analogue, is administered as vaginal suppositories. It directly affects the collagenase of the cervix and also stimulates the contraction of the uterus. The usual dose is 20 mg repeated at 3- to 5-hour intervals depending on the response of the uterus. Abortion is usually achieved within 90 hours, but nearly 25% of cases are incomplete and require additional intervention.

The use of PGE analogues for "menstrual regulation" or very early abortions—within 1–2 weeks after the last menstrual period—has been explored extensively. There are two major problems: prolonged vaginal bleeding and severe menstrual cramps.

Antiprogestins (eg, RU 486) have been combined with an oral oxytocic prostaglandin to produce early abortion, currently available in France. The ease and effectiveness of this combination has aroused considerable opposition in some quarters (see Chapter 39). The major toxicities are cramping pain and diarrhea.

B. Facilitation of Labor: Numerous studies have shown that PGE_2, $PGF_{2\alpha}$, and their analogues effectively initiate and stimulate labor. However, this is an unlabeled use. There appears to be no difference in the efficacy of the two drugs when they are administered intravenously, but $PGF_{2\alpha}$ is one-tenth as potent as PGE_2. These agents and oxytocin have similar success rates and comparable induction-to-delivery intervals. The adverse effects of the prostaglandins are moderate, with a slightly higher incidence of nausea, vomiting, and diarrhea than that produced by oxytocin. $PGF_{2\alpha}$ has more gastrointestinal toxicity than PGE_2. Neither drug has significant maternal cardiovascular toxicity in the recommended doses. In fact, PGE_2 must be infused at a rate about 20 times that used for induction of labor to decrease blood pressure and increase heart rate. $PGF_{2\alpha}$ is a bronchoconstrictor and should be used with caution in asthmatics; however, neither asthmatic attacks nor bronchoconstriction has been observed during the induction of labor. Although both PGE_2 and $PGF_{2\alpha}$ pass the fetoplacental barrier, fetal toxicity is uncommon.

The effects of oral PGE_2 administration (0.5–1.5 mg/h) have been compared to those of intravenous oxytocin and oral demoxytocin, an oxytocin derivative, in the induction of labor. Oral PGE_2 is superior to the oral oxytocin derivative and in most studies is as efficient as intravenous oxytocin. However, the only available form of PGE_2 at present is dinoprostone (vaginal suppositories), though its route of administration is slightly less effective than that of oxytocin. Vaginal PGE_2 is also used to soften the cervix before inducing labor. Oral $PGF_{2\alpha}$ has too much gastrointestinal toxicity to be useful for this indication.

Theoretically, PGE_2 and $PGF_{2\alpha}$ should be superior to oxytocin for inducing labor in women with preeclampsia or cardiac and renal diseases because, unlike oxytocin, they have no antidiuretic effect. In addition, PGE_2 has natriuretic effects. However, the clinical benefits of these effects have not been documented. In cases of intrauterine fetal death, the prostaglandins alone or with oxytocin seem to cause delivery effectively. In some cases of postpartum bleeding, 15-methyl-$PGF_{2\alpha}$ will successfully control hemorrhage when oxytocin and methylergonovine fail to do so.

C. Dysmenorrhea: Primary dysmenorrhea is attributed to increased endometrial synthesis of PGE_2 and $PGF_{2\alpha}$ during menstruation, with contractions of the uterus that lead to ischemic pain. NSAIDs successfully inhibit the formation of these prostaglandins (see Chapter 35) and so relieve dysmenorrhea in 75–85% of cases. Some of these drugs are available over the counter. Aspirin is also effective in dysmenorrhea, but because it has low potency and is quickly hydrolyzed, large doses and frequent administration are necessary.

Cardiovascular System

The vasodilator effects of PGE and PGA compounds have been studied extensively in hypertensive patients. These compounds also promote sodium diuresis.

Prostacyclin lowers peripheral and coronary resistance. It has been used to treat both primary pulmonary hypertension and secondary pulmonary hypertension (which sometimes occurs after mitral valve surgery). However, its pulmonary vasodilator effects are not specific enough, so the patient's blood pressure must also be supported with pressor drugs.

A number of studies have investigated the use of PGE and PGI_2 compounds to treat Raynaud's phenomenon and peripheral atherosclerosis. In the latter case, prolonged infusions have been used to permit "remodeling" of the vessel wall and to enhance regression of ischemic ulcers.

A. Thrombosis: Eicosanoids are involved in thrombosis mainly because TXA_2 promotes platelet aggregation and PGI_2 inhibits it. Aspirin inhibits platelet cyclooxygenase to produce a mild clotting defect. The mildness of this defect is supported by the fact that very modest hemostatic defects are noted in patients with diseases involving deficiencies of platelet cyclooxygenase and thromboxane synthase—ie, these patients have no history of increased or decreased bleeding. Blockade of either of these two enzymes inhibits secondary aggregation of platelets induced by ADP, by low concentrations of thrombin and collagen, or by epinephrine. Thus, these platelet enzymes are not necessary for platelet function but may amplify an aggregating stimulus. Clearly, the most important physiologic factors act through other pathways.

Epidemiologic studies in the USA and UK indicate that low doses of aspirin reduce the risk of death due to infarction but perhaps increase overall mortality rates and produce a higher incidence of stroke (see Chapter 33). It is now difficult to find patients at risk for thromboembolism—as in orthopedic surgery or angioplasty for coronary artery stenosis—who do not take aspirin. However, the beneficial effects of aspirin may relate to its other acetylating properties and not to acetylation of cyclooxygenase.

During the development of deep vein thrombosis, thromboxane and its metabolites are excreted in the urine, probably because the whole platelet pool is activated. This phenomenon is seen to a lesser extent in kidney transplant patients experiencing organ rejection. Elevated excretion of thromboxane metabolites is also seen in patients before infarction and during unstable angina.

Prostacyclin is not a circulating hormone, as originally claimed; it inhibits platelet aggregation but does not inhibit platelet adhesion to the endothelium, platelet spreading, or granule release. PGI_2 and PGE_2 analogues can inhibit the development of atherosclerosis in cholesterol-fed animals, but hypotension is an adverse effect.

B. Patent Ductus Arteriosus: Patency of the fetal ductus arteriosus is now generally believed to be dependent on local PGE_2 and PGI_2 synthesis. In certain types of congenital heart disease (transposition of the great arteries, pulmonary atresia, pulmonary artery stenosis), it is important to maintain the patency of the neonate's ductus arteriosus before surgery. This is done with alprostadil, PGE_1. Like PGE_2, PGE_1 is a vasodilator and an inhibitor of platelet aggregation, and it contracts uterine and intestinal smooth muscle. There are no absolute contraindications for the use of this drug, but in cases of respiratory distress syndrome it is not recommended. Adverse effects include apnea, bradycardia, hypotension, and hyperpyrexia. Because of rapid pulmonary clearance, the drug must be continuously infused at an initial dose of 0.05–0.1 µg/kg/min, which may be increased to 0.4 µg/kg/min. Prolonged treatment has been associated with ductal fragility and rupture.

In delayed closure of the ductus arteriosus, cyclooxygenase inhibitors can be used to inhibit synthesis of the vasodilators PGE_2 and PGI_2 and so close the ductus. Premature infants who develop respiratory distress due to failure of ductus closure can be treated with a high degree of success with indomethacin. This treatment precludes the need for surgical closure of the ductus.

C. Impotence or Erectile Dysfunction: Intracavernosal injection therapy with the vasodilator alprostadil (PGE_1) has become important in the treatment of impotence. This agent has not received approval for this indication by the Food and Drug Administration. Alprostadil may be used as monotherapy or in combination with either papaverine or phentolamine.

Respiratory System

PGE$_2$ is a powerful bronchodilator when given in aerosol form. Unfortunately, it also promotes coughing, and an analogue that possesses only the bronchodilator properties has been difficult to obtain.

PGF$_{2\alpha}$ and TXA$_2$ are both strong bronchoconstrictors and were once thought to be primary mediators in asthma. However, the identification of the leukotrienes (LTC$_4$, LTD$_4$, and LTE$_4$) with the slow-reacting substance of anaphylaxis (SRS-A) expanded the role of eicosanoids as important mediators in asthma and other immune responses. The leukotrienes increase mucus secretion as well as promote bronchoconstriction. In addition, leukotrienes may be partially responsible for the adult respiratory distress syndrome. Other pathologic mediators such as PAF not only possess direct bronchoconstrictor effects but also (depending on species) can release PGF$_{2\alpha}$, thromboxane, and leukotrienes. Consequently, considerable effort has been focused on PAF antagonists for treating asthma. Unfortunately, these approaches have not yet been successful. However, LT antagonists and lipoxygenase inhibitors may become useful in treating acute asthmatic attacks and hypersensitivity reactions. Recent clinical trials indicate that leukotriene antagonists have a bronchodilator effect in humans, indicating that leukotrienes modulate pulmonary airway tone.

Corticosteroids and cromolyn are still the major eicosanoid-related drugs used in asthma (see Chapter 19). Corticosteroids inhibit eicosanoid synthesis and thus limit the amounts of eicosanoid mediator available for release. Cromolyn probably inhibits the release of eicosanoids and other mediators such as histamine and PAF.

Renal System

Both the renal medulla and the renal cortex synthesize prostaglandins, but the synthetic capacity of the medulla is substantially greater than that of the cortex. These functional areas synthesize several hydroxyeicosatetraenoic acids, leukotrienes, cytochrome P450 products, and epoxides that play an important autoregulatory role in renal function. These compounds modify both renal hemodynamics and glomerular and tubular function. This regulatory role is especially important in marginally functioning kidneys, as shown by the decline in kidney function associated with the use of cyclooxygenase inhibitors in elderly patients or those with renal disease.

The major eicosanoid products of the renal cortex are PGE$_2$ and PGI$_2$. Both compounds increase renin release; however, renin release is normally under β_1-adrenoceptor control. The glomeruli also synthesize small amounts of TXA$_2$. This very potent vasocon-

strictor does not appear to be responsible for regulating glomerular function in healthy humans.

PGE$_1$, PGE$_2$, and PGI$_2$ increase glomerular filtration through their vasodilatory effects. These prostaglandins also increase water and sodium excretion. The increase in water clearance is probably caused by attenuating the action of antidiuretic hormone (ADH) on adenylyl cyclase. It is uncertain whether the natriuretic effect is caused by the direct inhibition of sodium resorption in the distal tubule or by increased medullary blood flow. The loop diuretic furosemide produces some of its effect by stimulating cyclooxygenase activity. In the normal kidney, this increases the synthesis of the vasodilator prostaglandins. Therefore, patient response to the loop diuretic will be diminished if a cyclooxygenase inhibitor is concurrently administered.

Like ADH, TXA$_2$ appears to increase water transport in the toad bladder. This finding led to the suggestion that ADH may exert part of its effect by increasing TXA$_2$ synthesis. The normal kidney synthesizes only small amounts of TXA$_2$. In renal conditions involving inflammatory cell infiltration of the interstitium (such as glomerulonephritis and renal transplant rejection), the inflammatory cells (monocyte-macrophages) release substantial amounts of TXA$_2$. This increased concentration causes intrarenal vasoconstriction (and perhaps an ADH-like effect), leading to a decline in renal function. Administration of TXA$_2$-synthase inhibitors or antagonists (when available) to these patients and to those with preeclampsia may improve renal function.

Hypertension reportedly is associated with increased TXA$_2$ and decreased PGE$_2$ and PGI$_2$ synthesis in animals. These changes may be either primary contributing factors or secondary responses. Similarly, TXA$_2$ formation has been reported in cyclosporine-induced nephrotoxicity but no causal relationship has yet been established.

PGE$_2$ may also be involved in renal phosphate excretion, because exogenous PGE$_2$ antagonizes the inhibition of phosphate resorption by parathyroid hormone (PTH) in the proximal tubule. However, the physiologic role of this eicosanoid may be limited because the proximal tubule, the major site for phosphate transport, produces few prostaglandins.

The roles of leukotrienes and cytochrome P450 products in the human kidney are currently speculative. More information is needed to suggest any specific renal functions for these compounds. Recently, the -5,6-epoxide has been shown to be a powerful vasodilator in animal experiments. Another recent discovery is that free radicals attack arachidonic acid-containing phospholipids to yield an 8-iso-PGF$_{2\alpha}$ which has powerful thromboxane-like properties. Synthesis is *not* blocked by cyclooxygenase inhibitors but can be blocked by antioxidants. This vasoconstrictor, which is present in humans, is thought to be the mediator causing renal failure in the hepatorenal syndrome.

Gastrointestinal System

The word "cytoprotection" was coined to signify the protective effect of the E prostaglandins against gastric ulcers in animals at doses that do not reduce acid secretion. These prostaglandins were independently discovered to inhibit gastric acid secretion. Since then, numerous experimental and clinical investigations have shown that PGE and its analogues protect against gastric ulcers produced by either steroids or NSAIDs. Misoprostol is an orally active synthetic analogue of PGE_1 available in Europe and the USA for anti-ulcer treatment. The FDA-approved indication is for prevention of NSAID-induced gastric ulcers only. This and other PGE analogues (eg, enprostil) are cytoprotective at low doses and inhibit gastric acid secretion at higher doses. The adverse effects are abdominal discomfort and occasional diarrhea; both effects are dose-related.

Increased leukotriene formation in colonic mucosa has been demonstrated in patients with inflammatory bowel diseases. Whether these products play a significant pathophysiologic role has not yet been established.

Immune System

Monocyte-macrophages are the only principal cells of the immune system that can synthesize all the eicosanoids. T and B lymphocytes are interesting exceptions to the general rule that all nucleated cells produce eicosanoids. However, in a B lymphoma cell line, there is nonreceptor-mediated uptake of LTB_4 and 5-HETE. Interaction between lymphocytes and monocyte-macrophages may cause the lymphocytes to release arachidonic acid from their cell membranes. The arachidonic acid is then used by the monocyte-macrophages for eicosanoid synthesis. In addition to these cells, there is evidence for eicosanoid cell-cell interaction by platelets, erythrocytes, PMNs, and endothelial cells.

The eicosanoids modulate the effects of the immune system, as illustrated by the cell-mediated immune response. As shown in Figure 18–7, PGE_2 and PGI_2 affect T cell proliferation as corticosteroids do. They inhibit T cell clonal expansion by inhibiting interleukin-1 and -2, and class II antigen expression on macrophages or other antigen-presenting cells. The leukotrienes, TXA_2, and PAF stimulate T cell clonal expansion. These compounds stimulate the formation of interleukin-1 and -2 as well as the expression of interleukin-2 receptors. The leukotrienes also promote interferon-gamma release and can replace interleukin-2 as a stimulator of interferon-gamma. These in vitro effects of the eicosanoids and PAF agree with in vivo findings in animals with acute organ transplant rejection, as described below. The association between the use of the anti-inflammatory steroids and increased risk of infection is well established; how-

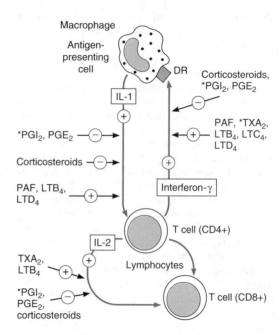

Figure 18–7. Modulation of macrophage and lymphocyte interactions by eicosanoids, platelet activating factor, and corticosteroids. Corticosteroids, PGE_2, and possibly PGI_2 inhibit the expression of interleukin-1 (IL-1) and its effect on T lymphocytes. Platelet-activating factor (PAF), LTB_4, and LTD_4 increase IL-1 expression. Similar inhibitory and stimulant effects are exerted on the action of interferon-gamma on the macrophage and on the action of interleukin-2 (IL-2). Agents marked with an asterisk are suspected, but not yet proved, to have the effects indicated. (DR, class II MHC [major histocompatibility complex] receptor; T, T lymphocytes.) (Modified and reproduced, with permission, from Foegh ML, Ramwell PW: PAF and transplant immunology. In: Braquet P [editor]: *The Role of Platelet Activating Factor in Immune Disorders.* Karger, 1988.)

ever, the nonsteroidal anti-inflammatory drugs do not seem to alter patient responses to infection.

A. Cell-Mediated Organ Transplant Rejection: Acute organ transplant rejection is a cell-mediated immune response. Administration of PGI_2 to renal transplant patients has reversed the rejection process in some cases. Experimental in vitro and in vivo data show that PGE_2 and PGI_2 can prevent T cell proliferation and rejection, whereas prevention of TXA_2 and leukotriene formation attenuates organ graft rejection. In kidney transplant patients, excretion of TXB_2 in the urine increases during acute rejection. This eicosanoid has not yet been proved to cause organ transplant rejection; however, corticosteroids are still the primary means for dealing with acute organ rejection.

B. Inflammation: Aspirin has been used to treat arthritis for nearly a century, but its mechanism of action—inhibition of cyclooxygenase activity—was not discovered until 1971. Aspirin and other anti-inflammatory agents that inhibit cyclooxygenase are discussed in Chapter 35. Cox II appears to be the form of the enzyme associated with cells involved in the inflammatory process. The prostaglandins are not chemoattractants, but the leukotrienes and some of the HETEs, eg, 12-HETE, are strong chemoattractants. Thus, researchers are currently trying to develop drugs that inhibit cyclooxygenase II, 5-lipoxygenase, and 12-lipoxygenase. PGE_2 inhibits both antigen-driven and mitogen-induced B lymphocyte proliferation and differentiation to plasma cells, resulting in inhibition of immunoglobulin M (IgM) synthesis (Figure 18–8). The concomitant elevation of serum IgE and monocyte PGE_2 synthesis which are seen in severe trauma patients and patients with Hodgkin's disease is explained by PGE_2 enhancing immunoglobulin class switching to immunoglobulin E (IgE).

C. Rheumatoid Arthritis: In rheumatoid arthritis, immune complexes are deposited in the affected joints, causing an inflammatory response that is amplified by eicosanoids and PAF. Lymphocytes and macrophages accumulate in the synovium, while polymorphonuclear leukocytes (PMNs) localize mainly in the synovial fluid. The major eicosanoids produced by PMNs are leukotrienes, which facilitate T cell proliferation and act as chemoattractants. Human macrophages synthesize the cyclooxygenase products PGE_2 and TXA_2, in addition to PAF and large amounts of leukotrienes.

DIETARY MANIPULATION OF ARACHIDONIC ACID METABOLISM

Because arachidonic acid is derived from dietary linoleic and linolenic acids, the effects of dietary manipulation on arachidonic acid metabolism are currently being studied. Two approaches have been used. The first adds corn, safflower, and sunflower oils, which contain linoleic acid (C18-polyenoic acid), to the diet. The second approach adds oils containing C20- and C22-polyenoic acids from oils of coldwater fish. Both types of diet change the phospholipid composition of cell membranes by replacing arachidonic acid with the dietary fatty acids. It has been claimed that the synthesis of both TXA_2 and

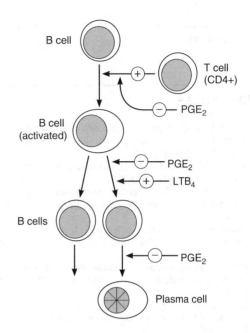

Figure 18–8. The activation and proliferation of B lymphocytes by T lymphocytes (CD4+) are inhibited by PGE_2. Both mitogen- and antigen-induced B cell proliferation is inhibited by PGE_2 and stimulated by LTB_4. PGE_2 inhibits the differentiation of B cells into plasma cells and thus indirectly inhibits immunoglobulin M (IgM) synthesis.

PGI_2 is reduced and that changes in platelet aggregation, vasomotor spasm, and cholesterol metabolism follow. However, none of these interventions have been convincingly shown to modify the natural history of the disease that they address.

As indicated above, there are many documented and possible oxidation products of the different polyenoic acids. It is probably naive to ascribe the effects reported thus far to related metabolites. Carefully controlled clinical studies will be needed before these questions can be satisfactorily answered. However, subjects on diets containing highly saturated fatty acids clearly show increased platelet aggregation when compared with other study groups. Such diets (eg, in Finland and the USA) are associated with higher rates of myocardial infarction than are more polyunsaturated diets (eg, in Italy).

PREPARATIONS AVAILABLE

Alprostadil (Prostin VR Pediatric)
    Parenteral: 500μg/mL in 1 mL ampule
Carboprost tromethamine (Prostin/15 M)
    Parenteral: 250 μg carboprost and 83 μg tromethamine per mL in 1 mL ampule

Dinoprostone (Prostin E2)
    Vaginal: 20 mg suppository
Epoprostenol [prostacyclin] (Flolan, Cycloprostin)
    Orphan drug available from manufacturers for

replacement of heparin in some hemodialysis patients.

Misoprostol (Cytotec)

Oral: 100, 200 μg tablets

REFERENCES

Bønaa KH et al: Effect of eicosapentenoic and docosahexenoic acids on blood pressure in hypertension. N Engl J Med 1990;322:795.

Brain SD, Williams TJ: Leukotrienes and inflammation. Pharmacol Ther 1990;46:57

Chang J, Musser JH, McGregor H: Phospholipase A_2: Function and pharmacological regulation. Biochem Pharmacol 1987;36:2429.

Claesson HE, Odlander B, Jakobsson PJ: Leukotriene B_4 in the immune system. Int J Immunopharmacol 1992;14:441.

Dennis EA: Phospholipase A_2 mechanism: Inhibition and role in arachidonic acid release. Drug Devel Res 1987;10:205.

Foegh ML: Obstetrics and gynecology. In: *Prostaglandins in Clinical Practice.* Watkins WD et al (editors). Raven Press, 1989.

Foegh ML et al (editors): First international Alexis Carrel conference on lipid mediators in organ transplantation: April 8–10, 1986, Washington DC. Transplant Proc 1986;18(5 Suppl 4):1.

Giles H: More selective ligands at eicosanoid receptor subtypes improve prospects in inflammatory and cardiovascular research. Trends Pharmacol Sci 1990;11:301.

Giles H, Leff P: The biology and pharmacology of PGD_2. Prostaglandins 1988;35:277.

Halushka PV et al: Thromboxane, prostaglandin, and leukotriene receptors. Annu Rev Pharmacol Toxicol 1989;29:213.

Hayashi RH: Pharmacological application of prostaglandins, their analogues, and their inhibitors in obstetrics. In: *Uterine Function: Molecular and Cellular Aspects.* Carsten ME, Miller JD (editors). Plenum, 1990.

Holtzman MJ: Arachidonic acid metabolism in airway epithelial cells. Annu Rev Physiol 1992;54:303.

Lands WEM: *Biochemistry of Arachidonic Acid Metabolism.* Martinus Nijhoff, 1985.

Lands WEM: Proceedings of the AOCS: *Short Course on Polyunsaturated Fatty Acids and Eicosanoids.* American Oil Chemists Society, 1987.

Lands WEM: Biochemistry and physiology of n-3 fatty acids. FASEB J 1992;6:2530.

Lewis RA, Austen KF, Soberman RJ: Leukotrienes and other products of the 5-lipoxygenase pathway: Biochemistry and relation to pathobiology in human diseases. N Engl J Med 1990;323:645.

Malle E et al: Lipoxygenases and hydroperoxy/hydroxyeicosatetraenoic acid formation. Int J Biochem 1987;19:1013.

McGiff JC: Cytochrome P-450 metabolism of arachidonic acid. Annu Rev Pharmacol Toxicol 1991;31:339.

Monk JP, Clissold SP: Misoprostol: A preliminary review of its pharmacodynamic and pharmacokinetic properties, and therapeutic efficacy in the treatment of peptic ulcer disease. Drugs 1987;33:1.

Needleman P et al: Arachidonic acid metabolism. Annu Rev Biochem 1986;55:69.

Ohia SE, Jumblatt JE: Prejunctional inhibitory effects of prostanoids on sympathetic neurotransmission in the rabbit iris-ciliary body. J Pharmacol Exp Ther 1990;255:11.

Phipps RP, Stein SH, Roper RL: A new view of prostaglandin E regulation of the immune response. Immunol Today 1991;12:349.

Samuelsson B, Paoletti R, Ramwell PW (editors): *Prostaglandins and Related Compounds.* Vol 17 of: *Advances in Prostaglandin, Thromboxane, and Leukotriene Research.* Raven Press, 1987.

Samuelsson B et al: Leukotrienes and lipoxins: Structures, biosynthesis, and biological effects. Science 1987;237:1171.

Sebaldt RJ et al: Inhibition of eicosanoid biosynthesis by glucocorticoids in humans. Proc Natl Acad Sci USA 1990;87:6974.

Shimizu T, Wolfe LS: Arachidonic acid cascade and signal transduction. J Neurochem 1990;55:1.

Snyder DW, Fleisch JH: Leukotriene receptor antagonists as potential therapeutic agents. Annu Rev Pharmacol Toxicol 1989;29:123.

Stenson WF: Role of eicosanoids as mediators of inflammation in inflammatory bowel disease. Scand J Gastroenterol 1990;25(Suppl 172):13.

Xie W, Robertson DL, Simmons DL: Mitogen-inducible prostaglandin G/H synthase: A new target for nonsteroidal anti-inflammatory drugs. Drug Devel Res 1992;25:249.

Bronchodilators & Other Agents Used in Asthma

19

Homer A. Boushey, MD

Asthma is characterized by increased responsiveness of the trachea and bronchi to various stimuli and by widespread narrowing of the airways that changes in severity either spontaneously or as a result of therapy. The clinical hallmarks of asthma are recurrent, episodic bouts of coughing, shortness of breath, chest tightness, and wheezing. Its pathologic features are contraction of airway smooth muscle, mucosal thickening from edema and cellular infiltration, and inspissation in the airway lumen of abnormally thick, viscid plugs of mucus. Of these causes of airway obstruction, contraction of smooth muscle is most easily reversed by current therapy; reversal of the edema and cellular infiltration requires sustained treatment with anti-inflammatory agents.

The most widely used bronchodilators are β-adrenoceptor stimulants (Chapter 9) and theophylline, a methylxanthine drug. Reversal of airway constriction can also be brought about by the use of antimuscarinic agents (Chapter 8). Two other types of drugs important in asthma are the so-called anti-inflammatory agents; putative inhibitors of mast cell degranulation, cromolyn and nedocromil, inhibitors of mast cell degranulation; and corticosteroids. Recent studies using small numbers of patients suggest that chronic treatment with methotrexate or gold, both of which are effective in rheumatoid arthritis, may be effective for severe, steroid-dependent asthma.

This chapter presents the basic pharmacology of cromolyn and methylxanthines—agents whose medical use is almost exclusively for pulmonary disease. The other classes of drugs listed above are discussed in relation to the therapy of asthma.

Pathogenesis of Asthma

A rational approach to the pharmacotherapy of asthma depends on an understanding of a conceptual model for the pathogenesis of the disease. In the classic immunologic model, asthma is a disease mediated by reaginic (IgE) antibodies bound to mast cells in the airway mucosa (Figure 19–1). On reexposure to an antigen, antigen-antibody interaction takes place on the surface of the mast cells, triggering both the release of mediators stored in the cells' granules and the synthesis and release of other mediators. The agents released include histamine, tryptase and other neutral proteases, leukotrienes C_4 and D_4, prostaglandin D_2, eosinophil chemotactic factor (ECF), neutrophil chemotactic factor (NCF), neutral proteases, and other compounds. These agents diffuse throughout the airway wall and cause contraction of muscle, edema, cellular infiltration, and a change in mucous secretion either by their direct actions or by altering neurohumoral regulatory mechanisms.

There are several features of asthma, however, that cannot be accounted for by this model. Many adults with asthma have no evidence of immediate hypersensitivity to antigens, and most attacks cannot be related to recent exposure to an unusual quantity of antigen. Even in patients with a history of asthma during the ragweed season and positive cutaneous and bronchial responses to ragweed antigen, the severity of symptoms correlates poorly with the quantity of antigen in the atmosphere. Furthermore, bronchospasm can be provoked by nonantigenic stimuli, such as distilled water, exercise, cold air, sulfur dioxide, and rapid respiratory maneuvers.

In healthy nonasthmatic people, inhalation of small doses of mediators of anaphylaxis (eg, histamine) does not provoke bronchoconstriction. In people with asthma, however, inhalation of even smaller doses of the same mediator provokes intense symptomatic bronchospasm. The response can be quantitated by measurement of the fall in forced expiratory volume in 1 second (FEV_1). This exaggerated sensitivity of the airways is sometimes called "nonspecific bronchial hyperreactivity" to distinguish it from the bronchospasm provoked by specific antigens. Bronchial hyperactivity appears to be fundamental to asthma's pathogenesis, for it is nearly ubiquitous in patients with asthma; its degree correlates with the symptomatic severity of the disease; and the events that increase bronchial reactivity (viral respiratory infections, exposure to oxidizing pollutants) have often been noted to cause symptomatic worsening of disease.

The mechanisms underlying bronchial hyperactivity are unknown but may be related to inflammation of the airway mucosa. This hypothesis is supported by the observation that the agents that increase bron-

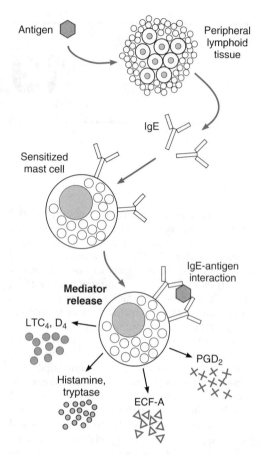

Figure 19–1. Immunologic model for pathogenesis of immediate hypersensitivity. Exposure to antigen causes synthesis of IgE, which binds to mast cells in the target organ. On reexposure to antigen, antigen-antibody interaction on mast cell surfaces triggers release of mediators of anaphylaxis. (LTC$_4$ and LTD$_4$, leukotrienes C$_4$ and D$_4$; PGD$_2$, prostaglandin D$_2$; ECF-A, eosinophil chemotactic factor.) (Modified and reproduced, with permission, from Gold WW: Cholinergic pharmacology in asthma. In: *Asthma Physiology, Immunopharmacology, and Treatment.* Austen KF, Lichtenstein LM [editors]. Academic Press, 1974.)

chial reactivity, such as ozone exposure, allergen inhalation, and infection with respiratory viruses, also cause airway inflammation. In both dogs and humans, the increase in bronchial reactivity induced by ozone is associated with an increase in the number of polymorphonuclear leukocytes found in fluid obtained by bronchial lavage or from bronchial mucosal biopsies. The increase in reactivity due to allergen inhalation is associated with an increase in both eosinophils and polymorphonuclear leukocytes in bronchial lavage fluid. The increase in reactivity that is associated with the late asthmatic response to allergen inhalation (Figure 19–2) is sustained, and it is now considered to be caused by airway inflammation.

How the increase in airway reactivity is linked to inflammation is uncertain, but accumulating evidence points to the eosinophil as importantly involved. The concentrations of an eosinophil granule protein—major basic protein—in expectorated sputum or in fluid lavaged from the lungs correlate with the degree of bronchial hyperreactivity. The most consistent difference in bronchial mucosal biopsies obtained from asthmatic and healthy nonasthmatic subjects is an increase in the number of eosinophils found within and beneath the airway epithelium. Immunohistochemical staining shows increased levels of another eosinophil product—eosinophil cationic protein—beneath the epithelium, indicating activation of the cells. Eosinophil products have in turn been shown to cause epithelial sloughing and an increase in contractile responsiveness of airway smooth muscle. The products of other cells in the airways, such as macrophages, mast cells, sensory nerves, and epithelial cells, have also been shown to alter airway smooth muscle function, however, so it may not be the case that a specific antagonist to a single mediator or class of mediators would be effective antiasthmatic therapy. It is nonetheless encouraging that leukotriene antagonists and lipoxygenase inhibitors have appeared to be effective in controlling asthma in early clinical trials (Cloud, 1989; Israel, 1993).

Whatever the mechanisms responsible for the overall increase in bronchomotor responsiveness of the asthmatic airway, the bronchoconstriction itself seems to be a function of the direct effect of the mediators released and of the amplification of this effect by neural or humoral pathways activated by the mediators. Evidence for the importance of neural pathways stems largely from studies of laboratory animals. Thus, the bronchospasm provoked in dogs by histamine can be greatly reduced by pretreatment with an inhaled topical anesthetic agent, by blockade of the vagus nerves, and by pretreatment with atropine, a competitive antagonist of acetylcholine, in doses that have no effect on the responses of airway smooth muscle to histamine in vitro. Studies of humans, however, provide equivocal data. Pharmacologic blockade of vagal efferent pathways with aerosolized hexamethonium, a drug that inhibits transmission through parasympathetic ganglia (Chapter 8), or with atropine sulfate, a postganglionic muscarinic antagonist, causes reduction but not abolition of the bronchospastic responses to both antigenic and nonantigenic stimuli (eg, exercise, inhalation of cold air, sulfur dioxide, and distilled water). While it is possible that activity in some other neural pathway (eg, the nonadrenergic, noncholinergic system; Chapter 6) contributes to bronchomotor responses, the fact that responses are also partially blocked by cromolyn, a drug that appears to inhibit mast cell degranulation, suggests that both antigenic and nonantigenic stimuli may provoke the release of mediators that contract airway smooth muscle both through direct effects and

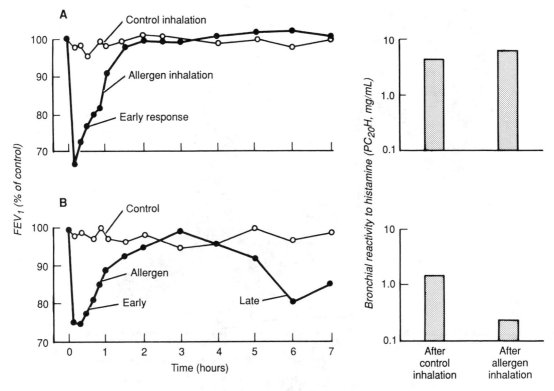

Figure 19–2. Comparison of responses to control and allergen inhalation in two subjects, one with only early responses *(panel A)* and one with both early and late bronchial responses *(panel B)*. Forced expiratory volume in 1 second (FEV$_1$) is shown on the left as a percentage of the control value. Bronchoconstriction results in a fall in FEV$_1$. The doses (mg/mL) of inhaled histamine required to cause a 20% fall in FEV$_1$ (PC$_{20}$H) 8 hours after the control inhalation and 8 hours after the allergen inhalation are shown in the bar graphs on the right. An increase in responsiveness is shown by a decrease in the dose of histamine required. The subject shown in panel A had a transient drop in FEV$_1$ immediately after inhaling allergen but recovered rapidly and showed no later fall in this variable. He showed no increase in responsiveness to histamine 8 hours later (panel A). In contrast, the subject who showed a late bronchoconstriction response to the inhaled allergen (panel B, dip at 6 hours in the graph at left) also showed a marked reduction in the dose of histamine required to cause a further bronchoconstrictor response (bar graph, after allergen inhalation). (Redrawn from Cockcroft DW et al: Allergen-induced increase in non-allergic bronchial reactivity. Clin Allergy 1977;7:503.)

through activation of parasympathetic efferent activity (Figure 19–3).

The hypothesis suggested by these studies—that asthmatic bronchospasm results from a combination of release of mediators and an exaggeration of responsiveness to their effects—holds that asthma may be effectively treated by drugs with different modes of action. (See Figure 19–4.) Asthmatic bronchospasm might be reversed or prevented, for example, by drugs that prevent mast cell degranulation (cromolyn or nedocromil, beta agonists, calcium channel blockers), inhibit the effect of acetylcholine released from vagal motor nerves (muscarinic antagonists), or directly relax airway smooth muscle (sympathomimetic agents, theophylline).

Another approach to the treatment of asthma is aimed not just at preventing or reversing acute bronchospasm but at reducing the level of responsiveness itself. Because increased responsiveness appears to be linked to airway inflammation and because airway inflammation is a feature of late asthmatic responses, this strategy is implemented by prolonged therapy with agents that prevent late responses, such as cromolyn and corticosteroids. Agents effective in other chronic inflammatory conditions, such as methotrexate and gold, may also be useful in this treatment approach.

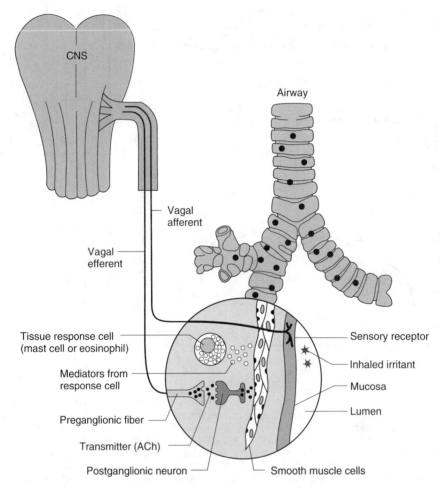

Figure 19–3. Mechanisms of response to inhaled irritants. The airway is represented microscopically by a cross section of the wall with branching vagal sensory endings lying adjacent to the lumen. Afferent pathways in the vagus nerves travel to the central nervous system; efferent pathways from the central nervous system travel to efferent ganglia. Postganglionic fibers release acetylcholine (ACh), which binds to muscarinic receptors on airway smooth muscle. Inhaled materials may provoke bronchoconstriction by several possible mechanisms. First, they may trigger the release of chemical mediators from mast cells. Second, they may stimulate afferent receptors to initiate reflex bronchoconstriction or to release tachykinins (eg, substance P) that directly stimulate smooth muscle contraction.

I. BASIC PHARMACOLOGY OF AGENTS USED IN THE TREATMENT OF ASTHMA

CROMOLYN & NEDOCROMIL

Cromolyn sodium (disodium cromoglycate) and nedocromil sodium differ from most antiasthmatic medications in that they are only of value when taken prophylactically. They are stable but extremely insoluble salts (see structures below). When used as aerosols (metered-dose inhalers), they effectively inhibit both antigen- and exercise-induced asthma, and chronic use (4 times daily) may reduce the overall level of bronchial reactivity; however, these drugs have no effect on airway smooth muscle tone and are ineffective in reversing asthmatic bronchospasm.

Cromolyn is poorly absorbed from the gastrointestinal tract. For use in asthma, it must be applied topically, by inhalation of a microfine powder or aerosolized solution as described below. When given by inhalation or orally, less than 10% is absorbed, and most is excreted unchanged. Nedocromil also has a very low bioavailability and is only available in metered-dose aerosol form.

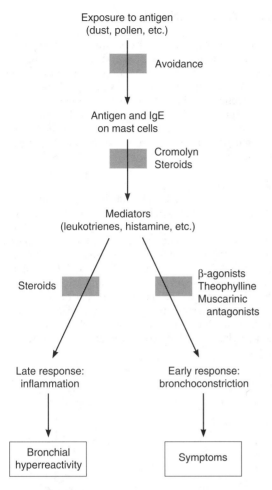

Exposure to antigen
(dust, pollen, etc.)

Avoidance

Antigen and IgE
on mast cells

Cromolyn
Steroids

Mediators
(leukotrienes, histamine, etc.)

Steroids

β-agonists
Theophylline
Muscarinic
antagonists

Late response:
inflammation

Early response:
bronchoconstriction

Bronchial
hyperreactivity

Symptoms

Figure 19–4. Summary of strategies for treatment of asthma. Therapeutic interventions are indicated by shaded bars. (Redrawn from Cockcroft DW: The bronchial late response in the pathogenesis of asthma and its modulation by therapy. Ann Allergy 1985;55:857.)

ferent sites. For example, mast cells from human lung and skin differ in their neutral protease content. Lung mast cells contain only tryptase, while cutaneous mast cells contain both tryptase and chymase.

Studies of asthmatic subjects support the concept that cromolyn inhibits mediator release from airway mast cells. Pretreatment with cromolyn inhibits not only the bronchospasm provoked by antigen inhalation or by exercise; it inhibits also the coincident appearance of neutrophil chemotactic factor (NCF)—a putative marker of mast cell activation—in circulating blood. This mechanism of action of cromolyn is considered by some investigators to be so well established that cromolyn has been used as a tool in studies of the mechanisms of bronchial responses. Thus, if bronchoconstriction is inhibited by cromolyn, the release of mediators from mast cells is presumed to be involved.

Other evidence, however, suggests that cromolyn's mechanism of action may not be so straightforward. The search for more effective agents has yielded many with greater potency in inhibiting mast cell degranulation in vitro, but most of these have been ineffective in inhibiting bronchomotor responses in vivo. Other experimental work also suggests that cromolyn may inhibit phosphodiesterase, thus increasing intracellular cAMP, and that it may alter neural pathways that influence airway smooth muscle tone.

Clinical Use of Cromolyn & Nedocromil

In patients, the efficacy of cromolyn has been demonstrated in several circumstances. When used before exposure, the drug inhibits the immediate and delayed reactions to inhalation of antigen. Pretreatment with cromolyn also blocks exercise- and aspirin-induced bronchoconstriction and protects against the bronchospasm provoked by a variety of industrial agents, including toluene diisocyanate, wood dusts, soldering fluxes, piperazine hydrochloride, and certain enzymes. This acute protective effect of a single

Mechanism of Action

Cromolyn has been more extensively studied than nedocromil, but the two agents probably share a similar mechanism of action. In vitro studies show that both prevent antigen-induced release of histamine and leukotrienes from sensitized mast cells and lung fragments, apparently by preventing the transmembrane influx of calcium provoked by IgE antibody-antigen interaction on the mast cell surface (Dahlén, 1989; Bruijnzeel, 1990). This inhibitory effect appears to be specific for both cell and antibody type, since cromolyn has little inhibitory effect on mediator release from human basophils or on IgG-mediated degranulation of mast cells. It may also be specific for different organs, since cromolyn inhibits anaphylaxis in human and primate lung but not in skin. This in turn may reflect differences in mast cells found in dif-

Cromolyn sodium

Nedocromil sodium

treatment makes cromolyn useful for administration shortly before exercise or before unavoidable exposure to an allergen.

Cromolyn is also effective in reducing the symptomatic severity and the need for bronchodilator medications in patients with perennial asthma. Not all patients benefit from chronic therapy, and although young patients with extrinsic asthma are most likely to respond favorably, some older patients with intrinsic disease are also improved. At present, the only way of determining whether a patient will respond is by a therapeutic trial for 4 weeks. In those who respond, the effectiveness of regular use of cromolyn in controlling asthmatic symptoms appears to be roughly equal to that of maintenance theophylline therapy.

It has been proposed that chronic treatment with cromolyn causes a decrease in bronchial hyperreactivity, perhaps by protecting the airway against the inflammatory effects of the chemical mediators of anaphylaxis. At present, cromolyn appears to effectively prevent seasonal increases in bronchial reactivity in patients with allergic asthma, but it seems to be less effective than inhaled corticosteroids in reducing bronchial reactivity.

Cromolyn is absorbed poorly from the gastrointestinal tract and therefore is effective only when deposited directly into the airways. Two methods of administration are currently used. In adults, the drug is given by metered-dose inhaler. The usual dose is 2–4 mg inhaled 4 times daily. In children, who may have difficulty coordinating the use of the inhaler device, cromolyn may be given by aerosol of a 1% solution.

Cromolyn solution is also useful in reducing symptoms of allergic rhinitis. Applying the solution by nasal spray or eye drops several times a day is effective in about 75% of patients with hay fever, even during the peak pollen season.

Because it is so poorly absorbed, adverse effects of cromolyn are minor and are localized in the sites of deposition. These include such symptoms as throat irritation, cough, mouth dryness, chest tightness, and wheezing. Some of these symptoms can be prevented by inhaling a β_2-agonist drug before cromolyn treatment. Serious adverse effects are rare. Reversible dermatitis, myositis, or gastroenteritis occurs in about 2% of patients, and few cases of pulmonary infiltration with eosinophilia or of anaphylaxis have been reported.

Nedocromil appears to have greater inhibitory action on primate lung mast cells in vitro and has given promising results in large clinical trials. Nedocromil may offer greater antiasthmatic potency than cromolyn.

Neither cromolyn nor nedocromil can fully replace inhaled steroids in patients who require the latter drugs for control of asthma (Ruffin, 1987).

METHYLXANTHINE DRUGS

The three important methylxanthines are theophylline, theobromine, and caffeine. Their major source is, of course, beverages (tea, cocoa, and coffee, respectively). The importance of theophylline as a therapeutic agent in the treatment of asthma is waning as the greater effectiveness of inhaled sympathomimetic agents for acute asthma and of inhaled anti-inflammatory agents for chronic asthma has been established.

Chemistry

As shown below, theophylline is 1,3-dimethylxanthine; theobromine is 3,7-dimethylxanthine; and caffeine is 1,3,7-trimethylxanthine. The theophylline preparation most commonly used for therapeutic purposes is the theophylline-ethylenediamine complex **aminophylline.** A synthetic analogue of theophylline (dyphylline) is both less potent and shorter-acting than theophylline. The pharmacokinetics of theophylline are discussed below (see Clinical Use of Methylxanthines). The metabolic products, partially demethylated xanthines (not uric acid), are excreted in the urine.

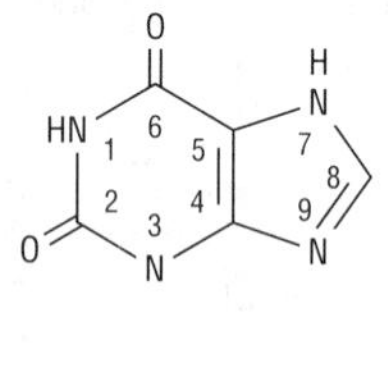

Xanthine

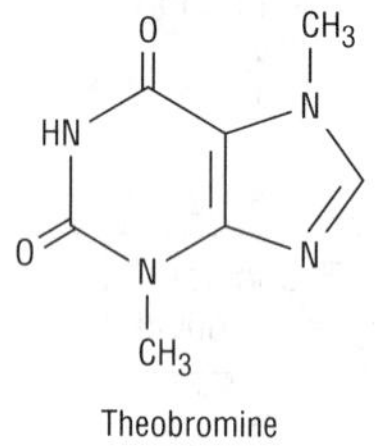

Theobromine

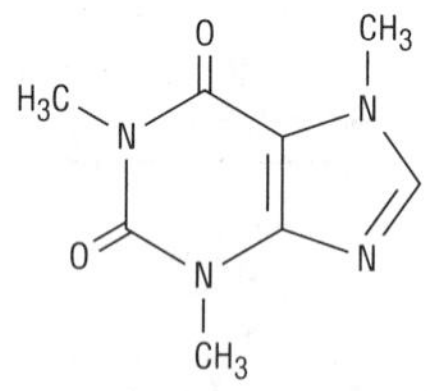

Caffeine

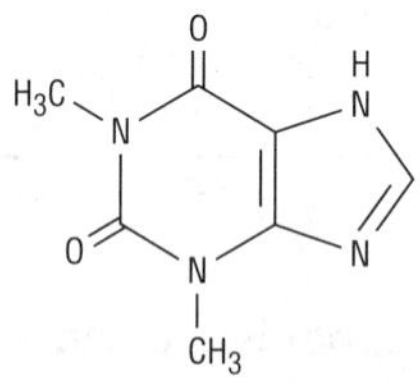

Theophylline

Mechanism of Action

Several mechanisms have been proposed for the action of the methylxanthines, but none have been established as responsible for their bronchodilating effect. At high concentrations, they can be shown in vitro to inhibit the enzyme phosphodiesterase (Figure 19–5). Since phosphodiesterase hydrolyzes cyclic nucleotides, this inhibition results in higher concentrations of intracellular cAMP. This effect could explain the cardiac stimulation and smooth muscle relaxation produced by these drugs, but it is not certain that sufficiently high concentrations are achieved in vivo to inhibit phosphodiesterase. Another proposed mecha-

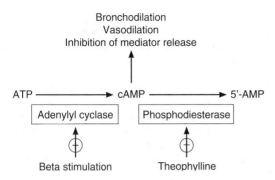

Figure 19–5. Intracellular levels of cAMP can be increased by beta-adrenoceptor agonists, which increase the rate of its synthesis by adenylyl cyclase; or by phosphodiesterase inhibitors, such as theophylline, which slow the rate of its degradation.

nism is the inhibition of cell surface receptors for adenosine. These receptors modulate adenylyl cyclase activity, and adenosine has been shown to cause contraction of isolated airway smooth muscle and to enhance histamine release from cells present in the lung. These effects are antagonized by theophylline, an agent generally regarded as a universal antagonist of cell surface adenosine receptors. It has also been shown, however, that xanthine derivatives devoid of adenosine-antagonistic properties (eg, enprofylline) may be many times more potent than theophylline in inhibiting bronchoconstriction in asthmatic subjects.

Pharmacodynamics of Methylxanthines

The methylxanthines have effects on the central nervous system, kidney, and cardiac and skeletal muscle as well as smooth muscle. Of the three agents, theophylline is most selective in its smooth muscle effects, while caffeine has the most marked central nervous system effects.

A. Central Nervous System Effects: In low and moderate doses, the methylxanthines—especially caffeine—cause mild cortical arousal with increased alertness and deferral of fatigue. In unusually sensitive individuals, the caffeine contained in beverages, eg, 100 mg in a cup of coffee, is sufficient to cause nervousness and insomnia. At very high doses, medullary stimulation and convulsions may occur. Nervousness and tremor are primary side effects in patients taking large doses of aminophylline for asthma.

B. Cardiovascular Effects: The methylxanthines have direct positive chronotropic and inotropic effects on the heart. At low concentrations, these effects appear to result from increased catecholamine release that is caused by inhibition of presynaptic adenosine receptors. At higher concentrations (> 10 μmol/L), calcium influx may be increased directly through the increase in cAMP that results from inhibition of phosphodiesterase. At very high (> 100

μmol/L) concentrations, sequestration of calcium by the sarcoplasmic reticulum is impaired. In unusually sensitive individuals, consumption of a few cups of coffee may result in arrhythmias; but in most people, parenteral administration of higher doses of the methylxanthines produces only sinus tachycardia and increased cardiac output. Methylxanthines have occasionally been used in the treatment of pulmonary edema associated with heart failure (Chapter 13). In large doses, these agents also relax vascular smooth muscle except in cerebral blood vessels, where they cause contraction. Ordinary consumption of coffee and other methylxanthine-containing beverages, however, usually raises the peripheral vascular resistance and blood pressure slightly, probably through the release of catecholamines.

Methylxanthines decrease blood viscosity and may improve blood flow under certain conditions. The mechanism that causes this action is not well defined, but the effect is exploited in the treatment of intermittent claudication with pentoxifylline, a dimethylxanthine agent. However, no evidence suggests that this therapy is superior to other approaches.

C. Effects on Gastrointestinal Tract: The methylxanthines stimulate secretion of both gastric acid and digestive enzymes. However, even decaffeinated coffee has a potent stimulant effect on secretion, which means that the primary secretagogue in coffee is not caffeine.

D. Effects on Kidney: The methylxanthines—especially theophylline—are weak diuretics. This effect may involve both increased glomerular filtration and reduced tubular sodium reabsorption. The diuresis is not of sufficient magnitude to be therapeutically useful.

E. Effects on Smooth Muscle: The bronchodilation produced by the methylxanthines is the major therapeutic action. Tolerance does not develop, and adverse effects, especially in the central nervous system, may limit the dose (see below). In addition to this direct effect on the airway smooth muscle, these agents—in sufficient concentration—inhibit antigen-induced release of histamine from lung tissue; their effect on mucociliary transport is unknown.

F. Effects on Skeletal Muscle: The therapeutic actions of the methylxanthines may not be confined to the airways, for they also strengthen the contractions of isolated skeletal muscle in vitro and have potent effects in improving contractility and in reversing fatigue of the diaphragm in patients with chronic obstructive lung diseases. This effect on diaphragmatic performance, rather than an effect on the respiratory center, may account for theophylline's ability to improve the ventilatory response to hypoxia and to diminish dyspnea even in patients with irreversible airflow obstruction.

Clinical Use of Methylxanthines

Of the xanthines, theophylline is the most effective

bronchodilator, and it has been shown repeatedly both to relieve airflow obstruction in acute asthma and to reduce the severity of symptoms and time lost from work or school in chronic asthma. Theophylline base is only slightly soluble in water, so it has been administered as a number of different salts containing varying amounts of theophylline base. The two commonly used theophylline salts are aminophylline, which contains 86% theophylline by weight; and oxtriphylline, which contains 64% by weight. Corrections must be made to ensure equivalent doses of theophylline for different preparations. Most preparations are well absorbed from the gastrointestinal tract; their absorption is not affected significantly by food. The absorption of rectal suppositories, however, is unreliable, and these preparations should be used only in special circumstances.

Improvements in theophylline preparations have come from alterations in the physical state of the drugs rather than from new chemical formulations. For example, several companies now provide anhydrous theophylline in a microcrystalline form in which the increased surface area facilitates solubilization for complete and rapid absorption after oral administration. In addition, several sustained-release preparations (eg, Slo-Phyllin, Theo-Dur) are available and can produce therapeutic blood levels of theophylline for up to 12 hours. These preparations offer the advantages of less frequent drug administration, less fluctuation of theophylline blood levels, and, in many cases, more effective treatment of nocturnal bronchospasm.

An important advance in the use of theophylline is the availability of theophylline blood level measurements to monitor therapy. Therapeutic and toxic effects of theophylline are related to the plasma concentrations of the drug. Improvement in pulmonary function is well correlated with plasma concentration in the range of 5–20 mg/L. Anorexia, nausea, vomiting, abdominal discomfort, headache, and anxiety begin to occur at concentrations of 15 mg/L in some patients and become common at concentrations greater than 20 mg/L. Higher levels (> 40 mg/L) may cause seizures or arrhythmias; these may not be preceded by gastrointestinal or neurologic warning symptoms. Rational administration of theophylline, therefore, requires knowledge of its pharmacokinetics.

As described in Chapter 3, the initial or loading dose of a drug is determined by its volume of distribution (V_d) and the subsequent or maintenance dose by the rate of plasma clearance. The V_d for theophylline is proportionate to lean body weight but otherwise varies only slightly among individuals. On the average, V_d = 0.5 L/kg, so a plasma concentration of 10 mg/L will be achieved by a loading dose of 5 mg of theophylline per kilogram of body weight. Because aminophylline contains 86% theophylline by weight, this is approximately equivalent to 6 mg/kg of aminophylline. If administered intravenously, the loading

dose should be given over 30 minutes, since rapid injection ("IV push") may result in transient toxic plasma levels with the risk of seizures or cardiac arrhythmias.

The plasma clearance of theophylline has been shown to vary widely among healthy subjects and even more so among asthma patients. Because theophylline is metabolized by the liver, changes in hepatic function can alter the drug's half-life. For example, a decrease in hepatic function from cirrhosis or decrease in hepatic blood flow from heart failure may decrease plasma clearance and lead to toxic concentrations of the drug. Induction of hepatic enzymes by cigarette smoking or by changes in diet may increase plasma clearance and cause inadequate concentrations of drug. In normal adults, the mean plasma clearance is 0.69 mL/kg/min (0.041 L/kg/h). Children appear to clear theophylline faster than adults (1–1.5 mL/kg/min; 0.06–0.09 L/kg/h). Neonates and young infants have the slowest clearance (Chapter 61). Even when maintenance doses are altered to correct for the above factors, plasma concentrations vary widely.

Intravenous maintenance therapy is now given only in unusual circumstances, for theophylline has been shown to add insignificantly to the bronchodilation achieved with frequent administration of aerosolized sympathomimetics. When it is given, an infusion rate of 0.7 mg/kg/h may be used in stable patients; but in acutely ill patients, it should be decreased to approximately 0.6 mg/kg/h. In the presence of liver disease or heart failure, the dose should be decreased further (approximately 0.3 mg/kg/h). Theophylline levels should be measured 24 hours after starting treatment. For oral therapy, an initial dose equivalent to 3–4 mg/kg of theophylline every 6 hours is appropriate. Changes in dosage will result in a new steady-state concentration of theophylline in 1–2 days, so the dose may be increased at intervals of 2–3 days until therapeutic plasma concentrations are achieved (10–20 mg/L) or until adverse effects develop.

SYMPATHOMIMETIC AGENTS

The adrenoceptor agonists, discussed in detail in Chapter 9, have several pharmacologic actions that are important in the treatment of asthma—ie, they relax airway smooth muscle and inhibit release of bronchoconstricting substances from mast cells. They may also increase mucociliary transport by increasing ciliary activity or by affecting the composition of mucous secretions. As in other tissues, the beta agonists stimulate adenylyl cyclase and catalyze the formation of cAMP in the airway tissues.

The best-characterized action of the adrenoceptor agonists on airways is relaxation of airway smooth muscle, resulting in bronchodilation. Although there is no evidence for direct sympathetic innervation of human airway smooth muscle, there is ample evidence for the presence of adrenoceptors on airway smooth muscle. In general, stimulation of β_2 receptors relaxes airway smooth muscle, inhibits mediator release, and causes skeletal muscle tremor as a toxic effect.

The sympathomimetic agents that have been widely used in the treatment of asthma include epinephrine, ephedrine, isoproterenol, and a number of β_2-selective agents (Figure 19–6). Because epinephrine and isoproterenol cause more cardiac stimulation (mediated by β_1 receptors), they should probably be reserved for special situations (see below). Ephedrine has no advantages over more selective agents except low cost, and it should be avoided if possible.

Epinephrine is an effective, rapidly acting bronchodilator when injected subcutaneously (0.4 mL of 1:1000 solution) or inhaled as a microaerosol from a pressurized canister (320 µg per puff). Maximal bronchodilation is achieved 15 minutes after inhalation and lasts 60–90 minutes. Because epinephrine stimulates β_1 as well as β_2 receptors, tachycardia, arrhythmias, and worsening of angina pectoris are troublesome adverse effects.

Ephedrine probably has the longest history of any drug used in treating asthma, for it was used in China for more than 2000 years before it was introduced into Western medicine in 1924. Compared with epinephrine, ephedrine has a longer duration, oral activity, more pronounced central effects, and much lower potency. Because of the development of more efficacious and β_2-selective agonists, ephedrine is now used infrequently in treating asthma. It was formerly prescribed in fixed-dose combination with theophylline and a sedative in commercial preparations. These fixed-dose combinations make adjustment of dosage of the individual agents impossible and should be avoided.

Isoproterenol is a potent bronchodilator; when inhaled as a microaerosol from a pressurized canister, 80–120 µg causes maximal bronchodilation within 5 minutes. When the drug is given as an aerosolized solution from a nebulizer, the larger particle size generated results in a smaller quantity being delivered to the tracheobronchial tree, so larger doses must be given to achieve the same effect. Isoproterenol has a 60- to 90-minute duration of action. An increase in the asthma mortality rate that occurred in the United Kingdom in the mid 1960s has been attributed to cardiac arrhythmias resulting from the use of high doses of inhaled isoproterenol, though this attribution remains a subject of controversy.

Beta$_2$-Selective Drugs

The beta$_2$-selective adrenoceptor agonist drugs are the most widely used sympathomimetics for the treatment of asthma at the present time (Figure 19–6).

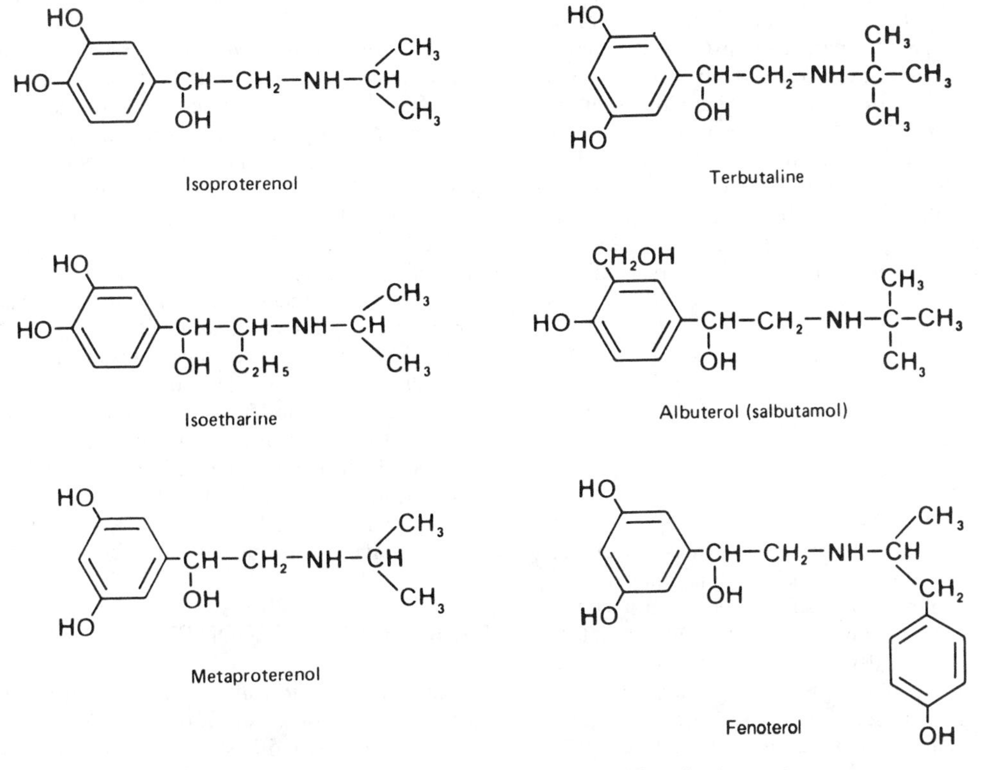

Figure 19–6. Structures of isoproterenol and several β_2-selective analogues.

They are effective after oral administration and have a long duration of action and significant β_2 selectivity. These agents differ structurally from epinephrine in having a larger substitution on the amino group and in the position of the hydroxyl groups on the aromatic ring. **Metaproterenol, albuterol, terbutaline,** and **bitolterol** are available as metered-dose inhalers; 0.3–0.5 mL of metaproterenol solution (5%) and albuterol solution (0.5%) can be diluted in 0.3–1.5 mL of saline for delivery from a hand-held nebulizer. When given by inhalation, these agents cause bronchodilation equivalent to that produced by isoproterenol. Bronchodilation is maximal by 30 minutes and persists for 3–4 hours.

Metaproterenol and terbutaline are also prepared in tablet form. One tablet 3 times daily is the usual regimen; the principal adverse effects of skeletal muscle tremor, nervousness, and occasional weakness may be reduced by starting the patient on half-strength tablets for the first 2 weeks of therapy.

Only terbutaline is available for subcutaneous injection (0.25 mg). The indications for this route are similar to those for subcutaneous epinephrine—severe asthma requiring treatment under a physician's observation—but it should be remembered that terbutaline's longer duration of action means that cumulative effects may be seen after repeated injections.

Newer beta$_2$-selective agonists include formoterol and salmeterol. These agents were developed for an increased duration of action (12 hours or more) compared with the older beta$_2$ agonists (4–6 hours). Both drugs are highly selective and potent beta$_2$ agonists; salmeterol may be a partial agonist at beta receptors in some tissues. They appear to achieve their long duration of action as a result of high lipid solubility rather than resistance to metabolism. Their high lipid solubility permits them to dissolve in the smooth muscle cell membrane in high concentration. It is postulated that this dissolved drug functions as a "slow release depot" that provides drug to adjacent beta receptors over a long period (Anderson, 1993).

Formoterol

Although adrenoceptor agonists may be administered by inhalation or by the oral or parenteral routes, delivery by inhalation results in the greatest local effect on airway smooth muscle with the least systemic toxicity. Aerosol deposition depends on the particle size, the pattern of breathing (tidal volume and rate of airflow), and the geometry of the airways. Even with particles in the optimal size range of 2–5 μm, 80–90% of the total dose of aerosol is deposited in the mouth or pharynx. Particles under 1–2 μm in size remain suspended and may be exhaled. Deposition can be increased by holding the breath in inspiration.

Undesirable effects of beta agonists. Use of sympathomimetic agents by inhalation at first raised fears about possible tachyphylaxis or tolerance to beta agonists, cardiac arrhythmias from β_1-adrenoceptor stimulation and hypoxemia, and arrhythmias from fluorinated hydrocarbons in Freon aerosol propellants. The concept that beta-agonist drugs cause worsening of clinical asthma by inducing tachyphylaxis to their own action remains unestablished. Most studies have shown only a small change in airway smooth muscle response to beta stimulation after prolonged treatment with beta-agonist drugs, but one well-designed controlled study has shown that regular use of inhaled formoterol was associated with slight worsening of asthmatic symptoms and of bronchial reactivity when compared with use of the agent only on an "as-needed" basis.

Another highly publicized epidemiologic study reported an association between the use of two or more inhalers of fenoterol per month and the risk of death or near-death from asthma (Spitzer, 1992). This study was not able to distinguish whether increased beta agonist use was a risk factor or simply a marker of disease severity. A later meta-analysis of several published studies of the relationship could find no association between risk of death from asthma and use of beta agonists by either oral or metered dose inhaler administration (Mullen, 1993).

Other experiments have demonstrated that arterial oxygen tension (PaO$_2$) may decrease after administration of beta agonists if ventilation/perfusion ratios in the lung worsen. This effect is usually small, however, and may occur with any bronchodilator drug, and the significance of such an effect will depend on the initial PaO$_2$ of the patient. Supplemental oxygen may be necessary if the initial PaO$_2$ is decreased markedly or if there is a large decrease in PaO$_2$ during treatment with bronchodilators. Finally, there is concern over myocardial toxicity from Freon propellants contained in all of the commercially available metered-dose canisters. While fluorocarbons may sensitize the heart to toxic effects of catecholamines, such an effect occurs only at very high myocardial concentrations, which are not achieved if inhalers are used as recommended. In general, β_2-adrenoceptor agonists are safe and effective bronchodilators when given in doses that avoid systemic adverse effects.

MUSCARINIC ANTAGONISTS

Leaves from *Datura stramonium* have been used in treating asthma for hundreds of years. Interest in the potential value of antimuscarinic agents has recently been increased by demonstration of the importance of the vagus nerves in bronchospastic responses of laboratory animals and by the development of a potent antimuscarinic agent that is poorly absorbed after aerosol administration to the airways and is therefore unassociated with systemic atropine effects.

Mechanism of Action

Muscarinic antagonists competitively inhibit the effect of acetylcholine at muscarinic receptors (Chapter 8). In the airways, acetylcholine is released from efferent endings of the vagus nerves, and muscarinic antagonists can effectively block the contraction of airway smooth muscle and the increase in secretion of mucus that occurs in response to vagal activity. Very high concentrations—well above those achieved even with maximal therapy—are required to inhibit the response of airway smooth muscle to nonmuscarinic stimulation. This selectivity of muscarinic antagonists accounts for their usefulness as investigative tools in examining the role of parasympathetic pathways in bronchomotor responses but limits their usefulness in preventing bronchospasm. In the doses given, antimuscarinic agents inhibit only that portion of the response mediated by muscarinic receptors, and the involvement of parasympathetic pathways in bronchospastic responses appears to vary among individuals.

Clinical Use of Muscarinic Antagonists

Antimuscarinic agents are effective bronchodilators. When given intravenously, atropine, the prototypical muscarinic antagonist (Chapter 8), causes bronchodilation at a lower dose than that needed to cause an increase in heart rate. The selectivity of atropine's effect can be increased further by administering the drug by inhalation. Studies of atropine sulfate aerosol have shown that it can cause an increase in baseline airway caliber—nearly equivalent to that achieved with beta-agonist agents—and that this effect persists for 5 hours. In patients with emphysema, the bronchodilation achieved may exceed what is obtainable with beta-agonist agents. The dose required depends on the particle size of the aerosol used. Using a nebulizer producing particles with a diameter of 1–1.5 μm, systemic effects commonly occur when 2 mg is inhaled. The initial dose, then, should be 1 mg or less. Deposition of the aerosol in the mouth frequently causes a local drying effect. Adverse effects due to systemic absorption include urinary retention, tachycardia, loss of visual accommodation, and agitation.

The dose of an antimuscarinic drug causing maximal change in resting airway caliber is smaller than the dose needed to maximally inhibit bronchospastic responses (Figure 19–7), probably because the quantity of acetylcholine released under resting conditions

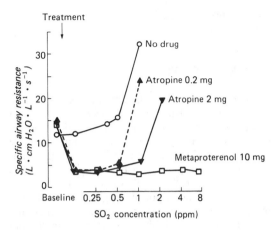

Figure 19–7. Inhibition of bronchomotor response to sulfur dioxide by two doses of atropine sulfate and by 10 mg of metaproterenol aerosol in one asthmatic subject. Specific airway resistance was measured after 5 minutes of eucapnic hyperpnea (40 L/min) of filtered air containing increasing amounts of SO_2. Note that all treatments caused equal changes in baseline specific resistance but different degrees of inhibition of the response to SO_2.

is smaller than the quantity released in response to an inhaled irritant. This is an important consideration in treating patients with asthma, for asthma is characterized by episodic bouts of bronchospasm, often occurring in response to exercise or to inhalation of antigens or irritants.

Systemic adverse effects limit the quantity of atropine sulfate that can be given, but the development of a more selective quaternary ammonium derivative of atropine, **ipratropium bromide,** permits delivery of high doses to muscarinic receptors in the airways because the compound is poorly absorbed and does not enter the central nervous system readily. Studies with this agent have shown that the degree of involvement of parasympathetic pathways in bronchomotor responses varies among subjects. In some, bronchoconstriction is inhibited effectively. In others, bronchoconstriction is inhibited only modestly. That administration of higher doses of the muscarinic antagonist fails to inhibit the response further implies that mechanisms other than parasympathetic reflex pathways must be involved.

Even in the subjects least protected by this antimuscarinic agent, however, the degree of bronchodilation and inhibition of provoked bronchoconstriction are of potential clinical value, and antimuscarinic agents may be valuable for patients intolerant of inhaled beta-agonist agents. While antimuscarinic agents generally appear to be slightly less potent than beta-agonist agents in reversing asthmatic bronchospasm, they appear to be equally or more potent in patients with chronic obstructive pulmonary disease (COPD) that includes a partially reversible component.

CORTICOSTEROIDS

Although corticosteroids have been used to treat asthma since 1950, their precise mechanism of action remains unknown. Like cromolyn, these drugs do not relax airway smooth muscle directly, but they may produce marked increases in airway caliber if administered for some time to asthmatic patients. Some studies suggested that corticosteroids may decrease airway obstruction by potentiating the effects of beta-receptor agonists, but most recent studies suggest that they also work by inhibiting or otherwise modifying the inflammatory response in airways. For example, corticosteroids may inhibit the release of arachidonic acid from cell membranes and thereby inhibit the first step in the production of eicosanoid products from arachidonic acid. Some of these products have potent effects on airway function and may be responsible for some of the abnormalities of airway function in asthmatic patients (Chapter 18). Indeed, acute severe bronchospasm may be provoked in a small percentage of asthmatic patients by aspirin or other nonsteroidal anti-inflammatory drugs that inhibit cyclooxygenase activity, thereby diverting arachidonic acid derivatives into the leukotriene pathway.

Clinical Use of Corticosteroids

In spite of increasing evidence of their efficacy, there is still controversy over the indications for corticosteroids in the treatment of asthma and their appropriate dosage schedule. Because of severe adverse effects when given chronically, oral corticosteroids are generally reserved for patients who do not improve adequately with bronchodilators or who experience worsening symptoms despite maintenance bronchodilator therapy. Treatment is often begun with an oral dose of 30–60 mg of prednisone per day or an intravenous dose of 1 mg/kg of methylprednisolone every 6 hours; the daily dose is decreased gradually after airway obstruction has improved. In most patients, corticosteroid therapy can be discontinued in a week or 10 days, but in other patients symptoms may worsen as the dose is decreased to lower levels. Because adrenal suppression by corticosteroids is related to dose and because secretion of corticosteroids has a diurnal variation, low doses of corticosteroids may cause less adrenal suppression if taken early in the morning. Adrenal suppression can be better avoided by alternate-day treatment. This schedule is best achieved by gradually tapering one day's dose while increasing the alternate day's dose by the same amount.

The most effective method of decreasing systemic adverse effects due to corticosteroid therapy is to administer the drug as an aerosol. The introduction of lipid-soluble corticosteroids such as **beclomethasone, triamcinolone, budesonide,** and **flunisolide** offers an effective method of delivering corticosteroids to the airways with minimal systemic absorption and reduced adverse effects. An average daily dose of two puffs 4 times daily or four puffs twice daily is often as effective as oral corticosteroids in mild to moderate asthma and appears to be equivalent to about 10–15 mg/d of prednisone in the control of asthma, with far fewer systemic effects. Larger doses of inhaled steroid preparations appear to be more effective, and doses up to 8–12 puffs 4 times daily have been prescribed in attempts to wean patients from chronic high-dose oral prednisone therapy. While these high doses of inhaled steroids may have systemic steroid effects, the effects are still negligible compared with those of the oral prednisone they replace. A special problem caused by inhaled topical corticosteroids is the occurrence of oropharyngeal candidiasis. This risk can be reduced by having patients gargle plain water and spit after each inhalation. The drug is remarkably free of other complications, but when switching from chronic oral therapy to inhaled beclomethasone, the oral therapy must be tapered slowly to avoid precipitation of adrenal insufficiency.

Chronic use of inhaled corticosteroids effectively reduces symptoms and improves pulmonary function in patients with mild asthma. Such use also reduces or eliminates the need for oral corticosteroids in patients with more severe disease. Unlike beta-stimulant agents and theophylline, chronic use of inhaled corticosteroids reduces bronchial reactivity. This important effect, which usually becomes apparent after 2–4 weeks, is both dose- and time-dependent. Bronchial reactivity is greatly reduced in some individuals, and the maximal reduction may not be achieved until the ninth to twelfth months of therapy. Because of the efficacy and safety of inhaled corticosteroids, they are now often prescribed for patients who require more than occasional inhalations of a beta agonist for relief of symptoms. Others give them as first-line therapy for mild asthma in combination with use of a beta agonist when needed. This therapy is continued for 10–12 weeks and then withdrawn to determine if more prolonged therapy is needed.

OTHER DRUGS IN THE TREATMENT OF ASTHMA

Calcium Channel Blockers

Each of the cell functions that may become abnormal in patients with asthma—contraction of airway smooth muscle, secretion of mucus and of various mediators, and transmission along airway nerves—depends to some degree on the movement of calcium into cells. The calcium channel blockers agents have no effect on baseline airway diameter but do significantly inhibit the airway narrowing that is induced by various stimuli. In patients, nifedipine and verapamil given by inhalation each significantly inhibited the bronchoconstriction induced by exercise, hyperventilation, or inhalation of aerosolized histamine, methacholine, or antigen. In only one study, however, was protection against bronchoconstriction completely effective. Other studies showed only partial protection and considerable variability in drug effect between subjects. The reasons for the small effects of calcium channel blockers are uncertain.

Leukotriene Antagonists & Lipoxygenase Inhibitors

Because of the evidence of leukotriene involvement in many inflammatory diseases (Chapter 18) and in anaphylaxis, considerable effort has been expended on the development of drugs that block the synthesis of these arachidonic acid derivatives or their receptors. Several leukotriene antagonists have entered early clinical trials and have shown some efficacy in asthmatic patients (Cloud, 1989; Israel, 1993). In some studies, the drug has blocked both the early and the late components of the asthmatic response to antigenic provocation (Friedman, 1993). Studies of these agents are continuing.

Nitric Oxide Donors

Preliminary studies in animals suggest that airway smooth muscle, like that in the vasculature, is effectively relaxed by nitric oxide. This very lipophilic drug can be inhaled as a gas in acute asthma and dilates the pulmonary blood vessels as well as the airway smooth muscle. Although nitric oxide itself—or nitric oxide donors—may prove of value in acute severe asthma, it appears more likely that they will be used in pulmonary hypertension.

Potassium Channel Openers

Cromakalim is an investigational drug with vasodilating actions that are ascribed partly to alpha-adrenoceptor blockade and direct hyperpolarization of smooth muscle cells by activation of potassium channels. A similar hyperpolarization may occur in the smooth muscle of the airways. Although relaxation of airway smooth muscle can be readily demonstrated in vitro, conflicting results have been obtained in asthma patients (Williams, 1990; Kidney, 1993).

II. CLINICAL PHARMACOLOGY OF AGENTS USED IN THE TREATMENT OF ASTHMA

BRONCHODILATORS

Patients with mild asthma and only occasional symptoms generally require no more than an inhaled beta-receptor agonist (eg, metaproterenol or albuterol) on an "as-needed" basis. If symptoms occur more frequently and the patient requires frequent aerosol inhalations—or if nocturnal symptoms occur—additional treatment is needed, preferably with an inhaled anti-inflammatory agent such as cromolyn or an inhaled corticosteroid. Theophylline should be reserved for patients in whom symptoms remain poorly controlled despite the combination of regular treatment with an inhaled anti-inflammatory agent and as-needed use of a β_2 agonist. If the addition of theophylline fails to improve symptoms or if adverse effects become bothersome, it is important to check the plasma level of theophylline to be sure it is in the therapeutic range (10–20 mg/L).

CORTICOSTEROIDS

If airway obstruction remains severe despite bronchodilator therapy, oral corticosteroids may be started. After initial treatment with high doses of corticosteroids (eg, 30 mg/d of prednisone for 3 weeks), these drugs should be given in the lowest dose necessary to control symptoms. If possible, patients should then be converted to therapy with an inhaled corticosteroid or, if that fails, continued on oral corticosteroid therapy at the lowest dosage necessary. If possible, patients receiving chronic oral therapy should then be converted to alternate-day therapy.

Numerous recent studies suggest that inhaled corticosteroids should be considered as the first drug in newly diagnosed asthma, ie, that they may be as effective as and less toxic than inhaled β_2 agonists (Juniper, 1990, 1991; Haahtela, 1991; Guidelines, 1991). During 1–2 years of observation, patients who inhaled the topical corticosteroid budesonide had fewer acute asthmatic attacks and fewer drug-induced toxicities than matched groups who inhaled beta-agonists alone.

CROMOLYN & NEDOCROMIL

A therapeutic trial of cromolyn or nedocromil is warranted in patients who require maintenance therapy with oral theophylline and an inhaled agent and in those whose symptoms occur seasonally or after clear-cut inciting stimuli such as exercise or exposure to animal dander or irritants. In a patient whose symptoms are continuous or occur without an obvious inciting stimulus, the value of these drugs can only be established with a therapeutic trial of inhaled drug 4 times a day for 4 weeks. If the patient responds to this therapy, the dose can be reduced. Maintenance therapy with cromolyn appears to be as effective as maintenance therapy with theophylline and has become widely used for treating children.

MUSCARINIC ANTAGONISTS

The role of inhaled muscarinic antagonists in the treatment of asthma has not been defined. When adequate doses are given, their effect on baseline airway resistance is as nearly great as that of the sympathomimetic drugs. The airway effects of antimuscarinic and sympathomimetic drugs given in full doses are not additive ie, administration of a sympathomimetic drug does not cause further bronchodilation in a person who has been treated with an antimuscarinic agent. The converse is also true: The addition of an antimuscarinic agent causes only slight additional bronchodilation beyond that achieved with treatment with an inhaled sympathomimetic agent. Antimuscarinic agents appear to be of significant value in chronic obstructive pulmonary disease—perhaps more so than in asthma.

When muscarinic antagonists are used for long-term treatment, they appear to be effective bronchodilators. Although it was predicted that muscarinic antagonists might "dry up" airway secretions, direct measurements of fluid volume secretion from single airway submucosal glands in animals show that atropine decreases secretory rates only slightly; however, the drug does prevent excessive secretion caused by vagal reflex stimulation. No cases of inspissation of mucus have been reported following administration of these drugs.

ANTI-INFLAMMATORY THERAPY

Some recent reports suggest that agents commonly used to treat rheumatoid arthritis might also be used to treat patients with chronic steroid-dependent asthma. The development of an alternative treatment is important, since chronic treatment with oral corticosteroids may cause osteoporosis, cataracts, glucose intolerance, worsening of hypertension, and cushingoid changes in appearance. Two double-blind prospective studies of prednisone-dependent asthmatic patients showed that the use of methotrexate (15–50 mg/wk) permitted a reduction in prednisone dosage (Mullarkey, 1990; Shiner, 1990). However, a third study showed no such effect (Erzurum, 1991). An open study of 20 patients with prednisone-dependent asthma reported that a dose of 3 mg of oral gold (auranofin) twice daily for 24 weeks reduced symptoms, bronchial reactivity, and prednisone requirements. These promising results offer hope for the small proportion of patients whose asthma can be managed only with high doses of oral prednisone. However, these results must be confirmed by larger studies before either treatment can be recommended, and at least one prospective trial has failed to confirm methotrexate's effectiveness.

MANAGEMENT OF ACUTE ASTHMA

The treatment of acute attacks of asthma in patients reporting to the hospital requires more continuous assessment and objective measurement of lung function than is necessary for chronic outpatient therapy. Repeated measurements of arterial blood gas tensions and spirometry are generally necessary. For patients with mild attacks, inhalation of a beta-receptor agonist is as effective as subcutaneous injection of epinephrine. Both of these treatments are more effective than intravenous administration of aminophylline. Severe attacks require treatment with oxygen, bronchodilators, and corticosteroids. For example, the combination of β_2 agonist drugs given subcutaneously and by aerosol, aminophylline given by continuous intravenous infusion, and intravenous corticosteroids may all be necessary in severe attacks.

PREPARATIONS AVAILABLE

Sympathomimetics Used in Asthma

Albuterol (Proventil, Ventolin, generic)
   Inhalant: 90 μg/puff aerosol; 0.083, 0.5% solution for nebulization; 200 μg capsules for inhalation

   Oral: 2, 4 mg tablets; 2 mg/5 mL syrup
   Oral sustained-release (Proventil Repetabs): 4 mg tablets

Bitolterol (Tornalate)
Inhalant: 0.37 mg/puff aerosol in 300 dose container

Ephedrine (generic)
Oral: 25, 50 mg capsules
Parenteral: 25, 50 mg/mL for injection

Epinephrine (generic, Adrenalin, others)
Inhalant: 1, 1.25, 2.25% for nebulization; 0.16, 0.2, 0.27 mg epinephrine base aerosol in 233 and 350 dose containers
Parenteral: 1:1000 (1 mg/mL), 1:200 (5 mg/mL) for injection

Ethylnorepinephrine (Bronkephrine)
Parenteral: 2 mg/mL for injection

Isoetharine (generic, others)
Inhalant: 0.062, 0.08, 0.1, 0.125, 0.167, 0.17, 0.2, 0.25, 1% for nebulization; 340 µg/puff aerosol

Isoproterenol (generic, Isuprel, others)
Inhalant: 0.25, 0.5, 1% for nebulization; 80, 131 µg/puff aerosols
Oral: 10, 15 mg sublingual tablets
Parenteral: 0.2 mg/mL for injection

Metaproterenol (Alupent, Metaprel, generic)
Inhalant: 0.65 mg/puff aerosol in 75, 150 mg container; 0.6, 5% for nebulization;
Oral: 10, 20 mg tablets; 10 mg/5 mL syrup

Pirbuterol (Maxair)
Inhalant: 0.2 mg/puff aerosol in 300 dose container

Salmeterol (Serevent)
Inhalant: 42µg/puff in 120 dose container

Terbutaline (Brethine, Bricanyl)
Inhalant: 0.2 mg/puff aerosol
Oral: 2.5, 5 mg tablets
Parenteral: 1 mg/mL for injection

Antimuscarinic Drugs Used in Asthma
Ipratropium (Atrovent)
Aerosol: 18 µg/puff in 200 metered-dose inhaler

Cromolyn Sodium & Nedocromil Sodium
Cromolyn sodium
Pulmonary aerosol (Intal): 800 µg/puff in 200 dose container; 20 mg capsules for inhalation; 20 mg/2 mL for nebulization (for asthma)
Nasal aerosol (Nasalcrom): 5.2 mg/puff (for hay fever)
Oral (Gastrocrom): 100 mg capsules (for gastrointestinal allergy)
Nedocromil sodium (Tilade)
Pulmonary aerosol: 1.75 mg/puff in 112 metered-dose container

Aerosol Corticosteroids
(See also Chapter 38.)
Beclomethasone (Beclovent, Vanceril)
Aerosol: 42 µg/puff in 200 dose container
Dexamethasone (Decadron Phosphate Respihaler)
Aerosol: 84 µg/puff in 170 dose container
Flunisolide (AeroBid)
Aerosol: 250 µg/puff in 50 dose container
Triamcinolone acetonide (Azmacort)
Aerosol: 100 µg/puff in 240 dose container

Methylxanthines: Theophylline & Derivatives
Aminophylline (theophylline ethylenediamine, 79% theophylline) (generic, others)
Oral: 105 mg/5 mL liquid; 100, 200 mg tablets,
Oral sustained-release: 225 mg tablets
Rectal: 250, 500 mg suppositories
Parenteral: 250 mg/10 mL for injection
Oxtriphylline, choline theophyllinate (64% theophylline) (generic, Choledyl)
Oral: 50 mg/5 mL mg syrup, 100 mg/5 mL elixir; 100, 200 mg tablets;
Oral sustained-release: 400, 600 mg tablets
Theophylline (generic, Elixophyllin, Slo-Phyllin, Uniphyl, Theo-Dur, Theo-24, others)
Oral: 100, 125, 200, 250, 300 mg tablets; 100, 200 mg capsules; 26.7, 50 mg/5 mL elixirs, syrups, and solutions
Oral sustained-release, 8–12 hours: 50, 60, 65, 75, 100, 125, 130, 200, 250, 260, 300 mg capsules
Oral sustained-release, 8–24 hours: 100, 200, 300, 450 mg tablets
Oral sustained-release, 12 hours: 50, 75, 125, 130, 200, 250, 260 mg capsules
Oral sustained-release, 12–24 hours: 100, 200, 250, 300, 450, 500 tablets
Oral sustained-release, 24 hours: 100, 200, 300, 400 mg tablets and capsules
Parenteral: 200, 400, 800 mg/container, theophylline and 5% dextrose for injection

Other Methylxanthines

Dyphylline (generic, other)
Oral: 200, 400 mg tablets; 33.3, 53.3 mg/5 mL elixir
Parenteral: 250 mg/mL for injection
Pentoxifylline (Trental)
Oral: 400 mg controlled-release tablets

REFERENCES

Pathophysiology of Airway Disease

Barnes PJ, Chung KF, Page CP: Inflammatory mediators and asthma. Pharmacol Rev 1988;40:49.

Bigby TD, Nadel JA: Asthma. Chapter 44 in: *Inflammation: Basic Principles and Clinical Correlations. Gallin JI, Goldstein IM (editors). Raven 1992.*

Boushey H, Holtzman M: Experimental airway inflammation and hyperreactivity. Am Rev Respir Dis 1985; 131:312.

Busquet J et al: Eosinophilic inflammation in asthma. N Engl J Med 1990;323:1033.

Cockcroft DW: Mechanism of perennial allergic asthma. Lancet 1983;2:253.

Cockcroft DW: The bronchial late response in the pathogenesis of asthma and its modulation by therapy. Ann Allergy 1985;55:857.

Djukanović R et al: Mucosal inflammation in asthma. Am Rev Respir Dis 1990;142:434.

Gleich GJ, Loegering DA, Adolphson CR: Eosinophils and bronchial inflammation. Chest 1985;87(Suppl): 10S.

Goldie RG: Receptors in asthmatic airways. Am Rev Respir Dis 1990;141(Suppl):S151.

Gross NJ, Skorodin MS: Role of the parasympathetic system in airway obstruction due to emphysema. N Engl J Med 1984;311:421.

Lewis RA, Austen KF, Soberman RJ: Leukotrienes and other products of the 5-lipoxygenase pathway: Biochemistry and relation to pathobiology in human diseases. N Engl J Med 1990;323:645.

Weitzman M et al: Recent trends in the prevalence and severity of childhood asthma. JAMA 1992;268:2673.

Methylxanthines

Aubier M et al: Aminophylline improves diaphragmatic contractility. N Engl J Med 1981;305:249.

Becker AB et al: The bronchodilator effects and pharmacokinetics of caffeine in asthma. N Engl J Med 1984;310:743.

Benowitz N: Clinical pharmacology of caffeine. Annu Rev Med 1990;41:277.

Brackett LE, Shamim MT, Daly JW: Activities of caffeine, theophylline, and enprofylline analogs as tracheal relaxants. Biochem Pharmacol 1990;39:1897.

Hirsh K: Central nervous system pharmacology of the dietary methylxanthines. In: *The Methylxanthine Beverages and Foods: Chemistry, Consumption, and Health Effects.* Spiller GA (editor). Alan Liss, 1984.

Murciano D et al: Effects of theophylline on diaphragmatic strength and fatigue in patients with chronic obstructive pulmonary disease. N Engl J Med 1984; 311:349.

Murphy DG et al: Aminophylline in the treatment of acute asthma when β_2-adrenergics and steroids are provided. Arch Intern Med 1993;153:1784.

Persson CGA: The pharmacology of anti-asthmatic xanthines and the role of adenosine. Asthma Rev 1987; 1:61.

Pincomb GA et al: Effects of caffeine on vascular resistance, cardiac output, and myocardial contractility in young men. Am J Cardiol 1985;56:119.

Thelle DS, Arnesen E, Førde OH: The Tromsö heart study: Does coffee raise serum cholesterol? N Engl J Med 1983;308:1454.

Cromolyn & Nedocromil

Aalbers R et al: The effect of nedocromil sodium on the early and late reaction and allergen-induced bronchial hyperresponsiveness. J Allergy Clin Immunol 1991; 87:993.

Bergmann K-Ch, Bauer CP, Overlack A: A placebo-controlled blinded comparison of nedocromil sodium and beclomethasone dipropionate in bronchial asthma. Lung 1990;168(Suppl):230.

Brogden RN, Sorkin EM: Nedocromil sodium: An updated review of its pharmacological properties and therapeutic efficacy in asthma. Drugs 1993;45:693.

Bruijnzeel PLB et al: Inhibition of neutrophil and eosinophil induced chemotaxis by nedocromil sodium and sodium cromoglycate. Br J Pharmacol 1990;99:798.

Dahlén S-E et al: Dual inhibitory action of nedocromil sodium on antigen-induced inflammation. Drugs 1989;37(Suppl 1):63.

Neale MG et al: The pharmacokinetics of nedocromil sodium, a new drug for the treatment of reversible obstructive airways disease, in human volunteers and patients with reversible airways disease. Br J Clin Pharmacol 1987;24:493.

Neale MG et al: The pharmacokinetics of sodium cromoglycate in man after intravenous and inhalation administration. Br J Clin Pharm 1986;22:373.

Pelikan Z, Knotterus I: Inhibition of the late response asthmatic response by nedocromil sodium administered more than two hours after antigen challenge. J Allergy Clin Immunol 1993;92:19.

Rebuck AS et al: A 3-month evaluation of the efficacy of nedocromil sodium in asthma: A randomized, double-blind, placebo-controlled trial of nedocromil sodium conducted by a Canadian multicenter study group. J Allergy Clin Immunol 1990;85:612.

Ruffin RE et al: The efficacy of nedocromil sodium (Tilade) in asthma. Aust N Z J Med 1987;17:557.

Svendsen UG et al: A comparison of the effects of sodium cromoglycate and beclomethasone dipropionate on pulmonary function and bronchial hyperreactivity in subjects with asthma. J Allergy Clin Immunol 1987;80:68.

Corticosteroids

Check WA, Kaliner MA: Pharmacology and pharmacokinetics of topical corticosteroids used for asthma therapy. Am Rev Respir Dis 1990;141(Suppl):S44.

Juniper EF et al: Effect of long-term treatment with an inhaled corticosteroid (budesonide) on airway hyperresponsiveness and clinical asthma in nonsteroid-dependent asthmatics. Am Rev Respir Dis 1990;142: 832.

Stein LM, Cole RP: Early administration of corticosteroids in emergency room treatment of acute asthma. Ann Intern Med 1990;112:822.

Toogood JH: Bronchial asthma and glucocorticoids. In: *Anti-inflammatory Steroid Action: Basic And Clinical Aspects.* Schleimer RP, Claman HN, Oronsky AL (editors). Academic Press, 1989.

Woolcock AJ et al: Effect of therapy on bronchial hyper-responsiveness in the long-term management of asthma. Clin Allergy 1988;18:165.

Beta Agonists

Anderson GP: Formoterol: Pharmacology, molecular basis of agonism, and mechanism of long duration of a highly potent and selective β_2-adrenoceptor agonist bronchodilator. Life Sci 1993;52:2145.

Coleman JJ et al: Cardiac arrhythmias during the combined use of β-adrenergic agonist drugs and theophylline. Chest 1986;89:45.

Mullen M, Mullen B, Carey M: The association between β-agonist use and death from asthma. A meta-analytic integration of case-control studies. JAMA 1993 270:1842.

Schatz M et al: The safety of inhaled β-agonist bronchodilators during pregnancy. J Allergy Clin Immunol 1988;82:686.

Spitzer WO et al: The use of β-agonists and the risk of death and near death from asthma. N Engl J Med 1992;326:501.

Svedmyr N: The current place of β_2-agonists in the management of asthma. Lung 1990;168(Suppl):105.

Antimuscarinic Drugs

Gross NJ: Ipratropium bromide. N Engl J Med 1988;319:486.

Karpel JP et al: A comparison of the effects of ipratropium bromide and metaproterenol sulfate in acute exacerbations of COPD. Chest 1990;98:835.

Schleuter DP: Ipratropium bromide in asthma: A review of the literature. Am J Med 1986;81(Suppl 5A):55.

Tashkin DP et al: Comparison of the anticholinergic bronchodilator ipratropium bromide with metaproterenol in chronic obstructive pulmonary disease. Am J Med 1986;81(Suppl 5A):81.

Other Drugs for Asthma

Bernstein DI et al: An open study of auranofin in the treatment of steroid-dependent asthma. J Allergy Clin Immunol 1988;81:6.

Cloud ML et al: A specific LTD_4/LTE_4-receptor antagonist improves pulmonary function in patients with mild, chronic asthma. Am Rev Respir Dis 1989;140:1336.

Dupuy PM et al: Bronchodilator action of inhaled nitric oxide in guinea pigs. J Clin Invest 1992;90:421.

Erzurum SC et al: Lack of effect of methotrexate in severe, steroid-dependent asthma: A double-blind, placebo-controlled study. Ann Intern Med 1991;114:353.

Friedman BS et al: Oral leukotriene inhibitor (MK-886) blocks allergen-induced airway responses. Am Rev Respir Dis 1993;147:839.

Garty M et al: Effect of nifedipine and theophylline in asthma. Clin Pharmacol Ther 1986;40:195.

Israel E et al: The effect of inhibition of 5-lipoxygenase by zileuton in mild-to-moderate asthma. Ann Intern Med 1993;119:1059.

Kidney JC et al: Effect of an oral potassium channel activator, BRL 38227, on airway function and responsiveness in asthmatic patients: comparison with oral salbutamol. Thorax 1993;48:130.

Manning PJ et al: Inhibition of exercise-induced bronchoconstriction by MK-571, a potent leukotriene D_4-receptor antagonist. N Engl J Med 1990;323:1736.

Mullarkey MF, Lammert JK, Blumenstein BA: Long-term methotrexate treatment in corticosteroid-dependent asthma. Ann Intern Med 1990;112:577.

Ozenne G et al: Nifedipine in chronic bronchial asthma: A randomized double-blind crossover trial against placebo. Eur J Respir Dis 1985;67:238.

Shiner RJ et al: Randomised, double-blind, placebo-controlled trial of methotrexate in steroid-dependent asthma. Lancet 1990;336:137.

Williams AJ et al: Attenuation of nocturnal asthma by cromakalim. Lancet 1990;336:334.

Clinical Management of Airway Disease

Barnes PJ: A new approach to the treatment of asthma. N Engl J Med 1989;321:1517.

Haahtela T et al: Comparison of a β_2-agonist, terbutaline, with an inhaled corticosteroid, budesonide, in newly detected asthma. N Engl J Med 1991;325:388.

Guidelines for the diagnosis and management of asthma: National Heart, Lung, and Blood Institute National Asthma Education Program Expert Panel Report. J Allergy Clin Immunol 1991;88:425.

Juniper EF et al: Reduction of budesonide use after a year of increased use: A randomized controlled trial to evaluate whether improvements in airway responsiveness and clinical asthma are maintained. J Allergy Clin Immunol 1991;87:483.

Kesten S, Rebuck AS: Management of chronic obstructive pulmonary disease. Drugs 1989;38:160.

Sears MR et al: Asthma mortality: comparison between New Zealand and England. Br Med J 1986;293:1342.

Szefler SJ: Anti-inflammatory drugs in the treatment of allergic disease. Med Clin North Am 1992;76:953.

Section V.
Drugs That Act in the Central Nervous System

Introduction to the Pharmacology of CNS Drugs

20

Roger A. Nicoll, MD

Drugs acting in the central nervous system (CNS) were among the first to be discovered by primitive human beings and are still the most widely used group of pharmacologic agents. In addition to their use in therapy, drugs acting on the CNS are used without prescription to increase one's sense of well-being. Caffeine, alcohol, and nicotine are socially accepted drugs in many countries, and their consumption is practiced worldwide. Because some of the drugs in this group are addictive and cause severe personal, social, and economic dysfunction, societies have found it necessary to control their use and availability.

The mechanisms by which various drugs act in the CNS have not always been clearly understood. Since the causes of many of the conditions for which these drugs are used (schizophrenia, anxiety, etc) are themselves poorly understood, it is not surprising that in the past much of CNS pharmacology has been purely descriptive. In the last 2 decades, however, dramatic advances have been made in the methodology of CNS pharmacology. It is now possible to study the action of a drug on individual cells and even single ion channels within synapses. The information obtained from such studies is the basis for several major developments in studies of the CNS.

First, it is clear that nearly all drugs with CNS effects act on specific receptors that modulate synaptic transmission. A very few agents such as general anesthetics and alcohol may have nonspecific actions on membranes (although these exceptions are not fully accepted), but even these non-receptor-mediated actions result in demonstrable alterations in synaptic transmission.

Second, drugs are among the most important tools for studying all aspects of the physiology of CNS, from the mechanism of convulsions to the laying down of long-term memory. As will be described below, agonists that mimic natural transmitters (and in many cases are more selective than the endogenous substances) and antagonists are both extremely useful in such studies.

Third, unraveling the actions of drugs with known clinical efficacy has led to some of the most fruitful hypotheses regarding the mechanisms of disease. For example, information on the action of antipsychotic drugs on dopamine receptors has provided the basis for important hypotheses regarding the pathophysiology of schizophrenia. Studies of the effects of a variety of agonists and antagonists on γ-aminobutyric acid (GABA) receptors are resulting in new concepts pertaining to the pathophysiology of several diseases, including anxiety and epilepsy.

This chapter provides an introduction to the functional organization of the CNS and its synaptic transmitters as a basis for understanding the actions of the drugs described in the following chapters.

Methods for the Study of CNS Pharmacology

Although scientists (and the public) have always been interested in the action of drugs in the CNS, a detailed description of synaptic transmission was not possible until glass microelectrodes, which permit intracellular recording, were developed. Detailed electrophysiologic studies of the action of drugs on both voltage- and transmitter-operated channels were greatly facilitated by the introduction of the patch clamp technique, which permits the recording of current through single channels. Histochemical, immunologic, and radioisotopic methods are widely used to map the distribution of specific transmitters, their associated enzyme systems, and their receptors. Molecular cloning is now having a major impact on our understanding of CNS receptors. These techniques make it possible to determine the precise molecular structure of the receptors and their associated channels.

ION CHANNELS

The membranes of nerve cells contain two types of channels defined on the basis of the mechanisms controlling their gating (opening and closing). The first mechanism is that of membrane *voltage-sensitive* gating; the second is that of *chemically activated* gating. The voltage-sensitive sodium channel described in Chapter 14 for the heart is an example of the first type and is very important in the CNS. In nerve cells, these channels are concentrated on the initial segment and the axon and are responsible for the fast action potential, which transmits the signal from cell body to nerve terminal. There are many types of voltage-sensitive calcium and potassium channels on the cell body, dendrites, and initial segment, which act on a much slower time scale and modulate the rate at which the neuron discharges. For example, some types of potassium channels opened by depolarization of the cell result in slowing of further depolarization and act as a brake to limit further action potential discharge.

Chemically activated channels, also called receptor-operated channels, are opened by the action of neurotransmitters and other chemical agents. The channel is thought to be an integral part of the receptor protein. These channels are insensitive or only weakly sensitive to membrane potential. Neurotransmitter receptors and their ion channels are concentrated on subsynaptic membranes, eg, the nicotinic neuromuscular receptor of the skeletal muscle end plate.

Recent evidence suggests that the traditional view of completely separate electrically gated and chemically gated channels requires modification. In particular, many neurotransmitter receptors are coupled to voltage-sensitive channels via second messenger systems.

THE SYNAPSE & SYNAPTIC POTENTIALS

It is now well established that communication between neurons in the CNS occurs through chemical synapses in the vast majority of cases. (A few instances of electrical coupling between neurons have been documented, and such coupling may play a role in synchronizing neuronal discharge. However, it is unlikely that these electrical synapses are an important site of drug action.) The events involved in the release of transmitter from the presynaptic terminal have been studied most extensively at the vertebrate neuromuscular junction and at the giant synapse of the squid. An action potential in the presynaptic fiber propagates into the synaptic terminal and activates voltage-sensitive calcium channels in the membrane of the terminal (Figure 6–3). The calcium channels responsible for the release of transmitter are generally resistant to the calcium channel-blocking agents discussed in Chapter 12 (verapamil, etc) but are sensitive to blockade by certain marine toxins and metal ions. Calcium flows into the terminal, and the increase in intraterminal calcium concentration promotes the fusion of synaptic vesicles with the presynaptic membrane. The transmitter contained in the vesicles is released into the synaptic cleft and diffuses to the receptors on the postsynaptic membrane. Binding of the transmitter to its receptor causes a brief change in membrane conductance (permeability to ions) of the postsynaptic cell. The time delay from the arrival of the presynaptic action potential to the onset of the postsynaptic response is approximately 0.5 ms. Most of this delay is consumed by the release process, particularly the time required for calcium channels to open.

The first systematic analysis of synaptic potentials in the CNS was by Eccles et al, who recorded intracellularly from spinal motoneurons in the early 1950s. When a microelectrode enters a cell, there is a sudden change in the potential recorded by the electrode, which is typically about –70 mV (Figure 20–1). This is the resting membrane potential of the neuron. Two types of pathways, excitatory and inhibitory, impinge on the motoneuron. When an excitatory pathway is stimulated, a small depolarization or excitatory postsynaptic potential (EPSP) is recorded. This potential is due to the excitatory transmitter activating a large increase in sodium and potassium permeability. The duration of these potentials is quite brief, usually less than 20 ms. Changing the stimulus intensity to the pathway and therefore the number of presynaptic fibers activated results in a graded change in the size of the depolarization. This indicates that the contribution a single fiber makes to the EPSP is quite small. When a sufficient number of excitatory fibers are activated, the EPSP depolarizes the postsynaptic cell to

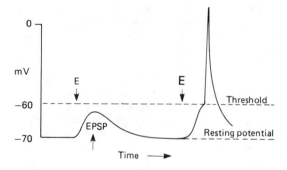

Figure 20–1. Excitatory synaptic potentials and spike generation. The figure shows a resting membrane potential of –70 mV in a postsynaptic cell. Stimulation of an excitatory pathway *(E)* generates transient depolarization. Increasing the stimulus strength (second *E*) increases the size of the depolarization, so that the threshold for spike generation is reached.

threshold, and an all-or-none action potential is generated.

When an inhibitory pathway is stimulated, the postsynaptic membrane is hyperpolarized, producing an inhibitory postsynaptic potential (IPSP) (Figure 20–2). A number of inhibitory synapses must be activated simultaneously to appreciably alter the membrane potential. This hyperpolarization is due to a selective increase in membrane permeability to chloride ions that flow into the cell during the IPSP. If an EPSP that under resting conditions would evoke an action potential in the postsynaptic cell (Figure 20–2) is elicited during an IPSP, it no longer evokes an action potential, because the IPSP has moved the membrane potential farther away from the threshold for action potential generation. A second type of inhibition is termed presynaptic inhibition. In the CNS, this is limited to the sensory fibers entering the brain stem and spinal cord. The excitatory synaptic terminals of these sensory fibers receive synapses called axoaxonic synapses (Figure 20–4B). When activated, the axoaxonic synapses reduce the amount of transmitter released from the synapses of sensory fibers. Synaptic inhibition in an unanesthetized subject lasts tens of milliseconds.

SITES OF DRUG ACTION

Virtually all of the drugs that act in the CNS produce their effects by modifying some step in chemical synaptic transmission. Figure 20–3 illustrates some of the steps that can be altered. These transmitter-dependent actions can be divided into presynaptic and postsynaptic categories.

Drugs acting on the synthesis, storage, metabolism, and release of neurotransmitters fall into the presy-

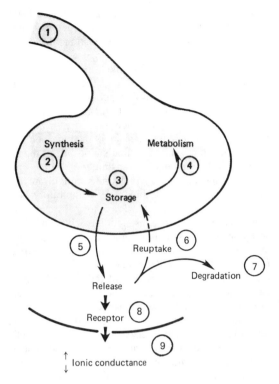

Figure 20–3. Sites of drug action. Schematic drawing of steps at which drugs can alter synaptic transmission. (1) Action potential in presynaptic fiber; (2) synthesis of transmitter; (3) storage; (4) metabolism; (5) release; (6) reuptake; (7) degradation; (8) receptor for the transmitter; (9) receptor-induced increase or decrease in ionic conductance.

naptic category. Synaptic transmission can be depressed by blockade of transmitter synthesis or storage. For example, *p*-chlorophenylalanine blocks the synthesis of serotonin, and reserpine depletes the synapses of monoamines by interfering with intracellular storage. Blockade of transmitter catabolism can increase transmitter concentrations and has been reported to increase the amount of transmitter released per impulse. Drugs can also alter the release of transmitter. The stimulant amphetamine induces the release of catecholamines from adrenergic synapses. Capsaicin causes the release of the peptide substance P from sensory neurons, and tetanus toxin blocks the release of inhibitory amino acid transmitters. After the transmitter has been released into the synaptic cleft, its action is terminated either by uptake or degradation. For most neurotransmitters, there are uptake mechanisms into the synaptic terminal and also into surrounding neuroglia. Cocaine, for example, blocks the uptake of catecholamines at adrenergic synapses and thus potentiates the action of these amines. However, acetylcholine is inactivated by enzymatic degradation. Anticholinesterases block the degradation of acetylcholine and thereby prolong its action. No up-

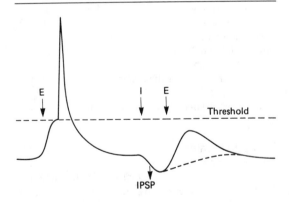

Figure 20–2. Interaction of excitatory and inhibitory synapses. On the left, a suprathreshold stimulus is given to an excitatory pathway *(E)*. On the right, this same stimulus is given shortly after stimulating an inhibitory pathway *(I)*, which prevents the excitatory potential from reaching threshold.

take mechanism has been found for any of the numerous CNS peptides, and it has yet to be demonstrated whether specific enzymatic degradation terminates the action of peptide transmitters.

In the postsynaptic region, the transmitter receptor provides the primary site of drug action. Drugs can act either as neurotransmitter agonists, such as the opiates, which mimic the action of enkephalin, or they can block receptor function. Receptor antagonism is a common mechanism of action for CNS drugs. An example is strychnine's blockade of the receptor for the inhibitory transmitter glycine. This block, which underlies strychnine's convulsant action, illustrates how the blockade of inhibitory processes results in excitation. Receptors are generally coupled to one of two transduction mechanisms. The receptors at most synapses in the central nervous system are coupled to ion channels, and receptor activation typically results in a brief (a few milliseconds to tens of milliseconds) opening of the channel. Drugs can act directly on the ion channel. For example, barbiturates enter and block the channel coupled to many excitatory neurotransmitter receptors. In other cases, receptors are coupled to enzymes, and receptor activation can lead to metabolic changes in the postsynaptic cell. Such metabolic changes can alter neuronal function by blocking voltage-sensitive ion channels. These effects can persist long after the transmitter has left the receptor, ie, tens of seconds to minutes. The methylxanthines are the best-known examples of drugs that can modify neurotransmitter responses mediated through cAMP. At high concentrations, the methylxanthines elevate the level of cAMP by blocking its metabolism and thereby prolong its action in the postsynaptic cell.

General anesthetics and ethanol are not thought to produce their effects by binding to specific receptors. Their actions are closely correlated with their lipophilicity. These drugs are believed to alter transmitter release and postsynaptic responsiveness by interacting with membrane lipids as well as membrane proteins.

The selectivity of drug action is based almost entirely on the fact that different transmitters are used by different groups of neurons. Furthermore, these various transmitters are often segregated into neuronal systems that subserve broadly different CNS functions. Without such segregation, it would be impossible to selectively modify CNS function even if one had a drug that operated on a single neurotransmitter system. It is not entirely clear why the CNS has relied on so many neurotransmitters and segregated them into different neuronal systems, since the primary function of a transmitter is either excitation or inhibition; this could be accomplished with two transmitter substances or perhaps even one. That such segregation does occur has provided neuroscientists with a powerful pharmacologic approach for analyzing CNS function and treating pathologic conditions.

IDENTIFICATION OF CENTRAL NEUROTRANSMITTERS

Since drug selectivity is based on the fact that different pathways utilize different transmitters, it is a primary goal of neuropharmacologists to identify the transmitters in CNS pathways. Establishing that a chemical substance is a transmitter has been far more difficult for central synapses than for peripheral synapses. In theory, to identify a transmitter it is sufficient to show that stimulation of a pathway releases enough of the substance to produce the postsynaptic response. In practice, this experiment cannot be done satisfactorily for at least two reasons. First, the anatomic complexity of the CNS prevents the selective activation of a single set of synaptic terminals. Second, available techniques for measuring the released transmitter and applying the transmitter are not sufficiently precise to satisfy the quantitative requirements. Therefore, the following criteria have been established for transmitter identification.

Localization

A number of approaches have been used to prove that a suspected transmitter resides in the presynaptic terminal of the pathway under study. These include biochemical analysis of regional concentrations of suspected transmitters, often combined with interruption of specific pathways, and microcytochemical techniques. Immunocytochemical techniques have proved very useful in localizing peptides and enzymes that synthesize or degrade nonpeptide transmitters.

Release

To determine whether the substance can be released from a particular region, local collection (in vivo) of the extracellular fluid can sometimes be accomplished. In addition, slices of brain tissue can be electrically or chemically stimulated in vitro and the released substances measured. To determine if the release is relevant to synaptic transmission, it is important to establish that the release is calcium-dependent. As mentioned above, anatomic complexity often prevents identification of the synaptic terminals responsible for the release, and the amount collected in the perfusate is a small fraction of the amount actually released.

Synaptic Mimicry

Finally, application of the suspected substance should produce a response that mimics the action of the transmitter released by nerve stimulation. Microiontophoresis, which permits highly localized drug administration, has been a valuable technique in assessing the action of suspected transmitters. In practice, this criterion has two parts: physiologic and pharmacologic identity. To establish physiologic identity of action, the substance must be shown to initiate the same change in ionic conductance in the postsynaptic cell as synaptically released transmitter. This requires intracellular recording and determination of the reversal potential and ionic dependencies of the responses. However, since different transmitters can elicit identical ionic conductance changes, this finding is not sufficient. Thus, selective pharmacologic antagonism is used to further establish that the suspected transmitter is acting in a manner identical to synaptically released transmitter. Because of the complexity of the CNS, specific pharmacologic antagonism of a synaptic response provides a particularly powerful technique for transmitter identification.

CELLULAR ORGANIZATION OF THE BRAIN

Neuronal systems in the CNS can be divided in many instances into two broad categories: hierarchical systems and nonspecific or diffuse neuronal systems.

Hierarchical Systems

These systems include all of the pathways directly involved in sensory perception and motor control. The pathways are generally clearly delineated, being composed of large myelinated fibers that can often conduct action potentials in excess of 50 m/s. The information is typically phasic, and in sensory systems the information is processed sequentially by successive integrations at each relay nucleus on its way to the cortex. A lesion at any link will incapacitate the system. Within each nucleus and in the cortex, there are two types of cells: relay or projection neurons and local circuit neurons (Figure 20–4A). The projection neurons that form the interconnecting pathways transmit signals over long distances. The cell bodies are relatively large, and their axons emit collaterals that arborize extensively in the vicinity of the neuron. These neurons are excitatory, and their synaptic influences are very short-lived. The excitatory transmitter released from these cells is, in most instances, glutamate. Local circuit neurons are typically smaller than projection neurons, and their axons arborize in the immediate vicinity of the cell body. The vast majority of these neurons are inhibitory, and they release either GABA or glycine. They synapse primarily on the cell body of the projection neurons but can also synapse on the dendrites of projection neurons as well as with each other. A special class of local circuit neurons in the spinal cord forms axoaxonic synapses on the terminals of sensory axons (Figure 20–4B). Two common types of pathways for these neurons (Figure 20–4A) include recurrent feedback pathways and feed-forward pathways. In many sensory pathways, local circuit neurons may actually lack an axon and release neurotransmitter from dendritic synapses

in a graded fashion in the absence of action potentials. Some pathways involving presynaptic dendrites of local circuit neurons are shown in Figure 20–4C.

Although there is a great variety of synaptic connections in these hierarchical systems, the fact that a limited number of transmitters are utilized by these neurons indicates that any major pharmacologic manipulation of this system will have a profound effect on the overall excitability of the CNS. For instance, selectively blocking GABA receptors with a drug such as picrotoxin results in generalized convulsions. Thus, while the mechanism of action of picrotoxin is quite specific in blocking the effects of GABA, the overall functional effect appears to be quite nonspecific, since GABA-mediated synaptic inhibition is so widely utilized.

Nonspecific or Diffuse Neuronal Systems

Those neuronal systems that contain one of the monoamines—norepinephrine, dopamine, or 5-hydroxytryptamine (serotonin)—provide examples in this category. Certain other pathways emanating from the reticular formation and possibly some peptide-containing pathways also fall into this category. These systems differ in fundamental ways from the hierarchical systems, and the noradrenergic systems will serve to illustrate the differences.

Noradrenergic cell bodies are found primarily in a compact cell group called the locus ceruleus located in the caudal pontine central gray matter. The number of neurons in this cell group is quite small, approximately 1500 on each side of the brain in the rat. The axons of these neurons are very fine and unmyelinated. Indeed, they were entirely missed with classic anatomic techniques. It was not until the mid 1960s, when the formaldehyde fluorescence histochemical technique was applied to the study of CNS tissues, that the anatomy of the monoamine-containing systems was described. Because these axons are fine and unmyelinated, they conduct very slowly, in the range of 0.5 m/s. The axons branch repeatedly and are extraordinarily divergent. Branches from the same neuron can innervate several functionally different parts of the CNS. In the neocortex, these fibers have a tangential organization and therefore can monosynaptically influence large areas of cortex. The pattern of innervation in the cortex and nuclei of the hierarchical systems is diffuse, and the noradrenergic fibers form a very small percentage of the total number in the area. In addition, the axons are studded with periodic enlargements called varicosities that contain large numbers of vesicles. In some instances, these varicosities do not form synaptic contacts, suggesting that norepinephrine may be released in a rather diffuse manner, as occurs with the noradrenergic innervation of smooth muscle. This indicates that the cellular targets of these systems will be determined largely by the location of the receptors rather than the loca-

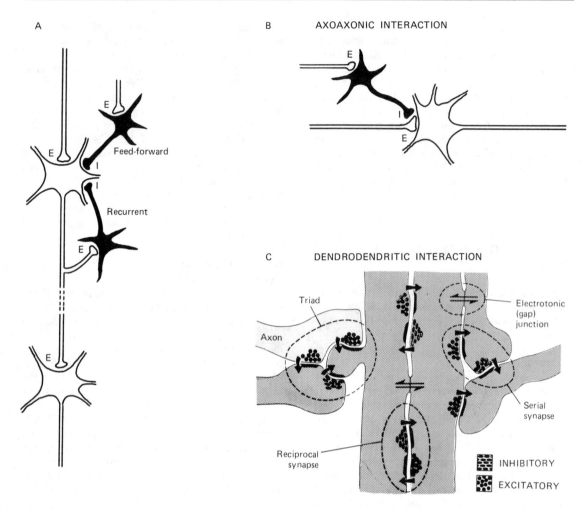

Figure 20–4. Pathways in the central nervous system. *A* shows two relay neurons and two types of inhibitory pathways, recurrent and feed-forward. The inhibitory neurons are shown in black. *B* shows the pathway responsible for presynaptic inhibition in which the axon of an inhibitory neuron synapses on the axon terminal of an excitatory fiber. *C:* Diagram illustrating that dendrites may be both pre- and postsynaptic to each other, forming reciprocal synapses, two of which are shown between the same dendrite pair. In triads, an axon synapses on two dendrites, and one of these dendrites synapses on the second. In serial synapses, a dendrite may be postsynaptic to one dendrite and presynaptic to another, thus connecting a series of dendrites. Dendrites also interact through low-resistance electrotonic ("gap") junctions (two of which are shown). Except for one axon, all structures shown in *C* are dendrites. (Reproduced, with permission, from Schmitt FO, Dev P, Smith BH: Electrotonic processing of information by brain cells. Science 1976;193:114. Copyright © 1976 by the American Association for the Advancement of Science.)

tion of the release sites. Based on all of these observations, it is clear that the monoamine systems cannot be conveying specific topographic types of information–rather, vast areas of the CNS must be affected simultaneously and in a rather uniform way. It is not surprising, then, that these systems have been implicated in such global functions as sleeping and waking, attention, appetite, and emotional states.

CENTRAL NEUROTRANSMITTERS

A number of small molecules have been isolated from brain (Table 20–1), and studies using a variety of approaches suggest that these agents may be neurotransmitters. A brief summary of the evidence for some of these compounds follows.

Amino Acids

The amino acids of primary interest to the pharmacologist fall into two categories: the neutral amino acids **glycine** and **GABA** and the acidic amino acids

Table 20–1. Summary of nonpeptide neurotransmitter pharmacology in the central nervous system.

Transmitter	Anatomy	Receptor Subtypes and Preferred Agonists	Antagonists	Receptor Mechanisms
Acetylcholine	Cell bodies at all levels; long and short connections	Muscarinic (M_1): muscarine, McN-A-343	Pirenzepine, atropine	Excitatory: decrease in K^+ conductance.
		Muscarinic (M_2): muscarine, bethanechol	Atropine	Inhibitory: increase in K^+ conductance.
	Motoneuron-Renshaw cell synapse.	Nicotinic: nicotine	Dihydro-β-erythroidine	Excitatory: increase in cation conductance.
Dopamine	Cell bodies at all levels; short, medium, and long connections.	D_1: SKF 38393	Phenothiazines, SCH 23390	Inhibitory: (?)increases cAMP
		D_2: apomorphine	Phenothiazines, butyrophenones	Inhibitory: increase in K^+ conductance.
GABA	Supraspinal interneurons; spinal interneurons involved in presynaptic inhibition.	$GABA_A$: muscimol	Bicuculline, picrotoxin	Inhibitory: increase in Cl^- conductance.
		$GABA_B$: baclofen	2-OH saclofen, CGP 35348	Inhibitory (presynaptic): decrease in Ca^{2+} conductance. Inhibitory (postsynaptic): increase in K^+ conductance.
Glutamate; aspartate	Relay neurons at all levels.	N-Methyl-D-aspartate (NMDA)	2-Amino-5-phosphonovalerate, CPP	Excitatory: increase in cation conductance, particularly Ca^{2+}.
		AMPA, quisqualate, kainate	CNQX	Excitatory: increase in cation conductance but not Ca^{2+} in most cases.
		ACPD, quisqualate	MCPG	Excitatory: decrease in K^+ conductance.
Glycine	Spinal interneurons and some brain stem interneurons.	Taurine, β-alanine	Strychnine	Inhibitory: increase in Cl^- conductance.
5-Hydroxytryptamine (serotonin)	Cell bodies in midbrain and pons project to all levels.	$5\text{-}HT_{1A}$: LSD, 8-OH-DPAT	Metergoline, spiperone	Inhibitory: increase in K^+ conductance.
		$5\text{-}HT_{2A}$: LSD, DOB	Ketanserin	Excitatory: decrease in K^+ conductance.
		$5\text{-}HT_3$: 2-methyl-5-HT, phenylbiguanide	ICS 205930, ondansetron	Excitatory: increase in cation conductance.
		$5HT_4$: BIMU8	GR 1138089	Excitatory: decrease in K^+ conductance; mediated by cAMP
Norepinephrine	Cell bodies in pons and brain stem project to all levels.	$Alpha_1$: phenylephrine	Prazosin	Excitatory: decrease in K^+ conductance.
		$Alpha_2$: clonidine	Yohimbine	Inhibitory: increase in K^+ conductance.
		$Beta_1$: isoproterenol, dobutamine	Atenolol, practolol	Excitatory: decrease in K^+ conductance; mediated by cAMP
		$Beta_2$: salbutamol	Butoxamine	Inhibitory: may involve increase in electrogenic sodium pump.

Abbreviations: ACPD, *trans*-1-amino-cyclopentyl-1,3-dicarboxylate; **AMPA,** DL-α-amino-3-hydroxy-5-methylisoxazole-4-propionate; **BIMU8,** (endo-*N*-8-methyl-8-azabicyclo[3.2.1]oct-3-yl)-2,3-dihydro-3-isopropyl-2-oxo-1*H*-benzimidazol-1-carboxamide hydrochloride; **CGP 35348,** 3-aminopropyl(diethoxymethyl)phosphinic acid; **CNQX,** 6-cyano-7-nitroquinoxaline-2,3-dione; **CPP,** 3-(2-carboxypiperazin-4-yl)propyl-1-phosphonic acid; **DOB,** 5-bromo-2,5-dimethoxyamphetamine; **GR 113808,** [1-[2-[(methylsulfonyl)amino]ethyl]-4-piperidinyl]methyl-1-methyl-1*H*-indole-3-carboxylate; **8-OH DPAT,** 8-hydroxy-2(di-*n*-propylamino)tetralin; **MCPG,** ($\pm$)-α-methyl-4-carboxyphenylglycine.

glutamate and **aspartate.** All of these compounds are present in high concentrations in the CNS and are extremely potent modifiers of neuronal excitability.

A. Neutral Amino Acids: The neutral amino acids are inhibitory and increase membrane permeability to chloride ions, thus mimicking the IPSP. Glycine concentrations are particularly high in the gray matter of the spinal cord, and destruction of the neurons in this area results in a marked decrease in the concentration of glycine. In addition, strychnine, which is a potent spinal cord convulsant and has been used in some rat poisons, selectively antagonizes both the action of glycine and the IPSPs recorded in spinal cord neurons. Thus, it is generally agreed that glycine is released from spinal cord inhibitory local circuit neurons involved in postsynaptic inhibition.

GABA receptors are divided into two types: $GABA_A$ and $GABA_B$. $GABA_A$ receptors open chloride channels and are antagonized by picrotoxin and bicuculline, which both cause generalized convulsions. $GABA_B$ receptors, which can be selectively activated by the antispastic drug baclofen, are coupled to potassium channels in the postsynaptic membrane. In most regions of the brain, IPSPs have a fast and slow component. Good evidence suggests that GABA is the inhibitory transmitter mediating both components. The fast IPSPs are blocked by $GABA_A$ antagonists, while the slow IPSPs are blocked by $GABA_B$ antagonists. Immunohistochemical studies indicate that a large majority of the local circuit neurons synthesize GABA. A special class of local circuit neuron localized in the dorsal horn of the spinal cord also synthesizes GABA. These neurons form axoaxonic synapses with primary sensory nerve terminals and are responsible for presynaptic inhibition (Figure 20–4B).

B. Acidic Amino Acids: Both glutamate and aspartate are present in very high concentrations in the CNS. Virtually all neurons that have been tested are strongly excited by these two amino acids. This excitation is caused by the activation of receptors that can be divided into two classes: *ionotropic* and *metabotropic,* which have been extensively characterized by molecular cloning. As their name suggests, the ionotropic receptors directly gate cation-selective channels and are further divided into three subtypes based on the action of the selective agonists kainate (K), α-amino-3-hydroxy-5-methylisoxazole-4-propionate (AMPA), and N-methyl-D-aspartate (NMDA). The AMPA- and K-activated channels are permeable to sodium and potassium ions and, for certain subtypes, calcium as well. They are often grouped together and referred to as non-NMDA channels. The NMDA-activated channel is highly permeable to sodium, potassium, and calcium ions.

The metabotropic glutamate receptors act not on ion channels but on intracellular enzymes. They are selectively activated by *trans*-1-amino-cyclopentyl-1,3-dicarboxylate (ACPD). These G protein-coupled receptors are positively coupled to (ie, stimulate) phospholipase C or negatively coupled to adenylyl cyclase. Biochemical studies have shown that either (1) glutamate concentrations in a particular region fall when specific excitatory pathways to the region are cut, or (2) the calcium-dependent release of glutamate is reduced. Although it is unclear whether the ACPD receptor is involved in synaptic transmission, pharmacologic studies indicate that both NMDA and non-NMDA receptors are so involved.

The role of NMDA receptors has recently received considerable attention. These receptors play a critical role in synaptic plasticity, which is thought to underlie certain forms of learning and memory. They are very selectively blocked by the dissociative anesthetic ketamine and the hallucinogenic drug phencyclidine. They exert their effects by entering and blocking the open channel. Drugs that block this receptor channel have potent antiepileptic activity in animal models, though these drugs have yet to be tested clinically. A particularly exciting finding is that blocking the NMDA receptor can attenuate the neuronal damage caused by anoxia in experimental animals. The potential therapeutic benefits of this action are considerable.

Acetylcholine

Acetylcholine was the first compound to be identified pharmacologically as a transmitter in the CNS. Eccles showed in the early 1950s that excitation of Renshaw cells by motor axon collaterals was blocked by nicotinic antagonists. Furthermore, Renshaw cells were extremely sensitive to nicotinic agonists. These experiments were remarkable for two reasons. First, this early success at identifying a transmitter for a central synapse was followed by disappointment, because it remained the sole central synapse for which the transmitter was known until the late 1960s, when comparable data became available for the neutral amino acids. Second, the motor axon collateral synapse remains the only clearly documented example of a cholinergic nicotinic synapse in the mammalian CNS, despite the rather widespread distribution of nicotinic receptors as defined by in situ hybridization studies. Most CNS responses to acetylcholine are mediated by a large family of G protein-coupled muscarinic receptors. At a few sites, acetylcholine causes slow inhibition of the neuron by activating the M_2 subtype of receptor, which opens potassium channels. A far more widespread muscarinic action in response to acetylcholine is a slow excitation that in some cases may be mediated by M_1 receptors. These muscarinic effects are much slower than either nicotinic effects on Renshaw cells or the effect of amino acids. Furthermore, this muscarinic excitation is unusual in that acetylcholine produces it by *decreasing* the membrane permeability to potassium, ie, the opposite of conventional transmitter action.

A number of pathways contain acetylcholine, including neurons in the neostriatum, the medial septal nucleus, and the reticular formation. The introduction of monoclonal antibodies that bind to choline acetyltransferase has greatly improved the histochemical localization of this transmitter. Cholinergic pathways appear to play an important role in cognitive functions, especially memory. Presenile dementia of the Alzheimer type is reportedly associated with a profound loss of cholinergic neurons. However, the specificity of this loss has been questioned since the levels of other putative transmitters, eg, somatostatin, are also decreased.

Monoamines

Monoamines include the catecholamines (dopamine and norepinephrine) and 5-hydroxytryptamine. Although these compounds are present in very small amounts in the CNS, they can be localized using extremely sensitive histochemical methods. These include formaldehyde-induced fluorescence of the monoamines and immunohistochemical methods for localizing the individual synthetic enzymes. These pathways are the site of action of many drugs; for example, the CNS stimulants cocaine and amphetamine are believed to act primarily at catecholamine synapses. Cocaine blocks the reuptake of dopamine and norepinephrine, while amphetamines cause presynaptic terminals to release these transmitters.

A. Dopamine: The major pathways containing dopamine are the projection linking the substantia nigra to the neostriatum and the projection linking the ventral tegmental region to limbic structures, particularly the limbic cortex. The therapeutic action of the antiparkinsonism drug levodopa is associated with the former area, whereas the therapeutic action of the antipsychotic drugs is thought to be associated with the latter area. Dopamine-containing neurons in the tuberobasal ventral hypothalamus play an important role in regulating hypothalamohypophysial function. Dopamine generally exerts a slow inhibitory action on CNS neurons. This action has been best characterized on dopamine-containing substantia nigra neurons, where D_2 receptor activation opens potassium channels.

B. Norepinephrine: This system has already been discussed. Most noradrenergic neurons are located in the locus ceruleus or the lateral tegmental area of the reticular formation. Although the density of fibers innervating various sites differs considerably, most regions of the central nervous system receive diffuse noradrenergic input. When applied to neurons, norepinephrine can hyperpolarize them by increasing potassium conductance. This effect is mediated by alpha$_2$ receptors and has been characterized most thoroughly on locus ceruleus neurons. In many regions of the CNS, norepinephrine actually enhances excitatory inputs by both indirect and direct mechanisms. The indirect mechanism involves disinhibition, ie, inhibitory local circuit neurons are inhib-

ited. The direct mechanism is blockade of potassium conductances that slow neuronal discharge. Depending on the type of neuron, this effect is mediated by either alpha$_1$ or beta receptors. Facilitation of excitatory synaptic transmission is in accordance with many of the behavioral processes thought to involve noradrenergic pathways–attention, arousal, and so on.

C. 5-Hydroxytryptamine: Most 5-hydroxytryptamine (5-HT) pathways originate from neurons in the raphe or midline regions of the pons and upper brain stem. 5-Hydroxytryptamine is contained in unmyelinated fibers that diffusely innervate most regions of the CNS, but the density of the innervation varies. In most areas of the central nervous system, 5-hydroxytryptamine has a strong inhibitory action. This action is mediated by 5-HT$_{1A}$ receptors and is associated with membrane hyperpolarization caused by an increase in potassium conductance. It has been found that 5-HT$_{1A}$ receptors and GABA$_B$ receptors share the same potassium channels. These receptors and the potassium channels are coupled using a GTP-binding protein. Some cell types are slowly excited by 5-hydroxytryptamine owing to its blockade of potassium channels via 5-HT$_2$ receptors. Both excitatory and inhibitory actions can occur on the same neurons. It has often been speculated that 5-hydroxytryptamine pathways may be involved in the hallucinations induced by LSD, since this compound can antagonize the peripheral actions of 5-hydroxytryptamine. However, LSD does not appear to be a 5-hydroxytryptamine antagonist in the central nervous system, and typical LSD-induced behavior is still seen in animals after raphe nuclei are destroyed. Other proposed regulatory functions of 5-hydroxytryptamine-containing neurons include sleep, temperature, appetite, and neuroendocrine control.

Peptides

A great many CNS peptides have been discovered that produce dramatic effects both on animal behavior and on the activity of individual neurons. Many of the peptides have been mapped with immunohistochemical techniques and include opioid peptides (enkephalin, endorphins, etc), neurotensin, substance P, somatostatin, cholecystokinin, vasoactive intestinal polypeptide, neuropeptide Y, and thyrotropin-releasing hormone. As in the peripheral autonomic nervous system, peptides often coexist with a conventional nonpeptide transmitter in the same neuron. A good example of the approaches used to define the role of these peptides in the central nervous system comes from studies on substance P and its association with sensory fibers. Immunohistochemical studies have found substance P to be present in some of the small unmyelinated primary sensory neurons of the spinal cord and brain stem. In addition, stimulation of the sensory neurons releases substance P from the spinal cord. Application of substance P to neurons in the spinal cord excites neurons that are activated by painful stimuli. Painful stimuli are known to selectively activate unmyelinated sensory fibers. Thus, it is believed that substance P may be an excitatory transmitter released from unmyelinated fibers that respond to painful stimulation. Substance P is certainly involved in many other functions, since it is found in many areas of the central nervous system that are unrelated to pain pathways.

REFERENCES

Bloom FE: The endorphins: A growing family of pharmacologically pertinent peptides. Annu Rev Pharmacol Toxicol 1983;23:344.

Bloom FE: Neurotransmitters: Past, present, and future directions. FASEB J 1988;2:32.

Bowery NG, Bittiger H, Olpe H-R: *GABA*_B *Receptors in Mammalian Function.* Wiley, 1990.

Catterall WA: Structure and function of voltage-sensitive ion channels. Science 1988;242:50.

Cooper JR, Bloom FE, Roth RH: *The Biochemical Basis of Neuropharmacology,* 6th ed. Oxford Univ Press, 1991.

Costa E et al: Coexistence of neuromodulators: Biochemical and pharmacological consequences. (Symposium.) Fed Proc 1983;42:2910.

Cotman CW, Iversen LL: Excitatory amino acids in the brain: Focus on NMDA receptors. Trends Neurosci 1987;10:263.

Coyle JT, Price DL, DeLong MR: Alzheimer's disease: A disorder of cortical cholinergic innervation. Science 1983;219:1184.

Creese I: Dopamine receptors explained. Trends Neurosci 1982;5:40.

Eccles JC: *The Physiology of Synapses.* Academic Press, 1964.

Gasic GP, Hollman M: Molecular neurobiology of glutamate receptors. Annu Rev Physiol 1992;54:507.

Grandy DK, Civelli O: G-protein-coupled receptors: the new dopamine receptor subtypes. Curr Biol 1992;2:275.

Hille B: *Ionic Channels of Excitable Membranes,* 2nd ed. Sinauer Associates, 1992.

Hokfelt T: Neuropeptides in perspective: The last ten years. Neuron 1991;7:867.

Iversen LL: Nonopioid neuropeptides in mammalian CNS. Annu Rev Pharmacol Toxicol 1983;23:1.

Iversen SD, Iversen, LL: *Behavioral Pharmacology,* 2nd ed. Oxford Univ Press, 1979.

Julius D: Molecular biology of serotonin receptors. Annu Rev Neurosci 1991;14:335.

Krnjević K: Acetylcholine receptors in vertebrate CNS. In: *Handbook of Psychopharmacology,* vol 6. Iversen LL, Iversen SD, Snyder SH (editors). Plenum Press, 1975.

Llinas RR: The intrinsic electrophysiologic properties of mammalian neurons: Insights into CNS function. Science 1988;242:1654.

Meltzer HY (editor): *Psychopharmacology: The Third Generation of Progress.* Raven Press, 1987.

Miller RJ: Multiple Ca channels and neuronal function. Science 1987;235:46.

Moore RY, Bloom FE: Central catecholamine neuron systems: Anatomy and physiology. Annu Rev Neurosci 1978;2:113.

Nakanishi S: Molecular diversity of glutamate receptors and implications for brain function. Science 1992;258:597.

Nicoll RA: The coupling of neurotransmitter receptors to ion channels in the brain. Science 1988;241:545.

Nicoll RA, Schenker C, Leeman SE: Substance P as a transmitter candidate. Annu Rev Neurosci 1980;3:227.

Peroutka SJ: 5-Hydroxytryptamine receptor subtypes. Annu Rev Neurosci 1988;7:45.

Rakic P: Local circuit neurons. Neurosci Res Program Bull 1975;13:293.

Robinson MB, Coyle JT: Glutamate and related acidic excitatory transmitters: From basic science to clinical application. FASEB J 1987;1:446.

Rogawski MA, Barker JL (editors): *Neurotransmitter Actions in the Vertebrate Nervous System.* Plenum Press, 1985.

Shepherd GM: *Neurobiology,* 2nd ed. Oxford Univ Press, 1988.

Snyder SH: Drug and neurotransmitter receptors in the brain. Science 1984;224:22.

Tecott LH, Julius D: A new wave of serotonin receptors. Curr Biol 1993;3:310.

Walaas SI, Greengard P: Protein phosphorylation and neuronal function. Pharmacol Rev 1991;43:299.

Watkins JC, Krogsgaard-Larsen P, Honoré T: Structure-activity relationships in the development of excitatory amino acid receptor agonists and antagonists. Trends Pharmacol Sci 1990;11:25.

Wisden W, Seeburg PH: Mammalian ionotropic glutamate receptors. Curr Biol 1993;3:291.

Sedative-Hypnotic Drugs

21

Anthony J. Trevor, PhD, & Walter L. Way, MD

Assignment of a particular compound to the sedative-hypnotic class of drugs indicates that its major therapeutic use is to cause sedation (with concomitant relief of anxiety) or to encourage sleep. There is considerable chemical variation within this group, so this is an example of drug classification based on clinical uses rather than on similarities in chemical structures or mechanisms of action. These clinical uses are very extensive, and sedative-hypnotics are among the most widely prescribed drugs worldwide.

I. BASIC PHARMACOLOGY OF SEDATIVE-HYPNOTICS

An effective **sedative** (anxiolytic) agent should reduce anxiety and exert a calming effect with little or no effect on motor or mental functions. The degree of central nervous system depression caused by a sedative should be the minimum consistent with therapeutic efficacy. A **hypnotic** drug should produce drowsiness and encourage the onset and maintenance of a state of sleep that as far as possible resembles the natural sleep state. Hypnotic effects involve more pronounced depression of the central nervous system than sedation, and this can be achieved with most sedative drugs simply by increasing the dose.

Graded dose-dependent depression of central nervous system function is a characteristic of sedative-hypnotics. However, individual drugs differ in the relationship between the dose and the degree of central nervous system depression. Two examples of such dose-response relationships are shown in Figure 21–1. The linear slope for drug A is typical of many of the older sedative-hypnotics, including the barbiturates and alcohols. With such drugs, an increase in dose above that needed for hypnosis may lead to a state of general anesthesia. At still higher doses, sedative-hypnotics may depress respiratory and vasomotor centers in the medulla, leading to coma and death. Deviations from a linear dose-response relationship, as shown for drug B, will require proportionately

greater dosage increments in order to achieve central nervous system depression more profound than hypnosis. This appears to be the case for most drugs of the benzodiazepine class, and the greater margin of safety this offers is an important reason for their extensive clinical use to treat anxiety states and sleep disorders.

CHEMICAL CLASSIFICATION

The benzodiazepines (Figure 21–2) are the most important sedative-hypnotics. All of the structures shown are 1,4-benzodiazepines, and most contain a carboxamide group in the 7-membered heterocyclic ring structure. A substituent in the 7 position, such as a halogen or a nitro group, is required for sedative-hypnotic activity. The structures of triazolam and alprazolam include the addition of a triazole ring at the 1,2-positions, and such drugs are sometimes referred to as triazolobenzodiazepines.

The chemical structures of some older and less commonly used sedative-hypnotics are shown in Figure 21–3. The barbiturates have been regarded as prototypes of the class because of their extensive use in the past. The motivation to develop the benzodiaze-

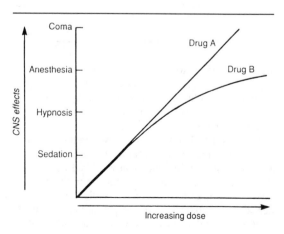

Figure 21–1. Theoretical dose-response curves for sedative-hypnotics.

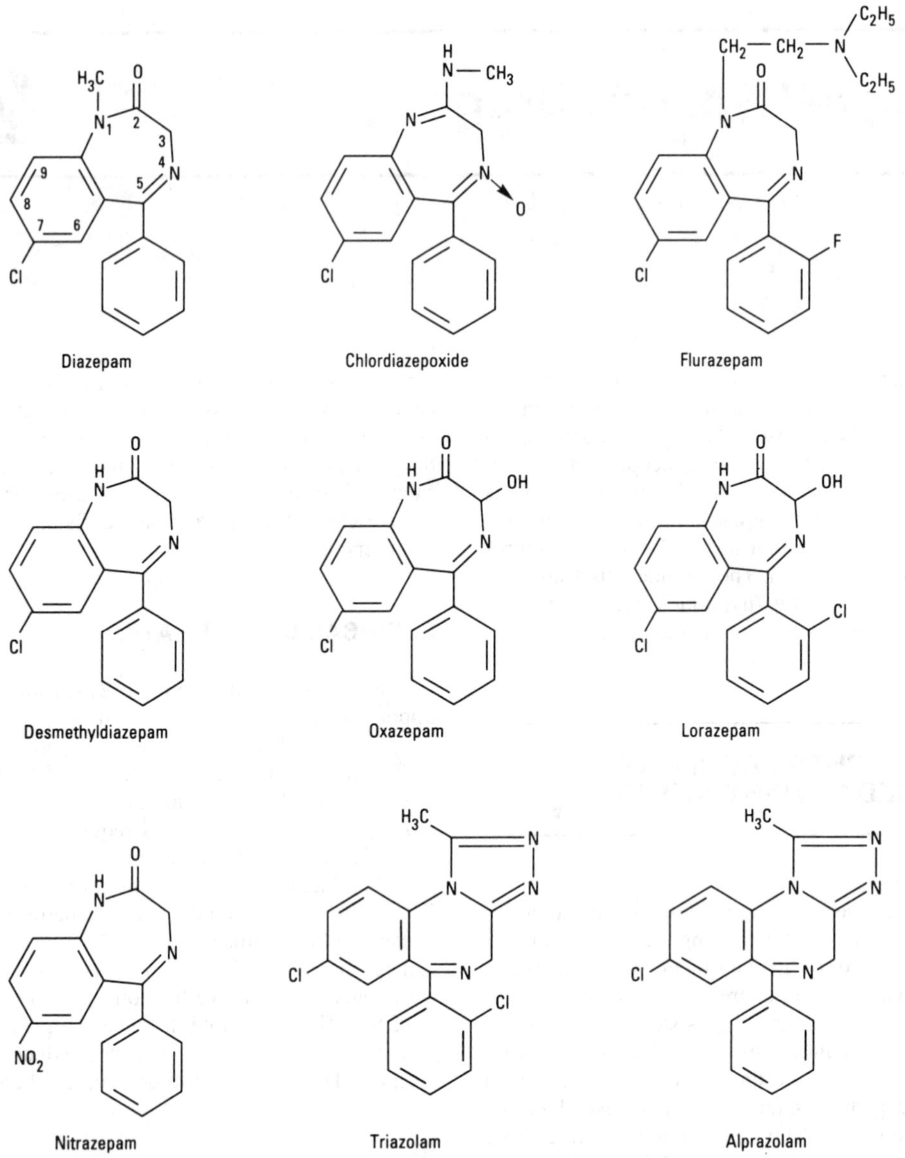

Figure 21–2. Chemical structures of benzodiazepines.

pines and other newer sedative-hypnotics can be attributed to efforts to avoid undesirable features of the barbiturates, including their potential for inducing psychologic and physical dependence. Unfortunately, such efforts have not always been successful. For example, the piperidinediones such as glutethimide and methyprylon, introduced as "nonbarbiturate sedative-hypnotics," are in fact chemically related and virtually indistinguishable from barbiturates in their pharmacologic properties. The propanediol carbamates such as meprobamate are of distinctive chemical structure but are practically equivalent to barbiturates in their pharmacologic effects, and their clinical use is rapidly declining. The sedative-hypnotic class also includes compounds of simple chemical structure, including alcohols (ethanol, chloral hydrate) and the cyclic ethers. Chloral hydrate and its congeners, such as trichloroethanol, together with paraldehyde (not shown), continue to be used, particularly in institutionalized patients. Several drugs with novel chemical structures have been introduced recently. Buspirone, an azaspirodecanedione, is an anxiolytic agent that has actions different from those of conventional sedative-hypnotic drugs. Zolpidem is an imidazopyridine hypnotic, structurally unrelated to benzodiazepines but with similar pharmacologic properties.

Other classes of drugs not included in Figure 21–3

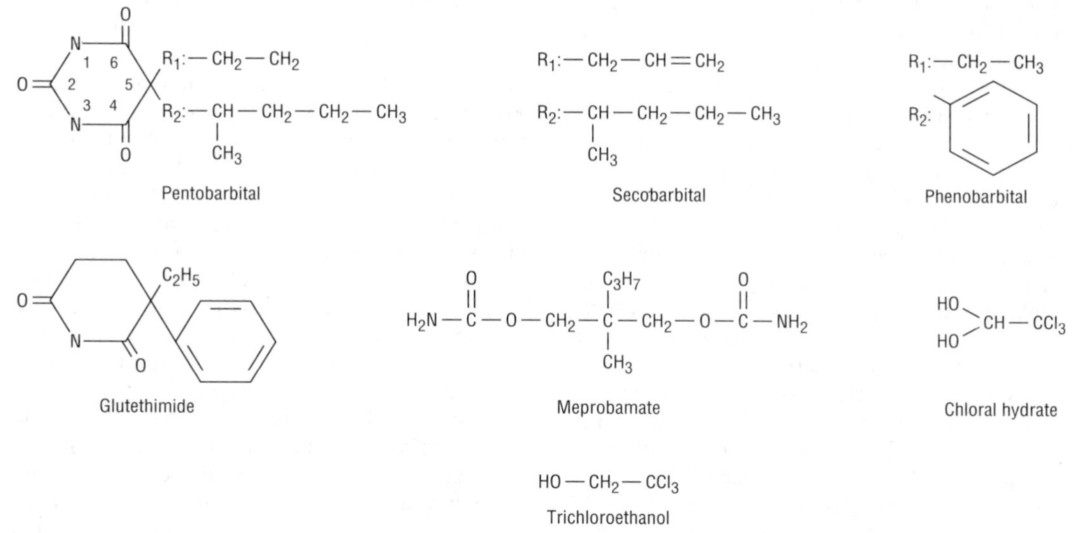

Figure 21–3. Chemical structures of barbiturates and other sedative-hypnotics.

may exert sedative effects. For example, beta-blocking drugs are effective in certain anxiety states and functional disorders, particularly those in which somatic and autonomic symptoms are prominent. Clonidine, a partial agonist at alpha$_2$ receptors, including presynaptic adrenoceptors in the brain, also has anxiolytic properties. Sedative effects can also be obtained with the antipsychotic tranquilizers, the tricyclic antidepressant drugs, and antihistaminic agents. As discussed in other chapters, these agents differ from conventional sedative-hypnotics in both their effects and their major therapeutic uses. Most importantly, they do not produce general anesthesia, and they have low abuse liability. Since they commonly exert marked effects on the peripheral autonomic nervous system, they are sometimes referred to as "sedative-autonomic" drugs. Compounds of the antihistaminic type are present in a number of over-the-counter sleep preparations, in which their autonomic properties as well as their long duration of action can result in unwanted side effects.

THE BENZODIAZEPINES & BARBITURATES

Pharmacokinetics

A. Absorption: When used to treat anxiety or sleep disorders, sedative-hypnotics are usually given orally. The benzodiazepines are weakly basic drugs and are absorbed most effectively at the high pH found in the duodenum. The rates of oral absorption of benzodiazepines differ depending on a number of factors, including lipophilicity. Oral absorption of triazolam is extremely rapid, and that of diazepam and the active metabolite of clorazepate is more rapid

than that of the other commonly used benzodiazepines. Clorazepate is converted to its active form, desmethyldiazepam, by acid hydrolysis in the stomach. Oxazepam and temazepam are absorbed at slower rates than other benzodiazepines. The bioavailability of several benzodiazepines, including chlordiazepoxide and diazepam, may be unreliable after intramuscular injection. The barbiturates and the piperidinediones are weak acids and are usually absorbed very rapidly into the blood from the stomach as well as the small intestine.

B. Distribution: Transport of a sedative-hypnotic in the blood is a dynamic process in which drug molecules enter and leave tissues at rates dependent upon blood flow, concentration gradients, and permeabilities. Lipid solubility plays a major role in determining the rate at which a particular sedative-hypnotic enters the central nervous system. For example, diazepam and triazolam are more lipid-soluble than chlordiazepoxide and lorazepam; thus, the central nervous system actions of the latter drugs are slower in onset. The thiobarbiturates (eg, thiopental), in which the oxygen on C2 is replaced by sulfur, are very lipid-soluble, and a high rate of entry into the central nervous system contributes to the rapid onset of their central effects (see Chapter 24), whereas meprobamate has quite low solubility in lipids and penetrates the brain slowly even when given intravenously.

Redistribution of drug from the central nervous system to other tissues is an important feature of the biodisposition of sedative-hypnotics. Classic studies on the thiobarbiturates have shown that they are rapidly redistributed from the brain, first to highly perfused tissues such as skeletal muscle and subsequently to poorly perfused adipose tissue. These processes contribute to the termination of their major central nervous system effects. This may also be the case for other sedative-hypnotics, including the benzodiazepines, where the rate of metabolic transformation and elimination in humans is much too slow to account for the relatively short time required for dissipation of major pharmacologic effects.

Administration of benzodiazepines and other sedative-hypnotics during pregnancy should be done with the recognition that the placental barrier to lipid-soluble drugs is incomplete and that all of these agents are capable of reaching the fetus. The rate at which maternal and fetal blood concentrations equilibrate is slower than that for the maternal blood and central nervous system, partly because of lower blood flow to the placenta. Nonetheless, if sedative-hypnotics are given in the predelivery period, they may contribute to the depression of neonatal vital functions.

Benzodiazepines and most other sedative-hypnotics bind extensively to plasma proteins. For example, plasma albumin binding of benzodiazepines ranges from 60% to over 95%. Since only free (nonbound) drug molecules have access to the central nervous system, the displacement of a sedative-hypnotic from plasma binding sites by another drug could modify its effects and possibly lead to drug interactions between this class and other pharmacologic agents. However, few clinically significant interactions involving sedative-hypnotic drugs appear to be based on competition for common binding sites on the plasma proteins. One exception is chloral hydrate, which increases the anticoagulant effects of warfarin by displacement of the anticoagulant from such binding sites.

C. Biotransformation: As noted above, redistribution to tissues other than the brain may be as important as biotransformation in terminating the central nervous system effects of many sedative-hypnotics. However, metabolic transformation to more water-soluble metabolites is necessary for clearance from the body of almost all drugs in this class. The microsomal drug-metabolizing enzyme systems of the liver are most important in this regard. Since few sedative-hypnotics are excreted from the body unchanged, the elimination half-life ($t_{1/2\beta}$) depends mainly on the rate of their metabolic transformation.

1. Benzodiazepines—Hepatic metabolism accounts for the clearance or elimination of all benzodiazepines. The patterns and rates of metabolism depend on the individual drugs. Most benzodiazepines undergo microsomal oxidation (phase I reactions), including N-dealkylation and aliphatic hydroxylation. The metabolites are subsequently conjugated (phase II reactions) by glucuronosyltransferases to form glucuronides that are excreted in the urine. However, many phase I metabolites of benzodiazepines are active, with half-lives greater than the parent drugs.

As shown in Figure 21–4, desmethyldiazepam, which has an elimination half-life of 40–140 hours, is an active metabolite of chlordiazepoxide, diazepam, prazepam, and clorazepate. Desmethyldiazepam in turn is biotransformed to the active compound oxazepam. Other active metabolites of chlordiazepoxide include desmethylchlordiazepoxide and demoxepam. While diazepam is metabolized mainly to desmethyldiazepam, it is also converted to temazepam (not shown in Figure 21–4), which is further metabolized in part to oxazepam. Flurazepam, which is used mainly for hypnosis, is oxidized by hepatic enzymes to three active metabolites, desalkylflurazepam, hydroxyethylflurazepam, and flurazepam aldehyde (not shown), which have elimination half-lives ranging from 30 to 100 hours. This may result in unwanted central nervous system depression, including daytime sedation. The triazolobenzodiazepines alprazolam and triazolam undergo alpha-hydroxylation, and the resulting metabolites appear to exert short-lived pharmacologic effects since they are rapidly conjugated to form inactive glucuronides.

The formation of active metabolites has complicated studies on the pharmacokinetics of the benzodiazepines in humans because the elimination half-life of the parent drug may have little relationship to the time course of pharmacologic effects. Those benzodiazepines for which the parent drug or active metabolites have long half-lives are more likely to cause cumulative effects with multiple doses. Cumulative and residual effects such as excessive drowsiness appear to be less of a problem with such drugs as oxazepam and lorazepam, which have shorter half-lives and are metabolized directly to inactive glucuronides. Some pharmacokinetic properties of selected benzodiazepines are listed in Table 21–1.

2. Barbiturates—With the exception of phenobarbital, only insignificant quantities of the barbiturates are excreted unchanged. The major metabolic pathways involve oxidation by hepatic enzymes of chemical groups attached to C5, which are different for the individual barbiturates. The alcohols, acids, and ketones formed appear in the urine as glucuronide conjugates. With very few exceptions, the metabolites of the barbiturates lack pharmacologic activity. The overall rate of hepatic metabolism in humans depends on the individual drug but (with the exception of the thiobarbiturates) is usually slow. The elimination half-lives of secobarbital and pentobarbital range from 18 to 48 hours in different individuals. The elimination half-life of phenobarbital in humans is 4–5 days. Multiple dosing with these agents can lead to cumulative effects.

D. Excretion: The water-soluble metabolites of benzodiazepines and other sedative-hypnotics are excreted mainly via the kidney. In most cases, changes in renal function do not have a marked effect on the elimination of parent drugs. Phenobarbital is excreted unchanged in the urine to a certain extent (20–30% in humans), and its elimination rate can be increased

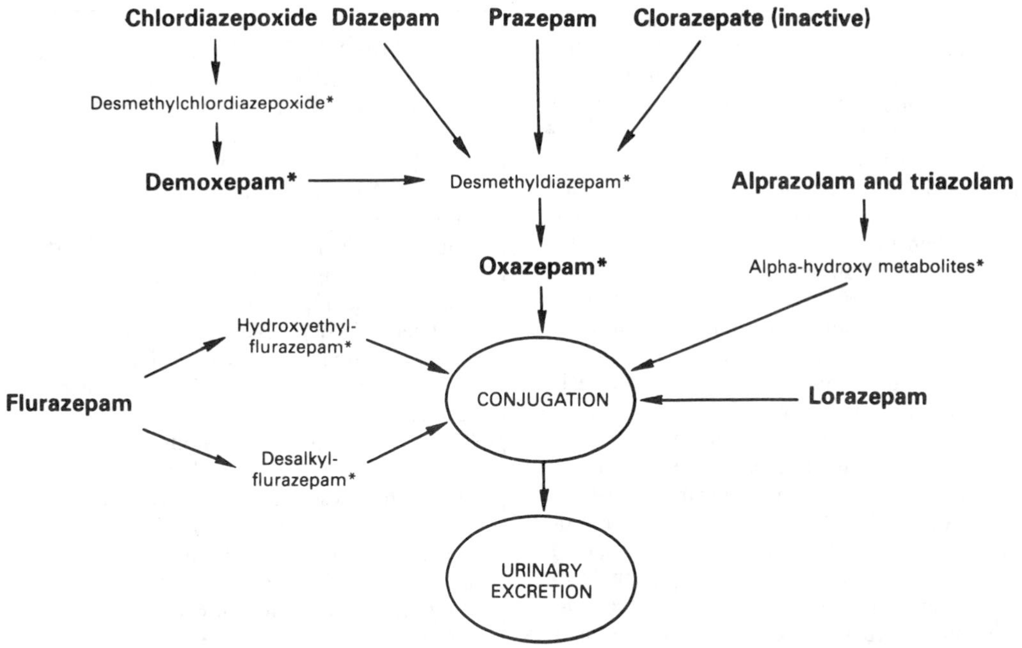

Figure 21–4. Biotransformation of benzodiazepines. (**Boldface,** drugs available for clinical use; *, active metabolite.)

significantly by alkalinization of the urine. This is partly due to increased ionization at alkaline pH, since phenobarbital is a weak acid with a pK_a of 7.2. Only trace amounts of the benzodiazepines and less than 10% of a hypnotic dose of meprobamate appear in the urine unchanged.

E. Factors Affecting Biodisposition: The biodisposition of sedative-hypnotics can be influenced by several factors, particularly alterations in hepatic function resulting from disease, old age, or drug-induced increases or decreases in microsomal enzyme activities.

Generally, decreased hepatic function results in reduction of the clearance rates of drugs metabolized via oxidative pathways. This group includes many of the benzodiazepines, almost all of the barbiturates,

Table 21–1. Pharmacokinetic properties of benzodiazepines in humans.

Drug	Elimination Half-Life Range (hours)	Metabolites	Comments
Alprazolam	12–15	Active: α-hydroxyalprazolam	Rapid oral absorption.
Chlordiazepoxide	5–30	Active: desmethyl derivative, demoxepam, oxazepam	Poor intramuscular bioavailability.
Chlorazepate	50–100 (metabolites)	Active: desmethyldiazepam, oxazepam	Hydrolyzed to active form in stomach.
Diazepam	50–150	Active: desmethyldiazepam, temazepam, oxazepam	Poor intramuscular bioavailability.
Flunitrazepam	12–24	Active: desmethylflunitrazepam	Large volume of distribution.
Flurazepam	24–100 (metabolites)	Active: desalkyl derivative and others	Long elimination half-lives of active metabolites.
Lorazepam	10–18	Inactive: glucuronides	Elimination not much affected by age or liver disease.
Nitrazepam	24–36	Probably inactive	Large volume of distribution.
Oxazepam	4–10	Inactive: glucuronides	Slow oral absorption may delay onset of effects.
Prazepam	30–120	Active: desmethyldiazepam	Slow oral absorption.
Temazepam	5–8	Possibly active	Slow oral absorption.
Triazolam	3–5	Active: α-hydroxytriazolam	Rapid oral absorption.

the piperidinediones, and meprobamate. In very old patients and in patients with severe liver disease, the elimination half-lives of these drugs are usually increased significantly. In such cases, multiple normal doses of these sedative-hypnotics often result in excessive central nervous system effects. Thus, it is common practice to reduce the dosage of such sedative-hypnotics in patients who are elderly or who may have limited hepatic function. Metabolism involving glucuronide conjugation appears to be less affected by old age or liver disease than oxidative metabolism.

The activity of hepatic microsomal drug-metabolizing enzymes may be increased in patients exposed to certain older sedative-hypnotics on a chronic basis (enzyme induction; see Chapter 4). Drugs with long elimination half-lives such as phenobarbital and meprobamate are most likely to cause this effect and result in an increase in their own hepatic metabolism as well as that of certain other drugs. Self-induction of metabolism is a possible but poorly documented mechanism that contributes to the development of tolerance to sedative-hypnotics. Increased biotransformation of other pharmacologic agents by barbiturates is a potential mechanism underlying drug interactions. (See Appendix II.) The benzodiazepines do not change hepatic drug-metabolizing enzyme activity with continuous use.

Pharmacodynamics of Benzodiazepines & Barbiturates

A. Molecular Pharmacology of the GABA$_A$ Receptor: The benzodiazepines, the barbiturates, and the new sedative-hypnotic zolpidem bind to the chloride channel molecule that functions as the GABA$_A$ receptor but not to the GABA binding site itself.

Molecular cloning techniques show the GABA$_A$ receptor to be a hetero-oligomeric glycoprotein (200–400 kDa) that consists of at least three different subunits (alpha, beta, and gamma) in a still unknown stoichiometry. Several different subunits of each type have been found, ie, six different alpha, four beta, and three gamma. In addition, delta, epsilon, and rho subunits have been proposed. Although alpha subunits alone or beta units alone can form chloride channels with weak GABA responsiveness, a combination of at least three types of units—alpha, beta, and gamma—appears to be essential for normal physiologic and pharmacologic function of the molecule. Receptors in different areas of the CNS may contain different versions of the essential subunits (eg, $\alpha_1\beta_1\gamma_2$ versus $\alpha_3\beta_1\gamma_2$), conferring different pharmacologic properties on them. Like the subunits of the nicotinic ACh receptor (with which the GABA$_A$ alpha and beta subunits share a 15–20% homology), each subunit has four membrane-spanning domains.

Reconstitution of channels with various combinations of the subunits indicates that GABA can bind to receptor sites on the alpha or beta subunits, and this

---

THE VERSATILITY OF THE CHLORIDE CHANNEL GABA RECEPTOR COMPLEX

The chloride channel molecule that contains the GABA receptor is one of the most versatile drug-responsive machines in the body. In addition to the benzodiazepines and barbiturates, many other drugs with CNS effects bind to this important channel.

Other CNS depressants include propofol (an important intravenous anesthetic), alfaxolone (a steroid anesthetic), certain gaseous anesthetics, and ivermectin (an anthelmintic agent). These agents facilitate or mimic the action of GABA. (It must be noted that it has not been shown that these drugs act exclusively or even primarily by this mechanism.) CNS excitatory agents that act on the chloride channel include picrotoxin and bicuculline. These convulsant drugs block the channel directly (picrotoxin) or interfere with GABA binding (bicuculline).

Binding of these diverse ligands appears to involve multiple distinct sites on the channel molecule. Some of the drugs interact allosterically. For example, the benzodiazepines appear to increase the affinity of GABA for its binding site, even though the binding sites are probably on different subunits. Barbiturates enhance benzodiazepine binding with a potency ranking that parallels their anesthetic potency.

---

interaction initiates gating of the chloride channel current. Sensitivity of the complex to benzodiazepines requires a gamma$_2$ subunit, suggesting that the benzodiazepine (BDZ) receptor site is probably located on or near this structure. Different combinations of the several types of alpha, beta, and gamma subunits appear to significantly alter benzodiazepine and zolpidem sensitivity. A hypothetical model of the GABA-BDZ receptor–chloride ion channel complex is shown in Figure 21–5.

B. Neuropharmacology: Gamma-aminobutyric acid (GABA) is the major inhibitory neurotransmitter in the CNS. Electrophysiologic studies have shown that benzodiazepines potentiate GABAergic neurotransmission at all levels of the neuraxis, including the spinal cord, hypothalamus, hippocampus, substantia nigra, cerebellar cortex, and cerebral cortex. Benzodiazepines appear to increase the efficiency of GABAergic synaptic inhibition (via membrane hyperpolarization), which leads to a decrease in the firing rate of critical neurons in many regions of the brain. The benzodiazepines do not substitute for GABA but appear to *enhance* GABA's effects without direct activation of GABA receptors or the associ-

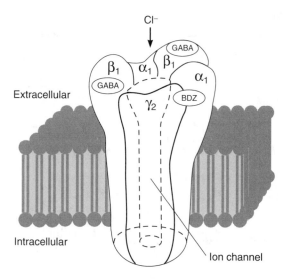

Figure 21–5. A hypothetical model of the GABA$_A$ receptor–chloride ion channel macromolecular complex (many others could be proposed). A hetero-oligomeric glycoprotein, the complex probably consists of five or more membrane-spanning subunits. GABA can interact with alpha or beta subunits triggering chloride channel opening with resultant membrane hyperpolarization. Binding of benzodiazepines to gamma subunits or to an area of the alpha unit influenced by the gamma unit facilitates the process of channel opening but does not directly initiate chloride current. (Modified and reproduced, with permission, from Zorumsky CF, Isenberg KE: Insights into the structure and function of GABA-benzodiazepine receptors: Ion channels and psychiatry. Am J Psychiatry 1991;148:162.)

ated chloride channels. The enhancement in chloride ion conductance induced by the interaction of benzodiazepines with GABA takes the form of an increase in the *frequency* of channel-opening events (Figure 21–6). This effect may be due in part to enhanced affinity for GABA.

Barbiturates also facilitate the actions of GABA at multiple sites in the CNS, but—in contrast to benzodiazepines—they appear to increase the *duration* of the GABA-gated channel openings (Figure 21–6). At high concentrations, the barbiturates may also be GABA-mimetic, directly activating chloride channels. These effects involve a binding site or sites distinct from the BDZ binding site. Barbiturates are less selective in their actions than benzodiazepines, since they also depress the actions of excitatory neurotransmitters and exert nonsynaptic membrane effects in parallel with their effects on GABA neurotransmission. This multiplicity of sites of action of barbiturates may be the basis for their ability to induce full surgical anesthesia (see Chapter 24) and for their more pronounced central depressant effects (which result in their low margin of safety) compared to benzodiazepines. The actions of other sedative-hypnotics

such as meprobamate have been less well studied electrophysiologically but do not appear to be related to GABA neurotransmission.

C. Benzodiazepine Receptor Ligands: Three types of ligand-benzodiazepine receptor interactions have been reported: (1) **Agonists** facilitate GABA action. These effects are typically produced by the clinically useful benzodiazepines, which exert anxiolytic and anticonvulsant effects. Endogenous agonist ligands for these receptors have been proposed, since benzodiazepine-like chemicals have been isolated from brain tissue of animals never exposed to these drugs, and benzodiazepine-like immunoreactivity has been detected in human brains stored in paraffin 15 years before the first benzodiazepine drug was synthesized. Nonbenzodiazepine molecules that have affinity for BDZ receptors have also been detected in human brain. Such "endozepines" facilitate GABA-mediated chloride channel gating in cultured neurons. (2) **Antagonists** are typified by the synthetic benzodiazepine derivative **flumazenil,** which blocks the actions of benzodiazepines but does not affect the actions of barbiturates, meprobamate, or ethanol. Certain endogenous compounds, eg, diazepam-binding inhibitor (DBI), are also capable of blocking the interaction of benzodiazepines with BDZ receptors. (3) **Inverse agonists** produce anxiety and seizures, an action that has been demonstrated for several compounds, especially the β-carbolines, eg, *n*-butyl-β-carboline-3-carboxylate (β-CCB). In addition to their direct actions, these molecules can block the effects of benzodiazepines.

D. Organ Level Effects:

1. Sedation–Sedation can be defined as a suppression of responsiveness to a constant level of stimulation, with decreased spontaneous activity and ideation. These behavioral changes occur at the lowest effective doses of the sedative-hypnotics. It is not yet clear whether antianxiety actions seen clinically are equivalent to or different from sedative effects. In experimental animal models, benzodiazepines and the older sedative-hypnotic drugs are able to release punishment-suppressed behavior, and this disinhibition has been equated with antianxiety effects. However, the release of previously suppressed behavior may be more relevant to behavioral disinhibitory effects of these drugs, including euphoria, impaired judgment, and loss of self-control, which can occur at dosages in the range of those used for management of anxiety. While most sedative-hypnotic drugs are capable of releasing punishment-suppressed behavior in animals, the benzodiazepines exert such effects at dosages that cause only minor central nervous system depression. Although they have sedative actions, antipsychotic drugs and tricyclic antidepressants are not effective in this experimental model. The benzodiazepines also exert anterograde amnesic effects (inability to remember events occurring during the drug's action) at sedative dosages.

Control

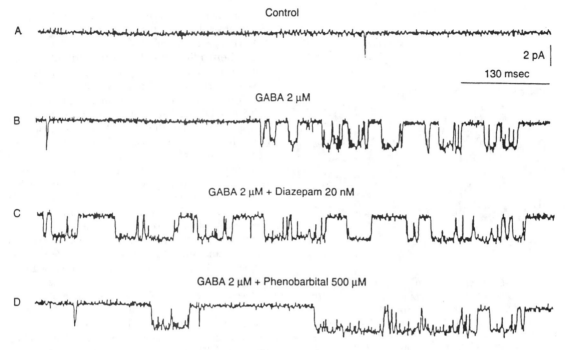

Figure 21–6. Patch-clamp recording of single-channel GABA-evoked currents in mouse spinal cord neurons. *A:* Control. *B:* Channel opening (downward deflections) elicited by GABA. *C:* Diazepam increases the frequency of channel opening without marked effects on duration of openings. *D:* Phenobarbital prolongs the duration of channel openings without marked effects on frequency. (Reproduced, with permission from, Twyman RE et al: Differential regulation of GABA receptor channels by diazepam and phenobarbital. Ann Neurol 1989;25:213.)

2. Hypnosis–By definition, all of the sedative-hypnotics will induce sleep if high enough doses are given. Normal sleep consists of distinct stages, based on three physiologic measures: the electroencephalogram, the electromyogram, and the electronystagmogram (a measure of lateral movements of the eye). Based on the latter, two major categories can be distinguished: non-rapid eye movement (NREM) sleep, which represents approximately 70–75% of total sleep; and rapid eye movement (REM) sleep. REM and NREM sleep occur cyclically over an interval of about 90 minutes. The REM sleep stage is that in which most recallable dreams occur. NREM sleep progresses through four stages (1–4), with the greatest proportion (50%) of sleep being spent in stage 2. This is followed by delta or slow-wave sleep (stages 3 and 4), in which somnambulism and night terrors have been noted to occur.

The effects of drugs on the sleep stages have been studied extensively, though often with normal volunteer subjects rather than patients with sleep disorders. In the case of sedative-hypnotics, effects depend on several factors, including the specific drug, the dose, and the frequency of its administration. While some exceptions exist, the effects of sedative-hypnotics on patterns of normal sleep are as follows: (1) the latency of sleep onset is decreased (time to fall asleep); (2) the duration of stage 2 NREM sleep is increased; (3) the duration of REM sleep is decreased; and (4) the duration of slow-wave sleep is decreased.

More rapid onset of sleep and prolongation of stage 2 are presumably clinically useful effects. However, the significance of effects on REM and slow-wave sleep is not clear. Use of sedative-hypnotics for more than a week leads to some tolerance to their effects on sleep patterns. Withdrawal after continued use can result in a "rebound" increase in the frequency of occurrence and duration of REM sleep.

3. Anesthesia–As shown in Figure 21–1, certain sedative-hypnotics in high doses will depress the central nervous system to the point known as stage III or general anesthesia (see Chapter 24). However, the suitability of a particular agent as an adjunct in anesthesia depends mainly on the physicochemical properties that determine its rapidity of onset and duration of effect. Among the barbiturates, thiopental and methohexital are very lipid-soluble, penetrating brain tissue rapidly following intravenous administration. Rapid tissue redistribution accounts for the short duration of action of these drugs, which are therefore useful in anesthesia practice.

Certain benzodiazepines, including diazepam and midazolam, are used intravenously in anesthesia (see Chapter 24) but have not proved to be fully successful as induction agents capable of producing surgical anesthesia by themselves. This statement is supported by the fact that the MAC (minimum alveolar anesthetic concentration) of another anesthetic cannot be reduced to zero by the substitution of a benzodiazepine. Not surprisingly, benzodiazepines given in large doses as adjuncts to general anesthetics may contribute to a persistent postanesthetic respiratory depression. This is probably related to their relatively long half-lives and the formation of active metabolites.

4. Anticonvulsant effects–Most of the sedative-hypnotics are capable of inhibiting the development and spread of epileptiform activity in the central nervous system. Some selectivity exists in that certain drugs can exert anticonvulsant effects without marked central nervous system depression, so that mentation and physical activity are relatively unaffected. Several benzodiazepines, including clonazepam, nitrazepam, lorazepam, and diazepam, have selective actions that are clinically useful in the management of seizure states (see Chapter 23). Of the barbiturates, phenobarbital and metharbital (converted to phenobarbital in the body) are effective in the treatment of grand mal and jacksonian epilepsy.

5. Muscle relaxation–Some sedative-hypnotics, particularly members of the carbamate and benzodiazepine groups, exert inhibitory effects on polysynaptic reflexes and internuncial transmission and at high doses may depress transmission at the skeletal neuromuscular junction. Selective actions of this type leading to muscle relaxation can be readily demonstrated in animals, and this has led to claims of usefulness for relaxing contracted voluntary muscle in joint disease or muscle spasm (see Clinical Pharmacology.

6. Effects on respiration and cardiovascular function–At hypnotic doses in healthy patients, the effects of sedative-hypnotics on respiration are comparable to changes during natural sleep. However, sedative-hypnotics even at therapeutic doses can produce significant respiratory depression in patients with obstructive pulmonary disease. Effects on respiration are dose-related, and depression of the medullary respiratory center is the usual cause of death due to overdose of sedative-hypnotics.

At doses up to those causing hypnosis, no significant effects on the cardiovascular system are observed in healthy patients. However, in hypovolemic states, congestive heart failure, and other diseases impairing cardiovascular function, normal doses of sedative-hypnotics may cause cardiovascular depression, probably as a result of actions on the medullary vasomotor centers. At toxic doses, myocardial contractility and vascular tone may both be depressed by central and peripheral effects, leading to circulatory collapse. Respiratory and cardiovascular effects become more apparent when sedative-hypnotics are given intravenously.

Tolerance; Psychologic & Physical Dependence

Tolerance, a decrease in responsiveness to a drug following continuous exposure, is a common feature of sedative-hypnotic use. In some instances, it may result in a need to increase the dose to maintain symptomatic improvement or to promote sleep. It is important to recognize that partial cross-tolerance occurs between the sedative-hypnotics described here and also with ethanol (Chapter 22)—a feature of some clinical importance, as explained below. The mechanisms of development of tolerance to sedative-hypnotics are not well understood. An alteration in rates of metabolic inactivation with chronic administration may be partly responsible (metabolic tolerance) in the case of barbiturates, but changes in responsiveness of the central nervous system (pharmacodynamic tolerance) are more important for most sedative-hypnotics.

The perceived desirable properties of relief of anxiety, euphoria, disinhibition, and promotion of sleep have led to the compulsive misuse of virtually all of the drugs classed as sedative-hypnotics. (See Chapter 31 for a detailed discussion of drug abuse.) The consequences of abuse of these agents can be defined in both psychologic and physiologic terms. The psychologic component may initially parallel simple neurotic behavior patterns difficult to differentiate from those of the inveterate coffee drinker or cigarette smoker. When the pattern of sedative-hypnotic use becomes compulsive, more serious complications develop, including physical dependence and tolerance.

Physical dependence can be described as an altered physiologic state that requires continuous drug administration to prevent the appearance of an abstinence or withdrawal syndrome. As described more fully later, in the case of sedative-hypnotics this syndrome is characterized by states of increased anxiety, insomnia, and CNS excitability that may progress to convulsions. All sedative-hypnotics are capable of causing physical dependence when used on a chronic basis. However, the severity of withdrawal symptoms differs between individual drugs and depends also on the magnitude of the dose used immediately prior to cessation of use. When higher doses of sedative-hypnotics are used, abrupt withdrawal will lead to more serious withdrawal signs. Differences in the severity of withdrawal symptoms between individual sedative-hypnotics relate in part to half-life, since drugs with long half-lives are eliminated slowly enough to accomplish gradual withdrawal with few physical symptoms. The use of drugs with very short half-lives for hypnotic effects may lead to signs of withdrawal even between doses. For example, triazolam, a benzodiazepine with a half-life of about 4 hours, has been reported to cause daytime anxiety when used to treat sleep disorders.

BENZODIAZEPINE ANTAGONISTS: FLUMAZENIL

Flumazenil is one of several 1,4-benzodiazepine derivatives with high affinity for the BDZ receptor that act as competitive antagonists. It is the only BDZ receptor antagonist available for clinical use at present. It blocks many of the actions of benzodiazepines but does not antagonize the CNS effects of other sedative-hypnotics, ethanol, opioids, or general anesthetics. Flumazenil is approved for use in reversing the CNS depressant effects of benzodiazepine overdose and following use of these drugs in anesthetic and diagnostic procedures. While the drug reverses the sedative effects of benzodiazepines, antagonism of benzodiazepine-induced respiratory depression is less predictable. Transient improvement in mental status has been reported with flumazenil when used in patients with hepatic encephalopathy. When given intravenously, flumazenil acts rapidly but has a short half-life (0.7–1.3 hours) due to rapid hepatic clearance. Since all benzodiazepines have a longer duration of action than flumazenil, sedation commonly recurs, requiring repeated administration of the antagonist. Adverse effects of flumazenil include agitation, confusion, dizziness, and nausea. Flumazenil may cause a severe precipitated abstinence syndrome in patients who have developed physical benzodiazepine dependence. In patients who have ingested benzodiazepines with tricyclic antidepressants, seizures and cardiac arrhythmias may occur following flumazenil administration.

NEWER SEDATIVE-HYPNOTIC DRUGS

Although the benzodiazepines continue to be the agents of choice in the treatment of anxiety and insomnia, their pharmacologic effects include sedation and drowsiness, synergistic CNS depression with other drugs (especially alcohol), and dependence with continuous use. Anxiolytic drugs that act through non-GABAergic systems might have a reduced propensity for such actions. Several new nonbenzodiazepines with this characteristic have been investigated, including buspirone. Zolpidem acts through the BDZ receptor, though its structure differs from that of the benzodiazepines.

Buspirone

Buspirone relieves anxiety without marked sedation. Unlike benzodiazepines, the drug has no hypnotic, anticonvulsant, or muscle relaxant properties. Buspirone does not interact directly with GABAergic systems but appears to exert its anxiolytic effects by acting as a partial agonist at 5-HT$_{1A}$ receptors. It is not effective in blocking the withdrawal syndrome resulting from cessation of use of benzodiazepines or other sedative-hypnotics, and the drug has minimal abuse liability. Buspirone does not potentiate the CNS depressant effects of conventional sedative-hypnotic drugs, ethanol, or tricyclic antidepressants. In contrast to the benzodiazepines, buspirone's anxiolytic effects may take more than a week to become established, making this drug suitable mainly for generalized anxiety states. It is not effective in panic disorders.

Buspirone is rapidly absorbed from the gastrointestinal tract but undergoes extensive first-pass metabolism. Its elimination half-life is 2–4 hours, with virtually no free drug appearing in the urine. Liver enzymes metabolize buspirone via hydroxylation and N-dealkylation reactions, resulting in formation of several metabolites that may retain slight pharmacologic activity. Liver dysfunction may decrease the clearance of buspirone.

Buspirone causes less psychomotor impairment than diazepam and does not affect driving skills. Tachycardia, palpitations, nervousness, gastrointestinal distress, and paresthesias may occur more fre-

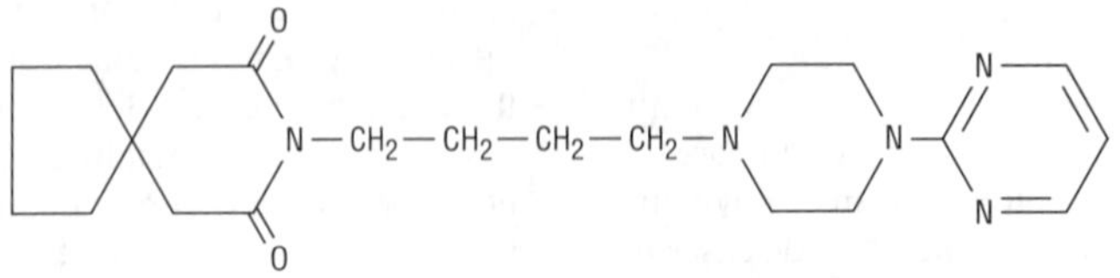

Buspirone

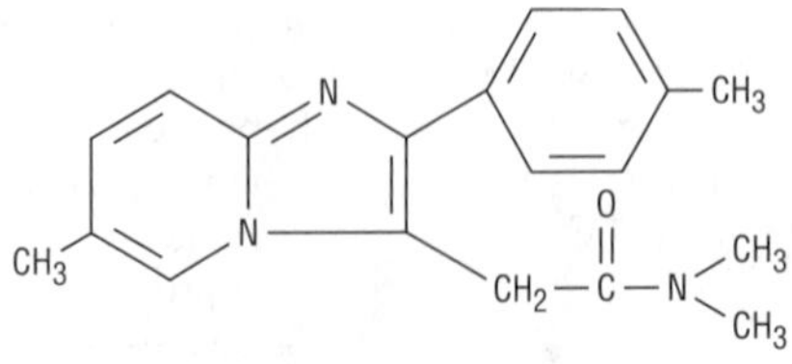

Zolpidem

quently than with benzodiazepines. Blood pressure may be elevated in patients receiving MAO inhibitors.

A number of buspirone analogues have been developed (eg, ipsapirone, gepirone, tandospirone) and are under study.

Zolpidem

Zolpidem is an imidazopyridine derivative, structurally unrelated to benzodiazepines. However, the drug binds to BDZ receptors and appears to have a similar mechanism of action to facilitate GABA-mediated inhibition. When used for the short-term treatment of insomnia, zolpidem has an efficacy and side effect profile similar to that of triazolam. No information is available on the development of tolerance and dependence with prolonged use of zolpidem. The drug is rapidly metabolized by the liver and has a half-life of approximately 2.4 hours. Dosage reductions are recommended in hepatic dysfunction and in the elderly patient.

OLDER SEDATIVE-HYPNOTICS

These drugs include alcohols (ethchlorvynol, chloral hydrate), piperidinediones (glutethimide, methyprylon), and carbamates (meprobamate) and even inorganic bromide ion. They are rarely used in therapy, though the low cost of chloral hydrate makes it attractive for institutional use. Little is known about their molecular mechanisms of action. Most of these drugs are biotransformed to more water-soluble compounds by hepatic enzymes. Trichloroethanol is the pharmacologically active metabolite of chloral hydrate and has a half-life of 6–10 hours. However, its toxic metabolite, trichloroacetic acid, is cleared very slowly and can accumulate with the nightly administration of chloral hydrate. Furthermore, recurrent concerns regarding the possible carcinogenicity of chloral hydrate itself—or its metabolites—suggest that this drug should not be used until more data are available.

II. CLINICAL PHARMACOLOGY OF SEDATIVE-HYPNOTICS

TREATMENT OF ANXIETY STATES

The psychologic, behavioral, and physiologic responses that characterize anxiety can take many forms. Classically, the psychic awareness of anxiety is accompanied by enhanced vigilance, motor tension, and autonomic hyperactivity. Before prescribing sedative-hypnotics, one should analyze the pa-

tient's symptoms carefully. Anxiety is in many cases secondary to organic disease states—acute myocardial infarction, angina pectoris, gastrointestinal ulcers, etc—which themselves require specific therapy. Another class of secondary anxiety states (situational anxiety) results from circumstances that may have to be dealt with only once or only a few times, including anticipation of frightening medical or dental procedures and family illness or other tragedy. Even though situational anxiety tends to be self-limiting, the *short-term use* of sedative-hypnotics may be appropriate for the treatment of this and certain disease-associated anxiety states. Similarly, the use of a sedative-hypnotic as premedication prior to surgery or some unpleasant medical procedure is rational and proper (Table 21–2). If the patient presents with chronic anxiety as the primary complaint, it may be appropriate to review the diagnostic criteria set forth in the *Diagnostic & Statistical Manual of Mental Disorders (DSM III-R)* to determine whether the diagnosis is correct and treatment should include drug therapy. For example, excessive or unreasonable anxiety about life circumstances (generalized anxiety disorder), panic disorders, and agoraphobia are amenable to drug therapy, usually in conjunction with psychotherapy. In some cases, anxiety may be a symptom of other psychiatric problems that may warrant the use of pharmacologic agents such as the tricyclic antidepressants or antipsychotic drugs.

The benzodiazepines are the drugs most commonly used for treatment of anxiety. In 1991, for example, alprazolam was the fifth most frequently prescribed proprietary drug in the United States, while lorazepam and diazepam ranked 18th and 20th, respectively, in terms of generic prescriptions. Although anxiety symptoms may be relieved by many sedatives, it is not always easy to demonstrate superiority of one drug over another. Thus, a preference for a particular drug in a specific situation is often based on factors other than anxiolytic efficacy. An exception to this generalization is alprazolam, which is particularly effective in the treatment of panic disorders and agoraphobia and is more selective in this regard than other benzodiazepines. The choice of benzodiazepines is based on several sound pharmacologic principles: (1) a relatively high therapeutic index (see drug

Table 21–2. Clinical uses of sedative-hypnotics.
For relief of anxiety.
Hypnosis.
For sedation and amnesia before medical and surgical procedures.
Treatment of epilepsy and seizure states.
Intravenous administration, as a component of balanced anesthesia.
For control of ethanol or other sedative-hypnotic withdrawal states.
For muscle relaxation in specific neuromuscular disorders.
As diagnostic aids or for treatment in psychiatry.

B in Figure 21–1), plus availability of flumazenil for treatment of overdose; (2) a low risk of drug interactions based on liver enzyme induction; (3) slow elimination rates, which may favor persistence of useful central nervous system effects; and (4) a low risk of physical dependence, with minor withdrawal symptoms.

Disadvantages of the benzodiazepines include the tendency to develop psychologic dependence, the formation of active metabolites, amnesic effects, and their higher cost. *The benzodiazepines exert additive central nervous system depression when administered with other drugs, including ethanol. This is true of all drugs of the sedative-hypnotic class except buspirone.* The patient should be warned of this possibility to avoid impairment of performance of any task requiring mental alertness and motor coordination.

Perhaps the most important guide to therapy is to use the drug selected with appropriate restraint to minimize adverse effects. A dose should be prescribed that does not impair mentation or motor functions during working hours. Some patients may tolerate the drug better if most of the daily dose is given at bedtime, with smaller doses during the day. Prescriptions should be written for short periods, since there is little justification for long-term therapy. The physician should make an effort to assess the efficacy of therapy from the patient's subjective responses. Plasma drug concentrations are too variable to be useful as a guide to dosage. Combinations of antianxiety agents should be avoided, and people taking sedatives should be cautioned about drinking alcohol and concurrent use of over-the-counter medications (see Chapter 65).

Although phenobarbital, meprobamate, and sedative-autonomic drugs (hydroxyzine, diphenhydramine) continue to be used occasionally as antianxiety agents, they have been almost completely—and justifiably—supplanted by the benzodiazepines.

The clinical use of beta-blocking drugs (eg, propranolol) as antianxiety agents has been suggested in a number of situations. The sympathetic nervous system overactivity associated with anxiety appears to be satisfactorily relieved by the beta-blockers, and a slight improvement in the nonsomatic components of anxiety may also occur. Studies comparing the effects of beta-blocking drugs with those of benzodiazepines have not demonstrated any significant therapeutic differences in efficacy for this indication. Adverse CNS effects of propranolol include lethargy, vivid dreams, and hallucinations.

The antihypertensive drug clonidine has also been used in the treatment of anxiety states, including panic attacks. Concomitant treatment with drugs that exert alpha-adrenoceptor-blocking actions (including tricyclic antidepressants) may decrease the effects of clonidine. Withdrawal from clonidine after protracted use, especially at high doses, has led to life-threatening hypertensive crisis (See Chapter 11).

TREATMENT OF SLEEP PROBLEMS

The complaint of insomnia embraces a wide variety of sleep problems that include difficulty in falling asleep, frequent awakenings, short duration of sleep, and "unrefreshing" sleep. Insomnia is a serious complaint calling for careful evaluation to uncover possible causes (organic, psychologic, situational, etc) that can perhaps be managed without hypnotic drugs. Nonpharmacologic therapies sometimes useful include proper diet and exercise, avoiding stimulants before retiring, ensuring a comfortable sleeping place, and retiring at a regular time each night. In some cases, however, the patient will need and should be given a sedative-hypnotic for a limited period. It should be noted that the discontinuance of any drug in this class can lead to rebound insomnia.

Claims have often been made for superiority of one sedative-hypnotic over another based on differential actions on one stage of sleep or another. Since little is known about the function of any sleep stage, statements about the desirability of a particular drug based on its effects on sleep patterns have no validity. Clearly, clinical criteria of efficacy in alleviating a particular sleeping problem are more useful. The ideal hypnotic drug that would promote sleep without any change in its natural pattern has yet to be introduced. The drug selected should be one that provides sleep of fairly rapid onset (decreased sleep latency) and sufficient duration, with minimal "hangover" effects such as drowsiness, dysphoria, and mental or motor depression the following day. While older drugs such as chloral hydrate, secobarbital, and pentobarbital are still used, a benzodiazepine is generally preferred. Daytime sedation is more common with benzodiazepines that have slow elimination rates and are biotransformed to active metabolites, eg, flurazepam. Conversely, early morning awakening may occur with a short-acting drug such as triazolam, the most frequently prescribed hypnotic drug in the United States. If hypnotics are used every night, tolerance can occur, leading to dose increases by the patient to produce the desired effect. It should be recalled that if physical dependence develops, the shorter-acting drugs are associated with more intense withdrawal signs when discontinued. These can include rebound anxiety and insomnia, restlessness, increased reflex activity, and possibly seizures. Anterograde amnesia occurs to some degree with all hypnotic benzodiazepines. The drugs commonly used for sedation and hypnosis are listed in Table 21–3 together with recommended doses. *Note: Long-term use of hypnotics is irrational and dangerous medical practice.*

Table 21–3. Dosages of drugs used commonly for sedation and hypnosis.

Sedation		Hypnosis	
Drug	Dosage	Drug	Dosage (at Bedtime)
Alprazolam (Xanax)	0.25–0.5 mg 2–3 times daily	Chloral hydrate	500–1000 mg
Chlordiazepoxide (Librium)	10–20 mg 2–3 times daily	Flurazepam (Dalmane)	15–30 mg
Clorazepate (Tranxene)	5–7.5 mg twice daily	Lorazepam (Ativan)	2–4 mg
Diazepam (Valium)	5 mg twice daily	Pentobarbital	100–200 mg
Lorazepam (Ativan)	1–2 mg once or twice daily	Secobarbital	100–200 mg
Oxazepam (Serax)	15–30 mg 3–4 times daily	Temazepam (Restoril)	10–30 mg
Phenobarbital	15–30 mg 2–3 times daily	Triazolam (Halcion)	0.125–0.5 mg
Prazepam (Centrax)	10–20 mg 2–3 times daily		

OTHER THERAPEUTIC USES

Table 21–2 summarizes several other important clinical uses of drugs in the sedative-hypnotic class. Drugs used in the management of seizure disorders and for intravenous anesthesia are discussed in Chapters 23 and 24.

For sedative and possible amnesic effects during medical or surgical procedures such as endoscopy and bronchoscopy—as well as premedication prior to anesthesia—oral formulations of shorter-acting drugs are preferred. When drug administration is under close supervision, the danger of accidental or intentional overdosage is less than in the outpatient situation, and a barbiturate may be as appropriate as any sedative-hypnotic.

Long-acting drugs such as diazepam and, to a lesser extent, chlordiazepoxide or phenobarbital are administered in progressively decreasing doses to patients during withdrawal from physical dependence on ethanol or other sedative-hypnotics.

Meprobamate and, more recently, the benzodiazepines have frequently been used as central muscle relaxants, though evidence for general efficacy without accompanying sedation is lacking. A possible exception is diazepam, which has useful relaxant effects in skeletal muscle spasticity of central origin (see Chapter 26).

Psychiatric uses of benzodiazepines other than treatment of anxiety states include the initial management of mania and perhaps the treatment of major depressive disorders with alprazolam. Sedative-hypnotics are also used occasionally as diagnostic aids in neurology and psychiatry.

CLINICAL TOXICOLOGY OF SEDATIVE-HYPNOTICS

Direct Toxic Actions

Many of the common adverse effects of drugs in this class are those resulting from dose-related depression of central nervous system functions. In am-bulatory patients, relatively low doses may lead to drowsiness, impaired judgment, and diminished motor skills, sometimes with a significant impact on driving skills, job performance, and personal relationships. Benzodiazepines cause a significant dose-related anterograde amnesia. These drugs can significantly impair ability to learn new information, particularly that involving effortful cognitive processes, while leaving the retrieval of previously learned information intact. (The effect is utilized to advantage in uncomfortable procedures, eg, endoscopy, since the appropriate dose leaves the patient able to cooperate during the procedure but amnesic regarding it afterward.) Hangover effects are not uncommon following use of drugs with long half-lives for sleep problems in such patients. Because elderly patients are more sensitive to the effects of sedative-hypnotics, doses approximately half those used conventionally are usually effective. The most common reversible cause of confusional states in the elderly is overuse of sedative-hypnotics. At higher doses, toxicity may present as lethargy or a state of exhaustion or, alternatively, in the form of gross symptoms equivalent to those of ethanol intoxication. The titration of useful therapeutic effects against such side effects is usually more difficult with sedative-hypnotics that exhibit steep dose-response relationships of the type shown in Figure 21–1 (drug A), including the barbiturates and piperidinediones. Unwanted depression of the CNS also occurs more frequently when therapy is continued for longer periods and when drugs with long half-lives and active metabolites are used. The physician should be aware of variability among patients in terms of doses causing adverse effects. A relatively small dose in one individual may result in a level of central nervous system depression that would require two or three times that dose in another patient. Variability is even more common in patients with cardiovascular or respiratory disease and hepatic impairment and in older patients.

Sedative-hypnotics are the drugs most frequently involved in deliberate overdoses, in part because of their general availability as very commonly prescribed pharmacologic agents. The benzodiazepines are considered to be "safer" drugs in this respect, since they have flatter dose-response curves. Epidemiologic studies on the incidence of drug-related deaths support this general assumption—eg, 0.3 deaths per million tablets of diazepam prescribed versus 11.6 deaths per million capsules of secobarbital in one study. Of course, many factors other than the specific sedative-hypnotic could influence such data—particularly the presence of other central nervous system depressants, including ethanol. In fact, most serious cases of drug overdosage, intentional or accidental, do involve polypharmacy; and when combinations of agents are taken, the practical safety of benzodiazepines may be less than the foregoing would imply.

The lethal dose of any sedative-hypnotic varies with the patient and the circumstances (Chapter 60). If discovery of the ingestion is made early and a conservative treatment regimen is started, the outcome is rarely fatal, even following very high doses. On the other hand, for most sedative-hypnotics—with the exception of benzodiazepines—a dose as low as ten times the hypnotic dose may be fatal if the patient is not discovered or does not seek help in time. With severe toxicity, the respiratory depression from central actions of the drug may be complicated by aspiration of gastric contents in the unattended patient—an even more likely occurrence if ethanol is present. Loss of brain stem vasomotor control, together with direct myocardial depression, further complicates successful resuscitation. In such patients, treatment consists of mechanical ventilation; maintenance of plasma volume, renal output, and cardiac function; and perhaps use of a positive inotropic drug such as dopamine, which preserves renal blood flow. Hemodialysis or hemoperfusion may be used to hasten elimination of some of these drugs (see Table 60–4). Flumazenil reverses the sedative actions of benzodiazepines. However, its duration of action is short and its antagonism of respiratory depression unpredictable. Therefore, the use of flumazenil in benzodiazepine overdose *must* be accompanied by adequate monitoring and support of respiratory function.

Adverse effects of the sedative-hypnotics that are not referable to their CNS actions occur infrequently. Hypersensitivity reactions, including skin rashes, occur only occasionally with most drugs of this class. Reports of teratogenicity leading to fetal deformation following use of piperidinediones and certain benzodiazepines justify caution in the use of these drugs during pregnancy. Because barbiturates enhance porphyrin synthesis, they are absolutely contraindicated in patients with a history of acute intermittent porphyria, variegate porphyria, hereditary coproporphyria, or symptomatic porphyria.

Alterations in Drug Response

Depending on the dosage and the duration of use,

tolerance occurs in varying degrees to many of the pharmacologic effects of sedative-hypnotics. This can be demonstrated experimentally during chronic use in humans by changes in the effects of these drugs on the electroencephalogram and other characteristics of the stages of sleep. Clearly, it must occur with respect to other effects, since it is known that chronic abusers sometimes ingest quantities of sedative-hypnotics many times the conventional dosage without experiencing severe toxicity. However, it should not be assumed that the degree of tolerance achieved is identical for all pharmacologic effects: There is evidence that lethal dose ranges are not altered significantly by the chronic use of sedative-hypnotics. Cross-tolerance between the different sedative-hypnotics, including ethanol, can lead to an unsatisfactory therapeutic response when standard doses of a drug are used in a patient with a recent history of excessive use of these agents.

With the chronic use of sedative-hypnotics, especially if doses are increased, a state of physical dependence can occur. This may develop to a degree unparalleled by any other drug group, *including the opioids.* Withdrawal from a sedative-hypnotic can have severe and life-threatening manifestations. Withdrawal symptoms range from restlessness, anxiety, weakness, and orthostatic hypotension to hyperactive reflexes and generalized seizures. The severity of withdrawal symptoms depends to a large extent on the dosage range used immediately prior to discontinuance but also on the particular drug. For example, barbiturates such as secobarbital or pentobarbital (in doses < 400 mg/d) or diazepam (at < 40 mg/d) may produce only mild symptoms of withdrawal when discontinued. On the other hand, the use of more than 800 mg/d of barbiturates or 50–60 mg/d of diazepam for 60–90 days is likely to result in seizures if abrupt withdrawal is attempted. Symptoms of withdrawal are usually more severe following discontinuance of sedative-hypnotics with shorter half-lives. Symptoms are less pronounced with longer-acting drugs, which may partly accomplish their own withdrawal by virtue of their slow elimination. Cross-dependence, defined as the ability of one drug to suppress abstinence symptoms from discontinuance of another drug, is quite marked among sedative-hypnotics. This provides the rationale for therapeutic regimens in the management of withdrawal states: Longer-acting drugs such as phenobarbital and diazepam can be used to alleviate withdrawal symptoms of shorter-acting drugs, including ethanol.

Drug Interactions

The most frequent drug interactions involving sedative-hypnotics are interactions with other central nervous system depressant drugs, leading to additive effects. These interactions have some therapeutic utility with respect to the use of these drugs as premedicants or anesthetic adjuvants. However, if not anticipated, they can lead to serious consequences, including enhanced depression with concomitant use of many other drugs. Obvious additive effects can be predicted with use of alcoholic beverages, narcotic analgesics, anticonvulsants, phenothiazines, and other sedative-hypnotic drugs. Less obvious but just as important is enhanced central nervous system depression with a variety of antihistamines, antihypertensive agents, and antidepressant drugs of the tricyclic class.

Interactions involving changes in the activity of hepatic drug-metabolizing enzyme systems can occur, especially following continuous use of barbiturates and meprobamate. For example, in humans, barbiturates have been shown to increase the rate of metabolism of dicumarol, phenytoin, digitalis compounds, and griseofulvin—effects that could lead to decrease in response to these agents. This type of drug interaction has not been reported following continuous use of benzodiazepines. Cimetidine, which is known to inhibit hepatic metabolism of many drugs, doubles the elimination half-life of diazepam, presumably via inhibition of its metabolism. As mentioned above, chloral hydrate may displace warfarin from plasma proteins to cause enhanced anticoagulant effects.

PREPARATIONS AVAILABLE

Benzodiazepines
Alprazolam (Xanax)
  Oral: 0.25, 0.5, 1, 2 mg tablets
Chlordiazepoxide (generic, Librium, others)
  Oral: 5, 10, 25 mg tablets, capsules
  Parenteral: 100 mg powder for injection
Clorazepate (Tranxene)
  Oral: 3.75, 7.5, 15 mg tablets and capsules
  Oral sustained-release: 11.25, 22.5 mg tablets
  Parenteral: 100 mg powder to reconstitute for injection
Clonazepam (Klonopin)
  Oral: 0.5, 1, 2 mg tablets
Diazepam (generic, Valium, others)
  Oral: 2, 5, 10 mg tablets; 5 mg/5 mL, 5 mg/mL solutions
  Oral sustained-release: 15 mg capsules
  Parenteral: 5 mg/mL for injection
Estazolam (ProSom)
  Oral: 1, 2 mg tablets
Flurazepam (generic, Dalmane)
  Oral: 15, 30 mg capsules
Halazepam (Paxipam)
  Oral: 20, 40 mg tablets
Lorazepam (generic, Ativan, Alzapam)
  Oral: 0.5, 1, 2 mg tablets
  Parenteral: 2, 4 mg/mL for injection
Midazolam (Versed)
  Parenteral: 1, 5 mg/mL in 1, 2, 5, 10 mL vials for injection
Oxazepam (generic, Serax)
  Oral: 10, 15, 30 mg capsules, 15 mg tablets
Prazepam (Centrax)
  Oral: 5, 10, 20 mg capsules, 10 mg tablets
Quazepam (Doral)
  Oral: 7.5,15 mg tablets
Temazepam (generic, Restoril)
  Oral: 15, 30 mg capsules
Triazolam (Halcion)
  Oral: 0.125, 0.25 mg tablets

Benzodiazepine Antagonist
Flumazenil (Romazicon)
  Parenteral: 0.1 mg/mL for IV injection

Barbiturates
Amobarbital (generic, Amytal)
  Oral: 30, 50, 100 mg tablets (base); 65, 200 mg capsules (sodium salt)
  Parenteral: powder in 250, 500 mg vials to reconstitute for injection
Aprobarbital (Alurate)
  Oral: 40 mg/5 mL elixir
Butabarbital sodium (generic, Butisol, others)
  Oral: 15, 30, 50, 100 mg tablets; 15, 30 mg capsules; 30, 33.3 mg/5 mL elixirs
Mephobarbital (Mebaral)
  Oral: 32, 50, 100 mg tablets
Metharbital (Gemonil)
  Oral: 100 mg tablets
Pentobarbital (generic, Nembutal Sodium)
  Oral: 50, 100 mg capsules; 18.2 mg/5 mL elixir
  Rectal: 30, 60, 120, 200 mg suppositories
  Parenteral: 50 mg/mL for injection
Phenobarbital (generic, Luminal Sodium, others)
  Oral: 8, 16, 32, 65, 100 mg tablets; 16 mg capsules; 15, 20 mg/5 mL elixirs
  Parenteral: 30, 60, 65, 130 mg/mL for injection; powder in 120 mg ampules to reconstitute for injection
Secobarbital (generic, Seconal)
  Oral: 50, 100 mg capsules; 100 mg tablets
  Rectal: 50 mg/mL
  Parenteral: 50 mg/mL for injection
Talbutal (Lotusate)
  Oral: 120 mg tablets

Miscellaneous Drugs
Buspirone (BuSpar)
  Oral: 5, 10 mg tablets
Chloral hydrate (generic, Noctec, Aquachloral Supprettes)

Oral: 250, 500 mg capsules; 250, 500 mg/5 mL syrups

Rectal: 324, 500, 648 mg suppositories

Ethchlorvynol (Placidyl)

Oral: 200, 500, 750 mg capsules

Ethinamate (Valmid Pulvules)

Oral: 500 mg capsules

Glutethimide (generic, Doriden)

Oral: 250, 500 mg tablets

Hydroxyzine (generic, Atarax, Vistaril)

Oral: 10, 25, 50, 100 mg tablets; 25, 50, 100 mg capsules; 10 mg/5 mL syrup; 25 mg/5 mL suspension

Parenteral: 25, 50 mg/mL for injection

Meprobamate (generic, Miltown, Equanil, others)

Oral: 200, 400, 600 mg tablets

Oral sustained-release: 200, 400 mg capsules

Methyprylon (Noludar)

Oral: 200 mg tablets; 300 mg capsules

Paraldehyde (generic)

Oral, rectal liquids

Zolpidem (Ambien)

Oral: 5, 10 mg tablets

REFERENCES

Ballenger JC: Pharmacotherapy of the panic disorders. J Clin Psychiatry 1986;47(Suppl):27.

Barrett JE, Vanover KE: 5-HT receptors as targets for the development of novel anxiolytic drugs: Models, mechanisms, and future directions. Psychopharmacology 1993; 112:1.

Bansky G et al: Effects of the benzodiazepine antagonist flumazenil in hepatic encephalopathy in humans. Gastroenterology 1989;97:744.

Basile AS et al: Elevated brain concentrations of 1,4-benzodiazepines in fulminant hepatic failure. N Engl J Med 1991;325:473.

Colburn WA, Jack ML: Relationships between CSF drug concentrations, receptor binding characteristics, and pharmacokinetic and pharmacodynamic properties of selected 1,4-substituted benzodiazepines. Clin Pharmacokinet 1987;13:179.

Dubovsky SL: Generalized anxiety disorder: New concepts and psychopharmacologic therapies. J Clin Psychiatry 1990;51(Suppl):3.

Eison AS, Temple DL Jr: Buspirone: Review of its pharmacology and current perspectives on its mechanism of action. Am J Med 1986;80 (Suppl 3B):1.

Garzone PD, Kroboth PD: Pharmacokinetics of the newer benzodiazepines. Clin Pharmacokinet 1989;16:337.

Ghonheim MM, Mewaldt SP: Benzodiazepines and human memory: A review. Anesthesiology 1990;72:926.

Gillin JC et al: Rebound insomnia: A critical review. J Clin Psychopharmacol 1989;9:161.

Gillin JC, Byerly WF: The diagnosis and management of sleep disorders. N Engl J Med 1990;322:239.

Gottlieb GL: Sleep disorders and their management. Special considerations in the elderly. Am J Med 1990;88(Suppl 3B):29S.

Greenblatt DJ, Harmatz JS, Shader RI: Clinical pharmacokinetics of anxiolytics and hypnotics in the elderly. Clin Pharmacokinet 1991;21:165.

Greenblatt DJ et al: Pharmacokinetic determinants of dynamic differences among three benzodiazepine hypnotics. Arch Gen Psychiatry 1989;46:326.

Horne AL et al: The influence of the γ_2L subunit on the modulation of responses to GABA$_A$ receptor activation. Br J Pharmacol 1993;108:711.

Jochemsen R et al: Kinetics of five benzodiazepine hypnotics in healthy subjects. Clin Pharmacol Ther 1983;34:42.

Kales A et al: Diazepam: Effects on sleep and withdrawal phenomena. J Clin Psychopharmacol 1988;8:340.

Lader M: Long-term anxiolytic therapy: The issue of drug withdrawal. J Clin Psychiatry 1987;48 (Suppl):12.

Lader M: Rebound insomnia and newer hypnotics. Psychopharmacology 1990;108:248.

Langtry HD, Benfield P: Zolpidem: A review of its pharmacodynamic and pharmacokinetic properties and therapeutic potential. Drugs 1990;40:291.

Lin L-H, Whiting P, Harris RA: Molecular determinants of general anesthetic action: Role of GABA$_A$ receptor structure. J Neurochem 1993;60:1548

Lydiard RB et al: A fixed dose study of alprazolam 2 mg, alprazolam 6 mg, and placebo in panic disorder. J Clin Psychopharmacol 1992;12:96.

Melander A et al: Anxiolytic-hypnotic drugs: Relationships between prescribing, abuse and suicide. Eur J Clin Pharmacol 1991;41:525.

Mohler H, Richards JG: The benzodiazepine receptor: A pharmacological control element of brain function. Eur J Anaesthesiol 1988;2(Suppl):15.

Novas ML et al: Proconvulsant and "anxiogenic" effects of N-butyl-carboline-3-carboxylate, a potent benzodiazepine binding inhibitor. Pharmacol Biochem Behav 1988; 30:331.

Olsen RW, Tobin AJ: Molecular biology of GABA$_A$ receptors. FASEB J 1990;4:1469.

Prinz PN et al: Geriatrics: Sleep disorders and aging. N Engl J Med 1990;323:520.

Pritchett D et al: Importance of a novel GABA$_A$ subunit for benzodiazepine pharmacology. Nature (Lond) 1989;338: 582.

Rickels K: Buspirone in clinical practice. J Clin Psychiatry 1990; 5(Suppl):51.

Rothstein JD et al: Purification and characterization of naturally occurring benzodiazepine receptor ligands in rat and human brain. J. Neurochem 1992; 58:2102.

Scharf MB, Saschais BA: The pharmacology of disordered sleep. In: *Textbook of Clinical Neuropharmacology and Therapeutics*. Klawans HL et al (editors). Raven Press, 1992.

Sheehan DV: Benzodiazepines in panic disorder and agoraphobia. J Affective Disord 1987;13:169.

Sieghart W: GABA$_A$ receptors: Ligand-gated Cl$^-$ ion channels modulated by multiple drug-binding sites. Trends Pharmacol Sci 1992;13:446.

Sloan JW, Martin WR, Wala E: Effect of the chronic dose of diazepam on the intensity and characteristics of the precipitated abstinence syndrome in the dog. J Pharmacol Exp Therap 1993;265:1152.

Smith MC, Riskin BJ: The clinical use of barbiturates in neurological disorders. Drugs 1991;42:365.

Taylor DP: Buspirone: A new approach to the treatment of anxiety. FASEB J 1988;2:2445.

Taylor DP, Moon SL: Buspirone and related compounds as alternative anxiolytics. Neuropeptides 1991;19(Suppl): 15.

Twyman RE et al: Differential regulation of GABA receptor channels by diazepam and phenobarbital. Ann Neurol 1989;25:213.

Unseld E et al: Occurrence of "natural" diazepam in human brain. Biochem Pharmacol 1990;38:2473.

van Laar MW, Volkerts ER, van Willigenburg PP: Therapeutic effects and effects on actual driving performance of chronically administered buspirone and diazepam in anxious outpatients. J Clin Psychopharmacol 1992; 12:86.

Votey SR et al: Flumazenil: A new benzodiazepine antagonist. Ann Emerg Med 1991;20:181.

Wafford KA, Whiting PJ, Kemp JA: Differences in affinity and efficacy of benzodiazepine receptor ligands at recombinant γ-aminobutyric acid-A receptor subtypes. Mol Pharmacol 1993;43:240.

Woods JH et al: Abuse liability of benzodiazepines. Pharmacol Rev 1987;39:251.

Woods JH et al: Use and abuse of benzodiazepines: Issues relevant to prescribing. JAMA 1988;260:3476.

Wysowsky DK, Baum C: Outpatient use of prescription sedative-hypnotic drugs in the United States, 1970 through 1989. Arch Intern Med 1991;151:1779.

Zorumsky CF, Isenberg KE: Insights into the structure and function of GABA-benzodiazepine receptors: Ion channels and psychiatry. Am J Psychiatry 1991;148:162.

22

The Alcohols

Nancy M. Lee, PhD, & Charles E. Becker, MD

Ethyl alcohol (ethanol) is a sedative-hypnotic consumed as a social drug. Alcohol abuse (alcoholism) is a complex disorder whose natural history and basic causes are not well defined. It is a major medical and public health problem in many societies.

Ethanol and many other alcohols with potentially toxic effects are used in industry, some in enormous quantities. In addition to ethanol, methanol and ethylene glycol toxicity occur with sufficient frequency to warrant discussion in this chapter.

I. BASIC PHARMACOLOGY OF ETHANOL

ETHANOL

Pharmacokinetics

Ethanol (C_2H_5OH) is a small water-soluble molecule that is absorbed rapidly and completely from the gastrointestinal tract. Ethanol vapor can also be readily absorbed in the lungs. After ingestion of alcohol in the fasting state, peak blood levels are reached within 30 minutes. The presence of food in the gut delays absorption. Distribution is rapid, with tissue levels approximating the blood concentration. The volume of distribution is approximately 0.7 L/kg.

Over 90% of alcohol consumed is oxidized in the liver; the rest is excreted through the lungs and in urine. At usual clinical doses, the rate of oxidation follows zero-order kinetics, ie, it is independent of time and concentration of the drug. The amount of alcohol oxidized per unit time is approximately proportionate to body weight or liver weight, and the rate of disappearance of alcohol from the body is markedly reduced or halted entirely by hepatectomy or liver damage. However, the typical adult can metabolize 7–10 g (0.15–0.22 mol) of alcohol per hour. Two pathways of alcohol metabolism to acetaldehyde

have been proposed. Acetaldehyde is then oxidized by a third metabolic process (Geokas, 1984).

A. Alcohol Dehydrogenase Pathway: The main pathway for alcohol metabolism involves alcohol dehydrogenase, a cytosolic enzyme that contains zinc and catalyzes the conversion of alcohol to acetaldehyde, according to the following reaction:

$$C_2H_5OH + NAD^+ \xrightarrow{\text{Alcohol dehydrogenase}} CH_3CHO + NADH + H^+$$

This enzyme is located mainly in the liver; however, it can also be found in other organs such as brain and stomach.

A significant amount of ethanol metabolism by gastric alcohol dehydrogenase occurs in the stomach in men but a much smaller amount in women, who appear to have lower levels of this enzyme. As a result, women have higher blood alcohol levels than men after oral doses of ethanol, but after intravenous injection the sexes do not differ (Frezza et al, 1990).

In the reaction shown above, hydrogen ion is transferred from alcohol to the cofactor nicotinamide adenine dinucleotide (NAD) to form NADH. As a net result, alcohol oxidation generates an excess of reducing equivalents in the liver, chiefly as NADH. There is some controversy over whether chronic alcohol consumption affects the activities of hepatic alcohol dehydrogenase. Actually, alcohol dehydrogenase itself is not rate-limiting, but the velocity of oxidation may depend on the availability of the cofactor NAD; therefore, the increased rate of blood alcohol clearance in alcoholics is probably not due to increased alcohol dehydrogenase activity. 4-Methylpyrazole (fomepizole), a compound with orphan drug status as an antidote in methanol and ethylene glycol poisoning, is a potent inhibitor of alcohol dehydrogenase (Baud et al, 1986).

B. Microsomal Ethanol Oxidizing System (MEOS): This enzyme system, also known as the mixed function oxidase system (Chapter 4), uses

NADPH instead of NAD as cofactor in the following reaction:

$$C_2H_5OH + NADPH + H^+ + O_2 \xrightarrow{\boxed{\text{MEOS}}} CH_3CHO + NADP^+ + 2 H_2O$$

Since the K_m varies from 0.26 to 2 mmol/L for alcohol dehydrogenase and from 8 to 10 mmol/L for microsomal ethanol oxidizing system, it is thought that at concentrations of alcohol below 100 mg% (22 mmol/L), alcohol dehydrogenase is the main oxidizing system while at higher alcohol concentrations MEOS plays the more significant role. During chronic alcohol consumption, MEOS activity increases significantly. As described in Chapter 4, this induction of enzyme activity is associated with an increase in various constituents of the smooth fraction of the membranes involved in drug metabolism. As a result, chronic alcohol consumption can result in significant increases in the clearance of drugs that are eliminated by hepatic microsomal enzyme systems. Similarly, other "inducing" drugs such as barbiturates may also enhance the rate of blood alcohol clearance slightly. However, the effect of other drugs on ethanol clearance is less important, because the MEOS is not the primary pathway for ethanol.

C. Acetaldehyde Metabolism: It is now generally accepted that over 90% of the acetaldehyde formed from alcohol is also oxidized in the liver. While several enzyme systems may be responsible for this reaction, observations that acetaldehyde levels in the liver after ethanol administration are only 100–350 μmol/L have led to the conclusion that mitochondrial NAD-dependent aldehyde dehydrogenase (the apparent K_m for acetaldehyde is about 10 μmol/L) is the main pathway for acetaldehyde oxidation. The product of this reaction is acetate, which can be further metabolized to CO_2 and water. Chronic alcohol consumption results in a decreased rate of acetaldehyde oxidation in intact mitochondria, though the enzyme activity is unaffected.

Tolerance & Physical Dependence

The consumption of alcohol in high doses over a long period results in tolerance and physical dependence. Tolerance to the intoxicating effects of alcohol is a complex process involving changes in metabolism and poorly understood changes in the nervous system. Some recent studies suggest that tolerance may be associated with alterations in an adenosine transporter, resulting in a change in receptor-stimulated cAMP levels (Nagy et al, 1990). Acute tolerance may occur after a few hours of drinking; this may occur in both alcoholics and social drinkers. Although minor degrees of metabolic tolerance after chronic alcohol use have been demonstrated in which the subject's capacity to metabolize the drug increases, the maximal increase in alcohol metabolism is insufficient to account for the magnitude of the observed clinical tolerance. Finally, as with other sedative-hypnotic drugs, there is a limit to tissue tolerance, so that only a relatively small increase in the lethal dose occurs with increasing exposure.

Chronic alcohol drinkers, when forced to reduce or discontinue alcohol, experience a withdrawal syndrome, which indicates the existence of physical dependence. Although the mechanism of physical dependence for sedative-hypnotic drugs and alcohol is not known, it is recognized that the dose, rate, and duration of alcohol consumption determine the intensity of the withdrawal syndrome. When consumption has been very high, merely reducing the rate of consumption may lead to signs of withdrawal. Although tolerance and physical dependence are important components of alcohol abuse, the spectrum of illness associated with abuse of alcohol is so broad that it is difficult to create a simple definition of the phenomenon.

Pharmacodynamics of Acute Ethanol Consumption

A. Central Nervous System: The central nervous system is markedly affected by acute alcohol consumption. Alcohol can lead to sedation and relief of anxiety, slurred speech, ataxia, impaired judgment, uninhibited behavior, usually called drunkenness. These effects are most marked as the blood level is rising.

Ethanol may affect a large number of molecular processes, but it is now generally accepted that two of its most significant sites of action are the cell membranes and enzymes found in the brain. It has been pointed out that small organic molecules such as ethanol can readily dissolve in the lipid bilayer of cell membranes. Studies have confirmed that ethanol reduces the viscosity of ("fluidizes") the membrane of many types of cells and even of artificial systems such as liposomes. Fluidization is thus a general response to ethanol of virtually all biologic membranes and one that is likely to contribute to the great diversity of the drug's effects. It is not surprising that the fluidizing effect of ethanol has been related to changes in a broad variety of membrane functions, including neurotransmitter receptors for dopamine, norepinephrine, glutamate, and opioids; enzymes such as Na^+/K^+ ATPase, Ca^{2+} ATPase, 5'-nucleotidase, acetylcholinesterase, and adenylyl cyclase; the mitochondrial electron transport chain; and ion channels such as those for Ca^{2+} (Lee, 1986). Chronic alcohol use in humans has been reported to alter the activity of two enzymes, monoamine oxidase and adenylyl cyclase, in platelets (Tabakoff et al, 1988). These alterations may be valuable markers of excess alcohol consumption and perhaps of predisposition to alcoholism.

Ethanol may also have direct effects on receptor-operated ion channels and transport molecules associated with the cell membrane. For example, acute ethanol exposure has been reported to increase the number of GABA receptors, which is consistent with the ability of GABA-mimetics to intensify many of the acute effects of alcohol. Ethanol also inhibits the NMDA subtype of glutamate receptors in mammalian brain cells and activates a phosphoinositide-specific phospholipase C in hepatocytes.

Alcohol also has diverse effects at the cellular and tissue levels, particularly in the nervous system. In trigeminal motoneurons, both intracellular and extracellular application of ethanol depress action potentials and excitatory and inhibitory postsynaptic potentials (EPSPs and IPSPs); intracellular application also depolarizes the membrane, while extracellular application results in biphasic potential shifts. Similarly, ethanol has been reported to both reduce and enhance function at the neuromuscular junction.

In cerebellar Purkinje cells and in the dopamine-containing neurons in the substantia nigra, pars compacta, and striate nucleus, low concentrations of ethanol enhance the firing rate while higher doses inhibit it. In other systems, including the lateral geniculate nucleus, the locus ceruleus, the midbrain raphe nucleus, and hippocampal neurons in culture, only inhibitory effects have been observed. More complex neuronal responses are similarly affected. For example, both the after-discharge following high-frequency stimulation of hippocampal neurons and the frog spinal reflex are enhanced by low doses of ethanol and inhibited by higher doses (Lee, 1986).

B. Heart: Significant depression of myocardial contractility has been observed in individuals who consume moderate amounts of alcohol, ie, at a blood concentration above 100 mg/dL. Myocardial biopsies in humans before and after infusion of small amounts of alcohol have shown ultrastructural changes that may be associated with impaired myocardial function. Acetaldehyde is implicated as a cause of heart abnormalities by altering myocardial stores of catecholamines. Careful studies in animals also document the detrimental effects of ethanol on cardiac muscle. Interestingly, one such study also suggests that ethanol can reduce the injury sustained by myocardium during anoxia.

C. Smooth Muscle: Ethanol is a vasodilator, probably as a result of both central nervous system effects (depression of the vasomotor center) and direct smooth muscle relaxation caused by its metabolite, acetaldehyde. In cases of severe overdose, hypothermia consequent to vasodilation may be marked in cold environments. Ethanol also relaxes the uterus and was formerly used intravenously for the suppression of premature labor. However, the acute maternal toxicity of ethanol and the hazard to the fetus should relegate this therapeutic application to history, since other drugs (calcium blockers, magnesium ion, β_2-adrenoceptor stimulants, and other drugs) appear to be more effective.

Consequences of Chronic Alcohol Consumption

The literature on alcoholism contains only limited data relating to precise dose-response relationships between chronic alcohol ingestion and injury of vital organ systems. However, several major studies with appropriate controls have demonstrated that the threshold for increased mortality rate is in the range of admitted regular alcohol intake of three to five drinks a day. The risk rises sharply at six or more drinks a day. Deaths linked to alcohol consumption are caused by liver disease, cancer, accidents, and suicide.

A. Liver and Gastrointestinal Tract: Alcohol in large doses creates a metabolic cascade effect, resulting in liver and gastrointestinal tract injury. The increased NADH/NAD ratio described above is dependent on the availability of NAD. It has been proposed that this altered ratio of NADH to NAD leads to a number of metabolic abnormalities in the liver, including reduced gluconeogenesis, hypoglycemia and ketoacidosis, and accumulation of fat in the liver parenchyma. Other factors such as heredity, associated disease, and the amount and duration of alcohol intake probably determine the severity of liver injury. Acetaldehyde also adversely affects liver function. Since metabolism of acetaldehyde via aldehyde dehydrogenase results in the generation of NADH, some of the acetaldehyde effects may be attributable to NADH excess. Acetaldehyde, however, is a very reactive compound that may have toxic effects of its own.

In some cases, nutritional factors are critical in alcohol-induced liver disease. It has been suggested that essential factors such as glutathione may be decreased in a malnourished alcoholic, thus removing a valuable scavenger of toxic free radicals that otherwise will injure the liver. Hormonal factors may also contribute to this disease, because female alcoholics are at greater risk for alcohol-induced liver dysfunction than male alcoholics. Clinically significant alcoholic liver disease may be insidious in onset and progress without evidence of overt nutritional abnormalities. Alcoholic fatty liver may progress to alcoholic hepatitis and finally to cirrhosis. Hepatic failure may be the cause of death.

Other portions of the gastrointestinal tract may also be injured. Ingestion of alcohol increases gastric and pancreatic secretion and alters mucosal barriers that enhance the risk of gastritis and pancreatitis. Acute gastrointestinal bleeding is often caused by alcoholic gastritis. The acute effects of alcohol on the stomach are related primarily to the toxic effect of ethanol on the mucosal membranes and have relatively little to do with increased production of gastric acid. Chronic alcoholics are prone to develop gastritis and increased susceptibility to blood and plasma protein loss during drinking, which may contribute to anemia and protein malnutrition. Alcohol also reversibly injures the small intestine, leading to diarrhea, weight loss, and multiple vitamin deficiencies.

The statement sometimes made that malnutrition of alcoholic patients is due simply to dietary deficiency is probably not justified. Malabsorption of vitamins, especially water-soluble ones, contributes to the clinical abnormalities. Although deficiencies in water-soluble vitamins were proposed in the past to account for most of the pathologic effects of alcohol, replacement doses of the vitamins do not completely protect against the injurious effects of alcohol. Thiamine deficiency, associated with Wernicke-Korsa-koff syndrome, peripheral neuropathy, and beriberi heart disease, occurs in alcoholic patients, yet these severe nutritional deficiency syndromes are relatively rare in the alcoholic population.

B. Nervous System: As noted above, chronic ethanol consumption produces tolerance and physical dependence; when forced to reduce or discontinue the drug, the subject experiences withdrawal symptoms, which may consist of hyperexcitability in mild cases and convulsions, toxic psychosis, and delirium tremens in severe ones. Acute and chronic alcohol consumption often leads to impairment of recent memory. Consumption of large amounts of alcohol over extended periods (usually years) can also result in a number of neurologic deficits. The patient may have impairment of intellectual and motor functions, emotional lability, reduced perceptual acuity, and amnesia.

The most frequent neurologic abnormality in chronic alcoholism is a generalized symmetric peripheral nerve injury that begins with distal paresthesias of the hands and feet. While this is a diagnosis of exclusion requiring absence of other factors known to cause peripheral neuropathy, such neuropathies are commonly related to chronic alcohol use.

Wernicke-Korsakoff syndrome is a relatively uncommon but important entity characterized by paralysis of the external eye muscles, ataxia, and altered mentation, with amnesia and impairment of memory function. It is apparently associated with thiamine deficiency but is rarely seen in the absence of alcoholism. Wernicke-Korsakoff disease may be difficult to distinguish from the acute confusional state created by acute alcohol intoxication, which later blends in with the perceptual and behavioral problems associated with alcohol withdrawal. A distinguishing feature is the longer duration of the confusional state in Korsakoff's disease and the relative absence of the agitation that would be expected during withdrawal. Because of the importance of this pathologic condition, all patients suspected of Korsakoff's disease should receive thiamine therapy (50 mg intravenously once and 50 mg intramuscularly repeated daily until a normal diet is resumed).

Alcohol may also impair visual acuity, with painless bilateral blurring that occurs over several weeks of heavy alcohol consumption. Examination may reveal scotomas and reduced visual acuity for near and distant objects. Changes are usually bilateral and symmetric and may be followed by optic nerve degeneration. Ingestion of ethanol substitutes such as methanol (see page 358) causes severe visual disturbances.

C. Blood: Mild anemia resulting from alcohol-related folic acid deficiency is the most common hematologic disorder resulting from chronic alcohol abuse. Iron deficiency anemia may result from gastrointestinal bleeding, but sideroblastic anemia has also been described in alcoholic patients. Alcohol has also been implicated as a cause of several hemolytic syndromes, some of which are associated with hyperlipidemia and severe liver disease. Alcohol directly inhibits the proliferation of all cellular elements in bone marrow.

Abnormalities in platelets and leukocytes have been described in alcoholics. These effects may account for some of the hemostatic impairment and increased frequency of infection in these individuals.

D. Cardiovascular System: Alcohol alters the cardiovascular system in many ways. Direct injury to the myocardium resulting from alcohol abuse was thought to be caused by thiamine deficiency or by contaminants in alcoholic beverages. Alcohol cardiomyopathy is now thought to occur in men with a history of heavy drinking episodes over prolonged periods regardless of vitamin or other dietary deficiencies. Arrhythmias have been reported in association with "social" drinking and during the alcohol abstinence syndrome.

The amount of alcohol intake appears to be directly related to elevated blood pressure, independent of obesity, salt intake, coffee drinking, or cigarette smoking. Although magnesium deficiency has also been associated with changes in blood pressure and alcohol intake, convincing data are not yet available to link these two observations. Current data do not establish the threshold of alcohol administration that causes alterations of electrolyte balance.

Curiously, the incidence of coronary heart disease has been reported to be lower in modest consumers of alcohol (one to three drinks a day) than in those who totally abstain (Suh et al, 1992). Evidence also suggests that alcohol elevates plasma levels of the HDL_3 fraction of high-density lipoproteins (Haskell et al, 1984). However, HDL_2, which is less dense, is epidemiologically associated with reduction of heart disease risk, while the denser HDL_3 is not clearly related to heart disease. When alcohol use is associated with liver disease, HDL fractions decrease. The clinical significance of this information is not fully understood. The purported cardiovascular protective effects of specific beverages, eg, red wine, require further study.

Patients undergoing alcohol withdrawal can develop severe arrhythmias that may reflect abnormalities of potassium or magnesium metabolism. Seizures and syncope as well as sudden death during alcohol withdrawal may be due to these arrhythmias.

E. Endocrine System: Chronic alcohol use has important effects on the endocrine system and mineral and fluid electrolyte balance. Clinical reports of gynecomastia and testicular atrophy in alcoholics with cirrhosis suggest a derangement in steroid hormone balance. Gynecomastia and testicular atrophy have also been noted in alcoholics who have limited evidence of liver disease.

Alcoholics with chronic liver disease may have disorders of fluid and electrolyte balance, including ascites, edema, and effusions. These factors may be related to decreased protein synthesis and portal hypertension. Alterations of whole body potassium induced by vomiting and diarrhea, as well as severe secondary aldosteronism, may contribute to muscle weakness and can be worsened by diuretic therapy. Abnormalities of trace metals such as zinc may also contribute to metabolic difficulties and infertility. Some alcoholic patients develop hypoglycemia, probably as a result of impaired hepatic gluconeogenesis. Some alcoholics also develop ketosis, caused by excessive lipolytic factors, especially increased cortisol and growth hormone.

F. Fetal Alcohol Syndrome: Chronic maternal alcohol abuse during pregnancy is associated with important teratogenic effects on the offspring (Abel, 1981; Ernhart et al, 1987). The abnormalities that have been characterized as fetal alcohol syndrome include (1) retarded body growth; (2) microcephaly (small head size relative to body size); (3) poor coordination; (4) underdevelopment of midfacial region (appearing as a flattened face); and (5) minor joint anomalies. More severe cases may include congenital heart defects and mental retardation. It is likely that heavy drinking in the first trimester of pregnancy has the greatest effect on fetal maldevelopment; heavy alcohol consumption near term may have a greater effect on fetal nutrition and birth weight. Abel (1989) has reported that paternal alcohol consumption in rats decreases litter size and activity levels and testosterone levels in male pups; moreover, the paternal sperm showed altered characteristics in an electric field. However, these intriguing findings have not yet been extended to humans. Windham (1992) recently reported a study of spontaneous abortions in which there was no correlation with paternal alcohol consumption.

G. Immune System: A number of studies have indicated that chronic ethanol consumption can alter immune function. This could be a major factor underlying the increased incidence of certain forms of cancer in alcoholics (see below). The changes reported include alterations in chemotaxis of granulocytes, lymphocyte response to mitogens, T cell numbers, natural killer cell (NK) activity, and levels of tumor necrosis factor. Even a single dose of ethanol may alter some of these variables.

H. Increased Risk of Cancer: Chronic alcohol use increases the risk for cancer of the mouth, pharynx, larynx, esophagus, and liver. Some evidence suggests that there is an increase in the incidence of breast cancer that is alcohol intake-dependent (Schatzkin et al, 1987). Although the methodologic problems of studies relating cancer to alcohol use have been formidable, the consistency of results is impressive. Much more information is required before a threshold level for alcohol consumption as it relates to cancer can be established. In fact, alcohol itself does not appear to be a carcinogen in most test systems. However, alcoholic beverages may carry potential carcinogens produced in fermentation or processing and may alter liver function so that the activity of potential carcinogens is increased.

Alcohol-Drug Interactions

Interactions between ethanol and other drugs can have important clinical effects that result from alterations in the pharmacokinetics or pharmacodynamics of the second drug. The interaction with disulfiram is discussed on page 356.

The most frequent pharmacokinetic alcohol-drug interactions occur as a result of alcohol-induced proliferation ("induction") of the smooth endoplasmic reticulum of liver cells as described in Chapter 4. Thus, prolonged intake of alcohol without damage to the liver may enhance the metabolic biotransformation of other drugs. In contrast, *acute* alcohol use may *inhibit* metabolism of other drugs. This inhibition may be due to alteration of metabolism or alteration of liver blood flow. This acute alcohol effect may contribute to the commonly recognized danger of mixing alcohol with other drugs when performing activities requiring some skill, especially driving. Phenothiazines, tricyclic antidepressants, and sedative-hypnotic drugs are the most important drugs that may interact with alcohol by this mechanism.

Pharmacodynamic alcohol interactions are also of great clinical significance. Additive interaction with other sedative-hypnotics is most important. Alcohol also potentiates the pharmacologic effects of many nonsedative drugs including vasodilators and oral hypoglycemic agents. Alcohol also enhances the antiplatelet action of aspirin.

II. CLINICAL PHARMACOLOGY OF ETHANOL

Ethanol is one of the least potent drugs consumed by humans, yet it is the cause of more preventable morbidity and mortality than all other drugs combined with the exception of tobacco. This is true even though moderate consumption of ethanol is associated with sedative-hypnotic effects, reduction of the symptoms and hormonal changes associated with stress, and even, in some studies, with a reduction in the risk of heart attacks.

Although the disorder known as alcoholism is difficult to define precisely, epidemiologic studies of alcohol consumption provide important information for predicting health-related factors that predispose to physical and psychologic problems. Approximately 80% of adults in the USA consume alcoholic beverages. It is estimated that 5–10% of the adult male population have alcohol-related problems at some time in their lives. Women alcoholics have earlier onset of brain and liver damage than men, probably because, for the same intake, women have higher blood levels (see Alcohol Dehydrogenase Pathway, above). Recent studies in almost 90,000 men and women who participated in multiphasic health examinations and were observed over a 10-year period disclosed a twice-normal mortality rate in persons who admitted to having six or more drinks a day; those taking three to five drinks a day had a rate 40–50% higher than normal. Cancer, hepatic cirrhosis, and accidents contributed significantly to the excessive mortality rate of heavy drinkers. Smoking, which is common in alcoholics, is also a possible mortality risk factor in heavy drinkers. The results of the study suggest that there is a threshold for increased mortality risk in the range of two or three drinks a day and that this risk rises sharply at a level of six or more drinks a day. There is also evidence that small amounts of alcohol (one beer a day) place patients at less risk of myocardial infarction than individuals who never consume alcohol.

The search for specific etiologic factors or the identification of significant predisposing variables for alcohol abuse has generally given disappointing results. Personality type, severe life stresses, psychiatric disorders, and parental role models are not reliable predictors of alcohol abuse. Comparisons of differences in alcohol metabolism are unreliable, and markers of disordered alcohol metabolism are not sufficiently predictive. It is clear that alcohol abuse is not equally distributed in all social groups, and abuse appears to occur at a higher rate among relatives of alcoholics than in the general population (Devor, 1989). The rate of alcoholism in persons with an alcoholic biologic parent is almost four times that of a selected control group—a finding that has now been confirmed by several studies. It is difficult to distinguish between contributing factors of familial learning experiences and genetic variables, but current evidence suggests that genetic factors play a role in defining human alcohol use and medical complications. Genetic control of alcohol preference in animals has been clearly established. A surprisingly strong association between an allele of the dopamine D_2 gene and alcoholism has been reported for humans (Blum, 1990). Nevertheless, the detailed nature of the genetic factors involved is still unknown. Methods of tracking changes such as altered platelet enzymes (mentioned previously) or desialylated transferrin (Storey et al, 1987) may eventually provide laboratory markers predictive of heavy drinking.

MANAGEMENT OF ACUTE ALCOHOLIC INTOXICATION

Nontolerant individuals who consume alcohol in large quantities develop typical effects of acute sedative-hypnotic drug overdose, along with the cardiovascular effects described above (vasodilation, tachycardia) and gastrointestinal irritation. Since tolerance is not absolute, even chronic alcoholics may become severely intoxicated. The degree of intoxication depends upon three factors: the blood ethanol concentration, the rapidity of the rise of the alcohol level, and the time during which the blood level is maintained. The pattern of drinking, the state of the absorptive surface of the gastrointestinal tract, and the presence in the body of other medications also affect the apparent degree of intoxication.

The most important goals in the treatment of acute alcohol intoxication are to prevent severe respiratory depression and aspiration of vomitus. Even with very high blood ethanol levels, survival is probable as long as the respiratory and cardiovascular systems can be supported. The lethal dose of alcohol varies widely because of varying degrees of tolerance. A normal nontolerant adult individual can metabolize 7–10 g of alcohol per hour (the ethanol content of 30 mL [one "shot"] of 80-proof whiskey, one can of beer, or one glass of unfortified wine). The legal definition of intoxication in the USA varies in different states, but a blood level of 80 mg/dL (17 mmol/L) or higher is often regarded as evidence of impaired judgment and performance sufficient for conviction of driving while intoxicated. The average blood alcohol concentration in fatal cases is above 400 mg/dL.

Metabolic alterations may require treatment of hypoglycemia and ketosis by administration of glucose. Alcoholic patients who are dehydrated and vomiting should also receive electrolyte solutions. If vomiting is severe, large amounts of potassium may also be required as long as renal function is normal. Especially important is recognition of decreased phosphate stores, which may be aggravated by glucose administration. Low phosphate stores may contribute to poor wound healing, neurologic deficits, and increased risk of infection.

MANAGEMENT OF ALCOHOL WITHDRAWAL SYNDROME

When alcohol ingestion is abruptly discontinued, the characteristic syndrome of motor agitation, anxiety, insomnia, and reduction of seizure threshold occurs. The severity of the alcohol withdrawal syndrome is usually proportionate to the dose and the duration of alcohol abuse. However, this can be greatly modified by the use of other sedatives as well as by associated medical (eg, diabetes) or surgical factors (injury). In its mildest form, the alcohol withdrawal syndrome of tremor, anxiety, and insomnia occurs 6–8 hours after alcohol is stopped. These effects usually abate in 1–2 days. In some patients, more severe withdrawal reactions occur in which visual hallucinations, total disorientation, and marked abnormalities of vital signs occur. The more severe the withdrawal syndrome, the greater the need for meticulous investigation of possible underlying medical or surgical complications. The mortality risks of severe alcohol withdrawal have been overstated in the past. The prognosis is probably related chiefly to the underlying medical and surgical complications.

The major objective of drug therapy in the alcohol withdrawal period is prevention of seizures, delirium, and arrhythmias (Romach, 1991). Restoration of potassium, magnesium, and phosphate balance should be achieved rapidly if renal function is normal. Thiamine therapy is initiated in all cases. Persons in mild alcohol withdrawal do not need any other pharmacologic assistance.

Specific drug treatment for detoxification in severe cases involves two basic principles: substituting a long-acting sedative-hypnotic drug for alcohol and then gradually reducing ("tapering") the dose of the long-acting drug. Unfortunately, the most widely used "treatment" for alcohol withdrawal is renewed alcohol intake. Although alcohol can be slowly tapered, it is psychologically undesirable to maintain the patient on alcohol. Currently, benzodiazepines are preferred for this purpose. The benzodiazepines chlordiazepoxide and diazepam have pharmacologically active metabolites that may accumulate. Oxazepam is rapidly converted to inactive water-soluble metabolites that will not accumulate and is especially useful in alcoholic patients with liver disease. Most benzodiazepines are poorly absorbed from intramuscular sites; when rapid clinical effects are required, the intravenous route is preferred.

Phenothiazine medications for alcohol withdrawal have potentially serious adverse effects (eg, increasing seizures) that probably outweigh their benefits. Antihistaminic medications have been used but with little justification.

Phenytoin has been suggested by some to be effective in preventing seizures in alcoholic patients with a history of seizures. Since phenytoin is poorly absorbed from intramuscular sites, the drug should be given intravenously. A loading dose of 12–15 mg/kg is given, and the patient is maintained on 300 mg/d with monitoring of blood levels.

After the alcohol withdrawal syndrome has been treated acutely, sedative-hypnotic medications must be tapered slowly over several weeks. Complete detoxification is not achieved with just a few days of sobering up. Several months may be required for restoration of normal nervous system function, especially sleep. Because of the long period required for complete detoxification, other factors that may promote this process—or help prevent relapse—have been examined. In particular, it is now recognized that anxiety and alcoholism are closely related (Frances, 1993). Many alcoholics may drink at least in part to relieve anxiety, and, conversely, anxiety may increase in the absence of alcohol. Since specialists in alcoholism treatment are not necessarily highly knowledgeable about anxiety and its treatment, this is an area where collaboration with other professionals could be useful. Another possible approach is suggested by the observation that smoking is common among alcoholics and that quitting smoking improves the chances of giving up alcohol (Hughes, 1993).

Disulfiram & Other Drugs Used to Reduce Ethanol Intake

Disulfiram (tetraethylthiuram), a widely used antioxidant in the rubber industry, has been shown to cause extreme discomfort to patients who drink alcoholic beverages. Disulfiram given by itself to nondrinkers has little effect; however, flushing, throbbing headache, nausea, vomiting, sweating, hypotension, and confusion occur within a few minutes after taking a drink. The effect may last 30 minutes in mild cases or several hours in severe ones. After the symptoms wear off, the patient is usually exhausted and may sleep for several hours.

Disulfiram acts by inhibiting **aldehyde dehydrogenase.** Thus, alcohol is metabolized as usual, but acetaldehyde is accumulated. The symptoms resulting from disulfiram plus alcohol are typical for acetaldehyde toxicity; the reaction is reproduced by acetaldehyde infusion in humans.

Disulfiram is rapidly and completely absorbed from the gastrointestinal tract; however, a period of 12 hours is required for its full action. Its elimination rate is very slow, so that the action may persist for several days after the last dose. The drug interacts with many other therapeutic agents.

Disulfiram should be considered as a pharmacologic adjunct in the treatment of alcoholism and should only be used in concert with behavioral therapies (Chick et al, 1992). When the drug is prescribed, the alcohol content of common nonprescription medications should be communicated to the patient; some of these are listed in Table 65–3. Management with disulfiram should be initiated only when the patient has been free of alcohol for at least 24 hours. The drug may cause mild changes in liver function tests. The safety of disulfiram in pregnancy has not been demonstrated. The duration of disulfiram treatment should be individualized and determined by the patient's responsiveness and clinical improvement. The usual oral dose is 250 mg daily taken at bedtime. Mandated use of disulfiram by court order is probably not efficacious.

Many other drugs, eg, metronidazole, certain cephalosporins, sulfonylurea hypoglycemic drugs, and chloral hydrate, have disulfiram-like effects on ethanol metabolism (Stockley, 1983).

A great many drugs have been studied as potential "prophylactic" agents—drugs that would decrease the craving for ethanol without the aversive effect of disulfiram (Litten, 1991). Recent reports that chronic alcohol abuse results in decreased brain serotonin levels and altered angiotensin concentrations have prompted investigation into the therapeutic effects of serotonin uptake inhibitors and angiotensin-converting enzyme inhibitors in chronic alcoholics. There is preliminary evidence that chronic treatment with inhibitors of serotonin uptake, eg, fluoxetine, results in a decrease of alcohol consumption (Naranjo et al, 1990). The reduction in ethanol intake was not associated with any aversive effects such as those associated with disulfiram therapy. Dopamine agonists (eg, bromocriptine) and opioid antagonists (eg, naltrexone) have also been claimed to reduce alcohol craving and consumption in selected patients.

III. BASIC PHARMACOLOGY OF OTHER ALCOHOLS

Other alcohols related to ethanol have wide applications as industrial solvents and occasionally cause severe poisoning (Litovitz, 1986).

Methanol (CH_3OH; methyl alcohol, wood alcohol) is derived from the destructive distillation of wood. Methanol is used as a gasoline additive, home heating material, industrial solvent, solvent in xerographic copier solutions, and feedstock for bacterial synthesis of protein. Methanol is most frequently found in the home in the form of "canned heat" or in windshield-washing products. It can be absorbed through the skin or from the respiratory or gastrointestinal tract. It is rapidly absorbed from the gastrointestinal tract and distributed in body water. The primary mechanism of elimination of methanol in humans is by oxidation to formaldehyde, formic acid,

$$CH_3OH \rightarrow \overset{\overset{O}{\|}}{HCH} \rightarrow \overset{\overset{O}{\|}}{HCOH} \rightarrow CO_2 + H_2O$$

and CO_2:

Methanol may also be removed by induced vomiting, and small amounts are excreted in the breath, sweat, and urine. Methanol does not bind to charcoal.

Animal species show great variability in mean lethal doses of methanol. The special susceptibility of humans to methanol toxicity is probably due to folate-dependent production of the formate metabolite of methanol and not to methanol itself or to formaldehyde, the intermediate metabolite.

The enzyme chiefly responsible for methanol oxidation in the liver is alcohol dehydrogenase. Ethanol has a higher affinity than methanol for alcohol dehydrogenase; thus, saturation of alcohol dehydrogenase with ethanol can reduce formate production and is often used as treatment for acute methanol toxicity. An investigational orphan drug known to inhibit alcohol dehydrogenase, 4-methylpyrazole (fomepizole), alone or in combination with ethanol, appears to be of therapeutic value in methanol as well as ethylene glycol poisoning (see below).

Polyhydric alcohols such as **ethylene glycol** (CH_2OHCH_2OH) are used as heat exchangers, in antifreeze formulations, and as industrial solvents. Owing to the low volatility of the glycols, they produce little vapor hazard at ordinary temperatures. However, since they are used as antifreeze mixtures and as heat exchangers, they may be encountered in vapor or mist form, particularly if the temperature is high. Ethylene glycol appears to be considerably more toxic to humans than to many other animal species. As with other alcohols, ethylene glycol is metabolized by alcohol dehydrogenase to aldehydes, acids, and oxalate. The oxalate may be deposited in the renal tubules, causing acute renal failure. Prompt administration of ethanol or treatment with 4-methylpyrazole may prevent the development of metabolic acidosis (Baud et al, 1986).

IV. CLINICAL PHARMACOLOGY OF OTHER ALCOHOLS

Management of Methanol Intoxication

Severe methanol poisoning is usually encountered in chronic alcoholics and may not be recognized unless characteristic symptoms are noted in a group of patients. Because methanol and its metabolite formate are much more potent toxins than ethanol, it is essential that patients with methanol poisoning be recognized and treated as soon as possible.

The most important initial symptom in methanol poisoning is a visual disturbance frequently described as "like being in a snowstorm." Visual disturbances are a universal complaint in epidemics of methanol poisoning. A complaint of blurred vision with a relatively clear sensorium should strongly suggest the diagnosis of methanol poisoning. In severe cases, the odor of formaldehyde may be present on the breath or in the urine. The development of bradycardia, prolonged coma, seizures, and resistant acidosis all indicate a poor prognosis.

Physical findings in methanol poisoning are generally nonspecific. Fixed dilated pupils have been described in severe cases. Optic atrophy is a late finding. The cause of death in fatal cases is sudden cessation of respiration.

It is critical that the blood methanol level be determined as soon as possible if the diagnosis is suspected. If the clinical suspicion of methanol poisoning is high, treatment should not be delayed. Methanol levels in excess of 50 mg/dL are thought to be an absolute indication for hemodialysis and ethanol treatment, although formate blood levels are a better indication of clinical pathology. Additional laboratory evidence includes metabolic acidosis with an elevated anion gap and osmolar gap (see Chapter 60). Ethylene glycol, paraldehyde, and salicylates may also cause an anion gap. A decrease in serum bicarbonate is a uniform feature of severe methanol poisoning. Ethylene glycol toxicity (see below) usually results in central nervous system excitation, increase in muscle enzymes, and hypocalcemia but not visual symptoms. Salicylate intoxication can be readily determined from salicylate levels in the blood.

The first treatment for methanol poisoning, as in all critical poisoning situations, is to establish respiration, with intubation of the trachea if necessary. Emesis can be induced if the patient is not comatose, is not having seizures, and has not lost the gag reflex. If any of these contraindications exists, the patient should be endotracheally intubated and gastric lavage carried out with a large-bore tube after the airway has been protected.

There are three "specific" modalities of treatment for severe methanol poisoning: suppression of metabolism by alcohol dehydrogenase to toxic products, dialysis to enhance removal of methanol and its toxic products, and alkalinization to counteract metabolic acidosis.

Because ethanol competes for alcohol dehydrogenase, which is responsible for metabolizing methanol to formic acid, it is essential to saturate this enzyme with the less toxic ethanol. The dose-dependent characteristics of ethanol metabolism and the variability induced by chronic ethanol intake require frequent monitoring of blood ethanol levels to ensure appropriate alcohol concentration. Ethanol may be given intravenously as a 10% solution. 4-Methylpyrazole, a potent inhibitor of alcohol dehydrogenase, may also be a useful adjunct in methanol poisoning when it becomes fully available for human use. It is currently an orphan drug.

With initiation of dialysis procedures, ethanol will also be eliminated in the dialysate, requiring alterations in the dose of ethanol. Hemodialysis is discussed in Chapter 60.

Because of profound metabolic acidosis in methanol poisoning, treatment with bicarbonate may be necessary. Quantities of bicarbonate to be administered should be based on estimated sodium intake, potassium balance, cardiovascular status, and changes in urine pH.

Since folate-dependent systems are responsible for the oxidation of formic acid to CO_2 in humans, it is probably useful to administer folic acid to patients poisoned with methanol, though this has never been fully tested in clinical studies.

A special diagnostic problem occurs if a patient has a relatively low methanol level but visual symptoms are present. In this situation, laboratory tests for methanol itself should be repeated and confirmed with osmolality estimates. If visual impairment is present, hemodialysis should be started in spite of low methanol levels.

Management of Ethylene Glycol Intoxication

Few clinical cases of ethylene glycol poisoning have been reported in detail. As with methanol poisoning, there may be a delay in the onset of acidosis and renal insufficiency. Three stages of ethylene glycol overdose have been recognized. Initially, there is transient excitation followed by central nervous system depression. Severe acidosis then develops, and finally delayed renal insufficiency occurs. Ophthalmoscopic examination is usually normal, although occasional cases of papilledema have been described. Oxalate crystals are usually present in urine. Ethylene glycol-intoxicated patients have no detectable odor of alcohol on their breath. In severe cases, increased muscle enzyme and decreased calcium have been found in the plasma. The key to the diagnosis of ethylene glycol poisoning is the recognition of anion gap acidosis, osmolar gap, and oxalate crystals in the urine in a patient without visual symptoms. As with methanol poisoning, early alcohol infusion and dialy-sis are required. 4-Methylpyrazole therapy will also be of use in this situation when that drug becomes commercially available.

PREPARATIONS AVAILABLE

Drugs for the Treatment of
Acute Alcohol Withdrawal Syndrome
    Diazepam (generic, Valium, others)
        Parenteral: 5 mg/mL for injection
    Thiamine (generic, Betalin S, Beamine)
        Parenteral: 100, 200 mg/mL for IV injection

Drugs for the Prevention of Alcohol Intake
    Disulfiram (generic, Antabuse)
        Oral: 250, 500 mg tablets

Drugs for the Treatment of Acute Methanol
or Ethylene Glycol Poisoning
    Ethanol (generic)
        Parenteral: 5% or 10% ethanol and 5% dextrose
        in water for IV infusion

REFERENCES

Abel EL (editor): *Fetal Alcohol Syndrome.* CRC Press, 1981.

Abel EL: Paternal behavioral mutagenesis. Neurotoxicology 1989;10:335.

Abel EL: Paternal and maternal alcohol consumption: Effects on offspring in two strains of rats. Alcoholism 1989;13:533.

Aldo-Benson M: Mechanisms of alcohol-induced suppression of B-cell response. Alcoholism: Clin Exp Res 1989;13:469.

Ballard HS: Hematological complications of alcoholism. Alcoholism: Clin Exp Res 1989;13:706.

Baud FJ et al: 4-Methylpyrazole may be an alternative to ethanol therapy for ethylene glycol intoxication in man. J Toxicol Clin Toxicol 1986;24:463.

Baud FJ et al: Treatment of ethylene glycol poisoning with intravenous 4-methylpyrazole. N Engl J Med 1988; 319:97.

Becker CE: Alcohol and drug use: Is there a "safe" amount? West J Med 1984;141:884.

Becker CE: The alcoholic patient is a toxic emergency. Emerg Med Clin North Am 1983;1:51.

Becker CE: Methanol poisoning. J Emerg Med 1983;2:47.

Becker CE, Roe RL, Scott RA: *Alcohol as a Drug: A Curriculum on Pharmacology, Neurology and Toxicology.* RE Kreiger, 1979.

Blum K, Noble EP, Sheridan PJ: Allelic association of human dopamine receptor gene and alcoholism. JAMA 1990;263:2055.

Brien JF, Loomis CW: Pharmacology of acetaldehyde. Can J Physiol Pharmacol 1983;61:1.

Charness ME, Simon RP, Greenberg DA: Ethanol and the nervous system. N Engl J Med 1989;321:442.

Chick J et al: Disulfiram treatment of alcoholism. Br J Psychiatry 1992;161:84.

Devor EJ, Cloninger CR: Genetics of alcoholism. Annu Rev Genet 1989;23:19.

Dietrich RA et al: Mechanism of action of ethanol: Initial central nervous system actions. Pharmacol Rev 1989; 41:489.

Ernhart CB et al: Alcohol teratogenicity in the human: A detailed assessment of specificity, critical period, and threshold. Am J Obstet Gynecol 1987;156:33.

Frances RJ, Borg L: The treatment of anxiety in patients with alcoholism. J Clin Psychiatry 1993;54 (Suppl): 37.

Frezza M et al: High blood alcohol levels in women: The role of decreased gastric alcohol dehydrogenase activity and first-pass metabolism. N Engl J Med 1990;322:95.

Friedman JD, Klatsky AR: Is alcohol good for your health? N Engl J Med 1993;329:1882.

Gandhi CR, Ross DH: Influence of ethanol on calcium, inositol phospholipids, and intracellular signalling mechanisms. Experientia 1989;45:407.

Geokas MC (editor): Ethyl alcohol and disease. (Symposium.) Med Clin North Am 1984;68:1.

Gustavsson L, Alling C: Effects of chronic alcohol exposure on fatty acids of rat brain glycerophospholipids. Alcohol 1989;6:139.

Harris RA, Allan AM: Alcohol intoxication: Ion channels and genetics. FASEB J 1989;3:1689.

Haskell WL et al: The effect of cessation and resumption of moderate alcohol intake on serum high-density-lipoprotein subfractions: A controlled study. N Engl J Med 1984;310:805.

Holford NH: Clinical pharmacokinetics of ethanol. Clin Pharmacokinet 1987;13:273.

Hughes JR: Treatment of smoking cessation in smokers with past alcohol/drug problems. J Subst Abuse Treat 1993;10:181.

Irwin M et al: Testosterone in chronic alcoholic men. Br J Addict 1988;83:949.

Klatsky AR, Friedman JD, Siegelaub AB: Alcohol and mortality: A ten year Kaiser Permanente experience. Ann Intern Med 1981;95:139.

Kotake H et al: Membrane actions of ethanol on rabbit sinoatrial node studied by voltage clamp method. Pharmacol Toxicol 1989;65:343.

Lee NM, Smith AS: Ethanol. In: *Toxicology of CNS Depressants.* Ho IK (editor). CRC Press, 1986.

Levallois C et al: Effects of ethanol in vitro on some parameters of the immune system. Drug Alcohol Depend 1989;24:239.

Lieber CS: Interaction of ethanol with drugs, hepatotoxic agents, carcinogens, and vitamins. Alcohol Alcohol 1990;25:157.

Litovitz T: The alcohols: Ethanol, methanol, isopropanol, ethylene glycol. Pediatr Clin North Am 1986;33:311.

Litten RZ, Allen JP: Pharmacotherapies for alcoholism: Promising agents and clinical issues. Alcoholism: Clin Exp Res 1991;15:620.

Lovinger DM, White G, Weight FF: Ethanol inhibits NMDA-activated ion current in hippocampal neurons. Science 1989;243:1721.

Martensson E, Olofsson U, Heath A: Clinical and metabolic features of ethanol-methane poisoning in chronic alcoholics. Lancet 1988;1:327.

Meagher RC, Sieber F, Spivak JL: Suppression of hematopoietic-progenitor-cell proliferation by ethanol and acetaldehyde. N Engl J Med 1982;307:845.

Mufti SI, Darban HR, Watson RR: Alcohol, cancer, and immunomodulation. Crit Rev Oncol Hematol 1989;9:243.

Nagy LE et al: Ethanol increases extracellular adenosine by inhibiting adenosine uptake via the nucleoside transporter. J Biol Chem 1990;265:1946.

Naranjo CA et al: Fluoxetine differentially alters alcohol intake and other consummatory behaviors in problem drinkers. Clin Pharmacol Ther 1990;47:490.

Neurobiological correlates of intoxication and physical dependence upon ethanol. (Symposium.) Fed Proc 1981; 40:2048.

O'Malley SS et al: Naltrexone and coping skills therapy for alcohol dependence: A controlled study. Arch Gen Psychiatry 1992;49:881.

Romach MK, Sellers EM: Management of the alcohol withdrawal syndrome. Annu Rev Med 1991;42:323.

Rooney TA et al: Short chain alcohols activate guanine nucleotide-dependent phosphoinositidase C in turkey erythrocyte membranes. J Biol Chem 1989;264:6817.

Schatzkin A et al: Alcohol consumption and breast cancer in the epidemiologic follow-up study of the First National Health and Nutrition Examination Survey. N Engl J Med 1987;316:1169.

Schenker S et al: Fetal alcohol syndrome: Current status of pathogenesis. Alcoholism: Clin Exp Res 1990;14:635.

Spinosa G et al: Angiotensin-converting enzyme inhibitors: Animal experiments suggest a new pharmacological treatment for alcohol abuse in humans. Alcoholism: Clin Exp Res 1988;12:65.

Steinberg W, Tenner S: Acute pancreatitis. N Engl J Med 1994;330:1198.

Stockley IH: Drugs, foods, and environmental chemical agents which can initiate Antabuse-like reactions with alcohol. Pharmacy Int 1983;4:12.

Storey FL et al: Desialylated transferrin as a serological marker of chronic excessive alcohol ingestion. Lancet 1987;1:1292.

Suh I et al: Alcohol use and mortality from coronary heart disease: The role of high-density lipoprotein cholesterol. Ann Intern Med 1992;116:881.

Sullivan LW et al: 7th Special Report to U.S. Congress on Alcohol and Health from the Secretary of Health and Human Services. U.S. Department of Health and Human Services, 5600 Fishers Lane, Rockville MD 20857.

Suzdak PD et al: A selective imidazobenzodiazepine antagonist of ethanol in the rat. Science 1986;234:1243.

Tabakoff B et al: Differences in platelet enzyme activity between alcoholics and nonalcoholics. N Engl J Med 1988;318:134.

Windham GC, Fenster L, Swan SH: Moderate maternal and paternal alcohol consumption and the risk of spontaneous abortion. Epidemiology 1992;3:364.

Wood WG, Gorka C, Schroeder F: Acute and chronic effects of ethanol on transbilayer membrane domains. J Neurochem 1989;52:1925.

Wright C, Moore RD: Disulfiram treatment of alcoholism. Am J Med 1990;88:647.

Antiepileptic Drugs*

23

Roger J. Porter, MD, & Brian S. Meldrum, MB, PhD

Approximately 1% of the population of the USA has epilepsy, the second most common neurologic disorder after stroke. Although standard therapy permits control of seizures in 80% of these patients, 500,000 people in the USA have uncontrolled epilepsy. Epilepsy is a heterogeneous symptom complex—a chronic disorder characterized by recurrent seizures. Seizures are finite episodes of brain dysfunction resulting from abnormal discharge of cerebral neurons. The causes of seizures are many and include the full range of neurologic diseases, from infection to neoplasm and head injury. In a few subgroups, heredity has proved to be a major contributing factor.

The antiepileptic drugs described in this chapter are also used in patients with febrile seizures or with seizures occurring as part of an acute illness such as meningitis, even though the term "epilepsy" is not usually applied to such patients unless they later develop chronic seizures. Seizures are occasionally caused by an acute underlying toxic or metabolic disorder, in which case appropriate therapy should be directed toward the specific abnormality, eg, hypocalcemia. In most cases of epilepsy, however, the choice of medication depends on the empirical seizure classification.

History

Before the antiepileptic drugs were discovered and developed, treatment of epilepsy consisted of trephining, cupping, and the administration of herbal medicines and animal extracts. In 1857, Sir Charles Locock reported the successful use of potassium bromide in the treatment of what is now known as catamenial epilepsy. In 1912, phenobarbital was first used for epilepsy, and in the next 25 years, 35 analogues of phenobarbital were studied as anticonvulsants. In 1938, phenytoin was found to be effective against experimental seizures in cats.

Between 1935 and 1960, tremendous strides were made both in the development of experimental models and in methods for screening and testing new an-

tiepileptic drugs. During that period, 13 new antiepileptic drugs were developed and marketed. Following the enactment of requirements for proof of drug efficacy in 1962, antiepileptic drug development slowed dramatically, and only a few new antiepileptic drugs were marketed in the next 3 decades. However, several new compounds are becoming available in the 1990s.

Present Status of Drug Development For Epilepsy

For a long time it was assumed that a single drug could be developed for treatment of all forms of epilepsy. It now appears unlikely that the wide variety of epileptic seizures can be managed successfully with just one drug. More than one mechanism may be responsible for the various seizures, and drugs useful for one seizure type may occasionally aggravate other types. Drugs used in the treatment of the two major types of seizures (partial and generalized; Table 23–1) are quite distinct in their clinical effects and also fall into two pharmacologic classes, even though seizures may be induced experimentally by a wide variety of methods. The clinical aspects of certain generalized seizures—especially absence seizures—are highly correlated with experimental seizures produced in animals by subcutaneous administration of pentylenetetrazol. Likewise, partial seizures in humans correlate positively with experimental seizures elicited by the maximal electroshock (MES) test. In general, antiepileptic drugs effective against maximal electroshock seizures alter ionic transport across excitable membranes. Phenytoin, for example, is effective against partial seizures and maximal electroshock but with the exception of generalized tonic-clonic seizures is not effective against generalized seizures or those induced by subcutaneous pentylenetetrazol. Phenytoin affects cell firing through its action on Na^+ conductance mechanisms. On the other hand, ethosuximide and trimethadione, which are active against pentylenetetrazol and certain generalized seizures, diminish Ca^{2+} entry (through T-type, or low-threshold calcium channels). It is notable that the two distinct classes of antiepileptic drugs have different mechanisms of action in spite of marked structural similarities between many of the drugs in the two groups.

*The authors wish to thank Harold Boxenbaum, PhD, for his assistance in reviewing the pharmacokinetic data in this chapter.

Table 23–1. Classification of seizure types.

Partial seizures
    Simple partial seizures.
    Complex partial seizures.
    Partial seizures secondarily generalized.

Generalized seizures
    Generalized tonic-clonic (grand mal) seizures.
    Absence (petit mal) seizures.
    Tonic seizures.
    Atonic seizures.
    Clonic and myoclonic seizures.
    Infantile spasms.[1]

[1]Infantile spasms is an epileptic syndrome rather than a specific seizure type; drugs useful in infantile spasms will be reviewed separately.

New antiepileptic drugs are being sought not only by the screening tests noted above but also by more rational approaches. Compounds are sought that act by one of three mechanisms: (1) enhancement of GABAergic (inhibitory) transmission, (2) diminution of excitatory (usually glutamatergic) transmission, or (3) modification of ionic conductances.

I. BASIC PHARMACOLOGY OF ANTIEPILEPTIC DRUGS

Chemistry

Up to 1990, approximately 16 antiepileptic drugs were available, and 13 of them have been classified into five very similar chemical groups: barbiturates, hydantoins, oxazolidinediones, succinimides, and acetylureas. These groups have in common a similar heterocyclic ring structure with a variety of substituents (Figure 23–1). For drugs with this basic structure, the substituents on the heterocyclic ring determine the pharmacologic class, either anti-MES or antipentylenetetrazol. Very small changes in structure can dramatically alter the mechanism of action and clinical properties of the compound. The remaining drugs–carbamazepine, valproic acid, and the ben-

zodiazepines–are structurally dissimilar, as are the newer compounds of the 1990s such as vigabatrin, oxcarbazepine, lamotrigine, gabapentin, and felbamate.

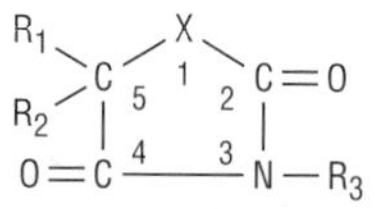

Pharmacokinetics

The antiepileptic drugs exhibit many similar pharmacokinetic properties–even those whose structural and chemical properties are quite diverse. Although many of these compounds are only sparingly soluble, absorption is usually good, with 80–100% of the dose reaching the circulation. Bioavailability is a problem with phenytoin, in which both the rate and extent of absorption are highly dependent on the formulation.

Except for phenytoin, the benzodiazepines, and valproic acid, antiepileptic drugs are not highly bound to plasma proteins. Only phenytoin and valproic acid are able to displace other highly bound drugs, including other anticonvulsants. Benzodiazepine concentrations are too low to affect the binding of other drugs.

Antiepileptic drugs have low extraction ratios (see Chapter 3). An increase in the percentage of free drug will not change free concentrations but will reduce total drug concentrations and may lead the clinician to increase the dose; this increase in dose will result in higher free drug levels and possible drug toxicity. Sodium valproate is unique in that the fraction of drug bound is a function of the concentrations of both the drug and the free fatty acids in plasma.

Antiepileptic drugs are cleared chiefly by hepatic mechanisms. Many, such as primidone and the benzodiazepines, are converted to active metabolites that are also cleared by the liver. The intrinsic ability of the liver to metabolize anticonvulsant drugs is generally low and, with the exception of phenytoin, independent of concentration. These drugs are predominantly distributed into total body water. Plasma clearance is relatively slow; many anticonvulsants are therefore considered to be medium- to long-acting. For most, half-lives are greater than 12 hours. Phenobarbital and carbamazepine are potent inducers of hepatic microsomal enzyme activity.

DRUGS USED IN PARTIAL SEIZURES & GENERALIZED TONIC-CLONIC SEIZURES

The major drugs for partial and generalized tonic-clonic seizures are phenytoin (and congeners), carbamazepine, and the barbiturates. However, the addition of oxcarbazepine, vigabatrin, and lamotrigine is altering clinical practice in countries where these newer compounds are available.

Figure 23–1. Antiepileptic heterocyclic ring structure. The "X" varies as follows: hydantoin derivatives, $-N-$; barbiturates, $-C-N-$; oxazolidinediones, $-O-$; succinimides, $-C-$; acetylureas, $-NH_2$ (N connected to C2). R_1, R_2, and R_3 vary within each subgroup.

PHENYTOIN

Phenytoin is the oldest nonsedative antiepileptic drug, introduced in 1938 following a systematic evaluation of compounds such as phenobarbital that altered electrically induced seizures in laboratory animals. It was known for decades as diphenylhydantoin (DPH).

Chemistry

Phenytoin is a diphenyl-substituted hydantoin with the structure shown below. It has much lower sedative properties than compounds with alkyl substituents at the 5 position.

Phenytoin

Mechanism of Action

Phenytoin has major effects on several physiologic systems. It alters Na^+, K^+, and Ca^{2+} conductances, membrane potentials, and the concentrations of amino acids and the neurotransmitters norepinephrine, acetylcholine, and γ-aminobutyric acid (GABA). Phenytoin blocks posttetanic potentiation in spinal cord preparations, but the role of this effect in suppressing seizure spread is not yet defined.

Studies with neurons in cell culture show that phenytoin blocks sustained high-frequency repetitive firing of action potentials (Figure 23–2). This effect is seen at therapeutically relevant concentrations. It is a use-dependent effect (see Chapter 14) on Na^+ conductance, arising from preferential binding to—and prolongation of—the inactivated state of the Na^+ channel (Macdonald, 1989). This effect is also seen with therapeutically relevant concentrations of carbamazepine and valproate and probably contributes to their antiepileptic action in the electroshock model and in partial seizures.

At high concentrations, phenytoin also inhibits the release of serotonin and norepinephrine, promotes the uptake of dopamine, and inhibits monoamine oxidase activity. The drug interacts with membrane lipids; this binding might promote the stabilization of the membrane. In addition, phenytoin paradoxically causes excitation in some cerebral neurons. A reduction of calcium permeability, with inhibition of calcium influx across the cell membrane may explain the ability of phenytoin to inhibit a variety of calcium-induced secretory processes, including release of hormones and neurotransmitters. The significance of these biochemical actions and their relationship to phenytoin activity are unclear.

The mechanism of phenytoin's action probably involves a combination of actions at several levels. Evidence indicates that at therapeutic concentrations, the major action of phenytoin is to block sodium channels and inhibit the generation of repetitive action potentials.

Clinical Use

Phenytoin is one of the most effective drugs against partial seizures and generalized tonic-clonic seizures. In the latter, it appears to be effective against attacks that are either primary or secondary to another seizure type.

Pharmacokinetics

Absorption of phenytoin is highly dependent on the formulation of the dosage form. Particle size and pharmaceutical additives affect both the rate and extent of absorption. Absorption of phenytoin sodium

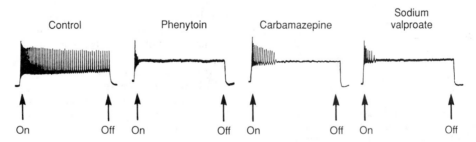

Figure 23–2. Effects of three antiepileptic drugs on sustained high-frequency firing of action potentials by cultured neurons. Intracellular recordings were made from neurons while depolarizing current pulses, approximately 0.75 s in duration, were applied (on-off step changes indicated by arrows). In the absence of drug, a series of high-frequency repetitive action potentials filled the entire duration of the current pulse. Phenytoin, carbamazepine, and sodium valproate all markedly reduced the number of action potentials elicited by the current pulses. (Modified and reproduced, with permission, from Macdonald RL, Meldrum BS: Principles of antiepileptic drug action. In: *Antiepileptic Drugs,* 3rd ed. Levy RH et al [editors]. Raven Press 1989.)

from the gastrointestinal tract is nearly complete in most patients, though the time to peak may range from 3 hours to 12 hours. Absorption after intramuscular injection is unpredictable, and some drug precipitation in the muscle occurs; this route of administration is not recommended.

Phenytoin is highly bound to plasma proteins. It appears certain that the total plasma level decreases when the percentage that is bound decreases, as in uremia or hypoalbuminemia, but correlation of free levels with clinical states remains uncertain. Drug concentration in cerebrospinal fluid is proportionate to the free plasma level. Phenytoin accumulates in and becomes bound to the endoplasmic reticulum of cells in brain, liver, muscle, and fat.

Phenytoin is metabolized primarily by parahydroxylation to 5-(p-hydroxyphenyl)-5-phenylhydantoin (HPPH), which is subsequently conjugated with glucuronic acid. The metabolites are clinically inactive and are excreted in the urine. Only a very small portion of phenytoin is excreted unchanged.

The elimination pharmacokinetics of phenytoin are dose-dependent. At very low blood levels, phenytoin metabolism is proportionate to the rate at which the drug is presented to the liver, ie, first-order metabolism. However, as blood levels rise within the therapeutic range, the maximum capacity of the liver to metabolize phenytoin is approached (Figure 23–3). Further increases in dose, even though relatively small, may produce very large changes in phenytoin concentrations. In such cases, the half-life of the drug

increases markedly, steady state is not achieved (since the plasma level continues to rise), and patients quickly develop symptoms of toxicity.

The half-life of phenytoin varies from 12 hours to 36 hours, with an average of 24 hours for most patients in the low- to mid-therapeutic range. Much longer half-lives are observed at higher concentrations. At low blood levels, it takes 5–7 days to reach steady state blood levels after every dosage change; at higher levels it may be 4–6 weeks before blood levels are stable.

Therapeutic Levels & Dose

The therapeutic plasma level of phenytoin for most patients is between 10 and 20 μg/mL. A loading dose can be given either orally or intravenously; the latter is the method of choice for convulsive status epilepticus (discussed later). When oral therapy is started, it is common to begin adults at a dosage of 300 mg/d regardless of body weight. While this may be acceptable in some patients, it frequently yields steady state blood levels below 10 μg/mL, the minimum therapeutic level for most patients. If seizures continue, higher doses are usually necessary to achieve plasma levels in the upper therapeutic range. Because of its dose-dependent kinetics, some toxicity may occur with only small increments in dose; the phenytoin dosage should be increased each time by only 25–30 mg in adults, and ample time should be allowed for the new steady state to be achieved before further increasing the dose. A common clinical error is to increase the dose directly from 300 mg/d to 400 mg/d; toxicity frequently occurs at a variable time thereafter. In children, a dose of 5 mg/kg/d should be followed by readjustment after steady state plasma levels are obtained.

Two types of oral phenytoin sodium are currently available in the USA, differing in their respective rates of dissolution; one is absorbed rapidly and one more slowly. Only the latter can be given in a single daily dose, and care must be used when changing brands (see Preparations Available). Although a few patients being given phenytoin on a chronic basis have been proved to have low blood levels either from poor absorption or rapid metabolism, the most common cause of low levels is poor compliance.

Drug Interactions & Interference With Laboratory Tests

Drug interactions involving phenytoin are primarily related to protein binding or to metabolism. Since phenytoin is bound to plasma protein, other highly bound drugs, such as phenylbutazone or sulfonamides, can displace phenytoin from its binding site. In theory, such displacement may cause a transient increase in free drug. A decrease in protein binding—eg, in hypoalbuminemia—results in a decrease in the *total* plasma concentration of drug but not the *free* concentration; intoxication may occur if efforts

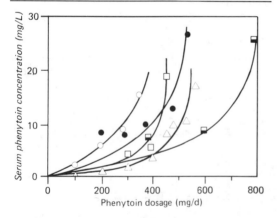

Figure 23–3. Nonlinear effect of phenytoin dosage on plasma concentration. Five different patients (identified by different symbols) received increasing dosages of phenytoin by mouth, and the steady-state serum concentration was measured at each dosage. The curves are not linear, since, as the dosage increases, the first-pass effect is proportionately less marked. Note also the marked variation among patients in the serum levels achieved at any dosage. (Modified, with permission, from Jusko WJ: Bioavailability and disposition kinetics of phenytoin in man. In: *Quantitative Analytic Studies in Epilepsy.* Kellaway P, Peterson I [editors]. Raven Press, 1977.)

are made to maintain total drug levels in the therapeutic range by increasing the dose. The protein binding of phenytoin is decreased in the presence of renal disease. The drug has an affinity for thyroid-binding globulin (TBG), which confuses some tests of thyroid function; the most reliable screening test of thyroid function in patients taking phenytoin appears to be measurement of TSH.

Phenytoin has been shown to induce microsomal enzymes responsible for the metabolism of a number of drugs. Autostimulation of its own metabolism, however, appears to be insignificant. Other drugs, notably phenobarbital and carbamazepine, cause decreases in phenytoin steady state concentrations through induction of hepatic microsomal enzymes. On the other hand, isoniazid inhibits the metabolism of phenytoin, resulting in increased steady state concentrations when the two drugs are given together.

Toxicity

Dose-related adverse effects caused by phenytoin are unfortunately similar to other antiepileptic drugs in this group, making differentiation difficult in patients receiving multiple drugs. Nystagmus occurs early, as does loss of smooth extraocular pursuit movements, but neither is an indication for decreasing the dose. Diplopia and ataxia are the most common dose-related adverse effects requiring dosage adjustment; sedation usually occurs only at considerably higher levels. Gingival hyperplasia and hirsutism occur to some degree in most patients; the latter can be especially unpleasant in females. Long-term chronic use is associated in some patients with coarsening of facial features and with mild peripheral neuropathy, usually manifested by diminished deep tendon reflexes in the lower extremities. Chronic use may also result in abnormalities of vitamin D metabolism, leading to osteomalacia. Low folate levels and megaloblastic anemia have been reported, but the clinical importance of this observation is unknown.

Idiosyncratic reactions to phenytoin are relatively rare. Most commonly, a typical skin rash heralds the hypersensitivity of the patient to the drug, which is then appropriately discontinued. Fever may also occur, and in rare cases the skin lesions may be severe and exfoliative. Lymphadenopathy may be difficult to distinguish from malignant lymphoma, and although some studies suggest a causal relationship between phenytoin and Hodgkin's disease, the data are far from conclusive. Hematologic complications are exceedingly rare, though agranulocytosis has been reported in combination with fever and rash.

MEPHENYTOIN, ETHOTOIN, & PHENACEMIDE

Many congeners of phenytoin have been synthesized, but only three are marketed in the USA, and

these are used to a limited extent. Mephenytoin has a methyl group at the 3 position of the heterocyclic ring, and one of the phenyl groups at the 5 position is replaced by an ethyl group (Figure 23–1). Ethotoin has an ethyl group at the 3 position of the heterocyclic ring and only one phenyl group at the 5 position. The third analogue, phenacemide, is similar to phenytoin except that only one phenyl ring is present at carbon 5 and the heterocyclic ring has been opened to form a straight-chain phenylacetylurea compound.

Mephenytoin and ethotoin, like phenytoin, appear to be most effective against generalized tonic-clonic seizures and partial seizures. No well-controlled clinical trials have documented their effectiveness. The incidence of severe reactions such as dermatitis, agranulocytosis, or hepatitis is higher for mephenytoin than for phenytoin.

Ethotoin may be recommended for patients hypersensitive to phenytoin, but larger doses are required. The adverse effects and toxicity are generally less severe than those associated with phenytoin, but the drug appears to be less effective.

Both ethotoin and mephenytoin share with phenytoin the property of saturable metabolism within the therapeutic dosage range. Careful monitoring of the patient during dosage alterations with either drug is essential. Mephenytoin is metabolized to 5,5-ethylphenylhydantoin via demethylation. This metabolite, nirvanol, contributes most of the antiepileptic activity of mephenytoin. Both mephenytoin and nirvanol are hydroxylated and undergo subsequent conjugation and excretion. Therapeutic levels for mephenytoin range from 5 to 16 μg/mL, and levels above 20 μg/mL are considered toxic.

Therapeutic blood levels of nirvanol are between 25 and 40 μg/mL. A therapeutic range for ethotoin has not been established.

Phenacemide, the straight-chain analogue of phenytoin, is a toxic drug of last resort for refractory partial seizures. It is active against both maximal electroshock and pentylenetetrazol seizures. Its mechanism of action is unknown. It is well absorbed and completely metabolized. The relationship between blood levels and effect has not been established. Serious and sometimes fatal adverse effects have been reported in association with the use of phenacemide. Dose-related effects include behavioral changes, eg, psychosis and depressive reactions. Reactions of an idiosyncratic nature—hepatitis, nephritis, aplastic anemia, and others—appear to be more frequent than with other antiepileptic drugs.

CARBAMAZEPINE

Closely related to imipramine and other antidepressants, carbamazepine is a tricyclic compound effective in treatment of bipolar depression. It was initially marketed for the treatment of trigeminal neuralgia but has proved useful for epilepsy as well.

Chemistry

Although not obvious from a two-dimensional representation of its structure (Figure 23–4), carbamazepine has many similarities to phenytoin. The ureide moiety (–N–CO–NH$_2$) present in the heterocyclic ring of most antiepileptic drugs is also present in carbamazepine. Three-dimensional structural studies indicate that its spatial conformation is similar to that of phenytoin.

Mechanism of Action

The mechanism of action of carbamazepine appears to be similar to that of phenytoin. Like phenytoin, carbamazepine shows activity against maximal electroshock seizures. Studies on membrane permeability indicate that carbamazepine, like phenytoin, blocks sodium channels at therapeutic concentrations and inhibits high-frequency repetitive firing in neurons in culture (Figure 23–2). It also acts presynapti-

cally to decrease synaptic transmission. These effects probably account for the anticonvulsant action of carbamazepine. Binding studies show that carbamazepine interacts with adenosine receptors, but the functional significance of this observation is not known. Carbamazepine also inhibits uptake and release of norepinephrine from brain synaptosomes but does not influence GABA uptake in brain slices or postsynaptic inhibition induced by GABA, suggesting that its action is probably independent of the GABAergic system.

Clinical Use

Carbamazepine is considered the drug of choice for partial seizures, and many physicians also use it first for generalized tonic-clonic seizures. It is used with phenytoin in many patients who are difficult to control. Carbamazepine is not sedative in its usual therapeutic range. The drug is also very effective in some patients with trigeminal neuralgia, though older patients may tolerate higher doses poorly, with ataxia and unsteadiness.

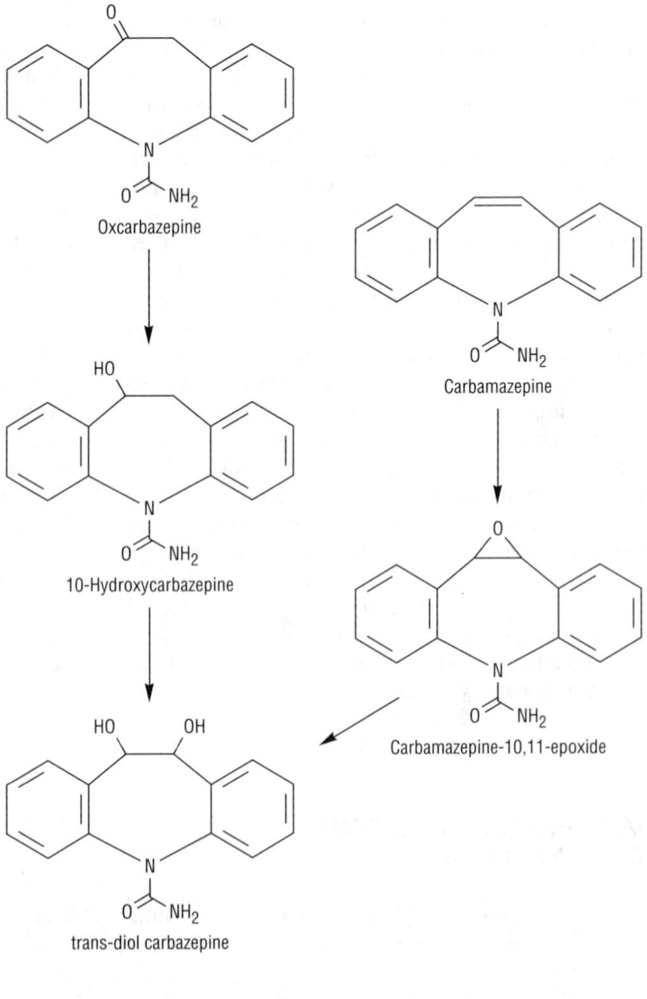

Figure 23–4. Carbamazepine and oxcarbazepine and their metabolites. Carbamazepine is oxidized to an epoxy intermediate, which opens to form the dihydroxy derivative. Oxcarbazepine does not have an epoxide metabolite but is rapidly converted to 10-hydroxycarbazepine, which also eventually converts to the same dihydroxy derivative.

Oxcarbazepine

Carbamazepine

10-Hydroxycarbazepine

Carbamazepine-10,11-epoxide

trans-diol carbazepine

Pharmacokinetics

The rate of absorption of carbamazepine varies widely among different patients, though almost complete absorption apparently occurs in all. Peak levels are usually achieved 6–8 hours after administration. Slowing absorption by giving the drug after meals helps the patient tolerate larger total daily doses.

Distribution is slow, and the volume of distribution is roughly 1 L/kg. The drug is only 70% bound to plasma proteins; no displacement of other drugs from protein binding has been observed.

Carbamazepine has a very low systemic clearance of approximately 1 L/kg/d at the start of therapy. The drug has a notable ability to induce microsomal enzymes. In several studies of epileptic patients or volunteers on dosage regimens exceeding 1 month, the clearance of carbamazepine increased twofold over initial treatment. Typically, the half-life of 36 hours observed in subjects following an initial single dose decreases to much less than 20 hours in subjects receiving continuous therapy. Considerable dosage adjustments are thus to be expected during the first weeks of therapy. These changes in dose may further alter the microsomal enzyme capacity. Carbamazepine also alters the clearance of other drugs (see below).

Carbamazepine is completely metabolized in humans, in part to the 10,11-dihydro derivative, which is subsequently conjugated. The dihydro derivative is formed by way of a stable epoxide, carbamazepine-10,11-epoxide, which has been shown to have anticonvulsant activity (Figure 23–4). The contribution of this and other metabolites to the clinical activity of carbamazepine is unknown.

Therapeutic Levels & Dose

Carbamazepine is considered the drug of choice in partial seizures. It is available only in oral form. The drug is effective in children, in whom a dose of 15–25 mg/kg/d is appropriate. In adults, daily doses of 1 g or even 2 g are tolerated. Higher doses are achieved by giving multiple divided doses daily. In patients receiving three or four daily doses in whom the blood is drawn just before the morning dose (trough level), the therapeutic level is usually 4–8 µg/mL; although many patients complain of diplopia at drug levels above 7 µg/mL, others can tolerate levels above 10 µg/mL, especially with monotherapy. When blood samples are drawn randomly, levels are frequently above 8 µg/mL, but fluctuations related to absorption make long-term comparisons difficult.

Drug Interactions

Drug interactions involving carbamazepine are almost exclusively related to the drug's enzyme-inducing properties. As noted previously, the increased metabolic capacity of the hepatic enzymes may cause a reduction in steady state carbamazepine concentrations and an increased rate of metabolism of primi-done, phenytoin, ethosuximide, valproic acid, and clonazepam. Other drugs such as propoxyphene, troleandomycin, and valproic acid may inhibit carbamazepine clearance and increase steady state carbamazepine blood levels. Other anticonvulsants, however, such as phenytoin and phenobarbital, may decrease steady state concentrations of carbamazepine through enzyme induction. No clinically significant protein-binding interactions have been reported.

Toxicity

The most common dose-related adverse effects of carbamazepine are diplopia and ataxia. The diplopia often occurs first and may last less than an hour during a particular time of day. Rearrangement of the divided daily dose can often remedy this complaint. Other dose-related complaints include mild gastrointestinal upsets, unsteadiness, and, at much higher doses, drowsiness. Hyponatremia and water intoxication have occasionally occurred and may be dose-related.

Considerable concern exists regarding the occurrence of idiosyncratic blood dyscrasias with carbamazepine, including fatal cases of aplastic anemia and agranulocytosis. Most of these have been in elderly patients with trigeminal neuralgia, and most have occurred within the first 4 months of treatment. The mild and persistent leukopenia seen in some patients is not necessarily an indication to stop treatment but requires careful monitoring. The most common idiosyncratic reaction is an erythematous skin rash; other responses such as hepatic dysfunction are unusual.

OXCARBAZEPINE

Oxcarbazepine is a newer drug closely related to carbamazepine and useful in the same seizure types, but it may have an improved toxicity profile. The activity of the drug resides almost exclusively in the 10-hydroxy metabolite (Figure 23–4), to which it is rapidly converted. The latter has a half-life similar to carbamazepine, ie, 8–12 hours. The drug is less potent than carbamazepine, both in animal models of epilepsy and in epileptic patients; clinical doses of oxcarbazepine may need to be 50% higher than that of carbamazepine to obtain equivalent seizure control. Some studies report fewer hypersensitivity reactions to oxcarbazepine. Also, the drug appears to induce hepatic enzymes to a lesser extent than carbamazepine, minimizing drug interactions. Those adverse effects that do occur with oxcarbazepine are similar in character to reactions reported with carbamazepine. The drug is marketed in some European countries but not in the USA.

PHENOBARBITAL

Aside from the bromides, phenobarbital is the oldest of the currently available antiepileptic drugs. Although it has long been considered one of the safest of the antiepileptic agents, the use of other medications with lesser sedative effects has been urged. Many consider the barbiturates the drugs of choice for seizures only in infants.

Chemistry

The four derivatives of barbituric acid clinically useful as antiepileptic drugs are phenobarbital, mephobarbital, metharbital, and primidone. The first three are so similar that they will be considered together. Metharbital is methylated barbital, and mephobarbital is methylated phenobarbital; both are demethylated in vivo. The pK_a's of these three weak acid compounds range from 7.3 to 7.9. Slight changes in the normal acid-base balance, therefore, can cause significant fluctuation in the ratio of the ionized to the un-ionized species. This is particularly important for phenobarbital, the most commonly used barbiturate, whose pK_a is similar to the plasma pH of 7.4.

The three-dimensional conformations of phenobarbital and N-methylphenobarbital are virtually identical to that of phenytoin. Both compounds possess a phenyl ring and are active against partial seizures.

Mechanism of Action

The exact mechanism of action of phenobarbital is unknown, but enhancement of inhibitory processes and diminution of excitatory transmission probably contribute importantly. Recent data indicate that phenobarbital may selectively suppress abnormal neurons, inhibiting the spread and suppressing firing from the foci. Like phenytoin, phenobarbital suppresses high-frequency repetitive firing in neurons in culture through an action on Na^+ conductance, but only at high concentrations. Also at high concentrations, barbiturates block some Ca^{2+} currents (L- and N-types). Phenobarbital binds to an allosteric regulatory site on the GABA-benzodiazepine receptor, and it enhances the GABA receptor-mediated current by prolonging the openings of the Cl^- channels. Phenobarbital also blocks excitatory responses induced by glutamate, principally those mediated by activation of the AMPA receptor (see Chapter 20). Both the enhancement of GABA-mediated inhibition and the reduction of glutamate-mediated excitation are seen with therapeutically relevant concentrations of phenobarbital.

Clinical Use

Phenobarbital is useful in the treatment of partial seizures and generalized tonic-clonic seizures, though the drug is often tried for virtually every seizure type, especially when attacks are difficult to control. There is little evidence for its effectiveness in generalized seizures such as absence, atonic attacks, or infantile spasms; it may worsen certain patients with these seizure types.

Some physicians prefer either metharbital or mephobarbital—especially the latter—to phenobarbital because of supposed decreased adverse effects. Only anecdotal data are available to support such comparisons.

Pharmacokinetics
See Chapter 21.

Therapeutic Levels & Dose
The therapeutic levels of phenobarbital in most patients range from 10 to 40 μg/mL. Documentation of effectiveness is best in febrile seizures, and levels below 15 μg/mL appear ineffective for prevention of febrile seizure recurrence. The upper end of the therapeutic range is more difficult to define, as many patients appear to tolerate chronic levels above 40 μg/mL.

Drug Interactions & Toxicity
See Chapter 21.

PRIMIDONE

Primidone, or 2-desoxyphenobarbital (Figure 23–5), was marketed in the early 1950s. It was later reported that primidone was metabolized to phenobarbital and phenylethylmalonamide (PEMA). All three compounds are active anticonvulsants.

Mechanism of Action
Although primidone is converted to phenobarbital, the mechanism of action of primidone itself may be more like that of phenytoin.

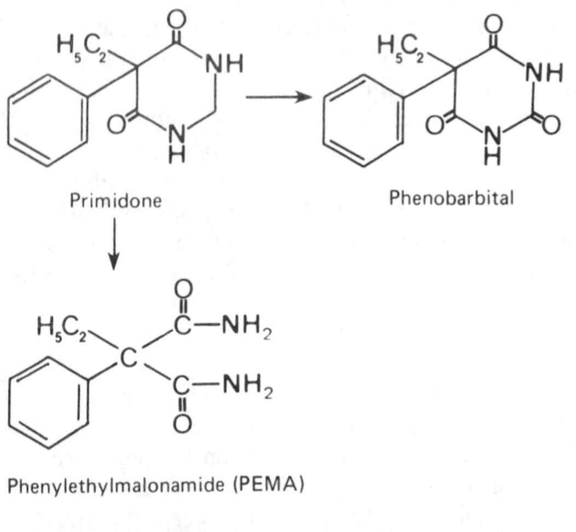

Primidone

Phenobarbital

Phenylethylmalonamide (PEMA)

Figure 23–5. Primidone and its active metabolites.

Clinical Use

Primidone, like its metabolites, is effective against partial seizures and generalized tonic-clonic seizures and may be more effective than phenobarbital. It was previously considered to be the drug of choice for complex partial seizures, but the latest studies of partial seizures in adults strongly suggest that carbamazepine and phenytoin are superior to primidone. Recent attempts to determine the relative potencies of the parent drug and its two metabolites have concentrated on newborn infants, in whom drug-metabolizing enzyme systems are very immature and in whom primidone is only slowly metabolized. Primidone has been shown to be effective in controlling seizures in this group and in older patients beginning treatment with primidone; the latter show seizure control before phenobarbital concentrations reach the therapeutic range. Finally, studies of maximal electroshock seizures in animals suggest that primidone has an anticonvulsant action independent of its conversion to phenobarbital and PEMA (but weaker than that of phenobarbital).

Pharmacokinetics

Primidone is absorbed completely, reaching peak concentrations usually in about 3 hours after oral administration, though considerable variation has been reported. Primidone is generally confined to total body water, with a volume of distribution of 0.6 L/kg. It is not highly bound to plasma proteins; approximately 70% circulates as unbound drug.

Primidone is metabolized by oxidation to phenobarbital, which accumulates very slowly, and by scission of the heterocyclic ring to form PEMA (Figure 23–5). Both primidone and phenobarbital are also hydroxylated at the para position of the phenyl ring and undergo subsequent conjugation and excretion.

Primidone has a larger clearance than most other antiepileptic drugs (2 L/kg/d), corresponding to a half-life of 6–8 hours. PEMA clearance is approximately half that of primidone, but phenobarbital has a very low clearance. The appearance of phenobarbital corresponds to the disappearance of primidone. Phenobarbital therefore accumulates very slowly but eventually reaches therapeutic concentrations in most patients when therapeutic doses of primidone are administered. Phenobarbital levels derived from primidone are usually two to three times higher than primidone levels. PEMA, which probably makes a minimal contribution to the efficacy of primidone, has a half-life of 8–12 hours and therefore reaches steady state more rapidly than phenobarbital.

Therapeutic Levels & Dose

Primidone is most efficacious when plasma levels are in the range of 8–12 µg/mL. Concomitant levels of its metabolite, phenobarbital, at steady state will usually vary from 15 to 30 µg/mL. Doses of 10–20 mg/kg/d are necessary to obtain these levels. It is very important, however, to start primidone at low doses and gradually increase over days to a few weeks to avoid prominent sedation and gastrointestinal complaints. When adjusting doses of the drug, it is important to remember that the parent drug will rapidly reach steady state (30–40 hours), but the active metabolites phenobarbital (20 days) and PEMA (3–4 days) will reach steady state much more slowly.

Toxicity

The dose-related adverse effects of primidone are similar to those of its metabolite, phenobarbital, except that drowsiness occurs early in treatment and may be prominent if the initial dose is too large; gradual increments are indicated when starting the drug in either children or adults.

VIGABATRIN

Current investigations that seek drugs to enhance the effects of GABA include efforts to find GABA agonists and prodrugs, GABA transaminase inhibitors, and GABA uptake inhibitors. Vigabatrin (γ-vinyl-GABA) is the most promising of these new drugs and was recently released in Europe and South America; its discovery and successful development validates enhancement of the inhibitory effects of GABA as a rational approach to epilepsy treatment. The drug is not yet available in the USA.

$$CH_2=CH\diagdown_{CH}\diagup^{CH_2}\diagdown_{CH_2}\diagup^{COOH}$$
$$|$$
$$NH_2$$

Vigabatrin

Mechanism of Action

Vigabatrin is an irreversible inhibitor of GABA aminotransferase (GABA-T), the enzyme responsible for the degradation of GABA. It may act by increasing GABA at synaptic sites, enhancing inhibitory effects and thereby—in a manner yet to be determined—diminishing the hyperexcitability required for the generation and propagation of an epileptic seizure. It is effective in a number of seizure models.

Clinical Use

Vigabatrin is indicated particularly for partial seizures and for West's syndrome. In adults, vigabatrin should be started at a dosage of 500 mg twice daily; a total of 1.5 g (or more) daily may be required for full effectiveness. Typical toxicities include drowsiness, dizziness, and weight gain. Less common but more troublesome adverse reactions are agitation, confusion, and psychosis; preexisting mental illness is a relative contraindication. The drug was delayed in its worldwide introduction by the appearance in rats and dogs of a reversible intramyelinic edema; thousands of patients have now been exposed to vigabatrin with no evidence that this edema occurs in humans.

Pharmacokinetics

Absorption of vigabatrin is rapid, and peak levels are attained in 1–3 hours. The half-life is approximately 6–8 hours, but considerable evidence suggests that the pharmacodynamic activity of the drug is more prolonged and not well correlated with the plasma level. The drug has linear kinetics, no active metabolites, and binds minimally to plasma proteins; elimination is predominantly by the kidneys.

LAMOTRIGINE

Lamotrigine was developed when some investigators thought that the antifolate effects of certain antiepileptic drugs (eg, phenytoin) may contribute to their effectiveness. Several phenyltriazines were developed, and although their antifolate properties were weak, some were active in seizure screening tests, in which this drug resembles phenytoin. Lamotrigine's mechanism of action is not well understood, but, like phenytoin, it prevents rapid repetitive firing by prolonging inactivation of the sodium channel. It has a half-life of approximately 24 hours, and most of the drug is excreted in the urine as the glucuronide. The half-life is shortened by enzyme-inducing drugs. Lamotrigine is effective against partial seizures in adults, with doses typically between 100 and 300 mg/d and with a therapeutic blood level near 3 μg/mL. It is also active against absence and myoclonic seizures in children. The drug is marketed in some European countries but not yet in the USA.

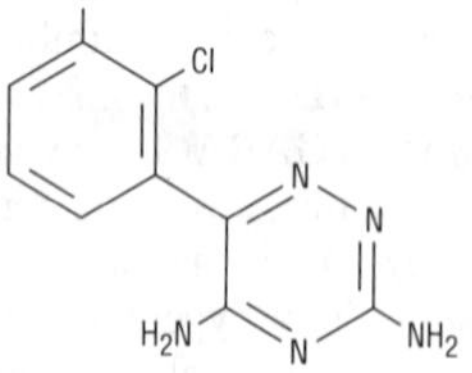

Lamotrigine

FELBAMATE & GABAPENTIN

Two other new drugs are worthy of mention, as they seem likely to be marketed worldwide in the next few years. Felbamate was approved and marketed briefly in the USA but has been withdrawn because of the occurrence of aplastic anemia. It is effective in some patients with partial seizures, has a half-life of 20 hours and is eliminated by hepatic metabolism. The drug increases plasma phenytoin and valproic acid levels but decreases levels of carbamazepine.

Gabapentin is an analogue of GABA and is also effective against partial seizures. Its half-life is 6 hours, and it is eliminated by renal mechanisms (Rogawski, 1990).

DRUGS USED IN GENERALIZED SEIZURES

ETHOSUXIMIDE

Ethosuximide was introduced in 1960 as the third of three marketed succinimides in the USA. Ethosuximide has very little activity against maximal electroshock but considerable efficacy against pentylenetetrazol seizures and was introduced as a "pure petit mal" drug. Its popularity continues, based on its safety and efficacy; its role as the "first choice" antiabsence drug remains undiminished, in part because of the idiosyncratic hepatotoxicity of the alternative drug, valproic acid.

Chemistry

Ethosuximide is the last antiepileptic drug to be marketed whose origin is in the cyclic ureide structure. The three antiepileptic succinimides marketed in the USA are ethosuximide, phensuximide, and methsuximide. All three are substituted at the 2 position. (See structure below, and note difference in numbering relative to Figure 23–1.) Methsuximide and phensuximide have phenyl substituents, while ethosuximide is 2-ethyl-2-methylsuccinimide.

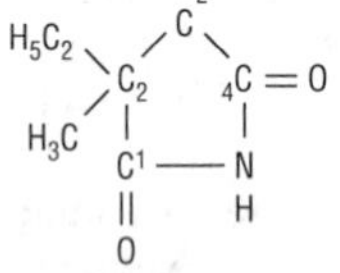

Ethosuximide

Mechanism of Action

The mechanism of action of the succinimides probably involves calcium channels. Ethosuximide also inhibits Na^+/K^+ ATPase, depresses the cerebral metabolic rate, and inhibits GABA aminotransferase. However, none of these actions are seen at therapeutic concentrations. Ethosuximide has an important effect on Ca^{2+} currents, reducing the low-threshold (T-type) current. This effect is seen at therapeutically relevant concentrations in thalamic neurons. The T-type calcium currents are thought to provide a pacemaker current in thalamic neurons responsible for generating the rhythmic cortical discharge of an absence attack. Inhibition of this current could therefore account for the specific therapeutic action of etho-suximide.

Clinical Use

Ethosuximide is particularly effective against absence seizures, as predicted from its activity in laboratory models. Documentation of its effectiveness required specific advances in quantitation of absence seizures; this was accomplished in the 1970s, when the characteristic generalized 3/s spike-wave electroencephalographic abnormality was correlated with a decrement in consciousness even when the abnormality occurs for only a few seconds. Long-term electroencephalographic recordings, therefore, provided the necessary quantitative method for determining the frequency of absence attacks and allowed rapid and effective evaluation of the efficacy of anti-absence drugs. Although ethosuximide was marketed in advance of the federal requirements for efficacy, these techniques were applied to later drugs such as clonazepam and valproic acid in documentation of their efficacy. This was accomplished by comparison with ethosuximide.

Pharmacokinetics

Absorption is complete following administration of the oral dosage forms. Peak levels are observed 3–7 hours after oral administration of the capsules. Animal studies indicate that chronic administration of the solution may prove irritating to the gastric mucosa.

Ethosuximide is uniformly distributed throughout perfused tissues but does not penetrate fat. The volume of distribution approximates that of total body water, ie, 0.7 L/kg. It is not protein-bound, and spinal fluid concentrations are therefore equal to plasma concentrations.

Ethosuximide is completely metabolized, principally by hydroxylation. Four hydroxylated metabolites have been identified. These metabolites undergo subsequent conjugation and excretion. There is no evidence that they are pharmacologically active.

Ethosuximide has a very low total body clearance (0.25 L/kg/d). This corresponds to a half-life of approximately 40 hours, though values from 18 to 72 hours have been reported.

Therapeutic Levels & Dose

Therapeutic levels of 60–100 μg/mL can be achieved in adults with doses of 750–1500 mg/d, though lower or higher doses may be necessary. Some authors report that higher levels (up to 125 μg/mL) are needed in certain patients to achieve efficacy; such patients may tolerate the drug without apparent toxicity at these levels. Ethosuximide has a linear relationship between dose and steady state plasma levels. The drug might be administered as a single daily dose were it not for its adverse gastrointestinal effects; twice-a-day dosage is common. The time of

day at which the level is measured is not particularly critical for ethosuximide, as its half-life is relatively long. No parenteral dosage form for ethosuximide is available.

Drug Interactions

Administration of ethosuximide with valproic acid results in a decrease in ethosuximide clearance and higher steady state concentrations due to inhibition of metabolism. No other important drug interactions have been reported for the succinimides.

Toxicity

The most common dose-related adverse effect of ethosuximide is gastric distress, including pain, nausea, and vomiting. This can often be avoided by starting therapy at a low dose, with gradual increases into the therapeutic range. When the adverse effect does occur, temporary dosage reductions may allow adaptation. Ethosuximide is a highly efficacious and safe drug for absence seizures; the appearance of relatively mild, dose-related adverse effects should not immediately call for its abandonment. Other dose-related adverse effects include transient lethargy or fatigue and, much less commonly, headache, dizziness, hiccup, and euphoria. Behavioral changes are usually in the direction of improvement.

Non-dose-related or idiosyncratic adverse effects of ethosuximide are extremely uncommon. Skin rashes have been reported, including at least one case of Stevens-Johnson syndrome. A few patients have had eosinophilia, thrombocytopenia, leukopenia, or pancytopenia; it is not entirely certain that ethosuximide was the causal agent. The development of systemic lupus erythematosus has also been reported, but other drugs may have been involved.

PHENSUXIMIDE & METHSUXIMIDE

Phensuximide and methsuximide are phenylsuccinimides that were developed and marketed before ethosuximide. They are used primarily as anti-absence drugs. Methsuximide is generally considered more toxic—and phensuximide less effective—than ethosuximide. Unlike ethosuximide, these two compounds have some activity against maximal electroshock seizures, and methsuximide has been used for partial seizures by some investigators. The desmethyl metabolite of methsuximide has a half-life of 25 hours or more and exerts the major antiepileptic effect. The toxicity and lack of effectiveness of phensuximide when compared with methsuximide has been investigated, and the failure of the desmethyl metabolite to accumulate in the former probably explains its relatively weak effect.

VALPROIC ACID & SODIUM VALPROATE

Sodium valproate, also used as the free acid, valproic acid, was found to have antiepileptic properties when it was used as a solvent in the search for other drugs effective against seizures. It was marketed in France in 1969 but was not licensed in the USA until 1978. Valproic acid is fully ionized at body pH, thus the active form of the drug may be assumed to be the valproate ion regardless of whether valproic acid or a salt of the acid is administered.

Chemistry

Valproic acid is one of a series of fatty or carboxylic acids that have antiepileptic activity; this activity appears to be greatest for carbon chain lengths of five to eight atoms. Branching and unsaturation do not significantly alter the drug's activity but may increase its lipophilicity, thereby increasing its duration of action. The amides and esters of valproic acid are also active antiepileptic agents.

$$CH_3 - CH_2 - CH_2$$
$$CH_3 - CH_2 - CH_2 > CH - COOH$$

Valproic acid

Mechanism of Action

The time course of anticonvulsant activity appears to be poorly correlated with blood or tissue levels of the parent drug, an observation giving rise to considerable speculation regarding both the active species and the mechanism of action of valproic acid. Valproate is active against both pentylenetetrazol and maximal electroshock seizures. Like phenytoin and carbamazepine, valproate blocks sustained high-frequency repetitive firing of neurons in culture at therapeutically relevant concentrations. Its action against partial seizures is probably a consequence of this effect on Na^+ currents. Much attention, however, has been paid to the effects of valproate on GABA. Several studies have shown increased levels of GABA in the brain after administration of valproate, though the mechanism for this increase remains unclear. Doubt about the relevance of this increase in GABA to the therapeutic effect is raised by the fact that anticonvulsant effects are observed before GABA brain levels are elevated. If the effect of valproate is related to the enzymes necessary for either the production or breakdown of GABA, the drug may have a greater effect on inhibiting GABA-aminotransferase (GABA-T, responsible for GABA breakdown) than on facilitating glutamic acid decarboxylase (GAD, responsible for GABA synthesis). At very high concentrations, valproate inhibits GABA-T in the brain, thus increasing levels of GABA by blocking conversion of GABA to succinic semialdehyde. However, at the relatively low doses of valproate needed to abolish pentylenetetrazol seizures, brain GABA levels may remain unchanged. Valproate produces a reduction in the aspartate content of rodent brain, but the relevance of this effect to its anticonvulsant action is not known.

At high concentrations, valproate has been shown to increase membrane potassium conductance. Furthermore, low concentrations of valproate tend to hyperpolarize membrane potentials. These findings have led to speculation that valproate may exert an action through a direct effect on the potassium channels of the membrane.

Valproate probably owes its broad spectrum of action to more than one molecular mechanism. Its action against absence attacks remains to be explained.

Clinical Use

Valproate is very effective against absence seizures. Although ethosuximide is the drug of choice when absence seizures occur alone, valproate is preferred if the patient has concomitant generalized tonic-clonic attacks. The reason for preferring ethosuximide for uncomplicated absence seizures is valproate's idiosyncratic hepatotoxicity, described below. Valproate is unique in its ability to control certain types of myoclonic seizures; in some cases the effect is very dramatic. The drug is effective in generalized tonic-clonic seizures, especially those which are primarily generalized. A few patients with atonic attacks may also respond, and some evidence suggests that the drug is effective in partial seizures.

Pharmacokinetics

Valproate is well absorbed following an oral dose, with bioavailability greater than 80%. Peak blood levels are observed within 2 hours. Food may delay absorption, and decreased toxicity may result if the drug is given after meals.

Valproic acid has a pK_a of 4.7 and is therefore virtually completely ionized at physiologic plasma pH. The drug is also 90% bound to plasma proteins, though the fraction bound is somewhat reduced at blood levels greater than 150 μg/mL. Since it is both highly ionized and highly protein-bound, its distribution is essentially confined to extracellular water, with a volume of distribution of approximately 0.15 L/kg.

Approximately 20% of the drug is excreted as a direct conjugate of valproate. The remainder is metabolized by beta and omega oxidation to a number of compounds; these are also subsequently conjugated and excreted.

Clearance for valproate is very low; its half-life varies from 9 hours to 18 hours. At very high blood levels, the clearance of valproate is dose-dependent. There appear to be offsetting changes in the intrinsic clearance and protein binding at higher doses.

The sodium salt of valproate is marketed in Europe as a tablet protected by aluminum foil, as it is quite hygroscopic. In Central and South America, the magnesium salt is available, which is considerably less hygroscopic. The free acid of valproate was first marketed in the USA in a capsule containing corn oil; the sodium salt is also available in syrup, primarily for pediatric use. An enteric-coated tablet of *divalproex sodium* is now marketed in the USA. This improved product, a 1:1 "coordination compound" of valproic acid and sodium valproate, is as bioavailable as the capsule but is absorbed much more slowly and is preferred by most patients. Peak concentrations following administration of the enteric-coated tablets are seen in 3–4 hours.

Therapeutic Levels & Dose

Doses of 25–30 mg/kg/d may be adequate in some patients, but others may require 60 mg/kg or even more. Therapeutic levels of valproate range from 50 to 100 μg/mL. In testing efficacy, this drug should not be abandoned until morning "trough" levels of at least 80 μg/mL have been attained; some patients may require and tolerate levels in excess of 100 μg/mL.

Drug Interactions

As noted above, the clearance of valproate is dose-dependent, caused by changes in both the intrinsic clearance and protein binding. Valproate inhibits its own metabolism at low doses, thus decreasing intrinsic clearance. At higher doses, there is an increased free fraction of valproate, resulting in lower total drug levels than expected. It may be clinically useful, therefore, to measure both total and free drug levels. Valproate also displaces phenytoin from plasma proteins. In addition to binding interactions, valproate inhibits the metabolism of several drugs, including phenobarbital, phenytoin, and carbamazepine, leading to higher steady state concentrations of these agents. The inhibition of phenobarbital metabolism may cause levels of the barbiturate to rise precipitously, causing stupor or coma.

Toxicity

The most common dose-related adverse effects of valproate are nausea, vomiting, and other gastrointestinal complaints such as abdominal pain and "heartburn." The drug should be started gradually to avoid these symptoms; a temporary reduction in dose can usually alleviate the problems, and the patient will eventually tolerate higher doses. Sedation is uncommon with valproate alone but may be striking when valproate is added to phenobarbital. A fine tremor is frequently seen at higher levels. Other reversible adverse effects, seen in a small number of patients, include weight gain, increased appetite, and hair loss.

The idiosyncratic toxicity of valproate is largely limited to hepatotoxicity, but this may be severe; there seems little doubt that the hepatotoxicity of valproate has been responsible for more than 50 fatalities in the USA alone. The risk is greatest for patients under the age of 2 years and for those taking multiple medications. Initial AST (SGOT) values may not be elevated in susceptible patients, though these levels do eventually become abnormal. Most fatalities have occurred within 4 months after initiation of therapy. Careful monitoring of liver function is recommended when starting the drug; the hepatotoxicity is reversible in some cases if the drug is withdrawn. The other observed idiosyncratic response with valproate is thrombocytopenia, though documented cases of abnormal bleeding are lacking. It should be noted that valproate is an effective and popular antiepileptic drug and that only a very small number of patients have had severe toxic effects from its use.

Studies of valproate suggest an increased incidence of spina bifida in the offspring of women who took the drug during pregnancy. In addition, an increased incidence of cardiovascular, orofacial, and digital abnormalities has been reported. These observations, although based on a small number of cases, must be strongly considered in the choice of drugs during pregnancy.

OXAZOLIDINEDIONES

Trimethadione, the first oxazolidinedione, was introduced as an antiepileptic drug in 1945 and remained the drug of choice for absence seizures until the introduction of succinimides in the 1950s. The use of the oxazolidinediones (trimethadione, paramethadione, and dimethadione) is now very limited.

Chemistry

The oxazolidinediones contain as a heterocyclic ring the oxazolidine ring (Figure 23–1) and are similar in structure to other antiepileptic drugs introduced before 1960. The structure includes only short-chain alkyl substituents on the heterocyclic ring, with no attached phenyl group.

Trimethadione

Mechanism of Action

These compounds are active against pentylenetetrazol-induced seizures. Trimethadione raises the threshold for seizure discharges following repetitive thalamic stimulation. It has the same effect on thalamic Ca^{2+} currents as ethosuximide (reducing the T-type calcium current). Thus, suppression of absence seizures is likely to depend on inhibiting the pacemaker action of thalamic neurons.

Pharmacokinetics

Trimethadione is rapidly absorbed, with peak levels reached within an hour after drug administration. It is distributed to all perfused tissues, with a volume of distribution that approximates that of total body water. It is not bound to plasma proteins. Trimethadione is completely metabolized in the liver by demethylation to 5,5-dimethyl-2,4-oxazolidinedione (dimethadione), which may exert the major antiepileptic activity. The drug has a relatively low clearance (1.6 L/kg/d), corresponding to a half-life of approximately 16 hours. The demethylated metabolite, however, is very slowly cleared and accumulates to a much greater extent than the parent drug. The clearance of dimethadione is 0.08 L/kg/d; this metabolite has an extremely long half-life (240 hours).

Therapeutic Levels & Dose

The therapeutic plasma level range for trimethadione has never been established, though trimethadione blood levels above 20 µg/mL and dimethadione levels above 700 µg/mL have been suggested. A dose of 30 mg/kg/d of trimethadione is necessary to achieve these levels in adults.

Drug Interactions

Relatively few drug interactions involving the oxazolidinediones have been reported, though trimethadione may competitively inhibit the demethylation of other drugs such as metharbital.

Toxicity

The most notable dose-related adverse effect of the oxazolidinediones is sedation. An unusual adverse effect is hemeralopia, a glare effect in which visual adaptation is impaired; it is reversible upon withdrawal of the drug. Accumulation of dimethadione has been reported to cause a very mild metabolic acidosis. Trimethadione has been associated with idiosyncratic dermatologic reactions, including rashes and exfoliative dermatitis, as well as toxic reactions involving the blood-forming organs; these have ranged from mild alterations in cell counts to fulminating pancytopenia. Other reactions include reversible nephrotic syndrome, which may involve an immune reaction to the drug, as well as a myasthenic syndrome. These drugs should not be used during pregnancy.

OTHER DRUGS USED IN MANAGEMENT OF EPILEPSY

Some drugs not classifiable by application to seizure type are discussed in this section.

BENZODIAZEPINES
(See also Chapter 21.)

Six benzodiazepines play prominent roles in the therapy of epilepsy. Although many benzodiazepines are quite similar chemically, subtle structural alterations result in differences in activity. They have two different mechanisms of antiepileptic action, which are shown to different degrees by the six compounds. This is evident from the fact that diazepam is relatively more potent against electroshock and clonazepam against pentylenetetrazol (the latter effect correlating with an action at the GABA-benzodiazepine allosteric receptor site). Possible mechanisms of action are discussed in Chapter 21.

Diazepam given intravenously is highly effective for stopping continuous seizure activity, especially generalized tonic-clonic status epilepticus (see page 378). The drug is marketed as an adjunct to therapy and is occasionally given orally on a chronic basis, though it is not considered very effective in this application, probably because of the rapid development of tolerance.

Lorazepam is a newer benzodiazepine that, when given intravenously, appears in some studies to be more effective and longer-acting than diazepam in the treatment of status epilepticus.

Clonazepam is a long-acting drug with documented efficacy against absence seizures; it is one of the most potent antiepileptic agents known. It is also effective in some cases of myoclonic seizures and has been tried in infantile spasms. Sedation is prominent, especially on initiation of therapy; starting doses should be small. Maximal tolerated doses are usually in the range of 0.1–0.2 mg/kg, but many weeks of gradually increasing daily dosage may be needed to achieve these doses in some patients. Therapeutic blood levels are usually less than 0.1 µg/mL and are not routinely measured in most laboratories.

Clorazepate dipotassium is a benzodiazepine approved in the USA as an adjunct to treatment of complex partial seizures in adults. Drowsiness and lethargy are common adverse effects, but as long as the drug is increased gradually, doses as high as 45 mg/d can be given.

Nitrazepam is not marketed in the USA but is used in many other countries, especially for infantile spasms and myoclonic seizures. It is less potent than clonazepam, and whether it has any clinical advantages over clonazepam remains unclear.

Clobazam is not available in the USA but is marketed in most countries. It is a 1,5-benzodiazepine (unlike other marketed compounds, all of which are 1,4-benzodiazepines) and reportedly has less sedative potential than marketed benzodiazepines. Whether the drug has significant clinical advantages is not clear.

The pharmacokinetic properties of the benzodiazepines in part determine their clinical use. In general, the drugs are well absorbed, widely distributed, and extensively metabolized, with many active metabolites. The rate of distribution of benzodiazepines within the body is different from that of other antiepileptic drugs. Diazepam and lorazepam in particular are rapidly and extensively distributed to the tissues, with volumes of distribution between 1 and 3 L/kg. The onset of action is very rapid. Total body clearances of the parent drug and its metabolites are low, corresponding to half-lives of 20–40 hours.

Two prominent aspects of benzodiazepines limit their usefulness. The first is their pronounced sedative effect, which is unfortunate both in the treatment of status epilepticus and in chronic therapy. Children may manifest a paradoxical hyperactivity, as with barbiturates. The second problem is tolerance, in which seizures may initially respond, but within a few months the initial improvement may diminish. The remarkable antiepileptic potency of these compounds often cannot be realized because of these limiting factors.

ACETAZOLAMIDE

Acetazolamide is a diuretic whose main action is the inhibition of carbonic anhydrase (see Chapter 15). The accumulation of carbon dioxide in the brain may be the mechanism by which the drug exerts its antiepileptic activity; alternatively, it may act by a direct neuronal effect. Acetazolamide has been used for all types of seizures but is severely limited by the rapid development of tolerance, with return of seizures usually within a few weeks. The drug may have a special role in epileptic women who experience seizure exacerbations at the time of menses; seizure control may be improved and tolerance may not develop because the drug is not administered continuously. The usual dose is approximately 10 mg/kg up to a maximum of 1000 mg/d.

Another carbonic anhydrase inhibitor, sulthiame, was not found to be effective in clinical trials in the USA. It is marketed in some other countries.

BROMIDE

Bromide was introduced by Locock in 1857 and was the first antiepileptic drug with any measurable efficacy. Though largely discarded in favor of phenobarbital after the turn of the century, bromide is still occasionally useful, such as in management of epilepsy in patients with porphyria, in whom other drugs may be contraindicated. Its half-life is approximately 12 days, and it is given in doses of 3–6 g/d in adults to obtain plasma levels of 10–20 meq/L. The mechanism of action of bromide as an antiepileptic agent is unknown. Major toxic problems are unfortunately frequent and include skin rashes, sedation, and behavioral changes. It is not currently available in the USA.

II. CLINICAL PHARMACOLOGY OF ANTIEPILEPTIC DRUGS

SEIZURE CLASSIFICATION

The type of medication utilized for epilepsy is dependent upon the empirical nature of the seizure. For this reason, considerable effort has been made to classify seizures so that clinicians will be able to make a "seizure diagnosis" and thereby prescribe appropriate therapy. Errors in seizure diagnosis cause use of the wrong drugs, and an unpleasant cycle ensues in which poor seizure control is followed by increasing drug doses and medication toxicity. As noted above, seizures are divided into two groups: partial and generalized. Drugs used for partial seizures are more or less the same for the entire group, but drugs used for generalized seizures are determined by the individual seizure type. A shortened version of the international classification of epileptic seizures is presented in Table 23–1.

Partial Seizures

Partial seizures are those in which a localized onset of the attack can be ascertained, either by clinical observation or by electroencephalographic recording; the attack begins in a specific locus in the brain. There are three types of partial seizures, determined to some extent by the degree of brain involvement by the abnormal discharge.

The least complicated partial seizure is the **simple partial seizure,** characterized by minimal spread of the abnormal discharge such that normal consciousness and awareness are preserved. For example, the patient may have a sudden onset of clonic jerking of an extremity lasting 60–90 seconds; residual weakness may last for 15–30 minutes after the attack. The patient is completely aware of the attack and can describe it in detail. The EEG may show an abnormal discharge highly localized to the involved portion of the brain.

The **complex partial seizure** also has a localized onset, but the discharge becomes more widespread (usually bilateral) and almost always involves the limbic system. Most (not all) complex partial seizures arise from one of the temporal lobes, possibly because of the susceptibility of this area of the brain to insults such as hypoxia or infection. Clinically, the patient may have a brief warning followed by an alteration of consciousness during which some patients may stare and others may stagger or even fall. Most, however, demonstrate fragments of integrated motor behavior called automatisms for which the patient has no memory. Typical automatisms are lip smacking, swallowing, fumbling, scratching, or even walking about. After 30–120 seconds, the patient makes a gradual recovery to normal consciousness but may feel tired or ill for several hours after the attack.

The last type of partial seizure is the secondarily generalized attack, in which a partial seizure immediately precedes a generalized tonic-clonic (grand mal) seizure. This seizure type is described below.

Generalized Seizures

Generalized seizures are those in which there is no evidence of localized onset. The group is quite heterogeneous.

Generalized tonic-clonic (grand mal) seizures are the most dramatic of all epileptic seizures and are characterized by tonic rigidity of all extremities, followed in 15–30 seconds by a tremor that is actually an interruption of the tonus by relaxation. As the relaxation phases become longer, the attack enters the clonic phase, with massive jerking of the body. The clonic jerking slows over 60–120 seconds, and the patient is usually left in a stuporous state. The tongue or cheek may be bitten, and urinary incontinence is common. Primary generalized tonic-clonic seizures begin without evidence of localized onset, whereas secondary generalized tonic-clonic seizures are preceded by another seizure type, usually a partial seizure. The medical treatment of both primary and secondary generalized tonic-clonic seizures is the same and utilizes drugs appropriate for *partial* seizures.

The **absence (petit mal) seizure** is characterized by both sudden onset and abrupt cessation. Its duration is usually less than 10 seconds and rarely more than 45 seconds. Consciousness is altered; the attack may also be associated with mild clonic jerking of the eyelids or extremities, with postural tone changes, autonomic phenomena, and automatisms. The occurrence of automatisms can complicate the clinical differentiation from complex partial seizures in some patients. Absence attacks begin in childhood or adolescence and may occur up to hundreds of times a day. The EEG during the seizure shows a highly characteristic 2.5–3.5 Hz spike-and-wave pattern. Atypical absence patients have seizures with postural changes that are more abrupt, and the patients are often mentally retarded; the EEG may show a slower spike-and-wave discharge, and the seizures may be more refractory to therapy.

Myoclonic jerking is seen, to a greater or lesser extent, in a wide variety of seizures, including generalized tonic-clonic seizures, partial seizures, absence seizures, and infantile spasms. Treatment of seizures that include myoclonic jerking should be directed at the primary seizure type rather than at the myoclonus. Some patients, however, have myoclonic jerking as the major seizure type, and some have frequent myo-

clonic jerking and occasional generalized tonic-clonic seizures without overt signs of neurologic deficit. Many kinds of myoclonus exist, and much effort has gone into attempts to classify this entity.

Atonic seizures are those in which the patient has sudden loss of postural tone. If standing, the patient falls suddenly to the floor and may be injured. If seated, the head and torso may suddenly drop forward. Although most often seen in children, this seizure type is not unusual in adults. Many patients with atonic seizures wear helmets to prevent head injury.

Infantile spasms are an epileptic syndrome and not a seizure type. The attacks, though sometimes fragmentary, are most often bilateral and are included for pragmatic purposes with the generalized seizures. These attacks are most often characterized clinically by brief, recurrent myoclonic jerks of the body with sudden flexion or extension of the body and limbs; the forms of infantile spasms are, however, quite heterogeneous. Ninety percent of affected patients have their first attack before the age of 1 year. Most patients are mentally retarded, presumably from the same cause as the spasms. The cause is unknown in many patients, but such widely disparate disorders as infection, kernicterus, tuberous sclerosis, and hypoglycemia have been implicated. In some cases, the EEG is characteristic. Drugs used to treat infantile spasms are effective only in some patients; there is little evidence that the mental retardation is alleviated by therapy, even when the attacks disappear.

THERAPEUTIC STRATEGY

For antiepileptic drugs, relationships between blood levels and therapeutic effects have been characterized to a particularly high degree. The same is true for the pharmacokinetics of these drugs. These relationships provide significant advantages in the development of therapeutic strategies for the treatment of epilepsy. The therapeutic index for most antiepileptic drugs is low, and toxicity is not uncommon. Thus, effective treatment of seizures requires an awareness of the therapeutic levels and pharmacokinetic properties as well as the characteristic toxicities of each agent. Measurements of antiepileptic drug plasma levels are extremely useful when combined with clinical observations and pharmacokinetic data (Table 23–2).

Table 23–2. Effective plasma levels of 6 antiepileptic drugs.[1]

Drug	Effective Level (μg/mL)	High Effective Level[2] (μg/mL)	Toxic Level (μg/mL)
Carbamazepine	4–12	7	>8
Primidone	5–15	10	>12
Phenytoin	10–20	18	>20
Phenobarbital	10–40	35	>40
Ethosuximide	50–100	80	>100
Valproate	50–100	80	>100

[1]Reprinted, with permission, from Porter RJ: *Epilepsy: 100 Elementary Principles,* 2nd ed. Saunders, 1989.

[2]Level that should be achieved, if possible, in patients with refractory seizures, assuming that the blood samples are drawn before administration of the morning medication. Higher levels are often possible—without toxicity—when the drugs are used alone, ie, as monotherapy.

MANAGEMENT OF EPILEPSY

PARTIAL SEIZURES & GENERALIZED TONIC-CLONIC SEIZURES

Until recently, the choice of drugs was usually limited to phenytoin, carbamazepine, or barbiturates. There has been a strong tendency in the past few years to limit the use of sedative antiepileptic drugs such as barbiturates and benzodiazepines to patients who cannot tolerate other medications. In the 1980s, the trend was to increase the use of carbamazepine. More recently, the use of oxcarbazepine has been increasing, and the addition of vigabatrin and lamotrigine has made decisions more complex.

GENERALIZED SEIZURES

The drugs used for generalized tonic-clonic seizures are the same as for partial seizures; in addition, valproate is clearly useful.

Three drugs are effective against absence seizures. Two are nonsedative and therefore preferred: ethosuximide and valproate. Clonazepam is also highly effective but has disadvantages of dose-related adverse effects and development of tolerance. The drug of choice is ethosuximide, though valproate is effective in some ethosuximide-resistant patients.

Specific myoclonic syndromes are usually treated with valproate. It is nonsedative and can be dramatically effective. Other patients respond to clonazepam

or other benzodiazepines, though high doses may be necessary, with accompanying sedation and drowsiness. A highly specific myoclonic syndrome, "intention myoclonus," which occurs after severe hypoxia, is characterized by myoclonus associated with volitional activity. Improvement in some patients with this unusual disorder has been reported using 5-hydroxytryptophan.

Atonic seizures are often refractory to all available medications, though some reports suggest that valproate may be beneficial, as may lamotrigine. Benzodiazepines have been reported to improve seizure control in some of these patients but may worsen the attacks in others. A new drug, felbamate, may eventually prove useful. If the loss of tone appears to be part of another seizure type (such as absence or complex partial seizures), every effort should be made to treat the other seizure type vigorously, hoping for simultaneous alleviation of the atonic component of the seizure.

DRUGS USED IN INFANTILE SPASMS

The treatment of infantile spasms is unfortunately limited to improvement of control of the seizures rather than other features of the disorder, such as retardation. Most patients receive a course of intramuscular corticotropin, though some clinicians note that prednisone may be equally effective and can be given orally. Clinical trials have thus far been unable to settle the matter. In either case, therapy must often be discontinued because of adverse effects. If seizures recur, repeat courses of corticotropin or corticosteroids can be given, or other drugs may be tried. Other drugs widely used are the benzodiazepines such as clonazepam or nitrazepam; their efficacy in this heterogeneous syndrome may be nearly as good as corticosteroids. Vigabatrin may also be effective. The mechanism of action of corticosteroids or corticotropin in the treatment of infantile spasms is unknown.

In spite of more than 30 years experience with corticosteroids and corticotropin for infantile spasms, the optimal dosage and duration of therapy have not been established. Currently, a broad range of dosages are utilized, although most patients are treated with 25–40 units of corticotropin daily. A very few investigators recommend up to 240 units daily. In the 60% of patients who respond, seizure reduction is usually reported within 1–5 weeks. Corticotropin therapy may be continued for 3 months or more unless toxicity requires cessation. For corticosteroids, doses of 2 mg/kg of prednisolone or 0.3 mg/kg of dexamethasone have been utilized.

The toxic effects of corticotropin are characteristic of corticosteroid excess and include hypertension, cushingoid obesity, gastrointestinal disturbances, skin changes, osteoporosis, and electrolyte imbalance.

STATUS EPILEPTICUS

There are many forms of status epilepticus. The most common, generalized tonic-clonic status epilepticus, is a life-threatening emergency, requiring immediate cardiovascular, respiratory, and metabolic management as well as pharmacologic therapy. The latter virtually always requires intravenous administration of antiepileptic medications. Diazepam is the most effective drug in most patients for stopping the attacks and is given directly by intravenous push to a maximum total dose of 20–30 mg in adults. Intravenous diazepam may depress respiration (less frequently cardiovascular function), and facilities for resuscitation must be immediately at hand during its administration. The effect of diazepam is not lasting, but the 30- to 40-minute seizure-free interval allows more definitive therapy to be initiated. For patients who are not actually in the throes of a seizure, diazepam therapy can be omitted and the patient treated at once with a long-acting drug such as phenytoin. Some physicians prefer lorazepam, which is equivalent to diazepam in effect and perhaps somewhat longer-acting.

The mainstay of continuing therapy for status epilepticus is intravenous phenytoin, which is effective and nonsedative. It should be given as a loading dose of 13–18 mg/kg in adults; the usual error is to give too little. Administration should be at a maximum rate of 50 mg/min. It is safest to give the drug directly by intravenous push, but it can also be diluted in saline; it precipitates rapidly in the presence of glucose. Careful monitoring of cardiac rhythm and blood pressure is necessary, especially in elderly people. At least part of the cardiotoxicity is from the propylene glycol in which the phenytoin is dissolved.

In previously treated epileptic patients, the administration of a large loading dose of phenytoin may cause some dose-related toxicity such as ataxia. This is usually a relatively minor problem during the acute status episode and is easily alleviated by later adjustment of plasma levels.

For patients who do not respond to phenytoin, phenobarbital can be given in large doses: 100–200 mg intravenously to a total of 400–800 mg. Respiratory depression is a common complication, especially if benzodiazepines have already been given, and there should be no hesitation in instituting intubation and ventilation.

Although other drugs such as lidocaine have been recommended for the treatment of generalized tonic-clonic status epilepticus, general anesthesia is usually necessary in highly resistant cases.

SPECIAL ASPECTS OF THE TOXICOLOGY OF ANTIEPILEPTIC DRUGS

TERATOGENICITY

The potential teratogenicity of antiepileptic drugs is a controversial and important area. It is important because teratogenicity resulting from chronic drug treatment of millions of people throughout the world may have a profound effect even if the effect occurs in only a small percentage of cases. It is controversial because both epilepsy and antiepileptic drugs are heterogeneous, and few epileptic patients are available for study who are not receiving these drugs. Furthermore, patients with severe epilepsy, in whom genetic factors rather than drug factors may be of greater importance in the occurrence of fetal malformations, are often receiving multiple antiepileptic drugs in high doses.

In spite of these limitations, it appears—from whatever cause—that children born to mothers taking antiepileptic drugs have an increased risk, perhaps twofold, of congenital malformations. One drug, phenytoin, has been implicated in a specific syndrome called **fetal hydantoin syndrome,** though not all investigators are convinced of its existence and a similar syndrome has been attributed both to phenobarbital and to carbamazepine. Valproate, as noted above, has also been implicated in a specific malformation, spina bifida. It is estimated that a pregnant woman taking valproic acid or sodium valproate has a 1–2% risk of having a child with spina bifida (Valproate, 1983).

In dealing with the clinical problem of a pregnant woman with epilepsy, most epileptologists agree that while it is important to minimize exposure to antiepileptic drugs, both in numbers and dosages, it is also important not to allow maternal seizures to go unchecked.

WITHDRAWAL

Withdrawal of antiepileptic drugs, whether by accident or by design, can cause increased seizure frequency and severity. There are two factors to consider: the effects of the withdrawal itself and the need for continued drug suppression of seizures in the individual patient. In many patients, both factors must be considered. It is important to note, however, that the abrupt discontinuance of antiepileptic drugs ordinarily does not cause seizures in nonepileptic patients provided that the drug levels are not above the usual therapeutic range when the drug is stopped.

Some drugs are more easily withdrawn than others. In general, withdrawal of anti-absence drugs is easier than withdrawal of drugs needed for partial or generalized tonic-clonic seizures. Barbiturates and benzodiazepines are the most difficult to discontinue; weeks or months may be required, with very gradual dosage decrements, to accomplish their complete removal, especially if the patient is not hospitalized.

Because of the heterogeneity of epilepsy, consideration of the complete removal of antiepileptic drugs is an especially difficult problem. If a patient is seizure-free for 3 or 4 years, gradual discontinuance is usually warranted.

OVERDOSE

Antiepileptic drugs are real or potential central nervous system depressants but are rarely lethal. Very high blood levels are usually necessary before overdoses can be considered life-threatening. The most dangerous effect of antiepileptic drugs after large overdoses is respiratory depression, which may be potentiated by other agents, such as alcohol. Treatment of antiepileptic drug overdose is supportive; stimulants should not be used. Efforts to hasten removal of antiepileptic drugs, such as urine alkalinization, are usually ineffective. Lipid dialysis has also been attempted; the data are too scanty to interpret its efficacy.

PREPARATIONS AVAILABLE

Carbamazepine (generic, Tegretol)
Oral: 200 mg tablets; 100 mg chewable tablets; 100 mg/5 mL suspension
Clonazepam (Klonopin)
Oral: 0.5, 1, 2 mg tablets
Clorazepate dipotassium (generic, Tranxene)
Oral: 3.75, 7.5, 15 mg tablets, capsules;
Oral sustained-release (Tranxene-SD): 11.25, 22.5 mg tablets
Diazepam (generic, Valium, others)
Oral: 2, 5, 10 mg tablets; 5 mg/5 mL, 5 mg/mL solutions
Oral sustained-release: 15 mg capsules
Parenteral: 5 mg/mL for injection
Ethosuximide (Zarontin)
Oral: 250 mg capsules; 250 mg/5 mL syrup
Ethotoin (Peganone)
Oral: 250, 500 mg tablets
Gabapentin (Neurontin)
Oral: 100, 300, 400 mg capsules
Lorazepam (generic, Ativan)
Oral: 0.5, 1, 2 mg tablets
Parenteral: 2, 4 mg/mL for injection
Mephenytoin (Mesantoin)
Oral: 100 mg tablets
Mephobarbital (Mebaral)
Oral: 32, 50, 100 mg tablets
Metharbital (Gemonil)
Oral: 100 mg tablets
Methsuximide (Celontin Kapseals)

Oral: 150, 300 mg capsules
Paramethadione (Paradione)
Oral: 150, 300 mg tablets
Pentobarbital sodium (generic, Nembutal)
Parenteral: 50 mg/mL for injection
Phenacemide (Phenurone)
Oral: 500 mg tablets
Phenobarbital (generic, Luminal Sodium, others)
Oral: 8, 16, 32, 65, 100 mg tablets; 16 mg capsules; 15, 20 mg/5 mL elixirs
Parenteral: 30, 60, 65, 130 mg/mL for injection
Phensuximide (Milontin Kapseals)
Oral: 500 mg capsules
Phenytoin (generic, Dilantin, others)
Oral: 30, 100 mg capsules; 50 mg chewable tablets; 30, 125 mg/5 mL suspension;
Oral extended-action: 30, 100 mg capsules
Parenteral: 50 mg/mL for IV injection
Primidone (generic, Mysoline)
Oral: 50, 250 mg tablets; 250 mg/5 mL suspension
Trimethadione (Tridione)
Oral: 150 mg chewable tablets; 300 mg capsules; 40 mg/mL solution
Valproic acid (generic, Depakene, Myproic Acid)
Oral: 250 mg capsules; 250 mg/5 mL syrup (sodium valproate)
Oral sustained-release (Depakote): 125, 250, 500 mg tablets (as divalproex sodium)

REFERENCES

Bialer M: Comparative pharmacokinetics of the newer antiepileptic drugs. Clin Pharmacokinet 1993;24:441.

Brodie MJ: Drug interactions in epilepsy. Epilepsia 1992; 33(Suppl):S13.

Brodie MJ: Lamotrigine. Lancet 1992;339:1397.

Brodie MJ, Porter RJ: New and potential anticonvulsants. Lancet 1990;336:425.

Browne TR et al: Multicenter long-term safety and efficacy study of vigabatrin for refractory complex partial seizures: an update. Neurology 1991;41:363.

Callaghan N, Garrett A, Goggin T: Withdrawal of anticonvulsant drugs in patients free of seizures for two years. N Engl J Med 1988;318:942.

Dam M, Gram L: *Comprehensive Epileptology.* Raven Press, 1991.

Dalessio DJ: Current concepts: Seizure disorders and pregnancy. N Engl J Med 1985;312:559.

Dreifuss FE, Langer DH: Hepatic considerations in the use of antiepileptic drugs. Epilepsia 1987;28(Suppl 2):S23.

Emerson R et al: Stopping medication in children with epilepsy: Predictors of outcome. N Engl J Med 1981;304:1125.

Jones KL et al: Pattern of malformations in the children of women treated with carbamazepine during pregnancy. N Engl J Med 1989;320:1661.

Macdonald RL, Meldrum BS: Principles of antiepileptic drug action. In: *Antiepileptic Drugs,* 3rd ed. Levy RH et al (editors). Raven Press, 1989.

Mattson RH et al: Comparison of carbamazepine, phenobarbital, phenytoin, and primidone in partial and secondarily generalized tonic-clonic seizures. N Engl J Med 1985;313:145.

Mattson RH et al: A comparison of valproate with carbamazepine for the treatment of complex partial seizures and secondarily generalized tonic-clonic seizures in adults. N Engl J Med 1992;327:765.

Meldrum BS: GABAergic mechanisms in the pathogenesis and treatment of epilepsy. Br J Pharmacol 1989;27:3S.

Meldrum BS, Porter RJ (editors): *New Anticonvulsant Drugs.* John Libbey, 1986.

Porter RJ: *Epilepsy: 100 Elementary Principles,* 2nd ed. Saunders, 1989.

Porter RJ: Recognizing and classifying epileptic seizures and epileptic syndromes. In: *Neurologic Clinics: Epilepsy.* Porter RJ, Theodore WH (editors). Saunders, 1986.

Porter RJ, Nadi NS: Investigations in the pharmacotherapy of the focal epilepsies. In: *The Epileptic Focus.* Weiser HG, Speckmann EJ, Engel J (editors). John Libbey, 1987.

Porter RJ: New antiepileptic agents: Strategies for drug development. Lancet 1990;336:423.

Ramsay RE: Treatment of status epilepticus. Epilepsia 1993;34 (Suppl 1):S71.

Rogawski MA: The NMDA receptor, NMDA antagonists and epilepsy therapy: A status report. Drugs 1992;44:279.

Rogawski MA, Porter RJ: Antiepileptic drugs: Pharmacological mechanisms and clinical efficacy with consideration of promising developmental stage compounds. Pharmacol Rev 1990;42:223.

Sivenius J et al: Vigabatrin in drug-resistant partial epilepsy: A 5-year follow-up study. Neurology 1991;41:562.

Theodore WH, Porter RJ, Raubertas RF: Seizures during barbiturate withdrawal: Relation to blood level. Ann Neurol 1987;22:644.

Theodore WH et al: Barbiturates reduce human cerebral glucose metabolism. Neurology 1986;36:60.

Thomson AH, Brodie MJ: Pharmacokinetic optimisation of anticonvulsant therapy. Clin Pharmacokinet 1992;23:216.

Treiman DM: The role of benzodiazepines in the management of status epilepticus. Neurology 1990;40 (Suppl 2):32.

Treiman DM: Gamma vinyl GABA: Current role in the management of drug-resistant epilepsy. Epilepsia 1989;30 (Suppl 3):S31.

Yerby MS: Risks of pregnancy in women with epilepsy. Epilepsia 1992;33(Suppl 1):S23.

Valproate: A new cause of birth defects: Report from Italy and follow-up from France. MMWR Morb Mortal Wkly Rep 1983;32:438.

General Anesthetics

24

Anthony J. Trevor, PhD, & Ronald D. Miller, MD

Attempts to suppress the pain of surgical procedures by the use of drugs date from ancient times and have included the oral administration of ethanol and opiates. The first scientific demonstration of drug-induced anesthesia during surgery was in 1846, when William Morton used diethyl ether in Boston. Within a year, chloroform was introduced by James Simpson in Scotland. This was followed 20 years later by the successful demonstration of the anesthetic properties of nitrous oxide, which had been first suggested by Davy in the 1790s. Modern anesthesia dates from the 1930s, when the intravenous barbiturate thiopental was introduced. A decade later, curare was used in anesthesia to achieve skeletal muscle relaxation. The first modern halogenated hydrocarbon, halothane, was introduced as an inhaled anesthetic in 1956 and soon became the standard for comparison for newer inhaled anesthetic drugs.

The state of "general anesthesia" usually includes analgesia, amnesia, loss of consciousness, inhibition of sensory and autonomic reflexes, and, in many cases, skeletal muscle relaxation. The extent to which any individual anesthetic drug can exert these effects varies with the drug, the dosage, and the clinical circumstances.

An ideal anesthetic drug would induce anesthesia smoothly and rapidly and permit rapid recovery as soon as administration ceased. The drug would also possess a wide margin of safety and be devoid of adverse effects. No single anesthetic agent is capable of achieving all of these desirable effects without some disadvantages when used alone. The modern practice of anesthesia most commonly involves the use of combinations of drugs, taking advantage of their individual favorable properties while attempting to minimize their potential for harmful actions.

A number of anesthesia protocols are available for different surgical interventions. For minor procedures, **conscious sedation** may be used, involving the use of benzodiazepines in conjunction with local anesthetics. **Balanced anesthesia,** using short-acting barbiturates with nitrous oxide and intravenous opioids, is often appropriate for more extensive procedures. For major surgery, the anesthesia procedure frequently includes the administration of medications preoperatively for sedation and analgesia, the induc-

tion of anesthesia with thiopental or other rapidly acting intravenous agent, and the provision of deep anesthesia with inhalational agents alone or in combination with intravenous drugs. In many cases, such protocols include the use of skeletal muscle relaxing drugs. For "day surgery" (surgery performed on ambulatory patients who go home the same day) and for sedation-anesthesia used in patients in intensive care units who must be mechanically ventilated, intravenous agents such as benzodiazepines and propofol are often used.

TYPES OF GENERAL ANESTHETICS

General anesthetics are usually given by inhalation or by intravenous injection.

Inhalational Agents

The chemical structures of the inhalational agents are shown in Figure 24–1. Nitrous oxide, a gas at ambient temperature and pressure, continues to be an important component of many anesthesia regimens. Halothane, enflurane, isoflurane, desflurane, and methoxyflurane are volatile liquids. Sevoflurane is a newer inhalational agent that is not yet approved for use in the USA. The older inhalational agents such as ether, cyclopropane, and chloroform are no longer used in developed countries for reasons that include potential flammability (ether, cyclopropane) and organ toxicity (chloroform).

Intravenous Agents

Several drugs are used intravenously, alone or with other drugs, to achieve anesthesia, as components of balanced anesthesia, or to sedate patients in intensive care units who must be mechanically ventilated for prolonged periods. They include the following: (1) barbiturates (thiopental, methohexital), (2) benzodiazepines (midazolam, diazepam), (3) opioid analgesics and neuroleptics, (4) miscellaneous drugs (propofol, etomidate), and (5) ketamine, an arylcyclohexylamine, which produces a state called dissociative anesthesia.

Figure 24–2 shows the structures of commonly used intravenous anesthetics.

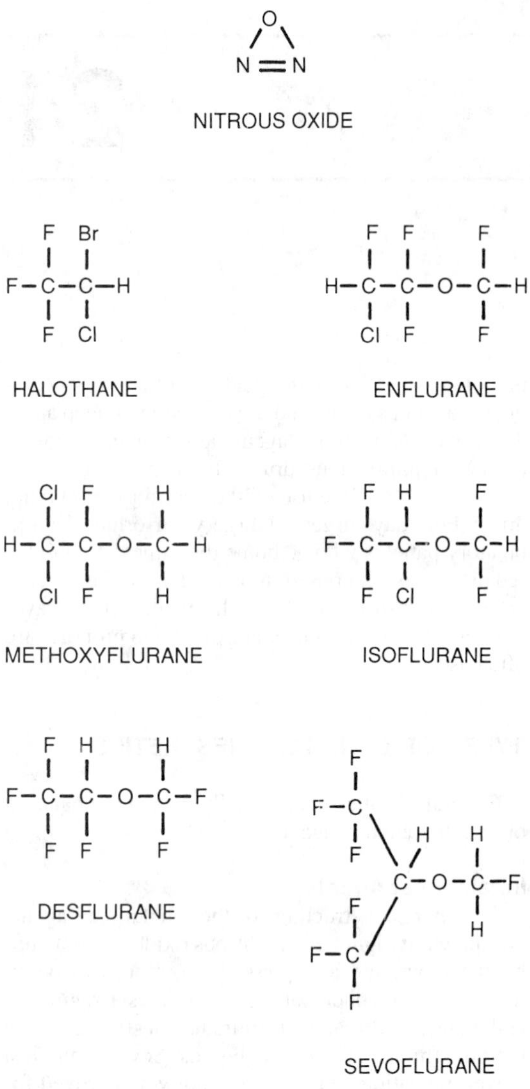

Figure 24–1. Inhalational anesthetics.

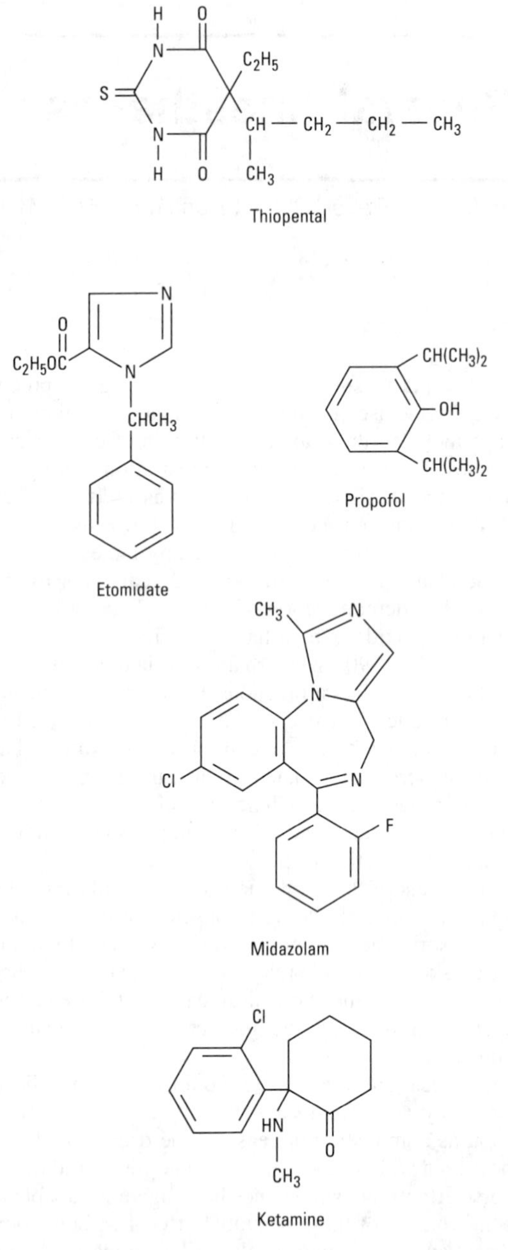

Figure 24–2. Intravenous anesthetics.

SIGNS & STAGES OF ANESTHESIA

Since the introduction of general anesthetics, attempts have been made to correlate their observable effects or signs with the *depth* of anesthesia. A traditional description of the signs and stages of anesthesia (Guedel's signs) derives mainly from observations of the effects of diethyl ether, which has a slow onset of central action owing to its high solubility in blood. The intermediate stages and signs are rarely observed with the more rapidly acting modern inhaled anesthetics and intravenous agents. Furthermore, most anesthetic protocols for major procedures now consist of a combination of inhaled and intravenous agents. Nevertheless, the signs of diethyl ether anesthesia still provide the basis for assessing anesthetic effect for all general anesthetics. Many of these signs refer to the effects of anesthetic agents on respiration, reflex activity, and muscle tone. Traditionally, anesthetic effects are divided into four stages of increasing depth of central nervous system depression.

I. Stage of Analgesia: The patient initially experiences analgesia without amnesia. Later in stage I, both analgesia and amnesia ensue.

II. Stage of Excitement: During this stage, the patient often appears to be delirious and excited but definitely is amnesic. Respiration is irregular both in volume and rate, and retching and vomiting may occur. Incontinence and struggling sometimes occur. For these reasons, efforts are made to limit the duration and severity of this stage, which ends with the reestablishment of regular breathing.

III. Stage of Surgical Anesthesia: This stage begins with the recurrence of regular respiration and extends to complete cessation of spontaneous respiration. Four planes of stage III have been described in terms of changes in ocular movements, eye reflexes, and pupil size, which under specified conditions may represent signs of increasing depth of anesthesia.

IV. Stage of Medullary Depression: When spontaneous respiration ceases, stage IV is present. This stage of anesthesia includes severe depression of the vasomotor center in the medulla as well as the respiratory center. Without full circulatory and respiratory support, death rapidly ensues.

In modern anesthesia practice, the distinctive signs of each of the four stages described above are often obscured. Reasons for this include the relatively rapid onset of action of many inhaled anesthetics compared to that of diethyl ether and the fact that respiratory activity is often controlled with the aid of a mechanical ventilator. In addition, the presence of other pharmacologic agents given preoperatively or intraoperatively can also influence the signs of anesthesia. Atropine, used to decrease secretions, also dilates pupils; drugs such as tubocurarine and succinylcholine affect muscle tone; and the opioid analgesics exert depressant effects on respiration. The most reliable indications that stage III (surgical anesthesia) has been achieved are loss of the eyelash reflex and establishment of a respiratory pattern that is regular in rate and depth. The adequacy of ensuing depth of anesthesia for the specific surgical requirements is assessed mainly by changes in respiratory and cardiovascular responses to stimulation.

INHALED ANESTHETICS

PHARMACOKINETICS

Depth of anesthesia is determined by the concentrations of anesthetics in the central nervous system. The rate at which an effective brain concentration is reached (the rate of induction of anesthesia) depends on multiple pharmacokinetic factors that influence the uptake and distribution of the anesthetic. These factors determine the different rates of transfer of the inhaled anesthetic from the lung to the blood and from the blood to the brain and other tissues. These factors also influence the rate of recovery from anesthesia when inhalation of the anesthetic is terminated.

Uptake & Distribution

The **concentration** of an individual gas in a mixture of gases is proportionate to its **partial pressure** or **tension.** These terms are often used interchangeably in discussing the various transfer processes of anesthetic gases in the body. Achievement of a brain concentration of an anesthetic adequate to cause anesthesia requires transfer of that anesthetic from the alveolar air to blood and then to brain. The rate at which a given concentration of anesthetic in the brain is reached depends on the solubility properties of the anesthetic, its concentration in the inspired air, pulmonary ventilation rate, pulmonary blood flow, and the concentration (partial pressure) gradient of the anesthetic between arterial and mixed venous blood.

A. Solubility: One of the most important factors influencing the transfer of an anesthetic from the lungs to the arterial blood is its solubility. The blood:gas partition coefficient is a useful index of solubility and defines the relative affinity of an anesthetic for the blood compared to air. The partition coefficient may be as low as 0.5 for anesthetics such as nitrous oxide or cyclopropane, which are quite insoluble in blood. At the other extreme, the value may be higher than 10 for agents such as methoxyflurane, which is very soluble in blood (Table 24–1). When an anesthetic with low blood solubility diffuses from the lung into the arterial blood, relatively few molecules are required to raise its partial pressure, and the arterial tension rises quickly (Figure 24–3, top, nitrous oxide). Conversely, for anesthetics with moderate to high solubility, more molecules dissolve before partial pressure changes significantly, and arterial tension of the gas increases less rapidly (Figure 24–3, bottom, halothane). This inverse relationship between the blood solubility of an anesthetic and the rate of rise of its tension in arterial blood is illustrated in Figure 24–4. The blood:gas partition coefficients for ni-

Table 24–1. Properties of inhalational anesthetics.

Anesthetic	Blood: Gas Partition Coefficient[1]	Brain: Blood Partition Coefficient[1]	Minimum Alveolar Concentration[2] (percent)
Nitrous oxide	0.47	1.1	>100
Desflurane	0.42	1.3	6–7
Sevoflurane	0.69	1.7	2.0
Isoflurane	1.40	2.6	1.40
Enflurane	1.80	1.4	1.68
Halothane	2.30	2.9	0.75
Methyoxyflurane	12.00	2.0	0.16

[1]Partition coefficients (at 37 °C) are from multiple literature sources.
[2]Minimum alveolar concentration (MAC) is the anesthetic concentration that produces immobility in 50% of patients exposed to a noxious stimulus.

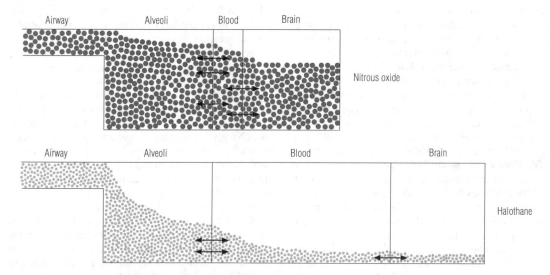

Figure 24–3. Why induction of anesthesia is slower with more soluble anesthetic gases. In this schematic diagram, solubility in blood is represented by the relative size of the blood compartment (the more soluble, the larger the compartment). Relative partial pressures of the agents in the compartments are indicated by the degree of filling of each compartment. For a given concentration or partial pressure of the two anesthetic gases in the inspired air, it will take much longer for the blood partial pressure of the more soluble gas (halothane) to rise to the same partial pressure as in the alveoli. Since the concentration of the anesthetic agent in the brain can rise no faster than the concentration in the blood, the onset of anesthesia will be slower with halothane than with nitrous oxide.

trous oxide, halothane, and methoxyflurane are 0.47, 2.3, and 12, respectively. Nitrous oxide, with low solubility in blood, reaches high arterial tensions rapidly, which in turn results in more rapid equilibrium with the brain and faster induction of anesthesia. In

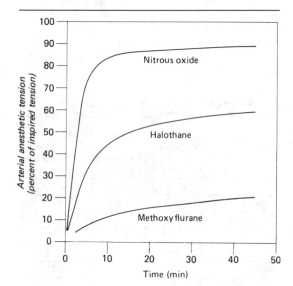

Figure 24–4. Tensions of three anesthetic gases in arterial blood as a function of time after beginning inhalation. Nitrous oxide is relatively insoluble (blood:gas partition coefficient = 0.47); methoxyflurane is much more soluble (coefficient = 12).

contrast, even after 40 minutes, methoxyflurane has reached only 20% of the equilibrium concentration.

B. Anesthetic Concentration in the Inspired Air: The concentration of an inhaled anesthetic in the inspired gas mixture has direct effects on both the maximum tension that can be achieved in the alveoli and the rate of increase in its tension in arterial blood. Increases in the inspired anesthetic concentration will increase the rate of induction of anesthesia by increasing the rate of transfer into the blood according to Fick's law (see Chapter 1). Advantage is taken of this effect in anesthetic practice with inhaled anesthetics of moderate blood solubility such as enflurane, isoflurane, and halothane, which have a relatively slow onset of anesthetic effect. For example, a 3–4% concentration of halothane may be administered initially to increase the rate of induction; this is reduced to 1–2% for maintenance when adequate anesthesia is achieved.

C. Pulmonary Ventilation: The rate of rise of anesthetic gas tension in arterial blood is directly dependent on both the rate and depth of ventilation, ie, minute ventilation. The magnitude of the effect varies according to the blood:gas partition coefficient. An increase in pulmonary ventilation is accompanied by only a slight increase in arterial tension of an anesthetic with low blood solubility or low coefficient but can significantly increase tension of agents with moderate or high blood solubility (Figure 24–5). For example, a fourfold increase in ventilation rate almost doubles the arterial tension of halothane during the

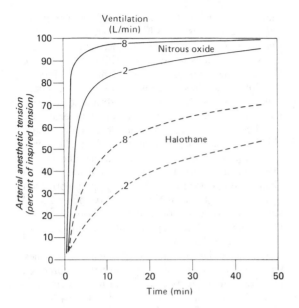

Figure 24–5. Ventilation rate and arterial anesthetic tensions. Increased ventilation (8 versus 2 L/min) has a much greater effect on equilibration of halothane than nitrous oxide.

first 10 minutes of anesthesia but increases the arterial tension of nitrous oxide by only 15%. Hyperventilation by mechanical control of respiration increases the speed of induction of anesthesia with inhaled anesthetics that would normally have a slow onset. Depression of respiration by other pharmacologic agents, including opioid analgesics, may slow the onset of anesthesia of some inhaled anesthetics if ventilation is not controlled.

D. Pulmonary Blood Flow: Changes in the rates of blood flow to and from the lungs influence transfer processes of the anesthetic gases. An increase in pulmonary blood flow (increased cardiac output) slows the rate of rise in arterial tension, particularly for those anesthetics with moderate to high blood solubility. This is because increased pulmonary blood flow exposes a larger volume of blood to the anesthetic; thus, blood "capacity" increases and tension rises slowly. A decrease in pulmonary blood flow has the opposite effect and increases the rate of rise of arterial tension of inhaled anesthetics. In a patient with circulatory shock, the combined effects of decreased cardiac output (decreased pulmonary flow) and increased ventilation may accelerate the induction of anesthesia with some anesthetics. This is least likely to occur with nitrous oxide because of its low solubility.

E. Arteriovenous Concentration Gradient: The anesthetic concentration gradient between arterial and mixed venous blood is dependent mainly on uptake of the anesthetic by the tissues; depending on the rate and extent of tissue uptake, venous blood re-

turning to the lungs may contain significantly less anesthetic than that present in arterial blood. The greater this difference in tensions, the more time it takes to achieve equilibrium. Anesthetic entry into tissues is influenced by factors similar to those that determine transfer from lung to blood, including tissue:blood partition coefficient, rates of blood flow to the tissues, and concentration gradients.

During the induction phase of anesthesia, the tissues that exert greatest influence on the arterial-venous anesthetic concentration gradient are those which are highly perfused. These include the brain, heart, liver, kidneys, and splanchnic bed, which together receive over 75% of the resting cardiac output. In the case of anesthetics with relatively high solubility in these tissues, venous blood concentration will initially be very low, and equilibrium with arterial blood is achieved slowly.

During maintenance of anesthesia with inhaled anesthetics, these drugs may continue to be transferred between various tissues at rates dependent on solubility and blood flow. Muscle and skin, which together constitute 50% of body mass, accumulate anesthetics more slowly than the richly vascularized tissues, since they receive only one-fifth the blood flow of the latter group. Although most anesthetic gases have high solubility in adipose tissues, low blood perfusion rates to these tissues delay accumulation, and equilibrium is unlikely to occur with anesthetics such as halothane and enflurane during the time anesthetics are usually required for surgery.

Elimination

The time to recovery from inhalational anesthesia depends on the rate of elimination of anesthetics from the brain after the inspired concentration of anesthetic has been decreased. Many of the processes of anesthetic transfer during recovery are similar to those that occur during induction of anesthesia. Factors controlling rate of recovery include the pulmonary blood flow and the magnitude of ventilation as well as solubility of the anesthetic in the tissues and the blood and in the gas phase in the lung. Two features of recovery, however, are quite different from what happens during induction of anesthesia. First, while transfer of an anesthetic from the lungs to blood can be enhanced by increasing its concentration in inspired air, the reverse transfer process cannot be enhanced, since the concentration in the lungs cannot be reduced below zero. Second, at the beginning of recovery, the anesthetic gas tension in different tissues may be quite variable, depending on the specific agent and the duration of anesthesia. With induction of anesthesia, the initial anesthetic tension in all tissues is zero.

Inhaled anesthetics that are relatively insoluble in blood and brain are eliminated at faster rates than more soluble anesthetics. For example, the "washout" of nitrous oxide and desflurane occurs at a rapid rate, which leads to rapid recovery from their anesthetic effects. Halothane is approximately twice as soluble in brain tissue and five times more soluble in blood than nitrous oxide; its elimination therefore takes place more slowly, and recovery from halothane anesthesia is less rapid. The duration of exposure to the anesthetic can have a marked effect on the time of recovery, especially in the case of more soluble anesthetics such as methoxyflurane. Accumulation of agents in tissues, including muscle, skin, and fat, increases with continuous inhalation, and blood tension may decline slowly during recovery as the anesthetic gradually leaves such tissues. Thus, if exposure to the anesthetic is short, recovery may be rapid. After prolonged anesthesia, recovery may be delayed even with anesthetics of modest solubility such as halothane.

Clearance of inhaled anesthetics by the lungs into the expired air is the major route of their elimination from the body. However, metabolism by enzymes of the liver and other tissues may also contribute to the elimination of anesthetics. For example, the washout of halothane during recovery is more rapid than that of enflurane, which would not be predicted from their respective solubilities. However, 15–20% of inspired halothane is metabolized during an average anesthetic procedure, while only 2–3% of enflurane is metabolized over the same period. Oxidative metabolism of halothane results in the formation of trifluoroacetic acid and release of bromide and chloride ions. Under conditions of low oxygen tension, halothane is metabolized to the chlorotrifluoroethyl free radical, which is capable of reacting with hepatic membrane components. Isoflurane and desflurane are the most slowly metabolized of the fluorinated anesthetics, only traces of trifluoroacetic acid appearing in the urine. The slow rate of metabolism of enflurane results in the formation of difluoromethoxyfluoroacetic acid and fluoride ion, which do not reach toxic levels. Methoxyflurane is metabolized by the liver at a much faster rate than any other inhaled anesthetic and releases fluoride ions at levels that can be nephrotoxic. Nitrous oxide is probably not metabolized by human tissue.

PHARMACODYNAMICS

Mechanism of Action

An important neurophysiologic action common to most general anesthetics is to increase the cellular threshold for firing (Aloia, 1991). With the increase in threshold, there is a decrease in neuronal activity. The inhalational anesthetic agents—as well as the intravenous barbiturates and benzodiazepines—depress spontaneous and evoked activity of neurons in many regions of the brain. Such actions are exerted on both axonal and synaptic transmission, but synaptic processes are more sensitive to the effects. The ionic

mechanisms thought to be involved are varied. Inhaled gaseous anesthetics have been reported to cause hyperpolarization of neurons via activation of K^+ currents, which leads to decreased ability to initiate action potentials, ie, an increase in threshold. Electrophysiologic studies of cells in culture, using patch clamp analysis, have shown that isoflurane decreases the duration of opening of nicotinic receptor-activated cation channels—an action that would presumably decrease synaptic transmission at cholinergic synapses. The effects of benzodiazepines and barbiturates on the $GABA_A$ receptor-mediated chloride channel affect opening and cause hyperpolarization, again leading to decreased firing (Chapter 21). A similar action to facilitate the inhibitory effects of GABA has also been reported for propofol and certain inhalational agents.

The molecular mechanism by which gaseous anesthetics modify ion currents in neuronal membranes is not clear. Such effects could result from direct interaction between anesthetic molecules and hydrophobic sites on specific membrane protein channels. This type of mechanism has been suggested from studies on gas anesthetic interactions with nicotinic cholinoceptor channels—interactions that appear to stabilize the channel in its closed state. Alternative interpretations, which attempt to take into account the marked structural differences among the anesthetics, invoke less specific interactions of these agents with the lipid matrix of the membrane, with secondary changes in channel function. These interpretations are supported by older observations of the close correlation of anesthetic potency with lipid solubility (Meyer-Overton principle). The concept of indirect interactions mediated via solution in membrane lipid is supported by studies of anesthetics on artificial lipid membranes. These studies show that as an anesthetic gas dissolves in the lipid, there is an increase in membrane fluidity suggestive of a reduction in the "orderliness" of the lipid structure. Such effects on the lipid could be reflected in changes in the function of the channels floating in the lipid membrane.

In experimental animals, general anesthesia can be reversed by placing the animal in a high-pressure chamber. Very high pressures—eg, 50–100 atm—cause reversal of the anesthetic state. High pressure is known to increase the orderliness (decrease the fluidity) of lipid membranes. Such experiments have led to suggestions that solution of anesthetic molecules in the membrane lipid—and the resulting decrease in order—causes a small expansion that distorts ion channels. However, hypotheses based on increased membrane fluidity fail to explain why small elevations of temperature, which increase membrane fluidity to an extent comparable to the effect of clinical concentrations of anesthetics, actually *decrease* anesthetic potency. In addition, such hypotheses are not congruent with the clinical observation that older patients often have a reduced anesthetic requirement despite the fact that the fluidity of neuronal membranes tends to decrease with age.

The neuropharmacologic basis for the effects that characterize the stages of anesthesia appears to be **differential sensitivity** to the anesthetic of specific neurons or neuronal pathways. Cells of the substantia gelatinosa in the dorsal horn of the spinal cord are very sensitive to relatively low anesthetic concentration in the central nervous system. A decrease in the activity of neurons in this region interrupts sensory transmission in the spinothalamic tract, including transmission of nociceptive stimuli. These effects contribute to stage I, or analgesia. The disinhibitory effects of general anesthetics (stage II), which occur at higher brain concentrations, result from complex neuronal actions including blockade of many small inhibitory neurons such as Golgi type II cells, together with a paradoxical facilitation of excitatory neurotransmitters. A progressive depression of ascending pathways in the reticular activating system occurs during stage III, or surgical anesthesia, together with suppression of spinal reflex activity, which contributes to muscle relaxation. Neurons in the respiratory and vasomotor centers of the medulla are relatively insensitive to the effects of the general anesthetics, but at high concentrations their activity is depressed, leading to cardiorespiratory collapse (stage IV).

Dose-Response Characteristics: The Minimum Alveolar Anesthetic Concentration (MAC)

Inhaled anesthetics are delivered to the lungs in gas mixtures in which concentrations and flow rates are easy to measure and control. However, dose-response characteristics of gaseous anesthetics are particularly difficult to measure. First, achievement of an anesthetic state depends on the concentration of the anesthetic in the brain, and that concentration is impossible to measure under clinical conditions. Second, neither the lower nor the upper ends of the graded dose-response curve can be ethically determined, since at very low concentrations severe pain might be experienced while at high concentrations there would be a high risk of fatal cardiovascular and respiratory depression. Nevertheless, a useful estimate of anesthetic potency can be obtained using quantal dose-response principles.

During general anesthesia, the partial pressure of an inhaled anesthetic in the brain equals that in the lung when steady state is reached. At a given level of anesthesia, the measurement of the steady state alveolar concentrations of different anesthetics provides a comparison of their relative potencies. The minimum alveolar anesthetic concentration (MAC) of an anesthetic is defined as the concentration (ie, the percentage of the alveolar gas mixture, or partial pressure of the anesthetic as a percentage of 760 mm Hg) that results in immobility in 50% of patients when exposed to a noxious stimulus such as surgical incision. Thus, it represents one point (the ED50) on a conventional quantal dose-response curve (see Figure 2–17). Table 24–1 shows concentrations for the common inhaled anesthetics, permitting comparison of their relative anesthetic potencies. The MAC value greater than 100% for nitrous oxide shows that it is the least potent, since at normal barometric pressure even 760 mm Hg partial pressure of nitrous oxide (100% of the inspired gas) is not equal to 1 MAC.

The dose of anesthetic gas that is administered can be stated in multiples of MAC. While a dose of 1 MAC of any agent prevents movement in response to surgical incision in 50% of patients, individual patients may require 0.5–1.5 MAC. (The MAC gives no information about the slope of the dose-response curve.) In general, however, the dose-response relationship for inhaled anesthetics is steep; thus, over 95% of patients may fail to respond to a noxious stimulus at 1.1 MAC. The measurement of MAC values under controlled conditions has permitted quantitation of the effects of a number of variables on anesthetic requirements. For example, MAC values decrease in elderly patients but are not affected greatly by sex, height, and weight. Of particular importance is the presence of adjuvant drugs, which can change anesthetic requirements greatly. For example, when drugs such as the opioid analgesics or sedative-hypnotics are present, MAC is decreased, which means that the inspired concentration of anesthetic should be decreased accordingly.

A variety of other techniques, such as measurement of changes in the electroencephalogram, have been tried in an effort to delineate graded dose-response curves for inhaled anesthetics in humans. However, because many other variables unrelated to anesthesia can influence the results, these attempts have not succeeded to date.

Organ System Effects of Inhaled Anesthetics

A. Effects on Cardiovascular System: Halothane, desflurane, enflurane, and isoflurane all decrease mean arterial pressure in direct proportion to their alveolar concentration. With halothane and enflurane, the reduced arterial pressure appears to be caused by a reduction in cardiac output, because there is little change in systemic vascular resistance despite marked changes in individual vascular beds (eg, increase in cerebral blood flow). In contrast, isoflurane and desflurane have a depressant effect on arterial pressure as a result of a marked decrease in systemic vascular resistance; they have little effect on cardiac output.

Inhaled anesthetics change heart rate either by directly altering the rate of sinus node depolarization or by shifting the balance of autonomic nervous system activity. Bradycardia is often seen with halothane and may be a result of direct depression of atrial rate. In contrast, methoxyflurane and enflurane have little effect, and isoflurane increases heart rate. Most of these changes in heart rate have been determined in normal volunteer subjects rather than in patients undergoing surgery. The patient's preoperative excited state or the stimulation of surgery will often alter the heart rate response to inhaled anesthetics.

All inhaled anesthetics tend to increase right atrial pressure in a dose-related fashion that reflects depression of myocardial function. In general, enflurane and halothane have marked myocardial depressant effects, and isoflurane to a lesser extent. Inhaled anesthetics reduce myocardial oxygen consumption, primarily by decreasing those variables that control oxygen demand, such as arterial blood pressure and contractile force. Although certainly less depressant than the other inhaled anesthetics, nitrous oxide has also been found to depress the myocardium in a dose-dependent manner. However, nitrous oxide—alone or in combination with potent inhaled anesthetics—produces sympathetic stimulation that may obscure any cardiac depressant effects of the inhaled anesthetic. The combination of nitrous oxide plus halothane or enflurane, for example, appears to produce less depression at a given level of anesthesia than either of the more potent anesthetics given alone.

Several factors influence the cardiovascular effects of inhaled anesthetics. Surgical stimulation, hypercapnia, and increasing duration of anesthesia will lessen the depressant effects of these drugs. Hypercapnia releases catecholamines, which attenuate the decrease in blood pressure. The blood pressure decrease after 5 hours of anesthesia is less than it is after 1 hour; propranolol blocks this adaptive effect. Halothane sensitizes the myocardium to catecholamines, and ventricular arrhythmias may occur in patients with cardiac disease who are given either direct-acting or indirect-acting sympathomimetic drugs or who have high circulating levels of endogenous catecholamines (eg, patients with pheochromocytoma). Other modern inhalational agents are less likely to be arrhythmogenic.

B. Effects on Respiratory System: With the exception of nitrous oxide, all inhaled anesthetics in current use cause a decrease in tidal volume and an increase in respiratory rate. However, the increase in rate is insufficient to compensate for the decrease in volume, resulting in a decrease in minute ventilation. All inhaled anesthetics are respiratory depressants, as gauged by the reduced response to various levels of carbon dioxide. The degree of ventilatory depression varies with anesthetic agents, with isoflurane and enflurane being the most depressant. All inhaled anesthetics in current use increase the resting level of $PaCO_2$ (the partial pressure of carbon dioxide in arterial blood).

Inhaled anesthetics increase the apneic threshold ($PaCO_2$ level below which apnea occurs through lack of CO_2-driven respiratory stimulation) and decrease the ventilatory response to hypoxia. The latter effect is especially important because subanesthetic concentrations (ie, those that exist during recovery) depress the normal compensating increase in ventilation that occurs during hypoxia. All of these respiratory depressant effects of anesthetics are overcome by assisting or controlling ventilation via a mechanical ventilator during surgery. Furthermore, the ventilatory depressant effects of the inhaled anesthetics are lessened by surgical stimulation and increasing duration of anesthesia.

Inhaled anesthetics also depress mucociliary function in the airway. Thus, prolonged anesthesia may lead to pooling of mucus and then result in atelectasis and respiratory infections. However, inhaled anesthetics tend to be bronchodilators. This effect has been used in the treatment of status asthmaticus. Airway irritation, which may provoke coughing or breath holding, is rarely a problem with most inhalational agents. However, it is relatively common with desflurane, and induction may be more difficult to accomplish with this agent despite its low blood:gas partition coefficient. Similarly, the pungency of enflurane may elicit breath holding, which can limit speed of induction.

C. Effects on Brain: Inhaled anesthetics decrease the metabolic rate of the brain. Nevertheless, most of them *increase* cerebral blood flow because they decrease cerebral vascular resistance. The increase in cerebral blood flow is often clinically undesirable. For example, in patients who have an increased intracranial pressure because of brain tumor or head injury, administration of an inhaled anesthetic may increase cerebral blood flow, which in turn will increase cerebral blood volume and further increase intracranial pressure.

Of the inhaled anesthetics, nitrous oxide increases cerebral blood flow the least, although when 60% nitrous oxide is added to halothane anesthesia, cerebral blood flow usually increases more than with halothane alone. At low doses, all of the halogenated agents have similar effects to increase cerebral blood flow. At higher doses, enflurane and isoflurane increase cerebral blood flow less than does halothane. If the patient is hyperventilated before the anesthetic is given (to reduce $PaCO_2$), the increase in intracranial pressure from inhaled anesthetics can be minimized.

Halothane, isoflurane, and enflurane have similar effects (eg, burst suppression) on the EEG up to doses of 1–1.5 MAC. At higher doses, the cerebral irritant effects of enflurane may lead to the development of a spike-and-wave pattern during which auditory stimuli can precipitate mild generalized muscle twitching that is augmented by hyperventilation. This seizure activity has never been shown to have any adverse clinical consequences. The effect is not seen clinically with the other inhaled anesthetics. Though nitrous oxide has low anesthetic potency, it does exert marked analgesic and amnesic actions, desirable properties when used in combination with other agents in general anesthesia and dental anesthesia.

D. Effects on Kidney: To varying degrees, all inhaled anesthetics decrease glomerular filtration rate and effective renal plasma flow and increase filtration fraction. All the anesthetics tend to increase renal vascular resistance. Since renal blood flow decreases during general anesthesia in spite of well-maintained or even increased perfusion pressures, autoregulation of renal flow is probably impaired.

E. Effects on Liver: All inhaled anesthetics cause a decrease in hepatic blood flow, ranging from 15% to 45% of the preanesthetic flow. Despite transient changes in liver function tests intraoperatively, rarely does permanent change of liver function occur from the use of these agents. The possible hepatotoxicity of halothane is discussed below.

F. Effects on Uterine Smooth Muscle: Nitrous oxide appears to have little effect on uterine musculature. However, isoflurane, halothane, and enflurane are potent uterine muscle relaxants. This pharmacologic effect can be used to advantage when profound uterine relaxation is required for intrauterine fetal manipulation during delivery. In contrast, during dilatation and curettage for therapeutic abortion, these anesthetics may cause increased bleeding.

Toxicity

A. Hepatotoxicity (Halothane): Postoperative hepatitis is usually associated with factors such as blood transfusions, hypovolemic shock, and other surgical stresses rather than anesthetic toxicity. However, halocarbon drugs such as halothane can cause liver damage, and chloroform was identified as a hepatotoxin in the first decade of this century. Halothane was introduced into clinical practice in 1956; by 1963, several cases of postoperative jaundice and liver necrosis associated with halothane had been reported. However, several retrospective studies in which halothane was compared with other anesthetics showed no increased incidence in postoperative hepatic damage with halothane. In 1966, the United States National Halothane Study undertook a retrospective review of the incidence of fatal massive hepatic necrosis in a population of about 850,000 surgical patients. Results of the study were inconclusive and did not identify halothane clearly as a hepatotoxin. The incidence of massive necrosis associated with halothane was 7 out of 250,000 halothane administrations, or about 1 in 35,000 (not 1 in 10,000, as sometimes reported). Because halothane is such a valuable anesthetic, it is important to establish whether it is indeed a significant hepatotoxin before limiting its use. Unlike chloroform and fluroxene, which can produce fatty infiltration, centrilobular necrosis, and elevated aminotransferase concentrations, prolonged exposure of animals to halothane produces little evidence of liver damage. Several animal models have been developed to help define possible ha-

lothane-mediated hepatotoxicity. When rats are pretreated with phenobarbital and then exposed to hypoxic conditions with an inspired oxygen concentration of 7–14%, hepatotoxicity from halothane (as well as some other inhalational agents) will occur. The mechanism underlying hepatotoxicity in the animals remains unclear, though these models suggest that it may depend on the production of a reactive metabolite (eg, a free radical) that either causes direct hepatocellular damage or initiates an immune-mediated response. Although this model is reproducible and well defined, its clinical applicability is uncertain because hypoxia is a necessary precondition for production of liver damage.

Recently, it has been found that some individuals have a defect in their hepatic cell membranes that make these cells more susceptible to halothane-induced injury. These individuals are at a higher risk for halothane-induced hepatic necrosis. A test is being developed that would identify such individuals preoperatively.

B. Nephrotoxicity (Methoxyflurane): In 1966, vasopressin-resistant polyuric renal insufficiency was first reported in 13 of 41 patients receiving methoxyflurane anesthesia for abdominal surgery. Subsequently, the causative agent was shown to be inorganic fluoride, an end product of the biotransformation of methoxyflurane.

C. Malignant Hyperthermia: Although occurrences are rare, genetically susceptible patients exposed to inhalational anesthetics may develop this potentially lethal syndrome, which includes tachycardia and hypertension progressing to acidosis, hyperkalemia, muscle rigidity, and hyperthermia. The onset is more dramatic if succinylcholine is used for muscle relaxation. Treatment involves intravenous dantrolene with appropriate measures to lower elevated temperature and to restore electrolyte and acid-base balance.

D. Chronic Toxicity:

1. Mutagenicity–Under normal conditions, most modern and many older inhaled anesthetics are not mutagens and probably not carcinogens. However, older anesthetics that contain the vinyl moiety (fluroxene and divinyl ether) may be mutagens. These agents are rarely or never used.

2. Carcinogenicity–Several epidemiologic studies have suggested an increase in the cancer rate in operating room personnel who may be exposed to trace concentrations of anesthetic agents. However, no study has demonstrated the existence of a cause-and-effect relationship between anesthetics and cancer. Many other factors might account for the questionably positive results seen after a careful review of epidemiologic data. Most operating room theaters remove trace concentrations of anesthetics released from anesthetic machines via vents to the atmosphere.

3. Effects on reproduction–The most consistent finding reported from surveys conducted to determine the reproductive performance of female operating room personnel has been a higher than expected incidence of miscarriages. There are several problems in interpreting these studies, but in general it can be asserted that the evidence is not strong.

However, the association of obstetric problems with surgery and anesthesia in pregnant patients is not open to question. In the USA, at least 50,000 pregnant women each year undergo anesthesia and surgery for indications unrelated to pregnancy. The risk of abortion is clearly higher following this experience. It is not obvious whether the underlying disease, surgery, anesthesia, or a combination of these factors is the cause of the increased risk. Another concern not yet substantiated is that anesthetics during pregnancy may lead to an increased incidence of congenital anomalies. If anesthetics are teratogenic, the risk may be very small.

4. Hematotoxicity–Prolonged exposure to nitrous oxide decreases methionine synthetase activity and causes megaloblastic anemia. This is a potential occupational hazard for staff working in poorly ventilated dental operating suites.

Clinical Use of Inhaled Anesthetics

Of the inhaled anesthetics available, nitrous oxide, desflurane, and isoflurane are most commonly used in the USA. Although not often used in adults, halothane is frequently used in pediatric anesthesia. As indicated previously, nitrous oxide lacks sufficient potency to produce surgical anesthesia by itself and therefore is usually used with another inhaled or intravenous anesthetic to produce complete anesthesia. Methoxyflurane is occasionally used—especially in obstetric anesthesia—but not for prolonged procedures because of its nephrotoxicity, which is described above. Chloroform is not used because of its hepatotoxicity. Although cyclopropane and diethyl ether were the most commonly used anesthetics before 1960, they are no longer used because of their flammable and explosive characteristics.

INTRAVENOUS ANESTHETICS

ULTRA-SHORT-ACTING BARBITURATES

Although several ultra-short-acting barbiturates are available, **thiopental** is the one most commonly used for induction of anesthesia, often in combination with inhaled anesthetics. The general pharmacology of the barbiturates is discussed in Chapter 21.

Following intravenous administration, thiopental rapidly crosses the blood-brain barrier and, if given in sufficient dosage, produces hypnosis in one circulation time. Similar effects occur with other ultra-short-acting barbiturates, eg, thiamylal and methohexital. With all of these barbiturates, plasma:brain equilibrium occurs rapidly (in approximately 1 minute) because of high lipid solubility. Thiopental rapidly diffuses out of the brain and other highly vascular tissues and is redistributed to muscle, fat, and eventually all body tissues (Figure 24–6). It is because of this rapid removal from brain tissue that a single dose of thiopental is so short-acting.

Metabolism of thiopental is much slower than its redistribution and takes place primarily in the liver. Less than 1% of an administered dose of thiopental is excreted unchanged by the kidney. Thiopental is metabolized at the rate of 12–16% per hour in humans following a single dose.

With large doses, thiopental causes dose-dependent decreases in arterial blood pressure, stroke volume, and cardiac output. This is due primarily to its myocardial depressant effect and increased venous capacitance; there is little change in total peripheral resistance.

Thiopental, like other barbiturates, is a potent respiratory depressant, lowering the sensitivity of the medullary respiratory center to carbon dioxide.

Cerebral metabolism and oxygen utilization are decreased after thiopental administration in proportion to the degree of cerebral depression. Cerebral blood flow is also decreased but much less so than oxygen consumption. This makes thiopental a much more desirable drug for use in patients with cerebral swelling than the inhaled anesthetics, since intracranial pressure and blood volume are not increased.

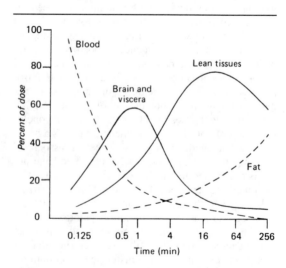

Figure 24–6. Redistribution of thiopental after an intravenous bolus administration. Note that the time axis is not linear.

Thiopental may reduce hepatic blood flow and glomerular filtration rate, but it produces no lasting effects on hepatic and renal function. Barbiturates may exacerbate acute intermittent porphyria (see Chapter 21).

BENZODIAZEPINES

Certain members of this class of sedative-hypnotic drugs, including diazepam, lorazepam, and midazolam, are used in anesthetic procedures. (The basic pharmacology of benzodiazepines is discussed in Chapter 21.) Diazepam and lorazepam are not water-soluble, and their intravenous use necessitates nonaqueous vehicles, which may cause local irritation. Midazolam formulations are water-soluble and thus produce less irritation, but they become lipid-soluble at physiologic pH and readily cross the blood-brain barrier. Compared with intravenous barbiturates, benzodiazepines produce a slower onset of central nervous system effects and induce a plateau of central depression that appears to be below that of a true anesthetic state. Used intravenously, benzodiazepines prolong the postanesthetic recovery period (an undesirable effect) but also cause a high incidence of anterograde amnesia (amnesia for events occurring after the drug is administered), which is useful. Because it causes a high incidence of amnesia (> 50%), midazolam is frequently given intravenously 15–60 minutes before induction of general anesthesia. Midazolam has a more rapid onset, a shorter elimination half-life ($t_{1/2\beta}$ 2–4 hours), and a steeper dose-response curve than do the other benzodiazepines used in anesthesia. The benzodiazepines are useful in anesthesia as premedication; they can also be used for intraoperative sedation and, with other drugs, as part of balanced anesthesia. The benzodiazepine antagonist flumazenil is now used to accelerate recovery from the sedative actions of intravenous benzodiazepines, but its reversal of respiratory depression is less predictable. Its short duration of action may necessitate multiple doses.

OPIOID ANALGESIC ANESTHESIA

Large doses of opioid analgesics have been used to achieve general anesthesia, particularly in patients undergoing cardiac surgery or other major surgery when circulatory reserve is minimal. Intravenous morphine, 1–3 mg/kg, and the high-potency drug fentanyl, 50–100 μg/kg, have been used in such situations with minimal evidence of circulatory deterioration. More recently, sufentanyl, a congener of fentanyl, has also been used. Despite such high doses (see Table 30–2 for conventional analgesic doses), awareness during anesthesia and unpleasant postoperative recall have occurred. Intravenous opioids can increase chest wall rigidity, which may impair ventilation, and postoperative respiratory depression may occur, requiring assisted ventilation and the administration of opioid antagonists, eg, naloxone. Postoperative respiratory effects may be reduced by lowering the opioid analgesic dose and simultaneously administering short-acting barbiturates or benzodiazepines, usually with nitrous oxide to achieve balanced anesthesia. Alfentanyl, a short-acting congener of fentanyl, is available for use as intravenous agent in shorter surgical procedures. Fentanyl and droperidol (a butyrophenone derivative) together produce analgesia and amnesia and are sometimes used with nitrous oxide to provide **neuroleptanesthesia**.

Narcotics are also given intrathecally and epidurally. While this approach cannot prevent pain caused by surgical incision, it does provide profound postoperative analgesia.

PROPOFOL

2,6-Diisopropylphenol—propofol or disoprofol—is an extremely important intravenous anesthetic. It produces anesthesia at a rate similar to that of the intravenous barbiturates, and recovery is more rapid. In particular, patients are able to ambulate sooner after propofol. Furthermore, patients "feel better" in the immediate postoperative period after propofol as compared with other intravenous anesthetics. Postoperative vomiting is uncommon, and propofol is reported to have antiemetic actions. The drug does not appear to cause cumulative effects or delayed arousal following prolonged infusion. These favorable properties are responsible for the extensive use of propofol as a component of balanced anesthesia and for its great popularity as an anesthetic for use in "day surgery." The drug is also effective in producing prolonged sedation in patients in critical care settings. However, resistance to its effects occurs after a few days, so this application is of limited duration.

After intravenous administration, distribution occurs with a half-life ($t_{1/2\alpha}$) of 2–8 minutes; the elimination half-life ($t_{1/2\beta}$) of propofol is approximately 1–3 hours. The drug is rapidly metabolized in the liver by conjugation to glucuronide and sulfate and excreted in the urine. Less than 1% of the drug is excreted unchanged. Total body clearance of the anesthetic is greater than hepatic blood flow, suggesting that its elimination includes other mechanisms in addition to metabolism by liver enzymes. This property is useful in patients with impaired ability to metabolize other sedative-anesthetic drugs such as midazolam.

Effects on respiration are similar to those of thiopental at usual anesthetic doses. However, propofol causes a marked decrease in systemic blood pressure during induction of anesthesia, primarily through decreased peripheral resistance. Apnea and pain at the site of injection also occur. Muscle movements, hypotonus, and (rarely) tremors have also been reported following its use. Hypersensitivity reactions involving hypotension, flushing, and bronchospasm have occurred with preparations of propofol dissolved in the original vehicle (Cremophor), but these do not occur when Intralipid (intravenous fat emulsion) is used as a vehicle. An important disadvantage of prolonged use of propofol is its cost, which exceeds that of the benzodiazepines and barbiturates.

ETOMIDATE

Etomidate is a carboxylated imidazole used for induction of anesthesia and in techniques of balanced anesthesia that do not require its prolonged administration. Its major advantage over other agents is that it causes minimal cardiovascular and respiratory depressant effects. Etomidate produces loss of consciousness within seconds, with slight hypotension, no effect on heart rate, and a low frequency of apnea. The drug has no analgesic effects, and premedication with opioids may be required to decrease cardiac responses during tracheal intubation and to lessen spontaneous muscle movements. Following an induction dose, recovery occurs within 3 minutes.

Distribution of etomidate is rapid, with a biphasic plasma concentration curve showing distribution half-lives of 3 and 29 minutes. Redistribution of the drug from brain to highly perfused tissues appears to be responsible for the short duration of its anesthetic effects. Etomidate is hydrolyzed in the liver and plasma to inactive metabolites. Studies in humans indicate that almost 90% of the drug–of which only 2% is unchanged–eventually appears in the urine. Unfortunately, etomidate causes a high incidence of nausea and vomiting, pain on injection, and myoclonus. The myoclonic movements are not associated with epileptiform discharges on the EEG. Etomidate may also cause adrenocortical suppression via inhibitory effects on steroidogenesis. Prolonged infusion may result in hypotension, electrolyte imbalance, and oliguria.

KETAMINE

Ketamine (Figure 24–2) produces **dissociative anesthesia,** which is characterized by catatonia, amnesia, and analgesia. Its mechanism of action involves blockade of the membrane effects of the excitatory neurotransmitter glutamic acid at the NMDA receptor subtype. Although it is a desirable anesthetic in many respects, ketamine has been associated with disorientation, sensory and perceptual illusions, and vivid dreams following anesthesia, effects that are termed "emergence phenomena." Diazepam, 0.2–0.3 mg/kg intravenously 5 minutes before administration of ketamine, reduces the incidence of these phenomena.

Ketamine, a lipophilic drug, is rapidly distributed into highly vascular organs, including the brain, and subsequently redistributed to less perfused tissues with concurrent hepatic metabolism and both urinary and biliary excretion.

Besides being a powerful analgesic, ketamine is the only intravenous anesthetic that routinely produces cardiovascular stimulation. Heart rate, arterial blood pressure, and cardiac output are usually significantly increased. The peak increases in these variables occur 2–4 minutes after intravenous injection and then slowly decline to normal over the next 10–20 minutes. Ketamine produces its cardiovascular stimulation by excitation of the central sympathetic nervous system and possibly by inhibition of the reuptake of norepinephrine at sympathetic nerve terminals. Increases in plasma epinephrine and norepinephrine levels occur as early as 2 minutes after intravenous ketamine and return to control levels 15 minutes later.

Ketamine markedly increases cerebral blood flow, oxygen consumption, and intracranial pressure. Like most inhaled anesthetics, this intravenous agent is therefore a potentially dangerous drug when intracranial pressure is elevated.

In most patients, ketamine decreases the respiratory rate slightly for 2–3 minutes. Upper airway muscle tone is well maintained, and upper airway reflexes are usually (not always) active. Ketamine produces little other change in organ systems.

Because of the high incidence of postoperative psychic phenomena associated with its use, ketamine is not commonly used in general surgery in the USA. It is considered useful for poor-risk geriatric patients and patients in shock, because of its cardiostimulatory properties. It is also used in outpatient anesthesia and in children undergoing painful procedures such as dressing changes on burned tissue.

PREPARATIONS AVAILABLE
(See Chapter 30 for formulations of opioid agents used in anesthesia.)

Desflurane (Suprane)
  Liquid: 240 mL for inhalation
Diazepam (generic, Valium, others)

Oral: 2, 5, 10 mg tablets; 5 mg/5 mL and 5 mg/mL solution
Oral sustained release: 15 mg capsules

Parenteral: 5 mg/mL for injection
Enflurane (Ethrane)
Liquid: 125, 250 mL for inhalation
Etomidate (Amidate)
Parenteral: 2 mg/mL for injection
Halothane (generic, Fluothane)
Liquid: 125, 250 mL for inhalation
Isoflurane (Forane)
Liquid: 100 mL for inhalation
Ketamine (Ketalar)
Parenteral: 10, 50, 100 mg/mL for injection
Lorazepam (generic, Ativan, Alzapam)
Oral: 0.5, 1, 2 mg tablets
Parenteral: 2, 4 mg/mL for injection
Methohexital (Brevital Sodium)
Parenteral: 0.5, 2.5, 5 g powders to reconstitute for injection

Methoxyflurane (Penthrane)
Liquid: 15, 125 mL for inhalation
Midazolam (Versed)
Parenteral: 1, 5 mg/mL for injection in 1, 2, 5, 10 mL vials
Nitrous oxide (gas, supplied in blue cylinders)
Propofol (Diprivan)
Parenteral: 10 mg/mL in 20 mL vials for injection
Thiamylal (Surital)
Parenteral: solutions for injection in 1, 5, 10 g vials
Thiopental (Pentothal)
Parenteral: 250, 400, 500 mg in preloaded syringes; 500 mg, 1 g solutions with diluent; 1, 2.5, 5 g kits
Rectal: 400 mg solution in preloaded syringes

REFERENCES

Albanese J et al: Pharmacokinetics of long-term propofol infusion used for sedation in ICU patients. Anesthesiology 1990;73:214.

Albin MS, Bunegin L, Garcia C: Ketamine and postanesthetic emergence reaction. In: *Status of Ketamine in Anesthesiology*, Domino EF (editor). NPP Books, 1990.

Aloia RC, Curtain CC, Gordon LM (editors): *Drug and Anesthetic Effects on Membrane Structure and Function.* Wiley-Liss, 1991.

Baden JM, Rice, SA: Metabolism and toxicity of inhaled anesthetics. In: *Anesthesia,* 4th ed. Miller RD (editor). Churchill Livingstone, 1994.

Berg-Johnson J, Langmoen IA: Isoflurane hyperpolarizes neurons in rat and human cerebral cortex. Acta Physiol Scand 1987;130:679.

Brett RS, Dilger JP, Yland KF: Isoflurane causes flickering of the acetylcholine receptor channel: Observations using the patch clamp. Anesthesiology 1988;69:161.

Carpenter RL et al: Extent of metabolism of inhaled anesthetics in humans. Anesthesiology 1986;65:201.

Christ DD et al: Enflurane metabolism produces covalently bound liver adducts recognized by antibodies from patients with halothane hepatitis. Anesthesiology 1988; 69:885.

Davis PJ, Cook DR: Clinical pharmacokinetics of the newer intravenous anaesthetic agents. Clin Pharmacokinet 1986;11:18.

Dilger JP, Firestone LL: More models described for molecular "target" of anesthetics and alcohols. Trends Pharmacol Sci 1990;11:431.

Eger EI II: Uptake and distribution. In: *Anesthesia,* 4th ed. Miller RD (editor). Churchill Livingstone, 1994.

Eger EI II: Desflurane animal and human pharmacology: Aspects of kinetics, safety, and MAC. Anesth Analg 1992;75:S3.

Eger EI II, Saidman LJ, Brandstater B: Minimum alveolar anesthetic concentration: A standard of anesthetic potency. Anesthesiology 1965;26:756.

Firestone LL et al: Actions of general anesthetics on acetyl-choline receptor-rich membranes from *Torpedo californica.* Anesthesiology 1986;64:694.

Flacke JW et al: Comparison of morphine, meperidine, fentanyl, and sufentanil in balanced anesthesia: A double-blind study. Anesth Analg 1985;64:897.

Franks NP, Lieb WR: Volatile general anesthetics activate a novel neuronal K^+ current. Nature 1988;333:662.

Grounds RM et al: The hemodynamic effects of thiopentone and propofol. Anaesthesia 1985;40:735.

Harris RA, Bruno P: Membrane disordering by anesthetic drugs: Relationship to synaptosomal sodium and calcium fluxes. J Neurochem 1985;44:1274.

Herregods L et al: Propofol combined with nitrous oxide-oxygen for induction and maintenance of anaesthesia. Anaesthesia 1987;42:360.

Koblin DD: Mechanisms of action. In: *Anesthesia,* 4th ed. Miller RD (editor). Churchill Livingstone, 1994.

Langley MS, Heel RC: Propofol: Review of its pharmacodynamic and pharmacokinetic properties and use as an intravenous anesthetic. Drugs 1988;35:334.

Laster M et al: Comparison of kinetics of sevoflurane and isoflurane in humans. Anesth Analg 1991;72:316.

Lebovic S et al: Comparison of propofol versus ketamine for anesthesia in pediatric patients undergoing cardiac catheterization. Anesth Analg 1992;74:490.

Nakahiro M et al: General anesthetics modulate GABA receptor channel complex in rat dorsal root ganglions. FASEB J 1989;3:1850.

Prys-Roberts C, Hug CC Jr: *Pharmacokinetics of Anesthesia.* Blackwell, 1984.

Reves JG et al: Midazolam: Pharmacology and uses. Anesthesiology 1985;62:310.

Roth SH, Miller KW: *Molecular and Cellular Mechanisms of Anesthetics.* Plenum Press, 1986.

Saidman LJ: The role of desflurane in the practice of anesthesia. Anesthesiology 1991;74:399.

Sebel PS, Lowdon JD: Propofol: New intravenous anesthetic. Anesthesiology 1989; 71:260.

Smiley R et al: Desflurane and isoflurane in surgical patients: Comparison of emergence time. Anesthesiology 1991;74:425.

Sweeney B et al: Toxicity of bone marrow in dentists exposed to nitrous oxide. Br Med J 1985;291:567.

Swerdlow BN, Holley FO: Intravenous anesthetic agents. Pharmacokinetic-pharmacodynamic relationships. Clin Pharmacokinet 1987;12:79.

Vessey MP: Epidemiological studies of the occupational hazards of anaesthesia. Anaesthesia 1978;33:430.

Votey SR et al: Flumazenil: A new benzodiazepine antagonist. Ann Emerg Med 1991;20:181.

White PF: Ketamine update: Its clinical uses in anesthesia. Semin Anesth 1988;7:113.

Yasuda N et al: Desflurane, isoflurane and halothane pharmacokinetics in humans. Anesth Analg 1990;70:S444.

Local Anesthetics

25

Ronald D. Miller, MD, & Luc M. Hondeghem, MD, PhD

Local anesthetics reversibly block impulse conduction along nerve axons and other excitable membranes that utilize sodium channels as the primary means of action potential generation. This action can be used clinically to block pain sensation from—or sympathetic vasoconstrictor impulses to—specific areas of the body. Cocaine, the first such agent, was isolated by Niemann in 1860. It was introduced into clinical use by Koller in 1884 as an ophthalmic anesthetic. It was soon found to have strongly addicting central nervous system actions but was widely used, nevertheless, for 30 years, since it was the only local anesthetic drug available. In an attempt to improve the properties of cocaine, Einhorn in 1905 synthesized procaine, which became the dominant local anesthetic for the next 50 years. Since 1905, many local anesthetic agents have been synthesized. The goals of these efforts were reduction of local irritation and tissue damage, minimization of systemic toxicity, faster onset of action, and longer duration of action. Lidocaine, currently the most popular agent, was synthesized in 1943 by Löfgren and may be considered the prototype local anesthetic agent.

None of the currently available local anesthetics are ideal, and development of newer agents continues. However, while it is relatively easy to synthesize a chemical with local anesthetic effects, it is very difficult to reduce the toxicity significantly below that of the current agents. The major reason for this difficulty is the fact that the most serious toxicity of local anesthetics represents extensions of the therapeutic effect on the brain and the circulatory system.

I. BASIC PHARMACOLOGY OF LOCAL ANESTHETICS

Chemistry

Most local anesthetic agents consist of a lipophilic group (frequently an aromatic ring) connected by an intermediate chain (commonly including an ester or amide) to an ionizable group (usually a tertiary amine; Table 25–1). Optimal activity requires a delicate balance between the lipophilic and hydrophilic strengths of these groups. In addition to the general physical properties of the molecules, specific stereochemical configurations can also be important; ie, differences in the potency of stereoisomers have been documented for a few compounds. Since ester links (as in procaine) are more prone to hydrolysis than amide links, esters usually have a shorter duration of action.

Local anesthetics are weak bases. For therapeutic application, they are usually made available as salts for reasons of solubility and stability. In the body, they exist either as the uncharged base or as a cation. The relative proportions of these two forms is governed by their pK_a and the pH of the body fluids according to the Henderson-Hasselbalch equation:

$$\log \frac{\text{Cationic form}}{\text{Uncharged form}} = pK_a - pH$$

Since the pK_a of most local anesthetics is in the range of 8.0–9.0, the larger fraction in the body fluids at physiologic pH will be the charged, cationic form. The cationic form is thought to be the most active form at the receptor site (cationic drug cannot readily leave closed channels), but the uncharged form is very important for rapid penetration of biologic membranes: The local anesthetic receptor is not accessible from the external side of the cell membrane (Figure 14–2). This partly explains why dentists and surgeons observe that local anesthetics are much less effective in infected tissues; these tissues have a low extracellular pH, so that a very low fraction of nonionized local anesthetic is available for diffusion into the cell.

Pharmacokinetics

Local anesthetics are usually administered by injection into the area of the nerve fibers to be blocked. Thus, absorption and distribution are not as important in controlling the onset of effect as in determining the rate of offset of anesthesia and the likelihood of central nervous system and cardiac toxicity. Topical application of local anesthetics, however, requires drug diffusion for both onset and offset of anesthetic effect.

A. Absorption: Systemic absorption of injected

Table 25–1. Structure and properties of some ester and amide local anesthetics.[1]

	Lipophillic Group	Intermediate Chain	Amine Substituents	Potency (Procaine = 1)	Duration of Action
Esters					
Cocaine				2	Medium
Procaine (Novocain)	H_2N-〔benzene〕	$\overset{O}{\overset{\|}{C}}-O-CH_2-CH_2-N$	$\begin{smallmatrix}C_2H_5\\C_2H_5\end{smallmatrix}$	1	Short
Tetracaine (Pontocaine)	$HN-$〔benzene〕, $\|$, C_4H_9	$\overset{O}{\overset{\|}{C}}-O-CH_2-CH_2-N$	$\begin{smallmatrix}CH_3\\CH_3\end{smallmatrix}$	16	Long
Benzocaine	H_2N-〔benzene〕	$\overset{O}{\overset{\|}{C}}-O-CH_2-CH_3$		Surface use only	
Amides					
Lidocaine (Xylocaine, etc)	〔benzene with 2 CH_3〕	$NH-\overset{O}{\overset{\|}{C}}-CH_2-N$	$\begin{smallmatrix}C_2H_5\\C_2H_5\end{smallmatrix}$	4	Medium
Mepivacaine (Carbocaine, Isocaine)	〔benzene with 2 CH_3〕	$NH-\overset{O}{\overset{\|}{C}}$	piperidine N–CH₃	2	Medium
Bupivacaine (Marcaine)	〔benzene with 2 CH_3〕	$NH-\overset{O}{\overset{\|}{C}}$	piperidine N–C_4H_9	16	Long
Etidocaine (Duranest)	〔benzene with 2 CH_3〕	$NH-\overset{O}{\overset{\|}{C}}-\underset{C_2H_5}{\overset{\|}{CH}}-N$	$\begin{smallmatrix}C_2H_5\\C_3H_7\end{smallmatrix}$	16	Long
Prilocaine (Citanest)	〔benzene with CH_3〕	$NH-\overset{O}{\overset{\|}{C}}-\underset{CH_3}{\overset{\|}{CH}}-NHC_3H_7$		3	Medium

[1]Other chemical types are available including ethers (pramoxine), ketones (dyclonine), and phenetidin derivatives (phenacaine).

local anesthetic from the site of administration is modified by several factors, including dosage, site of injection, drug-tissue binding, the presence of vasoconstricting substances, and the physicochemical properties of the drug. Application of a local anesthetic to a highly vascular area such as the tracheal mucosa results in more rapid absorption and thus higher blood levels than if the local anesthetic had been injected into a poorly perfused area, such as tendon. For regional anesthesia involving block of large nerves, maximum blood levels of local anesthetic decrease according to site of administration in the following order: intercostal (highest) > caudal > epidural > brachial plexus > sciatic nerve (lowest).

Vasoconstrictor substances such as epinephrine reduce systemic absorption of local anesthetics from the depot site by decreasing blood flow in these areas. This is especially true for drugs with intermediate and short durations of action such as procaine, lidocaine, and mepivacaine (but not prilocaine). Neuronal uptake of the drug is presumably enhanced by the higher local drug concentration, and the systemic toxic effects of the drug are reduced, since blood levels are lowered by as much as one-third. The combination of reduced systemic absorption and enhanced uptake by the nerve is responsible for prolonging the local anesthetic effect by about 50%. Vasoconstrictors are less effective in prolonging anesthetic properties of the more lipid-soluble, long-acting drugs (bupivacaine, etidocaine), possibly because these molecules are highly tissue-bound. In addition, catecholamines may also alter neuronal function in such a way as to promote analgesia, especially in the spinal cord. As noted below, cocaine is a special case owing to its sympathomimetic properties (Table 6–5).

B. Distribution: The amide local anesthetics are widely distributed after intravenous bolus administration. There is evidence that sequestration occurs in storage sites, possibly fat tissue. After an initial rapid distribution phase, which probably indicates uptake into highly perfused organs such as the brain, liver, kidney, and heart, a slower distribution phase occurs with uptake into moderately well perfused tissues, such as muscle and gut. Because of the extremely short plasma half-lives of the ester type agents (see below), their tissue distribution has not been studied.

C. Metabolism and Excretion: The local anesthetics are converted in the liver or in plasma to more water-soluble metabolites and then excreted in the urine. Since local anesthetics in the uncharged form diffuse readily through lipid, little or no urinary excretion of the neutral form occurs. Acidification of urine will promote ionization of the tertiary base to the more water-soluble charged form, which is more readily excreted since it is not so easily reabsorbed by renal tubules.

Ester type local anesthetics are hydrolyzed very rapidly in the blood by butyrylcholinesterase (pseudocholinesterase). Therefore, they typically have very short plasma half-lives, eg, less than 1 minute for procaine and chloroprocaine.

The amide linkage of amide local anesthetics is hydrolyzed by liver microsomal enzymes. There is considerable variation in the rate of liver metabolism of individual amide compounds, the approximate order being prilocaine (fastest) > etidocaine > lidocaine > mepivacaine > bupivacaine (slowest). As a result, toxicity from the amide type of local anesthetic is more likely to occur in patients with liver disease. For example, the average half-life of lidocaine may be increased from 1.8 hours in normal patients to over 6 hours in patients with severe liver disease.

Decreased hepatic removal of local anesthetics should also be anticipated in patients with reduced hepatic blood flow. For example, the hepatic elimination of lidocaine in animals anesthetized with halothane is slower than that measured in animals receiving nitrous oxide and curare. The reduced elimination may be related to decreased hepatic blood flow and to halothane-induced depression of hepatic microsomes. Propranolol may also prolong the half-life of amide local anesthetics.

Pharmacodynamics

A. Mechanism of Action: The excitable membrane of nerve axons, like the membrane of cardiac muscle (see Chapter 14) and neuronal cell bodies (see Chapter 20), maintains a transmembrane potential of –90 to –60 mV. During excitation, the sodium channels open, and a fast inward sodium current quickly depolarizes the membrane toward the sodium equilibrium potential (+40 mV). As a result of depolarization, the sodium channels close (inactivate) and potassium channels open. The outward flow of potassium repolarizes the membrane toward the potassium equilibrium potential (about –95 mV); repolarization returns the sodium channels to the rested state. The transmembrane ionic gradients are maintained by the sodium pump. These characteristics are similar to those of heart muscle, and local anesthetics have similar effects in both tissues.

The function of sodium channels can be disrupted in several ways. Biologic toxins such as **batrachotoxin, aconitine, veratridine,** and some **scorpion venoms** bind to receptors within the channel and prevent inactivation. This results in prolonged influx of sodium through the channel rather than block of conduction, with the result that some investigators consider these agents *agonists* at the sodium channel. The marine toxins **tetrodotoxin** and **saxitoxin** block these channels by binding to channel receptors near the extracellular surface. Their clinical effects superficially resemble those of local anesthetics even though their receptor site is quite different. Local anesthetics bind to receptors near the intracellular end of the channel (Figure 14–2) and block the channel in a time- and voltage-dependent fashion (see below).

When progressively increasing concentrations of a local anesthetic are applied to a nerve fiber, the threshold for excitation increases, impulse conduction slows, the rate of rise of the action potential declines, the action potential amplitude decreases, and, finally, the ability to generate an action potential is abolished. These incremental effects result from binding of the local anesthetic to more and more sodium channels; in each channel, binding results in blockade of the sodium current. If the sodium current is blocked over a critical length of the nerve, propagation across the blocked area is no longer possible. At the minimum dose required to block propagation, the resting potential is not significantly affected.

The blockade of sodium channels by most local anesthetics is *voltage-* and *time-dependent:* Channels in the rested state (which predominate at more negative membrane potentials) have a much lower affinity for local anesthetics than activated (open state) and inactivated channels (which predominate at more positive membrane potentials; Figure 14–8). Thus, the effect of a given drug concentration is more marked in rapidly firing axons than in resting fibers (Figure 25–1).

Between depolarizations of the axon, a portion of the sodium channels recover from local anesthetic block (Figure 14–8). The recovery from drug-induced block is 10–1000 times slower than the recovery of channels from normal inactivation, as shown for the cardiac membrane in Figure 14–4. As a result, the refractory period is lengthened and the nerve can conduct fewer impulses.

Elevated extracellular calcium partially antagonizes the action of local anesthetics. This reversal is caused by the calcium-induced increase of the surface potential on the membrane, which favors the low-affinity rested state. Conversely, increase of extracellular potassium depolarizes the membrane potential and favors the inactivated state (Figure 14–9). This enhances the effect of local anesthetics.

Although local anesthetics can be shown to block a variety of other channels, including chemically gated synaptic channels, there is no convincing evidence that such actions play an important role in the clinical effects of these drugs. However, experimental studies in both nerve fibers and cardiac muscle cells indicate that drugs which prolong the action potential can significantly increase the sensitivity of sodium channels to local anesthetic blockade (Drachman, 1991). This can be explained by the observations described above, ie, that the affinity of activated and inactivated channels for local anesthetics is greater than the affinity of channels in the rested state.

Structure-activity characteristics of local anesthetics. The smaller and more lipophilic the molecule, the faster the rate of interaction with the sodium channel receptor. Potency is also positively correlated with lipid solubility as long as the agent retains sufficient water solubility to diffuse to the site of action. Lidocaine, procaine, and mepivacaine are more water-soluble than tetracaine, etidocaine, and bupivacaine. The latter agents are more potent and have longer durations of action. They also bind more extensively to proteins and will displace or be displaced from these binding sites by other drugs.

B. Actions on Nerves: Since local anesthetics are capable of blocking all nerves, their actions are not usually limited to the desired loss of sensation. Although motor paralysis may at times be desirable, it may also limit the ability of the patient to cooperate, eg, during obstetric delivery. During spinal anesthesia, motor paralysis may impair respiratory activity and autonomic nerve blockade may lead to hypotension. However, different types of nerve fibers differ significantly in their susceptibility to local anesthetic blockade on the basis of size and myelination (Table 25–2). Upon application of a local anesthetic to a nerve root, the smaller B and C fibers are blocked first. The small type A delta fibers are blocked next. Thus, pain fibers are blocked first; other sensations disappear next; and motor function is blocked last.

1. Effect of fiber diameter—Local anesthetics preferentially block small fibers because the distance over which such fibers can passively propagate an electrical impulse (related to the space constant) is

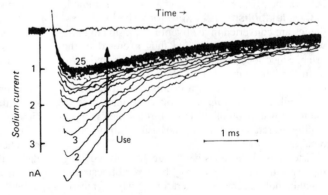

Figure 25–1. Effect of repetitive activity on the block of sodium current produced by a local anesthetic in a myelinated axon. A series of 25 pulses was applied, and the resulting sodium currents are superimposed. Note that the current produced by the pulses rapidly decreased from the first to the 25th pulse. A long rest period following the train resulted in recovery from block, but the block could be reinstated by a subsequent train. (nA, nanoamperes.) (Modified slightly and reproduced, with permission, from Courtney KR: Mechanism of frequency-dependent inhibition of sodium currents in frog myelinated nerve by the lidocaine derivative GEA. J Pharmacol Exp Ther 1975; 195: 225.)

Table 25–2. Relative size and susceptibility to block of types of nerve fibers.

Fiber Type	Function	Diameter (μm)	Myelination	Conduction Velocity (m/s)	Sensitivity to Block
Type A					
Alpha	Proprioception, motor	12–20	Heavy	70–120	+
Beta	Touch, pressure	5–12	Heavy	30–70	++
Gamma	Muscle spindles	3–6	Heavy	15–30	++
Delta	Pain, temperature	2–5	Heavy	12–30	+++
Type B	Preganglionic autonomic	<3	Light	3–15	++++
Type C					
Dorsal root	Pain	0.4–1.2	None	0.5–2.3	++++
Sympathetic	Postganglionic	0.3–1.3	None	0.7–2.3	++++

shorter. During the onset of local anesthesia, when short sections of nerve are blocked, the small-diameter fibers are the first to fail to conduct. For myelinated nerves, three successive nodes must be blocked by the local anesthetic to halt impulse propagation. The thicker the nerve fiber, the farther apart the nodes tend to be—which explains, in part, the greater resistance to block of large fibers. Myelinated nerves tend to become blocked before unmyelinated nerves of the same diameter. For this reason, the preganglionic B fibers may be blocked before the smaller unmyelinated C fibers.

2. Effect of firing frequency–Another important reason for preferential blockade of sensory fibers follows directly from the state-dependent mechanism of action of local anesthetics. Block by these drugs is more marked at higher frequencies of depolarization and with longer depolarizations. Sensory fibers, especially pain fibers, have a high firing rate and a relatively long action potential duration (up to 5 ms). Motor fibers fire at a slower rate and have a shorter action potential duration (< 0.5 ms). A delta and C fibers are small-diameter fibers that participate in high-frequency pain transmission. They therefore are blocked sooner with low concentrations of local anesthetics than are the A alpha fibers.

3. Effect of fiber position in the nerve bundle–An anatomic circumstance that sometimes creates exceptions to the above rules for differential nerve block is the location of the fiber in the peripheral bundle. In large nerve trunks, motor nerves are usually located circumferentially, and for that reason they are exposed first to the drug when it is administered by injection into the tissue surrounding the nerve. Therefore, it is not uncommon that motor nerve block occurs before sensory block in large mixed nerves. In the extremities, proximal sensory fibers are located in the mantle of the nerve trunk, whereas the distal sensory innervation is in the core of the nerve. Thus, during infiltration block of a large nerve, anesthesia first develops proximally and then spreads distally as the drug penetrates the core of the nerve.

C. Effects on Other Excitable Membranes:

Local anesthetics have weak neuromuscular blocking effects that are of little clinical importance. However, their effects on cardiac cell membranes are of major clinical significance. Some are useful antiarrhythmic agents (see Chapter 14) at concentrations lower than those required to produce nerve block, and all can cause arrhythmias in high enough concentration.

II. CLINICAL PHARMACOLOGY OF LOCAL ANESTHETICS

Local anesthetics can provide temporary but complete analgesia of well-defined parts of the body. The usual routes of administration include topical application, injection in the vicinity of peripheral nerve endings and major nerve trunks, and instillation within the epidural or subarachnoid spaces surrounding the spinal cord (Figure 25–2). In addition, block of autonomic sympathetic fibers can be used to evaluate the role of sympathetic tone in patients with peripheral vasospasm.

The choice of local anesthetic for a specific procedure is usually based on the duration of action required. Procaine and chloroprocaine are short-acting; lidocaine, mepivacaine, and prilocaine have an intermediate duration of action; tetracaine, bupivacaine, and etidocaine are long-acting drugs (Table 25–1).

As noted above, the anesthetic effect of the agents with short and intermediate durations of action can be prolonged by increasing the dose or by adding a vasoconstrictor agent, such as epinephrine or phenylephrine. The vasoconstrictor retards the removal of drug from the injection site. In addition, it decreases the blood level and hence the chance of toxicity.

The onset of local anesthesia is sometimes accelerated by the use of solutions saturated with carbon dioxide ("carbonated"). The high tissue level of CO_2 results in intracellular acidosis (CO_2 crosses membranes readily), which in turn results in intracellular

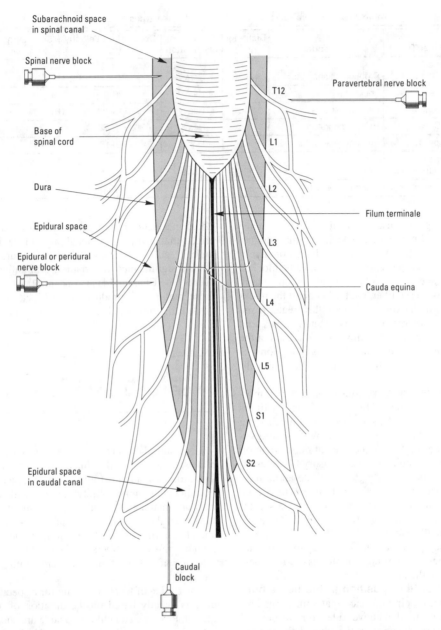

Figure 25–2. Schematic diagram of sites of injection of local anesthetics in and near the spinal canal.

accumulation of the cationic form of the local anesthetic.

Repeated injection of local anesthetics during epidural anesthesia results in loss of effectiveness (tachyphylaxis). This is probably a consequence of local extracellular acidosis. Local anesthetics are commonly marketed as hydrochloride salts (pH 4.0–6.0). After injection, the salts are buffered in the tissue to physiologic pH, thereby providing sufficient free base for diffusion through axonal membranes. However, repeated injections deplete the local available buffer. The ensuing acidosis increases the ex-

tracellular cationic form, which diffuses poorly into axons. The clinical result is apparent tachyphylaxis, especially in areas of limited buffer reserve, such as the cerebrospinal fluid.

Toxicity

Ultimately, local anesthetic agents are absorbed from the site of administration. If blood levels rise too high, effects on several organ systems may be observed.

A. Central Nervous System: Since prehistoric times, the natives of Peru have chewed the leaves of the indigenous plant *Erythroxylon coca,* the source of cocaine, to obtain a feeling of well-being and reduce fatigue. Intense central nervous system effects can be achieved by sniffing cocaine powder and smoking cocaine base. Cocaine has become one of the most widely used drugs of abuse (see Chapter 31). Other local anesthetics have been thought to lack the euphoriant effects of cocaine. However, some studies indicate that some habitual cocaine users cannot differentiate between intranasal cocaine and lidocaine given by the same route.

Other central nervous system effects include sleepiness, light-headedness, visual and auditory disturbances, and restlessness. At higher concentrations, nystagmus and shivering may occur. Finally, overt tonic-clonic convulsions followed by central nervous system depression and death may occur with all local anesthetics, including cocaine. Local anesthetics apparently lead to depression of cortical inhibitory pathways, thereby allowing unopposed activity of excitatory components. This transitional stage of unbalanced excitation may be followed by generalized central nervous system depression if higher blood levels of local anesthetic are reached.

Most serious toxic reactions to local anesthetics are due to convulsions from excessive blood levels. These are best prevented by administering the smallest dose of local anesthetic required for adequate anesthesia. When large doses must be administered, premedication with a benzodiazepine, eg, diazepam, 0.1–0.2 mg/kg parenterally, probably provides significant prophylaxis against seizures. If seizures do occur, it is essential to prevent hypoxemia and acidosis. Although administration of oxygen does not prevent seizure activity, hyperoxemia after onset of seizures appears to be beneficial. Conversely, hypercapnia and acidosis appear to promote the occurrence of seizures. Thus, hyperventilation is recommended during treatment of seizures. Hyperventilation elevates blood pH, which in turn lowers extracellular potassium. This hyperpolarizes the transmembrane potential of axons, which favors the rested or low-affinity state of the sodium channels, resulting in decreased local anesthetic toxicity.

Seizures induced by local anesthetics can also be treated with small doses of short-acting barbiturates, eg, thiopental, 1–2 mg/kg intravenously, or diazepam, 0.1 mg/kg intravenously. The muscular manifestations can be suppressed by a short-acting neuromuscular blocking agent, eg, succinylcholine, 0.5–1 mg/kg intravenously. It should be emphasized that succinylcholine does not obliterate cortical manifestations on the EEG. In especially severe cases of convulsions, intubation of the trachea combined with succinylcholine administration and mechanical ventilation can prevent pulmonary aspiration of gastric contents and facilitate hyperventilation therapy.

B. Peripheral Nervous System (Neurotoxicity): When applied at excessively high concentra-

tions, all local anesthetics can be toxic to nerve tissue. Several case reports document prolonged sensory and motor deficits following accidental spinal anesthesia with large volumes of chloroprocaine. Whether chloroprocaine is more neurotoxic than other local anesthetics has not been determined.

C. Cardiovascular System: The cardiovascular effects of local anesthetics result partly from direct effects upon the cardiac and smooth muscle membranes and from indirect effects upon the autonomic nerves. As described in Chapter 14, local anesthetics block cardiac sodium channels and thus depress abnormal cardiac pacemaker activity, excitability, and conduction. With the exception of cocaine, they also depress the strength of cardiac contraction and cause arteriolar dilation, both effects leading to hypotension. Although cardiovascular collapse and death usually occur only after large doses, they may result occasionally from the small amounts used for infiltration anesthesia.

As noted above, cocaine differs from the other local anesthetics in its cardiovascular effects. The blockade of norepinephrine reuptake results in vasoconstriction and hypertension. It may also precipitate cardiac arrhythmias. The vasoconstriction produced by cocaine can lead to ischemia of the nasal mucosa and, in chronic users, to ulceration of the mucous membrane and even damage to the septum. This vasoconstrictor property of cocaine can be used clinically to decrease bleeding from mucosal damage in the nasopharynx.

Bupivacaine is more cardiotoxic than other local anesthetics. Several case reports have appeared indicating that accidental intravenous injection of bupivacaine may lead not only to seizures but also to cardiovascular collapse, from which resuscitation may be extremely difficult or unsuccessful. Several experimental animal studies have confirmed the idea that bupivacaine is indeed more toxic when given intravenously than most other local anesthetics. This reflects the fact that bupivacaine block of sodium channels is greatly potentiated by the very long action potential duration of cardiac cells (as compared to nerve fibers) and, unlike lidocaine blockade, cumulates markedly at normal heart rates. Subsequent studies have shown that the most common electrocardiographic finding in patients with bupivacaine intoxication is slow idioventricular rhythm with broad QRS complexes and electromechanical dissociation. Resuscitation has been successful with standard cardiopulmonary support—including the prompt correction of acidosis by hyperventilation and administration of bicarbonate—and aggressive administration of epinephrine, atropine, and bretylium. **Ropivacaine** is a new investigational amide local anesthetic with local anesthetic effects similar to those of bupivacaine. Preliminary evidence suggests that it may have lower cardiovascular toxicity than bupivacaine.

D. Blood: The administration of large doses

(> 10 mg/kg) of prilocaine during regional anesthesia may lead to accumulation of the metabolite *o*-toluidine, an oxidizing agent capable of converting hemoglobin to methemoglobin. When sufficient methemoglobin is present (3–5 mg/dL), the patient may appear cyanotic and the blood chocolate-colored. Such levels of methemoglobinemia are tolerated by healthy individuals but may cause decompensation in patients with cardiac or pulmonary disease and require immediate treatment. Reducing agents such as methylene blue or, less satisfactorily, ascorbic acid may be given intravenously to rapidly convert methemoglobin to hemoglobin.

E. Allergic Reactions: The ester type local anesthetics are metabolized to *p*-aminobenzoic acid derivatives. These metabolites are responsible for allergic reactions in a small percentage of the population. Amides are not metabolized to *p*-aminobenzoic acid, and allergic reactions to agents of the amide group are extremely rare.

PREPARATIONS AVAILABLE

Benzocaine (generic, others)
Topical: 5, 6% creams; 6, 20% gels; 5% ointments; 0.5% lotion; 20% spray
Bupivacaine (generic, Marcaine, Sensorcaine)
Parenteral: 0.25, 0.5, 0.75% for injection; 0.25, 0.5, 0.75% with 1:200,000 epinephrine
Butamben picrate (Butesin Picrate)
Topical: 1% ointment
Chloroprocaine (Nesacaine)
Parenteral: 1, 2, 3% for injection
Cocaine (generic)
Topical: 40, 100, mg/mL solutions; 5, 25 g powder; 135 mg soluble tablets
Dibucaine (generic, Nupercainal)
Topical: 0.5% cream; 1% ointment
Dyclonine (Dyclone)
Topical: 0.5, 1% solution
Etidocaine (Duranest)
Parenteral: 1% for injection; 1, 1.5% with 1:200,000 epinephrine for injection
Lidocaine (generic, Xylocaine, others)
Parenteral: 0.5, 1, 1.5, 2, 4, 10, 20% for injection; 0.5, 1, 1.5, 2% with 1:200,000 epinephrine;

1, 2% with 1:100,000 epinephrine, 2% with 1:50,000 epinephrine
Topical: 2.5, 5% ointments; 0.5% cream; 2% jelly and solution; 2, 4, 10% solutions
Mepivacaine (generic, Carbocaine, others)
Parenteral: 1, 1.5, 2, 3% for injection; 2% with 1:20,000 levonordefrin
Pramoxine (Tronothane, Prax)
Topical: 0.5, 1% cream; 1% lotion and gel
Prilocaine (Citanest)
Parenteral: 4% for injection; 4% with 1:200,000 epinephrine
Procaine (generic, Novocain)
Parenteral: 1, 2, 10% for injection
Propoxycaine and procaine (Ravocaine and Novocain)
Parenteral: 7.2 mg propoxycaine with 36 mg procaine and norepinephrine or cobefrin per 1.8 mL dental injection unit
Tetracaine (Pontocaine)
Parenteral: 1% for injection; 0.2, 0.3% with 6% dextrose for spinal anesthesia
Topical: 0.5% ointment; 0.5% solution (ophthalmic); 1% cream; 2% solution for sore throat

REFERENCES

Albright GA: Cardiac arrest following regional anesthesia with etidocaine or bupivacaine. Anesthesiology 1979;51: 285.

Arthur GR, Feldman HS, Covino BG: Comparative pharmacokinetics of bupivacaine and proparacaine, a new amide local anesthetic. Anesth Analg 1988;67:1053.

Butterworth JF, Strichartz GR: Molecular mechanisms of local anesthesia: A review. Anesthesiology 1990;72:711.

Catterall WA: Structure and function of voltage-sensitive ion channels. Science 1988;242:50.

Clarkson CW, Hondeghem LM: Evidence for a specific receptor site for lidocaine, quinidine, and bupivacaine associated with cardiac sodium channels in guinea pig ventricular myocardium. Circ Res 1985;56:496.

Concepcion M et al: A new local anesthetic, ropivacaine. Its epidural effects in humans. Anesth Analg 1990;70:80.

Covino BG: Pharmacology of local anaesthetic agents. Br J Anaesth 1986;58:701.

Drachman D, Strichartz G: Potassium channel blockers potentiate impulse inhibition by local anesthetics. Anesthesiology 1991;75:1051.

Fleming JA, Byck R, Barash PG: Pharmacology and therapeutic applications of cocaine. Anesthesiology 1990;73: 518.

Hille B: Local anesthetics: Hydrophilic and hydrophobic pathways for the drug-receptor reactions. J Gen Physiol 1977;69:497.

Kendig JJ, Courtney KR: New modes of nerve block. Anesthesiology 1991;74:207.

Ravindran RS et al: Prolonged neural blockade following regional anesthesia with 2-chloroprocaine. Anesth Analg 1980;59:447.

Reiz S, Nath S: Cardiotoxicity of local anesthetic agents. Br J Anaesth 1986;58:736.

Scott DB et al: Acute toxicity of ropivacaine compared to that of bupivacaine. Anesth Analg 1989;69:563.

Strichartz GR et al: Fundamental properties of local anesthetics: II. Measured octanol:buffer partition coefficients and pK$_a$ values of clinically used drugs. Anesth Analg 1990;71:158.

Strichartz GR: Pharmacology of local anesthetics. In: *Anesthesia,* 4th ed. Miller RD (editor). Churchill Livingstone, 1994.

Tucker GT: Pharmacokinetics of local anaesthetics. Br J Anaesth 1986;58:717.

26

Skeletal Muscle Relaxants

Ronald D. Miller, MD

Drugs that affect skeletal muscle function fall into two major therapeutic groups: those used during surgical procedures and in intensive care units to cause paralysis, ie, **neuromuscular blockers,** and those used to reduce spasticity in a variety of neurologic conditions, ie, **spasmolytics.** Members of the first group, as their name implies, interfere with transmission at the neuromuscular endplate and are not CNS-active drugs. However, because they are used primarily as adjuncts to general anesthesia, they are often discussed in connection with central nervous system agents. Drugs in the second group have traditionally been called "centrally acting" muscle relaxants. However, at least one of its important members (dantrolene) has no central effects, so the traditional name is now inappropriate.

NEUROMUSCULAR BLOCKING DRUGS

History

During the 16th century, European explorers found that natives of the Amazon Basin of South America were using an arrow poison that produced death by skeletal muscle paralysis. This poison later became the subject of intense investigation. **Curare,** the active crude material, formed the basis for some of the earliest scientific studies in pharmacology. The active principle from curare, **tubocurarine (d-tubocurarine),** and its synthetic derivatives have had a tremendous influence on the practice of anesthesia and surgery and have been useful also in defining normal neuromuscular physiologic mechanisms.

Normal Neuromuscular Function

Theoretically, muscular relaxation and paralysis can occur from interruption of function at several sites, including the central nervous system, myelinated somatic nerves, unmyelinated motor nerve terminals, the acetylcholine receptor, the motor endplate, and the muscle membrane or contractile apparatus (Figure 26–1). The mechanism of neuromuscular transmission at the endplate is similar to that described in Chapter 6, with arrival of an impulse at the motor nerve terminal, influx of calcium, and release of acetylcholine. Acetylcholine then diffuses across the synaptic cleft to the nicotinic receptor located on the motor endplate. When the receptor and acetylcholine interact, permeability of the membrane in the endplate region increases—to sodium primarily, but also to potassium. Sodium moves from outside to inside the cell, depolarizing the membrane. This change in voltage is termed the endplate potential. The magnitude of the endplate potential is directly related to the amount of acetylcholine released. If the potential is small, the permeability and the endplate potential return to normal without an impulse being propagated from the endplate region to the rest of the muscle membrane. However, if the endplate potential is large, the muscle membrane is depolarized to its threshold, and an action potential will be propagated along the entire muscle fiber. Muscle con-

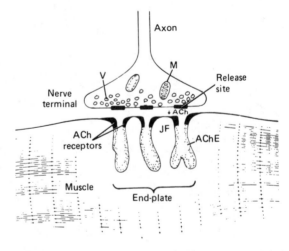

Figure 26–1. Schematic representation of the neuromuscular junction. (V, transmitter vesicle; M, mitochondrion; ACh, acetylcholine; AChE, acetylcholinesterase; JF, junctional folds.) (Reproduced, with permission, from Drachman DB: Myasthenia gravis. N Engl J Med 1978;298:135.)

traction is then initiated by excitation-contraction coupling. The released acetylcholine is removed from the endplate region by diffusion and rapid enzymatic destruction by acetylcholinesterase.

Blockade of normal endplate function can occur by two mechanisms. Pharmacologic blockade of the agonist, acetylcholine, is characteristic of *antagonist* drugs. These drugs prevent access of the transmitter to its receptor and prevent depolarization. The prototype of this **nondepolarizing** subgroup is tubocurarine. Block of transmission can also be produced by an excess of depolarizing *agonist.* (This paradoxical effect also occurs at the ganglionic nicotinic acetylcholine receptor.) The prototype **depolarizing** blocking drug is succinylcholine. A similar depolarizing block can be produced by acetylcholine itself if very high local concentrations are reached (eg, in cholinesterase inhibitor intoxication), by nicotine, and by other nicotinic agonists. However, because the block produced by these agents cannot be controlled adequately, they are of no clinical value in this application.

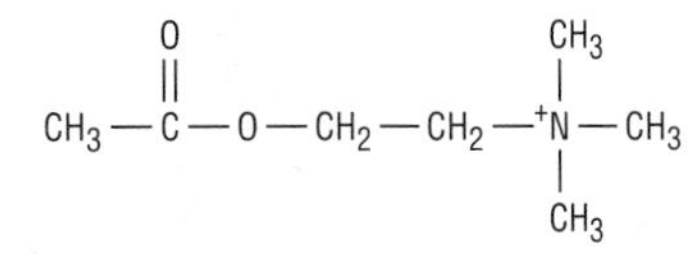

I. BASIC PHARMACOLOGY OF NEUROMUSCULAR BLOCKING DRUGS

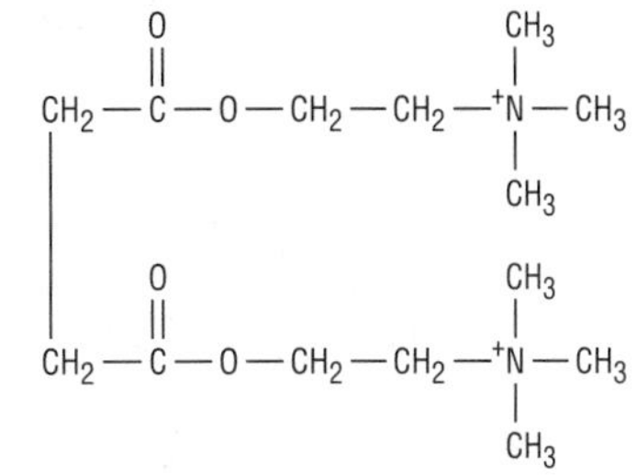

Chemistry

All of the neuromuscular blocking drugs bear a structural resemblance to acetylcholine. In fact, succinylcholine is two acetylcholine molecules linked end-to-end (Figure 26–2). In contrast to the single linear structure of succinylcholine and other depolarizing drugs, the nondepolarizing agents conceal the "double-acetylcholine" structure in one of two types of bulky, relatively rigid ring systems (eg, pancuronium; Figure 26–2). The two major families of nondepolarizing blocking drugs (isoquinoline derivatives and steroids) are shown in Figures 26–3 and 26–4. Another feature common to all useful drugs in this class is the presence of one or two quaternary nitrogens, which makes them poorly soluble in lipid and prevents entry into the central nervous system.

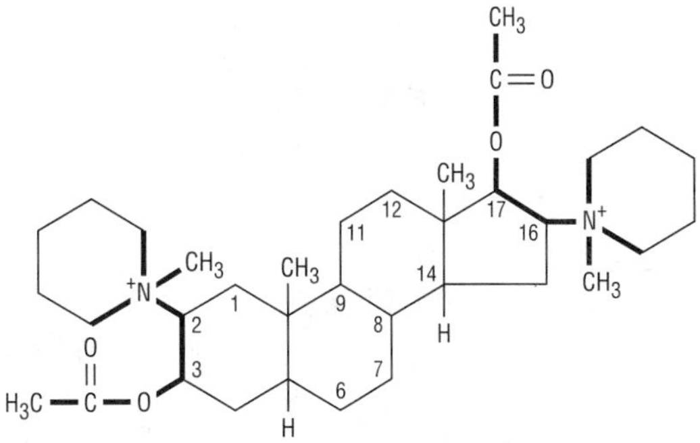

Pharmacokinetics of Neuromuscular Blocking Drugs

All of the neuromuscular blocking drugs are highly polar and inactive when administered by mouth. They are always administered intravenously.

A. Nondepolarizing Drugs: The rate of disappearance of a nondepolarizing neuromuscular blocking drug from blood is characterized by a rapid initial distribution phase followed by a slower elimination phase. Because neuromuscular blocking drugs are

Figure 26–2. Structural relationship of succinylcholine, a depolarizing agent, and pancuronium, a nondepolarizing agent, to acetylcholine, the neuromuscular transmitter. Succinylcholine, originally called diacetylcholine, is simply two molecules of acetylcholine linked through the acetate methyl groups. Pancuronium may be viewed as two acetylcholine-like fragments (outlined in dark print) oriented on a steroid nucleus.

highly ionized, they do not cross membranes well and have a limited volume of distribution of 80–140 mL/kg—not much larger than blood volume.

Tubocurarine (Figure 26–3), metocurine (dimethyltubocurarine), and gallamine (not shown) are not metabolized. Gallamine is entirely dependent on the kidney for its elimination (Table 26–1). In contrast, only about 50–60% of an injected dose of tubocurarine or metocurine is excreted in the urine over a 24-hour period in humans. The exact route of excretion of the remainder of these agents in humans is unclear, though it is presumed that biliary excretion accounts for most of it. All steroidal muscle relaxants are metabolized to their 3-hydroxy, 17-hydroxy, and

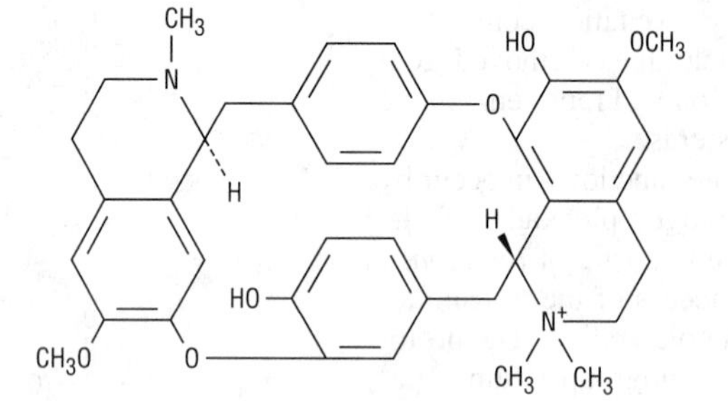

Tubocurarine

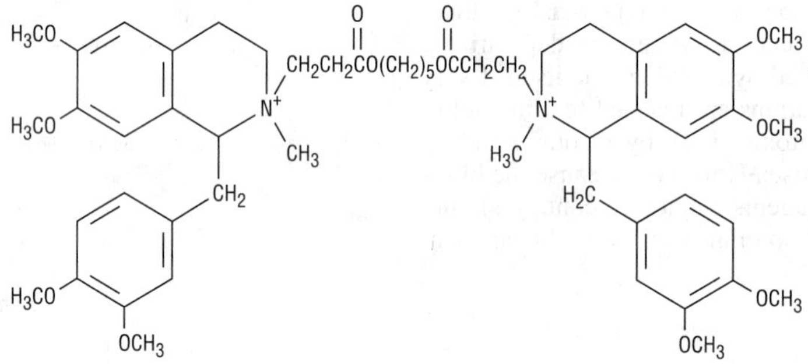

Atracurium

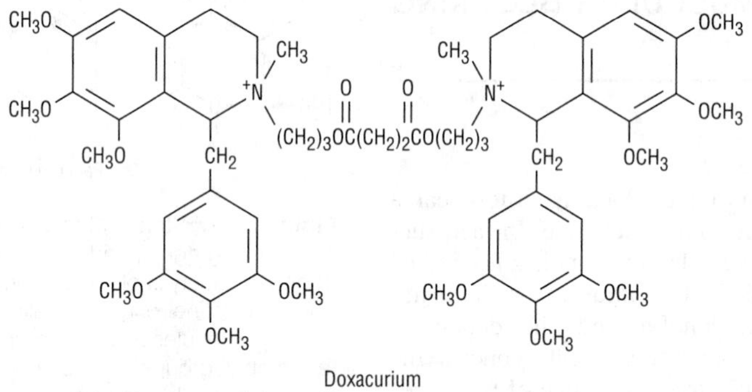

Doxacurium

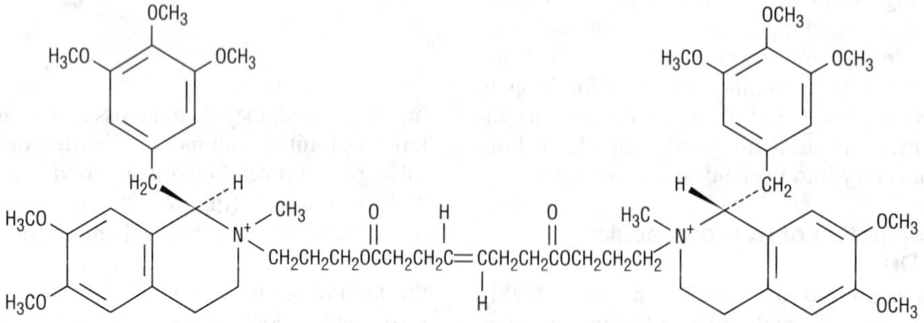

Mivacurium

Figure 26–3. Structures of some isoquinoline neuromuscular blocking drugs. These agents are all nondepolarizing in their action.

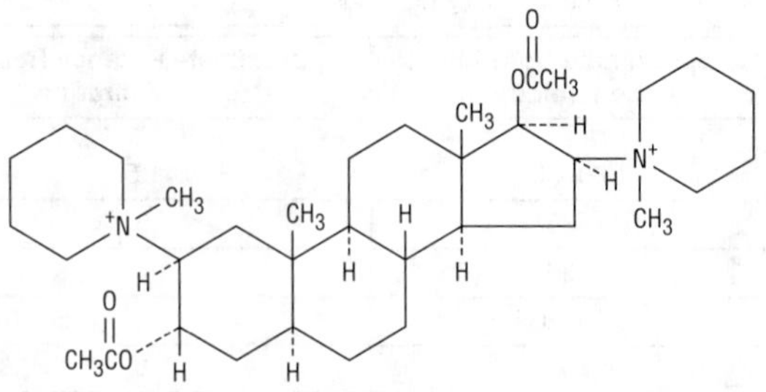

Pancuronium

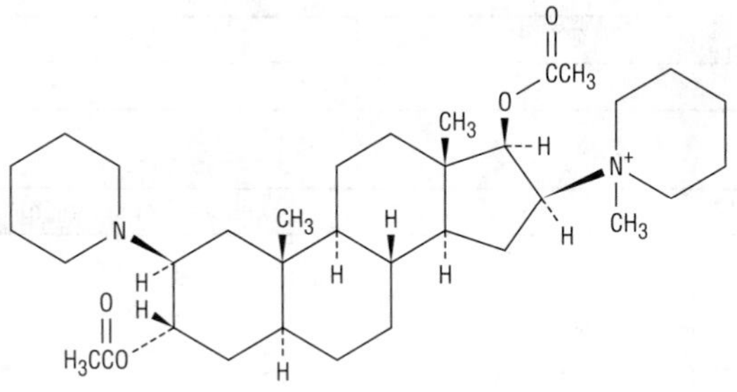

Vecuronium

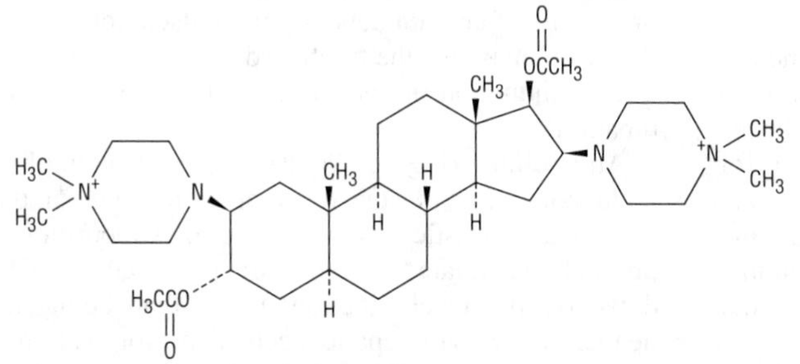

Pipecuronium

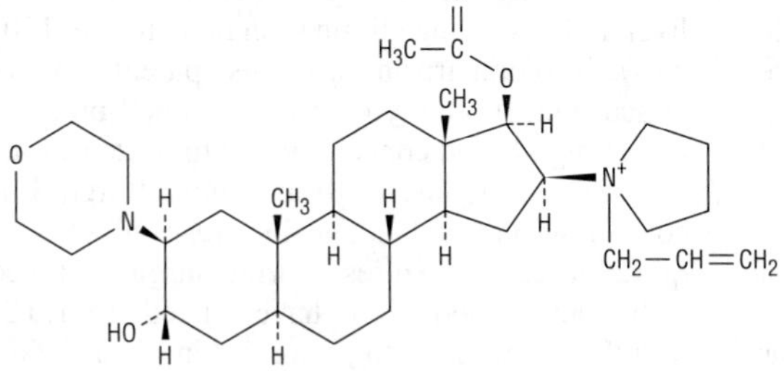

Rocuronium

Figure 26–4. Structures of some steroid neuromuscular blocking drugs. These agents are all nondepolarizing in their action.

Table 26–1. Some properties of neuromuscular blocking drugs.

Drug	Elimination via	Approximate Duration of Action (minutes)	Approximate Potency Relative to Tubocurarine
Isoquinoline derivatives			
Atracurium	Spontaneous[1]	20–35	1.5
Doxacurium	Kidney	>35	6
Metocurine	Kidney (40%)	>35	4
Mivacurium	Plasma ChE[2]	10–20	4
Tubocurarine	Kidney (40%)	>35	1
Steroid derivatives			
Pancuronium	Liver and kidney	>35	6
Pipecuronium	Kidney (60%) and liver	>35	6
Rocuronium	Liver (75–90%) and kidney	20–35	0.8
Vecuronium	Liver (75–90%) and kidney	20–35	6
Other agents			
Gallamine	Kidney (100%)	>35	0.2
Succinylcholine	Plasma ChE[2] (100%)	<8	Different mechanism[3]

[1]Nonenzymatic and enzymatic hydrolysis of ester bonds.
[2]Butyrylcholinesterase (pseudocholinesterase).
[3]A depolarizing cholinoceptor agonist.

3,17-dihydroxy products, mainly in the liver. The 3-hydroxy metabolites are usually 40–80% as potent as the parent drug. These metabolites are not formed in sufficient quantities to cause significant additional neuromuscular block during surgical anesthesia. However, if the parent compound is being given for several days, as may be done in the intensive care unit, the 3-hydroxy metabolite may accumulate and cause prolonged paralysis (Segredo, 1992). Although the remaining metabolites also have neuromuscular blocking properties, they are very weak.

Like tubocurarine, the other long-acting muscle relaxants (doxacurium, metocurine, pancuronium, and pipecuronium) are dependent mainly on the kidney for their elimination (about 60–90% of a dose; Table 26–1). In contrast, the intermediate-duration muscle relaxants (vecuronium and rocuronium) tend to be more dependent on biliary excretion or hepatic metabolism for their elimination. These drugs are more commonly used clinically than the long-acting drugs. Vecuronium has a steroid nucleus like that of pancuronium (Figure 26–4), differing only in that one of the nitrogens is tertiary rather than quaternary. Despite this small structural difference, vecuronium has distinctly different pharmacologic properties. Vecuronium has a shorter duration of action (approximately 20–35 minutes versus 60 minutes) and minimal cardiovascular effects, and is not as dependent upon the kidney for its elimination. Only about 15% of an injected dose of vecuronium is eliminated by the kidney; the remaining 85% is eliminated into the bile as either the unchanged drug or its 3-hydroxy metabolite. Rocuronium is the newest of the steroid derivatives and has a pharmacokinetic profile similar to

that of vecuronium. Rocuronium has the most rapid onset time of any nondepolarizing muscle relaxant. It therefore may be the preferred drug for rapid-sequence induction of anesthesia and endotracheal intubation.

Atracurium (Figure 26–3) is an isoquinoline nondepolarizing muscle relaxant with many of the same characteristics as vecuronium. Atracurium is probably inactivated by a form of spontaneous breakdown (Hofmann elimination) rather than being dependent on renal or hepatic mechanisms for the termination of its action. The main breakdown products are laudanosine and a related quaternary acid, neither of which has neuromuscular blocking properties. However, laudanosine is very slowly metabolized by the liver and has a long elimination half-life (ie, 150 minutes) in comparison with its parent compound, atracurium. It readily crosses the blood-brain barrier and at high blood concentrations may cause seizures. In dogs and rabbits, 17 μg/mL and 3.9 μg/mL blood concentrations of laudanosine, respectively, are required to cause seizures. During surgical procedures in humans, blood levels have ranged from 0.2 to 1 μg/mL. However, with prolonged infusions of atracurium in the intensive care unit, blood levels of laudanosine as high as 5.5 μg/mL have been reported. At much lower blood concentrations (0.2–0.8 μg/mL), laudanosine causes about a 30% increase in anesthetic requirement.

Mivacurium has the shortest duration of action of any nondepolarizing muscle relaxant (Table 26–1). It is metabolized entirely by plasma cholinesterase and is not dependent on the liver or kidney for its elimination. However, because patients with renal failure have decreased plasma cholinesterase levels, the duration of action of mivacurium may be prolonged in patients with impaired renal function.

B. Depolarizing Drugs: The extremely brief duration of action of succinylcholine (5–10 minutes) is due chiefly to its rapid hydrolysis by plasma cholinesterase (butyrylcholinesterase, pseudocholinesterase), an enzyme of the liver and plasma. Apparently, plasma cholinesterase metabolizes succinylcholine more rapidly than mivacurium, since the duration of action of succinylcholine is shorter than that of mivacurium (Table 26–1). The initial metabolite, succinylmonocholine, is a much weaker neuromuscular blocker. It in turn is metabolized to succinic acid and choline. Plasma cholinesterase has an enormous capacity to hydrolyze succinylcholine at a very rapid rate; as a result, only a small fraction of the original intravenous dose reaches the neuromuscular junction. Since there is little or no plasma cholinesterase at the motor endplate, the neuromuscular blockade of succinylcholine is terminated by its diffusion away from the endplate into extracellular fluid. Plasma cholinesterase, therefore, influences the duration of action of succinylcholine by determining the amount of the drug that reaches the endplate.

Neuromuscular blockade by both succinylcholine and mivacurium may be prolonged in patients with an abnormal variant of plasma cholinesterase of genetic origin. The "dibucaine number"—a test for ability to metabolize succinylcholine—can be used to identify such patients. Under standardized test conditions, dibucaine inhibits the normal enzyme about 80% and abnormal enzyme only 20%. Many genetic variants of plasma cholinesterase have been identified, although the dibucaine-related variants are the most important.

Mechanism of Action

The interactions of drugs with the acetylcholine receptor and the endplate channel have been described at the molecular level. Several modes of action of drugs on the receptor appear to be possible and are illustrated in Figure 26–5.

A. Nondepolarizing Blocking Drugs: All of the neuromuscular blocking drugs in use in the USA except succinylcholine are classified as nondepolarizing agents. Tubocurarine is the prototype. They produce a surmountable blockade. In low clinical doses and at low frequencies of stimulation, nondepolarizing muscle relaxants act predominantly at the **nicotinic receptor site** to compete with acetylcholine. At higher doses, some of these drugs also enter the pore of the ion channel to cause blockade. This further weakens neuromuscular transmission and diminishes the ability of acetylcholinesterase inhibitors (eg, neostigmine) to antagonize nondepolarizing muscle relaxants. Nondepolarizing relaxants may also block prejunctional sodium—but probably not calcium—channels. As a result, these muscle relaxants also interfere with the mobilization of acetylcholine at the nerve ending.

One consequence of the surmountable nature of the postsynaptic blockade produced by these agents is the fact that tetanic stimulation, by releasing a large quantity of acetylcholine, is followed by a transient posttetanic breakthrough or relief of the block. An important clinical consequence of the same principle is the ability of cholinesterase inhibitors to reverse the blockade.

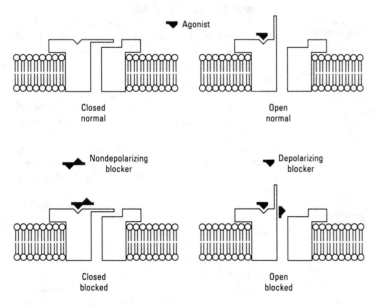

Figure 26–5. Schematic diagram of the interactions of drugs with the acetylcholine receptor on the endplate channel (structures are purely symbolic). **Top:** The action of the normal agonist, acetylcholine, in opening the channel. **Bottom: Left,** A nondepolarizing blocker, eg, tubocurarine, is shown as preventing the opening of the channel when it binds to the receptor. **Right,** a depolarizing blocker, eg, succinylcholine, both occupying the receptor and blocking the channel. Normal closure of the channel gate is prevented. Depolarizing blockers may "desensitize" the endplate by occupying the receptor and causing persistent depolarization. An additional effect of drugs on the endplate channel may occur through changes in the lipid environment surrounding the channel (not shown). General anesthetics and alcohols may impair neuromuscular transmission by this mechanism.

Agonist

Closed normal

Open normal

Nondepolarizing blocker

Depolarizing blocker

Closed blocked

Open blocked

The characteristics of a nondepolarizing neuromuscular blockade are summarized in Table 26–2 and Figure 26–6.

B. Depolarizing Drugs:

1. Phase I block (depolarizing)–Succinylcholine is the only depolarizing neuromuscular blocking drug used clinically in the USA. Its neuromuscular effects are almost identical to those of acetylcholine, except that succinylcholine produces a longer effect. Succinylcholine reacts with the nicotinic receptor to open the channel and cause depolarization of the endplate, and this in turn spreads to and depolarizes adjacent membranes, causing generalized disorganized contraction of muscle motor units. Results from single-channel recordings indicate that depolarizing blockers can enter the channel to produce a prolonged "flickering" of the ion conductance (Figure 26–7). Because succinylcholine is not metabolized effectively at the synapse, the depolarized membranes remain depolarized and unresponsive to additional impulses. Furthermore, because excitation-concentration coupling requires endplate repolarization ("repriming") and repetitive firing to maintain muscle tension, a flaccid paralysis results. Phase I block is augmented, not reversed, by cholinesterase inhibitors. The characteristics of a depolarizing neuromuscular blockade are summarized in Table 26–2 and Figure 26–6.

2. Phase II block (desensitizing)–With continued exposure to succinylcholine, the initial endplate depolarization decreases and the membrane becomes repolarized. Despite this repolarization, the membrane cannot be depolarized again by acetylcholine as long as succinylcholine is present. The mechanism for the development of a phase II block is still unclear, but recent evidence (Marshall, 1990) indicates that channel block may become more important than agonist action in this phase of succinylcholine's action. Another hypothesis is that an inexcitable area develops in the muscle membrane immediately surrounding the endplate. This inexcitable area presumably impedes centrifugal spread of impulses initiated by the action of acetylcholine on the receptor. Because the endplate is partially repolarized and still does not respond to acetylcholine, the membrane is said to be desensitized to the effects of acetylcholine. Therefore, this block has also been called a "desensitization block." Whatever the mechanism, the channels behave as if they are in a prolonged closed state (Figure 26–5).

Later in phase II, the characteristics of the blockade become nearly identical to those of a nondepolarizing block, ie, a nonsustained response to a tetanic stimulus (Figure 26–6) and reversal by acetylcholinesterase inhibitors.

II. CLINICAL PHARMACOLOGY OF NEUROMUSCULAR BLOCKING DRUGS

Skeletal Muscle Paralysis

Before the introduction of neuromuscular blocking drugs, adequate skeletal muscle relaxation could only be achieved by deep anesthesia that was often associated with hazardous depressant effects on various organ systems, especially the cardiorespiratory system. The neuromuscular blocking drugs have made it possible to achieve adequate muscle relaxation for all surgical requirements without the depressant effects of deep anesthesia.

Monitoring of the effect of muscle relaxants during surgery may be carried out by means of transdermal stimulation of one of the nerves to the hand and recording of the evoked twitches (Figure 26–6). The "train of four" pattern of stimulation is the one most commonly used.

A. Nondepolarizing Drugs: During anesthesia, the intravenous administration of tubocurarine, 0.12–0.4 mg/kg, will first cause motor weakness; ultimately, skeletal muscles become totally flaccid and inexcitable to stimulation (Figure 26–8). Muscles capable of rapid movement, such as those of the jaw and

Table 26–2. Comparison of a typical nondepolarizing muscle relaxant (tubocurarine) and a depolarizing muscle relaxant (succinylcholine).

	Tubocurarine	Succinylcholine	
		Phase I	Phase II
Administration of tubocurarine	Additive	Antagonistic	Augmented[1]
Administration of succinylcholine	Antagonistic	Additive	Augmented[1]
Effect of neostigmine	Antagonistic	Augmented[1]	Antagonistic
Initial excitatory effect on skeletal muscle	None	Fasciculations	None
Response to a tetanic stimulus	Unsustained	Sustained[2]	Unsustained
Posttetanic facilitation	Yes	No	Yes
Rate of recovery	30–60 min[3]	4–8 min	>20 min[3]

[1]It is not known whether this interaction is additive or synergistic (superadditive).
[2]The amplitude is decreased, but the response is sustained.

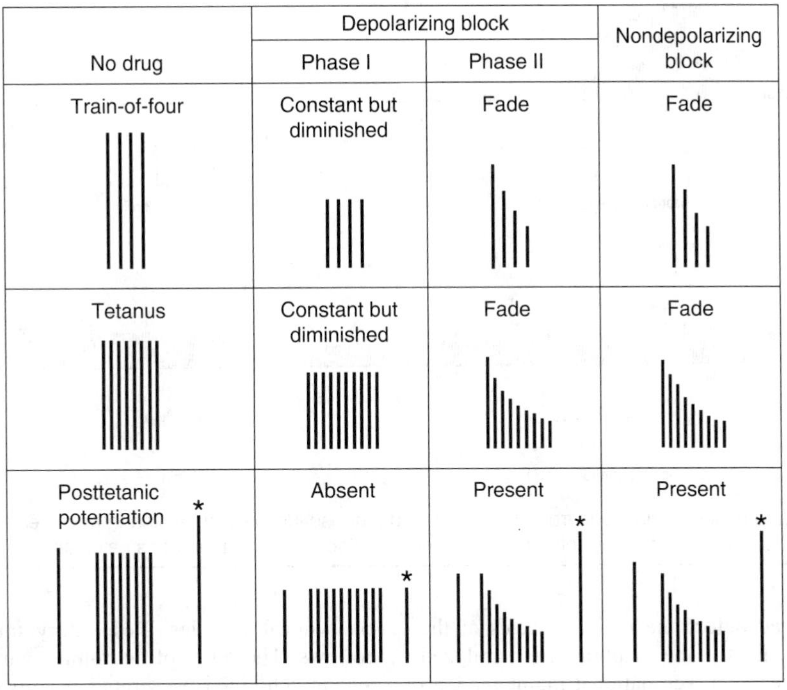

No drug	Depolarizing block		Nondepolarizing block
	Phase I	Phase II	
Train-of-four	Constant but diminished	Fade	Fade
Tetanus	Constant but diminished	Fade	Fade
Posttetanic potentiation *	Absent	Present *	Present *

Figure 26–6. Muscle responses to different patterns of nerve stimulation used in monitoring skeletal muscle relaxation. The alterations produced by depolarizing and desensitizing blockade by succinylcholine and by a nondepolarizing blocker are shown. (*, posttetanic contraction.) (Modified and reproduced, with permission, from Morgan GE, Mikhail MS: *Clinical Anesthesiology.* Appleton & Lange, 1992.

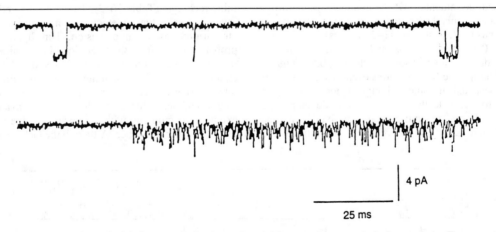

4 pA

25 ms

Figure 26–7. Action of succinylcholine on single-channel endplate receptor currents in frog muscle. The upper trace was recorded in the presence of a low concentration of succinylcholine; the downward deflections represent two openings of the channel and passage of inward (depolarizing) current. The lower trace was recorded in the presence of a much higher concentration of succinylcholine and shows prolonged "flickering" of the channel as it repetitively opens and closes or is "plugged" by the drug. (Reproduced, with permission, from Marshall CG, Ogden DC, Colquhoun D: The actions of suxamethonium (succinyldicholine) as an agonist and channel blocker at the nicotinic receptor of frog muscle. J Physiol [Lond] 1990;428:155.)

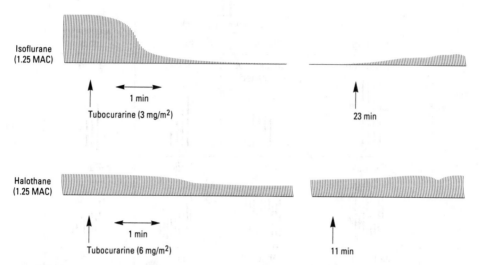

Figure 26–8. Neuromuscular blockade from tubocurarine during isoflurane and halothane anesthesia in patients. Note that at equivalent levels of anesthesia, isoflurane augments the block far more than does halothane.

eye, are paralyzed before the larger muscles of the limbs and trunk. Lastly, the diaphragm is paralyzed and respiration ceases. If ventilation is maintained, no adverse effects occur. When the drug is withdrawn, recovery of muscles usually occurs in reverse order, with the diaphragm regaining function first. The effects of the above dose of tubocurarine usually last 30–60 minutes by gross evaluation; more subtle evidence of paralysis may last for another hour. Potency and duration of action of the other nondepolarizing drugs are shown in Table 26–1. Other than the duration of action, the most important property distinguishing the nondepolarizing relaxants is the time to onset of effect, which determines how soon the patient can be intubated. Of the nondepolarizing drugs currently available or under investigation, rocuronium has the fastest onset (1–2 minutes).

B. Depolarizing Drugs: Following the intravenous administration of succinylcholine, 0.5–1 mg/kg, transient muscle fasciculations occur, especially over the chest and abdomen, though general anesthesia tends to attenuate them. As paralysis develops, the arm, neck, and leg muscles are involved at a time when there is only slight weakness of the facial and pharyngeal muscles. Respiratory muscle weakness follows. The onset of neuromuscular blockade from succinylcholine is very rapid, usually within 1 minute (Figure 26–9). Because of its rapid hydrolysis by cholinesterase in the plasma and liver, the duration of neuromuscular block from this dose usually is 5–10 minutes (Table 26–1).

Cardiovascular Effects

Vecuronium, pipecuronium, doxacurium, and rocuronium have little or no cardiovascular effect. All of the other currently used nondepolarizing muscle relaxants produce some cardiovascular effects. Many of these effects are mediated by autonomic and histamine receptors (Table 26–3). Tubocurarine and, to a much lesser extent, metocurine, mivacurium, and atracurium produce hypotension. This hypotension probably results from the liberation of histamine and, in larger doses, from ganglionic blockade. Premedication with an antihistamine drug will attenuate tubocurarine-induced hypotension. Pancuronium causes a moderate increase in heart rate and to a lesser extent cardiac output, with little or no change in systemic vascular resistance. Although the tachycardia is

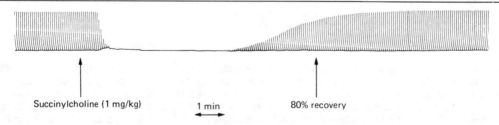

Figure 26–9. Neuromuscular blockade from succinylcholine during anesthesia in patients. Fasciculations are not seen, because the anesthetic obliterated them.

Table 26–3. Effects of neuromuscular blocking drugs on other tissues.

Drug	Effect on Autonomic Ganglia	Effect on Cardiac Muscarinic Receptors	Tendency to Cause Histamine Release
Isoquinoline derivatives			
Atracurium	None	None	Slight
Doxacurium	None	None	None
Metocurine	Weak block	None	Slight
Mivacurium	None	None	Slight
Tubocurarine	Weak block	None	Moderate
Steroid derivatives			
Pancuronium	None	Moderate block	None
Pipecuronium	None	None	None
Rocuronium	None	None	None
Vecuronium	None	None	None
Other agents			
Gallamine	None	Strong block	None
Succinylcholine	Stimulation	Stimulation	Slight

primarily due to a vagolytic action, release of norepinephrine from adrenergic nerve endings and blockade of neuronal uptake of norepinephrine have been suggested as secondary mechanisms. Gallamine increases heart rate by both vagolytic (antimuscarinic) action and sympathetic stimulation. The latter involves the release of norepinephrine from adrenergic nerve endings in the heart by an unknown mechanism.

Succinylcholine causes various cardiac arrhythmias. The drug stimulates all autonomic cholinoceptors: nicotinic receptors in both sympathetic and parasympathetic ganglia and muscarinic receptors in the sinus node of the heart. In low doses, negative inotropic and chronotropic responses occur that can be attenuated by administration of atropine. With large doses, positive inotropic and chronotropic effects may result. Bradycardia has been repeatedly observed when a second dose of the drug is given approximately 5 minutes after the first dose. This bradycardia can be prevented by thiopental, atropine, ganglionic blocking drugs, and nondepolarizing muscle relaxants. Direct myocardial effects, increased muscarinic stimulation, and ganglionic stimulation may all be involved in the bradycardia response.

Other Effects

These effects are seen exclusively with depolarizing blockade.

A. Hyperkalemia: Some patients respond to succinylcholine by an exaggerated release of potassium into the blood, occasionally of such magnitude that cardiac arrest occurs. Patients with burns, nerve damage or neuromuscular disease, closed head injury and other trauma, peritoneal infections, and renal failure are especially susceptible. The mechanism of the hyperkalemic response has not been established, but it

may be related to the increased number of nicotinic receptors that occur extrajunctionally in a denervated muscle or one that is not used. These extrajunctional receptors tend to be more sensitive to succinylcholine and therefore more prone to release potassium than junctional receptors.

B. Intraocular Pressure: Administration of succinylcholine is followed by an increase in intraocular pressure that is manifested 1 minute after injection, maximal at 2–4 minutes, and subsides after 5 minutes. The mechanism for this effect has not been clearly defined, but it may involve contraction of tonic myofibrils or transient dilation of choroidal blood vessels. Despite the increase in pressure, the use of succinylcholine for eye operations is not contraindicated unless the anterior chamber is to be opened.

C. Intragastric Pressure: In some patients, especially muscular ones, the fasciculations associated with succinylcholine will cause an increase in intragastric pressure ranging from 5 to 40 cm of water. This may make emesis more likely, with the potential hazard of aspiration of gastric contents.

D. Muscle Pain: This is an important postoperative complaint of patients who have received succinylcholine. Because of subjective factors and differences in study design, the true incidence of this symptom is difficult to establish, but it has been reported in 0.2–20% of patients in different studies. It occurs more frequently in ambulatory than in bedridden patients. The pain is thought to be secondary to damage produced in muscle by the unsynchronized contractions of adjacent muscle fibers just before the onset of paralysis. Muscle damage has been verified by the occurrence of myoglobinuria following the use of succinylcholine.

Interactions With Other Drugs

A. Anesthetics: Inhaled anesthetics augment the neuromuscular blockade from nondepolarizing muscle relaxants in dose-dependent fashion. Of the drugs that have been studied, inhaled anesthetics augment the effects of muscle relaxants in the following order: Isoflurane (Figure 26–8), desflurane, and enflurane augment more than halothane, which in turn augments more than nitrous oxide-barbiturate-benzodiazepine-opioid anesthesia. The most important factors involved in this interaction are the following: (1) Depression at sites proximal to the neuromuscular junction, ie, the central nervous system. (2) Increased muscle blood flow, which allows a larger fraction of the injected muscle relaxant to reach the neuromuscular junction. This is probably a factor only with isoflurane. (3) Decreased sensitivity of the postjunctional membrane to depolarization.

B. Antibiotics: Over 140 reports of enhancement of neuromuscular blockade by antibiotics, especially aminoglycosides, have appeared in the literature. Many of the antibiotics have been shown to cause a depression of evoked release of acetylcholine similar to that caused by magnesium. The same antibiotics also have postjunctional activity.

C. Local Anesthetics and Antiarrhythmic Drugs: In large doses, most local anesthetics block neuromuscular transmission; in smaller doses, they enhance the neuromuscular block from both nondepolarizing and depolarizing muscle relaxants.

In low doses, local anesthetics depress posttetanic potentiation, and this is thought to be a neural prejunctional effect. With higher doses, local anesthetics block acetylcholine-induced muscle contractions. This stabilizing effect is the result of blockade of the nicotinic receptor ion channels.

Experimentally, similar effects can be demonstrated with antiarrhythmic drugs such as quinidine. However, this interaction is of little or no clinical significance.

D. Other Neuromuscular Blocking Drugs: Depolarizing muscle relaxants are antagonized by nondepolarizing blockers. To prevent the fasciculations associated with succinylcholine administration, a small, nonparalyzing dose of tubocurarine is often given before succinylcholine. While this dose usually reduces fasciculations and postoperative pain, it also increases the amount of succinylcholine required for relaxation by 50–90%.

Effects of Disease & Aging on Drug Response

Several diseases can diminish or augment the neuromuscular blockade produced by nondepolarizing muscle relaxants. Myasthenia gravis markedly augments the neuromuscular blockade from these drugs. Advanced age is often associated with a prolonged duration of action from nondepolarizing relaxants, probably owing to decreased clearance of drugs by the liver and kidneys. As a result, the dose of neuromuscular blocking drugs should probably be reduced in elderly patients.

Conversely, patients with severe burns and those with upper motor neuron disease are resistant to nondepolarizing muscle relaxants. This is probably because of proliferation of extrajunctional receptors, which requires additional nondepolarizing relaxant to block a sufficient number of receptors to produce neuromuscular blockade.

Reversal of Nondepolarizing Neuromuscular Blockade

The cholinesterase inhibitors effectively antagonize the neuromuscular blockade caused by nondepolarizing drugs. Their general pharmacology is discussed in Chapter 7. Neostigmine and pyridostigmine antagonize nondepolarizing neuromuscular blockade by increasing the availability of acetylcholine at the muscle endplate, mainly by inhibition of acetylcholinesterase. To a lesser extent, these agents also increase release of transmitter from the motor nerve terminal. In contrast, edrophonium antagonizes neuromuscular blockade purely by inhibiting acetylcholinesterase.

Neostigmine also decreases the activity of plasma cholinesterase. Because mivacurium is metabolized by plasma cholinesterase, the interaction between these drugs is unpredictable. On one hand, the neuromuscular blockade is antagonized because of increased acetylcholine concentrations in the synapse. On the other hand, mivacurium concentration may be higher because of decreased plasma cholinesterase concentration. The former effect usually dominates clinically.

Other Uses of Neuromuscular Blocking Drugs

A. Control of Ventilation: In patients who have ventilatory failure from various causes, such as obstructive airway disease, it is often desirable to control ventilation to provide adequate volumes and expansion of lungs. Paralysis is sometimes induced by administration of neuromuscular blocking drugs to eliminate chest wall resistance and ineffective spontaneous ventilation.

B. Treatment of Convulsions: Neuromuscular blocking drugs are sometimes used to attenuate or eliminate the peripheral manifestations of convulsions from such causes as epilepsy or local anesthetic toxicity. Although this approach is effective in eliminating the muscular manifestations of the seizures, it has no effect on the central processes involved, since neuromuscular blocking drugs do not cross the blood-brain barrier in significant amounts when used in clinical doses.

SPASMOLYTIC DRUGS

Bertram G. Katzung, MD, PhD

Spasticity is characterized by an increase in tonic stretch reflexes and flexor muscle spasms together with muscle weakness. It is often associated with cerebral palsy, multiple sclerosis, and stroke. These conditions often involve abnormal function of the bowel and bladder as well as of skeletal muscle. In this section, only skeletal muscle spasticity is considered. The mechanisms underlying clinical spasticity appear to involve not the stretch reflex arc itself but higher centers ("upper motor neuron lesion"), with damage to descending pathways that results in hyperexcitability of alpha motoneurons in the cord. Nevertheless, drug therapy may ameliorate some of the symptoms of spasticity by modifying the stretch reflex arc or by interfering directly with skeletal muscle excitation-contraction coupling. The components involved in these processes are shown in Figure 26–10.

Drugs modifying this reflex arc may modulate excitatory or inhibitory synapses (Chapter 20). Thus, to reduce the hyperactive stretch reflex, it is desirable to reduce the activity of the Ia fibers that excite the primary motoneuron or to enhance the activity of the inhibitory internuncial neurons. These structures are shown in greater detail in Figure 26–11.

A variety of compounds used in the past can be loosely described as depressants of spinal "polysynaptic" reflex arcs (barbiturates: phenobarbital; glycerol ethers: mephenesin). A number of similar com-

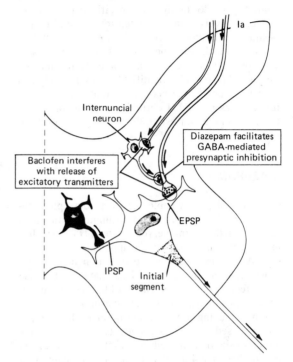

Figure 26–11. Postulated sites of spasmolytic action of diazepam and baclofen in the spinal cord. (Reproduced, with permission, from Young RR, Delwaide PJ: Drug therapy: Spasticity. N Engl J Med 1981;304:28.)

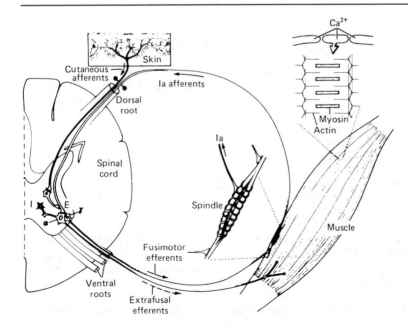

Figure 26–10. Diagram of the structures involved in the stretch reflex arc. *I* is an inhibitory interneuron; *E* indicates an excitatory presynaptic terminal; *Ia* is a primary intrafusal afferent fiber, Ca^{2+} denotes activator calcium stored in the sarcoplasmic reticulum of skeletal muscle. (Reproduced, with permission, from Young RR, Delwaide PJ: Drug therapy: Spasticity. N Engl J Med 1981;304:28.)

pounds are still promoted (see Drugs Used For Acute Local Muscle Spasm, below). However, it is clear from Figure 26–11 that nonspecific depression of synapses involved in the stretch reflex could reduce desirable inhibitory activity as well as excitatory transmission. During the past 2 decades, more specific therapy has become available. Unfortunately, the lack of a precisely quantifiable measure of clinical response—or, alternatively, an accurate experimental model—has prevented definitive comparison of the agents promoted for use in this heterogeneous group of conditions.

DIAZEPAM

As described in Chapter 21, benzodiazepines facilitate the action of gamma-aminobutyric acid (GABA) in the central nervous system. Diazepam has useful antispastic activity. It apparently acts at all GABA synapses, but its site of action in reducing spasticity is at least partly in the spinal cord, because it is effective in patients with cord transection. It can be used in patients with muscle spasm of almost any origin, including local muscle trauma. However, it produces sedation in most patients at the doses required to significantly reduce muscle tone. Dosage is usually begun at 4 mg/d and gradually increased to a maximum of 60 mg/d.

BACLOFEN

Baclofen (*p*-chlorophenyl GABA) was designed to be an orally active GABA-mimetic agent. The structure is shown below.

$$Cl \text{—} \langle \text{phenyl} \rangle \text{—} CH \text{—} CH_2 \text{—} NH_2$$
$$| \\ CH_2 \text{—} COOH$$

Baclofen

Baclofen is an active spasmolytic and acts as a GABA agonist at $GABA_B$ receptors. Activation of receptors in the brain by baclofen results in hyperpolarization, probably by increased K^+ conductance. It has been suggested that this hyperpolarization (in the cord as well as the brain) serves a presynaptic inhibitory function (Figure 26–11), probably by reducing calcium influx, to reduce the release of excitatory transmitters in both the brain and the spinal cord. Baclofen may also reduce pain in patients with spasticity, perhaps by inhibiting the release of substance P in the spinal cord.

Baclofen is at least as effective as diazepam in reducing spasticity and causes much less sedation. In addition, it does not reduce general muscle strength, as does dantrolene. It is rapidly and completely absorbed after oral administration and has a plasma half-life of 3–4 hours. Dosage is started at 15 mg twice daily, increasing, if tolerated, to as much as 100 mg daily. Toxicity of this drug includes drowsiness, to which the patient may become tolerant. Increased seizure activity has been reported in epileptic patients.

Short-term double-blind and long-term nonblind studies, using implanted programmable infusion pumps, have shown that *intrathecal* administration of baclofen may control severe spasticity and pain that is not responsive to medication by oral or other parenteral routes. Because of poor egress of baclofen from the spinal cord, peripheral symptoms are few, and higher central concentrations of the drug may be tolerated. Although dramatic beneficial responses have been reported, several cases of somnolence, respiratory depression, and even coma have also been recorded. Physostigmine, though claimed to be effective as an antidote for these depressant effects, is probably more dangerous and no more effective than conservative management.

OTHER DRUGS THAT ACT IN THE SPINAL CORD

Progabide and **glycine** have been found in preliminary studies to reduce spasticity in some patients. Progabide is a $GABA_A$ and $GABA_B$ agonist and has active metabolites, including GABA itself. Glycine is another inhibitory amino acid neurotransmitter (Chapter 20). It appears to be active when given orally and readily passes the blood-brain barrier. These drugs are investigational. Idrocilamide and tizanidine are newer agents under investigation.

DANTROLENE

Dantrolene is a hydantoin derivative (like phenytoin) but with a unique mechanism of spasmolytic action outside the central nervous system. Its structure is shown below.

$$HN \text{—} \text{ring} \text{—} N \text{—} N \text{=} CH \text{—} \text{(furan)} \text{—} \langle \text{phenyl} \rangle \text{—} NO_2$$

Dantrolene

Dantrolene reduces skeletal muscle strength by interfering with excitation-contraction coupling in the muscle fiber. The normal contractile response involves release of activator calcium from its stores in the sarcoplasmic reticulum of the sarcomere. This calcium brings about the tension-generating interaction of actin with myosin. Dantrolene interferes with the release of activator calcium from the sarcoplasmic reticulum. Thus, the action of this drug involves neither central synapses nor the neuromuscular junction; it is intracellular at the effector organ. Motor units that contract rapidly are more sensitive to the drug than are slow units. Cardiac muscle and smooth muscle are depressed only slightly, perhaps because the release of calcium from their sarcoplasmic reticulum involves a somewhat different process.

Only about one-third of an oral dose of dantrolene is absorbed; the half-life of the drug is about 8 hours. Treatment is usually begun with 25 mg daily as a single dose, increasing to a maximum of 100 mg 4 times daily if necessary and tolerated. Major adverse effects are generalized muscle weakness, sedation, and occasionally hepatitis.

A special application of dantrolene is in the treatment of **malignant hyperthermia,** a rare disorder that can be triggered by a variety of stimuli, including general anesthesia and neuromuscular blocking drugs. Patients with this condition have a hereditary impairment of the ability of the sarcoplasmic reticulum to sequester calcium. A trigger event results in sudden and prolonged release of calcium, with massive muscle contraction, lactic acid production, and increased body temperature. Prompt treatment is essential to control acidosis and body temperature and to reduce calcium release. The latter is accomplished with intravenous dantrolene, starting with 1 mg/kg and repeating as necessary to a maximum of 10 mg/kg.

DRUGS USED FOR ACUTE LOCAL MUSCLE SPASM

A large number of drugs are promoted for the relief of acute temporary muscle spasm caused by local trauma or strain. Most act as sedatives or at the level of the spinal cord or brain stem. Cyclobenzaprine may be regarded as a prototype of the latter group. Cyclobenzaprine is structurally related to the tricyclic antidepressants and has some properties in common with them, eg, antimuscarinic effects. It is believed to act at the level of the brain stem. Cyclobenzaprine is ineffective in muscle spasm due to cerebral palsy or spinal cord injury. The drug has strong antimuscarinic actions in most patients and causes significant sedation, confusion, and transient visual hallucinations in some. Dosage for acute spasm due to injury is 20–40 mg/d in three divided doses.

PREPARATIONS AVAILABLE

Neuromuscular Blocking Drugs
Atracurium (Tracrium)
  Parenteral: 10 mg/mL for injection
Doxacurium (Nuromax)
  Parenteral: 1 mg/mL for IV injection
Gallamine (Flaxedil)
  Parenteral: 20 mg/mL for injection
Metocurine (Metubine Iodide, generic)
  Parenteral: 2 mg/mL for injection
Mivacurium (Mivacron)
  Parenteral: 0.5, 2 mg/mL for injection
Pancuronium (Pavulon)
  Parenteral: 1, 2 mg/mL for injection
Pipecuronium (Arduan)
  Parenteral: 1 mg/mL for IV injection
Rocuronium (Zemuron)
  Parenteral: 10 mg/mL for IV injection
Succinylcholine (Anectine, others)
  Parenteral: 20, 50, 100 mg/mL for injection; 100, 500 mg per vial powders to reconstitute for injection

Tubocurarine (generic)
  Parenteral: 3 mg (20 units)/mL for injection
Vecuronium (Norcuron)
  Parenteral: 10 mg/mL powder to reconstitute for injection

Muscle Relaxants (Spasmolytics)
Baclofen (Lioresal, generic)
  Oral: 10, 20 mg tablets
  Intrathecal: 10 mg/20 mL, 10 mg/5 mL ampules
Cyclobenzaprine (Flexeril, generic)
  Oral: 10 mg tablets
Dantrolene (Dantrium)
  Oral: 25, 50, 100 mg capsules
  Parenteral: 20 mg per vial powder to reconstitute for injection
Diazepam (generic, Valium, others)
  Oral: 2, 5, 10 mg tablets; 15 mg sustained-release capsules; 5 mg/5 mL, 5 mg/mL solutions
  Parenteral: 5 mg/mL for injection

REFERENCES

Neuromuscular Blockers

Adams PR: Acetylcholine receptor kinetics. J Membr Biol 1981;58:161.

Adt M, Baumert J-H, Reimann H-J: The role of histamine in the cardiovascular effects of atracurium. Br J Anaesth 1992;68:155.

Agoston S et al: Clinical pharmacokinetics of neuromuscular blocking drugs. Clin Pharmacokinet 1992;22:94.

Bartkowski RR et al: Rocuronium onset of action: A comparison with atracurium and vecuronium. Anesth Analg 1993;77:574.

Bevan DR et al: Reversal of neuromuscular blockade. Anesthesiology 1992;77:785.

Canfell PC et al: The metabolic disposition of laudanosine in dog, rabbit, and man. Drug Metab Dispos Biol Fate Chem 1986;14:703.

Eldefrawi AT, Miller ER, Eldefrawi ME: Binding of depolarizing drugs to ionic channel sites of the nicotinic acetylcholine receptor. Biochem Pharmacol 1982; 31:1819.

Gibb AJ, Marshall IG: Pre- and postjunctional effects of tubocurarine and other nicotinic antagonists during repetitive stimulation in the rat. J Physiol 1984;351:275.

Hansen-Flaschen JH et al: Use of sedating drugs and neuromuscular blocking agents in patients requiring mechanical ventilation for respiratory failure: A national survey. JAMA 1991;266:2870.

Lambert JJ, Durant NN, Henderson EG: Drug-induced modification of ionic conductance at the neuromuscular junction. Annu Rev Pharmacol Toxicol 1983; 23:505.

Marshall CG, Ogden DC, Colquhoun D: The actions of suxamethonium (succinyldicholine) as an agonist and channel blocker at the nicotinic receptor of frog muscle. J Physiol (Lond) 1990;428:155.

Miller RD, Agoston S, Booij LDHJ: The comparative potency and pharmacokinetics of pancuronium and its metabolites in anesthetized man. J Pharmacol Exp Ther 1978;207:539.

Miller RD, Savarese JJ: Pharmacology of muscle relaxants and their antagonists. In: Anesthesia, 4th ed. Miller RD (editor). Churchill Livingstone, 1994.

Miller RD et al: Clinical pharmacology of vecuronium and atracurium. Anesthesiology 1984;61:444.

Nigrovic V, Fox JL: Atracurium decay and the formation of laudanosine in humans. Anesthesiology 1991; 74:446.

Owen RT: Resistance to competitive neuromuscular blocking agents in burn patients: A review. Methods Find Exp Clin Pharmacol 1985;7:203.

Phillips BJ, Hunter JM: Use of mivacurium chloride by constant infusion in the anephric patient. Br J Anaesth 1992;68:494.

Scuka M, Mozrzymas JW: Postsynaptic potentiation and desensitization at the vertebrate end-plate receptors. Prog Neurobiol 1992;38:19.

Segredo V et al: Persistent paralysis in critically ill patients after long-term administration of vecuronium. N Engl J Med 1992;327:524.

Sine SM, Taylor P: Relationship between reversible antagonist occupancy and the functional capacity of the acetylcholine receptor. J Biol Chem 1981;256:6692.

Stroud RM: Acetylcholine receptor structure. Neurosci Comment 1983;1:124.

Szenshradsky J et al: Pharmacokinetics of rocuronium bromide (ORG 9426) in patients with normal renal function or patients undergoing cadaver renal transplantation. Anesthesiology 1992;77:899.

Spasmolytics

Albright AL, Cervi A, Singletary J: Intrathecal baclofen for spasticity in cerebral palsy. JAMA 1991;265: 1418.

Davidoff RA: Antispasticity drugs: Mechanisms of action. Ann Neurol 1985;17:107.

Dolphin AC, Scott RH: Activation of calcium channel currents in rat sensory neurons by large depolarizations: Effect of guanine nucleotides and (−)-baclofen. Eur J Neurosci 1990;2:104.

Giesser B: Multiple sclerosis: Current concepts in management. Drugs 1985;29:88.

Lazorthes Y et al: Chronic intrathecal baclofen administration for control of severe spasticity. J Neurosurg 1990;72:393.

Lopez JR et al: Effects of dantrolene on myoplasmic free $[Ca^{2+}]$ measured in vivo in patients susceptible to malignant hyperthermia. Anesthesiology 1992;76:711.

Newberry NR, Nicoll RA: Direct hyperpolarizing action of baclofen on hippocampal pyramidal cells. Nature 1984;308:450.

Ochs G et al: Intrathecal baclofen for long-term treatment of spasticity: A multi-centre study. J Neurol Neurosurg Psychiat 1989;52:933.

Penn RD et al: Intrathecal baclofen for severe spinal spasticity. N Engl J Med 1989;320:1517.

Pinder RM et al: Dantrolene sodium: A review of its pharmacological properties and therapeutic efficacy in spasticity. Drugs 1977;3:3.

Young RR, Delwaide PJ: Drug therapy: Spasticity. (Two parts.) N Engl J Med 1981;304:28, 96.

Young RR, Wiegner AW: Spasticity. Clin Orthop 1987; 219:50.

Pharmacologic Management of Parkinsonism & Other Movement Disorders

27

Michael J. Aminoff, MD, FRCP

Several different types of abnormal movement are recognized. **Tremor** consists of a rhythmic oscillatory movement around a joint and is best characterized by its relation to activity. Tremor present at rest is characteristic of parkinsonism, when it is often associated with rigidity and an impairment of voluntary activity. Tremor may occur during maintenance of sustained posture (postural tremor) or during movement (intention tremor). A conspicuous postural tremor is the cardinal feature of benign essential or familial tremor. Intention tremor occurs in patients with a lesion of the brain stem or cerebellum, especially when the superior cerebellar peduncle is involved, and may also occur as a manifestation of toxicity from alcohol or certain other drugs.

Chorea consists of irregular, unpredictable, involuntary muscle jerks that occur in different parts of the body and impair voluntary activity. In some instances, the proximal muscles of the limbs are most severely affected, and because the abnormal movements are then particularly violent, the term ballismus has been used to describe them. Chorea may be hereditary or may occur as a complication of a number of general medical disorders and of therapy with certain drugs.

Abnormal movements may be slow and writhing in character (**athetosis**) and in some instances are so sustained that they are more properly regarded as abnormal postures (**dystonia**). Athetosis or dystonia may occur with perinatal brain damage, with focal or generalized cerebral lesions, as an acute complication of certain drugs, as an accompaniment of diverse neurologic disorders, or as an isolated phenomenon of uncertain cause known as idiopathic torsion dystonia or dystonia musculorum deformans. Its pharmacologic basis is uncertain, and treatment is unsatisfactory.

Tics are sudden coordinated abnormal movements that tend to occur repetitively, particularly about the face and head, especially in children, and can be suppressed voluntarily for short periods of time. Common tics include, for example, repetitive sniffing or shoulder shrugging. Tics may be single or multiple and transient or chronic. Gilles de la Tourette's syndrome is characterized by chronic multiple tics; its pharmacologic management is discussed at the end of this chapter.

Many of the movement disorders have been attributed to disturbances of the basal ganglia, but the precise function of these anatomic structures is not yet fully understood, and it is not possible to relate individual symptoms to involvement at specific sites.

PARKINSONISM
(Paralysis Agitans)

Parkinsonism is characterized by a combination of rigidity, bradykinesia, tremor, and postural instability that can occur for a wide variety of reasons but is usually idiopathic. The pathophysiologic basis of the idiopathic disorder may relate to exposure to some unrecognized neurotoxin or to the occurrence of oxidation reactions with the generation of free radicals. Parkinson's disease is generally progressive, leading to increasing disability unless effective treatment is provided. The normally high concentration of dopamine in the basal ganglia of the brain is reduced in parkinsonism, and pharmacologic attempts to restore dopaminergic activity with levodopa and dopamine agonists have been successful in alleviating many of the clinical features of the disorder. An alternative but complementary approach has been to restore the normal balance of cholinergic and dopaminergic influences on the basal ganglia with antimuscarinic drugs. The pathophysiologic basis for these therapies is that in idiopathic parkinsonism, dopaminergic neurons in the substantia nigra that normally inhibit the output of GABAergic cells in the corpus striatum are lost (Figure 27–1). (In contrast, Huntington's chorea involves the loss of some cholinergic neurons and an even greater loss of the

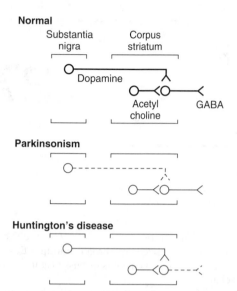

Normal

Substantia nigra | Corpus striatum

Dopamine

Acetyl choline | GABA

Parkinsonism

Huntington's disease

Figure 27–1. Schematic representation of the sequence of neurons involved in parkinsonism and Huntington's chorea. *Top:* Dopaminergic neurons originating in the substantia nigra normally inhibit the GABAergic output from the striatum, whereas cholinergic neurons exert an excitatory effect. ***Middle:*** In parkinsonism, there is a selective loss of dopaminergic neurons. ***Bottom:*** In Huntington's chorea, some cholinergic neurons may be lost, but even more GABAergic neurons degenerate.

GABAergic cells that exit the corpus striatum.) Drugs that *induce* parkinsonian syndromes either are dopamine receptor antagonists (eg, antipsychotic agents, Chapter 28) or lead to the destruction of the dopaminergic nigrostriatal neurons (eg, MPTP; see page 427).

LEVODOPA

Dopamine does not cross the blood-brain barrier and if given into the peripheral circulation has no therapeutic effect in parkinsonism. However, (−)-3-(3,4-dihydroxyphenyl)-L-alanine (levodopa), the immediate metabolic precursor of dopamine, does penetrate the brain, where it is decarboxylated to dopamine. Several dopamine agonists have also been developed and may lead to clinical benefit, as discussed below.

Dopamine receptors can be classified according to various biochemical and pharmacologic features. They have, for example, been subdivided according to whether they are linked to an adenylyl cyclase. Cyclic adenosine monophosphate (cAMP) is formed with activation of this cyclase and may well be responsible for mediating certain tissue-specific responses to dopamine. Other responses to dopamine apparently do not involve the stimulation of adenylyl

cyclase or accumulation of cAMP. The designation D_1 has been proposed for the receptors that stimulate adenylyl cyclase and D_2 for those that do not (Table 6–2).

Dopamine receptors of the D_1 type are located in the zona compacta of the substantia nigra and presynaptically on striatal axons coming from cortical neurons and from dopaminergic cells in the substantia nigra. The D_2 receptors are located postsynaptically on striatal neurons and presynaptically on axons in the substantia nigra belonging to neurons in the basal ganglia. The benefits of dopaminergic antiparkinsonism drugs appear to depend mostly on stimulation of the D_2 receptors, but D_1-receptor stimulation may also be required for maximal benefit. Dopamine agonist or partial agonist ergot derivatives such as lergotrile and bromocriptine that are powerful stimulators of the D_2 receptors have antiparkinsonism properties, whereas certain dopamine blockers that are selective D_2 antagonists can induce parkinsonism.

Chemistry

As discussed in Chapter 6, dopa is the precursor of dopamine and norepinephrine. Its structure is shown in Figure 27–2. Levodopa is the levorotatory stereoisomer of dopa.

Pharmacokinetics

Levodopa is rapidly absorbed from the small intestine, but its absorption depends on the rate of gastric emptying and the pH of the gastric contents. Food will delay the appearance of levodopa in the plasma. Moreover, certain amino acids from ingested food can compete with the drug for absorption from the gut and for transport from the blood to the brain. Plasma concentrations usually peak between 1 and 2 hours after an oral dose, and the plasma half-life is usually between 1 and 3 hours, though it varies considerably between individuals. About two-thirds of the dose appears in the urine as metabolites within 8 hours of an oral dose, the main metabolic products being 3-methoxy-4-hydroxyphenylacetic acid (homovanillic acid, HVA) and dihydroxyphenylacetic acid (DOPAC). Unfortunately, only about 1–3% of administered levodopa actually enters the brain unaltered, the remainder being metabolized extracerebrally, predominantly by decarboxylation to dopamine, which does not penetrate the blood-brain barrier. This means that levodopa must be given in large amounts when it is used alone. However, when it is given in combination with a dopa decarboxylase inhibitor that does not penetrate the blood-brain barrier, the peripheral metabolism of levodopa is reduced, plasma levels of levodopa are higher, plasma half-life is longer, and more dopa is available for entry into the brain (Figure 27–3). Indeed, concomitant administration of a peripheral dopa decarboxylase inhibitor may reduce the daily requirements of levodopa by approximately 75%.

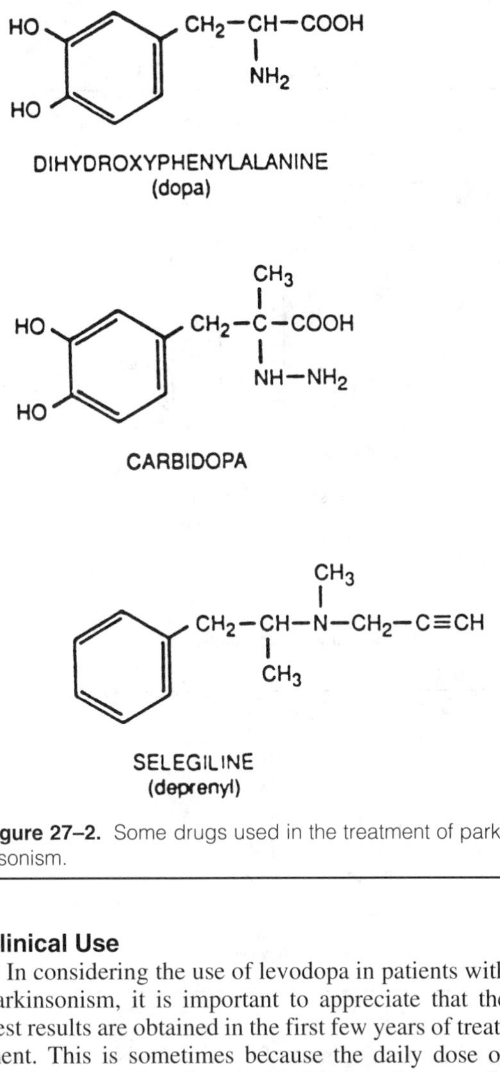

Figure 27–2. Some drugs used in the treatment of parkinsonism.

Clinical Use

In considering the use of levodopa in patients with parkinsonism, it is important to appreciate that the best results are obtained in the first few years of treatment. This is sometimes because the daily dose of levodopa must be reduced with time in order to avoid side effects at doses that were well tolerated at the outset. The reason that adverse effects develop in this way is unclear, but selective denervation or drug-induced supersensitivity may be responsible. Some patients also become less responsive to levodopa, so that previously effective doses eventually fail to produce any therapeutic benefit. It is not clear whether this relates to disease progression or to duration of treatment, although the evidence is increasing that disease progression is primarily responsible for the declining response. Responsiveness to levodopa may ultimately be lost completely, perhaps because of the disappearance of dopaminergic nigrostriatal nerve terminals or some pathologic process directly involving the striatal dopamine receptors. For such reasons, the benefits of levodopa treatment often begin to diminish after about 3 or 4 years of therapy irrespective of the initial therapeutic response. Although levodopa therapy does not stop the progression of parkinsonism, recent evidence suggests that the early initiation of levodopa therapy lowers the mortality rate due to Parkinson's disease. However, long-term therapy may lead to a number of problems in management such as development of the on-off phenomenon discussed below. The most appropriate time to introduce levodopa therapy must therefore be determined individually.

When levodopa is used, it is generally given in combination with carbidopa (Figure 27–2), a peripheral dopa decarboxylase inhibitor, for the reasons set forth above. **Sinemet** is a dopa preparation containing carbidopa and levodopa in fixed proportion (1:10 or 1:4). Treatment is started with a small dose, eg, Sinemet-25/100 (carbidopa 25 mg, levodopa 100 mg) 3 times daily, and gradually increased depending upon the therapeutic response and development of adverse effects. Most patients ultimately require Sinemet-25/250 (carbidopa 25 mg, levodopa 250 mg) 3 or 4 times daily. It may be preferable to keep treatment with this agent at a low level (eg, Sinemet-25/100 3 times daily) and to increase dopaminergic therapy by the addition of a dopamine agonist if necessary, in order to reduce the risk of development of response fluctuations, as discussed below. A controlled-release formulation of Sinemet is now available and may be helpful in patients with established response fluctuations or as a means of reducing dosing frequency.

Levodopa can ameliorate all of the clinical features of parkinsonism, but it is particularly effective in relieving bradykinesia and any disabilities resulting from it. When it is first introduced, about one-third of patients respond very well and one-third less well. Most of the remainder either are unable to tolerate the medication or simply fail to respond at all.

Adverse Effects

A. Gastrointestinal Effects: When levodopa is given without a peripheral decarboxylase inhibitor, anorexia and nausea and vomiting occur in about 80% of patients. These adverse effects can be minimized by taking the drug in divided doses, with or immediately after meals, and by increasing the total daily dose very slowly; antacids taken 30–60 minutes before levodopa may also be beneficial. The vomiting has been attributed to stimulation of an emetic center located in the brain stem but outside the blood-brain barrier to dopamine and to peripheral decarboxylase inhibitors. Fortunately, tolerance to this emetic effect develops in many patients after several months. Antiemetics such as phenothiazines are sometimes given but may reduce the antiparkinsonism effects of levodopa.

When levodopa is given in combination with carbidopa to reduce its extracerebral metabolism, adverse gastrointestinal effects are much less frequent and troublesome, occurring in fewer than 20% of cases, so that patients can tolerate proportionately higher doses.

B. Cardiovascular Effects: A variety of car-

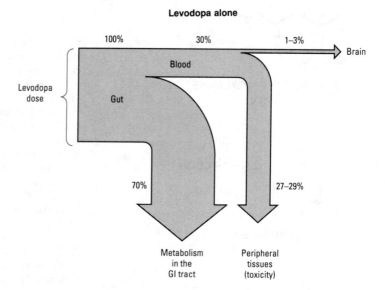

Levodopa alone

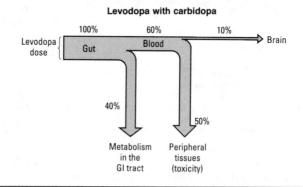

Levodopa with carbidopa

Figure 27–3. Fate of orally adminis-tered levodopa and the effect of carbi-dopa, estimated from animal data. The width of each pathway indicates the ab-solute amount of the drug present at each site, while the percentages shown denote the relative proportion of the administered dose. The benefits of co-administration of carbidopa include re-duction of the amount of levodopa diverted to peripheral tissues and an increase in the fraction of the dose that reaches the brain. (Data from Nutt and Fellman, 1984.)

diac arrhythmias have been described in patients re-ceiving levodopa, including tachycardia, ventricular extrasystoles, and, rarely, atrial fibrillation. This ef-fect has been attributed to increased catecholamine formation peripherally. The incidence of such ar-rhythmias is low, even in the presence of established cardiac disease, and may be reduced still further if the levodopa is taken in combination with a peripheral decarboxylase inhibitor. In parkinsonism patients who also have heart disease, the anticipated benefits of levodopa, especially when combined with carbi-dopa, generally outweigh the slight risk of inducing a cardiac arrhythmia.

Postural hypotension is common and often asymp-tomatic, and tends to diminish with continuing treat-ment. Hypertension may also occur, especially in the presence of nonselective monoamine oxidase inhibi-tors or sympathomimetics or when massive doses of levodopa are being taken.

C. Dyskinesias: Dyskinesias occur in up to 80% of patients receiving levodopa therapy for long peri-ods. The development of dyskinesias is dose-related, but there is considerable individual variation in the dose required to produce them. Dyskinesias seem to occur more commonly in patients receiving levodopa combined with a peripheral decarboxylase inhibitor than in those receiving levodopa alone. Moreover, with continuing treatment, dyskinesias may develop at a dose of levodopa that previously was well toler-ated. They can be alleviated or reversed by lowering the daily dose of levodopa, but usually at the expense of reduced antiparkinsonism benefit; many patients are therefore willing to tolerate even a marked dyski-nesia, because their mobility is so greatly improved by the medication. In some instances dyskinesias are less marked if levodopa is prescribed alone rather than in combination with carbidopa; in other in-stances, a drug holiday (see below) may help control the problem. Pharmacologic attempts to counteract the dyskinesia with drugs used to treat chorea have generally not been successful or require the use of drugs that tend to worsen the parkinsonism.

The form and nature of dopa dyskinesias vary widely in different patients but tend to remain constant in character in individual patients. Chorea, ballismus, athetosis, dystonia, myoclonus, tics, and tremor may occur individually or in any combination in the face, trunk, or limbs. Choreoathetosis of the face and distal extremities is the most common presentation.

D. Behavioral Effects: A wide variety of adverse mental effects have been reported including depression, anxiety, agitation, insomnia, somnolence, confusion, delusions, hallucinations, nightmares, euphoria, and other changes in mood or personality. Such adverse effects are more common in patients taking levodopa in combination with a decarboxylase inhibitor rather than levodopa alone, presumably because higher levels are reached in the brain. They may be precipitated by intercurrent illness or operation. The only treatment is to reduce or withdraw the medication if necessary. A drug holiday (see below) may also lead to improvement of adverse mental effects.

E. Fluctuations in Response: Certain fluctuations in clinical response to levodopa occur with increasing frequency as treatment continues. In some patients, these fluctuations relate to the timing of levodopa intake, and they are then referred to as wearing-off reactions or end-of-dose akinesia. In other instances, fluctuations in clinical state are unrelated to the timing of doses (on-off phenomenon). In the on-off phenomenon, off-periods of marked akinesia alternate over the course of a few hours with on-periods of improved mobility but often marked dyskinesia. The phenomenon is most likely to occur in patients who responded well to treatment initially. The exact mechanism is unknown, but the off-period can sometimes be shown to relate to falling plasma levels of levodopa. Patients may benefit from taking their medication at more frequent intervals in smaller doses during the day or from the addition of dopamine agonists such as bromocriptine (see below) to the drug regimen. Reduction in dietary intake of protein to the minimum recommended daily allowance and adjustment of the daily routine so that the main protein meal is taken in the evening is also helpful. Controlled-release formulations of Sinemet may also be useful. A brief holiday from levodopa under careful medical supervision may occasionally help in restoring its effectiveness, but this practice is generally unwarranted because any benefit is usually temporary.

F. Miscellaneous Adverse Effects: Mydriasis may occur and may precipitate an attack of acute glaucoma in some patients. Other reported but rare adverse effects include various blood dyscrasias; a positive Coombs test with evidence of hemolysis; hot flushes; aggravation or precipitation of gout; abnormalities of smell or taste; brownish discoloration of saliva, urine, or vaginal secretions; priapism; and mild—usually transient—elevations of blood urea nitrogen and of serum transaminases, alkaline phosphatase, and bilirubin.

Drug Holidays

A drug holiday may help in alleviating some of the neurologic and behavioral adverse effects of levodopa but is usually of little help in the management of the on-off phenomenon. Patients must be under close medical supervision. Levodopa medication must be withdrawn gradually, since abrupt cessation of treatment may lead to a severely akinetic state. The optimal duration of a break in treatment with levodopa is unclear but has varied from 3 to 21 days in different studies. Up to about two-thirds of patients show improved responsiveness to levodopa when the drug is reinstituted, and—because they can be managed on lower doses than before—adverse mental effects and dyskinesias are less troublesome. The medication can be either restarted at half the previous dose or built up gradually from an even lower level. Fluctuations in response (on-off phenomenon) are reduced in many instances, but any benefit in this regard is usually short-lived. Unfortunately, there is no way of predicting which patients will respond satisfactorily to the holiday. Furthermore, a drug holiday carries the risks of aspiration pneumonia, venous thrombosis, pulmonary embolism, and depression resulting from the immobility accompanying severe parkinsonism.

Drug Interactions

Pharmacologic doses of pyridoxine (vitamin B_6) enhance the extracerebral metabolism of levodopa and may therefore prevent its therapeutic effect unless a peripheral decarboxylase inhibitor is also taken. Levodopa should not be given to patients taking monoamine oxidase A inhibitors or within 2 weeks of their discontinuance, because such a combination can lead to hypertensive crises.

Contraindications

Levodopa should not be given to psychotic patients, as it may exacerbate the mental disturbance. It is also contraindicated in patients with angle-closure glaucoma, but those with chronic open-angle glaucoma may be given levodopa if intraocular pressure is well controlled and can be monitored. It is best given combined with carbidopa to patients with cardiac disease, but even so there is a slight risk of cardiac dysrhythmia. Patients with active peptic ulcer must also be managed carefully, since gastrointestinal bleeding has occasionally occurred with levodopa. Because levodopa is a precursor of skin melanin and conceivably may activate malignant melanoma, its use should be avoided in patients with a history of melanoma or with suspicious undiagnosed skin lesions.

DOPAMINE AGONISTS

The enzymes responsible for synthesizing dopamine are depleted in the brains of parkinsonism patients, and drugs acting directly on dopamine receptors may therefore have a beneficial effect additional to that of levodopa. Unlike levodopa, they do not require enzymatic conversion to an active metabolite, have no potentially toxic metabolites, and do not compete with other substances for active transport into the blood and across the blood-brain barrier. Moreover, drugs specifically affecting certain (but not all) dopamine receptors may have more limited adverse effects than levodopa. There are a number of dopamine agonists with antiparkinsonism activity. Some, such as apomorphine, piribedil, and lergotrile, have such serious adverse effects that they cannot be used clinically, but others may have a role in treatment of parkinsonism.

BROMOCRIPTINE

Several ergot derivatives are dopamine agonists (Chapter 16) and have been used in the treatment of parkinsonism; unlike other dopamine-like drugs, these drugs appear to be partial agonists at presynaptic dopamine D_2 receptors. Bromocriptine (structure shown in Table 16–5) is the most widely used in the USA. It has also been used to treat certain endocrinologic disorders, especially hyperprolactinemia (see Chapters 16 and 36), but in lower doses than those required to counteract parkinsonism. The drug is absorbed to a variable extent from the gastrointestinal tract, peak plasma levels being reached within 1–2 hours after an oral dose. It is excreted in the bile and feces.

There is some evidence that bromocriptine has a role as a first-line drug in the treatment of parkinsonism and that its use in this disease is associated with a lower incidence of the response fluctuations and dyskinesias commonly seen with long-term levodopa therapy. In consequence, dopaminergic therapy may best be initiated with a low dose of carbidopa plus levodopa (eg, Sinemet 25/100 3 times daily) and then increased by the addition of bromocriptine. Some physicians, however, reserve bromocriptine for parkinsonism patients taking levodopa who have end-of-dose akinesia or on-off phenomena or who are becoming refractory to treatment with levodopa. Partial replacement of levodopa with bromocriptine may then be valuable. Optimal results are obtained by a combination of levodopa and bromocriptine in doses less than the maximum tolerated doses of each. The results of bromocriptine treatment are generally disappointing in patients totally unresponsive to levodopa, and addition of bromocriptine to patients receiving optimal levodopa therapy may cause intolerable adverse effects. Bromocriptine does not complicate treatment with antimuscarinic drugs or amantadine, and these drugs can be continued without change in dosage in patients who are to be given bromocriptine as well.

Clinical Use

The usual daily dose of bromocriptine in parkinsonism is between 7.5 and 30 mg, but in some patients these doses either fail to provide sustained benefit or cannot be tolerated. In order to minimize adverse effects, the dose of bromocriptine should be built up slowly over about 2 or 3 months from a starting level of 1.25 mg twice daily after meals; the daily dose is then increased by 2.5 mg every 2 weeks depending on the response or the development of adverse reactions. The dose of levodopa taken concurrently may have to be gradually lowered to about half of that previously required. However, because occasional patients are very sensitive to the hypotensive effect of bromocriptine and may even collapse within an hour of the first dose, a test dose of 1 mg should be given initially, with food and with the patient in bed. If vascular collapse occurs, recovery is usually rapid and spontaneous, and patients often tolerate subsequent doses well. Treatment with bromocriptine should be stopped if it leads to psychiatric disturbances, cardiac dysrhythmia, erythromelalgia, ergotism, or other intolerable adverse effects.

Adverse Effects

A. Gastrointestinal Effects: Anorexia and nausea and vomiting are especially common when bromocriptine therapy is introduced and can be minimized by taking the medication with meals. Other adverse gastrointestinal effects include constipation, dyspepsia, and symptoms suggestive of reflux esophagitis. Bleeding from peptic ulceration has also been reported.

B. Cardiovascular Effects: Postural hypotension is fairly common, especially at the initiation of therapy. Painless digital vasospasm is a complication of long-term treatment that can be reversed by lowering the dose. Cardiac arrhythmias may also occur with bromocriptine and are an indication for discontinuing treatment.

C. Dyskinesias: Abnormal movements similar to those introduced by levodopa can be produced by bromocriptine. Treatment consists of reducing the total dose of dopaminergic drugs being taken.

D. Mental Disturbances: Confusion, hallucinations, delusions, and other psychiatric reactions are established complications of dopaminergic treatment of parkinsonism. They are more common and severe with bromocriptine than with levodopa itself. Such effects clear on withdrawal of the offending medication.

E. Miscellaneous Adverse Effects: Headache, nasal congestion, increased arousal, pulmonary infiltrates, and erythromelalgia are other reported side effects of bromocriptine. Erythromelalgia consists of red, tender, painful, swollen feet and, occasionally, hands, at times associated with arthralgia; symptoms and signs clear within a few days of withdrawal of bromocriptine.

Contraindications

Bromocriptine treatment is contraindicated in patients with a history of psychotic illness or recent myocardial infarction. It is best avoided in patients with peripheral vascular disease or peptic ulceration.

PERGOLIDE

Pergolide is a dopamine agonist that directly stimulates both D_1 and D_2 receptors. The drug may benefit patients not receiving levodopa, and it also prolongs the response to levodopa in patients with response fluctuations. It is generally well tolerated, but adverse effects are frequent at the initiation of therapy and resemble those of bromocriptine. Pergolide tends to lose its efficacy with time, probably owing to the down-regulation of dopamine receptors. It is not clear whether the use of pergolide at an early stage of Parkinson's disease—either alone or in combination with low-dose levodopa—will delay the onset of dopa-induced adverse effects.

The average therapeutic dose of pergolide is 3 mg daily; patients are generally started on 0.05 mg daily, and the dose is built up by increments until benefit occurs or toxicity limits further increments. The dose of levodopa taken concurrently may have to be reduced.

MONOAMINE OXIDASE INHIBITORS

Two types of monoamine oxidase have been distinguished. Monoamine oxidase A metabolizes norepinephrine and serotonin; monoamine oxidase B metabolizes dopamine. **Selegiline** (deprenyl) (Figure 27–2), a selective inhibitor of monoamine oxidase B, retards the breakdown of dopamine; in consequence, it enhances and prolongs the antiparkinsonism effect of levodopa (thereby allowing the dose of levodopa to be reduced) and may reduce mild on-off or wearing-off phenomena. It is therefore used as adjunctive therapy for patients with a declining or fluctuating response to levodopa. The standard dose is 5 mg with breakfast and 5 mg with lunch. The adverse effects of levodopa may be increased by selegiline. Selegiline has only a minor therapeutic effect on parkinsonism when given alone, but studies in animals suggest that it may reduce disease progression. Such an effect of antioxidative therapy on disease progression may be expected if Parkinson's disease is associated with the oxidative generation of free radicals. However, studies to test the effect of selegiline on the progression of

parkinsonism in humans have yielded ambiguous results. The findings in a recent large multicenter study have been taken to suggest a beneficial effect in slowing disease progression but may simply have reflected a symptomatic response.

The combined administration of levodopa and an inhibitor of both forms of monoamine oxidase must be avoided, since it may lead to hypertensive crises, probably because of the peripheral accumulation of norepinephrine.

CATECHOL-O-METHYLTRANSFERASE INHIBITORS

Inhibition of dopa decarboxylase is associated with compensatory activation of other pathways of levodopa metabolism, especially catechol-O-methyltransferase (COMT), and this increases plasma levels of 3-methyldopa (3OMD). Elevated levels of 3OMD have been associated with a poor therapeutic response to levodopa, perhaps in part because 3OMD competes with levodopa for an active carrier mechanism that governs its transport across the intestinal mucosa and the blood-brain barrier. For this reason, selective COMT inhibitors are currently being evaluated as adjunctive therapy for parkinsonian patients receiving levodopa.

AMANTADINE

Amantadine, an antiviral agent, was by chance found to have antiparkinsonism properties. Its mode of action in parkinsonism is unclear, but it may potentiate dopaminergic function by influencing the synthesis, release, or reuptake of dopamine. Release of catecholamines from peripheral stores has been documented.

Pharmacokinetics

Peak plasma concentrations of amantadine are reached 1–4 hours after an oral dose. The plasma half-life is between 2 and 4 hours, most of the drug being excreted unchanged in the urine.

Clinical Use

Amantadine is less efficacious than levodopa and its benefits may be short-lived, often disappearing after only a few weeks of treatment. Nevertheless, during that time it may favorably influence the bradykinesia, rigidity, and tremor of parkinsonism. The standard dose is 100 mg orally twice daily.

Adverse Effects

Amantadine has a number of undesirable central nervous system effects, all of which can be reversed by stopping the drug. These include restlessness, depression, irritability, insomnia, agitation, excitement, hallucinations, and confusion. Overdosage may produce an acute toxic psychosis. With doses several times higher than recommended, convulsions have occurred.

Livedo reticularis sometimes occurs in patients taking amantadine and usually clears within a month after the drug is withdrawn. Other dermatologic reactions have also been described. Peripheral edema, another well-recognized complication, is not accompanied by signs of cardiac, hepatic, or renal disease and responds to diuretics. Other adverse reactions include headache, congestive heart disease, postural hypotension, urinary retention, and gastrointestinal disturbances (eg, anorexia, nausea, constipation, and dry mouth).

Contraindications

The drug should be used with caution in patients with a history of seizures or congestive heart failure.

ACETYLCHOLINE-BLOCKING DRUGS

A number of centrally acting antimuscarinic preparations are available that differ in their potency and in their efficacy in different patients.

Clinical Use

Treatment is started with a low dose of one of the drugs in this category, the level of medication gradually being increased until benefit occurs or adverse effects limit further increments. Antimuscarinic drugs may improve the tremor and rigidity of parkinsonism but have little effect on bradykinesia. If patients fail to respond to one drug, a trial with another is certainly warranted and may be successful. Some of the more commonly used drugs are listed in Table 27–1.

Adverse Effects

Antimuscarinic drugs have a number of central nervous system effects, including drowsiness, mental slowness, inattention, restlessness, confusion, agitation, delusions, hallucinations, and mood changes. Such effects are sometimes precipitated by intercurrent infections and usually subside within a few days

Table 27–1. Some drugs with antimuscarinic properties used in parkinsonism.

Drug	Usual Daily Dose (mg)
Benztropine mesylate	1–6
Biperiden	2–12
Chlorphenoxamine	150–400
Orphenadrine	150–400
Procyclidine	7.5–30
Trihexyphenidyl	6–20

after withdrawal of the drug. Other common effects include dryness of the mouth, blurring of vision, mydriasis, urinary retention, nausea and vomiting, constipation, tachycardia, tachypnea, increased intraocular pressure, palpitations, and cardiac arrhythmias. Dyskinesias occur in rare cases. Acute suppurative parotitis sometimes occurs as a complication of dryness of the mouth.

If medication is to be withdrawn, this should be accomplished gradually rather than abruptly in order to prevent acute exacerbation of parkinsonism.

Contraindications

Acetylcholine-blocking drugs should be avoided in patients with prostatic hypertrophy, obstructive gastrointestinal disease (eg, pyloric stenosis or paralytic ileus), or angle-closure glaucoma. In parkinsonism patients receiving antimuscarinic medication, concomitant administration of other drugs with antimuscarinic properties (eg, tricyclic antidepressants or antihistamines) may precipitate some of the complications mentioned above.

D,L-*THREO*-3,4-DIHYDROXY-PHENYLSERINE (DOPS)

Regional cerebral deficits of norepinephrine (as well as of dopamine) have been found in patients with parkinsonism, and it has been proposed that norepinephrine lack is responsible for the clinical phenomenon of sudden transient freezing-up or arrest of movement observed in some patients with advanced disease who respond unpredictably to levodopa. Administration of D,L-*threo*-3,4-dihydroxyphenylserine (DOPS), a precursor of norepinephrine, has been reported to improve such phenomena in some studies but not in others.

OTHER EXPERIMENTAL APPROACHES TO THE TREATMENT OF PARKINSON'S DISEASE

A therapeutic role has been suggested for vitamin E, a scavenger of free radicals, in slowing disease progression. A recent large multicenter study, however, found no evidence of benefit when tocopherol (2000 IU) was taken daily.

In nonhuman primates with experimentally induced parkinsonism, treatment with G_{MI} ganglioside increased striatal dopamine levels and enhanced the dopaminergic innervation of the striatum. This suggests a potential new therapeutic strategy for Parkinson's disease in humans.

The effect of transplantation of dopaminergic tissue (autologous adrenal medullary tissue or fetal substantia nigra tissue) is currently under study. The results have been conflicting, and the mechanism for any benefit is uncertain.

GENERAL COMMENTS ON DRUG MANAGEMENT OF PATIENTS WITH PARKINSONISM

Parkinson's disease generally follows a progressive course. Moreover, the benefits of levodopa therapy often seem to diminish with time and certain adverse effects may complicate long-term levodopa treatment. Nevertheless, evidence is accumulating that dopaminergic therapy at a relatively early stage may be most effective in alleviating symptoms of parkinsonism and may also favorably affect the mortality rate due to the disease. Symptomatic treatment of mild parkinsonism is probably best avoided until there is some degree of disability or until symptoms begin to have a significant impact on the patient's life-style. When treatment becomes necessary, levodopa is usually prescribed in combination with carbidopa as Sinemet, and amantadine or an antimuscarinic drug (or both) may be necessary as well for optimal benefit. Some of the long-term adverse effects of levodopa (such as response-fluctuations and dyskinesias) can probably be avoided or minimized if the total daily dose of Sinemet is kept low and dopaminergic therapy is increased by adding bromocriptine or pergolide. Physical therapy is helpful in improving mobility. In patients with severe parkinsonism and long-term complications of levodopa therapy, such as the on-off phenomena, a trial of treatment with bromocriptine or pergolide may be worthwhile. Regulation of dietary protein intake may also improve response fluctuations.

Treatment with selegiline of patients who are young or have mild parkinsonism may delay disease progression and merits serious consideration.

DRUG-INDUCED PARKINSONISM

Reserpine and the related drug tetrabenazine deplete biogenic monoamines from their storage sites, while haloperidol and the phenothiazines block dopamine receptors. These drugs may therefore produce a parkinsonian syndrome, usually within 3 months after introduction, which is related to high dosage and clears over a few weeks or months after withdrawal. If treatment is necessary, antimuscarinic agents are preferred. Levodopa is of no help if neuroleptic drugs are continued and may in fact aggravate the mental disorder for which antipsychotic drugs were prescribed originally.

In 1983, a drug-induced form of parkinsonism was discovered in individuals who attempted to synthesize and use a narcotic drug related to meperidine but actually synthesized and self-administered 1-methyl-4-phenyl-1,2,5,6-tetrahydropyridine. This compound (MPTP) leads to the selective destruction of dopaminergic neurons in the substantia nigra and induces a severe form of parkinsonism in animals as well as in humans. The experimental use of this drug has provided a model that could assist in the development of new drugs for this disease. The toxicity of MPTP is related to its oxidation by monoamine oxidase B to 1-methyl-4-phenylpyridinium (MPP^+).

OTHER MOVEMENT DISORDERS

Tremor

Tremor consists of rhythmic oscillatory movements. Physiologic postural tremor, which is a normal phenomenon, is enhanced in amplitude by anxiety, fatigue, thyrotoxicosis, and intravenous epinephrine or isoproterenol. Propranolol reduces its amplitude, and, if administered intra-arterially, prevents the response to isoproterenol in the perfused limb, presumably through some peripheral action. Certain drugs—especially the bronchodilators, tricyclic antidepressants, and lithium—may produce a dose-dependent exaggeration of the normal physiologic tremor that is readily reversed by discontinuing the drug. Although the tremor produced by sympathomimetics such as terbutaline (a bronchodilator) is blocked by propranolol, which antagonizes both β_1 and β_2 receptors, it is not blocked by metoprolol, a β_1-selective antagonist, suggesting that such tremor is mediated mainly by the β_2 receptors.

Essential tremor is a postural tremor, sometimes familial, that is clinically similar to physiologic tremor. Dysfunction of β_1 receptors has been implicated in some instances, since the tremor may respond dramatically to standard doses of metoprolol as well as to propranolol. The most useful approach is with propranolol, but whether the response depends on a central or peripheral action is unclear. The pharmacokinetics, pharmacologic effects, and adverse reactions of propranolol are discussed in Chapter 10. Daily doses of propranolol on the order of 120 mg (range, 60–240 mg) are usually required, and reported adverse effects have been few. Propranolol should be used with caution in patients with congestive cardiac failure, heart block, asthma, and hypoglycemia. Patients can be instructed to take their own pulse and call the physician if significant bradycardia develops. Metoprolol is sometimes useful in treating tremor when patients have concomitant pulmonary disease that contraindicates use of propranolol. Primidone (an antiepileptic drug; see Chapter 23), in gradually increasing doses up to 250 mg 3 times daily, is also effective in providing symptomatic control in some cases. Patients with tremor are very sensitive to primidone and often cannot tolerate the doses used to treat seizures; they should be started on 50 mg once daily and the daily dose increased by 50 mg every 2 weeks depending on response. Small quantities of alcohol may suppress essential tremor, but only for a short time and by an unknown mechanism. Diazepam, chlordiazepoxide, mephenesin, and antiparkinsonism agents have been advocated in the past but are generally worthless. Isoniazid (in doses up to 1200 mg daily, with pyridoxine, 300 mg) is helpful in occasional patients.

Intention tremor—tremor present during movement but not at rest—sometimes occurs as a toxic manifestation of alcohol or drugs such as phenytoin. Withdrawal or reduction in dosage provides dramatic relief. There is no satisfactory pharmacologic treatment for intention tremor due to other neurologic disorders.

Rest tremor is usually due to parkinsonism.

Huntington's Disease

This dominantly inherited disorder is characterized by progressive chorea and dementia that usually begin in adulthood. The development of chorea seems to be related to an imbalance of dopamine, acetylcholine, GABA, and perhaps other neurotransmitters in the basal ganglia (Figure 27–1). Pharmacologic studies indicate that chorea results from functional overactivity in dopaminergic nigrostriatal pathways, perhaps because of increased responsiveness of postsynaptic dopamine receptors or deficiency of a neurotransmitter that normally antagonizes dopamine. Drugs that impair dopaminergic neurotransmission, either by depleting central monoamines (eg, reserpine, tetrabenazine) or by blocking dopamine receptors (eg, phenothiazines, butyrophenones), often alleviate chorea, whereas dopamine-like drugs such as levodopa tend to exacerbate it.

Both GABA and the enzyme (glutamic acid decarboxylase) concerned with its synthesis are markedly reduced in the basal ganglia of patients with Huntington's disease, and GABA receptors are usually implicated in inhibitory pathways. There is also a significant decline in concentration of choline acetyltransferase, the enzyme responsible for synthesizing acetylcholine, in the basal ganglia of these patients. These findings may be of pathophysiologic significance and have led to attempts to alleviate chorea by enhancing central GABA or acetylcholine activity. Unfortunately, such pharmacologic manipulations have been disappointing, yielding no consistently beneficial response, and as a consequence the most commonly used drugs for controlling dyskinesia in patients with Huntington's disease are still those that interfere with dopamine activity. With all of the latter drugs, however, reduction of abnormal movements may be associated with iatrogenic parkinsonism.

Reserpine depletes cerebral dopamine by preventing intraneuronal storage; it is introduced in low doses (eg, 0.25 mg daily), and the daily dose is then built up gradually (eg, by 0.25 mg every week) until benefit occurs or adverse effects become troublesome. A daily dose of 2–5 mg is often effective in suppressing abnormal movements, but adverse effects may include hypotension, depression, sedation, diarrhea, and nasal congestion. Tetrabenazine resembles reserpine in depleting cerebral dopamine and has less troublesome adverse effects, but it is not available in the USA. Treatment with postsynaptic dopamine receptor blockers such as phenothiazines and butyrophenones may also be helpful. Haloperidol is started in a small dose, eg, 1 mg twice daily, and increased every 4 days depending upon the response. If haloperidol is not helpful, treatment with increasing doses of perphenazine up to a total of about 20 mg daily sometimes helps. The pharmacokinetics and clinical properties of these drugs are considered in greater detail elsewhere in this book.

Other Forms of Chorea

Treatment is directed at the underlying cause when chorea occurs as a complication of general medical disorders such as thyrotoxicosis, polycythemia vera rubra, systemic lupus erythematosus, hypocalcemia, and hepatic cirrhosis. Drug-induced chorea is managed by withdrawal of the offending substance, which may be levodopa, an antimuscarinic drug, amphetamine, lithium, phenytoin, or an oral contraceptive. Neuroleptic drugs may also produce an acute or tardive dyskinesia (discussed below). Sydenham's chorea is temporary and usually so mild that pharmacologic management of the dyskinesia is unnecessary, but dopamine-blocking drugs are effective in suppressing it.

Ballismus

The biochemical basis of ballismus is unknown, but the pharmacologic approach to management is the same as for chorea. Treatment with haloperidol, perphenazine, or other dopamine-blocking drugs may be helpful.

Athetosis & Dystonia

The pharmacologic basis of these disorders is unknown, and there is no satisfactory medical treatment for them. Occasional patients with dystonia may respond to diazepam, amantadine, antimuscarinic drugs (in high dosage), levodopa, carbamazepine, baclofen, haloperidol, or phenothiazines. A trial of these pharmacologic approaches is worthwhile even though often not successful. Patients with focal dystonias such as blepharospasm or torticollis may benefit from injection of botulinum toxin into the overactive muscles.

Tics

The pathophysiologic basis of tics is unknown. Chronic multiple tics (Gilles de la Tourette's syndrome) may require treatment if the disorder is severe or is having a significant impact on the patient's life. The most effective pharmacologic approach is with haloperidol, and patients are better able to tolerate this drug if treatment is started with a small dosage (eg, 0.25 or 0.5 mg daily) and then increased very gradually over the following weeks. Most patients ultimately require a total daily dose of 3–8 mg. If haloperidol is not helpful, fluphenazine, clonazepam, clonidine, or carbamazepine should be tried. The pharmacologic properties of these drugs are discussed elsewhere in this book. Pimozide, an oral dopamine blocker, may help patients intolerant or unresponsive to haloperidol, but the long-term safety of the drug is unclear.

Drug-Induced Dyskinesias

The pharmacologic basis of the acute dyskinesia or dystonia sometimes precipitated by the first few doses of a phenothiazine is not clear. In most instances, parenteral administration of an antimuscarinic drug such as benztropine (2 mg intravenously) or biperiden (2–5 mg intravenously or intramuscularly) is helpful, while in other instances diazepam (10 mg intravenously) alleviates the abnormal movements.

Tardive dyskinesia is a disorder characterized by a variety of abnormal movements that develop after long-term neuroleptic drug treatment. A reduction in dose of the offending medication, a dopamine receptor blocker, commonly worsens the dyskinesia, while an increase in dose may suppress it. These clinical observations, and the exacerbation in the movement disorder that is produced by levodopa, suggest that tardive dyskinesia relates to increased dopaminergic function, but its precise pharmacologic basis is unclear. It would seem, therefore, that phenothiazines cause a short-term reversible blockade of dopamine receptors but that over the long term they increase dopaminergic function. Whether this latter effect depends upon the development of denervation supersensitivity, increased dopamine synthesis, or diminished reuptake of dopamine at central synapses is not known.

There is some evidence that GABA is involved in a striatonigral feedback loop modulating the activity of dopaminergic cells in the substantia nigra, and GABA efferents also pass from the striatum to the globus pallidus and thalamus. GABA-mediated activity may diminish the activity of nigrostriatal dopaminergic cells and thereby decrease involuntary movements. **Muscimol,** a semirigid structural analogue of GABA, has been given to a small number of patients with tardive dyskinesia, and at oral doses of 5–9 mg daily consistently attenuated their involuntary movements in one study. However, muscimol has adverse behavioral effects that limit any role for it in the treatment of tardive dyskinesia. Other attempts to increase central GABA activity (eg, with benzodiazepines or sodium valproate) have not yielded consistent benefit. Attempts to restore the balance between dopaminergic and cholinergic activity by increasing the latter with oral choline or lecithin have been helpful in some instances but not in others, and the same was true of treatment with deanol acetamidobenzoate, a drug related to acetylcholine and now discontinued. The drugs most likely to provide immediate symptomatic benefit are those interfering with dopaminergic function, either by depletion (eg, reserpine, tetrabenazine) or receptor blockade (eg, phenothiazines, butyrophenones). Paradoxically, the receptor-blocking drugs are the very ones that also cause the dyskinesia, and they are probably best avoided to prevent the development of a spiral phenomenon in which continuing aggravation of the dyskinesia by the drugs used to control it necessitates increasingly higher doses for its temporary suppression.

Because tardive dyskinesia developing in adults is usually irreversible and has no satisfactory treatment, care must be taken to reduce the likelihood of its occurrence. Antipsychotic medication should be prescribed only when necessary and should be withheld periodically to assess the need for continued treatment and to unmask incipient dyskinesia. Thioridazine, a phenothiazine with a piperidine side chain, is an effective antipsychotic that seems less likely than most to cause extrapyramidal reactions, perhaps because it has little effect on dopamine receptors in the striatal system. Finally, antimuscarinic drugs should not be prescribed routinely in patients receiving neuroleptics, since the combination may increase the likelihood of dyskinesia.

Wilson's Disease

Wilson's disease, a recessively inherited disorder of copper metabolism, is characterized biochemically by reduced serum copper and ceruloplasmin concentrations, pathologically by markedly increased concentration of copper in the brain and viscera, and clinically by signs of hepatic and neurologic dysfunction. Treatment involves the removal of excess copper, followed by maintenance of copper balance. The most satisfactory agent currently available for this purpose is **penicillamine** (dimethylcysteine), a chelating agent that forms a ring complex with copper. It is readily absorbed from the gastrointestinal tract and rapidly excreted in the urine. A common starting dose in adults is 500 mg 3 or 4 times daily. After remission occurs, it may be possible to lower the maintenance dose, generally to not less than 1 g daily, which must thereafter be continued indefinitely. Adverse effects include nausea and vomiting, nephrotic syndrome, a lupus-like syndrome, pemphigus, myasthenia, arthropathy, optic neuropathy, and various blood dyscrasias. Treatment should be monitored by frequent urinalysis and complete blood counts. Dietary copper should also be kept below 2 mg daily by the exclusion of chocolate, nuts, shellfish, liver, mushrooms, broccoli, and cereals; and distilled or demineralized water may have to be provided if tap water contains more than 0.1 mg of copper per liter. Potassium disulfide, 20 mg 3 times daily with meals, reduces the intestinal absorption of copper and should also be prescribed.

For those patients who are unable to tolerate penicillamine, **trientine,** a newer chelating agent, may be used in a daily dose of 1–1.5 g. Trientine appears to have few adverse effects other than mild anemia due to iron deficiency in a few patients.

PREPARATIONS AVAILABLE

Amantadine (Symmetrel)
  Oral: 100 mg capsules; 10 mg/mL syrup
Benztropine (Cogentin, others)
  Oral: 0.5, 1, 2 mg tablets
  Parenteral: 1 mg/mL for injection
Biperiden (Akineton)
  Oral: 2 mg tablets
  Parenteral: 5 mg/mL for injection
Bromocriptine (Parlodel)
  Oral: 2.5 mg tablets; 5 mg capsules
Carbidopa (Lodosyn)
  Oral: 25 mg tablets
Carbidopa/levodopa (Sinemet)
  Oral: 10 mg carbidopa and 100 mg levodopa, 25 mg carbidopa and 100 mg levodopa, 25 mg carbidopa and 250 mg levodopa tablets
  Oral sustained-release (Sinemet CR): 50 mg carbidopa and 200 mg levodopa
Levodopa (Dopar, Larodopa)

  Oral: 100, 250, 500 mg tablets, capsules
Orphenadrine (Disipal)
  Oral: 100 mg tablets
  Oral sustained-release: 100 mg tablets
  Parenteral: 30 mg/mL for injection
Penicillamine (Cuprimine, Depen)
  Oral: 125, 250 mg capsules; 250 mg tablets
Pergolide (Permax)
  Oral: 0.05, 0.25, 1 mg tablets
Procyclidine (Kemadrin)
  Oral: 5 mg tablets
Selegiline (deprenyl) (Eldepryl)
  Oral: 5 mg tablets
Trientine (Cuprid)
  Oral: 250 mg capsules
Trihexyphenidyl (Artane, others)
  Oral: 2, 5 mg tablets; 2 mg/5 mL elixir
  Oral sustained-release (Artane Sequels): 5 mg capsules

REFERENCES

Agid Y: Parkinson's disease: Pathophysiology. Lancet 1991;337:1321.

Campanella G et al: Drugs affecting movement disorders. Annu Rev Pharmacol Toxicol 1987;27:113.

Carter JH, et al: Amount and distribution of dietary protein affects clinical response to levodopa in Parkinson's disease. Neurology 1989;39:552.

Cedarbaum JM: Clinical pharmacokinetics of anti-parkinsonian drugs. Clin Pharmacokinet 1987;13:141.

Diamond SG et al: Multi-center study of Parkinson mortality with early versus later dopa treatment. Ann Neurol 1987;22:8.

Goetz CG et al: Neurosurgical horizons in Parkinson's disease. Neurology 1993;43:1.

Hallett M et al: A double-blind trial of isoniazid for essential tremor and other action tremors. Mov Disord 1991; 6:253.

Hubble JP et al: Essential tremor. Clin Neuropharmacol 1989;12:453.

Hutton JT et al: Multicenter controlled study of Sinemet CR vs Sinemet (25/100) in advanced Parkinson's disease. Neurology 1989;39 (Suppl 2):67.

Jankovic J: Pergolide: Short-term and long-term experience in Parkinson's disease. In: *Recent Developments in Parkinson's Disease.* Fahn S et al (editors). Raven Press, 1986.

Jankovic J: Recent advances in the management of tics. Clin Neuropharmacol 1986;9(Suppl 2):S100.

Kopin IJ: The pharmacology of Parkinson's disease therapy: An update. Annu Rev Pharmacol Toxicol 1993; 32:467.

Langston JW et al: Selective nigral toxicity after systemic administration of 1-methyl-4-phenyl-1,2,5,6-tetrahydropyridine (MPTP) in the squirrel monkey. Brain Res 1984;292:390.

Lieberman AN, Goldstein M: Bromocriptine in Parkinson disease. Pharmacol Rev 1985;37:217.

Markham CH, Diamond SG: Long-term follow-up of early dopa treatment in Parkinson's disease. Ann Neurol 1986;19:365.

Mannisto O, Kaakola S: New selective COMT inhibitors: Useful adjuncts for Parkinson's disease? Trends Pharmacol Sci 1989;10:54.

Nakanishi T et al: Second interim report of the nation-wide collaborative study on the long-term effects of bromocriptine in the treatment of parkinsonian patients. Eur Neurol 1989;29 (Suppl 1):3.

Nutt JG: On-off phenomenon: Relation to levodopa pharmacokinetics and pharmacodynamics. Ann Neurol 1987; 22:535.

Nutt JG, Fellman JH: Pharmacokinetics of levodopa. Clin Neuropharmacol 1984;7:35.

Nygaard TG et al: Dopa-responsive dystonia: Long-term treatment response and prognosis. Neurology 1991;41: 174.

Obeso JA et al: Overcoming pharmacokinetic problems in the treatment of Parkinson's disease. Mov Disord 1989; 4 (Suppl 1):70.

Parkinson Study Group: Effects of tocopherol and deprenyl on the progression of disability in early Parkinson's disease. N Engl J Med 1993;328:176.

Rinne UK: Long-term combination therapy with bromocriptine and levodopa. In: *Recent Developments in Parkinson's Disease II*. Macmillan, 1987.

Ross RT: Drug-induced parkinsonism and other movement disorders. Can J Neurol Sci 1990;22:155.

Scheinberg IH, Jaffe ME, Sternlieb I: The use of trientine in preventing the effects of interrupting penicillamine therapy in Wilson's disease. N Engl J Med 1987;317:209.

Schneider JS et al: Recovery from experimental parkinsonism in primates with G_{M1} ganglioside treatment. Science 1992;256:843.

Shapiro AK et al: Pimozide treatment of tic and Tourette disorders. Pediatrics 1987;79:6.

Stoof JC et al: Regulation of the activity of striatal cholinergic neurons dopamine. Neuroscience 1992;47:755.

28

Antipsychotic Agents & Lithium

Leo E. Hollister, MD

I. ANTIPSYCHOTIC AGENTS

The terms **antipsychotic** and **neuroleptic** are used interchangeably to denote a group of drugs that have been used mainly for treating schizophrenia but are also effective in some other psychoses and agitated states.

History

Antipsychotic drugs have been used clinically for almost 40 years. Reserpine and chlorpromazine were the first drugs found to be useful in schizophrenia. Although chlorpromazine is still sometimes used for the treatment of psychoses, these forerunner drugs have been superseded by many newer agents. Their impact on psychiatry, however—especially on the treatment of schizophrenia—has been enormous: The number of patients requiring hospitalization in mental institutions has markedly decreased, and psychiatric thinking has shifted to a more biologic basis. Unfortunately, neither of these developments has been as rewarding in human or medical-economic terms as initially hoped.

Nature of Psychosis
& Schizophrenia

The term "psychosis" denotes a variety of mental disorders. Schizophrenia is a particular kind of psychosis characterized mainly by a clear sensorium but a marked thinking disturbance.

The pathogenesis is unknown. Largely as a result of research stimulated by the discovery of antipsychotic drugs, a genetic predisposition has been proposed as a necessary but not always sufficient condition underlying the psychotic disorder. To some extent, this assumption has been supported by the familial incidence of schizophrenia. Actual determination of chromosomal linkages using the techniques of molecular genetics has been more difficult to establish firmly, mainly because the phenotype is not accurately diagnosable. The molecular basis for schizophrenia still eludes full definition, but a great deal of effort has been expended in attempting to link the dis-

order with abnormalities of amine neurotransmitter function, especially dopamine function (see accompanying box). The defects of this hypothesis are significant, however, and suggest that the disorder is even more complex than originally supposed.

An additional factor indicating heterogeneity among schizophrenic patients is the presence or absence of anatomic changes. A number of studies using brain imaging techniques (CT or MRI) in living subjects have shown atrophy of various brain structures in some schizophrenics as compared with age-matched normals. Such patients tend to show predominantly "negative" symptoms (emotional blunting, poor socialization, cognitive deficit), which are unresponsive to drugs. Furthermore, positron emission tomography (PET) scanning has shown areas of decreased metabolism in various parts of the brain in some patients.

BASIC PHARMACOLOGY OF ANTIPSYCHOTIC AGENTS

Chemical Types

A number of chemical structures have been associated with antipsychotic properties. The drugs can be classified into several groups as shown in Figure 28–1.

A. Phenothiazine Derivatives: Three subfamilies of phenothiazines, based primarily on the side chain of the molecule, are currently used. Aliphatic derivatives (eg, chlorpromazine) and piperidine derivatives (eg, thioridazine) are the least potent. Piperazine derivatives are more potent in the sense that they are effective in lower doses. The piperazine derivatives are also more selective in their pharmacologic effects (Table 28–1).

B. Thioxanthene Derivatives: This group of drugs is exemplified primarily by thiothixene. In general, these compounds are slightly less potent than their phenothiazine analogues.

C. Butyrophenone Derivatives: This group, of

THE DOPAMINE HYPOTHESIS

The dopamine hypothesis for schizophrenia is the most fully developed of several hypotheses and is the basis for much of the rationale for drug therapy. Several lines of circumstantial evidence suggest that excessive dopaminergic activity underlies the disorder: (1) most antipsychotic drugs strongly block postsynaptic D_2 receptors in the central nervous system, especially in the mesolimbic-frontal system; (2) drugs that increase dopaminergic activity, such as levodopa (a precursor), amphetamines (releasers of dopamine), or apomorphine (a direct dopamine receptor agonist), either aggravate schizophrenia or produce it de novo in some patients; (3) dopamine receptor density has been found, postmortem, to be increased in the brains of schizophrenics who have not been treated with antipsychotic drugs; (4) positron emission tomography (PET) has shown increased dopamine receptor density in both treated and untreated schizophrenics when compared with such scans of nonschizophrenic persons; and (5) successful treatment of schizophrenic patients has been reported to change the amount of homovanillic acid (HVA), a metabolite of dopamine, in the cerebrospinal fluid, plasma, and urine.

The dopamine hypothesis is far from complete, however. If an abnormality of dopamine physiology were completely responsible for the pathogenesis of schizophrenia, antipsychotic drugs would do a much better job of treating patients—but they are only partially effective for most and ineffective for some patients. The recent cloning and characterization of multiple dopamine receptor types may permit more widespread acceptance of the dopamine hypothesis if drugs can be developed that act selectively on each receptor type. The traditional antipsychotics bind D_2 50 times more avidly than D_1 or D_3 receptors. Until recently, the main thrust in drug development was to find agents that were more potent and more selective in blocking D_2 receptors. The fact that several of the atypical antipsychotic drugs have much less effect on D_2 receptors and yet are effective in schizophrenia has redirected attention to the role of other dopamine receptors and to nondopamine receptors, especially the $5\text{-}HT_2$ receptor. Some studies suggest that even among the traditional phenothiazines, the correlation of clinical efficacy with α-adrenoceptor-blocking potency is better than with dopamine-blocking potency. As a result of these considerations, the direction of research has changed to a greater focus on compounds that may act on several transmitter-receptor systems. The great hope is to produce drugs with greater efficacy and fewer adverse effects, especially extrapyramidal toxicity.

which haloperidol is the most widely used, has a very different structure from those of the two preceding groups. Diphenylbutylpiperidines are closely related compounds. These agents tend to be more potent and to have fewer autonomic effects.

D. Miscellaneous Structures: These newer drugs include the diphenylbutylpiperidines (pimozide), dihyroindolones (molindone), dibenzoxazepines (loxapine), dibenzodiazepines (clozapine), and benzamides (remoxipride).

Pharmacokinetics

A. Absorption and Distribution: Most antipsychotic drugs are readily but incompletely absorbed. Furthermore, many of these drugs undergo significant first-pass metabolism. Thus, oral doses of chlorpromazine and thioridazine have systemic availability from 25% to 35%, while haloperidol, which is less likely to be metabolized, has an average systemic availability of about 65%.

Most antipsychotics are highly lipid-soluble and protein-bound (92–99%). They tend to have large volumes of distribution (usually > 7 L/kg). Probably because these drugs are sequestered in lipid compartments of the body, they generally have a much longer clinical duration of action than could be estimated from their plasma half-lives. Metabolites of chlorpromazine may be excreted in the urine weeks after the last dose of chronically administered drug.

B. Metabolism: Most antipsychotics are almost completely metabolized by a variety of processes. Although some metabolites retain activity, eg 7-hydroxychlorpromazine and reduced haloperidol, metabolites are not considered to be highly important to the action of these drugs. The sole exception is mesoridazine, the major metabolite of thioridazine, which is more potent than the parent compound and accounts for most of the effect. This compound has been marketed as a separate entity.

C. Excretion: Very little of any of these drugs is excreted unchanged, as they are almost completely metabolized to more polar substances. The elimination half-lives (as determined by metabolic clearance) vary from 10 to 24 hours.

Pharmacologic Effects

The first phenothiazine antipsychotic drugs, with chlorpromazine as the prototype, proved to have a

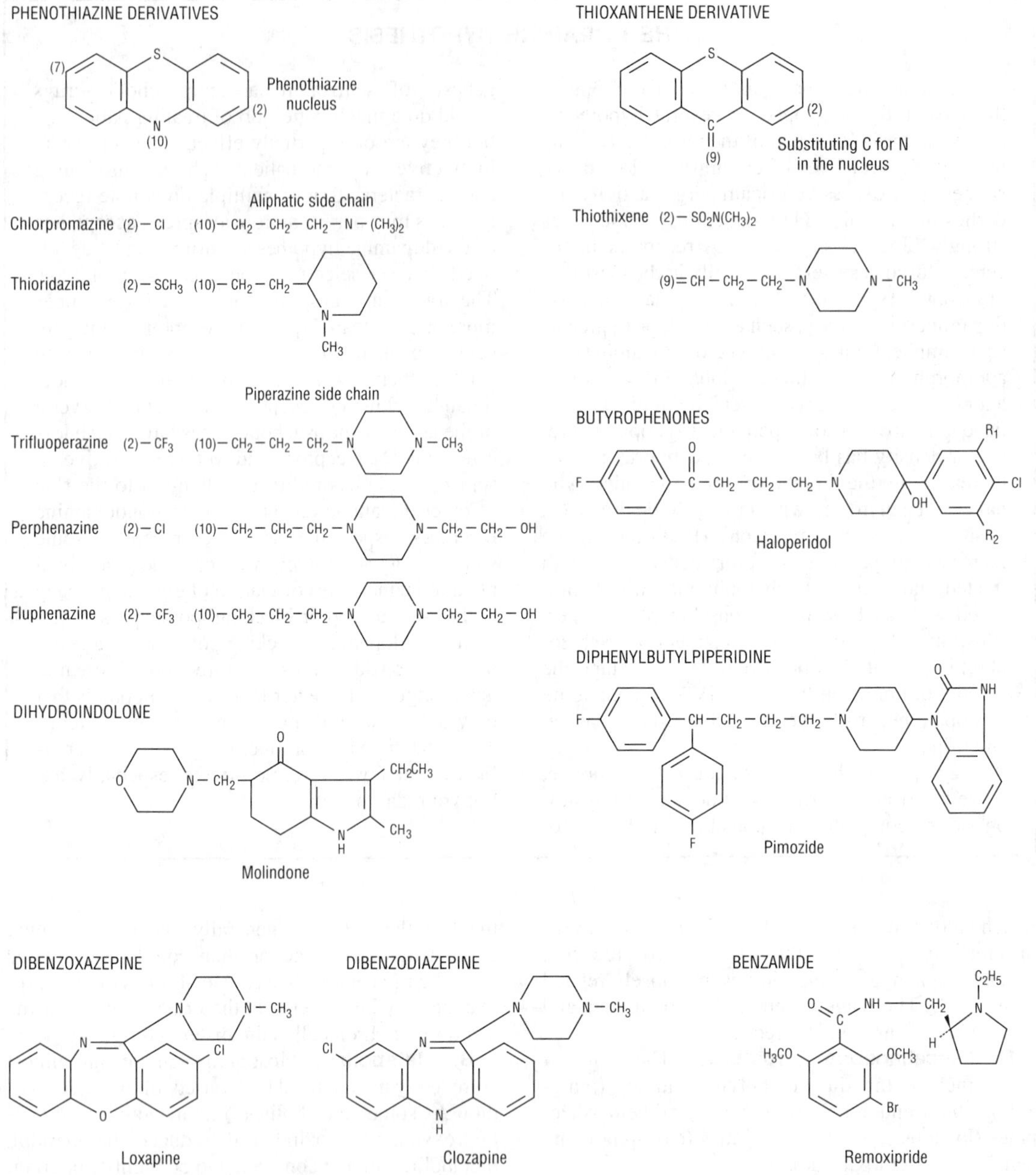

PHENOTHIAZINE DERIVATIVES

THIOXANTHENE DERIVATIVE

Figure 28–1. Structural formulas of phenothiazines, thioxanthenes, butyrophenones, and a miscellaneous group of antipsychotics. Only representative members of each type are shown.

wide variety of CNS, autonomic, and endocrine effects. These actions were traced to blocking effects at a remarkable number of receptors. These include dopamine and alpha-adrenoceptor, muscarinic, H_1 histaminic, and serotonin ($5\text{-}HT_2$) receptors. Of these, the dopamine receptor effects quickly became the major focus of interest.

A. Dopaminergic Systems: Until 1959, dopamine was not recognized as a neurotransmitter in the central nervous system but was simply regarded as a precursor for norepinephrine. Now five important dopaminergic systems or pathways are recognized in the brain. The first pathway—the one most closely related to behavior—is the **mesolimbic-mesocortical** pathway, which projects from cell bodies near the substantia nigra to the limbic system and neocortex. The second system—the **nigrostriatal** pathway—consists of neurons that project from the

Table 28–1. Antipsychotic drugs: Relation of chemical structure to potency and toxicities.

Chemical Class	Drug	Clinical Potency	Extrapyramidal Toxicity	Sedative Action	Hypotensive Actions
Phenothiazines					
Aliphatic	Chlorpromazine	Low	Medium	High	High
Piperazine	Fluphenazine	High	High	Low	Very low
Thioxanthine	Thiothixene	High	Medium	Medium	Medium
Butyrophenone	Haloperidol	High	Very high	Low	Very low
Dibenzodiazepine	Clozapine	Medium	Very low	Low	Very low

substantia nigra to the caudate and putamen; it is involved in the coordination of voluntary movement. The third pathway—the **tuberoinfundibular** system—connects arcuate nuclei and periventricular neurons to the hypothalamus and posterior pituitary. Dopamine released by these neurons physiologically inhibits prolactin secretion. The fourth dopaminergic system—the **medullary-periventricular** pathway—consists of neurons in the motor nucleus of the vagus whose projections are not well defined. This system may be involved in eating behavior. The fifth pathway—the **incertohypothalamic** pathway—forms connections within the hypothalamus and to the lateral septal nuclei. Its functions are not yet defined.

After dopamine was recognized as a neurotransmitter, various experiments showed that its effects on electrical activity in central synapses and on production of cAMP by adenylyl cyclase could be blocked by most antipsychotic drugs. This evidence led to the conclusion in the early 1960s that these drugs should be considered **dopamine antagonists.** The antipsychotic action is now thought to be produced by their ability to block dopamine in the mesolimbic and mesofrontal systems. Furthermore, the antagonism of dopamine in the nigrostriatal system explains the unwanted effect of parkinsonism produced by these drugs. The hyperprolactinemia that follows treatment with antipsychotics is caused by blockade of dopamine's tonic inhibitory effect on prolactin release from the pituitary. Finally, the changes in eating behavior observed in many patients taking antipsychotic drugs may be due to the drugs' effects on the medullary-periventricular pathway. Thus, the same pharmacodynamic action may have distinct psychiatric, neurologic, and endocrinologic consequences.

B. Dopamine Receptors and Their Effects: At present, five different dopamine receptors have been described, consisting of two separate families, the D_1-like and D_2-like receptor groups. The D_1 receptor is coded by a gene on chromosome 5, increases cAMP by activation of adenylyl cyclase, and is located mainly in the putamen, nucleus accumbens, and olfactory tubercle. The second member of this family, D_5, is coded by a gene on chromosome 4, also increases cAMP, and is found in the hippocampus and hypothalamus. The therapeutic potency of antipsychotic drugs does not correlate with their affinity for binding the D_1 receptor (Figure 28–2, top). The D_2 receptor is coded on chromosome 11, decreases cAMP (by inhibition of adenylyl cyclase), and blocks calcium channels but opens potassium channels. It is found both pre- and postsynaptically on neurons in the caudate-putamen, nucleus accumbens, and olfactory tubercle. A second member of this family, the D_3 receptor, is coded by a gene on chromosome 11, is thought to decrease cAMP, and is located in the frontal cortex, medulla, and midbrain. D_4 receptors, the newest members of the D_2-like family, also decrease cAMP. All dopamine receptors have seven transmembrane domains and are G protein-coupled.

The activation of D_2 receptors by a variety of direct or indirect agonists (eg, amphetamines, levodopa, apomorphine) causes increased motor activity and stereotyped behavior in rats, a model that has been extensively used for antipsychotic drug screening. When given to humans, the same drugs aggravate schizophrenia. The antipsychotic agents block D_2 receptors stereoselectively, and their binding affinity is very strongly correlated with clinical antipsychotic and extrapyramidal potency (Figure 28–2, bottom), an observation that has led to a profusion of receptor binding studies.

Continuous treatment with antipsychotic drugs has been reported in some (but not all) studies to produce a transient increase in levels of a dopamine metabolite, homovanillic acid (HVA), in the cerebrospinal fluid, plasma, and urine. After 1–3 weeks, HVA levels decrease to lower than normal levels, and this decrease persists. These changes may be explained as follows. The initial period of receptor blockade causes a compensatory increase in transmitter turnover, resulting in increased levels of HVA. With chronic therapy, feedback inhibition caused by the increased synaptic levels of dopamine results in decreased dopamine release and turnover.

As noted above, these findings have been incorporated into the dopamine hypothesis of schizophrenia. However, many questions have not yet been satisfactorily answered, and many observations have not been fully confirmed. For example, dopamine receptors exist in both high- and low-affinity forms, and it is not yet known whether schizophrenia or the anti-

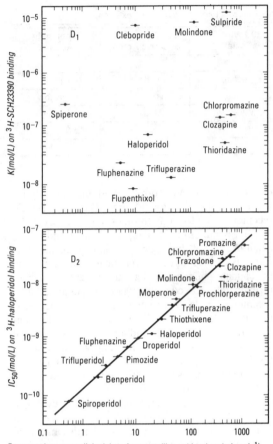

Figure 28–2. Correlations between the therapeutic potency of antipsychotic drugs and their affinity for binding to dopamine D_1 *(top)* or D_2 receptors *(bottom)*. Potency is indicated on the horizontal axes; it decreases to the right. Binding affinity for D_1 receptors was measured by displacing the selective D_1 ligand SCH 23390; affinity for D_2 receptors was similarly measured by displacing the selective D_2 ligand haloperidol. Binding affinity decreases upward. (Modified and reproduced, with permission, from Seeman P: Synapse 1987;1:133.)

psychotic drugs alter the proportions of receptors in these two forms. Furthermore, the drug-induced progression of extrapyramidal changes—from diminished function (resembling parkinsonism) to increased activity (manifested by dyskinesias)—often occurs over a period of months to years. This time scale is much longer than that described for other drug-induced changes in receptor function.

It has not yet been possible to test whether antagonism of any receptor other than the D_2 receptor plays any role in the action of antipsychotic drugs. Selective D_3 receptor antagonists are not yet available. Specific D_1 receptor antagonists are available but have not yet been used in clinical trials. Selective D_1

antagonists interfere with the action of D_2 agonists, suggesting some interaction between the two receptors. Answers to these questions should be forthcoming in the near future. Participation of glutamate, GABA, and other receptors in the pathophysiology of schizophrenia or the action of antipsychotic drugs has also been proposed. Definitive answers to these proposals may require a much longer time.

C. Differences Among Antipsychotic Drugs: Although all effective antipsychotic drugs block D_2 receptors, the degree of this blockade in relation to other actions on receptors varies considerably between drugs. Vast numbers of ligand-receptor binding experiments have been performed in an effort to discover a single receptor action that would best predict antipsychotic efficacy. For example, in vitro binding studies indicate that chlorpromazine and thioridazine block α_1 adrenoceptors more potently than D_2 receptors. They also block serotonin 5-HT$_2$ receptors relatively strongly. However, their affinity for D_1 receptors as measured by displacement of a selective D_1 ligand, SCH 23390, is relatively weak (Figure 28–2). Drugs such as perphenazine and haloperidol act mainly on D_2 receptors; they have some effect on 5-HT$_2$ and α_1 receptors but negligible effects on D_1 receptors. Pimozide and remoxipride act almost exclusively on D_2 receptors. The atypical antipsychotic clozapine, which shows marked clinical differences from the others, binds more to D_4, 5-HT$_2$, α_1, and histamine H$_1$ receptors than to either D_2 or D_1 receptors. Risperidone is about equally potent in blocking D_2 and 5-HT$_2$ receptors. A summary of the relative receptor-binding potencies of three key agents in such comparisons illustrates the difficulty in drawing simple conclusions from such experiments:

Chlorpromazine: $\alpha_1 = 5\text{-HT}_2 \geq D_2 > D_1$
Haloperidol: $D_2 > D_1 = D_4 > \alpha_1 > 5\text{-HT}_2$
Clozapine: $D_4 = \alpha_1 > 5\text{-HT}_2 > D_2 = D_1$

It appears that binding to D_1 receptors is the *least* predictive of significant clinical efficacy, but other receptor affinities are more difficult to interpret. Current research is directed toward discovering atypical antipsychotic compounds that are either more selective for the mesolimbic system (to reduce their effects on the extrapyramidal system) or have a broad spectrum of action on central neurotransmitter receptors.

In contrast to the search for *efficacy*, such differences in the receptor effects of various antipsychotics do explain many of their *adverse* effects (Tables 28–1 and 28–2). In particular, extrapyramidal toxicity appears to be associated with high D_2 potency. It is hoped that some combination of various receptor actions may be found to mitigate these unwanted effects as well as increase antipsychotic efficacy.

D. Psychologic Effects: Most antipsychotic drugs cause unpleasant subjective effects in nonpsychotic individuals; the combination of sleepiness, restlessness, and autonomic effects creates experiences unlike those associated with more familiar sedatives or hypnotics. Nonpsychotic persons also experience impaired performance as judged by a number of psychomotor and psychometric tests. Psychotic individuals, however, may actually show improvement in their performance as the psychosis is alleviated.

E. Neurophysiologic Effects: Antipsychotic drugs produce shifts in the pattern of electroencephalographic frequencies, usually slowing them and increasing their synchronization. The slowing (hypersynchrony) is sometimes focal or unilateral, which may lead to erroneous diagnostic interpretations. Both the frequency and the amplitude changes induced by psychotropic drugs are readily apparent and can be quantitated by sophisticated electronic techniques.

Electroencephalographic changes associated with antipsychotic drugs appear first in subcortical electrodes, supporting the view that they exert their main action at subcortical sites. The hypersynchrony produced by these drugs may account for their activating effect on the EEG in epileptic patients as well as their occasional elicitation of seizures in patients with no history of seizure disorders.

F. Endocrine Effects: Antipsychotic drugs produce striking adverse effects on the reproductive system. Amenorrhea-galactorrhea, false-positive pregnancy tests, and increased libido have been reported in women, whereas men have experienced decreased libido and gynecomastia. Some of these effects are secondary to blockade of dopamine's tonic inhibition of prolactin secretion; others may be due to increased peripheral conversion of androgens to estrogens.

G. Cardiovascular Effects: Orthostatic hypotension and high resting pulse rates frequently result from use of the "high-dose" (low potency) phenothiazines. Mean arterial pressure, peripheral resistance, and stroke volume are decreased, and pulse rate is increased. These effects are predictable from the autonomic actions of these agents (Table 28–2). Abnormal ECGs have been recorded, especially with thioridazine. Changes include prolongation of QT interval and abnormal configurations of the ST segment and T waves, the latter being rounded, flattened, or notched. These changes are readily reversed by withdrawing the drug.

H. Animal Screening Tests: Inhibition of conditioned (but not unconditioned) avoidance behavior is one of the most predictive tests of antipsychotic action. Another is the inhibition of amphetamine- or apomorphine-induced stereotyped behavior. This inhibition is undoubtedly related to the D_2 receptor-blocking action of the drugs, countering these two dopamine agonists. Other tests that may predict antipsychotic action are reduction of exploratory behavior without undue sedation, induction of a cataleptic state, inhibition of intracranial stimulation of reward

Table 28–2. Adverse pharmacologic effects of antipsychotic drugs.

Type	Manifestations	Mechanism
Autonomic nervous system	Loss of accommodation, dry mouth, difficulty urinating, constipation.	Muscarinic cholinoceptor blockade.
	Orthostatic hypotension, impotence, failure to ejaculate.	Alpha adrenoceptor blockade.
Central nervous system	Parkinson's syndrome, akathisia, dystonias.	Dopamine receptor blockade.
	Tardive dyskinesia.	Supersensitivity of dopamine receptors.
	Toxic-confusional state.	Muscarinic blockade.
Endocrine system	Amenorrhea-galactorrhea, infertility, impotence.	Dopamine receptor blockade resulting in hyperprolactinemia.

areas, and prevention of apomorphine-induced vomiting. Most of these tests are difficult to relate to any model of clinical psychosis.

CLINICAL PHARMACOLOGY OF ANTIPSYCHOTIC AGENTS

Indications

A. Psychiatric Indications: Schizophrenia is the primary indication for these drugs, which are presently the mainstay of treatment for this condition. Unfortunately, some patients do not respond at all and virtually none show a complete response. Because some schizophrenics have a favorable course with prolonged remission after an initial episode, most physicians recommend discontinuing drug therapy in this situation after remission has been achieved.

Schizoaffective disorders may be more similar to affective disorders than to schizophrenia. Nonetheless, the psychotic aspects of the illness require treatment with antipsychotic drugs, which may be used with other drugs such as antidepressants or lithium. The manic episode in bipolar affective disorder is most effectively treated with antipsychotic agents, though lithium alone may suffice in milder cases. As mania subsides, the antipsychotic drug may be withdrawn. Nonmanic excited states may also be managed by antipsychotics, often in combination with benzodiazepines, but attempts to define the diagnosis should not be abandoned.

Other psychiatric indications for the use of antipsychotics include Tourette's syndrome and the need to control disturbed behavior in patients with senile dementia of the Alzheimer type. The drugs may also be used with antidepressants to control agitation or psychosis in depressed patients. Such patients tend to develop tardive dyskinesia more readily, so they must be dosed sparingly. Antipsychotics are not indicated for the treatment of various withdrawal syndromes, eg, opioid withdrawal.

Antipsychotics in small doses have been (wrongly) promoted for the relief of anxiety associated with minor emotional disorders. The antianxiety sedatives (see Chapter 21) are far better in every respect, including safety and acceptability to patients.

B. Nonpsychiatric Indications: Most antipsychotic drugs, with the exception of thioridazine, have a strong antiemetic effect. This action is due to dopamine receptor blockade, both centrally (in the chemoreceptor trigger zone of the medulla) and peripherally (on receptors in the stomach). Some drugs, such as prochlorperazine and benzquinamide, are promoted solely as antiemetics. Phenothiazines with shorter side chains have considerable H_1 receptor-blocking action and have been used for relief of pruritus or, in the case of promethazine, as preoperative sedatives. The butyrophenone droperidol is used in combination with a meperidine-like drug, fentanyl, in "neuroleptanesthesia." The use of these drugs for anesthesia is described in Chapter 24.

Drug Choice

A rational choice of antipsychotic drugs may be based on differences between chemical structures and the attendant pharmacologic differences, since the differences between groups are greater than the differences within groups. Thus, one might choose to be familiar with one member of each of the three sub-

families of phenothiazines, a member of the thioxanthene and butyrophenone group, and perhaps two members of the miscellaneous group. A possible selection is shown in Table 28–3.

No basis exists for choosing drugs for use against selected "target symptoms," as there is no evidence of specificity in their effects. Although new antipsychotic drugs under development are alleged to be more effective than older ones for treating negative symptoms (emotional blunting, social withdrawal, lack of motivation), such claims have not been verified. It is not necessary for practitioners to know all of the drugs intimately, but they should be familiar with the effects—including the adverse effects—of one or two drugs in each class. The best guide for selecting a drug for an individual patient is the patient's past responses to drugs. The trend in recent years has been away from the "low-potency" agents such as chlorpromazine and thioridazine to the "high-potency" drugs such as thiothixene, haloperidol, and fluphenazine. At present, use of clozapine is limited to those patients who have failed to respond to substantial doses of conventional antipsychotic drugs or those who have disabling tardive dyskinesia. The agranulocytosis and seizures associated with this drug prevent more widespread use.

Dosage

The range of effective dosages among various antipsychotics is quite broad. Therapeutic margins are substantial. Assuming that dosages are equivalent, most antipsychotics, with the exception of clozapine, are of equal efficacy in groups of patients. However, some patients who fail to respond to one drug may respond to another, and for this reason several drugs

Table 28–3. Some representative antipsychotic drugs.

Drug Class	Drug	Advantages	Disadvantages
Phenothiazines Aliphatic	Chlorpromazine[1] (Thorazine)	Generic.	Many adverse effects.
Piperidine	Thioridazine[2] (Mellaril)	Slight extrapyramidal syndrome; generic	800 mg/d limit; no parenteral form; cardiotoxicity.
Piperazine	Fluphenazine[3] (Permitil, Prolixin)	Depot form also available (enanthate, decanoate).	(?) Increased tardive dyskinesia.
Thioxanthene	Thiothixene[4] (Navane)	Parenteral form also available; (?) decreased tardive dyskinesia.	Uncertain.
Butyrophenone	Haloperidol (Haldol)	Parenteral form also available; generic.	Severe extrapyramidal syndrome.
Dibenzoxazepine	Loxapine (Loxitane)	(?) No weight gain.	Uncertain.
Dihydroindolone	Molindone (Moban)	(?) No weight gain.	Uncertain.
Dibenzodiazepine	Clozapine (Clozaril)	May benefit treatment-resistant patients; little extrapyramidal toxicity.	May cause agranulocytosis in up to 3% of patients.

[1]Other aliphatic phenothiazines: promazine, triflupromazine.
[2]Other piperidine phenothiazines: piperacetazine, mesoridazine.
[3]Other piperazine phenothiazines: acetophenazine, perphenazine, carphenazine, prochlorperazine, trifluoperazine.
[4]Other thioxanthenes: chlorprothixene.

may have to be tried to find the one most effective for an individual patient. Quite possibly, this phenomenon might be due to the differing profiles of receptor actions of the various drugs. Patients who have become refractory to two or three antipsychotics given in substantial doses now become candidates for treatment with clozapine. This drug, in dosages up to 900 mg/d, salvages about 30–50% of patients previously refractory to 60 mg/d of haloperidol. In such cases, the increased risk of clozapine can well be justified.

Some dosage relationships between various antipsychotic drugs, as well as possible therapeutic ranges, are shown in Table 28–4.

Plasma Concentrations & Clinical Effects

Attempts to define a therapeutic range of plasma concentrations of antipsychotic agents are beset by many difficulties. Ranges of 2–20 ng/mL have been suggested for haloperidol, though such a wide range is not very helpful clinically. Clinical monitoring of plasma concentrations of these drugs, though technically feasible, is not warranted at this time.

Pharmaceutical Preparations

Well-tolerated parenteral forms of the high-potency drugs are available for rapid initiation of treatment as well as for maintenance treatment in noncompliant patients. Since the parenterally administered drugs may have much greater bioavailability than the oral forms, doses should be only a fraction of what might be given orally. Fluphenazine decanoate and haloperidol decanoate are suitable for long-term parenteral maintenance therapy in patients who cannot or will not take oral medication.

Table 28–4. Dose relationships of antipsychotics.

	Minimum Effective Therapeutic Dose (mg)	Usual Range of Daily Doses (mg)
Chlorpromazine (Thorazine)	100	100–1000
Thioridazine (Mellaril)	100	100–800
Mesoridazine (Lidanar, Serentil)	50	50–400
Piperacetazine (Quide)	10	20–160
Trifluoperazine (Stelazine)	5	5–60
Perphenazine (Trilafon)	10	8–64
Fluphenazine (Permitil, Prolixin)	2	2–60
Thiothixene (Navane)	2	2–120
Haloperidol (Haldol)	2	2–60
Loxapine (Loxitane)	10	20–160
Molindone (Lidone, Moban)	10	20–200
Clozapine (Clozaril)	50	25–600
Risperidone (Risperdal)	4	4–16

Dosage Schedules

Antipsychotics may be given in divided daily doses initially while an effective dosage level is being sought. They need not always be equally divided doses, even when given orally. After an effective daily dosage has been defined for an individual patient, doses can be given less frequently. Once-daily doses, usually given at night, are feasible for many patients during chronic maintenance treatment. Simplification of dosage schedules leads to better compliance. Maximum dose sizes of many drugs are being increased by manufacturers to meet the needs of once-daily dosing.

Maintenance Treatment

A small minority of schizophrenic patients may remit from an acute episode and require no further drug therapy for prolonged periods. In most cases the choice is between "as needed" treatment for recurrent episodes versus continual maintenance treatment with the smallest possible doses. The choice will depend on social factors such as the availability of family or friends familiar with the symptoms of early relapse and ready access to care.

Drug Combinations

Combining antipsychotic drugs confounds evaluation of the efficacy of the drugs being used. Tricyclic antidepressants may be used with antipsychotics but only for clear symptoms of depression complicating schizophrenia. They are of no proved efficacy for alleviating the social withdrawal and blunted affect of the psychotic. Lithium is sometimes added to antipsychotic agents with benefit to patients who fail to respond to the latter drugs alone. It is uncertain whether such instances represent misdiagnosed cases of mania. Sedative drugs may be added for relief of anxiety or insomnia not controlled by antipsychotics.

The drugs most frequently combined with antipsychotics are antiparkinsonism agents (see below).

Adverse Reactions

Most of the unwanted effects of antipsychotics are extensions of their known pharmacologic actions (Tables 28–1 and 28–2), but a few are allergic and some are idiosyncratic.

A. Behavioral Effects: Antipsychotic drugs are unpleasant to take—the more so the less psychotic the patient. Many patients stop taking these drugs because of the adverse effects, which may be mitigated by giving small doses during the day and the major portion at bedtime. A "pseudodepression" that may be due to drug-induced akinesia usually responds to treatment with antiparkinsonism drugs. Other "pseudodepressions" may be due to using higher doses than needed in a partially remitted patient, in which case decreasing the dose may relieve the symptoms. Toxic-confusional states may occur with very high doses of drugs that have prominent antimuscarinic actions.

B. Neurologic Effects: Extrapyramidal reactions occurring early during treatment include typical **Parkinson's syndrome, akathisia** (uncontrollable restlessness), and **acute dystonic reactions** (spastic retrocollis or torticollis). Parkinson's syndrome can be treated, when necessary, with conventional antiparkinsonism drugs of the antimuscarinic type or, in rare cases, with amantadine. Parkinson's syndrome may be self-limiting, so that an attempt to withdraw antiparkinsonism drugs should be made every 3–4 months. Akathisia and dystonic reactions will also respond to such treatment, but many prefer to use a sedative antihistamine with anticholinergic properties, eg, diphenhydramine, which can be given either parenterally or orally as capsules or elixir.

Tardive dyskinesia, as the name implies, is a late-occurring syndrome of abnormal choreoathetoid movements. It is the most important unwanted effect of antipsychotic drugs. It has been proposed that it is caused by a relative cholinergic deficiency secondary to supersensitivity of dopamine receptors in the caudate-putamen. Older women treated for long periods are most susceptible to the disorder, though it can occur at any age and in either sex. The prevalence varies enormously, but tardive dyskinesia is estimated to occur in 20–40% of chronically treated patients. Early recognition is important, since advanced cases may be difficult to reverse. Many treatments have been proposed, but their evaluation is confounded by the fact that the course of the disorder is variable and sometimes self-limited. Most authorities agree that the first step would be to try to decrease dopamine receptor sensitivity by discontinuing the antipsychotic drug or by reducing the dose. A logical second step would be to eliminate all drugs with central anticholinergic action, particularly antiparkinsonism drugs and tricyclic antidepressants. These two steps are often enough to bring about improvement. If they fail, the addition of diazepam in doses as high as 30–40 mg/d may add to the improvement by enhancing GABAergic activity. The use of reserpine may also be considered, though one runs the risk of increasing receptor sensitivity or precipitating a depressive reaction.

Seizures, while recognized as a complication from chlorpromazine, were so rare with the high-potency drugs as to merit little consideration. However, de novo seizures may occur in 2–5% of patients treated with clozapine.

C. Autonomic Nervous System Effects: Most patients become tolerant to the antimuscarinic adverse effects of antipsychotic drugs. Those who are made too uncomfortable or who are impaired, as with urinary retention, should be given bethanechol, a peripherally acting cholinomimetic. Orthostatic hypotension or impaired ejaculation—common complications of therapy with chlorpromazine or mesoridazine—should be managed by switching to drugs with less marked adrenoceptor-blocking actions.

D. Metabolic and Endocrine Effects: Weight gain is common and requires monitoring of food intake. Hyperprolactinemia in women results in the amenorrhea-galactorrhea syndrome and infertility; in men, loss of libido, impotence, and infertility may result.

E. Toxic or Allergic Reactions: Agranulocytosis, cholestatic jaundice, and skin eruptions occur rarely with the high-potency antipsychotic drugs currently used.

In contrast to other antipsychotic agents, clozapine causes agranulocytosis in a small but significant number of patients–approximately 1–2% of those treated. This serious, potentially fatal effect can develop rapidly, usually between the sixth and 18th weeks of therapy. It is not known whether it represents an immune reaction, but it appears to be reversible upon discontinuance of the drug. *Because of the risk, weekly blood counts are mandatory for patients receiving clozapine.*

F. Ocular Complications: Deposits in the anterior portion of the eye (cornea and lens) are a common complication of chlorpromazine therapy. They may accentuate the normal processes of aging of the lens. Thioridazine is the only antipsychotic drug that causes retinal deposits, which in advanced cases may resemble retinitis pigmentosa. The deposits are usually associated with "browning" of vision. The maximum daily dose of thioridazine has been limited to 800 mg/d to reduce the possibility of this complication.

G. Cardiac Toxicity: Thioridazine in doses exceeding 300 mg daily is almost always associated with minor abnormalities of T waves that are easily reversible. Overdoses of thioridazine are associated with major ventricular arrhythmias, cardiac conduction block, and sudden death; it is not certain whether thioridazine can cause these same disorders when used in therapeutic doses. In view of possible additive antimuscarinic and quinidine-like actions with various tricyclic antidepressants, thioridazine should be combined with the latter drugs only with great care.

H. Use in Pregnancy; Dysmorphogenesis: Although the antipsychotic drugs appear to be relatively safe in pregnancy, a small increase in risk could be missed. Questions about whether to use these drugs during pregnancy and whether to abort a pregnancy in which the fetus has already been exposed must be decided individually.

I. Neuroleptic Malignant Syndrome: This life-threatening disorder occurs in patients who are extremely sensitive to the extrapyramidal effects of antipsychotics. The initial symptom is marked muscle rigidity. If sweating is impaired, as it often is during treatment with anticholinergic drugs, fever may ensue, often reaching dangerous levels. The stress leukocytosis and high fever associated with this syndrome may erroneously suggest an infectious process. Autonomic instability, with altered blood pressure and pulse rate, is another midbrain manifestation. Creatine kinase (CK) isozymes are usually elevated, reflecting muscle damage. This syndrome is believed to result from an excessively rapid blockade of postsynaptic dopamine receptors. A severe form of extrapyramidal syndrome follows. Early in the course, vigorous treatment of the extrapyramidal syndrome with antiparkinsonism drugs is worthwhile. Muscle relaxants, particularly diazepam, are often helpful. The use of other muscle relaxants, such as dantrolene, or dopamine agonists, such as bromocriptine, has been reported to be helpful. If fever is present, cooling by physical measures should be tried. Various minor forms of this syndrome are now recognized.

Drug Interactions

Antipsychotics produce more important pharmacodynamic than pharmacokinetic interactions because of their multiple effects. Additive effects may occur when these drugs are combined with others that have sedative effects, alpha adrenoceptor-blocking action, anticholinergic effects, and—for thioridazine—quinidine-like action.

A variety of pharmacokinetic interactions have been reported, but none are of major clinical significance.

Overdoses

Poisonings with antipsychotics are rarely fatal, with the exception of those due to mesoridazine and thioridazine. In general, drowsiness proceeds to coma, with an intervening period of agitation. Neuromuscular excitability may be increased and proceed to convulsions. Pupils are miotic, and deep tendon reflexes are decreased. Hypotension and hypothermia are the rule, though fever may be present later in the course. The lethal effects of mesoridazine and thioridazine are related to induction of ventricular tachyarrhythmias.

Patients should be monitored in an intensive care setting for the usual vital signs, venous pressure, arterial blood gases, and electrolytes. Attempts at gastric lavage should be made even if several hours have elapsed since the drug was taken, because gastrointestinal motility is decreased and tablets may still be present in the stomach. Activated charcoal effectively binds most of these drugs, following which a saline cathartic may be given. Hypotension often responds to fluid replacement. If a pressor agent is to be used, norepinephrine or dopamine is preferred to epinephrine, whose unopposed beta adrenoceptor-stimulant action in the presence of alpha blockade may cause vasodilation. Seizures may be treated with either diazepam or phenytoin, the latter being given with an initial loading dose. Management of overdoses of thioridazine and mesoridazine, which are compli-

cated by cardiac arrhythmias, is similar to that for tricyclic antidepressants (see Chapter 29).

New Approaches

Remoxipride and raclopride are antagonists at both D_2 and D_3 receptors. They are effective and produce less extrapyramidal toxicity than traditional drugs. However, several cases of agranulocytosis have been reported in clinical trials with remoxipride. Risperidone blocks not only D_2 receptors but 5-HT_2 receptors as well. Zotepine has a similar pharmacologic profile. Thus, they are among the new antipsychotic drugs with mixed (dopamine and nondopamine) actions. Their clinical utility relative to other drugs remains to be ascertained.

The psychosis produced by phencyclidine (PCP) is a good model for schizophrenia. As this drug is an antagonist of the NMDA glutamate receptor, attempts have been made to develop antipsychotics that work as NMDA agonists. Thus far, success has been elusive. Nonetheless, it is encouraging to see the many approaches to development of antipsychotic drugs. Some agents now under study may represent real advances.

Unconventional Drugs

The efficacy of propranolol as treatment for schizophrenia remains uncertain after 30 years of study. Patients with marked agitation, hostility, and belligerence may be controlled by the addition of propranolol to a regimen of conventional antipsychotic drugs. High-dose treatment with benzodiazepines may control disturbed behavior, just as barbiturates did 35 years ago. Levodopa, thyrotropin-releasing hormone, endorphins, and apomorphine have been ineffective. Megavitamin therapy has been discredited scientifically, but adherents still persist.

Benefits & Limitations of Drug Treatment

As noted at the beginning of this chapter, these drugs have had a major impact on psychiatry and psychiatric patients. First, they have shifted the care of patients from mental institutions to the community . For many patients, this shift has provided a better life under more humane circumstances and in some cases has made possible life without constant physical restraints. For others, the tragedy of an aimless existence is now being played out in the streets of our inner cities rather than in mental institutions.

Second, these drugs have markedly shifted psychiatric thinking to a more biologic orientation. Partly because of research stimulated by the effects of these drugs on schizophrenia, we now know much more about CNS physiology and pharmacology than we did before the introduction of these agents. However, despite a great amount of research done by highly competent scientists from many disciplines, schizophrenia remains a scientific mystery and a personal disaster. While most schizophrenic patients obtain some degree of benefit from these drugs, none are made well by them.

II. LITHIUM & OTHER MOOD-STABILIZING DRUGS

Lithium carbonate is often referred to as an "antimanic" drug, but in many parts of the world it is considered a "mood-stabilizing" agent because of its primary action of preventing mood swings in patients with bipolar affective (manic-depressive) disorder. Its discovery in 1949 was based on an incorrect hypothesis and extremely good fortune in choosing the correct dosage. Carbamazepine has also been recognized as an effective mood stabilizer despite not being formally approved for such use. It was introduced during the 1970s, based on the tenuous assumption that since manic attacks, like epilepsy, are episodic, an anticonvulsant might help. Valproate and clonazepam, both GABA-mimetic anticonvulsants, have also been found to be helpful.

Nature of Bipolar Affective Disorder

Bipolar affective (manic-depressive) disorder is a frequently diagnosed and very serious emotional disorder. Patients with cyclic attacks of mania have many symptoms of paranoid schizophrenia (grandiosity, bellicosity, paranoid thoughts, and overactivity). The gratifying response to lithium therapy of patients with bipolar disorder has made such diagnostic distinctions important.

The episodes of mood swings characteristic of this condition are generally unrelated to life events. The exact biologic disturbance has not been identified, but a preponderance of catecholamine-related activity is thought to be present. Drugs that increase this activity tend to exacerbate mania, whereas those that reduce activity of dopamine or norepinephrine relieve mania. Acetylcholine may also be involved. The nature of the abrupt switch from mania to depression experienced by some patients is uncertain. Bipolar disorder has a strong familial component. Genetic studies have identified at least three possible linkages to different chromosomes.

BASIC PHARMACOLOGY OF LITHIUM

Pharmacokinetics

Lithium is a small monovalent cation. Its pharmacokinetics are summarized in Table 28–5.

Pharmacodynamics

Despite considerable investigation, the mode of action of lithium remains unclear. The major possibilities being investigated include (1) its effects on electrolytes and ion transport; (2) its effects on neurotransmitters and their release; and (3) its effects on second messengers that mediate transmitter action. The last of these three approaches appears to be the most promising.

A. Effects on Electrolytes and Ion Transport: Lithium is closely related to sodium in its properties. It can substitute for sodium in generating action potentials and in Na^+/Na^+ exchange across the membrane. It inhibits the latter process, ie, Li^+/Na^+ exchange is gradually slowed after lithium is introduced into the body. At therapeutic concentrations (around 1 mmol/L), it does not significantly affect the Na^+/Ca^{2+} exchange process or the Na^+/K^+ ATPase sodium pump.

B. Effects on Neurotransmitters: Lithium appears to enhance some of the actions of serotonin, though findings have been contradictory. Its effects on norepinephrine are variable. The drug may decrease norepinephrine and dopamine turnover, and these effects, if confirmed, might be relevant to its antimanic action. Lithium also appears to block the development of dopamine receptor supersensitivity that may accompany chronic therapy with antipsychotic agents. Finally, lithium may augment the synthesis of acetylcholine, perhaps by increasing choline uptake into nerve terminals. Some clinical studies have suggested that increasing cholinergic activity may mitigate mania. However, as noted below, a second messenger effect of lithium may obviate any effect of increased acetylcholine release.

Table 28–5. Pharmacokinetics of lithium.

Absorption	Virtually complete within 6–8 hours; peak plasma levels in 30 minutes to 2 hours.
Distribution	In total body water; slow entry into intracellular compartment. Initial volume of distribution 0.5 L/kg, rising to 0.7–0.9 L/kg; some sequestration in bone. No protein binding.
Metabolism	None.
Excretion	Virtually entirely in urine. Lithium clearance about 20% of creatinine. Plasma half-life about 20 hours.

C. Effects on Second Messengers: Currently, the best-defined effect of lithium is its action on inositol phosphates. Early studies of lithium demonstrated changes in brain inositol phosphate levels, but the significance of these changes was not appreciated until the second messenger roles of inositol-1,4,5-trisphosphate (IP_3) and diacylglycerol (DAG) were discovered. As described in Chapter 2, IP_3 and DAG are important second messengers for both alpha-adrenergic and muscarinic transmission. Lithium inhibits several important enzymes in the normal recycling of membrane phosphoinositides, including conversion of IP_2 to IP_1 (IP, inositol monophosphate) and the conversion of IP to inositol (Figure 28–3). This block leads to a depletion of phosphatidylinositol-4,5-bisphosphate (PIP_2), the membrane precursor of IP_3 and DAG. Over time, the effects of transmitters on the cell will diminish in proportion to the amount of activity in the PIP_2-dependent pathways. Such activity might be greatly increased in mania, resulting in the selective depression of the overactive circuits. For example, recent studies suggest that persistent activation of muscarinic receptors can prevent the normal inhibitory action of adenosine on certain hippocampal neurons. This excitatory cholinergic action can be prevented by therapeutic concentrations of lithium, as would be predicted from the proposed mechanism of selective depression.

Studies of noradrenergic effects in isolated brain tissue indicate that lithium can inhibit norepinephrine-sensitive adenylyl cyclase. Such an effect could relate to both its antidepressant and antimanic effects. The relationship of these effects to lithium's actions on IP_3 mechanisms is currently unknown.

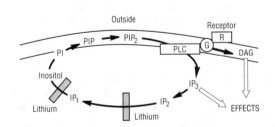

Figure 28–3. Effect of lithium on the IP_3 and DAG second messenger system. The schematic diagram shows the synaptic membrane of a neuron. (PIP_2, phosphatidylinositol-4,5-bisphosphate; PLC, phospholipase-C; G, coupling protein; EFFECTS, activation of protein kinase C, mobilization of intracellular Ca^{2+}, etc.) Lithium, by inhibiting the recycling of inositol substrates, may cause the depletion of the second messenger source PIP_2 and therefore reduce the release of IP_3 and DAG. Lithium may also act by other mechanisms.

CLINICAL PHARMACOLOGY OF LITHIUM

Bipolar Affective Disorder

Agreement is almost universal that lithium carbonate is the preferred treatment for bipolar disorder, especially in the manic phase. Because its onset of action is slow, concurrent use of antipsychotic drugs may be required for severely manic patients. The overall success rate for achieving remission from the manic phase of bipolar disorder has been reported to be 60–80%. However, among patients who require hospitalization, success rates are considerably lower. A similar situation applies to maintenance treatment, which is about 60% effective overall but less in severely ill patients. These considerations have led to increased use of combined treatment in severe cases.

When mania is mild, lithium alone may be effective treatment. In more severe cases, it is almost always necessary to give one of the antipsychotic drugs also. After mania is controlled, the antipsychotic drug may be stopped and lithium continued as maintenance therapy.

The depressive phase of manic-depressive disorder requires concurrent use of an antidepressant drug (Chapter 29). Tricyclic antidepressant agents have been linked to precipitation of mania, with more rapid cycling of mood swings. Nevertheless, the tricyclic antidepressants may still be first-choice agents, as this unwanted effect occurs in only a few cases. It is difficult to choose among the newer antidepressants, because most of them may also activate mania. Carbamazepine may be useful in such situations or in patients whose manic episodes are not controlled by lithium alone.

Unlike antipsychotic or antidepressant drugs, which exert several actions on the central or autonomic nervous system, lithium ion produces only mild sedation and is devoid of autonomic blocking effects. Since it is a small inorganic ion, lithium is distributed in body water and is not metabolized. It is easily measured in body fluids such as plasma, urine, or saliva. Thus, its kinetics can be studied easily, and plasma or tissue concentrations can be correlated with clinical effects.

Another attribute of considerable interest has been the prophylactic use of lithium in preventing both mania and depression. It is indeed remarkable that a so-called functional psychosis can be controlled so easily by such a simple chemical as lithium carbonate.

Other Applications

Acute endogenous depression is not generally considered to be an indication for treatment with lithium. However, recurrent endogenous depressions with a cyclic pattern are controlled by either lithium or imipramine, both of which are superior to a placebo.

Schizoaffective disorders are characterized by a mixture of schizophrenic symptoms and altered affect in the form of depression or excitement. Antipsychotic drugs alone or combined with lithium are used in the excited phase; tricyclic antidepressants are used if depression is present.

Alcoholism is commonly believed to have a high association with bipolar illness. When the two conditions coexist, lithium may be useful in reducing drinking. Lithium has no established efficacy in the absence of affective symptoms.

While lithium alone is rarely successful in treating schizophrenia, adding it to an antipsychotic may salvage an otherwise treatment-resistant patient. Carbamazepine may work equally well when added to an antipsychotic.

An interesting application of lithium currently being investigated is the management of aggressive, violent behavior in prisoners. This indication, while potentially important, does not have strong scientific support.

Dosage Schedules

Before treatment is started, one should obtain laboratory data such as a complete blood count, urinalysis, common biochemical tests, and an ECG in older patients and those with a history of cardiac disorders. These tests serve as baseline measurements in assessing possible complications of treatment.

The patient's age, body weight, and renal function should be considered in determining appropriate initial doses of lithium carbonate. The initial volume of distribution of lithium will be the same as that of body water, or about 0.5–0.6 L/kg body weight for women and 0.55–0.7 L/kg for men. As lithium is excreted solely by the kidneys, the dosage should be reduced if creatinine clearance is impaired, as it may be in elderly patients.

A daily lithium dose of 0.5 meq/kg will produce the desired serum lithium concentration in the range of 0.6–1.4 meq/L after a week of treatment if renal function is normal. Each 300 mg dose unit of lithium carbonate contains approximately 8 meq of lithium. Daily doses of lithium may range between 600 and 3600 mg among different individuals. The majority require between 1500 and 1800 mg/d.

It is almost always necessary to give lithium in divided doses to avoid gastric distress. Medication is best taken with or shortly after meals. Slow-release dosage forms may also be tried.

Monitoring Treatment

Clinicians have relied heavily on measurements of serum concentrations for assessing both the dosage required for satisfactory treatment of acute mania and the adequacy of maintenance treatment. These measurements are customarily taken 10–12 hours after the last dose, so all data in the literature pertaining to these concentrations reflect this interval.

An initial determination of serum lithium concentration should be obtained about 5 days after the start of treatment, at which time steady state conditions should obtain for the dosage chosen. If the clinical response suggests a change in dosage, simple arithmetic (new dose equals present dose times desired blood level divided by present blood level) should produce the desired level. The serum concentration attained with the adjusted dosage can be checked in another 5 days. Once the desired concentration has been achieved, levels can be measured at increasing intervals unless the schedule is influenced by intercurrent illness or the introduction of a new drug into the treatment program.

Maintenance Treatment

The decision to use lithium as *prophylactic* treatment depends on many factors: the frequency and severity of previous episodes, a crescendo pattern of appearance, and the degree to which the patient is willing to follow a program of indefinite maintenance therapy. If the present attack was the patient's first or if the patient is unreliable, one might prefer to terminate treatment after the attack has subsided. Patients who have one or more episodes of illness per year are candidates for maintenance treatment. While some patients can be maintained with serum levels as low as 0.6 meq/L, the best results in groups of patients have been obtained with higher levels, such as 0.9 meq/L.

Drug Interactions

Renal clearance of lithium is reduced about 25% by diuretics (eg, thiazides), and doses may need to be reduced by a similar amount. A similar reduction in lithium clearance has been noted with several of the newer nonsteroidal anti-inflammatory drugs that block synthesis of prostaglandins. This interaction has not been reported for either aspirin or acetaminophen. All neuroleptics may produce more severe extrapyramidal syndromes when combined with lithium.

Adverse Effects & Complications

Many adverse effects associated with lithium treatment occur at varying times after treatment is started. Some are harmless, but it is important to be alert to adverse effects that may signify impending serious toxic reactions.

A. Neurologic and Psychiatric Adverse Effects: Tremor is one of the most frequent adverse effects of lithium treatment, occurring at therapeutic dosage levels. Propranolol, which has been reported to be effective in essential tremor, also alleviates lithium-induced tremor. Other reported neurologic abnormalities include choreoathetosis, motor hyperactivity, ataxia, dysarthria, and aphasia. Psychiatric disturbances are generally marked by mental confusion and withdrawal or bizarre motor movements. Appearance of any new neurologic or psychiatric symptoms or signs is a clear indication for temporarily stopping treatment with lithium and close monitoring of serum levels.

B. Effects on Thyroid Function: Lithium probably decreases thyroid function in most patients exposed to the drug, but the effect is reversible or nonprogressive. Few patients develop frank thyroid enlargement, and fewer still show symptoms of hypothyroidism. Although initial thyroid testing with regular monitoring of thyroid function has been proposed, such procedures are not cost-effective.

C. Renal Adverse Effects: Polydipsia and polyuria are frequent but reversible concomitants of lithium treatment, occurring at therapeutic serum concentrations. The principal physiologic lesion involved is loss of the ability of the collecting tubule to conserve water under the influence of antidiuretic hormone, resulting in excessive free water clearance (**nephrogenic diabetes insipidus**). Lithium-induced diabetes insipidus is resistant to vasopressin but responds to amiloride.

An extensive literature has accumulated concerning other forms of renal dysfunction during long-term lithium therapy, including **chronic interstitial nephritis** and **minimal change glomerulopathy** with nephrotic syndrome. Some instances of decreased glomerular filtration rate have been encountered but no instances of marked azotemia or renal failure.

Patients receiving lithium should avoid dehydration and the associated increased concentration of lithium in urine. Periodic tests of renal concentrating ability should be performed to detect changes.

D. Edema: Edema is a frequent adverse effect of lithium treatment and may be related to some effect of lithium on sodium retention. Although weight gain may be expected in patients who become edematous, water retention alone probably does not account for all of it.

E. Cardiac Adverse Effects: The bradycardia-tachycardia ("sick sinus") syndrome is a definite contraindication to the use of lithium because the ion further depresses the sinus node. T wave flattening is often observed on the ECG but is of questionable significance.

F. Use During Pregnancy: Renal clearance of lithium increases during pregnancy and reverts to lower levels immediately after delivery. A patient whose serum lithium concentration is in a good therapeutic range during pregnancy may develop toxic levels following delivery. Special care in monitoring lithium levels is needed at these times. Lithium is transferred to nursing children through breast milk, in which it has a concentration about one-third to one-half that of serum. Lithium toxicity in newborns is manifested by lethargy, cyanosis, poor suck and Moro reflexes, and perhaps hepatomegaly.

The issue of dysmorphogenesis is not settled. One report suggests an alarming increase in the frequency of cardiac anomalies, especially Ebstein's anomaly, in lithium babies.

G. Miscellaneous Adverse Effects: Transient acneiform eruptions have been noted early in lithium treatment. Some of them subside with temporary discontinuance of treatment and do not recur with its resumption. Folliculitis is less dramatic and probably occurs more frequently. Leukocytosis is always present during lithium treatment, probably reflecting a direct effect on leukopoiesis rather than mobilization from the marginal pool. This "adverse effect" has now become a therapeutic effect in patients with low leukocyte counts. Disturbed sexual function has been reported in men treated with lithium.

Overdoses

Therapeutic overdoses are more common than those due to deliberate or accidental ingestion of the drug. Therapeutic overdoses are usually due to accumulation of lithium resulting from some change in the patient's status, such as diminished serum sodium, use of diuretics, fluctuating renal function, or pregnancy. Since the tissues will have already equilibrated with the blood, the plasma concentrations of lithium may not be excessively high in proportion to the degree of toxicity; any value over 2 meq/L must be considered as indicating potential toxicity. As lithium is a small ion, it is dialyzed readily. Both peritoneal dialysis and hemodialysis are effective, though the latter is preferred. Dialysis should be continued until the plasma concentrations fall below the usual therapeutic range.

CARBAMAZEPINE

Carbamazepine has emerged as a reasonable alternative to lithium when the latter is less than optimal. It may be used to treat acute mania and also for prophylactic therapy. Adverse effects are no greater and sometimes are less than those associated with lithium. It may be used alone or, in refractory patients, in combination with lithium. The mode of action of carbamazepine is unclear, but it may reduce the sensitization of the brain to repeated episodes of mood swing. Such a mechanism might be similar to its anticonvulsant effect.

The use of carbamazepine as a mood stabilizer is similar to its use as an anticonvulsant (see Chapter 23). Dosage usually begins with 200 mg twice daily with increases as needed. Maintenance dosage is similar to that used for treating epilepsy, ie, 800–1200 mg/d. Plasma concentrations between 3 and 14 mg/L are considered desirable, though no therapeutic range has been established. Although blood dyscrasias have figured prominently in the adverse effects of carbamazepine when it is used as an anticonvulsant, they have not been a major problem with its use as a mood stabilizer. Overdoses of the drug are a major emergency and should be managed in general like overdoses of tricyclic antidepressants.

VALPROIC ACID & CLONAZEPAM

These agents have not been as fully studied as lithium and carbamazepine in the treatment of bipolar disorder. Preliminary studies suggest that sodium valproate is useful in the prophylaxis of recurrences. Like carbamazepine, it is administered as in epilepsy, with dosage starting at 100 mg 3 or 4 times daily and increasing gradually to antiepileptic levels. Clonazepam is considered inadequate as monotherapy by most authors but appears to be of prophylactic value in some cases not adequately controlled by lithium alone. It is used in the conventional anticonvulsant dosage of 0.5–20 mg/d.

PREPARATIONS AVAILABLE

Antipsychotic Agents
Acetophenazine (Tindal) Oral: 20 mg tablets
Chlorpromazine (generic, Thorazine, others)
Oral: 10, 25, 50, 100, 200 mg tablets; 10 mg/5 mL syrup; 30, 100 mg/mL concentrate
Oral sustained-release: 30, 75, 150, 200, 300 mg capsules
Rectal: 25, 100 mg suppositories
Parenteral: 25 mg/mL for IM injection
Chlorprothixene (Taractan)
Oral: 10, 25, 50, 100 mg tablets; 100 mg/5 mL concentrate
Parenteral: 12.5 mg/mL for IM injection
Clozapine (Clozaril)
Oral: 25, 100 mg tablets
Fluphenazine (generic, Permitil, Prolixin)
Oral: 1, 2.5, 5, 10 mg tablets; 2.5 mg/5 mL elixir; 5 mg/mL concentrate
Parenteral: 2.5 mg/mL for IM injection
Fluphenazine esters (generic [decanoate only], Prolixin Enanthate, Prolixin Decanoate)
Parenteral: 25 mg/mL
Haloperidol (generic, Haldol)
Oral: 0.5, 1, 2, 5, 10, 20 mg tablets; 2 mg/mL concentrate
Parenteral: 5 mg/mL for IM injection
Haloperidol ester (Haldol Decanoate)
Parenteral: 50, 100 mg/mL for IM injection
Loxapine (Loxitane)
Oral: 5, 10, 25, 50 mg capsules; 25 mg/mL concentrate
Parenteral: 50 mg/mL for IM injection
Mesoridazine (Serentil)
Oral: 10, 25, 50, 100 mg tablets; 25 mg/mL concentrate
Parenteral: 25 mg/mL for IM injection
Molindone (Moban)
Oral: 5, 10, 25, 50, 100 mg tablets; 20 mg/mL concentrate
Perphenazine (generic, Trilafon)
Oral: 2, 4, 8, 16 mg tablets; 16 mg/5 mL concentrate

Parenteral: 5 mg/mL for IM or IV injection
Pimozide (Orap)
Oral: 2 mg tablets
Prochlorperazine (generic, Compazine)
Oral: 5, 10, 25 mg tablets; 5 mg/5 mL syrup
Oral sustained-release: 10, 15, 30 mg capsules
Rectal: 2.5, 5, 25 mg suppositories
Parenteral: 5 mg/mL for IM injection
Promazine (generic, Sparine)
Oral: 25, 50, 100 mg tablets
Parenteral: 25, 50 mg/mL for IM injection
Risperidone (Risperdal)
Oral: 1, 2, 3, 4 mg tablets
Thioridazine (generic, Mellaril, others)
Oral: 10, 15, 25, 50, 100, 150, 200 mg tablets; 30, 100 mg/mL concentrate; 25, 100 mg/5 mL suspension
Thiothixene (generic, Navane)
Oral: 1, 2, 5, 10, 20 mg capsules; 5 mg/mL concentrate
Parenteral: 2 mg/mL for IM injection; powder to reconstitute for 5 mg/mL for injection
Trifluoperazine (generic, Stelazine, Suprazine)
Oral: 1, 2, 5, 10 mg tablets; 10 mg/mL concentrate
Parenteral: 2 mg/mL for IM injection
Triflupromazine (Vesprin)
Parenteral: 10, 20 mg/mL for IM injection

Mood Stabilizers
Carbamazepine (generic, Tegretol)
Oral: 200 mg tablets, 100 mg chewable tablets; 100 mg/5 mL oral suspension.
Clonazepam (Klonopin)
Oral: 0.5, 1, 2 mg tablets
Lithium carbonate(generic, Eskalith) (*Note:* 300 mg lithium carbonate = 8.12 meq Li$^+$.)
Oral: 150, 300, 600 mg capsules; 300 mg tablets; 8 meq/5 mL syrup
Oral sustained-release: 300, 450 mg tablets
Valproic acid (generic, Depakene)
Oral: 250 mg capsules; 250 mg/5 mL oral syrup

REFERENCES

Antipsychotics

Ad Hoc Committee on Schizophrenia: Friedhoff AJ et al: Report on schizophrenia of the American College of Neuropsychopharmacology. Neuropsychopharmacology 1987;1:89.

Baldessarini RJ, Frankenburg FR: Clozapine: A novel antipsychotic agent. N Engl J Med 1991;324:746.

Deutsch AY et al: Mechanisms of action of atypical antipsychotic drugs: Implications for novel therapeutic strategies for schizophrenia. Schizophr Res 1991; 4:121.

Dickey W. The neuroleptic malignant syndrome. Prog Neurobiol 1991;36:423.

Farde L et al: Central D_2-dopamine receptor occupancy in schizophrenic patients treated with antipsychotic drugs. Arch Gen Psychiatry 1987;45:71.

Gingrich JA, Caron MG: Recent advances in the molecular biology of dopamine receptors. Annu Rev Neurosci 1993;16:299.

Grace AA: Phasic versus tonic dopamine release and the modulation of dopamine system responsivity: A hypothesis for the etiology of schizophrenia. Neuroscience 1991;41:1.

Hashimoto F, Sherma CB, Jeffery WH: Neuroleptic malignant syndrome and dopaminergic blockade. Arch Intern Med 1984;144:629.

Healy D: D_1 and D_2 and D_3. Br J Psychiatry 1991; 159:319.

Hollister LE, Csernansky JG: Antipsychotic drugs. In: *Clinical Pharmacology of Psychotherapeutic Drugs,* 3rd ed. Churchill Livingstone, 1990.

Jacobsen E: The early history of psychotherapeutic drugs. Psychopharmacology 1986;89:138.

Kane JM et al: Clozapine for the treatment of treatment-resistant schizophrenia: Results of a US multicenter trial. Psychopharmacology 1989;99:560.

Lehmann HE, Wilson WH, Deutsch M: Minimal maintenance medication: Effects of three dose schedules on relapse rates and symptoms in chronic schizophrenic outpatients. Compr Psychiatry 1983;24:293.

Pickar D et al: Longitudinal measurement of plasma homovanillic acid levels in schizophrenic patients: Correlation with psychosis and response to neuroleptic treatment. Arch Gen Psychiatry 1986;43:669.

Reynolds GP: Beyond the dopamine hypothesis: The neurochemical pathology of schizophrenia. Br J Psychiatry 1989;155:305.

Seeman P: Dopamine receptors and the dopamine hypothesis of schizophrenia. Synapse 1987;1:133.

Sibley DR, Monsma FJ Jr: Molecular biology of dopamine receptors. Trends Pharmacol Sci 1992; 13:61.

Sokoloff P et al: Molecular cloning and characterization of a novel dopamine receptor (D_3) as a target for neuroleptics. Nature 1990;347:146.

Tarsy D, Baldessarini RJ: The pathophysiologic basis of tardive dyskinesia. Biol Psychiatry 1977;12:431.

Thompson LT, Moran MG, Nies AS: Psychotropic drug use in the elderly. (Two parts.) N Engl J Med 1983;308:134, 194.

Tricklebank MD, Bristow LJ, Hutson PH: Alternative approaches to the discovery of novel antipsychotic agents. Prog Drug Res 1992;38:299.

Wong DF et al: Positron emission tomography reveals elevated D_2 dopamine receptors in drug-naive schizophrenics. Science 1986;234:1558.

Mood Stabilizers

Amdisen A: History of lithium. (Letter.) Biol Psychiatry 1987;22:522.

Baraban JM, Worley PF, Snyder SH: Second messenger systems and psychoactive drug action: Focus on the phosphoinositide system and lithium. Am J Psychiatry 1989;146:1251.

Berridge MJ: Inositol trisphosphate, calcium, lithium, and cell signaling. JAMA 1989;262:1834.

Bunney WE Jr, Garland-Bunnery BL: Mechanisms of action of lithium in affective illness: Basic and clinical implications. In: *Psychopharmacology: The Third Generation of Progress.* Meltzer HY (editor) Raven Press, 1987.

Consensus Development Conference: *Mood disorder: Pharmacologic Prevention of Recurrences.* Vol 5, No 4. National Institutes of Health, 1984.

Elphick M: The clinical uses and pharmacology of carbamazepine in psychiatry. Int Clin Psychopharmacol 1988;3:185.

Hodgkinson S: Molecular genetic evidence for heterogeneity in manic depression. Nature 1987;325:805.

Jefferson JW, Greist JH: *Primer of Lithium Therapy.* Williams & Wilkins, 1977.

Kishimoto A et al: Long-term prophylactic effects of carbamazepine in affective disorder. Br J Psychiatry 1983;143:327.

McElroy SL, Keck PE Jr, Pope HG Jr: Sodium valproate: its use in primary psychiatric disorders. J Clin Psychopharmacol 1987;7:16.

Mitchell PB, Parker GB: Treatment of bipolar disorder. Med J Australia 1991;155:488.

Page C, Benaim S, Lappin F: A long-term retrospective follow-up of patients treated with prophylactic lithium carbonate. Br J Psychiatry 1987;150:175.

Post RM et al: Correlates of antimanic response to carbamazepine. Psychiatry Res 1987;21:71.

Prien RF, Galenberg AJ: Alternatives to lithium for preventive treatment of bipolar disorder. Am J Psychiatry 1989;146:840.

Sillence DJ, Downes CP: Lithium treatment of affective disorders: Effects of lithium on the inositol phospholipid and cyclic AMP signalling pathways. Biochim Biophys Acta 1992;1138:46.

VanValkenburg C, Kluznik JC, Merrill R: New uses of anticonvulsant drugs in psychosis. Drugs 1992; 44:326.

Vestergaard P, Amdisen A, Schou M: Clinically significant side effects of lithium treatment: A survey of 237 patients in long-term treatment. Acta Psychiatr Scand 1980;62:193.

Wood AJ, Goodwin GM: A review of the biochemical and neuropharmacological actions of lithium. Psychol Med 1987;17:579.

29

Antidepressant Agents

Leo E. Hollister, MD

Depression is one of the most common psychiatric disorders. At any given moment, about 5–6% of the population is depressed (point prevalence), and an estimated 10% of people may become depressed during their lives (lifetime prevalence). The symptoms of depression are subtle and often unrecognized by both patients and physicians. Patients with vague complaints that resist explanation as manifestations of somatic disorders and those who might be simplistically called "neurotics" should be suspected of being depressed.

Depression is a heterogeneous disorder that has been characterized and classified in a variety of ways. According to the American Psychiatric Association's revised third edition (1987) of the *Diagnostic and Statistical Manual of Mental Disorders (DSM-III-R)*, several diagnoses of affective disorders are possible. Major depression and dysthymia (minor) are pure depressive syndromes, whereas bipolar disorder and cyclothymic disorder signify depression in association with mania. A simplified classification based on presumed origin is as follows: (1) "reactive" or "secondary" depression (most common; over 60%), occurring in response to real stimuli such as grief, illness, etc; (2) "endogenous" depression, a genetically determined biochemical disorder manifested by inability to cope with ordinary stress (about 25%); and (3) depression associated with bipolar affective (manic-depressive) disorder (about 10–15%). Drugs discussed in this chapter are used chiefly in management of the second type. Table 29–1 indicates how the three types may be differentiated.

Psychiatrically depressed patients were treated only with electroconvulsive therapy before the antidepressant drugs became available. These drugs are not central nervous system stimulants and are actually contraindicated in organic or drug-induced central nervous system depression. Studies of the mode of action of antidepressants have largely focused on their effects on various amine neurotransmitters in the brain.

The Pathogenesis of Major Depression: The Amine Hypothesis

Soon after the introduction of reserpine in the early 1950s, it became apparent that the drug could induce depression in patients being treated for hypertension and schizophrenia as well as in normal subjects. Within the next few years, pharmacologic studies revealed that the principal mechanism of action of reserpine was to inhibit the storage of amine neurotransmitters such as serotonin and norepinephrine in the vesicles of presynaptic nerve endings. Reserpine induced depression and depleted stores of amine neurotransmitters; therefore, it was reasoned, depression must be associated with decreased functional amine-dependent transmission. This simple syllogism provided the basis for what became known as the amine hypothesis of depression. A major puzzle in applying this hypothesis was the fact that although the pharmacologic actions of both tricyclic and MAO inhibitor classes of antidepressants are prompt, the clinical effects require weeks or even months to become manifest. Attempts have been made to explain this observation by invoking slow compensatory responses to the initial blockade of reuptake or MAO inhibition (see below).

While the amine hypothesis is undoubtedly too simplistic, it has provided the major experimental models for the discovery of new antidepressant drugs. As a result, all the currently available antidepressant drugs except bupropion have their primary actions on the storage, metabolism, or reuptake of serotonin or norepinephrine.

I. BASIC PHARMACOLOGY OF ANTIDEPRESSANTS

Chemistry

A variety of different chemical structures have been found to have antidepressant activity. The number is constantly growing, but as yet no group has been found to have a clear therapeutic advantage over the others.

A. Tricyclics: (Figure 29–1.) Tricyclic antidepressants—so called because of the characteristic three-ring nucleus—have been used clinically for over three decades. They closely resemble the phenothiazines chemically and, to a lesser extent, phar-

Table 29–1. Differentiation of types of depression.		
Type	**Diagnostic Features**	**Comments**
Reactive	Loss (adverse life events). Physical illness (myocardial infarct, cancer). Drugs (antihypertensives, alcohol, hormones). Other psychiatric disorders (senility).	More than 60% of all depressions. Core depressive syndrome: depression, anxiety, bodily complaints, tension, guilt. May respond spontaneously or to a variety of ministrations.
Major depressive (endogenous)	Precipitating life event not adequate for degree of depression. Autonomous (unresponsive to changes in life). May occur at any age (childhood to old age). Biologically determined (family history).	About 25% of all depressions. Core depressive syndrome plus "vital" signs: abnormal rhythms of sleep, motor activity, libido, appetite. Usually responds specifically to antidepressants or electroconvulsive therapy. Tends to recur throughout life.
Bipolar affective (manic-depressive)	Characterized by episodes of mania. Cyclic; mania alone, rare; depression alone, occasional; mania-depression, usual.	About 10–15% of all depressions. May be misdiagnosed as endogenous if hypomanic episodes are missed. Lithium carbonate stabilizes mood. Mania may require antipsychotic drugs as well; depression managed with antidepressants.

macologically. Like the latter drugs, they were first thought to be useful as antihistamines and later as antipsychotics. The discovery of their antidepressant properties was a fortuitous clinical observation. Imipramine and amitriptyline are the prototypical drugs of the class.

B. Heterocyclics, Second Generation Drugs: Since 1980, a number of new "second-generation" or "heterocyclic" antidepressants have been introduced. Five of these agents are available for clinical use in the USA and four are shown in Figure 29–2. Amoxa-

pine and maprotiline resemble the structure of the tricyclic agents, while trazodone and bupropion are distinctive. The heterocyclic agents are not notably different from the older agents in potency. Venlafaxine is a newer and chemically unrelated second generation agent.

C. Selective Serotonin Reuptake Inhibitors (SSRI): One of the drawbacks of many existing antidepressants has been the multitude of pharmacologic actions, a trait inherited from the phenothiazine antipsychotic agents. As far as we know, the anti-

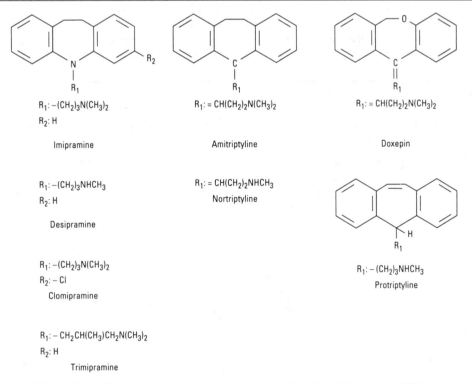

Figure 29–1. Structural relationships between various tricyclic antidepressants (TCA).

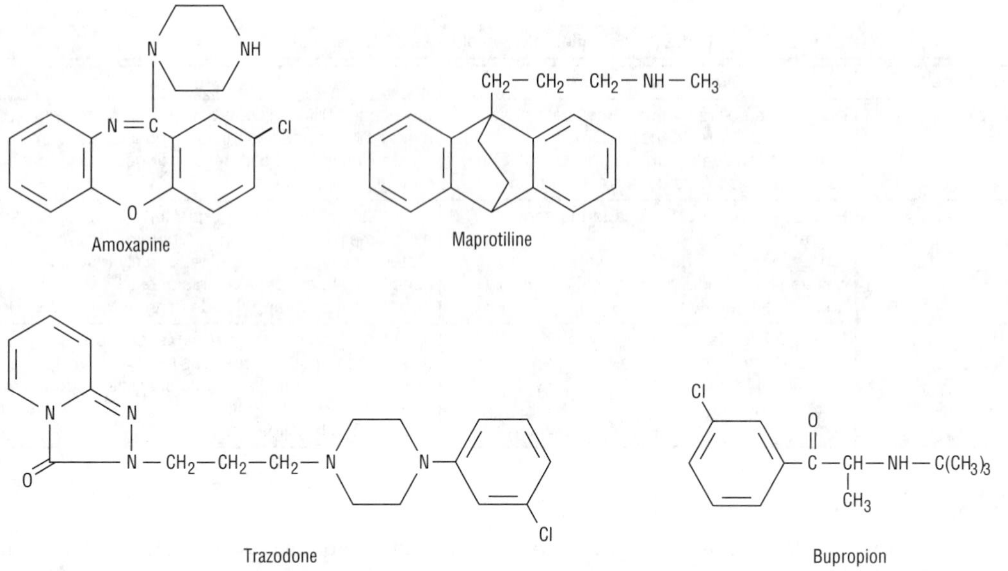

Figure 29–2. Some heterocyclic (second-generation) antidepressants.

muscarinic, antihistaminic, and alpha adrenoceptor-blocking actions of tricyclic antidepressants contribute only to the toxicity of these agents. Ever since it was found that fluoxetine, an antidepressant with minimal autonomic toxicity, was a highly selective serotonin reuptake inhibitor, a major effort has been under way to find molecules with similar actions. Three selective serotonin reuptake inhibitors are currently available, and more are undergoing clinical trials. All are clearly unlike the tricyclic molecules (Figure 29–3).

D. Monoamine Oxidase (MAO) Inhibitors: MAO inhibitors may be classified as hydrazides, exemplified by the C–N–N moiety, as in the case of phenelzine and isocarboxazid; or nonhydrazides, which lack such a moiety, as in tranylcypromine (Figure 29–4). Tranylcypromine closely resembles dextroamphetamine, which is itself a weak inhibitor of MAO. Tranylcypromine retains some of the sympathomimetic characteristics of the amphetamines. The hydrazides appear to combine irreversibly with the enzyme, while tranylcypromine has a prolonged

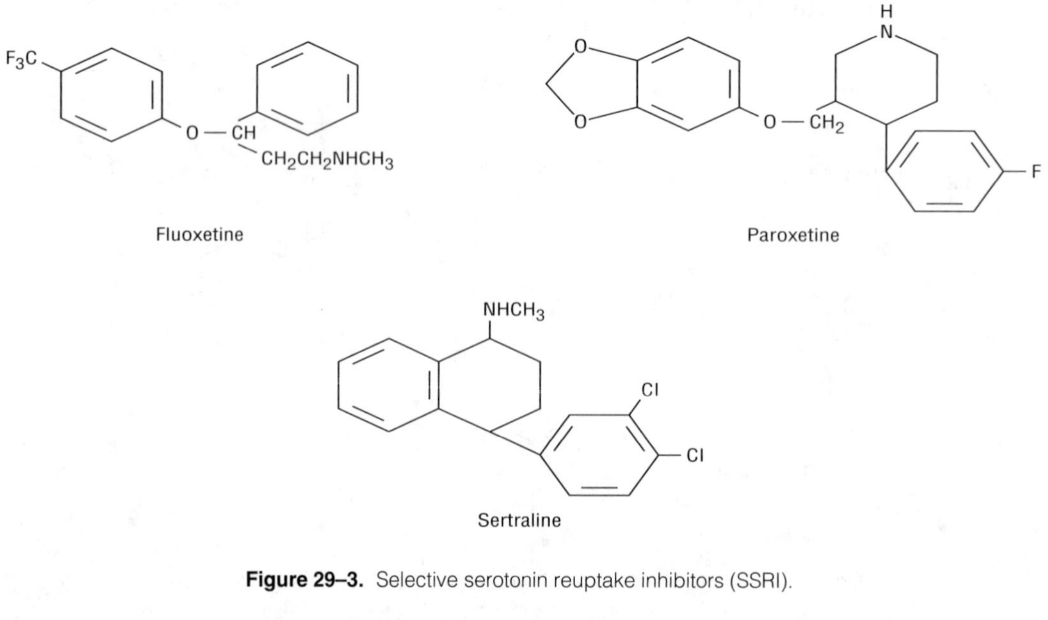

Figure 29–3. Selective serotonin reuptake inhibitors (SSRI).

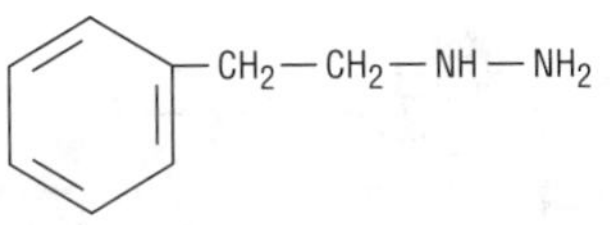

Phenelzine

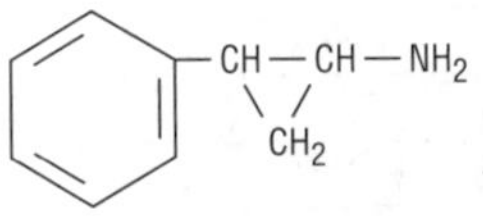

Tranylcypromine

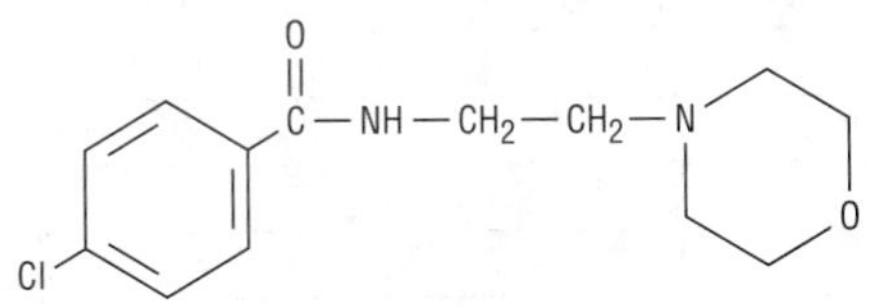

Moclobemide

Figure 29–4. Some monoamine oxidase inhibitors. Phenelzine is the hydrazide of phenylethylamine (Figure 9–3), while tranylcypromine has a cyclopropyl amine side chain and closely resembles dextroamphetamine (see Figure 9–4). These agents are unselective and produce an extremely long-lasting inhibition of the enzyme. Moclobemide is a new short-acting reversible inhibitor of MAO-A (RIMA) and bears the least structural resemblance to sympathomimetics.

duration of effect even though it is not bound irreversibly. These older MAO inhibitors are nonselective inhibitors of both MAO-A and MAO-B. Moclobemide is a new, short-acting, selective MAO-A inhibitor. Though not yet available, it appears likely to be approved in the near future. Many similar reversible inhibitors of MAO-A (RIMAs) are under study.

E. Sympathomimetic Stimulants: Dextroamphetamine, other amphetamines, and amphetamine surrogates such as methylphenidate are occasionally used as antidepressants. Although the action of amphetamines in blocking MAO has generally been regarded as too weak to confer significant antidepressant action, it may contribute to an antidepressant action in some people.

Pharmacokinetics

A. Tricyclics: Most tricyclics are incompletely absorbed and undergo significant first-pass metabolism. As a result of high protein binding and relatively high lipid solubility, volumes of distribution tend to be very large. Tricyclics are metabolized by two major routes: transformation of the tricyclic nucleus and alteration of the aliphatic side chain. The former route involves ring hydroxylation and conjugation to form glucuronides; the latter, primarily demethylation of

the nitrogen. Monodemethylation of tertiary amines leads to active metabolites, such as desipramine and nortriptyline (which are themselves available as drugs; Figure 29–1). The proportion of monodemethylated metabolites formed varies from one patient to another. In general, the proportion of amitriptyline to its metabolite nortriptyline favors the parent drug. The converse is the case with imipramine and its metabolite desipramine. The pharmacokinetic parameters of various antidepressants are summarized in Table 29–2.

B. Heterocyclics: The pharmacokinetics of these drugs and of the tricyclics are similar. As can be seen from Table 29–2, data are less complete for these agents. Still, they tend to have variable bioavailability, high protein binding, variable and large volumes of distribution, and, perhaps, active metabolites. Trazodone and venlafaxine have the shortest plasma half-lives, which mandates divided doses during the day.

C. Selective Serotonin Reuptake Inhibitors (SSRIs): The pharmacokinetic parameters of these drugs are summarized in Table 29–2. Fluoxetine is well absorbed, and peak plasma concentrations are attained within 4–8 hours. Its demethylated active metabolite, norfluoxetine, has a half-life of 7–9 days at steady state; the parent drug has a slightly shorter half-life. Fluoxetine inhibits various drug-metabolizing enzymes, which has led to a number of significant drug-drug interactions with other antidepressants and with other drugs as well. Sertraline and paroxetine have pharmacokinetic parameters similar to those of tricyclics.

D. MAO Inhibitors: The MAO inhibitors are readily absorbed from the gastrointestinal tract. The hydrazide inhibitors (phenelzine and isocarboxazid) are acetylated in the liver and manifest differences in elimination depending on the acetylation phenotype of the individual (see Chapter 4). However, inhibition of MAO persists even after the older MAO inhibitors are no longer detectable in plasma. Therefore, conventional pharmacokinetic parameters (half-life, etc) are not very helpful in governing dosage. Instead, measuring the inhibition of MAO activity has been used to predict the level of effect, though such measurements are not employed clinically. In practice, it is prudent to assume that the effect will persist for from 7 days (tranylcypromine) to 2 or 3 weeks (phenelzine, isocarboxazid) after discontinuance of the drug. Moclobemide is rapidly absorbed and excreted, with over 90% of the drug appearing as metabolites in the urine within 12 hours.

Pharmacodynamics

A. Action of Antidepressants on Biogenic Amine Neurotransmitters: The amine hypothesis was buttressed by studies on the mechanism of action of various types of antidepressant drugs (Figure 29–5). Tricyclics block the amine (norepinephrine or

Table 29–2. Pharmacokinetic parameters of various antidepressants.[1]

Drug	Bioavailability (percent)	Protein Binding (percent)	Plasma $t_{1/2}$ (hours)	Active Metabolites	Volume of Distribution (L/kg)	Therapeutic Plasma Concentrations (ng/mL)
Amitriptyline	31–61	82–96	31–46	Nortriptyline	5–10	80–200 total
Amoxapine	nd	nd	8	7-,8-Hydroxy	nd	nd
Bupropion	60–80	85	11–14	?	20–30	25–100
Clomipramine	nd	nd	22–84	Desmethyl	7–20	240–700
Desipramine	60–70	73–90	14–62	nd	22–59	145[2]
Doxepin	13–45	nd	8–24	Desmethyl	9–33	30–150
Fluoxetine	70	94	24–96	Norfluoxetine	12–97	nd
Imipramine	29–77	76–95	9–24	Desipramine	15–30	>180 total
Maprotiline	66–75	88	21–52	Desmethyl	15–28	200–300
Nortripyline	32–79	93–95	18–93	10-Hydroxy	21–57	50–150
Paroxetine	50	95	24	None	28–31	nd
Protriptyline	77–93	90–95	54–198	nd	19–57	70–170
Sertraline	nd	98	22–35	Desmethyl	20	nd
Trazodone	nd	nd	4–9	m-Chlorophenyl-piperazine	nd	nd

[1]nd = no data.
[2]Lower concentrations may be effective, but no data are available.

serotonin) reuptake pumps, the "off switches" of amine neurotransmission (see Table 29–2 and Chapter 6). Such an action presumably permits a longer sojourn of neurotransmitter at the receptor site. MAO inhibitors block a major degradative pathway for the amine neurotransmitters, which permits more amines to accumulate in presynaptic stores and more to be released. Amphetamine-like sympathomimetics also block the amine pump but are thought to act chiefly by increasing the release of catecholamine neurotransmitters. Thus, these three classes of antidepressant drugs might remedy a deficiency in amine neurotransmission, though by somewhat different mechanisms. Some of the second-generation antidepressants have similar effects on amine neurotransmitters, while others have mild or minimal effects. The apparent ability of trazodone and selective serotonin reuptake inhibitors to block serotonin uptake by nerve endings without inhibiting norepinephrine uptake contrasts with the ability of most of the tricyclic agents to block norepinephrine uptake at doses that have negligible effects on serotonin uptake. Since both groups of drugs are antidepressant, a dual mechanism, involving both transmitter systems, is suggested. It has been postulated that norepinephrine is the final common pathway and that serotonin uptake inhibition interacts with this system to produce a similar result.

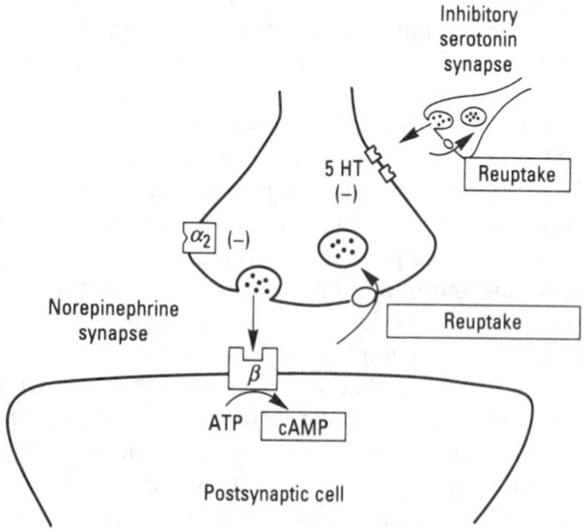

B. Receptor and Postreceptor Effects: More attention has recently been paid to the ultimate effects of the increase in neurotransmitter in the synapse on postsynaptic receptors. In tests of postsynaptic activity, cAMP concentrations have consistently decreased rather than increased. In addition, the number of postsynaptic beta adrenoceptors also shows a measurable decrease that follows the same delayed time course as clinical improvement in patients. Thus, the initial increase in neurotransmitter appears to produce, over time, a compensatory decrease in receptor activity, ie, down-regulation of receptors. Decreases in norepinephrine-stimulated cAMP and in beta-ad-

Figure 29–5. Schematic diagram showing some of the potential sites of action of antidepressant drugs. Chronic therapy with these drugs has been proved to reduce reuptake of norepinephrine or serotonin (or both), reduce the number of postsynaptic beta receptors, and reduce the generation of cAMP. The MAO inhibitors act on MAO in the nerve terminals and cause the same effects on beta receptors and cAMP generation.

renoceptor binding have been conclusively shown for selective norepinephrine uptake inhibitors, those with mixed action on norepinephrine and serotonin, monoamine oxidase inhibitors, and even electroconvulsive therapy. To a lesser extent, such findings have been reported for selective serotonin uptake inhibitors, α_2-receptor antagonists, and beta agonists. A decrease in serotonin receptor activity has been shown more conclusively for drugs that inhibit serotonin uptake.

Demonstrating alterations in either beta adrenoceptors or serotonin receptors in depressed patients has been difficult. Thus, the relationship of receptor changes produced by drugs to their therapeutic action on depression is still unclear. In the search for an explanation of how antidepressants work, the emphasis has shifted from the changes in neurotransmitters to the subsequent alterations in receptor function.

C. Effects of Specific Antidepressants:

1. Tricyclics–The first generation antidepressants demonstrate varying degrees of selectivity for the reuptake pumps for norepinephrine and serotonin (Table 29–3). A characteristic electrophysiologic effect is a prompt reduction of firing rate in central noradrenergic neurons. This is followed later (when the clinical response is becoming manifest) by a return to normal or above-normal firing frequency. They also have numerous autonomic actions, as described below under Adverse Effects.

2. Heterocyclics–Amoxapine is a metabolite of the antipsychotic drug loxapine and retains some of its antipsychotic action. A combination of antidepressant and antipsychotic actions might make it a suitable drug for depression in psychotic patients. However, the antipsychotic action may cause akathisia, parkinsonism, amenorrhea-galactorrhea syndrome, and perhaps tardive dyskinesia.

Maprotiline (a "tetracyclic" drug) is most like desipramine, including some structural resemblance. Like the latter drug, it may have fewer sedative and antimuscarinic actions than the older tricyclics.

Clinical experience with trazodone has indicated unpredictable efficacy: Some patients do remarkably well, while others obtain scarcely any benefit.

Bupropion has a chemical structure reminiscent of amphetamine and cathinone, a central stimulant much used in the Middle East (in the form of khat). At high doses, bupropion inhibits the dopamine reuptake pump in central neurons in animals. It may work primarily through dopaminergic effects.

3. Selective Serotonin Reuptake Inhibitors–Fluoxetine was the first SSRI to reach general clinical use. Paroxetine and sertraline differ mainly in having somewhat shorter half-lives. While they have not been shown to be more effective overall than prior drugs, they lack many of the toxicities of the tricyclics and other antidepressants. Thus, patient acceptance has been high despite new adverse effects such as headache, nausea, and restlessness.

An important pharmacodynamic interaction may occur when fluoxetine or one of the newer selective serotonin reuptake inhibitors is used in the presence of a monoamine oxidase inhibitor. The combination of increased stores of the monoamine plus inhibited reuptake after release are thought to result in marked increases of serotonin in the synapses, leading to a **"serotonin syndrome."** This syndrome includes hyperthermia, muscle rigidity, myoclonus, and rapid changes in mental status and vital signs.

4. MAO inhibitors–MAO-A is the amine oxidase primarily responsible for norepinephrine, serotonin, and tyramine metabolism. MAO-B is more selective for dopamine. If noradrenergic and serotonergic synapses—but not dopaminergic ones—are involved in depression, selective block of MAO-A might be more selective for this condition. Furthermore, irreversible block of MAO, characteristic of the older MAO inhibitors, allows significant accumulation of tyramine and loss of the first-pass metabolism that protects against tyramine in foods. As a result, the irreversible MAO inhibitors are subject to a very high risk of hypertensive reactions to tyramine ingested in food. From the evidence available to date, the reversible, short-acting MAO inhibitor moclobemide appears to be relatively free of this interaction. (The selective MAO-B inhibitor selegiline loses selectivity at antidepressant dosage. Because its action is on the enzyme that metabolizes dopamine, it is most useful in the treatment of Parkinson's disease [see Chapter 27].)

II. CLINICAL PHARMACOLOGY OF ANTIDEPRESSANTS

Clinical Indications

The major indication for these drugs is to treat depression, but a number of other uses have been established by clinical experience.

A. Depression: This indication has been kept broad deliberately, even though evidence from clinical studies strongly suggests that the drugs are specifically useful only in major depressive episodes. Major depressive episodes are diagnosed not so much by their severity as by their quality. Formerly, they were referred to as "endogenous," "vital," or "vegetative"—reflecting the characteristic disturbances of major body rhythms of sleep, hunger and appetite, sexual drive, and motor activity. The diagnosis of major depression may be uncertain in individual patients, so that on balance this condition is underdiagnosed and undertreated.

B. Panic disorder: Imipramine was first shown in 1962 to have a beneficial effect in the acute episodes of anxiety that have come to be known as panic attacks. Recent studies have shown it to be as effective as MAO inhibitors and benzodiazepines. In general, the latter drugs are preferred, as they are better tolerated and their clinical effects become evident promptly.

C. Obsessive-Compulsive Disorders: The serotonin reuptake inhibitors have been exploited for treating these disorders. Recent studies have focused on fluoxetine and other selective serotonin reuptake inhibiting drugs.

D. Enuresis: Enuresis is an established indication for tricyclics. Proof of efficacy for this indication is substantial, but drug therapy is not the preferred approach. The beneficial effect of drug treatment lasts only as long as drug treatment is continued.

E. Chronic Pain: Clinicians in pain clinics have found tricyclics to be especially useful for treating a variety of chronically painful states that often cannot be definitively diagnosed. Whether such painful states represent depressive equivalents or whether such patients become secondarily depressed after some initial pain-producing insult is not clear. It is even possible that the tricyclics work directly on pain pathways. Phenothiazines are also sometimes used in combination.

F. Other Indications: Less well established indications for antidepressants are eating disorders, such as bulimia and anorexia nervosa, cataplexy associated with narcolepsy, school phobia, and attention deficit disorder.

Drug Choice

Controlled comparisons of the available antidepressants have usually led to the conclusion that they are roughly equivalent drugs. Although this may be true for groups of patients, individual patients may for uncertain reasons fare better on one drug than on another. Thus, finding the right drug for the individual patient must be accomplished empirically. The past history of the patient's drug experience is the most valuable guide. At times such a history may lead to the exclusion of tricyclics, as in the case of patients who have responded well in the past to MAO inhibitors.

Antidepressant drugs are apt to be most successful in patients with clearly "vegetative" characteristics, including psychomotor retardation, sleep disturbance, poor appetite and weight loss, and loss of libido.

Tricyclic and heterocyclic agents differ mainly in the degree of sedation (amitriptyline, doxepin, and trazodone cause the most, protriptyline the least) and the amount of antimuscarinic effects (amitriptyline and doxepin have the greatest, trazodone the least) (Table 29–3). Although it is often argued that more sedative drugs are preferable for markedly anxious or agitated depressives while the least sedative drugs are preferable for patients with psychomotor withdrawal, this hypothesis has not been tested.

None of the heterocyclic antidepressants have been shown to be more effective overall than the tricyclics with which they have been compared. The major claims are (1) a faster onset of action, (2) less adverse sedative and autonomic effects, and (3) less toxicity when overdoses are taken. Solid evidence to support a claim of more rapid onset of action has been difficult to obtain. Amoxapine and maprotiline seem to have as many sedative and autonomic actions as most tricyclics; some of the other drugs, such as trazodone, bupropion, and fluoxetine, have fewer. Amoxapine and maprotiline are at least as dangerous as the tricyclics when taken in overdoses; the other newer agents seem to be safer.

No special indications for particular types of de-

Table 29–3. Pharmacologic differences among several antidepressants.[1]

Drug	Sedative	Antimuscarinic	Block of Amine Pump for: Serotonin	Block of Amine Pump for: Norepinephrine	Block of Amine Pump for: Dopamine
Amitriptyline	+++	+++	+++	+	0
Amoxapine	++	++	+	++	+
Bupropion	0	0	+,0	+,0	?
Desipramine	+	+	0	+++	0
Doxepin	+++	+++	++	+	0
Fluoxetine	+	+	+++	0,+	0,+
Imipramine	++	++	+++	++	0
Maprotiline	++	++	0	+++	0
Nortriptyline	++	++	+++	++	0
Paroxetine	+	0	+++	0	0
Protriptyline	0	++	?	+++	?
Sertraline	+	0	+++	0	0
Trazodone	+++	0	++	0	0

[1]0 = none; + = slight; ++ = moderate; +++ = high; ? = uncertain.

pression have been found for the selective serotonin reuptake inhibitors. As yet, there is no way to determine which depression might be due to an underlying abnormality of serotonergic versus noradrenergic neurotransmission. The popularity of these drugs, despite their higher cost, is due principally to their greater acceptance by patients. The early claims by some that fluoxetine use increased suicidal or aggressive ideation or behavior remain to be documented; such thoughts are part of the depressive syndrome.

MAO inhibitors are helpful in patients described as having "atypical" depressions—a nonspecific designation scarcely helpful in their identification. Depressed patients with considerable attendant anxiety, phobic features, and hypochondriasis are the ones who respond best to these drugs.

Few clinicians use lithium, an antimanic agent, as primary treatment for depression. However, some have found that lithium along with one of the other antidepressants may achieve a favorable response not obtained by the antidepressant alone. Another potential use of lithium is to prevent relapses of depression.

Dosages

The usual daily dose ranges of antidepressants are shown in Table 29–4. Doses are almost always determined empirically; the patient's acceptance of adverse effects is the usual limiting factor. Tolerance to some of the objectionable effects may develop, so that the usual pattern of treatment has been to start with small doses, increasing either to a predetermined daily dose, or to one that produces relief of depression, or to the maximum tolerated dose. The effective dose of an antidepressant varies widely depending upon many factors.

Table 29–4. Usual daily doses of antidepressant drugs.

Drug	Dose (mg)
Tricyclics	
Amitriptyline	75–200
Clomipramine	75–300
Desipramine	75–200
Doxepin	75–300
Imipramine	75–200
Nortriptyline	75–150
Protriptyline	20–40
Trimipramine	75–200
Second-generation drugs	
Amoxapine	150–300
Bupropion	200–400
Maprotiline	75–300
Trazodone	50–600
Venlafaxine	75–225
Monoamine oxidase inhibitors	
Isocarboxazid	20–50
Phenelzine	45–75
Tranylcypromine	10–30
Selective serotonin reuptake inhibitors	
Fluoxetine	10–60
Paroxetine	20–50
Sertraline	50–200

Dosage Schedules for Treating the Acute Episode

When patients are treated as outpatients, as many can be, initial doses of tricyclics may vary from 10 mg to 75 mg on the first day of treatment, depending on the patient's size and tolerance for the acute effects. Such conservative dosing regimens are not required for hospitalized patients, in whom initial doses should be around 100 mg. After 2 or 3 days at these levels, doses may be increased in increments of 25 mg every second or third day until a maximum daily dose of 150 mg is reached. Such a dose will place most patients within the presumed range of therapeutic plasma concentration of the drug. However, for patients who do not respond at this dosage, further increments up to 300 mg/d may be made.

A similar pattern may be used with most of the heterocyclic drugs and the selective serotonin reuptake inhibitors. Trazodone, which has a short half-life, is often given in two or three doses per day. With fluoxetine, it is customary to begin with a dose of 20 mg/d and maintain this level for several weeks until the patient's response can be estimated. Only infrequently are higher doses needed, and elderly patients may be treated with 20 mg every other day.

Phenelzine has been the most carefully studied of the MAO inhibitors. Approximately 80% inhibition of the enzyme is desirable, a goal usually attained with a dosage of 1 mg/kg/d. Dosages of the other MAO inhibitors should be gradually titrated to levels that produce a mild degree of orthostatic hypotension.

The MAO inhibitors, bupropion, fluoxetine, sertraline, and paroxetine are customarily given early in the day, as they tend to be somewhat stimulating and may cause insomnia if given late. Virtually all the other antidepressants have varying degrees of sedative effects and are best given near bedtime. Autonomic adverse effects also tend to be less troublesome if the dose is given late.

Maintenance Treatment

Whether or not to undertake long-term maintenance treatment of a depressed patient depends entirely on the natural history of the disorder. If the depressive episode was the patient's first and if it responded quickly and satisfactorily to drug therapy, it is rational to gradually withdraw treatment over a period of a few months. If relapse does not occur, drug treatment can be stopped until the next attack occurs, which is unpredictable but nearly certain. However, a patient who has had several previous attacks of depression—especially if each succeeding attack was more severe and more difficult to treat—is a candidate for maintenance therapy. In general, maintenance therapy is more effective if full dosage is used rather than partial dosage. The duration of treatment varies, though many patients require maintenance treatment indefinitely.

Monitoring Plasma Concentrations

Routine monitoring of plasma concentrations of antidepressants, while technically feasible for most drugs, is still of uncertain value. Experience with monitoring of plasma concentrations of tricyclics suggests that about 20% of patients become noncompliant at some time or other. Thus, a "poor response" in a patient for whom an adequate dosage of drug has been prescribed may be shown by measurement of the plasma drug concentration to be due merely to failure to take the drug. Blood for plasma drug level determination should be obtained in the postabsorptive state, about 10–12 hours after the last dose. Even when sampling time is constant, the same patient may show variation in both the total plasma concentration and the proportion of parent drug versus metabolites while on a constant dose at steady state conditions. Under no circumstances should the laboratory test results be permitted to overrule the physician's clinical judgment.

Unresponsive Patients

Almost one-third of patients receiving tricyclic antidepressants fail to respond. In evaluating a patient's resistance to treatment, one should consider the five *d*'s: diagnosis, drug, dose, duration of treatment, and different treatment.

Diagnosis might be reassessed if the patient shows little response over a period of 2–3 weeks of adequate dosage or plasma concentrations. If the patient is actually bipolar, lithium might be added; if psychotic, treatment might be augmented with an antipsychotic. Some clinicians believe that several weeks or months of treatment should be tried before giving up on a drug. The morbidity of depression is such that long delays in attaining relief are demoralizing.

Besides adding drugs more appropriate to the diagnosis, one must consider other types of antidepressants. It might be worthwhile to start patients on one of the tricyclics. If that fails, the trend has been to move directly to selective serotonin reuptake inhibitors, bypassing MAO inhibitors and heterocyclic drugs. Most clinicians would prefer to move through various antidepressant drug classes in the search for the right drug rather than through various drugs within a class.

Dose and duration of treatment must be considered. Most treatment failure is due to inadequate dosage, which should be pushed to the limits of the patient's tolerance in refractory cases. The duration of treatment before giving up on a drug is a matter of clinical judgment.

Finally, some patients may need a completely different type of treatment, such as electroconvulsive therapy. Electroconvulsive therapy (ECT) is often viewed as a treatment of last resort for endogenous depressions, but it should not be withheld from patients with this disorder who cannot be helped by drug therapy.

Noncompliance is an important cause of lack of response. Patients should be warned also that noticeable improvement may be slow, perhaps taking 3 weeks or more. Inability to tolerate adverse effects and discouragement with treatment are two major causes for noncompliance and for failure of tricyclics to relieve depression.

Combination therapy using tricyclics and MAO inhibitors has been recommended, though recent controlled trials do not suggest any special virtues for such combinations. Antidepressants should be combined with lithium or antipsychotics for treatment of psychotic depressions or the depressed phase of bipolar affective (manic-depressive) disorder.

Adverse Effects

Adverse effects of various antidepressants are summarized in Table 29–5. Most common unwanted effects are minor, but they may seriously affect patient compliance; the more seriously depressed the patient is, the more likely it is that unwanted effects will be tolerated. Most normal persons find that even moderate doses of these drugs cause disagreeable symptoms.

Drug Interactions

A. Pharmacodynamic Interactions: Many of the pharmacodynamic interactions of antidepressants with other drugs have already been discussed. Sedative effects may be additive with other sedatives, especially alcohol. Patients taking tricyclics should be warned that use of alcohol may lead to greater than expected impairment of driving ability. MAO inhibitors, by increasing stores of catecholamines, sensitize the patient to indirectly acting sympathomimetics such as tyramine, which is found in some fermented foods and beverages, and to sympathomimetic drugs that may be administered therapeutically, such as diethylpropion or phenylpropanolamine. Such sensitization can result in dangerous hypertensive emergencies. Evidence from clinical trials of moclobemide suggests that this selective and reversible MAO-A inhibitor is not associated with tyramine sensitivity. The serious interaction between MAO inhibitors and selective serotonin reuptake inhibitors has been mentioned; the "serotonin syndrome" is potentially lethal and must be avoided.

B. Pharmacokinetic Interactions: Reversal of the antihypertensive action of guanethidine is a dramatic interaction produced by tricyclics (see Chapter 11). The blood pressure not only returns quickly to high levels but may overshoot to dangerously high levels. Guanethidine is concentrated in sympathetic nerve endings by the same amine pump that is blocked by tricyclics. Thus, it is prevented from reaching its site of action. A similar reversal of action of other antihypertensives, such as methyldopa and clonidine, has been described. Although doxepin is less likely than other tricyclics to produce this inter-

Table 29–5. Adverse effects of antidepressants.

Tricyclics	
Sedation	Sleepiness, additive effects with other sedative drugs
Sympathomimetic	Tremor, insomnia
Antimuscarinic	Blurred vision, constipation, urinary hesitancy, confusion
Cardiovascular	Orthostatic hypotension, conduction defects, arrhythmias
Psychiatric	Aggravation of psychosis, withdrawal syndrome
Neurologic	Seizures
Metabolic-endocrine	Weight gain, sexual disturbances
Monoamine oxidase inhibitors	Headache, drowsiness, dry mouth, weight gain, postural hypotension, sexual disturbances
Amoxapine	Similar to the tricyclics with the addition of some effects associated with the antipsychotics (Chapter 28)
Maprotiline	Similar to tricyclics; seizures dose-related
Trazodone, venlafaxine	Drowsiness, dizziness, insomnia, headache, weight loss
Bupropion	Dizziness, dry mouth, sweating, tremor, aggravation of psychosis, potential for seizures at high doses
Fluoxetine and other serotonin reuptake inhibitors	Anxiety, insomnia, asthenia, tremor, sweating, gastrointestinal symptoms, rashes

action, because it is less potent in blocking the amine pump, interaction can occur with high doses of the drug. MAO inhibitors predictably prolong the half-lives of the many drugs that are oxidatively deaminated. Fluoxetine, by blocking metabolism of several drugs, may increase their plasma concentrations to the point of toxicity. Paroxetine and sertraline appear to lack this effect.

Overdoses

A. Tricyclics: Tricyclics are extremely dangerous when taken in overdose quantities, and depressed patients are more likely than others to be suicidal. Prescriptions should therefore be limited to amounts less than 1.25 g, or 50 dose units of 25 mg, on a "no refill" basis. If suicide is a serious possibility, the tablets should be entrusted to a family member. The drugs must be kept away from children. Both accidental and deliberate overdoses are frequent and are a serious medical emergency. Major effects include (1) coma with shock and sometimes metabolic acidosis; (2) respiratory depression with a tendency to sudden apnea; (3) agitation or delirium both before and after consciousness is obtunded; (4) neuromuscular irritability and seizures; (5) hyperpyrexia; (6) bowel and bladder paralysis; and (7) a great variety of cardiac manifestations, including conduction defects and arrhythmias.

Management of cardiac problems is difficult. Antiarrhythmic drugs having the least depressant effect on cardiac conduction should be used. Lidocaine, propranolol, and phenytoin have been used successfully, but quinidine and procainamide are contraindicated. Physostigmine given in small (0.5 mg) intravenous boluses to a total dose of 3–4 mg may awaken the patient and reverse a rapid supraventricular arrhythmia. It is *unlikely* to be effective for ventricular arrhythmias. Poison control centers no longer consider physostigmine to be appropriate treatment for this condition. Continuous cardiac monitoring is essential, and facilities must be at hand for resuscitation if needed. Arterial blood gases and pH should be measured frequently, since both hypoxia and metabolic acidosis predispose to arrhythmias. Sodium bicarbonate and intravenous potassium chloride may be required to restore acid-base balance and to correct hypokalemia. Electrical pacing must be used in refractory cases. Other treatment is entirely supportive. (See Chapter 60.)

B. Heterocyclic Drugs: Overdoses of amoxapine are characterized by severe neurotoxicity with seizures that are difficult to control. Overdoses of maprotiline also have a tendency to cause seizures as well as cardiotoxicity. Overdoses of the other heterocyclic drugs appear to create only minor problems and can usually be managed with purely supportive measures.

C. MAO Inhibitors: Intoxication with MAO inhibitors is unusual. Agitation, delirium, and neuromuscular excitability are followed by obtunded consciousness, seizures, shock, and hyperthermia. Supportive treatment is usually all that is required, though sedative phenothiazines with alpha adrenoceptor-blocking action, such as chlorpromazine, may be useful.

D. Selective Serotonin Reuptake Inhibitors: A few deaths have occurred during overdosage of fluoxetine, usually when other drugs were also being taken. Only supportive treatment can be offered, since the high volume of distribution, as with other antidepressants, rules out removal of drug by dialysis. Seizures have been a prominent feature of overdosage and may respond to diazepam. As much as 2.6 g of sertraline has been taken with survival. Overdoses of paroxetine are relatively benign: Up to 850 mg has been taken, with no evidence of cardiotoxicity.

PREPARATIONS AVAILABLE

Tricyclics

Amitriptyline (generic, Elavil, others)
Oral: 10, 25, 50, 75, 100, 150 mg tablets
Parenteral: 10 mg/mL for IM injection

Clomipramine (Anafranil, labeled only for obsessive-compulsive disorder)
Oral: 25, 50, 75 mg capsules

Desipramine (generic, Norpramin, Pertofrane)
Oral: 10, 25, 50, 75, 100, 150 mg tablets; 25, 50 mg capsules

Doxepin (generic, Sinequan, others)
Oral: 10, 25, 50, 75, 100, 150 mg capsules; 10 mg/mL concentrate

Imipramine (generic, Tofranil, others)
Oral: 10, 25, 50 mg tablets (as hydrochloride); capsules (as pamoate)
Parenteral: 25 mg/2 mL for IM injection

Nortriptyline (Aventyl, Pamelor)
Oral: 10, 25, 50, 75 mg capsules; 10 mg/5 mL solution

Protriptyline (Vivactil)
Oral: 5, 10 mg tablets

Trimipramine (Surmontil)
Oral: 25, 50, 100 mg capsules

Heterocyclics

Amoxapine (generic, Asendin)
Oral: 25, 50, 100, 150 mg tablets

Bupropion (Wellbutrin)
Oral: 75, 100 mg tablets

Maprotiline (generic, Ludiomil)
Oral: 25, 50, 75 mg tablets

Trazodone (generic, Desyrel)
Oral: 50, 100, 150, 300 mg tablets

Venlafaxine (Effexor)
Oral: 25, 37.5, 50, 75, 100 mg tablets

Selective Serotonin Reuptake Inhibitors

Fluoxetine (Prozac)
Oral: 20 mg pulvules, 20 mg/5 mL liquid

Paroxetine (Paxil)
Oral: 20, 30 mg tablets

Sertraline (Zoloft)
Oral: 50, 100 mg tablets

Monoamine Oxidase Inhibitors

Isocarboxazid (Marplan)
Oral: 10 mg tablets

Phenelzine (Nardil)
Oral: 15 mg tablets

Tranylcypromine (Parnate)
Oral: 10 mg tablets

REFERENCES

Aberg-Wistedt A: The antidepressant effects of 5-HT uptake inhibitors. Br J Psychiatry 1989;155(Suppl 8):32.

APA Task Force on Use of Laboratory Tests in Psychiatry: Tricyclic antidepressants—Blood level measurements and clinical outcome: An APA Task Force Report. Am J Psychiatry 1985;142:155.

American Psychiatric Association: *Diagnostic and Statistical Manual of Mental Disorders (DSM-III-R),* 3rd ed, revised. American Psychiatric Association, 1987.

Baldessarini RJ: Current status of antidepressants: Clinical pharmacology and therapy. J Clin Psychiatry 1989; 50:117.

Blackwell B: Side effects of antidepressant drugs. In: *American Psychiatric Association Annual Review,* vol 6. Hales RE, Frances AJ (editors). American Psychiatric Press, 1987.

Cesura AM, Pletscher A: The new generation of monoamine oxidase inhibitors. Prog Drug Res 1992;38:171.

Dechant KL, Clissold SP: Paroxetine. A review of its pharmacodynamic and pharmacokinetic properties, and therapeutic potential in depressive illness. Drugs 1991; 41:225.

Derby LE, Jick H, Dean AD: Antidepressant drugs and suicide. J Clin Psychopharmacol 1992;12:235.

Dzuikas LJ, Vohra J: Tricyclic antidepressant poisoning. Med J Aust 1991;154:344.

Frommer DA et al: Tricyclic antidepressant overdose: A review. JAMA 1987;257:521.

Garver DL, Davis JM: Biogenic amine hypothesis of affective disorders. Life Sci 1979;24:383.

Heninger GR, Charney DS: Mechanism of action of antidepressant treatments: Implications for the etiology and treatment of depressive disorders. In: *Psychopharmacology: The Third Generation of Progress.* Meltzer HY (editor). Raven Press, 1987.

Hollister LE: Current antidepressants. Annu Rev Pharmacol Toxicol 1986;26:23.

Hollister LE, Claghorn JL: New antidepressants. Annu Rev Pharmacol Toxicol 1993;32:165.

Jick SS et al: Antidepressants and convulsions. J Clin Psychopharmacol 1992;12:241.

Lemberger L, Fuller RW, Zerbe RL: Use of specific serotonin uptake inhibitors as antidepressants. Clin Neuropharmacol 1985;8:299.

McDaniel KD: Clinical pharmacology of monamine oxidase inhibitors. Clin Neuropharmacol 1986;9:207.

McGrath PJ et al: Phenelzine treatment of melancholia. J Clin Psychiatry 1986;47:420.

NIH Consensus Development Conference: Mood disorders: Pharmacologic prevention of recurrences. Vol 5, No. 4, 1982.

Potter WZ: Psychotherapeutic drugs and biogenic amines:

Current concepts and therapeutic implications. Drugs 1984;28:127.

Reimherr FW et al: Antidepressant efficacy of sertraline: A double blind placebo and amitriptyline-controlled multicenter comparison study in outpatients with major depression. J Clin Psychiatry 1990;51(Suppl 12B):18.

Rothschild AJ: Biology of depression. Med Clin North Am 1988;72:765.

Rudorfer MV, Potter WZ: Pharmacokinetics of antidepressants. In: *Psychopharmacology: The Third Generation of Progress.* Meltzer HY (editor). Raven Press, 1987.

Schopf J: Treatment of depressions resistant to tricyclic antidepressants, related drugs, or MAO-inhibitors by lithium addition: Review of the literature. Pharmacopsychiatry 1989;22:174.

Sommi RW, Crismon ML, Bowden CL: Fluoxetine: A serotonin-specific, second-generation antidepressant. Pharmacotherapy 1987;7:1.

Snyder SH: Second messengers and affective illness. Focus on the phosphoinositide cycle. Pharmacopsychiatry 1992;25:25.

Sulser F: Serotonin-norepinephrine receptor interactions in the brain: Implications for the pharmacology and pathophysiology of affective disorders. J Clin Psychiatry 1987;48(Suppl):12.

van Harten J: Clinical pharmacokinetics of selective serotonin reuptake inhibitors. Clin Pharmacokinet 1993;24:203.

Zemlan FP, Garver DL: Depression and antidepressant therapy: Receptor dynamics. Prog Neuropsychopharmacol Biol Psychiatry 1990;14:503.

30 Opioid Analgesics & Antagonists

Walter L. Way, MD, E. Leong Way, PhD, & Howard L. Fields, MD, PhD

One hundred years ago, there were no antibiotics, hormonal drugs, or antipsychotic agents. Indeed, few truly useful drugs of any kind were available, but morphine effectively relieved severe pain of several types. It could also control diarrhea, cough, anxiety, and insomnia. For these reasons, Sir William Osler called morphine "God's own medicine."

The term "narcotic," often used in connection with this drug group, is an imprecise one, since "narcosis" connotes a stuporous or somnolent state; the terms "opiate" and "opioid analgesic" are more appropriate because they imply the production of analgesia without causing sleep or loss of consciousness. *Opioid* analgesics are usually understood to include all of the natural and semisynthetic alkaloid derivatives from opium as well as their synthetic surrogates with actions that mimic those of morphine. *Opiates* are taken to be those opioid drugs that are derived from alkaloids of the opium poppy. In recent years, analgesics that also possess morphine *antagonist* properties (mixed agonist-antagonists) have found applications in clinical situations where morphine might otherwise be used. Moreover, the existence of endogenous peptides with analgesic properties suggests that synthetic peptides with opioid characteristics may in the future also be included in this group. Among the opioids we therefore include the **opiates** (derived from the opium alkaloids), **synthetic opioids** (agonists, mixed agonist-antagonists, and antagonists), and the **opiopeptins** (such as β-endorphin and the enkephalins). Morphine is considered the prototypical agonist.

History

The source of opium, the crude substance, and morphine, one of its purified constituents, is the opium poppy, *Papaver somniferum.* The plant may have been in use for over 6000 years, and there are accounts of its use in ancient Egyptian, Greek, and Roman documents. Interestingly, it was not until the 18th century that the addiction liability of opium began to cause concern.

The modern basis of pharmacology was established by Sertürner, a German pharmacist, who isolated a pure active alkaline substance from opium in 1803. This was a landmark event in that it made it possible to derive a standardized potency for a natural product. After testing the compound on himself and some friends, Sertürner proposed the name "morphine" for the compound–after Morpheus, the Greek god of dreams.

I. BASIC PHARMACOLOGY OF THE OPIOID ANALGESICS

Source

Opium is obtained from the opium poppy by incision of the seed pod after the petals of the flower have dropped. The white latex that oozes out turns brown and hardens on standing. This sticky brown gum is opium. It contains about 20 alkaloids, including morphine, codeine, thebaine, and papaverine. Thebaine and papaverine are not analgesic agents, but thebaine is the precursor of several semisynthetic opiate agonists (eg, etorphine, a veterinary agent 500–1000 times as potent as morphine) and antagonists (naloxone). Papaverine is a vasodilator with no established clinical applications that nevertheless inspired the development of verapamil, an important calcium channel-blocking drug (see Chapter 12). The principal alkaloid in opium is morphine, present in a concentration of about 10%. Codeine is present in less than 0.5% concentration; it is synthesized commercially from morphine. Cultivation of the opium poppy is now restricted by international agreement, but illicit production of opium is widespread and difficult to control.

Chemistry

In Table 30–1, compounds are listed according to their agonist, mixed agonist-antagonist, or antagonist properties. Some of their pharmacologic properties are summarized in Table 30–2. Relatively small molecular alterations may drastically change the action of these compounds, converting an agonist to an antagonist or to a compound with both agonist and antagonist effects—a "mixed agonist-antagonist."

Antagonist properties are associated with replace-

Table 30–1. Chemical structures of opioid analgesics and antagonists.

Basic Structure	Strong Agonists	Mild to Moderate Agonists	Mixed Agonist-Antagonists	Antagonists
Phenanthrenes	Morphine Hydromorphone Oxymorphone	Codeine Oxycodone Hydrocodone	Nalbuphine Buprenorphine	Nalorphine [1] Naloxone Naltrexone
Phenylheptylamines	Methadone	Propoxyphene		

Table 30-1. Chemical structures of opioid analgesics and antagonists. (continued)

Basic Structure	Strong Agonists	Mild to Moderate Agonists	Mixed Agonist-Antagonists	Antagonists
Phenylpiperidines	Meperidine	Diphenoxylate		
	Fentanyl			
Morphinans	Levorphanol		Butorphanol	Levallorphan [1]
Benzomorphans			Pentazocine	

[1] Not a pure antagonist. See text for explanation.

462

Table 30–2. Common opioid analgesics.

Generic Name	Product Name	Approximate Dose (mg)	Oral:Parenteral Potency Ratio	Duration of Analgesia (hours)	Maximum Efficacy	Addiction/Abuse Liability
Morphine		10	Low	4–5	High	High
Hydromorphone	Dilaudid	1.5	Low	4–5	High	High
Oxymorphone	Numorphan	1.5	Low	3–4	High	High
Methadone	Dolophine	10	High	4–6	High	High
Meperidine	Demerol	60–100	Medium	2–4	High	High
Fentanyl	Sublimaze	0.1	Parenteral use only	1–1½	High	High
Sufentanil	Sufenta	0.02	Parenteral use only	1–1½	High	High
Alfentanil	Alfenta	Titrated	Parenteral use only	¼–¾	High	High
Levorphanol	Levo-Dromoran	2–3	High	4–5	High	High
Codeine		30–60[2]	High	3–4	Low	Medium
Oxycodone[1]	Percodan	4.5[2]	Medium	3–4	Moderate	Medium
Dihydrocodeine[1]	Drocode	16[2]	Medium	3–4	Moderate	Medium
Propoxyphene	Darvon	60–120[2]	Oral use only	4–5	Very low	Low
Pentazocine	Talwin	30–50[2]	Medium	3–4	Moderate	Low
Nalbuphine	Nubain	10	Parenteral use only	3–6	High	Low
Buprenorphine	Buprenex	0.3	Parenteral use only	4–8	High	Low
Butorphanol	Stadol	2	Parenteral use only	3–4	High	Low

[1]Available only in tablets containing aspirin, etc.
[2]Analgesic efficacy at this dose not equivalent to 10 mg of morphine. See text for explanation.

ment of the methyl substituent on the nitrogen atom with larger groups—allyl in the case of nalorphine and naloxone; methylcyclopropane or methylcyclobutane for several other agents.

Substitutions at the C3 and C6 hydroxyl groups of morphine significantly alter pharmacokinetic properties. Methyl substitution at the phenolic hydroxyl at C3 reduces susceptibility to first-pass hepatic metabolism of the molecule by glucuronide conjugation at this position. Therefore, drugs such as codeine and oxycodone have a higher ratio of oral:parenteral potency. Acetylation of both hydroxyl groups of morphine yields heroin, which penetrates the blood-brain barrier much more rapidly than morphine. It is then rapidly hydrolyzed in the brain to monoacetylmorphine and morphine.

Pharmacokinetics

A. Absorption: Most opioid analgesics are well absorbed from subcutaneous and intramuscular sites as well as from the mucosal surfaces of the nose or mouth and gastrointestinal tract. In addition, transdermal absorption of fentanyl has become an important route of administration (see below). However, although absorption from the gastrointestinal tract may be rapid, the bioavailability of some compounds taken by this route may be considerably reduced because of significant first-pass metabolism by glucuronidation in the liver. Therefore, the oral dose required to elicit a therapeutic effect may be much higher than that required when parenteral administration is used. Since the amount of the enzyme responsible for this reaction varies considerably in different individuals, the effective oral dose of a compound may be difficult to predict. As noted above, codeine and oxycodone have high oral:parenteral potency ratios because their conjugation is prevented by a methyl group on the aromatic hydroxyl group.

B. Distribution: The uptake of opioids by various organs and tissues is a function of both physiologic and chemical factors. Although all opioids bind to plasma proteins with varying degrees of affinity, the compounds rapidly leave the blood and localize in highest concentrations in tissues that are highly perfused, such as the lungs, liver, kidneys, and spleen. Although drug concentrations in skeletal muscle may be much lower, this tissue serves as the main reservoir for the drug because of its greater bulk. However, accumulation in fatty tissue can also become important, particularly after frequent high-dose administration of highly lipophilic opioids that are slowly metabolized, eg, fentanyl. Brain concentrations of opioids are usually relatively low in comparison to most other organs because of the blood-brain barrier. However, the blood-brain barrier is traversed more readily by compounds in which the aromatic hydroxyl at C3 is substituted, as in heroin and codeine. Difficulty in gaining access to the brain appears to be greater with amphoteric agents (ie, drugs possessing both acidic and basic properties) such as morphine. However, this barrier is lacking in neonates. Since the opioid analgesics also traverse the placenta, their use for obstetric analgesia can result in delivery of an infant with depressed respiration.

C. Metabolism: The opioids are converted in large part to polar metabolites, which are then readily excreted by the kidneys. Compounds that have free hydroxyl groups are readily conjugated with glucuronic acid; examples are morphine and levorphanol. Esters (eg, meperidine, heroin) are rapidly hydrolyzed by common tissue esterases. Heroin (diacetylmorphine) is hydrolyzed to monoacetylmorphine and finally to morphine, which is then conjugated with glucuronic acid. These polar glucuronidated metabolites were thought to be inactive, but recent findings indicate that morphine-6-glucuronide possesses analgesic properties perhaps even greater than those of morphine itself. Accumulation of these active metabolites may occur in patients in renal failure and may lead to prolonged and more profound analgesia even though CNS entry is limited. The opioids are also N-demethylated by the liver, but this is a minor pathway. Accumulation of a metabolite of meperidine, normeperidine, may occur in patients with decreased renal function or those receiving multiple high doses of the drug. In sufficiently high concentrations, this metabolite may cause seizures, especially in children.

D. Excretion: The polar metabolites of the opioids are excreted mainly in the urine. Small amounts of the unchanged drug may also be excreted in the urine. Glucuronide conjugates are also excreted in the bile, but enterohepatic circulation represents only a small portion of the excretory process.

Pharmacodynamics

A. Mechanism of Action: Morphine and its surrogates bind selectively at many recognition sites throughout the body to produce pharmacologic effects. Brain loci involved in the transmission of pain and in the alteration of reactivity to nociceptive (painful) stimuli appear to be primary but not the only sites at which opioids act. In general, sites that display a high affinity for exogenous opioid ligands such as morphine also contain high concentrations of several endogenous peptides having opiate-like properties. There are many shared features in the chemistry and pharmacology of these peptides, but there are distinct differences with respect to their biochemical and neuronal pathways. The generic name used for these substances has been **endorphins** ("endogenous morphine"). However, this term has caused considerable confusion because of its association with one principal opioid peptide prototype, β-endorphin. Of all the native peptides, the pharmacologic profile of β-endorphin appears to be most similar to that of morphine. As a consequence, the term **"opiopeptins"** has been suggested as the generic name for the native opioid peptides, and the term endorphin is being reserved for the peptide type closely related to β-endorphin.

The smallest peptides possessing direct opioid activity are two pentapeptides: **methionine-enkephalin** (met-enkephalin) and **leucine-enkephalin** (leu-enkephalin). With the exception of the methionine or leucine terminal group, the amino acid sequences of the enkephalins are identical (tyrosine-glycine-glycine-phenylalanine). One or both of these two peptides are contained in three principal precursor proteins having between 257 and 265 amino acids with different repetitive peptide sequences.

The three principal precursor peptides are pro-opiomelanocortin (POMC), proenkephalin (proenkephalin A), and prodynorphin (proenkephalin B). Pro-opiomelanocortin contains met-enkephalin, β-endorphin, and several nonopioid peptides, including ACTH, β-lipotropin, and melanocyte-stimulating hormone. Proenkephalin contains six copies of met-enkephalin and one copy of leu-enkephalin. Prodynorphin yields several active opioid peptides that contain leu-enkephalin as a fragment. These are dynorphin A, dynorphin B (rimorphin), and alpha and beta neoendorphins. Each of these endogenous opioid peptide precursor molecules is present at brain sites that have been implicated in pain modulation, and there is evidence that they can be activated during stress such as that produced by pain or the anticipation of pain. It is important to note that these precursor peptides are found not only in the central nervous system but also in many other tissues. The presence of such compounds has led to experiments showing that both endogenous and exogenous opioids can produce opioid receptor-mediated analgesia at sites outside the CNS. This antinociceptive action may occur because mu (μ), kappa (κ), and delta (δ) receptors (see below) located on primary afferent neurons are activated. Another interesting aspect of these observations is that pain associated with inflammation seems especially sensitive to these peripheral opioid actions (Barber, 1992). Peripheral mechanisms, although probably not opioid receptor-mediated, are also important in the analgesia produced by potent NSAID drugs such as ketorolac (see Chapter 35). Recent studies suggest that several phenanthrene opioids (morphine and codeine) may also be found as endogenous substances in mammalian tissue.

1. Receptor types—Several types of opioid receptors have been identified at various sites in the nervous system and other tissues. Exogenous and endogenous ligands bind at these loci to varying degrees, and the predominance and nature of the combination between a particular substance and a specific receptor give rise to a characteristic pharmacologic profile.

Analgesia at the supraspinal level as well as the euphoriant, respiratory depressant, and physical dependence properties of morphine (typical agonist effects) result principally from combination with mu and delta receptors. These receptors also mediate spinal opioid analgesia. In addition, kappa receptors contribute to analgesia at the spinal level. These three receptor types have been isolated and cloned. A fourth receptor, the sigma (σ) receptor, is more controversial but may be related to the dysphoric, hallucinogenic, and cardiac stimulant effects of opioids. Recent research suggests that each receptor type may have subtypes (μ_1, μ_2, etc). Since an opioid drug might function with different potencies as an agonist, partial agonist, or antagonist with each of these multiple receptor types, it is not surprising that these agents are capable of such diverse effects.

Despite their heterogeneity, all three primary receptor types appear to elicit their actions via receptors that are closely linked with the cAMP system and changes in Ca^{2+} and K^+ flux.

2. Receptor distribution–Opioid binding or recognition sites have been identified by radioligand-binding, autoradiographic, and immunohistochemical techniques. A high density of binding sites is present in the dorsal horn of the spinal cord (B, Figure 30–1) and certain subcortical regions of the brain (C, thalamus; D, midbrain periaqueductal gray; and E, rostral ventral medulla sites; see Figure 30–1).

Opioid binding sites are present on both spinal cord pain transmission neurons and upon the primary afferents that relay the pain message to them (Figure 30–1, left). Opioids and opiopeptins have been shown to inhibit the release of excitatory transmitters from these primary afferents. Some of the brain opioid binding sites that are concerned with pain modulation via *descending* pathways (Figure 30–1, right) include the nucleus raphe magnus in the rostral ventral medulla and locus ceruleus of the brain stem, the midbrain periaqueductal gray area, and several hypothalamic and thalamic nuclei. The presence of opioids at the periaqueductal gray and rostral ventral medulla sites activates neurons that send processes to the spinal cord and inhibit pain transmission neurons. Thus, binding of an opioid at these supraspinal sites greatly augments the opioid effect at the spinal level to reduce nociceptive transmission and raise the pain threshold.

The modulatory brain sites involved in altering reactivity to pain are less well identified than those con-

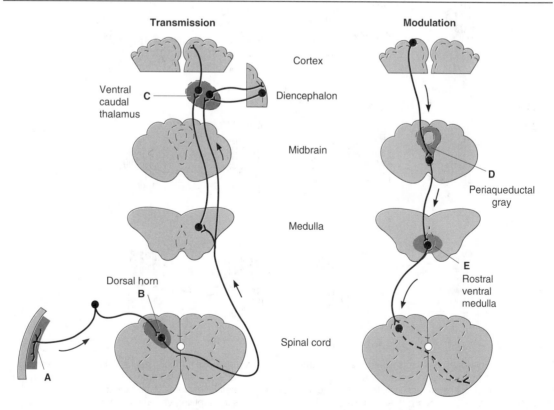

Figure 30–1. Putative sites of action of opioid analgesics (color). On the left, sites of action on the pain transmission pathway from the periphery to the higher centers are shown. At **A,** possible direct action of opioids on inflamed peripheral tissues. **B:** Inhibition occurs in the spinal cord. **C:** Possible site of action in the thalamus. On the right, actions on pain-modulating neurons in the midbrain (site **D**) and medulla (site **E**) secondarily affect pain transmission pathways.

cerned with pain transmission. It has been suggested that the limbic system, which includes the anterior temporal and orbital frontal cortex, as well as parts of the hypothalamus and amygdala are involved since opioid analgesics reduce fear and anxiety and may produce euphoria. Support for such a postulate is provided by the fact that some limbic structures have a high density of opioid-binding sites.

3. Cellular effects–The opioids appear to exert their effects either by hyperpolarizing and inhibiting postsynaptic neurons (probably by increasing K^+ efflux) or by reducing Ca^{2+} influx into presynaptic nerve endings and thereby reducing transmitter release. Figure 30–2 illustrates the postsynaptic inhibitory effect of opioids acting at the mu receptor. The presynaptic action—depressed transmitter release—has been demonstrated for a large number of neurotransmitters, including acetylcholine, norepinephrine, dopamine, serotonin, and substance P. It is likely that several of these transmitters are involved in the action of opioids, since no one transmitter system can account for all of the effects of the opioids. At the mo-

lecular level, opioid receptors are linked to G proteins and are therefore able to affect ion gating, intracellular calcium disposition, and protein phosphorylation (see Chapter 2).

4. Tolerance and physical dependence– With frequently repeated administration of therapeutic doses of morphine or its surrogates, there is a gradual loss in effectiveness, ie, tolerance. To reproduce the original response, a larger dose must be administered. With the development of tolerance, physical dependence occurs, so that continued administration of the drug becomes necessary to prevent a characteristic withdrawal or abstinence syndrome (Chapter 31).

The mechanism of development of tolerance and physical dependence is not related to pharmacokinetic factors but is a true cellular adaptive response that is associated with changes in second messenger systems related to Ca^{2+} flux, adenylyl cyclase inhibition, and G protein synthesis. Chronic exposure and tolerance to opioids is associated with an elevation of intracellular Ca^{2+} content—unlike acute exposure,

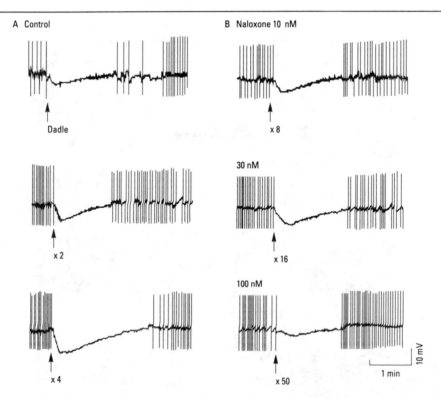

Figure 30–2. Enkephalin interacts with a naloxone-sensitive receptor on locus ceruleus neurons. Figure shows intracellular recordings from a spontaneously firing locus ceruleus neuron in a tissue slice cut from rat pons and maintained in vitro. Upward deflections are action potentials (truncated); downward deflections are action potential afterhyperpolarizations. [D-Ala^2, D-Leu^5]enkephalin (DADLE) was administered at *arrows* by applying various numbers of pressure pulses (55 kPa, 24 ms, number indicated) to a micropipette containing the peptide positioned above the slice. **A:** Control responses. **B:** Selected records taken in the presence of different amounts of naloxone (added to the superfusing solution, concentration indicated). (Reproduced, with permission, from Williams JT, Egan TM, North RA: Enkephalin opens potassium channels on mammalian central neurons. Nature [Sept 2] 1982; 299:74.)

which often causes a decrease. The effect appears to be related to a change in the receptor's ability to associate with G coupling proteins, increased level of G proteins, and an up-regulated cAMP system. In addition, the number of receptors may be reduced by internalization and by reduced synthesis.

The clinical aspects of tolerance and physical dependence are discussed below.

B. Organ System Effects of Morphine and Its Surrogates: The actions given below for morphine, the prototype agonist opioid, are also observed with all of the other agonists (Table 30–1). The mixed agonist-antagonist agents, when given to a patient who has *not* recently received an agonist agent, also produce analgesia, but with minor variations in effects as noted below. Characteristics of specific members of these two groups are discussed below.

The pure antagonists and the mixed agonist-antagonists, when given to a subject who has received an agonist, will have very different effects, as noted at the end of this chapter.

1. Central nervous system effects–The principal effects of the opioid analgesics with affinity for mu receptors are on the central nervous system; the more important ones include analgesia, euphoria, sedation, and respiratory depression. With repeated use, a high degree of tolerance occurs to all of these effects (Table 30–3).

a. Analgesia–A painful sensation, no matter what its origin, consists of the noxious input plus the reaction of the organism to the stimulus. The analgesic properties of the opioids are related to their ability to change both pain *perception* and the *reaction* of the patient to pain. Experimental and clinical studies indicate that opioid analgesics can effectively raise the threshold for pain, but their effects on the reactive component can only be inferred from subjective effects reported by the patient. In the presence of effective analgesia, pain may still be perceived by the patient, but even very severe pain is no longer an all-consuming and destructive sensory input.

b. Euphoria–After a dose of morphine, a typical patient in pain or an addict experiences a pleasant floating sensation and freedom from anxiety and distress. However, other patients and some normal subjects (not in pain) experience dysphoric rather than pleasant effects after a dose of opioid analgesic. Dysphoria is a disquieted state accompanied by both restlessness and a feeling of malaise. In general, if a real indication exists for administration of an opioid analgesic, the most common affective response is euphoria.

c. Sedation–Drowsiness and clouding of mentation are frequent concomitants of opioid action, and there may be some impairment of reasoning ability. There is little or no amnesia. Sleep is induced by opiates more frequently in the elderly than in young, healthy individuals. Ordinarily, the patient can be easily aroused from sleep. However, the combination of morphine with other central depressant drugs, such as the sedative-hypnotics, may result in profound depression. Marked sedation occurs more frequently with compounds closely related to the phenanthrene derivatives and less frequently with the synthetic agents such as meperidine and fentanyl. Morphine (a phenanthrene) in standard analgesic doses disrupts normal REM and NREM sleep patterns. This effect is probably characteristic of all opioids. In contrast to humans, a number of species (cats, horses, cows, pigs) may manifest excitation rather than sedation when given opioids. These paradoxical effects are at least partially dose-dependent.

d. Respiratory depression–All of the opioid analgesics can produce significant respiratory depression by inhibiting brain stem respiratory mechanisms. Alveolar PCO_2 may increase, but the most significant aspect of this depression is a depressed response to a carbon dioxide challenge. The respiratory depression is dose-related and is influenced significantly by the degree of other sensory input occurring at the same time. For example, it is possible to partially overcome the opioid-induced respiratory depression by stimulation of various sorts. When strongly painful stimuli that have prevented the depressant action of a large dose of an opioid are relieved, respiratory depression may suddenly become marked. A small to moderate decrease in respiratory function, as measured by PCO_2 elevation, may be well tolerated in the patient without prior respiratory impairment. However, in individuals with increased intracranial pressure, asthma, chronic obstructive pulmonary disease, or cor pulmonale, this decrease in respiratory function may not be tolerated.

e. Cough suppression–Suppression of the cough reflex is a well-recognized action of opioids. Codeine in particular has been used to advantage in persons suffering from pathologic cough and in patients in whom it is necessary to maintain ventilation via an endotracheal tube. However, cough suppression by opioids may allow accumulation of secretions and thus lead to airway obstruction and atelectasis. Tolerance develops to the cough suppressant action of opioid analgesics (Table 30–3).

f. Miosis–Constriction of the pupils is seen with

Table 30–3. Extent of tolerance developed to some of the effects of the opioids.

High Degree of Tolerance	Moderate Degree of Tolerance	Minimal or No Tolerance
Analgesia Euphoria, dysphoria Mental clouding Sedation Respiratory depression Antidiuresis Nausea and vomiting Cough suppression	Bradycardia	Miosis Constipation Convulsions Antagonist actions

virtually all of the opioid agonists. Miosis is also a pharmacologic action to which little or no tolerance develops; thus, it is valuable in the diagnosis of opioid overdose, since even highly tolerant addicts will have miosis. The action can be blocked by atropine and by opioid antagonists.

g. Truncal rigidity–An intensification of tone in the large trunk muscles has been noted with a number of opioids. It was believed that truncal rigidity was the result of an action of the opioids at the spinal cord level, but there is now evidence that it results from an action at supraspinal levels. Truncal rigidity reduces thoracic compliance and thus interferes with ventilation. It is most apparent when high doses of the highly lipid-soluble or nonpolar opioids (fentanyl, sufentanil, alfentanil) are rapidly administered intravenously. This action may be overcome by administration of an opioid antagonist.

h. Nausea and vomiting–The opioid analgesics can activate the brain stem chemoreceptor trigger zone to produce nausea and vomiting. There may be another component to these effects in that ambulation seems to increase the incidence of nausea and vomiting, perhaps by an action on the vestibular apparatus.

2. Peripheral effects–

a. Cardiovascular system–Most opioids have no significant direct effects on the heart and no major effects on cardiac rhythm (except bradycardia) or blood pressure. Exceptions to this generalization will be noted below as the specific drugs are discussed. Blood pressure is usually well maintained in subjects receiving opioids unless the cardiovascular system is stressed, in which case hypotension may occur. This hypotensive effect is probably due to peripheral arterial and venous dilation, which has been attributed to a number of mechanisms including release of histamine and central depression of vasomotor-stabilizing mechanisms. No consistent effect on cardiac output is seen, and the ECG is not significantly affected. However, caution should be exercised in patients with decreased blood volume, since the above mechanisms make these patients quite susceptible to blood pressure decreases. Opioid analgesics affect cerebral circulation minimally except when PCO_2 rises as a consequence of respiratory depression. Increased PCO_2 leads to cerebral vascular dilation and a concomitant decrease in cerebral vascular resistance, increase in cerebral blood flow, and increase in intracranial pressure.

b. Gastrointestinal tract–Constipation has long been recognized as an effect of opioids. Opioid receptors exist in high density in the gastrointestinal tract, and the constipating effects of the opioids are mediated through an action on the local enteric nervous system (Chapter 6) as well as the CNS (Kromer, 1988). In the stomach, motility may be decreased but tone may increase—particularly in the central portion; gastric secretion of hydrochloric acid is decreased. Small intestine resting tone is increased, with periodic spasms, but the amplitude of nonpropulsive contractions is markedly decreased. In the large intestine, propulsive peristaltic waves are diminished and tone is increased; this delays passage of the fecal mass and allows increased absorption of water, which leads to constipation. The large bowel actions are the basis for the use of opioids in management of diarrhea. There is a clinical impression that the benzomorphans (eg, pentazocine) cause less constipation than other opioids.

c. Biliary tract–The opioids constrict biliary smooth muscle, which may result in biliary colic. The sphincter of Oddi may constrict, resulting in reflux of biliary and pancreatic secretions and elevated plasma amylase and lipase levels.

d. Genitourinary tract–Renal function is depressed by opioids. It is believed that in humans this is chiefly due to decreased renal plasma flow. This contrasts with animal studies, in which reduced urine output seems to result from increased secretion of antidiuretic hormone as well as reduced renal perfusion. Ureteral and bladder tone are increased by therapeutic doses of the opioid analgesics. Increased urethral sphincter tone may precipitate urinary retention, especially in postoperative patients. Occasionally, ureteral colic caused by a renal calculus is made worse by opioid-induced increase in ureteral tone.

e. Uterus–The opioid analgesics may prolong labor. The mechanism for this action is unclear, but both peripheral and central effects of the opioids may reduce uterine tone.

f. Neuroendocrine–Opioid analgesics stimulate the release of antidiuretic hormone, prolactin, and somatotropin but inhibit the release of luteinizing hormone. These effects are of importance in that they may reflect regulatory roles in these systems by endogenous opioid peptides and are probably mediated by effects in the hypothalamus.

g. Miscellaneous–Therapeutic doses of the opioid analgesics produce flushing and warming of the skin accompanied sometimes by sweating and itching; central effects and histamine release may be responsible for these reactions.

C. Effects of Mixed Agonist-Antagonists: Pentazocine and other opioids with agonist actions at some opioid receptors and antagonist actions at others usually produce sedation in addition to analgesia when given in therapeutic doses. At higher doses, sweating, dizziness, and nausea are common, but severe respiratory depression may be less common than with pure agonists. When it does occur, respiratory depression may be reversed by naloxone but not reliably by other agonist-antagonists such as nalorphine. Psychotomimetic effects, with hallucinations, nightmares, and anxiety, have been reported following use of the mixed agonist-antagonist agents.

II. CLINICAL PHARMACOLOGY OF THE OPIOID ANALGESICS

Management of pain is essential to good medical practice and requires careful consideration of proper dose, type of drug, and the disease being treated. There are many situations in which analgesia must be provided before a definitive diagnosis can be reached. Indeed, in some acute situations relief of pain may actually facilitate history taking and physical examination and thus speed the diagnostic process.

Use of opioid drugs in acute situations may be contrasted to their use in chronic pain management, where other factors must be considered—particularly tolerance and physical dependence. In all instances, the factors that should enter into the decision about choice of drug include the following: (1) Is analgesia needed? (2) Will the opioid analgesic obscure or alter the signs and symptoms of the underlying disorder? (3) Are the pharmacologic effects of the opioid liable to worsen the condition for which the drug is being used, eg, by increasing cerebrospinal fluid pressure or producing respiratory depression? (4) Do the opioid agent's adverse effects impose a significant hazard? (See Table 30–4.) (5) Is there a possibility of significant drug interaction between the opioid agent and other drugs the patient is receiving? (See Table 30–5.) (6) Are tolerance and drug dependence likely to develop?

Table 30–2 shows the range of agonist efficacy of different opioid drugs. It is therefore necessary to select a drug appropriate to the type and severity of pain being treated to make certain that adequate analgesia is provided. The level of pain associated with various disease states also varies; thus, the postoperative pain of a forearm fracture may be adequately treated with codeine; the severe pain of a kidney stone may not. Each drug has a therapeutic ceiling, and to attempt to raise the ceiling with higher doses creates a risk of significant adverse effects and therapeutic failure.

Clinical Use of Opioid Analgesics

A. Analgesia: Severe, *constant* pain is usually

Table 30–4. Toxic effects of the opioid analgesics.

Behavioral restlessness, tremulousness, hyperactivity (in dysphoric reactions).
Respiratory depression.
Nausea and vomiting.
Increased intracranial pressure.
Postural hypotension accentuated by hypovolemia.
Constipation.
Urinary retention.
Itching around nose, urticaria (more frequent with parenteral adminstration).

Table 30–5. Opioid drug interactions.

Sedative-hypnotics: Increased central nervous system depression, particularly respiratory depression.

Antipsychotic tranquilizers: Increased sedation. Variable effects on respiratory depression. Accentuation of cardiovascular effects (antimuscarinic and alpha-blocking actions).

MAO inhibitors: Relative contraindication to all opioid analgesics because of the high incidence of hyperpyrexic coma; hypertension has also been reported.

relieved with the more efficacious opioids, whereas sharp, intermittent pain does not appear to be as amenable to relief. An attempt should be made to quantify the pain; this information should be used to select the proper agent and to monitor its effects. In this evaluation and selection process, such considerations as route of administration (oral versus parenteral administration), duration of action, ceiling effect (maximal efficacy), duration of therapy, and past experience with opioids are of obvious importance.

The pain associated with cancer and other terminal illnesses must be treated adequately, and concerns about tolerance and dependence should be set aside in favor of making the patient as comfortable as possible. Research by workers in the hospice movement has demonstrated that fixed-interval administration of opioid medication (a regular dose at a regular time) is more effective in achieving pain relief than dosing on demand. New dosage forms of morphine that allow slower release of the alkaloid are now available (eg, MS-Contin). Their purported advantage is a longer and more stable level of analgesia. In addition, stimulant drugs such as the amphetamines have been shown to enhance the actions of the opioids and thus may be very useful adjuncts in the patient with chronic pain. Alpha$_2$-adrenoceptor agonists (eg, clonidine) have been shown in both laboratory and clinical studies to produce analgesia when given by a variety of routes of administration, but the place of these drugs in pain management is still unclear.

Opioid analgesics are often employed during obstetric labor. Because opioids cross the placental barrier and reach the fetus, care must be taken to minimize neonatal opioid depression. If this occurs, immediate injection of the antagonist, naloxone, will reverse the depression. The phenylpiperidine drugs (eg, meperidine) appear to produce less depression in newborn infants than does morphine; this may justify their use in obstetric practice.

The acute, severe pain of renal and biliary colic often requires a strong agonist opioid for adequate relief. However, the drug-induced increase in smooth muscle tone may cause a paradoxical *increase* in pain secondary to increased spasm. An increase in the dose of opioid is usually successful in providing analgesia.

B. Acute Pulmonary Edema: The relief produced by intravenous morphine in dyspnea from pulmonary edema associated with left ventricular failure is remarkable. The mechanism is not clear but probably involves a reduction in *perception* of shortness of breath and the anxiety associated with it as well as a reduction in cardiac preload (reduced venous tone) and afterload (decreased peripheral resistance).

C. Cough: Suppression of cough can be obtained at doses lower than those needed for analgesia. However, in recent years the use of opioid analgesics to allay cough has diminished largely because a number of effective synthetic compounds have been developed that are neither analgesic nor addictive. These agents are discussed in the section on antitussives.

D. Diarrhea: Diarrhea from almost any cause can be controlled with the opioid analgesics, but if diarrhea is associated with infection such use must not substitute for appropriate chemotherapy. Opium preparations (eg, paregoric) have long been used to control diarrhea, but in recent years synthetic surrogates with more selective gastrointestinal effects and few or no CNS effects have been developed, eg, diphenoxylate. Formulations are cited below that have been prepared specifically for this purpose.

E. Applications in Anesthesia: The opioids are frequently used as premedicant drugs before anesthesia and surgery because of their sedative, anxiolytic, and analgesic properties. The opioids are also used intraoperatively both as adjuncts to other anesthetic agents and, in high doses (eg, 1–3 mg/kg of morphine, or 0.02–0.075 mg/kg of fentanyl), as the primary anesthetic agent (see Chapter 24), most commonly in cardiovascular surgery and other types of high-risk surgery where a primary goal is to minimize cardiovascular depression. In such situations, mechanical respiratory assistance *must* be provided.

Because of their direct action on the spinal cord, opioids can also be used as regional analgesics by administration into the epidural or subarachnoid spaces of the spinal column. A number of studies have demonstrated that long-lasting analgesia with minimal adverse effects can be achieved by epidural administration of 3–5 mg of morphine, followed by slow infusion through a catheter placed in the epidural space. It was initially assumed that the epidural application of opioids might selectively produce analgesia without impairment of motor, autonomic, or sensory functions other than pain. However, respiratory depression may occur after the drug is injected into the epidural space and may require reversal with naloxone. Other effects such as pruritus and nausea and vomiting are common after epidural and subarachnoid administration of opioids and may also be reversed with naloxone if necessary. Currently, the epidural route is favored because adverse effects are less common. Morphine is the most frequently used agent, but current research is actively aimed at finding compounds that can produce good analgesia with even fewer adverse effects.

F. Alternative Routes of Administration:

Rectal suppositories of morphine and hydromorphone have long been used where oral and parenteral routes are undesirable. With the rapid progress in drug delivery systems, it is not surprising that the opioids would be adapted to such technology. The epidural route, for action at the spinal level, has been described above. Another example is the transdermal route for systemic effects, ie, a patch that provides stable blood levels of drug and better pain control while avoiding the need for repeated parenteral injections. Fentanyl has been most successful in this application and finds great use in providing pain relief for those with constant pain associated with cancer.

The **intranasal route** is another route of administration that is utilized on a very limited basis for patients unable to tolerate oral medications and in whom repeat parenteral drug injections are not practical.

Another type of pain control, called **patient-controlled analgesia,** is now being used more frequently. In this approach, the patient controls a parenteral (usually intravenous) injection device to provide the desired degree of pain control. Claims of better pain control using less opioid are supported by well-designed clinical trials, making this approach very useful in postoperative pain control. Some lingering problems are equipment malfunction and the risk of drug overdosage secondary to improper programming or set-up of the device.

Toxicity & Undesired Effects

Direct toxic effects of the opioid analgesics that are extensions of their acute pharmacologic actions include the adverse effects of respiratory depression, nausea, vomiting, and constipation (Table 30–4). In addition, the following must be considered.

A. Tolerance and Dependence: Drug dependence of the opioid type is marked by tolerance, a relatively specific withdrawal or abstinence syndrome reflecting physical dependence, and pronounced craving or psychologic dependence. Just as there are pharmacologic differences between the various opioids, there are also differences in abuse potential and the severity of withdrawal effects. For instance, withdrawal from dependence upon a strong agonist is associated with more severe withdrawal signs and symptoms than withdrawal from a mild or moderate agonist. Administration of an opioid *antagonist* to an opioid-dependent person is followed by severe withdrawal symptoms. Propoxyphene, a weak opioid agonist, may cause less marked dependence, but the withdrawal syndrome appears to be qualitatively similar to that of other opioids. The addiction liabilities of the mixed agonist-antagonist opioids appear to be less than those of the agonist drugs.

1. Tolerance–Although development of tolerance begins with the first dose of an opioid, tolerance generally does not become clinically manifest until after 2–3 weeks of frequent exposure to ordinary therapeutic doses. Tolerance develops most readily when large doses are given at short intervals and is minimized by giving small amounts of drug with longer intervals between doses.

Depending on the compound and the effect measured, the degree of tolerance may be as great as 35-fold. Marked tolerance usually develops to the analgesic, euphoriant, and respiratory depressant effects. It is possible to produce respiratory arrest in a nontolerant person with a dose of 60 mg of morphine, whereas in addicts maximally tolerant to opioids as much as 2000 mg of morphine taken over a 2- or 3-hour period may not produce significant respiratory depression. Tolerance also develops to the antidiuretic, emetic, and hypotensive effect but not to the miotic, convulsant, and constipating actions (Table 30–3).

Tolerance to the euphoriant and respiratory effects of the opioids dissipates within a few days after the drugs are discontinued. Tolerance to the emetic effects may persist for several months after withdrawal of the drug. The rates at which tolerance appears and disappears, as well as the degree of tolerance, may also differ considerably among the different opioid analgesics. For instance, tolerance to methadone develops more slowly and to a lesser degree than to morphine.

Cross-tolerance is an extremely important characteristic of the opioids, ie, patients tolerant to morphine are also tolerant to other agonist opioids. Morphine, meperidine, methadone, and their congeners exhibit cross-tolerance not only with respect to their analgesic actions but also to their euphoriant, sedative, and respiratory effects.

Tolerance develops also to the mixed agonist-antagonist analgesics but to a lesser extent than to the agonists. Such effects as hallucinations, sedation, hypothermia, and respiratory depression are reduced after repeated administration of the mixed agonist-antagonist drugs. However, tolerance to agonist-antagonist agents does not generally include cross-tolerance to the agonist opioids. It is also important to note that tolerance does not develop to the *antagonist* actions of the mixed agonist-antagonists nor to those of the pure antagonists.

2. Physical dependence–The development of physical dependence is an invariable accompaniment of tolerance to an opioid of the mu type after its repeated administration. Failure to continue administering the drug results in a characteristic withdrawal or **abstinence syndrome** that reflects an exaggerated rebound from the acute pharmacologic effects of the opioid. The signs and symptoms of withdrawal include rhinorrhea, lacrimation, yawning, chills, gooseflesh (piloerection), hyperventilation, hyperthermia, mydriasis, muscular aches, vomiting, diarrhea, anxiety, and hostility (see Chapter 31). The number and intensity of the signs and symptoms are largely dependent on the degree of physical dependence that

has developed. Administration of an opioid at this time suppresses abstinence signs and symptoms almost immediately. The time of onset, the intensity, and the duration of the abstinence effects depend on the drug used and may be related to its biologic half-life. With morphine or heroin, withdrawal signs usually start within 6–10 hours after the last dose. Peak effects are seen at 36–48 hours, after which most of the signs and symptoms gradually subside. By 5 days, most of the effects have disappeared, but some may persist for months. In the case of meperidine, the withdrawal syndrome largely subsides within 24 hours, whereas with methadone several days are required to reach the peak of abstinence syndrome, and it may last as long as 2 weeks. The slower subsidence of methadone effects is associated with a less intense immediate syndrome, and this is the basis for its use in the detoxification of heroin addicts. After the abstinence syndrome subsides, tolerance also disappears as evidenced by a restoration in sensitivity to the opioid agonist. However, despite the loss of physical dependence on the opioid, craving for it may persist for many months.

A transient, explosive abstinence syndrome—**antagonist-precipitated withdrawal**—can be induced in a subject physically dependent on opioids by administering naloxone or another antagonist. Within 3 minutes after injection of the antagonist, signs and symptoms similar to those seen after abrupt discontinuance appear, peaking in 10–20 minutes and largely subsiding after 1 hour. Even in the case of methadone, withdrawal of which results in a relatively mild abstinence syndrome, the antagonist-precipitated abstinence syndrome may be very severe.

In the case of the mixed agonist-antagonist agents, withdrawal signs and symptoms can be induced after repeated administration followed by abrupt discontinuance of pentazocine, cyclazocine, or nalorphine, but the syndrome appears to be somewhat different from that produced by morphine and other agonists. Anxiety, loss of appetite and body weight, tachycardia, chills, increase in body temperature, and abdominal cramps have been noted.

3. Psychologic dependence–The euphoria, indifference to stimuli, and sedation usually caused by the opioid analgesics, especially when injected intravenously, tend to promote their compulsive use. In addition, the addict experiences abdominal effects that have been likened to an intense sexual orgasm. These factors constitute the primary reasons for opioid abuse liability and are strongly reinforced by the development of physical dependence, since the drug user rationalizes continued use of the drug as the means of preventing abstinence symptoms, ie, to remain "normal."

Obviously, the danger of causing dependence is an important consideration in the therapeutic use of these drugs. However, *under no circumstances* should adequate pain relief ever be withheld simply because an opioid exhibits potential for abuse or because legislative control measures complicate the process of prescribing narcotics. However, certain principles can be observed by the clinician to avoid problems presented by tolerance and dependence when using opioid analgesics:

a. Establish therapeutic goals before starting opioid therapy. This tends to limit the potential for physical dependence. The patient should be included in this process.

b. Once a therapeutic dose is established, attempt to limit dosage to this level.

c. Instead of opioid analgesics—especially in chronic management—consider using other types of analgesics or compounds exhibiting less pronounced withdrawal symptoms on discontinuance.

d. Frequently evaluate continuing analgesic therapy and the patient's need for opioids.

B. Diagnosis and Treatment of Opioid Overdosage: The diagnosis of opioid overdosage may be very simple (known addict, needle marks, brought to hospital by friends who appear to be using drugs), or it may be very difficult—as in any comatose patient for whom no past history is available. Intravenous injection of naloxone, 0.2–0.4 mg, dramatically reverses coma due to opioid overdose but not that due to other CNS depressants. Treatment is with the same drug, 0.4–0.8 mg given intravenously, and repeated whenever necessary. In using naloxone in the severely depressed newborn, it is important to start with doses of 5–10 μg/kg and to consider a second dose of up to a total of 25 μg/kg if no response is noted. Use of the antagonist should not, of course, delay the institution of other therapeutic measures, especially respiratory support.

C. Contraindications and Cautions in Therapy:

1. Use of pure agonists with mixed agonist-antagonists–When a mixed agonist-antagonist agent such as pentazocine is given to a patient also receiving an agonist (eg, morphine), the possibility of diminishing analgesia or perhaps inducing a state of withdrawal is present; combining agonist with mixed agonist-antagonist opioids should be done cautiously, if at all.

2. Use in patients with head injuries–Carbon dioxide retention caused by respiratory depression results in cerebral vasodilation; in patients with elevated intracranial pressure, this may lead to lethal alterations in brain function.

3. Use during pregnancy–In pregnant women who are chronically using opioids, the fetus may become physically dependent in utero and manifest withdrawal symptoms in the early postpartum period. A daily dose as small as 6 mg of heroin (or equivalent) taken by the mother will result in a mild withdrawal syndrome in the infant, and twice that much may result in severe signs and symptoms, including irritability, shrill crying, diarrhea, or even seizures.

Recognition of the problem is aided by a careful history and physical examination. When withdrawal symptoms are judged to be relatively mild, treatment is aimed at control of these symptoms with such drugs as diazepam; with more severe withdrawal, camphorated tincture of opium (paregoric; 0.4 mg of morphine/mL) in an oral dose of 0.12–0.24 mL/kg is used. Oral doses of methadone (0.1–0.5 mg/kg) have also been used.

4. Use in patients with impaired pulmonary function–In patients with borderline respiratory reserve, the depressant properties of the opioid analgesics may lead to acute respiratory failure.

5. Use in patients with impaired hepatic or renal function–Morphine and its congeners are metabolized primarily by conjugation to glucuronides in the liver; their use in patients in prehepatic coma may thus be questioned. Half-life is prolonged in patients with impaired renal function, and morphine and its active metabolite, morphine 6-glucuronide, may accumulate; dosage can often be reduced in such patients.

6. Use in patients with endocrine disease–Patients with adrenal insufficiency (Addison's disease) and those with hypothyroidism (myxedema) may have prolonged and exaggerated responses to opioids.

Drug Interactions

Because seriously ill or hospitalized patients may require a large number of drugs, there is always a possibility of drug interactions when the opioid analgesics are administered. Table 30–5 lists some of these drug interactions and the reasons for not combining the named drugs with opioids.

SPECIFIC AGENTS

The following section describes the most important widely used opioid analgesics, along with features peculiar to specific agents. Data about doses approximately equivalent to 10 mg of intramuscular morphine, oral versus parenteral efficacy, duration of analgesia, maximum efficacy, and addiction and abuse liability are presented in Table 30–2.

STRONG AGONISTS

1. PHENANTHRENES

Morphine, hydromorphone, and **oxymorphone** are strong agonists useful in treating severe pain. These prototypic agents have been described in detail above. **Heroin** is potent and fast-acting, but its use is prohibited by legislation in the USA. In recent years there has been considerable agitation to revive its use. However, double-blind studies have not supported the claim that heroin is more effective than morphine in relieving severe chronic pain.

2. PHENYLHEPTYLAMINES

Methadone has a pharmacodynamic profile very similar to that of morphine but is somewhat longer acting. Acutely, its analgesic potency and efficacy are at least equal to those of morphine. Methadone gives reliable effects when administered orally. Tolerance and physical dependence develop more slowly with methadone than with morphine. As noted above, the withdrawal signs and symptoms occurring after abrupt discontinuance of methadone are milder, although more prolonged, than those of morphine. These properties make methadone a useful drug for detoxification and for maintenance of the chronic relapsing heroin addict. For detoxification of a heroin-dependent addict, low doses of methadone (5–10 mg orally) are given 2 or 3 times daily for 2 or 3 days. Upon discontinuing methadone, the addict experiences a mild but endurable withdrawal syndrome. For maintenance therapy of the opioid recidivist, tolerance to 50–100 mg/d of oral methadone is deliberately produced; in this state, the addict experiences cross-tolerance to heroin that prevents most of the addiction-reinforcing effects of heroin. A related compound, levomethadyl acetate (L-alpha-acetylmethadol), which has an even longer half-life than methadone, has been approved by the FDA for use in detoxification clinics. This agent may be given once every two to three days.

The rationale of maintenance programs is that blocking the reinforcement obtained from abuse of illicit opioids removes the drive to obtain them, thereby reducing criminal activity and making the addict more amenable to psychiatric and rehabilitative therapy. The pharmacologic basis for the use of methadone in maintenance programs is sound and the sociologic basis is rational, but some methadone programs fail because nonpharmacologic management is inadequate.

3. PHENYLPIPERIDINES

Meperidine and **fentanyl** are the most widely used agents in this family of synthetic opioids. Meperidine has significant antimuscarinic effects, which may be a contraindication if tachycardia would be a problem. It is also reported to have a negative inotropic action on the heart. The potential for producing seizures secondary to accumulation of normeperidine in patients receiving high doses of meperidine or with renal com-

promise must be considered. The fentanyl subgroup now includes sufentanil and alfentanil in addition to the parent compound, fentanyl. These opioids differ mainly in their potency and biodisposition. Sufentanil is five to seven times more potent than fentanyl. Alfentanil is considerably less potent than fentanyl, acts more rapidly, and has a markedly shorter duration of action.

4. MORPHINANS

Levorphanol is a synthetically prepared opioid analgesic closely resembling morphine in its action but offering no advantages.

MILD TO MODERATE AGONISTS

1. PHENANTHRENES

Codeine, oxycodone, dihydrocodeine, and **hydrocodone** are all somewhat less efficacious than morphine or have adverse effects that limit the maximum tolerated dose when one attempts to achieve analgesia comparable to that of morphine. These compounds are rarely used alone but are combined in formulations containing aspirin or acetaminophen and other drugs.

2. PHENYLHEPTYLAMINES

Propoxyphene is chemically related to methadone but has low analgesic activity. Various studies have reported its potency at levels ranging from no better than placebo to half as potent as codeine, ie, 120 mg propoxyphene = 60 mg codeine. Its true potency probably lies somewhere between these extremes, and its analgesic effect is additive to that of an optimal dose of aspirin. However, its low efficacy makes it unsuitable, even in combination with aspirin, for severe pain. Although propoxyphene has a low abuse liability, the increasing incidence of deaths associated with its misuse has caused it to be scheduled as a controlled substance with low potential for abuse.

3. PHENYLPIPERIDINES

Diphenoxylate and its metabolite, **difenoxin,** are not used for analgesia but for the treatment of diarrhea. They are scheduled for minimal control (difenoxin is schedule IV, diphenoxylate schedule V; see inside front cover) because the likelihood of their abuse is remote. The poor solubility of the compounds limits their use for parenteral injection. As antidiarrheal drugs, they are used in combination with atropine. The atropine is added in a concentration too low to have a significant antidiarrheal effect but is presumed to further reduce the likelihood of abuse.

Loperamide is another phenylpiperidine derivative used to control diarrhea. Its potential for abuse is low because of its limited ability to gain access to the brain.

The usual dose with all of these antidiarrheal agents is two tablets to start and then one tablet after each diarrheal stool.

MIXED AGONIST-ANTAGONISTS & PARTIAL AGONISTS

1. PHENANTHRENES

Nalbuphine is a strong kappa receptor *agonist* and mu receptor *antagonist*; it is given parenterally. At higher doses there seems to be a definite ceiling—not noted with morphine—to the respiratory depressant effect. Unfortunately, when respiratory depression does occur, it may be relatively resistant to naloxone reversal.

Buprenorphine is a potent and long-acting phenanthrene derivative that is a partial mu receptor agonist. Its long duration of action is due to its slow dissociation from mu receptors. This property renders its effects resistant to naloxone reversal. Its clinical applications are much like those of nalbuphine. In addition, some studies suggest that buprenorphine may be as effective as methadone in the detoxification and maintenance of heroin abusers (eg, Bickel, 1988).

2. MORPHINANS

Butorphanol produces analgesia equivalent to nalbuphine and buprenorphine but appears to produce more sedation at equianalgesic doses. Butorphanol is considered to be a kappa-agonist.

3. BENZOMORPHANS

Pentazocine is also a kappa-agonist with weak mu-antagonist properties. It is the oldest mixed agonist-antagonist available. It may be used orally or parenterally. However, because of its irritant properties, the injection of pentazocine subcutaneously is not recommended. As with all of the agonist-antagonists, care should be taken not to administer it to patients receiving pure agonist drugs because of the unpredictability of both drugs' effects.

Dezocine is a compound structurally related to pentazocine. It has its highest affinity for mu receptors and less interaction with kappa receptors. Although it is said to be equivalent in efficacy to morphine, its use is associated with the same problems observed with all agonist-antagonists.

ANTITUSSIVES

As noted above, the opioid analgesics are among the most effective drugs available for the suppression of cough. This effect is often achieved at doses below those necessary to produce analgesia. The receptors involved in the antitussive effect appear to differ from those associated with the other actions of opioids. For example, the antitussive effect is also produced by the stereoisomers of opioid molecules, which are devoid of analgesic effects and addiction liability.

The physiologic mechanism of a cough is a complex one, and little is known about the specific mechanism of action of the opioid antitussive drugs. It is likely that both central and peripheral effects play a role.

The opioid derivatives most commonly used as antitussives are dextromethorphan, codeine, levopropoxyphene, and noscapine. While these agents (other than codeine) are largely free of the adverse effects associated with the opioids, they should be used with caution in patients taking MAO inhibitors (see Table 30–5).

Dextromethorphan is the dextrorotatory stereoisomer of a methylated derivative of levorphanol. It is essentially free of analgesic and addictive properties and produces less constipation than codeine. The usual antitussive dose is 15–30 mg 3 or 4 times daily. It is available in many over-the-counter products.

Codeine, as noted above, has a useful antitussive action at doses lower than those required for analgesia. Thus, 15 mg is usually sufficient to relieve cough.

Levopropoxyphene is the stereoisomer of the weak opioid agonist dextropropoxyphene. It is devoid of opioid effects, although sedation has been described as a side effect. The usual antitussive dose is 50–100 mg every 4 hours.

THE OPIOID ANTAGONISTS

The pure opioid antagonist drugs **naloxone** and **naltrexone** are morphine derivatives with bulkier substituents at the N position. These agents have a relatively high affinity for opioid binding sites of the mu receptor type. They have less affinity for the other receptors.

Pharmacokinetics

Naloxone has poor efficacy when given by the oral route and a short duration of action (1–2 hours) when given by injection. Metabolic disposition is chiefly by glucuronide conjugation, like that of the agonist opioids with free hydroxyl groups. Naltrexone is well absorbed after oral administration but may undergo rapid first-pass metabolism. It has a half-life of 10 hours, and a single oral dose of 100 mg will block the effects of injected heroin for up to 48 hours.

Pharmacodynamics

When given in the absence of an agonist drug, these antagonists are almost inert at doses that produce marked antagonism of agonist effects.

When given to a morphine-treated subject, the antagonist will completely and dramatically reverse the opioid effects within 1–3 minutes. In individuals who are acutely depressed by an overdose of an opioid, the antagonist will effectively normalize respiration, level of consciousness, pupil size, bowel activity, etc. In dependent subjects who appear normal while taking opioids, naloxone or naltrexone will almost instantaneously precipitate an abstinence syndrome, as described previously.

There is no tolerance to the antagonistic action of these agents, nor does withdrawal after chronic administration precipitate an abstinence syndrome.

Clinical Use

Naloxone is a pure antagonist and is preferred over earlier weak agonist-antagonist agents that had been used primarily as antagonists, eg, nalorphine and levallorphan.

The major application of naloxone is in the treatment of acute opioid overdose, as described above (see also Chapter 60). It is very important that the relatively short duration of action of naloxone be borne in mind, because a severely depressed patient may recover after a single dose of naloxone and appear normal, only to relapse into coma after 1–2 hours. The usual dose of naloxone is 0.1–0.4 mg intravenously, repeated as necessary.

Because of its long duration of action, naltrexone has been proposed as a "maintenance" drug for addicts in treatment programs. A single dose given on alternate days blocks virtually all of the effects of a dose of heroin. It might be predicted that this approach to rehabilitation would not be popular with a large percentage of drug users unless they are motivated to become drug-free. More recently, considerable interest has been aroused by reports that naltrexone decreases craving for alcohol in chronic alcoholics (Volpicelli, 1992).

Opioid antagonists appear to be of value in several experimental models of spinal cord injury. Similarly, it has been claimed that the antagonists are of value in cerebrovascular disease, eg, stroke, where they may lessen regional ischemic effects. Unfortunately, controlled clinical studies have not confirmed the value of antagonists for such purposes.

PREPARATIONS AVAILABLE
(Antidiarrheal opioid preparations are listed in Chapter 64.)

Analgesic Opioids
Alfentanil (Alfenta)
Parenteral: 500 µg/mL for injection
Buprenorphine (Buprenex)
Parenteral: 0.3 mg/mL for injection
Butorphanol (Stadol)
Parenteral: 1, 2 mg/mL for injection
Nasal (Stadol NS): 10 mg/mL nasal spray
Codeine sulfate or phosphate (generic)
Oral: 15, 30, 60 mg tablets and soluble tablets
Parenteral: 30, 60 mg/mL for IM, SC, or IV injection
Dezocine (Dalgan)
Parenteral: 5, 10, 15 mg/mL for IM or IV injection
Fentanyl (Sublimaze)
Parenteral: 50 µg/mL for injection
Fentanyl Transdermal System (Duragesic): 25, 50, 75, 100, µg/h
Hydromorphone (generic, Dilaudid)
Oral: 1, 2, 3, 4 mg tablets
Parenteral: 1, 2, 3, 4, 10 mg/mL for injection
Rectal: 3 mg suppositories
Levomethadyl acetate (Orlaam)

Oral: 10 mg/mL solution. *Note:* Approved *only* for the treatment of narcotic addition.
Levorphanol (Levo-Dromoran)
Oral: 2 mg tablets
Parenteral: 2 mg/mL for injection
Meperidine (generic, Demerol)
Oral: 50, 100 mg tablets; 50 mg/5 mL syrup
Parenteral: 25, 50, 75, 100 mg per dose for SC, IM injection; 10 mg/mL for IV infusion; 50 mg/ in 30 mL, 100 mg/mL in 20 mL
Methadone (generic, Dolophine)
Oral: 5, 10 mg tablets; 40 mg dispersible tablets; 1, 2, 10 mg/mL solutions
Parenteral: 10 mg/mL for injection
Morphine sulfate (generic, others)
Oral: 10, 15, 30 mg tablets; 10, 20 mg/mL solution; 20, 100 mg/5 mL solution
Oral sustained release (MS-Contin): 30, 60 mg tablets
Parenteral: 0.5, 1, 2, 3, 4, 5, 8, 10, 15 mg/mL for injection
Rectal: 5, 10, 20, 30 mg suppositories
Nalbuphine (generic, Nubain)
Parenteral: 10, 20 mg/mL for injection

Oxycodone (generic)
Oral: 5 mg tablets; 1, 20 mg/mL solutions
Oxymorphone (Numorphan)
Parenteral: 1, 1.5 mg/mL for injection
Rectal: 5 mg suppositories
Pentazocine (Talwin)
Oral: 50 mg tablets
Parenteral: 30 mg/mL for injection
Propoxyphene (generic, Darvon Pulvules, others)
Oral: 32, 65 mg capsules *Note:* This product is not recommended.
Sufentanil (Sufenta)
Parenteral: 50 μg/mL for injection

Analgesic Combinations*

Codeine/acetaminophen (generic, Tylenol w/Codeine, others)
Oral: 7.5, 15, 30 mg codeine plus 300 mg acetaminophen tablets; 12 mg codeine plus 120 mg acetaminophen tablets
Codeine/aspirin (generic, Empirin Compound, others)
Oral: 15, 30, 60 mg codeine plus 325 mg aspirin tablets
Hydrocodone/acetaminophen (generic, Norcet, Vicodin, Lortab, others)

Oral: 5, 7.5 mg hydrocodone plus 500 mg acetaminophen tablets
Oxycodone/acetaminophen (generic, Percocet, Percodan, Tylox, others)
Oral: 5 mg oxycodone plus 325 or 500 mg acetaminophen tablets
Oxycodone/aspirin (generic, Percodan)
Oral: 4.9 mg oxycodone plus 325 mg aspirin
Propoxyphene/aspirin (Darvon Compound-65, others)
Oral: 65 mg propoxyphene plus 389 mg aspirin plus 32.4 mg caffeine
Note: This product is not recommended.

Antitussives

Codeine (generic, others)
Oral: 15, 30, 60 mg tablets; constituent of many proprietary syrups
Dextromethorphan (generic, Benylin DM, Delsym, others)
Oral: 5 mg lozenges; 5, 7.5, 10, 15 mg/5 mL syrup; 30 mg sustained-action liquid; 15 mg chewy squares; constituent of many proprietary syrups

---

REFERENCES

Akil H et al: Endogenous opioids: Biology and function. Annu Rev Neurosci 1984;7:233.

Barber A, Gottschlich R: Opioid agonists and antagonists: An evaluation of their peripheral actions in inflammation. Med Res Rev 1992;12:525.

Beaver WT (editor): Appropriate management of pain in primary care practice. Symposium. Am J Med 1984; 77(Suppl 3A):1.

Beaver WT: Impact of non-narcotic analgesics on pain management. Am J Med 1988;84 (Suppl 5A):3.

Benedetti C, Bonica JJ (editors): Recent advances in intraspinal pain therapy. Acta Anaesthesiol Scand 1987;31(Suppl 85):1.

Benedetti C, Premuda L: The history of opium and its derivatives. In: *Advances in Pain Research and Therapy,* vol 14. Benedetti C et al (editors). Raven Press, 1990.

Bickel WK et al: A clinical trial of buprenorphine: Comparison with methadone in the detoxification of heroin addicts. Clin Pharmacol Ther 1988;43:72.

Bloom FE: Neurotransmitters: Past, present, and future directions. FASEB J 1988;2:32.

Braga PC: Centrally acting opioid drugs. In: *Cough.* Braga PC, Allegra L (editors). Raven Press, 1989.

Crain SM, Shen K-F: Opioids can evoke direct receptor-mediated excitatory effects on sensory neurons. Trends Pharmacol Sci 1990;11:77.

Duggan AW, North RA: Electrophysiology of opioids. Pharmacol Rev 1983;35:219.

Evans CJ et al: Cloning of a delta opioid receptor by functional expression. Science 1992;258:1952.

Fields HL: Brain stem mechanisms of pain modulation: Anatomy and physiology. In *Handbook of Experimental Pharmacology.* Vol 104: *II. Opioids.* Herz A et al (editors). Springer Verlag, 1993.

Fields HL, Heinricher MM, Mason P: Neurotransmitters in nociceptive modulatory circuits. Annu Rev Neurosci 1991;14:219.

Frances B et al: Further evidence that morphine-6β-glucuronide is a more potent opioid agonist than morphine. J Pharmacol Exp Therap 1992;262:25.

Goldstein A, Naidu A: Multiple opioid receptors: Ligand selectivity profiles and binding site signatures. Molec Pharmacol 1989;36:265.

Griffin MT, Law PY, Loh HH: Involvement of both inhibitory and stimulatory guanine nucleotide-binding proteins in the expression of chronic opiate regulation of adenylate cyclase activity. J Neurochem 1985;45:1585.

Harmer M, Rosen M, Vickers MD: *Patient-Controlled Analgesia: Proceedings of the First International Workshop on Patient-Controlled Analgesia.* Blackwell, 1985.

Heijna MH et al: Opioid receptor-mediated inhibition of 3H-dopamine and 14C-acetylcholine release from rate nu-

---

*Dozens of combination products are available. Only a few of those most commonly prescribed are listed. Codeine combination products available in several strengths are usually denoted No. 1 (for 7.5 mg codeine), No. 2 (for 15 mg codeine), No. 3 (for 30 mg codeine), and No. 4 (for 60 or 65 mg codeine).

cleus accumbens slices: A study on the possible involvement of K^+ channels and adenylate cyclase. Naunyn Schmiedebergs Arch Pharmacol 1992;345:627.

Hill CS, Fields WS (editors): *Drug Treatment of Cancer Pain in a Drug Oriented Society. Advances in Pain Research and Therapy,* vol 11. Raven Press, 1989.

Höllt V: Opioid peptide genes: Structure and regulation In: *Neurobiology of Opioids.* Almeida OFX, Shippenberg TS (editors). Springer Verlag, 1991.

Houde RW: Analgesic effectiveness of the narcotic agonist-antagonists. Br J Clin Pharmacol 1979;7(Suppl 3):297S.

Johnson SM, Fleming WW: Mechanisms of cellular adaptive sensitivity changes: Applications to opioid tolerance and dependence. Pharmacol Rev 1989;41:435.

Kromer W: Endogenous and exogenous opioids in the control of gastrointestinal motility and secretion. Pharmacol Rev 1988;40:121.

Kuhar MJ, Pasternak GW (editors): *Analgesics: Neurochemical, Behavioral, and Clinical Perspectives.* Raven Press, 1984.

Louie AK, Way EL: Overview of opioid tolerance and physical dependence. In: *Neurobiology of Opioids.* Almeida OFX, Shippenberg TS (editors). Springer Verlag, 1991.

Millan MJ: κ-Opioid receptors and analgesia. Trends Pharmacol Sci 1990;11:70.

Neil A: Tolerance and dependence. In: *Advances in Pain Research and Therapy.* Benedetti C et al (editors). Raven Press, 1990.

North RA: Opioid receptors and ion channels. In: *Neurobiology of Opioids.* Almeida OFX, Shippenberg TS (editors). Springer Verlag, 1991.

Paul D et al: Pharmacological characterization of morphine 6-β glucuronide, a very potent morphine metabolite. J Pharmacol Exp Therap 1989;251:477.

Rasmussen K et al: Opiate withdrawal from the rat locus coeruleus [sic]: behavioral, electrophysiologic, and biochemical correlates. J Neurosci 1990;10:2308.

Razaka RS, Porreca F: Development of delta opioid peptides as nonaddicting analgesics. Pharm Res 1991 8:1.

Simonds WF: The molecular basis of opioid receptor function. Endocrine Rev 1988;9:200.

Smith NT et al: Seizures during opioid anesthetic induction: Are they opioid-induced rigidity? Anesthesiology 1989;71:852.

Stein C: Peripheral mechanisms of opioid analgesia. Anesth Analg 1993;76:182.

Thirlwell MP et al: Pharmacokinetics and clinical efficacy of oral morphine solution and controlled-release morphine tablets in cancer patients. Cancer 1989;63:2275.

Valentino RJ: Neurophysiological and neuropharmacological effects of opiates. Monogr Neural Sci 1987;13:91.

Volpicelli JR et al: Naltrexone in the treatment of alcohol dependence. Arch Gen Psychiatry 1992;49:876.

Way EL, Adler TK: The pharmacologic implications of the fate of morphine and its surrogates. Pharmacol Rev 1968;12:383.

Way EL: Opioid tolerance and physical dependence and their relationship. In: *Handbook of Experimental Pharmacology.* Vol 104: *II. Opioids.* Herz A et al (editors). Springer Verlag, 1993.

Yaksh TL: CNS mechanisms of pain and analgesia. Cancer Surv 1988;7:55.

Yaster M, Deshpande JK: Management of pediatric pain with opioid analgesics. J Pediatr 1988;113:421.

Yeadon M, Kitchen I: Opioids and respiration. Prog Neurobiol 1989;33:1.

31

Drugs of Abuse

Leo E. Hollister, MD

The term "drug abuse" is unfortunate because it connotes social disapproval and may have different meanings to different people. One must also distinguish drug *abuse* from drug *misuse*. Abuse of a drug might be construed as any use of a drug for nonmedical purposes, usually for altering consciousness but also for body-building, etc. To misuse a drug might be to take it for the wrong indication, in the wrong dosage, or for too long a period, to mention only a few obvious examples. In the context of drug abuse, the drug itself is of less importance than the pattern of use. For example, taking 50 mg of diazepam to heighten the effect of a daily dose of methadone is an abuse of diazepam. On the other hand, taking the same excessive daily dose of the drug but only for its anxiolytic effect is misusing diazepam.

Dependence is a biologic phenomenon often associated with "drug abuse." **Psychic dependence** is manifested by compulsive drug-seeking behavior in which the individual uses the drug repetitively for personal satisfaction, often in the face of known risks to health. Heavy cigarette smoking is an example. **Physical dependence** is present when withdrawal of the drug produces symptoms and signs that are frequently the opposite of those sought by the user. It has been suggested that the body adjusts to a new level of homeostasis during the period of drug use and reacts in opposite fashion when the new equilibrium is disturbed. Alcohol withdrawal syndrome is perhaps the best-known example, but milder degrees of withdrawal may be observed in people who drink a lot of coffee every day. Psychic dependence almost always precedes physical dependence but does not inevitably lead to it. **Addiction** is usually taken to mean a state of physical and psychic dependence, but the word is too imprecise to be useful.

Tolerance signifies a decreased response to the effects of the drug, necessitating ever larger doses to achieve the same effect. Tolerance is closely associated with the phenomenon of physical dependence. It is largely due to compensatory responses that mitigate the drug's pharmacodynamic action. **Metabolic tolerance** due to increased disposition of the drug after chronic use is occasionally reported. **Behavioral tolerance,** an ability to compensate for the drug's effects, is another possible mechanism of tolerance. **Functional tolerance,** which may be the most common type, is due to compensatory changes in receptors, effector enzymes, or membrane actions of the drug.

A number of experimental techniques have been devised to predict the ability of a drug to produce dependence and to assess its likelihood for abuse. Most of these techniques employ self-administration of the drug by animals. The rates of reinforcement can be altered so as to make the animal work harder for each dose of drug, providing a semiquantitative measure as well. Comparisons are made against a standard drug in the class, eg, morphine among the opioids. Withdrawal of dependent animals from drugs can be used to assess the nature of the withdrawal syndrome as well as to test drugs that might cross-substitute for the standard drug. Most agents with significant potential for psychic or physical dependence can be readily detected by these techniques. The actual abuse liability, however, is difficult to predict, since many variables enter into the decision to abuse drugs.

Cultural Considerations

Each society accepts certain drugs as licit and condemns others as illicit. In the USA and most of Western Europe, the "national drugs" are caffeine, nicotine, and alcohol. In the Middle East, cannabis may be added to the list of licit drugs, while alcohol is forbidden. Among certain Native American tribes, peyote, a hallucinogen, may be used licitly for religious purposes. In the Andes of South America, cocaine is used to allay hunger and enhance the ability to perform arduous work at high altitude. Thus, which drugs are licit or illicit or—to use other terminology—"used" or "abused" depends on a social judgment. A major social cost of relegating any substance to the illicit category is the criminal activity that often results, since purveyors of the substance are lured into illegal traffic by the opportunity to make enormous profits while dependent users may resort to robbery, prostitution, and other types of antisocial behavior to support their habits.

Current USA attitudes to drugs of this type are reflected in the Schedule of Controlled Substances (Table 65–2; Inside Front Cover). This schedule is quite similar to those published by international control bodies. Such schedules affect principally ethical and law-abiding manufacturers of the drugs and have had little deterrent effect on illicit manufacturers or suppliers. Such schedules have been circumvented by the synthesis of "designer" drugs that make small modifications of the chemical structures of drugs with little or no change in their pharmacodynamic actions. Thus, schedules must constantly be revised to include these attempts to produce compounds not currently listed.

Because of the high social cost of drug abuse, many countries attempt to interdict the entry of drugs. While some surveys have indicated that the use of drugs such as cocaine and marijuana is decreasing, it is difficult to credit such declines to law enforcement efforts. Little progress has been made in decreasing the demand for illicit drugs. Some have argued that the only reasonable solution to the problem is legalization of the drugs. Such proposals are obviously highly controversial.

Any use of mind-altering drugs is based on a complicated interplay between three factors: the user, the setting in which the drug is taken, and the drug. Thus, the personality of the user and the setting may have a strong influence on what the user experiences. Nonetheless, it is usually possible to identify a pharmacologic "core" of drug effects that will be experienced by almost anyone under almost any circumstances if the dosage is adequate.

OPIOIDS

History

The nepenthe (Gk "free from sorrow") mentioned in the *Odyssey* probably contained opium. Opium smoking was widely practiced in China and the Near East until recently. Isolation of active opium alkaloids as well as the introduction of the hypodermic needle, allowing parenteral use of morphine, increased opioid use in the West. The first of several "epidemics" of opioid use in the USA followed the Civil War. Relief of pain with liberal doses of opiates was one of the few forms of treatment army physicians could offer the gravely wounded, and those lucky enough to survive often found themselves physically dependent. About 4% of adults in the USA used opiates regularly during the postbellum period. By the 1900s, the number had dropped to about one in 400 people in the USA, but the problem was still considered serious enough to justify passage of the Harrison Narcotic Act just before World War I. A new epidemic of opioid use started around 1964 and has remained unabated ever since. Present estimates are that the number of opioid-dependent people in the USA has recently stabilized at around 400,000.

Chemistry & Pharmacology

The most commonly abused drugs in this group are heroin, morphine, oxycodone, and (among health professionals) meperidine. The chemistry and general pharmacology of these agents are presented in Chapter 30.

Tolerance to the mental effects of opioids develops with chronic use. The need for ever-increasing amounts of drugs to sustain the desired euphoriant effects—as well as avoid the discomfort of withdrawal—has the expected consequence of strongly reinforcing dependence once it has started. The role of endogenous opioids (endorphins) in opioid dependence is uncertain.

Clinical Aspects

Curiosity and social pressure are the strongest factors in initiating opioid use. Intravenous administration is routine not only because it is the most efficient route but also because it produces a bolus of high concentration of drug that reaches the brain to produce a "rush," followed by euphoria, a feeling of tranquility, and sleepiness ("the nod"). Most doses of heroin available on the street are less than 25 mg and produce effects that last 3–5 hours. Thus, several doses a day are required to forestall manifestations of withdrawal in dependent persons. The trouble and expense of meeting these dose requirements put the dependent person always "on the hustle," either to get money to buy the drug or to find a "connection" with something to sell. Since supplies of heroin are of widely varying potency, the risk of overdosage is always present. And sooner or later in the lives of most heroin abusers, the money runs out or the supplies run out, and the withdrawal syndrome then begins.

Symptoms of opioid withdrawal begin 8–10 hours after the last dose. Many of these symptoms resemble those of increased activity of the autonomic nervous system. Lacrimation, rhinorrhea, yawning, and sweating appear first. Restless sleep followed by weakness, chills, gooseflesh ("cold turkey"), nausea and vomiting, muscle aches, and involuntary movements ("kicking the habit"), hyperpnea, hyperthermia, and hypertension occur in later stages of the withdrawal syndrome. The acute course of withdrawal may last 7–10 days. A secondary phase of protracted abstinence lasts for 26–30 weeks and is characterized by hypotension, bradycardia, hypothermia, mydriasis, and decreased responsiveness of the respiratory center to carbon dioxide.

Heroin users in particular tend to be polydrug users, also using alcohol, sedatives, and stimulants. None of these other drugs serve as substitutes for opioids, but they have desired additive effects. One needs to be sure that the person undergoing a withdrawal reaction is not also withdrawing from alcohol or sedatives, which might be more dangerous and more difficult to manage.

Besides the ever-present risk of fatal overdose, a number of other serious complications are associated with opioid dependence. Hepatitis B and AIDS are among the many potential complications of sharing contaminated hypodermic syringes. Bacterial infections lead to septic complications such as meningitis, osteomyelitis, and abscesses in various organs. A novel complication of attempts to illicitly manufacture meperidine has been the production of parkinsonism in users of this product. The culprit is a highly specific neurotoxin, MPTP (see Chapter 27). Homicide, suicide, and accidents are more prevalent among heroin abusers than in the general population.

Treatment

Treatment of acute overdoses of opioids may be lifesaving and is described in Chapters 30 and 60.

Pharmacologic or psychosocial approaches may be used, either separately or together, in long-term treatment of opioid-dependent persons. Widely different opinions have been vigorously expounded about which is the preferred type of treatment. Because each treatment method has a self-selected patient population, it is difficult to compare results. Chronic users tend to prefer pharmacologic approaches; those with shorter histories of drug abuse are more amenable to psychosocial interventions.

Pharmacologic treatment is most often used for detoxification. The principles of detoxification are the same for all drugs: to substitute a longer-acting, orally active, pharmacologically equivalent drug for the abused drug, stabilize the patient on that drug, and then gradually withdraw the substituted drug. **Methadone** is admirably suited for such use in opioid-dependent persons. More recently, clonidine, a centrally acting sympatholytic agent, has been used for detoxification. By reducing central sympathetic outflow clonidine might be expected to mitigate many of the signs of sympathetic overactivity. A presumed advantage of clonidine is that it has no narcotic action and is not addicting.

While it is easy to detoxify patients, the recidivism rate (return to abuse of the agent) is extraordinarily high. Methadone maintenance therapy, which substitutes a long-acting orally active opioid for heroin, has been effective in some settings. A single dose can be given each day, with the possibility of even less frequent than once-a-day doses for long-term patients. Methadone saturates the opiate receptors and prevents the desired sudden onset of central nervous system effects normally produced by intravenous administration. An even longer-acting methadone homologue, L-alpha acetylmethadol, has been approved and may offer additional technical advantages.

Use of a narcotic antagonist is rational therapy because blocking the action of self-administered opiates should eventually extinguish the habit. **Naltrexone,** a long-acting orally active pure narcotic antagonist, has been extensively studied. It can be given 3 times a week once dosage reaches levels of 100–150 mg/d. The greatest drawback is that few addicts will accept naltrexone as permanent treatment. Unlike methadone, on which patients become dependent, naltrexone provides no such "hold" on them.

Psychosocial approaches include a variety of techniques. Drug-free communities are based on the assumption that drug use is a symptom of some emotional disturbance or inability to cope with life's stresses. The most common technique employs peer group pressures, emphasizing confrontation. Other techniques include variations on group or individual psychotherapy, didactic approaches, alternative lifestyles through work or communal living, and a variety of types of meditation. Treatment may have to be continued for months or years, with costs depending on the degree to which professional staff is used. Many users eventually tire of their habit or "burn out," even without therapy.

BARBITURATES & OTHER SEDATIVES

History

Barbiturates were introduced in 1903. Short-acting members of this group have been—and still are—widely abused. Meprobamate was introduced in 1954 as a nonbarbiturate sedative presumably lacking the disadvantages of the older drugs. It turned out to have more similarities to than differences from barbiturates. In fact, some of the nonbarbiturate sedative-hypnotics—examples are glutethimide and methaqualone—were worse than barbiturates in many respects, including abuse potential. The current era of **benzodiazepines** began in 1960. In the opinion of many authorities, these drugs are now the sedative-hypnotics of choice. Abuse and physical dependence have been reported but are probably less frequent than with barbiturates.

Chemistry & Pharmacology

The chemical relationships among this class of drugs are reviewed in Chapter 21.

Depending on the dose, these drugs produce sedation, hypnosis, anesthesia, coma, and death. The exact mechanism by which they produce psychic and physical dependence is unclear.

Both barbiturates and benzodiazepines can be classified pharmacokinetically into short- and long-acting compounds. Experience with barbiturates was that most nonmedical use involved short-acting drugs, eg, secobarbital or pentobarbital sodium, and not long-acting ones, eg, phenobarbital. To some extent, this pattern has been repeated with the benzodiazepines. What has become evident is that the abruptness of onset of withdrawal syndromes as well as their severity is a function of the half-life of the drug. Drugs with half-lives in the range of 8–24 hours produce a rapidly evolving, severe withdrawal syndrome, while those with longer half-lives, such as 48–96 hours, produce a withdrawal syndrome that is slower in onset and less severe but longer in duration. Drugs with half-lives longer than 96 hours usually have a built-in tapering-off action that reduces the possibility of withdrawal reactions. Drugs with very short half-lives (< 4 hours) generally cannot be taken frequently enough to sustain high concentrations of the drug and are rarely associated with withdrawal reactions.

Clinical Aspects

No one knows how many persons are dependent on sedatives. Much of the presumed dependence is psychologic, perhaps based on the need for these drugs as a form of "replacement therapy." Physical dependence of the classic type (see below) has been relatively rare with benzodiazepines considering the extensive use these agents have had. It usually occurs following long-term treatment with doses of 40 mg/d or more of diazepam or the equivalent dose of another drug. During the past several years, much interest has developed in the phenomenon of "therapeutic dose dependence." Many patients with this syndrome have never taken more than normal medical doses (15–30 mg/d of diazepam equivalents). Abrupt withdrawal of a benzodiazepine may be followed by some of the same symptoms observed in classic withdrawal but is characterized by weight loss, changes in perception, paresthesias, and headache. Such a syndrome almost always follows months or years of continual use. This phenomenon may be related to some adaptive change in benzodiazepine receptors following long-term exposure to the drug. All patients who have been taking these drugs for substantial periods of time should have them withdrawn slowly.

Several patterns of sedative abuse have emerged. People with severe emotional disorders may use these drugs to seek escape into oblivion. Most abusers of sedatives use them to produce an altered mental state with disinhibition in the same way other people—or they themselves—use alcohol. One sometimes sees a pattern of alternating use of sedatives and stimulants, one type of drug being used to counter the effects of the other. A growing trend has been to use sedatives in a pattern of polydrug abuse, which includes most drugs of abuse.

The effects sought by the user are similar to those produced by alcohol—an initial disinhibition followed by drowsiness. Speech may be slurred and incoordination evident. As the goal seems to be to repeat such intoxications frequently, drugs that are eliminated rapidly are preferred.

As these drugs are usually taken orally and the tablets or capsules are consistent in drug content, inadvertent fatal overdoses of single agents are rare. Tolerance may develop to the sedative effect but not to the respiratory depressant effect. Thus, if these drugs are used with large amounts of alcohol, another respiratory depressant, fatalities can occur.

The withdrawal syndrome from sedatives is so much like that from alcohol that the two types of dependence are classified together (alcohol-barbiturate type). Symptoms and signs of chronic intoxication from short-acting drugs may improve during the first 8 hours after withdrawal but are followed by increasing anxiety, tremors, twitches, and nausea and vomiting for the next 16 hours. Propranolol or clonidine may be of value in reducing some of these effects. Convulsions may occur 16–48 hours after withdrawal. Severe cases are associated with delirium, hallucinations, and other psychosis-like manifestations.

In the case of long-acting drugs, the withdrawal syndrome is attenuated. No symptoms may appear for 2–3 days, and initial symptoms may suggest a recrudescence of those originally treated. Only by the fourth or fifth day can one be sure that a withdrawal reaction is under way. Convulsions are a late manifestation when they do occur—often not until the eighth or ninth day. Following this, the syndrome subsides. This slow evolution may allow some patients to recognize what is happening and to abort the syndrome by resuming their drug. As withdrawal is generally mild, other patients may go through the syndrome, knowing that something is wrong but not being entirely sure what is happening.

Treatment

The time-honored principles of treating abstinence syndromes hold for sedative withdrawal as well. If short-acting drugs have been abused, phenobarbital is substituted as the pharmacologically equivalent agent. If long-acting drugs have been used, the same drug may be continued. The patient is stabilized on whatever dose is required to cause signs and symptoms to abate, and the drug is then gradually withdrawn. The rate of decrement may be 15–25% of the daily dose early in treatment, with later decrements of 5–10%. Complete detoxification can usually be achieved in less than 2 weeks.

No specific treatment programs have been developed for sedative abusers. The problem is so often complicated by abuse of other drugs that it may be more expeditious to enroll the patient in a program designed for alcoholics or opiate-dependent persons. Patients with psychiatric disorders that can be defined, especially those with depression, may be treated with specific drug treatment for the underlying disorder.

STIMULANTS

History

Caffeine is probably the most widely used social drug worldwide. Most people do not consider it to be a drug, though many, especially as they age, experience disturbing effects on sleep and heart rhythm from too much coffee. A withdrawal syndrome characterized by lethargy, irritability, and headache has been recognized in users of more than 600 mg/d (roughly six cups of coffee).

Nicotine is one of the most widely used licit drugs. It is now considered to be one of the most insidiously addicting substances because most users are not aware of strong feelings of reinforcement when consuming it but have extremely long-lasting cravings for it when trying to quit. Nicotine causes central electroencephalographic activation and euphoriant effects and release of catecholamines from peripheral adrenergic nerves. Tolerance develops rapidly. Despite compelling evidence of serious health hazards involving multiple organ systems (MMWR, 1993), about 28% of adults in the USA still smoke cigarettes because they have become dependent upon nicotine. Various techniques have been used to wean smokers from the drug, including substitution of nicotine in the form of nicotine-containing chewing gum and a slow-release transdermal form of nicotine. These preparations are designed to be used under medical supervision in gradually tapering dosage, so that the patient is gradually withdrawn from the drug. However, recruitment of new cigarette smokers seems to equal the number of those who quit. The use of smokeless tobacco products (snuff, chewing tobacco) has increased in recent years, especially in adolescents, apparently in response to new advertising campaigns directed at younger age groups. These products are subject to the same risks of cancer and addiction as smoked tobacco. A brief description of the pharmacology of nicotine is found in Chapter 7.

Cocaine has been used for at least 1200 years in the custom of chewing coca leaves by natives of the South American Andes. Coca was first imported to Europe from the Western Hemisphere in 1580. Cocaine was isolated as the active material in 1860. Its anesthetic properties, especially its topical anesthetic action, were discovered in the 1870s and 1880s. Sigmund Freud was intrigued by the drug and thought it might even be a panacea, but his enthusiasm was dampened by its disastrous effects on a friend who became addicted. A colleague of Freud's, Karl Koller, is credited with first using the drug as a topical anesthetic for eye surgery, a use that continues to this day.

Amphetamine was synthesized in the late 1920s and was introduced into medical practice in 1936. Dextroamphetamine is the major member of the class, though many other amphetamines and amphetamine surrogates, such as methamphetamine (Methedrine, "speed"), phenmetrazine (Preludin), and methylphenidate (Ritalin), were subsequently introduced. The number of amphetamine homologues with psychoactive effects continues to multiply. The first of these was 2,5-dimethoxy-4-methylamphetamine

(DOM, "STP"). More recently, methylene-dioxyamphetamine (MDA) and methylenedioxymethamphetamine (MDMA, "ecstasy") have been introduced. The latter drugs have more amphetamine-like than hallucinogenic effects. They have also been shown to be neurotoxic to serotonergic systems in the brains of animals, with uncertain adverse consequences in humans.

A closely related natural alkaloid, **cathinone,** is found in the leaves and stems of *Catha edulis,* or khat, a plant found and cultivated in the Middle East and Africa. Chewing of freshly harvested khat results in effects indistinguishable from those of the amphetamines.

Chemistry & Pharmacology

The chemical relationships of the various stimulants are shown in Figure 31–1. Despite their similar actions, caffeine, cocaine, and amphetamine have very different structures.

Caffeine, a methylxanthine compound, appears to exert its central actions (and perhaps its peripheral ones as well) by blocking adenosine receptors. Other methylxanthines, eg, theophylline, have the same actions. Adenosine modulates adenylyl cyclase activity, causing contraction of isolated airway smooth muscle as one of its peripheral actions. The same action probably accounts for the central stimulant actions of the methylxanthines. At high concentrations, the methylxanthines inhibit phosphodiesterase, thereby inhibiting the breakdown of cAMP and increasing its concentration inside cells. However, it is doubtful whether this is important at ordinary dosage. Cocaine binds to the dopamine reuptake transporter in the central nervous system, effectively inhibiting dopamine reuptake as well as that of norepinephrine. Dopamine is thought to be important in the reward system of the brain, and its increase may account for the high dependence potential of cocaine. Amphetamines may act in a variety of ways but probably mainly by increasing release of catecholaminergic neurotransmitters. They are also weak inhibitors of monoamine oxidase and, by virtue of structural similarity, possible direct catecholaminergic agonists in the brain.

Although psychic dependence is strong for many of these drugs (cocaine is one of the most strongly reinforcing drugs in self-administration paradigms in animals), it was thought for some time that physical dependence occurred only rarely. However, recent patterns of abuse of these drugs, especially amphetamine-like agents, have revealed a typical pattern of withdrawal manifested by signs and symptoms opposite to those produced by the drug. Users deprived of the drug become sleepy, have a ravenous appetite, are exhausted, and may suffer mental depression. This syndrome may last for several days after the drug is withdrawn. Tolerance develops quickly, so that abusers may take monumental doses compared with those used medically, eg, as anorexiants.

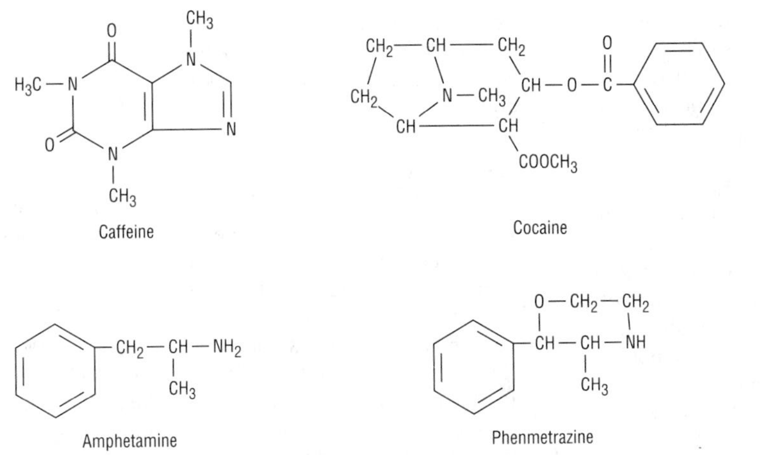

Figure 31–1. Chemical structures of some popular stimulants.

Clinical Aspects

Amphetamine abuse began in the 1940s. The substance was present in substantial amounts in inhalers promoted as nasal decongestants. During World War II, amphetamines were frequently used by military personnel. A huge supply of amphetamines became available to young people in Japan in the postwar period, resulting in an epidemic of abuse that was ultimately curbed by draconian punishments. Meanwhile, in the USA the drug continued to be used in relatively small oral doses, often alternating with barbiturates. In the 1960s, the pattern changed. Methamphetamine became the preferred drug (largely because it was more easily synthesized illicitly), and the preferred route of administration became intravenous injection.

One pattern of amphetamine abuse is called a "run." Repeated intravenous injections are self-administered to obtain a "rush"—an orgasm-like reaction—followed by a feeling of mental alertness and marked euphoria. Total daily doses as high as 4000 mg have been reported. After several days of such spree use, subjects may enter a paranoid schizophrenia-like state. Typically, they develop delusions that bugs are crawling under their skin, which leads to characteristic discrete excoriations. Finally, the spree is terminated by exhaustion from lack of sleep and lack of food, followed by the withdrawal syndrome mentioned above.

A new pattern of amphetamine abuse has evolved in which methamphetamine base crystals ("ice") are smoked—analogous to the use of "crack" cocaine (see below). Smoking delivers a rapid bolus of drug to the brain, somewhat similar to intravenous administration. Since the duration of action of methamphetamine is much longer than that of cocaine, intoxication may last for several hours after a single smoke. It remains to be seen whether "ice" will replace "crack" or merely add another form of abusable drug. It is a curious paradox that efforts to regulate the use

of drugs by law often lead to the introduction of more dangerous drugs. With the virtual outlawing of amphetamines from legitimate medical practice (based on adverse effects experienced by using doses two or three orders of magnitude larger than therapeutic doses), cocaine became the substitute. Cocaine may be construed as a highly potent amphetamine ("superspeed") with all of the effects of the latter drug magnified. It is far more likely to lead to dependence than amphetamines, and overdoses leading to death are possible.

Two types of administration of cocaine are current. One may "snuff" or "snort" the drug by sniffing a "line" (a measured amount of drug in a folded piece of paper applied to the nose), or one may smoke "free base." Cocaine is supplied as a hydrochloride salt, and free base (**"crack"**) is made by alkalinizing the salt and extracting with nonpolar solvents. When free base is smoked, entry through the lungs is almost as fast as by intravenous injection, so that effects are more accentuated than when the drug is snorted. Intravenous injection is rarely used, as the possibility of overdose is considerable. The purity and potency of cocaine available to users vary widely.

The plasma half-life of cocaine is short, so that effects following a single dose persist only for an hour or so. Consequently, the euphoric experience may be repeated many times during the course of a day or night.

Cocaine may be used sporadically, as at a party, or regularly by those with a self-imposed high level of activity, such as rock musicians. It may also be part of the repertoire of the polydrug abuser. A "speedball" is a combination of cocaine and heroin taken intravenously, presumably doubling the "rush" but extinguishing other effects. Patients in methadone maintenance programs who can no longer get much kick from heroin may turn to cocaine, whose euphoriant effects are not altered by methadone. An epidemic of "cocaine babies" born to mothers who are using cocaine heavily has posed a major new challenge to health care facilities in the inner cities (Volpe, 1992). There are clear-cut deleterious effects on the pregnancy, with increased fetal morbidity and mortality. Whether surviving babies will be impaired in the long term awaits further study.

Besides the paranoid psychosis associated with chronic use of amphetamines, intravenous injection using contaminated syringes leads to the same infectious complications as with heroin. A specific lesion associated with chronic amphetamine use is necrotizing arteritis, which may involve many small and medium-sized arteries and lead to fatal brain hemorrhage or renal failure. Overdoses of amphetamines are rarely fatal; they can usually be managed by sedating the patient with haloperidol. The powerful vasoconstrictive action of cocaine has led to an increasing number of patients with severe acute hypertensive episodes resulting in myocardial infarcts and strokes. The local anesthetic action of cocaine contributes to the production of seizures. Overdoses of cocaine are usually rapidly fatal, victims dying within minutes from arrhythmias, respiratory depression, or seizures. Those who survive for 3 hours usually recover fully. Intravenous administration of diazepam, propranolol, or calcium channel-blocking drugs may be the best treatment.

Long-Term Treatment

Subjects with residual emotional disorders, either schizophreniform psychosis or mental depression, may require treatment with antipsychotic or antidepressant drugs before or during weaning from stimulants. A number of drugs have been studied to assess their ability to mitigate withdrawal from cocaine, reduce craving during abstinence, and facilitate abstinence. Desipramine, carbamazepine, bromocriptine, amantadine, clonidine, buprenorphine, bupropion, and others are under investigation. No specific treatment programs have been devised for stimulant users. Those who administer these drugs intravenously have more in common with heroin users than any other group and may be suitable for some of the rehabilitative programs devised for opioid-dependent persons.

HALLUCINOGENS

History

Almost every society, however primitive, has found some bark, skin, leaf, vine, berry, or weed that contains "hallucinogenic" materials. Although the fortuitous discovery of the properties of lysergic acid diethylamide (LSD) occurred in a chemical laboratory during the 1940s, this was a case in which scientific art was merely imitating nature. Similar compounds have been found in morning glory seeds, and drugs such as mescaline and psilocybin had long been used by North and Central American Indians in the form of cactus buttons or magical mushrooms. Deliriants, such as the alkaloids in *Atropa belladonna* and *Datura stramonium,* were also known in ancient cultures.

Terminology

Although the term "hallucinogen" will be used here, it is not entirely accurate, since hallucinations may be uncommon effects or only part of the overall effects of these drugs. The term "psychotomimetic" is often used to connote the possible action of these drugs in mimicking naturally occurring psychoses. However, the state induced by these agents does not closely resemble that of schizophrenia. The term "psychedelic" was coined to denote a supposed "mind-revealing" aspect of such drug use, but the insights and revelations achieved are not much different from those that have been claimed with many other disinhibiting drugs, most commonly alcohol.

The drugs we here call hallucinogens are taken for many reasons. The one most widely given by users is that the drugs provide new ways of looking at the world and new insights into personal problems. The former claim implies varying degrees of perceptual distortion, while the latter implies changes in mood and increased introspection. LSD has become the prototypical hallucinogenic drug because of the extent of its use; because it represents a family of drugs that are similar; and because it has been most extensively studied.

Chemistry & Pharmacology

The LSD-like group of drugs includes **LSD, mescaline, psilocybin,** and their related compounds. Although these substances differ chemically, they share some chemical features and even more pharmacologic ones (Figure 31–2). LSD is a semisynthetic chemical not known to occur in nature. It is related to the ergot alkaloids (Chapter 16). The monoethyl—rather than the diethyl—amide is found in hallucinogenic morning glory seeds. Mescaline, a phenethylamine derivative, and psilocybin, an indolethylamine derivative, are found in nature. These drugs also have chemical resemblances to three major neurotransmitters: norepinephrine, dopamine, and serotonin.

The mode of action of hallucinogens of the LSD type is uncertain despite much experimental study. Measured electroencephalographically, their effects are to produce a state of hyperarousal of the central nervous system. LSD interacts with several serotonin (5-HT) receptor subtypes in the brain. Until recently it was thought to be a potent 5-HT_2 receptor antagonist. It appears to alter serotonin turnover, as indicated by increased brain concentrations of its major metabolite, 5-hydroxyindoleacetic acid. In addition, LSD displays agonist activity at 5-HT_{1A} and 5-HT_{1C} receptors. These actions may be more relevant to LSD's hallucinogenic action, because a number of

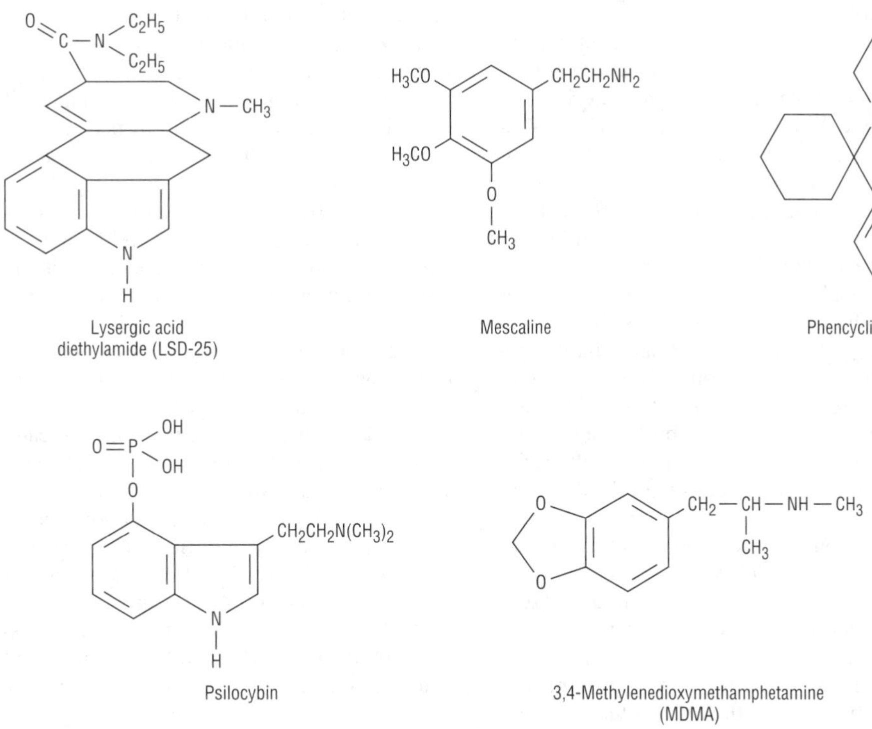

Figure 31–2. Chemical structures of lysergic acid diethylamide *(LSD)*, mescaline, phencyclidine, psilocybin, and the amphetamine analogue MDMA.

other drugs with good antagonist effects at central $5-HT_2$ receptors are not hallucinogenic.

The deliriant hallucinogens, exemplified by scopolamine (Chapter 8) and some synthetic centrally acting cholinoceptor-blocking agents, are different chemically as well as pharmacologically from the LSD group. Their effects seem to be entirely explainable by blockade of central muscarinic receptors. Similar mental effects may be seen during therapeutic or deliberate overdoses of commonly used medications with antimuscarinic action, such as anticholinergic antiparkinsonism drugs, tricyclic antidepressants, and antispasmodics. Occasional instances of abuse of these therapeutic agents have occurred.

Phencyclidine (PCP, "angel dust," many other names) is a synthetic phenylcyclohexylamine derivative. There is some question about how it should be classified, since it differs in many ways from other hallucinogens, but its primary use is to obtain hallucinogenic effects. The drug was originally introduced as a "dissociative anesthetic" in 1957. Such anesthetics were presumed to work by making patients insensitive to pain by "separating their bodily functions from their minds" without causing loss of consciousness. Hallucinogenic effects were noted in patients emerging from anesthesia. The drug was withdrawn from use in humans but retained in veterinary practice

under the name Sernylan. (The veterinary use has given the drug one of its street names—"hog.") **Ketamine,** a homologue, replaced phencyclidine as an anesthetic for use in humans (see Chapter 24). It too produces some emergent hallucinogenic effects. The first street use of PCP was in 1967, when it quickly gained a reputation as a bad drug. Over the next several years, it was mislabeled, being sold as LSD, tetrahydrocannabinol (THC), and other hallucinogens. Since the 1970s, PCP has become widely accepted and is now the most commonly used hallucinogenic agent. Phencyclidine may be smoked (by mixing the powder with tobacco), "snorted," taken orally, or injected intravenously. Fortunately, a recent trend toward less frequent use of the drug has been noted.

Some of the early investigators of PCP maintained that it provided a much better model of schizophrenia than LSD, mainly through its action in producing a form of sensory isolation. Receptors for PCP have been identified in the brain that are closely related, if not identical, to the opioid sigma receptor. The drug also acts on the NMDA subtype of glutamate receptors as an antagonist. Earlier work also suggested that PCP blocked uptake of dopamine as well. The drug is unique among hallucinogens in that animals will self-administer it.

Clinical Effects

LSD produces a series of somatic, perceptual, and psychic effects that overlap each other. Dizziness, weakness, tremors, nausea, and paresthesias are prominent somatic symptoms. Blurring of vision, distortions of perspective, organized visual illusions or "hallucinations," less discriminant hearing, and a change in sense of time are common perceptual abnormalities. Impaired memory, difficulty in thinking, poor judgment, and altered mood are prominent psychic effects. Physiologically, LSD produces signs of overactivity of the sympathetic nervous system and central stimulation, manifested by dilated pupils, increased heart rate, mild elevation of blood pressure, tremor, and alertness. Virtually identical effects are produced by mescaline and psilocybin when they are given in equivalent doses. The onset of effects is fairly rapid, but the duration varies with the dose and is usually measured in hours. Phenomena may vary considerably from one user to another owing to such factors as the personality and expectations of the user and the circumstances under which the drug is taken, but the above effects occur in almost everyone. Waxing and waning of effects is typical.

Usual doses of LSD in humans are approximately 1–2 μg/kg, making it one of the most potent pharmacologic agents known. The drug is equally effective parenterally or orally and consequently is almost always taken by mouth. Psilocybin is usually taken in doses of 250 μg/kg and mescaline in doses of 5–6 mg/kg. Despite these differences in potency, the effects are virtually indistinguishable.

Scopolamine and other antimuscarinic drugs produce delirium with fluctuating levels of awareness, disorientation, marked difficulty in thinking, marked loss of memory, and bizarre delusions. If doses are large, these impairments may last for more than a day, with some subjects claiming that several days may elapse before they once again feel confident about their memory. Most subjects, at least under experimental conditions, find these drugs to be unpleasant and have little desire to repeat the experience. Some become frightened during the period of drug effect. Others deliberately seek out and use such drugs repeatedly.

PCP produces detachment, disorientation, distortions of body image, and loss of proprioception. Somatic symptoms and signs include numbness, nystagmus, sweating, rapid heart rate, and hypertension. Effects are dose-dependent. Overdosage has been fatal, as contrasted with the absence of known fatalities directly caused by drugs of the LSD group.

Toxicity

Adverse psychologic consequences of hallucinogenic drugs are common. Panic reactions ("bad trips") may be related to excessive doses; they seem to be less common as the doses of street drugs have become more accurate. They are best managed by se-

dation with a barbiturate or benzodiazepine rather than with a phenothiazine. Simple "talking down" may suffice but is labor-intensive. Acute psychotic or depressive reactions have been precipitated by use of these drugs but usually only in persons with strong predispositions. Acute psychotic reactions are associated with PCP much more commonly than with any of the other hallucinogens. Errors of judgment may lead to reckless acts that threaten life; any person under the influence of one of these drugs should be provided with a nondrugged companion until the effect has dissipated.

Overdoses of the antimuscarinic agents can be treated with infusions of physostigmine, but supportive care is usually preferred.

Overdoses of PCP are dangerous but can be managed if recognized promptly. PCP is secreted into the stomach, so that removal may be hastened by continual nasogastric suction. Excretion of this basic drug may be hastened by acidification of the urine to pH 5.5 (but see Chapter 60). Diazepam can be given to protect against seizures or to curb excitation; antipsychotics aggravate matters at this point. If a prolonged schizophrenia-like illness follows acute intoxication, one may consider antipsychotics on a sustained basis.

Long-Term Treatment

No systematic program of treatment has been devised for abuse of this class of drugs. Users of hallucinogens are likely to stick to this class of drugs rather than proceed to a pattern of polydrug abuse. Separation of the user from the drug culture is probably the best treatment, but it must be voluntarily accepted.

Therapeutic Uses

No therapeutic indication has yet been accepted for any hallucinogen. LSD was promoted as a cure for alcoholism, but objective evidence of benefit is totally lacking. Facilitation of psychotherapy was another proposed use, again with no substantiation or comparison with other drugs. Although it has been tried in both schizophrenics and depressed individuals, LSD is more likely to precipitate or aggravate these disorders than to alleviate them. Use of the drug in chronic cancer patients was said to diminish the need for opioids, but this work has not been confirmed.

MARIJUANA

History

Use of cannabis has been recorded for thousands of years, especially in Eastern countries such as China and India. It was certainly known to the Greeks at the height of their civilization as well as to Arabic nations somewhat later. It is estimated that about 200–300 million people use cannabis in some form. Thus, it is not only one of the oldest but also one of the most widely used of mind-altering drugs. Since the 1960s, the rise in marijuana use in the USA has been remarkable. Although the drug was known in this country prior to that time, there were only a small number of users, mainly from minority groups. It is estimated now that 30–40 million persons in the USA have used the drug and that a substantial number are regular users. Recent reports suggest that the number of youngsters initiated into the use of this drug has declined after a steep rise and an increasingly lower age of first use.

Several species of cannabis (hemp) have been named, but botanists are not agreed that more than one species of the plant exists; many morphologic variants occur. Some plants are excellent for fiber, being a source of hemp, and rather poor producers of drug; and the converse also is true. These properties are due to genetic differences. The flowers and small leaves of *Cannabis sativa* supply most of the drug. **Marijuana** is a mixture of ground-up plant materials that resembles grass clippings thus the street name "grass." Extraction of the resin from the plant provides a more potent product: hashish.

Chemistry & Pharmacokinetics of Cannabinoids

Three major cannabinoids have been found in cannabis; cannabidiol (CBD), Δ^9-tetrahydrocannabinol (THC), and cannabinol (CBN). The biosynthetic pathway begins with CBD, proceeds to THC, and ends with CBN (Figure 31–3). Thus, one can deduce from the proportions of these cannabinoids in plant material the age of the plant. Many other variants of these structures have been found in cannabis, but with

the exception of THC and its homologues no other cannabinoids have definite psychoactivity. The content of THC varies considerably among plants, so that special genetic lines may produce as much as 4–6% THC content in very selected ("manicured") materials. Most plants have a THC content ranging from trace amounts to 1–2%.

The preferred route of administration in Western countries is by smoking. The high lipid solubility of THC causes it to be readily trapped on the surfactant lining of the lungs. Pharmacokinetic studies indicate that smoking is almost equivalent to intravenous administration except that lower peak plasma concentrations of THC are attained. In some Eastern countries, cannabis is taken orally in the form of various confections. The rate of absorption from this route is slow and highly variable, though the duration of action is longer.

THC is extensively metabolized, and new metabolites are still being discovered. One metabolite, 11-hydroxy-THC, is actually more active than the parent compound. However, it is not nearly as abundant, and one must assume that the major part of the activity of cannabis derives from THC itself. The high lipid solubility of the drug leads to extensive sequestration in the lipid compartments of the body, and metabolites may be excreted for as long as a week after a single dose. Whether accumulation of unchanged THC can occur is questionable.

Pharmacodynamics of Cannabinoids

The mechanism of action of THC has been the subject of intense investigation. A high degree of enantiomer selectivity—of both the natural and newer

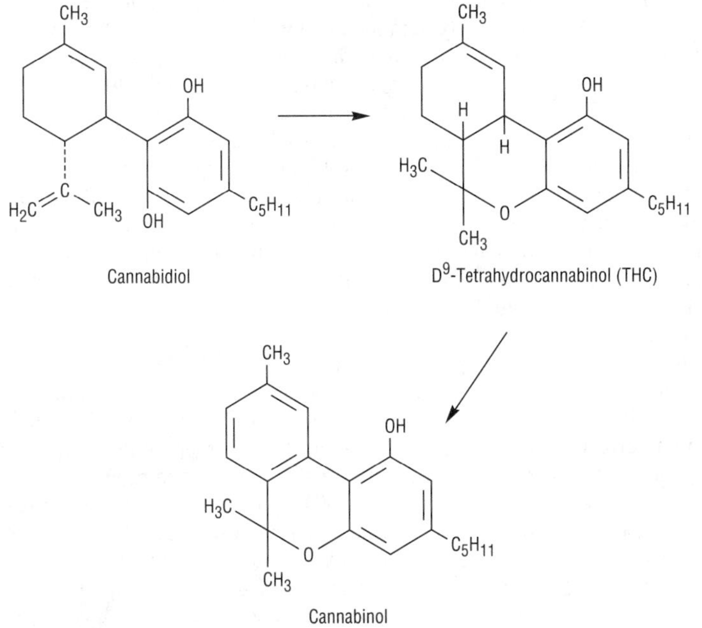

Figure 31–3. Structures of the three main cannabinoids in marijuana. Only THC has psychoactivity. C_5H_{11} is *n*-pentyl. Arrows indicate the biosynthetic sequence.

cannabinoids—has suggested a highly selective receptor. A putative endogenous ligand has already been reported (Devane, 1992). Synthetic cannabinoid agonists with high potency and stereoselectivity in behavioral assays have been used to characterize the cannabinoid binding site. The binding affinities correlate closely with the relative potencies in biologic assays, suggesting that the receptor also mediates the pharmacologic effects. Binding sites are most numerous in the outflow nuclei of the basal ganglia, the substantia nigra pars reticulata, globus pallidus, hippocampus, and brain stem. The receptor has been cloned and is G protein-coupled. Positron emission tomographic (PET) scan studies have revealed increases in metabolism following THC in the same areas in which receptors are localized, again suggesting that the receptors are closely involved in the clinical actions of the drug. Prostaglandins may play a mediator role in THC activity, but how this might occur is unclear. The high lipophilicity of THC has caused some investigators to propose a nonspecific membrane effect, but that would not explain the stereoselective action.

THC has a variety of pharmacologic effects that suggest actions like those of amphetamines, LSD, alcohol, sedatives, atropine, or morphine. Thus, the drug does not fit traditional pharmacologic classifications and must be considered as a separate class.

Small doses of THC may be associated with a rather definite placebo effect, but large doses are unequivocal in producing the expected range of effects. The expert smoker of marijuana is usually aware of a drug effect after two or three inhalations. As smoking continues, the effects increase, reaching a maximum about 20 minutes after the smoke has been finished. Most effects of the drug usually have vanished after 3 hours, by which time plasma concentrations are low. Peak effects after oral administration may be delayed until 3–4 hours after drug ingestion but may last for 6–8 hours.

The early stage is one of being "high" and is characterized by euphoria, uncontrollable laughter, alteration of time sense, depersonalization, and sharpened vision. Later, the user becomes relaxed and experiences introspective and dream-like states if not actual sleep. Thinking or concentrating becomes difficult, though by force of will the subject can attend.

Two characteristic physical signs of cannabis intoxication are increased pulse rate and reddening of the conjunctiva. The latter correlates well with the presence of detectable plasma concentrations. Pupil size is not changed. The blood pressure may fall, especially in the upright position. An antiemetic effect may be present. Muscle weakness, tremors, unsteadiness, and increased deep tendon reflexes may also be noted. Virtually any psychologic test shows impairment if the doses are large enough and the test difficult enough. No distinctive biochemical changes have been found in humans.

Tolerance has been demonstrated in virtually every animal species that has been tested. It is apparent in humans only among heavy long-term users of the drug. Different degrees of tolerance develop for different effects of the drug, with tolerance for the tachycardiac effect developing fairly rapidly. A mild withdrawal syndrome has been noted following chronic use at very high doses.

Health Hazards

Marijuana has raised concern about possible adverse effects on the health of users, probably because so many are very young. The hazards of use are still controversial and ambiguous, and there are many problems with the studies themselves. First, it is difficult to prove or disprove an adverse reaction for humans in an animal model. Second, users thus far have been mostly young people in excellent general health. Third, cannabis is often used in combination with alcohol or tobacco. And fourth, many investigators have biases for or against the drug.

Three epidemiologic studies in developing countries have failed to find definite evidence of impairment among heavy users of cannabis, but field studies may lack sensitivity. Experimental studies in which subjects have smoked heavily for varying periods have shown a lower serum testosterone level in men and airway narrowing. Effects on immune mechanisms, chromosomes, and cell metabolism are often contradictory. Effects on the fetus are still uncertain.

Heavy smokers of marijuana may be subject to some of the same problems of chronic bronchitis, airway obstruction, and squamous cell metaplasia as smokers of tobacco cigarettes. Angina pectoris may be aggravated by the speeding of the heart rate, orthostatic hypotension, and increased carboxyhemoglobin. Driving ability is likely to be impaired but is not easily demonstrated with usual testing. "Amotivational syndrome," in which promising young people with obvious social advantages lose interest in school and career and enter the drug culture, is a real phenomenon, but one cannot be sure whether drug use is the cause of the problem or simply a matter of personal choice. Acute panic reactions, toxic delirium, paranoid states, and frank psychoses are rare. Brain damage has not been confirmed in humans, though some suggestion of ultrastructural damage has been found in animals.

Therapeutic Uses

Cannabis was at one time listed in drug formularies but has not been used medically for some time. Recently, interest in cannabis for therapeutic purposes has revived. A finding of lowered intraocular pressure following oral THC administration has been repeatedly confirmed; it remains to be seen whether preparations of cannabis have any advantages over other forms of treatment for glaucoma. Amelioration of nausea and vomiting associated with cancer chemotherapy has also been studied. THC, now named **dronabinol** (Marinol), has been marketed for this indication. It seems able to reduce nausea and vomiting at doses that are associated with only moderate mental effects. **Levonantradol** is another homologue that may have medical use, possibly as an analgesic, as an agent for the relief of muscle spasm, or even as an anticonvulsant. It remains to be proved, however, that any of these homologues have advantages over standard agents.

Treatment

Few users seek treatment, though many who have stopped using the drug have been pleasantly surprised at the increased clarity of their thinking. Although marijuana has been alleged to be a substitute for alcohol, it is more commonly used along with alcohol; alcoholism complicating marijuana use is rare. Marijuana may be used in a pattern of multiple drug use, in which case treatment may be required for the more dangerous drugs being taken.

INHALANTS

History

The modern discovery of the intoxicant effects of inhalants began with Sir Humphry Davy in 1799, who administered nitrous oxide to himself and others. As other anesthetic gases were introduced, such as chloroform and ether, they were also used socially. Such use persists, with occasional instances of halothane inhalation being added to the anesthetic gases previously mentioned. In addition to these agents, three other patterns of inhalant use are now prevalent: (1) industrial solvents, including a variety of hydrocarbons, such as toluene; (2) aerosol propellants, such as various fluorocarbons; and (3) organic nitrites, such as amyl or butyl nitrite.

Chemistry & Pharmacology

The structures of some inhalants are shown in Figure 31–4. The mode of action of the inhalant anesthetics has been discussed in Chapter 24.

Clinical Aspects

Nitrous oxide, formerly not easily available, is now sold openly in so-called "head-shops." When self-administered, it produces difficulty in concentrating, dreaminess, euphoria, numbness and tingling, unsteadiness, and visual and auditory disturbances. It is usually taken as 35% N_2O mixed with oxygen; administration of 100% nitrous oxide may cause asphyxia and death.

Ether and **chloroform** are readily available through chemical supply houses. Cloths soaked with the material are used for inhalation of the fumes. After an initial period of exhilaration, the person often loses consciousness. Ether is highly flammable. Hal-

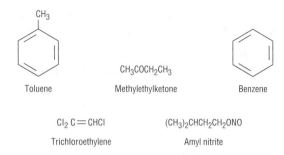

Figure 31–4. Structures of some commonly used inhalants.

othane is usually available only to medical or health care personnel.

A variety of **industrial solvents** that can be used as inhalants are on the market and virtually impossible to control. They include gasoline, paint thinner, glue, rubber cement, acrylic paint sprays, shoe polish, and degreasers. The toxic ingredients may be toluene, heptane, hexane, benzene, trichloroethylene, methylethylketone, and others. Because of their ready availability, this group of inhalants is widely used. Aerosol propellants have also been widely available, though manufacturers of products using propellants have recently changed from fluorocarbons to less hazardous materials.

Motives for use of inhalants include peer influence, low cost, ready availability, convenient packaging, quick intoxication of short duration, and mood enhancement. Boys in their early teen years from lower socioeconomic classes are the principal users. They generally also have worse than average problems at school and at home. Psychologic dependence perpetuates the use of inhalants.

The clinical effects of industrial solvent inhalation are short, lasting only 5–15 minutes. Rags or "toques" are soaked in the solvent and the fumes inhaled. Aerosol propellants are usually inhaled from a plastic bag. Euphoria and a relaxed "drunk" feeling are followed by disorientation, slow passage of time, and possibly hallucinations.

Organic nitrites have developed a reputation as a sexual enhancer, a sure avenue to popular acceptance. Amyl nitrite is used medically for angina in the form of fragile glass ampules covered with cloth. When these are broken, they make a popping sound—hence the nickname "poppers." Street forms of bottled isobutyl nitrite (Locker Room, Rush) are readily available in some areas. Inhalation causes dizziness, giddiness, rapid heart rate, lowered blood pressure, "speeding," and flushing of the skin. The effects last only a few minutes and can readily be repeated. The main effect the drug may have on sexual functioning is to diminish inhibition. Except for an occasional instance of methemoglobinemia associated with excessive use of nitrites, few significant adverse effects have been reported despite extensive use of this drug.

Toxicity

Chloroform has been implicated in liver and kidney damage. Industrial solvents have produced a variety of adverse effects: liver and kidney damage, peripheral nerve damage and possibly brain damage in animals, bone marrow suppression, and pulmonary disease. Fluorocarbon inhalation has resulted in sudden deaths, either due to ventricular arrhythmias or asphyxiation. Nitrites have been rather safe but might pose hazards for persons with preexisting cardiovascular problems.

REFERENCES

General

Bock GR, Whelan J (editors): *Cocaine: Scientific and Social Dimensions.* (Ciba Foundations Symposium 166.) Wiley, 1992.

Committee on Problems of Drug Dependence: *Testing Drugs for Physical Dependence Potential and Abuse Liability.* Brady JV, Lukas SE (editors). National Institute on Drug Abuse Research Monograph 52, US Government Printing Office, 1984.

Koob GF, Bloom FE: Cellular and molecular mechanisms of drug dependence. Science 1988;242:715.

Kulberg A: Substance abuse: Clinical identification and management. Pediatr Clin North Am 1986;33:325.

Musto DF: Opium, cocaine, and marijuana in American history. Sci Am 1991;265:40.

Nestler EJ: Molecular mechanisms of drug addiction. J Neurosci 1992;12:2439.

Ray OA: *Drugs, Society and Human Behavior,* 6th ed. Mosby, 1993.

Opioids

Agren H: Clonidine treatment of the opiate withdrawal syndrome: A review of clinical trials of a theory. Acta Psychiatr Scand 1986(Suppl);327:91.

Collier HOJ: Physiological basis of opiate dependence. Drug Alcohol Depend 1983;11:15.

Dole VP: Implications of methadone maintenance treatment for theories of narcotic addiction. JAMA 1988; 260:3025.

Kleber HD: The use of psychotropic drugs in the treatment of compulsive opiate abusers: The rationale for their use. Adv Alcohol Subst Abuse 1985;51:103.

Sedatives

Allgulander C: History and current status of sedative-hypnotic drug use and abuse. Acta Psychiatr Scand 1986;73:465.

Cowen PJ, Nutt DJ: Abstinence symptoms after withdrawal of tranquilizing drugs: Is there a common neurochemical mechanism? Lancet 1982;2:360.

Stimulants

Benowitz NL: Clinical pharmacology of caffeine. Annu Rev Med 1990;41:277.

Benowitz NL: Clinical pharmacology and toxicity of cocaine. Pharmacol Toxicol 1993;72:3.

Carroll ME et al: Buprenorphin's effects on self-administration of smoked cocaine base and orally delivered phencyclidine, ethanol, and saccharin in Rhesus monkeys. J Pharmacol Exp Therap 1992;261:26.

Cigarette smoking-attributable mortality and years of potential life lost—United States, 1990. MMWR Morb Mortal Wkly Rep 1993;42:645.

Cigarette smoking: A clinical guide to assessment and treatment. Med Clin North Am 1992;76(2):289.

Fiore MC et al: Tobacco dependence and the nicotine patch: Clinical guidelines for effective use. JAMA 1992;268:2687.

Grabowski J, Dworkin SI: Cocaine: An overview of current issues. Int J Addict 1985;20:1065.

Insel TR et al: 3,4-Methylenedioxymethamphetamine ("ecstasy") selectively destroys brain serotonin terminals in rhesus monkeys. J Pharmacol Exp Ther 1989; 249:713.

Johanson C-E, Fischman MW: The pharmacology of cocaine related to its abuse. Pharmacol Rev 1989;41:3.

Kalix P, Braenden O: Pharmacological aspects of the chewing of khat leaves. Pharmacol Rev 1985;37:149.

Kuhar MJ, Ritz MC, Boja JW: The dopamine hypothesis of the reinforcing properties of cocaine. Trends Neurosci 1991;14:299.

Mello NK et al: Buprenorphine suppresses cocaine self-administration by rhesus monkeys. Science 1989;245: 859.

Pomerleau OF: Nicotine and the central nervous system: Biobehavioral effects of cigarette smoking. Am J Med 1992;93(Suppl 1A):1A.

Silverman K et al: Withdrawal syndrome after double-blind cessation of caffeine consumption. N Engl J Med 1992;327:1109.

Smith DE et al (editors): *Amphetamine Use, Misuse and Abuse.* GK Hall, 1979.

Tennant FS, Sagherian AA: Double-blind comparison of amantadine and bromocriptine for ambulatory withdrawal from cocaine dependence. Arch Intern Med 1987;147:109.

Volpe JJ: Effect of cocaine use on the fetus. N Engl J Med 1992;327:399.

Hallucinogens

Dilsaver SC: Antimuscarinic agents as substances of abuse: A review. J Clin Psychopharmacol 1988;8:14.

Hollister LE: *Chemical Psychoses: LSD and Related Drugs.* Thomas, 1968.

Johnson KM, Jones SM: Neuropharmacology of phencyclidine: Basic mechanisms and therapeutic potential. Annu Rev Pharmacol Toxicol 1990;30:707.

Lewin L: Phantastica, *Narcotic and Stimulating Drugs.* Dutton, 1931.

Pierce PA, Peroutka SJ: Antagonist properties of d-LSD at 5-hydroxytryptamine$_2$ receptors. Neuropsychopharmacology 1990;3:503.

Strassman RJ: Adverse reactions to psychedelic drugs: A review of the literature. J Nerv Ment Dis 1984;172:577.

Cannabis

Bidaut-Russell M, Devane WA, Howlett AC: Cannabinoid receptors and modulation of cyclic AMP accumulation in the rat brain. J Neurochem 1990;55:21.

Block RI, Ghoneim MM: Effects of chronic marijuana use on human cognition. Psychopharmacology 1993;110:219.

Devane WA et al: Isolation and structure of a brain constituent that binds to the cannabinoid receptor. Science 1992;258:1946.

Herkenhamer M et al: Cannabinoid receptor localization in brain. Proc Natl Acad Sci USA 1990:87:1932.

Hollister LE: Health aspects of cannabis. Pharmacol Rev 1986;38:1.

Inhalants

Sharp CW, Carroll LT: *Voluntary Inhalation of Industrial Solvents.* DHEW Publication No. (ADM) 79–779, US Government Printing Office, 1979.

WHO: Report of the advisory group meeting on adverse health consequencews of volatile solvents/inhalants. Mexican Institute of Psychiatry, Mexico City, Mexico. 1986;April:21.

Section VI.
Drugs Used to Treat Diseases of the Blood, Inflammation, & Gout

Agents Used in Anemias; Hematopoietic Growth Factors

32

Curt A. Ries, MD, & Daniel V. Santi, MD, PhD

Iron, vitamin B_{12}, and folic acid are chemically unrelated essential nutrients that are required for normal erythropoiesis. Deficiency of any of these substances results in severe anemia. Iron is required for hemoglobin production; in the absence of adequate iron, small red cells with insufficient hemoglobin are formed, giving rise to microcytic hypochromic anemia. Vitamin B_{12} and folic acid are required for normal DNA synthesis, and deficiency of either of these vitamins results in impaired production and abnormal maturation of erythroid precursor cells, giving rise to the characteristic blood and bone marrow picture known as megaloblastic anemia.

Erythropoietin and colony-stimulating factors are hormones that regulate blood cell development and proliferation in the marrow. These substances are found in such minute quantities in human tissues that insufficient amounts were available for study until recently. Recombinant DNA technology has made useful quantities of these substances available and is revolutionizing the treatment of certain disorders.

IRON

Basic Pharmacology

Iron forms the nucleus of the iron-porphyrin ring heme, which when combined with appropriate globin chains forms hemoglobin. Hemoglobin is a protein whose structure allows for reversible binding of oxygen, providing the critical mechanism for oxygen transport from the lungs to other tissues. Although iron is also present in other important proteins (myoglobin, cytochromes, etc), the vast majority is normally present in hemoglobin; therefore, anemia is the most prominent clinical feature of iron deficiency.

Iron distribution in normal adults is shown in Table 32–1. About 70% of the total body iron content is in the form of hemoglobin in red blood cells, and 10–20% is in the form of storage iron as ferritin and he-

mosiderin. Women in the reproductive age group usually have less storage iron than men because of iron losses from menstruation and pregnancies. About 10% of the iron is in myoglobin, a heme-containing protein in muscle. The remainder (< 1%) is distributed in trace amounts in cytochromes and other iron-containing enzymes and as transport iron or transferrin.

Pharmacokinetics

Iron is normally available in the diet from a wide variety of foods; dietary iron is usually in the form of heme or iron complexed to various organic compounds. Therapeutic iron, on the other hand, is usually given in the form of iron salts or iron complexed to inorganic substances. These different forms of iron differ widely in the amount of iron available for absorption, as discussed below.

A. Absorption: Iron is normally absorbed in the duodenum and proximal jejunum, though more distal small bowel sites can absorb iron if necessary. The average diet in the USA contains 10–15 mg of elemental iron daily. A normal individual without iron deficiency absorbs 5–10% of this iron, or about 0.5–1 mg daily. Iron absorption is increased in response to low iron stores or increased iron requirements. Total iron absorption increases to 1–2 mg/d in normal menstruating women and may be as high as 3–4 mg/d in pregnant women. Infants and adolescents also have increased iron requirements during rapid growth periods. Iron is available in a wide variety of foods but is especially abundant in meat protein. The iron in meat protein is also more available for absorption and can be more efficiently absorbed, since heme iron in meat hemoglobin and myoglobin can be absorbed intact as hemin (the ferric form of heme) without first having to be broken down into elemental iron. Iron in other foods is often tightly bound to phytates or other complexing agents and may be much less available for absorption. Nonheme iron in foods and iron in inorganic

Table 32–1. Iron distribution in normal adults.[1,2]

	Iron Content (mg)	
	Men	Women
Hemoglobin	3050	1700
Myoglobin	430	300
Enzymes	10	8
Transport (transferrin)	8	6
Storage (ferritin and hemosiderin)	750	300
Total	4248	2314

[1]Adapted, with permission, from Brown EB: Iron deficiency anemia. In: *Cecil Textbook of Medicine,* 16th ed. Wyngaarden JB, Smith LH (editors). Saunders, 1982.

[2]Values are based on data from various sources and assume "normal" men weigh 80 kg and have a hemoglobin of 16 g/dL and "normal" women weigh 55 kg and have a hemoglobin of 14 g/dL.

iron salts and complexes must be converted to ferrous iron before it can be absorbed by the intestinal mucosal cells. Such absorption is decreased by the presence of chelators or complexing agents in the intestinal lumen and is increased in the presence of hydrochloric acid and vitamin C. Gastric resection decreases iron absorption by decreasing or eliminating hydrochloric acid production—and perhaps, even more importantly, by removing the site where food is digested to make dietary iron more available for absorption by the iron-absorbing areas in the duodenum and proximal jejunum.

Iron is transported across the intestinal mucosal cell by active transport. Absorbed ferrous iron is converted to ferric iron within the mucosal cell. Together with ferric iron split from hemin, the newly absorbed iron can be made available for immediate transport from the mucosal cell to the plasma via transferrin or can be converted to ferritin and stored in the mucosal cell. In general, when total body iron stores are high and iron requirements by the body are low, newly absorbed iron is diverted into ferritin in the intestinal mucosal cells rather than being transported to other sites. When iron stores are low or iron requirements are high, however, newly absorbed iron is immediately transported from the mucosal cells to the bone marrow for the production of hemoglobin.

B. Distribution: Iron is transported in the plasma bound to transferrin, a β-globulin that specifically binds ferric iron. Iron can thus be transported from intestinal mucosal cells or from storage sites in liver or spleen to the developing erythroid cells in bone marrow. The transferrin-ferric iron complex is delivered to maturing erythroid cells by a specific receptor mechanism. Transferrin receptors, which are integral membrane glycoproteins present in large numbers on proliferating erythroid cells, bind the transferrin-iron complex and internalize the iron, releasing it within the cell. The transferrin and transferrin receptor are then recycled, providing an efficient mechanism for

incorporating iron into hemoglobin in developing red blood cells.

C. Storage: Iron can be stored in two forms: ferritin and hemosiderin. Ferritin, the most readily available form of storage iron, is a water-soluble complex consisting of a core crystal of ferric hydroxide covered by a protein shell of apoferritin. Hemosiderin is a particulate substance consisting of aggregates of ferric core crystals partially or completely stripped of apoferritin. Both ferritin and hemosiderin are stored in macrophages in the liver, spleen, and bone marrow; ferritin is also present in intestinal mucosal cells and in plasma. Since the ferritin present in plasma is in equilibrium with storage ferritin in reticuloendothelial tissues, the plasma (or serum) ferritin level can be used to estimate total body iron stores.

D. Elimination: There is no mechanism for excretion of iron. Small amounts of iron are lost by exfoliation of intestinal mucosal cells into the stool, and trace amounts are excreted in bile, urine, and sweat. These losses, however, can account for no more than 1 mg of iron per day. Because the body's ability to increase excretion of iron is so limited, regulation of iron balance must be achieved by changing intestinal absorption of iron, depending on the body's needs.

E. Regulation of Iron Pharmacokinetics: Iron absorption is regulated by the amount of storage iron present, especially the amount of ferritin present in the intestinal mucosal cells, and by the rate of erythropoiesis. Increased erythropoiesis is associated with an increase in the number of transferrin receptor sites on developing erythroid cells, and the availability of these receptor sites in some way directly increases the rate of iron absorption. Transferrin and ferritin are both present in intestinal mucosal cells, and both appear to regulate iron absorption. Transferrin is increased and ferritin decreased in iron deficiency, promoting increased iron absorption, while transferrin is decreased and ferritin increased in iron overload states, inhibiting further iron absorption.

Clinical Pharmacology

A. Indications for the Use of Iron: The only clinical indication for the use of iron preparations is the treatment or prevention of iron deficiency anemia. Iron deficiency is commonly seen in infants, especially premature infants; in children during rapid growth periods; and in pregnant and lactating women. These situations are all associated with increased iron requirements, and individuals in these settings are often given dietary supplements of oral iron to meet the increased need. Iron deficiency also occurs frequently after gastrectomy and in patients with severe small bowel disease that results in generalized malabsorption. Iron deficiency in these situations is due to inadequate iron absorption.

The most common cause of iron deficiency in adults, however, is blood loss. Menstruating women lose about 30 mg of iron with each menstrual period;

women with heavy menstrual bleeding may lose much more. The most common site of unrecognized or occult blood loss is in the gastrointestinal tract. Patients with unexplained iron deficiency anemia must therefore always be evaluated for occult gastrointestinal bleeding, especially to exclude early gastrointestinal cancer, which may present with occult bleeding and anemia at a time when the cancer is still surgically curable. Simple nutritional iron deficiency due to inadequate diet is rare in adults and should never be accepted as an explanation of iron deficiency in a patient until a careful search has ruled out occult blood loss and other causes of iron deficiency.

Individuals suspected of being iron-deficient should generally have the diagnosis confirmed before being treated with iron preparations. As iron deficiency develops, storage iron decreases and then disappears; next, serum ferritin decreases; and then serum iron decreases and iron-binding capacity (transferrin) increases, resulting in a decrease in iron-binding saturation. Thereafter, anemia begins to develop. Red cell indices (mean corpuscular volume [MCV]: normal = 80–100 fL; mean corpuscular hemoglobin concentration [MCHC]: normal = 32–36 g/dL) are usually low normal when iron deficiency anemia is mild, but cells become progressively more microcytic and hypochromic as anemia becomes more severe. By the time iron deficiency is diagnosed, serum iron is usually less than 40 μg/dL; total iron-binding capacity (TIBC) is greater than 400 μg/dL; iron-binding saturation is less than 10%; and serum ferritin is less than 10 μg/L. One of the most sensitive ways to detect early iron deficiency is to examine bone marrow stained to detect the presence or absence of storage iron.

B. Treatment: The treatment of iron deficiency anemia consists of administration of oral or parenteral iron preparations. Oral iron corrects the deficiency just as rapidly and completely as parenteral iron in most cases if iron absorption from the gastrointestinal tract is normal.

1. Oral iron therapy–A wide variety of oral iron preparations are available. Since ferrous iron is most efficiently absorbed, only ferrous salts should be used. Ferrous sulfate, ferrous gluconate, and ferrous fumarate are all effective and inexpensive and are recommended for the treatment of most patients. Supplementation with vitamin C and other nutrients is generally not necessary. Sustained-release and enteric-coated iron preparations should not be used, since iron is best absorbed in the duodenum and proximal jejunum.

Different iron salts provide different amounts of elemental iron, as shown in Table 32–2. In an iron-deficient individual, about 50–100 mg of iron can be incorporated into hemoglobin daily, and about 25% of oral iron given as ferrous salt can be absorbed. Therefore, 200–400 mg of elemental iron should be given daily to correct iron deficiency most rapidly.

Table 32–2. Some commonly used oral iron preparations.

Preparation	Tablet Size	Elemental Iron per Tablet	Usual Adult Dose (Tablets per Day)
Ferrous sulfate, hydrated	325 mg	65 mg	3–4
Ferrous sulfate, desiccated	200 mg	65 mg	3–4
Ferrous gluconate	320 mg	37 mg	3–4
Ferrous fumarate	200 mg	66 mg	3–4
Ferrous fumarate	325 mg	106 mg	2–3

Patients unable to tolerate such large doses of iron can be given lower daily doses of iron, which results in slower but still complete correction of iron deficiency.

Treatment with oral iron should be continued for 3–6 months. This will not only correct the anemia but will replenish iron stores. The first measurable response to successful iron therapy can be seen in less than a week, when brisk reticulocytosis occurs, as newly formed hemoglobin-filled red cells from bone marrow enter the bloodstream. The hemoglobin level should increase significantly in 2–4 weeks and should reach normal levels (men = 14–18 g/dL; women = 12–16 g/dL) in 1–3 months. Failure to respond to oral iron therapy may be due to incorrect diagnosis (anemia due to causes other than iron deficiency), continued iron loss (usually secondary to continued blood loss), concurrent chronic inflammation or other illness that suppresses marrow function, or failure of the patient to take or absorb the oral iron.

Common adverse effects of oral iron therapy include nausea, epigastric discomfort, abdominal cramps, constipation, and diarrhea. These effects are usually dose-related and can often be overcome by lowering the daily dose of iron or by taking the tablets immediately after or with meals. Some patients have less severe gastrointestinal adverse effects with one iron salt than another and benefit from changing preparations. Patients taking oral iron develop black stools; this itself has no clinical significance but may obscure the diagnosis of continued gastrointestinal blood loss.

2. Parenteral iron therapy–Parenteral therapy should be reserved for patients with documented iron deficiency unable to tolerate or absorb oral iron and patients with extensive chronic blood loss who cannot be maintained with oral iron alone. This includes patients with various postgastrectomy conditions and previous small bowel resection, inflammatory bowel disease involving the proximal small bowel, malabsorption syndromes, and chronic heavy bleeding from nonresectable lesions, as may occur in hereditary hemorrhagic telangiectasia.

Iron dextran is a stable complex of ferric hydroxide and low-molecular-weight dextran containing 50 mg of elemental iron per milliliter of solution. It can be given either by deep intramuscular injection (using the "Z track" injection technique to avoid local tissue staining) or by intravenous infusion. Adverse effects of parenteral iron therapy include local pain and tissue staining (brown discoloration of the tissues overlying the injection site), headache, light-headedness, fever, arthralgias, nausea and vomiting, back pain, flushing, urticaria, bronchospasm, and, rarely, anaphylaxis and death.

The total amount of parenteral iron required to correct iron deficiency anemia and to replenish iron stores in a 70 kg adult can be calculated as follows: grams of iron required = 0.25 × (normal hemoglobin – patient's hemoglobin). Most adults with iron deficiency anemia thus require 1–2 g of replacement iron, or 20–40 mL of iron dextran. Although this amount of parenteral iron can be given as 10–20 daily intramuscular injections, most physicians now prefer to give the entire calculated dose in a single intravenous infusion in several hundred milliliters of normal saline over 1–2 hours. Intravenous administration eliminates the local pain and tissue staining that often occur with the intramuscular route and allows delivery of the entire dose of iron necessary to correct the iron deficiency at one time. There is no clear evidence that any of the adverse effects, including anaphylaxis, are more likely to occur with intravenous than with intramuscular administration.

A small test dose of iron dextran should always be given before full intramuscular or intravenous doses are given. A dose of 0.25–0.5 mL can be given by deep intramuscular injection or slow intravenous infusion of very dilute solution over 30–60 minutes before proceeding with full therapy. If signs or symptoms of an immediate hypersensitivity reaction occur, additional parenteral iron should not be given, and alternative therapy must be considered. Patients with a strong history of allergy and patients who have previously received parenteral iron are more likely to have hypersensitivity reactions following treatment with parenteral iron dextran than those who have not.

Clinical Toxicity

A. Acute Iron Toxicity: Acute iron toxicity is seen almost exclusively in young children who have ingested a number of iron tablets. Although adults appear to be able to tolerate large doses of oral iron without serious consequences, as few as ten tablets of any of the commonly available oral iron preparations can be lethal in young children. Oral iron preparations should therefore always be stored in "childproof" containers and kept out of the reach of children.

Large amounts of oral iron cause necrotizing gastroenteritis, with vomiting, abdominal pain, and bloody diarrhea followed by shock, lethargy, and dyspnea. Subsequently, improvement is often noted,

but this may be followed by severe metabolic acidosis, coma, and death. Urgent treatment of acute iron toxicity is necessary, especially in young children. Gastric aspiration should be performed, followed by lavage with carbonate solutions to form insoluble iron salts. Deferoxamine, a potent iron chelating compound, should be given systemically by intermittent intramuscular injection or by continuous intravenous infusion to bind iron that has already been absorbed and to promote its excretion in urine and feces. Some investigators advise also instilling deferoxamine into the stomach to bind any remaining free iron in the gut, but this is controversial. Appropriate supportive therapy for gastrointestinal bleeding, metabolic acidosis, and shock must also be provided (see Chapter 60).

B. Chronic Iron Toxicity: Chronic iron toxicity (iron overload), also known as hemochromatosis and hemosiderosis, results when excess iron is deposited in the heart, liver, pancreas, and other organs. It can lead to organ failure and death. It most commonly occurs in patients with hemochromatosis, an inherited disorder characterized by excessive iron absorption, and in patients who receive many red cell transfusions (each transfusion containing 250 mg of iron) over a long period of time. It is doubtful that clinically significant iron overload can occur in normal individuals who chronically ingest excess iron, because of the protective mechanisms that normally regulate iron absorption and because of the very large amounts of total body iron needed before clinical iron overload becomes apparent. However, continued ingestion of excess iron probably contributes to the development of iron overload in patients who have a higher than normal baseline iron absorption, whether due to inherited factors (subclinical hemochromatosis, etc) or to the presence of anemias other than those due to iron deficiency (anemia of chronic disease, hemolytic anemias, etc).

Chronic iron overload in the absence of anemia is most efficiently treated by intermittent phlebotomy. One unit of blood (containing 250 mg of iron) can be removed every week or so until all of the excess iron is removed. Iron chelation therapy using parenteral deferoxamine is much less efficient as well as more complicated, expensive, and hazardous, but it can be useful for severe iron overload that cannot be managed by phlebotomy.

VITAMIN B$_{12}$ & FOLIC ACID

Basic Pharmacology

Vitamin B$_{12}$ and folic acid are chemically unrelated vitamins essential for normal DNA synthesis. Deficiencies lead to impaired DNA synthesis, inhibition of normal mitosis, and abnormal maturation and function of the cells produced. These changes are most apparent in tissues where cells undergo rapid cell division, such as the bone marrow and the gastrointestinal epithelium, but all dividing cells are affected to some degree. Severe anemia is the chief finding in patients with vitamin B_{12} or folic acid deficiency, but pancytopenia (diminished production of red blood cells, white blood cells, and platelets) may occur, and gastrointestinal symptoms are common. Neurologic abnormalities may also occur in vitamin B_{12} deficiency but not in folic acid deficiency (see Clinical Pharmacology).

Anemias caused by vitamin B_{12} and folic acid deficiency have a characteristic appearance of peripheral blood and bone marrow called megaloblastic anemia. Since the underlying defect in megaloblastic anemias is impaired DNA synthesis, there is diminished cell division in the face of continued RNA and protein synthesis. This leads to production of large (macrocytic) red blood cells that have a high RNA:DNA ratio and are defective in the sense that they are highly susceptible to destruction. Morphologically, the bone marrow is hypercellular, with a marked increase in the number of large abnormal early red cell precursors (megaloblasts) but with very few cells maturing beyond this stage to become circulating red cells. The red cells that do form in the bone marrow characteristically show normal cytoplasmic maturation, including normal hemoglobin formation; it is nuclear maturation and cell division that are impaired in the megaloblastic anemias.

Although megaloblastic anemia can theoretically result from any event that impairs DNA synthesis, in practice almost all cases are due to deficiencies of vitamin B_{12} or folic acid. The biochemical and physiologic bases of these deficiencies are now well understood, and it is possible to describe the mechanisms causing these anemias at the molecular level.

Chemistry

A. Vitamin B_{12}: Vitamin B_{12} is made up of a porphyrin-like ring with a central cobalt atom attached to a nucleotide (Figure 32–1). Various ligands may be covalently bound to the cobalt atom, forming different cobalamins. Deoxyadenosylcobalamin and methylcobalamin are the active forms of the vitamin in humans. **Cyanocobalamin** and **hydroxocobalamin** (both available for therapeutic use) and other cobalamins found in food sources must be converted to the above active forms. The ultimate source of vitamin B_{12} is from microbial synthesis; the vitamin is not synthesized by animals or plants. The chief dietary source of vitamin B_{12} is microbially derived vitamin B_{12} in meat (especially liver), eggs, and dairy products. Vitamin B_{12} is sometimes called **extrinsic factor** to differentiate it from intrinsic factor, a substance normally secreted by the stomach.

B. Folic Acid: Folic acid (pteroylglutamic acid) is a compound composed of a pteridine heterocycle, p-aminobenzoic acid, and glutamic acid (Figure 32–2). Various numbers of glutamic acid moieties may be attached to the pteroyl portion of the mole-

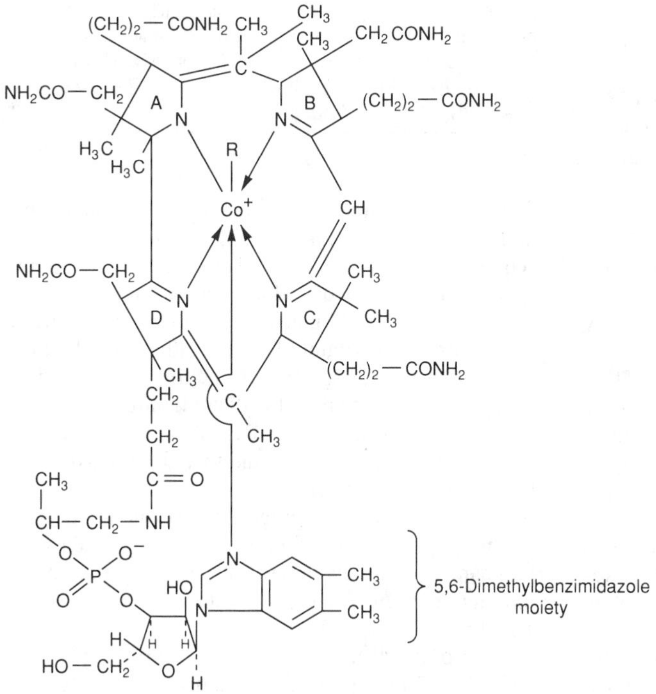

Figure 32–1. Cyanocobalamin; vitamin B_{12} (R, CN). (Reproduced, with permission, from Martin DW Jr et al: *Harper's Review of Biochemistry,* 22nd ed. Appleton & Lange, 1990.)

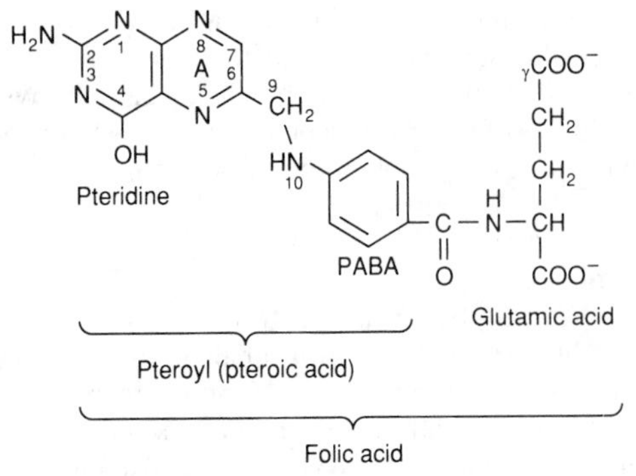

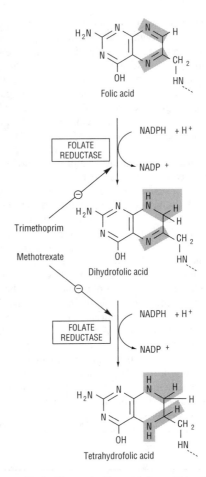

Figure 32–2. The structure and numbering of atoms of folic acid. (Reproduced, with permission, from Martin DW Jr et al: *Harper's Review of Biochemistry,* 22nd ed. Appleton & Lange, 1990.)

cule, resulting in monoglutamates, triglutamates, or polyglutamates. The fully oxidized pteridine ring of folic acid can undergo reduction, catalyzed by the enzyme dihydrofolate reductase, to give 7,8-dihydrofolic acid (H_2folate) and then to the fully reduced 5,6,7,8-tetrahydrofolic acid (H_4folate) (Figure 32–3). H_4folate can subsequently be transformed to folate cofactors possessing one-carbon units attached to the 5-nitrogen (5-CH_3–H_4folate and 5-CHO–H_4folate), the 10-nitrogen (10-CHO–H_4folate), or both positions (5,10-CH_2–H_4folate and 5,10-CH^+ = H_4folate) (Figure 32–4). The folate cofactors are interconvertible by various enzymatic reactions and serve the important biochemical function of donating one-carbon units at various levels of oxidation. In most instances, H_4folate is regenerated in these reactions and is available for reutilization. Various forms of folic acid are present in a wide variety of plant and animal tissues; the richest sources are yeast, liver, kidney, and green vegetables.

Pharmacokinetics

A. Vitamin B_{12}: The average diet in the USA contains 5–30 μg of vitamin B_{12} daily, 1–5 μg of which is usually absorbed. The vitamin is avidly stored, primarily in the liver, with an average adult having a total vitamin B_{12} storage pool of 3000–5000 μg. Only trace amounts of vitamin B_{12} are normally lost in urine and stool. Since the normal daily requirements of vitamin B_{12} are only about 2 μg, it would take about 5 years for all of the stored vitamin B_{12} to be exhausted and for megaloblastic anemia to develop if B_{12} absorption stopped. Vitamin B_{12} in physiologic amounts is absorbed only after it complexes with intrinsic factor. Intrinsic factor is a glycoprotein with a molecular weight of about 50,000 that is secreted by the parietal cells of the gastric mucosa. Intrinsic factor combines with vitamin B_{12} liberated

Figure 32–3. The reduction of folic acid to dihydrofolic acid and dihydrofolic acid to tetrahydrofolic acid by the enzyme dihydrofolate reductase. (Reproduced, with permission, from Martin DW Jr et al: *Harper's Review of Biochemistry,* 22nd ed. Appleton & Lange, 1990.)

from dietary sources in the stomach and duodenum, and the intrinsic factor–vitamin B_{12} complex is subsequently absorbed in the distal ileum by a highly specific receptor-mediated transport system. Vitamin B_{12} deficiency in humans most often results from malabsorption of vitamin B_{12}, due either to lack of intrinsic factor or to loss or malfunction of the specific absorptive mechanism in the distal ileum.

Once absorbed, vitamin B_{12} is transported to the various cells of the body bound to a plasma glycoprotein, transcobalamin II. Excess vitamin B_{12} is transported to the liver for storage. Significant amounts of vitamin B_{12} are excreted in the urine only when very large amounts are given parenterally, overcoming the binding capacities of the transcobalamins (50–100 μg).

B. Folic Acid: The average diet in the USA contains 500–700 μg of folates daily, 50–200 μg of

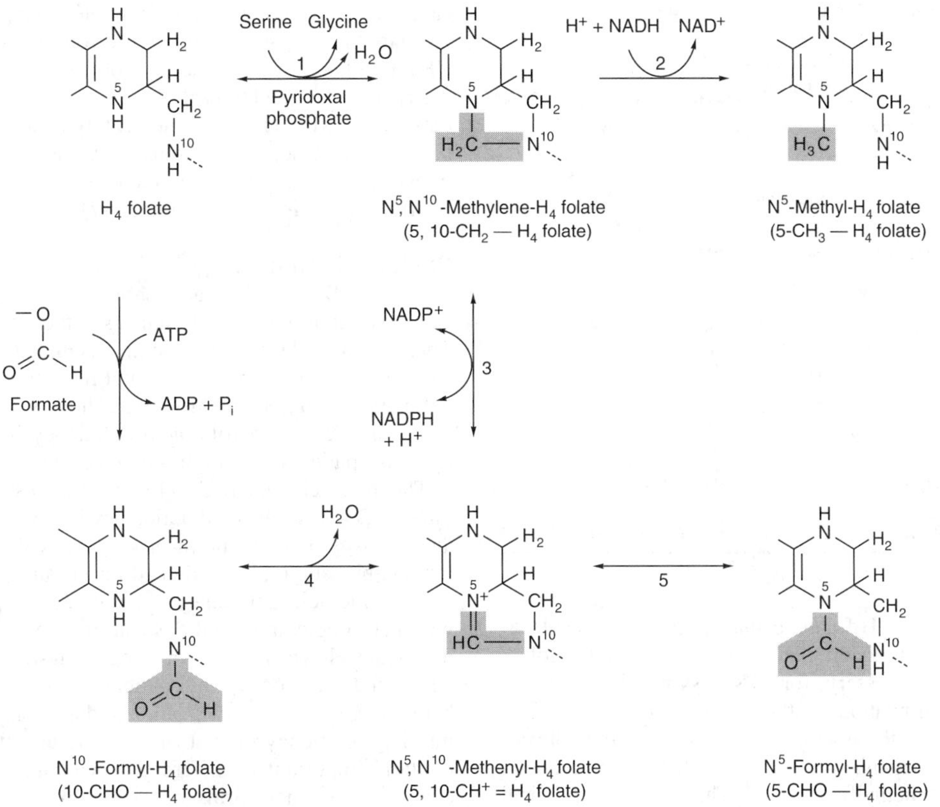

Figure 32–4. The interconversions of one-carbon moieties attached to tetrahydrofolate. (Reproduced, with permission, from Martin DW Jr et al: *Harper's Review of Biochemistry,* 20th ed. Lange, 1985.)

which is usually absorbed, depending on metabolic requirements (pregnant women may absorb as much as 300–400 μg of folic acid daily). Normally, 5–20 mg of folates is stored in the liver and other tissues. Folates are excreted in the urine and stool and are also destroyed by catabolism, so serum levels fall within a few days when intake is diminished. Since body stores of folates are relatively low and daily requirements high, folic acid deficiency and megaloblastic anemia can develop within 1–6 months after the intake of folic acid stops, depending on the patient's nutritional status and the rate of folate utilization.

Unaltered folic acid is readily and completely absorbed in the proximal jejunum. Dietary folates, however, consist primarily of polyglutamate forms of 5-CH₃–H₄folate, with very little unmodified folate present. Before absorption, all but one of the glutamyl residues of the polyglutamates must be hydrolyzed by the enzyme α-L-glutamyl transferase ("conjugase") within the brush border of the intestinal mucosa. The monoglutamate 5-CH₃–H₄folate is subsequently transported into the bloodstream, both by active and passive transport, and then widely distributed throughout the body.

Pharmacodynamics

A. Vitamin B₁₂: There are two essential enzymatic reactions in humans that require vitamin B₁₂ (Figure 32–5). In one reaction, deoxyadenosylcobalamin is a required cofactor in the conversion of methylmalonyl-CoA to succinyl-CoA by the enzyme methylmalonyl-CoA mutase. In vitamin B₁₂ deficiency, this conversion cannot take place, and the substrate, methylmalonyl-CoA, accumulates. As a result, abnormal fatty acids are synthesized and incorporated into cell membranes. It is believed that incorporation of such nonphysiologic fatty acids into cell membranes of the central nervous system is responsible for the neurologic manifestations of vitamin B₁₂ deficiency.

The other enzymatic reaction that requires vitamin B₁₂ is conversion of 5-CH₃–H₄folate and homocysteine to H₄folate and methionine by the enzyme 5-CH₃–H₄folate-homocysteine methyltransferase (Figure 32–5B). In this reaction, cobalamin and methylcobalamin are interconverted, and the vitamin may be considered a true catalyst. When vitamin B₁₂ deficiency occurs, conversion of the major dietary and storage folate, 5-CH₃–H₄folate, to the precursor of fo-

A. Methylmalonyl-CoA mutase

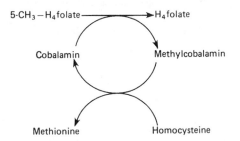

B. 5-CH₃ – H₄folate-homocysteine methyltransferase

Figure 32–5. Enzymatic reactions that use vitamin B_{12}.

late cofactors, H_4folate, cannot occur. As a result, 5-CH_3–H_4folate accumulates, and a deficiency of folate cofactors necessary for DNA synthesis develops. This accumulation of the body's folate as 5-CH_3–H_4folate and the associated inability to form folate cofactors in vitamin B_{12} deficiency have been referred to as the "methylfolate trap." This is the biochemical step whereby vitamin B_{12} and folic acid metabolism are linked and explains why the megaloblastic anemia of vitamin B_{12} deficiency (but not the neurologic abnormalities) can be partially corrected by folic acid.

B. Folic Acid: As noted above, the ultimate role of the folates is the formation of folate cofactors essential for one-carbon transfer reactions necessary for DNA synthesis. The de novo synthesis of the purine heterocycle involves two enzymatic reactions that use folate cofactors. In these, 10-CHO–H_4folate and 5,10-CH^+=H_4folate (Figure 32–4) donate their one-carbon units to ultimately form carbons 2 and 8 of the purine heterocycle. In both of these reactions, H_4folate is regenerated and can again accept a one-carbon unit and reenter the H_4folate cofactor pool.

Another essential reaction in which a folate cofactor is necessary is the synthesis of thymidylic acid (2′-deoxythymidine monophosphate; dTMP), an essential precursor of DNA. In this reaction, the enzyme thymidylate synthase catalyzes the transfer of the one-carbon unit of 5,10-CH_2–H_4folate to the 5-position of 2′-deoxyuridine monophosphate (dUMP) to form dTMP (Figure 32–6). Unlike all of the other enzymatic reactions that utilize folate cofactors, in this reaction the cofactor is oxidized to H_2folate, and for each mole of dTMP produced, a mole of H_4folate is consumed. In rapidly proliferating tissues, considerable amounts of H_4folate can be consumed in this reaction, and continued DNA synthesis requires continued regeneration of H_4folate by reduction of H_2folate,

catalyzed by the enzyme dihydrofolate reductase. The H_4folate thus produced can then re-form the cofactor CH_2–H_4folate by the action of serine transhydroxymethylase and thus allow for the continued synthesis of dTMP. The combined catalytic activities of dTMP synthetase, dihydrofolate reductase, and serine transhydroxymethylase are often referred to as the **dTMP synthesis cycle** (Figure 32–7).

Clinical Pharmacology

Vitamin B_{12} and folic acid should be used specifically to treat or prevent deficiencies of these vitamins. There is no evidence that vitamin B_{12} injections have any benefit in persons who do not have vitamin B_{12} deficiency. Supplemental folic acid, however, may be useful in preventing folic acid deficiency in certain high-risk patients with high folate requirements.

The most characteristic clinical manifestation of vitamin B_{12} and folic acid deficiency is megaloblastic anemia. Any patient with macrocytosis, with or without anemia, should be evaluated for possible vitamin B_{12} or folic acid deficiency. Although most patients with neurologic abnormalities caused by vitamin B_{12} deficiency have full-blown megaloblastic anemia when first seen, occasional patients have few if any hematologic abnormalities, and the diagnosis of vitamin B_{12} deficiency may at first be obscure. It is particularly important to differentiate vitamin B_{12} deficiency from other forms of megaloblastic anemia, since treatment with vitamin B_{12} must be continued for life in most cases and the hematologic abnormalities in vitamin B_{12} deficiency may be partially corrected by treatment with large doses of folic acid while the neurologic damage progresses and may become irreversible.

The typical clinical findings in megaloblastic anemia are macrocytic anemia (MCV usually > 120 fL), often with associated mild or moderate leukopenia or thrombocytopenia (or both), and a characteristic hypercellular bone marrow with megaloblastic maturation of erythroid and other precursor cells. Once a diagnosis of megaloblastic anemia is made, it must be determined whether vitamin B_{12} or folic acid deficiency is the cause. (Other causes of megaloblastic anemia are very rare.) This can usually be accomplished by measuring serum levels of the vitamins, though these measurements occasionally give false-positive or false-negative results. Red blood cell folic acid levels are often of greater diagnostic value than serum levels, since serum folic acid levels tend to be quite labile and do not necessarily reflect tissue levels. The Schilling test, which measures absorption and urinary excretion of radioactively labeled vitamin B_{12}, can be used to further define the mechanism of vitamin B_{12} malabsorption when this is found to be the cause of the megaloblastic anemia.

A. Vitamin B_{12} Deficiency: Vitamin B_{12} deficiency is almost always caused by malabsorption of vitamin B_{12}, due either to deficiency of intrinsic factor

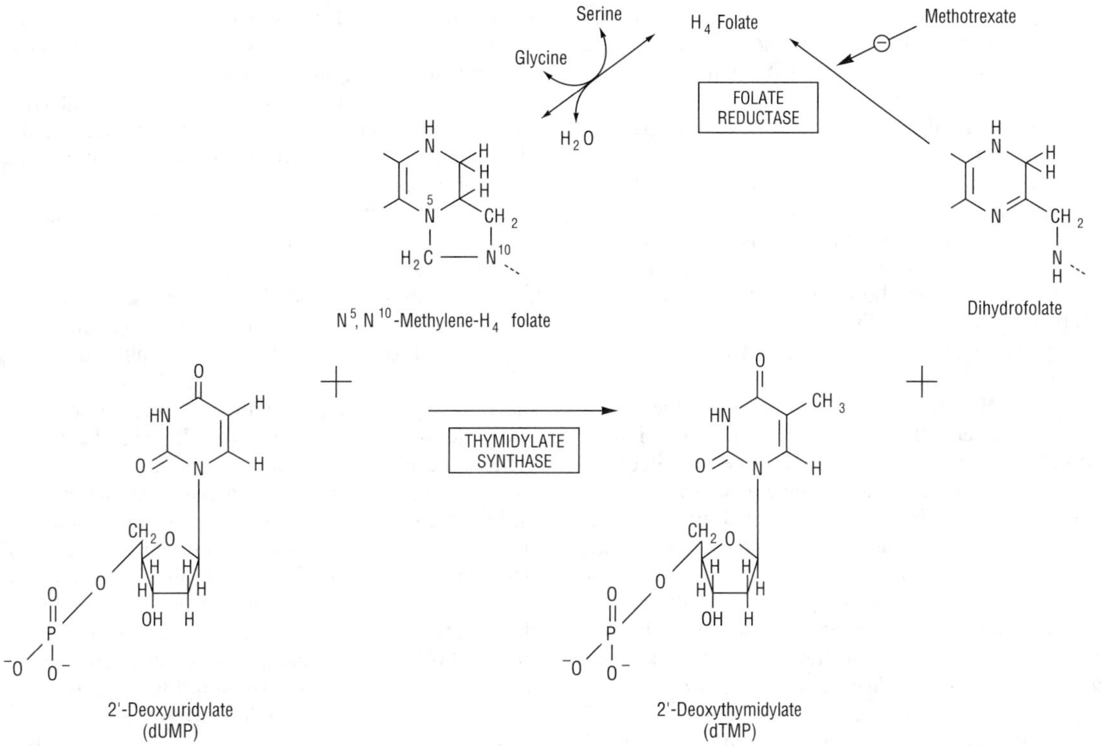

Serine

Glycine

H$_2$O

H$_4$ Folate

Methotrexate

⊖

FOLATE
REDUCTASE

N^5, N^{10}-Methylene-H$_4$ folate

Dihydrofolate

THYMIDYLATE
SYNTHASE

2'-Deoxyuridylate
(dUMP)

2'-Deoxythymidylate
(dTMP)

Figure 32–6. The transfer of a methyl moiety from N^5, N^{10}-methylene-H$_4$folate to deoxyuridylate to generate deoxythymidylate and dihydrofolate (H$_2$folate). (Reproduced, with permission, from Martin DW Jr et al: *Harper's Review of Biochemistry,* 20th ed. Lange, 1985.)

or to defects in the absorption of the vitamin B$_{12}$–intrinsic factor complex in the distal ileum. The most common causes of vitamin B$_{12}$ deficiency are pernicious anemia, partial or total gastrectomy, and diseases that affect the distal ileum, such as malabsorption syndromes, inflammatory bowel disease, or small bowel resection. Nutritional deficiency of vitamin B$_{12}$ is rare but may be seen in strict vegetarians after many years without meat, eggs, or dairy products.

Pernicious anemia results from defective secretion of **intrinsic factor** by the gastric mucosal cells. It is most common in older individuals of northern European extraction, but it may occur at any age and in all races. Patients with pernicious anemia have gastric atrophy and fail to secrete hydrochloric acid (as well as intrinsic factor). The Schilling test shows diminished absorption of radioactively labeled vitamin B$_{12}$, which is corrected when hog intrinsic factor is admin-

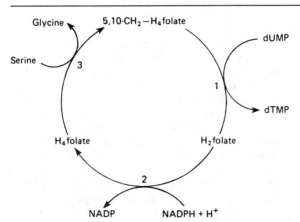

Figure 32–7. dTMP synthesis cycle. (1) dTMP synthetase; (2) H$_2$folate reductase; (3) serine transhydroxymethylase.

istered with radioactive B_{12}, since the vitamin can then be normally absorbed. Pernicious anemia is a lifelong disease, and treatment with vitamin B_{12} injections must be continued indefinitely.

Total or partial gastrectomy removes the parietal cell-containing portion of the stomach that secretes intrinsic factor, resulting in vitamin B_{12} malabsorption similar to that seen in pernicious anemia. Since vitamin B_{12} stores may not be exhausted until 5 years after gastrectomy, megaloblastic anemia will not develop until that time; however, many clinicians routinely start patients on vitamin B_{12} injections after gastrectomy to avoid any chance that vitamin B_{12} deficiency will develop later.

Vitamin B_{12} deficiency also occurs when the region of the distal ileum that absorbs the vitamin B_{12}–intrinsic factor complex is damaged, as when the ileum is involved with inflammatory bowel disease or sprue, or when the ileum is surgically resected. In these situations, radioactively labeled vitamin B_{12} is not absorbed in the Schilling test, even when intrinsic factor is added. Other rare causes of vitamin B_{12} deficiency include bacterial overgrowth of the small bowel, blind loop syndrome, fish tapeworm, chronic pancreatitis, and thyroid disease. Rare cases of vitamin B_{12} deficiency in children have been found to be secondary to congenital deficiency of intrinsic factor and congenital selective vitamin B_{12} malabsorption due to defects of the receptor sites in the distal ileum.

Since almost all cases of vitamin B_{12} deficiency are caused by malabsorption of the vitamin, parenteral injections of vitamin B_{12} are required for therapy. For patients with potentially reversible diseases (fish tapeworm, sprue, blind loops), the underlying disease should be treated after initial treatment with parenteral vitamin B_{12}. Most patients, however, do not have curable deficiency syndromes and require lifelong treatment with vitamin B_{12} injections.

Vitamin B_{12} for parenteral injection is available as cyanocobalamin or hydroxocobalamin. Hydroxocobalamin is preferred because it is more highly protein-bound and therefore remains longer in the circulation. Initial therapy should consist of 100–1000 μg of vitamin B_{12} intramuscularly daily or every other day for 1–2 weeks to replenish body stores. Maintenance therapy consists of 100–1000 μg intramuscularly once a month for life. If neurologic abnormalities are present, vitamin B_{12} injections should be given every 1–2 weeks for 6 months before switching to monthly injections. Oral vitamin B_{12}–intrinsic factor mixtures and liver extracts should not be used to treat vitamin B_{12} deficiency; however, oral doses of 1000 μg of vitamin B_{12} daily are usually sufficient to treat patients with pernicious anemia who refuse or cannot tolerate the injections.

The hematologic response to treatment with vitamin B_{12} is rapid. The bone marrow usually returns to normal within 48 hours. Reticulocytosis begins on the second or third day and is usually maximal by the fifth to tenth days. Hemoglobin begins to increase in the first week and returns to normal by 1–2 months. Incomplete correction of the anemia may be due to persistence of other deficiencies (ie, combined vitamin B_{12} and iron deficiency) or the presence of inflammatory disease or other disorders that inhibit erythropoiesis.

B. Folic Acid Deficiency: Folic acid deficiency, unlike vitamin B_{12} deficiency, is often caused by inadequate dietary intake of folates. Elderly patients, poor patients, and food faddists whose diets lack vegetables, eggs, and meat often develop folic acid deficiency. Prolonged cooking of vegetables destroys folates and can lead to folic acid deficiency if this is the only dietary source of this vitamin. Alcoholics and patients with liver disease develop folic acid deficiency because of poor diet and diminished hepatic storage of folates. There is also evidence that alcohol and liver disease interfere with absorption and metabolism of folates. Pregnant women and patients with hemolytic anemia have increased folate requirements and may become folic acid-deficient, especially if their diets are marginal. Recent evidence implicates maternal folic acid deficiency in the occurrence of fetal neural tube defects, eg, spina bifida. Patients with sprue and other malabsorption syndromes also frequently develop folic acid deficiency, perhaps because of a lack of intestinal conjugase. Folic acid deficiency is occasionally associated with cancer, leukemia, myeloproliferative disorders, certain chronic skin disorders, and other chronic debilitating diseases. Patients who require renal dialysis also develop folic acid deficiency, because folates are removed from the plasma each time the patient is dialyzed.

Folic acid deficiency can also be caused by drugs that interfere with folate absorption or metabolism. Phenytoin, some other anticonvulsants, oral contraceptives, and isoniazid can cause folic acid deficiency by interfering with folic acid absorption, possibly by inhibiting intestinal folate conjugases. Other drugs such as methotrexate and, to a lesser extent, trimethoprim and pyrimethamine, inhibit dihydrofolate reductase and may result in a deficiency of folate cofactors and ultimately in megaloblastic anemia (Figure 32–3).

Parenteral administration of folic acid is rarely necessary, since oral folic acid is well absorbed even in patients with malabsorption syndromes. A dose of 1 mg of folic acid orally daily is sufficient to reverse megaloblastic anemia, restore normal serum folate levels, and replenish body stores of folates in almost all patients. Therapy should be continued until the underlying cause of the deficiency is removed or corrected. Therapy may be required indefinitely for patients with malabsorption or dietary inadequacy. Folic acid supplementation to prevent folic acid deficiency should be considered in high-risk patients, including pregnant women, alcoholics, and patients with hemolytic anemia, liver disease, certain skin diseases, and patients on renal dialysis.

The response of patients with folate deficiency to treatment with oral folic acid is rapid and complete and similar to the response of the vitamin B_{12}–deficient patient given parenteral vitamin B_{12}. The hemoglobin level should begin to rise within the first week, and the anemia should be completely corrected in 1–2 months.

Clinical Toxicology

Vitamin B_{12} and folic acid have no known toxic effects even when administered in very large amounts. Large doses of both vitamins are promptly excreted in urine and to a lesser extent in stool, so that prolonged tissue exposure to very high levels does not occur. There is no evidence that cyanocobalamin, even in huge doses, causes cyanide poisoning.

HEMATOPOIETIC GROWTH FACTORS

The hematopoietic growth factors are glycoprotein hormones that regulate the proliferation and differentiation of hematopoietic progenitor cells in the bone marrow. The first growth factors identified were called colony-stimulating factors because they could stimulate the growth of colonies of various bone marrow progenitor cells in vitro. In the past decade, many of these growth factors have been purified and cloned, and their effects on hematopoiesis have been extensively studied (Table 32–3). Quantities of these growth factors sufficient for clinical use have been produced by recombinant DNA technology.

Of the known hematopoietic growth factors, **erythropoietin**, **granulocyte colony-stimulating factor** (G-CSF), and **granulocyte-macrophage colony-stimulating factor** (GM-CSF) are currently available and in clinical use. Interleukin-3 (IL-3), stem cell factor (SCF), and monocyte-macrophage colony-stimulating factor (M-CSF) are currently undergoing clinical trials and will probably become available in the next year or so. The other potentially useful hematopoietic growth factors listed in Table 32–3 are still in preclinical development.

ERYTHROPOIETIN

Chemistry & Pharmacokinetics

Erythropoietin was the first human hematopoietic growth factor to be isolated. It was first purified from the urine of patients with severe anemia. Recombinant human erythropoietin (rHuEpo, epoetin alfa) is produced in a mammalian cell expression system using recombinant DNA technology. It is a heavily glycosylated polypeptide of 165 amino acids with a molecular weight of 30,400. After intravenous administration, Erythropoietin has a serum half-life of 4–13 hours in patients with chronic renal failure. It is not cleared by dialysis. It is measured in international units (IU).

Pharmacodynamics

Erythropoietin stimulates erythroid proliferation and differentiation by interacting with specific erythropoietin receptors on red cell progenitors in the bone marrow. Endogenous erythropoietin is produced by the kidney in response to tissue hypoxia. When anemia occurs, more erythropoietin is pro-

Table 32–3. Hematopoietic growth factors.

Growth Factor	Progenitor Cell Lines Stimulated				
	Red Cells	Granulocytes	Monocytes-Macrophages	Megakaryocytes-Platelets	Other
EPO	3				
G-CSF		3			
M-CSF			3		
GM-CSF	3	3	3	3	Eosinophils
IL-3	3	3	3	3	Eosinophils, basophils
SCF	3	3	3	3	Eosinophils, basophils, lymphocytes
IL-6		3	3	3	Lymphocytes
IL-9, IL-11				3	Lymphocytes

Key:

EPO	=	erythropoietin
G-CSF	=	granulocyte colony-stimulating factor (filgrastim)
M-CSF	=	monocyte-macrophage colony-stimulating factor
GM-CSF	=	granulocyte-macrophage colony-stimulating factor (sargramostim)
IL	=	interleukin
SCF	=	stem cell factor

duced by the kidney, signaling the bone marrow to produce more red blood cells. This results in correction of the anemia provided that bone marrow response is not impaired by red cell nutritional deficiency (especially iron deficiency), primary bone marrow disorders (see below), or bone marrow suppression from drugs or chronic diseases.

Normally there is an inverse relationship between the hematocrit or hemoglobin level and the serum erythropoietin level. Nonanemic individuals have serum erythropoietin levels of less than 20 IU/L. As the hematocrit and hemoglobin level fall and anemia becomes more severe, the serum erythropoietin level rises exponentially. Patients with moderately severe anemias usually have erythropoietin levels in the 100–500 IU/L range, and patients with severe anemias may have levels of thousands of IU/L. The most important exception to this inverse relationship is in the anemia of chronic renal failure. In patients with renal disease, erythropoietin levels are usually low because the kidneys cannot produce the growth factor. These patients are the most likely to respond to treatment with exogenous erythropoietin. In most primary bone marrow disorders (aplastic anemia, leukemias, myeloproliferative and myelodysplastic disorders, etc) and most nutritional and secondary anemias, endogenous erythropoietin levels are high, so there is less likelihood of a response to erythropoietin (but see below).

Clinical Pharmacology

Erythropoietin is indicated in the treatment of renal failure patients with significant anemia. Erythropoietin consistently improves the hematocrit and hemoglobin level and usually eliminates the need for transfusions in these patients. An increase in reticulocyte count is usually observed in about 10 days and an increase in hematocrit and hemoglobin levels in 2–6 weeks. Most patients can maintain a hematocrit of about 35% with erythropoietin doses of 50–150 IU/kg intravenously or subcutaneously 3 times a week. Failure to respond to erythropoietin is most commonly due to concurrent iron deficiency, which can be corrected by giving oral iron. Folate supplementation may also be necessary in some patients.

Erythropoietin may also be useful for the treatment of anemia with primary bone marrow disorders and secondary anemias in selected patients. This includes patients with aplastic anemia and other bone marrow failure states, myeloproliferative and myelodysplastic disorders, multiple myeloma and perhaps other chronic bone marrow malignancies, and the anemias associated with chronic inflammation, AIDS, and cancer. Patients with these disorders who have disproportionately low serum erythropoietin levels for their degree of anemia are most likely to respond to treatment with this growth factor. Patients with endogenous erythropoietin levels of less than 100 IU/L have the best chance of response, though patients

with erythropoietin levels between 100 and 500 IU/L respond occasionally. These patients generally require higher erythropoietin doses (150–300 IU/kg 3 times a week) to achieve a response, and responses are often incomplete.

Erythropoietin has also been used successfully to offset the anemia produced by zidovudine treatment in patients with HIV infection and in the treatment of the anemia of prematurity. It can also be used to accelerate erythropoiesis after phlebotomies, when blood is being collected for autologous transfusion for elective surgery, or for treatment of iron overload (hemochromatosis).

Toxicity

The most common side effects of erythropoietin are associated with a rapid increase in hematocrit and hemoglobin and include hypertension and thrombotic complications. These difficulties can be minimized by raising the hematocrit and hemoglobin slowly and by adequately monitoring and treating hypertension. Allergic reactions have been infrequent and mild.

MYELOID GROWTH FACTORS

Chemistry & Pharmacokinetics

G-CSF and GM-CSF, the only myeloid growth factors currently available for clinical use, were originally purified from cultured human cell lines. Recombinant human G-CSF (rHuG-CSF; filgrastim) is produced in a bacterial expression system using recombinant DNA technology. It is a nonglycosylated polypeptide of 175 amino acids, with a molecular weight of 18,800. Recombinant human GM-CSF (rHuGM-CSF; sargramostim) is produced in a yeast expression system using recombinant DNA technology. It is a partially glycosylated polypeptide of 127 amino acids, with three molecular species with molecular weights of 15,500, 15,800, and 19,500. These preparations have serum half-lives of 2–4 hours after intravenous administration.

Monocyte-macrophage CSF (M-CSF), interleukin-3 (IL-3), stem cell factor (SCF), and the other interleukins with myeloid growth factor activity (Table 32–3) have also been purified, cloned, and produced in various expression systems by recombinant DNA technology. These growth factors are not yet available for clinical use.

Pharmacodynamics

The myeloid growth factors stimulate proliferation and differentiation of their respective cell lines by interacting with specific receptors found on various myeloid progenitor cells. G-CSF and M-CSF are lineage-specific growth factors that support proliferation and differentiation of progenitors already committed to neutrophil and monocyte-macrophage lineages, respectively. GM-CSF and IL-3 are multipotential hematopoietic growth factors that stimulate proliferation and differentiation of early and late granulocytic progenitor cells as well as erythroid and megakaryocyte progenitors. SCF is the earliest hematopoietic growth factor, acting on the earliest pluripotent stem cells and early committed granulocytic, erythroid, megakaryocytic, and lymphoid progenitors. The early growth factors potentiate the action of the later growth factors, producing synergy in their proliferative response. Both the early and the late myeloid growth factors (except SCF) also have direct effects on the mature target cells in the blood and tissues, enhancing neutrophil and monocyte-macrophage function.

Clinical Pharmacology

G-CSF and GM-CSF accelerate the rate of granulocyte recovery after dose-intensive myelosuppressive chemotherapy and after bone marrow transplantation. This can result in fewer infections and fewer days of hospitalization for these patients. G-CSF, 5 μg/kg/d, or GM-CSF, 250 μg/m²/d, is usually started within a few days after completing chemotherapy or the day after bone marrow transplantation and is continued until the absolute neutrophil count is approximately 2000–5000/μL. Although GM-CSF is a multilineage growth factor, it does not significantly accelerate red blood cell or platelet recovery in this setting.

G-CSF and GM-CSF in similar or higher doses may also be effective in treating granulocytopenia associated with myelodysplasia, aplastic anemia, congenital neutropenia, cyclic neutropenia, hairy cell leukemia and other chronic bone marrow malignancies, HIV infection, zidovudine-induced leukopenia, and other neutropenic disorders. Many patients respond with a prompt and sometimes dramatic increase in granulocyte count, and in some cases this results in a decrease in the frequency of infections. Again, few if any patients with anemia or thrombocytopenia have a significant increase in hematocrit and hemoglobin or platelet count.

Combinations of myeloid growth factors, particularly combinations acting on both early and late progenitors, can markedly enhance the proliferative effects on granulocytic as well as on erythroid and megakaryocytic progenitors. IL-3 and SCF will probably be used in this way, and there is hope that this will result in multilineage blood cell recovery. Interleukins-6, 9, and 11 are of particular interest because of their ability to stimulate megakaryocyte proliferation and platelet production. However, the interleukins (except IL-3) also have complex effects on the immune system, which may restrict or preclude their use as megakaryocyte or platelet growth factors in some clinical situations.

Toxicity

The adverse effects of treatment with G-CSF and GM-CSF have generally been infrequent and mild. G-CSF can cause bone pain, which clears when the drug is discontinued. GM-CSF can cause more severe side effects, particularly at higher doses. These include fevers, malaise, arthralgias, myalgias, and a capillary leak syndrome characterized by peripheral edema and pleural or pericardial effusions. Allergic reactions can occur but are infrequent.

PREPARATIONS AVAILABLE

Epoetin alfa (erythropoietin, Epo) (Epogen, Procrit)
Parenteral: 2000, 3000, 4000, and 10,000 IU/mL vials for IV or SC injection
Deferoxamine (Desferal)
Parenteral: 500 mg vials for IM, SC, or IV injection
Filgrastim (G-CSF) (Neupogen)
Parenteral: 300, 480 μg vials for IV or SC injection
Folic acid (folacin, pteroylglutamic acid) (generic)
Oral: 0.1, 0.4, 0.8, 1 mg tablets
Parenteral: 5, 10 mg/mL for injection
Iron (generic)

Oral: See Table 32–2
Parenteral (Iron Dextran) (InFeD): 50 mg elemental iron/mL
Sargramostim (GM-CSF) (Leukine, Prokine)
Parenteral: 250, 500 μg vials for IV infusion
Vitamin B₁₂ (generic cyanocobalamin or hydroxocobalamin)
Oral (cyanocobalamin): 25, 50, 100, 250, 500, 1000 μg tablets
Parenteral (cyanocobalamin): 30, 100, 1000 μg/mL for IM or SC injection
Parenteral (hydroxocobalamin): 1000 μg/mL for IM injection only

REFERENCES

Anthony AC: Megaloblastic anemias. In: *Hematology: Basic Principles and Practice,* Hoffman R et al (editors). Churchill Livingstone, 1991.

Brittenham GM: Disorders of iron metabolism: Iron deficiency and overload. In: *Hematology: Basic Principles and Practice.* Hoffman R et al (editors). Churchill Livingstone, 1991.

Crosier PS, Clark SC: Basic biology of the hematopoietic growth factors. Semin Oncol 1992;19:349.

Demetri GD, Antman KHS: Granulocyte-macrophage colony stimulating factor (GM-CSF): Preclinical and clinical investigations. Semin Oncol 1992;19:362.

Erslev AJ: Erythropoietin. N Engl J Med 1991;324:1339.

Glaspy JA, Golde DW: Granulocyte colony stimulating factor (G-CSF): Preclinical and clinical studies. Semin Oncol 1992;19:386.

Jandl JH: Iron deficiency anemia. In: *Blood: Textbook of Hematology.* Little, Brown, 1987.

Drugs Used in Disorders of Coagulation

33

Robert A. O'Reilly, MD

Bleeding and thrombosis are altered states of hemostasis. Impaired hemostasis results in spontaneous bleeding; stimulated hemostasis results in thrombus formation. The drugs used to arrest bleeding and to inhibit thrombosis are the subjects of this chapter.

MECHANISMS OF BLOOD COAGULATION

Thrombogenesis

Hemostasis is the spontaneous arrest of bleeding from a damaged blood vessel. The normal vascular endothelial cell is not thrombogenic, and circulating blood platelets and clotting factors do not adhere to it. The immediate hemostatic response of a damaged vessel is **vasospasm.** Within seconds, platelets stick to the exposed collagen of the damaged endothelium **(platelet adhesion)** and to each other **(platelet aggregation).** Platelets then lose their individual membranes and form a gelatinous mass during **viscous metamorphosis.** This platelet plug quickly arrests bleeding but must be reinforced by fibrin for long-term effectiveness. Fibrin reinforcement results from local stimuli to blood coagulation: the exposed collagen of damaged vessels and the membranes and released contents of platelets (Figure 33–1). The local production of thrombin not only releases platelet ADP, a powerful inducer of platelet aggregation, but also stimulates the synthesis of prostaglandins from the arachidonic acid of platelet membranes. These powerful substances are composed of two groups of eicosanoids (Chapter 18) that have opposite effects on thrombogenesis. **Thromboxane A$_2$** (TXA$_2$) is synthesized within platelets and induces thrombogenesis and vasoconstriction. **Prostacyclin** (PGI$_2$) is synthesized within vessel walls and inhibits thrombogenesis. Serotonin (5-HT) is also released from the platelets, stimulating further aggregation and vasoconstriction.

The **platelet** is central to normal hemostasis and to all thromboembolic disease. A **white thrombus** forms initially in high-pressure arteries by adherence of circulating platelets to areas of abnormal endothelium as described above. The growing thrombus of aggregated platelets reduces arterial flow. This localized stasis triggers fibrin formation, and a red thrombus forms around the nidal white thrombus.

A **red thrombus** can form around a white thrombus as described above or de novo in low-pressure veins, initially by adherence of platelets (as in arteries) but followed promptly by the other processes of hemostasis so that the bulk of the thrombus forms a long tail consisting of a fibrin network in which red cells are enmeshed. These tails become detached easily and travel as emboli to the pulmonary arteries. Although all thrombi are mixed, the platelet nidus dominates the arterial thrombus and the fibrin tail the venous thrombus. Arterial thrombi cause serious disease by producing local occlusive ischemia; venous thrombi, by giving rise to distant embolization.

Blood Coagulation

Blood coagulates by the transformation of soluble fibrinogen into insoluble fibrin. Several circulating proteins interact in a cascading series of limited proteolytic reactions. At each step, a clotting factor zymogen (eg, factor VII) undergoes limited proteolysis and becomes an active protease (eg, factor VIIa). This protease activates the next clotting factor (factor IX), until finally a solid fibrin clot is formed. Fibrinogen (factor I), the soluble precursor of fibrin, is the substrate for the enzyme thrombin (factor IIa). This protease is formed during coagulation by activation of its zymogen, prothrombin (factor II). Prothrombin is bound by calcium to a platelet phospholipid (PL) surface, where activated factor X (Xa), in the presence of factor Va, converts it into circulating thrombin. Several of the blood clotting factors are targets for drug therapy (Table 33–1).

The details of coagulation are still not fully understood. In a recently advanced theory of blood coagulation, the system is activated by a complex of tissue factor (TF) and factor VII (Figure 33–2). This com-

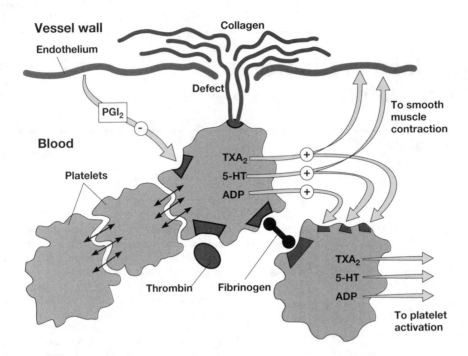

Figure 33–1. Formation of a platelet clot is a rapid multistep process. Platelets adhere to exposed collagen and are activated at the site of endothelial damage in the blood vessel. Activated platelets release adenosine diphosphate (ADP), serotonin (5-HT), and thromboxane A_2 (TXA_2), which activate additional platelets. Binding of thrombin further activates the platelets. Three adjoining platelets are shown in the process of viscous metamorphosis. Increased intracellular calcium facilitates binding of fibrinogen. These agents and other substances (not shown) bind to specific receptors on the platelet surface.

plex is inhibited and regulated by tissue factor pathway inhibitor (TFPI). Oral anticoagulant drugs inhibit the hepatic synthesis of several clotting factors. Heparin inhibits the activity of several of these *activated* clotting factors. The endogenous anticoagulants protein C and S down-regulate the amplification of blood clotting by proteolysis of factors Va, VIIIa, and XIa.

Regulation of Coagulation & Fibrinolysis

Blood coagulation and thrombus formation must be confined to the smallest possible area to achieve local hemostasis in response to bleeding from trauma or surgery without disseminated coagulation or impaired blood flow. Two major systems regulate and delimit these processes: **fibrin inhibition** and **fibrinolysis.**

Plasma contains protease inhibitors that rapidly inactivate the coagulation proteins as they escape from the site of vessel injury. The most important proteins of this system are α_1-antiprotease, α_2-macroglobulin, α_2-antiplasmin, and antithrombin III. If this system is overwhelmed, generalized intravascular clotting may occur. This process is called **disseminated intravascular coagulation (DIC)** and may follow massive

tissue injury, cell lysis in malignant neoplastic disease, obstetric emergencies such as abruptio placentae, or bacterial sepsis.

The central process of fibrinolysis is conversion of inactive plasminogen to the proteolytic enzyme **plasmin.** Injured cells release activators of plasminogen. Plasmin remodels the thrombus and limits the extension of thrombosis by proteolytic digestion of fibrin.

Regulation of the fibrinolytic system is useful in therapeutics. Increased fibrinolysis is effective therapy for thrombotic disease. **Tissue plasminogen activator (t-PA), urokinase,** and **streptokinase** all activate the fibrinolytic system (Figure 33–3). Conversely, decreased fibrinolysis protects clots from lysis and reduces the bleeding of hemostatic failure. **Aminocaproic acid** is a clinically useful inhibitor of fibrinolysis. Heparin and the oral anticoagulant drugs do not affect the fibrinolytic mechanism.

Table 33–1. Blood clotting factors and drugs that affect them.[1]

Component or Factor	Common Synonym	Drugs Targeting The Factor
I	Fibrinogen	
II	Prothrombin	Heparin (IIa); warfarin (synthesis)
III	Tissue thromboplastin	
IV	Calcium	
V	Proaccelerin	
VII	Proconvertin	Heparin (VIIa); warfarin (synthesis)
VIII	Antihemophilic globulin (AHG)	
IX	Christmas factor, plasma thromboplastin component (PTC)	Heparin (IXa); warfarin (synthesis)
X	Stuart-Prower factor	Heparin (Xa); warfarin (synthesis)
XI	Plasma thromboplastin antecedent (PTA)	
XII	Hageman factor	
XIII	Fibrin-stabilizing factor	
Proteins C and S		Warfarin (synthesis)
Plasminogen		Thrombolytic enzmes, aminocaproic acid

[1]See Figure 33–2 and text for additional details.

I. BASIC PHARMACOLOGY OF THE ANTICOAGULANT DRUGS

HEPARIN

Chemistry & Mechanism of Action

Heparin is a heterogeneous mixture of sulfated mucopolysaccharides. It binds to endothelial cell surfaces. Its biologic activity is dependent upon the plasma protease inhibitor **antithrombin III.** Antithrombin inhibits clotting factor proteases by forming equimolar stable complexes with them. In the absence of heparin, these reactions are slow; in the presence of heparin, they are accelerated 1000-fold. Only a third of the molecules in commercial heparin preparations have an accelerating effect and therefore anticoagulant activity. The active heparin molecules bind tightly to antithrombin and cause a conformational change in this inhibitor. The conformational change of antithrombin exposes its active site for more rapid interaction with the proteases—the activated clotting factors. Heparin catalyzes the antithrombin-protease reaction without being consumed. Once the antithrombin-protease complex is formed, heparin is released intact for renewed binding to more antithrombin.

The antithrombin binding region of commercial heparin consists of repeating sulfated disaccharide units composed of D-glucosamine-L-iduronic acid and D-glucosamine-D-glucuronic acid (Figure 33–4). High-molecular-weight fractions (HMW) of heparin with high affinity for antithrombin markedly inhibit blood coagulation. These fractions have an MW range of 5000–30,000. Low-molecular-weight (LMW) fractions of heparin inhibit activated factor X but have less effect on thrombin and on coagulation in general than the HMW species. **Enoxaparin,** one of many LMW heparin fractions, has been approved by the FDA for the primary prevention of deep venous thrombosis after hip replacement surgery. Enoxaparin has an MW range of 2000–6000. Several LMW heparins, upon comparison with regular heparin, have shown equal or greater efficacy, lower rates of bleeding, increased bioavailability from the subcutaneous site of injection, less need for laboratory monitoring, and less frequent dosing (once or twice daily is sufficient).

Because commercial heparin consists of a family of molecules of different molecular weights, the correlation between the concentration of a given heparin preparation and its effect on coagulation often is low. Therefore, regular (HMW) heparin is standardized as units of activity by bioassay. Heparin sodium USP must contain at least 120 USP units per milligram. Heparin is generally used as the sodium salt, but calcium heparin is equally effective. Lithium heparin is used in vitro as an anticoagulant for blood samples. Commercial heparin is extracted from porcine intestinal mucosa and bovine lung. Enoxaparin is obtained from the same sources as regular heparin, but doses are specified in milligrams.

Toxicity

The major adverse effect of heparin is bleeding. This risk can be decreased by scrupulous patient selection, careful control of dosage, and close monitoring of the partial thromboplastin time (PTT). Elderly women and patients with renal failure are prone to hemorrhage. Heparin is of animal origin and should be used cautiously in patients with allergy. Increased loss of hair and transient reversible alopecia have been reported. Long-term heparin therapy is associated with osteoporosis and spontaneous fractures. Heparin accelerates the clearing of postprandial lipemia by effecting the release of lipoprotein lipase from tissues.

Heparin causes transient thrombocytopenia in 25% of patients and severe thrombocytopenia in 5%. Mild platelet reduction results from heparin-induced aggregation and severe reduction from heparin-induced antiplatelet antibodies. Paradoxical thromboembolism may result from heparin-induced platelet aggregation. The following points should be considered in all patients receiving heparin: Platelet counts

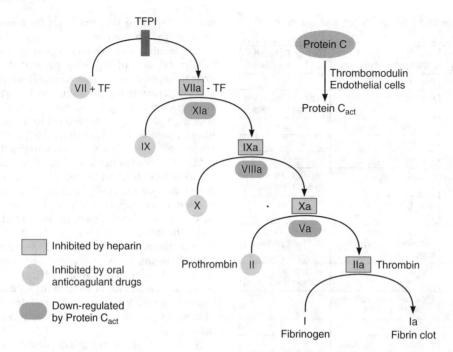

Figure 33–2. A model of blood coagulation. With tissue factor (TF), factor VII forms an activated complex (VIIa-TF) that catalyzes the activation of factor IX to factor IXa. Activated factor XIa also catalyzes this reaction. Tissue factor pathway inhibitor (TFPI) inhibits the catalytic action of the VIIa-TF complex. The cascade proceeds as shown, resulting ultimately in the conversion of fibrinogen to fibrin, an essential component of a functional clot. The two major anticoagulant drugs, heparin and warfarin (an oral anticoagulant), have very different actions. Heparin, acting in the blood, directly activates anticlotting factors—especially antithrombin III, which inactivate the factors enclosed in rectangles. Warfarin, acting in the liver, inhibits the synthesis of the factors enclosed in circles. Proteins C and S exert anticlotting effects by destroying activated factors Va, VIIIa, and XIa.

should be performed frequently; thrombocytopenia serious enough to cause bleeding should be considered to be heparin-induced; any new thrombus can be the result of heparin; and thromboembolic disease thought to be heparin-induced should be treated by discontinuance of heparin and administration of an oral anticoagulant if clinically warranted.

Contraindications

Heparin is contraindicated in patients who are hypersensitive to the drug, are actively bleeding, or have hemophilia, thrombocytopenia, purpura, severe hypertension, intracranial hemorrhage, infective endocarditis, active tuberculosis, ulcerative lesions of the gastrointestinal tract, threatened abortion, visceral carcinoma, or advanced hepatic or renal disease. Heparin should not be given to patients during or after surgery of the brain, spinal cord, or eye or to patients undergoing lumbar puncture or regional anesthetic blocks. Heparin should be used in pregnant women only when clearly indicated despite the apparent lack of placental transfer.

Administration & Dosage

The indications for the use of heparin are described in the section on clinical pharmacology. A plasma concentration of heparin of 0.2 unit/mL usually prevents pulmonary emboli in patients with established venous thrombosis. This concentration of heparin will prolong the partial thromboplastin time (PTT) to 2–$2\frac{1}{2}$ times that of the control value. This degree of anticoagulant effect should be maintained throughout the course of *continuous* intravenous heparin therapy. When *intermittent* heparin administration is used, the PTT should be measured just before the next heparin dose to adjust this dose so as to maintain prolongation of the PTT to 2–$2\frac{1}{2}$ times that of the control value.

The continuous intravenous administration of heparin is accomplished via an infusion pump. After an initial bolus injection of 5000–10,000 units, a continuous infusion of about 900 units/h or 10–15 units/kg/h is required to maintain the PTT at 2–$2\frac{1}{2}$ times control. Patients with acute pulmonary emboli often require larger doses than these during the first few days because of increased heparin clearance. With intermittent intravenous administration of heparin, 75–100 units/kg is administered every 4 hours. Subcutaneous administration of heparin, as in low-dose prophylaxis, is achieved with 5000 units every 8 or 12 hours. Heparin must never be administered in-

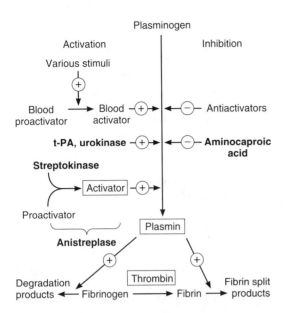

Figure 33–3. Schematic representation of the fibrinolytic system. Plasmin is the active fibrinolytic enzyme. Several clinically useful activators are shown on the left in bold. Anistreplase is a combination of streptokinase and the proactivator plasminogen. Aminocaproic acid (right) inhibits the activation of plasminogen to plasmin and is useful in some bleeding disorders.

tramuscularly, because of the danger of hematoma formation at the injection site. Enoxaparin is given in a dosage of 30 mg twice daily after hip surgery.

Reversal of Heparin Action

Excessive anticoagulant action of heparin is treated by discontinuance of the drug. If bleeding occurs, administration of a specific antagonist such as protamine sulfate is indicated. Protamine is a highly basic peptide that combines with heparin as an ion pair to form a stable complex devoid of anticoagulant activity. For every 100 units of heparin remaining in the patient, administer 1 mg of protamine sulfate intravenously; the rate of infusion should not exceed 50 mg

in any 10-minute period. Excess protamine must be avoided; it also has an anticoagulant effect.

HIRUDIN

For a number of years, surgeons have used medicinal leeches *(Hirudo medicinalis)* to prevent thrombosis in the fine vessels of reattached digits. Hirudin is a powerful and specific thrombin inhibitor from the leech which is now being prepared by recombinant DNA technology. Its action is independent of antithrombin III, which means it can reach and inactivate fibrin-bound thrombin in thrombi. Hirudin has little effect on platelets or the bleeding time. Like heparin, it must be administered parenterally and is monitored by the PTT. It has undergone extensive animal testing and is now in clinical trials.

WARFARIN & THE COUMARIN ANTICOAGULANTS

Chemistry & Pharmacokinetics

The clinical use of the coumarin anticoagulants can be traced to the discovery of an anticoagulant substance formed in spoiled sweet clover silage. It produced a deficiency of plasma prothrombin and a consequent hemorrhagic disease in cattle. The toxic agent was identified as bishydroxycoumarin and synthesized as dicumarol. This drug and its congeners, most notably warfarin (Figure 33–5), are widely used as rodenticides in addition to their application as antithrombotic agents in humans. These drugs are often referred to as "oral anticoagulants" because, unlike heparin, they are administered orally. Warfarin is the most reliable member of this group, and the other coumarin anticoagulants are almost never used in the USA.

Warfarin is generally administered as the sodium salt and has 100% bioavailability. Over 99% of racemic warfarin is bound to plasma albumin, which may contribute to its small volume of distribution (the albumin space), its long half-life in plasma (36 hours), and the lack of urinary excretion of un-

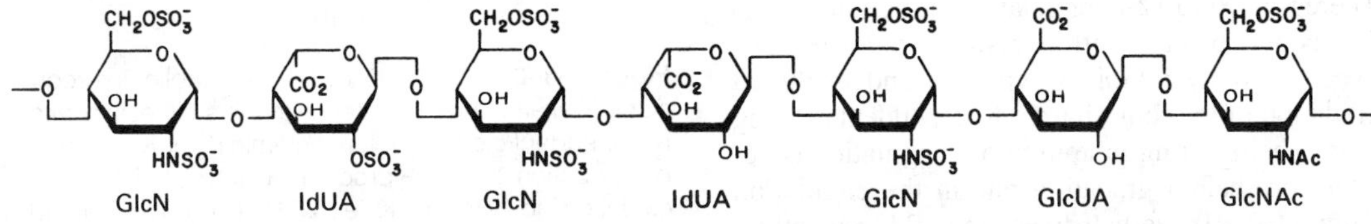

Figure 33–4. Structure of heparin. The polymer section illustrates structural features typical of heparin; however, the sequence of variously repeating disaccharide units has been arbitrarily selected. In addition, non-O-sulfated or 3-O-sulfated glucosamines may also occur. Heparin is a strongly acidic molecule because of its high content of anionic sulfate and carboxylic acid. GlcN, glucosamine; IdUA, iduronic acid; GlcUA, glucuronic acid. (Modified, redrawn, and reproduced, with permission, from Lindahl U et al: Structure and biosynthesis of heparinlike polysaccharides. Fed Proc 1977;36:19.)

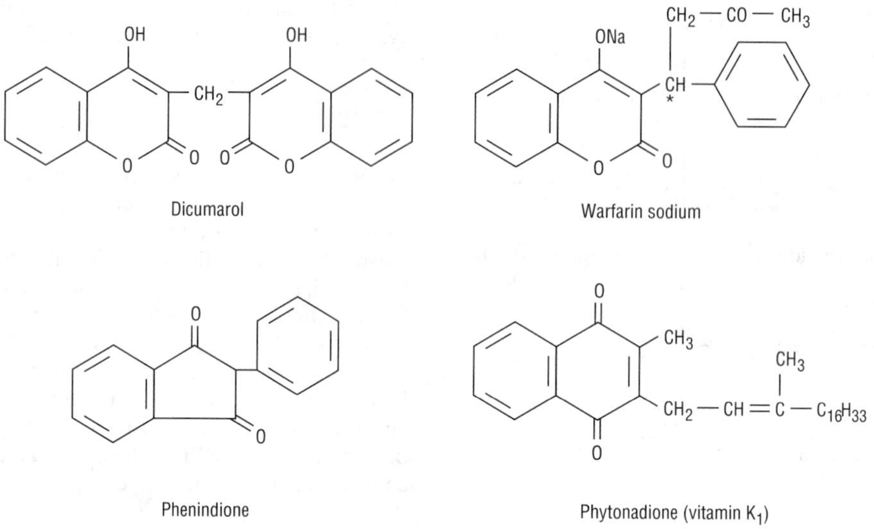

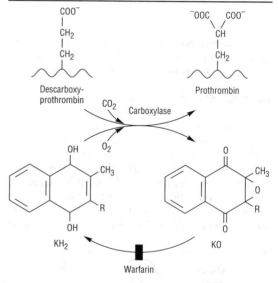

Dicumarol

Warfarin sodium

Phenindione

Phytonadione (vitamin K$_1$)

Figure 33–5. Structural formulas of several oral anticoagulant drugs and of vitamin K. The carbon atom of warfarin shown at the asterisk is an asymmetric center.

changed drug. Warfarin used clinically is a racemic mixture composed of equal amounts of two optical isomers. The levorotatory S-warfarin is four times more potent than the dextrorotatory R-warfarin. This observation is useful in understanding the stereoselective nature of several drug interactions involving warfarin.

Mechanism of Action

Coumarin anticoagulants block the γ-carboxylation of several glutamate residues in prothrombin and factors VII, IX, and X as well as the endogenous anticoagulant protein C (Figure 33–2). The blockade results in incomplete molecules that are biologically inactive in coagulation. This protein carboxylation is physiologically coupled with the oxidative deactivation of vitamin K. The anticoagulant prevents the reductive metabolism of the inactive vitamin K epoxide back to its active hydroquinone form (Figure 33–6). Mutational change of the responsible enzyme, vitamin K epoxide reductase, can give rise to genetic resistance to warfarin in humans and especially in rats.

There is an 8- to 12-hour delay in the action of warfarin. Its anticoagulant effect results from a balance between partially inhibited synthesis and unaltered degradation of the four vitamin K-dependent clotting factors. The resulting inhibition of coagulation is dependent on their degradation rate in the circulation (Figure 33–7). These half-lives are 6, 24, 40, and 60 hours for factors VII, IX, X, and II, respectively. Larger initial doses of warfarin—up to about 0.75 mg/kg—hasten the onset of the anticoagulant effect. Beyond this dosage, the speed of onset is independent

Figure 33–6. Vitamin K cycle—metabolic interconversions of vitamin K associated with the synthesis of vitamin K-dependent clotting factors. Vitamin K$_1$ or K$_2$ is activated by reduction to the hydroquinone form (KH$_2$). Stepwise oxidation to vitamin K epoxide (KO) is coupled to prothrombin carboxylation by the enzyme carboxylase. The reactivation of vitamin K epoxide is the warfarin-sensitive step (warfarin). The R on the vitamin K molecule represents a 20-carbon phytyl side chain in vitamin K$_1$ and a 30- to 65-carbon polyprenyl side chain in vitamin K$_2$.

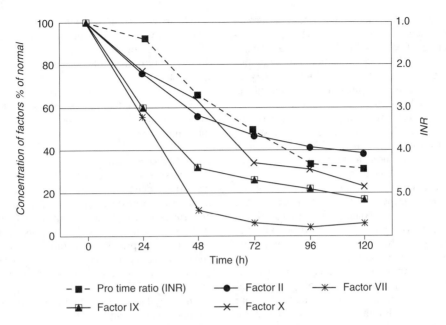

Figure 33–7. The activity of the four vitamin K-dependent clotting factors and the prothrombin time expressed in INR units as a function of time after starting administration of warfarin. True prothrombin, factor II, has a half-life of 60 hours; several days of therapy are required for its activity to reach the therapeutic range.

of the dose size. The only effect of a larger loading dose is to prolong the time that the plasma concentration of drug remains above that required for suppression of clotting factor synthesis. The 1- to 3-day delay between the peak drug concentration in plasma and its maximum hypoprothrombinemic effect can be described by a model based on the relationship of the plasma concentration of drug and the reduced synthesis of clotting factors. The only difference among oral anticoagulants in producing and maintaining hypoprothrombinemia is the half-life of each drug.

Toxicity

Warfarin crosses the placenta readily and can cause a hemorrhagic disorder in the fetus. Furthermore, fetal proteins with γ-carboxyglutamate residues found in bone and blood may be affected by warfarin; the drug can cause a serious birth defect characterized by abnormal bone formation. Thus, warfarin should never be administered during pregnancy. Cutaneous necrosis with reduced activity of protein C sometimes occurs during the first weeks of therapy. Rarely, the same process causes frank infarction of breast, fatty tissues, intestine, and extremities. The pathologic lesion associated with the hemorrhagic infarction is venous thrombosis, suggesting that it is caused by warfarin-induced depression of protein C synthesis.

Administration & Dosage

Treatment with warfarin should be initiated with small daily doses of 2–5 mg rather than the large loading doses formerly used. The initial adjustment of the prothrombin time takes about 1 week, which usually results in a maintenance dose of 5–7 mg/d. The prothrombin time should be increased to a level representing 25% of normal activity and maintained there for long-term therapy. When the activity is less than 20%, the warfarin dosage should be reduced or omitted until the activity rises above 20%.

The therapeutic range for oral anticoagulant therapy has recently been defined in terms of an international normalized ratio (INR). The INR is the prothrombin time ratio (test/control) obtained if the more sensitive international reference thromboplastin made from human brain is used rather than the less sensitive rabbit-brain thromboplastin used in North America (Poller, 1992). Randomized prospective studies with the INR system have resulted in use of lower doses of anticoagulant drug and less bleeding, yet the efficacy is equal to the regimens with higher doses. These less intensive and lower dose regimens are efficacious for many therapeutic indications. Analysis of several clinical trials has led to the recommendation that dosage be adjusted to achieve an INR of 2.5–3.5 (Eckman, 1993). (An INR of 3 corresponds to a prothrombin time ratio of 1.6 in the average North American laboratory.)

Drug Interactions

The oral anticoagulants often interact with other

drugs and with disease states. These interactions can be broadly divided into **pharmacokinetic** and **pharmacodynamic** effects (Table 33–2). Pharmacokinetic mechanisms for drug interaction with oral anticoagulants are mainly **enzyme induction, enzyme inhibition,** and **reduced plasma protein binding.** Pharmacodynamic mechanisms for interactions with warfarin are **synergism** (impaired hemostasis, reduced clotting factor synthesis, as in hepatic disease), **competitive antagonism** (vitamin K), and an **altered physiologic control loop for vitamin K** (hereditary resistance to oral anticoagulants).

The most serious interactions with warfarin are those that *increase* the anticoagulant effect and the risk of bleeding. The most dangerous of these interactions are the pharmacokinetic interactions with the pyrazolones phenylbutazone and sulfinpyrazone. These drugs not only augment the hypoprothrombinemia but also inhibit platelet function and may induce peptic ulcer disease (Chapter 35). The mechanisms for their hypoprothrombinemic interaction are a stereoselective inhibition of oxidative metabolic transformation of S-warfarin and displacement of albumin-bound warfarin, increasing the free fraction. Metronidazole, miconazole, and trimethoprim-sulfamethoxazole also stereoselectively inhibit the metabolic transformation of S-warfarin, whereas amiodarone, disulfiram, and cimetidine inhibit metabolism of both enantiomorphs of warfarin. Aspirin, hepatic disease, and hyperthyroidism augment warfarin pharmacodynamically: aspirin by its effect on platelet function and the latter two by increasing the turnover rate of clotting factors. The third-generation cephalosporins eliminate the bacteria in the intestinal tract that produce vitamin K, and, like warfarin, also directly inhibit vitamin K epoxide reductase. Heparin directly prolongs the prothrombin time by inhibiting the activity of several clotting factors.

Barbiturates and rifampin cause a marked *decrease* of the anticoagulant effect by induction of the hepatic enzymes that transform racemic warfarin. Cholestyramine binds warfarin in the intestine and reduces its absorption and bioavailability.

Pharmacodynamic reductions of anticoagulant effect occur with vitamin K (increased synthesis of clotting factors), the diuretics chlorthalidone and spironolactone (clotting factor concentration), hereditary resistance (mutation of vitamin K reactivation cycle), and hypothyroidism (decreased turnover rate of clotting factors).

Drugs with *no* significant effect on anticoagulant therapy include ethanol, phenothiazines, benzodiazepines, acetaminophen, narcotics, indomethacin, and most antibiotics.

Reversal of Action

Excessive anticoagulant effect and bleeding from warfarin can be reversed by stopping the drug and administering large doses of vitamin K_1 (phytonadione) and fresh-frozen plasma or factor IX concentrates such as Konyne and Proplex that also contain large amounts of the prothrombin complex. This disappearance of effect is not correlated with plasma warfarin concentrations but rather with reestablishment of normal activity of the clotting factors. A modest excess of anticoagulant effect without bleeding may require no more than cessation of the drug. Serious bleeding requires large amounts of vitamin K_1 intravenously in 50 mg infusions, factor IX concentrates, and sometimes even transfusion of whole blood.

Analogues & Variants

Vitamin K antagonists other than warfarin are seldom used because they have less favorable pharmacologic properties or greater toxicity. **Dicumarol** is incompletely absorbed and frequently causes gastrointestinal symptoms. **Phenprocoumon** has a long half-life of 6 days. The indanedione group, which includes phenindione and diphenadione, has potentially serious adverse effects in the kidney and liver and is of little clinical use.

Table 33–2. Pharmacokinetic and pharmacodynamic drug and body interactions with oral anticoagulants.

Increased Prothrombin Time		Decreased Prothrombin Time	
Pharmacokinetic	Pharmacodynamic	Pharmacokinetic	Pharmacodynamic
Amiodarone	**Drugs**	Barbiturates	**Drugs**
Cimetidine	Aspirin (high doses)	Cholestyramine	Diuretics
Disulfiram	Cephalosporins, third-generation	Rifampin	Vitamin K
Metronidazole[1]	Heparin		**Body factors**
Miconazole[1]	**Body factors**		Hereditary resistance
Phenylbutazone[1]	Hepatic disease		Hypothyroidism
Sulfinpyrazone[1]	Hyperthyroidism		
Trimethoprim-sulfamethoxazole[1]			

[1]Stereoselectively inhibits the oxidative metabolism of the S-warfarin enantiomorph of racemic warfarin.

II. BASIC PHARMACOLOGY OF THE FIBRINOLYTIC DRUGS

Fibrinolytic drugs rapidly lyse thrombi by catalyzing the formation of the serine protease **plasmin** from its precursor zymogen, plasminogen (Figure 33–3). These drugs create a generalized lytic state when administered intravenously. Thus, both protective hemostatic thrombi and target thromboemboli are broken down. Two new approaches have been proposed to reduce the nonselective systemic effects. First, intra-arterial use of a fibrinolytic drug, as in intracoronary injection, may reduce systemic bleeding by localizing the drug. Second, a new generation of prothrombolytic drugs, **tissue plasminogen activators,** may induce thrombolysis with less systemic fibrinolysis or fibrinogen breakdown. Unfortunately, the difference from the first-generation drugs (streptokinase) is clinically insignificant.

STREPTOKINASE, ANISTREPLASE, TISSUE PLASMINOGEN ACTIVATOR, & UROKINASE

Pharmacology

Streptokinase is a protein synthesized by streptococci that combines with the proactivator plasminogen. This enzymatic complex catalyzes the conversion of inactive plasminogen to active plasmin. **Urokinase** is a human enzyme synthesized by the kidney that directly converts plasminogen to active plasmin. While the naturally occurring inhibitors of plasmin in plasma preclude its direct use, the absence of inhibitors for urokinase and the streptokinase-proactivator complex permit their use clinically. Plasmin formed inside a thrombus by these activators is protected from plasma antiplasmins, which allows it to lyse the thrombus from within. **Anistreplase** (anisoylated plasminogen streptokinase activator complex; APSAC) consists of a complex of purified human plasminogen and bacterial streptokinase that has been acylated to protect the enzyme's active site. When administered, the acyl group spontaneously hydrolyzes, freeing the activated streptokinase-proactivator complex. This product allows for rapid intravenous injection, greater clot selectivity (ie, more activity on plasminogen associated with clots than on free plasminogen in the blood), and more thrombolytic activity.

Plasminogen can also be activated endogenously by **tissue plasminogen activators (t-PA).** These activators preferentially activate plasminogen that is bound to fibrin, which (in theory) confines fibrinolysis to the formed thrombus and avoids systemic activation. Human t-PA is manufactured by means of recombinant DNA technology.

Indications & Dosage

Use of fibrinolytic drugs by the intravenous route is indicated in cases of **multiple pulmonary emboli** that are not massive enough to require surgical intervention. Intravenous fibrinolytic drugs are also indicated in cases of **central deep venous thrombosis** such as the superior vena caval syndrome and ascending thrombophlebitis of the iliofemoral vein. They have also been used intra-arterially, especially for peripheral vascular disease.

Thrombolytic therapy in the management of **acute myocardial infarction** requires careful patient selection, the use of a specific thrombolytic agent, and the benefit of adjuvant therapy. Considerable controversy surrounds the question of greater safety or efficacy of t-PA compared with the other thrombolytic agents. In different large randomized clinical trials t-PA was (Topol, 1993) and was not (ISIS-3, 1992) more efficacious acutely than streptokinase in terms of restenosis, ventricular function, and mortality outcomes (Cobbe, 1992). Furthermore, the incidence of hemorrhagic strokes with t-PA was over twice that with streptokinase. Thus, it is still not obvious that one drug is superior to the others. However, it is clear that streptokinase is one-tenth to one-fifth as expensive as the other drugs (see below). Beta-blockers and aspirin both improve the results of thrombolytic therapy, but heparin given subcutaneously does not.

Streptokinase is administered by intravenous infusion of a loading dose of 250,000 units, followed by 100,000 units/h for 24–72 hours. Patients with antistreptococcal antibodies can develop fever, allergic reactions, and therapeutic resistance. Urokinase requires a loading dose of 300,000 units given over 10 minutes and a maintenance dose of 300,000 units/h for 12 hours. Alteplase (t-PA) is given by intravenous infusion of 60 mg over the first hour and then 40 mg at a rate of 20 mg/h. Anistreplase is given as a single intravenous injection of 30 units over 3–5 minutes. A course of fibrinolytic drugs is expensive: hundreds of dollars for streptokinase and thousands for urokinase, anistreplase, and t-PA. When thrombolytic enzyme therapy is completed, it should be followed by administration of heparin and then warfarin. The efficacy of thrombolytic therapy in reducing long-term mortality and the need for subsequent percutaneous coronary angioplasty are yet undetermined. Intracoronary administration of thrombolytic drugs delays therapy, complicates logistics, and may reduce efficacy.

III. BASIC PHARMACOLOGY OF ANTITHROMBOTIC DRUGS

Platelet function is regulated by three categories of substances. The first group consists of agents generated outside the platelet that interact with platelet membrane receptors, eg, catecholamines, collagen, thrombin, and prostacyclin. The second category contains agents generated within the platelet that interact with the membrane receptors, eg, ADP, prostaglandin D_2, prostaglandin E_2, and serotonin (Figure 33–1). The third contains agents generated within the platelet that act within the platelet, eg, prostaglandin endoperoxides and thromboxane A_2, the cyclic nucleotides cAMP and cGMP, and calcium ion. From this list of agents, two targets for platelet inhibitory drugs have been identified: inhibition of prostaglandin metabolism (aspirin) and inhibition of ADP-induced platelet aggregation (ticlopidine).

ASPIRIN

The prostaglandin **thromboxane A_2** is an arachidonate product that causes platelets to change shape, to release their granules, and to aggregate (Chapter 18). Drugs that antagonize this pathway interfere with platelet aggregation in vitro and prolong the bleeding time in vivo. **Aspirin** is the prototype of this class of drugs. Drugs that modulate the intraplatelet concentration of cAMP do not prolong the bleeding time. However, dietary therapy can be useful in the prophylaxis of thrombosis. Ingestion of the unsaturated fatty acid **eicosapentaenoic acid,** which is high in the diets of Eskimos, generates prostaglandin I_3, an antiaggregating substance like prostacyclin.

Aspirin inhibits the synthesis of thromboxane A_2 by irreversible acetylation of the enzyme cyclooxygenase (Chapter 18). Because the anuclear platelet cannot synthesize new proteins, it cannot manufacture new enzyme during its 10-day lifetime. Other salicylates and other nonsteroidal anti-inflammatory drugs also inhibit cyclooxygenase but have a shorter duration of inhibitory action because they cannot acetylate cyclooxygenase, ie, their action is reversible.

Two large prospective, randomized trials in healthy American and British physicians were conducted to evaluate the use of aspirin for 4–5 years in the *primary prophylaxis* of cardiovascular mortality, ie, prevention of first heart attacks. The American study showed a significant reduction in the incidence of nonfatal myocardial infarctions (and was prematurely terminated because of this finding), while the British study showed no significant change. Furthermore, the British study confirmed previous evidence

that at a dose of 500 mg/d, aspirin increases the incidence of peptic ulcer disease and gastrointestinal bleeding. Thus, the risk-versus-benefit measure of aspirin as an over-the-counter prophylactic drug is questionable for patients with hypertension or peptic ulcer disease.

The FDA has approved the use of 325 mg/d for *primary* prophylaxis of myocardial infarction but urges caution in this use of aspirin by the general population except when prescribed as an adjunct to risk factor management by smoking cessation and lowering of blood cholesterol and blood pressure. The striking eightfold reduction in expected cardiovascular deaths for both the control and the aspirin groups in the placebo-controlled, double-blinded American study suggested the importance of life-style in highly motivated, health-conscious physicians. Meta-analysis of many published trials of aspirin and other antiplatelet agents confirms the value of this intervention in the *secondary* prevention of vascular events among patients with a history of vascular events.

TICLOPIDINE

Ticlopidine reduces platelet aggregation by inhibiting the ADP pathway of platelets. Unlike aspirin, the drug has no effect on prostaglandin metabolism. Randomized clinical trials with ticlopidine report efficacy in the prevention of vascular events among patients with transient ischemic attacks, completed strokes, and unstable angina pectoris. Adverse effects include nausea, dyspepsia, and diarrhea in up to 20% of patients, hemorrhage in 5%, and leukopenia in 1%. The leukopenia is detected by regular monitoring of the white blood cell count during the first 3 months of treatment. The dosage of ticlopidine is 250 mg twice daily. It is particularly useful in patients who cannot tolerate aspirin. Doses of ticlopidine less than 500 mg/d may be efficacious with fewer adverse effects.

BETA-ADRENOCEPTOR-BLOCKING DRUGS

Many clinical trials have been performed with beta-blocking drugs for secondary prophylaxis of myocardial infarction or other cardiac events (eg, arrhythmia) following a first infarction. The Norwegian Multicenter Study of **timolol** was methodologically and statistically sound. It showed that use of timolol resulted in a highly significant reduction of total numbers of deaths (Figure 10–8), and the drug was approved by the FDA for use as a prophylactic agent following myocardial infarction. It is not certain whether these positive results reflect a direct effect on coagulation.

IV. CLINICAL PHARMACOLOGY OF DRUGS USED TO TREAT THROMBOSIS

The history of pharmacologic treatment of thromboembolism is one of broken promises resulting from the abuse of antithrombotic drugs. Drugs have been used and discarded before being properly evaluated, eg, oral anticoagulants in management of myocardial infarction and hip surgery. Use of prophylactic low-dose heparin during general surgery was undermined by overuse almost as soon as its efficacy had been rigorously established. The antiplatelet drugs were widely used before any proof of their efficacy was obtained.

VENOUS THROMBOSIS

Antithrombotic Management

A. Prevention: Primary prevention of venous thrombosis reduces the incidence of and mortality rate from pulmonary emboli. Heparin is used to prevent venous thrombosis. Intermittent administration of low-dose heparin subcutaneously provides effective prophylaxis. Oral anticoagulants are also effective, but the risk of bleeding and the necessity for laboratory monitoring of the prothrombin time limit their use for prophylaxis except in patients with prosthetic heart valves. Early ambulation postoperatively reduces venous stasis. Intermittent external pneumatic compression of the legs also is an effective form of postoperative prophylaxis. At the present time, enoxaparin (LMW heparin) is approved only for prophylaxis in patients undergoing hip replacement. Platelets have a lesser role in venous than in arterial disease; antiplatelet drugs are not consistently effective in prevention of venous disease.

B. Treatment of Established Disease: Established venous thrombosis is treated with maximal dosages of heparin and warfarin. Heparin is used for the first 7–10 days, with a 3- to 5-day overlap with warfarin. Therapy with warfarin is continued after hospital discharge for 6 weeks (first episode) to 6 months (recurrent episodes). Pulmonary embolism is treated the same way. Small thrombi confined to the calf veins are often managed without anticoagulants. The risk, expense, and inconvenience of unnecessary anticoagulant treatment far exceed those of venography, the definitive diagnostic test. Only a third of patients suspected of having deep venous thrombosis actually have the disease.

Deficiencies of proteins C or S are important diagnostic considerations in patients with recurrent thrombi who have a positive family history. Anti-thrombin III concentrate may be useful in deficient patients. Heparin resistance associated with antithrombin III deficiency can be overcome with this concentrate.

Pregnancy

Warfarin readily crosses the placenta. It can cause hemorrhage at any time during pregnancy, as well as developmental defects when administered during the first trimester. Therefore, venous thromboembolic disease in pregnant women should be treated with heparin, best administered by subcutaneous injection. Laboratory monitoring of the anticoagulant effect during pregnancy is mandatory.

Fibrinolytic Therapy

Early treatment with fibrinolytic drugs of a less than massive pulmonary embolus may improve survival and may preserve long-term pulmonary function. The standard course of fibrinolytic therapy should be followed by anticoagulant therapy with heparin and warfarin. Concomitant invasive procedures must be avoided, since bleeding may occur. Therapy is contraindicated after recent surgery or in patients with metastatic cancer, stroke, or underlying hemorrhagic disorders.

ARTERIAL THROMBOSIS

In patients with arterial thrombi, consumption of platelets is excessive. Thus, treatment with platelet-inhibiting drugs such as aspirin and ticlopidine is indicated in patients with transient ischemic attacks and strokes or unstable angina and acute myocardial infarction. In angina and infarction, these drugs are often used in conjunction with beta-blockers or calcium channel blockers and fibrinolytic drugs.

V. DRUGS USED IN BLEEDING DISORDERS

VITAMIN K

Vitamin K confers biologic activity upon prothrombin and factors VII, IX, and X by participating in their postribosomal modification. Severe hepatic failure results in loss of protein synthesis and a hemorrhagic diathesis that is unresponsive to vitamin K.

Vitamin K is a fat-soluble substance found primarily in leafy green vegetables. The dietary requirement is low, because the vitamin is additionally synthesized by bacteria that colonize the human intestine.

Two natural forms exist: vitamins K_1 and K_2. Vitamin K_1 (Figure 33–5) is found in food and is called phytonadione. Vitamin K_2 is found in human tissues, is synthesized by intestinal bacteria, and is called menaquinone.

Vitamins K_1 and K_2 require bile salts for absorption from the intestinal tract. Vitamin K_1 is available clinically in 5 mg tablets and 50 mg ampules. The effect is delayed for 6 hours but is complete by 24 hours when treating depression of prothrombin activity by excess warfarin or vitamin K deficiency. Intravenous administration of vitamin K_1 should be slow, because rapid infusion can produce dyspnea, chest and back pain, and even death. Vitamin K_1 is currently administered to all newborns to prevent the hemorrhagic disease of vitamin K deficiency, which is especially common in premature infants. The water-soluble salt of vitamin K_3 (menadione) should never be used in therapeutics. It is particularly ineffective in the treatment of warfarin overdosage. Vitamin K deficiency frequently occurs in hospitalized patients in intensive care units because of poor diet, parenteral nutrition, recent surgery, multiple antibiotic therapy, and uremia.

PLASMA FRACTIONS

Deficiencies in plasma coagulation factors can cause bleeding (Table 33–3). Spontaneous bleeding occurs when factor activity is less than 5% of normal. Factor VIII deficiency (classic hemophilia, or hemophilia A) and factor IX deficiency (Christmas disease, or hemophilia B) account for most of the heritable coagulation defects. Concentrated plasma fractions are available for the treatment of these deficiencies. However, the fear of viral hepatitis and of AIDS is tempering the use of these concentrates in patients with hemophilia. The best use of these therapeutic materials requires diagnostic specificity of the deficient factor and quantitation of its activity in plasma. There are many uncommon inherited and acquired disorders of platelet function. Recombinant factor VIII has been synthesized and has undergone successful clinical trial but has not yet been approved for clinical use. Its expense may overbalance the benefit of freedom from risk of transmission of viral disease.

1. FACTOR VIII

There are two preparations of concentrated human factor VIII. **Cryoprecipitate** is a plasma protein fraction and is obtainable from whole blood. It is used to treat deficiencies of factor VIII in patients with hemophilia and von Willebrand's disease and occasionally to provide fibrinogen. For infusion, the frozen cryoprecipitate unit is thawed and dissolved in a small volume of sterile citrate-saline solution and pooled

Table 33–3. Therapeutic products for the treatment of coagulation disorders.[1]

Factor	Deficiency State	Concentration (Percent) Relative to Normal Plasma Required for Hemostasis[2]	Half-Life (Days) of Infused Factor	Therapeutic Material
I	Afibrinogenemia, defibrination syndrome	40	4	Plasma fibrinogen, cryoprecipitate.
II	Prothrombin deficiency	40	3	Concentrate (factor IX-prothrombin complex).
V	Factor V deficiency	20	1	Fresh-frozen plasma.
VII	Factor VII deficiency	Unknown	$\frac{1}{4}$	Concentrate (some preparations of factor IX).
VIII	Hemophilia A (classic)	25–35	$\frac{1}{2}$	Plasma, cryoprecipitate, and other factor VIII concentrates.[3]
	von Willebrand's disease	30	Unknown	
IX	Hemophilia B (Christmas disease)	25	1	Plasma, factor IX–prothrombin complex.
X	Stuart-Prower defect	25	$1\frac{1}{2}$	Plasma, concentrate (some preparations of factor IX).
XI	PTA deficiency	Unknown	3	Fresh-frozen plasma.
XII	Hageman defect	Not required	Unknown	Treatment not needed.
XIII	Fibrin-stabilizing factor deficiency	2	6	Fresh-frozen plasma.
AT III	Antithrombin III	80	3	Concentrate (AT III-specific)

[1]Reproduced, with permission, from Biggs R (editor): *Human Blood Coagulation, Haemostasis, and Thrombosis,* 2nd ed. Blackwell, 1976.

[2]The immediate postinfusion level may need to be much higher and varies according to the degree of trauma.

[3]Highly purified preparations of factor VIII should not be used in the treatment of von Willebrand's disease without specific evidence of their efficacy.

with other units. Rh-negative women with potential for childbearing should receive only Rh-negative cryoprecipitate because of possible contamination of the product with Rh-positive blood cells. **Lyophilized factor VIII concentrates** are prepared from large pools of plasma. Cryoprecipitate prepared from individual donors is probably safer. Transmission of viral diseases such as hepatitis B and C and AIDS is reduced or eliminated by pasteurization and by extraction of plasma with solvents and detergents. Similarly, treatment of factor VIII concentrates with ultraviolet irradiation may reduce the danger of transmission of AIDS. Ultrapure factor VIII concentrates prepared by monoclonal antibody and recombinant DNA techniques are very expensive. Commercial freeze-dried concentrates may not suffice for treatment of patients with von Willebrand's disease, because the polymeric structure of factor VIII in the von Willebrand protein that supports platelet adhesion may be lost in the manufacturing process.

An uncomplicated hemorrhage into a joint should be treated with sufficient factor VIII replacement to maintain a level of at least 5% of the normal concentration for 24 hours. Soft tissue hematomas require a minimum of 10% activity for 7 days. Hematuria requires at least 10% activity for 3 days. Surgery and major trauma require a minimum of 30% activity for 10 days after an initial loading dose of 50 units/kg of body weight to achieve 100% activity of factor VIII (Table 33–3). Each unit per kilogram of factor VIII raises its activity in plasma 2%. Replacement should be administered every 12 hours.

Desmopressin acetate (arginine vasopressin) increases the factor VIII activity of patients with mild hemophilia A or von Willebrand's disease. It can be used in preparation for minor surgery such as tooth extraction without any requirement for infusion of clotting factor replacement. **Danazol**, an attenuated androgen that also elevates factor VIII activity, has been used experimentally with success in mild hemophiliacs.

Factor VIII concentrates and cryoprecipitate must not be used to treat deficiencies of vitamin K-dependent factors.

2. FACTOR IX

Freeze-dried concentrates of plasma containing prothrombin, factors IX and X, and varied amounts of factor VII (Proplex and Konÿne) are commercially available for treating deficiencies of these factors (Table 33–3). Each unit per kilogram of factor IX raises its activity in plasma 1.5%. Heparin is often added to inhibit coagulation factors activated by the manufacturing process. However, addition of heparin does not eliminate thromboembolic events. Nevertheless, patients managed with high-purity preparations of factor IX that were virally inactivated by the solvent-detergent method had fewer thrombotic episodes following surgery.

Some preparations of factor IX concentrate contain *activated* clotting factors, which has led to their use in treating patients with inhibitors or antibodies to factor VIII or IX. Two products are available expressly for this purpose: **Autoplex** (with factor VIII correctional activity) and **Feiba** (with factor VIII inhibitor bypassing activity). These products are not uniformly successful in arresting hemorrhage, and the inhibitor titers often rise after treatment with them.

3. FIBRINOGEN

Fibrinogen may be administered to patients as plasma, cryoprecipitate of factor VIII, or lyophilized concentrates of factor VIII. A single unit of cryoprecipitate contains 300 mg of fibrinogen. Lyophilized concentrates of factor VIII are rich in fibrinogen.

FIBRINOLYTIC INHIBITORS: AMINOCAPROIC ACID

Aminocaproic acid (EACA), which is chemically similar to the amino acid lysine, is a synthetic inhibitor of fibrinolysis. It competitively inhibits plasminogen activation (Figure 33–3). It is rapidly absorbed orally and is cleared from the body by the kidney. The usual oral dose of EACA is 6 g 4 times a day. When the drug is administered intravenously, a 5 g loading dose should be infused over 30 minutes to avoid hypotension. **Tranexamic acid** is an analogue of aminocaproic acid and has the same properties. It is administered orally with a 15 mg/kg loading dose followed by 30 mg/kg every 6 hours.

Clinical uses of aminocaproic acid are as adjunctive therapy in hemophilia, as therapy for bleeding from fibrinolytic therapy, and as prophylaxis for rebleeding from intracranial aneurysms. Treatment success has also been reported in patients with postsurgical gastrointestinal bleeding and postprostatectomy bleeding and bladder hemorrhage secondary to radiation- and drug-induced cystitis. Adverse effects of the drug include intravascular thrombosis from inhibition of plasminogen activator, hypotension, myopathy, abdominal discomfort, diarrhea, and nasal stuffiness.

PREPARATIONS AVAILABLE

Aminocaproic acid (generic, Amicar)
Oral: 500 mg tablets; 250 mg/mL syrup
Parenteral: 250 mg/mL for IV injection

Alteplase recombinant [t-PA] (Activase)
Parenteral: 20, 50 mg lyophilized powders to reconstitute for IV injection

Anistreplase (Eminase)
Parenteral: 30 units lyophilized powder to reconstitute for IV injection

Antihemophilic factor [Factor VIII, AHF] (Hemofil M, Koāte-HS, Koāte-HT, Monoclate)
Parenteral: in vials

Anti-inhibitor coagulant complex (Autoplex T, Feiba VH Immuno)
Parenteral: in vials

Antithrombin III (ATnativ)
500 IU powder to reconstitute for IV injection

Dipyridamole (Persantine)
Oral: 25, 50, 75 mg tablets

Enoxaparin (Low-molecular-weight heparin, Lovenox)
Parenteral: 30 mg/0.3 mL for SC injection only

Factor IX complex, human (Konȳne-HT, Profilnine Heat-Treated, Proplex T, Proplex SX-T)
Parenteral: in vials

Heparin sodium (generic, Liquaemin)
Parenteral: 1000, 5000, 10,000, 20,000, 40,000 units/mL for injection

Heparin calcium (Calciparine)
Parenteral: 5000 units/unit dose

Phytonadione [K_1] (Mephyton, AquaMephyton, Konakion)
Oral: 5 mg tablets
Parenteral: 2, 10 mg/mL aqueous colloidal solution or suspension for injection

Protamine (generic)
Parenteral: 10 mg/mL for injection

Streptokinase (Kabikinase, Streptase)
Parenteral: 250,000, 600,000, 750,000, 1,500,000 IU per vial powders to reconstitute for injection

Ticlopidine (Ticlid)
Oral: 250 mg tablets

Tranexamic acid (Cyklokapron)
Oral: 500 mg tablets
Parenteral: 100 mg/mL for injection

Urokinase (Abbokinase)
Parenteral: 250,000 IU per vial; powder to reconstitute for 5000 IU/mL for injection

Warfarin (generic, Coumadin)
Oral: 2, 2.5, 5, 7.5, 10 mg tablets
Parenteral: 50 mg per vial with 2 mL ampule diluent for injection

REFERENCES

Blood Coagulation

Furie B, Furie BC: Molecular and cellular biology of blood coagulation. N Engl J Med 1992;326:800.

Nemerson Y: The tissue factor pathway of blood coagulation. Semin Hematol 1992;29:170.

Rodgers GM, Chandler WL: Laboratory and clinical aspects of inherited thrombotic disorders. Am J Hematol 1992;41:113.

Anticoagulant Drugs

Eckman MH, Levine HJ, Pauker SG: Effect of laboratory variation in the prothrombin-time ratio on the results of oral anticoagulant therapy. N Engl J Med 1993; 329:696.

Hull RD, Pineo GF: Treatment of venous thromboembolism with low molecular weight heparins. Hematol Oncol Clin North Am 1992;6:1095.

Loeliger EA: Therapeutic target values in oral anticoagulation: Justification of Dutch policy and a warning against the so-called moderate-intensity regimens. Ann Hematol 1992;64:60.

O'Reilly RA et al: Mechanism of the stereoselective interaction between miconazole and racemic warfarin in human subjects. Clin Pharmacol Ther 1992;51:656.

Poller L: Therapeutic ranges for oral anticoagulation in different thromboembolic disorders. Ann Hematol 1992;64:52.

Singer DE: Randomized trials of warfarin for atrial fibrillation. N Engl J Med 1992;327:1451.

Stringer KA, Lindenfeld J: Hirudins: Antithrombin anticoagulants. Ann Pharmacother 1992;26:1535.

Thromboembolic Risk Factors (THRIFT) Consensus Group: Risk and prophylaxis for venous thromboembolism in hospital patients. Br Med J 1992;305:567.

Fibrinolytic Drugs

Anderson HV, Willerson JT: Thrombolysis in acute myocardial infarction. N Engl J Med 1993;329:703.

Cobbe SM: ISIS-3: The last word on thrombolytics? Streptokinase and aspirin sweep the field. Br Med J 1992;304:1454.

Eisenberg PR: Current concepts in coronary thrombolysis. Hematol Oncol Clin North Am 1992;6:1161.

ISIS-3 (Third International Study of Infarct Survival): A randomized comparison of streptokinase vs tissue plasminogen activator vs anistreplase and of aspirin plus heparin vs aspirin alone among 41,299 cases of suspected acute myocardial infarction. Lancet 1992; 339:753.

Kase CS et al: Intracranial hemorrhage after coronary

thrombolysis with tissue plasminogen activator. Am J Med 1992;92:384.

Topol E, for the GUSTO Investigators: An international randomized trial comparing four thrombolytic strategies for acute myocardial infarction. N Engl J Med 1993;329:673.

Antithrombotic Drugs

Antman EM et al: Comparison of results of meta-analysis of randomized control trials and recommendations of clinical experts: Treatments for myocardial infarction. JAMA 1992;268:240.

Dalen JE, Hirsh J: Third ACCP consensus conference on antithrombotic therapy. Chest 1992(Supp);102:303S.

Fuster V et al: American Heart Association medical/scientific statement: Aspirin as a therapeutic agent in cardiovascular disease. Circulation 1993;87:659.

Goodnight SH: Antiplatelet therapy. (2 parts) West J Med 1993;158:385, 506.

Haynes RB et al: Critical appraisal of ticlopidine, a new antiplatelet agent. Arch Intern Med 1992;152:1376.

Manson JE et al: Primary prevention of myocardial infarction. N Engl J Med 1992;326:1406.

Sandercock PAG et al: Antithrombotic therapy in acute ischemic stroke: An overview of the completed randomized trials. J Neurol Neurosurg Psychiatry 1993;56:17.

Bleeding Disorders

Julius C, Westphal RG: Safety of blood components and derivatives. Hematol Oncol Clin North Am 1992;6:1057.

Lusher JM et al: Recombinant factor VIII for the treatment of previously untreated patients with hemophilia A: Safety, efficacy, and development of inhibitors. N Engl J Med 1993;328:453.

Rose EH, Aledort LM: Nasal spray desmopressin (DDAVP) for mild hemophilia A and von Willebrand disease. Ann Intern Med 1991;114:563.

Singh I, Laungani GB: Intravesical epsilon aminocaproic acid in management of intractable bladder hemorrhage. J Urol 1992;40:227.

34

Agents Used in Hyperlipidemia

Mary J. Malloy, MD, & John P. Kane, MD, PhD

Virtually all the lipids of human plasma are transported as complexes with proteins. Except for fatty acids, which are bound chiefly to albumin, the lipids are carried in special macromolecular complexes termed **lipoproteins.** A number of metabolic disorders that involve elevations in plasma lipoprotein concentrations are thus termed **hyperlipoproteinemias.** The term **hyperlipemia** is restricted to conditions that involve increased levels of triglycerides in plasma. The **hyperlipidemias** include both groups of conditions.

The two major clinical sequelae of the hyperlipoproteinemias are acute pancreatitis and atherosclerosis. Acute pancreatitis occurs in patients with marked hyperlipemia. In such persons, control of triglyceride levels can prevent recurrent attacks of this life-threatening disease.

Atherosclerosis is the leading cause of death in the USA and other Western countries. Certain plasma lipoproteins are linked to accelerated atherogenesis. The lipoproteins that contain **apolipoprotein (Apo) B-100** have been identified as the vehicles in which cholesterol is transported into the artery wall. These atherogenic lipoproteins are the **low-density (LDL), intermediate-density (IDL), very low density (VLDL),** and **Lp(a) lipoproteins. Cholesteryl esters,** which are found in foam cells in the atheroma, also appear in the extracellular matrix and induce collagen production by fibroblasts. Macrophages and smooth muscle cells play a key role in atherogenesis. Oxidation of lipoproteins leads to their uptake by special receptors ("scavenger receptors") on these cells, forming foam cells in which cholesteryl esters accumulate. Other factors also contribute to formation of the atheroma. These include hypertension; low levels of **high-density lipoproteins (HDL),** which appear to be involved in removal of cholesterol from the atheroma; smoking and diabetes.

Atherosclerotic disease of both coronary and peripheral arteries appears to be a dynamic process. Recent trials in humans have demonstrated by angiographic methods that net regression of coronary lesions was associated with lipid-lowering therapy. The incidence of new coronary events was also de-

creased by treatment. Therefore, the timely diagnosis and treatment of hyperlipidemia can be expected to decrease morbidity and mortality due to coronary disease.

Many of the hyperlipidemic states are associated with the development of xanthomas. These lesions, which are produced by deposition of lipid in tendons or skin, may be painful or cosmetically unacceptable to the patient. Because xanthomas regress with lipid-lowering therapy, this provides another indication for treatment.

An understanding of the biology of the lipoproteins and the pathophysiology of the various hyperlipidemic states is essential to the rational choice of treatment regimens.

ACRONYMS USED IN THIS CHAPTER

ACAT	Acyl-CoA:cholesterol acyl-transferase
Apo	Apolipoprotein
CETP	Cholesteryl ester transfer protein
HDL	High-density lipoprotein
HMG-CoA	3-Hydroxy-3-methylglutaryl-coenzyme A
IDL	Intermediate-density lipoprotein
LCAT	Lecithin:cholesterol acyl-transferase
LDL	Low-density lipoprotein
Lp(a)	Lipoprotein(a)
LPL	Lipoprotein lipase
VLDL	Very low density lipoprotein

PATHOPHYSIOLOGY OF HYPERLIPOPROTEINEMIA

NORMAL LIPOPROTEIN METABOLISM

Structure

The major lipoproteins of plasma are spherical particles with hydrophobic core regions containing cholesteryl esters and triglycerides. A monolayer of unesterified cholesterol and phospholipids surrounds the core. Specific proteins (apolipoproteins) are located on the surface. Certain lipoproteins contain very high molecular weight apolipoproteins (B proteins) that do not migrate from one particle to another, as do smaller apolipoproteins. There are two primary forms of ApoB: B-48, which is formed in the intestine and found in chylomicrons and their remnants; and B-100, which is synthesized in the liver and found in VLDL, VLDL remnants (intermediate-density lipoproteins, or IDL), LDL (which are formed from VLDL), and the Lp(a) lipoproteins.

Smaller apolipoproteins distribute variably among the lipoproteins. ApoA-I is a cofactor for lecithin: cholesterol acyltransferase (LCAT). ApoC-II is a required cofactor for lipoprotein lipase. Several isoforms of ApoE, based on single amino acid substitutions, are recognized. Isoforms of this protein that are recognized by hepatic receptors are required for uptake of lipoprotein remnants by the liver.

The characteristics of various lipoprotein complexes are shown in Table 34–1.

Synthesis & Catabolism

A. Chylomicrons: Chylomicrons, the largest of the lipoproteins, are formed in the intestine and carry triglycerides of dietary origin. Some cholesterol esterified by the acyl-CoA:cholesterol acyltransferase (ACAT) system also appears in the chylomi-

cron core. Phospholipids and free cholesterol—together with newly synthesized ApoB-48, A-I, A-II, and other proteins—form the surface monolayer. The nascent chylomicron enters the extracellular lymph space and travels via the intestinal lymphatics and thoracic duct to the bloodstream.

Triglycerides are removed from the chylomicrons in extrahepatic tissues through a pathway shared with VLDL that involves hydrolysis by the lipoprotein lipase (LPL) system. Heparin and ApoC-II are cofactors for this reaction. A progressive decrease in particle diameter occurs as triglycerides in the core are depleted. Surface lipids, ApoA-I, ApoA-II, and ApoC are transferred to HDL. The resultant chylomicron "remnants" are taken up by receptor-mediated endocytosis into hepatocytes. The cholesteryl esters are hydrolyzed in lysosomes, and cholesterol is then excreted in bile, oxidized and excreted as bile acids, or secreted into plasma in lipoproteins.

B. Very Low Density Lipoproteins (VLDL): VLDL are secreted by liver and carry triglycerides synthesized there (Figure 34–1). VLDL contain ApoB-100 and some ApoC. More ApoC is acquired from HDL in plasma. After leaving the liver, the triglycerides are hydrolyzed by lipoprotein lipase, yielding free fatty acids for storage in adipose tissue and for oxidation in tissues such as cardiac and skeletal muscle. The resulting depletion of triglycerides produces smaller particles or remnants termed intermediate-density lipoproteins (IDL). Some of the IDL particles are endocytosed directly by the liver. The remainder are converted to LDL by further removal of triglycerides. This process explains the clinical phenomenon of the "beta shift," the increase of LDL (beta-lipoprotein) in serum as a hypertriglyceridemic state subsides. Increased levels of LDL in plasma can result from increased secretion of its precursor VLDL as well as from decreased LDL catabolism.

C. Low-Density Lipoproteins (LDL): A major pathway by which LDL are catabolized in hepatocytes and most other nucleated cells involves high-affinity receptor-mediated endocytosis. Cholesteryl esters from the LDL core are then hydrolyzed, yield-

Table 34–1. Major lipoproteins of human serum.

	Electrophoretic Mobility in Agarose Gel	Density Interval (g/cm^3)	Core Lipids	Diameter (nm)	Apolipoproteins in Order of Quantitative Importance
High-density (HDL)	Alpha	1.063–1.21	Cholesteryl esters	7.5–10.5	A-I, A-II, C, E, D
Low-density (LDL)	Beta	1.019–1.063	Cholesteryl esters	21–22	B-100
Intermediate-density (IDL)	Beta	1.006–1.019	Cholesteryl esters, triglycerides	25–30	B-100, E, C
Very low density (VLDL)	Prebeta, some "slow prebeta"	<1.006	Triglycerides, some cholesteryl esters	30–100	C species, B-100, E
Chylomicrons	Remain at origin	<1.006	Triglycerides, some cholesteryl esters	80–500	B-48, C, E, A-I, A-II
Lp(a) lipoproteins	Prebeta	1.04–1.08	Cholesteryl esters	21–30	B-100, Lp(a)

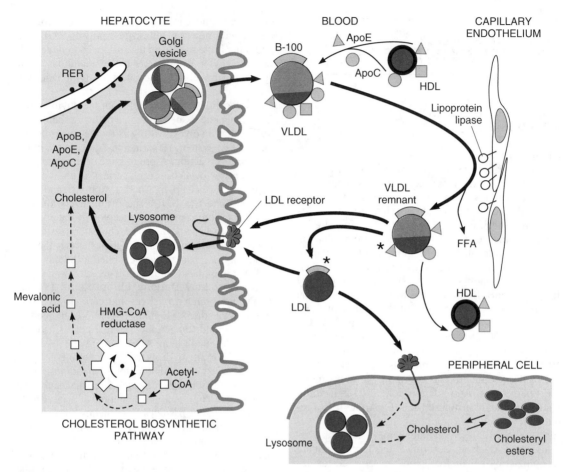

Figure 34–1. Metabolism of lipoproteins of hepatic origin. The heavy arrows show the primary pathways. Nascent VLDL are secreted via the Golgi apparatus. They acquire additional C lipoproteins and ApoE from HDL. VLDL are converted to VLDL remnants (IDL) by lipolysis via lipoprotein lipase in the vessels of peripheral tissues. In the process, C apolipoproteins and a portion of the ApoE are given back to HDL. Some of the VLDL remnants are converted to LDL by further loss of triglycerides and loss of ApoE. A major pathway for LDL degradation involves the endocytosis of LDL by LDL receptors in the liver and the peripheral tissues, for which ApoB-100 is the ligand. (Dark color denotes cholesteryl esters; light color, triglycerides; the asterisk denotes a functional ligand for LDL receptors; triangles indicate apolipoprotein E; circles and squares represent C apolipoproteins.) (Modified and redrawn, with permission, from Kane J, Malloy M: Disorders of lipoproteins. In: *The Molecular and Genetic Basis of Neurological Disease*. Rosenberg RN et al (editors). Butterworth-Heinemann, 1993.

ing free cholesterol for the synthesis of cell membranes. Cells also obtain cholesterol by de novo synthesis via a pathway involving the formation of mevalonic acid by HMG-CoA reductase. Production of this enzyme and of LDL receptors is regulated at the transcriptional level by the content of cholesterol in the cell.

D. High-Density Lipoproteins (HDL): The apolipoproteins of HDL are secreted by liver and intestine. Much of the lipid in HDL comes from the surface monolayers of chylomicrons and VLDL during lipolysis. HDL also acquires cholesterol from peripheral tissues in a pathway that protects the cholesterol retrieval homeostasis of cells. In this process, free

cholesterol absorbed from cell membranes is acquired by a small particle termed prebeta HDL. The cholesterol is then esterified by lecithin:cholesterol acyltransferase (LCAT), leading to the formation of larger HDL species. The cholesteryl esters are transferred to VLDL, IDL, LDL, and chylomicron remnants with the aid of cholesteryl ester transfer protein (CETP). Much of the cholesteryl ester thus transferred is ultimately delivered to the liver by endocytosis of the acceptor lipoproteins (Figure 34–1).

THE HYPERLIPOPROTEINEMIC STATES

The presence of hyperlipoproteinemia is established by measuring the content of lipids in serum after an overnight fast. The risk of atherosclerotic heart disease increases with the LDL cholesterol level and is modified by other risk factors (Table 34–2). Ideally, triglyceride levels should be below 150 mg/dL. Differentiation requires identification of the species of lipoproteins that account for the observed increases (Table 34–3). Diagnosis of a specific primary lipoprotein disorder usually necessitates gathering further clinical and genetic data as well as ruling out disorders that can cause secondary hyperlipidemia (Table 34–4). The various patterns of abnormal lipoprotein distribution are described in the next section. Drugs mentioned for use in these conditions are described in the section on basic and clinical pharmacology.

THE PRIMARY HYPERTRIGLYCERIDEMIAS

Although epidemiologic studies have shown only a modest relationship between hypertriglyceridemia and coronary heart disease, atherosclerosis appears to be strongly linked to hypertriglyceridemia in certain kindreds. Therefore, patients in these families should receive drug treatment, whereas such treatment is probably not necessary for other patients unless their levels of triglycerides exceed about 500 mg/dL.

Primary Chylomicronemia

Chylomicrons are not normally present in the serum of individuals who have fasted. The autosomal recessive traits of lipoprotein lipase deficiency and lipoprotein lipase cofactor deficiency are usually associated with severe lipemia (2000–25,000 mg/dL triglycerides when the patient is consuming a typical American diet). These disorders may not be diagnosed until an attack of acute pancreatitis occurs. Patients may have eruptive xanthomas, hepatosplenomegaly, hypersplenism, and lipid-laden foam cells in bone marrow, liver, and spleen. The lipemia is aggravated by estrogens, since they stimulate VLDL pro-

Table 34–2. National Cholesterol Education Program: Adult Treatment Guidelines (1993).

	Total Cholesterol	LDL Cholesterol
Desirable	<200	<130
Borderline-high[1]	200–239	130–159
High	≥240	≥160

[1]Consider as high if coronary heart disease or more than 2 risk factors are present. A level of HDL cholesterol below 35 mg/dl is considered a major risk factor. The LDL cholesterol goal in patients with coronary artery disease is 100 mg/dl or less.

Table 34–3. The primary hyperlipoproteinemias and their drug treatment.

Disorder	Manifestations	Single Drug[1]	Drug Combination
Primary chylomicronemia (familial lipoprotein lipase or cofactor deficiency)	Chylomicrons, VLDL increased	Dietary management	
Familial hypertriglyceridemia Severe	VLDL, chylomicrons increased	Niacin, gemfibrozil	Niacin plus gemfibrozil
Moderate	VLDL increased; chylomicrons may be increased	Niacin, gemfibrozil	
Familial combined hyperlipoproteinemia	VLDL increased	Niacin, gemfibrozil	
	LDL increased	Niacin, reductase inhibitor, resin	Niacin plus resin or reductase inhibitor
	VLDL, LDL increased	Niacin, reductase inhibitor	Niacin plus resin or reductase inhibitor
Familial dysbetalipoproteinemia	VLDL remnants, chylomicron remnants increased	Niacin, gemfibrozil	Gemfibrozil plus niacin or niacin plus reductase inhibitor
Familial hypercholesterolemia Heterozygous	LDL increased	Resin, reductase inhibitor, niacin	Two or 3 of the individual drugs
Homozygous	LDL increased	Probucol, niacin	Resin plus niacin plus reductase inhibitor; probucol plus agents above
Lp(a) hyperlipoproteinemia	Lp(a) increased	Niacin	Niacin plus reductase inhibitor
Unclassified hypercholesterolemia	Resin, niacin, reductase, inhibitorl		

[1]Single-drug therapy should be evaluated before drug combinations are used.

Table 34–4. Secondary causes of hyperlipoproteinemia.

Hypertriglyceridemia	Hypercholesterolemia
Diabetes mellitus	Hypothyroidism
Alcohol ingestion	Early nephrosis
Severe nephrosis	Resolving lipemia
Estrogens	Immunoglobulin-lipoprotein
Uremia	complex disorders
Corticosteroid excess	Anorexia nervosa
Hypothyroidism	Cholestasis
Glycogen storage disease	Hypopituitarism
Hypopituitarism	Corticosteroid excess
Acromegaly	
Immunoglobulin-lipoprotein	
complex disorders	

duction in the liver, and pregnancy may cause marked increases in triglyceride levels despite strict dietary control. Although these patients have a predominant chylomicronemia, they may also have moderately elevated VLDL, presenting with a pattern of mixed lipemia (fasting chylomicronemia and elevated VLDL). Lipoprotein lipase deficiency is diagnosed by in vitro assay of lipolytic activity in plasma after intravenous injection of heparin; cofactor deficiency is diagnosed by isoelectric focusing of the VLDL proteins. A presumptive diagnosis of these disorders is made by demonstrating a pronounced decrease in levels of plasma triglycerides a few days after sharp restriction of oral fat intake. Marked restriction of the total fat content in the diet provides effective long-term treatment. No drug treatment is indicated.

Familial Hypertriglyceridemia

A. Severe (Usually Mixed Lipemia): A pattern of mixed lipemia usually results from impaired removal of triglyceride-rich lipoproteins, though factors that increase VLDL production aggravate the lipemia because VLDL and chylomicrons are competing substrates for lipoprotein lipase. The primary mixed lipemias probably represent a variety of modes of inheritance. Most patients have the centripetal pattern of obesity with impaired effectiveness of insulin. In addition to obesity, other factors that lead to increased rate of secretion of VLDL also worsen the lipemia. Eruptive xanthomas, lipemia retinalis, epigastric pain, and overt pancreatitis are variably present, depending on the severity of the lipemia. Treatment is primarily dietary, with restriction of total fat, avoidance of alcohol, and weight reduction to ideal levels. Some patients may require treatment with gemfibrozil or niacin.

B. Moderate (Endogenous Lipemia): Primary increases of VLDL levels probably reflect a number of genetic determinants and are worsened by factors that increase the rate of VLDL secretion from liver, ie, hypertrophic obesity, alcohol ingestion, diabetes, and exogenous estrogens. A major indication for treatment is the presence of atherosclerosis in the patient or the patient's family. Treatment includes

weight reduction to ideal levels, restriction of all types of dietary fat, and avoidance of alcohol. Gemfibrozil or niacin usually produces further reduction in triglyceride levels if dietary measures do not reduce them below 500 mg/dL.

Familial Combined Hyperlipoproteinemia

In kindreds with this disorder, individuals may have elevated levels of VLDL, LDL, or both, and the pattern may change with time. Factors that increase levels of triglycerides in serum in other disorders do so in this one as well. Elevations of serum cholesterol and triglycerides are generally moderate, and xanthomas are usually absent. However, drug treatment is warranted because the risk of coronary atherosclerosis is increased, and diet alone usually does not normalize lipid levels. Patients with elevated VLDL usually respond to niacin.

Familial Dysbetalipoproteinemia

In familial dysbetalipoproteinemia, remnants of chylomicrons and VLDL accumulate. Levels of LDL are usually decreased. Because the remnants are rich in cholesteryl esters, the level of serum cholesterol may be as high as that of triglycerides. Diagnosis is confirmed by the absence of the E_3 and E_4 isoforms of ApoE. Patients often develop tuberous or tuberoeruptive xanthomas or characteristic planar xanthomas of the palmar creases. Patients tend to be obese, and some have impaired glucose tolerance. These factors, together with hypothyroidism, aggravate the lipemia. Coronary and peripheral atherosclerosis occur with increased frequency. A weight reduction diet, together with decreased cholesterol and alcohol consumption, often is sufficient treatment. Gemfibrozil or niacin is needed in some cases. Frequently, low doses are sufficient.

THE PRIMARY HYPERCHOLESTEROLEMIAS

Familial Hypercholesterolemia

This disorder is transmitted as an autosomal dominant trait. Although levels of LDL tend to increase throughout childhood, the diagnosis can often be made on the basis of elevated umbilical cord blood cholesterol. In most heterozygous adults, serum cholesterol levels commonly range from about 280 to 500 mg/dL. Triglyceride levels are usually normal, tendinous xanthomatosis is often present, and arcus corneae and xanthelasma may appear in the third decade. Coronary atherosclerosis tends to occur prematurely. Homozygous familial hypercholesterolemia, which can lead to coronary disease in childhood, is characterized by very high levels of cholesterol in serum (often exceeding 1000 mg/dL) and early tuberous and tendinous xanthomatosis. These patients may also develop elevated plaque-like xanthomas of the digital webs, buttocks, and extremities.

Defects of high-affinity receptors for LDL underlie this disorder. Heterozygotes have about half the usual number, and some individuals have combined heterozygosity for alleles producing nonfunctional and kinetically impaired receptors. Levels of LDL in compliant heterozygous patients can be normalized with combined drug regimens (Figure 34–2).

Individuals whose receptors retain even minimal function may partially respond to resins or reductase inhibitors. Niacin or probucol may benefit patients with no receptor function.

Familial Ligand-Defective Apolipoprotein B

Defects in the ligand domain of ApoB-100 (the region that binds to the LDL receptor) impair the endocytosis of LDL, leading to hypercholesterolemia of moderate severity. Tendon xanthomas may occur. It is anticipated that LDL levels will respond to niacin. Response to HMG-CoA reductase inhibitors is variable.

Familial Combined Hyperlipoproteinemia

As described above, some persons in kindreds with this disorder have only an elevation in LDL levels. Levels of serum cholesterol usually are less than 350

mg/dL. Premature onset of coronary disease is common. Dietary and drug treatment, usually with niacin or a reductase inhibitor, is indicated. It is frequently necessary to add niacin to normalize LDL levels or to lower triglycerides if treatment is initiated with a resin.

Lp(a) Hyperlipoproteinemia

This familial disorder, which is associated with increased atherogenesis, appears to be determined in part by genes that dictate increased production of the Lp(a) lipoprotein. Defects that inhibit the removal of LDL seem to augment plasma levels of Lp(a). Preliminary studies indicate that niacin may reduce levels of Lp(a) in some patients.

Unclassified Hypercholesterolemia

Other poorly defined types of hypercholesterolemia occur that are often familial but less severe than the disorders described above. Individuals in some kindreds who have elevated LDL levels have strikingly favorable responses to dietary management.

HDL DEFICIENCY

Certain rare genetic disorders are associated with extremely low levels of HDL in serum. These include Tangier disease and disorders of LCAT. Familial hypoalphalipoproteinemia is a more common disorder of HDL in which levels of HDL cholesterol are usually below 35 mg/dL, with apparent codominant transmission. These patients tend to have premature coronary atherosclerosis, and the low HDL levels may be the only identified risk factor. Treatment currently consists only of special attention to avoidance of other risk factors for coronary disease. Niacin increases HDL cholesterol levels in many of these patients.

In the presence of hypertriglyceridemia, HDL cholesterol levels are low because of exchange of cholesteryl esters from HDL into triglyceride-rich lipoproteins. This may contribute to the atherogenic effect of hypertriglyceridemia. In most patients, treatment of the hypertriglyceridemia will result in normalization of HDL cholesterol levels.

SECONDARY HYPERLIPOPROTEINEMIA

Before primary hyperlipoproteinemia can be diagnosed, secondary causes of the specific phenotype must be considered. The more common conditions that may be associated with hyperlipoproteinemia are summarized in Table 34–4. The lipoprotein abnormality usually resolves if the underlying disorder can be treated successfully.

Certain persons, often with a preexisting mild lipemia, develop severe hypertriglyceridemia when

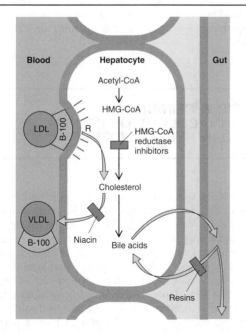

Figure 34–2. Sites of action of HMG-CoA reductase inhibitors, niacin, and resins used in treating hyperlipidemias. LDL receptors *(R)* are increased by treatment with resins and HMG-CoA reductase inhibitors.

given even small doses of estrogens, such as those in oral contraceptives. This effect is smaller when very low doses of estrogen are combined with a progestational agent. If estrogen therapy is clinically necessary, transdermal administration would be expected to have somewhat less hypertriglyceridemic effect by avoiding first pass extraction by the liver.

Treatment of the hyperlipidemia associated with chronic nephrotic syndrome is indicated, since coronary vascular disease is prevalent in these patients. Diet has little effect. Gemfibrozil must be used cautiously because it may precipitate myopathy in patients with hypoalbuminemia. Currently, the drugs of choice are bile acid-binding resins combined with niacin. Reductase inhibitors may also be useful. Tryptophan supplementation ameliorates hypertriglyceridemia in some nephrotic patients who may be deficient in this amino acid.

The hyperlipidemia associated with cholestasis involves abnormal lipoproteins, including LP-X, vesicular particles rich in unesterified cholesterol and phospholipid; and LP-Y, which contains triglycerides and carries ApoB. Neuropathy, caused by xanthomatous involvement of nerves, is an indication for treatment of this hyperlipidemia. Although plasmapheresis is most effective, bile acid-binding resins may be of some value. Gemfibrozil is contraindicated, since it can cause an increase in serum cholesterol in these patients.

DIETARY MANAGEMENT OF HYPERLIPOPROTEINEMIA

When the decision is made to treat hyperlipoproteinemia, dietary measures are always initiated first and may obviate the need for drugs. Exceptions are patients with familial hypercholesterolemia or familial combined hyperlipidemia in whom diet and drug therapy should be started simultaneously. Cholesterol and saturated fats are the principal dietary factors that influence lipoprotein levels in plasma. Dietary cholesterol and saturated fats increase the concentration of LDL independently.

Lipoprotein levels are also affected, but to a lesser extent, by other dietary factors. Transient increases in VLDL occur when carbohydrate intake is acutely increased. Sucrose and other simple sugars may raise VLDL levels in an occasional hypertriglyceridemic patient. Some forms of dietary fiber such as oat or rice bran may reduce LDL levels modestly. Alcohol can cause significant hypertriglyceridemia by increasing hepatic secretion of VLDL. Synthesis and secretion of VLDL are increased by excess caloric intake. Caloric restriction, especially in obese subjects, reduces

VLDL triglycerides and may also reduce levels of LDL somewhat. While the patient is losing weight, LDL and VLDL levels may be much lower than those that can be maintained during neutral caloric balance. Therefore, the conclusion that diet alone suffices for management can only be made after the patient's weight has stabilized for at least 1 month.

Most patients with hyperlipidemia can be managed appropriately with a diet that is restricted in cholesterol and saturated fat and provides calories to achieve and maintain ideal body weight. Total fat calories should be 20–25%, with saturated fats less than 8% of total calories and cholesterol less than 200 mg/d. Reductions in serum cholesterol range from 10% to 20% on this regimen. Increases in complex carbohydrates and fiber are recommended, and monounsaturated fats should predominate within the fat allowance. Weight reduction and caloric restriction are especially important for patients with elevated VLDL and IDL. Patients with hypertriglyceridemia should avoid alcohol.

The effect of dietary fats in patients with hypertriglyceridemia is highly dependent upon the disposition of double bonds in the fatty acid carbon chain. Omega-3 fatty acids found in fish oils can induce profound lowering of triglycerides in some patients with endogenous or mixed lipemia. In contrast, the omega-6 fatty acids present in vegetable oils may cause levels of triglycerides to rise in these patients.

Patients with primary chylomicronemia and some individuals with mixed lipemia must consume a diet severely restricted in total fat: 10–15 g/d, of which 5 g should be vegetable oils rich in essential fatty acids. Supplementation of fat-soluble vitamins should be given.

BASIC & CLINICAL PHARMACOLOGY OF DRUGS USED IN HYPERLIPIDEMIA

Decisions to use drug therapy for hyperlipidemia must be based on the specific metabolic defect and its potential for causing atherosclerosis or pancreatitis. Suggested drug treatments for the principal lipoprotein disorders are presented in Table 34–3. Diet is a necessary adjunct to drug therapy and should be continued for achievement of the full potential of the drug regimen. Drug treatment of hyperlipidemia should be avoided in women who are likely to become pregnant or who are lactating. Children with heterozygous familial hypercholesterolemia may be treated with a bile acid-binding resin, usually after 7 or 8 years of age, when myelination of the central nervous system is essentially complete. The decision to treat an individual child should be based on the level of plasma LDL, the family history, and the child's age.

NIACIN
(Nicotinic Acid)

Niacin (but not niacinamide) decreases VLDL and LDL levels in the plasma of patients with a variety of hyperlipidemias.

Chemistry & Pharmacokinetics

Niacin is a water-soluble vitamin. It is converted in the body to the amide, which is incorporated into niacinamide adenine dinucleotide (NAD). It is excreted unmodified in the urine and as niacinamide, N-methyl-2-pyridone-3-carboxamide, N-methyl-2-pyridone-5-carboxamide, and other less abundant metabolites.

Mechanism of Action

The primary mechanism of action of niacin probably involves inhibition of VLDL secretion, in turn decreasing production of LDL (Figure 34–2). Decreased incorporation of amino acids into VLDL apolipoproteins has been demonstrated. Increased clearance of VLDL via the lipoprotein lipase pathway contributes to the triglyceride-lowering effect of niacin. The drug has no effect on bile acid production. Excretion of neutral sterols in the stool is increased acutely as cholesterol is mobilized from tissue pools. A new steady state is then reached during chronic administration of the drug. Cholesterogenesis is inhibited, an effect that persists when bile acid-binding resins are given. Decreased synthesis of cholesterol in liver can increase hepatic uptake of LDL in support of increased bile acid synthesis induced by the resin. The catabolic rate for HDL is decreased, with an associated increase in the HDL_2 subfraction and high levels of HDL cholesterol and ApoA-I in plasma. The processes of atherogenesis or thrombosis may be influenced by the substantial reduction of circulating fibrinogen levels produced by niacin, and levels of tissue plasminogen activator appear to increase. Niacin is a potent inhibitor of the intracellular lipase system of adipose tissue, possibly reducing VLDL production by decreasing the flux of free fatty acids to liver. Sustained inhibition of lipolysis has not been established, however.

Therapeutic Uses & Dosage

In combination with a bile acid-binding resin, niacin has been found to normalize levels of LDL in most patients with heterozygous familial hypercholesterolemia. This drug combination is also indicated in some cases of nephrosis. In severe mixed lipemia that is incompletely responsive to dietary measures, niacin often produces marked reduction of triglyceride levels in plasma. It is also useful in patients with combined hyperlipoproteinemia and in those with familial dysbetalipoproteinemia. It can be used effectively alone or in combination with reductase inhibitors or neomycin to treat hypercholesterolemia. Niacin is clearly the most effective agent in increasing levels of HDL cholesterol.

For combined drug treatment of heterozygous familial hypercholesterolemia, most patients require 2–6.5 g of niacin daily orally; more than this should not be given. For other types of hypercholesterolemia and for hypertriglyceridemia, 1.5–3.5 g daily orally is often sufficient. The drug should be given in divided doses with meals, starting with 100 mg 2 or 3 times daily and increasing gradually.

Toxicity

Most persons experience a harmless cutaneous vasodilation and an uncomfortable sensation of warmth after each dose when the drug is started or the dose is increased. Taking 0.3 g of aspirin about half an hour beforehand blunts this prostaglandin-mediated effect. Ibuprofen, taken once daily, also mitigates the flush. Tachyphylaxis to this adverse effect usually occurs within a few days at any dose level. The physician should warn the patient to expect the flush and should explain that it is a harmless vasodilation of skin capillaries. Pruritus, rashes, dry skin, and acanthosis nigricans have been reported. Some patients experience nausea and abdominal discomfort. Many can continue the drug at reduced dosage or with the use of antacids not containing aluminum, but this drug should be avoided in patients with severe peptic disease. Moderate elevations in levels of aminotransferases or alkaline phosphatase may occur, usually not associated with serious liver toxicity. However, liver function should be monitored regularly. This effect is reversible and is minimized if the daily dose is increased by no more than 2.5 g in a month. Rarely, severe hepatotoxicity may occur and is an indication for discontinuing the drug. The association of severe hepatic dysfunction—including acute necrosis—with the use of *sustained-release* preparations of niacin contraindicates their use. Carbohydrate tolerance may be moderately impaired, but this is also reversible. In some patients with latent diabetes, however, this effect may be more evident and incompletely reversible. Hyperuricemia occurs in about one-fifth of patients and occasionally precipitates gout. Rarely described conditions associated with the use of niacin include arrhythmias, mostly atrial, and a reversible toxic amblyopia. Patients should be instructed to report blurring of distance vision if it occurs. Hypotension may occur, especially in patients receiving antihypertensive therapy.

GEMFIBROZIL

Gemfibrozil is a congener of the first-generation fibric acid derivative clofibrate. It resembles the parent drug pharmacologically in reducing VLDL levels and increasing the activity of lipoprotein lipase.

Chemistry & Pharmacokinetics

The gemfibrozil molecule differs from clofibrate in its aliphatic chain and in the presence of two methyl groups rather than a chlorine atom on the phenoxy group. It is supplied as the free carboxylic acid. Gemfibrozil is absorbed quantitatively from the intestine and is tightly bound to plasma proteins. It undergoes enterohepatic circulation and readily passes the placenta. Its plasma half-life is $1\frac{1}{2}$ hours. Seventy percent is eliminated through the kidneys, mostly unmodified. However, the liver modifies some of the drug at the methyl groups to hydroxymethyl or carboxyl derivatives and some of the compound to a quinol.

Gemfibrozil

Clofibrate

Mechanism of Action

Gemfibrozil appears to increase lipolysis of lipoprotein triglyceride via lipoprotein lipase. Intracellular lipolysis in adipose tissue is decreased. There is a decrease in levels of VLDL in plasma, perhaps in part due to decreased secretion by the liver. Only modest reductions of LDL levels occur in most patients. However, in others—especially those with combined hyperlipidemia—LDL levels often increase as triglycerides are reduced. HDL cholesterol levels increase moderately. Part of the apparent increase of HDL cholesterol levels is a direct consequence of decreasing the content of triglycerides in plasma, with reduction in exchange of triglycerides into HDL in place of cholesteryl esters. Some increase in HDL protein has been reported as well.

Therapeutic Uses & Dosage

This drug is useful in hypertriglyceridemias in which VLDL predominate and in dysbetalipoproteinemia. The usual dose of gemfibrozil is 600 mg orally once or twice daily.

Toxicity

Skin rashes, gastrointestinal and muscular symptoms, arrhythmias, hypokalemia, and high levels of aminotransferases or alkaline phosphatase in blood have been reported. A few patients show decreases in white blood count or hematocrit. Gemfibrozil potentiates the action of coumarin and indanedione anticoagulants. Doses of these agents should be adjusted during therapy with gemfibrozil. There is a risk of myopathy when gemfibrozil is given to patients receiving lovastatin. Rhabdomyolysis has occurred rarely. Gemfibrozil should be avoided in patients with hepatic or renal dysfunction. A modest increase in the incidence of gallstones is associated with this agent. It should be used with caution in patients with biliary tract disease or in those at high risk such as women, obese patients, or Native Americans. Data from the Helsinki Heart Study extension and its ancillary study resulted in the recommendation that gemfibrozil should not be used in patients with combined hyperlipidemia who have symptoms of atherosclerotic heart disease (Manninen, 1992).

OTHER FIBRIC ACID DERIVATIVES

Clofibrate is seldom used because of its association with a small increase in risk of gastrointestinal and hepatobiliary neoplasia. **Fenofibrate** is very similar in action to clofibrate and gemfibrozil, but it may be somewhat more potent in reducing LDL levels. It is hydrolyzed to the anion and is excreted mainly by the kidneys. It is given in doses of 100 mg 3 times a day.

Bezafibrate also resembles clofibrate and gemfibrozil in its effect on VLDL, and, like fenofibrate, it may be somewhat more potent in reducing LDL levels. It is given in doses of 200 mg 3 times daily.

BILE ACID-BINDING RESINS

Colestipol and cholestyramine are useful only in hyperlipoproteinemias involving elevated levels of LDL. In patients who have hypertriglyceridemia as well as elevated LDL levels, VLDL levels may be further increased during treatment with the resins.

Chemistry & Pharmacokinetics

Colestipol and cholestyramine are very large polymeric cationic exchange resins that are insoluble in water. They bind bile acids in the intestinal lumen and prevent their reabsorption. Chloride is released from cationic quaternary ammonium binding sites in exchange for bile acids, but the resin itself is not absorbed.

Mechanism of Action

The bile acids, metabolites of cholesterol, are normally reabsorbed in the jejunum and ileum with about 95% efficiency (Figure 34–2). Their excretion is increased up to tenfold when the resins are given. The increased clearance results in enhanced conversion of cholesterol to bile acids in liver via 7α-hydroxylation, normally controlled by negative feedback by bile acids. Increased uptake of LDL from plasma in patients treated with the resins results from upregulation of high-affinity LDL receptors on cell membranes, particularly in the liver. Hence, the resins are without effect in patients with homozygous familial hypercholesterolemia who have no functioning receptors, but they may be useful in patients with receptor-defective combined heterozygous states.

Therapeutic Uses & Dosage

The resins are used in treatment of patients with heterozygous familial hypercholesterolemia, producing approximately 20% reduction in LDL cholesterol when used in maximal dosage. Larger reductions at lower dosages may be expected in patients with less severe forms of hypercholesterolemia. If the resins are used to treat LDL elevations in persons with combined hyperlipidemia, they may cause an increase in levels of VLDL that would require the addition of a second agent such as niacin. The resins are also used in combination with other drugs to achieve further hypocholesterolemic effect (see below). In addition to their use in hyperlipidemia, they may be helpful in relieving itching in patients who have cholestasis and bile salt accumulation. Since they also bind digitalis glycosides, the resins may be used to increase the rate of removal of digitalis from the gastrointestinal tract in severe digitalis toxicity.

Colestipol and cholestyramine are granular preparations available in packets of 5 g and 4 g, respectively, in bulk or as tablets. A gradual increase of dosage from 5 or 4 g/d to 20 g/d orally is recommended. Total doses of 30–32 g/d may be needed for maximum effect. The usual dose for a child is 10–20 g/d. The resins are mixed with juice or water and allowed to hydrate for 1 minute. They should be taken in two or three doses, with meals.

Toxicity

The most common complaints are constipation and a bloating sensation, usually easily relieved by increasing dietary fiber or mixing psyllium seed with the resin. Heartburn and diarrhea are occasionally reported. In patients who have preexisting bowel disease or cholestasis, steatorrhea may occur. Malabsorption of vitamin K may occur rarely, leading to hypoprothrombinemia. Prothrombin time should be measured frequently in patients who are taking resins and anticoagulants. Malabsorption of folic acid has been reported rarely. Increased formation of gallstones, particularly in obese persons, was an anticipated adverse effect but has rarely occurred in practice. Another occasional problem is dry flaking skin,

which is relieved by application of lanolin. Absorption of certain drugs, including those with neutral or cationic charge as well as anions, may be impaired by the resins. These include digitalis glycosides, thiazides, hydrochlorothiazide, warfarin, tetracycline, vancomycin, thyroxine, iron salts, pravastatin, fluvastatin, folic acid, phenylbutazone, and aspirin and ascorbic acid. Any additional medication (except niacin) should be given 1 hour before or at least 2 hours after the resin to ensure adequate absorption.

NEOMYCIN

Pharmacokinetics & Mechanism of Action

This poorly absorbed aminoglycoside antibiotic inhibits reabsorption of cholesterol as well as bile acids, producing moderate reductions in levels of LDL. Bile acid excretion is increased, and the total body pool of cholesterol is decreased. The small amounts that are absorbed are cleared from plasma by the kidney. Neomycin has not been approved by the FDA for the treatment of hyperlipidemia.

Therapeutic Uses & Dosage

Neomycin is perhaps of greatest value when used in combination with other agents in treating primary hypercholesterolemias (see below). It is of no value in reducing levels of triglycerides. The total daily dose is 0.5–2 g, usually in two divided doses with meals.

Toxicity

The dosage of neomycin is limited by severe adverse effects. Even at low doses, nausea, abdominal cramps, diarrhea, and malabsorption have been reported. Overgrowth of resistant microorganisms may lead to enterocolitis. In patients with bowel disease, absorption of the drug may be enhanced, so that otic, hepatic, and hematopoietic toxicity will occur with greater frequency. In patients with normal bowel function, these effects are unusual at doses under 2 g/d. Neomycin also impairs absorption of digitalis glycosides. It should not be given to patients with renal disease.

COMPETITIVE INHIBITORS OF HMG-CoA REDUCTASE (Reductase Inhibitors)

These compounds are structural analogues of HMG-CoA (3-hydroxy-3-methylglutaryl-coenzyme A). The first drug in this class was compactin. A close congener, **lovastatin,** is widely used (Figure 34–3). **Simvastatin, pravastatin,** and **fluvastatin** are similar drugs.

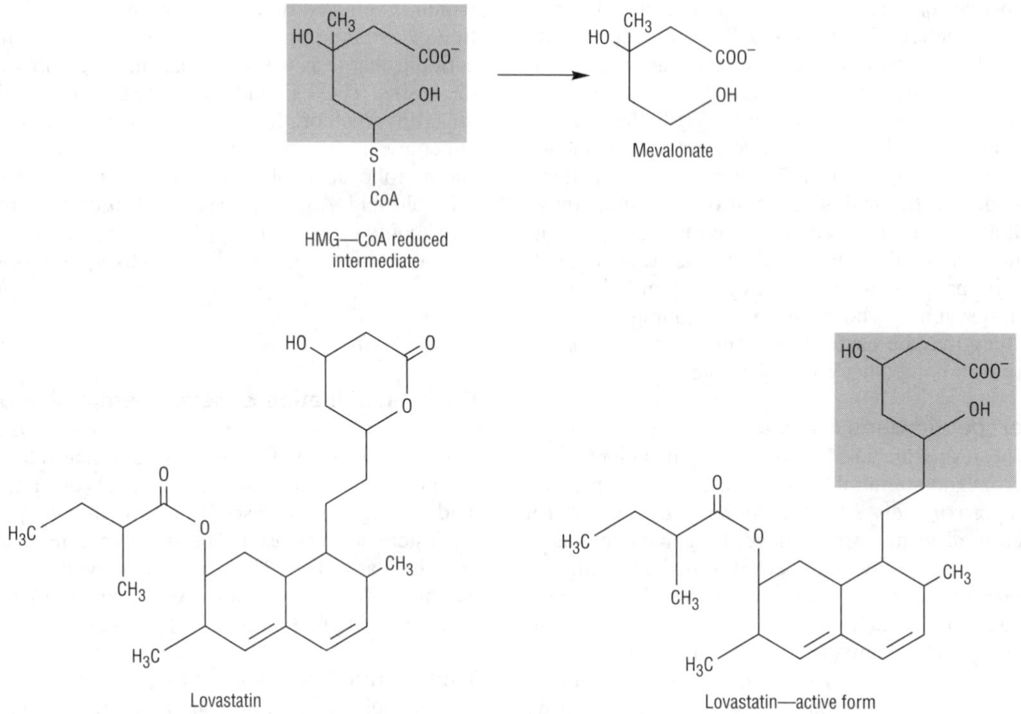

Figure 34-3. Inhibition of HMG-CoA reductase. ***Top:*** The HMG-CoA intermediate that is the immediate precursor of mevalonate, a critical compound in the synthesis of cholesterol. ***Bottom:*** The structure of lovastatin and its active form, showing the similarity to the normal HMG-CoA intermediate (shaded areas).

Chemistry & Pharmacokinetics

Lovastatin and simvastatin are inactive lactone prodrugs that are hydrolyzed in the gastrointestinal tract to the active beta-hydroxyl derivatives. Pravastatin and fluvastatin are active drugs as given. About 30–50% of the ingested dose of lovastatin and pravastatin are absorbed in contrast to fluvastatin, which is almost completely absorbed. All reductase inhibitors have high first pass extraction by the liver. Most of the absorbed dose is excreted in the bile; about 5–20% is excreted in the urine.

Mechanism of Action

HMG-CoA reductase mediates the first committed step in sterol biosynthesis. The active forms of lovastatin and its congeners are structural analogues of the HMG-CoA intermediate (Figure 34–3) that is formed by HMG-CoA reductase in the synthesis of mevalonate. The partial inhibition of the enzyme that these analogues causes may impair the synthesis of isoprenoids such as ubiquinone and dolichol, and the prenylation of proteins, but it is not known whether this will prove to have biologic significance. However, the reductase inhibitors clearly induce an increase in high-affinity LDL receptors. This effect increases both the fractional catabolic rate of LDL and the liver's extraction of LDL precursors (VLDL remnants), thus reducing the plasma pool of LDL (Figure 34–2). Because of the marked first-pass hepatic extraction of these drugs, the major effect of this drug is on the liver. Preferential activity in liver of some congeners appears to be attributable to tissue-specific differences in uptake. Modest decreases in plasma triglycerides and small increases in HDL cholesterol levels also occur during treatment with these agents.

Therapeutic Uses & Dosage

The HMG-CoA inhibitors are useful alone or with bile acid-binding resins or niacin in treating disorders involving elevated plasma levels of LDL. Women who are pregnant, lactating, or likely to become pregnant should not be given these agents. Furthermore, they should not be given to children except those with homozygous familial hypercholesterolemia who have some residual receptor activity.

Because of the diurnal pattern of cholesterol biosynthesis, reductase inhibitors should be given in the evening if a single daily dose is used. Absorption is enhanced by taking the dose with food. Daily doses of lovastatin vary from 10 mg to 80 mg. Moderately elevated LDL levels often respond to a single daily dose of 20 mg, preferably in the evening. In patients with heterozygous familial hypercholesterolemia, doses of 20 mg once or twice daily reduce total cholesterol levels by as much as 19% and 34%, respectively. Pravastatin is equipotent on a mass basis with lovastatin up to the maximum recommended daily dose, 40 mg. Simvastatin is twice as potent and is given in doses of 5–40 mg daily. Fluvastatin appears to be about half as potent as lovastatin on a mass basis and is given in doses of 10–40 mg daily.

Toxicity

Mild elevations of serum aminotransferase activity (up to three times the normal level) occur in some patients receiving reductase inhibitors. These increases are often intermittent and are not associated with other evidence of hepatic toxicity. Therapy may be continued in such patients if aminotransferase levels are measured frequently. In about 2% of patients, some of whom have underlying liver disease or a history of alcohol abuse, aminotransferase levels may exceed three times the normal limit. This effect, which may occur at any time after beginning therapy, may portend more severe hepatic toxicity. Medication should be discontinued in patients whose aminotransferase activity is persistently elevated more than three times the normal limit. Dosage of reductase inhibitors should be reduced in patients with hepatic parenchymal disease. In general, aminotransferase activity should be measured at baseline and at 2- to 4-month intervals during therapy.

Minor increases in creatine kinase activity in plasma are observed, usually intermittently, in about 10% of patients receiving lovastatin. Such increases are frequently associated with heavy physical activity. Rarely, patients receiving lovastatin, simvastatin, or pravastatin may experience marked elevations, often accompanied by generalized pain in skeletal muscles. If the drug is not discontinued, rhabdomyolysis may result with myoglobinuria, even leading to renal shutdown. Although not yet reported with fluvastatin, myopathy should be anticipated. Myopathy may occur with monotherapy, but there appears to be an increased incidence in patients receiving a reductase inhibitor concurrently with cyclosporine, fibric acid derivatives, erythromycin, and possibly niacin. Most patients receiving cyclosporine may be successfully treated with 10 mg of lovastatin or pravastatin daily. Creatine kinase activity should be measured frequently in such patients. Other drugs used with reductase inhibitors may also precipitate myopathy; general caution is advised until more experience with these combinations is obtained. Creatine kinase levels should be measured before treatment and then about every 4 months during therapy. If significant muscle pain, tenderness, or weakness appears, creatine kinase activity should be measured immediately and the drug should be discontinued if creatine kinase activity exceeds twice normal. The myopathy reverses promptly upon cessation of therapy. If the association is unclear, the patient can be rechallenged under close surveillance. Rarely, hypersensitivity syndromes have been reported that include a lupus-like disorder. Because of close structural and mechanistic similarities, hypersensitivity syndromes might be expected with all reductase inhibitors.

These drugs should be temporarily discontinued in the event of serious illness, trauma, or major surgery.

PROBUCOL

The chemical structure of probucol does not resemble the structures of any of the other agents used to lower lipoprotein levels. Its mechanisms of action are unclear, but it may inhibit sterol biosynthesis and improve transport of cholesterol from the periphery to the liver. Probucol is lipophilic and distributes into adipose tissue, persisting in tissues for a long time. Probucol substantially reduces HDL cholesterol and ApoA-I levels in plasma. This may primarily reflect increased efficiency of transfer of cholesteryl esters from HDL to acceptor lipoproteins attendant upon increased activity of cholesteryl ester transfer protein (CETP). LDL cholesterol levels are reduced only marginally in most patients. Some individuals with mildly elevated LDL levels may show a moderate reduction. The usual dose is 500 mg twice daily.

Recent observations in animal models suggest that probucol may help to inhibit atherogenesis by a mechanism other than lipid lowering. Its antioxidant properties protect lipoproteins from hydroperoxidation, thus inhibiting the formation of foam cells in the arterial intima. Because it is effective in reducing atherogenesis in rabbits genetically deficient in LDL receptors and in patients with homozygous familial hypercholesterolemia, it may also prove useful in other severe forms of hypercholesterolemia with aggressive atherogenesis. Because serious toxicity has been demonstrated in animals (arrhythmias, prolonged QT interval) and because more knowledge is needed about its HDL-lowering effect, probucol should probably not be used in less severe forms of hyperlipidemia until more information is available. In humans, prolongation of the QT interval is also observed. Probucol should not be given to patients who already have prolonged QT intervals or who are taking agents that induce QT prolongation. These include digitalis, quinidine, sotalol, and erythromycin. Uncommon adverse effects of probucol include abnormal liver function tests, myopathies, hyperuricemia, hyperglycemia, thrombocytopenia, and neuropathy. Mild gastrointestinal complaints are more frequently reported.

TREATMENT WITH DRUG COMBINATIONS

Combined drug therapy is useful when (1) VLDL levels are significantly increased during treatment of hypercholesterolemia with a bile acid-binding resin;

(2) LDL and VLDL levels are both elevated initially; and (3) LDL levels are not normalized with a single agent.

1. GEMFIBROZIL & BILE ACID-BINDING RESIN

This combination is sometimes useful in treating familial combined hyperlipidemia. However, it increases the risk of cholelithiasis.

2. HMG-CoA REDUCTASE INHIBITORS & BILE ACID-BINDING RESIN

HMG-CoA reductase inhibitors work with bile acid-binding resins in a highly synergistic manner. This combination is useful for treatment of familial hypercholesterolemia but may not control levels of VLDL in some patients with familial combined hyperlipidemia. Pravastatin and fluvastatin should be given at least one hour before or four hours after the resin to ensure their absorption.

3. NIACIN & BILE ACID-BINDING RESIN

This combination effectively controls VLDL levels during resin therapy of familial combined hyperlipidemia or other disorders involving increased VLDL and LDL levels. When VLDL and LDL levels are both initially increased, doses of niacin as low as 1–3 g/d may be sufficient for treatment in combination with a resin.

The niacin-colestipol combination is highly effective for treating heterozygous familial hypercholesterolemia. This probably reflects the combined effects of (1) increased catabolism of LDL due to the resin, (2) decreased synthesis of its precursor VLDL attributable to niacin, and perhaps also (3) the ability of niacin to inhibit cholesterol biosynthesis in the liver. Niacin also significantly elevates levels of HDL cholesterol.

In three major atherosclerosis regression trials, quantitative evidence of reversal of coronary disease was demonstrated with this regimen. Effects on lipoprotein levels are sustained, and no additional adverse effects beyond those encountered when the drugs are used singly have developed. Because the resin has acid-neutralizing properties, the gastric irritation produced by niacin in some patients is relieved when they take the drugs in combination. The drugs may be taken together, because niacin does not bind to the resins. LDL levels in patients with heterozygous familial hypercholesterolemia are usually normalized with daily doses of up to 6.5 g of niacin with 24–30 g of resin.

4. NIACIN & REDUCTASE INHIBITORS

This regimen appears to be more effective than either agent alone in treating familial combined hyperlipidemia and familial hypercholesterolemia. Experience with this combination is limited, however, and serum aminotransferase and creatine kinase should be monitored frequently.

5. NEOMYCIN & NIACIN

Neomycin and niacin appear to be highly complementary in the treatment of hypercholesterolemic patients with familial hypercholesterolemia or familial combined hyperlipidemia. Therefore, this combination may be considered for patients who tolerate other regimens poorly.

6. TERNARY COMBINATION OF RESIN, NIACIN, & REDUCTASE INHIBITORS

These agents act in a complementary fashion to reduce serum cholesterol levels into the low normal range in patients with severe disorders involving elevated LDL levels. The effects are sustained, and little compound toxicity has been observed. Effective doses of the individual drugs may be lower than when each is used alone, eg, as little as 1–2 g of niacin may substantially increase the effects of the other two agents.

PREPARATIONS AVAILABLE

Cholestyramine
Oral: 4 g cholestyramine resin per 5 g powder (Questran Light); in 9 g packets and 378 g cans (Questran); as chewable bar, 4 g/bar (Cholybar)
Clofibrate (generic, Atromid-S)
Oral: 500 mg capsules

Colestipol (Colestid)
Oral: granules, 5 g packets; 300, 500 g bottles
Fenofibrate (Lipidil)
Oral: 100 mg
Fluvastatin (Lescol)
Oral: 20, 40 mg capsules
Gemfibrozil (Lopid)

Oral: 300 mg capsules, 600 mg tablets
Lovastatin (Mevacor)
Oral: 10, 20, 40 mg tablets
Neomycin (generic)
Oral: 500 mg tablets
Niacin, nicotinic acid, vitamin B$_3$ (generic, others)

Oral: 25, 50, 100, 250, 500, 1000 mg tablets
Pravastatin (Pravachol)
Oral: 10, 20 mg tablets
Probucol (Lorelco)
Oral: 250, 500 mg tablets
Simvastatin (Zocor)
Oral: 5, 10, 20, 40 mg tablets

REFERENCES

Atherosclerosis: Mechanisms & Epidemiology

Fuster V et al: Mechanisms of disease: The pathogenesis of coronary artery disease and the acute coronary syndrome. (Two parts.) N Engl J Med 1992;326:242, 310.

Kannel WB et al: Overall and coronary heart disease mortality rates in relation to major risk factors in 325, 348 men screened for the MRFIT: Multiple Risk Factor Interventional Trial. Am Heart J 1986;112:825.

Kannel WB et al: Serum cholesterol, lipoproteins, and the risk of coronary heart disease: The Framingham Study. Ann Intern Med 1971;74:1.

Steinberg D et al: Beyond cholesterol: Modifications of low density lipoprotein that increase its atherogenicity. N Engl J Med 1989;320:915.

Atherosclerosis: Regression

Brown G et al: Regression of coronary artery disease as a result of intensive lipid-lowering therapy in men with high levels of apolipoprotein B. N Engl J Med 1990;323:1289.

Cashin-Hemphill J et al: Beneficial effects of colestipol-niacin on coronary atherosclerosis. A 4-year follow-up. JAMA 1990;264:3013.

Kane JP et al: Regression of coronary atherosclerosis during treatment of familial hypercholesterolemia with combined drug regimens. JAMA 1990;264:3007.

Watts GF et al: Effects on coronary artery disease of lipid-lowering diet, or diet plus cholestyramine in the St. Thomas Atherosclerosis Regression Study. Lancet 1992;339:563.

Hyperlipidemia

Kane JP, Havel RJ: In: *The Metabolic Basis of Inherited Disease,* 7th ed. Scriver CR et al (editors). McGraw-Hill, 1994, chapter 57.

Kane JP, Malloy MJ: Disorders of lipoprotein metabolism. In: *Basic & Clinical Endocrinology,* 4th ed. Greenspan FS (editor). Appleton & Lange, 1993.

Mahley RW: In: *The Metabolic Basis of Inherited Disease,* 7th ed. Scriver CR et al (editors). McGraw-Hill, 1993.

Dietary Treatment

Connor WE, Connor SL: The dietary treatment of hyperlipidemia: Rationale, technique, and efficacy. Med Clin North Am 1982;66:485.

Drug Treatment

Adult Treatment Panel II: Summary of the second report on detection, evaluation, and treatment of high blood cholesterol. JAMA 1993;269:3015.

Grundy SM: HMG-CoA reductase inhibitors for treatment of hypercholesterolemia. N Engl J Med 1988; 319:24.

Illingworth DR: Mevinolin plus colestipol in therapy for severe heterozygous familial hypercholesterolemia. Ann Intern Med 1984;101:598.

Malloy MJ, Kane JP: Medical management of hyperlipidemic states. Adv Intern Med 1994;39:603.

Malloy MJ et al: Complementarity of colestipol, niacin, and lovastatin in treatment of severe familial hypercholesterolemia. Ann Intern Med 1987;107:616.

35

Nonsteroidal Anti-inflammatory Drugs; Nonopioid Analgesics; Drugs Used in Gout

Donald G. Payan, MD & Bertram G. Katzung, MD, PhD

THE INFLAMMATORY RESPONSE

Inflammation is commonly divided into three phases: acute inflammation, the immune response, and chronic inflammation. Acute inflammation is the initial response to tissue injury; it is mediated by the release of autacoids and usually precedes the development of the immune response. Some of the autacoids involved are listed in Table 35–1. The immune response occurs when immunologically competent cells are activated in response to foreign organisms or antigenic substances liberated during the acute or chronic inflammatory response. The outcome of the immune response for the host may be beneficial, as when it causes invading organisms to be phagocytosed or neutralized. On the other hand, the outcome may be deleterious if it leads to chronic inflammation without resolution of the underlying injurious process. Chronic inflammation involves the release of a number of mediators that are not prominent in the acute response. Some of these are listed in Table 35–2. One of the most important conditions involving these mediators is rheumatoid arthritis, in which chronic inflammation results in pain and destruction of bone and cartilage that can lead to severe disability and in which systemic changes occur that can result in shortening of life.

The cell damage associated with inflammation acts on cell membranes to cause leukocytes to release lysosomal enzymes; arachidonic acid is then liberated from precursor compounds, and various eicosanoids are synthesized (see Chapter 18).

Prostaglandins have a variety of effects on blood vessels, on nerve endings, and on cells involved in inflammation. Leukotrienes have a powerful chemotactic effect on eosinophils, neutrophils, and macrophages and promote bronchoconstriction and alterations in vascular permeability. Recent evidence suggests that the cyclooxygenase isozyme (COX II) responsible for prostaglandin production by cells involved in inflammation is not identical to the cyclooxygenase present in most other cells in the body (COX I). A selective blocker of COX II would be desirable in the treatment of inflammation since it would leave undisturbed the other functions of the prostaglandins. It has been suggested that the corticosteroids are such selective blockers (see below).

Kinins, neuropeptides, and histamine are also released at the site of tissue injury, as are complement components, cytokines, and other products of leukocytes and platelets. Stimulation of the neutrophil membranes produces oxygen-derived free radicals. Superoxide anion is formed by the reduction of molecular oxygen, which may stimulate the production of other reactive molecules such as hydrogen peroxide and hydroxyl radicals. The interaction of these substances with arachidonic acid results in the generation of chemotactic substances, thus perpetuating the inflammatory process.

THERAPEUTIC STRATEGIES

The treatment of patients with inflammation involves two primary goals: first, the relief of pain, which is often the presenting symptom and the major continuing complaint of the patient; and second, the slowing or—in theory—arrest of the tissue-damaging process. Reduction of inflammation with anti-inflammatory drugs often results in relief of pain for significant periods. Furthermore, most of the nonopioid analgesics (aspirin, etc) also have anti-inflammatory effects, so they are appropriate for the treatment of both acute and chronic inflammatory conditions.

The glucocorticoids also have powerful anti-inflammatory effects and when first introduced were considered to be the ultimate answer to the treatment

Table 35–1. Some of the mediators of acute inflammation and their effects.

Mediator	Vasodilation	Vascular Permeability	Chemotaxis	Pain
Histamine	++	↑↑↑	−	−
Serotonin	+/−	↑	−	−
Bradykinin	+++	↑	−	+++
Prostaglandins	+++	↑	+++	+
Leukotrienes	−	↑↑↑	+++	−

of inflammatory arthritis. Unfortunately, the severe toxicity associated with chronic corticosteroid therapy prevents their use except in the control of acute flare-ups of joint disease. Therefore, the nonsteroidal anti-inflammatory drugs have assumed the major role in the treatment of arthritis.

Another important group of agents are characterized as slow-acting antirheumatic drugs (SAARDs) or disease-modifying antirheumatic drugs (DMARDs). Very little is known about their mechanisms of action. Unfortunately, they are considerably more toxic than the nonsteroidal anti-inflammatory agents.

I. NONSTEROIDAL ANTI-INFLAMMATORY DRUGS

Salicylates and other agents used to treat rheumatic disease share the capacity to suppress the signs and symptoms of inflammation. Some of the drugs also exert antipyretic and analgesic effects, but it is their

Table 35–2. Some of the mediators of chronic inflammation, eg, in rheumatoid arthritis.

Mediator	Sources	Primary Effects
Interleukins 1, 2, and 3	Macrophages, T lymphocytes	Lymphocyte activation, prostaglandin production
GM-CSF[1]	T lymphocytes, endothelial cells, fibroblasts	Macrophage and granulocyte activation
TNF-α[2]	Macrophages	Prostaglandin production
Interferons	Macrophages, endothelial cells, T lymphocytes	Multiple
PDGF[3]	Macrophages, endothelial cells, fibroblasts, platelets	Fibroblast chemotaxis, proliferation

[1]Granulocyte-macrophage colony-stimulating factor.
[2]Tumor necrosis factor alpha.
[3]Platelet-derived growth factor.

anti-inflammatory properties that make them useful in the management of disorders in which pain is related to the intensity of the inflammatory process. Several of the newer NSAIDs are used for special indications. These include indomethacin, phenylbutazone, and ketorolac. They are discussed separately.

ASPIRIN & OTHER SALICYLATES

Aspirin and all but one of the newer nonsteroidal anti-inflammatory drugs (NSAIDs) (ibuprofen, naproxen, etc) are related chemically in that they are weak organic acids; nabumetone is a ketone prodrug that is metabolized to an acidic active drug. They share the important property of inhibiting prostaglandin biosynthesis. They may also decrease the production of free radicals and of superoxide and may interact with adenylyl cyclase to alter the cellular concentration of cAMP. Although these drugs effectively inhibit inflammation, there is no evidence that—in contrast to drugs such as methotrexate and penicillamine—they alter the course of an arthritic disorder. Aspirin's long history of use and availability without prescription diminishes its glamour compared to that of the newer NSAIDs. However, because of its low cost and long history of safety, aspirin remains the initial drug of choice for treating the majority of articular and musculoskeletal disorders. Aspirin is also the standard against which all anti-inflammatory agents are measured (Table 35–3), and it should not be abandoned unless a specific contraindication exists or another NSAID offers a clearly demonstrable advantage.

History
Quinine from cinchona bark is one of the oldest remedies for relief of mild pain and fever. Willow bark was used in folk medicine for years for similar indications. In 1763, Reverend Edmund Stone, in a letter to the president of the Royal Society, described his success in treating fever with a powdered form of the bark of the willow. He had noted that the bitterness of willow bark was reminiscent of the taste of cinchona bark, the source of quinine. The active in-

Table 35–3. Properties of aspirin and some newer nonsteroidal anti-inflammatory drugs.

Drug	Half-life (hours)	Urinary Excretion of Unchanged Drug	Recommended Anti-inflammatory Dosage
Aspirin	0.25	<2%	1200–1500 mg tid
Salicylate[1]	2–19	2–30%	See footnote 2
Apazone	15	62%	600 mg bid
Diclofenac	1.1	<1%	50–75 mg qid
Diflunisal	13	3–9%	500 mg bid
Etodolac	6.5	<1%	200–300 mg qid
Fenoprofen	2.5	30%	600 mg qid
Flurbiprofen	3.8	<1%	300 mg tid
Ibuprofen	2	<1%	600 mg qid
Indomethacin	4–5	16%	50–70 mg tid
Ketoprofen	1.8	<1%	70 mg tid
Ketorolac	4–10	58%	10 mg qid[3]
Meclofen-amate	3	2–4%	100 mg qid
Nabumetone[4]	26	1%	1000–2000 mg qd[5]
Naproxen	14	<1%	375 mg bid
Oxaprozin	58	1–4%	1200–1800 mg qd[5]
Phenylbuta-zone[6]	68	1–3%	100 mg qid
Piroxicam	57	4–10%	20 mg qd[5]
Sulindac	8	7%	200 mg bid
Tolmetin	1	7%	400 mg qid

[1]Major anti-inflammatory metabolite of aspirin.
[2]Salicylate is usually given in the form of aspirin.
[3]Recommended for treatment of acute (eg, surgical) pain only.
[4]Nabumetone is a prodrug; the half-life and urinary excretion are for its active metabolite
[5]A single daily dose is sufficient because of the long half-life.
[6]Phenylbutazone is not recommended for chronic use. The dose listed is for treatment of acute gouty arthritis and should not be given for more than one week. It may be preceded by a single loading dose of 400 mg.

gredient of willow bark, salicin, which on hydrolysis yields salicylic acid, was later found in other natural sources. Acetylsalicylic acid was synthesized in 1853, but the drug was not used until 1899, when it was found to be effective in arthritis and well tolerated. The name aspirin was coined from the German word for the compound, *acetylspirsäure* (*Spirea,* the genus of plants from which it was obtained, and *Säure,* the German word for acid). Because of its greater efficacy and lower cost, aspirin rapidly replaced the natural products then in use and has remained one of the most widely employed remedies for over 90 years.

Chemistry & Pharmacokinetics

Salicylic acid is a simple organic acid with a pK_a of 3.0. Aspirin (acetylsalicylic acid; ASA) has a pK_a of 3.5 (see Table 1–2). It is about 50% more potent than sodium salicylate, although the latter compound causes less gastric irritation.

The salicylates (Figure 35–1) are rapidly absorbed from the stomach and upper small intestine, yielding a peak plasma salicylate level within 1–2 hours. The acid medium in the stomach keeps a large fraction of the salicylate in the nonionized form, promoting absorption. However, when high concentrations of salicylate enter the mucosal cell, the drug may damage the mucosal barrier. If the gastric pH is raised by a suitable buffer to 3.5 or higher, gastric irritation is minimized.

Aspirin is absorbed as such and is hydrolyzed to acetic acid and salicylate by esterases in tissue and blood. Salicylate is bound to albumin, but, as the serum concentration of salicylate increases, a greater fraction remains unbound and available to tissues. Ingested salicylate and that generated by the hydrolysis of aspirin may be excreted unchanged, but most is converted to water-soluble conjugates that are rapidly cleared by the kidney (Figure 35–1). When this pathway becomes saturated, a small increase in aspirin dose results in a large increase in plasma levels. Alkalinization of the urine increases the rate of excretion of free salicylate. When aspirin is used in low doses (600 mg), elimination is in accordance with first-order kinetics and the serum half-life is 3–5 hours. With higher dosage, zero-order kinetics prevail; at anti-inflammatory dosage (≥ 4 g/d), the half-life increases to 15 hours or more. This effect occurs in about a week and is related to saturation of hepatic enzymes that catalyze the formation of salicylate metabolites, salicylphenylglucuronide and salicyluric acid.

Pharmacodynamics

A. Mechanism of Action: The effectiveness of aspirin is largely due to its capacity to inhibit prostaglandin biosynthesis (see Chapter 18). It does this by irreversibly blocking the enzyme cyclooxygenase (prostaglandin synthase), which catalyzes the conversion of arachidonic acid to endoperoxide compounds; at appropriate doses, the drug decreases the formation of both the prostaglandins and thromboxane A_2 but not the leukotrienes (Figure 35–2). There is no evidence that aspirin is a selective inhibitor of COX II. Most of an anti-inflammatory dose of aspirin is rapidly deacetylated to form salicylate as the active metabolite. Salicylate reversibly inhibits prostaglandin synthesis.

B. Anti-inflammatory Effects: In addition to reducing the synthesis of eicosanoid mediators, aspirin also interferes with the chemical mediators of the kallikrein system (see Chapter 17). As a result, aspirin inhibits granulocyte adherence to damaged vasculature, stabilizes lysosomes, and inhibits the migration of polymorphonuclear leukocytes and macrophages into the site of inflammation.

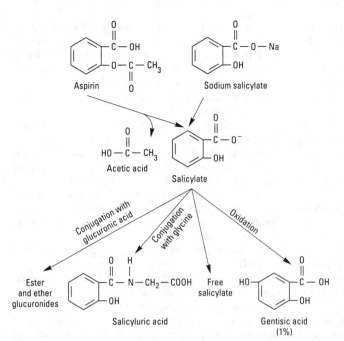

Figure 35–1. Structure and metabolism of the salicylates. (Modified and reproduced, with permission, from Meyers FH, Jawetz E, Goldfien A: *Review of Medical Pharmacology,* 7th ed. Lange, 1980.)

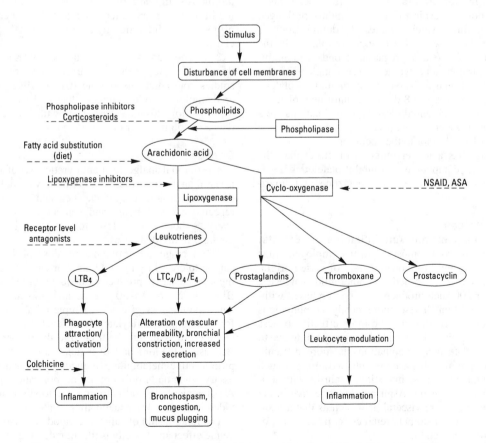

Figure 35–2. Scheme for mediators derived from arachidonic acid and sites of drug action.

C. Analgesic Effects: Aspirin is most effective in reducing pain of mild to moderate intensity. It alleviates pain of varying causes, such as that of muscular, vascular, and dental origin, postpartum states, arthritis, and bursitis. Aspirin acts peripherally through its effects on inflammation but probably also inhibits pain stimuli at a subcortical site.

D. Antipyretic Effects: Aspirin reduces elevated temperature, whereas normal body temperature is only slightly affected. The fall in temperature is related to increased dissipation of heat caused by vasodilation of superficial blood vessels. The antipyresis may be accompanied by profuse sweating.

The fever associated with infection is thought to result from two actions. The first is the production of prostaglandins in the central nervous system in response to bacterial pyrogens. The second is the effect of interleukin-1 on the hypothalamus. Interleukin-1 is produced by macrophages and is released during inflammatory responses, when its principal role is to activate lymphocytes (Table 35–2). Aspirin blocks both the pyrogen-induced production of prostaglandins and the central nervous system response to interleukin-1 and so may reset the "temperature control" in the hypothalamus, thereby facilitating heat dissipation by vasodilation.

E. Platelet Effects: Aspirin affects hemostasis. Single doses of aspirin produce a slightly prolonged bleeding time, which doubles if administration is continued for a week. The change is explained by the inhibition of platelet aggregation secondary to inhibition of thromboxane synthesis (see Chapter 33). Because its action is irreversible, aspirin inhibits platelet aggregation for up to 8 days—ie, until new platelets are formed. If potential bleeding complications are a concern in association with surgery, aspirin should be stopped 1 week prior to the operation.

Aspirin has a longer duration of effect than the many other compounds that inhibit platelet aggregation such as ticlopidine, phenylbutazone, and dipyridamole.

Clinical Uses

A. Analgesia and Anti-inflammatory Effects: Aspirin is one of the most frequently employed drugs for relieving mild to moderate pain of varied origin. Aspirin is often combined with other mild analgesics, and over 200 such products may be purchased without prescription. These more costly combinations have never been shown to be more effective or less toxic than aspirin alone, and treating poisoning due to overdoses of such combinations is more difficult. Furthermore, the phenacetin contained in many such compounds may cause interstitial nephritis with serious renal impairment. Aspirin is not effective in the treatment of severe visceral pain such as that associated with acute abdomen, renal colic, pericarditis, or myocardial infarction.

The anti-inflammatory properties of salicylates in high doses are responsible for their recommendation as initial therapy for rheumatoid arthritis, rheumatic fever, and other inflammatory joint conditions. In mild arthritis, many patients can be managed using salicylates as their sole medication.

B. Other Indications:

1. Antipyresis–Except for a few diseases (eg, neurosyphilis, chronic brucellosis), there is no evidence that elevation of body temperature is a useful defense mechanism. On the other hand, there is rarely any great need to reduce a mild or moderate fever, especially in adults (Styrt, 1990). Aspirin is the best available drug for reducing fever when doing so is desirable and when there are no contraindications to its use (see below).

2. Inhibition of platelet aggregation (see also Chapter 33)–Aspirin has been shown to decrease the incidence of transient ischemic attacks and unstable angina in men and has been used as a prophylactic agent in these conditions. It may also be effective in reducing the incidence of thrombosis in coronary artery bypass grafts. The results of several clinical studies of patients at risk for or recovering from myocardial infarction have provided evidence that aspirin reduces the incidence of coronary artery thrombosis. In one large study, the ingestion of 325 mg of aspirin every other day reduced the incidence of myocardial infarction by over 40% in male physicians.

3. Other uses–Several studies have suggested that aspirin may reduce cataract formation; other studies contradict this finding (Chew, 1992). Other epidemiologic studies suggest that long-term use of aspirin at low dosage is associated with a lower incidence of colon cancer (Thun, 1991).

Dosage

The optimal analgesic or antipyretic dose of aspirin is less than the 0.6 g oral dose commonly used. Larger doses may prolong the effect. The usual dose may be repeated every 4 hours and smaller doses (0.3 g) every 3 hours. The dose for children is 50–75 mg/kg/d in divided doses.

The average anti-inflammatory dose of 4 g daily can be tolerated by most adults. For children, 50–75 mg/kg/d usually produces adequate blood levels. Blood levels of 15–30 mg/dL are associated with anti-inflammatory effects. A simple reliable method for determining salicylate blood levels is available, and the drug can thus be titrated to the proper level. Because of the long half-lives (about 12 hours) of aspirin's active metabolites, frequent dosing is not necessary when daily doses of 4 g or more are required. A convenient method is to give the total amount divided into three doses taken after meals.

The relationship of salicylate blood levels to therapeutic effect and toxicity is illustrated in Figure 35–3.

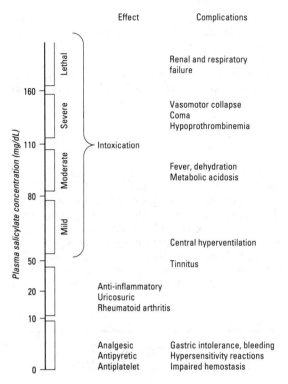

Figure 35–3. Approximate relationships of plasma salicylate levels to pharmacodynamics and complications. (Modified and reproduced, with permission, from Hollander J, McCarty D Jr: *Arthritis and Allied Conditions.* Lea & Febiger, 1972.)

Drug Selection

Aspirin is available from many different manufacturers, and although it may vary in texture and appearance, the content of aspirin is constant. A disintegration test is part of the official standard, and there is little evidence that differences among tablets have clinical significance. The most popular buffered aspirin does not contain sufficient alkali to modify gastric irritation, and there is no evidence that these more expensive preparations are associated with higher blood levels, greater clinical effectiveness, or a lower incidence of adverse effects. Enteric-coated aspirin may be suitable for patients in whom buffering fails to control gastritis, since the coating prevents the tablets from dissolving in the stomach and the drug is absorbed adequately in the small intestine. Therapeutic blood levels with this preparation may be similar to those achieved with the same doses of regular aspirin. Enteric coating increases the cost of aspirin, but these products are still less costly than the newer NSAIDs. The concomitant use of H_2 blockers and other drugs used in the treatment and prevention of acid-peptic disease has not been shown to reduce the incidence of NSAID-induced gastrointestinal damage. A pros-

taglandin E_1 derivative, misoprostol, has been shown to reduce NSAID-induced ulceration, but this drug is expensive and causes diarrhea in many patients (see below).

Adverse Effects

A. Gastrointestinal Effects: At the usual dosage, the main adverse effect is gastric upset (intolerance). This effect can be minimized with suitable buffering (taking aspirin with meals followed by a glass of water or antacids). The gastritis that occurs with aspirin may be due to irritation of the gastric mucosa by the undissolved tablet, to absorption in the stomach of nonionized salicylate, or to inhibition of protective prostaglandins. In animals, ulceration can be produced by the parenteral administration of aspirin, and administration of prostaglandins has prevented aspirin-induced gastric erosions; these observations suggest that the absence of a prostaglandin may make the gastric mucosa more vulnerable. As noted above, misoprostol does reduce the frequency of recurrence of peptic ulceration in patients taking large doses of NSAIDs but causes its own toxicities.

Although aspirin has never been shown to cause peptic ulcers in humans, experimental and epidemiologic studies overwhelmingly document an increased incidence of gastric ulcers and, to a lesser extent, duodenal ulcers with heavy aspirin or newer NSAID use (Ivey, 1986). Upper gastrointestinal bleeding associated with aspirin use is usually related to erosive gastritis. A small increase in fecal blood loss is routinely associated with aspirin administration; about 1 mL of blood normally lost in the stool daily increases to about 4 mL daily in persons using ordinary aspirin doses and more for higher doses. On the other hand, with appropriate therapy, ulcers have been shown to heal while aspirin was taken concomitantly. Nevertheless, aspirin should be avoided or taken with effective buffers or prostaglandins by individuals with peptic ulcer disease.

Vomiting may occur as a result of central nervous system stimulation after absorption of large doses of aspirin.

B. Central Nervous System Effects: With higher doses, patients may experience "salicylism"— tinnitus, decreased hearing, and vertigo—reversible by reducing the dosage. Still larger doses of salicylates cause hyperpnea through a direct effect on the medulla. At low toxic salicylate levels, respiratory alkalosis may occur as a result of the increased ventilation. Later, acidosis supervenes from accumulation of salicylic acid derivatives and depression of the respiratory center.

C. Other Adverse Effects: Aspirin in a daily dose of 2 g or less usually increases serum uric acid levels, whereas doses exceeding 4 g daily decrease urate levels below 2.5 mg/dL. (See Drugs Used in Gout, below.)

Aspirin may cause mild, usually asymptomatic hepatitis, especially in patients with underlying disorders such as systemic lupus erythematosus and juvenile and adult rheumatoid arthritis.

Salicylates may cause reversible decrease of glomerular filtration rate in patients with underlying renal disease, and this may also occur (though rarely) in persons with normal kidneys.

Aspirin in usual doses has a negligible effect on glucose tolerance. Toxic amounts affect the cardiovascular system directly and may depress cardiac function and dilate peripheral blood vessels. Large doses directly affect smooth muscles.

Hypersensitivity reactions may occur after ingestion of aspirin by patients with asthma and nasal polyps and may be associated with bronchoconstriction and shock. These reactions are probably mediated by leukotrienes.

Aspirin is contraindicated in patients with hemophilia. Aspirin is not recommended for pregnant women. However, some studies have suggested that low-dose aspirin may be valuable in certain pregnant patients with a high risk of hypertension and other complications of pregnancy (Schiff, 1989).

Use of aspirin in children during or immediately after a viral infection has been associated with an increase in the incidence of Reye's syndrome (Hurwitz, 1987, 1989). Acetaminophen should be used in place of aspirin in this situation.

Overdosage Toxicity

Aspirin is such a common household drug that it has been a frequent cause of poisoning in young children. Serious intoxication results when the amount ingested exceeds 150–175 mg/kg of body weight. Since the introduction of child-resistant containers, there has been a significant decrease in fatal aspirin-induced poisonings in children.

Most aspirin is sold and used without prescription. The drug must be kept out of reach of children and in the child-resistant container in which it is dispensed. Colorful, flavored, and liquid preparations should be kept in locked cabinets.

When overdosing occurs, either accidentally or with suicidal intent, gastric lavage is advised (Chapter 60). Hyperthermia may be treated with alcohol sponges or ice packs. It is important to maintain a high urine volume and to treat acid-base abnormalities. In severe toxic reactions, ventilatory assistance may be required. Sodium bicarbonate infusions may be employed to alkalinize the urine, which will increase the amount of salicylate excreted.

Drug Interactions

Drugs that enhance salicylate intoxication include acetazolamide and ammonium chloride. Alcohol increases gastrointestinal bleeding produced by salicylates. Aspirin displaces a number of drugs from protein binding sites in the blood. These include tolbutamide, chlorpropamide, nonsteroidal anti-inflammatory agents, methotrexate, phenytoin, and probenecid. Corticosteroids may decrease salicylate concentration. Aspirin reduces the pharmacologic activity of spironolactone, competes with penicillin G for renal tubular secretion, and inhibits the uricosuric effect of sulfinpyrazone and probenecid.

DIFLUNISAL

Diflunisal is a newer NSAID chemically derived from salicylic acid. The drug has a plasma half-life approaching that of salicylate, and blood levels reach a steady state after several days of dosing. Like aspirin, it has analgesic and anti-inflammatory effects; unlike aspirin, it has little antipyretic activity.

The indications for use of diflunisal include pain, osteoarthritis, and rheumatoid arthritis. Adverse reactions are similar to those of other NSAIDs.

OTHER NONSTEROIDAL ANTI-INFLAMMATORY DRUGS

The adverse effects of aspirin and other salicylates—especially the gastric irritation that occurs when large doses are employed—have led to the search for alternative compounds. Starting with phenylbutazone in 1949, many drugs with aspirin-like properties (designated newer nonsteroidal anti-inflammatory drugs) have been approved for use in the USA for the treatment of rheumatoid arthritis or osteoarthritis (Table 35–3). In addition to their use in joint disease, several newer NSAIDs have been approved for other indications as described below.

Chemistry

The NSAIDs are grouped in several chemical classes, some of which are shown in Figure 35–4. This chemical diversity yields such a broad range of pharmacokinetic characteristics that these properties are best discussed in connection with the individual agents.

Pharmacodynamics

The anti-inflammatory activity of the newer NSAIDs is similar in mechanism to that of aspirin and is mediated chiefly through inhibition of biosynthesis of prostaglandins. Unlike aspirin, these drugs are reversible inhibitors of cyclooxygenase. Selectivity for COX I versus COX II is variable and incomplete. For example, in testing against the mouse enzymes, aspirin, indomethacin, piroxicam, and sulindac were considerably more effective in inhibiting COX I; ibupro-

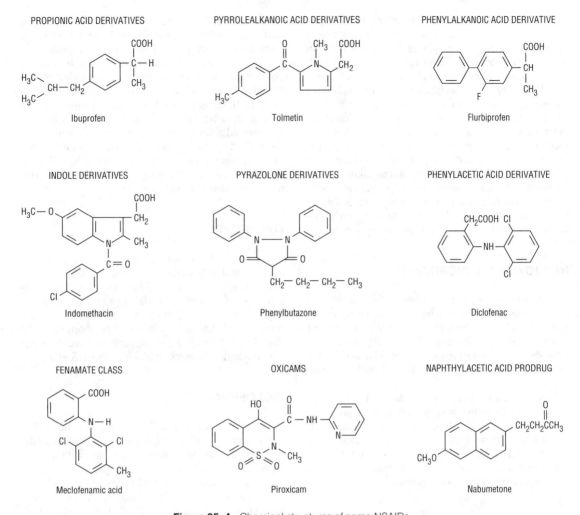

Figure 35–4. Chemical structures of some NSAIDs.

fen and meclofenamate inhibited the two isozymes about equally; and the active metabolite of nabumetone was somewhat selective for COX II (Meade, 1993). Inhibition of lipoxygenase synthesis by the newer NSAIDs, a desirable effect for an anti-inflammatory drug, is limited but may be greater than with aspirin. Benoxaprofen, another newer NSAID, was shown to significantly inhibit leukotriene synthesis but was withdrawn because of toxicity. Of the currently available NSAIDs, indomethacin and diclofenac have been reported to reduce the synthesis of both prostaglandins and leukotrienes. It is likely that development of newer NSAIDs will continue until the clinical significance of inhibition of COX II and of lipoxygenase can be fully evaluated with more selective inhibitors.

During therapy with these drugs, inflammation is reduced by decreasing the release of mediators from granulocytes, basophils, and mast cells. The NSAIDs decrease the sensitivity of vessels to bradykinin and histamine, affect lymphokine production from T lymphocytes, and reverse vasodilation. To varying degrees, all newer NSAIDs are analgesic, anti-inflammatory, and antipyretic, and all inhibit platelet aggregation. They are all gastric irritants as well, though as a group they tend to cause less gastric irritation than aspirin. Nephrotoxicity has increasingly been observed for all of the drugs for which extensive experience has been reported.

IBUPROFEN

Ibuprofen is a simple derivative of phenylpropionic acid. In doses of about 2400 mg daily, ibuprofen is equivalent to 4 g of aspirin in anti-inflammatory effect. The drug is often prescribed in lower doses, at which it is analgesic but inferior as an anti-inflammatory agent. It is available over the counter in lower dosage under several trade names.

Ibuprofen is extensively metabolized in the liver, and little is excreted unchanged. Gastrointestinal irritation and bleeding occur, though less frequently than with aspirin. The use of ibuprofen concomitantly with aspirin may decrease the total anti-inflammatory effect. The drug is contraindicated in individuals with nasal polyps, angioedema, and bronchospastic reactivity to aspirin. In addition to the gastrointestinal symptoms (which can be modified by ingestion with meals), rash, pruritus, tinnitus, dizziness, headache, anxiety, aseptic meningitis, and fluid retention have been reported. Interaction with anticoagulants is uncommon. Serious hematologic effects include agranulocytosis and aplastic anemia; effects on the kidney (as with all NSAIDs) include acute renal failure, interstitial nephritis, and nephrotic syndrome.

NAPROXEN & FENOPROFEN

Naproxen is a naphthylpropionic acid that binds to plasma protein and has a long half-life (Table 35–3). Antacids delay its absorption. Naproxen is excreted in the urine as an inactive glucuronide metabolite. Like ibuprofen, naproxen competes with aspirin for plasma protein binding sites. It also prolongs prothrombin time.

Fenoprofen, another propionic acid derivative, has a short half-life so that multiple dosing is required.

Adverse effects and drug interactions of naproxen and fenoprofen are similar to those of ibuprofen, ie, nephrotoxicity, jaundice, nausea, dyspepsia, peripheral edema, rash, pruritus, central nervous system and cardiovascular effects, and tinnitus.

FLURBIPROFEN

Flurbiprofen is another propionic acid derivative with an intermediate half-life. It is readily absorbed and achieves high synovial concentration. Following extensive metabolic degradation, it may undergo some enterohepatic recirculation before it is excreted by the kidneys. The efficacy of flurbiprofen is comparable to that of aspirin and other NSAIDs in clinical trials for patients with rheumatoid arthritis, ankylosing spondylitis, and osteoarthritis. It is also available in a topical ophthalmic formulation for inhibition of intraoperative miosis.

As with other NSAIDs, gastrointestinal symptoms are encountered in 15–20% of patients who take the oral preparation. No significant age-related increase in adverse reactions has been reported.

KETOPROFEN

Ketoprofen is a propionic acid derivative that has some ability to inhibit both cyclooxygenase and lipoxygenase. The drug is rapidly absorbed, but its half-life is short. It is metabolized completely in the liver. Despite being 99% bound to plasma proteins, it does not alter warfarin or digoxin activity. In contrast, concurrent administration of probenecid elevates ketoprofen levels and prolongs its plasma half-life.

The effectiveness of ketoprofen is equivalent to that of other NSAIDs and aspirin in the treatment of rheumatoid arthritis and osteoarthritis. In spite of its dual effect on prostaglandins and leukotrienes, it has not been shown to be superior to other NSAIDs. Its major adverse effects are on the central nervous system and gastrointestinal tract.

OXAPROZIN

Oxaprozin is one of the newest of the propionic acid derivative NSAIDs. As noted in Table 35–3, its major difference from the other members of this subgroup is a very long half-life; it can be given once a day. Because of this long half-life, dosage adjustments should be made at intervals no shorter than 10 days to 2 weeks. The drug appears to have the same benefits and risks associated with other NSAIDs.

DICLOFENAC

Diclofenac is a simple phenylacetic acid derivative that resembles both flurbiprofen and meclofenamate. It is a potent cyclooxygenase inhibitor with anti-inflammatory, analgesic, and antipyretic properties. The drug is rapidly absorbed following oral administration and has a short half-life. Like flurbiprofen, it accumulates in the synovial fluid. The potency of diclofenac is greater than that of naproxen. The drug is recommended for chronic inflammatory conditions such as rheumatoid arthritis and osteoarthritis and for the treatment of acute musculoskeletal pain. Adverse effects occur in approximately 20% of patients and include gastrointestinal distress, occult gastrointestinal bleeding, and gastric ulceration.

An ophthalmic preparation is available that is recommended for prevention of postoperative ophthalmic inflammation.

SULINDAC

Sulindac, a sulfoxide, is a prodrug. Its active metabolite is, like diclofenac, an acetic acid derivative. The drug is effective only after it is converted by liver enzymes to a sulfide, which is excreted in bile and then reabsorbed from the intestine. The enterohepatic cycling prolongs the duration of action to about 16 hours.

The indications and adverse reactions are similar to those of other NSAIDs. Among the more severe reactions, Stevens-Johnson epidermal necrolysis syndrome, thrombocytopenia, agranulocytosis, and nephrotic syndrome have all been observed.

TOLMETIN

Tolmetin, a pyrroleacetic acid derivative, is similar to aspirin in effectiveness in juvenile and adult rheumatoid arthritis and osteoarthritis. The drug has a short half-life and must be given frequently.

ETODOLAC

Etodolac is newer acetic acid derivative with an intermediate half-life (Table 35–3). Like some other NSAIDs, it is a racemic mixture of R and S forms, the R form being inactive. The drug is well absorbed, with a bioavailability of about 80%, and is strongly bound to plasma proteins (> 90%). There are no data to suggest that etodolac differs significantly from other NSAIDs except in its pharmacokinetic parameters.

NABUMETONE

Nabumetone is a prodrug. It is given as a ketone (Figure 35–4) and converted to an acetic acid derivative in the body. Its half-life of more than 24 hours (Table 35–3) permits once-daily dosing. Otherwise, its properties are very similar to those of other NSAIDs.

MECLOFENAMATE & MEFENAMIC ACID

Meclofenamate, a fenamic acid derivative, reaches a peak plasma level in 30–60 minutes and has a short half-life. It is excreted in the urine, largely as the glucuronide conjugate. Although long-term experience is lacking, meclofenamate appears to have adverse effects similar to those of other newer NSAIDs and to have no advantage over them. This drug enhances the effect of oral anticoagulants. Meclofenamate is contraindicated in pregnancy; its efficacy and safety have not been established for young children.

Mefenamic acid, another fenamate, possesses analgesic properties but is probably less effective than aspirin as an anti-inflammatory agent and is clearly more toxic. It should not be used for longer than 1 week and never in children.

PIROXICAM

Piroxicam, an oxicam, is an NSAID of novel structure (Figure 35–4). It has a long half-life, permitting

once-daily dosing, which should favor compliance. It is rapidly absorbed in the stomach and upper small intestine and reaches 80% of its peak plasma concentration in 1 hour. It is excreted as the glucuronide conjugate and to a small extent unchanged.

Gastrointestinal symptoms are encountered in 20% of patients. Other adverse reactions include dizziness, tinnitus, headache, and rash. The drug may be used in the treatment of rheumatoid arthritis, ankylosing spondylitis, and osteoarthritis.

APAZONE & CARPROFEN

These drugs are available in many other countries but are not sold in the USA. Apazone (azapropazone), a pyrazolone derivative, is structurally related to phenylbutazone but appears less likely to cause agranulocytosis. Its half-life is 12–16 hours. In patients with decreased renal function—eg, elderly patients—its half-life may be doubled. Carprofen is a propionic acid derivative with a similar half-life of 10–16 hours. The indications and adverse effects of apazone and carprofen are similar to those of other NSAIDs.

NSAIDs FOR SPECIAL INDICATIONS

INDOMETHACIN

Indomethacin, introduced in 1963, is an indole derivative (Figure 35–4). It is more toxic but in certain circumstances more effective than aspirin or any of the other NSAIDs. In the laboratory, it is the most potent of the inhibitors of prostaglandin synthesis. Indomethacin is well absorbed after oral administration and highly bound to plasma proteins. Metabolism occurs in the liver, and unchanged drug and inactive metabolites are excreted in bile and urine.

Clinical Uses

Indomethacin is not suggested for general use as an analgesic. Except for the treatment of patent ductus arteriosus (discussed below), it should not be used in children. It is useful in special situations, including acute gouty arthritis, ankylosing spondylitis, and osteoarthritis of the hip and has also been effective in extra-articular inflammatory conditions such as pericarditis and pleurisy and in Bartter's syndrome. In acute gout, indomethacin has virtually replaced colchicine as the initial medication (see Drugs Used in Gout, below).

A special application of indomethacin is in the management of patent ductus arteriosus in premature infants. Because this structure is kept patent in the fetus by the continuous production of prostaglandins, closure can be accelerated in a premature newborn by intravenous infusion of this drug. The production of prostaglandin in this situation is not an inflammatory process and is probably dependent upon COX I rather than COX II. As noted above, indomethacin is relatively selective for COX I. In many cases, surgery can be avoided by the use of indomethacin.

Indomethacin has been recommended for use as a tocolytic in preterm labor at less than 32 weeks gestation (Morales, 1989); inhibition of prostaglandin synthesis reduces the frequency and strength of uterine contractions. However, others dispute this application on the basis of the recognized fetal and maternal toxicity of the drug (Norton, 1993). Calcium channel blockers (Chapter 12) are receiving more attention in this application.

Adverse Reactions

Indomethacin produces a high incidence of dose-related toxic effects. At higher dosage levels, at least a third of patients have reactions requiring discontinuance of the medication. The gastrointestinal effects may include abdominal pain, diarrhea, gastrointestinal hemorrhage, and pancreatitis. Severe headache is experienced by 20–25% of patients and may be associated with dizziness, confusion, and depression. Rarely, psychosis with hallucinations has been reported. Hepatic abnormalities are rare. Serious hematologic reactions have been noted, including thrombocytopenia and aplastic anemia. Coronary vasoconstriction has been demonstrated. Hyperkalemia has been reported and is related to inhibition of the synthesis of prostaglandins in the kidney. A number of interactions with other drugs have been reported (see Appendix II). Use of indomethacin should be avoided in patients with nasal polyps or angioedema, in whom asthma may be precipitated. The drug is contraindicated in pregnancy and should be used with caution in persons with psychiatric disorders or peptic ulcer disease.

PHENYLBUTAZONE

Phenylbutazone, a pyrazolone derivative, rapidly gained favor after its introduction in 1949 for the treatment of rheumatoid arthritis, ankylosing spondylitis, acute gouty arthritis, and various musculoskeletal disorders. It has potent anti-inflammatory properties and is thus still commonly prescribed, even though aspirin and newer NSAIDs are superior in most applications. Oxyphenbutazone is an active metabolite of phenylbutazone with similar properties. It is available separately.

Phenylbutazone has a large number of serious adverse effects. The most serious are agranulocytosis and aplastic anemia, which have led to a number of deaths. Phenylbutazone has also caused hemolytic anemia, nephrotic syndrome, optic neuritis, deafness, serious allergic reactions, exfoliative dermatitis, and hepatic and renal tubular necrosis. The main indications for phenylbutazone are for the short-term therapy of such painful conditions as acute gouty arthritis and superficial thrombophlebitis. Safer drugs, such as indomethacin, appear to be equally efficacious for these specialized indications.

KETOROLAC

Ketorolac is an NSAID of intermediate duration of action that is promoted for systemic use mainly as a analgesic, not an anti-inflammatory drug (though it has typical NSAID properties). The drug does appear to have significant analgesic efficacy and has been used successfully to replace morphine in some situations involving mild to moderate postsurgical pain. It is most often given parenterally, but an oral dose-form is available. An ophthalmic preparation is available for anti-inflammatory applications.

CLINICAL PHARMACOLOGY OF THE NSAIDs

Most patients with inflammatory joint disorders benefit from aspirin when administered in sufficient doses (4 g or more) and when special attention is given to lessening gastric irritation by proper buffering. About 15% of patients develop adverse effects from aspirin; it is primarily for these patients that newer NSAIDs are indicated. As a group, these newer agents tend to cause less gastric irritation, and the dosing schedule of some is simpler (one tablet once or twice daily). In choosing an agent, it is worth remembering that the cost to the patient is $60–$200 for a 60-day supply of the newer agents compared to about $10 for generic over-the-counter aspirin. In addition, a reliable method for determining salicylate blood levels is available to establish therapeutic range, which is not true for the newer drugs. These advantages must be weighed against easier dosage schedules, better compliance, and lower incidence of gastric irritation with some of the newer agents. Surveys show that most patients with inflammatory arthritis receive NSAIDs without an adequate trial of salicylates, yet none of these newer drugs have proved more effective than aspirin in controlled studies. Moreover, although less gastrointestinal irritation has been shown for most of them, some are proving more toxic in other ways.

Because of the importance of gastric ulceration in

patients taking anti-inflammatory doses of the NSAIDs, considerable effort has gone into preventing this complication or reducing its severity. The prostaglandin E_1 analogue misoprostol inhibits gastric acid secretion at some doses and probably increases secretion of gastric mucosal protective factors such as bicarbonate as well (see Chapters 18 and 64). Misoprostol is labeled for use with NSAIDs in patients prone to development of peptic ulcers.

The newer NSAIDs have been responsible for many instances of acute renal failure and nephrotic syndrome, which develops insidiously and is neither dose-dependent nor related to duration of drug use. Patients rarely have symptoms suggestive of a hypersensitivity reaction, so the condition may go undetected until advanced.

If the decision is made to use a newer NSAID, it is important to consider adverse effects, cost, and dosing schedules. It is not possible to know which patient will respond in a specific way to which NSAID, for some patients derive benefit from one and not from another. How much of this variability of response is related to the agent per se, to individual differences in metabolism of the drug, or to a placebo effect is difficult to evaluate. When compliance is a problem, drugs such as piroxicam, naproxen, sulindac, and oxaprozin are useful because only one or two doses are required daily. If a patient is taking a hypoglycemic agent or warfarin, ibuprofen or tolmetin might be considered, since, unlike sulindac, they do not potentiate the effect of the hypoglycemic drugs or warfarin. Hypersensitivity to one of the phenylpropionic or phenylacetic acids, however, should preclude use of the others in that group. Dosing schedules listed for the drugs are those recommended by the manufacturer, but it is becoming clear that some patients require and may tolerate higher doses. Until blood level assays become available, it is probably safest to use the dosages as listed.

SLOW-ACTING ANTI-RHEUMATIC DRUGS (SAARDs)

Careful clinical and epidemiologic studies have shown that rheumatoid arthritis causes significant systemic effects that shorten life in addition to the joint disease that reduces mobility and quality of life. NSAIDs appear to offer mainly symptomatic relief; they reduce inflammation and the pain it causes but have little effect on the progression of bone and cartilage destruction. In recent years, therefore, interest has been renewed in treatments that might arrest—or at least slow—this progression by modifying the disease itself. The effects of disease-modifying drugs

(DMARDs) typically take 4 weeks to 1 year to become evident, ie, they are slow-acting compared with NSAIDs. Members of the group include immunosuppressant agents (methotrexate, azathioprine), chelators (penicillamine), antimalarials (hydroxychloroquine and chloroquine), and others. Considerable controversy surrounds the long-term efficacy of these drugs. The discovery that numerous cytokines are present in joints affected by the disease process (Table 35–2) suggests that one or more of these may be useful targets of disease-modifying drug therapy.

METHOTREXATE & OTHER IMMUNOSUPPRESSIVE DRUGS

The immunosuppressive agents (see Chapter 57) have been employed for many decades in the therapy of rheumatic diseases, but their use has been largely restricted to seriously crippling disease with reversible lesions after conventional therapy has failed. More aggressive early treatment with methotrexate has been suggested as one way of preventing the major manifestations of rheumatoid arthritis before irreversible damage occurs. Because of their toxic potential, however, immunosuppressive drugs should be employed only by physicians completely familiar with their actions. Reliable methods of selecting one drug instead of another are not available, and acceptable controlled studies demonstrating efficacy in humans are lacking for most of the drugs. However, several clinical studies suggest that of all the slow-acting antirheumatic drugs, methotrexate has the best benefit-to-risk ratio, ie, fewer patients drop out of therapy with this drug—for reasons of toxicity or lack of benefit—than with any other SAARD (Felson, 1990; Wolfe, 1990).

Immunosuppressive agents are useful in lupus nephritis, in seropositive progressive rheumatoid arthritis, and occasionally in other rheumatic diseases. They have also been shown to be effective in vasculitis syndromes, such as Wegener's granulomatosis and panarteritis. Because of the severity of toxic effects—especially the oncogenic effects, hepatotoxicity, and bone marrow depression—immunosuppressive drugs should be given only after safer agents have been tried.

Methotrexate, a dihydrofolate reductase inhibitor with potent immunosuppressive activity (see Chapter 57), is effective in rheumatoid arthritis when given in small weekly oral doses ("low-dose pulse therapy"). A maximum dose of 7.5 mg per week is recommended. Even at this low dosage, the drug has significant toxicity. Nausea and mucosal ulcers were the most common toxicities recorded in a large study comparing SAARDs in rheumatoid arthritis (Singh, 1991). Progressive dose-related hepatotoxicity in the form of enzyme changes, fibrosis, and cirrhosis affects up to 40% of patients receiving long-term methotrexate therapy. Recent evidence suggests that methotrexate toxicity can be reduced without decreasing its efficacy in rheumatoid arthritis by means of leucovorin given 24 hours after each weekly dose of methotrexate (Shiroky, 1993).

Other immunosuppressive drugs for which there is some experience in the treatment of arthritis include the alkylators mechlorethamine, cyclophosphamide, and chlorambucil and the purine antagonist azathioprine, which is FDA-approved for treatment in rheumatoid arthritis.

ANTIMALARIAL DRUGS
(Chloroquine, Hydroxychloroquine)

The pharmacology of the 4-aminoquinoline derivatives is more fully discussed in Chapter 54. Chloroquine and hydroxychloroquine have been used in the treatment of rheumatoid arthritis and systemic lupus erythematosus since the 1950s, and their efficacy in inducing remission has been confirmed in carefully controlled studies. Rheumatoid factor, a marker for disease intensity in many patients, declines after prolonged chloroquine use; however, there is no evidence that chloroquine decreases the progression of erosive bone lesions.

The mechanism of anti-inflammatory action of chloroquine and hydroxychloroquine in rheumatic disorders is unclear. They suppress the responsiveness of T lymphocytes to mitogens, decrease leukocyte chemotaxis, stabilize lysosomal membranes, inhibit DNA and RNA synthesis, and trap free radicals; one or more of these effects might be relevant. The actions of these agents are not apparent until after a latent period of 4–12 weeks. The drugs are often useful as adjuncts to treatment with NSAIDs and have no adverse interactions with other antirheumatic agents.

Indications

Antimalarials are often administered to patients with rheumatoid arthritis who have not responded optimally to salicylates and NSAIDs. In addition to their use in rheumatoid arthritis, antimalarials have been used successfully for their anti-inflammatory effect in juvenile chronic arthritis, Sjögren's syndrome, and systemic lupus erythematosus (in which they have a beneficial effect on both joint and skin findings). The antimalarial drugs should not be used in psoriatic arthritis because of the possible development of exfoliative dermatitis.

Adverse Effects

These are described in detail in Chapter 54.

Dosage

Hydroxychloroquine sulfate is the preferred drug. Initial dosage is 400 mg orally daily. Once clinical improvement is established, the dose can often be decreased to 200 mg daily.

GOLD

Gold compounds were introduced for treatment of rheumatoid arthritis in the 1920s, but it was not until 1960, in a report of a large double-blind trial, that the gold salts were shown to have a useful—though very modest—effect. Subsequent controlled studies have generally (not universally) supported the view that parenteral gold reduces symptoms and slows progression of the disease. Some studies have demonstrated that these agents retard the progression of bone and articular destruction determined roentgenographically. Further impetus to the popularity of gold salts has been the demonstration that the drug may be continued for years, allaying earlier fears of toxicity from accumulation. Nevertheless, careful analyses of the studies mentioned above have indicated numerous weaknesses in their design and have raised questions about the value of parenteral gold in rheumatoid arthritis (Epstein, 1991). A particular disadvantage of gold therapy is the high rate of discontinuance; the probability of remaining on gold therapy is less than 60% after 2 years and less than 10% after 7 years. Most of these dropouts are due to toxicity.

Introduction of an oral gold preparation (auranofin) stimulated a number of large clinical studies during the 1980s. Most of these studies suggest that this preparation has modest effects at best and that its benefits may not differ significantly from those of NSAIDs in some types of arthritis, though its toxicity is greater (Carette et al, 1989; Giannini et al, 1990).

Chemistry

The parenterally administered gold preparations are aurothiomalate and aurothioglucose. Both are administered intramuscularly as water-soluble gold salts containing 50% elemental gold. Auranofin is a substituted gold thioglucose derivative (29% gold) that can be given by mouth.

Pharmacokinetics

Gold salts are approximately 95% bound to plasma protein during transport by the blood. Although they tend to concentrate in synovial membranes, gold salts are also concentrated in the liver, kidney, spleen, adrenal glands, lymph nodes, and bone marrow. Following intramuscular injection of the parenteral forms, peak levels are reached in 2–6 hours; 40% is excreted within a week—about two-thirds in the urine and one-third in the feces. One month after intramuscular injection of 50 mg, 75–80% of the drug has been eliminated. After oral administration of auranofin, only about 25% is absorbed. Certain tissue compartments such as the epithelial cells of the renal tubules, which have a particular affinity for gold, show its presence many years after therapy has ceased. Most studies have failed to show a correlation between serum gold concentration and either therapeutic effect or toxicity.

Pharmacodynamics

The precise manner in which gold salts produce their beneficial effects in patients with rheumatoid arthritis and allied disorders is unknown. Gold alters the morphology and functional capabilities of human macrophages; this may be its major mode of action. Other effects ascribed to gold include inhibition of lysosomal enzyme activity, reduction of histamine release from mast cells, inactivation of the first component of complement, suppression of phagocytic activity of the polymorphonuclear leukocytes, and inhibition of the Shwartzman phenomenon. In addition, aurothiomalate reduces the number of circulating lymphocytes, and auranofin inhibits the release of prostaglandin E_2 from synovial cells and the release of leukotriene B_4 and leukotriene C_4 from polymorphonuclear leukocytes.

Indications & Contraindications

Gold therapy is indicated for active rheumatoid arthritis in patients who have been given an adequate trial of therapy with NSAIDs for a period of 3–4 months and continue to show active synovitis. Patients who later in the course of their disease show active inflammation and erosive changes are also candidates for gold. Patients with rheumatoid arthritis in the presence of Sjögren's syndrome and those with juvenile rheumatoid arthritis may also be considered, whereas the usefulness of gold in the treatment of psoriatic arthritis is less clear.

The major contraindications to gold are a confirmed history of previous toxicity from the drug, pregnancy, serious impairment of liver or renal function, and blood dyscrasias. Gold is not given in conjunction with penicillamine, because this chelator will remove much of the administered gold.

Adverse Effects

Approximately one-third of patients receiving gold salts experience some form of toxicity. Dermatitis, which is usually pruritic, is the most common adverse effect, occurring in 15–20% of patients. Eosinophilia may precede or be associated with cutaneous lesions. Hematologic abnormalities, including thrombocytopenia, leukopenia, and pancytopenia, occur in 1–10% of patients. Aplastic anemia, although rare, may be fatal. About 8–10% of patients develop proteinuria that may progress to nephrotic syndrome in a few cases. Other adverse effects include stomatitis, a metallic taste in the mouth, skin pigmentation, enterocolitis, cholestatic jaundice, peripheral neuropathy, pulmonary infiltrates, and corneal deposition of gold. Nitritoid reactions (sweating, faintness, flushing, and headaches) may occur, especially with gold thio-

malate, and are presumably due to the vehicle rather than the gold salts themselves. Transient aggravation of arthritis symptoms may occur after injections of gold. Gastrointestinal disturbances (especially diarrhea) and dermatitis are the most common adverse effects of oral gold therapy.

Dosage

Parenteral gold is usually given as a 50 mg dose intramuscularly weekly until a total of 1000 mg has been injected (unless there is no response by the time 600–700 mg has been given, in which case the drug can be stopped). If 1 g is given without serious adverse effects and a favorable response is observed, the drug can be continued indefinitely in lengthening intervals of 2, 3, then 4 weeks. Oral gold is given as a 6 mg dose daily, increasing to 9 mg/d if a response is not seen after 3 months. Clinical response usually requires a few months to become evident and may be delayed for as long as 4 months. Careful clinical and laboratory monitoring is mandatory.

PENICILLAMINE

Penicillamine, a metabolite of penicillin, is an analogue of the amino acid cysteine. The drug can be resolved into D and L isomers; the D form is used clinically.

$$HS-\overset{\overset{\displaystyle CH_3}{|}}{\underset{\underset{\displaystyle CH_3}{|}}{C}}-\overset{\overset{\displaystyle H}{|}}{\underset{\underset{\displaystyle NH_2}{|}}{C}}-COOH$$

Penicillamine

Pharmacokinetics

About half of an orally administered dose of penicillamine is absorbed. Absorption is enhanced if the drug is administered $1\frac{1}{2}$ hours after meals. Free penicillamine and its metabolites may be found in urine and feces. About 60% of the drug is excreted in 24 hours. No satisfactory method is available for determining blood levels.

Pharmacodynamics

The mechanism of penicillamine's action in rheumatoid arthritis is unclear. The drug suppresses arthropathy in experimental animal models and has been shown to interact with lymphocyte membrane receptors. It may interfere with the synthesis of DNA, collagen, and mucopolysaccharides. Rheumatoid factor titer falls following administration of drug, probably reflecting disruption of disulfide bonds of macroglobulins but perhaps also reflecting a basic action of the drug on the immune system. Penicillamine is similar to gold in its latency period (3–4 months) and in its anti-inflammatory properties. Like gold, it may retard the progression of bone and articular destruction.

Indications

Penicillamine is reserved for patients with active, progressive erosive rheumatoid disease not controlled by conservative therapy. Penicillamine is usually prescribed for patients who have not responded to gold therapy. Penicillamine is not useful in seronegative arthropathies. Caution is required when administering other drugs simultaneously, because penicillamine impedes absorption of many drugs and prevents them from reaching therapeutic levels.

Adverse Effects

The toxic effects of penicillamine limit its usefulness. Animal studies have shown inhibition of wound healing and evidence of muscle and blood vessel damage. In humans, adverse effects are reduced by giving lower doses and by slow progression to maintenance dosages. Proteinuria is encountered in 20% of patients. Immune complex nephritis has been seen in 4% of patients; it is often reversible when the drug is withdrawn. Leukopenia and thrombocytopenia may occur at any time and may herald aplastic anemia. Most deaths related to penicillamine are due to aplastic anemia. Skin and mucous membrane reactions, the most common adverse effects, may occur at any time during therapy and may respond to lowering the dose. Drug fever, which may be seen as an early response to penicillamine, is often associated with cutaneous eruptions.

A variety of autoimmune diseases, including myasthenia gravis, Goodpasture's syndrome, lupus erythematosus, hemolytic anemia, and thyroiditis may be seen. The drug must be discontinued permanently when any of these conditions is encountered.

Loss of taste perception or a metallic taste may develop. The blunting of taste perception relates to zinc chelation. Anorexia, nausea, and vomiting occur. Mammary hyperplasia, alopecia, and psychologic changes have also been observed.

Penicillamine is contraindicated in pregnancy and in the presence of renal insufficiency and should not be given in combination with gold, cytotoxic drugs, or phenylbutazone.

Adverse effects necessitating cessation of the drug occur in about 40% of patients. Blood counts (including platelet count) and urinalysis are performed twice a month for 4–6 months, then monthly. The drug should be stopped if the platelet count falls below 100,000/μL or the white count below 3000/μL. A history of penicillin allergy is not a contraindication to penicillamine. Patients who develop renal involvement, drug fever, autoimmune syndromes, and hematologic problems should not be rechallenged with the drug.

Dosage

Penicillamine is taken orally 1½ hours after meals. If clinical benefits are to occur, they should be apparent by 6 months. Treatment begins with 125 mg or 250 mg daily for 1–3 months; if no adverse effects are seen and improvement does not occur, the dose is doubled. If therapeutic effects are absent after 3–4 months, the dose is increased at monthly intervals up to 750 mg daily (250 mg 3 times daily), which it is rarely necessary to exceed. When therapy is discontinued after improvement, most patients relapse within 6 months.

SULFASALAZINE

Sulfasalazine, originally introduced for the treatment of ulcerative colitis, has been shown to be effective in some patients with rheumatoid arthritis. It appears to as effective as penicillamine but less likely to cause serious adverse effects (Felson, 1990). This is an unlabeled application.

Toxicity, which occurs more frequently in patients with rheumatoid arthritis than in those with ulcerative colitis, includes gastrointestinal upset, dizziness, and photosensitivity. Rarely, neutropenia may require discontinuation of the drug.

The usual dosage is 2 g/d, given in four divided doses.

LEVAMISOLE

Levamisole, a drug employed for the treatment of helminthic infections (especially with *Ascaris lumbricoides*), was found to have immunostimulant properties that led to its trial in rheumatic diseases, in which immune enhancement was considered (paradoxically) to be of potential benefit. Levamisole restored impaired cellular immune responses in arthritis induced by adjuvant injection in rats. The drug increases chemotaxis and phagocytosis of macrophages and polymorphonuclear leukocytes and appears to enhance T lymphocyte function, especially in situations where delayed hypersensitivity is impaired.

Levamisole has proved in randomized double-blind studies to be effective in rheumatoid arthritis but is unlabeled for this indication.

Rash is the most common adverse effect, but more serious toxic reactions include leukopenia, agranulocytosis, and thrombocytopenia. Influenza-like illnesses, mouth ulcers, and nausea and vomiting also occur. Reversible immune complex glomerulonephritis has been reported.

The usual dosage schedule for levamisole is 40–50 mg orally daily for the first week, increased to 80–100 mg daily for the second week and 120–150 mg daily thereafter. Like gold and penicillamine, there is a latent period of 3–4 months before clinical improvement is observed.

GLUCOCORTICOID DRUGS

The pharmacology of corticosteroids and their other applications are discussed in Chapter 38.

The effect of prednisone and other glucocorticoids on rheumatoid arthritis is prompt and dramatic. Glucocorticoids are known to inhibit phospholipase A_2, the enzyme responsible for the liberation of arachidonic acid from membrane lipids (Chapter 18). In addition, glucocorticoids have recently been shown to selectively inhibit the expression of COX II (Kujubu, 1992; Winn, 1993). However, prolonged use of these drugs leads to serious, disabling toxic effects. Corticosteroids do not alter the course of the disease, and bone and cartilage destruction continue while inflammation is decreased. Corticosteroids may be administered for certain serious extra-articular manifestations such as pericarditis or eye involvement or during periods of exacerbation. When prednisone is required for long-term therapy, the dosage should not exceed 10 mg daily, and gradual reduction of the dose should be encouraged. Alternate-day corticosteroid therapy is unsuccessful in arthritis: Patients become symptomatic on the day they do not take the drug.

Intra-articular corticosteroids are often helpful to alleviate painful symptoms and, when successful, are preferable to increasing the dosage of systemic medication.

DIETARY MANIPULATION OF INFLAMMATION

Arachidonic acid is an eicosatetraenoic acid metabolized by the cyclooxygenase and lipoxygenase pathways. In this process arachidonic acid is released from membrane phospholipids of stimulated cells and oxygenated, yielding several mediators. These mediators have potent effects on the development and function of smooth muscles, blood vessels, epithelial surfaces, secretory glands, leukocytes, and elements of the nervous system (Chapter 18).

It may be beneficial to alter or supplement a patient's diet to provide unsaturated fatty acids (such as eicosapentaenoic acid, which is found in marine fish)

similar to arachidonic acid. This dietary change causes the alternative fatty acids to be metabolized with arachidonic acid, changing the final products of the process. For example, eicosapentaenoic acid inhibits the uptake and incorporation of arachidonic acid into membrane phospholipids of some cells, and dilutes free arachidonic acid as a substrate for oxygenation. The products of eicosapentaenoic acid oxygenation are less potent than the corresponding mediators derived from arachidonic acid (sometimes by orders of magnitude), and they diminish the activities of these mediators by competing with them for shared target-cell receptors.

Ingestion of unpurified eicosapentaenoic acid by humans causes the attenuation of platelet aggregation and decreased chemotactic activity and adherence of polymorphonuclear leukocytes evoked by leukotriene B_4. The results of early clinical studies suggest that therapy with eicosapentaenoic acid decreases both morning stiffness and the number of tender joints in patients with rheumatoid arthritis and erythema associated with psoriasis. These preliminary results and the near absence of significant adverse effects suggest that dietary alteration or supplementation to provide 1–4 g/d of eicosapentaenoic acid may be a beneficial addition to conventional treatment of these conditions.

II. OTHER ANALGESICS

Acetaminophen is one of the most important drugs used for the treatment of mild to moderate pain when an anti-inflammatory effect is not necessary. Phenacetin, a prodrug that is metabolized to acetaminophen, is more toxic than its active metabolite and has no rational indications.

ACETAMINOPHEN

Acetaminophen is the metabolite of phenacetin that is responsible for its analgesic effect. It is a weak prostaglandin inhibitor in peripheral tissues and possesses no significant anti-inflammatory effects.

Pharmacokinetics

Acetaminophen is administered orally. Absorption is related to the rate of gastric emptying, and peak blood concentrations are usually reached in 30–60 minutes. Acetaminophen is slightly bound to plasma proteins and is partially metabolized by hepatic microsomal enzymes and converted to acetaminophen sulfate and glucuronide, which are pharmacologically inactive (Figure 4–4). Less than 5% is excreted unchanged. A minor but highly active metabolite (N-acetyl-*p*-benzoquinone) is important in large doses because of its toxicity to both liver and kidney. The half-life of acetaminophen is 2–3 hours and is relatively unaffected by renal function. With toxic quantities or liver disease, the half-life may be increased twofold or more.

Phenacetin
(acetophenetidin)

N-acetyl-*p*-amino-
phenol (acetaminophen)

Indications

Although equivalent to aspirin as an effective analgesic and antipyretic agent (Styrt, 1990), acetaminophen differs by its lack of anti-inflammatory properties. It does not affect uric acid levels and lacks platelet-inhibiting properties. The drug is useful in mild to moderate pain such as headache, myalgia, postpartum pain, and other circumstances in which aspirin is an effective analgesic. Acetaminophen alone is inadequate therapy for inflammatory conditions such as rheumatoid arthritis, though it may be used as an analgesic adjunct to anti-inflammatory therapy. For mild analgesia, acetaminophen is the preferred drug in patients allergic to aspirin or when salicylates are poorly tolerated. It is preferable to aspirin in patients with hemophilia or a history of peptic ulcer and in those in whom bronchospasm is precipitated by aspirin. Unlike aspirin, acetaminophen does not antagonize the effects of uricosuric agents; it may be used concomitantly with probenecid in the treatment of gout. It is preferred to aspirin in children with viral infections.

Adverse Effects

In therapeutic doses, a mild increase in hepatic enzymes may occasionally occur in the absence of jaundice: this is reversible when the drug is withdrawn. With larger doses, dizziness, excitement, and disorientation are seen. Ingestion of 15 g of acetaminophen may be fatal, death being caused by severe hepatotoxicity with central lobular necrosis, sometimes associated with acute renal tubular necrosis (Chapters 4 and 60). Early symptoms of hepatic damage include

nausea, vomiting, diarrhea, and abdominal pain. Therapy is much less satisfactory than for aspirin overdose. In addition to supportive therapy, measures that have proved extremely useful are the provision of sulfhydryl groups to neutralize the toxic metabolites. Acetylcysteine is used for this purpose (see Chapters 4 and 60).

Hemolytic anemia and methemoglobinemia, reported with the use of phenacetin, have rarely been noted with acetaminophen. Interstitial nephritis and papillary necrosis, serious complications of phenacetin, although anticipated with widespread chronic use of acetaminophen, have not occurred despite the fact that about 80% of phenacetin is rapidly metabolized to acetaminophen. Gastrointestinal bleeding does not occur. Caution should be exercised in patients with liver disease.

Dosage

Acute pain and fever may be managed by 325–500 mg 4 times daily and proportionately less for children. Steady-state conditions are attained within a day.

PHENACETIN

Phenacetin can no longer be prescribed in the USA and has been removed from many over-the-counter analgesic combinations such as Anacin and Empirin Compound. However, it is still present in a number of proprietary analgesics in this country and is in common use in many other parts of the world. The association between the excessive use of analgesic combinations—especially those that contain phenacetin—and the development of renal failure has been recognized for almost 30 years. Estimates of the percentage of patients with end-stage renal disease resulting from this kind of analgesic abuse range from 5% to 15%. After prohibition of the use of phenacetin in proprietary analgesics in Finland, Scotland, and Canada, the number of new cases of analgesic nephropathies in those countries decreased significantly.

III. DRUGS USED IN GOUT

Gout is a familial metabolic disease characterized by recurrent episodes of acute arthritis due to deposits of monosodium urate in joints and cartilage. Formation of uric acid calculi in the kidneys may also occur. Gout is associated with high serum levels of uric acid, a poorly soluble substance that is the major end product of purine metabolism. In most mammals, uricase converts uric acid to the more soluble allantoin; this enzyme is absent in humans.

The treatment of gout is aimed at relieving the acute gouty attack and preventing recurrent gouty episodes and urate lithiasis. Therapy for an attack of acute gouty arthritis is based on our current understanding of the pathophysiologic events that occur in this disease (Figure 35–5). Urate crystals are initially phagocytosed by synoviocytes, which then release prostaglandins, lysosomal enzymes, and interleukin-1. Attracted by these chemotactic mediators, polymorphonuclear leukocytes migrate into the joint space and amplify the ongoing inflammatory process. In the later phases of the attack, increased numbers of mononuclear phagocytes (macrophages) appear, ingest the urate crystals, and release more inflammatory mediators. This sequence of events suggests that the most effective agents for the management of acute urate crystal-induced inflammation are those that suppress different phases of leukocyte activation.

Before starting chronic therapy for gout, patients in whom hyperuricemia is associated with gout and urate lithiasis must be clearly distinguished from those who have only hyperuricemia. In an asymptomatic person with hyperuricemia, the efficacy of long-term drug treatment is unproved. Uric acid levels may be elevated up to 2 standard deviations above the mean for a lifetime without adverse consequences in some individuals.

COLCHICINE

Colchicine is an alkaloid isolated from the autumn crocus, *Colchicum autumnale*. Its structure is shown in Figure 35–6.

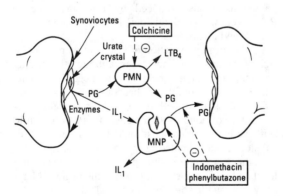

Figure 35–5. Pathophysiologic events in a gouty joint. Synoviocytes phagocytose urate crystals and then secrete inflammatory mediators, which attract and activate polymorphonuclear leukocytes *(PMN)* and mononuclear phagocytes *(MNP)* (macrophages). Drugs active in gout inhibit crystal phagocytosis and polymorphonuclear leukocyte and macrophage release of inflammatory mediators. (PG, prostaglandin; IL_1, interleukin-1; LTB_4, leukotriene B_4.)

Pharmacokinetics

Colchicine is absorbed readily after oral administration and reaches peak plasma levels within 2 hours. Metabolites of the drug are excreted in the intestinal tract and urine.

Pharmacodynamics

Colchicine dramatically relieves the pain and inflammation of gouty arthritis in 12–24 hours without altering the metabolism or excretion of urates and without other analgesic effects. Colchicine produces its anti-inflammatory effects by binding to the intracellular protein tubulin, thereby preventing its polymerization into microtubules and leading to the inhibition of leukocyte migration and phagocytosis. It also inhibits the formation of leukotriene B_4. Several of colchicine's adverse effects are produced by its inhibition of tubulin polymerization and cell mitosis.

Indications

Colchicine has been the traditional drug used for alleviating the inflammation of acute gouty arthritis. Although colchicine is more specific in gout than the NSAIDs, other agents (eg, indomethacin) are often employed because of the troublesome diarrhea associated with colchicine therapy. Colchicine is preferred for the prophylaxis of recurrent episodes of gouty arthritis, is effective in preventing attacks of acute Mediterranean fever, and may have a mild beneficial effect in sarcoid arthritis and in hepatic cirrhosis.

Adverse Effects

Colchicine often causes diarrhea and may occasionally cause nausea, vomiting, and abdominal pain. Colchicine may rarely cause hair loss and bone marrow depression as well as peripheral neuritis and myopathy.

Acute intoxication after ingestion of large (nontherapeutic) doses of the alkaloid is characterized by burning throat pain, bloody diarrhea, shock, hematuria, and oliguria. Fatal ascending central nervous system depression has been reported. Treatment is supportive.

Dosage

For terminating an attack of gout, the initial dose of colchicine is usually 0.5 or 1 mg, followed by 0.5 mg every 2 hours until pain is relieved or nausea and diarrhea appear. The total dose can be given intravenously, if necessary, but it should be remembered that as little as 8 mg in 24 hours may be fatal. The prophylactic dose of colchicine is 0.5 mg 1–3 times daily.

NSAIDs IN GOUT

In addition to inhibiting prostaglandin synthase, indomethacin and phenylbutazone also inhibit urate

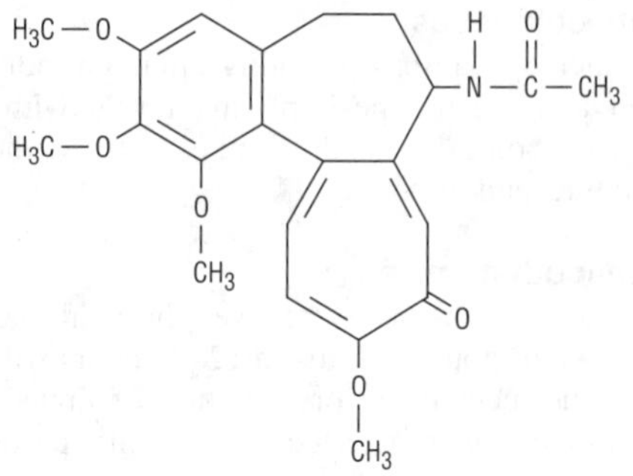

Colchicine

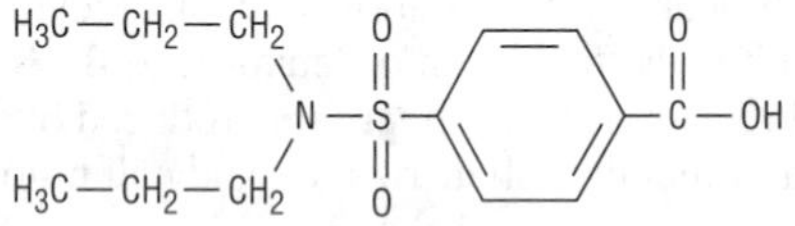

Probenecid

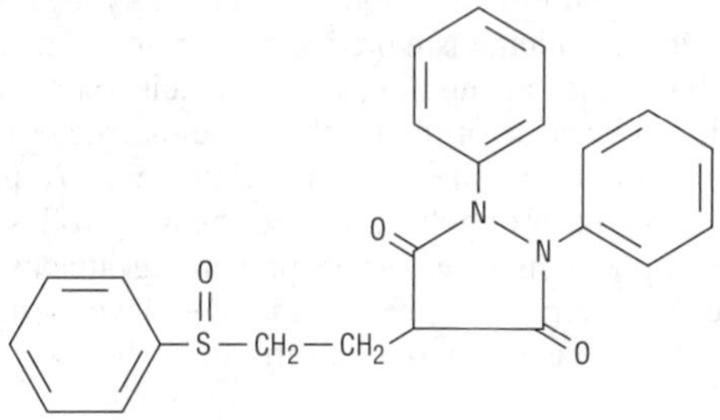

Sulfinpyrazone

Figure 35–6. Colchicine and uricosuric drugs.

crystal phagocytosis. Indomethacin may be used as initial treatment of gout or as an alternative drug when colchicine is unsuccessful or causes too much discomfort. Indomethacin is the agent most often used today to treat acute gout. Three to four doses of 50 mg every 6 hours are given; when a response occurs the dosage is reduced to 25 mg 3 or 4 times daily for about 5 days.

Phenylbutazone also is effective in the treatment of acute attacks of gout. Because the drug is used for a few days only, the serious adverse effects of phenylbutazone are rarely a problem in this application. The usual initial dose is 400 mg followed by 200 mg every 6 hours until the attack subsides. Phenylbutazone should not be continued after 3 days.

Other newer NSAIDs are also being used with success in the acute episode. Ibuprofen in doses of 2400 mg daily has alleviated attacks. These agents appear to be as effective and safe as the older drugs.

URICOSURIC AGENTS

Probenecid and sulfinpyrazone are uricosuric drugs employed to decrease the body pool of urate in patients with tophaceous gout or in those with increasingly frequent gouty attacks. In a patient who excretes large amounts of uric acid, the uricosuric agents should be avoided so as not to precipitate the formation of uric acid calculi.

Chemistry

Uricosuric drugs are organic acids (Figure 35–6) and, as such, act at the anion transport sites of the renal tubule (Chapter 15). Sulfinpyrazone is a metabolite of an analogue of phenylbutazone.

Pharmacokinetics

Probenecid is completely reabsorbed by the renal tubules and is metabolized very slowly. Sulfinpyrazone or its active hydroxylated derivative is rapidly excreted by the kidneys. Even so, the duration of its effect after oral administration is almost as long as that of probenecid.

Pharmacodynamics

Uric acid is freely filtered at the glomerulus. Like many other weak acids, it is also both reabsorbed and secreted in the middle segment of the proximal tubule. Uricosuric drugs—probenecid, sulfinpyrazone, and large doses of aspirin—affect these active transport sites so that net reabsorption of uric acid in the proximal tubule is decreased. Because aspirin in small (analgesic or antipyretic) doses causes net retention of uric acid by inhibiting the secretory transporter, it should not be used for analgesia in patients with gout. The secretion of other weak acids, eg, penicillin, is also reduced by uricosuric agents. Probenecid was originally developed to prolong penicillin blood levels.

As the urinary excretion of uric acid increases, the size of the urate pool decreases, although the plasma concentration may not be greatly reduced. In patients who respond favorably, tophaceous deposits of urate will be reabsorbed, with relief of arthritis and remineralization of bone. With the ensuing increase in uric acid excretion, a predisposition to the formation of renal stones is augmented rather than decreased; therefore, the urine volume should be maintained at a high level and at least early in treatment the urine pH kept above 6.0 by the administration of alkali.

Indications

Uricosuric therapy should be initiated if several acute attacks of gouty arthritis have occurred, when evidence of tophi appears, or when plasma levels of uric acid in patients with gout are so high that tissue damage is almost inevitable. Therapy should not be started until 2–3 weeks after an acute attack.

Adverse Effects

Adverse effects do not provide a basis for preferring one or the other of the uricosuric agents. Both of these organic acids cause gastrointestinal irritation, but sulfinpyrazone is more active in this regard. Probenecid is more likely to cause allergic dermatitis, but a rash may appear after the use of either compound. Nephrotic syndrome has resulted from the use of probenecid. Both sulfinpyrazone and probenecid may (though rarely) cause aplastic anemia.

Contraindications & Cautions

It is essential to maintain a large urine volume to minimize the possibility of stone formation.

Dosage

Probenecid is usually started at a dosage of 0.5 g orally daily in divided doses, progressing to 1 g daily after 1 week. Sulfinpyrazone is started at a dosage of 200 mg orally daily, progressing to 400–800 mg daily. It should be given in divided doses with food to reduce adverse gastrointestinal effects.

ALLOPURINOL

An alternative to increasing uric acid excretion in the treatment of gout is to reduce its synthesis by inhibiting xanthine oxidase with allopurinol.

Chemistry

The structure of allopurinol, an isomer of hypoxanthine, is shown in Figure 35–7.

Pharmacokinetics

Allopurinol is approximately 80% absorbed after oral administration. Like uric acid, allopurinol is itself metabolized by xanthine oxidase. The resulting compound, alloxanthine, retains the capacity to inhibit xanthine oxidase and has a long enough duration of action so that allopurinol need be given only once a day.

Pharmacodynamics

Dietary purines are not an important source of uric acid. The quantitatively important amounts of purine are formed from amino acids, formate, and carbon dioxide in the body. Those purine ribonucleotides not incorporated into nucleic acids and those derived from the degradation of nucleic acids are converted to xanthine or hypoxanthine and oxidized to uric acid (Figure 35–7). When this last step is inhibited by allopurinol, there is a fall in the plasma urate level and a decrease in the size of the urate pool with a concurrent rise in the more soluble xanthine and hypoxanthine.

Indications

Treatment of gout with allopurinol, as with uricosuric agents, is begun with the expectation that it will be continued for years if not for life. Allopurinol for the treatment of gout is indicated in the following circumstances: (1) in chronic tophaceous gout, in which reabsorption of tophi is more rapid than with uricosuric agents; (2) in patients with gout whose 24-hour urinary uric acid on purine-free diet exceeds 1.1 g; (3) when probenecid or sulfinpyrazone cannot be used because of adverse effects or allergic reactions, or when they are providing less than optimal therapeutic effect; (4) for recurrent renal stones; (5) in patients with renal functional impairment; or (6) when serum urate levels are grossly elevated. One should attempt

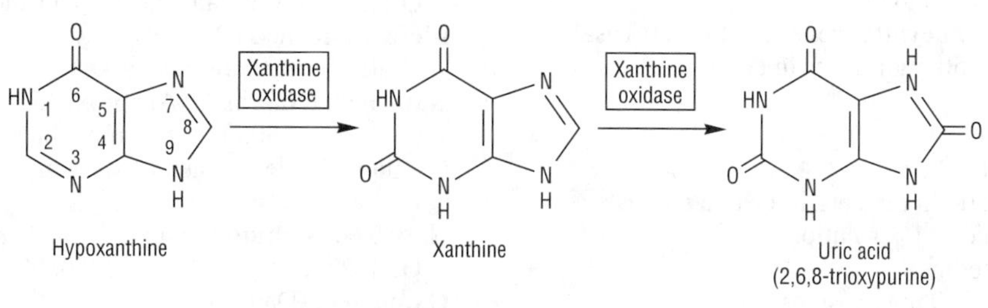

Figure 35–7. Inhibition of uric acid synthesis by allopurinol. (Modified and reproduced, with permission, from Meyers FH, Jawetz E, Goldfien A: *Review of Medical Pharmacology,* 7th ed. Lange, 1980.)

to lower serum urate levels to less than 6.5 mg/dL. Aside from gout, allopurinol is used as an antiprotozoal (Chapter 54) and is indicated to prevent the massive uricosuria following therapy of blood dyscrasias that could otherwise lead to renal calculi.

Adverse Effects

Acute attacks of gouty arthritis occur early in treatment with allopurinol when urate crystals are being withdrawn from the tissues and plasma levels are below normal. To prevent acute attacks, colchicine should be given during the initial period of therapy with allopurinol unless allopurinol is being used in combination with probenecid or sulfinpyrazone. Gastrointestinal intolerance, including nausea, vomiting, and diarrhea, may occur. Peripheral neuritis and necrotizing vasculitis, depression of bone marrow elements, and, rarely, aplastic anemia may also occur. Hepatic toxicity and interstitial nephritis have been reported. An allergic skin reaction characterized by pruritic maculopapular lesions develops in 3% of patients. Isolated cases of exfoliative dermatitis have been reported. Allopurinol may become bound to the lens, resulting in cataracts.

Interactions & Cautions

When chemotherapeutic mercaptopurines are being given concomitantly, their dose must be reduced to about 25%. Allopurinol may also increase the effect of cyclophosphamide. Allopurinol inhibits the metabolism of probenecid and oral anticoagulants and may increase hepatic iron concentration. Safety in children and during pregnancy has not been established.

Dosage

The initial dose of allopurinol is 100 mg daily. A daily dose of 300 mg is reached in 3 weeks and is adequate for most patients.

Colchicine or indomethacin should be given during the first weeks of allopurinol therapy to prevent the gouty arthritis episodes that sometimes occur.

PREPARATIONS AVAILABLE

Salicylates

Aspirin, acetylsalicylic acid (generic, A.S.A. Enseals, Easprin, others)
Oral (regular or enteric coated): 65, 81, 324, 325, 486, 500 mg tablets; 325, 500 mg capsules; 650, 800 mg timed-release tablets
Rectal: 60, 120, 125, 130, 195, 200, 300, 325, 600, 650, 1200 mg suppositories
Choline salicylate (Arthropan)
Oral: 870 mg/5 mL liquid
Diflunisal (Dolobid)
Oral: 250, 500 mg tablets
Magnesium salicylate (Doan's Pills, Magan, Mobidin)
Oral: 325, 545, 600 mg tablets
Salsalate, salicylsalicylic acid (generic, Disalcid)
Oral: 500, 750 mg tablets; 500 mg capsules
Sodium salicylate (generic, Uracel 5)
Oral: 324, 325, 650 mg tablets; 325, 650 mg enteric coated tablets
Sodium thiosalicylate (generic, Thiocyl, Tusal)
Parenteral: 50 mg/mL for injection

Newer NSAIDs

Diclofenac (Voltaren)
Oral: 25, 50, 75 mg enteric-coated tablets
Ophthalmic: 0.1% solution
Etodolac (Lodine)
Oral: 200, 300 mg capsules
Fenoprofen (Nalfon)
Oral: 200, 300, 600 mg capsules; 600 mg tablets
Flurbiprofen (Ansaid, Froben, Ocufen)
Oral: 50, 100 mg tablets
Ophthalmic: 0.03% solution
Ibuprofen (generic, Motrin, Rufen, Advil [OTC], Nuprin [OTC], others)
Oral: 200, 300, 400, 600, 800 mg tablets
Indomethacin (generic, Indocin, others)
Oral: 10, 25, 50, 75 mg capsules; 75 mg sustained-release capsules; 25 mg/5 mL suspension
Rectal: 50 mg suppositories
Ketoprofen (Orudis)
Oral: 25, 50, 75 mg capsules
Ketorolac (Toradol)
Oral: 10 mg tablets
Parenteral: 15, 30 mg/mL for IM injection
Ophthalmic: 0.5% solution
Meclofenamate sodium (generic, Meclomen)
Oral: 50, 100 mg tablets and capsules
Mefenamic acid (Ponstel)
Oral: 250 mg capsules
Naproxen (Naprosyn, Anaprox, Aleve [OTC])
Oral: 200, 250, 375, 500 mg tablets; 550 mg sustained release tablets; 125 mg/5 mL suspension
Naproxen sodium (Anaprox)
Oral: 275, 550 mg tablets (250, 500 mg base)
Oxaprozin (Daypro)
Oral: 600 mg tablets

Phenylbutazone (generic, Butazolidin, Azolid)
Oral: 100 mg tablets and capsules
Piroxicam (Feldene)
Oral: 10, 20 mg capsules
Sulindac (Clinoril)
Oral: 150, 200 mg tablets
Tolmetin (Tolectin)
Oral: 200, 600 mg tablets; 400 mg capsules

Slow-Acting Anti-inflammatory Agents
Auranofin (Ridaura)
Oral: 3 mg capsules
Aurothioglucose (Solganal)
Parenteral: 50 mg/mL suspension for injection
Gold sodium thiomalate (Myochrysine)
Parenteral: 25, 50 mg/mL for injection
Hydroxychloroquine (Plaquenil)
Oral: 200 mg tablets
Methotrexate (generic, Rheumatrex)
Oral: 2.5 mg tablets
Penicillamine (Cuprimine, Depen)
Oral: 125, 250 mg capsules; 250 mg tablets
Sulfasalazine (generic, Azulfidine)

Oral: 500 mg tablets, 500 mg enteric coated tablets, 250 mg/5 mL oral suspension

Drugs Used in Gout
Allopurinol (generic, Zyloprim, others)
Oral: 100, 300 mg tablets
Colchicine (generic)
Oral: 0.5, 0.6 mg tablets
Parenteral: 1 mg/2 mL for injection
Probenecid (generic, Benemid, Probalan)
Oral: 500 mg tablets
Sulfinpyrazone (generic, Anturane)
Oral: 100 mg tablets; 200 mg capsules

Acetaminophen
Acetaminophen (generic, Tylenol, Tempra, Panadol, Acephen, Acetaminophen, Uniserts, others)
Oral: 325, 500 mg tablets and capsules; 650 mg tablets; 120, 160, 325 mg/5 mL elixir; 500 mg/15 mL elixir; 100 mg/mL solution; 120 mg/2.5 mL solution
Rectal: 120, 125, 325, 600, 650 mg suppositories

REFERENCES

General

Chandrasoma P, Taylor CR: *Concise Pathology,* 2nd ed. Appleton & Lange, 1994.

Harris ED, Jr: Rheumatoid arthritis. Pathophysiology and implications for therapy. N Engl J Med 1990;322:1277.

Hellman DB: Arthritis and musculoskeletal disorders. In: *Current Medical Diagnosis & Treatment 1994.* Tierney LM, McPhee ST, Papadakis MA (editors). Appleton & Lange, 1994.

Kidd BL et al: Neurogenic influences in arthritis. Ann Rheum Dis 1990;49:649.

Shiroky JB et al: Experimental basis of innovative therapies of rheumatoid arthritis. In: *Therapy of Autoimmune Diseases* Cruse JM, Lewis RE Jr (editors). Karger, 1989.

Singh G et al: Toxicity profiles of disease modifying antirheumatic drugs in rheumatoid arthritis. J Rheumatol 1991;18:188.

Starkebaum G: Review of rheumatoid arthritis: Recent developments. Immunol Allergy Clin North Am 1993; 13:273.

Symposium: Arachidonic acid metabolism and inflammation. Therapeutic implications. Drugs 1987;33 (Suppl):1.

Tsokos GC: Immunomodulatory treatment in patients with rheumatic diseases: Mechanisms of action. Semin Arthritis Rheum 1987;17:24.

Vane J, Botting R: Inflammation and the mechanism of action of anti-inflammatory drugs. FASEB J 1987; 1:89.

Walson PD, Mortensen ME: Pharmacokinetics of common analgesics, anti-inflammatories and antipyretics in children. Clin Pharmacokinet 1989;17(Suppl 1): 116.

Wilkens RF: New perspectives of secondary and tertiary therapy for rheumatoid arthritis. Drugs 1989;37:739.

Williams KM, Day RO, Briet SN: Biochemical actions and clinical pharmacology of anti-inflammatory drugs. Adv Drug Res 1993;24:121.

Salicylates

Chew EY et al: Aspirin effects on the development of cataracts in patients with diabetes mellitus. Early treatment diabetic retinopathy study report 16. Arch Ophthalmol 1992;110:339.

Gordon IJ et al: Algorithm for modified alkaline diuresis in salicylate poisoning. Br Med J 1984;289:1039.

Henry J, Volans G: ABC of poisoning. Analgesic poisoning: I Salicylates. Br Med J 1984;289:820.

Hurwitz ES et al: Public Health Service Study of Reye's syndrome and medications. Report of the main study. JAMA 1987;257:1905.

Hurwitz ES: Reye's syndrome. Epidemiologic Rev 1989; 11:249.

Ivey KJ: Gastrointestinal intolerance and bleeding with non-narcotic analgesics. Drugs 1986;32(Suppl 4):71.

Miners JO: Drug interactions involving aspirin (acetylsalicylic acid) and salicylic acid. Clin Pharmacokinet 1989;17:327.

Pedersen AK, Fitzgerald GA: Dose-related kinetics of aspirin: Presystemic acetylation of platelet cyclooxygenase. N Engl J Med 1984;311:1206.

Schiff E et al: The use of aspirin to prevent pregnancy-induced hypertension and lower the ratio of thromboxane A_2 to prostacyclin in relatively high risk pregnancies. N Engl J Med 1989;321:351.

Steering Committee of The Physicians' Health Study Research Group: Final report on the aspirin component of the ongoing physicians' health study. N Engl J Med 1989;321:129.

Thun MJ, Namboodiri MM, Heath CW Jr: Aspirin use and reduced risk of fatal colon cancer. N Engl J Med 1991;325:1593.

van Heyningen R, Harding JJ: Do aspirin-like analgesics protect against cataract? Lancet 1986;1:1111.

Other Nonsteroidal Drugs (NSAIDs)

Bonney SL et al: Renal safety of two analgesics used over the counter: ibuprofen and aspirin. Clin Pharmacol Ther 1986;40:373.

Chan WY: Prostaglandins and nonsteroidal anti-inflammatory drugs in dysmenorrhea. Annu Rev Pharmacol Toxicol 1983;23:131.

Douidar SM, Richardson J, Snodgrass WR: Role of indomethacin in ductus closure: An update evaluation. Dev Pharmacol Ther 1988;11:196.

Meade EA, Smith WL, DeWitt DL: Differential inhibition of prostaglandin endoperoxide synthase (cyclooxygenase) isozymes by aspirin and other nonsteroidal anti-inflammatory drugs. J Biol Chem 1993; 268:6610.

Morales WJ et al: Efficacy and safety of indomethacin versus ritodrine in the management of preterm labor: A randomized study. Obstet Gynecol 1989;74:567.

Murray MD, Brater DC: Renal toxicity of the nonsteroidal anti-inflammatory drugs. Annu Rev Pharmacol Toxicol 1993;32:435.

Norton ME et al: Neonatal complications after the administration of indomethacin for preterm labor. N Engl J Med 1993;329:1602.

Paulus HE, Furst DE: Aspirin and other non-steroidal anti-inflammatory drugs. In: *Arthritis and Allied Conditions,* 10th ed. McCarty DJ (editor). Lea & Febiger, 1985.

Rainsford KD: Novel non-steroidal anti-inflammatory drugs. Bailliere's Clin Rheumatol 1988;2:485.

Roth SH: Misoprostol in the prevention of NSAID-induced gastric ulcer: A multicenter, double-blind, placebo-controlled trial. J Rheumatol 1990;17(Suppl 20):20.

Verbeeck RK: Pharmacokinetic drug interactions with nonsteroidal anti-inflammatory drugs. Clin Pharmacokinet 1990;19:44.

Eicosapentaenoic Acid

Kremer JM et al: Effects of manipulation of dietary fatty acids on clinical manifestations of rheumatoid arthritis. Lancet 1985;1:184.

Lee TH et al: Effect of dietary enrichment with eicosapentaenoic and docosahexaenoic acids on in vitro neutrophil and monocyte leukotriene generation and neutrophil function. N Engl J Med 1985;312:1217.

Maurice PDL et al: Effects of dietary supplementation with eicosapentaenoic acid in patients with psoriasis. In: *Advances in Prostaglandin, Thromboxane, and Leukotriene Research.* Samuelsson B, Paoletti R, Ramwell P (editors). Raven Press, 1987.

Slow-Acting Anti-inflammatory Drugs & Glucocorticoids

Arend WP, Dayer J-M: Cytokines and cytokine inhibitors or antagonists in rheumatoid arthritis. Arthritis Rheum 1990;33:305.

Arnold M, Schreiber L, Brooks P: Immunosuppressive drugs and corticosteroids in the treatment of rheumatoid arthritis. Drugs 1988;36:340.

Barnes PJ, Adcock I: Anti-inflammatory actions of steroids: Molecular mechanisms. Trends Pharmacol Sci 1993;14:436.

Carette S et al: A double blind placebo-controlled study of auranofin in patients with psoriatic arthritis. Arthritis Rheum 1989;32:158.

Cash JM, Klippel JH: Second-line drug therapy for rheumatoid arthritis. N Engl J Med 1994;330:1368.

Epstein WV et al: Effect of parenterally administered gold therapy on the course of adult rheumatoid arthritis. Ann Intern Med 1991;114:437.

Felson DT, Anderson JJ, Meenan RF: The comparative efficacy and toxicity of second-line drugs in rheumatoid arthritis: Results of two metaanalyses. Arthritis Rheum 1990;33:1449.

Fox DA, McCune WJ: Immunologic and clinical effects of cytotoxic drugs used in the treatment of rheumatoid arthritis and systemic lupus erythematosus. Concepts Immunopathol 1989;7:20.

Fries JF et al: The relative toxicity of disease-modifying antirheumatic drugs. Arthritis Rheum 1993;36:297.

Furst DE: Rational use of disease-modifying antirheumatic drugs. Drugs 1990;39:19.

Giannini EH et al: Auranofin in the treatment of juvenile rheumatoid arthritis. Results of the USA-USSR double blind, placebo-controlled trial. Arthritis Rheum 1990;33:466.

Hurst NP et al: Chloroquine and hydroxychloroquine inhibit multiple sites in metabolic pathways leading to neutrophil superoxide release. J Rheumatol 1988;15: 23.

Iannuzzi L et al: Does drug therapy slow radiographic deterioration in rheumatoid arthritis? N Engl J Med 1983;309:1023.

Kremer JM, Phelps CT: Long-term prospective study of the use of methotrexate in the treatment of rheumatoid arthritis. Update after a mean of 90 months. Arthritis Metab 1992;35:138.

Kujubu DA, Herschman HR: Dexamethasone inhibits the mitogen induction of TIS10 prostaglandin synthase/cyclooxygenase gene. J Biol Chem 1992;267:7991.

Lipsky PE: Remission-inducing therapy in rheumatoid arthritis. Am J Med 1983;75(Suppl 4B):40.

Sharp JT, Lidsky MD, Duffy J: Clinical responses during gold therapy for rheumatoid arthritis: Changes in synovitis, radiologically detectable erosive lesions, serum proteins, and serologic abnormalities. Arthritis Rheum 1982;25:540.

Shiroky JB et al: Low-dose methotrexate with leucovorin (folinic acid) in the management of rheumatoid arthritis. Results of a multicenter randomized, double-blind, placebo-controlled trial. Arthritis Rheum 1993; 36:795.

Tugwell P, Bennett R, Gent M: Methotrexate in rheumatoid arthritis. Ann Int Med 1987;107:358.

Weinblatt ME et al: Efficacy of low-dose methotrexate in rheumatoid arthritis. N Engl J Med 1985;312: 818.

Winn VD, O'Banion MK, Young DA: Anti-inflammatory action: inhibition of griPGHS, a new cyclooxygenase. J Lipid Mediators 1993;6:101.

Wolfe F, Hawley DJ, Cathey MA: Termination of slow acting antirheumatic therapy in rheumatoid arthritis: A 14-year prospective evaluation of 1017 consecutive starts. J Rheumatol 1990;17:994.

Yocum DE et al: Cyclosporin A in severe, treatment-refractory rheumatoid arthritis. A randomized study. Ann Int Med 1988;109:863.

Other Analgesics

Black M: Acetaminophen hepatotoxicity. Annu Rev Med 1984;35:577.

Linden CH, Rumack BH: Acetaminophen overdose. Emerg Med Clin North Am 1984;2:103.

Styrt B, Sugarman B: Antipyresis and fever. Arch Intern Med 1990;150:1589.

Drugs Used in Gout

Famey JP: Colchicine in therapy: State of the art and new perspectives for an old drug. Clin Exp Rheum 1988; 6:305.

Lerman S, Megaw JM, Gardner K: Allopurinol therapy and cataract progenesis in humans. Am J Ophthalmol 1982;94:141.

Pascual E, Castellano JA: Treatment with colchicine decreases white cell counts in synovial fluid of asymptomatic knees that contain monosodium urate crystals. J Rheumatol 1992;19:600.

Star VL, Hochberg MC: Prevention and management of gout. Drugs 1993;45:212.

Terkeltaub RA: Gout and mechanisms of crystal-induced inflammation. Curr Opinion Rheumatol 1993;5:510.

Section VII.
Endocrine Drugs

Hypothalamic & Pituitary Hormones

36

David C. Klonoff, MD, & John H. Karam, MD

Neuroendocrine control of metabolism, growth, and certain aspects of reproduction is mediated by a combination of neural and endocrine systems located in the hypothalamus and pituitary gland. The pituitary gland weighs an average of about 0.6 g and rests in the bony sella turcica under a layer of dura mater. It is connected to the overlying hypothalamus by a stalk containing neurosecretory fibers surrounded by a complex of blood vessels, including a portal venous system that drains the hypothalamus and perfuses the anterior pituitary.

The pituitary gland consists of an anterior lobe (adenohypophysis), an intermediate lobe, and a posterior lobe (neurohypophysis), which under hypothalamic influence release a number of hormones that either control the secretion of other endocrine glands or affect the metabolic actions of target tissues directly.

The secretion of anterior lobe hormones is regulated by hormones formed in the median eminence of the hypothalamus and carried to the adenohypophysis by the hypothalamic-hypophysial portal venous system (Table 36–1). These hormones are small peptides that function as releasing or inhibiting hormones. The structures of several of these peptides have been determined, thus permitting the synthesis of the natural hormones as well as of experimentally modified forms.

The posterior lobe hormones are synthesized in the hypothalamus and transported via the neurosecretory fibers in the stalk of the pituitary to the posterior lobe, from which they are released into the circulation.

The hormones of the intermediate lobe have melanocyte-stimulating properties that are important in animals that utilize skin color changes as adaptive mechanisms. They have not been identified as discrete hormones in humans and therefore have no role at present in clinical pharmacology.

Therapeutic preparations of pituitary and hypothalamic peptide hormones are usually synthetic; a few are purified from human sources or produced in mi-

ACRONYMS USED IN THIS CHAPTER	
ACTH	Adrenocorticotrophic hormone
CRH	Corticotropin-releasing hormone
FSH	Follicle-stimulating hormone
GH	Growth hormone
GHRH	Growth hormone-releasing hormone
GnRH	Gonadotropin-releasing hormone
LH	Luteinizing hormone
LHRH	Luteinizing hormone-releasing hormone
β-LPH	Beta-lipoprotein
PIH	Prolactin-inhibiting hormone (dopamine)
PRH	Prolactin-releasing hormone
PRL	Prolactin
SRIH	Somatotropin-release-inhibiting hormone (somatostatin)
T_4	Thyroxine
TRH	Thyrotropin-releasing hormone (protirelin)
TSH	Thyroid-stimulating hormone (thyrotropin)

croorganisms through recombinant DNA technology. Their applications lie in three areas: (1) as replacement therapy for hormone deficiency states; (2) as drug therapy for a variety of disorders using pharmacologic doses to elicit a hormonal effect that is not present at physiologic blood levels; and (3) as diagnostic tools for performing stimulation tests to diagnose hypo- or hyperfunctional endocrine states.

Table 36–1. Links between hypothalamic, pituitary, and target gland hormones.[1]

Hypothalamic Hormone	Pituitary Hormone	Target Organ	Target Organ Hormone
Growth hormone-releasing hormone (GHRH)(+)	Growth hormone (somatotropin) (GH)(+)	Liver	Somatomedins
Somatotropin release-inhibiting hormone (SRIH, somatostatin)(−)			
Corticotropin-releasing hormone (CRH) (+)	Adrenocorticotropin (ACTH) (+)	Adrenal cortex	Glucocorticoids, mineralocorticoids, androgens
Thyrotropin-releasing hormone (TRH)(+)	Thyroid-stimulating hormone (TSH)(+)	Thyroid	Thyroxine (T_4), triiodothyronine (T_3)
Gonadotropin-releasing hormone (GnRH or LHRH)(+)	Follicle-stimulating hormone (FSH) (+)	Gonads	Estrogen, progesterone, testosterone
	Luteinizing hormone (LH)(+)		
Prolactin-releasing hormone (PRH)(+)	Prolactin (PRL)(+)	Lymphocytes	Lymphokines
Prolactin-inhibiting hormone (PIH, dopamine)(−)		Breast	

[1](+) = stimulant; (−) = inhibitor.

HYPOTHALAMIC & ANTERIOR PITUITARY HORMONES

Hypothalamic regulatory hormones that have been identified and (in most cases) synthesized include growth hormone-releasing hormone (GHRH), a growth hormone-inhibiting hormone (somatostatin), thyrotropin-releasing hormone (TRH), corticotropin-releasing hormone (CRH), gonadotropin-releasing hormone (GnRH), also called luteinizing hormone-releasing hormone (LHRH), a prolactin-releasing hormone (PRH), and prolactin-inhibiting hormone (PIH, now believed to be dopamine).

Six anterior pituitary hormones are recognized: growth hormone (GH), thyrotropin (TSH), adrenocorticotropin (ACTH), follicle-stimulating hormone (FSH), luteinizing hormone (LH), and prolactin (PRL). Another polypeptide, beta-lipotropin (β-LPH), is derived from the same prohormone, pro-opiomelanocortin, as adrenocorticotropin. Beta-lipotropin is secreted from the pituitary along with adrenocorticotropin, but its hormonal function is unknown. It is a precursor of the opioid polypeptide beta-endorphin (see Chapter 30).

The release of hypothalamic releasing hormones is influenced by many factors. Depending on the particular hormone, these may include impulses from the cerebrum, stress, temperature, and drugs. Certain hormones from the thyroid, adrenal cortex, and gonads inhibit hypophysial-pituitary release of their respective tropic hormones in a negative feedback loop, while neurotransmitters such as serotonin, norepinephrine, and dopamine directly influence the secretion of the hypothalamic hormones by the peptidergic neurons of the median eminence.

In the discussion below, the hypothalamic control peptides are paired with their pituitary target hormones in the order in which they are listed in Table 36–1.

GROWTH HORMONE-RELEASING HORMONE (GHRH) (Sermorelin)

Growth hormone-releasing hormone is the hypothalamic hormone that stimulates pituitary production of growth hormone (GH).

Chemistry & Pharmacokinetics

A. Structure: In 1982, separate laboratories isolated a 40-amino-acid peptide and a carboxyl terminal longer sequence with 44 amino acids, both of which stimulated GH release. The activity of the molecule was found to reside in the first 29 amino acids. $GHRH_{40}$, $GHRH_{44}$, and analogues of $GHRH_{29}$ have all been investigated.

B. Absorption, Metabolism, and Excretion: GHRH may be administered intravenously, subcutaneously, or intranasally, and the relative potencies (defined as incremental growth hormone release) by these three routes are 300, 10, and 1, respectively. Intravenous GHRH has a half-life of 7 minutes.

Pharmacodynamics

GHRH stimulates anterior pituitary secretion only of growth hormone. With continuous somatotroph stimulation by GHRH, the secretion of growth hormone is preserved without receptor down-regulation.

Clinical Pharmacology

A. Diagnostic Uses: The growth hormone response to GHRH infusion can be used to evaluate short children with subnormal GH responses to conventional stimuli such as insulin-induced hypoglycemia, oral levodopa, or intravenous arginine. In such children, a normal response suggests GH deficiency due to hypothalamic dysfunction. A subnormal response may occur with dysfunction of either the pituitary or the hypothalamus. A rise in the growth hormone level demonstrates the ability of the somatotroph to produce GH and predicts a favorable response to GHRH therapy. In surgically treated acromegalic patients there is evidence that an absent growth hormone response to GHRH may predict a cure.

B. Experimental Therapeutic Uses: A growth hormone-deficient patient whose pituitary somatotrophs are responsive to GHRH could be a candidate for GHRH therapy. Potential advantages of GHRH over growth hormone for selected growth hormone-deficient patients include preservation of feedback on the pituitary, possible restoration of normal pituitary regulation leading to improved growth even after treatment, and the theoretically lower cost of synthesizing GHRH, which is a much smaller molecule than growth hormone. Factors favoring growth hormone include the need for certainty in selecting growth hormone-deficient children who can respond to GHRH as well as the inconvenience of multiple daily GHRH injections compared with daily or alternate-day growth hormone injections. There are insufficient data comparing these two treatments.

Preparations & Dosage

A single intravenous injection of $GHRH_{1-29}$, 1 µg/kg, with growth hormone measurements at 0, 15, 30, 45, and 60 minutes, will determine the somatotroph's ability to produce growth hormone. A normal response does not exclude growth hormone deficiency, because such a deficiency is frequently due to hypothalamic dysfunction with intact somatotrophic function. GHRH for therapy is investigational. An effective dose is 2–5 µg/kg subcutaneously every 3–12 hours.

Toxicity

There may be facial flushing or injection site pain.

SOMATOSTATIN
(Growth Hormone-Inhibiting
Hormone, Somatotropin Release-
Inhibiting Hormone)

Somatostatin, a tetradecapeptide, has been isolated from the hypothalamus and other parts of the central nervous system. It has been sequenced (Figure 36–1) and synthesized. This substance has been shown to inhibit growth hormone release in response to a wide variety of stimuli in normal individuals. It produces a decrease in circulating insulin levels and interferes

with the ability of thyrotropin-releasing hormone to cause thyrotropin release. Somatostatin has also been identified in the pancreas and other sites in the gastrointestinal tract. It has been shown to inhibit the release of glucagon, insulin, and gastrin.

The actions of somatostatin occur at the cell membrane. Molecular cloning has revealed the presence of four structurally related integral membrane glycoproteins that are high-affinity somatostatin receptors (Bell, 1993).

A 28-amino-acid peptide called prosomatostatin isolated from intestine and hypothalamus is believed to be the precursor of somatostatin. It is ten times more potent than somatostatin in inhibiting insulin secretion in rats, but its effect on glucagon secretion is only twice that of somatostatin. Its greater potency and prolonged action make prosomatostatin more useful than somatostatin in testing hormonal control mechanisms.

Exogenously administered somatostatin is rapidly cleared from the circulation, with an initial half-life of 1–3 minutes. The kidney appears to play an important role in its metabolism and excretion.

Somatostatin can effectively inhibit growth hormone release in patients with acromegaly. However, it is of no use in the treatment of this disorder because of its lack of specificity and short duration of action. Octreotide has a longer half-life and is used instead of somatostatin.

Peptides have been synthesized that partially separate the various properties of somatostatin. A 7-aminoheptanoic acid derivative containing only four of the 14 amino acids of somatostatin has been found to block the effect of somatostatin.

Clinical Pharmacology
of Octreotide
(Somatostatin Analogue, SMS 201–995)

The tetradecapeptide somatostatin has limited therapeutic usefulness because of its short duration of action and its multiple effects on many secretory systems. Among several analogues developed, octreotide has been the most effective in management of a variety of clinical disorders (Figure 36–1).

Octreotide is 45 times more potent than somato-

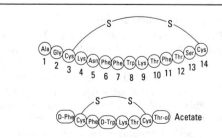

Figure 36–1. *Above:* Amino acid sequence of somatostatin. *Below:* Sequence of the synthetic analogue, octreotide (SMS 201-995).

statin in inhibiting growth hormone release in intact subjects but only twice as potent in reducing insulin secretion. Because of this relatively reduced effect on pancreatic B cells, octreotide has been particularly useful in treating acromegaly and other hormone-secreting tumor disorders without provoking hyperglycemia due to reduced insulin concentrations. The much greater potency of octreotide as compared with somatostatin is not due to differences in affinity for somatostatin receptors. Rather, it appears to be due to octreotide's much lower clearance rate and longer half-life. The plasma elimination half-life of octreotide is about 80 minutes, ie, 30 times longer in humans than the half-life of somatostatin. The difference between somatostatin and octreotide in their GH suppression:insulin suppression ratios has not been explained.

Octreotide, in doses of 50–100 μg given subcutaneously every 12 hours, has been reported to reduce symptoms of a variety of hormone-secreting tumors in patients with acromegaly; the carcinoid syndrome; gastrinoma; glucagonoma; nesidioblastosis; the watery diarrhea, hypokalemia, and achlorhydria (WDHA) syndrome; and of "diabetic diarrhea." Orally administered octreotide has been reported to effectively reduce growth hormone levels in acromegaly, but doses of up to 24 mg/d were required, in contrast to microgram quantities given parenterally.

Adverse effects of therapy include nausea with or without vomiting, abdominal cramps, flatulence, and steatorrhea with bulky bowel movements. Biliary sludge and gallstones may occur after 6 months of use in as many as 18% of patients. Patients may have a transient deterioration in glucose tolerance at the start of therapy, but this subsequently improves.

GROWTH HORMONE
(Somatotropin, GH)

Growth hormone is a peptide hormone produced by the anterior pituitary. Growth hormone has direct metabolic effects on lipolysis in adipose tissue and on insulin action and indirect anabolic effects mediated through another class of factors known as somatomedins.

Chemistry & Pharmacokinetics
A. Structure: Growth hormone is a 191-amino-acid peptide with two sulfhydryl bridges. Its structure closely resembles that of prolactin and the placental hormone human chorionic somatomammotropin. Growth hormone for pharmacologic use is produced with recombinant DNA technology and contains either the 191-amino-acid sequence of growth hormone proper (**somatotropin**) or 192 amino acids consisting of the 191 amino acids of growth hormone plus an extra methionine residue at the amino terminal end (**somatrem**).

B. Absorption, Metabolism, and Excretion:
Circulating endogenous growth hormone has a half-life of 20–25 minutes and is predominantly cleared by the liver. Human growth hormone can be administered intramuscularly, with peak levels occurring in 2–4 hours and active blood levels persisting for 36 hours.

Pharmacodynamics
Growth hormone binds to cell membrane receptors and brings about its actions without apparently utilizing any of the currently recognized second messengers (cAMP, Ca^{2+}, etc). These actions include both direct (metabolic) and indirect (anabolic) effects. By all the indices measured in short-term studies, biosynthetic methionyl human growth hormone is equipotent with native and biosynthetic pituitary growth hormone. The metabolic consequence of a pharmacologic dose of growth hormone is an initial insulin-like effect with increased tissue uptake of both glucose and amino acids and decreased lipolysis. Within a few hours, there is a peripheral insulin-antagonistic effect with impaired glucose uptake and increased lipolysis.

The major anabolic consequence of a pharmacologic dose of growth hormone is longitudinal growth. The anabolic effects of growth hormone are mediated indirectly via another class of peptide hormones, the somatomedins, or insulin-like growth factors (IGFs). Growth hormone stimulates synthesis of somatomedins IGF-I and IGF-II (predominantly in the liver); somatomedins promote uptake of sulfate into cartilage and are probably the actual mediators of the cellular processes associated with bone growth. This growth can be traced back to the molecular level, where increased incorporation of thymidine into DNA and uridine into RNA occurs (indicating cellular proliferation) along with increased conversion of proline to hydroxyproline (indicating cartilage synthesis).

It has long been recognized that growth hormone deficiency leads to inadequate somatomedin production and dwarfism. There are also states of dwarfism in which elevated plasma growth hormone levels fail to induce adequate production of somatomedins.

Clinical Pharmacology
A. Growth Hormone Deficiency: Timely growth hormone replacement therapy will permit achievement of full predicted adult height in children with growth hormone deficiency. Criteria for diagnosis of growth hormone deficiency usually include (1) a growth rate below 4 cm per year and (2) the absence of a serum growth hormone response to two growth hormone secretagogues. The prevalence of congenital growth hormone deficiency is approximately 1:4000. Congenital growth hormone deficiency can result from diseases of the hypophysial-pituitary region such as craniopharyngiomas but is most often

due to lack of hypothalamic growth hormone-releasing factors, resulting in pituitary dwarfism. In the newborn, hypoglycemia and even seizures can occur if growth hormone is absent.

In addition to isolated growth hormone deficiency, congenital deficiencies of multiple pituitary hormones occur with approximately equal frequency. Such patients—as well as those with acquired growth hormone deficiency, which is often accompanied by multiple hormone deficiencies—may also respond well to growth hormone plus other hormone replacements as needed, provided the underlying disease process can be controlled.

B. Growth Hormone-Responsive States: Some non-growth hormone-deficient short children with a delayed bone age and a slow growth rate achieve increased growth with short-term growth hormone therapy. It is not known whether their adult heights can be increased with prolonged therapy. Selected "normal variant short stature" children can be offered a trial of growth hormone following a baseline period of measurement to confirm a subnormal growth rate. During the first 6 months of treatment, the height velocity must increase by 2 cm per year for treatment to continue. The National Institute for Child Health and Human Development is conducting a 10-year study (to run until 1999) that will evaluate long-term effects and final adult height in growth hormone-treated short children without classic growth hormone deficiency. Girls with Turner's syndrome frequently respond to growth hormone therapy with increased growth velocity and increased height as adults.

C. Experimental Uses: Growth hormone is currently being tested for production of growth in short children with intrauterine growth retardation and chronic renal failure and for muscle preservation in catabolic states such as corticosteroid therapy, burns, and caloric restriction.

Short-term treatment of GH-deficient adults has resulted in increased lean body mass, decreased fat mass, and improved psychologic well-being. The safety of long-term GH treatment of adults is under investigation.

In 1993, the FDA approved the use of recombinant bovine growth hormone (rbGH) in dairy cattle to increase milk production. Although milk and meat from rbGH-treated cows appears to be safe, these cows have a higher frequency of mastitis, which could increase antibiotic use and result in greater antibiotic residues in milk and meat. This potential indirect health effect is being studied.

Dosage

Animal preparations of growth hormone are ineffective in humans. In the past, treatment of children with human growth hormone was limited by the scarcity of the hormone as well as its expense. Until 1985, all commercially available growth hormone (soma-

tropin) was freeze-extracted from human pituitaries. Use of human-derived growth hormone ceased in 1985 because of possible contamination (see below). Biosynthetic growth hormone has replaced these human-derived preparations.

In 1985, somatrem became the second biosynthetic pharmaceutical product (following human insulin) to be approved by the FDA. In 1987, somatropin was also approved by the FDA. The recommended dosage of biosynthetic growth hormone is up to 0.1 mg/kg (0.26 IU/kg) subcutaneously or intramuscularly 3 times weekly. The two biosynthetic growth hormones have not been studied in comparison to each other, but they appear to have similar potencies. The annual cost of treatment for a GH-deficient child depends upon the child's weight and is typically $10,000–$30,000.

Toxicity & Contraindications

In 1985, the National Hormone and Pituitary Program halted distribution of growth hormone derived from human pituitaries because of reports that three patients treated with the human-derived preparation—several years earlier—had died of Creutzfeldt-Jakob disease. Thirteen similar cases have subsequently been reported worldwide. It is considered possible that they had been infected by the neurotropic virus in the growth hormone preparations.

Antibody formation may occur in 30% of patients treated with biosynthetic growth hormone; however, these antibodies rarely interfere with the activity of this hormone. Rapid growth induced by successful hormone therapy may result in slipped capital femoral epiphyses, leading to a limp or lower extremity pain. A very slight increase in leukemia incidence has been reported in association with growth hormone therapy; however, it is not clear whether there is a causal relationship.

Growth hormone is contraindicated in patients with closed epiphyses or an expanding intracranial mass. Patients receiving growth hormone should be screened regularly for hypothyroidism or diabetes. If growth slows in the absence of rising antibody titers, hypopituitarism should be ruled out. Untreated hypothyroidism or excessive glucocorticoid replacement therapy can impair growth.

THYROTROPIN-RELEASING HORMONE (Protirelin, TRH)

Thyrotropin-releasing hormone, or protirelin, is a tripeptide hormone found in the hypothalamus as well as in other parts of the brain. TRH is secreted into the portal venous system and stimulates the pituitary to produce thyrotropin (TSH), which in turn stimulates the thyroid to produce thyroxine (T_4). TRH stimulation of thyrotropin is blocked by thyroxine and potentiated by lack of thyroxine such that the extent of thyrotropin response to TRH stimulation forms the basis for using TRH as a diagnostic agent in the evaluation of hyperthyroid and hypothyroid states.

Chemistry & Pharmacokinetics

TRH is (pyro)Glu-His-Pro-NH$_2$. TRH is usually administered intravenously. Rapid plasma inactivation occurs, with a half-life of 4–5 minutes.

Pharmacodynamics

TRH stimulates pituitary production of thyrotropin, probably through activation of a membrane receptor linked via a G protein to the inositol trisphosphate cascade (Chapter 2). TRH stimulation of thyrotropin may be blocked by pretreatment with thyroxine, corticosteroids, and somatostatin, whereas TRH stimulation of prolactin production is not blocked by thyroxine pretreatment. TRH may also function as a central nervous system neurotransmitter.

Peak serum thyrotropin levels occur 20–30 minutes after intravenous TRH injection in healthy individuals. In hyperthyroidism, high serum thyroxine levels blunt the thyrotropin response to TRH. In primary hypothyroidism, thyrotropin levels start high and the pituitary response to TRH may be accentuated, with a particularly brisk outpouring of additional thyrotropin. In secondary (pituitary) hypothyroidism, serum thyrotropin levels start low and fail to rise after TRH administration. In tertiary (hypothalamic) hypothyroidism, the baseline serum thyrotropin level may be low or normal and the thyrotropin response to TRH may be delayed.

TRH infusion leads to stimulation of prolactin release by the pituitary in healthy individuals but has no effect on cells producing growth hormone or ACTH. In certain types of pituitary tumors, however, the neoplastic cells may respond abnormally to TRH by releasing growth hormone (in acromegaly), by releasing ACTH (in Cushing's disease), or by failing to release prolactin (in prolactinoma). Timely high-dose TRH infusion may improve the outcome of spinal cord injuries (Ceylan, 1992). This property of TRH is currently being investigated. The mechanism is unknown.

Clinical Pharmacology

TRH is currently used only for diagnostic purposes: In hyperthyroidism, the TSH elevation that results following its administration is blunted, whereas in hypothyroidism, the response is exaggerated. A TRH infusion test is the most sensitive method for diagnosing mild hyper- and hypothyroidism in the minimally symptomatic patient with equivocal serum thyroxine or thyrotropin levels. In spite of overlap in the responses between various hyper- and hypothyroidism states and normals, the test is quite valuable in some patients.

TSH assays have evolved from first-generation radioimmunoassays to second-generation immunometric assays in the mid 1980s to third- and fourth-generation immunochemiluminometric assays (IMCAs) and modified IMCAs in the early 1990s, eliminating the need for TRH testing in some patients with previously undetectable baseline TSH levels. Newer assays may distinguish hyperthyroid patients with undetectable TSH levels from sick euthyroid patients with usually detectable TSH levels.

A blunted thyrotropin response to TRH may also occur in unipolar (contrasted with bipolar) depression and other mental disorders. However, for most psychiatric patients, this test lacks sensitivity, specificity, or value.

Dosage

The dose of protirelin is 500 μg for adults and 7 μg/kg for children aged 6 years or older but not to exceed the adult dose. A baseline thyrotropin level should be obtained, followed by three further determinations at 15, 30, and 60 minutes postinfusion.

Toxicity

Up to 50% of patients tested may note adverse effects lasting for a few minutes: an urge to urinate, a metallic taste, nausea, or light-headedness. Transient hypertension may occur.

THYROID-STIMULATING HORMONE (Thyrotropin, TSH)

Thyrotropin is an anterior pituitary hormone that regulates thyroid function by stimulating production of thyroxine. Diagnostic use of thyrotropin in various states of borderline thyroid function has been largely supplanted by measurement of the baseline thyrotropin concentration and its response to TRH. Therapeutic use of thyrotropin in conjunction with ^{131}I ablation is established in selected cases of thyroid carcinoma to enhance thyroid radioiodine uptake.

Chemistry & Pharmacokinetics

A. Structure: Thyrotropin consists of two peptides (alpha and beta), both of which contain branched carbohydrate side chains that are important for hormone activity. Therapeutic thyrotropin is prepared from bovine anterior pituitaries. There is 70% homology between human and bovine TSH-α subunits and 90% homology between human and bovine TSH-β subunits. The TSH-α subunit sequence in humans is virtually identical to that of the alpha subunit of FSH, LH, and hCG.

B. Absorption, Metabolism, and Excretion: Thyrotropin is administered intramuscularly or subcutaneously. Its half-life is approximately 1 hour, with degradation occurring in the kidneys. Little unchanged thyrotropin appears in the urine.

Pharmacodynamics

Thyrotropin stimulates thyroid cell adenylyl cyclase activity. Increased cAMP production causes increased iodine uptake and, ultimately, increased production of thyroid hormones. Increased thyroid size and vascularity follow thyrotropin administration.

Clinical Pharmacology

A. Diagnostic Uses: In hypothyroidism, thyrotropin administration may stimulate minimal (in the case of primary hypothyroidism) or substantial (in secondary or tertiary hypothyroidism) radioiodine uptake. This test has been replaced by the TRH stimulation test, which is faster and cheaper.

B. Therapeutic Uses: Thyrotropin has a role in the therapy of metastatic thyroid carcinoma. Following a tumoricidal dose of ^{131}I, the patient receives triiodothyronine for 10 weeks and is then taken off hormone replacement for 3 weeks. Finally, the patient receives thyrotropin to elicit iodine uptake by the metastatic tissue. Additional ^{131}I may be administered at that time.

Dosage

Thyrotropin is derived from beef pituitaries and is intended for intramuscular or subcutaneous administration. A dose of 5–10 units/d for 3 days is used for diagnostic purposes; 5–10 units/d for 3–7 days is used in conjunction with ^{131}I for ablation of thyroid carcinoma.

Toxicity

Local soreness at the injection site is common. Nausea, vomiting, thyroid tenderness, allergic symptoms, and symptoms of hyperthyroidism may occur. This drug should be used cautiously in the presence of heart disease or adrenocortical insufficiency.

CORTICOTROPIN-RELEASING HORMONE (CRH)

CRH is a hypothalamic hormone that stimulates release of ACTH and beta-endorphin from the pituitary.

Chemistry & Pharmacokinetics

A. Structure: Human CRH is a 41-amino-acid peptide. An analogue of human CRH is sheep CRH, which also contains 41 amino acids. These molecules differ in seven amino acids.

B. Absorption, Metabolism, and Excretion: CRH is administered intravenously. The first-phase half-lives of human and ovine CRH are 9 minutes and 18 minutes, respectively. The peptide is metabolized in various tissues, and less than 1% is excreted in the urine.

Pharmacodynamics

CRH stimulates secretion of ACTH and beta-endorphin from cultured pituitary cells. This effect is associated with cAMP generation. Pretreatment of these cells with dexamethasone inhibits the hormone-releasing response.

Clinical Pharmacology

CRH is used only for diagnostic purposes. In Cushing's syndrome, CRH has been used to distinguish Cushing's disease from ectopic ACTH secretion. ACTH-producing tumor cells of the pituitary—but not of ectopic locations—demonstrate a degree of responsiveness to physiologic suppression and stimulation. Whereas high-dose dexamethasone generally suppresses corticosteroid production in Cushing's disease but not in the ectopic ACTH syndrome, CRH elicits an increase in ACTH and cortisol secretion in Cushing's disease but not in the ectopic ACTH syndrome. A concordant positive or negative response to combined CRH and dexamethasone testing is extremely suggestive of Cushing's disease or the ectopic ACTH syndrome, respectively. However, an occasional ectopic ACTH-producing tumor of the lung may paradoxically increase output in response to CRH as well as show suppression in response to high-dose dexamethasone, and an occasional patient with Cushing's disease may fail to respond to CRH stimulation. Simultaneous bilateral inferior petrosal sinus and peripheral vein ACTH sampling, in conjunction with CRH stimulation, has shown Cushing's disease patients to consistently demonstrate a greater central-to-peripheral ratio than patients with ectopic ACTH syndrome.

Psychiatric depression is associated—in some patients—with elevation of cortisol secretion. In some of these patients, the hypercortisolism can be distinguished from that of Cushing's disease with CRH stimulation in that ACTH and cortisol levels usually rise in Cushing's disease but not in depression. CRH stimulation of ACTH secretion in Cushing's disease may distinguish successfully operated patients (blunted or normal response) from unsuccessfully operated patients (exaggerated response) and, in adrenal insufficiency, hypothalamic disease (normal response) from pituitary disease (blunted response).

Preparation & Dosage

Synthetic human and sheep CRH are available for investigational use. Sheep CRH is used more frequently because of its longer half-life and slightly greater potency. CRH may be dissolved in water or dilute acid but not in saline. A dose of 1 µg/kg is used for diagnostic testing.

Toxicity

Intravenous bolus doses of 1 µg/kg produce transient facial flushing and, rarely, cause dyspnea.

ADRENOCORTICOTROPIN
(Corticotropin, ACTH)

Adrenocorticotropin is a peptide hormone produced in the anterior pituitary. Its primary endocrine function is to stimulate synthesis and release of adrenocortical hormones. Pharmacologic administration of corticotropin results in increased production not only of cortisol but of adrenal androgens and mineralocorticoids as well. Corticotropin can be used therapeutically, but its primary usefulness is in the assessment of adrenocortical responsiveness. A substandard adrenocortical response to exogenous corticotropin administration indicates adrenocortical insufficiency.

Chemistry & Pharmacokinetics

A. Structure: Human ACTH is a single polypeptide chain of 39 amino acids (Figure 36–2). The amino terminal portion containing amino acids 1–24 is necessary for full biologic activity. The remaining amino acids (25–39) confer species specificity. Therapeutic ACTH preparations are derived from porcine pituitaries and differ in structure from human ACTH only in the nonessential 25–39 region. Synthetic human $ACTH_{1-24}$ is known as **cosyntropin.** The amino terminal amino acids 1–13 are identical to melanocyte-stimulating hormone (α-MSH), which has been found in animals but not in humans. In states of excessive pituitary ACTH secretion, hyperpigmentation—caused by the α-MSH activity intrinsic to ACTH—may be noted.

ACTH from animal sources is assayed biologically by measuring the depletion of adrenocortical ascorbic acid that follows subcutaneous administration of the ACTH. Synthetic ACTH can be assayed by weight. The steroidogenic activity of 1 unit of porcine ACTH is approximately equal to that of 10 μg of cosyntropin.

B. Absorption, Metabolism, and Excretion: Both porcine and synthetic corticotropin are well absorbed by the intramuscular route. Corticotropin cannot be administered orally because of gastrointestinal proteolysis.

The biologic half-lives of $ACTH_{1-39}$ and $ACTH_{1-24}$ are under 20 minutes. Tissue uptake occurs in the liver and kidneys. $ACTH_{1-39}$ is transformed into a biologically inactive substance, probably by modification of a side chain. ACTH is not excreted in the urine in significant amounts. The effects of long-acting repository forms of porcine corticotropin persist for up to 18 hours with a gelatin complex of the polypeptide and up to several days with a zinc hydroxide complex.

Pharmacodynamics

ACTH binds to G protein-coupled receptors in the adrenal cortex and increases cAMP. This stimulates the adrenal cortex to produce glucocorticoids, mineralocorticoids, and androgens. ACTH increases the activity of cholesterol esterase, the enzyme that catalyzes the rate-limiting step of steroid hormone production: cholesterol → pregnenolone. ACTH also stimulates adrenal hypertrophy and hyperplasia. In pharmacologic doses, corticotropin may cause adipose tissue lipolysis and increased skin pigmentation.

Clinical Pharmacology

A. Diagnostic Uses: ACTH stimulation of the adrenals will fail to elicit an appropriate response in states of adrenal insufficiency. A rapid test for ruling out adrenal insufficiency employs cosyntropin (see below). Plasma cortisol levels are measured before and either 30 or 60 minutes following an intramuscular or intravenous injection of 0.25 mg of cosyntropin. A normal plasma cortisol response is a stimulated increment exceeding 7 μg/dL and a peak level exceeding 18 μg/dL. A subnormal response indicates primary or secondary adrenocortical insufficiency that can be differentiated using endogenous plasma ACTH levels (which are increased in primary adrenal insufficiency and decreased in the secondary form). An incremental rise in plasma aldosterone generally occurs in secondary but not primary adrenal insufficiency after cosyntropin stimulation.

Many women with hirsutism have abnormal steroidogenic function in spite of normal adrenal androgen levels. ACTH stimulation may distinguish three forms of late-onset (nonclassic) congenital adrenal hyperplasia from states of ovarian hyperandrogenism, all of which may be associated with hirsutism. In patients with deficiency of 21-hydroxylase, ACTH stimulation results in an incremental rise in plasma 17-hydroxyprogesterone. Patients with 11-hydroxylase deficiency manifest a rise in 11-deoxycortisol, while those with 3β-hydroxy-Δ5 steroid dehydrogenase deficiency show an increase of 17-hydroxypregnenolone in response to ACTH stimulation.

B. Therapeutic Uses: Corticotropin may be prescribed for patients with normal adrenal function

1	2	3	4	5	6	7	8	9	10	11	12	13	-------	25	26	27	28	29	30	31	32	33	34	35	36	37	38	39
Ser	Tyr	Ser	Met	Glu	His	Phe	Arg	Trp	Gly	Lys	Pro	Val	(human)	Asp	Ala	Gly	Glu	Asp	Gln	Ser	Ala	Glu	Ala	Phe	Pro	Leu	Glu	Phe
Ser	Tyr	Ser	Met	Glu	His	Phe	Arg	Trp	Gly	Lys	Pro	Val	(pig)	Asp	Gly	Ala	Glu	Asp	Gln	Leu	Ala	Glu						
Ser	Tyr	Ser	Met	Glu	His	Phe	Arg	Trp	Gly	Lys	Pro	Val	(beef)	Asp	Gly	Glu	Ala	Glu	Asp	Ser	Ala	Gln						
Ser	Tyr	Ser	Met	Glu	His	Phe	Arg	Trp	Gly	Lys	Pro	Val	(sheep)	Ala	Gly	Glu	Asp	Asp	Glu	Ala	Ser	Glu						

Figure 36–2. Amino acid sequences of human, pig, beef, and sheep adrenocorticotropin. Amino acids 1–13 are also present in α-MSH. Amino acids 14–24 (not shown) are identical in all four species.

when increased glucocorticoid concentrations are desired. In choosing between ACTH and glucocorticoids, adverse effects should be considered since their effectiveness is similar. On balance, the disadvantages of ACTH (especially the need for parenteral administration) appear to outweigh its advantages, making glucocorticoids the drugs of choice in chronic conditions where anti-inflammatory or immunosuppressive therapy is warranted. An $ACTH_{4-9}$ analogue has been reported to prevent neuropathy induced by cisplatin or *Vinca* alkaloids used in cancer chemotherapy.

Dosage

Cosyntropin is the preferred preparation for diagnostic use. The standard diagnostic test dose of 0.25 mg is equivalent to 25 units of porcine corticotropin. ACTH may be used therapeutically in doses of 10–20 units 4 times daily. Repository ACTH, 40–80 units, may be administered every 24–72 hours.

Toxicity & Contraindications

The toxicity of ACTH resembles that of the glucocorticoids. The occasional development of antibodies to animal ACTH or to depot cosyntropin (a preparation not currently available in the USA) has produced anaphylactic reactions or refractoriness to ACTH therapy in a few individuals. Painful swelling occurs at the injection site more often with the zinc hydroxide depot preparation than with the gelatin preparation. Contraindications are similar to those of glucocorticoids. Use of ACTH during pregnancy should be minimized. When immediate effects are desired, glucocorticoids are preferable.

GONADOTROPIN-RELEASING HORMONE
(GnRH; Luteinizing Hormone-Releasing Hormone [LHRH]; Gonadorelin Hydrochloride)

Gonadotropin-releasing hormone is produced in the arcuate nucleus of the hypothalamus and controls release of the gonadotropins FSH and LH from three pituitary cell types: FSH-, LH-, and FSH/LH-gonadotrophs. One mechanism by which divergent production of two gonadotropins occurs is that the frequency of pulsatile GnRH secretion selectively regulates gonadotropin gene transcription.

Chemistry & Pharmacokinetics

A. Structure: GnRH is a decapeptide found in all mammals. Pharmaceutical GnRH is synthetic. Analogues (eg, leuprolide, nafarelin, buserelin, goserelin, and histrelin) with D-amino acids at position 6 and with ethylamide substituted for glycine at position 10 are more potent and longer-lasting than native GnRH.

5-O-Pro-His-Trp-Ser-Tyr-Gly-Leu-Arg-Pro-Gly-NH2
GnRH

5-O-Pro-His-Trp-Ser-Tyr-D-Leu-Leu-Arg-Pro-NHCH$_2$CH$_3$
Leuprolide

5-O-Pro-His-Trp-Ser-Tyr-D-Nal-*Leu-Arg-Pro-Gly-NH$_2$
Nafarelin

5-O-Pro-His-Trp-Ser-Tyr-D-Ser(*t*-Bu)-Leu-Arg-Pro-NHNHCONH$_2$
Goserelin

5-O-Pro-His-Trp-Ser-Tyr-D-His(N$^\tau$-PhCH$_2$-)-Leu-Arg-Pro-NHCH$_2$CH$_3$
Histrelin

*D-Nal = D-3-(2-naphthyl)-alanine.

B. Absorption, Metabolism, and Excretion: GnRH may be administered intravenously or subcutaneously. GnRH analogues may be administered subcutaneously, intramuscularly, or via nasal spray. The half-life of intravenous GnRH is 4 minutes, and the half-lives of subcutaneous and intranasal GnRH analogues are 3 hours. Degradation occurs in the hypothalamus and pituitary. GnRH analogues have increased affinity for GnRH receptors and reduced susceptibility to degradation.

Pharmacodynamics

GnRH binds to receptors on pituitary gonadotropes. Pulsatile intravenous administration every 1–4 hours stimulates FSH and LH secretion. In contrast, GnRH administered continuously or GnRH analogues administered in depot formulations *inhibit* gonadotropin release.

Clinical Pharmacology

A. Diagnostic Uses: Delayed puberty in a hypogonadotropic adolescent may be due to a constitutional delay or to hypogonadotropic hypogonadism. The LH response (but not the FSH response) to GnRH can distinguish between these two conditions. Serum LH levels are measured before and then 15, 30, 45, 60, and 120 minutes after a 100 µg intravenous or subcutaneous bolus of GnRH. A peak LH response exceeding 15.6 mIU/mL is normal and suggests impending puberty, whereas an impaired LH response suggests hypogonadotropic hypogonadism due to either pituitary or hypothalamic disease.

B. Therapeutic Uses:

1. Stimulation–GnRH can stimulate pituitary function and is used in hypogonadotropic hypogonadism of both sexes, delayed puberty, and cryptorchidism. A system for intravenous GnRH administration was approved by the FDA in 1990. A kit containing a battery-powered programmable pump and intravenous tubing allows pulsatile GnRH therapy every 90 minutes throughout the follicular and luteal phases.

2. Suppression–Leuprolide, nafarelin, goserelin, and histrelin are GnRH analogue agonists that—when given continuously—induce biochemical castration in adults with prostate cancer, uterine fibroids, endometriosis, and polycystic ovary syndrome and in children with precocious puberty. Many in vitro fertilization programs sequentially use a GnRH analogue to suppress endogenous gonadotropin release, followed by exogenous gonadotropins to achieve synchronous follicular development.

GnRH analogue therapy for the purpose of producing pituitary suppression leads to a transient rise in sex hormone concentration during the first 2 weeks of treatment. This can be deleterious in some disorders, such as prostate cancer. Several GnRH analogue *antagonists* are under investigation. These agents produce immediate pituitary suppression through complete receptor blockade.

Dosage

The recommended dose of leuprolide is 1 mg/d subcutaneously (Lupron) or 7.5 mg/month intramuscularly (Lupron Depot) for prostate cancer or 3.75 mg/month intramuscularly for endometriosis. Nafarelin is administered as one or two sprays (200 μg/spray) intranasally twice daily. Goserelin is injected from a preloaded syringe subcutaneously as a 3.6 mg implant every 28 days. Histrelin is injected subcutaneously in a dosage of 10 μg/kg daily.

Gonadorelin is administered intravenously, 5 μg every 90 minutes for 14–21 days, until ovulation occurs or the dose is increased. A corpus luteum can be maintained either by adding 14 more days of gonadorelin or by a series of hCG injections. Regular changes of the intravenous site and pelvic ultrasound examinations are necessary.

Toxicity

GnRH used for diagnosis rarely produces headache, abdominal discomfort, or flushing. GnRH analogues can acutely worsen bone pain in prostate cancer patients and may cause hot flushes in both sexes. Their use in women should be limited to 6 months because of the risk of osteoporosis. Intravenous GnRH for induction of ovulation is associated with a lower incidence of ovarian hyperstimulation and multiple births than is human menopausal gonadotropins (see below).

FOLLICLE-STIMULATING HORMONE (FSH)

Follicle-stimulating hormone is a glycoprotein hormone produced in the anterior pituitary that, along with LH, regulates gonadal function by increasing cAMP in the target tissue. It is composed of two linked peptide chains. The principal function of FSH is to stimulate gametogenesis and follicular development in women and spermatogenesis in men. FSH acts on the immature follicular cells of the ovary and induces development of the mature follicle and oocyte. Both LH and FSH are needed for proper ovarian steroidogenesis. LH stimulates androgen production by these cells, and FSH stimulates androgen conversion into estrogens by the granulosa cells. In the testes, FSH acts on the Sertoli cells and stimulates their production of an androgen-binding protein.

A naturally modified form of FSH is available for therapeutic use. The urine of postmenopausal women contains a substance with FSH-like properties (but with 4% of the potency) and an LH-like substance. The FSH-LH combination is known as menotropins. Another preparation of human FSH extracted from the urine of postmenopausal women contains virtually no LH and is known as urofollitropin. The use of these two gonadotropin preparations is discussed below.

LUTEINIZING HORMONE (LH)

Luteinizing hormone is a glycoprotein hormone consisting of two chains and, like FSH, is produced by the anterior pituitary. LH is primarily responsible for regulation of gonadal steroid hormone production. LH acts on testicular Leydig cells to stimulate testosterone production. In the ovary, LH acts in concert with FSH to stimulate follicular development. LH acts on the mature follicle to induce ovulation, and it stimulates the corpus luteum in the luteal phase of the menstrual cycle to produce progesterone and androgens.

There is no LH preparation presently available for clinical use. Human chorionic gonadotropin—with an almost identical structure—is available and can be used as a luteinizing hormone substitute in many gonadotropin-deficient states.

GONADOTROPINS
(hMG, Menotropins & FSH, Urofollitropin)

Human menopausal gonadotropins (hMG) are a mixture of partially catabolized human FSH and LH extracted from the urine of postmenopausal women. The commercial preparations of hMG, or menotropins, as well as human FSH, or urofollitropin, are biologically standardized for FSH and LH content.

They are used in states of infertility to stimulate ovarian follicle development in women and spermatogenesis in men. In both sexes, they must be used in conjunction with a luteinizing hormone, ie, human chorionic gonadotropin (hCG), to permit ovulation and implantation in women and testosterone production and full masculinization in men.

Pharmacokinetics

Over a 7 to 12 day course of daily hMG or urofollitropin administration intended to mimic the follicular phase of the ovarian cycle in women with hypothalamic amenorrhea, FSH levels gradually rise to twice their baseline level. LH levels increase to $1\frac{1}{2}$ times their baseline with hMG, but they do not rise with urofollitropin.

Pharmacodynamics

Ovarian follicular growth and maturation will occur during hMG or FSH treatment of gonadotropin-deficient women. Ovulation requires administration of chorionic gonadotropin when adequate follicular maturation has occurred.

In men with gonadotropin deficiencies, pretreatment with chorionic gonadotropin produces external sexual maturation; addition of a subsequent course of hMG will stimulate spermatogenesis and lead to fertility.

Clinical Pharmacology

Human menopausal gonadotropin is indicated for pituitary or hypothalamic hypogonadism with infertility. Anovulatory women with the following conditions may benefit from hMG: primary amenorrhea, secondary amenorrhea, polycystic ovary syndrome, and anovulatory cycles. Both hMG and FSH are used by in vitro fertilization programs for controlled ovarian hyperstimulation.

Over 50% of men with hypogonadotropic hypogonadism become fertile after hMG administration.

Dosage

An ampule of menotropins contains 75 IU or 150 IU of FSH and an equal amount of LH. One IU of LH is approximately equivalent to 0.5 IU of hCG. An ampule of urofollitropin contains 75 IU of FSH and less than 1 IU of LH. Human menopausal gonadotropins, FSH, and hCG are administered intramuscularly.

A. Women: In hypothalamic hypogonadism and for in vitro fertilization, 1–2 ampules are administered daily for 5–12 days until evidence of adequate follicular maturation is present. Serum estradiol levels should be measured and a cervical examination performed every 1–2 days. When appropriate follicular maturation has occurred, hMG or FSH is discontinued; the following day, hCG (5000–10,000 IU) is administered intramuscularly to induce ovulation.

B. Men: Following pretreatment with 5000 IU of hCG 3 times weekly for up to 6 months to achieve

masculinization and a normal serum testosterone level, menotropins is administered as 1 ampule 3 times weekly in combination with hCG, 2000 IU twice weekly. At least 4 months of combined treatment are usually necessary before spermatozoa appear in the ejaculate. If there is no response, the menotropins dose may be doubled with no change in the hCG dose.

Toxicity & Contraindications

Overstimulation of the ovary with hMG can lead to uncomplicated ovarian enlargement in approximately 20% of patients. This usually resolves spontaneously. A more serious complication, the "hyperstimulation syndrome," occurs in 0.5–4% of patients. It is characterized by hMG-induced ovarian enlargement, ascites, hydrothorax, and hypovolemia, sometimes to the point of shock. Hemoperitoneum (from a ruptured ovarian cyst), fever, or arterial thromboembolism can occur. The frequency of multiple births is approximately 20%. A reported 25% incidence of spontaneous abortions may be due to earlier diagnosis of pregnancy in treated than in untreated patients, with recognition of very early abortion. There may, however, be abnormal development and premature degeneration of corpus luteum in some treated patients. Gynecomastia occasionally occurs in men. An association between ovarian cancer and fertility drugs has been reported (Spirtas, 1993). However, it is not known which, if any, fertility drug is causally related to cancer.

Human menopausal gonadotropin and urofollitropin should be administered only by a physician experienced in treating infertility. Before treatment of women, a thorough gynecologic evaluation must be performed to rule out uterine, tubal, or ovarian diseases as well as pregnancy. In cases of irregular bleeding, uterine cancer should be ruled out.

HUMAN CHORIONIC GONADOTROPIN (hCG)

Human chorionic gonadotropin is a hormone produced by the human placenta and excreted into the urine, whence it can be extracted and purified. The function of hCG is to stimulate the ovarian corpus luteum to produce progesterone and maintain the placenta. It is very similar to LH in structure and is used to treat both men and women with LH deficiency.

Human chorionic gonadotropin is a glycoprotein consisting of a 92-amino acid alpha chain virtually identical to that of FSH, LH, and TSH and a beta chain of 145 amino acids that resembles that of LH except for the presence of a carboxyl terminal sequence of 30 amino acids not present in LH.

Pharmacokinetics

Human chorionic gonadotropin is well absorbed

after intramuscular administration and has a biologic half-life of 8 hours, compared with 30 minutes for LH. The difference may lie in the high sialic acid content of hCG compared with that of LH. It is apparently modified in the body prior to urinary excretion, because the half-life measured by immunoassay far exceeds that measured by bioassay.

Pharmacodynamics

Human chorionic gonadotropin stimulates production of gonadal steroid hormones. The interstitial and corpus luteal cells of the female produce progesterone, and the Leydig cells of the male produce testosterone. hCG can be used to mimic a midcycle LH surge and trigger ovulation in a hypogonadotropic woman.

Human chorionic gonadotropin has no established effect on appetite or fat mobilization and distribution. It has been advocated without justification as an adjunct to dietary management in obese patients.

Clinical Pharmacology

A. Diagnostic Uses: In prepubertal boys with undescended gonads, hCG can be used to distinguish a truly retained (cryptorchid) testis from a retracted (pseudocryptorchid) one. Testicular descent during a course of hCG administration usually foretells permanent testicular descent at puberty, when circulating LH levels rise. Lack of descent usually means that orchiopexy will be necessary at puberty to preserve spermatogenesis.

Patients with constitutional delay in onset of puberty can be distinguished from those with hypogonadotropic hypogonadism using repeated hCG stimulation. Serum testosterone and estradiol levels rise in the former but not in the latter group.

B. Therapeutic Uses: As described above, hCG can be used in combination with human menotropins to induce ovulation in women with secondary hypogonadism or as part of an in vitro fertilization program, as well as in men with secondary hypogonadism.

Dosage

The dosages for female and male infertility are described under hMG dosage. For prepubertal cryptorchidism, a dosage of 500–4000 units 3 times weekly for up to 6 weeks has been advocated.

Toxicity & Contraindications

Reported adverse effects include headache, depression, edema, precocious puberty, gynecomastia, or (rarely) production of antibodies to hCG.

Human chorionic gonadotropin should be administered for infertility only by a physician with experience in this field. Androgen-dependent neoplasia and precocious puberty are contraindications to its use.

PROLACTIN

Prolactin is a 198-amino-acid peptide hormone produced in the anterior pituitary. Its structure resembles that of growth hormone. Prolactin is the principal hormone responsible for lactation. Milk production is stimulated by prolactin when appropriate circulating levels of estrogens, progestins, corticosteroids, and insulin are present. Prolactin also induces mitogenesis in lymphocytes and has been postulated to play a role in autoimmune diseases. A deficiency of prolactin—which can occur in states of pituitary deficiency—is manifested by failure to lactate or by a luteal phase defect. In hypothalamic destruction, prolactin levels may be elevated as a result of impaired transport of prolactin-inhibiting hormone (dopamine) to the pituitary. Hyperprolactinemia can produce galactorrhea and hypogonadism and may be associated with symptoms of a pituitary mass. No preparation is available for use in prolactin-deficient patients. For patients with symptomatic hyperprolactinemia, inhibition of prolactin secretion can be achieved with bromocriptine, a dopamine agonist.

BROMOCRIPTINE

Although bromocriptine is not a hormone, it has important inhibitory effects on the pituitary that warrant discussion here.

Bromocriptine is an ergot derivative with dopamine agonist properties that lowers circulating prolactin levels. Its chemical structure and pharmacokinetic features are presented in Chapter 16.

Bromocriptine decreases pituitary prolactin secretion through a dopamine-mimetic action on the pituitary at two central nervous system loci: (1) It decreases dopamine turnover in the tuberoinfundibular neurons of the arcuate nucleus, generating increased hypothalamic dopamine; and (2) it acts directly on pituitary dopamine receptors to inhibit spontaneous prolactin release and that evoked by thyrotropin-releasing hormone.

Bromocriptine stimulates pituitary growth hormone release in normal subjects and—paradoxically and for unknown reasons—suppresses growth hormone release in acromegalics. Bromocriptine is the only FDA-approved medication for hyperprolactinemia. Pergolide, another dopamine agonist that has been approved by the FDA for Parkinson's disease, has been used as once-daily treatment for hyperprolactinemia. Cabergoline, an ergot derivative that is administered once or twice a week, and quinagolide, (CV 205502) a nonergot dopamine agonist that is administered once daily, are investigational medications for hyperprolactinemia.

Clinical Pharmacology

A. Prolactin-Secreting Adenomas: Bromocriptine has gained wide acceptance as initial treatment for prolactinomas. Significant reduction in both tumor size and serum prolactin levels can be demonstrated with bromocriptine treatment. For definitive therapy of such tumors, eventual surgical excision with or without radiation therapy probably remains necessary because the effects of long-term bromocriptine therapy are not known, and expansion of these tumors may occur if bromocriptine is discontinued.

B. Amenorrhea-Galactorrhea: Bromocriptine is approved for treatment of dysfunctions associated with hyperprolactinemia, including amenorrhea, galactorrhea, infertility, and hypogonadism. Both prolactin-secreting pituitary adenomas and idiopathic hyperprolactinemia respond well to bromocriptine. Upon cessation of therapy, hyperprolactinemia and galactorrhea generally recur.

C. Physiologic Lactation: Bromocriptine suppresses the prolactin secretion that occurs after parturition or abortion and is used to prevent breast engorgement when breast feeding is not desired.

D. Acromegaly: Bromocriptine alone or in combination with pituitary surgery or irradiation may be used for acromegaly. Acromegalic patients demonstrate improvement of symptoms less frequently than those with prolactinomas and rarely achieve clinical remissions. The role of bromocriptine in acromegaly remains to be determined.

E. Parkinson's Disease: The use of bromocriptine in Parkinson's disease is discussed in Chapter 27.

F. Cocaine Withdrawal: Cocaine withdrawal symptoms may be due to supersensitivity of inhibitory receptors on dopaminergic neurons. In experimental settings, bromocriptine has reduced cocaine craving.

Preparations & Dosage

Bromocriptine has a half-life of 3 hours and should be administered in divided doses with meals. Most hyperprolactinemic states, as well as physiologic lactation, respond to 2.5–7.5 mg per day. Daily requirements may reach 20 mg with large prolactinomas and 30 mg with acromegaly. Long-acting oral (Parlodel SRO) and intramuscular (Parlodel L.A.R.) bromocriptine formulations are available in Europe.

Toxicity & Contraindications

Dosages up to 10 mg/d may cause nausea, lightheadedness, orthostatic hypotension, or constipation. Dosages above 10 mg/d may cause cold-induced peripheral digital vasospasm, neuropsychiatric symptoms, or, rarely, peptic ulcer.

Although bromocriptine therapy during the first 3 weeks of pregnancy has not been associated with an increased risk of spontaneous abortion or congenital malformations, there are few data on the drug's safety if it is used throughout gestation. Therefore, bromocriptine should not be used in a woman known to be pregnant. If a woman who is receiving bromocriptine is late in having her period, a pregnancy test is necessary, and if she is amenorrheic, pregnancy tests should be performed regularly because ovulation may occur before menstruation resumes.

POSTERIOR PITUITARY HORMONES

Two posterior pituitary hormones are known: vasopressin and oxytocin. Their structures are very similar and they probably have a common phylogenetic precursor. Secretion of posterior pituitary hormones is not regulated by hypothalamic releasing hormones, as is the case with anterior pituitary hormones. Posterior pituitary hormones are synthesized in the hypothalamus and then transported to the posterior pituitary, where they are stored and then released into the circulation.

OXYTOCIN

Oxytocin is a peptide secreted by the posterior pituitary that elicits milk ejection in lactating women. In pharmacologic doses, oxytocin can be used to induce uterine contractions and maintain labor; however, at physiologic blood levels, the contribution of this hormone to parturition is probably small.

Chemistry & Pharmacokinetics

A. Structure: (Figure 36–3.) Oxytocin is a nine amino acid peptide composed of a six amino acid disulfide ring and a three-membered tail containing the carboxyl terminus. Oxytocin and vasopressin differ from vasotocin—the only posterior pituitary hormone

```
      ┌─S────────S─┐
Cys-Tyr-Phe-Gln-Asn-Cys-Pro-Arg-Gly-NH₂
 1   2   3   4   5   6   7   8   9
```

Arginine vasopressin

```
      ┌─S────────S─┐
Cys-Tyr-Ile-Gln-Asn-Cys-Pro-Leu-Gly-NH₂
 1   2   3   4   5   6   7   8   9
```

Oxytocin

Figure 36–3. Arginine vasopressin and oxytocin. In some species, lysine is substituted for arginine in position 8 of the vasopressin molecule. (Reproduced, with permission, from Ganong WF: *Review of Medical Physiology,* 15th ed. Appleton & Lange, 1991.)

found in nonmammalian vertebrates—by only one amino acid residue each.

B. Absorption, Metabolism, and Excretion: Oxytocin is usually administered intravenously for stimulation of labor, though buccal absorption is possible. It is inactive if swallowed, because it is destroyed in the stomach and intestine. Oxytocin is not bound to plasma proteins and is catabolized by the kidneys and liver, with a circulating half-life of 5 minutes.

Pharmacodynamics

Oxytocin alters transmembrane ionic currents in myometrial smooth muscle cells to produce sustained uterine contraction. The sensitivity of the uterus to oxytocin increases during pregnancy. Oxytocin-induced myometrial contractions can be inhibited by beta-adrenoceptor agonists, magnesium sulfate, or inhalation anesthetics. Oxytocin also causes contraction of myoepithelial cells surrounding mammary alveoli, which leads to milk ejection. Without oxytocin-induced contraction, normal lactation cannot occur. Oxytocin has weak antidiuretic and pressor activity.

Clinical Pharmacology

A. Diagnostic Uses: Oxytocin infusion near term will produce uterine contractions that decrease the fetal blood supply. The fetal heart rate response to a standardized oxytocin challenge test provides information about placental circulatory reserve. An abnormal response suggests intrauterine growth retardation and may warrant immediate cesarean delivery.

B. Therapeutic Uses: Oxytocin is used to induce labor and augment dysfunctional labor for (1) conditions requiring early vaginal delivery (eg, Rh problems, maternal diabetes, or preeclampsia), (2) uterine inertia, and (3) incomplete abortion. Oxytocin can also be used for control of postpartum uterine hemorrhage. Impaired milk ejection may respond to oxytocin.

Synthetic peptide and nonpeptide oxytocin antagonists that can prevent premature labor are being investigated.

Dosage

For induction of labor, oxytocin should be administered intravenously via an infusion pump with appropriate fetal monitoring. An initial infusion rate of 1 mU/min is gradually increased to 5–20 mU/min until a physiologic contraction pattern is established. For postpartum uterine bleeding, 10–40 units is added to 1 L of 5% dextrose, and the infusion rate is titrated to control uterine atony. Alternatively, 10 units can be given intramuscularly after delivery of the placenta. To induce milk let-down, one puff is sprayed into each nostril in the sitting position 2–3 minutes before nursing.

Toxicity & Contraindications

When oxytocin is used properly, serious toxicity is rare. Among the reported adverse reactions are maternal deaths due to hypertensive episodes, uterine rupture, and water intoxication and fetal deaths. Afibrinogenemia has also been reported.

Contraindications include fetal distress, prematurity, abnormal fetal presentation, cephalopelvic disproportion, and other predispositions for uterine rupture. Sympathomimetic agents should not be used with oxytocin.

VASOPRESSIN
(Antidiuretic Hormone, ADH)

Vasopressin is a peptide hormone released by the posterior pituitary in response to rising plasma tonicity or falling blood pressure. Vasopressin possesses antidiuretic and vasopressor properties. A deficiency of this hormone results in diabetes insipidus (see Chapters 15 and 17).

Chemistry & Pharmacokinetics

A. Structure: Vasopressin is a nonapeptide with a six amino acid ring and a three amino acid side chain. The residue at position 8 is arginine in humans and in most other mammals except pigs and related species, whose vasopressin contains lysine at position 8 (Figure 36–3).

B. Absorption, Metabolism, and Excretion: Vasopressin must be administered parenterally. Intravenous, intramuscular, or intranasal routes of administration may be selected. The half-life of circulating ADH is approximately 20 minutes, with renal and hepatic catabolism via reduction of the disulfide bond and peptide cleavage. A small amount of vasopressin is excreted as such in the urine, but urinary clearance is less than 5% of that of creatinine and does not reflect plasma levels.

Pharmacodynamics

Vasopressin interacts with two types of receptors. V_1 receptors are found on vascular smooth muscle cells and mediate vasoconstriction. V_2 receptors are found on renal tubule cells and mediate antidiuresis through increased water permeability and water resorption in the collecting tubules. Extrarenal V_2-like receptors mediate release of coagulation factor VIII_c and von Willebrand factor as well as a decrease in blood pressure and peripheral resistance.

Desmopressin acetate (DDAVP, 1-desamino-8-D-arginine vasopressin) is a long-acting synthetic analogue of vasopressin with minimal V_1 activity and an antidiuretic-to-pressor ratio 4000 times that of vasopressin.

Clinical Pharmacology

Vasopressin and desmopressin are the alternative

treatments of choice for pituitary diabetes insipidus. Bedtime desmopressin therapy ameliorates nocturnal enuresis by decreasing nocturnal urine production. A desmopressin challenge can assess renal concentrating capacity after long-term lithium therapy. Vasopressin infusion is effective in some cases of esophageal variceal bleeding and colonic diverticular bleeding. It is much less effective in bleeding caused by gastric or small intestine mucosal damage. Unfortunately, vasopressin infusion may also cause coronary artery vasoconstriction.

Synthetic vasopressin antagonists are being investigated for use in states of vasopressin-induced water retention.

Dosage

Four preparations are in common use.

A. Aqueous Vasopressin: Synthetic aqueous vasopressin is a short-acting preparation for intramuscular, subcutaneous, or intravenous administration. The dose is 5–10 units subcutaneously or intramuscularly every 36 hours for transient diabetes insipidus and 0.1–0.5 units/min intravenously for gastrointestinal bleeding.

B. Vasopressin Tannate in Oil: Vasopressin tannate in oil is a long-acting form for intramuscular injection. The dosage is 2.5–5 units every 24–72 hours.

C. Lysine Vasopressin: Lypressin is a short-acting nasal spray. The dosage is 2 units sprayed deeply into one or both nostrils every 4–6 hours.

D. Desmopressin Acetate: This is the preferred treatment for most patients with chronic diabetes insipidus. Desmopressin may be administered intranasally, intravenously, or subcutaneously. The nasal dosage is 10–40 µg (0.1–0.4 mL) daily in two or three divided doses. Injectable desmopressin is approximately ten times more bioavailable than intranasal desmopressin. The dosage by injection is 2–4 µg (0.5–1 mL) daily in two divided doses.

For nocturnal enuresis, desmopressin, 10–20 µg (0.1–0.2 mL) intranasally at bedtime is used. Renal concentrating capacity can be tested with a desmopressin challenge of 20 µg to each nostril. A urine osmolality above 800 mosm/kg within 8 hours is a normal response.

Desmopressin is also approved for the treatment of coagulopathy in hemophilia A and von Willebrand's disease (see Chapter 33).

Toxicity & Contraindications

Headache, nausea, abdominal cramps, and allergic reactions have been reported. Overdosage can result in hyponatremia.

Vasopressin should be used cautiously in patients with coronary artery disease. Drugs known to potentiate the effects of vasopressin include chlorpropamide, clofibrate, and carbamazepine. Inhalation of vasopressin may be ineffective when nasal congestion is present.

PREPARATIONS AVAILABLE

Bromocriptine (Parlodel)
  Oral: 2.5 mg tablets, 5 mg capsules
Chorionic gonadotropin [hCG] (generic, Profasi, A.P.L., Pregnyl, others)
  Parenteral: powder to reconstitute for injection: 200, 500, 1000, 2000 units/mL
Corticotropin (generic, ACTH, Acthar, H.P. Acthar Gel, others)
  Parenteral: 25, 40 units/vial for SC, IM injection
  Repository preparations: 40, 80 units/mL gel for injection; 40 units/mL corticotropin
Cosyntropin (Cortrosyn)
  Parenteral: 0.25 mg/vial with diluent for IV or IM injection
Desmopressin (DDAVP, Concentraid)
  Nasal: 100 µg/mL solution
  Nasal spray pump: 500 µg in 5 mL; 50 doses of 10 µg each
  Parenteral: 4 µg/mL, 40 µg/10 mL solution for injection
Gonadorelin hydrochloride [GnRH] (Factrel)

  Parenteral: powders to reconstitute for injection: 100, 500 µg/vial)
Gonadorelin acetate [GnRH] (Lutrepulse)
  Parenteral: powder to reconstitute for injection via Lutrepulse pump (0.8, 3.2 mg/vial)
Goserelin acetate (Zoladex)
  Parenteral: 3.6 mg SC implant
Histrelin (Supprelin)
  Parenteral: 120, 300, 600 µg in 0.6 mL vials for SC injection
Leuprolide (Lupron,)
  Parenteral: 5 mg/mL for SC injection
  Parenteral depot suspension (Lupron Depot): lyophilized microspheres to reconstitute for IM injection (3.75, 7.5 mg/vial)
Lypressin (Diapid)
  Nasal: 50 pressor units or 0.185 mg/mL spray
Menotropins [hMG] (Pergonal)
  Parenteral: 75 IU FSH and 75 IU LH activity, 150 IU FSH and 150 IU LH activity, each with diluent

Nafarelin (Synarel)
Nasal: 2 mg/mL; 200 µg/spray
Octreotide (Sandostatin)
Parenteral: 50, 100, 500 µg in 1 mL ampules and 200, 1000 µg/mL in 5 mL vials for SC or IV administration and 200, 1000 µg in 5 mL multidose vials for injection
Oxytocin (generic, Pitocin, Syntocinon)
Parenteral: 10 units/mL for injection
Nasal: 40 units/mL spray
Protirelin (Thypinone, Relefact TRH)
Parenteral: 500 µg/mL for injection
Sermorelin [GHRH] (Geref)
Parenteral: powder to reconstitute for injection (50 µg per vial)
Somatrem (Protropin)

Parenteral: 5, 10 mg/vial with diluent for SC or IM injection
Somatropin (Humatrope)
Parenteral: 5 mg/vial with diluent for SC or IM injection
Thyrotropin [TSH] (Thytropar)
Parenteral: 10 IU/vial with diluent for injection
Urofollitropin (Metrodin)
Parenteral: powder to reconstitute for injection (0.83 mg per ampule; 75 IU FSH activity)
Vasopressin (Pitressin Synthetic)
Parenteral: 20 pressor units/mL for IM or SC administration
Vasopressin Tannate (Pitressin Tannate in Oil)
Parenteral: 5 pressor units/mL for IM injection only

REFERENCES

Hypothalamic Releasing Hormones

Bell GI, Reisine T: Molecular biology of somatostatin receptors. Trends Neurosci 1993;16:34.

Bevan JS et al: Dopamine agonists and pituitary tumor shrinkage. Endocr Rev 1992;13:220.

Ceylan S et al: Treatment of acute spinal cord injuries: Comparison of thyrotropin-releasing hormone and nimodipine. Res Exp Med 1992;192:23.

Chrousos GP: Regulation and dysregulation of the hypothalamic-pituitary-adrenal axis: The corticotropin-releasing hormone perspective. Endocrinol Metab Clin North Am 1992;21:833.

Duck SC et al: Subcutaneous growth hormone-releasing hormone therapy in growth hormone-deficient children: First year of therapy. J Clin Endocrinol Metab 1992;75:1115.

Ezzat S et al: Octreotide treatment of acromegaly: A randomized, multicenter study. Ann Intern Med 1992; 117:711.

Klingmuller D et al: Hormonal responses to the new potent GnRH antagonist Cetrorelix. Acta Endocrinol 1993;128:15.

Lifshitz F et al: Sustained improvement in growth velocity and recovery from suboptimal growth hormone (GH) secretion after treatment with human pituitary GH-releasing hormone-(1–44)-NH$_2$. J Clin Endocrinol Metab 1992;75:1255.

Marbach P et al: From somatostatin to Sandostatin: Pharmacodynamics and pharmacokinetics. Metabolism 1992;41(Suppl 2):7.

Maton PN, Jensen RT: Use of gut peptide receptor agonists and antagonists in gastrointestinal diseases. Gastroenterol Clin North Am 1992;21:551.

Moghissi KS: Clinical applications of gonadotropin-releasing hormones in reproductive disorders. Endocrinol Metab Clin North Am 1992;21:125.

Molitch ME: Pathologic hyperprolactinemia. Endocrinol Metab Clin North Am 1992;21:877.

Orth DN: Corticotropin-releasing hormone in humans. Endocr Rev 1992;13:164.

Spencer CA et al: Thyrotropin (TSH)-releasing hormone stimulation test responses employing third and fourth generation TSH assays. J Clin Endocrinol Metab 1993;76:494.

Tjerk WA et al: Clinically monitoring pituitary adenoma and octreotide response to long term high dose treatment and studies in vitro. J Clin Endocrinol Metab 1992;75:1310.

Anterior Pituitary Hormones

Bengtsson B-A et al: Treatment of adults with growth hormone (GH) deficiency with recombinant human GH. J Clin Endocrinol Metab 1993;76:309.

Blacker CM: Ovulation stimulation and induction. Endocrinol Metab Clin North Am 1992;21:57.

Chappel SC, Howles C: Reevaluation of the roles of luteinizing hormone and follicle-stimulating hormone in the ovulatory process. Human Reprod 1991;6:1206.

Christiansen P et al: Hormonal treatment of cryptorchidism-hCG or GnRH: A multicentre study. Acta Paediatr 1992;81:605.

Fava M et al: The thyrotropin response to thyrotropin-releasing hormone as a predictor of response to treatment in depressed outpatients. Acta Psychiatr Scand 1992;86:42.

Lavalie C: Prolactin: A hormone with immunoregulatory properties that leads to new therapeutic approaches in rheumatic diseases. J Rheumatol 1992;19:839.

Oelkers W et al: Diagnosis and therapy surveillance in Addison's disease: Rapid adrenocorticotropin (ACTH) test and measurement of plasma ACTH, renin activity, and aldosterone. J Clin Endocrinol Metab 1992; 75:259.

Peabody CA et al: Prolactin bioassay and hyperprolactinemia. J Endocrinol Invest 1992;15:497.

Spirtas R et al: Fertility drugs and ovarian cancer: Red alert or red herring? Fertil Steril 1993;59:291.

Tapanainen P, Knip M: Evaluation of growth hormone secretion and treatment. Ann Med 1992;24:237.

Thotakura NR et al: The role of the oligosaccharide

chains of thyrotropin α- and β-subunits in hormone action. Endocrinol 1992;131:82.

van Kooten B et al: A pilot study on the influence of a corticotropin (4–9) analogue on *Vinca* alkaloid-induced neuropathy. Arch Neurol 1992;49:1027.

Posterior Pituitary Hormones

Blevins LS Jr, Wand GS: Diabetes insipidus. Crit Care Med 1992;20:69.

Chelmow D, Laros RK Jr: Maternal and neonatal outcomes after oxytocin augmentation in patients undergoing a trial of labor after prior cesarean delivery. Obstet Gynecol 1992;80:966.

Evans BE et al: Orally active, nonpeptide oxytocin antagonists. J Med Chem 1992;35:3919.

Key DW et al: Low-dose DDAVP in nocturnal enuresis. Clin Pediatr 1992;31:299.

37

Thyroid & Antithyroid Drugs

Francis S. Greenspan, MD, & Betty J. Dong, PharmD

Because of its anatomic prominence, the thyroid was one of the first of the endocrine glands to be correctly associated with the clinical conditions caused by its malfunction. This gland releases two very different types of hormones. This chapter discusses the pharmacology of the thyroid hormones essential for growth and development and for regulation of energy metabolism: thyroxine and triiodothyronine. The second type of thyroid hormone, calcitonin, is important in the regulation of calcium metabolism and is discussed in Chapter 41.

THYROID PHYSIOLOGY

The normal thyroid gland secretes sufficient amounts of the thyroid hormones—triiodothyronine (T_3) and tetraiodothyronine (T_4, thyroxine)—to maintain normal growth and development, normal body temperature, and normal energy levels. These hormones contain 59% and 65% (respectively) of iodine as an essential part of the molecule.

Iodide Metabolism

Nearly all of the iodide (I^-)[*] intake is via the gastrointestinal tract from food, water, or medication. The recommended daily adult intake is 150 µg. This ingested iodide is rapidly absorbed and enters an extracellular fluid pool. The thyroid gland removes about 75 µg a day from this pool for hormone secretion, and the balance is excreted in the urine. If iodide intake is increased, the fractional iodine uptake by the thyroid is diminished.

Biosynthesis of Thyroid Hormones

Once taken up by the thyroid gland, iodide undergoes a series of enzymatic reactions that convert it into active thyroid hormone (Figure 37–1). The first step is the transport of iodide into the thyroid gland, called **iodide trapping.** This can be inhibited by such

anions as SCN^-, BF_4^-, NO_3^-, and ClO_4^-. Iodide is then oxidized by thyroidal peroxidase to iodine, in which form it rapidly iodinates tyrosine residues within the thyroglobulin molecule to form monoiodotyrosine (MIT) and diiodotyrosine (DIT). This process is called **iodide organification.** Two molecules of DIT combine within the thyroglobulin molecule to form L-thyroxine (T_4). One molecule of MIT and one molecule of DIT combine to form T_3. In addition to thyroglobulin, other proteins within the gland may be iodinated, but these iodoproteins do not have hormonal activity. Thyroid hormones are released from thyroglobulin by exocytosis and proteolysis of thyroglobulin at the apical colloid border. The colloid droplets of thyroglobulin merge with lysosomes containing proteolytic enzymes, which hydrolyze thyroglobulin and release T_4, T_3, MIT, and DIT. The MIT and DIT are deiodinated within the gland, and the iodine is reutilized. In addition to T_4 and T_3, small amounts of thyroglobulin, tyrosine, and iodide are secreted. The ratio of T_4 to T_3 within thyroglobulin is approximately 5:1, so that most of the hormone released is thyroxine. Most of the T_3 circulating in the blood is derived from peripheral metabolism of thyroxine (see below).

Transport of Thyroid Hormones

T_4 and T_3 in plasma are reversibly bound to protein, primarily thyroxine-binding globulin (TBG). About 0.04% of total T_4 and 0.4% of T_3 exist in the free form.

Many physiologic and pathologic states and drugs affect T_4, T_3, and thyroid transport. However, the actual levels of free hormone generally remain normal, reflecting feedback control.

Peripheral Metabolism of Thyroid Hormones

A small amount of thyroxine is biologically inactivated by deamination, decarboxylation, or conjugation and excretion as a glucuronide or sulfate. The primary pathway for the peripheral metabolism of thyroxine, however, is deiodination. Deiodination of T_4 may occur by monodeiodination of the outer ring,

---

[*]In this chapter, the term "iodine" denotes all forms of the element; the term "iodide" denotes only the ionic form, I^-.

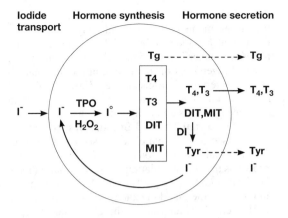

Figure 37–1. Thyroid hormone synthesis in a thyroid follicle (including the thyroid cell and the lumen of the follicle). (I⁻,iodide ion; I°, active I; DI, deiodinase; MIT, monoiodotyrosine; DIT, diiodotyrosine; T_3, triiodothyronine; T_4, thyroxine; TPO, thyroidal peroxidase; Tg, thyroglobulin; Tyr, tyrosine.) (Reproduced, with permission, from Greenspan FS. In: *Basic and Clinical Endocrinology*, 4th ed. Greenspan FS [editor]. Appleton & Lange, 1993.)

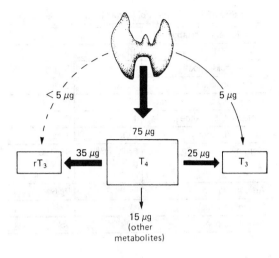

Figure 37–3. Quantitative aspects of thyroid hormone production and metabolism (per day) in normal adults.

producing 3,5,3′-triiodothyronine (T_3), which is three to four times more potent than T_4. Alternatively, deiodination may occur in the inner ring, producing 3,3′,5′triiodothyronine (reverse T_3, or rT_3), which is metabolically inactive (Figure 37–2).

Figure 37–3 shows the amounts of thyroid hormone produced and metabolized per day in normal adults. Normal levels of thyroid hormone in the serum are listed in Table 37–1. The low serum levels of

T_3 and rT_3 in normal individuals are due to the high metabolic clearances of these two compounds.

Control of Thyroid Function

The tests used to evaluate thyroid function are listed in Table 37–2.

A. Thyroid-Pituitary Relationships: Control of thyroid function via the thyroid-pituitary feedback is also discussed in Chapter 36. Briefly, hypothalamic

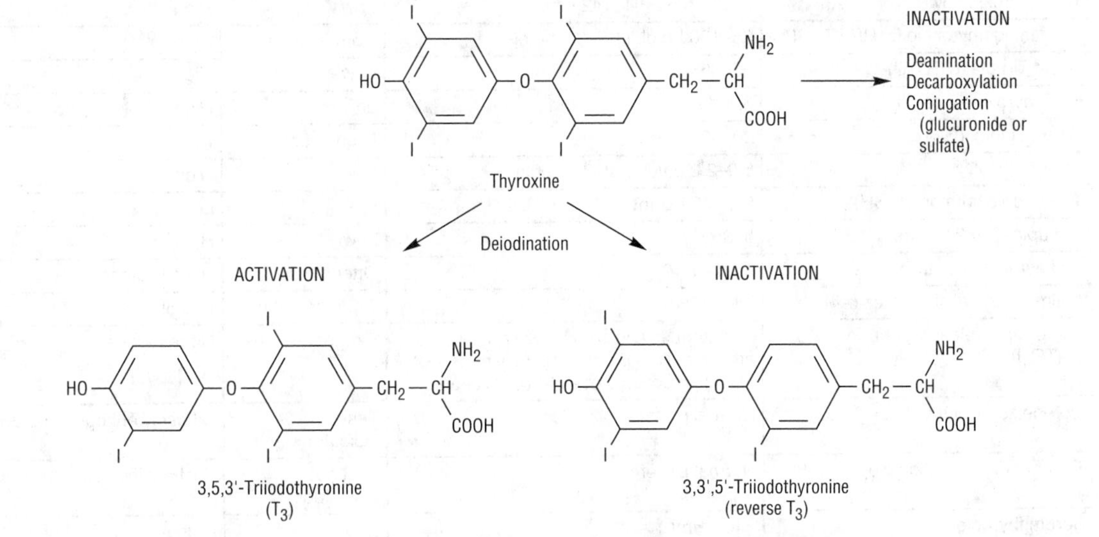

Figure 37–2. Peripheral metabolism of thyroxine. (Modified and reproduced, with permission, from Greenspan FS. In: *Gynecologic Endocrinology*, 3rd ed. Gold JJ, Josimovich JB [editors]. Harper & Row, 1980.)

Table 37–1. Summary of thyroid hormone kinetics.

Kinetic Variable	T_4	T_3
Volume of distribution	10 L	40 L
Extrathyroidal pool	800 µg	54 µg
Daily production	80 µg	30 µg
Fractional turnover per day	10%	60%
Metabolic clearance per day	1.1 L	24 L
Half-life (biologic)	7 days	1 day
Serum levels	5–11 µg/dL (64–142 nmol/L)	95–190 ng/dL (1.5–2.9 nmol/L)
Amount bound	99.96%	99.6%
Biologic potency	1	4
Oral absorption	75–90%	95%

cells secrete thyrotropin-releasing hormone (TRH) (Figure 37–4). TRH is secreted into capillaries of the pituitary portal venous system, and in the pituitary gland TRH stimulates the synthesis and release of thyroid-stimulating hormone (TSH). TSH in turn stimulates an adenylyl cyclase mechanism in the thyroid cell to increase the synthesis and release of T_4 and T_3. These thyroid hormones, in a negative feedback fashion, act in the pituitary to block the action of TRH and in the hypothalamus to inhibit the synthesis and secretion of TRH. Other hormones or drugs may also affect the release of TRH or TSH.

B. Autoregulation of the Thyroid Gland: The thyroid gland also regulates its uptake of iodide and thyroid hormone synthesis by intrathyroidal mechanisms that are independent of TSH. These mechanisms are primarily related to the level of iodine in the blood. Large doses of iodine inhibit iodide organification. In certain disease states (eg, Hashimoto's thyroiditis), this can result in inhibition of thyroid hormone synthesis and in hypothyroidism.

C. Abnormal Thyroid Stimulators: In Graves' disease (see below), lymphocytes secrete a TSH receptor-stimulating antibody (TSH-R Ab[stim]), also known as thyroid-stimulating immunoglobulin (TSI). This immunoglobulin binds to the TSH receptor site and turns on the gland in exactly the same fashion as TSH itself. The duration of the effect, however, is much longer than that of TSH.

I. BASIC PHARMACOLOGY OF THYROID & ANTITHYROID DRUGS

THYROID HORMONES

Chemistry

The structural formulas of thyroxine (T_4) and triiodothyronine (T_3) as well as reverse triiodothyronine

Table 37–2. Normal values for thyroid function tests.

Name	Normal Value[1]	Results in Hypothyroidism	Results in Hyperthyroidism
Total thyroxine by RIA (T_4[RIA])	5–11 µg/dL (64–142 nmol/L)	Low	High
Total triiodothyronine by RIA (T_3[RIA])	95–190 ng/dL (1.5–2.9 nmol/L)	Normal or low	High
Resin T_3 uptake (RT$_3$U)	25–35%	Low	High
Free thyroxine index (FT$_4$I)[1]	6.5–12.5	Low	High
Free T_3 index (FT$_3$I)	20–63	Normal or low	High
Free T_4 (FT$_4$D)[2]	0.9–2.0 pg/dL (12–26 pmol/L)	Low	High
Thyrotropic hormone (TSH)	0.3–5.0 µU/mL (0.3–5.0 mU/L)	High	Low
^{123}I uptake at 24 hours	5–35%	Low	High
Antithyroglobulin antibodies (Atg-ab)	Titer <1:10	Often present	Usually present
Antimicrosomal antibodies (AM-ab)	Titer <1:100	Often present	Usually present
Thyrotropin-releasing hormone (TRH)	>6 µU/mL rise in serum TSH 45 minutes after injection. Blunted TSH response <2 µU/mL in patients over 40 years of age.	Exaggerated rise	No response
Isotope scan with ^{123}I or ^{99m}TcO$_4$	Normal pattern	Test not indicated	Diffusely enlarged gland
Thin-needle aspiration biopsy (TNA)	Normal pattern	Test not indicated	Test not indicated
Serum thyroglobulin	<40 ng/mL	Low	High

[1]Results may vary with different laboratories.
[2]Free thyroxine by dialysis.

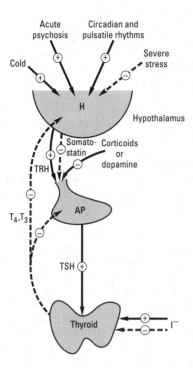

Figure 37–4. The hypothalamic-pituitary-thyroid axis. Acute psychosis or prolonged exposure to cold may activate the axis. Hypothalamic TRH stimulates pituitary TSH release, while somatostatin and dopamine inhibit it. TSH stimulates T_4 and T_3 synthesis and release from the thyroid, and they in turn inhibit both TRH and TSH synthesis and release. Small amounts of iodide are necessary for hormone production, but large amounts inhibit T_3 and T_4 production and release. (Solid arrows, stimulatory influence; dashed arrows, inhibitory influence.)

(rT_3) are shown in Figure 37–2. All of these naturally occurring molecules are levo (L) isomers. The synthetic dextro (D) isomer of thyroxine, dextrothyroxine, has approximately 4% of the biologic activity of the L isomer as evidenced by its ability to suppress TSH secretion and correct hypothyroidism.

Pharmacokinetics

Data on oral absorption of thyroid hormones are derived from administration of exogenous hormones. T_4 is absorbed best in the duodenum and ileum; absorption is modified by intraluminal factors such as food, drugs (eg, aluminum-containing antacids, iron), and intestinal flora. Oral absorption of earlier preparations of L-thyroxine ranged from 35% to 65%; current preparations are better-absorbed, averaging 80% (Table 37–1). In contrast, T_3 is almost completely absorbed (95%) and minimally interfered with by intraluminal binding proteins. T_4 and T_3 absorption appears not to be affected by mild hypothyroidism but may be impaired in severe myxedema with ileus. These factors are important in switching from oral to parenteral therapy. For parenteral use, the intravenous route is preferred for both hormones.

In patients with hyperthyroidism, the metabolic clearance rates of T_4 and T_3 are increased and the half-lives decreased; the opposite is true in patients with hypothyroidism. Drugs that induce hepatic microsomal enzymes (eg, rifampin, phenobarbital, carbamazepine, phenytoin) increase the metabolism of both T_4 and T_3. Despite this change in clearance, the normal hormone concentration is maintained in euthyroid patients as a result of compensatory hyperfunction of the thyroid. However, patients receiving T_4 replacement medication may require increased dosages to maintain clinical effectiveness. A similar compensation occurs if binding sites are altered. If TBG sites are increased by pregnancy, estrogens, or oral contraceptives, there is an initial shift of hormone from the free to the bound state and a decrease in its rate of elimination until the normal hormone concentration is restored. Thus, the concentration of total and bound hormone will increase, but the concentration of free hormone and the steady state elimination will remain normal. The reverse occurs when thyroid binding sites are decreased.

Mechanism of Action

A model of thyroid hormone action is depicted in Figure 37–5. In this model, thyroid hormone T_3 binds to a receptor protein in the cell membrane and increases the uptake of glucose and amino acids into the cell. T_3 can also enter the cell by diffusion. Once within the cell, T_3 binds to cytosol-binding protein (CBP) and exists in equilibrium with free T_3. In the cell, free T_3 may bind to receptors in the inner mitochondrial membrane or to receptors in the nuclear chromatin. The nuclear thyroid hormone receptor belongs to a family of receptors that are homologous with the c-*erb*-A oncogene; other members of this family include the steroid hormone receptors and the receptors for vitamins A and D. The T_3 receptor exists in two forms, a and b, which may function differently in different tissues; this may account for variations in T_3 effects on different tissues.

The responses that follow these hormone-receptor interactions are quite diverse. In the nucleus, an increase in RNA polymerase activity and transcription of DNA results in increased mRNA synthesis, leading to stimulation of protein synthesis and subsequent enzyme and cell activity. Interactions with the mitochondrial receptor may affect regulation of energy metabolism directly and protein synthesis indirectly. Thyroid hormones directly stimulate membrane Na^+/K^+ ATPase, increasing Na^+ and K^+ transport (the sodium pump) and oxygen utilization.

Most of the effects of thyroid on metabolic processes appear to be mediated by activation of nuclear receptors that lead to increased formation of RNA and subsequent protein synthesis. For example, increased formation of the protein Na^+/K^+ ATPase and

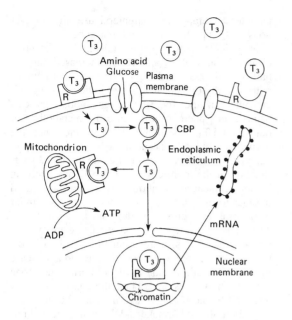

Figure 37–5. Proposed mechanisms of thyroid hormone action. Thyroid hormone (in this case triiodothyronine or T_3) binds to receptor proteins *(R)* on the cell surface and increases the uptake of glucose and amino acids. T_3 also enters the cell where it reacts with cytoplasmic binding proteins *(CBP)* and receptors on chromatin and mitochondria. In the nucleus, the T_3-receptor complex leads to the synthesis of new protein. (Courtesy of JA Williams.)

the consequent increase in ATP turnover and oxygen consumption are responsible for some of the calorigenic effects of thyroid hormones. This is consistent with the observation that the action of thyroid is manifested in vivo with a time lag of hours or days after its administration.

Large numbers of thyroid hormone receptors are found in the most hormone-responsive tissues (pituitary, liver, kidney, heart, skeletal muscle, lung, and intestine), while few receptor sites occur in hormone-unresponsive tissues (spleen, testes). The brain, which lacks an anabolic response to T_3, contains an intermediate number of receptors. In congruence with their biologic potencies, the affinity of the receptor site for T_4 is about ten times lower than that for T_3. The number of nuclear receptors may be altered to preserve body homeostasis. For example, starvation lowers both circulating T_3 hormone and cellular T_3 receptors.

Effects of Thyroid Hormones

The thyroid hormones are responsible for optimal growth, development, function, and maintenance of all body tissues (Table 37–3). Since T_3 and T_4 are qualitatively similar, they may be considered as one hormone in the discussion that follows.

Thyroid hormone is critical for nervous, skeletal, and reproductive tissues. Its effects depend upon protein synthesis as well as potentiation of the secretion and action of growth hormone. Thyroid deprivation in early life results in irreversible mental retardation and dwarfism—symptoms typical of congenital cretinism.

Effects on growth and calorigenesis are accompanied by a pervasive influence on metabolism of drugs as well as carbohydrates, fats, proteins, and vitamins. Many of these changes are dependent upon or modified by activity of other hormones. Conversely, the secretion and degradation rates of virtually all other hormones, including catecholamines, cortisol, estrogens, testosterone, and insulin, are affected by thyroid status.

Many of the manifestations of thyroid hyperactivity resemble sympathetic nervous system overactivity, though catecholamine levels are not increased. Possible explanations have included an increased number of beta receptor sites or enhanced amplification of the beta receptor signal without an increase in the number of receptor sites. Changes in catecholamine-stimulated adenylyl cyclase activity as measured by cAMP are found with changes in thyroid activity. The most dramatic effects of this catecholamine hyperactivity are seen in the cardiovascular system. Other clinical symptoms reminiscent of excessive epinephrine activity and partially alleviated by adrenoceptor antagonists include lid lag and retraction, tremor, excessive sweating, anxiety, nervousness, and muscle weakness. The opposite constellation of symptoms is seen in hypothyroidism (Table 37–3).

Thyroid Preparations

See the Preparations Available section at the end of this chapter for a list of available preparations. Available preparations may be synthetic (levothyroxine, liothyronine, liotrix) or of animal origin (desiccated thyroid).

Synthetic levothyroxine is the preparation of choice for thyroid replacement and suppression therapy because of its stability, content uniformity, low cost, lack of allergenic foreign protein, easy laboratory measurement of serum levels, and long half-life (7 days), which permits once-daily administration. In addition, T_4 is converted to T_3 intracellularly; thus, administration of T_4 produces both hormones. Generic levothyroxine preparations can be used because they provide comparable efficacy and are more cost-effective than branded preparations.

Although liothyronine is three to four times more active than levothyroxine, it is not recommended for routine replacement therapy because of its shorter half-life (24 hours), which requires multiple daily doses; its higher cost; and the greater difficulty of monitoring its adequacy of replacement by conventional laboratory tests. Furthermore, because of its greater hormone activity and consequent greater risk

Table 37–3. Summary of thyroid hormone effects.

System	Thyrotoxicosis	Hypothyroidism
Skin and appendages	Warm, moist skin; sweating; heat intolerance; fine, thin hair; Plummer's nails; pretibial dermopathy (Graves' disease).	Pale, cool, puffy skin; dry and brittle hair; brittle nails.
Eyes, face	Retraction of upper lid with wide stare; periorbital edema; exophthalmos; diplopia (Graves' disease).	Drooping of eyelids; periorbital edema; loss of temporal aspects of eyebrows; puffy, nonpitting facies; large tongue.
Cardiovascular system	Increased peripheral vascular resistance, heart rate, stroke volume, cardiac output, pulse pressure; high-output congestive heart failure; increased inotropic/chronotropic effects; arrhythmias; angina.	Decreased peripheral vascular resistance, heart rate, stroke volume, cardiac output, pulse pressure; low-output congestive heart failure; ECG: bradycardia, prolonged PR interval, flat T wave, low voltage; pericardial effusion.
Respiratory system	Dyspnea; decreased vital capacity.	Pleural effusions; hypoventilation and CO_2 retention.
Gastrointestinal system	Increased appetite; increased frequency of bowel movements; hypoproteinemia.	Decreased appetite; decreased frequency of bowel movements; ascites.
Central nervous system	Nervousness; hyperkinesia; emotional lability.	Lethargy; general slowing of mental processes; neuropathies.
Musculoskeletal system	Weakness and muscle fatigue; increased deep tendon reflexes; hypercalcemia; osteoporosis.	Stiffness and muscle fatigue; decreased deep tendon reflexes; increased alkaline phosphatase, LDH, AST.
Renal system	Mild polyuria; increased renal blood flow; increased glomerular filtration rate.	Impaired water excretion; decreased renal blood flow; decreased glomerular filtration rate.
Hematopoietic system	Increased erythropoiesis; anemia.[1]	Decreased erythropoiesis; anemia.[1]
Reproductive system	Menstrual irregularities; decreased fertility; increased gonadal steroid metabolism.	Hypermenorrhea; infertility; decreased libido; impotency; oligospermia; decreased gonadal steroid metabolism.
Metabolic system	Increased basal metabolic rate; negative nitrogen balance; hyperglycemia; increased free fatty acids; decreased cholesterol and triglycerides; increased hormone degradation; increased requirements for fat- and water-soluble vitamins; increased drug detoxification.	Decreased basal metabolic rate; slight positive nitrogen balance; delayed degradation of insulin, with increased sensitivity; increased cholesterol and triglycerides; decreased hormone degradation; decreased requirements for fat- and water-soluble vitamins; decreased drug detoxification.

[1]The anemia of hyperthyroidism is usually normochromic and caused by increased RBC turnover. The anemia of hypothyroidism may be normochromic, hyperchromic, or hypochromic and may be due to decreased production rate, decreased iron absorption, decreased folic acid absorption, or to autoimmune pernicious anemia.

of cardiotoxicity, T_3 should be avoided in patients with cardiac disease. It is best used as a diagnostic agent in the T_3 suppression test and in short-term suppression of TSH. Because oral administration of T_3 is unnecessary, use of the more expensive liotrix instead of levothyroxine is never required. It is also important to note that Euthroid is 20% more potent than Thyrolar when the effects of corresponding amounts are compared.

The use of desiccated thyroid rather than synthetic preparations is never justified, since the disadvantages of protein antigenicity, product instability, variable hormone concentrations, and difficulty in laboratory monitoring far outweigh the advantage of low cost. Significant amounts of T_3 found in some thyroid extracts and liotrix may produce significant elevations in T_3 levels and toxicity. Equivalent dosages are 100 mg ($1\frac{1}{2}$ grain) of thyroglobulin or desiccated thyroid, 100 μg of levothyroxine, and 37.5 μg of liothyronine.

The shelf life of synthetic hormone preparations is about 2 years, particularly if they are stored in dark

bottles to minimize spontaneous deiodination. The shelf life of desiccated thyroid is not well known, but if it is kept dry and free from moisture, its potency is better preserved.

ANTITHYROID AGENTS

Reduction of thyroid activity and hormone effects can be accomplished by agents that interfere with the production of thyroid hormones; by agents that modify the tissue response to thyroid hormones; or by glandular destruction with radiation or surgery. "Goitrogens" are agents that suppress secretion of T_3 and T_4 to subnormal levels and thereby increase TSH, which in turn produces glandular enlargement (goiter). The antithyroid compounds used clinically include the thioamides, iodides, and radioactive iodine, which will be discussed later.

1. THIOAMIDES

The thioamides methimazole and propylthiouracil are major drugs for treatment of thyrotoxicosis. In the United Kingdom, carbimazole, which is converted to methimazole in vivo, is widely used. Methimazole is about ten times more active than propylthiouracil.

The chemical structures of these compounds are shown in Figure 37–6. The thiocarbamide group is essential for antithyroid activity:

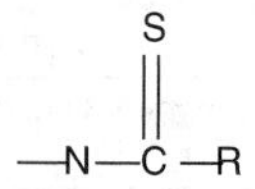

$$\underset{\Large\|}{\overset{\Large S}{\underset{}{}}}$$

$$-N-C-R$$

Pharmacokinetics

Propylthiouracil is rapidly absorbed, reaching peak serum levels after 1 hour. The bioavailability of 50–80% may be due to incomplete absorption or a large first-pass effect in the liver. The volume of distribution approximates total body water with accumulation in the thyroid gland. Most of an ingested dose of propylthiouracil is excreted by the kidney as the inactive glucuronide within 24 hours.

In contrast, methimazole is completely absorbed but at variable rates. It is readily accumulated by the thyroid gland and has a volume of distribution similar to that of propylthiouracil. Excretion is slower than with propylthiouracil; 65–70% of a dose is recovered in the urine in 48 hours.

The short plasma half-life of these agents ($1\frac{1}{2}$ hours for propylthiouracil and 6 hours for methimazole) has little influence on the duration of the antithyroid action or the dosing interval because both agents are accumulated by the thyroid gland. For propylthiouracil, giving the drug every 6 hours is reasonable since a single 100 mg dose can inhibit 60% of iodine organification for 7 hours. Since a single 30 mg dose of methimazole exerts an antithyroid effect for longer than 24 hours, a single daily dose is effective in the management of mild to moderate hyperthyroidism.

Both thioamides cross the placental barrier and are concentrated by the fetal thyroid, so that caution must be employed while using these drugs in pregnancy. Of the two, propylthiouracil is preferable in pregnancy because it is more strongly protein-bound and therefore crosses the placenta less readily. In addition, it is not secreted in sufficient quantity in breast milk to preclude breast feeding.

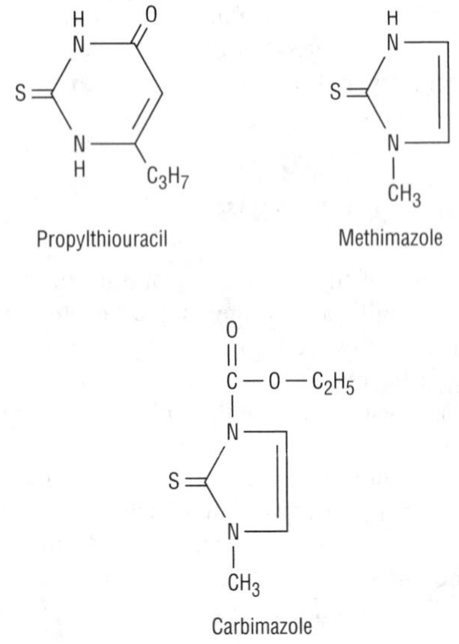

Pharmacodynamics

The thioamides act by multiple mechanisms. The major action is to prevent hormone synthesis by inhibiting the thyroid peroxidase-catalyzed reactions to block iodine organification. In addition, they block coupling of the iodotyrosines. They do not block uptake of iodide by the gland. Propylthiouracil and (to a much lesser extent) methimazole inhibit the peripheral deiodination of T_4 and T_3. Since the synthesis rather than the release of hormones is affected, the onset of these agents is slow, often requiring 3–4 weeks before stores of T_4 are depleted.

Toxicity

Adverse reactions to the thioamides occur in 3–12% of treated patients. Most reactions occur early. The most common adverse effect is a maculopapular pruritic rash, at times accompanied by systemic signs such as fever. Rare adverse effects include an urticarial rash, vasculitis, arthralgia, a lupus-like reaction, cholestatic jaundice, hepatitis, lymphadenopathy, hypoprothrombinemia, and polyserositis. The most dangerous complication is agranulocytosis, an infrequent but potentially fatal adverse reaction. It occurs in 0.3–0.6% of patients taking thioamides, but the risk is increased in older patients and in those receiving high-dose methimazole therapy (over 40 mg/d). The reaction is usually rapidly reversible when the drug is discontinued, but antibiotic therapy may be necessary for complicating infections. The cross-sensitivity between propylthiouracil and methimazole is about 50%; therefore, switching drugs in patients with severe reactions is not recommended.

2. ANION INHIBITORS

Monovalent anions such as perchlorate (ClO_4^-), pertechnetate (TcO_4^-), and thiocyanate (SCN^-) can block uptake of iodide by the gland through competitive inhibition of the iodide transport mechanism. Since these effects can be overcome by large doses of

Propylthiouracil   Methimazole

Carbimazole

Figure 37–6. Structure of thioamides.

iodides, their effectiveness is somewhat unpredictable.

Most of these agents, because of their toxicity, are used clinically only for diagnostic purposes. Potassium perchlorate was used clinically in the treatment of thyrotoxicosis until it was shown to cause aplastic anemia.

3. IODIDES

Iodides have been known since the 1920s to have multiple effects on the thyroid gland. Prior to the introduction of the thioamides in the 1940s, iodides were the major antithyroid agents; today they are rarely used as sole therapy.

Pharmacodynamics

Iodides have several actions on the thyroid. They inhibit organification and hormone release and decrease the size and vascularity of the hyperplastic gland. In susceptible individuals, iodides can induce hyperthyroidism (jodbasedow) or precipitate hypothyroidism.

In pharmacologic doses (> 6 mg daily), the major action of iodides is to inhibit hormone release, possibly through inhibition of thyroglobulin proteolysis. Rapid improvement in thyrotoxic symptoms occurs within 2–7 days—hence the value of iodide therapy in thyroid storm. In addition, iodides decrease the vascularity, size, and fragility of a hyperplastic gland, making the drugs valuable as preoperative preparation for surgery.

Clinical Use of Iodide

Disadvantages of iodide therapy include an increase in intraglandular stores of iodine, which may delay onset of thioamide therapy or prevent use of radioactive iodine therapy for several weeks. Thus, iodides should be initiated after onset of thioamide therapy and avoided if treatment with radioactive iodine seems likely. Iodide should not be used alone, because the gland will "escape" from the iodide block in 2–8 weeks, and its withdrawal may produce severe exacerbation of thyrotoxicosis in an iodine-enriched gland. Chronic use of iodides in pregnancy should be avoided, since they cross the placenta and can cause fetal goiter.

Toxicity

Adverse reactions to iodine (iodism) are uncommon and in most cases reversible upon discontinuance. They include acneiform rash (similar to that of bromism), swollen salivary glands, mucous membrane ulcerations, conjunctivitis, rhinorrhea, drug fever, metallic taste, bleeding disorders, and, rarely, anaphylactoid reactions.

4. IODINATED CONTRAST MEDIA

The iodinated contrast agents, ipodate and iopanoic acid, are valuable in the treatment of hyperthyroidism, though they are not approved by the FDA for this indication. These drugs rapidly inhibit the conversion of T_4 to T_3 in the liver, kidney, pituitary gland, and brain. This accounts for the dramatic improvement in both subjective and objective parameters. For example, a decrease in heart rate is seen after only 3 days of oral administration of 0.5–1 g/d. T_3 levels often return to normal during this time. The prolonged effect of suppressing T_4 as well as T_3 suggests that inhibition of hormone release due to the iodine released may be an additional mechanism of action. Fortunately, these agents are relatively nontoxic. They provide useful adjunctive therapy in the treatment of thyroid storm and offer valuable alternatives when iodides or thioamides are contraindicated. Surprisingly, these agents may not interfere with ^{131}I retention as much as iodides despite their large iodine content. Their toxicity is similar to that of the iodides, and their safety in pregnancy is undocumented.

5. RADIOACTIVE IODINE

[131]I is the only isotope used for treatment of thyrotoxicosis. Administered orally in solution as sodium ^{131}I, it is rapidly absorbed, concentrated by the thyroid, and incorporated into storage follicles. Its therapeutic effect depends on emission of beta rays with an effective half-life of 5 days and a penetration range of 400–2000 μm. Within a few weeks after administration, destruction of the thyroid parenchyma is evidenced by epithelial swelling and necrosis, follicular disruption, edema, and leukocyte infiltration. Advantages of radioiodine include easy administration, effectiveness, low expense, and absence of pain. Fears of radiation-induced genetic damage, leukemia, and neoplasia have caused some clinics to restrict the use of radioiodine in the treatment of hyperthyroidism to adults over some specified age such as 40 years. However, after more than 30 years of clinical experience with radioiodine, these fears have not been realized. Radioactive iodine should not be administered to pregnant women or nursing mothers, since it crosses the placenta and is excreted in breast milk.

6. ADRENOCEPTOR-BLOCKING AGENTS

Many of the symptoms of thyrotoxicosis mimic those associated with sympathetic stimulation, and sympathoplegic agents such as guanethidine or beta-blockers are useful therapeutic adjuncts. Beta-adrenoceptor-blocking drugs are the agents of choice because they are effective in patients refractory to guanethidine and reserpine. Propranolol has been the drug in this group most widely used and studied in the therapy of thyrotoxicosis.

II. CLINICAL PHARMACOLOGY OF THYROID & ANTITHYROID DRUGS

HYPOTHYROIDISM

Hypothyroidism is a syndrome resulting from deficiency of thyroid hormones and is manifested largely by a reversible slowing down of all body functions (Table 37–3). In infants and children, there is striking retardation of growth and development that results in dwarfism and irreversible mental retardation.

The etiology and pathogenesis of hypothyroidism are outlined in Table 37–4. Hypothyroidism can occur with or without thyroid enlargement (goiter). The laboratory diagnosis of hypothyroidism in the adult is easily made by the combination of a low free thyroxine (or low free thyroxine index) and elevated serum TSH (Table 37–2).

The most common cause of hypothyroidism in the USA at this time is probably Hashimoto's thyroiditis, an immunologic disorder in genetically predisposed individuals. In this condition, there is evidence of humoral immunity in the presence of antithyroid antibodies and lymphocyte sensitization to thyroid antigens.

Management of Hypothyroidism

Except for hypothyroidism caused by drugs (Table 37–4), which can be treated by simply removing the depressant agent, the general strategy of replacement therapy is appropriate. The most satisfactory preparation is levothyroxine. Infants and children require more T_4 per kilogram of body weight than adults. The average dose for an infant 1–6 months of age is 10–15 μg/kg/d, whereas the average dose for an adult is about 1.7 μg/kg/d. There is some variability in the absorption of thyroxine, so this dosage may vary from patient to patient. Because of the long half-life of thyroxine, the dose can be given once daily. Children should be monitored for normal growth and development. Serum TSH and the free thyroxine index should be measured at regular intervals and maintained within the normal range. It takes 6–8 weeks after starting a given dose of thyroxine to reach steady state levels in the bloodstream. Thus, dosage changes should be made slowly.

In long-standing hypothyroidism, in older patients, and in patients with underlying cardiac disease, it is imperative to start treatment with reduced dosage. In such adult patients, levothyroxine is given in a dose of 0.0125–0.025 mg/d for 2 weeks, increasing by 0.025 mg every 2 weeks until euthyroidism or drug toxicity is observed. In older patients, the heart is very sensitive to the level of circulating thyroxine, and if angina pectoris or cardiac arrhythmia develops, it is essential to stop or reduce the dose of thyroxine immediately. In younger patients or those with very mild disease, full replacement therapy may be started immediately.

The toxicity of thyroxine is directly related to the hormone level. In children, restlessness, insomnia, and accelerated bone maturation and growth may be signs of thyroxine toxicity. In adults, increased nervousness, heat intolerance, episodes of palpitation and tachycardia, or unexplained weight loss may be the presenting symptoms of thyroid toxicity. If these symptoms are present, it is important to monitor the free thyroxine index (Table 37–2), which will determine whether the symptoms are due to excess thyroxine blood levels.

Special Problems in Management of Hypothyroidism

A. Myxedema and Coronary Artery Disease: Since myxedema frequently occurs in older persons, it is often associated with underlying coronary artery disease. In this situation, the low levels of circulating thyroid hormone actually protect the heart against increasing demands that could result in angina pectoris or myocardial infarction. Correction of myxedema

Table 37–4. Etiology and pathogenesis of hypothyroidism.

Cause	Pathogenesis	Goiter	Degree of Hypothyroidism
Hashimoto's thyroiditis	Autoimmune destruction of thyroid.	Present early, absent later	Mild to severe
Drug-induced[1]	Blocked hormone formation.	Present	Mild to moderate
Dyshormonogenesis	Impaired synthesis of T_4 due to enzyme deficiency.	Present	Mild to severe
Radiation, ^{131}I, x-ray	Destruction of gland.	Absent	Severe
Congenital (cretinism)	Athyreosis or ectopic thyroid, iodine deficiency. TSH receptor blocking antibodies.	Absent or present	Severe
Secondary (TSH deficit)	Pituitary or hypothalamic disease.	Absent	Mild

[1]Iodides, lithium, fluoride, thionamides, aminosalicylic acid, phenylbutazone, amiodarone, etc.

must be done cautiously to avoid provoking arrhythmia, angina, or acute myocardial infarction. Complete restoration of the euthyroid state may not be possible in patients with severe coronary artery disease unless bypass coronary artery surgery restores a more adequate coronary circulation.

B. Myxedema Coma: Myxedema coma is an end state of untreated hypothyroidism. It is associated with progressive weakness, stupor, hypothermia, hypoventilation, hypoglycemia, hyponatremia, water intoxication, shock, and death. Symptoms usually develop quite slowly, with a gradual onset of lethargy, progressing to stupor or coma.

The pathophysiology of myxedema coma involves three major aspects: (1) CO_2 retention and hypoxia associated with decreased sensitivity of the respiratory center; (2) fluid and electrolyte imbalance with hyponatremia; and (3) marked hypothermia, with body temperatures as low as 24 °C (75 °F). Serum tests are consistent with severe hypothyroidism (see above).

Management of myxedema coma is a medical emergency. The patient should be treated in the intensive care unit, since tracheal intubation and mechanical ventilation may be required. Associated illnesses such as infection or heart failure must be treated by appropriate therapy. It is important to give all preparations intravenously, because patients with myxedema coma absorb drugs poorly from other routes. Intravenous fluids should be administered with caution to avoid excessive water intake. These patients have large pools of empty T_3 and T_4 binding sites in their sera that must be filled before there is adequate free thyroxine to affect tissue metabolism. Accordingly, the treatment of choice in myxedema coma is to give a loading dose of levothyroxine intravenously—usually 300–400 μg initially, followed by 50 μg daily. Intravenous T_3 can also be used but may be more cardiotoxic and more difficult to monitor. Intravenous hydrocortisone is indicated if the patient has associated adrenal or pituitary insufficiency but is probably not necessary in most patients with primary myxedema. Narcotics and sedatives must be used with extreme caution.

Clinically, improvement is evidenced by an increase in body temperature and arousal from the comatose state. Once the patient is able to breathe normally, assisted mechanical ventilation can be removed, and steady improvement will ensue.

C. Hypothyroidism and Pregnancy: Hypothyroid women frequently have anovulatory cycles and are therefore relatively infertile until restoration of the euthyroid state. This has led to the widespread use of thyroid hormone for infertility, though there is no evidence for its usefulness in infertile euthyroid patients. In a pregnant hypothyroid patient receiving thyroxine, it is extremely important that the daily dose of thyroxine be adequate because early development of the fetal brain is dependent on maternal thyroxine. In many hypothyroid patients, a modest increase in the thyroxine dose (about 20%) is required to normalize the serum TSH level during pregnancy. Because of the elevated maternal TBG, the free thyroxine index (FT_4I) or free thyroxine by dialysis (FT_4D) (Table 37–2) must be used to monitor maternal thyroxine dosages.

HYPERTHYROIDISM

Hyperthyroidism (thyrotoxicosis) is the clinical syndrome that results when tissues are exposed to high levels of thyroid hormone.

1. GRAVES' DISEASE

The most common form of hyperthyroidism is Graves' disease, or diffuse toxic goiter. The presenting signs and symptoms of Graves' disease are set forth in Table 37–3.

Pathophysiology

Graves' disease is considered to be an autoimmune disorder in which there is a genetic defect in suppressor T lymphocytes, and helper T lymphocytes stimulate B lymphocytes to synthesize antibodies to thyroidal antigens. One such antibody—TSH receptor-stimulating antibody (TSH-R Ab[stim]), also called thyroid-stimulating immunoglobulin (TSI)—is directed against the TSH receptor site in the thyroid cell membrane and has the capacity to stimulate the thyroid cell.

Laboratory Diagnosis

In most patients with hyperthyroidism, T_3, T_4, RT_3U, FT_4D, and FT_4I will all be elevated and TSH is suppressed (Table 37–2). Radioiodine uptake is usually markedly elevated as well. Antithyroglobulin antibodies, antimicrosomal antibodies, and TSH-R Ab[stim] are often present.

Management of Graves' Disease

The three primary methods for controlling hyperthyroidism are antithyroid drug therapy, surgical thyroidectomy, and destruction of the gland with radioactive iodine.

A. Antithyroid Drug Therapy: Drug therapy is most useful in young patients with small glands and mild disease. Methimazole or propylthiouracil is administered until the disease undergoes spontaneous remission, which may take from 1 year to 15 years. This is the only therapy that leaves an intact thyroid gland, but it does require a long period of treatment and observation (1–2 years), and there is a 60–70% incidence of relapse. The incidence of relapse is much lower when antithyroid drugs are used in combination with levothyroxine (see below).

Antithyroid drug therapy is usually begun with large divided doses, shifting to maintenance therapy with single daily doses when the patient becomes clinically euthyroid. However, mild to moderately severe thyrotoxicosis can often be controlled with methimazole given in a single morning dose of 30–40 mg; once-daily dosing may enhance compliance. Maintenance therapy requires 5–15 mg once daily. Alternatively, therapy is started with propylthiouracil, 100–150 mg every 6 hours, followed after 4–8 weeks by gradual reduction of the dose to the maintenance level of 50–150 mg once daily. In addition to inhibiting iodine organification, propylthiouracil also inhibits the conversion of T_4 to T_3, so it brings the level of activated thyroid hormone down more quickly than does methimazole. The best clinical guide to remission is reduction in the size of the goiter. Laboratory tests most useful in monitoring the course of therapy are serum T_3 by RIA, FT_4D or FT_4I, and serum TSH.

Reactivation of the autoimmune process occurs when the dosage of antithyroid drug is lowered during maintenance therapy and TSH begins to drive the gland. TSH release can be prevented by the daily administration of 0.05–0.15 mg of levothyroxine with 5–15 mg of methimazole or 50–150 mg of propylthiouracil for the second year of therapy. When antithyroid drug therapy is discontinued, levothyroxine is continued for an additional year. The relapse rate with this program may be as low as 20%.

Reactions to antithyroid drugs have been described above. A minor rash can often be controlled by antihistamine therapy. Because the more severe reaction of agranulocytosis is often heralded by sore throat or high fever, patients receiving antithyroid drugs must be instructed to discontinue the drug and seek immediate medical attention if these symptoms develop. White cell and differential counts and a throat culture are indicated in such cases, followed by appropriate antibiotic therapy. Rare adverse reactions to antithyroid drugs also requiring cessation of drug therapy include urticaria, cholestatic jaundice, hepatocellular toxicity, exfoliative dermatitis, and acute arthralgia.

B. Thyroidectomy: Subtotal thyroidectomy is the treatment of choice for patients with very large glands or multinodular goiters. Patients are treated with antithyroid drugs until euthyroid (about 6 weeks). In addition, for 2 weeks prior to surgery, they receive saturated solution of potassium iodide, 5 drops twice daily, to diminish vascularity of the gland and simplify surgery. About 50–60% of patients will require thyroid supplementation following subtotal thyroidectomy.

C. Radioactive Iodine: Radioiodine therapy utilizing ^{131}I is the preferred treatment for most patients over 21 years of age. In patients without heart disease, the therapeutic dose may be given immediately in a range of 80–120 μCi/g of estimated thyroid weight corrected for uptake. In patients with underlying heart disease or severe thyrotoxicosis and in elderly patients, it is desirable to treat with antithyroid drugs until the patient is euthyroid. The medication is then stopped for 5–7 days before the appropriate dose of ^{131}I is administered. Iodides should be avoided to ensure maximal ^{131}I uptake. Six to 12 weeks following the administration of radioiodine, the gland will shrink in size and the patient will usually become euthyroid. A second dose may be required in some patients. The major complication of radioiodine therapy is hypothyroidism, which occurs in about 80% of patients. Serum FT_4 and TSH levels should be monitored. When hypothyroidism develops, prompt replacement with levothyroxine, 0.1–0.15 mg orally daily, should be instituted.

D. Adjuncts to Antithyroid Therapy: During the acute phase of thyrotoxicosis, beta-adrenoceptor-blocking agents are extremely helpful. Propranolol, 20–40 mg orally every 6 hours, will control tachycardia, hypertension, and atrial fibrillation. Propranolol is gradually withdrawn as serum thyroxine levels return to normal. Diltiazem, 90–120 mg 3 or 4 times daily, can be used to control tachycardia in patients in whom beta-blockers are contraindicated, eg, those with asthma. Interestingly, other calcium channel blockers may not be effective. Adequate nutrition and vitamin supplements are essential. Barbiturates accelerate T_4 breakdown (by hepatic enzyme induction) and may be helpful both as a sedative and to lower T_4 levels.

2. TOXIC UNINODULAR GOITER & TOXIC MULTINODULAR GOITER

These forms of hyperthyroidism occur often in older women with nodular goiters. FT_4 is moderately elevated or occasionally normal, but T_3 by RIA is strikingly elevated. Single toxic adenomas can be managed with either surgical excision of the adenoma or with radioiodine therapy. Toxic multinodular goiter is usually associated with a large goiter and is best treated by preparation with methimazole or propylthiouracil followed by subtotal thyroidectomy.

3. SUBACUTE THYROIDITIS

During the acute phase of viral infection of the thyroid gland, thyroid hormones are produced that result in transient thyrotoxicosis. This syndrome has been called "spontaneously resolving hyperthyroidism." Supportive therapy is usually all that is necessary, such as propranolol for tachycardia and aspirin or NSAIDs to control local pain and fever. Corticosteroids may be necessary in severe cases to control the inflammation.

4. THYROTOXICOSIS FACTITIA

This is due to excessive ingestion of thyroid hormones, either accidentally or intentionally. Treatment consists of supportive therapy and discontinuing excessive medication.

5. SPECIAL PROBLEMS

Thyroid Storm

Thyroid storm, or thyrotoxic crisis, is sudden acute exacerbation of all of the symptoms of thyrotoxicosis, presenting as a life-threatening syndrome. The clinical manifestations are variable in intensity but reflect hypermetabolism and excessive adrenergic activity. Fever is present, often associated with flushing and sweating. Tachycardia is common, often with atrial fibrillation, high pulse pressure, and occasionally heart failure. Central nervous system symptoms include marked agitation, restlessness, delirium, and coma. Gastrointestinal symptoms include nausea, vomiting, diarrhea, and jaundice. Death may occur from heart failure and shock.

Vigorous management is mandatory. Propranolol, 1–2 mg slowly intravenously or 40–80 mg orally every 6 hours, is helpful to control the severe cardiovascular manifestations. If propranolol is contraindicated by the presence of severe heart failure or asthma, hypertension and tachycardia may be controlled with diltiazem, 90–120 mg orally 3 or 4 times daily or 5–10 mg/h by intravenous infusion (asthmatic patients only); or with reserpine, 1 mg orally every 6–12 hours; or with guanethidine, 1–2 mg/kg orally in divided doses. Release of thyroid hormones from the gland is retarded by the administration of saturated solution of potassium iodide, 10 drops orally daily, or sodium ipodate, 1 g orally daily. The latter medication will also block peripheral conversion of T_4 to T_3. Hormone synthesis is blocked by the administration of propylthiouracil, 250 mg orally every 6 hours. If the patient is unable to take propylthiouracil by mouth, a rectal formulation can be prepared and administered in a dosage of 400 mg every 6 hours as a retention enema. Methimazole may also be prepared for rectal administration in a dose of 25 mg every 6 hours.[*] Hydrocortisone, 50 mg intravenously every 6 hours, will protect the patient against shock and will block the conversion of T_4 to T_3,

___

[*]Preparation of rectal propylthiouracil: Dissolve 400 mg propylthiouracil in 60 mL of Fleet mineral oil for the first dose and then 400 mg in 60 mL of Fleet Phospho-soda for subsequent enemas. Preparation of rectal methimazole: Dissolve methimazole (1200 mg) in 12 mL of water to which has been added a mixture of 2 drops of Span 80 in 52 mL cocoa butter warmed to 37 °C. Stir the mixture to form a water-oil emulsion, pour into 2.6 mL suppository molds, and cool. (Nabil, 1982.)

bringing down the level of thyroactive material in the blood quickly.

Supportive therapy is essential to control fever, heart failure, and any underlying disease process that may have precipitated the acute storm. In rare situations, where the above methods are not adequate to control the problem, plasmapheresis or peritoneal dialysis has been used to lower the levels of circulating thyroxine.

Ophthalmopathy

Although severe ophthalmopathy is rare, it is difficult to treat. Management requires effective treatment of the thyroid disease, usually by total surgical excision or ^{131}I ablation of the gland. In addition, local therapy may be necessary, eg, elevation of the head to diminish periorbital edema and artificial tears to relieve corneal drying. Smoking cessation should be advised to prevent progression of the ophthalmopathy. For the severe, acute inflammatory reaction, a short course of prednisone, 60–100 mg orally daily for about a week and then 60–100 mg every other day, tapering the dose over a period of 6–12 weeks, may be effective. If steroid therapy fails or is contraindicated, irradiation of the posterior orbit, using well-collimated high-energy x-ray therapy, will frequently result in marked improvement of the acute process. Threatened loss of vision is an indication for surgical decompression of the orbit. Eyelid or eye muscle surgery may be necessary to correct residual problems after the acute process has subsided.

Dermopathy

Dermopathy or pretibial myxedema will often respond to topical corticosteroids applied to the involved area and covered with an occlusive dressing.

Thyrotoxicosis During Pregnancy

Ideally, women in the childbearing period with severe disease should have definitive therapy with ^{131}I or subtotal thyroidectomy prior to pregnancy in order to avoid an acute exacerbation of the disease during pregnancy or following delivery. If thyrotoxicosis does develop during pregnancy, radioiodine is contraindicated because it crosses the placenta and may injure the fetal thyroid. In the first trimester, the patient can be prepared with propylthiouracil and a subtotal thyroidectomy performed safely during the mid trimester. It is essential to give the patient a thyroid supplement during the balance of the pregnancy. However, most patients are treated with propylthiouracil during the pregnancy, and the decision regarding long-term management can be made after delivery. The dosage of propylthiouracil must be kept to the minimum necessary for control of the disease (ie, < 300 mg daily), because it may affect the function of the fetal thyroid gland. Methimazole is not recommended, because of the risk of fetal scalp defects.

Neonatal Graves' Disease

Graves' disease may occur in the newborn infant, either due to passage of TSH-R Ab[stim] through the placenta, stimulating the thyroid gland of the neonate, or to genetic transmission of the trait to the fetus. Laboratory studies reveal an elevated free thyroxine, a markedly elevated T_3, and a low TSH—in contrast to the normal infant, in whom TSH is elevated at birth. TSH-R Ab[stim] is usually found in the serum of both the child and the mother.

If caused by maternal TSH-R Ab[stim], the disease is usually self-limited and subsides over a period of 4–12 weeks, coinciding with the fall in the infant's TSH-R Ab[stim] level. However, treatment is necessary because of the severe metabolic stress the infant is subjected to. Therapy includes propylthiouracil in a dose of 5–10 mg/kg/d in divided doses at 8-hour intervals; Lugol's solution (8 mg of iodide per drop), 1 drop every 8 hours; and propranolol, 2 mg/kg/d in divided doses. Careful supportive therapy is essential. If the infant is very ill, prednisone, 2 mg/kg/d orally in divided doses, will help block conversion of T_4 to T_3. These medications are gradually reduced as the clinical picture improves and can be discontinued by 6–12 weeks.

NONTOXIC GOITER

Nontoxic goiter is a syndrome of thyroid enlargement without excessive thyroid hormone production. Enlargement of the thyroid gland is usually due to TSH stimulation from inadequate thyroid hormone synthesis. The most common cause of nontoxic goiter worldwide is iodide deficiency, but in the USA it is Hashimoto's thyroiditis. Less common causes include dietary goitrogens, dyshormonogenesis, and neoplasms (see below).

Goiter due to iodide deficiency is best managed by prophylactic administration of iodide. The optimal daily iodide intake is 150–300 μg. Iodized salt and iodate used as preservatives in flour and bread are excellent sources of iodine in the diet. In areas where it is difficult to introduce iodized salt or iodate preservatives, a solution of iodized poppyseed oil has been administered intramuscularly to provide a long-term source of inorganic iodine.

Goiter due to ingestion of goitrogens in the diet is managed by elimination of the goitrogen or by adding sufficient thyroxine to shut off TSH stimulation. Similarly, in Hashimoto's thyroiditis and dyshormonogenesis, adequate thyroxine therapy—0.15–0.2 mg/d orally—will suppress pituitary TSH and result in slow regression of the goiter as well as correction of hypothyroidism.

THYROID NEOPLASMS

Neoplasms of the thyroid gland may be benign (adenomas) or malignant. Thin-needle aspiration biopsy has proved effective for differentiation of benign from malignant disease. Some adenomas will regress following thyroxine therapy; those that do not should be rebiopsied or surgically removed. Management of thyroid carcinoma requires a near-total thyroidectomy, postoperative radioiodine therapy in selected instances, and lifetime replacement with levothyroxine.

PREPARATIONS AVAILABLE

Thyroid Agents

Levothyroxine (generic, Synthroid, Levothroid, Levoxine)
Oral: 0.025, 0.05, 0.075, 0.088, 0.1, 0.112, 0.125, 0.137, 0.15, 0.175, 0.2, 0.3 mg tablets
Parenteral: 200, 500 μg per vial (100 μg/mL when reconstituted) for injection

Liothyronine (generic, Cytomel, Triostat)
Oral: 5, 25, 50 μg tablets
Parenteral: 10 μg/mL

Liotrix [a 4:1 ratio of T4:T3] (Euthroid, Thyrolar)
Oral: tablets containing 12.5, 25, 30, 50, 60, 100, 120, 150, 180 μg T_4 and $\frac{1}{4}$ as much T_3

Thyroid desiccated [USP] (generic, Armour Thyroid, Thyroid Strong, Thyrar, S-P-T)
Oral: tablets containing 15, 30, 60, 90, 120, 180, 240, 300 mg; capsules (S-P-T) containing 120, 180, 300 mg

Antithyroid Agents

Iodide (^{131}I) sodium (Iodotope, Sodium Iodide I 131 Therapeutic)
Oral: available as capsules and solution

Iopanoic acid (Telepaque)
Oral: 500 mg tablets (unlabeled use)

Ipodate sodium (Oragrafin Sodium, Bilivist)
Oral: 500 mg capsules (unlabeled use)

Methimazole (Tapazole)
Oral: 5, 10 mg tablets

Potassium iodide solution
Oral solution (generic, SSKI): 1 g/mL
Oral solution (Lugol's solution): 100 mg/mL potassium iodide plus 50 mg/mL iodine
Oral syrup (Pima): 325 mg/5 mL
Oral controlled action tablets (Iodo-Niacin): 135 mg potassium iodide plus 25 mg niacinamide hydroiodide

Propylthiouracil [PTU](generic)
Oral: 50 mg tablets

REFERENCES

General

Burrow GN, Oppenheimer JH, Volpé R: *Thyroid Function and Disease.* Saunders,1989.

Braverman LE, Utiger RD (editors): *Werner and Ingbar's The Thyroid: A Fundamental and Clinical Text,* 6th ed. Lippincott, 1991.

Greer MA (editor): *The Thyroid Gland.* Comprehensive Endocrinology Series. Martini L (editor) Raven Press, 1990.

Greenspan FS: Thyroid gland. In: *Basic & Clinical Endocrinology,* 4th ed. Greenspan FS, Baxter JD (editors). Appleton & Lange, 1993.

Greenspan FS (editor): Thyroid disease. Med Clin North Am 1991;75:1.

Surks MI et al: American Thyroid Association guidelines for use of laboratory tests in thyroid disorders. JAMA 1990;263:1529.

Volpé R: Autoimmune thyroid disease. Endocrinol Metab Clin North Am 1991;20:565.

Hypothyroidism

Bastenie PA, Bonnyns M, Vanhaelst L: Natural history of primary myxedema. Am J Med 1985;79:91.

Evered D, Hall R: Hypothyroidism and goiter. Clin Endocrinol Metab 1979;8:1.

Fish LH et al: Replacement dose, metabolism, and bioavailability of levothyroxine in the treatment of hypothyroidism: Role of triiodothyronine in pituitary feedback in humans. N Engl J Med 1987;316:764.

Fisher DA, Foley BL: Early treatment of congenital hypothyroidism. Pediatrics 1989;83:785.

Helfand M, Crapo LM: Monitoring therapy in patients taking levothyroxine. Ann Intern Med 1990;113:450.

Hennessey JV et al: L-Thyroxine dosage: A reevaluation of therapy with contemporary preparations. Ann Intern Med 1986;105:11.

Mandel SJ et al: Increased need for thyroxine during pregnancy in women with primary hypothyroidism. N Engl J Med 1990;323:91.

Mandel SJ, Brent GA, Larsen PR: Levothyroxine therapy in patients with thyroid disease. Ann Intern Med 1993;119:492.

Robuschi G et al: Hypothyroidism in the elderly. Endocr Rev 1987;8:142.

Toft AD: Thyroxine replacement therapy. Clin Endocrinol 1991;34:103.

Hyperthyroidism

Bahn RS et al: Diagnosis and management of Graves' ophthalmopathy. (Clinical Reviews 13.) J Clin Endocrinol Metab 1990;71:559.

Becks GP, Burrow GN: Thyroid disease and pregnancy. Med Clin North Am 1991;75:121.

Cooper DS: Which antithyroid drug? Am J Med 1986; 80:1165.

Franklyn JA: The management of hyperthyroidism. N Engl J Med 1994;330:1731.

Hashizume K et al: Administration of thyroxine in treated Graves' disease: Effects on the level of antibodies to thyroid stimulating hormone receptors and on the risk of recurrence of hyperthyroidism. N Engl J Med 1991;324:947.

Hennemann G, Krenning EP, Senkerenereyenen K: Place of radioactive iodine in treatment of thyrotoxicosis. Lancet 1986;1:1369.

Nabil N, Miner DJ, Amatruda JM: Methimazole: An alternative route of administration. J Clin Endocrinol Metab 1982;54:180.

Noguchi K et al: Prolonged treatment of hyperthyroidism with sodium tyropanoate, an oral cholecystographic agent: A re-evaluation of its clinical utility. Clin Endocrinol 1986;25:293.

Toft AD (editor): Hyperthyroidism. (Symposium.) Clin Endocrinol Metab 1985;14:299.

Walter RM, Bartle WR: Rectal administration of propylthiouracil in the treatment of Graves' disease. Am J Med 1990;88:69.

Nontoxic Goiter, Nodules, & Cancer

Berghout A et al: Comparison of placebo with L-thyroxine alone or with carbimazole for treatment of sporadic nontoxic goiter. Lancet 1990;336:193.

Fenzi G et al: Clinical approach to goiter. Baillieres Clin Endocrinol Metab 1988;2:671.

Greenspan FS: The problem of the nodular goiter. Med Clin North Am 1991;75:195.

Kaplan MM (editor): Thyroid carcinoma. Endocrinol Metab Clin North Am 1990;19:469.

Lamberg BA: Endemic goiter-iodine deficiency disorders. Ann Med 1991;23:367.

Miller TR, Abele JS, Greenspan FS: Fine-needle aspiration biopsy in the management of thyroid nodules. West J Med 1981;134:198.

Adrenocorticosteroids
& Adrenocortical Antagonists

Alan Goldfien, MD

The natural adrenocortical hormones are steroid molecules produced and released by the adrenal cortex. Both natural and synthetic corticosteroids are used for diagnosis and treatment of disorders of adrenal function. They are also used—more often and in much larger doses—for treatment of a variety of inflammatory and immunologic disorders.

Secretion of adrenocortical steroids is controlled by the pituitary release of corticotropin (ACTH). Secretion of the salt-retaining hormone aldosterone is also under the influence of angiotensin. Corticotropin has some actions that do not depend upon its effect on adrenocortical secretion. However, its pharmacologic value as an anti-inflammatory agent and its use in testing adrenal function depend on its trophic action. Its pharmacology was discussed in Chapter 36 and will be reviewed with the adrenocortical hormones.

Antagonists of the synthesis or action of the adrenocortical steroids are important in the treatment of several tumors. These agents are described at the end of this chapter.

ADRENOCORTICOSTEROIDS

The adrenal cortex releases a large number of steroids into the circulation. Some have minimal biologic activity and function primarily as precursors, and there are some for which no function has been established. The hormonal steroids may be classified as those having important effects on intermediary metabolism (glucocorticoids), those having principally salt-retaining activity (mineralocorticoids), and those having androgenic or estrogenic activity (see Chapter 39). In humans, the major glucocorticoid is cortisol and the most important mineralocorticoid is aldosterone. Quantitatively, dehydroepiandrosterone (DHEA) is the major androgen, since about 20 mg is secreted daily, partly as the sulfate. However, both DHEA and androstenedione are very weak androgens. A small amount of testosterone is secreted by the adrenal and may be of greater importance as an androgen. Little is known about the estrogens secreted by the adrenal. However, it has been shown that the adrenal androgens such as testosterone and androstenedione can be converted to estrone in small amounts by nonendocrine tissues and that they constitute the major endogenous source of estrogen in women after menopause and in some patients in whom ovarian function is abnormal.

THE NATURALLY OCCURRING GLUCOCORTICOIDS; CORTISOL (Hydrocortisone)

Pharmacokinetics

The major glucocorticoid in humans is cortisol. It is synthesized from cholesterol (as shown in Figure 38–1) by the cells of the zona fasciculata and zona reticularis and released into the circulation under the influence of ACTH. The mechanisms controlling its secretion are discussed in Chapter 36.

In the normal adult in the absence of stress, 10–20 mg of cortisol is secreted daily. The rate of secretion changes in a circadian rhythm governed by irregular pulses of ACTH that peak in the early morning hours and after meals and that are also influenced by light (Figure 38–2). In plasma, cortisol is bound to plasma proteins. Corticosteroid-binding globulin (CBG), an α_2-globulin synthesized by the liver, binds 75% of the circulating hormone under normal circumstances. The remainder is free (about 20%) or loosely bound to albumin (about 5%) and is available to exert its effect on target cells. When plasma cortisol levels exceed 20–30 µg/dL, CBG is saturated, and the concentration of free cortisol rises rapidly. CBG is increased in pregnancy and with estrogen administration, which increases its synthesis by the liver, and in hyperthyroidism. It is decreased by hypothyroidism, genetic defects in synthesis, and protein deficiency states. Albumin has a large capacity but low affinity for cortisol. Synthetic corticosteroids such as dexamethasone are largely bound to albumin.

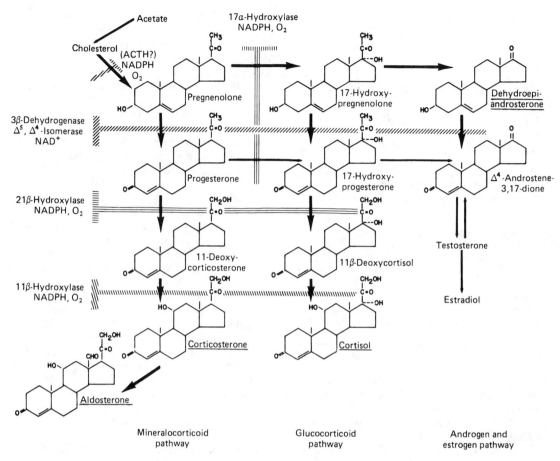

Figure 38–1. Outline of major pathways in adrenocortical hormone biosynthesis. The major secretory products are underlined. Pregnenolone is the major precursor of corticosterone and aldosterone, and 17-hydroxypregnenolone is the major precursor of cortisol. The enzymes and cofactors for the reactions progressing down each column are shown on the left and from the first to the second column at the top of the figure. When a particular enzyme is deficient, hormone production is blocked at the points indicated by the shaded bars. (Modified after Welikey et al; reproduced, with permission, from Ganong WF: *Review of Medical Physiology,* 15th ed. Appleton & Lange, 1991.)

The half-life of cortisol in the circulation is normally about 60–90 minutes; half-life may be increased when hydrocortisone (the pharmaceutical preparation of cortisol) is administered in large amounts or when stress, hypothyroidism, or liver disease is present. Only 1% of cortisol is excreted unchanged in the urine; about 20% of cortisol is converted to cortisone by 11-hydroxysteroid dehydrogenase in the kidney and other tissues with mineralocorticoid receptors (see below) before reaching the liver. Most of cortisone and the remaining cortisol is inactivated in the liver by reduction of the 4,5 double bond in the A ring and subsequent conversion to tetrahydrocortisol and tetrahydrocortisone by 3-hydroxysteroid dehydrogenase. Some is converted to cortol and cortolone by reduction of the C20 ketone. There are small amounts of other metabolites. The side chain (C20 and C21) is removed from about 5–

10% of the cortisol, and the resulting compounds are further metabolized and excreted into the urine as 11-oxy 17-ketosteroids. These metabolites are then conjugated with glucuronic acid or sulfate at the 3 and 21 hydroxyls, respectively, in the liver; reenter the circulation; and are excreted into the urine.

In some species (eg, the rat), corticosterone is the major glucocorticoid. It is less firmly bound to protein and therefore metabolized more rapidly. The pathways of its degradation are similar to those of cortisol.

Pharmacodynamics

A. Mechanism of Action: Upon entering tissues, glucocorticoids diffuse or are transported through cell membranes and bind to the cytoplasmic glucocorticoid receptor-heat-shock protein complex. The heat shock protein is released and the hormone-

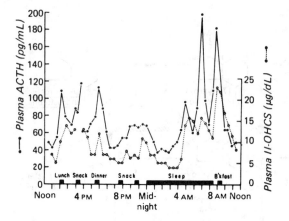

Figure 38–2. Fluctuations in plasma ACTH and glucocorticoids throughout the day in a normal girl (age 16). The ACTH was measured by immunoassay and the glucocorticoids as 11-oxysteroids *(11-OHCS)*. Note the greater ACTH and glucocorticoid rises in the morning, before awakening from sleep. (Reproduced, with permission, from Krieger DT et al: Characterization of the normal temporal pattern of plasma corticosteroid levels. J Clin Endocrinol Metab 1971;32:266.)

receptor complex is then transported into the nucleus, where it interacts with glucocorticoid response elements (GREs) on various genes and other regulatory proteins (which may be cell-specific) and stimulates or inhibits their expression. In the absence of hormone, the receptor protein is inhibited from binding to DNA; the hormone thus disinhibits the action of the receptor on DNA. The differences in glucocorticoid action in various tissues are thought to be governed by other tissue-specific proteins that must also bind to the gene to allow expression of particular glucocorticoid response elements.

In addition, glucocorticoids have some effects (eg, "fast-feedback inhibition") that occur too rapidly to be explained by gene expression. These effects may be mediated by nontranscriptional mechanisms.

B. Physiologic Effects: The glucocorticoids have widespread effects because they influence the function of most cells in the body. The major metabolic consequences of glucocorticoid secretion or administration are due to direct actions of these hormones in the cell. However, some important effects are the result of homeostatic responses by insulin and glucagon. Although many of the effects are dose-related and become magnified when large amounts are administered for therapeutic purposes, there are also "permissive" effects. In other words, many normal reactions that take place at a significant rate only in the presence of corticoids are not further stimulated in the presence of larger amounts of corticoids. For example, the response of vascular and bronchial muscle to catecholamines is diminished in the absence of cortisol and restored by physiologic

amounts of this glucocorticoid. The lipolytic responses of fat cells to catecholamines, ACTH, and growth hormone are also attenuated in the absence of glucocorticoid. The mechanisms of these effects have not been determined.

C. Metabolic Effects: The glucocorticoids have important dose-related effects on carbohydrate, protein, and fat metabolism. The same effects are responsible for some of the serious adverse effects associated with their use in therapeutic doses. Glucocorticoids stimulate and are required for gluconeogenesis in the fasted state and in diabetes. Glucocorticoids also increase amino acid uptake by the liver and kidney and increase the activity of enzymes required for gluconeogenesis.

In the liver, glucocorticoids increase glycogen deposition by stimulating glycogen synthase activity and increasing glucose production from protein. The increase in serum glucose levels stimulates insulin release.

Glucocorticoids inhibit the uptake of glucose by fat cells, leading to increased lipolysis. However the increased insulin secretion described above stimulates lipogenesis, leading to a net increase in fat deposition.

The net results of these actions are most apparent in the fasting state, when the supply of glucose from gluconeogenesis, the release of amino acids from muscle catabolism, the inhibition of peripheral glucose uptake, and the stimulation of lipolysis all contribute to the maintenance of an adequate glucose supply to the brain.

D. Catabolic Effects: Although glucocorticoids stimulate protein and RNA synthesis in the liver, they have catabolic effects in lymphoid and connective tissue, muscle, fat, and skin. Supraphysiologic amounts of glucocorticoids lead to decreased muscle mass and weakness. Catabolic effects on bone are the cause of osteoporosis in Cushing's syndrome and constitute a major limitation in the long-term therapeutic use of glucocorticoids. In children, the catabolic effects of excessive amounts of glucocorticoid reduce growth. This effect is not prevented by growth hormone.

E. Anti-inflammatory and Immunosuppressive Effects: Glucocorticoids have the capacity to dramatically reduce the manifestations of inflammation. This is due to their profound effects on the concentration, distribution, and function of peripheral leukocytes and to their inhibition of phospholipase A_2 activity. After a single dose of a short-acting glucocorticoid, the concentration of neutrophils increases while the lymphocytes (T and B cells), monocytes, eosinophils, and basophils in the circulation decrease in number. The changes are maximal at 6 hours and are dissipated in 24 hours. The increase in neutrophils is due both to the increased influx from the bone marrow and decreased migration from the blood vessels, leading to a reduction in the number of cells at the site of inflammation. The reduction in circulating lymphocytes, monocytes, eosinophils, and basophils is the result of their movement from the vascular bed to lymphoid tissue.

Glucocorticoids inhibit the functions of leukocytes and tissue macrophages. The ability of these cells to respond to antigens and mitogens is reduced. The effect on macrophages is particularly marked and limits their ability to phagocytose and kill microorganisms and to produce interleukin-1, pyrogen, collagenase, elastase, tumor necrosis factor, and plasminogen activator. Lymphocytes produce less interleukin-2. Although the evidence is conflicting, large doses of glucocorticoids have also been reported to stabilize lysosomal membranes, thereby reducing the concentration of proteolytic enzymes at the site of inflammation.

In addition to their effects on leukocyte function, glucocorticoids influence the inflammatory response by reducing the prostaglandin and leukotriene synthesis that results from activation of phospholipase A_2. Glucocorticoids increase the concentration of certain membrane phospholipids that appear to inhibit prostaglandin and leukotriene synthesis. Corticosteroids also increase the concentration of lipocortins, members of the annexin family of proteins that reduce the availability of the phospholipid substrates of phospholipase A_2. Finally, glucocorticoids may reduce expression of cyclooxygenase, thus reducing the amount of enzyme available to produce prostaglandins. Recent evidence suggests that genes exist for two isoforms of cyclooxygenase: COX I and COX II (Chapter 18). Glucocorticoids appear to inhibit expression of COX II, which may be the enzyme more involved in the inflammatory effects of eicosanoids. They have much less effect on the expression of COX I.

Glucocorticoids cause vasoconstriction when applied directly to vessels. They decrease capillary permeability by inhibiting the activity of kinins and bacterial endotoxins and by reducing the amount of histamine released by basophils.

The anti-immune effect of glucocorticoids is largely due to the effects described above. In humans, complement activation is unaltered, but its effects are inhibited. Antibody production can be reduced by large doses of steroids, though it is unaffected by moderate doses (eg, 20 mg/d of prednisone). However, inhibition of the production and effects of interleukin-2 and blockade of the effects of migration inhibition factor and macrophage inhibition factor impair delayed hypersensitivity reactions. The efficacy of these steroids in the control of transplant rejection is augmented by their ability to reduce antigen release from the grafted tissue, delay revascularization, and interfere with the sensitization of antibody-forming cells.

The anti-inflammatory and immunosuppressive effects of these agents are widely useful therapeutically but are also responsible for some of their most serious adverse effects (see below).

F. Other Effects: Glucocorticoids have impor-

tant effects on the nervous system. Adrenal insufficiency causes marked slowing of the alpha rhythm of the EEG. Increased amounts lower the threshold for electrically induced convulsions in rats and often produce behavioral disturbances in humans. Large doses of glucocorticoids may rarely increase intracranial pressure (pseudotumor cerebri).

Glucocorticoids suppress the pituitary release of ACTH and beta-lipotropin but do not decrease circulating levels of beta-endorphin (see Chapter 36). They also reduce secretion of TSH and FSH.

Large doses of glucocorticoids stimulate excessive production of acid and pepsin in the stomach and facilitate the development of peptic ulcer. They promote fat absorption and appear to antagonize the effect of vitamin D on calcium absorption. The glucocorticoids also have important effects on the hematopoietic system. In addition to their effects on leukocytes described above, they increase the number of platelets and red blood cells.

In the absence of physiologic amounts of cortisol, renal function (particularly glomerular filtration) is impaired and there is an inability to excrete a water load.

Glucocorticoids also have some effects on the development of the fetus. The structural and functional changes in the lungs near term, including the production of pulmonary surface-active material required for air breathing (surfactant), are stimulated by glucocorticoids.

SYNTHETIC ADRENOCORTICOSTEROIDS

ACTH and steroids having glucocorticoid activity have become important agents for use in the treatment of many inflammatory and allergic disorders. This has stimulated the development of many steroids with anti-inflammatory activity.

Pharmacokinetics

A. Source: Although the natural corticosteroids can be obtained from animal adrenals, they are usually synthesized from cholic acid (obtained from cattle) or steroid sapogenins, diosgenin in particular, that are found in plants of the Liliaceae and Dioscoreaceae families. Further modifications of these steroids have led to the marketing of a large group of synthetic steroids with special characteristics that are pharmacologically and therapeutically important (Table 38–1; Figure 38–3).

B. Metabolism: The metabolism of the naturally occurring adrenal steroids has been discussed above. The synthetic corticosteroids for oral use (Table 38–1) are in most cases rapidly and completely absorbed when given by mouth. Although they are transported and metabolized in a fashion similar to that of the endogenous steroids, important differences exist.

Table 38–1. Some commonly used natural and synthetic corticosteroids for general use.

Agent	Activity[1] Anti-inflammatory	Topical	Salt-Retaining	Equivalent Oral Dose (mg)	Forms Available
Short- to medium-acting glucocorticoids					
Hydrocortisone (cortisol)	1	1	1	20	Oral, injectable, topical.
Cortisone	0.8	0	0.8	25	Oral, injectable, topical.
Prednisone	4	0	0.3	5	Oral.
Prednisolone	5	4	0.3	5	Oral, injectable, topical.
Fluocortolone[2]				5	Oral, topical.
Methylprednisolone	5	5	0	4	Oral, injectable, topical.
Meprednisone[2]	5		0	4	Oral, injectable.
Intermediate-acting glucocorticoids					
Triamcinolone	5	5[3]	0	4	Oral, injectable, topical.
Paramethasone[2]	10		0	2	Oral, injectable.
Fluprednisolone	15	7	0	1.5	Oral.
Long-acting glucocorticoids					
Betamethasone	25–40	10	0	0.6	Oral, injectable, topical.
Dexamethasone	30	10	0	0.75	Oral, injectable, topical.
Mineralocorticoids					
Fludrocortisone	10	10	250	2	Oral, injectable, topical.
Desoxycorticosterone acetate	0	0	20		Injectable, pellets.

[1]Potency relative to hydrocortisone.
[2]Outside USA.
[3]Acetonide: Up to 100.

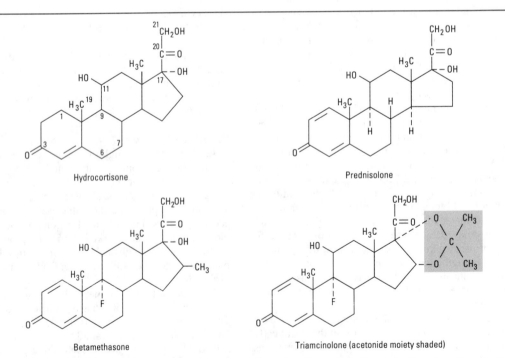

Figure 38–3. Chemical structures of several glucocorticoids. The acetonide-substituted derivatives (eg, triamcinolone acetonide) have increased surface activity and are useful in dermatology.

Alterations in the molecule influence its affinity for glucocorticoid and mineralocorticoid receptors as well as its protein-binding avidity, side chain stability, rate of reduction, and metabolic products. Halogenation at the 9 position, unsaturation of the $\Delta 1$–2 bond of the A ring, and methylation at the 2 or 16 position will prolong the half-life by more than 50%. The 11-hydroxyl group also appears to inhibit destruction, since the half-life of 11-deoxycortisol is half that of cortisol. The $\Delta 1$ compounds are excreted in the free form. In some cases, the agent given is a prodrug—eg, prednisone is rapidly converted to prednisolone in the body.

Pharmacodynamics

The actions of the synthetic steroids are similar to those of cortisol (see above). They bind to the specific intracellular receptor proteins and produce the same effects but have different ratios of glucocorticoid to mineralocorticoid potency (Table 38–1).

Clinical Pharmacology

A. Diagnosis and Treatment of Disturbed Adrenal Function:

1. Adrenocortical insufficiency–

a. Chronic (Addison's disease)–Chronic adrenocortical insufficiency is characterized by hyperpigmentation, weakness, fatigue, weight loss, hypotension, and inability to maintain the blood glucose level during fasting. In such individuals, minor noxious, traumatic, or infectious stimuli may produce acute adrenal insufficiency with shock and finally death.

In adrenal insufficiency, whether primary or following adrenalectomy, about 20–30 mg of cortisol must be given daily, with increased amounts during periods of stress. Although cortisol has some mineralocorticoid activity, this must be supplemented by an appropriate amount of salt-retaining hormone such as fludrocortisone. It is for this reason that glucocorticoids devoid of salt-retaining activity are not used in these patients.

b. Acute–When acute adrenocortical insufficiency is suspected, treatment must be instituted immediately. In addition to large amounts of parenteral cortisol, therapy includes correction of fluid and electrolyte abnormalities and treatment of precipitating factors.

Cortisol hemisuccinate or phosphate in doses of 100 mg intravenously is given every 6–8 hours until the patient is stable. The dose is then gradually reduced, achieving maintenance dosage in 5 days. The administration of salt-retaining hormone is resumed when the total cortisol dosage has been reduced to 50 mg/d.

2. Adrenocortical hyperfunction–

a. Congenital adrenal hyperplasia–This group of disorders is characterized by specific defects in the synthesis of cortisol. In pregnancies at high risk

for congenital adrenal hyperplasia, fetuses can be protected from genital abnormalities by administration of dexamethasone to the mother. The most common defect is a decrease in or lack of P450c21 (21β-hydroxylase) activity.* As can be seen in Figure 38–1, this would lead to a reduction in cortisol synthesis and produce a compensatory increase in ACTH release. If sufficient enzyme activity is present, a normal amount of cortisol will be produced in response to the increased level of ACTH, but the gland will become hyperplastic and produce abnormally large amounts of precursors such as 17-hydroxyprogesterone that can be diverted to the androgen pathway, leading to virilization. Metabolism of this compound in the liver leads to pregnanetriol, which is characteristically excreted into the urine in large amounts in this disorder and can be used to make the diagnosis.

If the defect is in 11-hydroxylation, large amounts of desoxycorticosterone are produced and hypertension is prominent. When 17-hydroxylation is defective in the adrenals and gonads, hypogonadism will be present. However, increased amounts of 11-desoxycorticosterone (DOC; see below) are formed, and the signs and symptoms associated with mineralocorticoid excess—such as hypertension and hypokalemia—are also found.

When first seen, the infant with congenital adrenal hyperplasia may be in an acute adrenal crisis and should be treated as described above using an intravenous preparation of cortisol, mineralocorticoid, and appropriate electrolyte solutions as required. Once the patient is stabilized, hydrocortisone, 12–18 mg/m²/d in three divided doses is begun. The dosage is then adjusted to allow normal growth and bone maturation and to prevent androgen excess. Alternate-day therapy with prednisone has also been used. Salt-losing patients also require fludrocortisone, 0.05–0.1 mg/d by mouth, and added salt to maintain normal blood pressure, plasma renin activity, and electrolytes.

b. Cushing's syndrome–Cushing's syndrome is usually the result of bilateral adrenal hyperplasia secondary to a pituitary adenoma (Cushing's disease) but occasionally is due to tumors or nodular hyperplasia of the adrenal gland or ectopic production of ACTH by other tumors. The manifestations are those associated with the presence of excessive glucocorticoids. When changes are marked, a rounded, plethoric face and trunk obesity are striking in appearance. In general, the manifestations of protein loss are found and include muscle wasting, thinning of the skin, striae, easy bruisability, poor wound

---

*Names for the adrenal steroid synthetic enzymes include the following:

P450c11 (11β-hydroxylase)
P450c17 (17α-hydroxylase)
P450c21 (21β-hydroxylase)

healing, and osteoporosis. Other serious disturbances include mental disorders, hypertension, and diabetes. This disorder is treated by surgical removal of the tumor producing the hormone, irradiation or removal of a pituitary microadenoma producing ACTH, or resection of hyperplastic adrenals. These patients must receive large doses of cortisol during and following the surgical procedure. Doses of 300 mg of soluble hydrocortisone are given as a continuous intravenous infusion on the day of surgery. The dose must be reduced slowly to normal replacement levels, since rapid reduction in dose may produce symptoms, including fever and joint pain. If adrenalectomy has been performed, long-term maintenance is similar to that outlined above for adrenal insufficiency.

c. Aldosteronism–Primary aldosteronism usually results from the excessive production of aldosterone by an adrenal adenoma. However, it may also result from abnormal secretion by hyperplastic glands or from a malignant tumor. The clinical findings of hypertension, polyuria, polydipsia, weakness, and tetany are related to the continued renal loss of potassium, which leads to hypokalemia, alkalosis, and hypernatremia. This syndrome can also be produced in disorders of adrenal steroid biosynthesis by excessive secretion of desoxycorticosterone, corticosterone, or 18-hydroxycorticosterone.

In contrast to patients with secondary aldosteronism (see below), these patients have low (suppressed) levels of plasma renin activity and angiotensin II. When treated with desoxycorticosterone acetate (20 mg/d intramuscularly for 3 days) or fludrocortisone (0.2 mg twice daily orally for 3 days), they fail to retain sodium and their secretion of aldosterone is not significantly reduced. They are generally improved when treated with spironolactone, and the response to this agent is of diagnostic and therapeutic value.

3. Use of glucocorticoids for diagnostic purposes–It is sometimes necessary to suppress the production of ACTH in order to identify the source of a particular hormone or to establish whether its production is influenced by the secretion of ACTH. In these circumstances, it is advantageous to employ a very potent substance such as dexamethasone because the use of small quantities reduces the possibility of confusion in the interpretation of hormone assays in blood or urine. For example, if complete suppression is achieved by the use of 50 mg of cortisol, the urinary 17-hydroxycorticosteroids will be 15–18 mg/24 h, since one-third of the dose given will be recovered in urine as 17-hydroxycorticosteroid. If an equivalent dose of 1.5 mg of dexamethasone is employed, the urinary excretion will be only 0.5 mg/24 h and blood levels will be low.

The **dexamethasone suppression test** is used for the diagnosis of Cushing's syndrome and has also been used in the differential diagnosis of depressive psychiatric states. Dexamethasone, 1 mg, is given orally at 11 PM, and a plasma sample is obtained in the morning. In normal individuals, the cortisol concentration is usually less than 5 μg/dL, whereas in Cushing's syndrome the level is usually greater than 10 μg/dL. The results are not reliable in the presence of depression, anxiety, illness, and other stressful conditions. However, in patients in whom the diagnosis of Cushing's syndrome has been established clinically and confirmed by a finding of elevated urine free cortisol, suppression with large doses of dexamethasone will help to distinguish patients with Cushing's disease from those with steroid-producing tumors of the adrenal cortex or with the ectopic ACTH syndrome. Dexamethasone is given in a dosage of 2 mg orally every 6 hours for 2 days and the urine assayed for cortisol or its metabolites—or dexamethasone is given as a single dose of 8 mg at 11 PM and the plasma cortisol is measured at 8 AM the following day. In patients with Cushing's disease, the suppressant effect of dexamethasone will usually produce a 50% reduction in hormone levels. In patients in whom suppression does not occur, the ACTH level will be low in the presence of a cortisol-producing adrenal tumor and elevated in patients with an ectopic ACTH-producing tumor.

Suppression of the adrenal with glucocorticoids and of the ovary with estrogens can be useful in locating the source of androgen production in a hirsute woman if the effect on androgen levels in blood can be measured before and during hormone administration.

B. Adrenocorticosteroids and Stimulation of Lung Maturation in the Fetus: Lung maturation in the fetus is regulated by the fetal secretion of cortisol. Treatment of the mother with large doses of glucocorticoid reduces the incidence of respiratory distress syndrome in infants delivered prematurely. When delivery is anticipated before 34 weeks of gestation, betamethasone, 12 mg, followed by an additional dose of 12 mg 18–24 hours later, is commonly used. Protein binding of this corticosteroid is less than that of cortisol, allowing increased transfer across the placenta to the fetus. Corticosteroid levels achieved in the fetus are equivalent to those observed when the fetus is stressed.

C. Adrenocorticosteroids and Nonadrenal Disorders: Cortisol and its synthetic analogues are useful in the treatment of a diverse group of diseases unrelated to any known disturbance of adrenal function (Table 38–2). The usefulness of corticosteroids in these disorders is a function of their ability to suppress inflammatory and immune responses, as described above. In disorders in which host response is the cause of the major manifestations of the disease, these agents are useful. In instances where the inflammatory or immune response is important in controlling the pathologic process, therapy with corticosteroids may be dangerous but justified to prevent irreparable damage from an inflammatory response—if used in conjunction with specific therapy for the disease process.

Table 38–2. Some therapeutic indications for the use of glucocorticosteroids in nonadrenal disorders.

Disorder	Examples
Allergic reactions	Angioneurotic edema, asthma, bee stings, contact dermatitis, drug reactions, allergic rhinitis, serum sickness, urticaria
Collagen-vascular disorders	Giant cell arteritis, lupus erythematosus, mixed connective tissue syndromes, polymyositis, polymyalgia rheumatica, rheumatoid arthritis, temporal arteritis
Eye diseases	Acute uveitis, allergic conjunctivitis, choroiditis, optic neuritis
Gastrointestinal diseases	Inflammatory bowel disease, nontropical sprue, subacute hepatic necrosis
Hematologic disorders	Acquired hemolytic anemia, acute allergic purpura, leukemia, autoimmune hemolytic anemia, idiopathic thrombocytopenic purpura, multiple myeloma
Infections	Gram-negative septicemia; occasionally helpful to suppress excessive inflammation
Inflammatory conditions of bones and joints	Arthritis, bursitis, tenosynovitis
Neurologic disorders	Cerebral edema (large doses of dexamethasone are given to patients following brain surgery, to minimize cerebral edema in the postoperative period), multiple sclerosis
Organ transplants	Prevention and treatment of rejection (immunosuppression)
Pulmonary diseases	Aspiration pneumonia, bronchial asthma, prevention of infant respiratory distress syndrome, sarcoidosis
Renal disorders	Nephrotic syndrome
Skin diseases	Atopic dermatitis, dermatoses, lichen simplex chronicus (localized neurodermatitis), mycosis fungoides, pemphigus, seborrheic dermatitis, xerosis
Thyroid diseases	Malignant exophthalmos, subacute thyroiditis
Miscellaneous	Hypercalcemia, mountain sickness

Since the corticosteroids are not usually curative, the pathologic process may progress while clinical manifestations are suppressed. Therefore, chronic therapy with these drugs should be undertaken with great care and only when the seriousness of the disorder warrants their use and less hazardous measures have been exhausted.

In general, attempts should be made to bring the disease process under control using short-acting glucocorticoids as well as all ancillary measures possible to keep the dose low. Where possible, alternate-day therapy should be utilized (see below). Therapy should not be decreased or stopped abruptly. When prolonged therapy is anticipated, it is helpful to obtain chest films and a tuberculin test. The presence of diabetes, peptic ulcer, osteoporosis, and psychologic disturbances should be excluded, and cardiovascular function should be assessed.

The following supplemental measures should be considered: The diet should be rich in potassium and low in sodium to prevent electrolyte disturbances. Caloric management to prevent obesity should be instituted. High protein intake is required to compensate for the loss due to the increased breakdown of protein from gluconeogenesis. Antacids should be used three or four times daily in patients prone to epigastric distress. Osteoporosis in these patients is difficult to prevent: It is caused by depressed bone formation in the presence of unaltered ongoing bone resorption, and parathyroid hormone and vitamin D changes are not involved. Physical therapy and an-

drogens have been recommended to limit glucocorticoid-induced osteoporosis but are not of proved value.

Toxicity

The benefits obtained from use of the glucocorticoids vary considerably. They must be carefully weighed in each patient against the widespread effects on every part of the organism. The major undesirable effects of the glucocorticoids are the result of their hormonal actions (see above) and lead to the clinical picture of iatrogenic Cushing's syndrome.

When the glucocorticoids are used for short periods (less than 1 week), it is unusual to see serious adverse effects even with moderately large doses. However, behavioral changes and acute peptic ulcers are occasionally observed even after a few days of treatment.

A. Metabolic Effects: Most patients who are given daily doses of 100 mg of cortisol or more (or the equivalent amount of synthetic steroid) for longer than 2 weeks undergo a series of changes that have been termed iatrogenic Cushing's syndrome. The rate of development is a function of the dose. The appearance of the face is altered by rounding, puffiness, and plethora. Fat tends to be redistributed from the extremities to the trunk and face. There is an increased growth of fine hair over the thighs and trunk and sometimes the face. Acne may increase or appear, and insomnia and increased appetite are noted. In the treatment of dangerous or disabling disorders, these changes may not require cessation of therapy. However, the underlying metabolic changes accompanying them can be very serious by the time they become obvious. The continuing breakdown of protein and diversion of amino acids to glucose production increase the need for insulin and over a period of time result in weight gain; fat deposition; muscle wasting; thinning of the skin, with striae and bruising; hyperglycemia; and eventually the development of osteoporosis, diabetes, and aseptic necrosis of the hip. Wound healing is also impaired under these circumstances. When diabetes occurs, it is treated by diet and insulin. These patients are often resistant to insulin but rarely develop ketoacidosis. In general, patients treated with corticosteroids should be on high-protein diets, and increased potassium and anabolic steroids should be used when required.

B. Other Complications: Other serious complications include the development of peptic ulcers and their complications. The clinical findings associated with other disorders, particularly bacterial and mycotic infections, may be masked by the corticosteroids, and patients must be carefully watched to avoid serious mishap when large doses are used. Some patients develop a myopathy the nature of which is unknown. The frequency of myopathy is greater in patients treated with triamcinolone. The administration of this drug as well as of methylprednisolone has been associated with nausea, dizziness, and weight loss in some patients. It is treated by changing drugs, reducing dosage, and increasing the potassium and protein intake.

Psychosis may occur, particularly in patients receiving large doses of corticosteroids. Long-term therapy is associated with the development of posterior subcapsular cataracts. Periodic slitlamp examination is indicated in such patients. Increased intraocular pressure is common, and glaucoma may be induced. Benign intracranial hypertension also occurs. In doses of 45 mg/m^2/d or more, growth retardation occurs in children.

When given in greater than physiologic amounts, steroids such as cortisone and hydrocortisone, which have mineralocorticoid effects in addition to glucocorticoid effects, cause some sodium and fluid retention and loss of potassium. In patients with normal cardiovascular and renal function, this leads to a hypokalemic, hypochloremic alkalosis and eventually a rise in blood pressure. In patients with hypoproteinemia, renal disease, or liver disease, edema may also occur. In patients with heart disease, even small degrees of sodium retention may lead to congestive heart failure. These effects can be minimized by sodium restriction and judicious use of potassium supplements.

C. Adrenal Suppression: When corticosteroids are administered for more than a few days, adrenal suppression occurs. If treatment extends over weeks to months, the patient should be given supplementary therapy at times of severe stress such as accidental trauma or surgery. If corticoid dosage is to be reduced, it should be tapered slowly. If therapy is to be stopped, the reduction process should be quite slow when the dose reaches replacement levels. It will take 2–3 months for the pituitary to become responsive, and cortisol levels may not return to normal for another 6–9 months. Treatment with ACTH does not significantly reduce the time required for the return of normal function.

If the dose is reduced too rapidly in such patients, the symptoms of the disorder may reappear or increase in intensity. However, patients without an underlying disorder (eg, with treated Cushing's disease) will also become symptomatic with rapid reductions in corticoid levels. These symptoms include anorexia, nausea or vomiting, weight loss, lethargy, headache, fever, joint or muscle pain, and postural hypotension. Although many of these symptoms suggest adrenal insufficiency, they may occur in the presence of normal or even elevated plasma cortisol levels.

Contraindications & Cautions

A. Special Precautions: Patients receiving these drugs must be observed carefully for the development of hyperglycemia, glycosuria, sodium retention with edema or hypertension, hypokalemia, peptic ulcer, osteoporosis, and hidden infections.

The dosage should be kept as low as possible and intermittent dosage (eg, alternate-day) employed when satisfactory therapeutic results can be obtained on this schedule. In patients being maintained on relatively low doses of corticosteroids, supplementary therapy may be required at times of stress such as when surgical procedures are performed or accidents occur.

B. Contraindications: These agents must be used with the greatest of caution in patients with peptic ulcer, heart disease or hypertension with congestive heart failure, infections, psychoses, diabetes, osteoporosis, glaucoma, or herpes simplex infection.

Selection of Drug & Dosage Schedule

Since these preparations differ with respect to relative anti-inflammatory and mineralocorticoid effect (Table 38–1), duration of action, cost, and dosage forms available, these factors should be taken into account in selecting the drug to be used.

A. ACTH Versus Adrenocortical Steroids: In patients with normal adrenals, ACTH has been used to induce the endogenous production of cortisol to obtain similar effects. However, except when the increase in androgens is desirable, the use of ACTH as a therapeutic agent is probably unjustified. Instances in which ACTH has been claimed to be more effective than glucocorticoids are probably due to the administration of smaller amounts of corticoids than were produced by the dosage of ACTH.

B. Dosage: In determining the dosage regimen

to be used, the physician must consider the seriousness of the disease, the amount of drug likely to be required to obtain the desired effect, and the duration of therapy. In some diseases, the amount required for maintenance of the desired therapeutic effect is less than the dose needed to obtain the initial effect, and the lowest possible dosage for the needed effect should be determined by gradually lowering the dose until an increase in signs or symptoms is noted.

Many types of dosage schedules have been used in administering glucocorticoids. When it is necessary to maintain continuously elevated plasma corticosteroid levels in order to suppress ACTH, a slowly absorbed parenteral preparation or small doses at frequent intervals are required. The opposite situation exists with respect to the use of corticosteroids in the treatment of inflammatory and allergic disorders. The same total quantity given in a few doses may be more effective than when given in many smaller doses or in a slowly absorbed parenteral form.

Severe autoimmune conditions involving vital organs must be treated aggressively, and undertreatment is as dangerous as overtreatment. In order to minimize the deposition of immune complexes and the influx of leukocytes and macrophages, 1 mg/kg/d of prednisone in divided doses is required initially. This dose is maintained until the serious manifestations respond. The dose can then be gradually reduced.

When large doses are required for prolonged periods of time, **alternate-day** administration of the compound may be tried after control is achieved. When used in this manner, very large amounts (eg, 100 mg of prednisone) can sometimes be administered with less marked adverse effects because there is a recovery period between each dose. The transition to an alternate-day schedule can be made after the disease process is under control. It should be done gradually and with additional supportive measures between doses. A typical schedule for a patient maintained on 50 mg of prednisone daily would be as follows:

Day	1:	50 mg	Day	7:	75 mg
	2:	40 mg		8:	5 mg
	3:	60 mg		9:	70 mg
	4:	30 mg		10:	5 mg
	5:	70 mg		11:	65 mg
	6:	10 mg		12:	5 mg, etc

When selecting a drug for use in large doses, a shorter-acting synthetic steroid with little mineralocorticoid effect is advisable. If possible, it should be given as a single morning dose.

Methylprednisolone in doses of 1 g given intravenously over 30–60 minutes at monthly intervals has been reported to be useful in treatment of rheumatoid arthritis in a few cases. The indications for this mode of therapy are not established.

C. Special Dosage Forms: The use of local therapy such as topical preparations for skin disease, ophthalmic forms for eye disease, intra-articular injections for joint disease, and hydrocortisone enemas for ulcerative colitis provides a means of delivering large amounts of steroid to the diseased tissue with reduced systemic effects.

Similarly, beclomethasone dipropionate and several other glucocorticoids administered as aerosols have been found to be effective in the treatment of asthma (see Chapter 19). The switch from therapy with systemic glucocorticoids to aerosol therapy must be undertaken with caution, since adrenal insufficiency will occur if adrenal function has been suppressed. In such patients, a slow, graded reduction of systemic therapy and monitoring of endogenous adrenal function should accompany the institution of aerosol administration.

Beclomethasone dipropionate, triamcinolone acetonide, and flunisolide are available as nasal sprays for the topical treatment of allergic rhinitis. They are effective at doses (one or two sprays 2 or 3 times daily) that in most patients result in plasma levels too low to influence adrenal function.

Corticosteroids incorporated in ointments, creams, lotions, and sprays are used extensively in dermatology. These preparations are discussed in more detail in Chapter 63.

MINERALOCORTICOIDS
(Aldosterone, Desoxycorticosterone, Fludrocortisone)

The most important mineralocorticoid in humans is aldosterone. However, small amounts of desoxycorticosterone (DOC) are also formed and released. Although the amounts are normally insignificant, DOC was of some importance therapeutically in the past. Its actions, effects, and metabolism are similar to those described below for aldosterone. Fludrocortisone, a synthetic corticosteroid, is the most commonly used salt-retaining hormone.

1. ALDOSTERONE

Aldosterone is synthesized mainly in the zona glomerulosa of the adrenal cortex. Its structure and synthesis are illustrated in Figure 38–1.

The rate of aldosterone secretion is subject to several influences. ACTH produces a moderate stimulation of its release, but this effect is not sustained for more than a few days in the normal individual. Although aldosterone is no less than one-third as effective as cortisol in suppressing ACTH, the quantities of aldosterone produced by the adrenal cortex are insufficient to participate in any significant feedback control of ACTH secretion.

After hypophysectomy and total elimination of

ACTH, aldosterone secretion gradually falls to about half the normal rate, which means that other factors, eg, angiotensin, are able to maintain and perhaps regulate its secretion (see Chapter 17). Independent variations between cortisol and aldosterone secretion can also be demonstrated by means of lesions in the nervous system such as decerebration, which decreases the secretion of hydrocortisone while increasing the secretion of aldosterone.

Physiologic & Pharmacologic Effects

Aldosterone and other steroids with mineralocorticoid properties promote the reabsorption of sodium from urine by the distal renal tubules, loosely coupled to the secretion of potassium and hydrogen ion. Sodium reabsorption in the sweat and salivary glands, gastrointestinal mucosa, and across cell membranes in general is also increased. Excessive levels of aldosterone produced by tumors or overdosage with other mineralocorticoids lead to hypernatremia, hypokalemia, metabolic alkalosis, increased plasma volume, and hypertension.

Mineralocorticoids act by binding to the mineralocorticoid receptor in the cytoplasm of target cells, especially principal cells of the collecting tubules of the kidney. It is of interest that this receptor has the same affinity for cortisol, which is present in higher concentrations in the extracellular fluid. The specificity for mineralocorticoids at this site appears to be conferred by the presence of the enzyme 11β-hydroxysteroid dehydrogenase, which converts cortisol to cortisone, which has low affinity for the receptor.

Metabolism

Aldosterone is secreted at the rate of 100–200 μg/d in normal individuals with a moderate dietary salt intake. The plasma level in males (resting supine) is about 0.007 μg/dL. The half-life of aldosterone injected in tracer quantities is 15–20 minutes, and it does not appear to be firmly bound to serum proteins.

The metabolism of aldosterone is similar to that of cortisol, about 50 μg/24 h appearing in the urine as conjugated tetrahydroaldosterone. Approximately 5–15 μg/24 h is excreted free or as the 3-oxo glucuronide.

2. DESOXYCORTICOSTERONE (DOC)

DOC, which also serves as a precursor of aldosterone (Figure 38–1), is normally secreted in amounts of about 200 μg/d. Its half-life when injected into the human circulation is about 70 minutes. Preliminary estimates of its concentration in plasma are approximately 0.03 μg/dL. The control of its secretion differs from that of aldosterone in that the secretion of DOC is primarily under the control of ACTH. Although the response to ACTH is enhanced by dietary sodium restriction, a low-salt diet does not increase DOC secretion. The secretion of DOC may be markedly increased in abnormal conditions such as adrenal carcinoma and congenital adrenal hyperplasia with reduced P450c11 or P450c17 activity.

3. FLUDROCORTISONE

This compound, a potent steroid with both glucocorticoid and mineralocorticoid activity, has become the most widely used mineralocorticoid. Doses of 0.1 mg 2–7 times weekly have potent salt-retaining activity and are used in the treatment of adrenocortical insufficiency but are too small to have important anti-inflammatory effects.

Fludrocortisone

ADRENAL ANDROGENS

The adrenal cortex secretes large amounts of dehydroepiandrosterone (DHEA) and smaller amounts of androstenedione and testosterone. Although these androgens are thought to contribute to the normal maturation process, they do not stimulate or support androgen-dependent pubertal changes in humans. Recent studies suggest that DHEA and DHEA sulfate (DHEAS) have other important metabolic effects mediated by liver enzymes. These effects inhibit weight gain and atherosclerosis and prolong life in experimental animals (rabbits) and possibly in humans. The therapeutic use of DHEA in humans is being explored.

ANTAGONISTS OF ADRENOCORTICAL AGENTS

SYNTHESIS INHIBITORS & GLUCOCORTICOID ANTAGONISTS

1. MITOTANE

Mitotane (Figure 38–4) produces adrenal atrophy in dogs and will interfere with biosynthetic pathways in the adrenal cortex. This drug is administered orally in divided doses of 6–12 mg daily. In 80% of patients, the toxic effects are sufficiently severe to require dose reduction. These include diarrhea, nausea, vomiting, depression, somnolence, and skin problems. About one-third of patients with adrenal carcinoma show a reduction in tumor mass. However, in two-thirds of patients, steroid production is decreased.

2. AMPHENONE B

Amphenone B (Figure 38–4) is a more potent inhibitor of synthesis than mitotane, blocking hydroxylation at the 11, 17, and 21 positions. It does not have a destructive effect on the tissue, and the block of steroid synthesis leads to increased production of ACTH and hyperplasia of the gland. It is considered too toxic for use in humans. Amphenone causes central nervous system depression and gastrointestinal tract and skin disorders and impairs liver and thyroid function.

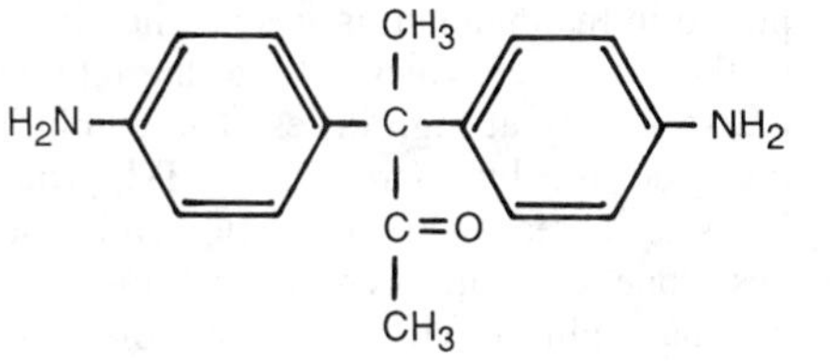

AMPHENONE B

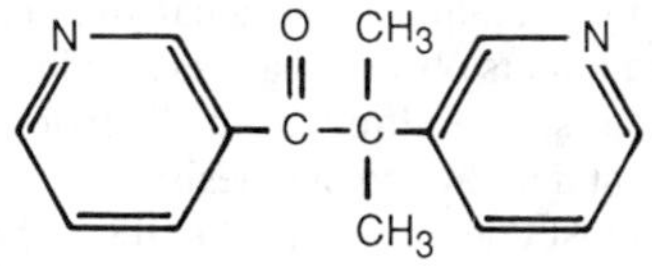

METYRAPONE (Su 4885)

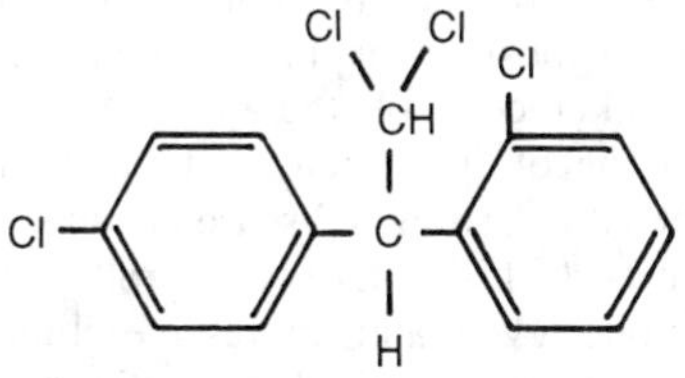

MITOTANE (*o,p'*-DDD; dichlorodiphenyldichloroethane)

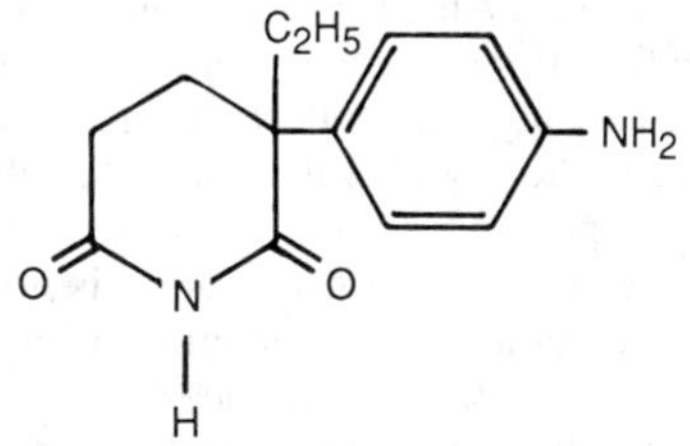

AMINOGLUTETHIMIDE

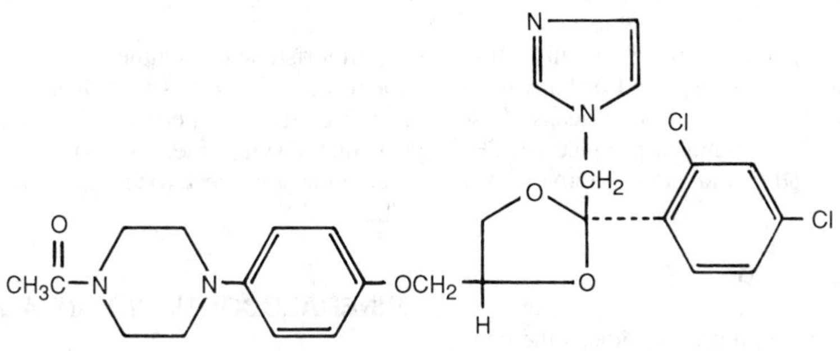

KETOCONAZOLE

Figure 38–4. Adrenocortical antagonists.

3. METYRAPONE

Metyrapone (Figure 38–4) has a more selective effect at low doses than either mitotane or amphenone B. It inhibits 11-hydroxylation, interfering with cortisol and corticosterone synthesis and leading to secretion of 11-deoxycortisol. In the presence of a normal pituitary gland, there is a compensatory increase in 11-deoxycortisol production. This response is a measure of the capacity of the anterior pituitary to produce ACTH and has been adapted for clinical use as a diagnostic test. Although the toxicity of metyrapone is much lower than that of the above agents, the drug does produce transient dizziness and gastrointestinal disturbances. This agent has not been widely used for the treatment of Cushing's syndrome. However, in doses of 0.25 g twice daily to 1 g 4 times daily, metyrapone can reduce cortisol production to normal levels in some patients with adrenal tumors, ectopic ACTH syndromes, and hyperplasia. It may be useful in the management of severe manifestations of cortisol excess while the cause is being determined or in conjunction with radiation or surgical treatment. The major adverse effects observed are salt and water retention and hirsutism resulting from diversion of precursor to DOC and androgen synthesis.

Metyrapone is most commonly used in tests of adrenal function. The blood levels of 11-deoxycortisol and the urinary excretion of 17-hydroxycorticoids are measured before and after administration of the compound. Normally, there is a twofold or greater increase in the urinary 17-hydroxycorticoid excretion. A dosage of 300–500 mg every 4 hours for six doses is commonly used, and urine collections are made on the day before and the day after treatment. In patients with Cushing's syndrome, a normal response to metyrapone indicates that the cortisol excess is not the result of adrenal carcinoma or autonomous adenoma, since secretion by such tumors produces suppression of ACTH and atrophy of normal adrenal cortex.

Adrenal function may also be tested by administering metyrapone, 2–3 g orally at midnight, and measuring the level of ACTH or 11-deoxycortisol in blood drawn at 8 AM, or by comparing the excretion of 17-hydroxycorticosteroids in the urine during the 24-hour periods preceding and following administration of the drug. In patients with suspected or known lesions of the pituitary, this procedure is a means of estimating the ability of the gland to produce ACTH. The response is inhibited by oral contraceptives.

4. AMINOGLUTETHIMIDE

Aminoglutethimide (Figure 38–4) blocks the conversion of cholesterol to pregnenolone and causes a reduction in the synthesis of all hormonally active steroids (Figure 38–1). It has been used in conjunction with dexamethasone to reduce or eliminate estrogen and androgen production in patients with carcinoma of the breast. In doses of 1 g/d it was well tolerated; however, with higher doses, lethargy was a common effect. This drug can be used in conjunction with ketoconazole to reduce steroid secretion in patients with Cushing's syndrome due to adrenocortical cancer who do not respond to mitotane.

Aminoglutethimide also apparently increases the clearance of some steroids. It has been shown to enhance the metabolism of dexamethasone, reducing its half-life from 264 minutes to 120 minutes.

5. KETOCONAZOLE

Ketoconazole, an antifungal imidazole derivative, is a potent and rather nonselective inhibitor of adrenal and gonadal steroid synthesis. This compound inhibits cholesterol side chain cleavage, P450c17, C17,20-lyase, 3β-hydroxysteroid dehydrogenase, and P450c11 enzymes required for glucocorticoid synthesis. The sensitivity of the P450 enzymes to this compound in mammalian tissues is much lower than that of the fungal enzymes, so that the inhibitory effects are seen only at high doses. This inhibition is compensated for by increased ACTH production and leads to increases in 17-deoxy steroids such as progesterone and aldosterone and to suppression of plasma renin activity. Ketoconazole also has other endocrine effects. It displaces estradiol and dihydrotestosterone from sex hormone-binding protein in vitro and increases the estradiol-testosterone ratio in plasma in vivo by a different mechanism. The latter may be responsible for the gynecomastia sometimes seen with ketoconazole therapy.

Ketoconazole has been used for the treatment of patients with Cushing's disease due to several causes. Doses of 200–1200 mg/d have produced a reduction in hormone levels and impressive clinical improvement in some patients in these preliminary studies.

6. MIFEPRISTONE (RU 486)

Mifepristone is a synthetic steroid that binds to glucocorticoid as well as to progesterone receptors and has been used experimentally in the treatment of Cushing's syndrome. Its pharmacology and use in women as a progesterone antagonist are discussed in Chapter 39.

MINERALOCORTICOID ANTAGONISTS

In addition to agents that interfere with aldosterone synthesis such as amphenone B (see above), there are steroids that compete with aldosterone for binding sites and decrease its effect peripherally. Progesterone is mildly active in this respect. However, it has been found that substitution of a 17-spirolactone group for the C20–C21 side chain of desoxycorticosterone results in a compound capable of blocking the sodium-retaining effect of aldosterone.

Spironolactone is a 7α-acetylthiospironolactone. Little is known about its metabolism. The onset of activity is slow, and the effects last for 2–3 days after the drug is discontinued. It is used in the treatment of primary aldosteronism in doses of 50–100 mg/d. This agent will reverse many of the findings of aldosteronism. It has been useful in establishing the diagnosis in some patients and in ameliorating the signs and symptoms when surgical removal of an adenoma is delayed. When used diagnostically for the detection of aldosteronism in hypokalemic patients with hypertension, doses of 400–500 mg/d for 4–8 days—with an adequate intake of sodium and potassium—will restore potassium levels to or toward normal. This agent is also useful in preparing these patients for surgery. Doses of 300–400 mg/d for 2 weeks are used for this purpose and may reduce the incidence of cardiac arrhythmias.

Spironolactone is also used in treatment of hirsutism in women. Doses of 50–200 mg/d cause a reduc-tion in the density, diameter, and rate of growth of facial hair in patients with idiopathic hirsutism or hirsutism secondary to androgen excess. The effect can usually be seen in 2 months and becomes maximal in about 6 months. It may be due to inhibition of androgen production and an action at the hair follicle.

Spironolactone

The use of spironolactone as a diuretic is discussed in Chapter 15. Adverse effects reported for spironolactone include hyperkalemia, menstrual abnormalities, gynecomastia, sedation, headache, gastrointestinal disturbances, and skin rashes.

PREPARATIONS AVAILABLE

Glucocorticoids for Aerosol Use: See Chapter 19.

Glucocorticoids for Dermatologic Use: See Chapter 63.

Glucocorticoids for Oral & Parenteral Use

Betamethasone (Celestone)
Oral: 0.6 mg tablets; 0.6 mg/5 mL syrup

Betamethasone sodium phosphate (generic, Celestone Phosphate, Cel-U-Jec)
Parenteral: 4 mg/mL for IV, IM, intralesional, or intra-articular injection

Cortisone (generic, Cortone Acetate)
Oral: 5, 10, 25 mg tablets

Dexamethasone (generic, Decadron, others)
Oral: 0.25, 0.5, 0.75, 1, 1.5, 2, 4, 6 mg tablets; 0.5 mg/5 mL elixir; 0.5 mg/5 mL, 0.5 mg/0.5 mL solution

Dexamethasone acetate (generic, Decadron-LA, others)
Parenteral: 8, 16 mg/mL suspension for IM, intralesional, or intra-articular injection

Dexamethasone sodium phosphate (generic, Decadron Phosphate, others)
Parenteral: 4, 10, 20, 24 mg/mL for IV, IM, intralesional, or intra-articular injection

Hydrocortisone [cortisol] (generic, Cortef)
Oral: 5, 10, 20 mg tablets

Hydrocortisone acetate (generic)
Parenteral: 25, 50 mg/mL suspension for intralesional, soft tissue, or intra-articular injection

Hydrocortisone cypionate (Cortef)
Oral suspension: 10 mg/5 mL

Hydrocortisone sodium phosphate
Parenteral: 50 mg/mL for IV, IM, or SC injection

Hydrocortisone sodium succinate (generic, Solu-Cortef, others)
Parenteral: 100, 250, 500, 1000 mg/vial for IV, IM injection

Methylprednisolone (generic, Medrol, Meprolone)
Oral: 2, 4, 8, 16, 24, 32 mg tablets

Methylprednisolone acetate (generic, Depo-Medrol, others)
Parenteral: 20, 40, 80 mg/mL for IM, intralesional, or intra-articular injection

Methylprednisolone sodium succinate (generic, Solu-Medrol, others)
Parenteral: 40, 125, 500, 1000, 2000 mg/vial for injection

Prednisolone (generic, Delta-Cortef, Prelone)

Oral: 5 mg tablets; 15 mg/5 mL syrup

Prednisolone acetate (generic, others)
Parenteral: 25, 50 mg/mL for injection

Prednisolone sodium phosphate
Oral: 5 mg/5 mL solution
Parenteral: 20 mg/mL for IV, IM, intra-articular, or intralesional injection

Prednisolone tebutate (generic, Hydeltra-T.B.A., others)
Parenteral: 20 mg/mL for intra-articular or intralesional injection

Prednisone (generic, Meticorten, others)
Oral: 1, 2.5, 5, 10, 20, 50 mg tablets; 5 mg/5 mL solution and syrup

Triamcinolone (generic, Aristocort, Kenacort, Atolone)
Oral: 1, 2, 4, 8 mg tablets; 4 mg/5 mL syrup

Triamcinolone acetonide (generic, Kenalog, others)
Parenteral: 3, 10, 40 mg/mL for IM, intra-articular, or intralesional injection

Triamcinolone diacetate (generic, Aristocort, others)

Parenteral: 25, 40 mg/mL for IM, intra-articular, or intralesional injection

Triamcinolone hexacetonide (Aristospan)
Parenteral: 5, 20 mg/mL for intra-articular, intralesional, or sublesional injection

Mineralocorticoids

Fludrocortisone acetate (Florinef Acetate)
Oral: 0.1 mg tablets

Adrenal Steroid Inhibitors

Aminoglutethimide (Cytadren)
Oral: 250 mg tablets

Ketoconazole (Nizoral)
Oral: 200 mg tablets (unlabeled use)

Metyrapone (Metopirone)
Oral: 250 mg tablets

Mitotane (Lysodren)
Oral: 500 mg tablets

Trilostane (Modrastane)
Oral: 30, 60 mg capsules

REFERENCES

Barnes PJ, Adcock I: Anti-inflammatory actions of steroids: Molecular mechanisms. Trends Pharmacol Sci 1993;14: 436.

Baulieu EE: The steroid hormone antagonist RU486: Mechanism at the cellular level and clinical applications. Endocrinol Metab Clin North Am 1991;20:873.

Baxter JD: Minimizing the effects of glucocorticoid therapy. Adv Intern Med 1990;35:173.

Berdanier CD: Role of the glucocorticoids in the regulation of lipogenesis. FASEB J 1989;3:2179.

Bikle DD et al: Elevated 1,25-dihydroxyvitamin D levels in patients with chronic obstructive pulmonary disease treated with prednisone. J Clin Endocrinol Metab 1993; 76:456

Blalock JE: A molecular basis of bidirectional communication between the immune and neuroendocrine systems. Physiol Rev 1989;69:1.

Bracken MB et al: A randomized, controlled trial of methylprednisolone or naloxone in the treatment of acute spinal-cord injury: Results of the Second National Acute Spinal Cord Injury Study. N Engl J Med 1990;322:1405.

Carella MJ et al: Hypothalamic-pituitary-adrenal function one week after a short burst of steroid therapy. J Clin Endocrinol Metab 1993;76:1188

Chin R: Adrenal crisis. Crit Care Clin 1991;7:23.

Chu PS, Buzdar AU, Hortobagyi GN: Trilostane with hydrocortisone in treatment of metastatic breast cancer. Breast Cancer Res Treat 1989;13:117.

Cleary MP: The antiobesity effect of dehydroepiandrosterone in rats. Proc Soc Exp Biol Med 1991;196:8.

Couch RM et al: Kinetic analysis of inhibition of human adrenal steroidogenesis by ketoconazole. J Clin Endocrinol Metab 1987;65:551.

Cumming DC et al: Treatment of hirsutism with spironolactone. JAMA 1982;247:1295.

Cummings JJ, D'Eugenio DB, Gross SJ: A controlled trial of dexamethasone in preterm infants at high risk for bronchopulmonary dysplasia. N Engl J Med 1989;320: 1505.

Cupps TR, Fauci AS: Corticosteroid-mediated immunoregulation in man. Immunol Rev 1982;65:133.

Davidson FF, Dennis EA: Biological relevance of lipocortins and related proteins as inhibitors of phospholipase A_2. Biochem Pharmacol 1989;38:3645.

Dixon RB, Christy NP: On the various forms of corticosteroid withdrawal syndrome. Am J Med 1980;68:224.

Dorr HG, Sippell WG: Prenatal dexamethasone treatment in pregnancies at risk for congenital adrenal hyperplasia due to 21-hydroxylase deficiency: Effect on midgestational amniotic fluid steroid levels. J Clin Endocrinol Metab 1993;76:117.

Farese RV Jr et al: Licorice induced hypermineralocorticoidism. N Engl J Med 1991;325:1223.

Farrell EE et al: Impact of antenatal dexamethasone administration on respiratory distress syndrome in surfactant-treated infants. Am J Obstet Gynecol 1989;161:628.

Feldman D: Ketoconazole and other imidazole derivatives as inhibitors of steroidogenesis. Endocr Rev 1985;7:409.

Frey BM, Frey FJ: Clinical pharmacokinetics of prednisone and prednisolone. Clin Pharmacokinet 1990:19:126.

Funder JW et al: Apparent mineralocorticoid excess, pseudohypoaldosteronism, and urinary electrolyte excretion: Toward a redefinition of mineralocorticoid action. FASEB J 1990;4:3234.

Gardiner P et al: Spironolactone metabolism: Steady-state serum levels of the sulfur-containing metabolites. J Clin Pharmacol 1989;29:324.

Godowski PJ, Picard D, Yamamoto KR: Signal transduction and transcriptional regulation by glucocorticoid receptor-LexA fusion proteins. Science 1988;241:812.

Gordon GB, Bush DE, Weisman HF: Reduction of athero-sclerosis by administration of dehydroepiandrosterone: A study in the hypercholesterolemic New Zealand white rabbit with intimal injury. J Clin Invest 1988;82:71.

Graber AL et al: Natural history of pituitary-adrenal recovery following long-term suppression with corticosteroids. J Clin Endocrinol Metab 1965;25:11.

Hammond GL: Molecular properties of corticosteroid binding globulin and the sex-steroid binding proteins. Endocr Rev 1990;11:65.

Helfer EL, Rose LI: Corticosteroids and adrenal suppression: Characterising and avoiding the problem. Drugs 1989;38:838.

Hyams JS, Carey DE: Corticosteroids and growth. J Pediatr 1988;113:249.

James VHT (editor): *The Adrenal Gland,* 2nd ed. Raven Press, 1992.

Johnson TS et al: Prevention of acute mountain sickness by dexamethasone. N Engl J Med 1984;310:683.

Kaye TB, Crapo L: The Cushing syndrome: An update on diagnostic tests. Ann Intern Med 1990;112:434.

Lacroix A et al: Gastric inhibitory polypeptide-dependent cortisol hypersecretion: A new cause of Cushing's syndrome. N Engl J Med 1992;327:974

Lamberts SWJ, Koper JW, de Jong FH: The endocrine effects of long-term treatment with mifepristone (RU 486). J Clin Endocrinol Metab 1991;73:187

LaRocca RV et al: Suramin in adrenal cancer: Modulation of steroid hormone production, cytotoxicity in vitro, and clinical antitumor effect. J Clin Endocrinol Metab 1990; 71:497.

Laue L: Glucocorticoid antagonists: Pharmacological attributes of a prototype antiglucocorticoid (RU 486). In: *Anti-inflammatory Steroid Action. Basic and Clinical Aspects.* Schleimer RP, Claman HN, Oronsky AL (editors). Academic Press, 1989.

Levine BD et al: Dexamethasone in the treatment of acute mountain sickness. N Engl J Med 1989;321:1707.

Libanati CR, Baylink DJ: Prevention and treatment of glucocorticoid-induced osteoporosis: A pathogenetic prospective. Chest 1992;102:1426.

Luton J-P et al: Clinical features of adrenocortical carcinoma, prognostic factors, and the effect of mitotane therapy. N Engl J Med 1990;322:1190.

Mao J, Regelson W, Kalimi M: Molecular mechanism of RU486 action: A review. Mol Cellular Biochem 1992; 109:1.

Meikle AW, Daynes RA, Araneo BA: Adrenal androgen secretion and biologic effects. Endocrinol Metab Clin North Am 1991;20:381.

Messer J et al: Association of adrenocorticosteroid therapy and peptic-ulcer disease. N Engl J Med 1983;309:21.

Miller WL: Molecular biology of steroid hormone synthesis. Endocr Rev 1988;9:295.

Muller M, Renkawitz R: The glucocorticoid receptor. Biochim Biophys Acta 1991;1088:171.

New ML: Prenatal diagnosis and treatment of congenital adrenal hyperplasia due to 21-hydroxylase deficiency. Development Pharmacol Therap 1990;15:200.

Ogirala RG et al: High dose intramuscular triamcinolone in severe, chronic, life-threatening asthma. N Engl J Med 1991;324:585.

Prummel MF et al: The course of biochemical parameters of bone turnover during treatment with corticosteroids. J Clin Endocrinol Metab 1991;72:382.

Samaan NA, Hickey RC: Adrenal cortical carcinoma. Semin Oncol 1987;14:262.

Sambrook P et al: Prevention of corticosteroid osteoporosis. N Engl J Med 1993;329:1747.

Schleimer RP: Effects of glucocorticosteroids on inflammatory cells relevant to their therapeutic applications in asthma. Am Rev Respir Dis 1990;141:S59.

Schurmeyer TH et al: Pituitary-adrenal responsiveness to corticotropin-releasing hormone in patients receiving chronic, alternate day glucocorticoid therapy. J Clin Endocrinol Metab 1985;61:22.

Semel JD: Fever on drug-free day of alternate-day steroid therapy. Am J Med 1984;76:315.

Smith DF, Toft DO: Steroid receptors and their associated proteins. Mol Endocrinol 1993;4:7.

Sonino N et al: Ketoconazole treatment in Cushing's syndrome: Experience in 34 patients. Clin Endocrinol 1991;35:347.

Sorenson DK et al: Corticosteroids stimulate an increase in phospholipase A_2 inhibitor in human serum. J Steroid Biochem 1988;2:271.

Tabarin A et al: Use of ketoconazole in the treatment of Cushing's disease and ectopic ACTH syndrome. Clin Endocrinol 1991;34:63.

Tyrell JB, Aron DC, Forsham PH: Glucocorticoids and adrenal androgens. In: *Basic & Clinical Endocrinology,* 3rd edition. Greenspan FS (editor). Appleton & Lange, 1991.

Ulick S, Tedde R, Wang ZW: Defective ring A reduction of cortisol as the major metabolic error in the syndrome of apparent mineralocorticoid excess. J Clin Endocrinol Metab 1992;74:593

White PC, New MI, Dupont B: Congenital adrenal hyperplasia. (Two parts.) N Engl J Med 1987;316:1519, 1580.

39

The Gonadal Hormones & Inhibitors

Alan Goldfien, MD

I. THE OVARY
(Estrogens, Progestins, Other Ovarian Hormones, Oral Contraceptives, Inhibitors & Antagonists, & Ovulation-Inducing Agents)

The ovary has important gametogenic functions that are integrated with its hormonal activity. In the human female, the gonad is relatively quiescent during the period of rapid growth and maturation. At puberty, the ovary begins a 30- to 40-year period of cyclic function called the **menstrual cycle** because of the regular episodes of bleeding that are its most obvious manifestation. It then fails to respond to gonadotropins secreted by the anterior pituitary gland, and the cessation of cyclic bleeding that occurs is called the **menopause.**

The mechanism responsible for the onset of ovarian function at the time of puberty is thought to be neural in origin, because the immature gonad can be stimulated by gonadotropins already present in the hypothalamus and because the pituitary is responsive to hypothalamic gonadotropin-releasing hormones. The maturation of centers such as the amygdala in the brain may withdraw an inhibition of the cells in the median eminence of the hypothalamus, allowing them to produce **gonadotropin-releasing hormone (GnRH)** in pulses with the appropriate frequency and amplitude, which stimulates the release of **follicle-stimulating hormone (FSH)** and **luteinizing hormone (LH)** (see Chapter 36). At first, small amounts of these latter two hormones are released, and the limited quantities of estrogen secreted in response cause breast development, alterations in fat distribution, and a growth spurt that culminates in epiphysial closure in the long bones.

After a year or so, sufficient estrogen is produced to induce endometrial changes and periodic bleeding. After the first few cycles, which may be anovulatory, normal cyclic function is established.

At the beginning of each cycle, a variable number of follicles (vesicular follicles), each containing an ovum, begin to enlarge in response to FSH. After 5 or 6 days, one of the follicles begins to develop more rapidly. The granulosa cells of this follicle multiply and, under the influence of LH, synthesize estrogens and release them at an increasing rate. The estrogens appear to inhibit FSH release and may lead to regression of the smaller, less mature follicles. The ovarian follicle consists of an ovum surrounded by a fluid-filled antrum lined by granulosa and theca cells. The estrogen secretion reaches a peak just before midcycle, and the granulosa cells begin to secrete progesterone. These changes stimulate the brief surge in LH and FSH release that precedes (and causes) ovulation. When the follicle ruptures, the ovum is released into the abdominal cavity near the uterine tube.

Following the above events, the cavity of the ruptured follicle fills with blood (corpus hemorrhagicum), and the luteinized theca and granulosa cells proliferate and replace the blood to form the corpus luteum. The cells of this structure produce estrogens and progesterone for the remainder of the cycle, or longer if pregnancy occurs.

If pregnancy does not occur, the corpus luteum begins to degenerate and ceases hormone production, eventually becoming a corpus albicans. The cause of luteolysis in humans is unknown. Most other hormonal events occurring during the normal ovarian cycle can be explained on the basis of feedback regulation. The endometrium, which proliferated during the follicular phase and developed its glandular structure during the luteal phase, is shed in the process of menstruation. These events are summarized in Figure 39–1.

The ovary normally ceases its gametogenic and endocrine function with time. This change is accompanied by a cessation in uterine bleeding (menopause) and occurs at a mean age of 52 years in the USA. Although the ovary ceases to secrete estrogen, significant levels of estrogen persist in many women as a result of conversion of adrenal steroids such as androstenedione to estrone and estradiol in adipose and possibly other nonendocrine tissues.

Disturbances in Ovarian Function

Disturbances of cyclic function are common even during the peak years of reproduction. A minority of these result from inflammatory or neoplastic processes that destroy the uterus, ovaries, or pituitary, but the causes of most menstrual problems are poorly understood. Many of the minor disturbances leading to periods of amenorrhea or anovulatory cycles are self-limited. They are often associated with emotional or environmental changes and are thought to represent temporary disorders in the centers in the brain that control the secretion of the hypothalamic releasing factors. Normal ovarian function can be modified by androgens produced by the adrenal cortex or tumors arising from it. The ovary also gives rise to androgen-producing neoplasms such as arrhenoblastomas and Leydig cell tumors as well as to estrogen-producing granulosa cell tumors.

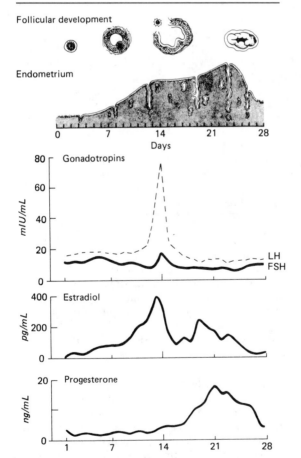

Figure 39–1. The menstrual cycle, showing plasma levels of pituitary and ovarian hormones and histologic changes.

THE ESTROGENS

Estrogenic activity is shared by a large number of chemical substances. In addition to the variety of steroidal estrogens derived from animal sources, numerous nonsteroidal estrogens have been synthesized. Many phenols are estrogenic, and estrogenic activity has been identified in such diverse forms of life as those found in the sediments of the seas and certain species of clover.

Natural Estrogens

The major estrogens produced by women are estradiol (estradiol-17β, E_2), estrone (E_1), and estriol (E_3) (Figure 39–2). Estradiol appears to be the major secretory product of the ovary. Although some estrone is produced in the ovary, most estrone and estriol are formed in the liver from estradiol or in peripheral tissues from androstenedione and other androgens. As noted above, during the first part of the menstrual cycle estrogens are produced in the ovarian follicle by the theca cells. After ovulation, the estrogens as well as progesterone are synthesized by the granulosa cells of the corpus luteum, and the pathways of biosynthesis are slightly different.

During pregnancy, a large amount of estrogen is synthesized by the fetoplacental unit. The estriol synthesized by the fetoplacental unit is released into the maternal circulation and excreted into the urine. Repeated assay of maternal urinary estriol excretion has been useful in the assessment of fetal well-being.

One of the most prolific natural sources of estro-

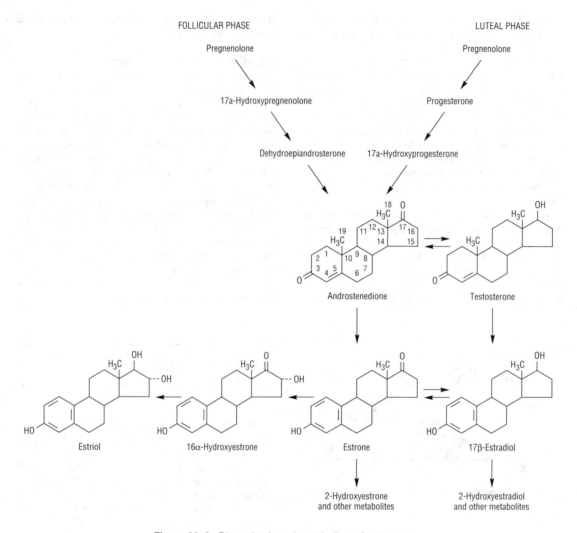

Figure 39–2. Biosynthesis and metabolism of estrogens.

genic substances is the stallion, which liberates more of this hormone than the pregnant mare or pregnant woman. The equine estrogens—equilenin and equilin—and their congeners are unsaturated in the B as well as the A ring and are excreted in large quantities in urine, from which they can be recovered and used for medicinal purposes.

In normal women, estradiol is produced at a rate that varies during the menstrual cycle, resulting in plasma levels as low as 50 pg/mL in the early follicular phase to as high as 350–850 pg/mL at the time of the preovulatory peak (Figure 39–1).

Synthetic Estrogens

A variety of chemical alterations have been produced in the natural estrogens. The most important effect of these alterations has been to increase the effectiveness of the estrogens when administered orally.

Some structures are shown in Figure 39–3. Those with therapeutic use are listed in Table 39–1.

In addition to the steroidal estrogens, a variety of nonsteroidal compounds with estrogenic activity have been synthesized and used clinically. These include dienestrol, diethylstilbestrol, benzestrol, hexestrol, methestrol, methallenestril, and chlorotrianisene (Figure 39–3).

Pharmacokinetics

When released into the circulation, estradiol binds strongly to an α_2-globulin (sex hormone-binding globulin [SHBG]) and to albumin with less affinity. Bound estrogen is relatively unavailable for diffusion into cells, so it is the free fraction that is physiologically active. Estradiol is converted by the liver and other tissues to estrone and estriol (which have low affinity for the estrogen receptor) and their 2-hy-

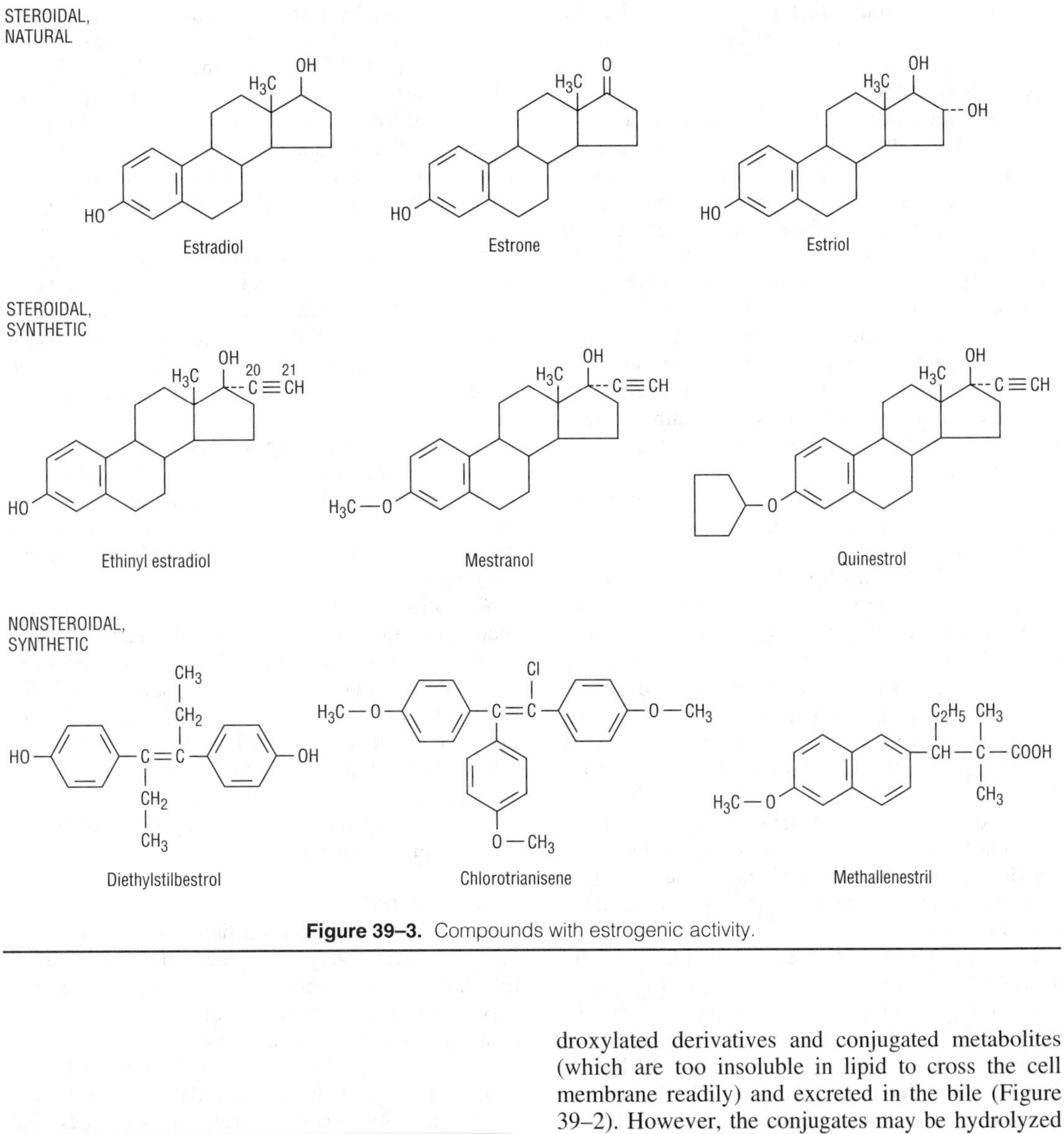

STEROIDAL,
NATURAL

Estradiol

Estrone

Estriol

STEROIDAL,
SYNTHETIC

Ethinyl estradiol

Mestranol

Quinestrol

NONSTEROIDAL,
SYNTHETIC

Diethylstilbestrol

Chlorotrianisene

Methallenestril

Figure 39–3. Compounds with estrogenic activity.

Table 39–1. Commonly used estrogens.

	Average Replacement Dosage
Ethinyl estradiol	0.005–0.02 mg/d
Micronized estradiol	1–2 mg/d
Estradiol cypionate	2–5 mg every 3–4 weeks
Estradiol valerate	2–20 mg every other week
Estropipate	1.25–2.5 mg/d
Conjugated, esterified, or mixed estrogenic substances:	
Oral	0.3–1.25 mg/d
Injectable	0.2–2 mg/d
Topical	Transdermal patch
Diethylstilbestrol	0.1–0.5 mg/d
Quinestrol	0.1–0.2 mg/week
Dienestrol	...
Chlorotrianisene	12–25 mg/d
Methallenestril	3–9 mg/d

droxylated derivatives and conjugated metabolites (which are too insoluble in lipid to cross the cell membrane readily) and excreted in the bile (Figure 39–2). However, the conjugates may be hydrolyzed in the intestine to active, reabsorbable compounds. The catechol estrogens serve as neurotransmitters in the central nervous system. They also compete for catechol-O-methyltransferase and in high concentration inhibit the inactivation of catecholamines by the enzyme. Estrogens are also excreted in small amounts in the breast milk of nursing mothers.

Because significant amounts of estrogens and their active metabolites are excreted in the bile and reabsorbed from the intestine, the resulting enterohepatic circulation ensures that orally administered estrogens will have a high ratio of hepatic to peripheral effects. As noted below, the hepatic effects are thought to be responsible for some undesirable actions such as synthesis of increased clotting factors and plasma renin substrate. When used for their peripheral effects—eg, in postmenopausal women—the hepatic effects can be minimized by routes that avoid first-pass hepatic exposure, ie, vaginal, transdermal, or by injection.

Physiologic Effects

A. Mechanism: Plasma estradiol is thought to enter its target cell by diffusion and is transported to the nucleus, where it binds to the estrogen receptors. The estrogen receptors are found in the nucleus bound to a number of different heat shock proteins that dissociate from the receptor when it binds to estradiol. The ligand-receptor complex forms a homodimer that binds to the estrogen response element on the gene and interacts with specific cellular proteins (transacting factors) to activate transcription and regulate the formation of specific messenger RNA. The effects described below may be the direct results of processes stimulated by induction of protein synthesis in the cell. However, some actions of estrogen appear to be the result of paracrine effects dependent upon growth factors and cytokines released by neighboring cells.

B. Female Maturation: Estrogens are required for the normal maturation of the female. They stimulate the development of the vagina, uterus, and uterine tubes as well as the secondary sex characteristics. They stimulate stromal development and ductal growth in the breast and are responsible for the accelerated growth phase and the closing of the epiphyses of the long bones that occur at puberty. They contribute to the growth of the axillary and pubic hair and alter the distribution of body fat so as to produce typical female body contours. Larger quantities also stimulate development of pigmentation in the skin, most prominent in the region of the nipples and areolae and in the genital region.

C. Endometrial Effects: In addition to its growth effects on the uterine muscle, estrogen also plays an important role in the development of the endometrial lining. Continuous exposure to estrogens for prolonged periods leads to an abnormal hyperplasia of the endometrium that is usually associated with abnormal bleeding patterns. When estrogen production is properly coordinated with the production of progesterone during the normal human menstrual cycle, regular periodic bleeding and shedding of the endometrial lining occur.

D. Metabolic Effects: Estrogens have a number of important metabolic effects. They seem to be partially responsible for maintenance of the normal structure of the skin and blood vessels in women. Estrogens decrease the rate of resorption of bone by antagonizing the effect of parathyroid hormone on bone but do not stimulate bone formation. Estrogens may have important effects on intestinal absorption because they reduce the motility of the bowel.

In addition to stimulating the synthesis of enzymes and growth factors leading to uterine growth and differentiation, estrogens alter the production and activity of many other proteins in the body. Metabolic alterations in the liver are especially important, so that there is a higher circulating level of proteins such as **transcortin (CBG), thyroxine-binding globulin (TBG), sex hormone-binding globulin (SHBG),** transferrin, renin substrate, and fibrinogen. This leads to increased circulating levels of thyroxine, estrogen, testosterone, iron, copper, and other substances.

E. Effects on Blood Coagulation: Estrogens enhance the coagulability of blood. Many changes in factors influencing coagulation have been reported, including increased circulating levels of factors II, VII, IX, and X and decreased antithrombin III, partially as a result of the hepatic effects mentioned above. Increased plasminogen levels and decreased platelet adhesiveness have also been found (see Hormonal Contraception).

Alterations in the composition of the plasma lipids caused by estrogens are characterized by an increase in the high-density lipoproteins, a slight reduction in the low-density lipoproteins, and a reduction in plasma cholesterol levels. Plasma triglyceride levels are increased.

F. Other Effects: Estrogens have many other effects. They induce the synthesis of progesterone receptors. They are responsible for estrous behavior in animals and influence libido in humans. They facilitate the loss of intravascular fluid into the extracellular space, producing edema. The resulting decrease in plasma volume causes a compensatory retention of sodium and water by the kidney. Estrogens also modulate sympathetic nervous system control of smooth muscle function.

Clinical Uses*

A. Primary Hypogonadism: Estrogens have been used extensively for replacement therapy in estrogen-deficient patients. The estrogen deficiency may be due to primary failure of development of the ovaries, castration, or menopause.

Treatment of primary hypogonadism is usually begun at 11–13 years of age in order to stimulate the development of secondary sex characteristics and menses, to stimulate optimal growth, and to avoid the psychologic consequences of delayed puberty. Treatment is initiated with small doses of estrogen (0.3 mg conjugated estrogens or 5–10 μg ethinyl estradiol) on days 1–21 each month. When growth is completed, chronic therapy consists mainly of the administration of estrogens and progestins, as described below.

B. Postmenopausal Hormonal Therapy: In addition to the signs and symptoms that follow closely upon the cessation of normal ovarian function—such as loss of periods, vasomotor symptoms, and genital atrophy—there are longer-lasting changes that influence the health and well-being of postmenopausal women. These include an acceleration of

---

*The use of estrogens in contraception is discussed below.

bone loss, which in susceptible women may lead to vertebral, hip, and wrist fractures; and lipid changes, which may contribute to the acceleration of cardiovascular disease noted in postmenopausal women. The effects of estrogens on bone have been extensively studied, and the effects of hormone withdrawal and replacement are well-characterized. However, the role of estrogen and progestins in the cause and prevention of cardiovascular disease, which is responsible for 350,000 deaths per year, and breast cancer, which causes 35,000 deaths per year, is less well understood.

When normal ovulatory function ceases and the estrogen levels fall after the menopause or oophorectomy, there is an accelerated rise in plasma cholesterol and LDL concentrations, and LDL receptors decline. HDL is not much affected, and levels remain higher than in men. VLDL and triglyceride levels are not much different. Since cardiovascular disorders account for most deaths in this age group, the risk for these disorders constitute a major consideration in deciding whether or not hormonal therapy is indicated and influences the selection of hormones to be administered. The effect of estrogen replacement therapy on circulating lipids and lipoproteins is associated with a reduction in myocardial infarction by about 50% and fatal strokes by as much as 40% percent. Progestins antagonize estrogen's effects on LDL and HDL to a variable extent.

Optimal management of the postmenopausal patient requires careful assessment of her symptoms as well as consideration of her age and the risk for cardiovascular disease, osteoporosis, breast cancer, and endometrial cancer. Bearing in mind the effects of the gonadal hormones on each of these disorders, the goals of therapy can then be defined and the risks of therapy assessed and discussed with the patient.

If the main indication for therapy is hot flushes, therapy with the lowest dose of estrogen required for symptomatic relief is recommended. Treatment may be required for only a limited period of time and the possible increased risk for breast cancer avoided. In women who have had a hysterectomy, estrogens alone can be given 5 days per week or continuously, since progestins are not required to reduce the risk for endometrial hyperplasia and cancer. Although hot flushes, sweating, insomnia, and atrophic vaginitis are generally relieved by estrogens and although many patients experience some increased sense of well-being, depression and other psychopathologic states are seldom improved.

The role of estrogens in the prevention and treatment of osteoporosis has been carefully studied (see Chapter 41). The amount of bone present is maximal in the young active adult and begins to decline in middle age in both men and women. The development of osteoporosis also depends on the amount of bone present at the start of this process, on calcium intake, and on the degree of physical activity. The risk of osteo-

porosis is highest in smokers who are thin, Caucasian, and inactive and have a low calcium intake and a strong family history of osteoporosis.

Estrogens should be used in the smallest dosage consistent with relief of symptoms. In women who have not undergone hysterectomy, it is most convenient to prescribe estrogen on the first 21–25 days of each month. The recommended dosages of estrogen are 0.3–1.25 mg/d of conjugated estrogen or 0.01–0.02 mg/d of ethinyl estradiol. Doses in the middle of this range have been shown to be maximally effective in preventing the decrease in bone density occurring at menopause. From this point of view, it is important to begin therapy as soon as possible after the menopause for maximum effect. In these patients and others not taking estrogen, calcium supplements, bringing the total daily calcium intake up to 1500 mg, are useful.

Patients at low risk of developing osteoporosis who manifest only mild atrophic vaginitis can be treated with topical preparations. The vaginal route of application is also useful in the treatment of urinary tract symptoms in these patients. It is important to realize, however, that although locally administered estrogens escape the first-pass effect (so that some undesirable hepatic effects are reduced), they are almost completely absorbed into the circulation, and these preparations should be given cyclically.

As noted below, the administration of estrogen is associated with an increased risk of endometrial carcinoma. The administration of a progestational agent with the estrogen prevents endometrial hyperplasia and markedly reduces the risk of cancer. When estrogen is given for the first 25 days of the month and the progestin medroxyprogesterone (10 mg/d) is added during the last 10–14 days, the risk is only half of that in women not receiving hormone replacement therapy. On this regimen, some women will experience a return of symptoms during the period off estrogen administration. In these patients, the estrogen can be given continuously. If the progestin produces sedation or other undesirable effects, its dose can be reduced to 2.5–5 mg for the last 10 days of the cycle with a slight increase in the risk for endometrial hyperplasia. These regimens are usually accompanied by bleeding at the end of each cycle. Some women experience migraine headaches during the last few days of the cycle. The use of a continuous estrogen regimen will often prevent their occurrence. Women who object to the cyclic bleeding associated with sequential therapy can also consider continuous therapy. Daily therapy with 0.625 mg of conjugated equine estrogens and 2.5–5 mg medroxyprogesterone will eliminate cyclic bleeding, control vasomotor symptoms, prevent genital atrophy, maintain bone density, and show a favorable lipid profile with a small decrease in LDL and an increase in HDL concentrations. These women have endometrial atrophy on biopsy. About half of these patients will experience breakthrough bleeding during the first few months of therapy. Seventy to 80 percent become amenorrheic after the first 4 months, and most remain so. The main disadvantage of continuous therapy is the need for uterine biopsy when bleeding occurs after the first few months.

As noted above, estrogens may also be administered vaginally or transdermally. When estrogens are given by these routes, the liver is bypassed on the first circulation, and the ratio of the liver effects to peripheral effects is reduced.

In patients in whom estrogen replacement therapy is contraindicated, such as those with estrogen-sensitive tumors, relief of vasomotor symptoms may be obtained by the use of progestational agents or clonidine.

C. Other Uses: Estrogens combined with progestins can be used to suppress ovulation in patients with intractable dysmenorrhea or when suppression of ovarian function is used in the treatment of hirsutism and amenorrhea due to excessive secretion of androgens by the ovary. Under these circumstances, greater suppression may be needed, and oral contraceptives containing 50–80 μg of estrogen or a combination of a low estrogen pill with GnRH suppression may be required.

Estrogens have been used to stop excessive uterine bleeding due to endometrial hyperplasia. Repeated doses of 20 μg of ethinyl estradiol every few hours or the administration of 20 mg of conjugated estrogens intravenously has been useful in arresting blood loss temporarily.

Adverse Effects

Adverse effects of variable severity have been reported with the therapeutic use of estrogens. Many other effects reported in conjunction with hormonal contraceptives may be related to their estrogen content. These are discussed below.

Estrogen therapy is a major cause of **postmenopausal bleeding.** Unfortunately, vaginal bleeding at this time of life may also be due to carcinoma of the endometrium. In order to avoid confusion, patients should be treated with the smallest amount of estrogen possible. It should be given cyclically so that bleeding, if it occurs, will be more likely to occur during the withdrawal period. As noted above, endometrial hyperplasia can be prevented by administration of a progestational agent with estrogen in each cycle.

Nausea and **breast tenderness** are common and can be minimized by using the smallest effective dose of estrogen. **Hyperpigmentation** also occurs. Estrogen therapy is associated with an increase in frequency of **migraine headaches** as well as **cholestasis, hypertension,** and gallbladder disease.

The relationship of estrogen therapy to **cancer** continues to be the subject of active investigation. Although no adverse effect of short-term estrogen ther-

apy on the incidence of breast cancer has been demonstrated, a small increase in the incidence of this tumor may occur with prolonged therapy. Although the risk factor is small (1.25), the impact is great since this tumor occurs in 10% of women. The effect of progesterone has not been determined as yet. Studies indicate that following unilateral excision of breast cancer, women receiving tamoxifen show a 35% decrease in contralateral breast cancer compared with controls. These studies also demonstrate that tamoxifen is well tolerated by most patients, produces estrogen-like alterations in plasma lipid levels, and stabilizes bone mineral loss. Studies bearing on the possible efficacy of tamoxifen in postmenopausal women at high risk for breast cancer are under way. Many studies show an increased risk of endometrial carcinoma in patients taking estrogens. The risk seems to vary with the dose and duration of treatment: 15 times as great in patients taking large doses of estrogen for 5 or more years, in contrast with two to four times greater in patients receiving lower doses for short periods. However, as noted above, the concomitant use of a progestin not only prevents this increased risk but actually reduces the incidence of endometrial cancer to less than that in the general population.

There have been a number of reports of adenocarcinoma of the vagina in young women whose mothers were treated with large doses of diethylstilbestrol early in pregnancy. These cancers are most common in young women (ages 14–44). The incidence is less than 1:1000 women exposed—too low to establish a cause-and-effect relationship with certainty. However, the risks for infertility, ectopic pregnancy, and premature delivery are also increased. It is now recognized that there is no indication for the use of diethylstilbestrol during pregnancy, and it should be avoided. It is not known whether other estrogens have a similar effect or whether the observed phenomena are peculiar to diethylstilbestrol. This agent should be used only for the treatment of cancer (eg, of the prostate) or as a "morning after" contraceptive (see Table 39–4).

Contraindications

Estrogens should not be used in patients with estrogen-dependent neoplasms such as carcinoma of the endometrium or in those with—or at high risk for—carcinoma of the breast. They should be avoided in patients with undiagnosed genital bleeding, liver disease, or a history of thromboembolic disorder.

Preparations & Dosages

The dosages of commonly used natural and synthetic preparations are listed in Table 39–1. Although the estrogens produce almost the same hormonal effects, their potencies vary both between agents and depending on the route of administration. As noted above, estradiol is the most active endogenous estrogen, and it has the highest affinity for the estrogen receptor. However, its metabolites estrone and estriol have weak uterotropic effects. Another important metabolite of estradiol, 2-hydroxyestrone (a catechol estrogen), has been shown to act as a neurotransmitter in the brain. It also competes with catecholamines for catechol-O-methyltransferase and inhibits tyrosine hydroxylase. Therefore, preparations with estrone and estradiol may produce more central effects than preparations with synthetic estrogens, which are metabolized differently.

For a given level of gonadotropin suppression, oral estrone and estradiol preparations have more effect on the circulating levels of CBG and SHBG than do synthetic preparations. This route of administration allows greater concentrations of hormone to reach the liver, thus increasing the synthesis of these binding proteins. Transdermal preparations were developed to avoid this effect. When administered transdermally, 50–100 μg of estradiol has effects similar to those of 0.625–1.25 mg of conjugated oral estrogens on gonadotropin concentrations, endometrium, and vaginal epithelium. Furthermore, the transdermal estrogen preparations do not significantly increase the concentrations of renin substrate, CBG, and TBG and do not produce the characteristic changes in serum lipids.

THE PROGESTINS

Natural Progestins: Progesterone

Progesterone is the most important progestin in humans. In addition to having important hormonal effects, it serves as a precursor to the estrogens, androgens, and adrenocortical steroids. It is synthesized in the ovary, testis, and adrenal from circulating cholesterol. Large amounts are also synthesized and released by the placenta during pregnancy.

In the ovary, progesterone is produced primarily by the corpus luteum. Normal males appear to secrete 1–5 mg of progesterone daily, resulting in plasma levels of about 0.03 μg/dL. The level is only slightly higher in the female during the follicular phase of the cycle, when only a few milligrams per day of progesterone are secreted. During the luteal phase, plasma levels range from 0.5 μg/dL to more than 2 μg/dL (Figure 39–1).

Synthetic Progestins

A variety of progestational compounds have been synthesized. Some are active when given by mouth. They are not a uniform group of compounds, and all of them differ from progesterone in one or more respects. Table 39–2 lists some of these compounds and

Table 39–2. Activities of progestational agents.

	Route	Duration of Action	Activities[1]				
			Estrogenic	Androgenic	Antiestrogenic	Antiandrogenic	Anabolic
Progesterone and derivatives							
Progesterone	IM	1 day	–	–	+	–	–
Hydroxyprogesterone caproate	IM	8–14 days	sl	sl	–	–	–
Medroxyprogesterone acetate	IM, PO	Tabs: 1–3 days; injection: 4–12 weeks	–	+	+		
Megestrol acetate	PO	1–3 days	–	+	–	+	–
17α-Ethinyl testosterone derivatives **Testosterone derivatives** Dimethisterone	PO	1–3 days	–	–	sl	–	–
19-Nortestosterone derivatives Norethynodrel[2]	PO	1–3 days	+	–	–	–	–
Lynestrenol[3]	PO	1–3 days	+	+	–	–	+
Norethindrone[2]	PO	1–3 days	sl	+	+	–	+
Norethindrone acetate[2]	PO	1–3 days	sl	+	+	–	+
Ethynodiol diacetate[2]	PO	1–3 days	sl	+	+	–	–
L-Norgestrel[2]	PO	1–3 days	–	+	+	–	+

[1]**Interpretation:** + = active; – = inactive; sl = slightly active. Activities have been reported in various species using various end points and may not apply to humans.
[2]See Table 39–3.
[3]Not available in USA

their effects. In general, the 21-carbon compounds (hydroxyprogesterone, medroxyprogesterone, megestrol, and dimethisterone) are the most closely related, pharmacologically as well as chemically, to progesterone. A new group of "third-generation" synthetic progestins has entered clincial trials, principally as components of oral contraceptives. These 19-nor, 13-ethyl steroid compounds include gestodene, norgestimate, and desogestrel. They are claimed to have lower androgenic activity than older progestins (Bringer, 1992).

Pharmacokinetics

Progesterone is rapidly absorbed following administration by any route. Its half-life in the plasma is approximately 5 minutes, and small amounts are stored temporarily in body fat. It is almost completely metabolized in one passage through the liver, and for that reason it is quite ineffective when administered orally.

In the liver, progesterone is metabolized to pregnanediol and conjugated with glucuronic acid. It is excreted into the urine as pregnanediol glucuronide (Figure 39–4). The amount of pregnanediol in the urine has been used as an index of progesterone secretion. It has been very useful in spite of the fact that the proportion of secreted progesterone converted to this compound varies from day to day and from individual to individual. In addition to progesterone, 20α- and 20β-hydroxyprogesterone (20α- and 20β-hydroxy-4-pregnene-3-one) are also found. These compounds have about one-fifth the progestational activity of progesterone in humans and other species. Little is known of their physiologic importance, but 20α-hydroxyprogesterone is produced in large amounts in some species and may be of some importance biologically.

The usual routes of administration and durations of action of the synthetic progestins are listed in Table 39–2. Most of these agents are extensively metabolized to inactive products that are excreted mainly in the urine.

Physiologic Effects

A. Mechanism: Progestins enter the cell and bind to progesterone receptors that are distributed between the nucleus and the cytoplasmic domains. The ligand-receptor complex binds to a response element to activate gene transcription. The response element for progesterone appears to be similar to the corticoid response element, and the specificity of the response depends upon which receptor is present in the cell as well as upon other cell-specific transcription factors. The progesterone-receptor complex forms a dimer before binding to DNA. However, in contrast to the estrogen receptor, it can form heterodimers as well as homodimers.

B. Effects of Progesterone: Progesterone has little effect on protein metabolism. It stimulates lipo-

protein lipase activity and seems to favor fat deposition. The effects on carbohydrate metabolism are more marked. Progesterone increases basal insulin levels and the insulin response to glucose. There is usually no manifest change in carbohydrate tolerance. In the liver, progesterone promotes glycogen storage, possibly by facilitating the effect of insulin. Progesterone also promotes ketogenesis.

Progesterone can compete with aldosterone at the renal tubule, causing a decrease in Na^+ reabsorption. This leads to an increased secretion of aldosterone by the adrenal cortex (eg, in pregnancy). Progesterone increases the body temperature in humans. The mechanism of this effect is not known, but an alteration of the temperature-regulating centers in the hypothalamus has been suggested. Progesterone also alters the function of the respiratory centers. The ventilatory response to CO_2 is increased (synthetic progestins with an ethinyl group do not have respiratory effects). This leads to a measurable reduction in arterial and alveolar P_{CO_2} during pregnancy and in the luteal phase of the menstrual cycle. Progesterone and related steroids also have depressant and hypnotic effects on the brain.

Progesterone is responsible for the alveolobular development of the secretory apparatus in the breast. It also causes the maturation and secretory changes in the endometrium that are seen following ovulation (Figure 39–1).

Progesterone decreases the plasma levels of many amino acids and leads to increased urinary nitrogen excretion. It has been found to induce changes in the structure and function of smooth endoplasmic reticulum in experimental animals.

Other effects are noted in the section on Hormonal Contraception.

C. Synthetic Progestins: The 21-carbon analogues antagonize aldosterone-induced sodium retention (see above) and have slight androgenic or estrogenic effects. The remaining compounds (19-carbon) produce a decidual change in the endometrial stroma, do not support pregnancy in test animals, are more effective gonadotropin inhibitors, and may have minimal estrogenic and androgenic or anabolic activity (Table 39–2). They are sometimes referred to as "impeded androgens."

Clinical Uses of Progestins

A. Therapeutic Applications: The major uses of progestational hormones are for hormone replacement therapy (see above) and hormonal contraception (see below). In addition, they are useful in producing long-term ovarian suppression for other purposes. When used alone in large doses parenterally (eg, medroxyprogesterone acetate, 150 mg intramuscularly every 90 days), prolonged anovulation and amenorrhea result. This therapy has been employed in the treatment of dysmenorrhea, endometriosis, hirsutism, and bleeding disorders when estrogens are contrain-

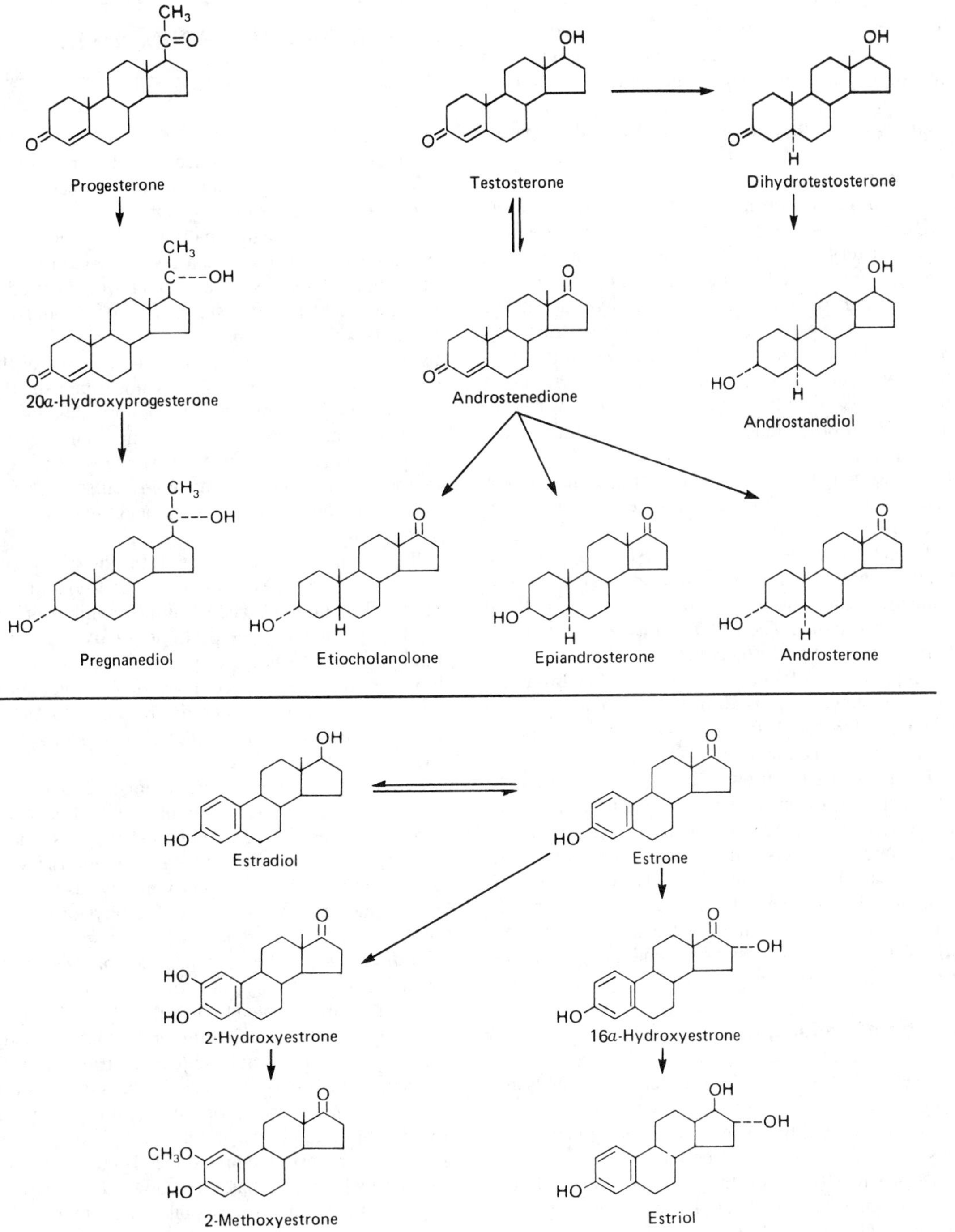

Figure 39–4. Synthetic and degradation pathways for progesterone, androgens, and estrogens. These pathways are similar in the ovary, testis, and adrenal. (Reproduced, with permission, from Greenspan FS [editor]: *Basic & Clinical Endocrinology,* 3rd ed. Appleton & Lange, 1991.)

dicated and for contraception. The major problem with this regimen is the prolonged time required in some patients for ovulatory function to return after cessation of therapy. It should not be used for patients planning a pregnancy in the near future. Similar regimens will relieve hot flushes in some menopausal women and can be used if estrogen therapy is contraindicated.

Medroxyprogesterone acetate, 10–20 mg orally twice weekly–or intramuscularly in doses of 100 mg/m^2 every 1–2 weeks—will arrest accelerated maturation in children with precocious puberty.

Progestins do not appear to have any place in the therapy of threatened or habitual abortion. Early reports of the usefulness of these agents resulted from the unwarranted assumption that after several abortions the likelihood of repeated abortions was over 90%. When progestational agents were administered to patients with previous abortions, a salvage rate of 80% was achieved. It is now recognized that similar patients abort only 20% of the time even when untreated.

Progesterone and medroxyprogesterone have been used in the treatment of women who have difficulty in conceiving and who demonstrate a slow rise in basal body temperature. There is no convincing evidence that this treatment is effective.

Preparations of progesterone and medroxyprogesterone have been used to treat premenstrual syndrome. Controlled studies have not confirmed the effectiveness of such therapy.

B. Diagnostic Uses: Progesterone can be used as a test of estrogen secretion. The administration of progesterone, 150 mg/d, or medroxyprogesterone, 10 mg/d for 5–7 days, is followed by withdrawal bleeding in amenorrheic patients only when the endometrium has been stimulated by estrogens. A combination of estrogen and progestin can be given to test the responsiveness of the endometrium in patients with amenorrhea.

Contraindications, Cautions, & Adverse Effects

Recent studies with progestational compounds and with combination oral contraceptives indicate that the progestin in these agents may increase blood pressure in some patients. The more potent progestins also reduce plasma HDL levels in women. Lower HDL levels are associated with an increased incidence of myocardial infarction. (See Hormonal Contraception.)

OTHER OVARIAN HORMONES

The normal ovary produces small amounts of **androgens,** including testosterone, androstenedione, and dehydroepiandrosterone. Of these, only testosterone has a significant amount of biologic activity, though androstenedione can be converted to estrone in peripheral tissues. The normal woman produces less than 200 μg of testosterone in 24 hours, and about one-third of this is probably formed in the ovary directly. The physiologic significance of these small amounts of androgens is not established, but they may be partly responsible for normal hair growth at puberty and may have other important metabolic effects. Androgen production by the ovary may be markedly increased in some abnormal states, usually in association with hirsutism and amenorrhea as noted above.

The ovary also produces **inhibin** and **activin.** These polypeptides consist of several combinations of α and β subunits. The αβ dimer (inhibin) inhibits FSH secretion while the ββ dimer (activin) increases FSH secretion. Studies in primates indicate that inhibin has no direct effect on ovarian steroidogenesis but that activin modulates the response to LH and FSH. For example, simultaneous treatment with activin and human FSH enhances FSH stimulation of progesterone synthesis and aromatase activity in granulosa cells. When combined with LH, activin suppressed the LH-induced progesterone response by 50% while markedly enhancing basal and LH-stimulated aromatase activity. Activin may also act as a growth factor in other tissues. The physiologic roles of these modulators are not fully understood.

Relaxin is another polypeptide that can be extracted from the ovary. The three-dimensional structure of relaxin is related to that of the growth-promoting polypeptides and is similar to that of insulin. Although the amino acid sequence differs from that of insulin, it consists of two chains linked by disulfide bonds, cleaved from a prohormone. It is found in the ovary, placenta, uterus, and blood. Relaxin synthesis has been demonstrated in luteinized granulosa cells of the corpus luteum. It has been shown to increase glycogen synthesis and water uptake by the myometrium and decreases uterine contractility. In some species, it changes the mechanical properties of the cervix and pubic ligaments, facilitating delivery.

In women, relaxin has been measured by immunoassay. Levels were highest immediately after the LH surge and during menstruation. A physiologic role for this hormone has not been established.

Clinical trials with relaxin have been conducted in patients with dysmenorrhea. Relaxin has also been administered to patients in premature labor and during prolonged labor. When applied to the cervix of women at term, it facilitates dilation and shortens labor.

HORMONAL CONTRACEPTION
(Oral & Implanted Contraceptives)

A large number of oral contraceptives containing estrogens or progestins (or both) are now available for clinical use (Table 39–3). These preparations vary chemically and, as might be expected, have many properties in common, but they exhibit definite differences.

Two types of preparations are used for oral contraception: (1) combinations of estrogens and progestins and (2) continuous progestin therapy without concomitant administration of estrogens. The preparations for oral use are all well absorbed, and in combination preparations, the pharmacokinetics of neither drug is significantly altered by the other.

Only one implantable contraceptive preparation is available at present. Norgestrel, also utilized as the progestin component of oral contraceptive preparations, is an effective suppressant of ovulation when it is released from subcutaneous implants.

Pharmacologic Effects

A. Mechanism of Action: The combinations of estrogens and progestins exert their contraceptive effect largely through selective inhibition of pituitary function that results in inhibition of ovulation. The combination agents also produce a change in the cervical mucus, in the uterine endometrium, and in motility and secretion in the uterine tubes, all of which decrease the likelihood of conception and implantation. The continuous use of progestins alone does not always inhibit ovulation. The other factors mentioned, therefore, play a major role in the prevention of pregnancy when these agents are used.

B. Effects on the Ovary: Chronic use of combination agents depresses ovarian function. Follicular development is minimal, and corpora lutea, larger follicles, stromal edema, and other morphologic features normally seen in ovulating women are absent. The ovaries usually become smaller even when enlarged before therapy.

The great majority of patients return to normal menstrual patterns when these drugs are discontinued. About 75% will ovulate in the first posttreatment cycle and 97% by the third posttreatment cycle. About 2% of patients remain amenorrheic for periods of up to several years after therapy has been concluded, and the prevalence of amenorrhea, often with galactorrhea, is higher in women who have used this form of contraception.

The cytologic findings on vaginal smears vary depending on the preparation used. However, with almost all of the combined drugs, a low maturation index is found because of the presence of progestational agents.

C. Effects on the Uterus: After prolonged use, the cervix may show some hypertrophy and polyp formation. There are also important effects on the cervical mucus, making it more like postovulation mucus, ie, thick and less copious.

Agents containing both estrogens and progestins produce a stromal deciduation toward the end of the cycle. The agents containing the 19-nor progestins—particularly those with the smaller amounts of estrogen—tend to produce more glandular atrophy and usually less bleeding.

D. Effects on the Breast: Stimulation of the breasts occurs in most patients receiving estrogen-containing agents. Some enlargement is generally noted. The administration of estrogens and combinations of estrogens and progestins tends to suppress lactation. When the doses are small, the effects on breast feeding are not appreciable. Preliminary studies of the transport of the oral contraceptives into the breast milk suggest that only small amounts of these compounds are found, and they have not been considered to be of importance.

E. Other Effects of Oral Contraceptives:

1. Effects on the central nervous system– The central nervous system effects of the oral contraceptives have not been well studied in humans. A variety of effects of estrogen and progesterone have been noted in animals. Estrogens tend to increase excitability in the brain, whereas progesterone tends to decrease it. The thermogenic action of progesterone and some of the synthetic progestins is also thought to be in the central nervous system.

It is very difficult to evaluate any behavioral or emotional effects of these compounds. Although the incidence of pronounced changes in mood, affect, and behavior appears to be low, milder changes are commonly reported.

2. Effects on endocrine function–The inhibition of pituitary gonadotropin secretion has been mentioned. Estrogens are known to alter adrenal structure and function. Estrogens increase the plasma concentration of the α_2-globulin that binds hydrocortisone (corticosteroid-binding globulin). This does not appear to lead to any chronic alteration in the rate of secretion of cortisol, but plasma concentrations may be more than double the levels found in untreated individuals. It has also been observed that the ACTH response to the administration of metyrapone is attenuated by estrogens and the oral contraceptives.

These preparations cause alterations in the angiotensin-aldosterone system. Plasma renin activity has

Table 39–3. Some oral and implantable contraceptive agents in use. The estrogen-containing compounds are arranged in order of increasing content of estrogen (ethinyl estradiol and mestranol have similar potencies).

	Estrogen (mg)		Progestin (mg)	
Monophasic combination tablets				
Loestrin 1/20	Ethinyl estradiol	0.02	Norethindrone acetate	1.0
Loestrin 1.5/30	Ethinyl estradiol	0.03	Norethindrone acetate	1.5
Desogen	Ethinyl estradiol	0.03	Desogestrel	0.15
Lo/Ovral	Ethinyl estradiol	0.03	DL-Norgestrel	0.3
Nordette	Ethinyl estradiol	0.03	L-Norgestrel	0.15
Brevicon, Modicon	Ethinyl estradiol	0.035	Norethindrone	0.5
Demulen 1/35	Ethinyl estradiol	0.035	Ethynodiol diacetate	1.0
Genora 1/35, Nelova 1/35 E, Norinyl 1/35, Ortho-Novum 1/35	Ethinyl estradiol	0.035	Norethindrone	1.0
Ortho-Cyclen	Ethinyl estradiol	0.035	Norgestimate	0.25
Ovcon 35	Ethinyl estradiol	0.035	Norethindrone	0.4
Demulen 1/50	Ethinyl estradiol	0.05	Ethynodiol diacetate	1.0
Norlestrin 1/50	Ethinyl estradiol	0.05	Norethindrone acetate	1.0
Norlestrin 2.5/50	Ethinyl estradiol	0.05	Norethindrone acetate	2.5
Ovcon 50	Ethinyl estradiol	0.05	Norethindrone	1.0
Ovral	Ethinyl estradiol	0.05	DL-Norgestrel	0.5
Genora 1/50, Norinyl 1/50, Ortho-Novum 1/50	Mestranol	0.05	Norethindrone	1.0
Enovid 5	Mestranol	0.075	Norethynodrel	5.0
Norinyl 1/80, Ortho-Novum 1/80	Mestranol	0.08	Norethindrone	1.0
Enovid E	Mestranol	0.1	Norethynodrel	2.5
Norinyl-2, Ortho-Novum-2	Mestranol	0.1	Norethindrone	2.0
Ovulen	Mestranol	0.1	Ethynodiol diacetate	1.0
Biphasic combination tablets				
Ortho-Novum 10/11 Days 1–10	Ethinyl estradiol	0.035	Norethindrone	0.5
Days 11–21	Ethinyl estradiol	0.035	Norethindrone	1.0
Triphasic combination tablets				
Triphasil Days 1–6	Ethinyl estradiol	0.03	L-Norgestrel	0.05
Days 7–11	Ethinyl estradiol	0.04	L-Norgestrel	0.075
Days 12–21	Ethinyl estradiol	0.03	L-Norgestrel	0.125
Ortho-Novum 7/7/7 Days 1–7	Ethinyl estradiol	0.035	Norethindrone	0.5
Days 8–14	Ethinyl estradiol	0.035	Norethindrone	0.75
Days 15–21	Ethinyl estradiol	0.035	Norethindrone	1.0
Tri-Norinyl Days 1–7	Ethinyl estradiol	0.035	Norethindrone	0.5
Days 8–16	Ethinyl estradiol	0.035	Norethindrone	1.0
Days 17–21	Ethinyl estradiol	0.035	Norethindrone	0.5
Ortho-Tri-Cyclen Days 1–7	Ethinyl estradiol	0.035	Norgestimate	0.18
Days 8–14	Ethinyl estradiol	0.035	Norgestimate	0.215
Days 15–21	Ethinyl estradiol	0.035	Norgestimate	0.25
Daily progestin tablets				
Micronor	. . .		Norethindrone	0.35
Nor-QD	. . .		Norethindrone	0.35
Ovrette	. . .		D,L-Norgestrel	0.075
Implantable progestin preparation				
Norplant	. . .		L-Norgestrel (6 tubes of 36 mg each)	

been found to increase, and there is an increase in aldosterone secretion.

Thyroxine-binding globulin is increased. As a result, plasma thyroxine (T_4) levels are increased to those commonly seen during pregnancy. Since more of the thyroxine is bound, the free thyroxine level in these patients is normal.

3. Effects on blood—Serious thromboembolic phenomena occurring in women taking oral contraceptives have given rise to a great many studies of the effects of these compounds on blood coagulation. A clear picture of such effects has not yet emerged. The oral contraceptives do not consistently alter bleeding or clotting times. The changes that have been observed are similar to those reported in pregnancy. There is an increase in factors VII, VIII, IX, and X. Increased amounts of coumarin derivatives may be required to prolong prothrombin time in patients taking oral contraceptives.

There is an increase in serum iron and total iron-binding capacity similar to that reported in patients with hepatitis.

Significant alterations in the cellular components of blood have not been reported with any consistency. A number of patients have been reported to develop folic acid deficiency anemias.

4. Effects on the liver—These hormones also have profound effects on the function of the liver. Some of these effects are deleterious and will be considered below in the section on adverse effects.

The effects on serum proteins result from the effects of the estrogens on the synthesis of the various α_2-globulins and fibrinogen. Serum haptoglobins that also arise from the liver are depressed rather than increased by estrogen.

Some of the effects on carbohydrate and lipid metabolism are probably influenced by changes in liver metabolism (see below).

Important alterations in hepatic drug excretion and metabolism also occur. Estrogens in the amounts seen during pregnancy or used in oral contraceptive agents delay the clearance of sulfobromophthalein and reduce the flow of bile. The proportion of cholic acid in bile acids is increased while the proportion of chenodeoxycholic acid is decreased. These changes may cause the observed increase in cholelithiasis associated with the use of these agents.

5. Effects on lipid metabolism—The available studies indicate that estrogens increase serum triglycerides and free and esterified cholesterol. Phospholipids are also increased, as are high-density lipoproteins. Low-density lipoproteins usually decrease. Although the effects are marked with doses of 100 μg of mestranol or ethinyl estradiol, doses of 50 μg or less have minimal effects. The progestins (particularly the 19-nortestosterone derivatives) tend to antagonize these effects of estrogen. Preparations containing small amounts of estrogen and a progestin may slightly decrease triglycerides and high-density lipoproteins.

6. Effects on carbohydrate metabolism—The administration of oral contraceptives produces alterations in carbohydrate metabolism similar to those observed in pregnancy. There is a reduction in the rate of absorption of carbohydrates from the gastrointestinal tract. Progesterone increases the basal insulin level and the rise in insulin induced by carbohydrate ingestion. Preparations with more potent progestins such as norgestrel may cause progressive decreases in carbohydrate tolerance over the years. However, the changes in glucose tolerance are reversible on discontinuing medication.

7. Effects on the cardiovascular system—These agents cause small increases in cardiac output associated with higher systolic and diastolic blood pressure and heart rate. Pathologic increases in blood pressure have been reported in a small number of patients. The pressure returns to normal when treatment is terminated. Although the magnitude of the pressure change is small in many patients, it is marked in others. It is important that blood pressure be followed in each patient. An increase in blood pressure has been reported to occur in few postmenopausal women treated with estrogens alone.

8. Effects on the skin—The oral contraceptives have been noted to increase pigmentation of the skin (chloasma). This effect seems to be enhanced in women who have dark complexions and by exposure to ultraviolet light. Some of the androgen-like progestins may increase the production of sebum, causing acne in some patients. However, since ovarian androgen is suppressed, many patients note decreased acne and terminal hair growth. The sequential oral contraceptive preparations as well as estrogens often decrease sebum production. This may be due to suppression of the ovarian production of androgens.

Clinical Uses

The most important use of combined estrogens and progestins is for oral contraception. A large number of preparations are available for this specific purpose, some of which are listed in Table 39–3. They are specially packaged for ease of administration. In general, they are very effective; when these agents are taken according to directions, the risk of conception is extremely small. The pregnancy rate with combination agents is estimated to be about 0.5–1 per 100 woman years at risk. Contraceptive failure has been observed in some patients taking phenytoin or antibiotics or when one or more doses are missed.

Progestins and estrogens are also useful in the treatment of endometriosis. When severe dysmenorrhea is the major symptom, the suppression of ovulation with estrogen may be followed by painless periods. However, in most patients this approach to therapy is inadequate. The long-term administration of large doses of progestins or combinations of progestins and estrogens prevents the periodic breakdown of the endometrial tissue and in some cases will lead to endometrial fibrosis and prevent the reactivation of implants for prolonged periods.

As is true with most hormonal preparations, many of the undesired effects are physiologic or pharmacologic effects that are objectionable only because they are not pertinent to the situation for which they are being used. Therefore, the product containing the smallest effective amounts of hormones should be selected for use.

Adverse Effects

The incidence of serious known toxicities associated with the use of these drugs is low. There are a number of reversible changes in intermediary metabolism. Minor adverse effects are frequent, but most are mild and many are transient. Continuing problems may respond to simple changes in pill formulation. Although it is not often necessary to discontinue medication for these reasons, as many as one-third of all patients started on oral contraception discontinue therapy for reasons other than a desire to become pregnant.

A. Mild Adverse Effects:

1. Nausea, mastalgia, breakthrough bleeding, and edema are related to the amount of estrogen in the preparation. These effects can often be alleviated by a shift to a preparation containing smaller amounts of estrogen or to agents containing progestins with more androgenic effects.

2. Changes in serum proteins and other effects on endocrine function (see above) must be taken into account when thyroid, adrenal, or pituitary function is being evaluated. Increases in sedimentation rate are thought to be due to increased levels of fibrinogen.

3. Headache is mild and often transient. Migraine is often made worse and has been reported to be associated with an increased frequency of cerebrovascular accidents. When this occurs or when migraine has its onset during therapy with these agents, treatment should be discontinued.

4. Withdrawal bleeding sometimes fails to occur—most often with combination preparations—and may cause confusion with regard to pregnancy. If this is disturbing to the patient, a different preparation may be tried or other methods of contraception used.

B. Moderate Adverse Effects: Any of the following may require discontinuance of oral contraceptives:

1. Breakthrough bleeding is the most common problem in using progestational agents alone for contraception. It occurs in as many as 25% of patients. It is more frequently encountered in patients taking low-dose preparations than in those taking combination pills with higher levels of progestin and estrogen. The biphasic and triphasic oral contraceptives (Table 39–3) decrease breakthrough bleeding without increasing the total hormone content.

2. Weight gain is more common with the combination agents containing androgen-like progestins. It

can usually be controlled by shifting to preparations with less progestin effect or by dieting.

3. Increased skin pigmentation may occur, especially in dark-skinned women. It tends to increase with time, the incidence being about 5% at the end of the first year and about 40% after 8 years. It is thought to be exacerbated by vitamin B deficiency. It is often reversible upon discontinuance of medication but may disappear very slowly.

4. Acne may be exacerbated by agents containing androgen-like progestins (see Table 39–2), whereas agents containing large amounts of estrogen usually cause marked improvement in acne.

5. Hirsutism may also be aggravated by the 19-nortestosterone derivatives, and combinations containing nonandrogenic progestins are preferred.

6. Ureteral dilation similar to that observed in pregnancy has been reported, and bacteriuria is more frequent.

7. Vaginal infections are more common and more difficult to treat in patients who are receiving oral contraceptives.

8. Amenorrhea–Following cessation of administration of oral contraceptives, 95% of patients with normal menstrual histories resume normal periods and all but a few resume normal cycles during the next few months. However, some patients remain amenorrheic for several years. Many of these patients also have galactorrhea. Patients who have had menstrual irregularities before taking oral contraceptives are particularly susceptible to prolonged amenorrhea when the agents are discontinued.

C. Severe Adverse Effects:

1. Vascular disorders–Thromboembolism was one of the earliest of the serious unanticipated effects to be reported and has been the most thoroughly studied.

a. Venous thromboembolic disease–Superficial or deep thromboembolic disease in women not taking oral contraceptives occurs in about one patient per 1000 woman years. The overall incidence of these disorders in patients taking low-dose oral contraceptives is about threefold higher. The risk for this disorder is increased during the first month of contraceptive use and remains constant for several years or more. The risk returns to normal within a month when use is discontinued. The risk of venous thrombosis or pulmonary embolism among women with predisposing conditions may be higher than that in normal women.

The incidence of this complication is related to the estrogen but not the progestin content of oral contraceptives and is not related to age, parity, mild obesity, or cigarette smoking. Decreased venous blood flow, endothelial proliferation in veins and arteries, and increased coagulability of blood resulting from changes in platelet coagulation and fibrinolytic systems contribute to the increased incidence of thrombosis. The major plasma inhibitor of thrombin, antithrombin III, is substantially decreased during oral contraceptive use. This change occurs in the first month of treatment and lasts as long as treatment persists, reversing within a month thereafter.

b. Myocardial infarction–The use of oral contraceptives is associated with a slightly higher risk of myocardial infarction in women who are obese, have a history of preeclampsia or hypertension, or have hyperlipoproteinemia or diabetes. There is a much higher risk in women who smoke. The risk attributable to oral contraceptives in women 30–39 years of age who do not smoke is about 4 cases per 100,000 users per year, as compared to 185 cases per 100,000 among women 40–44 who smoke heavily. The association with myocardial infarction is thought to involve acceleration of atherogenesis because of decreased glucose tolerance, decreased levels of HDLs, increased levels of LDLs, and increased platelet aggregation. However, facilitation of coronary arterial spasm may also play a role in some of these patients. The progestational component of oral contraceptives decreases HDL cholesterol levels, in proportion to the androgenic activity of the progestin. The net effect, therefore, will depend on the specific composition of the pill used and the patient's susceptibility to the particular effects. Recent studies suggest that risk of infarction is not increased in past users who have discontinued oral contraceptives.

c. Cerebrovascular disease–The risk of strokes is concentrated in women over age 35. It is increased in current users of oral contraceptives but not in past users. However, subarachnoid hemorrhages have been found to be increased among both current and past users and may increase with time. The risk of thrombotic or hemorrhagic stroke attributable to oral contraceptives (based on older, higher-dose preparations) has been estimated to about 37 cases per 100,000 users per year. Ten percent of these strokes were fatal, and most of the fatal ones were due to subarachnoid hemorrhage. Insufficient data are available on which to base an assessment of the effects of smoking and other risk factors.

Elevations in blood pressure may also increase the risk, since there is a three- to sixfold increase in the incidence of overt hypertension in women taking oral contraceptives.

In summary, available data indicate that oral contraceptives increase the risk of various cardiovascular disorders at all ages and among both smokers and nonsmokers. However, this risk appears to be concentrated in women 35 years of age or older who are heavy smokers. It is clear that these risk factors must be considered in each individual patient for whom oral contraceptives are considered.

2. Gastrointestinal disorders–Many cases of cholestatic jaundice have been reported in patients taking progestin-containing drugs. The differences in incidence of these disorders from one population to another suggest that genetic factors may be involved. The jaundice caused by these agents is similar to that produced by other 17-alkyl-substituted steroids. It is most often observed in the first three cycles and is particularly common in women with a history of cholestatic jaundice during pregnancy. Jaundice and pruritus disappear 1–8 weeks after the drug is discontinued.

These agents have also been found to increase the incidence of symptomatic gallbladder disease, including cholecystitis and cholangitis. This is probably the result of the alterations responsible for jaundice described above.

It also appears that the incidence of hepatic adenomas is increased in women taking oral contraceptives. Ischemic bowel disease secondary to thrombosis of the celiac and superior and inferior mesenteric arteries and veins has also been reported in women using these drugs.

3. Depression–Depression of sufficient degree to require cessation of therapy occurs in about 6% of patients treated with some preparations.

4. Cancer–The occurrence of malignant tumors in patients taking oral contraceptives has been studied extensively. It is now clear that these compounds *reduce* the risk of endometrial and ovarian cancer. The lifetime risk of breast cancer in the population as a whole does not seem to be affected by oral contraceptive use. Some studies have shown an increased risk in younger women, and it is possible that tumors that develop in younger women become clinically apparent sooner. The relationship of risk of cervical cancer to oral contraceptive use is still controversial.

In addition to the above effects, a number of other adverse reactions have been reported for which a causal relationship has not been established. These include alopecia, erythema multiforme, erythema nodosum, and other skin disorders.

Contraindications & Cautions

These drugs are contraindicated in patients with thrombophlebitis, thromboembolic phenomena, and cerebrovascular disorders or a past history of these conditions. They should not be used to treat vaginal bleeding when the cause is unknown. They should be avoided in patients with known or suspected tumor of the breast or other estrogen-dependent neoplasm. Since these preparations have caused aggravation of preexisting disorders, they should be avoided or used with caution in patients with liver disease, asthma, eczema, migraine, diabetes, hypertension, optic neuritis, retrobulbar neuritis, or convulsive disorders.

The oral contraceptives may produce edema, and for that reason they should be used with great caution in patients in congestive failure or in whom edema is otherwise undesirable or dangerous.

Estrogens may increase the rate of growth of fibroids. Therefore, for women with these tumors, agents with the smallest amounts of estrogen and the most androgenic progestins should be selected. The use of progestational agents alone for contraception might be especially useful in such patients (see below).

These agents are contraindicated in adolescents in whom epiphysial closure has not yet been completed.

Women using oral contraceptives must be made aware of an important interaction that occurs with antimicrobial drugs. Because the normal gastrointestinal flora *increases* the enterohepatic cycling of estrogens, antimicrobial drugs that interfere with these organisms may reduce the efficacy of oral contraceptives.

Contraception With Progestins Alone

Small doses of progestins administered orally or by implantation under the skin can be used for contraception. They are particularly suited for use in patients for whom estrogen administration is undesirable. They are about as effective as intrauterine devices or combination pills containing 20–30 μg of ethinyl estradiol. There is a high incidence of abnormal bleeding. Effective contraception can also be achieved by injecting 150 mg of depot medroxyprogesterone acetate monthly. The use of large doses of oral progestins at the time of intercourse is under study.

Hormonal contraception by progestin implants under the skin is available in the USA. This method utilizes the subcutaneous implantation of capsules containing a progestin (L-norgestrel). These capsules release one-fifth to one-third as much steroid as oral agents, are extremely effective, and last for 5–6 years. The low levels of hormone have little effect on lipoprotein and carbohydrate metabolism or blood pressure. The disadvantages include the need for surgical insertion and removal of capsules and some irregular bleeding rather than predictable menses.

Postcoital Contraceptives

Pregnancy can be prevented following coitus by the administration of estrogens alone or in combination with progestins ("morning after" contraception). When treatment is begun within 72 hours, it is effective 99% of the time. Some effective schedules are shown in Table 39–4. The hormones are often administered with antiemetics, since 40% of the patients have nausea or vomiting. Other adverse effects include headache, dizziness, breast tenderness, and abdominal and leg cramps.

Mifepristone (RU 486), an antagonist at progesterone (and glucocorticoid) receptors, has been shown to have a luteolytic effect and may be useful as a postcoital contraceptive (see below).

Beneficial Effects of Oral Contraceptives

It has become apparent during the last decade that reduction in the dose of the constituents of oral contraceptives has markedly reduced mild and severe adverse effects, providing a relatively safe and convenient method of contraception for many young women. Treatment with oral contraceptives has now been shown to be associated with many benefits unrelated to contraception. These include a reduced risk of ovarian cysts, ovarian and endometrial cancer, and benign breast disease. There is a lower incidence of pelvic inflammatory disease and ectopic pregnancy. Iron deficiency, duodenal ulcer, and rheumatoid arthritis are less common, and premenstrual symptoms, dysmenorrhea, and endometriosis are ameliorated with their use.

ESTROGEN & PROGESTERONE INHIBITORS & ANTAGONISTS

TAMOXIFEN

Tamoxifen is a competitive partial agonist inhibitor of estradiol at the receptor and is extensively used in the palliative treatment of advanced breast cancer in postmenopausal women. It is a nonsteroidal agent (see structure below) that is given orally. Peak plasma levels are reached in a few hours. Tamoxifen has an initial half-life of 7–14 hours in the circulation and is predominantly excreted by the liver. It is used in doses of 10–20 mg twice daily. Hot flushes and nausea and vomiting occur in 25% of patients, and many other minor adverse effects are observed. Studies of patients treated with tamoxifen as adjuvant therapy for early breast cancer have shown a 35% decrease in contralateral breast cancer. Prevention of the expected loss of lumbar spine bone density and plasma lipid changes consistent with a reduction in the risk for atherosclerosis have also been reported in these patients following spontaneous or surgical menopause.

CLOMIPHENE

Clomiphene citrate is a partial agonist, a weak estrogen that also acts as a competitive inhibitor of endogenous estrogens. It has found use as an ovulation-inducing agent (see below).

Table 39–4. Schedules for use of postcoital contraceptives.

Conjugated estrogens: 10 mg 3 times daily for 5 days
Ethinyl estradiol: 2.5 mg twice daily for 5 days
Diethylstilbestrol: 50 mg daily for 5 days
Norgestrel, 0.5 mg, with ethinyl estradiol, 0.05 mg (eg, Ovral): 2 tablets and 2 in 12 hours

MIFEPRISTONE

Mifepristone (RU 486) is a 19-norsteroid that binds strongly to the progesterone receptor and inhibits the activity of progesterone. Preliminary studies indicate that it has luteolytic properties in 80% of women when given in the midluteal period. The mechanism of this effect is unknown, but it may provide the basis for using mifepristone as a contraceptive (as opposed to an abortifacient). However, the compound has a long half-life; large doses of mifepristone may prolong the follicular phase of the subsequent cycle and so make it difficult to use continuously for this purpose. However, a single dose of 600 mg is an effective emergency postcoital contraceptive, though it may result in a delay in the following cycle. The drug also binds to the glucocorticoid receptor. Limited clinical studies suggest that mifepristone may be useful in the treatment of endometriosis, Cushing's syndrome, breast cancer, and other neoplasms that contain glucocorticoid or progesterone receptors.

Mifepristone's major use thus far has been to terminate early pregnancies. Doses of 400–600 mg/d for 4 days or 800 mg/d for 2 days successfully terminated pregnancy in 85% of the women studied. The major adverse effect was prolonged bleeding that did not require treatment. The combination of a single oral dose of 600 mg of mifepristone and a vaginal pessary containing 1 mg of prostaglandin E_1 or oral misoprostol has been found to effectively terminate pregnancy in 95% of patients treated during the first 7 weeks after conception. The adverse effects of the medications included vomiting, diarrhea, and pain. As many as 5% of patients have vaginal bleeding requiring intervention.

DANAZOL

Danazol, an isoxazole derivative of ethisterone (17α-ethinyl testosterone) with weak progestational and androgenic activities, is used to suppress ovarian function. Danazol inhibits the midcycle surge of LH and FSH and can prevent the compensatory increase in LH and FSH following castration in animals, but it does not significantly lower or suppress basal LH or FSH levels in normal women. Danazol binds to androgen, progesterone, and glucocorticoid receptors and can translocate the androgen receptor into the nucleus to initiate androgen-specific RNA synthesis. It does not bind to intracellular estrogen receptors, but it does bind to sex hormone-binding globulin (SHBG) and corticosteroid-binding globulins (CBG). It inhibits P450scc (the cholesterol side chain-cleaving enzyme), 3β-HSD (3-β-hydroxysteroid dehydrogenase), 17β-HSD (17-α-hydroxysteroid dehydrogenase), 17,21-lyase, P450c17 (17α-hydroxylase), P450c11 (11β-hydroxylase), and P450c21 (21-hydroxylase), but it does not inhibit aromatase. It increases the mean clearance rate of progesterone, probably by competing with the hormone for binding proteins, and may have similar effects on other active steroid hormones. Ethisterone, a major metabolite, has both progestational and mild androgenic effects.

Danazol is slowly metabolized in humans, having a half-life of over 15 hours. This results in stable circulating levels when the drug is administered twice daily. It has been found to be highly concentrated in the liver, adrenals, and kidneys and is excreted in both feces and urine.

Danazol has been employed as an inhibitor of gonadal function and has found its major use in the treatment of endometriosis. For this purpose, it can be given in a dosage of 600 mg/d. The dosage is reduced to 400 mg/d after 1 month and to 200 mg/d in 2 months. About 85% of patients show marked improvement in 3–12 months.

Danazol has also been used for the treatment of fibrocystic disease of the breast and hematologic disorders, including hemophilia, Christmas disease, and idiopathic thrombocytopenic purpura.

The major adverse effects are weight gain, edema, decreased breast size, acne and oily skin, increased hair growth, deepening of the voice, headache, hot flushes, changes in libido, and muscle cramps. Although mild adverse effects are very common, it is

Tamoxifen

Mifepristone

seldom necessary to discontinue the drug because of them.

Danazol should be used with great caution in patients with hepatic dysfunction, since it has been reported to produce mild to moderate hepatocellular damage in some patients, as evidenced by enzyme changes. It is also contraindicated during pregnancy and breast feeding, as it may produce urogenital abnormalities in the offspring.

GONADOTROPIN-RELEASING HORMONE (GnRH) ANALOGUES

As noted below, GnRH administered in pulses will stimulate ovarian function and induce ovulation in women with amenorrhea. However, continuous administration suppresses ovarian function by downregulation of the receptor and desensitization. The development of potent polypeptide analogues such as nafarelin and buserelin has made it possible to produce ovarian suppression by daily subcutaneous or intranasal administration of these agents. The marked suppression produced by large doses has found use in the treatment of precocious puberty and gonadal hormone-dependent tumors. Smaller doses have been found to be effective in the treatment of endometriosis.

Recently, GnRH *antagonists* with minimal histamine-releasing properties have been developed and show promise in preliminary studies. They have the advantage of rapidly suppressing gonadal function without the early period of stimulation caused by the GnRH agonist analogues and a potential for use as male contraceptives.

OVULATION-INDUCING AGENTS

CLOMIPHENE

Clomiphene citrate, a partial estrogen agonist, is closely related to the estrogen chlorotrianisene (Figure 39–3). This compound is active when taken orally, since it is readily absorbed. Very little is known about its metabolism, but about half of the compound is excreted in the feces within 5 days after administration. It has been suggested that clomiphene is slowly excreted from an enterohepatic pool.

Pharmacologic Effects

A. Mechanisms of Action: Clomiphene is a partial agonist at estrogen receptors. The estrogenic effects are best demonstrated in animals with marked gonadal deficiency. Clomiphene has also been shown to effectively inhibit the action of stronger estrogens. In humans it leads to an increase in the secretion of gonadotropins and estrogens.

B. Effects: The pharmacologic importance of this compound rests on its ability to stimulate ovulation in women with amenorrhea and other ovulatory disorders. The mechanism by which ovulation is produced is not known. It has been suggested that it blocks an inhibitory influence of estrogens on the hypothalamus and increases the production of gonadotropins.

Clinical Uses

Clomiphene is used for the treatment of disorders of ovulation in patients wishing to become pregnant. In general, a single ovulation is induced by a single course of therapy, and the patient must be treated repeatedly until pregnancy is achieved, since normal ovulatory function does not usually resume. The compound is of no use in patients with ovarian or pituitary failure.

When clomiphene is administered in doses of 100 mg daily for 5 days, a rise in plasma LH and FSH is observed after several days. In patients who ovulate, the initial rise is followed by a second rise of gonadotropin levels just prior to ovulation.

Adverse Effects

The most common adverse effects in patients treated with this drug are hot flushes, which resemble those experienced by menopausal patients. They tend to be mild, and disappear when the drug is discontinued. There have been occasional reports of eye symptoms due to intensification and prolongation of afterimages. These are generally of short duration. Headache, constipation, allergic skin reactions, and reversible hair loss have been reported occasionally.

The effective use of clomiphene is associated with some stimulation of the ovaries and usually with ovarian enlargement. The degree of enlargement tends to be greater and its incidence higher in patients who have enlarged ovaries at the beginning of therapy.

A variety of other symptoms such as nausea and vomiting, increased nervous tension, depression, fatigue, breast soreness, weight gain, urinary frequency, and heavy menses have also been reported. However, these appear to result from the hormonal changes associated with an ovulatory menstrual cycle rather than from the medication. The incidence of multiple pregnancy is approximately 10%. Clomiphene has not been shown to have an adverse effect when inadvertently given to women who are already pregnant.

Contraindications & Cautions

Special precautions should be observed in patients with enlarged ovaries. These women are thought to be more sensitive to this drug and should receive small doses. Any patient who complains of abdominal symptoms should be examined carefully. Maximum ovarian enlargement occurs after the 5-day course has been completed, and many patients can be shown to have a palpable increase in ovarian size by the seventh to tenth days.

Special precautions must also be taken in patients who have visual symptoms associated with clomiphene therapy, since these symptoms may make activities such as driving more hazardous.

Dosages

The recommended dosage of clomiphene citrate at the beginning of therapy is 50 mg/d for 5 days. If ovulation occurs, this same course may be repeated until pregnancy is achieved. If ovulation does not occur, the dosage is doubled to 100 mg/d for 5 days. If ovulation and menses occur, the next course can be started on the fifth day of the cycle. Experience to date suggests that patients who do not ovulate after three courses of 100 mg/d of clomiphene are not likely to respond to continued therapy. However, larger doses are effective in some individuals. Clomiphene is sometimes used in combination with menotropins.

About 80% of patients with anovulatory disorders or amenorrhea can be expected to respond by having ovulatory cycles. Approximately half of these patients will become pregnant.

BROMOCRIPTINE

In some amenorrheic women, an elevated level of prolactin appears to be the causative factor. These patients may have prolactin-secreting tumors or "empty sella" syndrome, which should be excluded before treatment is begun. The criteria for selecting medical, surgical, and radiation therapy for prolactinomas have not been firmly established.

Bromocriptine, an ergot derivative (Chapter 16), binds to dopamine receptors in the pituitary and inhibits prolactin secretion. In 90% or more of patients, treatment leads to the onset of menses in 3–5 weeks. The usual dose required is 2.5 mg 2 or 3 times a day. Prolactin levels should be depressed to normal if treatment is adequate. Some patients with polycystic ovary syndrome may also respond.

HUMAN MENOPAUSAL GONADOTROPIN (hMG, Menotropins)

Human menopausal gonadotropin—in conjunction with **human chorionic gonadotropin (hCG);**—is used to stimulate ovulation in patients who do not ovulate but have potentially functional ovarian tissue. It has been successful in the induction of ovulation in patients with hypopituitarism and other defects in gonadotropin secretion. It is also used in patients with amenorrhea or anovulatory cycles and in patients in whom ovulatory disturbances are associated with galactorrhea or hirsutism. In addition, it is used to prepare infertile patients for in vitro fertilization.

Preparations of human menopausal gonadotropin can stimulate spermatogenesis in males with isolated gonadotropin deficiency. Using hMG in conjunction with hCG (see Chapter 36), endocrine and gametogenic function can be restored in some of these patients.

GONADOTROPIN-RELEASING HORMONE (GnRH)

The pulsatile administration of GnRH is an effective means of inducing ovulation in patients with hypothalamic amenorrhea. It is cumbersome in that it requires the use of a pump that delivers a pulse of 1–10 µg of this hypothalamic hormone every 60–120 minutes. It has the advantage of maintaining the normal processes for the control of follicular development, thus avoiding the complications seen with menotropins and resulting in fewer multiple pregnancies.

II. THE TESTIS (Androgens & Anabolic Steroids, Antiandrogens, & Male Contraception)

The testis, like the ovary, has both gametogenic and endocrine functions. The gametogenic function of the testes is controlled largely by the secretion of FSH by the pituitary. High concentrations of androgens locally are also required for sperm production in the seminiferous tubules. The Sertoli cells in the seminiferous tubules may be the source of the estradiol produced in the testes. The androgens are produced in the interstitial or Leydig cells found in the spaces between the seminiferous tubules.

The Sertoli cells in the testis synthesize and secrete a variety of active proteins, including müllerian duct inhibitory factor, inhibin, and activin. As in the ovarian peptides, inhibin and activin appear to be the product of three genes that produce a common alpha subunit and two beta subunits, A and B. Activin is composed of the two beta subunits ($\beta_A\beta_B$). There are two inhibins (A and B), which contain the alpha subunit and one of the beta subunits. Activin stimulates pituitary FSH release and is structurally similar to transforming growth factor-β, which also increases FSH. The inhibins in conjunction with dihydrotestosterone are responsible for the feedback inhibition of pituitary FSH secretion.

ANDROGENS & ANABOLIC STEROIDS

In humans, the most important androgen secreted by the testis is testosterone. The pathways of synthesis of testosterone in the testes are similar to those previously described for the adrenal and ovary (Figures 38–1 and 39–2).

In the male, approximately 8 mg of testosterone is produced daily. About 95% is produced by the Leydig cells and only 5% by the adrenal. The testis also secretes small amounts of another potent androgen, dihydrotestosterone, as well as androstenedione and dehydroepiandrosterone, which are weak androgens. Pregnenolone and progesterone and their 17-hydroxylated derivatives are also released in small amounts. Plasma levels of testosterone in males are about 0.6 µg/dL after puberty and do not appear to vary significantly with age. Testosterone is also present in the plasma of women in concentrations of approximately 0.03 µg/dL and is derived in approximately equal parts from the ovaries, the adrenals, and by the peripheral conversion of other hormones.

About 65% of circulating testosterone is bound to sex hormone-binding globulin (SHBG), a specific protein produced by the liver. This protein is increased in plasma by estrogen, by thyroid hormone, and in patients with cirrhosis of the liver. It is decreased by androgen and growth hormone and is lower in obese individuals. Most of the remaining testosterone is bound to albumin. However, approximately 2% remains free and available to enter cells and bind to intracellular receptors.

Metabolism

In many target tissues, testosterone is converted to dihydrotestosterone by the enzyme 5α-reductase. In these tissues, dihydrotestosterone is the major androgen. The conversion of testosterone to estradiol also occurs in some tissues, including the hypothalamus, and may be of importance in regulating gonadal function.

The major pathway for the degradation of testosterone in humans is illustrated in Figure 39–4. In the liver, the reduction of the double bond and ketone in the A ring, as is seen in other steroids with a Δ^4-ketone configuration in the A ring, leads to the production of inactive substances such as androsterone and etiocholanolone that are then conjugated and excreted into the urine.

Androstenedione, dehydroepiandrosterone (DHEA), and dehydroepiandrosterone sulfate (DHEAS) are also produced in significant amounts in humans, though largely in the adrenal rather than in the testes. Although they are thought to contribute to the normal maturation process (adrenarche), they do not stimulate or support other androgen-dependent pubertal changes in the human. Recent studies suggest that DHEA and DHEAS may have other important metabolic effects that inhibit atherosclerosis and prolong life in rabbits and possibly in men. The therapeutic use of these hormones is currently being explored. They are to a large extent metabolized in the same fashion as testosterone. Both steroids—but particularly androstenedione—can be converted by peripheral tissues to estrone in very small amounts (1–5%). The P450 aromatase enzyme responsible for this conversion is also found in the brain and is thought to play an important role in development.

Physiologic Effects

In the normal male, testosterone is responsible for the many changes that occur in puberty. In addition to the general growth-promoting properties of androgens on the body tissues, these hormones are responsible for penile and scrotal growth. Changes in the skin include the appearance of pubic, axillary, and beard hair. The sebaceous glands become more active, and the skin tends to become thicker and oilier. The larynx grows and the vocal cords become thicker, leading to a lower-pitched voice. Skeletal growth is stimulated and epiphysial closure accelerated. Other effects include growth of the prostate and seminal vesicles, darkening of the skin, and increased skin circulation. Psychologic and behavioral changes also occur.

Synthetic Steroids With Androgenic & Anabolic Action

Testosterone, when administered by mouth, is rapidly absorbed. However, it is largely converted to inactive metabolites, and only about one-sixth of the dose administered is available in active form. Testosterone can be administered parenterally, but it has a more prolonged absorption time and greater activity when esterified. Methyltestosterone and fluoxymesterone are active when given by mouth.

Testosterone and its derivatives have been used for their anabolic effects as well as for the replacement of testosterone deficiency. Although testosterone and other known active steroids can be isolated in pure form and measured by weight, biologic assays are still used in the investigation of new compounds. In some of these studies in animals, the anabolic effects of the compound as measured by trophic effects on muscles or the reduction of nitrogen excretion may be dissociated from the other androgenic effects. This has led to the marketing of compounds claimed to have anabolic activity associated with only weak androgenic effects. Unfortunately, this dissociation is less marked in humans than in the animals used for testing (Table 39–5), and all are potent androgens.

Pharmacologic Effects

A. Mechanisms of Action: Like other steroids, testosterone acts intracellularly in target cells. In skin, prostate, seminal vesicles, and epididymis, it is converted to 5α-dihydrotestosterone by the enzyme 5α-reductase. In these tissues, dihydrotestosterone is the dominant androgen. The distribution of this enzyme in the fetus is different and has important developmental implications.

Testosterone and dihydrotestosterone bind to the cytosol androgen receptor, initiating a series of events leading to growth, differentiation, and synthesis of a variety of enzymes and other functional proteins.

B. Effects: In the male at puberty, androgens cause development of the secondary sex characteristics (see above). In the adult male, large doses of testosterone—when given alone—or its derivatives suppress the secretion of gonadotropins and result in some atrophy of the interstitial tissue and the tubules of the testes. Since fairly large doses of androgens are required to suppress gonadotropic secretion, it has been postulated that inhibin, in combination with androgens, is responsible for the feedback control of secretion. In women, androgens are capable of producing changes similar to those observed in the prepubertal male. These include growth of facial and body hair, deepening of the voice, enlargement of the clitoris, frontal baldness, and prominent musculature. The natural androgens stimulate erythrocyte production.

The administration of androgens reduces the excretion of nitrogen into the urine, indicating an increase in protein synthesis or a decrease in protein breakdown within the body. This effect is much more pronounced in women and children than in normal men.

Clinical Uses

A. Androgen Replacement Therapy in Men: Androgens are used to replace or augment endogenous androgen secretion in hypogonadal men (Table 39–6). Even in the presence of pituitary deficiency, androgens are used rather than gonadotropin except when normal spermatogenesis is to be achieved. When androgen deficiency occurs prior to completion of sexual maturation, large doses of androgens are required, and orally administered androgens are not sufficiently efficacious. In these patients, therapy should be started with long-acting agents such as testosterone enanthate or cypionate in doses of 200 mg intramuscularly every 1–2 weeks until maturation is complete. The dose can then be reduced to 200 mg at 2- to 3-week intervals. Testosterone propionate, though potent, has a short duration of action and is not practical for long-term use. The development of polycythemia or hypertension may require some reduction in dose.

In patients with hypopituitarism, androgens are not added to the treatment regimen until puberty, at which time they are instituted in gradually increasing doses to achieve the growth spurt and the development of secondary sex characteristics.

B. Gynecologic Disorders: Androgens are

Table 39–5. Androgens: Preparations available and relative androgenic/anabolic activity in animals

	Androgenic/ Anabolic Activity
Testosterone	1:1
Testosterone cypionate	1:1
Testosterone enanthate	1:1
Testosterone propionate	1:1
Methyltestosterone	1:1
Fluoxymesterone	1:2
Methandrostenolone (metandienone)	1:3
Oxymetholone	1:3
Ethylestrenol	1:4–1:8
Oxandrolone	1:3–1:13
Nandrolone phenpropionate	1:3–1:6
Nandrolone decanoate	1:2.5–1:4
Stanozolol	1:3–1:6
Dromostanolone propionate	1:3–1:4

Table 39–6. Androgen preparations for replacement therapy.

	Route of Administration	Dosage
Methyltestosterone	Oral	25–50 mg/d
	Sublingual (buccal)	5–10 mg/d
Fluoxymesterone	Oral	2–10 mg/d
Testosterone propionate	Sublingual (buccal)	5–20 mg/d
	Intramuscular	10–50 mg 3 times weekly
Testosterone enanthate	Intramuscular	200 mg every 1–2 weeks until maturation is complete, then every 2–3 weeks for maintenance.
Testosterone cypionate	Intramuscular	

used occasionally in the treatment of certain gynecologic disorders, but the undesirable effects in women are such that they must be used with great caution. Androgens have been used to reduce breast engorgement during the postpartum period, usually in conjunction with estrogens.

Androgens are sometimes given in combination with estrogens for replacement therapy in the postmenopausal period in an attempt to eliminate the endometrial bleeding that may occur when only estrogens are used. They are also used for chemotherapy of breast tumors in premenopausal women.

C. Use as Protein Anabolic Agents: Androgens and anabolic steroids have been used in conjunction with dietary measures and exercises in an attempt to reverse protein loss after trauma, surgery, or prolonged immobilization and in patients with debilitating diseases.

D. Anemia: Large doses of androgens have been employed in the treatment of refractory anemias and have resulted in some increase in reticulocytosis and hemoglobin levels. The large amounts required prevent this from being a useful method of therapy in women. It is expected that the availability of hematopoietic colony-stimulating factors will completely eliminate this application of androgens (see Chapter 32).

E. Osteoporosis: Androgens and anabolic agents have been used in the treatment of osteoporosis, either alone or in conjunction with estrogens.

F. Use as Growth Stimulators: These agents have been used to stimulate growth in prepubertal boys. If the drugs are used carefully, these children will probably achieve their expected adult height (and sooner than normal). If treatment is too vigorous, the patient may grow rapidly at first but will not achieve full stature because of the accelerated epiphysial closure that occurs. It is difficult to control this type of therapy adequately even with frequent x-ray examination of the epiphyses, since the action of the hormones on epiphysial centers may continue for many months after therapy is discontinued.

G. Anabolic Steroid and Androgen Abuse in Sports: The use of anabolic steroids by athletes has received worldwide attention. Many athletes and their coaches believe that anabolic steroids—in doses 10–200 times larger than normal—increase strength and aggressiveness, thereby improving competitive performance. Although such effects have been demonstrated in women, many studies have failed to unequivocally demonstrate them in men. Placebo effects and the potential impact of minimal changes in championship competitions make evaluation of these studies very difficult. However, the adverse effects of these drugs clearly make their use inadvisable.

Adverse Effects

The adverse effects of these compounds are due largely to their masculinizing actions and are most noticeable in women and prepubertal children. In women, the administration of more than 200–300 mg of testosterone per month is usually associated with hirsutism, acne, depression of menses, clitoral enlargement, and deepening of the voice. These effects may occur with even smaller doses in some women. Some of the androgenic steroids exert progestational activity leading to endometrial bleeding. These hormones also alter serum lipids and could conceivably increase susceptibility to atherosclerotic disease in women. Except under the most unusual circumstances, androgen should not be used in infants. Recent studies in animals suggest that administration of androgens in early life may have profound effects on maturation of central nervous system centers governing sexual development, particularly in the female. Administration of these drugs to pregnant females may lead to masculinization of the external genitalia in the infant. Although the above-mentioned effects may be less marked with the anabolic agents, they do occur.

Sodium retention and edema are not common but must be carefully watched for in patients with heart and kidney disease.

Most of the synthetic androgens and anabolic agents are 17-alkyl-substituted steroids. Administration of drugs with this structure is often associated with evidence of hepatic dysfunction, eg, increase in sulfobromophthalein retention and aspartate aminotransferase (AST) (SGOT) levels. Alkaline phosphatase values are also elevated. These changes usually occur early in the course of treatment, and the degree is proportionate to the dose. Bilirubin levels occasionally increase until clinical jaundice is apparent. The cholestatic jaundice is reversible upon cessation of therapy, and permanent changes do not occur. In older males, prostatic hyperplasia may develop, causing urinary obstruction.

Contraindications & Cautions

The use of androgenic steroids is contraindicated in pregnant women or women who may become pregnant during the course of therapy.

Androgens should not be administered to male patients with carcinoma of the prostate or breast. Until more is known about the effects of these hormones on the central nervous system in developing children, they should be avoided in infants and young children.

Special caution is required in giving these drugs to children to produce a growth spurt.

Care should be exercised in the administration of these drugs to patients with renal or cardiac disease predisposed to edema. If sodium and water retention occurs, it will respond to diuretic therapy.

Methyltestosterone therapy is associated with creatinuria, but the significance of this finding is not known.

Caution: Several cases of hepatocellular carcinoma have been reported in patients with aplastic anemia treated with androgen anabolic therapy.

ANDROGEN SUPPRESSION & ANTIANDROGENS

ANDROGEN SUPPRESSION

The treatment of advanced prostatic carcinoma often requires orchiectomy or large doses of estrogens to reduce available androgen. The psychologic effects of the former and gynecomastia produced by the latter make these approaches undesirable. As noted above, the gonadotropin-releasing hormone analogues such as goserelin, nafarelin, buserelin, and leuprolide acetate produce gonadal suppression when blood levels are continuous rather than pulsatile (see Chapter 36 and Figure 39–5). **Leuprolide acetate** is injected subcutaneously daily in doses of 1 mg for the treatment of prostatic carcinoma. Goserelin is administered once every 4 weeks as a subcutaneous slow-release injection. Although testosterone levels fall to 10% of their initial values after a month with either of these drugs, they increase significantly in the beginning. This increase is usually associated with a flare of tumor activity and an increase in symptoms. Recent studies suggest that the combination of a GnRH agonist and flutamide can prevent the initial stimulation and provide a more effective inhibition of androgenic activity.

GnRH antagonists have also been under study, since they would have the advantage of eliminating the surge of androgen secretion seen at the beginning of GnRH analogue therapy. Most of the compounds studied have the capacity to release histamine and are unsuitable for use. However, newer agents with less histamine releasing activity are being studied.

ANTIANDROGENS

The potential usefulness of antiandrogens for the treatment of patients producing excessive amounts of testosterone has led to the search for effective drugs that can be used for this purpose. Several approaches to the problem, especially inhibition of synthesis and receptor antagonism, have met with some success.

Steroid Synthesis

Ketoconazole, used primarily for the treatment of fungal disease, is an inhibitor of adrenal and gonadal steroid synthesis. This compound inhibits P450scc (cholesterol side chain cleavage enzyme), P450c17 (17α-hydroxylase and C17,20-lyase), 3β-hydroxysteroid dehydrogenase, and P450c11 (11β-hydroxylase) enzymes. The sensitivity of the P450 enzymes to this compound in mammalian tissues is much lower than the sensitivity of fungal enzymes, so that the inhibitory effects are seen only at high doses. Ke-

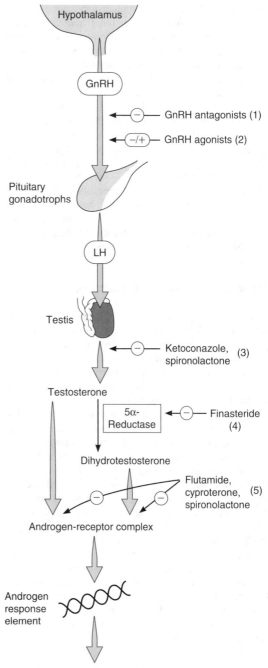

Figure 39–5. Control of androgen secretion and activity and some sites of action of antiandrogens. **(1)**, competitive inhibition of GnRH receptors; **(2)**, stimulation (+, pulsatile administration) or inhibition via desensitization of GnRH receptors (–, continuous administration); **(3)**, decreased synthesis of testosterone in the testis; **(4)**, decreased synthesis of dihydrotestosterone by inhibition of 5α-reductase; **(5)**, competition for binding to cytosol androgen receptors.

toconazole also has other endocrine effects. It does not affect ovarian aromatase, but it reduces human placental aromatase activity. It displaces estradiol and dihydrotestosterone from sex hormone-binding protein in vitro and increases the estradiol:testosterone ratio in plasma in vivo by a different mechanism. The latter effect may be responsible for the gynecomastia seen with ketoconazole therapy. This compound has been used with some success for the treatment of patients with Cushing's syndrome. However, it does not appear to be clinically useful in women with increased androgens because of the toxicity associated with prolonged use of the 400–800 mg/d required. The drug has also been used experimentally to treat prostatic carcinoma, but the results have not been encouraging. Men treated with ketoconazole often develop reversible gynecomastia during therapy; this may be due to the demonstrated increase in the estradiol:testosterone ratio.

Conversion of Steroid Precursors to Androgens

Several compounds have been developed that inhibit the 17-hydroxylation of progesterone or pregnenolone, thereby preventing the action of the side chain-splitting enzyme and the further transformation of these steroid precursors to active androgens. A few of these compounds have been tested clinically but have been too toxic for prolonged use.

Since dihydrotestosterone—not testosterone—appears to be the essential androgen in the prostate, androgen effects in this and similar dihydrotestosterone-dependent tissues can be reduced by an inhibitor of 5α-reductase (Figure 39–5). **Finasteride,** a steroid-like inhibitor of this enzyme, is orally active and produces a reduction in dihydrotestosterone levels within 8 hours after administration that lasts for about 24 hours. The half-life is about 8 hours (longer in elderly individuals). Forty to 50 percent of the dose is metabolized; more than half is excreted in the feces. It has been reported to be moderately effective in reducing prostate size in men with benign prostatic hypertrophy and is approved for this use in the USA. The dosage is 5 mg/d. Its use in advanced prostatic carcinoma is under study. The drug is not approved for use in women or children.

Receptor Inhibitors

Cyproterone and **cyproterone acetate** are effective antiandrogens that inhibit the action of androgens at the target organ. The acetate form has a marked progestational effect that suppresses the feedback enhancement of LH and FSH, leading to a more effective antiandrogen effect. These compounds have been used in women for the treatment of hirsutism and in men to decrease excessive sexual drive and are being studied in other conditions in which the reduction of androgenic effects would be useful. Cyproterone acetate in a dosage of 2 mg/d administered concurrently with an estrogen is used in the treatment of hirsutism in women; it has orphan drug status in the USA.

Flutamide, a substituted anilide, is a potent antiandrogen that has been used in the treatment of prostatic carcinoma. Though not a steroid, it behaves like a competitive antagonist at the androgen receptor. It is rapidly metabolized in humans. It frequently causes mild gynecomastia (probably by increasing testicular estrogen production) and occasionally causes mild reversible hepatic toxicity. Administration of this compound causes some improvement in most patients who have not had prior endocrine therapy.

Flutamide

Spironolactone, a competitive inhibitor of aldosterone (see Chapter 15), also competes with dihydrotestosterone for the androgen receptors in target tissues. It also reduces 17α-hydroxylase activity, lowering plasma levels of testosterone and androstenedione. It is used in doses of 50–200 mg/d for the treatment of hirsutism in women.

CHEMICAL CONTRACEPTION IN MEN

Although many studies have been conducted, an effective oral contraceptive for men has not yet been found. For example, various androgens, including testosterone and testosterone enanthate, in a dosage of 400 mg/mo, produced azoospermia in less than half the men treated. Minor adverse reactions, including gynecomastia and acne, were encountered. Testosterone in combination with danazol was well tolerated but no more effective than testosterone alone. Androgens in combination with a progestin such as medroxyprogesterone acetate were no more effective.

Finasteride

Cyproterone acetate, a very potent progestin and antiandrogen, will also produce oligospermia but has not produced reliable contraception.

At present, pituitary hormones—and potent antagonist analogues of GnRH—are receiving increased attention. A GnRH antagonist in combination with testosterone has been shown to produce a reversible azoospermia in nonhuman primates.

GOSSYPOL

Extensive trials of this cottonseed derivative have been conducted in China. This compound destroys elements of the seminiferous epithelium but does not alter the endocrine function of the testis.

In Chinese studies, large numbers of men were treated with 20 mg/d of gossypol or gossypol acetic acid for 2 months, followed by a maintenance dosage of 60 mg/wk. On this regimen, 99% of men devel-

Gossypol

oped sperm counts below 4 million/mL. Preliminary data indicate that recovery (return of normal sperm count) following discontinuance of gossypol administration is more apt to occur in men whose counts do not fall to extremely low levels and when administration is not continued for more than 2 years. Hypokalemia is the major adverse effect and may lead to transient paralysis. The drug has also been tried as an intravaginal spermicide contraceptive.

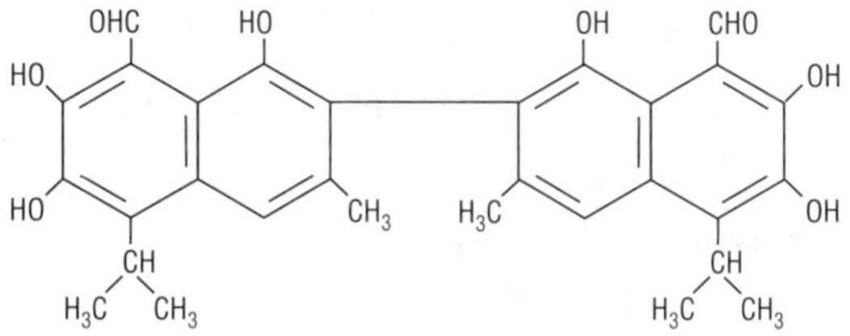

PREPARATIONS AVAILABLE
(Oral contraceptives are listed in Table 39–3.)

Estrogens
  Chlorotrianisene (TACE)
    Oral: 12, 25 mg capsules
  Conjugated estrogens (generic, Premarin)
    Oral: 0.3, 0.625, 0.9, 1.25, 2.5 mg tablets
    Parenteral: 25 mg/5 mL for IM, IV injection
    Vaginal: 0.625 mg/g cream base
  Dienestrol (Ortho Dienestrol, DV)
    Vaginal: 10 mg/g cream
  Diethylstilbestrol [DES] (generic)
    Oral: 1, 5 mg tablets
  Estradiol cypionate in oil (generic, Depo-Estradiol Cypionate)
    Parenteral: 5 mg/mL for IM injection
  Estradiol (Estrace)
    Oral: 1, 2 mg tablets
    Vaginal: 0.1 mg/g cream
  Estradiol transdermal (Estraderm)
    Transdermal: 4, 8 mg patches
  Estradiol valerate in oil (generic, others)
    Parenteral: 10, 20, 40 mg/mL for IM injection
  Estrone aqueous suspension (generic, Theelin Aqueous, others)
    Parenteral: 2, 5 mg/mL for injection
  Estropipate (Ogen)
    Oral: 0.625, 1.25, 2.5, 5 mg tablets
    Vaginal: 1.5 mg/g cream base
  Ethinyl estradiol (Estinyl, Feminone)
    Oral: 0.02, 0.05, 0.5 mg tablets
  Quinestrol (Estrovis)
    Oral: 100 µg tablets

Progestins
  Hydroxyprogesterone caproate (generic, Delalutin, others)
    Parenteral: 125, 250 mg/mL for IM injection
  Levonorgestrel (Norplant)
    Kit for subcutaneous implant: 6 capsules of 36 mg each
  Medroxyprogesterone acetate (Provera, others)
    Oral: 2.5, 5, 10 mg tablets
    Parenteral: 100, 400 mg/mL for IM injection
    Parenteral depot: 150 mg/mL for IM injection
  Megestrol (generic, Megace)
    Oral: 20, 40 mg tablets
  Norethindrone
    Oral: 5 mg tablets (Norlutin)
    Oral: 0.35 mg tablets (Micronor, Nor-Q.D.)
  Norethindrone acetate (Norlutate, Aygestin)
    Oral: 5 mg tablets
  Norgestrel (Ovrette)
    Oral: 0.075 mg tablets
  Progesterone in oil (generic, others)
    Parenteral: 50 mg/mL for IM injection

Androgens & Anabolic Steroids
  Fluoxymesterone (generic, Halotestin, others)
    Oral: 2, 5, 10 mg tablets
  Methyltestosterone (generic, Metandren, others)
    Oral: 10, 25 mg tablets; 10 mg capsules; 10 mg buccal tablets
  Nandrolone decanoate (generic, Deca-Durabolin, others)

Parenteral: 50, 100, 200 mg/mL in oil for injection

Nandrolone phenpropionate (generic, Durabolin, others)

Parenteral: 25, 50 mg/mL in oil for IM injection

Oxandrolone (Anavar)

Oral: 2.5 mg tablets

Oxymetholone (Androl-50)

Oral: 50 mg tablets

Stanozolol (Winstrol)

Oral: 2 mg tablets

Testolactone (Teslac)

Oral: 50 mg tablets

Testosterone aqueous (generic, others)

Parenteral: 25, 50, 100 mg/mL suspension for IM injection

Testosterone cypionate in oil (generic, others)

Parenteral: 100, 200 mg/mL for IM injection

Testosterone enanthate in oil (generic, others)

Parenteral: 100, 200 mg/mL for IM injection

Testosterone propionate in oil (generic, Testex)

Parenteral: 100 mg/mL for IM injection

**Antagonists & Inhibitors
(See also Chapter 36)**

Clomiphene (Clomid, Serophene)

Oral: 50 mg tablets

Danazol (Danocrine)

Oral: 50, 100, 200 mg capsules

Finasteride (Proscar)

Oral: 5 mg tablets

Flutamide (Eulexin)

Oral: 125 mg capsules

Goserelin (Zoladex)

Parenteral: 3.6 mg implant

Leuprolide

Parenteral (Lupron): 5 mg/mL for SC injection

Parenteral depot (Lupron Depot): 3.75, 7.5 mg/mL for IM injection

Tamoxifen (Nolvadex)

Oral: 10 mg tablets

REFERENCES

Estrogens & Progestins

Adashi EY: Intraovarian peptides: Stimulators and inhibitors of follicular growth and differentiation. Endocrinol Metab Clin North Am 1992;21:1.

Andreyko JL et al: Therapeutic uses of gonadotropin-releasing hormone analogs. Obstet Gynecol Surv 1987; 42:1.

Beato M: Gene regulation by steroid hormones. Cell 1989;56:335.

Belchetz PE: Hormonal treatment of postmenopausal women. N Engl J Med 1994;330:1062.

Bikle DD et al: Progestin antagonism of estrogen-stimulated 1,25-dihydroxyvitamin D levels. J Clin Endocrinol Metab 1992;75:519.

Bringer J: Norgestimate: A clinical overview of a new progestin. Am J Obstet Gynecol 1992;166:1969.

Casper RF, Chapdelaine A: Estrogen and interrupted progestin: A new concept for hormone replacement therapy. Am J Obstet Gynecol 1993;168:1186.

Chen CL: Inhibin and activin as paracrine/autocrine factors. Endocrinology 1993;132:4.

Colvin PL et al: Differential effects of oral estrone versus 17β-estradiol on lipoproteins in postmenopausal women. J Clin Endocrinol Metab 1990;70:1568.

Golditz GA, Egan KM, Stampfer MJ: Hormone replacement therapy and the risk of breast cancer: results from epidemiologic studies. Am J Obstet Gynecol 1993;168:1473.

Kalkhoff RK: Metabolic effects of progesterone. Am J Obstet Gynecol 1982;142:735.

Kaplan SN, Grumbach MM: Pathophysiology and treatment of sexual precocity. J Clin Endocrinol Metab 1990;71:785.

Mashchak AC et al: Comparison of pharmacodynamic properties of various estrogen formulations. Am J Obstet Gynecol 1982;144:511.

Melnick S et al: Rates and risks of diethylstilbestrol-related clear-cell adenocarcinoma of the vagina and cervix: An update. N Engl J Med 1987;316:514.

Miller-Bass K, Adashi EY: Current status and future prospects of transdermal estrogen replacement therapy. Fertil Steril 1990:53:961.

Mishell DR et al: Postmenopausal replacement with a combination estrogen-progestin regimen for five days per week. J Reprod Med 1991;36:351.

Mortola JF, Yen SSC: The effects of oral dehydroepiandrosterone on endocrine-metabolic parameters in postmenopausal women. J Clin Endocrinol Metab 1990;71:696.

Myeres LS et al: Effects of estrogen, androgen, and progestin on sexual psychophysiology and behavior in postmenopausal women. J Clin Endocrinol Metab 1990;70:1124.

Nabulsi AA et al: Association of hormone-replacement therapy with various cardiovascular risk factors in postmenopausal women. N Engl J Med 1993;328: 1069.

Naessén T et al: Hormone replacement therapy and the risk for first hip fracture: A prospective, population-based cohort study. Ann Intern Med 1990;113:95.

Sherwin BB: The impact of different doses of estrogen and progestin on mood and sexual behavior in postmenopausal women. J Clin Endocrinol Metab 1991; 72:336.

Spelsberg TC et al: Nuclear acceptor sites for steroid hormone receptors: Comparisons of steroids and antisteroids. J Steroid Biochem 1988;31:579.

Spicer LJ, Hammond JM: Regulation of ovarian function

by catecholestrogens: Current concepts. J Steroid Biochem 1989;33:489.

Symposium: Current perspectives in the management of the menopausal and postmenopausal patient. Obstet Gynecology 1990;75(No. 4 Suppl):1.

Venturoli S et al: Ketoconazole therapy for women with acne and/or hirsutism. J Clin Endocrinol Metab 1990; 71:335.

Walsh BW et al: Effects of postmenopausal estrogen replacement on the concentration and metabolism of plasma lipoproteins. N Engl J Med 1991;325:1196.

Weinstein L, Bewtra C, Gallagher JC: Evaluation of a continuous combined low-dose regimen of estrogen-progestin for treatment of the menopausal patient. Am J Obstet Gynecol 1990;162:1534.

Williams SR et al: A study of combined continuous ethinyl estradiol and norethindrone acetate for postmenopausal hormone replacement. Am J Obstet Gynecol 1990;162:438.

Wolf PH et al: Reduction of cardiovascular disease-related mortality among postmenopausal women who use hormones: Evidence from a national cohort. Am J Obstet Gynecol 1991;164:489.

Oral Contraceptives

Baird DT, Glasier AF: Hormonal contraception. N Engl J Med 1993;328:1543.

Boutaleb Y, Goldzieher J (editors): Toward a new standard in oral contraception. Am J Obstet Gynecol 1990; 163 (Suppl):1379.

Brinton LA et al: Oral contraceptive use and the risk of invasive cervical cancer. Int J Epidemiol 1990;19:4.

Centers for Disease Control Cancer and Steroid Hormone Study: Oral-contraceptive use and the risk of breast cancer. N Engl J Med 1986;315:405.

Centers for Disease Control Cancer and Steroid Hormone Study: Oral contraceptive use and the risk of endometrial cancer. JAMA 1983;249:1600.

Centers for Disease Control Cancer and Steroid Hormone Study: Oral contraceptive use and the risk of ovarian cancer. JAMA 1983;249:1596.

Gambrell RD, Maier RC, Sanders BI: Decreased incidence of breast cancer in postmenopausal estrogen-progestogen users. Obstet Gynecol 1983;62:435.

Godsland IF et al: The effects of different formulations of oral contraceptive agents on lipid and carbohydrate metabolism. N Engl J Med 1990;323:1375.

Grimes DA, Mishell DR Jr, Speroff L (editors): Contraceptive choices for women with medical problems. Am J Obstet Gynecol 1993;168(No. 6 Part 2):1979.

Knopp RH, Mishell DR Jr (editors): Prevention and management of cardiovascular risk in women. (Symposium.) Am J Obstet Gynecol 1988;158(Suppl 2): 1551.

Kuhl H, Goethe JW (editors): Pharmacokinetics of oral contraceptive steroids and drug interaction. Am J Obstet Gynecol 1990;163:2113.

Kuhnz W et al: Single and multiple administration of a new triphasic oral contraceptive to women: Pharmacokinetics of ethinyl estradiol and free and total testosterone levels in serum. Am J Obstet Gynecol 1991; 165:596.

Leemay A: Attenuation of mild hyperandrogenic activity in postpubertal acne by a triphasic oral contraceptive

containing low doses of ethynyl estradiol and DL-norgestrel. J Clin Endocrinol Metab 1990;71:8.

Mishell DR Jr: Noncontraceptive health benefits of oral contraceptives. Am J Obstet Gynecol 1982;142:809.

Mishell DR: Contraception. N Engl J Med 1989;320: 777.

Nieman LK et al: The progesterone antagonist RU 486: A potential new contraceptive agent. N Engl J Med 1987;316:187.

Skouby SO, Jesperson J (editors): Oral contraceptives in the nineties: Metabolic aspects—facts and fiction. Am J Obstet Gynecol 1990;163 (Suppl):276.

Weiss NS, Sayvetz TA: Incidence of endometrial cancer in relation to the use of oral contraceptives. N Engl J Med 1980;302:551.

Wynn V: Cardiovascular effects and progestins in oral contraceptives. Am J Obstet Gynecol 1982;142 (Suppl):718.

Wynn V: Effect of duration of low-dose oral contraceptive administration on carbohydrate metabolism. Am J Obstet Gynecol 1982;142 (No. 6 Part 2):739.

Androgens

Bardin W, Swerdloff RS, Santen RJ: Androgens: Risks and benefits. J Clin Endocrinol Metab 1991;73:4.

Bhasin S et al: A biodegradable testosterone microcapsule formulation provides uniform eugonadal levels of testosterone for 10–11 weeks in hypogonadal men. J Clin Endocrinol Metab 1992;74:75.

Bhasin S: Androgen treatment of hypogonadal men. J Clin Endocrinol Metab 1993;74:1221.

Bremner WJ, Bagatell CJ, Steiner RA: Gonadotropin-releasing hormone antagonist plus testosterone: A potential male contraceptive. J Clin Endocrinol Metab 1991;73:465.

Butler GE et al: Oral testosterone undecanoate in the management of delayed puberty in boys: Pharmacokinetics and effects on sexual maturation and growth. J Clin Endocrinol Metab 1992;75:37.

Conn MP, Crowley WF: Gonadotropin releasing hormone and its analogs. N Engl J Med 1991;324:93.

Cunningham GR, Cordero E, Thornby JI: Testosterone replacement with transdermal therapeutic systems: Physiologic serum testosterone and elevated dihydrotestosterone levels. JAMA 1989;261:2525.

Johnson FL et al: Association of androgenic-anabolic steroid therapy with development of hepatocellular carcinoma. Lancet 1972;2:1273.

Kopera H: The history of anabolic steroids and a review of clinical experience with anabolic steroids. Acta Endocrinol 1985;271(Suppl):11.

Linde R et al: Reversible inhibition of testicular steroidogenesis and spermatogenesis by a potent gonadotropin-releasing hormone agonist in normal men. N Engl J Med 1981;305:663.

Malarkey WB et al: Endocrine effects in female weight lifters who self administer testosterone and anabolic steroids. Am J Obstet Gynecol 1991;165:1385.

Matsumoto AM: Effects of chronic testosterone administration in normal men: Safety and efficacy of high dosage testosterone and parallel-dose dependent depression of luteinizing hormone, follicle-stimulating hormone, and sperm production. J Clin Endocrinol Metab 1990;70:282.

Meikle W et al: Enhanced transdermal delivery of testosterone across nonscrotal skin produces physiological concentrations of testosterone and its metabolites in hypogonadal men. J Clin Endocrinol Metab 1992;74: 623.

Mooradian AD, Morley JD, Korenman SG: Biological action of androgens. Endocr Rev 1987;8:1.

Mortola JF, Yen SSC: The effects of oral dehydroepian- drosterone on endocrine-metabolic parameters in postmenopausal women. J Clin Endocrinol Metab 1990;71:69.

Tenover JS: Effects of testosterone supplementation in the aging male. J Clin Endocrinol Metab 1992;75: 1092.

Thompson PD et al: Contrasting effects of testosterone and stanozolol on serum lipoprotein levels. JAMA 1989;261:1165.

Wilson JD: Androgen abuse by athletes. Endocr Rev 1988; 9:181.

Inhibitors

Bagdade JD et al: Effects of tamoxifen treatment on plasma lipids and lipoprotein lipid concentration. J Clin Endocrinol Metab 1990;70:1132

Barbieri RL, Ryan KJ: Danazol: Endocrine pharmacol- ogy and therapeutic applications. Am J Obstet Gyne- col 1981;141:453.

Baulieu E-E: Contragestion and other clinical applica- tions of RU 486, an antiprogesterone at the receptor. Science 1989;245:1351.

Conn MP, Crowley WF: Gonadotropin releasing hor- mone and its analogues. N Engl J Med 1991;324:93.

Davidson NE: Tamoxifen: Panacea or Pandora's box? (Editorial.) N Engl Med 1992;326:885.

DiMattina M et al: Ketoconazole inhibits multiple steroi- dogenic enzymes involved in androgen biosynthesis in the human ovary. Fertil Steril 1988;49:62.

Feldman D: Ketoconazole and other imidazole deriva- tives as inhibitors of steroidogenesis. Endocr Rev 1985;7:409.

Flack MR et al: Oral gossypol in the treatment of meta- static adrenal cancer. J Clin Endocrinol Metab 1993; 76:1019.

Glasier A et al: Mifepristone (RU 486) compared with high-dose estrogen and progestogen for emergency postcoital contraception. N Engl J Med 1992;327: 1041.

Love RR et al: Effects of tamoxifen on bone mineral den- sity in postmenopausal women with breast cancer. N Engl J Med 1992;326:852.

Filicori M et al: Comparison of the suppressive capacity

of different depot gonadotropin-releasing hormone analogues in women. J Clin Endocrinol Metab 1993; 77:130.

Friedman AJ et al: A prospective, randomized trial of go- nadotropin-releasing hormone agonist plus estrogen- progestin or progestin "add-back" regimens for women with leiomyomata uteri. J Clin Endocrinol Metab 1993;76:1439.

Gittes RF: Carcinoma of the prostate. N Engl J Med 1991;324:236.

Gormley GJ et al: Effects of finasteride (MK-906), a 5α- reductase inhibitor, on circulating androgens in male volunteers. J Clin Endocrinol Metab. 1990;70:1136.

Henzyl MR, Kwei L: Efficacy and safety of nafarelin in the treatment of endometriosis. Am J Obstet Gynecol 1990;162:570.

Hill NCW, Ferguson J, MacKenzie IZ: The efficacy of oral mifepristone (RU 38,486) with a prostaglandin E_1 analog vaginal pessary for the termination of early pregnancy: Complications and patient acceptability. Am J Obstet Gynecol 1990:162:414.

Martin KA et al: Comparison of exogenous gonado- tropins and pulsatile gonadotropin-releasing hormone for induction of ovulation in hypogonadotropic amenorrhea. J Clin Endocrinol Metab 1993;77:125.

McConnell JD et al: Finasteride, an inhibitor of 5α-re- ductase, suppresses prostatic dihydrotestosterone in men with benign prostatic hyperplasia. J Clin Endo- crinol Metab 1992;74:505.

Peyron R et al: Early termination of pregnancy with mifepristone (RU 486) and the orally active pros- taglandin misoprostol. N Engl J Med 1993;328:1509.

Porat O: Effects of gossypol on the motility of mammal- ian sperm. Mol Reprod Devel 1990;25:400.

Rabinovici J et al: Endocrine effects and pharmacoki- netic characteristics of a potent new gonadotropin-re- leasing hormone antagonist (Ganirelix) with minimal histamine-releasing properties: Studies in postmeno- pausal women. J Clin Endocrinol Metab 1992; 75: 1220.

Rittmaster RS: Finasteride. (Drug Therapy.) N Engl J Med 1993;330:120.

Sawaya ME, Hordinsky MK: The antiandrogens: When and how they should be used. Dermatol Ther 1993; 11:65.

Silvestre L et al: Voluntary interruption of pregnancy with mifepristone (RU 486) and a prostaglandin ana- logue: A large-scale French experience. N Engl J Med 1990;322:645.

Pancreatic Hormones & Antidiabetic Drugs

40

John H. Karam, MD

THE ENDOCRINE PANCREAS

The endocrine pancreas in the adult human consists of approximately 1 million islets of Langerhans interspersed throughout the pancreatic gland. Within the islets, at least four hormone-producing cells have been identified (Table 40–1). Their hormone products include **insulin,** the storage and anabolic hormone of the body; **islet-amyloid polypeptide (IAPP, or amylin),** whose metabolic function remains undefined; **glucagon,** the hyperglycemic factor that mobilizes glycogen stores; somatostatin, a universal inhibitor of secretory cells; and **pancreatic polypeptide,** a small protein that facilitates digestive processes by a mechanism not yet clarified.

Diabetes mellitus is the most important disease involving the endocrine pancreas. Its major manifestations include disordered metabolism and inappropriate hyperglycemia. A "therapeutic" classification presently recommended by the American Diabetes Association includes two major types: insulin-dependent (IDDM) and non-insulin-dependent (NIDDM) diabetes mellitus. An estimated 10 million people in the USA are known to have diabetes, and at least 800,000 have the insulin-dependent type.

Type I diabetes (IDDM) is a severe form associated with ketosis in the untreated state. It occurs most commonly in juveniles but occasionally in adults, especially the nonobese and those who are elderly when hyperglycemia first appears. It is a catabolic disorder in which circulating insulin is virtually absent, plasma glucagon is elevated, and the pancreatic B cells fail to respond to all insulinogenic stimuli. Exogenous insulin is therefore required to reverse the catabolic state, prevent ketosis, and reduce the hyperglucagonemia and the elevated blood glucose level.

Type I diabetes is thought to result from an infectious or toxic environmental insult in people whose immune system is genetically predisposed to develop a vigorous autoimmune response against pancreatic B cell antigens. Extrinsic factors that might affect B cell function include damage caused by viruses such as mumps virus and coxsackievirus B4, by toxic chemical agents, or by destructive cytotoxins and antibodies released from sensitized immunocytes. An underlying genetic defect relating to B cell replication or function may predispose to development of B cell failure after viral infection; in addition, specific HLA genes may increase susceptibility to a diabetogenic virus or may be linked to certain immune response genes that predispose patients to a destructive autoimmune response against their own islet cells (autoaggression). Recent observations that pancreatic B cell damage appears to be lessened when immunosuppressive drugs such as cyclosporine or azathioprine are given at the initial manifestations of type I diabetes support the importance of autoaggression by the immune system as a major factor in the pathogenesis of this type of diabetes.

Type II diabetes (NIDDM) represents a heterogeneous group comprising milder forms of diabetes that occur predominantly in adults but occasionally in adolescents. Circulating endogenous insulin is sufficient to prevent ketoacidosis but is often either subnormal or relatively inadequate because of tissue insensitivity. Obesity, which generally results in impaired insulin action, is a common risk factor for this type of diabetes, and most patients with NIDDM are obese.

In addition to tissue insensitivity to insulin, which has been noted in most NIDDM patients irrespective of weight, there is an accompanying deficiency of the pancreatic B cell's response to glucose. Both the tissue resistance to insulin and the impaired B cell response to glucose appear to be further aggravated by increased hyperglycemia, and both of these defects are ameliorated by therapeutic maneuvers that reduce the hyperglycemia.

When dietary treatment and attempts at weight reduction of obesity fail to correct hyperglycemia, sulfonylurea drugs are usually prescribed. Insulin therapy may be required to achieve satisfactory glycemic control even though it is not needed to prevent ketoacidosis in patients with NIDDM.

Table 40–1. Pancreatic islet cells and their secretory products.

Cell Types	Approximate Percent of Islet Mass	Secretory Products
A cell (alpha)	20	Glucagon, proglucagon.
B cell (beta)	75	Insulin, C-peptide, proinsulin, islet amyloid polypeptide.
D cell (delta)	3–5	Somatostatin.
F cell (PP cell)[1]	< 2	Pancreatic polypeptide (PP).

[1]Within pancreatic polypeptide-rich lobules of adult islets, located only in the posterior portion of the head of the human pancreas, glucagon cells are scarce (less than 0.5%), and F cells make up as much as 80% of the cells.

INSULIN

Chemistry

Insulin is a small protein with a molecular weight in humans of 5808. It contains 51 amino acids arranged in two chains (A and B) linked by disulfide bridges; there are species differences in the amino acids of both chains. Within the B cell, insulin precursor is produced by DNA- or RNA-directed synthesis. Proinsulin, a long single-chain protein molecule, is processed within the Golgi apparatus and packaged into granules, where it is hydrolyzed into insulin and a residual connecting segment called the C-peptide by removal of four amino acids (shown in dashed circles in Figure 40–1). Insulin and C-peptide are secreted in equimolar amounts in response to all insulin secretagogues; a small quantity of unprocessed or partially hydrolyzed proinsulin is released as well. While proinsulin may have some mild hypoglycemic action, C-peptide has no known physiologic function. Granules within the B cell store the insulin in the form of crystals consisting of two atoms of zinc and six molecules of insulin. The entire human pancreas contains up to 8 mg of insulin, representing approximately 200 biologic "units." Originally, the unit was defined on the basis of the hypoglycemic activity of insulin in rabbits. With improved purification techniques, the unit is presently defined on the basis of weight, and present insulin standards used for assay purposes are 28 units per milligram.

Insulin Secretion

Insulin is released from pancreatic B cells at a low basal rate and at a much higher stimulated rate in response to a variety of stimuli, especially glucose. Other stimulants such as other sugars (eg, mannose), certain amino acids (eg, leucine, arginine), and vagal activity are also recognized. One mechanism of stimulated insulin release is diagrammed in Figure 40–2. As shown in the figure, hyperglycemia results in increased intracellular ATP levels, which close the ATP-dependent potassium channels. Decreased outward potassium current through this channel results in depolarization of the B cell and opening of voltage-gated calcium channels. The resulting increased intracellular calcium triggers secretion of the hormone.

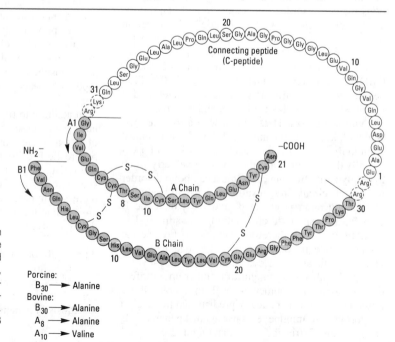

Figure 40–1. Structure of human proinsulin. Insulin is shown as the shaded polypeptide chains, A and B. Comparisons of human, porcine, and bovine C-peptides show considerable differences between species, with only about 40% homology. Species differences in the A and B chains are noted in the inset.

Porcine:
B$_{30}$ ⟶ Alanine
Bovine:
B$_{30}$ ⟶ Alanine
A$_8$ ⟶ Alanine
A$_{10}$ ⟶ Valine

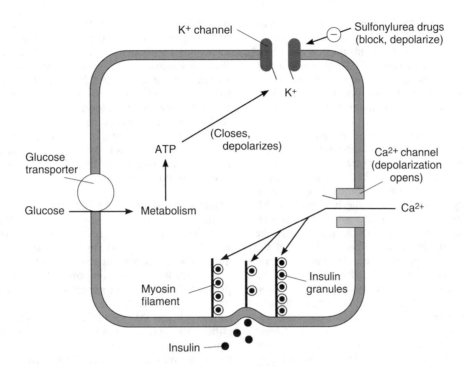

Figure 40–2. One model of control of insulin release from the pancreatic B cell by glucose and by sulfonylurea drugs. In the resting cell with normal (low) ATP levels, potassium diffuses down its concentration gradient through ATP-gated potassium channels (ATP *closes* the channels), maintaining the intracellular potential at a fully polarized, negative level. Insulin release is minimal. If glucose concentration rises, ATP production increases, potassium channels close, and depolarization of the cell results. As in muscle and nerve, voltage-gated calcium channels open in response to depolarization, allowing more calcium to enter the cell. Increased intracellular calcium results in increased insulin secretion. Sulfonylurea hypoglycemic drugs block the ATP-dependent potassium channel, thereby depolarizing the membrane and causing increased insulin release by the same mechanism. (Modified and reproduced, with permission, from Basic & Clinical Endocrinology, 3rd edition, Greenspan F [editor]. Appleton & Lange, 1994.)

The mechanism is undoubtedly more complex than this brief summary suggests, since several intracellular messengers are known to modulate the process (cAMP, inositol trisphosphate, diacylglycerol) and the insulin response to a monophasic rise in glucose is biphasic. As noted below, the sulfonylurea oral hypoglycemic drug group is thought to exploit parts of this mechanism.

Insulin Degradation

The liver and kidney are the two main organs that remove insulin from the circulation, presumably by hydrolysis of the disulfide connections between the A and B chains through the action of glutathione insulin transhydrogenase (insulinase). After this reductive cleavage, further degradation by proteolysis occurs. The liver normally clears the blood of approximately 60% of the insulin released from the pancreas by virtue of its location as the terminal site of portal vein blood flow, with the kidney removing 35–40% of the endogenous hormone. However, in insulin-treated diabetics receiving subcutaneous insulin injections,

this ratio is reversed, with as much as 60% of exogenous insulin being cleared by the kidney and the liver removing no more than 30–40%. The half-life of circulating insulin is 3–5 minutes.

Measurement of Circulating Insulin

The radioimmunoassay of insulin permits detection of insulin in picomolar quantities. The assay is based on antibodies developed in guinea pigs against bovine or pork insulin. Because of the similarities between these two insulins and human insulin, the assay successfully measures the human hormone.

With this assay, basal insulin values of 5–15 μU/mL (30–90 pmol/L) are found in normal humans, with a peak rise to 60–90 μU/mL (360–540 pmol/L) during meals. Similar assays for measuring all of the known hormones of the endocrine pancreas (including C-peptide and proinsulin) have been developed.

The Insulin Receptor

Once insulin has entered the circulation, it is bound

by specialized receptors that are found on the membranes of most tissues. However, the biologic responses promoted by these insulin-receptor complexes have been identified in only a few target tissues, eg, liver, muscle, and adipose tissue. The receptors bind insulin with high specificity and affinity in the picomolar range. The full insulin receptor consists of two heterodimers, each containing an alpha subunit, which is entirely extracellular and constitutes the recognition site, and a beta subunit that spans the membrane (Figure 40–3). The beta subunit contains a tyrosine kinase. When insulin binds to the alpha subunit at the outside surface of the cell, tyrosine kinase activity is stimulated in the beta portion. Although the αβ dimeric form is capable of binding insulin, it does so with much lower affinity than the tetrameric ααββ form. Self-phosphorylation of the beta portion of the receptor causes both increased aggregation of αβ heterodimers and stabilization of the activated state of the receptor tyrosine kinase. Phosphorylation of other proteins within the cell is the major effect and represents the "second message" because it results in translocation of certain proteins such as the glucose transporter from sequestered sites within the cell to exposed locations on the cell surface. Finally, the insulin-receptor complex is internalized. However, it remains controversial whether internalization contributes to further action of insulin or is merely a means of limiting further effects of the hormone by removing insulin and its receptor into scavenger lysosomes.

Various hormonal agents (eg, hydrocortisone) lower the affinity of insulin receptors to insulin; growth hormone in excess increases this affinity slightly. The concentration of these specific receptor molecules as well as their affinity for binding insulin seems to be affected by the concentration of insulin molecules to which they are exposed. Experimentally, desensitization of insulin receptors has been shown to occur with a time course of 4 hours (in vitro) to 24 hours (in vivo). In clinical situations associated with elevated blood levels of circulating insulin, such as obesity or insulinoma, the concentration of insulin receptors is reduced. This down-regulation of insulin receptors seems to provide an intrinsic mechanism whereby target cells limit their response to excessive hormone concentrations.

Effects of Insulin on Its Targets

Insulin promotes the storage of fat as well as glucose (both sources of energy) within specialized target cells (Figure 40–4) and influences cell growth and the metabolic functions of a wide variety of tissues.

A. Action of Insulin on Glucose Transporters: Insulin has an important effect on several transport molecules that facilitate glucose movement across cell membranes (Table 40–2). These transporters may play a role in the etiology as well as the manifestations of diabetes. GLUT 4, quantitatively the most important in terms of lowering blood glucose, is inserted into the membranes of muscle and adipose cells from intracellular storage vesicles by insulin. Defects in GLUT 2-mediated transport into pancreatic B cells may contribute to the reduced insulin secretion that characterizes NIDDM.

B. Action of Insulin on Liver: (Table 40–3.) The first major organ endogenous insulin reaches via the portal circulation is the liver, where it acts to increase storage of glucose as glycogen and to reset the liver to the fed state by reversing a number of cata-

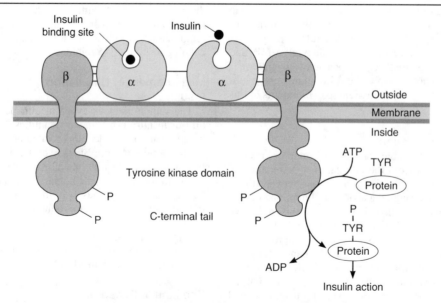

Figure 40–3. Schematic diagram of the probable structure of the insulin receptor tetramer in the activated state.

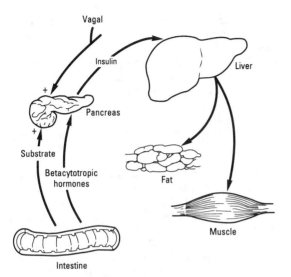

Figure 40–4. Insulin promotes synthesis (from circulating nutrients) and storage of glycogen, triglycerides, and protein in its major target tissues: liver, fat, and muscle. The release of insulin from the pancreas is stimulated by increased blood glucose, vagal nerve stimulation, and other factors (see text).

Table 40–3. Endocrine effects of insulin.

Effect on liver:
　Reversal of catabolic features of insulin deficiency
　　Inhibits glycogenolysis.
　　Inhibits conversion of fatty acids and amino acids to
　　　keto acids.
　　Inhibits conversion of amino acids to glucose.
　Anabolic action
　　Promotes glucose storage as glycogen (induces glu-
　　　cokinase and glycogen synthase, inhibits phosphory-
　　　lase).
　　Increases triglyceride synthesis and very low density
　　　lipoprotein formation.
Effect on muscle:
　Increased protein synthesis
　　Increases amino acid transport.
　　Increases ribosomal protein synthesis.
　Increased glycogen synthesis
　　Increases glucose transport.
　　Induces glycogen synthase and inhibits phosphorylase.
Effect on adipose tissue:
　Increased triglyceride storage
　　Lipoprotein lipase is induced and activated by insulin to
　　　hydrolyze triglycerides from lipoproteins.
　　Glucose transport into cell provides glycerol phosphate
　　　to permit esterification of fatty acids supplied by lipo-
　　　protein transport.
　　Intracellular lipase is inhibited by insulin.

bolic mechanisms associated with the postabsorptive state: glycogenolysis, ketogenesis, and gluconeogenesis. These effects are brought about in part through insulin-induced phosphorylations, which activate pyruvate kinase, phosphofructokinase, and glucokinase, while repressing gluconeogenic enzymes, including pyruvate carboxylase, phosphoenolpyruvate carboxykinase, fructose bisphosphatase, and glucose 6-phosphatase. In addition, insulin decreases urea production, protein catabolism, and cAMP in the liver, promotes triglyceride synthesis, and increases potassium and phosphate uptake by the organ.

C. Effect of Insulin on Muscle: (Table 40–3.) Insulin promotes protein synthesis by increasing amino acid transport and by stimulating ribosomal activity. It also promotes glycogen synthesis to replace glycogen stores expended by muscle activity. This is accomplished by increasing glucose transport into the muscle cell, inducing glycogen synthase, and inhibiting phosphorylase. Approximately 500–600 g of glycogen is stored in muscle tissue of a 70 kg male.

D. Effect of Insulin on Adipose Tissue: (Table 40–3.) The most efficient means of storing energy is in the form of triglyceride depots. This provides 9 kcal per gram of stored substrate and, unlike glycogen, does not require water to maintain it within cells. A normal 70 kg man has 12–14 kg of fat in storage, chiefly in adipose tissue.

Insulin acts to reduce circulating free fatty acids and to promote triglyceride storage in adipocytes by three primary mechanisms: (1) induction of lipoprotein lipase, which actively hydrolyzes triglycerides from circulating lipoproteins; (2) glucose transport into cells to generate glycerophosphate as a metabolic product, which permits esterification of fatty acids supplied by lipoprotein hydrolysis; and (3) reduction of intracellular lipolysis of stored triglyceride by a direct inhibition of intracellular lipase. These effects appear to involve suppression of cAMP production and dephosphorylation of the lipases in the fat cell.

Table 40–2. Glucose transporters.

Transporter	Tissues	Glucose K_m (mmol/L)	Function
GLUT 1	All tissues, especially red cells, brain	1–2	Basal uptake of glucose; transport across the blood-brain barrier
GLUT 2	B cells of pancreas, liver, kidney, gut	15–20	Regulation of insulin release, other aspects of glucose homeostasis
GLUT 3	Brain, kidney, placenta, other tissues	<1	Uptake into neurons, other tissues
GLUT 4	Muscle, adipose	≈5	Insulin-mediated uptake of glucose
GLUT 5	Gut, kidney	1–2	Intestinal absorption of fructose

Characteristics of Available Insulin Preparations

Commercial insulin preparations differ in a number of ways, including differences in the animal species from which they are obtained; their purity, concentration, and solubility; and the time of onset and duration of their biologic action. In the past 12 years, a number of human insulin preparations have been added to the list of available insulins, and some animal preparations have been removed. As a result, in 1994, approximately 30 different insulin formulations were available for purchase in the USA. If the use of human insulin continues to increase, the number of available insulins from animal sources should decline.

A. Principal Types and Duration of Action of Insulin Preparations: Three principal types of insulins are available: (1) short-acting, with rapid onset of action; (2) intermediate-acting; and (3) long-acting, with slow onset of action (Figure 40–5, Table 40–4). Short-acting insulin is a crystalline zinc-insulin complex dispensed as a clear solution at neutral pH. All other commercial insulins have been modified to provide prolonged action and are dispensed as turbid suspensions at neutral pH with either protamine in phosphate buffer (protamine zinc and NPH insulin) or varying concentrations of zinc in acetate buffer (ultralente, lente, and semilente insulins). Production of protamine zinc insulin and semilente preparations has recently been discontinued, since almost no clinical indications for their use exist. Conventional subcutaneous insulin therapy presently consists of split-dose injections of mixtures of short-acting and intermediate-acting insulins (NPH or lente) or multiple doses of short-acting insulin preprandially in association with any of three insulin suspensions (NPH, lente, or ultralente) whose prolonged duration of action provides overnight basal insulin levels.

1. Short-acting insulin–Regular insulin is a short-acting soluble crystalline zinc insulin whose ef-fect appears within 15 minutes of subcutaneous injection and generally lasts 5–7 hours. As with all insulin formulations, the duration of action as well as the intensity of peak action increases with the size of the dose. Short-acting soluble insulin is the only type of insulin that can be administered intravenously or by infusion pumps. It is particularly useful for intravenous therapy in the management of diabetic ketoacidosis and when the insulin requirement is changing rapidly, such as after surgery or during acute infections.

2. Lente and ultralente insulin–Lente insulin is a mixture of 30% semilente (an amorphous precipitate of insulin with zinc ions in acetate buffer that has a relatively rapid onset of action) with 70% ultralente insulin (a poorly soluble crystal of zinc insulin that has a delayed onset and prolonged duration of action). These two components provide a combination of relatively rapid absorption, with sustained long action making lente insulin a useful therapeutic agent. While beef, pork, and human insulins can readily form zinc crystals in acetate buffer under the conditions employed, only beef insulin has the proper hydrophobic alignment within the crystal to provide the delayed, sustained release of insulin characteristic of ultralente. Zinc crystals of pork insulin dissolve more rapidly, and while the appearance of the crystals is virtually identical to that of zinc crystals of beef insulin, the onset of action is earlier and the duration shorter. Accordingly, there is no ultralente insulin made of porcine insulin alone. Novo Nordisk continues to use beef insulin for its ultralente insulin. Eli Lilly has marketed an ultralente human insulin formulation that is claimed to have a time-action profile comparable to that of beef insulin, but this remains controvsial.

Lente insulin is the most widely used of the lente series of insulins, particularly in therapeutic combination with regular insulin, which has a more rapid on-

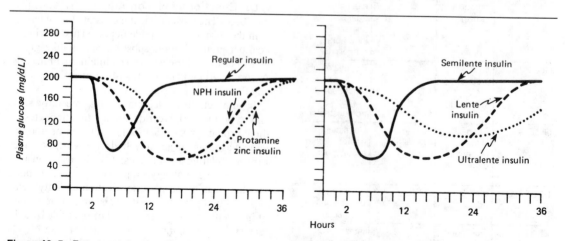

Figure 40–5. Extent and duration of action of various types of insulin (in a fasting diabetic). The durations of action shown are typical of average therapeutic doses; duration increases considerably when dosage is increased.

Table 40–4. Some insulin preparations available in the USA.[1,2]

Preparation	Species Source	Concentration
Short-acting insulins		
Standard[3]		
Regular (Novo Nordisk)	Pork	U100
Regular Iletin I (Lilly)	Beef and pork	U100
"Purified"[4]		
Regular (Novo Nordisk)[5]	Pork or human	U100
Regular Humulin (Lilly)	Human	U100
Regular Iletin II (Lilly)	Pork or beef	U100, U500[6]
Velosulin (Novo Nordisk)	Human	U100
Humulin BR[7]	Human	U100
Intermediate-acting insulins		
Standard[3]		
Isophane NPH (Novo Nordisk)	Beef	U100
Lente (Novo Nordisk)	Beef	U100
Lente Iletin I (Lilly)	Beef and pork	U100
NPH Iletin I (Lilly)	Beef and pork	U100
"Purified"[4]		
Lente Humulin (Lilly)	Human	U100
Lente Iletin II (Lilly)	Pork or beef	U100
Lente (Novo Nordisk)[5]	Pork or human	U100
NPH Humulin (Lilly)	Human	U100
NPH Iletin II (Lilly)	Pork or beef	U100
NPH (Novo Nordisk)[5]	Pork or human	U100
Premixed insulins (70% NPH, 30% regular)		
Novolin 70/30 (Novo Nordisk)[5]	Human	U100
Humulin 70/30 and 50/50 (Lilly)	Human	U100
Long-acting insulins		
Standard[3]		
Ultralente (Novo Nordisk)	Beef	U100
Ultralente Iletin I (Lilly)	Beef and pork	U40, U100
"Purified"[4]		
Ultralente (Novo Nordisk)	Beef	U100
Ultralente Humulin (Lilly)	Human	U100

[1]Modified and reproduced, with permission, from Katzung BG (editor): *Drug Therapy*, 2nd ed. Appleton & Lange, 1991.
[2]These agents are all available without a prescription. Wholesale prices for all preparations are similar.
[3]Greater than 10 but less than 25 ppm proinsulin.
[4] Less than 10 ppm proinsulin.
[5]Novo Nordisk human insulins are termed Novolin R, L, and N.
[6]U500 available only as pork insulin.
[7]Humulin BR (Buffered Regular) is recommended for use in pumps only. Its phosphate buffer reduces the risk of aggregation of insulin molecules in pump tubing.

set of action than the semilente component. Ultralente has a very slow onset of action with a prolonged duration, and its administration once or twice daily has been advocated to provide a basal level of insulin comparable to that achieved by basal endogenous insulin secretion or the overnight infusion rate programmed into insulin pumps. There has recently been a resurgence of use of ultralente insulin in combination with multiple injections of regular insulin as a means of attempting optimal control in patients with insulin-dependent diabetes.

3. NPH (neutral protamine Hagedorn, or isophane) insulin–NPH insulin is an intermediate-acting insulin wherein the onset of action is delayed by combining appropriate amounts of insulin and protamine so that neither is present in an uncomplexed form ("isophane"). Protamine isolated from the sperm of rainbow trout is a mixture of six major and some minor compounds of similar structure. They appear to be arginine-rich peptides with an average molecular weight of approximately 4400. To form an isophane complex (one in which neither component retains any free binding sites), approximately a 1:10 ratio by weight of protamine to insulin is required eg, 0.3–0.4 mg of protamine to 4 mg of insulin (100 units). This represents approximately six molecules of insulin per molecule of protamine. After subcutaneous injection, proteolytic enzymes degrade the protamine to permit absorption of insulin.

The onset and duration of action of NPH insulin is comparable to that of lente insulin (Table 40–4); it is usually mixed with regular insulin and given at least twice daily for insulin replacement in patients with insulin-dependent diabetes.

4. Mixtures of insulins–Since intermediate-acting insulins require several hours to reach adequate therapeutic levels, their use in insulin-dependent diabetic patients requires supplements of regular insulin preprandially. For convenience, these are often mixed together in the same syringe and injected subcutaneously in split dosage before breakfast and supper. NPH is preferred to lente insulin as the intermediate-acting component in these mixtures because increased proportions of lente to regular insulin may retard the rapid action of admixed regular insulin, particularly if not injected immediately after mixing. The excess zinc in lente and ultralente insulin can precipitate some of the soluble regular insulin when mixed in vitro (even at equal proportions) and can explain the slight retardation of regular insulin's absorption and biologic effect when mixed with lente or ultralente insulin.

So that NPH insulin does not retard the pharmacokinetic profile of admixed regular insulin, the protamine content of NPH insulin has been reduced by all manufacturers to levels at or below 0.4 mg per 4 mg insulin. It is therefore preferable to lente insulin as the intermediate component of a therapeutic mixture containing regular insulin.

B. Species of Insulin:

1. Beef/pork insulins–Most commercial insulin in the USA contains beef insulin as its chief component. Beef insulin differs by three amino acids from human insulin, whereas only a single amino acid distinguishes pork and human insulins (Figure 40–1). The beef hormone is slightly more antigenic than pork insulin in humans. The most commonly prescribed preparations in the USA are standard mixtures containing 70% beef and 30% pork insulin. However, supplies of "monospecies" pork or beef insulin are commercially available and are particularly useful in patients with conditions in which pure monospecies insulin may be indicated, such as insulin allergy or insulin resistance (see below).

2. Human insulins–Mass production of human insulin by recombinant DNA techniques is now carried out by inserting the human proinsulin gene cDNA into *E coli* or yeast and treating the extracted proinsulin to form the human insulin molecule.

Human insulin is available for clinical use as Humulin (Lilly) and dispensed as either regular, NPH, lente, or ultralente Humulin. Human insulin prepared biosynthetically in yeast is marketed by Novo Nordisk as human insulin injection (Novolin R), Monotard Human Insulin (Novolin L), and an isophane suspension of human insulin (Novolin N). The postscripts R, L, and N refer to the formulations: regular, lente, and NPH, respectively. The same company also produces a human insulin marketed as Velosulin (regular) that contains a phosphate buffer. This reduces aggregation of regular insulin molecules when used in infusion pumps, so that, like Humulin BR, it is recommended for pump use. However, because of the tendency of phosphate to precipitate zinc ions, these two preparations should not be mixed with any of the lente insulins.

A premixed formulation of 70% NPH and 30% regular human insulin is available for use in elderly patients and others who may have difficulties in mixing insulins: Novolin 70/30, Humulin 70/30, and Mixtard Human Insulin. Human insulin is also available in a premixed 50:50 formulation. Human insulins appear to be as effective as conventional animal insulins, and they appear to be considerably less immunogenic in diabetic patients than beef-pork insulins and slightly less immunogenic than pork insulin. However, a question has recently been raised regarding a higher risk of hypoglycemia with human preparations (see Complications).

Since threonine contains a hydroxyl group that makes it more polar—and thus more hydrophilic—than alanine, the presence of two threonines in place of two alanines in beef insulin and one such replacement in pork insulin (Figure 40–1) may explain why human insulin tends to be absorbed more rapidly and have a slightly shorter duration of action than animal insulins, regardless of the formulation in which it is administered.

C. Purity of Insulin:
Improvements in purification techniques (using gel columns) have greatly reduced contaminating proteins with molecular weights greater than that of insulin. These include proinsulin and partially cleaved proinsulins that are metabolically inactive yet capable of inducing anti-insulin antibodies. Further purification with chromatography can virtually eliminate these larger proteins and markedly lower the concentration of smaller peptide contaminants. Conventional formulations of insulin contain less than 50 ppm of proinsulin. When proinsulin content is less than 10 ppm, manufacturers are entitled by FDA regulations in the USA to label the insulin as "purified."

D. Concentration:
Currently, all insulins in the USA and Canada are available in a concentration of 100 units/mL (U100) and are dispensed in 10 mL vials. A limited supply of U500 regular porcine insulin is available for use in rare cases of severe insulin resistance in which large quantities of insulin are required.

E. Human Proinsulin:
Human proinsulin is now available from recombinant DNA synthesis and shows biologic activity in humans which is 8–12% that of human insulin. Since it has a circulating half-life four to six times longer than that of human insulin, it was proposed for use as an alternative form of longer-acting insulin. It has certain advantages over NPH and lente formulations of human insulin in that it provides prolonged insulin action without need for fish protamine additives or large concentrations of zinc acetate to precipitate the insulin. Moreover, some reports indicate that human proinsulin is less immunogenic than human insulin and has more reproducible absorption characteristics than do precipitated formulations of human insulin (NPH and lente) that have a comparable "intermediate" duration of action. However, clinical trials were suspended because of concern over an increased number of fatal cardiovascular events in a group of diabetic patients receiving human proinsulin. The ultimate role of proinsulin remains to be defined.

F. Insulin Analogues:
Among the many variables affecting the absorptive kinetics of insulin, an important one seems to be the tendency of insulin molecules to aggregate in hexameric form when formulated at pharmacologic concentrations. This causes lag periods of up to 30 minutes before insulin absorption is initiated from a subcutaneous depot site and results in a prolonged profile of absorption because the U100 injected regular insulin must be diluted more than 1000-fold by tissue fluids before it becomes monomeric and more readily absorbable into the circulation. The Novo Research Institute is currently developing insulin analogues such as one with two amino acid substitutions (Asp B9, Glu B27) that has the property of remaining monomeric even at therapeutic concentrations. This analogue and others are undergoing clinical trials at present with encour-

aging preliminary results: rapid absorption after subcutaneous injection, excellent biologic activity in vivo, and relatively low immunogenicity (Brange et al, 1990; Kang et al 1991).

Insulin Delivery Systems

The standard mode of insulin therapy is subcutaneous injection using conventional disposable needles and syringes. During the last 2 decades, much effort has gone into exploration of other means of administration.

A. Portable Pen Injectors: To facilitate multiple subcutaneous injections of insulin, particularly during intensive insulin therapy, portable pen-sized injectors have been developed (Novo Pen, Novolin Pen). These contain cartridges of U100 human insulin and retractable needles. Human insulin is available for these devices as cartridges of either regular insulin (Novolin R PenFill), NPH insulin (Novolin N PenFill), and premixed 70% NPH and 30% regular (Novolin 70/30 PenFill). These portable injectors have been well accepted by patients because they eliminate the need to carry syringes and bottles of insulin to the workplace and while traveling.

B. Closed-Loop Systems: Automated administration of soluble insulin by "closed-loop" systems (blood glucose-controlled insulin infusion systems) has been successful in acute situations such as management of diabetic ketoacidosis or maintenance of insulin balance in diabetics undergoing surgery. Chronic use of such systems is prevented by the need for uninterrupted aspiration of blood to reach an external glucose sensor and by the size of the computerized insulin pump system used on present models.

C. Open-Loop Systems (Insulin Pumps): Research into smaller "open-loop" methods of insulin delivery (insulin reservoir and pump programmed to deliver regular insulin at a calculated rate without a glucose sensor) has resulted in readily portable pumps for subcutaneous, intravenous, or intraperitoneal infusion. As methods for self-monitoring of blood glucose are increasingly accepted by patients, these pump systems are becoming less "open loop" and therefore potentially more useful for managing insulin-dependent diabetics. However, at present, intensive therapy using conventional daily administration of multiple subcutaneous injections of soluble, rapid-acting insulin and a single daily injection of long-acting insulin appears to provide blood glucose control as effective as either type of loop system for most patients.

D. Nasal Insulin Delivery: When insulin is combined with a detergent and administered as an aerosol to the nasal mucosa, effective circulating levels of insulin can be achieved almost as rapidly as when an intravenous bolus of insulin is administered. If this route can be shown to produce reliable and reproducible absorption over the long term without toxicity to the nasal mucosa, it may improve insulin delivery to the circulation while reducing the need for injections. However, current formulations have not achieved these goals.

Treatment With Insulin

The current classification of diabetes mellitus identifies a group of patients who have virtually no insulin secretion and whose survival is dependent on administration of exogenous insulin. This "insulin-dependent" group (type I) represents only about 8% of the diabetic population in the USA. Most type II diabetics do not require exogenous insulin for survival, but many need exogenous supplementation of their endogenous secretion to achieve optimum health. It is estimated that as many as 20% of type II diabetics in the USA (1–1.5 million people) are presently treated with insulin.

Benefit of Glycemic Control in Diabetes Mellitus

A long-term randomized prospective study involving 1441 IDDM patients in 29 medical centers reported in 1993 that "near normalization" of blood glucose resulted in a delay in onset and a major slowing of progression of microvascular and neuropathic complications of diabetes during follow-up periods of up to 10 years (Diabetes Control and Complications Trial [DCCT] Research Group, 1993).

Multiple insulin injections (66%) or insulin pumps (34%) were used in the intensively treated group who were trained to modify their therapy depending on frequent glucose monitoring. The conventionally treated groups used no more than two insulin injections, and clinical well-being was the goal with no attempt to modify management based on glycated hemoglobin or their glucose results.

In one-half of the subjects, a mean glycated hemoglobin of 7.2% (normal, < 6%) and a blood glucose of 155 mg/dL was achieved using intensive therapy, while in the conventionally treated group, glycated hemoglobin averaged 8.9% with an average blood glucose of 225 mg/dL. Over the study period, which averaged 7 years, there was an approximately 60% reduction in risk in the tight control group compared with the standard control group in regard to diabetic retinopathy, nephropathy, and neuropathy.

Intensively treated patients had a threefold greater risk of serious hypoglycemia as well as a greater tendency toward weight gain. However, there were no proven deaths from hypoglycemia in any subjects in the DCCT study, and no evidence of posthypoglycemic neurologic damage was detected.

The consensus of the American Diabetes Association is that intensive insulin therapy associated with comprehensive self-management training should become standard therapy in most IDDM patients after the age of puberty. Exceptions include those with advanced renal disease and the elderly, since, in these groups, the detrimental risks of hypoglycemia outweigh the benefit of tight glycemic control. In children under the age of 7 years, the extreme susceptibility of the developing brain to damage from hypoglycemia contraindicates attempts at tight glycemic control, particularly since diabetic complications do not seem to occur until some years after the onset of puberty.

While patients with NIDDM were not studied in the DCCT, there is no reason to believe that the effects of better control of blood glucose levels would not also apply to NIDDM. The eye, kidney, and nerve abnormalities are quite similar in both types of diabetes, and it is likely that similar underlying mechanisms apply. However, weight gain may be greater in obese NIDDM patients receiving intensive insulin therapy, and hypoglycemia may be more hazardous in older patients with NIDDM. For these reasons, common sense and clinical judgment on an individual basis should determine whether intensive insulin therapy is appropriate in NIDDM.

Complications of Insulin Therapy

A. Hypoglycemia:

1. Mechanisms and diagnosis–Hypoglycemic reactions are the most common complication of insulin therapy. They may result from a delay in taking a meal, unusual physical exertion, or a dose of insulin that is too large for immediate needs. With more patients attempting tight control without frequent capillary blood glucose home monitoring, hypoglycemia is likely to become an even more frequent complication.

It has been suggested (Berger et al, 1989) that there is less awareness of hypoglycemia (ie, fewer symptoms are generated) when human insulin rather than pork or beef insulin is used. This would increase the risk of potentially severe hypoglycemic reactions. Considerable controversy has been generated by this claim, and some data (Heine et al, 1989; Kern et al, 1990) give mechanistic support to the clinical impression, while others feel that the claim has not been substantiated. Moreover, preliminary data from the extensive DCCT trial—after more than 53,000 patient months of follow-up—showed no substantive differences in the proportion of patients with asymptomatic hypoglycemia who were using human insulin as compared with those receiving nonhuman insulin (Gorden, 1990). The consensus at present is to continue the use of human insulin while awaiting more definitive data from studies specifically directed at the question.

In older diabetics, in those taking longer-acting insulins (regardless of insulin species), and in those exposed to frequent hypoglycemic episodes during tight glycemic control, autonomic warning signals of hypoglycemia are less frequent, and the manifestations of insulin excess are mainly those of impaired function of the central nervous system, ie, mental confu-

sion, bizarre behavior, and ultimately coma. More rapid development of hypoglycemia from the effects of regular insulin causes signs of autonomic hyperactivity, both sympathetic (tachycardia, palpitations, sweating, tremulousness) and parasympathetic (nausea, hunger), that may progress to convulsions and coma if untreated.

An identification bracelet, necklace, or card in the wallet or purse should be carried by every diabetic who is receiving hypoglycemic drug therapy.

2. Treatment–All of the manifestations of hypoglycemia are rapidly relieved by glucose administration. In a case of mild hypoglycemia in a patient who is conscious and able to swallow, orange juice, glucose, or any sugar-containing beverage or food may be given. If more severe hypoglycemia has produced unconsciousness or stupor, the treatment of choice is to give 20–50 mL of 50% glucose solution by intravenous infusion over a period of 2–3 minutes. If intravenous therapy is not available, 1 mg of glucagon injected either subcutaneously or intramuscularly will usually restore consciousness within 15 minutes to permit ingestion of sugar. Family members or others in the household should be taught how to give glucagon when the need arises. If the patient is stuporous and glucagon is not available, small amounts of honey or syrup can be inserted into the buccal pouch. In general, however, oral feeding is contraindicated in unconscious patients.

B. Immunopathology of Insulin Therapy: At least five molecular classes of insulin antibodies may be produced during the course of insulin therapy in diabetes: IgA, IgD, IgE, IgG, and IgM. There are two major types of immune disorders in these patients:

1. Insulin allergy–Insulin allergy, an immediate type hypersensitivity, is a rare condition in which local or systemic urticaria is due to histamine release from tissue mast cells sensitized by anti-insulin IgE antibodies. In severe cases, anaphylaxis results. A subcutaneous nodule appearing several hours later at the site of insulin injection and lasting for up to 24 hours has been attributed to an IgG-mediated complement-binding Arthus reaction. Because sensitivity is often to noninsulin protein contaminants, the new highly purified insulins have markedly reduced the incidence of insulin allergy, especially local reactions; use of human insulin from the onset of therapy virtually eliminates allergic reactions. When allergy to beef insulin is present, a species change (eg, to pure pork or human insulin) may correct the problem. Antihistamines, corticosteroids, and even desensitization may be required, especially for systemic hypersensitivity. A special kit with serial dilutions of beef or pork insulin for desensitization is available from Eli Lilly.

2. Immune insulin resistance–Most insulin-treated patients develop a low titer of circulating IgG anti-insulin antibodies that neutralize the action of insulin to a small extent. In some diabetic patients, principally those with some degree of tissue insensitivity to insulin (such as occurs in obese diabetics) and a history of interrupted insulin therapy with preparations of less-than-pure beef insulin, a high titer of circulating IgG anti-insulin antibodies develops. This results in extremely high insulin requirements—often more than 200 units daily. With the advent of highly purified insulins, this complication has become exceedingly rare. Switching to a less antigenic (pork or human) purified insulin may make possible a dramatic reduction in insulin dosage or may at least shorten the duration of immune resistance. Other forms of therapy include sulfated beef insulin (a chemically modified form of beef insulin containing an average of six sulfate groups per molecule) and immunosuppression with corticosteroids. In some adults, the foreign insulin can be completely discontinued and the patient maintained on diet alone with oral sulfonylureas. This is possible only when the circulating antibodies do not effectively neutralize the patient's own insulin.

C. Lipodystrophy at Injection Sites: Atrophy of subcutaneous fatty tissue may occur at the site of injection. This type of immune complication has become rare since the development of highly concentrated, pure pork or human insulin preparations of neutral pH. Injection of these preparations directly into the atrophic area often results in restoration of normal contours. Hypertrophy of subcutaneous fatty tissue remains a problem, even with the purified insulins, if injected repeatedly at the same site. However, this is readily corrected with liposuction.

ORAL HYPOGLYCEMIC AGENTS

A large number of substances are capable of modifying insulin release (Table 40–5), including drugs that are useful in the treatment of diabetes. In the USA, the only oral medications currently available for treating hyperglycemia in non-insulin-dependent diabetics are the class of compounds known as sulfonylureas, which increase the release of endogenous insulin as well as improve its peripheral effectiveness. In other countries, a much wider choice of preparations is available, including a second class of compounds, the biguanides, that reduce blood glucose even in the absence of pancreatic B cell function. Biguanides were removed from the market in the USA in 1977 because the use of phenformin was reported to be associated with a relatively high incidence of lactic acidosis. However, clinical trials with metformin, a less toxic biguanide, are currently being completed in

Table 40–5. Regulation of insulin release in humans.[1]

Stimulants of insulin release
  Glucose, mannose
  Leucine
  Vagal stimulation
  Sulfonylureas
Amplifiers of glucose-induced insulin release
  1. Enteric hormones:
    Glucagon-like peptide 1(7–37)
    Gastrin inhibitory polypeptide
    Cholecystokinin
    Secretin, gastrin
  2. Neural amplifiers:
    β-Adrenoceptor stimulation
  3. Amino acids:
    Arginine
Inhibitors of insulin release
  Neural: α-Sympathomimetic effect of catecholamines
  Humoral: Somatostatin
  Drugs: Diazoxide, phenytoin, vinblastine, colchicine

[1]Modified and reproduced, with permission, from Greenspan FS (editor): *Basic & Clinical Endocrinology*, 3rd ed. Lange, 1991.

the USA, and the drug should be available here for clinical use in late 1994. A third class of drugs, the thiazolidinediones, is in early clinical trials.

SULFONYLUREAS

In 1955, sulfonylurea drugs became widely available for treatment of NIDDM. The compounds are arylsulfonylureas with substitutions on the benzene and urea groups. Table 40–6 depicts the chemical structures of the six sulfonylureas used in the USA, including two "second generation" preparations of higher potency.

Mechanism of Action

At least three mechanisms of sulfonylurea action have been proposed: (1) release of insulin from B cells, (2) reduction of serum glucagon levels, and (3) an extrapancreatic effect to potentiate the action of insulin on its target tissues.

A. Insulin Release From Pancreatic B Cells: (Figure 40–2.) Sulfonylureas bind to a specific receptor that is associated with a potassium channel in the B cell membrane. Binding of a sulfonylurea inhibits the efflux of potassium ion through the channel and results in depolarization. Depolarization, in turn, opens a voltage-gated calcium channel and results in calcium influx and the release of preformed insulin. Calcium channel blockers can prevent the action of sulfonylureas in vitro, but it takes calcium blocker concentrations 100–1000 times the usual therapeutic levels to achieve such blockade, probably because the calcium channels associated with B cells are not identical to the L-type calcium channels of the cardiovascular system (see Chapter 12). Moreover, diazoxide,

Table 40–6. Sulfonylureas.

Sulfonylurea	Chemical Structure	Daily Dose	Duration of Action (hours)
Tolbutamide (Orinase)	H_3C—⬡—SO_2—NH—$\overset{O}{\overset{\|}{C}}$—$NH$—$(CH_2)_3$—$CH_3$	0.5–2 g in divided doses	6–12
Tolazamide (Tolinase)	H_3C—⬡—SO_2—NH—$\overset{O}{\overset{\|}{C}}$—$NH$—$N$⬡	0.1–1 g as single dose or in divided doses	10–14
Acetohexamide (Dymelor)	H_3C—$\overset{O}{\overset{\|}{C}}$—⬡—$SO_2$—$NH$—$\overset{O}{\overset{\|}{C}}$—$NH$—⬡	0.25–1.5 g as single dose or in divided doses	12–24
Chlorpropamide (Diabinese)	Cl—⬡—SO_2—NH—$\overset{O}{\overset{\|}{C}}$—$NH$—$(CH_2)_2$—$CH_3$	0.1–0.5 g as single dose	Up to 60
Glyburide (Glibenclamide[1]) (Diaβeta, Micronase)	Cl ... $\overset{O}{\overset{\|}{C}}$—$NH$—$(CH_2)_2$—⬡—$SO_2$—$NH$—$\overset{O}{\overset{\|}{C}}$—$NH$—⬡ ($OCH_3$)	0.00125–0.02 g	10–24
Glipizide (Glydiazinamide[1]) (Glucotrol, Glucotrol XL)	$\overset{O}{\overset{\|}{C}}$—$NH$—$(CH_2)_2$—⬡—$SO_2$—$NH$—$\overset{O}{\overset{\|}{C}}$—$NH$—⬡ ($H_3C$—pyrazine)	0.005–0.03 g	10–24[2]

[1]Outside USA.
[2]Elimination half-life considerably shorter (see text).

a thiazide-like potassium channel opener (see Chapter 11), counteracts the insulinotropic effect of sulfonylureas (as well as that of glucose). This observation also provides one explanation for the hyperglycemic effects of thiazide diuretics.

Insulin synthesis is not stimulated and may even be reduced by sulfonylureas. Release of insulin in response to glucose is enhanced. There is some evidence, however, that after prolonged sulfonylurea therapy, serum insulin levels are no longer increased by the drug and may even be decreased. This observation is complicated by the fact that most such data are obtained from oral glucose tolerance testing—an unphysiologic measure of pancreatic response. After mixed meals containing protein as well as carbohydrate, the beneficial effect of chronic sulfonylurea treatment is generally associated with increased levels of serum insulin.

B. Reduction of Serum Glucagon Concentrations: It is now established that chronic administration of sulfonylureas to non-insulin-dependent diabetics reduces serum glucagon levels. This could contribute to the hypoglycemic effect of the drugs. The mechanism for this suppressive effect of sulfonylureas on glucagon levels is unclear but may involve indirect inhibition due to enhanced release of both insulin and somatostatin, which inhibit A cell secretion.

C. Potentiation of Insulin Action on Target Tissues: There is evidence that increased binding of insulin to tissue receptors occurs during sulfonylurea administration to patients with type II diabetes. As described in Chapter 2, an increase in receptor number can increase the effect achieved with a given concentration of agonist; such an action by the sulfnylureas would potentiate the effect of the patient's low levels of insulin as well as that of exogenous insulin. However, this in vivo effect has not been found to occur when insulin is added in vitro to insulin target tissues. Moreover, in insulin-dependent diabetics with no endogenous insulin secretion, therapy with sulfonylureas has yet to be shown to improve blood glucose control, enhance sensitivity to administered insulin, or increase receptor binding of insulin.

These observations argue strongly against a direct potentiating effect of sulfonylureas on insulin action. Rather, they suggest a secondary beneficial metabolic effect resulting from reduced glycemia or lower fatty acid levels as sulfonylureas increase insulin release.

Efficacy & Safety of the Sulfonylureas

In 1970, the University Group Diabetes Program (UGDP) reported that the number of deaths due to cardiovascular disease in diabetic patients treated with tolbutamide was excessive compared with either insulin-treated patients or those receiving placebos. Controversy persists about the validity of the conclusions reached by the UGDP, because of the heterogeneity of the population studied and certain features of the experimental design such as the use of a fixed dose of tolbutamide. However, in 1984 a package insert warning of a possible increased risk of death due to cardiovascular disease was placed in all sulfonylureas by order of the FDA. Because of doubts about the study and several qualifying statements in the package insert that considerably weaken the impact of the warning, sulfonylureas continue to be widely prescribed.

1. TOLBUTAMIDE

Tolbutamide is well absorbed but rapidly oxidized in the liver. Its duration of effect is relatively short (6–10 hours), and it is therefore the safest sulfonylurea for use in elderly diabetics. Tolbutamide is best administered in divided doses (eg, 500 mg before each meal and at bedtime); however, some patients require only one or two tablets daily. Acute toxic reactions are rare; skin rash occurs infrequently. Prolonged hypoglycemia has been reported rarely, mostly in patients receiving certain drugs (eg, dicumarol, phenylbutazone, or some of the sulfonamides). These drugs apparently compete for oxidative enzymes in the liver, resulting in higher levels of unmetabolized, active tolbutamide in the circulation.

2. CHLORPROPAMIDE

Chlorpropamide has a half-life of 32 hours and is slowly metabolized in the liver to products that retain some biologic activity; approximately 20–30% is excreted unchanged in the urine. Chlorpropamide also interacts with the drugs mentioned above that depend on hepatic oxidative catabolism, and it is contraindicated in patients with hepatic or renal insufficiency. The average maintenance dose is 250 mg daily, given as a single dose in the morning. Prolonged hypoglycemic reactions are more common than with tolbutamide, particularly in elderly patients, in whom chlorpropamide therapy should be monitored with special care. Doses in excess of 500 mg daily increase the risk of jaundice, which is uncommon at lower doses. Patients with a genetic predisposition who are taking chlorpropamide may experience a hyperemic flush when alcohol is ingested. Dilutional hyponatremia has been recognized as a complication of chlorpropamide therapy in some patients. This appears to result from both stimulation of vasopressin secretion and potentiation of its action at the renal tubule by chlorpropamide. The antidiuretic effect of chlorpropamide appears to be independent of the sulfonylurea part of its structure, since three other sulfonylureas (acetohexamide, tolazamide, and glyburide) have diuretic effects in humans. Hematologic toxicity (transient leukopenia, thrombocytopenia) occurs in less than 1% of patients.

3. TOLAZAMIDE

Tolazamide is comparable to chlorpropamide in potency but has a shorter duration of action, similar to that of acetohexamide. Tolazamide is more slowly absorbed than the other sulfonylureas, and its effect on blood glucose does not appear for several hours. Its half-life is about 7 hours. Tolazamide is metabolized to several compounds that retain hypoglycemic effects. If more than 500 mg/d is required, the dose should be divided and given twice daily. Doses larger than 1000 mg daily do not further improve the degree of blood glucose control.

4. ACETOHEXAMIDE

Acetohexamide has a duration of action of 10–16 hours (intermediate between that of tolbutamide and that of chlorpropamide). Therapeutic dosage consists of 0.25–1.5 g daily in one or two doses. The drug is metabolized in the liver to an active metabolite. Adverse effects are similar to those of the other sulfonylurea drugs.

5. SECOND-GENERATION SULFONYLUREAS

Two potent sulfonylurea compounds, glyburide and glipizide, are considered "second-generation" hypoglycemic agents. Initial use of glyburide in other countries was associated with a high rate of severe hypoglycemic reactions and even some deaths, due probably to lack of familiarity with its potent effects. These drugs should be used with caution in patients with cardiovascular disease or in elderly patients, in whom hypoglycemia would be especially dangerous.

Diabetes patients who have not responded to tolbutamide or tolazamide may respond to the more potent first-generation sulfonylurea chlorpropamide or to either of the second-generation sulfonylureas. It has not been established that the second-generation agents are more efficacious than chlorpropamide.

Glyburide is metabolized in the liver into products with very low hypoglycemic activity. Although assays specific for the unmetabolized compound suggest a short plasma half-life, the biologic effects of glyburide are clearly persistent 24 hours after a single morning dose in diabetic patients. The usual starting dose is 2.5 mg/d or less, and the average maintenance dose is 5–10 mg/d given as a single morning dose; maintenance doses higher than 20 mg/d are not recommended. A recently marketed formulation of "micronized" glyburide ("PresTab"), is currently available in tablet sizes of 1.5, 3, 4.5, and 6 mg. However, there is some question as to its bioequivalence as compared with nonmicronized formulations, so that the FDA recommends careful monitoring to retitrate dosage when switching from standard glyburide doses or from other sulfonylurea drugs.

Glyburide has few adverse effects other than its potential for causing hypoglycemia. Flushing has rarely been reported after ethanol ingestion. Glyburide does not cause water retention—as chlorpropamide does—but it slightly enhances free water clearance. Glyburide is particularly contraindicated in the presence of hepatic impairment and in patients with renal insufficiency.

Glipizide has the shortest half-life (2–4 hours) of the more efficacious agents. For maximum effect in reducing postprandial hyperglycemia, this agent should be ingested 30 minutes before breakfast, since rapid absorption is delayed when the drug is taken with food. The recommended starting dose is 5 mg/d, with up to 15 mg/d given as a single daily dose. When higher daily doses are required, they should be divided and given before meals. The maximum recommended dose is 30 mg/d. Recently an extended release preparation has been formulated (Glucotiol XL) that provides 24 hour action after a once-daily morning dose.

Because of its shorter half-life, glipizide is much less likely than glyburide to produce serious hypoglycemia. At least 90% of glipizide is metabolized in the liver to inactive products, and 10% is excreted unchanged in the urine. Glipizide therapy is therefore contraindicated in patients with hepatic or renal impairment, who would therefore be at high risk for hypoglycemia.

6. SECONDARY FAILURE TO SULFONYLUREAS & TACHYPHYLAXIS

Secondary failure (ie, failure to maintain a good response to sulfonylurea therapy) remains a disconcerting problem in the management of type II diabetes. While the inability to maintain dietary compliance may be responsible for many of these cases, it is possible that multiple-dose conventional therapy which produces sustained blood levels of long-acting sulfonylureas may induce a refractoriness in responding pancreatic B cells. This phenomenon has been observed during short-term studies of sulfonylurea-induced insulin release and has suggested clinical trials of intermittent or pulse therapy with sulfonylureas in which a single daily dose of a short-acting sulfonylurea is prescribed.

7. COMBINED THERAPY WITH SULFONYLUREAS & INSULIN

Since sulfonylurea drugs not only increase the pancreatic B cell secretion of insulin but also might restore peripheral tissue sensitivity to insulin, their use with insulin has been advocated to reduce the total insulin dose required to control hyperglycemia. Moreover, nighttime NPH insulin has been suggested as an adjunct to sulfonylurea therapy in those NIDDM patients who fail to respond adequately to maximal sulfonylurea dosage. Currently, however, data from clinical trials with appropriate controls and crossover studies are too limited to justify the expense of prescribing both insulin and sulfonylureas to treat NIDDM. However, if a patient fails to respond to more than 100 units of insulin per day, a trial of sulfonylureas with insulin has been preferred over continued increases in the total insulin dose.

BIGUANIDES

The structure of biguanides is shown in Table 40–7. Phenformin was discontinued in the USA because of its association with lactic acidosis and because there was no documentation of any long-term benefit from its use. Metformin, buformin, and phenformin continue to be used elsewhere, though in some areas the indications for biguanide therapy are being reevaluated. Clinical trials of metformin are currently nearing completion in the USA.

Mechanisms of Action

A full explanation of the biguanides' mechanism of action remains elusive. Their blood glucose-lowering action does not depend on the presence of functioning pancreatic B cells. Glucose is not lowered in normal subjects after an overnight fast, but postprandial

Table 40–7. Biguanides.

Biguanide $H_2N-C\underset{\overset{\|}{NH}}{C}\underset{\overset{\|}{NH}}{C}-R$		Daily Dose	Duration of Action (hours)
Phenformin (DBI, Meltrol-50)[1]	$-NH-(CH_2)_2-$⬡	0.025–0.15 g as single dose or in divided doses	4–6 8–14[2]
Buformin[1]	$-NH-(CH_2)_3-CH_3$	0.05–0.3 g in divided doses	10–12
Metformin[1]	$-N-(CH_3)_2$	1–3 g in divided doses	10–12

[1]In clinical use outside USA.
[2]Timed-disintegration capsules.

blood glucose levels are considerably lower during phenformin administration. Patients with NIDDM have considerably less fasting hyperglycemia as well as lower postprandial hyperglycemia after biguanides; however, hypoglycemia during biguanide therapy is essentially unknown. These agents might therefore be more appropriately termed "euglycemic" rather than hypoglycemic agents. Currently proposed mechanisms of action include (1) direct stimulation of glycolysis in peripheral tissues, with increased glucose removal from blood; (2) reduced hepatic gluconeogenesis; (3) slowing of glucose absorption from the gastrointestinal tract; (4) reduction of plasma glucagon levels; and (5) increased insulin binding to insulin receptors.

Metabolism & Excretion

Phenformin is bound to plasma protein, and therapeutic plasma levels range from 100 to 250 ng/mL. The half-life is approximately 11 hours. Phenformin is about one-third metabolized; the remainder is excreted unchanged in the urine. In patients with renal insufficiency, phenformin accumulates and thereby increases the risk of lactic acidosis, which appears to be a dose-related complication. Metformin is not metabolized and is excreted by the kidneys as the active compound. Lactic acidosis occurs with less frequency in patients treated with metformin compared with those treated with phenformin.

Clinical Use

Biguanides have been most often prescribed for patients with refractory obesity whose hyperglycemia is due to ineffective insulin action. Another indication for their use is in combination with sulfonylureas in non-insulin-dependent diabetics in whom sulfonylurea therapy alone is inadequate.

Biguanides are contraindicated in patients with renal disease, alcoholism, hepatic disease, or conditions predisposing to tissue anoxia (eg, chronic cardiopulmonary dysfunction), because of an increased risk of

lactic acidosis induced by these drugs (especially phenformin) in the presence of these diseases.

In the UGDP study, phenformin given in a dosage of 100 mg daily showed minimal therapeutic advantages in comparison with a control group of placebo-treated patients. A slight increase in heart rate and blood pressure was noted in the phenformin-treated diabetics, and an increased risk of cardiovascular mortality was reported.

The most frequent toxic effects of metformin are gastrointestinal (anorexia, nausea, vomiting, abdominal discomfort, diarrhea) and occur in up to 20% of patients. They are dose related, tend to occur at the onset of therapy, and are often transient. However, use of metformin may have to be discontinued in 3–5% of patients because of persistent diarrhea.

THIAZOLIDINEDIONE DERIVATIVES

This new class of oral antidiabetic drugs is presently undergoing clinical trials. The primary mechanism appears to be increased target tissue sensitivity to insulin. Animal studies have documented that these drugs potentiate the action of insulin to increase glucose uptake and glucose oxidation in both muscle and adipose tissue, while reducing hepatic glucose output as well as lipid synthesis in muscle and fat cells. These effects occur in vivo without any increase in insulin release (Hofman, 1992; Suter et al, 1992). Included in this class of drugs are ciglitazone, pioglitazone, englitazone, and CS-045. A recent report (Suter et al, 1992) demonstrated the efficacy of CS-045 during a trial of up to 12 weeks in which it lowered insulin resistance, reduced insulinemia, and improved both fasting and postprandial hyperglycemia in NIDDM subjects. Since insulin resistance and hyperinsulinism are considered by some to contribute to the presence of hypertension, hyperlipidemia, and atherosclerosis (Reaven, 1988), this class of agents would seem to offer a welcome therapeutic option for NIDDM therapy.

GLUCAGON

Chemistry & Metabolism

Glucagon is synthesized in the A cells of the pancreatic islets of Langerhans (Table 40–1). Glucagon is a polypeptide—identical in all mammals—consisting of a single chain of 29 amino acids (Figure 40–6), with a molecular weight of 3485. Selective proteolytic cleavage converts a large precursor molecule of approximately 18,000 MW to glucagon. One of the precursor intermediates consists of a 69-amino-acid polypeptide called **glicentin,** which contains the glucagon sequence interposed between peptide extensions.

Glucagon is extensively degraded in the liver and kidney as well as in plasma, and at its tissue receptor sites. Because of its rapid inactivation by plasma, chilling of the collecting tubes and addition of inhibitors of proteolytic enzymes are necessary when samples of blood are collected for immunoassay of circulating glucagon. Its half-life in plasma is between 3 and 6 minutes, which is similar to that of insulin.

"Gut Glucagon"

Glicentin immunoreactivity has been found in cells of the small intestine as well as in pancreatic A cells and in effluents of perfused pancreas. The intestinal cells secrete **enteroglucagon,** a family of glucagon-like polypeptides, of which glicentin is a member, along with glucagon-like peptides 1 and 2 (GLP-1 and GLP-2). Unlike the pancreatic A cell, these intestinal cells lack the enzymes to convert glucagon precursors to true glucagon by removing the carboxyl terminal extension from the molecule.

The function of the enteroglucagons has not been clarified, though smaller peptides can bind hepatic glucagon receptors where they exert partial activity. A derivative of the 37-amino-acid form of GLP-1 that lacks the first six amino acids (GLP-1[7–37]) is a potent stimulant of insulin release. It represents the predominant form of GLP in the human intestine and has been termed "insulinotropin."

Pharmacologic Effects of Glucagon

A. Metabolic Effects: The first six amino acids at the amino terminal of the glucagon molecule bind to specific receptors on liver cells. This leads to a G protein-linked increase in adenylyl cyclase activity and the production of cAMP, which facilitates catabolism of stored glycogen and increases gluconeogenesis and ketogenesis. The immediate pharmacologic result of glucagon infusion is to raise blood glucose at the expense of stored hepatic glycogen. There is no effect on skeletal muscle glycogen, presumably because of the lack of glucagon receptors on skeletal muscle. Pharmacologic amounts of glucagon cause release of insulin from normal pancreatic B cells, catecholamines from pheochromocytoma, and calcitonin from medullary carcinoma cells.

B. Cardiac Effects: Glucagon has a potent inotropic and chronotropic effect on the heart, mediated by the cAMP mechanism described above. Thus, it produces an effect very similar to that of beta-adrenoceptor agonists without requiring functioning beta receptors.

C. Effects on Smooth Muscle: Large doses of glucagon produce profound relaxation of the intestine. In contrast to the above effects of the peptide, this action on the intestine may be due to mechanisms other than adenylyl cyclase activation.

Clinical Uses

A. Severe Hypoglycemia: The major use of glucagon is for emergency treatment of severe hypoglycemic reactions in insulin-dependent patients when unconsciousness precludes oral feedings. It is currently available for parenteral use (Glucagon Emergency Kit). Nasal sprays have been developed for this purpose and are presently undergoing clinical trials.

B. Endocrine Diagnosis: Several diagnostic tests use glucagon to diagnose endocrine pathophysiologic processes. In patients with insulin-dependent diabetes mellitus, a standard test of pancreatic B cell secretory reserve utilizes 1 mg of glucagon administered as an intravenous bolus. Since insulin-treated patients develop circulating anti-insulin antibodies that interfere with radioimmunoassays of insulin, measurements of C-peptide are used to indicate B cell secretion. Normal persons achieve a standard serum concentration of pancreatic C-peptide within 10 minutes after injection, and in insulin-treated diabetics

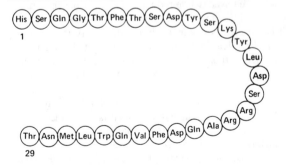

Figure 40–6. Amino acid sequence of glucagon polypeptide.

various degrees of B cell insufficiency can be quantitated. Most diabetics with long-standing IDDM show no C-peptide response to glucagon.

In patients with suspected endocrine tumors such as insulinoma, pheochromocytoma, or medullary carcinoma of the thyroid, a bolus of 0.5–1 mg of glucagon intravenously is occasionally effective in discharging hormonal products from a tumor, though negative tests may not rule out the diagnosis.

C. Beta-Blocker Poisoning: Glucagon is sometimes useful for reversing the cardiac effects of an overdose of beta-blocking agents because of its ability to increase cAMP production in the heart. However, it is not clinically useful in the treatment of congestive cardiac failure.

D. Radiology of the Bowel: Glucagon has been used extensively in radiology as an aid to x-ray visualization of the bowel because of its ability to relax the intestine.

Adverse Reactions

Transient nausea and occasional vomiting can result from glucagon administration. These are generally mild, and glucagon is relatively free of severe adverse reactions.

ISLET AMYLOID POLYPEPTIDE (IAPP, Amylin)

IAPP is a 37-amino-acid polypeptide originally derived from islet amyloid deposits in pancreas material from patients with long-standing NIDDM or insulinomas. It is produced by pancreatic B cells, packaged within B cell granules in a concentration 1–2% that of insulin, and secreted in response to B cell secretagogues. A physiologic effect has not been established; however, pharmacologic doses inhibit the action of insulin to promote muscle uptake of glucose. IAPP appears to be a member of the superfamily of neuroregulatory peptides, with 46% homology with the calcitonin gene-related polypeptide CGRP (see Chapter 17). Whereas CGRP inhibits insulin secretion, this has not been demonstrated at physiologic concentrations of IAPP. Clinical trials are planned to evaluate IAPP as an adjunct to insulin therapy in type I diabetic patients with recurrent episodes of severe insulin-induced hypoglycemia—episodes that are generally refractory to usual preventive measures.

PREPARATIONS AVAILABLE
(See Table 40–4 for insulin preparations.)

Sulfonylureas
Acetohexamide (generic, Dymelor)
Oral: 250, 500 mg tablets
Chlorpropamide (generic, Diabinese)
Oral: 100, 250 mg tablets
Glipizide (Glucotrol, Glucotrol XL)
Oral: 5, 10 mg tablets; 5, 10 mg extended release tablets
Glyburide (DiaβetA, Micronase, Glynase PresTab)
Oral: 1.25, 2.5, 5 mg tablets; 1.5, 3, 4.5, 6 mg "PresTab" tablets

Tolazamide (generic, Tolinase)
Oral: 100, 250, 500 mg tablets
Tolbutamide (generic, Orinase)
Oral: 250, 500 mg tablets

Glucagon
Glucagon (generic)
Parenteral: 1, 10 mg lyophilized powders to reconstitute for injection

REFERENCES

Bailey CJ: Biguanides and NIDDM. Diabetes Care 1992; 15:755.

Berger M et al: Absorption kinetics and biologic effects of subcutaneously injected insulin preparations. Diabetes Care 1982;5:77.

Binder C et al: Insulin pharmacokinetics. Diabetes Care 1984;7:188.

Bloom SR, Polak JM: Somatostatin. Br Med J 1987;295: 288.

Boyd AE III: Sulfonylurea receptors, ion channels, and fruit flies. Diabetes 1988;37:847.

Brange J et al: Monomeric insulins and their experimental and clinical implications. Diabetes Care 1990;13:923.

Bressler R, Johnson D: New pharmacological approaches to therapy of NIDDM. Diabetes Care 1992;15:792.

Charron MJ, Kahn BB: Divergent molecular mechanisms for insulin-resistant glucose transport in muscle and adipose cells in vivo. J Biol Chem 1990;265:7994.

Conlon JM: Proglucagon derived polypeptides: Nomenclature, biosynthetic relationships, and physiologic roles. Diabetologia 1988;31:563.

Diabetes Control and Complications Trial Research Group: Epidemiology of severe hypoglycemia in the diabetes control and complications trial. Am J Med 1991;90:450.

Diabetes Control and Complications Trial Research Group: The effect of intensive treatment of diabetes on the development and progression of long-term complications in insulin-dependent diabetes mellitus. N Engl J Med 1993;329:977.

Galloway JA et al: Biosynthetic human proinsulin: review of chemistry, in vitro and in vivo receptor binding, animal and human pharmacology studies, and clinical trial experience. Diabetes Care 1992;15:666.

Genuth S: Management of the adult onset diabetic with sulfonylurea failure. Endocrinol Metab Clin North Am 1992;21:351.

Gorden P: Human insulin use and hypoglycemia. (Letter.) N Engl J Med 1990;322:1007.

Groop L et al: Comparison of pharmacokinetics, metabolic effects and mechanisms of action of glyburide and glipizide during long-term treatment. Diabetes Care 1987; 10:671.

Heine RJ et al: Responses to human and porcine insulin in healthy subjects. Lancet 1989;2:946.

Hermann LS: Biguanides and sulfonylureas as combination therapy in NIDDM. Diabetes Care 1990;13(Suppl 3):37.

Hirsch IB, Farkas-Hirsch R, Skyler JS: Intensive insulin therapy for treatment of type I diabetes mellitus. Diabetes Care 1990;13:1265.

Hofman CA, Colca JR: New oral thiazolidinedione antidiabetic agents act as insulin sensitizers. Diabetes Care 1992;15:1075.

Kadowaki T et al: Chlorpropamide-induced hyponatremia: Incidence and risk factors. Diabetes Care 1983;6:468.

Kang S et al: Subcutaneous insulin absorption explained by insulin's physicochemical properties. Diabetes Care 1991;14:942.

Karam JH: Type II diabetes and syndrome X: Pathogenesis and glycemic management. Endocrinol Metab Clin North Am 1992;21:329.

Kasanicki MA, Pilch PF: Regulation of glucose transporter function. Diabetes Care 1990;13:219.

Kern W et al: Differential effects of human and pork insulin-induced hypoglycemia on neuronal functions in humans. Diabetes 1990;39:1091.

Klip A, Leitner L: Cellular mechanism of action of metformin. Diabetes Care 1990;13:696.

Klonoff DC: Association of hyperinsulinemia with chlorpropamide toxicity. Am J Med 1988;84:33.

Lane MD et al: Insulin-receptor tyrosine kinase and glucose transport. Diabetes Care 1990;13:565.

Lebovitz HE, Melander A (editors): Sulfonylurea drugs: Basic and clinical considerations. Diabetes Care 1990;13 (Suppl 3):1.

Lebovitz HE (editor): Therapy for Diabetes Mellitus and Related Disorders. American Diabetes Association, 1991.

Lipton R et al: Cyclosporin therapy for prevention and cure of IDDM: Epidemiologic perspective of benefits and risks. Diabetes Care 1990;13:776.

Malaisse WJ, Lebrun P: Mechanisms of sulfonylurea-induced insulin release. Diabetes Care 1990;13(Suppl 3):9.

Maran A et al: Double blind clinical and laboratory study of

hypoglycaemia with human and porcine insulin in diabetic patients reporting hypoglycaemia unawareness after transferring to human insulin. Br Med J 1993;306:167

Miller JL et al: Bedtime insulin added to daytime sulfonylureas improves glycemic control in uncontrolled type II diabetes. Clin Pharmacol Ther 1993;53:380.

Moller DE, Flier JS: Insulin resistance: Mechanism, syndromes, and implications. N Engl J Med 1991;325:938.

Muhlhauer I et al: Hypoglycemic symptoms and frequency of severe hypoglycemia in patients treated with human and animal insulin preparations. Diabetes Care 1991;14: 745.

Muhlhauser I, Koch J, Berger M: Pharmacokinetics and bioavailability of injected glucagon: Differences between intramuscular, subcutaneous, and intravenous administration. Diabetes Care 1984;8:39.

Nathan DM, Roussell A, Godine JE: Glyburide or insulin for metabolic control in non-insulin-dependent diabetes mellitus: A randomized, double-blind study. Ann Intern Med 1988;108:334.

Nolte MS et al: Biological activity of nasally administered insulin in normal subjects. Hormone Metab Res 1990; 22:170.

Nolte MS: Insulin therapy in insulin-dependent (type I) diabetes mellitus. Endocrinol Metab Clin North Am 1992; 21:281.

Olson PO, Hans A, Henning VS: Miscibility of human semisynthetic regular and lente insulin and human biosynthetic regular and NPH insulin. Diabetes Care 1987; 10:473.

Pilch PF, Waugh SM, O'Hare T: The structural basis for insulin receptor function. In: Advances in Regulation of Cell Growth, vol 1: Regulation of Cell Growth and Activation. Mond JJ, Cambier JC, Weiss A (editors). Raven Press, 1989.

Pontiroli AE, Alberetto M, Pozza G: Intranasal glucagon raises blood glucose concentrations in healthy volunteers. Br Med J 1983;287:462.

Rasmussen H et al: Physiology and pathophysiology of insulin secretion. Diabetes Care 1990;13:655.

Reaven GM: Role of insulin resistance in human disease. Diabetes 1988;37:1595.

Samols E, Bonner-Weir S, Weir GC: Intra-islet insulin-glucagon-somatostatin relationships. Clin Endocrinol Metab 1986;15:33.

Selam JL, Charles MA: Devices for insulin administration. Diabetes Care 1990;13:955.

Simonson DC et al: Effect of glyburide on glycemic control, insulin requirement, and glucose metabolism in insulin-treated diabetic patients. Diabetes 1987;36:136.

Stevenson RW et al: Similar dose responsiveness of hepatic glycogenolysis and gluconeogenesis to glucagon in vivo. Diabetes 1987;36:382.

Suter SL et al: Metabolic effects of new oral hypoglycemic agent CS-045 in NIDDM subjects. Diabetes Care 1992; 15:193.

Unger RH: Diabetic hyperglycemia: Link to impaired glucose transport in pancreatic β cells. Science 1991;251: 1200.

Westermark P et al: Islet amyloid polypeptide: A novel controversy in diabetes research. Diabetologia 1992;35:297.

Wu MS et al: Effect of metformin on carbohydrate and lipoprotein metabolism in NIDDM patients. Diabetes Care 1990;13:1.

Agents That Affect Bone Mineral Homeostasis

41

Daniel D. Bikle, MD, PhD

I. BASIC PHARMACOLOGY

Calcium and phosphate, the major mineral constituents of bone, are also two of the most important minerals for general cellular function. Accordingly, the body has evolved a complex set of mechanisms by which calcium and phosphate homeostasis are carefully maintained (Figure 41–1). Approximately 98% of the 1–2 kg of calcium and 85% of the 1 kg of phosphorus in the human adult are found in bone, the principal reservoir for these minerals. These functions are dynamic, with constant remodeling of bone and ready exchange of bone mineral with that in the extracellular fluid. Bone also serves as the principal structural support for the body and provides the space for hematopoiesis. Thus, abnormalities in bone mineral homeostasis can lead not only to a wide variety of cellular dysfunctions (eg, tetany, coma, muscle weakness) but also to disturbances in structural support of the body (eg, osteoporosis with fractures) and loss of hematopoietic capacity (eg, infantile osteopetrosis).

Calcium and phosphate enter the body from the intestine. The average American diet provides 600–1000 mg of calcium per day, of which approximately 100–250 mg is absorbed. This figure represents net absorption, since both absorption (principally in the duodenum and upper jejunum) and secretion (principally in the ileum) occur. The amount of phosphorus in the American diet is about the same as that of calcium. However, the efficiency of absorption (principally in the jejunum) is greater, ranging from 70% to 90% depending on intake. In the steady state, renal excretion of calcium and phosphate balances intestinal absorption. In general, over 98% of filtered calcium and 85% of filtered phosphate is reabsorbed by the kidney. The movement of calcium and phosphate across the intestinal and renal epithelia is closely regulated. Intrinsic disease of the intestine (eg, nontropical sprue) or kidney (eg, chronic renal failure) disrupts bone mineral homeostasis.

Two hormones serve as the principal regulators of calcium and phosphate homeostasis: the polypeptide parathyroid hormone (PTH) and the steroid vitamin D. Vitamin D is a prohormone rather than a true hormone, since it must be further metabolized to gain biologic activity. Other hormones—calcitonin, prolactin, growth hormone, insulin, thyroid hormone, glucocorticoids, and sex steroids—influence calcium and phosphate homeostasis under certain physiologic circumstances and can be considered secondary regulators. Deficiency or excess of these secondary regulators within a physiologic range does not produce the disturbance of calcium and phosphate homeostasis observed in situations of deficiency or excess of PTH and vitamin D. However, certain of these secondary regulators—especially calcitonin, glucocorticoids, and estrogens—are useful therapeutically and will be discussed in subsequent sections.

In addition to these hormonal regulators, calcium and phosphate themselves, other ions such as sodium and fluoride, and a variety of drugs (bisphosphonates, plicamycin, and diuretics) also alter calcium and phosphate homeostasis.

PRINCIPAL HORMONAL REGULATORS OF BONE MINERAL HOMEOSTASIS

PARATHYROID HORMONE

Parathyroid hormone (PTH) is a single-chain polypeptide hormone composed of 84 amino acids. It is produced in the parathyroid gland in a precursor form of 115 amino acids, the remaining 31 amino terminal amino acids being cleaved off prior to secretion. Within the gland is a calcium-sensitive protease capable of cleaving the intact hormone into fragments. Biologic activity resides in the amino terminal region such that synthetic 1–34 PTH is fully active.

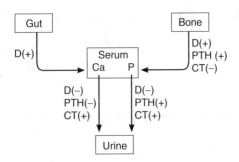

Figure 41–1. Some mechanisms contributing to bone mineral homeostasis. Calcium and phosphorus concentrations in the serum are controlled principally by two hormones, 1,25(OH)$_2$D$_3$ (D) and parathyroid hormone (PTH), through their action on absorption from the gut and from bone and on excretion in the urine. Both hormones increase input of calcium and phosphorus from bone into the serum; vitamin D also increases absorption from the gut. Vitamin D decreases urinary excretion of both calcium and phosphorus, while PTH reduces calcium but increases phosphorus excretion. Calcitonin (CT) is a less critical hormone for calcium homeostasis, but in pharmacologic concentrations CT can reduce serum calcium and phosphorus by inhibiting bone resorption and stimulating their renal excretion. Feedback effects are not shown.

Loss of the first two amino terminal amino acids eliminates most biologic activity.

The metabolic clearance rate of intact PTH in dogs has been estimated to be 20 mL/min/kg, with a half-time of disappearance measured in minutes. Most of the clearance occurs in the liver and kidney. The biologically inactive carboxyl terminal fragments produced during metabolism of the intact hormone have a much lower clearance rate, especially in renal failure. This accounts in part for the very high PTH values often observed in the past in patients with renal failure when measured by radioimmunoassays directed against the carboxyl terminal region of the molecule. However, most PTH assays currently in use measure the intact hormone by a double antibody method, so that this circumstance is less frequently encountered in clinical practice. The appearance of amino terminal fragments of PTH in the blood is difficult to demonstrate—consistent with the observation that only small amounts of such fragments are released into the blood and that their clearance is high.

PTH regulates calcium and phosphate flux across cellular membranes in bone and kidney, resulting in increased serum calcium and decreased serum phosphate. In bone, PTH increases the activity and number of osteoclasts, the cells responsible for bone resorption. However, it appears that this stimulation of osteoclasts is not a direct effect. Rather, PTH acts on the osteoblast (the bone-forming cell) and the

osteoblast somehow regulates the activity of the osteoclast. This action increases bone turnover or bone remodeling, a specific sequence of cellular events initiated by osteoclastic bone resorption and followed by osteoblastic bone formation. In addition, PTH stimulates the differentiation of osteoclast precursors to osteoclasts, thus increasing the number of osteoclasts. Although both bone resorption and bone formation are enhanced by PTH, the net effect of excess PTH is to increase bone resorption. PTH in low doses may actually increase bone formation without first stimulating bone resorption. Although cAMP is involved in the action of PTH on bone cells, other mediators (including calcium) probably play a role.

In the kidney, PTH increases the ability of the nephron to reabsorb calcium and magnesium but reduces its ability to reabsorb phosphate, amino acids, bicarbonate, sodium, chloride, and sulfate. Although PTH markedly stimulates the renal production and excretion of cAMP and cAMP reproduces a number of the renal actions of PTH, cAMP may not be the sole mediator of PTH action on the kidney. Another important action of PTH on the kidney is its stimulation of 1,25-dihydroxyvitamin D (1,25[OH]$_2$D) production.

Recent evidence has called attention to vasoactive and cardiotropic actions of PTH. These observations may explain the ability of PTH to increase the glomerular filtration rate acutely. Whether such actions are involved in the apparent association of hyperparathyroidism and hypertension remains to be determined.

Recently, a peptide containing the first 34 amino acids of PTH has become available for biologic testing. This material is currently being evaluated as a treatment for osteoporosis.

VITAMIN D

Vitamin D is a secosteroid produced in the skin from 7-dehydrocholesterol under the influence of ultraviolet irradiation. Vitamin D is also found in certain foods and is used to supplement dairy products. Both the natural form (vitamin D$_3$, cholecalciferol) and the plant-derived form (vitamin D$_2$, ergocalciferol) are present in the diet. These forms differ in that ergocalciferol contains a double bond (C22–23) and an additional methyl group in the side chain (Figure 41–2). In humans this difference apparently is of little physiologic consequence, and the following comments apply equally well to both forms of vitamin D.

Vitamin D is a prohormone that serves as precursor to a number of biologically active metabolites (Figure 41–2). Vitamin D is first hydroxylated in the liver to form 25-hydroxyvitamin D (25[OH]D). This metabolite is further converted in the kidney to a number of other forms, the best-studied of which are 1,25-dihydroxyvitamin D (1,25[OH]$_2$D) and 24,25-dihydroxy-

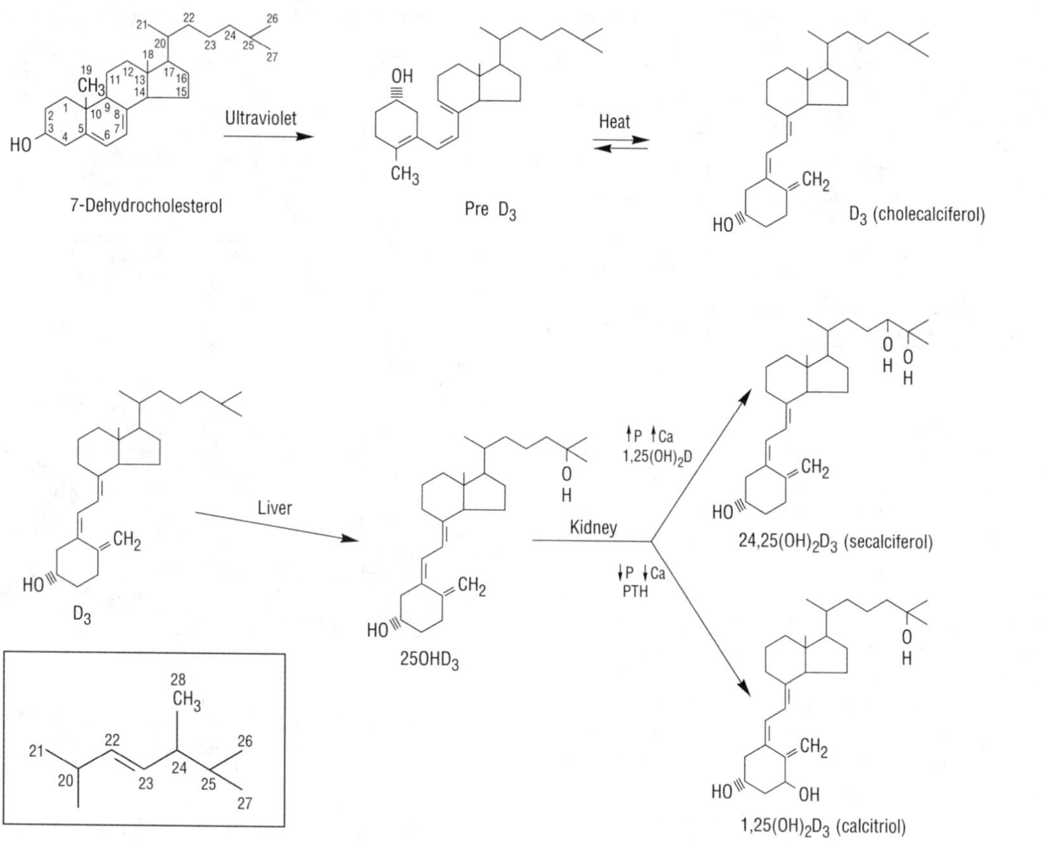

Figure 41–2. Conversion of 7-dehydrocholesterol to vitamin D_3 and metabolism of D_3 to $1,25(OH)_2D_3$ and $24,25(OH)_2D_3$. Control of the latter step is exerted primarily at the level of the kidney, where low serum phosphorus, low serum calcium, and high parathyroid hormone favor the production of $1,25(OH)_2D_3$. The inset shows the side chain for ergosterol. Ergosterol undergoes similar transformation to vitamin D_2 (ergocalciferol), which, in turn, is metabolized to $25OHD_2$, $1,25(OH)_2D_2$, and $24,25(OH)_2D_2$. In humans, corresponding D_2 and D_3 derivatives have equivalent effects and potency. They are therefore referred to in the text without a subscript.

vitamin D $(24,25[OH]_2D)$. Of the natural metabolites, only vitamin D, $25(OH)D$ (as calcifediol), and $1,25(OH)_2D$ (as calcitriol), are available for clinical use (see Table 41–1), though clinical studies with $24,25(OH)_2D$ are under way. Moreover, a number of analogues of $1,25(OH)_2$ are being synthesized in an effort to extend the usefulness of this metabolite to a variety of nonclassic conditions. Calcipotriol, for example, is currently being used to treat psoriasis, a hyperproliferative skin disorder. The regulation of vitamin D metabolism is complex, involving calcium, phosphate, and a variety of hormones, the most important of which is PTH.

Vitamin D and its metabolites circulate in plasma tightly bound to a carrier protein, the vitamin D-binding protein. This α-globulin binds $25(OH)D$ and $24,25(OH)_2D$ with comparable high affinity and vitamin D and $1,25(OH)_2D$ with lower affinity. In normal subjects, the terminal half-life of injected calcifediol is 23 days, whereas in anephric subjects it is longer

(42 days). The half-life of $24,25(OH)_2D$ is probably similar. Tracer studies with vitamin D have shown a rapid clearance from the blood. The liver appears to be the principal organ for clearance. Excess vitamin D is stored in adipose tissue. The metabolic clearance rate of calcitriol in humans indicates a rapid turnover, with a terminal half-life measured in hours. Several of the $1,25(OH)_2$ analogues are bound poorly by the vitamin D-binding protein. As a result, their clearance is very rapid, with a terminal half-life measured in minutes. Such analogues have little of the hypercalcemic, hypercalciuric effects of calcitriol, an important aspect of their use for the management of conditions such as psoriasis.

The mechanism of action of the vitamin D metabolites remains under active investigation. However, calcitriol is well established as the most potent agent with respect to stimulation of intestinal calcium and phosphate transport and bone resorption. Calcitriol appears to act on the intestine both by induction of

Table 41–1. Vitamin D and its clinically available metabolites and analogues.

Chemical Name	Abbreviation	Generic Name
Vitamin D_3	D_3	Cholecalciferol
Vitamin D_2	D_2	Ergocalciferol
25-Hydroxyvitamin D_3	$25(OH)D_3$	Calciferol
1,25-Dihydroxy-vitamin D_3	$1,25(OH)_2D_3$	Calcitriol
24,25-Dihydroxy-vitamin D_3	$24,25(OH)_2D_3$	Secalcifediol
Dihydrotachysterol	DHT	Dihydrotachysterol

Table 41–2. Actions of PTH and vitamin D on gut, bone, and kidney.

	PTH	Vitamin D
Intestine	Increased calcium and phosphate absorption (by increased $1,25[OH]_2D$ production).	Increased calcium and phosphate absorption (by $1,25[OH]_2D$).
Kidney	Decreased calcium excretion, increased phosphate excretion.	Calcium and phosphate excretion may be decreased by $25(OH)D$ and $1,25(OH)_2D$.
Bone	Calcium and phosphate resorption increased by high doses. Low doses may increase bone formation.	Increased calcium and phosphate resorption by $1,25(OH)_2D$. Bone formation may be increased by $24,25(OH)_2D$.
Net effect on serum levels	Serum calcium increased, serum phosphate decreased.	Serum calcium and phosphate both increased.

new proteins (eg, calcium-binding protein) and by modulation of calcium flux across the brush border and mitochondrial membranes by a means that does not require new protein synthesis. The molecular action of calcitriol on bone has received less attention. The metabolites $25(OH)D$ and $24,25(OH)_2D$ are far less potent stimulators of intestinal calcium and phosphate transport or bone resorption. However, $25(OH)D$ appears to be more potent than $1,25(OH)_2D$ in stimulating renal reabsorption of calcium and phosphate and may be the major metabolite regulating calcium flux and contractility in muscle. Recent evidence suggests that $24,25(OH)_2D$ stimulates bone formation. Specific receptors for $1,25(OH)_2D$ exist in target tissues. However, the role and even the existence of receptors for $25(OH)D$ and $24,25(OH)_2D$ remain controversial.

INTERACTION OF PTH & VITAMIN D

A summary of the principal actions of PTH and vitamin D on the three main target tissues—intestine, kidney, and bone—is presented in Table 41–2. The net effect of PTH is to raise serum calcium and reduce serum phosphate; the net effect of vitamin D is to raise both. Regulation of calcium and phosphate homeostasis is achieved through a variety of feedback loops. Calcium is the principal regulator of PTH secretion. It binds to a novel ion recognition site that is part of a G_q protein-coupled receptor which links changes in intracellular free calcium concentration to changes in extracellular calcium. As serum calcium levels rise and bind to this receptor, intracellular calcium levels increase and inhibit PTH secretion. Phosphate regulates PTH secretion indirectly, by forming complexes with calcium in the serum. Since it is the ionized concentration of calcium that is detected by the parathyroid gland, increases in serum phosphate levels reduce the ionized calcium and lead to enhanced PTH secretion. Such feedback regulation is appropriate to the net effect of PTH to raise serum calcium and reduce serum phosphate levels. Likewise, both calcium and phosphate at high levels reduce the amount of $1,25(OH)_2D$ produced by the kidney and increase the amount of $24,25(OH)_2D$ produced. Since $1,25(OH)_2D$ raises serum calcium and phosphate, whereas $24,25(OH)_2D$ has less effect, such feedback regulation is again appropriate. $1,25(OH)_2D$ itself directly inhibits PTH secretion (independently of its effect on serum calcium) by a direct action on PTH gene transcription. This provides yet another negative feedback loop, because PTH is a major stimulus for $1,25(OH)_2D$ production. This ability of $1,25(OH)_2D$ to inhibit PTH secretion directly is being evaluated using calcitriol analogues that do not raise serum calcium. Such drugs are likely to prove useful in the management of secondary hyperparathyroidism accompanying renal failure or even in selected cases of primary hyperparathyroidism.

SECONDARY HORMONAL REGULATORS OF BONE MINERAL HOMEOSTASIS

A number of hormones modulate the actions of PTH and vitamin D in regulating bone mineral homeostasis. Compared with that of PTH and vitamin D, the physiologic impact of such secondary regulation on bone mineral homeostasis is minor. However, in pharmacologic amounts, a number of these hormones have actions on the bone mineral homeostatic mechanisms that can be exploited therapeutically.

CALCITONIN

The calcitonin secreted by the parafollicular cells of the mammalian thyroid (and by piscine ultimobranchial bodies) is a single-chain polypeptide hormone with 32 amino acids and a molecular weight of 3600. A disulfide bond between positions 1 and 7 is essential for biologic activity. Calcitonin is produced in these glands from a precursor with MW 15,000. The circulating forms of calcitonin are multiple, ranging in size from the monomer (MW 3600) to forms with an apparent molecular weight of 60,000. Whether such heterogeneity includes precursor forms or covalently linked oligomers is not known. Because of its heterogeneity, calcitonin is standardized by bioassay in rats. Activity is compared to a standard maintained by the British Medical Research Council (MRC) and expressed as MRC units.

Human calcitonin monomer has a half-life of about 10 minutes with a metabolic clearance rate of 8–9 mL/kg/min. Salmon calcitonin has a longer half-life and a reduced metabolic clearance rate (3 mL/kg/min). Much of the clearance occurs in the kidney, although little intact calcitonin appears in the urine.

The principal effects of calcitonin are to lower serum calcium and phosphate by actions on bone and kidney. Calcitonin inhibits osteoclastic bone resorption. Although bone formation is not impaired at first after calcitonin administration, with time both formation and resorption of bone are reduced. Thus, the early hope that calcitonin would prove useful in restoring bone mass has not been realized. In the kidney, calcitonin reduces both calcium and phosphate reabsorption as well as reabsorption of other ions, including sodium, potassium, and magnesium. Although calcitonin stimulates cAMP formation in both bone and kidney, a requirement for cAMP in mediating its actions is not established. PTH also stimulates cAMP accumulation in these tissues, yet the effects of PTH and calcitonin are generally antagonistic.

Tissues other than bone and kidney are also affected by calcitonin. Calcitonin in pharmacologic amounts decreases gastrin secretion and reduces gastric acid output while increasing secretion of sodium, potassium, chloride, and water in the gut. Pentagastrin is a potent stimulator of calcitonin secretion (as is hypercalcemia), suggesting a possible physiologic relationship between gastrin and calcitonin. In the adult human, no readily demonstrable problem develops in cases of calcitonin deficiency (thyroidectomy) or excess (medullary carcinoma of the thyroid). However, the ability of calcitonin to block bone resorption and lower serum calcium makes it a useful drug for the treatment of Paget's disease, hypercalcemia, and osteoporosis.

GLUCOCORTICOIDS

Glucocorticoid hormones alter bone mineral homeostasis by antagonizing vitamin D-stimulated intestinal calcium transport, by stimulating renal calcium excretion, by blocking bone collagen synthesis, and by increasing PTH-stimulated bone resorption (although this last action is not universally accepted). Although these observations underscore the negative impact of glucocorticoids on bone mineral homeostasis, these hormones have proved useful in two situations involving bone mineral homeostasis: in the intermediate term treatment of hypercalcemia and as a diagnostic test for determining the cause of hypercalcemia. Prolonged admininistration of glucocorticoids is a common cause of osteoporosis in adults and poor skeletal development in children.

ESTROGENS

Estrogens can prevent accelerated bone loss during the immediate postmenopausal period and at least transiently increase bone in the postmenopausal subject. The prevailing hypothesis advanced to explain these observations is that estrogens reduce the bone-resorbing action of PTH. Estrogen administration leads to an increased $1,25(OH)_2D$ level in blood, but estrogens have no direct effect on $1,25(OH)_2D$ production in vitro. The increased $1,25(OH)_2D$ levels in vivo following estrogen treatment may result from decreased serum calcium and phosphate and increased PTH. Estrogen receptors have been found in bone, suggesting that estrogen may have direct effects on bone remodeling. The principal therapeutic application for estrogen administration in disorders of bone mineral homeostasis is the treatment or prevention of postmenopausal osteoporosis.

NONHORMONAL AGENTS AFFECTING BONE MINERAL HOMEOSTASIS

BISPHOSPHONATES

The bisphosphonates are analogues of pyrophosphate in which the P–O–P bond has been replaced with a nonhydrolyzable P–C–P bond (Figure 41–3). Both etidronate and pamidronate are available for clinical use, and newer forms are likely to be available soon. The bisphosphonates owe at least part of their clinical usefulness and toxicity to their ability to retard formation and dissolution of hydroxyapatite crystals within and outside the skeletal system. How-

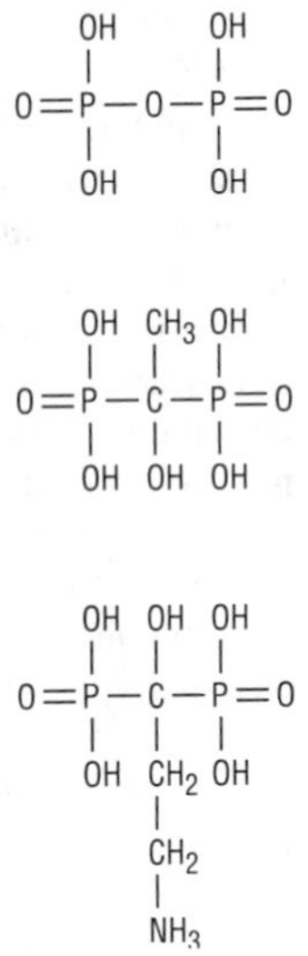

Inorganic pyrophosphoric acid

Ethane-1-hydroxy-1,1-bisphosphonate (EHDP, etidronate)

3-Amino-1-hydroxy-propylidene bisphosphonate (APD, pamidronate)

Figure 41–3. The structure of pyrophosphate and the two bisphosphonates, etidronate and pamidronate, that are currently approved for use in the USA.

ever, the exact mechanism by which they selectively inhibit bone resorption is not clear.

The results from animal studies indicate that 1–10% of an oral dose of etidronate is absorbed. Nearly half of the absorbed drug accumulates in bone; the remainder is excreted unchanged in the urine. The portion bound to bone is retained for weeks, depending on the turnover of bone itself.

Etidronate and the other bisphosphonates exert a variety of effects on bone mineral homeostasis. Their physicochemical properties of reducing hydroxyapatite formation and dissolution make them clinically useful. In particular, bisphosphonates are being evaluated for the treatment of hypercalcemia associated with malignancy, osteoporosis, and syndromes of ectopic calcification. Their usefulness in the management of Paget's disease is well established. The bisphosphonates exert a variety of other cellular effects, including inhibition of $1,25(OH)_2D$ production, inhibition of intestinal calcium transport, metabolic changes in bone cells such as inhibition of glycolysis, inhibition of cell growth, and changes in acid and alkaline phosphatase. These effects vary depending on the bisphosphonate being studied and may account for some of the clinical differences observed in the effects of the various bisphosphonates on bone mineral homeostasis.

PLICAMYCIN (Mithramycin)

Plicamycin is a cytotoxic antibiotic (see Chapter 56) that has been used clinically for two disorders of bone mineral metabolism: Paget's disease and hypercalcemia. The cytotoxic properties of the drug appear to involve its binding to DNA and interruption of DNA-directed RNA synthesis. The reasons for its usefulness in the treatment of Paget's disease and hypercalcemia are unclear but may relate to the need for protein synthesis to sustain bone resorption. The doses required to treat Paget's disease and hypercalcemia are about one-tenth the amounts required to achieve cytotoxic effects.

THIAZIDES

The chemistry and pharmacology of this family of drugs are covered in Chapter 15. The principal application of thiazides in the treatment of bone mineral disorders is in reducing renal calcium excretion. Thiazides may increase the effectiveness of parathyroid hormone in stimulating reabsorption of calcium by the renal tubules or may act on calcium reabsorption secondarily by increasing sodium reabsorption in the proximal tubule. In the distal tubule, thiazides block sodium reabsorption at the luminal surface, increasing the calcium-sodium exchange at the basolateral membrane and thus enhancing calcium reabsorption into the blood at this site. Thiazides have proved to be quite useful in reducing the hypercalciuria and incidence of stone formation in subjects with idiopathic hypercalciuria. Part of their efficacy in reducing stone formation may lie in their ability to decrease urine oxalate excretion and increase urine magnesium and zinc levels (both of which inhibit calcium oxalate stone formation).

FLUORIDE

Fluoride is well established as effective for the prophylaxis of dental caries and has been under investigation for the treatment of osteoporosis. Both therapeutic applications originated from epidemiologic observations that subjects living in areas with naturally fluoridated water (1–2 ppm) had less dental caries and fewer vertebral compression fractures than subjects living in nonfluoridated water areas. Fluoride is accumulated by bones and teeth, where it may stabilize the hydroxyapatite crystal. Such a mechanism may explain the effectiveness of fluoride in increasing the resistance of teeth to dental caries, but it does not explain new bone growth.

Fluoride in drinking water appears to be most effective in preventing dental caries if consumed prior to the eruption of the permanent teeth. The optimum concentration in drinking water supplies is 0.5–1 ppm. Topical application is most effective if done just as the teeth erupt. There is little further benefit to giving fluoride after the permanent teeth are fully formed. Excess fluoride in drinking water leads to mottling of the enamel proportionate to the concentration above 1 ppm.

Because of the general lack of effectiveness of other agents in stimulating new bone growth in patients with osteoporosis, interest in the use of fluoride for this disorder has been renewed (see Osteoporosis, page 666). Results of earlier studies indicated that fluoride alone without adequate calcium supplementation produced osteomalacia. More recent studies, in which calcium supplementation has been adequate, have demonstrated an improvement in calcium balance, an increase in bone mineral, and an increase in trabecular bone volume. However, two studies of the ability of fluoride to reduce fractures reached opposite conclusions (Riggs, 1990; Pak, 1989). Adverse effects observed—at the doses used for testing fluoride's effect on bone—include nausea and vomiting, gastrointestinal blood loss, arthralgias, and arthritis in a substantial proportion of patients. Such effects are usually responsive to reduction of the dose or giving fluoride with meals (or both). At present, fluoride is not approved by the Food and Drug Administration for use in osteoporosis.

Acute toxicity, generally due to ingestion of fluoride-containing rat poisons, includes gastrointestinal symptoms and neurologic signs of hypocalcemia presumably related to the calcium-binding properties of fluoride. Fluoride in acutely toxic doses may also cause cardiovascular collapse or respiratory failure. Chronic exposure to very high levels of fluoride dust in the inspired air results in **crippling fluorosis**, characterized by thickening of the cortex of long bones and bony exostoses, especially in the vertebrae.

II. CLINICAL PHARMACOLOGY

Disorders of bone mineral homeostasis generally present with abnormalities in serum or urine calcium levels (or both), often accompanied by abnormal serum phosphate levels. These abnormal mineral concentrations may themselves cause symptoms requiring immediate treatment (eg, coma in malignant hypercalcemia, tetany in hypocalcemia). More commonly, they serve as clues to an underlying disorder in hormonal regulators (eg, primary hyperparathyroidism), target tissue response (eg, chronic renal failure), or drug abuse (eg, vitamin D intoxication). In such cases, treatment of the underlying disorder is of prime importance.

Since bone and kidney play central roles in bone mineral homeostasis, conditions that alter bone mineral homeostasis usually affect either or both of these tissues secondarily. Effects on bone can result in osteoporosis (abnormal loss of bone; remaining bone histologically normal), osteomalacia (abnormal bone formation due to inadequate mineralization), or osteitis fibrosa (excessive bone resorption with fibrotic replacement of resorption cavities). Biochemical markers of skeletal involvement include changes in serum levels of the skeletal isoenzyme of alkaline phosphatase and osteocalcin (reflecting osteoblastic activity) and urine levels of hydroxyproline and pyridinoline cross-links (reflecting osteoclastic activity). The kidney becomes involved when the calcium-times-phosphate product in serum exceeds the point at which ectopic calcification occurs (often in renal parenchyma) or when the calcium-times-oxalate (or phosphate) product in urine exceeds saturation, leading to nephrocalcinosis and nephrolithiasis. Subtle early indicators of such renal involvement include polyuria, nocturia, and hyposthenuria. Radiologic evidence of nephrocalcinosis and stones is not generally observed until later. The degree of the ensuing renal failure is best followed by monitoring the decline in creatinine clearance.

ABNORMAL SERUM CALCIUM & PHOSPHATE LEVELS

HYPERCALCEMIA

Hypercalcemia causes central nervous system depression, including coma, and is potentially lethal. Its major causes (other than thiazide therapy) are hyperparathyroidism and cancer with or without bone metastases. Less common causes are hypervitaminosis D, sarcoidosis, thyrotoxicosis, milk-alkali syndrome, adrenal insufficiency, and immobilization. With the possible exception of hypervitaminosis D, these latter disorders seldom require emergency lowering of serum calcium. A number of approaches are used to manage the hypercalcemic crisis.

Saline Diuresis

In hypercalcemia of sufficient severity to produce symptoms, rapid reduction of serum calcium is required. The first steps include rehydration with saline and diuresis with furosemide. Most patients presenting with severe hypercalcemia have a substantial component of prerenal azotemia owing to dehydration, which prevents the kidney from compensating for the rise in serum calcium by excreting more calcium in the urine. Therefore, the initial infusion of 500–1000 mL/h of saline to reverse the dehydration and restore urine flow can by itself substantially lower serum calcium. The addition of a loop diuretic such as furosemide (Chapter 15) not only enhances urine flow but also inhibits calcium reabsorption in the ascending limb of the loop of Henle. Monitoring central venous pressure is important to forestall the development of congestive heart failure and pulmonary edema in predisposed subjects. In many subjects, saline diuresis will suffice to reduce serum calcium levels to a point at which more definitive diagnosis and treatment of the underlying condition can be achieved. If this is not the case or if more prolonged medical treatment of hypercalcemia is required, the following agents are available (discussed in order of preference).

Bisphosphonates

Etidronate, 7.5 mg/kg in 250–500 mL saline, infused over several hours each day for 3 days, has proved quite useful in treating hypercalcemia of malignancy. More recently, pamidronate, 60–90 mg in 500–750 mL saline, infused over 4–24 hours, has been approved for the same indication. This form of treatment is remarkably free of toxicity. The effects generally persist for weeks, but treatment can be repeated after a 7-day interval if necessary.

Calcitonin

Calcitonin has proved useful as ancillary treatment in a large number of patients. Calcitonin by itself seldom restores serum calcium to normal, and refractoriness frequently develops. However, its lack of toxicity permits frequent administration at high doses (200 MRC units or more). An effect on serum calcium is observed within 4–6 hours and lasts for 6–10 hours. Calcimar (salmon calcitonin) is available for parenteral administration only.

Gallium Nitrate

Gallium nitrate is approved by the Food and Drug Administration for the management of hypercalcemia of malignancy and is undergoing trials for the treatment of advanced Paget's disease. This drug acts by inhibiting bone resorption. At a dose of 200 mg/m^2 body surface area per day given as a continuous intravenous infusion in 5% dextrose for 5 days, gallium nitrate proved superior to calcitonin in reducing serum calcium in cancer patients. Because of potential nephrotoxicity, patients should be well-hydrated and have good renal output before starting the infusion.

Plicamycin
(Mithramycin)

Because of its toxicity, plicamycin (mithramycin) is not the drug of first choice for the treatment of hypercalcemia. However, when other forms of therapy fail, 25–50 μg/kg given intravenously usually lowers serum calcium substantially within 24–48 hours. This effect can last for several days. This dose can be repeated as necessary. The most dangerous toxic effect is sudden thrombocytopenia followed by hemorrhage. Hepatic and renal toxicity can also occur. Hypocalcemia, nausea, and vomiting may limit therapy.

Use of this drug must be accompanied by careful monitoring of platelet counts, liver and kidney function, and serum calcium levels.

Phosphate

Giving intravenous phosphate is probably the fastest and surest way to reduce serum calcium, but it is a hazardous procedure if not done properly. Intravenous phosphate should be used only after other methods of treatment (etidronate, calcitonin, saline diuresis with furosemide, and plicamycin) have failed to control symptomatic hypercalcemia. Phosphate must be given slowly (50 mmol or 1.5 g elemental phosphorus over 6–8 hours) and the patient switched to oral phosphate (1–2 g/d elemental phosphorus, as one of the salts indicated below) as soon as symptoms of hypercalcemia have cleared. The risks of intravenous phosphate therapy include sudden hypocalcemia, ectopic calcification, acute renal failure, and hypotension. Oral phosphate can also lead to ectopic calcification and renal failure if serum calcium and phosphate levels are not carefully monitored, but the risk is less and the time of onset much longer. Phosphate is available in oral and intravenous forms as the sodium or potassium salt. Amounts required to provide 1 g of elemental phosphorus are as follows:

> Intravenous:
>   In-Phos: 40 mL
>   Hyper-Phos-K: 15 mL
> Oral:
>   Fleet Phospho-Soda: 6.2 mL
>   Neutra-Phos: 300 mL

Glucocorticoids

Glucocorticoids have no clear role in the acute treatment of hypercalcemia. However, the chronic hypercalcemia of sarcoidosis, vitamin D intoxication, and certain cancers may respond within several days to glucocorticoid therapy. Prednisone in doses of 30–60 mg orally daily is generally used, though equivalent doses of other glucocorticoids are effective. The rationale for the use of glucocorticoids in these diseases differs, however. The hypercalcemia of sarcoidosis appears to be secondary to increased production of 1,25(OH)$_2$D, possibly by the sarcoid tissue itself. Glucocorticoid therapy directed at the reduction of sarcoid tissue results in restoration of normal serum calcium and 1,25(OH)$_2$D levels. The treatment of hypervitaminosis D with glucocorticoids probably does not alter vitamin D metabolism significantly but is thought to reduce vitamin D-mediated intestinal calcium transport. An action of glucocorticoids to reduce vitamin D-mediated bone resorption has not been excluded, however. The effect of glucocorticoids on the hypercalcemia of cancer is probably twofold. The malignancies responding best to glucocorticoids (ie, multiple myeloma and related lymphoproliferative diseases) are sensitive to the lytic action of glucocorticoids, so part of the effect may be related to decreased tumor mass and activity. Glucocorticoids have also been shown to inhibit the effectiveness of osteoclast-activating factor, a humoral substance or substances elaborated by multiple myeloma and related cancers that stimulate osteoclastic bone resorption. Other causes of hypercalcemia—particularly primary hyperparathyroidism—do not respond to glucocorticoid therapy.

This difference in response of the various forms of hypercalcemia to glucocorticoids forms the basis for the glucocorticoid suppression test, in which the response of serum calcium to a 10-day course of prednisone, 60 mg orally daily, helps differentiate the hypercalcemia of primary hyperparathyroidism from other causes such as sarcoidosis, vitamin D intoxication, and certain cancers. This test may be misleading and should not be used as a substitute for more specific tests for primary hyperparathyroidism such as serum immunoreactive PTH determinations.

HYPOCALCEMIA

The main features of hypocalcemia are neuromuscular—tetany, paresthesias, laryngospasm, muscle cramps, and convulsions. The major causes of hypocalcemia in the adult are hypoparathyroidism, vitamin D deficiency, renal failure, and malabsorption. Neonatal hypocalcemia is a common disorder that usually resolves without therapy. The roles of PTH, vitamin D, and calcitonin in the neonatal syndrome are under active investigation. Large infusions of citrated blood can produce hypocalcemia by the formation of citrate-calcium complexes. Calcium and vitamin D (or its metabolites) form the mainstay of treatment of hypocalcemia.

Calcium

A number of calcium preparations are available for intravenous, intramuscular, and oral use. Calcium gluceptate (0.9 meq calcium/mL), calcium gluconate (0.45 meq calcium/mL), and calcium chloride (0.68–1.36 meq calcium/mL) are available for intravenous therapy. Calcium gluconate is the preferred form because it is less irritating to veins. Oral preparations include calcium carbonate (40% calcium), calcium lactate (13% calcium), calcium phosphate (25% calcium), and calcium citrate (17% calcium). Calcium carbonate is often the preparation of choice because of its high percentage of calcium, ready availability (eg, Tums), low cost, and antacid properties. In achlorhydric patients, calcium carbonate should be given with meals to increase absorption. Combinations of vitamin D and calcium are available, but treatment must be tailored to the individual patient and individual disease, a flexibility lost by fixed-dosage combinations. Treatment of severe symptomatic hypocalcemia can be accomplished with slow infusion of 5–20 mL of 10% calcium gluconate. Rapid infusion can lead to cardiac arrhythmias. Less severe hypocalcemia is best treated with oral forms sufficient to provide approximately 400–800 mg of elemental calcium (1–2 g calcium carbonate per day). Dosage must be adjusted to avoid hypercalcemia and hypercalciuria.

Vitamin D

When rapidity of action is required, $1,25(OH)_2D_3$ (calcitriol), 0.25–1 µg daily, is the vitamin D metabolite of choice, since it is capable of raising serum calcium within 24–48 hours. Calcitriol also raises serum phosphate, though this action is usually not observed early in treatment. The combined effects of calcitriol and all other vitamin D metabolites and analogues on both calcium and phosphate make careful monitoring of these mineral levels especially important to avoid ectopic calcification secondary to an abnormally high serum calcium × phosphate product. Since the choice of the appropriate vitamin D metabolite or analogue for long-term treatment of hypocalcemia depends on the nature of the underlying disease, further discussion of vitamin D treatment will be found under the headings of the specific diseases.

HYPERPHOSPHATEMIA

Hyperphosphatemia is a frequent complication of renal failure but is also found in all types of hypoparathyroidism (idiopathic, surgical, and pseudo), vitamin D intoxication, and the rare syndrome of tumoral calcinosis. Emergency treatment of hyperphosphatemia is seldom necessary but can be achieved by dialysis or glucose and insulin infusions. In general, control of hyperphosphatemia involves restriction of dietary phosphate plus the use of phosphate binding gels such as $Al(OH)_3$-containing antacids and of calcium supplements. Because of their potential to induce aluminum-associated bone disease, aluminum-containing antacids should be used sparingly and only when other measures fail to control the hyperphosphatemia.

HYPOPHOSPHATEMIA

A variety of conditions are associated with hypophosphatemia, including primary hyperparathyroidism, vitamin D deficiency, idiopathic hypercalcemia, vitamin D-resistant rickets, various other forms of renal phosphate wasting (eg, Fanconi's syndrome), overzealous use of $Al(OH)_3$-containing antacids, and parenteral nutrition with inadequate phosphate content. Acute hypophosphatemia may lead to a reduction in the intracellular levels of high-energy organic phosphates (eg, ATP), interfere with normal hemoglobin-to-tissue oxygen transfer by decreasing red cell 2,3-diphosphoglycerate levels, and lead to rhabdomyolysis. However, clinically significant acute effects of hypophosphatemia are seldom seen, and emergency treatment is generally not indicated. The long-term effects of hypophosphatemia include proximal muscle weakness and abnormal bone mineralization (osteomalacia). Therefore, hypophosphatemia should be avoided during other forms of therapy and treated in conditions such as vitamin D-resistant rickets of which it is a cardinal feature. Oral forms of phosphate available for use are listed above in the section on hypercalcemia.

SPECIFIC DISORDERS INVOLVING THE BONE MINERAL REGULATING HORMONES

PRIMARY HYPERPARATHYROIDISM

This rather common disease, if associated with symptoms and significant hypercalcemia, is best treated surgically. Oral phosphate has been tried but cannot be recommended.

HYPOPARATHYROIDISM

In the absence of PTH (idiopathic or surgical hypoparathyroidism) or a normal target tissue response to PTH (pseudohypoparathyroidism), serum calcium falls and serum phosphate rises. In such patients, $1,25(OH)_2D$ levels are usually low, presumably reflecting the lack of stimulation by PTH of $1,25(OH)_2D$ production. The skeletons of patients with idiopathic or surgical hypoparathyroidism are normal except for a slow turnover rate. A number of patients with pseudohypoparathyroidism appear to have osteitis fibrosa, suggesting that the normal or high PTH levels found in such patients are capable of acting on bone but not on the kidney. The distinction between pseudohypoparathyroidism and idiopathic hypoparathyroidism is made on the basis of normal or high PTH levels but deficient renal response (ie, diminished excretion of cAMP or phosphate) in patients with pseudohypoparathyroidism.

The principal therapeutic concern is to restore normocalcemia and normophosphatemia. Under most circumstances, vitamin D (25,000–100,000 units 3 times per week) and dietary calcium supplements suffice. More rapid increments in serum calcium can be achieved with calcitriol, although it is not clear that this metabolite offers a substantial advantage over vitamin D itself for long-term therapy. Many patients treated with vitamin D develop episodes of hypercalcemia. This complication is more rapidly reversible with cessation of therapy using calcitriol rather than vitamin D. This would be of importance to the patient in whom such hypercalcemic crises are common. Dihydrotachysterol and 25(OH)D have not received much study as therapy for hypoparathyroidism, though both should be effective. Whether they offer advantages over vitamin D sufficient to justify their added expense remains to be seen.

NUTRITIONAL RICKETS

Vitamin D deficiency, once thought to be rare in this country, is being recognized more often, especially in the pediatric and geriatric populations on vegetarian diets and with reduced sunlight exposure. This problem can be avoided by daily intake of 400 units of vitamin D and treated by somewhat higher doses (4000 units per day). No other metabolite is indicated. The diet should also contain adequate amounts of calcium and phosphate.

CHRONIC RENAL FAILURE

The major problems of chronic renal failure that impact on bone mineral homeostasis are the loss of $1,25(OH)_2D$ and $24,25(OH)_2D$ production, the retention of phosphate that reduces ionized calcium levels, and the secondary hyperparathyroidism that results. With the loss of $1,25(OH)_2D$ production, less calcium is absorbed from the intestine and less bone is resorbed under the influence of PTH. As a result. hypocalcemia usually develops, furthering the development of hyperparathyroidism. The bones show a mixture of osteomalacia and osteitis fibrosa.

In contrast to the hypocalcemia that is more often associated with chronic renal failure, some patients may become hypercalcemic from two causes (in addition to overzealous treatment with calcium). The most common cause of hypercalcemia is the development of severe secondary (sometimes referred to as tertiary) hyperparathyroidism. In such cases, the PTH level in blood is very high. Serum alkaline phosphatase levels also tend to be high. Treatment often requires parathyroidectomy.

A less common circumstance leading to hypercalcemia is development of a form of osteomalacia characterized by a profound decrease in bone cell activity and loss of the calcium buffering action of bone. In the absence of kidney function, any calcium absorbed from the intestine accumulates in the blood. Therefore, such patients are very sensitive to the hypercalcemic action of $1,25(OH)_2D$. These individuals generally have a high serum calcium but nearly normal alkaline phosphatase and PTH levels. Recent evidence suggests that bone in such patients has a high aluminum content, especially in the mineralization front, which may block normal bone mineralization. These patients do not respond favorably to parathyroidectomy. Deferoxamine, an agent used to chelate iron (Chapter 59), also binds aluminum and is undergoing clinical trials as therapy for this disorder.

Use of Vitamin D Preparations

The choice of vitamin D preparation to be used in the setting of chronic renal failure in the dialysis patient depends on the type and extent of bone disease and hyperparathyroidism. No consensus has been reached regarding the advisability of using any vitamin D metabolite in the predialysis patient. $1,25(OH)_2D_3$ (calcitriol) will rapidly correct hypocalcemia and at least partially reverse the secondary hyperparathyroidism and osteitis fibrosa. Many patients with muscle weakness and bone pain gain an improved sense of well-being.

Dihydrotachysterol, an analogue of $1,25(OH)_2D$, is also available for clinical use. Dihydrotachysterol appears to be as effective as calcitriol, differing principally in its time course of action; calcitriol increases serum calcium in 1–2 days, whereas dihydrotachysterol requires 1–2 weeks. For an equipotent dose (0.2 mg dihydrotachysterol versus 0.5 μg calcitriol), dihydrotachysterol costs about one-fourth as much as calcitriol. A disadvantage of dihydrotachysterol is the inability to measure it in serum. Neither dihydrotachysterol nor calcitriol corrects the osteomalacic component of renal osteodystrophy in the majority of patients, and neither should be used in patients with hypercalcemia, especially if the bone disease is primarily osteomalacic.

Calcifediol ($25[OH]D_3$) may also be used to advantage. Calcifediol is less effective than calcitriol in stimulating intestinal calcium transport, so that hypercalcemia is less of a problem with calcifediol. Like dihydrotachysterol, calcifediol requires several weeks to restore normocalcemia in hypocalcemic individuals with chronic renal failure. Presumably because of the reduced ability of the diseased kidney to metabolize calcifediol to more active metabolites, high doses (50–100 μg daily) must be given to achieve the supraphysiologic serum levels required for therapeutic effectiveness.

Vitamin D has been used in treating renal osteodystrophy. However, patients with a substantial degree of renal failure who are thus unable to convert vitamin D to its active metabolites usually are refractory to vitamin D. Its use is decreasing as more effective alternatives become available.

Several nonhypercalcemic analogues of calcitriol are being tested for their ability to reduce the secondary hyperparathyroidism of chronic renal failure. Their biggest impact will be in patients in whom the use of calcitriol may lead to unacceptably high serum calcium levels.

Regardless of the drug employed, careful attention to serum calcium and phosphate levels is required.

Calcium supplements (dietary and in the dialysate) and phosphate restriction (dietary and with oral ingestion of phosphate binders) should be employed along with the use of vitamin D metabolites. Monitoring serum PTH and alkaline phosphatase levels is useful in determining whether therapy is correcting or preventing secondary hyperparathyroidism. Although not generally available, percutaneous bone biopsies for quantitative histomorphometry may help in choosing appropriate therapy and following the effectiveness of such therapy. Unlike the rapid changes in serum values, changes in bone morphology require months to years. Monitoring serum levels of the vitamin D metabolites is useful to determine compliance, absorption, and metabolism.

INTESTINAL OSTEODYSTROPHY

A number of gastrointestinal and hepatic diseases result in disordered calcium and phosphate homeostasis that ultimately leads to bone disease. The bones in such patients show a combination of osteoporosis and osteomalacia. Osteitis fibrosa does not occur (as it does in renal osteodystrophy). The common features that appear to be important in this group of diseases are malabsorption of calcium and vitamin D. Liver disease may, in addition, reduce the production of $25(OH)D$ from vitamin D, though the importance of this in all but patients with terminal liver failure remains in dispute. The malabsorption of vitamin D is probably not limited to exogenous vitamin D. The liver secretes into bile a substantial number of vitamin D metabolites and conjugates that are reabsorbed in (presumably) the distal jejunum and ileum. Interference with this process could deplete the body of endogenous vitamin D metabolites as well as limit absorption of dietary vitamin D.

In mild forms of malabsorption, vitamin D (25,000–50,000 units 3 times per week) should suffice to raise serum levels of $25(OH)D$ into the normal range. Many patients with severe disease do not respond to vitamin D. Clinical experience with the other metabolites is limited, but both calcitriol and calcifediol have been used successfully in doses similar to those recommended for treatment of renal osteodystrophy. Theoretically, calcifediol should be the drug of choice under these conditions, since no impairment of the renal metabolism of $25(OH)D$ to $1,25(OH)_2D$ and $24,25(OH)_2D$ exists in these patients. Both calcitriol and calcifediol may be of importance in reversing the bone disease. As in the other diseases discussed, treatment of intestinal osteodystrophy with vitamin D and its metabolites should be accompanied by appropriate dietary calcium supplementation and monitoring of serum calcium and phosphate levels.

OSTEOPOROSIS

Osteoporosis is defined as abnormal loss of bone predisposing to fractures. It is most common in postmenopausal women but may occur in older men. It may occur as a side effect of chronic administration of glucocorticoids or other drugs; as a manifestation of endocrine disease such as thyrotoxicosis or hyperparathyroidism; as a feature of malabsorption syndrome; as a consequence of alcohol abuse; or without obvious cause (idiopathic). The ability of some agents to reverse the bone loss of osteoporosis is shown in Figure 41–4. The postmenopausal form of osteoporosis may be accompanied by lower $1,25(OH)_2D$ levels and reduced intestinal calcium transport. This form of osteoporosis appears to be due to estrogen deficiency and is best treated with cyclic doses of estrogen. It is important to note that the most rapid loss of bone occurs within the first 5 years after menopause and that administration of estrogens after this time may be less effective. Furthermore, if estrogen therapy is discontinued, a period of accelerated bone loss may occur. Thus, treatment with estrogens should be started shortly after the onset of menopause and may need to be continued for life. Since continuous estrogen therapy is associated with increased risk of endometrial carcinoma, among other complications, the recommendation to treat all postmenopausal women with estrogens has not been universally accepted. With the advent of sensitive means of measuring vertebral bone mineral content (CT scan, dual energy x-ray absorptiometry), estrogen therapy may be reserved for women with reduced bone mineral content at the time of menopause or those who

lose bone rapidly in the first year after menopause. Recent evidence, however, indicates that cyclic estrogen therapy in combination with a progestational agent reduces or eliminates this added risk of cancer. Therefore, estrogens should be administered for 21 of 28 days in the lowest effective dose (eg, 0.625 mg of conjugated estrogens or 25–50 µg of ethinyl estradiol), with addition of a progestational agent on days 14–21 (eg, 10 mg of medroxyprogesterone acetate). This may reinitiate menstrual bleeding, so the patient must be advised of this in advance. Other complications of estrogen therapy such as hypertension and thrombophlebitis must also be kept in mind when such treatment is initiated.

To counter the reduced intestinal calcium transport associated with osteoporosis, vitamin D therapy is often employed in addition to dietary calcium supplementation. There is no clear evidence that pharmacologic doses of vitamin D are of much additional benefit beyond cyclic estrogens and calcium supplementation. However, calcitriol and its analogue $1\alpha OHD_3$ have been shown to increase bone mass and reduce fractures in several recent studies.

Despite early promise that fluoride might be useful in the prevention or treatment of postmenopausal osteoporosis, a recently completed study has indicated otherwise (Riggs, 1990). However, other recent studies continue to indicate a potential role for fluoride in this bone disease (Pak, 1989). Fluoride is the only known agent that can directly stimulate bone formation and lead to a progressive increase in bone density, at least in the spine (Figure 41–4).

Calcitonin has recently been approved for use in the treatment of postmenopausal osteoporosis.

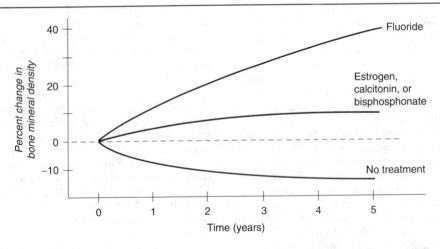

Figure 41–4. Typical changes in bone mineral density with time after the onset of menopause, with and without treatment. In the untreated condition, bone is lost during aging in both men and women. Fluoride promotes new bone formation and can increase bone mineral density in subjects who respond to it throughout the period of treatment. In contrast, estrogen, calcitonin, and bisphosphonates block bone resorption. This leads to a transient increase in bone mineral density because bone formation is not initially decreased. However, with time, both bone formation and bone resorption are decreased and bone mineral density reaches a new plateau.

Whether this agent, which reduces bone resorption acutely, will have a long-term effect on bone mass remains uncertain. It has few adverse effects.

Several studies have been published suggesting that intermittent short courses of etidronate (2 weeks per 12-week cycle) improve bone density and reduce spinal fractures (Watts 1990, Storm 1990). A number of new bisphosphonates are undergoing clinical trials, so this form of therapy seems certain to receive close study, especially because these agents have relatively few serious toxicities.

The cause of idiopathic osteoporosis in men is not known. Treatment usually consists of giving vitamin D and dietary calcium supplements, but little information is available about its efficacy. It is important to exclude more treatable forms of osteoporosis such as that accompanying corticosteroid therapy, alcohol abuse, hyperparathyroidism, thyrotoxicosis, malabsorption, or occult nutritional osteomalacia.

VITAMIN D-RESISTANT RICKETS

This X-linked recessive disorder is manifested by the appearance of rickets and hypophosphatemia in children. The disease can present in adulthood, presumably reflecting either less severe disease or a missed diagnosis in childhood. The main defect appears to be an abnormality in renal phosphate reabsorption. Phosphate is critical to normal bone mineralization; when phosphate stores are deficient, a clinical and pathologic picture resembling vitamin D-deficient rickets develops. However, such children fail to respond to the usual doses of vitamin D employed in the treatment of nutritional rickets. A defect in $1,25(OH)_2D$ production by the kidney has also been suggested by some investigators, because the serum $1,25(OH)_2D$ levels tend to be low relative to the degree of hypophosphatemia observed. This combination of low serum phosphate and low or low-normal serum $1,25(OH)_2D$ provides the rationale for treating such patients with oral phosphate (1–3 g daily) and large doses of vitamin D (25,000–100,000 units daily). Recently, some groups have used calcitriol with good effect (0.25–1 μg daily). Reports of such combination therapy are encouraging in this otherwise debilitating disease.

VITAMIN D-DEPENDENT RICKETS

This entity actually represents two different diseases (types I and II). Both present as childhood rickets that does not respond to conventional doses of vitamin D. Type I vitamin D-dependent rickets is due to an isolated deficiency of $1,25(OH)_2D$ production. This condition can be treated with vitamin D (4000 units daily) or calcitriol (0.25–0.5 μg daily). Type II vitamin D-dependent rickets is caused by a target tissue defect in response to $1,25(OH)_2D$. Recent studies have shown a number of point mutations in the gene for the $1,25(OH)_2D$ receptor, which disrupt the functions of this receptor and lead to this syndrome (Hughes, 1988). The serum levels of $1,25(OH)_2D$ are very high in type II but not in type I. Treatment with large doses of calcitriol has been claimed to be effective in restoring normocalcemia. Such patients are totally refractory to vitamin D. One recent report indicates a reversal of resistance to calcitriol when $24,25(OH)_2D$ was given. These diseases are rare.

NEPHROTIC SYNDROME

Patients with nephrotic syndrome can lose vitamin D metabolites into their urine, presumably by loss of the vitamin D-binding protein. Such patients may have very low 25(OH)D levels. Some of them develop bone disease. It is not yet clear what value vitamin D therapy has in such patients, since this complication of the nephrotic syndrome has only recently been recognized, and therapeutic trials with vitamin D (or any other vitamin D metabolite) have not yet been carried out. Since the problem is not related to vitamin D metabolism, one would not anticipate any advantage in using the more expensive vitamin D metabolites in place of vitamin D itself.

IDIOPATHIC HYPERCALCIURIA

This syndrome, characterized by hypercalciuria and nephrolithiasis with normal serum calcium and PTH levels, has been subdivided into three groups of patients: (1) hyperabsorbers, patients with increased intestinal absorption of calcium, resulting in high-normal serum calcium, low-normal PTH, and a secondary increase in urine calcium; (2) renal calcium leakers, patients with a primary decrease in renal reabsorption of filtered calcium, leading to low-normal serum calcium and high-normal serum PTH; and (3) renal phosphate leakers, patients with a primary decrease in renal reabsorption of phosphate, leading to stimulation of $1,25(OH)_2D$ production, increased intestinal calcium absorption, increased ionized serum calcium, low-normal PTH levels, and a secondary increase in urine calcium. There is some disagreement about this classification, and in many cases patients are not readily categorized. Many such patients present with mild hypophosphatemia, and oral phosphate has been used with some success to reduce stone formation. However, a clear role for phosphate in the treatment of this disorder has not been established. Therapy with hydrochlorothiazide, up to 50 mg twice daily, is recommended, although equivalent doses of other thiazide diuretics work as well. Loop diuretics such as furosemide and ethacrynic acid should not be used, since they increase urinary calcium excretion. The major toxicity of thiazide diuretics, besides hypokalemia, hypomagnesemia, and hyperglycemia, is hypercalcemia. This is seldom more than a biochemical observation unless the patient has a disease such as hyperparathyroidism in which bone turnover is accelerated. Accordingly, one should screen patients for such disorders before starting thiazide therapy and monitor serum and urine calcium when therapy has begun.

An alternative to thiazides is allopurinol. Some studies indicate that hyperuricosuria is associated with idiopathic hypercalcemia and that a small nidus of urate crystals could lead to the calcium oxalate stone formation characteristic of idiopathic hypercalcemia. Allopurinol, 300 mg daily, may reduce stone formation by reducing uric acid excretion.

OTHER DISORDERS OF BONE MINERAL HOMEOSTASIS

PAGET'S DISEASE OF BONE

Paget's disease is a localized bone disease characterized by uncontrolled osteoclastic bone resorption with secondary increases in bone formation. This new bone is poorly organized, however. The cause of Paget's disease is obscure, though recent studies suggest that a slow virus may be involved. The disease is fairly common, though symptomatic bone disease is less common. The biochemical parameters of elevated serum alkaline phosphatase and urinary hydroxyproline are useful for diagnosis. Along with the characteristic radiologic and bone scan findings, these biochemical determinations provide good markers by which to follow therapy. The goal of treatment is to reduce bone pain and stabilize or prevent other problems such as progressive deformity, hearing loss, high-output cardiac failure, and immobilization hypercalcemia. Calcitonin can be used as sole treatment or in combination with bisphosphonates for this disease. Treatment failures may respond to plicamycin. Calcitonin is administered subcutaneously or intramuscularly in doses of 50–100 MRC units every day or every other day. Higher or more frequent doses have been advocated when this initial regimen is ineffective. Improvement in bone pain and reduction in serum alkaline phosphatase and urine hydroxyproline levels require weeks to months. Often a patient who responds well initially will lose the re-

sponse to calcitonin. This refractoriness is not correlated with the development of antibodies.

Sodium etidronate is the only bisphosphonate currently approved for clinical use in this condition in the USA. However, other bisphosphonates including pamidronate are being used in other countries. The recommended dosage is 5 mg/kg of sodium etidronate daily by oral administration. Long-term (months to years) remission may be expected in patients who respond to etidronate. Treatment should not exceed 6 months per course but can be repeated after 6 months if necessary. The principal toxicity of etidronate is the development of osteomalacia and an increased incidence of fractures when the dose is raised substantially above 5 mg/kg. Other bisphosphonates such as pamidronate are less toxic in this regard. Some patients treated with etidronate develop bone pain similar in nature to the bone pain of osteomalacia. This subsides after stopping the drug.

The use of a potentially lethal cytotoxic drug such as plicamycin in a generally benign disorder such as Paget's disease is recommended only when other less toxic agents (calcitonin, etidronate) have failed and the symptoms are debilitating. Insufficient clinical data on long-term use of plicamycin are available to determine its usefulness for extended therapy. However, short courses involving 15–25 µg/kg intravenously for 5–10 days followed by 15 µg/kg intravenously each week have been used to control the disease.

ENTERIC OXALURIA

Patients with short bowel syndromes associated with fat malabsorption can present with renal stones composed of calcium and oxalate. Such patients characteristically have normal or low urine calcium levels but elevated urine oxalate levels. The reasons for the development of oxaluria in such patients are thought to be twofold: first, in the intestinal lumen, calcium (which is now bound to fat) fails to bind oxalate and no longer prevents its absorption; second, enteric flora, acting on the increased supply of nutrients reaching the colon, produce larger amounts of oxalate. Although one would ordinarily avoid treating a patient with calcium oxalate stones with calcium supplementation, this is precisely what is done in patients with enteric oxaluria. The increased intestinal calcium binds the excess oxalate and prevents its absorption. One to 2 g of calcium carbonate can be given daily in divided doses, with careful monitoring of urinary calcium and oxalate to be certain that urinary oxalate falls without a dangerous increase in urinary calcium.

PREPARATIONS AVAILABLE

Vitamin D & Metabolites
Calcifediol (Calderol)
Oral: 20, 50 µg capsules
Calcitriol
Oral (Rocaltrol): 0.25, 0.5 µg capsules
Parenteral (Calcijex): 1, 2 µg/mL for injection
Cholecalciferol [D₃] (vitamin D₃, Delta-D)
Oral: 400, 1000 IU tablets
Dihydrotachysterol [DHT] (DHT, Hytakerol)
Oral: 0.125 mg tablets, capsules; 0.2, 0.4 mg tablets; 0.2 mg/mL intensol solution; 0.25 mg/mL solution in oil
Ergocalciferol [D₂] (vitamin D₂, Calciferol, Drisdol)
Oral: 50,000 IU tablets, capsules; 8000 IU/mL drops
Parenteral: 500,000 IU/mL for injection

Calcium
Calcium acetate (Phos-Ex, PhosLo) 250 mg (62.5 mg calcium, 668 mg (167 mg calcium), 1000 mg (250 mg calcium) tablets; 500 mg (125 mg calcium) capsules
Calcium carbonate [40% calcium] (generic, Tums, Cal-Sup, Os-Cal 500, others)
Oral: Numerous forms available
Calcium chloride [27% calcium] (generic)
Parenteral: 10% solution for IV injection only
Calcium citrate [21% calcium] (generic, Citracal)
Oral: 950 mg (200 mg calcium), 2376 mg (500 mg calcium)
Calcium glubionate [6.5% calcium] (Neo-Calglucon)
Oral: 1.8 g (115 mg calcium)/5 mL syrup
Calcium gluceptate [8% calcium] (Calcium Gluceptate)
Parenteral: 1.1 g/5 mL solution for IM or IV injection
Calcium gluconate [9% calcium] (generic)
Oral: 500 mg (45 mg calcium), 650 mg (58.5 mg calcium), 975 mg (87.75 mg calcium), 1 g (90 mg calcium) tablets

Parenteral: 10% solution for IV or IM injection
Calcium lactate [13% calcium] (generic)
Oral: 325 mg (42.25 mg calcium), 650 mg (84.5 mg calcium) tablets
Dibasic calcium phosphate dihydrate [23% calcium] (generic)
Oral: 486 mg (112 mg calcium) tablets
Tricalcium phosphate [39% calcium] (Posture)
Oral: 300 mg calcium, 600 mg calcium tablets (as phosphate)

Phosphate
Phosphate (Fleet Phospho-Soda, Neutra-Phos)
Oral: solution containing 815 mg phosphate, 760 mg sodium per 5 mL (Fleet Phospho-Soda); capsules containing 250 mg phosphorus, 278 mg potassium, 164 mg sodium (Neutra-Phos); capsules containing 250 mg phosphorus, 556 mg potassium, 0 mg sodium (Neutra-Phos-K)
Parenteral (Sodium or potassium phosphate): 3 mM phosphate/mL solution for IV infusion only

Other Drugs
Calcitonin-Human (Cibacalcin)
Parenteral: 0.5 mg per vial for injection
Calcitonin-Salmon (Calcimar, Miacalcin)
Parenteral: 100, 200 IU/mL for injection
Etidronate (Didronel)
Oral: 200, 400 mg tablets
Parenteral: 300 mg/6 mL for IV injection
Gallium nitrate (Ganite)
Parenteral: 500 mg/20 mL vial
Pamidronate (Aredia)
Parenteral: 30 mg/vial
Plicamycin (mithramycin) (Mithracin)
Parenteral: 2.5 mg per vial powder to reconstitute for injection
Sodium fluoride (generic)
Oral: 0.55 mg (0.25 mg F), 1.1 mg (0.5 mg F), 2.2 mg (1.0 mg F) tablets

REFERENCES

Austin LA, Heath HH III: Calcitonin: Physiology and pathophysiology. N Engl J Med 1981;304:269.

Bikle DD: The vitamin D endocrine system. Adv Intern Med 1982;27:45.

Bikle DD: Vitamins D: New actions, new analogs, new therapeutic potential. Endocr Rev 1992;13:765.

Bikle DD et al: Bone disease in alcohol abuse. Ann Intern Med 1985;103:42.

Bilezikian JP: Management of acute hypercalcemia. N Engl J Med 1992;326:1196.

Brown A, Dusso A, Slatopolsky E: Vitamin D. In: *The Kidney: Physiology and Pathophysiology,* 2nd ed. Seldin DW, Giebisch G (editors). Raven Press, 1992.

Cauley JA et al: Effects of thiazide diuretic therapy on bone mass, fractures, and falls. Ann Intern Med 1993;118:666.

Chapuy MC et al: Vitamin D₃ and calcium to prevent hip

fractures in elderly women. N Engl J Med 1992;327: 1637.

Coburn JW, Massry SG (editors): Uses and actions of 1,25-dihydroxyvitamin D_3 in uremia. Contrib Nephrol 1980; 18:1.

Dambacher MD, Binswanger U, Fischer JA: Diagnosis and treatment of primary hyperparathyroidism. Urol Res 1979;7:171.

Dawson-Hughes B et al: A controlled trial of the effect of calcium supplementation on bone density in postmenopausal women. N Engl J Med 1990;323:878.

Delmas PD: Biochemical markers of bone turnover: Methodology and clinical use in osteoporosis. Am J Med 1991;91(Suppl 5B):59S.

Ettinger B, Genant HK, Cann CE: Long-term estrogen replacement therapy prevents bone loss and fractures. Ann Intern Med 1985;102:319.

Felson DT et al: The effect of postmenopausal estrogen therapy on bone density in elderly women. N Engl J Med 1993;329:1141.

Fleisch H: Bisphosphonates: Pharmacology and use in the treatment of tumour-induced hypercalcaemic and metastatic bone disease. Drugs 1991;42:919.

Forscher BK, Arnaud CD (editors): The Third F. Raymond Keating, Jr., Memorial Symposium: Parathyroid hormone, calcitonin and vitamin D. Am J Med 1974;56:743 and 57:1.

Gallagher JC, Goldgar D: Treatment of postmenopausal osteoporosis with high doses of synthetic calcitriol. Ann Intern Med 1990;113:649.

Gucalp R et al: Comparative study of pamidronate disodium and etidronate disodium in the treatment of cancer-related hypercalcemia. J Clin Oncol 1992;10:134.

Hasling C, Charles P, Mosekilde L: Etidronate disodium in the management of malignancy-related hypercalcemia. Am J Med 1987;82(Suppl 2A):51.

Hodsman AB, Drost DJ: The response of vertebral bone mineral density during the treatment of osteoporosis with sodium fluoride. J Clin Endocrinol Metab 1989;69:932.

Hughes MR et al: Point mutations in the human vitamin D receptor gene associated with hypocalcemic rickets. Science 1988;242:1702.

Kleerkoper M, Balena R: Fluorides and osteoporosis. Annu Rev Nutr 1991;11:309.

Lei DBM, Zawada ET, Kleeman CR: The pathophysiology and clinical aspects of hypercalcemic disorders. West J Med 1978;129:278.

Leyvraz S et al: Pharmacokinetics of pamidronate in patients with bone metastases. J Natl Cancer Inst 1992;84: 788.

Long RG: Hepatic osteodystrophy: Outlook good but some problems unsolved. Gastroenterology 1980;78:644.

Malluche HH et al: The use of deferoxamine in the management of aluminum accumulation in bone in patients with renal failure. N Engl J Med 1984;311:140.

Okamura WH et al: Vitamin D: Structure-function analyses and the design of analogs. J Cell Biochem 1992;49:10.

Pak CYC (editor): Symposium on urolithiasis. Kidney Int 1978;13:341.

Pak CYC et al: Safe and effective treatment of osteoporosis with intermittent slow release sodium fluoride: Augmentation of vertebral bone mass and inhibition of fracture. J Clin Endocrinol Metab 1989;68:150.

Parfitt AM: Bone and plasma calcium homeostasis. Bone 1987;8(Suppl 1):51.

Popopoulos SE et al: The use of bisphosphonates in the treatment of osteoporosis. Bone 1992;13(Suppl):S41.

Prince RL et al: Prevention of postmenopausal osteoporosis: A comparative study of exercise, calcium supplementation, and hormone-replacement therapy. N Engl J Med 1991;325:1189.

Riggs BL et al: Changes in bone mineral density of the proximal femur and spine with aging: Differences between the postmenopausal and senile osteoporosis syndromes. J Clin Invest 1982;70:716.

Riggs BL et al: Effect of fluoride treatment on the fracture rate in postmenopausal women with osteoporosis. N Engl J Med 1990;322:802.

Riggs BL, Melton LJ III: The prevention and treatment of osteoporosis. N Engl J Med 1992;327:620.

Storm T et al: Effect of intermittent cyclical etidronate treatment on bone mass and fracture rate in women with postmenopausal osteoporosis. N Engl J Med 1990;322:1265.

Suda T, Takahashi N, Abe E: Role of vitamin D in bone resorption. J Cell Biochem 1992;49:53.

Tilyard MW et al: Treatment of postmenopausal osteoporosis with calcitriol or calcium. N Engl J Med 1992;326: 357.

Wallach S: Treatment of Paget's disease. Adv Intern Med 1982;27:1.

Watts NB et al: Intermittent cyclical etidronate treatment of postmenopausal osteoporosis. N Engl J Med 1990;323: 73.

Section VIII.
Chemotherapeutic Drugs

Principles of Antimicrobial Drug Action

42

Ernest Jawetz, MD, PhD

An ideal antimicrobial drug exhibits **selective toxicity.** This term implies that the drug is harmful to a parasite without being harmful to the host. In many instances, selective toxicity is relative rather than absolute, meaning that a drug may damage a parasite in a concentration that can be tolerated by the host.

Selective toxicity usually depends on the inhibition of biochemical processes that exist in or are essential to the parasite but not to the host. For many of the antimicrobial drugs, the mechanism of action is not completely understood. However, for purposes of discussion, it is convenient to present antimicrobial mechanisms under four distinct headings:

(1) Inhibition of cell wall synthesis.

(2) Alteration in the permeability of cell membrane or active transport across cell membrane.

(3) Inhibition of protein synthesis (ie, inhibition of translation and transcription of genetic material).

(4) Inhibition of nucleic acid synthesis.

Antimicrobial drugs are often described as **bacteriostatic** or **bactericidal.** The term "bacteriostatic" describes a drug that temporarily inhibits the growth of a microorganism. The therapeutic success of these agents often depends upon the participation of host defense mechanisms. Furthermore, the effect may be reversible: When the drug is removed, the organism will resume growth, and infection or disease may recur. Typical bacteriostatic drugs are the tetracyclines and sulfonamides.

The term "bactericidal" is applied to drugs that cause the death of the microorganism. Typical bactericidal drugs are the beta-lactams (penicillins, cephalosporins) and the aminoglycosides.

In infections that cannot usually be controlled or eradicated by host mechanisms (eg, infective endocarditis), bactericidal drugs are typically required for cure, and treatment with bacteriostatic drugs results in relapse as soon as treatment is stopped. In a host with adequate defenses (immune, phagocytic, etc), a bacteriostatic effect may be sufficient to result in eradication of the infection.

However, the terms "bacteriostatic" and "bactericidal" are relative, not absolute. Sometimes prolonged treatment with bacteriostatic drugs can kill certain microbial populations (eg, chloramphenicol and meningococci), whereas bactericidal drugs may fail to do so (eg, penicillin G and enterococci), both in vitro and in vivo.

ANTIMICROBIAL ACTION THROUGH INHIBITION OF CELL WALL SYNTHESIS
(Bacitracin, Cephalosporins, Cycloserine, Penicillins, Vancomycin)

In contrast to animal cells, bacteria possess a rigid outer layer, the cell wall, that completely surrounds the cytoplasmic cell membrane. It maintains the shape of microorganisms and "corsets" the bacterial cell, which possesses an unusually high internal osmotic pressure. In gram-negative bacteria, the outermost portion of the cell wall is a lipid bilayer called the outer membrane (Figure 42–1). The internal pressure is three to five times greater in gram-positive than in gram-negative bacteria. Injury to the cell wall (eg, by lysozyme) or inhibition of its formation may lead to lysis of the cell. In a hypertonic environment (eg, 20% sucrose), impaired cell wall synthesis leads to formation of spherical bacterial protoplasts from gram-positive organisms or spheroplasts from gram-negative organisms, which are limited by the fragile cytoplasmic membrane. If such flexible cells are placed in an environment of ordinary tonicity, they take up fluid rapidly and may explode.

The cell wall contains a chemically distinct complex cross-linked polymer, **peptidoglycan** (murein, mucopeptide), consisting of polysaccharides and polypeptides. The polysaccharides regularly contain the amino sugars N-acetylglucosamine and acetylmuramic acid. The latter is found only in bacteria. To the amino sugars are attached short peptide chains. The final rigidity of the cell wall is imparted by cross-link-

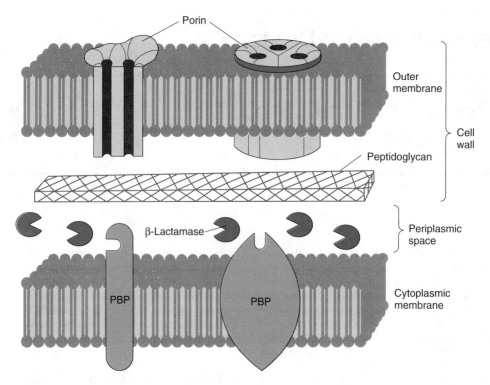

Figure 42–1. A highly simplified diagram of the cell envelope of a gram-negative bacterium. Many components have been omitted for clarity. The outer membrane, a lipid bilayer, is present in gram-negative but not gram-positive organisms. It is penetrated by porins, special proteins that provide hydrophilic access to the cytoplasmic membrane. The peptidoglycan layer is unique to bacteria and is much thicker in gram-positive organisms than in gram-negative organisms. Together, the outer membrane and the peptidoglycan layer constitute the cell wall. Penicillin-binding proteins *(PBPs)* are transmembrane or surface proteins in the cytoplasmic membrane and normally function in the synthetic process for building the peptidoglycan layer. Beta-lactamases, if present, reside in the periplasmic space or on the outer surface of the cytoplasmic membrane, where they may destroy beta-lactam antibiotics that penetrate the outer membrane.

ing of the peptide chains (eg, through pentaglycine bonds) as a result of **transpeptidation** reactions catalyzed by several enzymes (Figure 42–2). The peptidoglycan layer is much thicker in the cell walls of gram-positive than of gram-negative bacteria.

Inhibition of Transpeptidation (Beta-Lactams)

All penicillins and all cephalosporins (beta-lactam antibiotics) are selective inhibitors of bacterial cell wall synthesis. While this is only one of the activities of these drugs, it is perhaps understood better than the others. The initial step in drug action consists of binding of the drug to cell receptors. These **penicillin-binding proteins (PBPs)** number three to six (MW 40,000–120,000) in many bacteria. Different receptors (PBPs) may possess different affinities for a drug, and each may mediate a different mode of action. For example, attachment of penicillin to one PBP may result chiefly in abnormal elongation of the

cell, whereas attachment to another may lead to a cell wall defect at the periphery with resulting cell lysis.

PBPs are under chromosomal control, and mutations may alter their number and their affinities for specific beta-lactam drugs. After a beta-lactam drug has attached to its receptors, the transpeptidation reaction is inhibited and peptidoglycan synthesis is blocked. The next step probably involves the removal or inactivation of an inhibitor of autolytic enzymes (hydrolases) in the cell wall. This activates the lytic enzyme in some microorganisms and may result in lysis if the environment is isotonic. In a hypertonic environment (eg, 20% sucrose), the microbes may change to protoplasts or spheroplasts covered only by the fragile cell membrane. In such cells, synthesis of proteins and nucleic acids may continue for some time.

Inhibition of the transpeptidation enzymes by the penicillins and cephalosporins may be due to a structural similarity of these drugs to acyl-D-alanyl-D-alanine. The transpeptidation reaction involves loss of a D-alanine from the pentapeptide (Figure 42–2). The remarkable lack of toxicity of beta-lactam antibiotics to mammalian cells must be attributed to the absence of a bacterial type cell wall, with its peptidoglycan, in animal cells. The differences in susceptibility of gram-positive and gram-negative bacteria to various penicillins or cephalosporins probably depend on structural differences in their cell walls—eg, the amount of peptidoglycan; the presence of receptors, pores, and lipids; the nature of cross-linking; the activity of autolytic enzymes—that determine penetration, binding, and activity of the drugs.

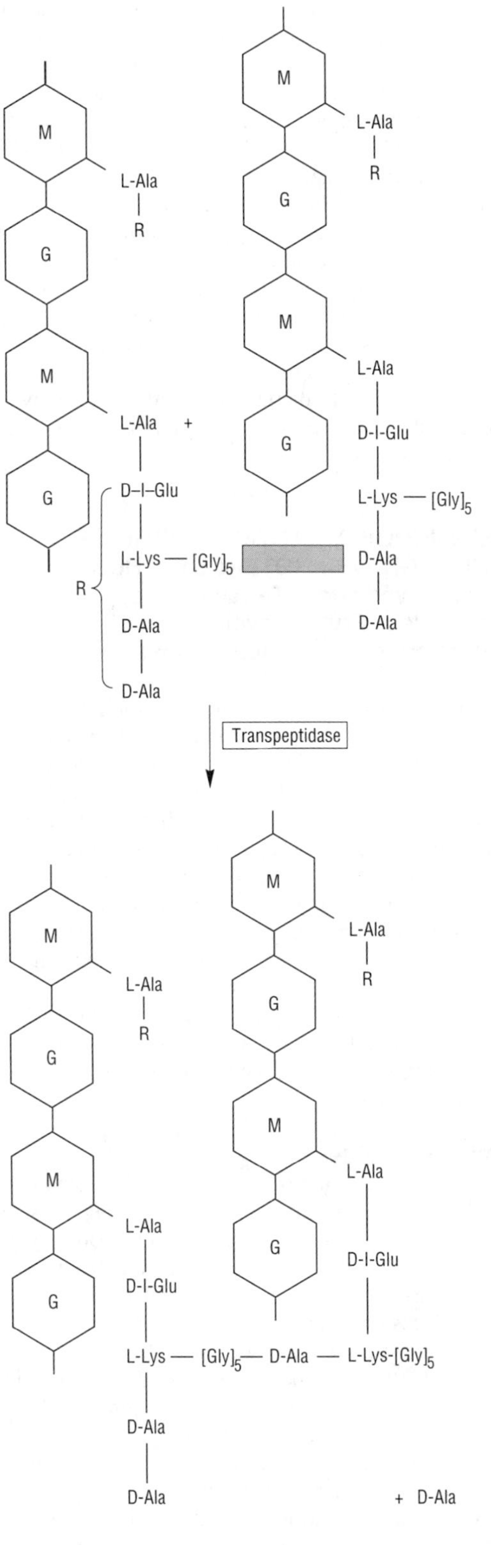

Susceptibility of bacteria to beta-lactam antibiotics depends on various structural and functional characteristics. In order to reach receptors, the drugs must permeate the outer layers of the cell envelope. In gram-negative bacteria, there is an outer phospholipid membrane that may hinder passage of these drugs. If they are able to pass through pore molecules (porins) in this outer barrier, hydrophilic molecules (eg, ampicillin, amoxicillin) may pass more readily than penicillin G. In gram-positive bacteria, the outer phospholipid membrane is lacking and its barrier function is absent.

Amdinocillin is an amidinopenicillanic acid derivative that binds *only* to PBP 2 and is more active against gram-negative than against gram-positive bacteria. Amdinocillin can act synergistically with other beta-lactam drugs that attach to other PBPs.

Some bacteria may be inhibited by beta-lactam drugs as peptidoglycan formation is inhibited, but they may fail to lyse. This tolerance may be due to a lack of activation of autolytic enzymes (hydrolases) in the cell wall. This in turn may be a function of the presence or absence of precursors or of the nature of the enzyme inhibitor.

The most important clinically encountered mechanism of resistance to beta-lactam drugs is the production by the bacteria of beta-lactamases (Figure 42–1). These enzymes break the beta-lactam ring and nullify the antibacterial effect of the drug.

There are many types of beta-lactamases, most of

Figure 42–2. The transpeptidation reaction in *Staphylococcus aureus* that is inhibited by beta-lactam antibiotics. The cell wall of gram-positive bacteria is made up of long peptidoglycan polymer chains consisting of the alternating aminohexoses N-acetylglucosamine *(G)* and N-acetylmuramic acid *(M)* with pentapeptide side chains linked (in *S aureus*) by pentaglycine bridges. The exact composition of the side chains varies among species. The diagram illustrates small segments of two such polymer chains and their amino acid side chains. These linear polymers must be cross-linked by transpeptidation of the side chains at the points indicated by the shaded box to achieve the strength necessary for cell viability. (D-I-Glu, D-isoglutamine.)

them under the genetic control of **plasmids.** Such gene-bearing plasmids are widespread among staphylococci and enteric gram-negative rods. Some beta-lactamases can be firmly bound by compounds such as clavulanic acid or sulbactam and can thus be prevented from attacking hydrolyzable penicillins. A mixture of amoxicillin or ticarcillin with clavulanic acid is used to treat beta-lactamase-producing *Haemophilus* infections. Certain beta-lactam antibiotics are resistant to beta-lactamases because their beta-lactam ring is protected by steric hindrance by methoxy or other groups (eg, methicillin, cefoxitin). Such antibiotics can attack beta-lactamase-producing bacteria, inhibit their transpeptidation, or lyse them. The basis for resistance of some bacteria (eg, methicillin-resistant staphylococci) to the latter type of drug is not well understood. It may depend on varying affinity of receptors for the drug or on the lack of required PBP.

Inhibition of Peptidoglycan Precursor Synthesis

Several drugs, including bacitracin, vancomycin, and ristocetin, inhibit early steps in the biosynthesis of the peptidoglycan (Figure 42–3). Since the early stages of synthesis take place inside the cytoplasmic membrane, these drugs must penetrate the membrane to be effective. For these drugs, the inhibition of peptidoglycan synthesis is not the sole mode of antibacterial action.

Cycloserine, an analogue of D-alanine, also interferes with peptidoglycan synthesis. This drug blocks the action of alanine racemase, an essential enzyme in the incorporation of D-alanine in the pentapeptide of peptidoglycan. Phosphonopeptides also inhibit enzymes needed for early steps in the synthesis of peptidoglycans.

ANTIMICROBIAL ACTION THROUGH INHIBITION OF CELL MEMBRANE FUNCTION (Amphotericin B, Azoles, Polyenes, Polymyxins)

The cytoplasm of all living cells is bounded by the cytoplasmic membrane, which serves as a selective permeability barrier, performs active transport functions, and thus controls the internal composition of the cell. If the functional integrity of the cytoplasmic membrane is disrupted, macromolecules and ions escape from the cell, and cell damage or death ensues. The cytoplasmic membrane of certain bacteria and fungi can be more readily disrupted by certain agents than can the membranes of animal cells. Consequently, selective chemotherapeutic activity is possible.

Examples of this mechanism are the polymyxins acting on gram-negative bacteria (polymyxins selectively act on membranes rich in phosphatidyl ethano-

lamine and act like cationic detergents) and the polyene antibiotics acting on fungi. However, polymyxins are inactive against fungi, and polyenes are inactive against bacteria. This is because ergosterol is present in the fungal cell membrane and absent in the bacterial cell membrane. Polyenes require ergosterol in the fungal cell membrane to exert their effect. Bacterial cell membranes do not contain that sterol and (presumably for this reason) are resistant to polyene action—a good example of cell individuality and of selective toxicity. Fungi that are resistant to polyenes exhibit a decrease in membrane ergosterol or a modification in its structure, so that it combines less well with the drug. The antifungal azoles (see Chapter 48) impair the integrity of fungal cell membranes by inhibiting the biosynthesis of membrane lipids, especially ergosterol.

ANTIMICROBIAL ACTION THROUGH INHIBITION OF PROTEIN SYNTHESIS (Aminoglycosides, Tetracyclines, Macrolides [Erythromycins], Chloramphenicol, Lincomycins)

It is established that aminoglycosides, tetracyclines, chloramphenicol, macrolides, and lincomycins can selectively inhibit protein synthesis through an action on ribosomes in bacteria (Figure 42–4).

Bacteria have 70S ribosomes, whereas mammalian cells have 80S ribosomes. The subunits of each type of ribosome, their chemical composition, and their functional specificities are sufficiently different to explain why antimicrobial drugs can inhibit protein synthesis in bacterial ribosomes without having a major effect on mammalian ribosomes.

In normal microbial protein synthesis, the mRNA message is simultaneously read by several ribosomes that are strung out along the mRNA strand. These are called polysomes.

Aminoglycosides

The mode of action of streptomycin has been studied far more than that of other aminoglycosides (kanamycin, neomycin, gentamicin, tobramycin, netilmicin, sisomicin, amikacin, etc), but probably all act similarly. The first step is the attachment of the aminoglycoside to a specific receptor protein (P 12 in the case of streptomycin) on the 30S subunit of the microbial 70S ribosome. Second, the aminoglycoside blocks the normal activity of the initiation complex of peptide formation (mRNA + formyl methionine + tRNA). Third, the mRNA message is misread on the recognition region of the ribosome, and, as a result, the wrong amino acid is inserted into the peptide, resulting in a nonfunctional protein. Fourth, aminoglycoside attachment results in the breakup of polysomes and their separation into monosomes incapable of protein synthesis. These activities occur more or less

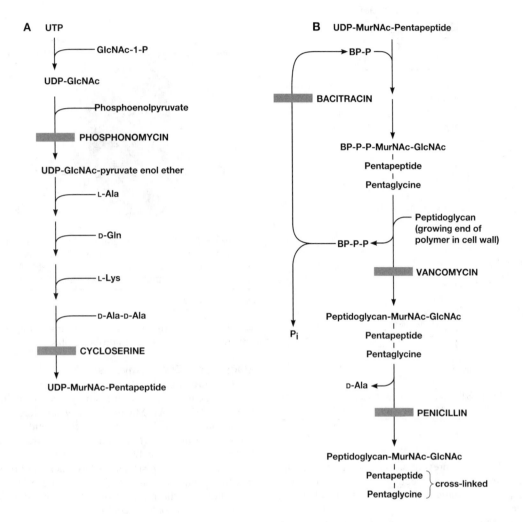

Figure 42–3. The biosynthesis of cell wall peptidoglycan, showing the sites of action of five antibiotics (shaded bars). (BP, bactoprenol; MurNAc, N-acetylmuramic acid; GlcNAc, N-acetylglucosamine.) **A:** Synthesis of UDP-acetylmuramic acid-pentapeptide. **B:** Synthesis of peptidoglycan from UDP-acetylmuramic acid-pentapeptide, UDP-N-acetylglucosamine, and glycyl residues.

simultaneously, and the overall effect is usually an irreversible event—killing the cell.

Chromosomal resistance of microbes to aminoglycosides depends principally on the deletion of a specific protein receptor on the 30S subunit of the ribosome. Plasmid-dependent resistance to aminoglycosides depends mainly on the production by the microorganism of adenylylating, phosphorylating, or acetylating enzymes that destroy the drugs. A third type of resistance consists of a permeability defect, an outer membrane change that reduces active transport of the aminoglycoside into the cell with the result that the drug cannot reach the ribosome. This is at least in some cases plasmid-mediated. The active transport of aminoglycosides into the cell is an energy-dependent, oxygen-dependent process. Therefore, strict anaerobes are relatively insusceptible to aminoglycosides.

Tetracyclines

Tetracyclines bind to the 30S subunit of microbial ribosomes (Figure 42–5). They inhibit protein synthesis by blocking the attachment of charged aminoacyl-

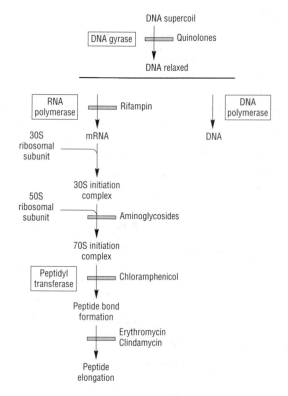

Figure 42–4. Sites of action of drugs that inhibit (shaded bars) microbial nucleic acid and protein synthesis.

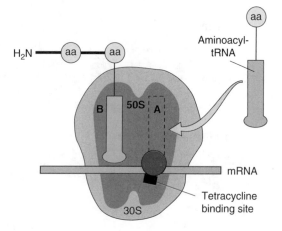

Figure 42–5. Schematic diagram of the site of action of tetracycline antibiotics. Binding to the 30S portion of the ribosome prevents docking of the aminoacyl-tRNA complex, thus inhibiting protein synthesis. (aa, amino acid.)

tRNA. Thus, they prevent introduction of new amino acids into the nascent peptide chain. The action is usually bacteriostatic and reversible upon withdrawal of the drug.

Resistance to tetracyclines results from changes in permeability of the microbial cell envelope. In susceptible cells, the drug is concentrated from the environment by an energy-dependent process of active transport and does not readily leave the cell. In resistant cells, the drug either is not actively transported into the cell or leaves it so rapidly that inhibitory concentrations are not maintained. This is often plasmid-controlled. Mammalian cells do not actively concentrate tetracyclines.

Chloramphenicol

Chloramphenicol attaches to the 50S subunit of the ribosome (Figure 42–6). It interferes with the binding of new amino acids to the nascent peptide chain, largely because chloramphenicol inhibits peptidyl transferase. Chloramphenicol is mainly bacteriostatic, and growth of microorganisms resumes (ie, drug action is reversible) when the drug is withdrawn.

Microorganisms resistant to chloramphenicol produce the enzyme chloramphenicol acetyltransferase,

which destroys drug activity. The production of this enzyme is usually under control of a plasmid.

Macrolides (Erythromycins)

These drugs bind to the 50S subunit of the ribosome and can compete with lincomycins for binding sites (a 23S rRNA). Macrolides may interfere with formation of initiation complexes for peptide chain synthesis or may interfere with aminoacyl translocation reactions (Figure 42–4).

Some macrolide-resistant bacteria lack the proper receptor conformation on the ribosome (through methylation of the receptor site); this may be under plasmid or chromosomal control.

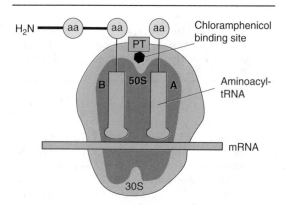

Figure 42–6. Schematic diagram of the site of action of chloramphenicol. Binding to the 50S portion of the ribosome prevents the action of transpeptidase, and blocks the linkage of the new amino acid to the growing peptide chain. (PT, peptidyl transferase; aa, amino acid.)

Lincomycins (Clindamycin)

Lincomycins bind to the 50S subunit of the microbial ribosome and resemble macrolides in binding site, antibacterial activity, and mode of action (Figure 42–4). There may be mutual interference between these drugs, presumably because they share the same receptor.

Chromosomal mutants are resistant to lincomycins by virtue of lacking the proper binding site on the 50S subunit.

ANTIMICROBIAL ACTION THROUGH INHIBITION OF NUCLEIC ACID SYNTHESIS
(Quinolones, Pyrimethamine, Rifampin, Sulfonamides, Trimethoprim)

Drugs such as the actinomycins are effective inhibitors of DNA synthesis. Actually, they form complexes with DNA by binding to the deoxyguanosine residues. The DNA-actinomycin complex inhibits the DNA-dependent RNA polymerase and blocks mRNA formation. Actinomycin also inhibits DNA virus replication. Mitomycins result in the firm cross-linking of complementary strands of DNA and subsequently block DNA replication. Both actinomycins and mitomycin inhibit bacterial as well as animal cells but are not sufficiently selective to be employed in antibacterial chemotherapy.

Rifampin inhibits bacterial growth by binding strongly to the DNA-dependent RNA polymerase of bacteria (Figure 42–4). Thus, it inhibits bacterial RNA synthesis. Rifampin resistance develops as a chromosomal mutation of high frequency that results in a change in RNA polymerase.

All **quinolones** and **fluoroquinolones** are potent inhibitors of nucleic acid synthesis. They block the action of DNA gyrase (topoisomerase II), the enzyme responsible for packing and unpacking supercoiled DNA.

For many microorganisms, p-aminobenzoic acid (PABA) is an essential metabolite. It is used by them as a precursor in the synthesis of folic acid in the pathway leading to the synthesis of nucleic acids. The specific mode of action of PABA probably involves an ATP-dependent condensation of a pteridine with PABA to yield dihydropteroic acid, which is subsequently converted to folic acid. Sulfonamides are structural analogues of PABA and inhibit dihydropteroate synthetase.

Sulfonamides can enter into the reaction in place of PABA in susceptible bacteria and compete for the active center of the enzyme. As a result, nonfunctional analogues of folic acid are formed, preventing further growth of the bacterial cell. The inhibiting action of sulfonamides on bacterial growth can be counteracted by an excess of PABA in the environment (competitive inhibition). Animal cells cannot synthesize folic acid and must depend upon exogenous sources; therefore, they are resistant to the action of sulfonamides. Some bacteria, like animal cells, are not inhibited by sulfonamides.

Tubercle bacilli are not inhibited markedly by sulfonamides, but their growth is inhibited by PAS (p-aminosalicylic acid). Conversely, most sulfonamide-susceptible bacteria are resistant to PAS. This suggests that the receptor site for PABA differs in different types of microorganisms.

Trimethoprim inhibits the dihydrofolic acid reductase of bacteria 50,000 times more efficiently than the same enzyme of mammalian cells. This enzyme reduces dihydrofolic to tetrahydrofolic acid, a stage in the sequence leading to the synthesis of purines and ultimately of DNA. Sulfonamides and trimethoprim produce sequential blocking of this pathway, resulting in marked enhancement (synergism) of activity. Such mixtures (sulfonamide 5 parts + trimethoprim 1 part) have been used in the treatment of *Pneumocystis carinii* pneumonia, *Shigella* enteritis, systemic *Salmonella* infections, and many others.

Pyrimethamine inhibits protozoal dihydrofolate reductase, but it is also somewhat active against the mammalian cell enzyme and therefore more toxic than trimethoprim. Pyrimethamine plus sulfonamides is the current treatment of choice in toxoplasmosis and some other protozoal infections.

Many different chemicals that can interfere with the synthesis of viral nucleic acids have been employed for chemoprophylaxis and chemotherapy of viral infections. These are discussed in Chapter 49, and their mechanism of action is presented there.

RESISTANCE TO ANTIMICROBIAL DRUGS

As described above, there are many different mechanisms by which microorganisms may exhibit resistance to drugs. They are reviewed briefly below.

(1) Microorganisms produce enzymes that destroy the active drug. *Examples:* Staphylococci resistant to penicillin G produce a beta-lactamase that destroys the drug. Other beta-lactamases are produced by gram-negative rods. Gram-negative bacteria resistant to aminoglycosides (usually mediated by a plasmid) produce adenylylating, phosphorylating, or acetylating enzymes that destroy the drug. Gram-negative bacteria may be resistant to chloramphenicol if they produce a chloramphenicol acetyltransferase.

(2) Microorganisms change their permeability to the drug. *Examples:* Tetracyclines accumulate in susceptible bacteria but not in resistant ones. Resistance to polymyxins is probably associated with a change in permeability to the drugs. Streptococci have a natural permeability barrier to aminoglycosides. This can be partly overcome by the simultaneous presence of a cell wall-active drug, eg, a penicillin. Resistance to amikacin and some other aminoglycosides may depend on a lack of permeability to the drugs, apparently due to an outer membrane change that impairs active transport into the cell.

(3) Microorganisms develop an altered structural target for the drug (see also ¶ [5]). *Examples:* Chromosomal resistance to aminoglycosides is associated with the loss (or alteration) of a specific protein on the 30S subunit of the bacterial ribosome that serves as a receptor in susceptible organisms. Erythromycin-resistant organisms have an altered receptor site on the 50S subunit of the bacterial ribosome, resulting from methylation of a 23S ribosomal RNA. Resistance to some penicillins and cephalosporins may be a function of the loss or alteration of PBPs.

(4) Microorganisms develop an altered metabolic pathway that bypasses the reaction inhibited by the drug. *Example:* Some sulfonamide-resistant bacteria do not require extracellular PABA but, like mammalian cells, can utilize preformed folic acid.

(5) Microorganisms develop an altered enzyme that can still perform its metabolic function but is much less affected by the drug than the enzyme in the susceptible organism. *Example:* In some sulfonamide-susceptible bacteria, dihydropteroate synthetase has a much higher affinity for sulfonamide than for PABA. In sulfonamide-resistant mutants, the opposite is the case.

Origin of Drug Resistance

The origin of drug resistance may be genetic or nongenetic.

A. Nongenetic Origin: Active replication of bacteria is usually required for most antibacterial drug actions. Consequently, microorganisms that are metabolically inactive (nonmultiplying) may be resistant to drugs. However, their offspring are fully susceptible. *Example:* Mycobacteria often survive in tissues for many years after infection yet are restrained by the host's defenses and do not multiply. Such persisting organisms are resistant to treatment and cannot be eradicated by drugs. However, if they start to multiply (eg, following loss of cellular immunity in the patient), their progeny are fully susceptible to the same drugs.

Microorganisms may lose the specific target structure for a drug for several generations and thus be resistant. *Example:* Penicillin-susceptible organisms may change to L forms (protoplasts) during penicillin administration. Lacking the cell wall, they are then resistant to cell wall-inhibitor drugs (penicillins, cephalosporins) and may remain so for several generations as "persisters." When these organisms revert to their bacterial parent forms by resuming cell wall production, they are again fully susceptible to penicillin.

B. Genetic Origin: The vast majority of drug-resistant microbes have emerged as a result of genetic changes and subsequent selection processes. Genetic changes may be chromosomal or extrachromosomal.

1. Chromosomal resistance–This develops as a result of spontaneous mutation in a locus on the bacterial chromosome that controls susceptibility to a given antimicrobial. The presence of the drug serves as a selecting mechanism to suppress susceptibles and promote the growth of drug-resistant mutants. Spontaneous mutation occurs with a frequency of 10^{-12} to 10^{-7} and thus is an infrequent cause for the emergence of clinical drug resistance within a given patient. However, chromosomal mutants for resistance to rifampin occur in many bacteria with a much higher frequency (10^{-7}–10^{-5}). Consequently, treatment of bacterial infections with rifampin as the sole drug generally fails.

Chromosomal mutants are commonly resistant by virtue of a change in a structural receptor for a drug. *Examples:* The P 12 protein on the 30S subunit of the bacterial ribosome serves as a receptor for streptomycin attachment. Mutation in the gene that controls the P 12 protein results in streptomycin resistance. A narrow region of the bacterial chromosome contains structural genes that code for a number of drug receptors, including those for erythromycin, tetracycline, lincomycin, aminoglycosides, etc. Mutation may also result in a loss of penicillin receptors in some microbial species, making the mutant penicillin-resistant. Mutation in the structure of DNA gyrase results in resistance to quinolones.

2. Extrachromosomal resistance–Bacteria also contain extrachromosomal genetic elements called plasmids. Plasmids are circular DNA molecules, have 1–3% of the weight of the bacterial chromosome, may exist free in the bacterial cytoplasm, or may be integrated into the bacterial chromosome. Some carry their own genes for replication and transfer. Others rely on genes in other plasmids.

R factors are a class of plasmids that carry genes for resistance to one or more antimicrobial drugs and heavy metals. Plasmid genes for antimicrobial resistance often control the formation of enzymes capable of destroying antimicrobial drugs. *Examples:* Plasmids determine resistance to penicillins and cephalosporins by carrying genes for the formation of beta-lactamases. Plasmids code for enzymes that destroy chloramphenicol (acetyltransferase); enzymes that acetylate, adenylylate, or phosphorylate various aminoglycosides; enzymes that determine the permeability of the cell envelope to tetracyclines; and others.

Genetic material and plasmids can be transferred by the following mechanisms:

a. Transduction–Plasmid DNA is enclosed in a bacterial virus and transferred by the virus to another bacterium of the same species.

b. Transformation–Naked DNA passes from one cell of a species to another cell, thus altering the genotype of the latter. This can occur through laboratory manipulation, such as in recombinant DNA technology, and perhaps spontaneously.

c. Bacterial conjugation–A unilateral transfer of genetic material between bacteria of the same or different genera occurs during a mating (conjugation) process. This is especially important for the spread of plasmid-mediated resistance.

d. Transposition–An exchange of short DNA sequences (transposons), which carry only a few genes, occurs between one plasmid and another or between a plasmid and a portion of the bacterial chromosome within a bacterial cell.

Cross-Resistance

Microorganisms resistant to a certain drug may also be resistant to other drugs that share a mechanism of action or attachment. Such relationships exist mainly between agents that are closely related chemically (eg, polymyxin B-colistin; erythromycin-oleandomycin; neomycin-kanamycin), but they may also exist between unrelated chemicals (erythromycin-lincomycin). In certain classes of drugs, the active nucleus of the chemical is so similar among many congeners (eg, tetracyclines) that full cross-resistance is to be expected.

REFERENCES

Archer GL, Dietrick DR, Johnston JL: Molecular epidemiology of transmissible gentamicin resistance among coagulase-negative staphylococci in a cardiac surgery unit. J Infect Dis 1985;151:243.

Buchanan CE, Strominger JL: Altered penicillin-binding components in penicillin-resistant mutants of *Bacillus subtilis.* Proc Natl Acad Sci USA 1976;73:1816.

Brooks GF et al: *Jawetz, Melnick, & Adelberg's Medical Microbiology, 20th edition.* Appleton & Lange, 1994.

Brumfitt W, Hamilton-Miller J: Methicillin-resistant *Staphylococcus aureus.* N Engl J Med 1989;320:1188.

Cohen ML: Epidemiology of drug resistance: Implications for a post-antimicrobial era. Science 1992;257:1050.

Datta N (editor): Antibiotic resistance in bacteria. Br Med Bull 1984;40:1.

Dever LA, Dermody TS: Mechanisms of bacterial resistance to antibiotics. Arch Intern Med 1991;151:886.

Donowitz GR, Mandell GL: Beta-lactam antibiotics. (Two parts.) N Engl J Med 1988;318:419,490.

Handwerger S, Tomasz A: Antibiotic tolerance among clinical isolates of bacteria. Rev Infect Dis 1985;7:368.

Jacoby GA, Archer GL: New mechanisms of bacterial resistance to antimicrobial agents. N Engl J Med 1991;324:601.

Kass EH, Lode H (editors): Enzyme-mediated resistance to β-lactam antibiotics: Symposium on sulbactam/ampicillin. Rev Infect Dis 1986;8(Suppl 5):S465.

Mandell GL, Douglas RG, Bennett JE (editors): *Principles and Practice of Infectious Diseases,* 3rd ed. Wiley, 1989.

Neu HC: Relation of structural properties of beta-lactam antibiotics to antibacterial activity. Am J Med 1985;79 (Suppl 2A):2.

Neu HC: The crisis in antibiotic resistance. Science 1992;257:1064.

O'Brien TF: Resistance of bacteria to antibacterial agents. Rev Infect Dis 1987;9(Suppl 3):S244.

Reynolds PE: Resistance of the antibiotic target site. Br Med Bull 1984;40:3.

Sanders CC, Weidemann B: Resistance to beta-lactam antibiotics among non-fastidious gram negative organisms. Rev Infect Dis 1988;10:679.

Spratt BG: Penicillin-binding proteins and the future of beta-lactam antibiotics. J Gen Microbiol 1983;129:1247.

Tomasz A: Penicillin-binding proteins in bacteria. Ann Intern Med 1982;96:502.

Ernest Jawetz, MD, PhD

PENICILLINS

In 1929, Fleming reported his observation that colonies of staphylococci lysed on a plate that had become contaminated with a *Penicillium* mold. His efforts to extract the bacteriolytic substance failed, but in 1940 Chain, Florey, and their associates succeeded in producing significant quantities of the first penicillins from cultures of *Penicillium notatum*. By 1949, virtually unlimited quantities of penicillin G were available for clinical use.

The two principal limitations of penicillin G were its susceptibility to destruction by beta-lactamase (penicillinase) and its relative inactivity against most gram-negative bacteria. A research assault on these problems organized by Chain, Rolinson, and Batchelor led, in 1957, to the isolation of 6-aminopenicillanic acid in bulk amounts. Thus began the development of a long series of semisynthetic penicillins. This resulted in the selective design of drugs resistant to beta-lactamase, stable to acid pH, and active against both gram-positive and gram-negative bacteria.

Penicillins and cephalosporins are large groups of drugs that share features of chemistry, mechanism of action, pharmacologic and clinical effects, and immunologic characteristics. These drugs are referred to as beta-lactam drugs because of their unique four-membered lactam ring.

Chemistry

All penicillins share the basic structure shown in Figure 43–1 (top). There is a thiazolidine ring (A) attached to a beta-lactam ring (B) that carries a secondary amino group (R–NH–). Acidic radicals (R, shown in Figure 43–2) can be attached to the amino group and cleaved by bacterial and other amidases. Similar basic structures incorporating the beta-lactam ring provide the cephalosporin, monobactam, and carbapenem families, as shown in Figure 43–1. The structural integrity of the 6-aminopenicillanic acid nucleus is essential to the biologic activity of the molecules. If the beta-lactam ring is enzymatically cleaved by bacterial beta-lactamases (penicillinases),

the resulting product, penicilloic acid, is devoid of antibacterial activity. However, it carries an antigenic determinant of the penicillins, acts as a sensitizing structure when attached to host proteins, and can be used as skin-testing material when attached to peptide chains. Products of alkaline hydrolysis of the penicillins also contribute to sensitization.

The attachment of different radicals (R) to the amino group of 6-aminopenicillanic acid determines the essential pharmacologic properties of the resulting molecules. Clinically important penicillins available in 1994 fall into several groups: (1) Highest activity against gram-positive organisms, little activity against gram-negative rods, and susceptibility to hydrolysis by beta-lactamases, eg, penicillin G. (2) Relatively resistant to staphylococcal beta-lactamases but of lower activity against gram-positive organisms and inactive against gram-negatives, eg, nafcillin, methicillin. (3) Relatively high activity against both gram-negative and gram-positive organisms but destroyed by beta-lactamases, eg, carbenicillin, ticarcillin. (4) Relatively stable to gastric acid and suitable for oral administration, eg, penicillin V, ampicillin, cloxacillin. Some representatives of each group are shown in Figure 43–2, with a few distinguishing characteristics.

Most penicillins are dispensed as the sodium or potassium salt of the free acid. Potassium penicillin G contains about 1.7 meq of K^+ per million units of penicillin (2.8 meq/g). Nafcillin contains Na^+, 2.8 meq/g. Procaine salts and benzathine salts provide repository forms for intramuscular injection.

In dry crystalline form, penicillin salts are stable for long periods (eg, for years at 4 °C). Solutions lose their activity rapidly (eg, 24 hours at 20 °C) and must be prepared fresh for administration.

Antimicrobial Activity of Beta-Lactam Drugs

Beta-lactam agents share general mechanisms of antibacterial action that involve damage to the cell wall of bacteria. These mechanisms are described in Chapter 42. Briefly, the steps are (1) attachment to specific penicillin-binding proteins (PBPs) that serve

Substituted 6-aminopenicillanic acid (PENICILLINS)

Substituted 7-aminocephalosporanic acid (CEPHALOSPORINS)

Substituted 3-amino-4-methylmonobactamic acid (aztreonam) (MONOBACTAMS)

Substituted 3-hydroxyethylcarbapenemic acid (imipenem) (CARBAPENEMS)

Clavulanic acid

as drug receptors on bacteria, (2) inhibition of cell wall synthesis by blocking transpeptidation of peptidoglycan, and (3) activation of autolytic enzymes in the cell wall, which result in lesions that cause bacterial death.

Penicillins and cephalosporins can be bactericidal only if active peptidoglycan synthesis takes place. Metabolically inactive cells are unaffected.

Different penicillins possess different quantitative activity against certain organisms. Whereas 0.002–0.5 µg/mL of penicillin G is lethal for a majority of susceptible gram-positive bacteria, nafcillin and other beta-lactamase-resistant penicillins are 10–100 times less active against the same organisms. The susceptibility of microorganisms is in part a function of the genus and in part a characteristic of individual strains. The difference in susceptibility of gram-positive and gram-negative organisms must depend in part on the number and type of drug receptors; on the relative amount of peptidoglycan present (gram-positive organisms usually possess far more); on the amount of lipids in the cell wall; and on other chemical differences that determine binding, penetration, and resistance to lysis or rupture. The gram-negative *Neisseriae* are as susceptible to penicillin G as many gram-positive organisms.

The activity of penicillin G was originally defined in units. Crystalline sodium penicillin G contains approximately 1600 units/mg (1 unit = 0.6 µg; 1 million units of penicillin = 0.6 g). Most semisynthetic penicillins are prescribed by weight rather than units.

Resistance

Resistance to penicillins falls into several distinct categories.

(1) Certain bacteria (eg, many *Staphylococcus aureus,* some *Haemophilus influenzae* and gonococci, most gram-negative enteric rods) produce beta-lactamases that inactivate some penicillins by breaking the beta-lactam ring. The genetic control of beta-lactamase production—there are about 50 different such enzymes—resides in transmissible plasmids (see Chapter 42). Other penicillins (eg, nafcillin) and cephalosporins are beta-lactamase-resistant because the beta-lactam ring is protected by parts of the R side

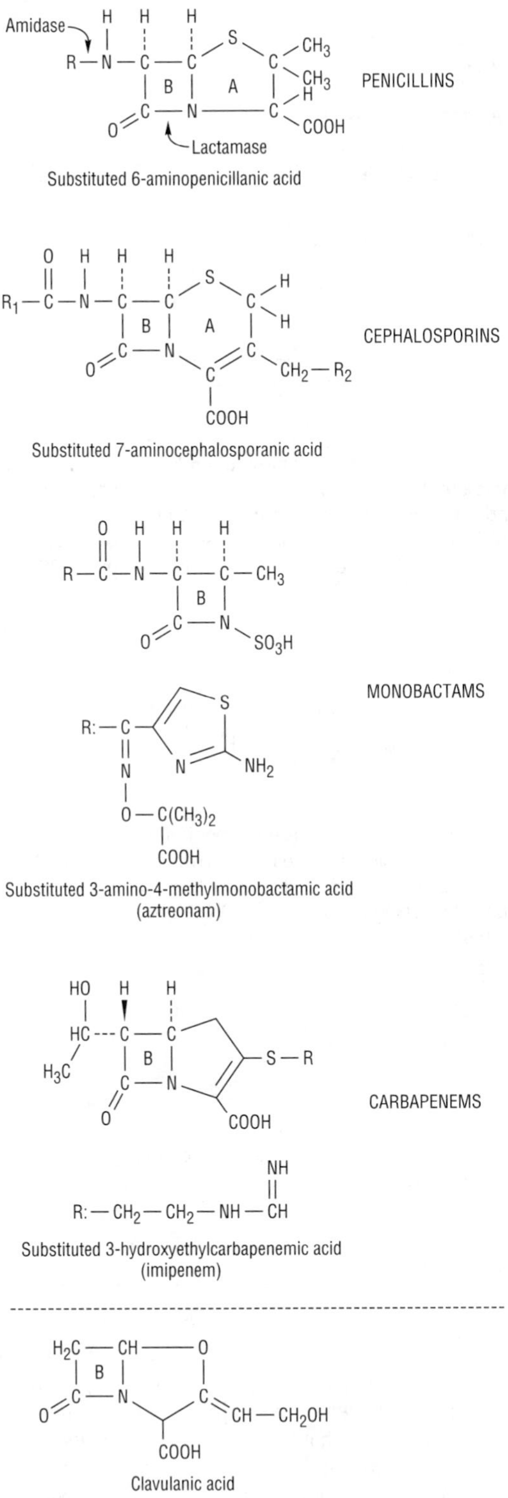

Figure 43–1. Core structures of four beta-lactam antibiotic families and of clavulanic acid. The ring marked B in each structure is the beta-lactam ring. The penicillins are susceptible to bacterial metabolism and inactivation by amidases and lactamases at the points shown. Note that the carbapenems have a different stereochemical configuration in the lactam ring that apparently imparts resistance to beta-lactamases. Substituents for the penicillin and cephalosporin families are shown in Figures 43–2 and 43–3, respectively.

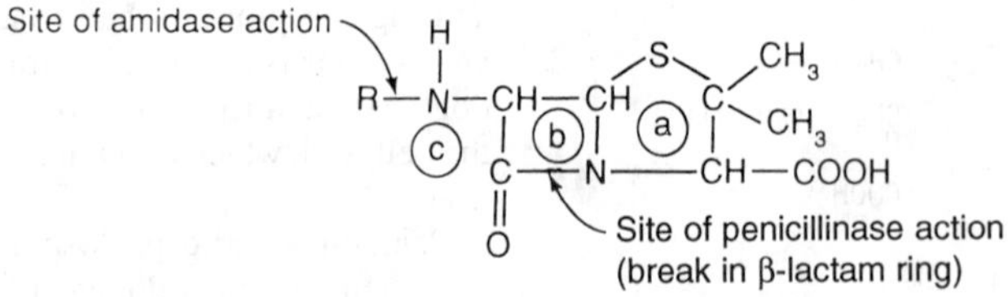

Site of amidase action

6-Aminopenicillanic acid

Site of penicillinase action
(break in β-lactam ring)

The following structures can each be substituted at the R to produce a new penicillin.

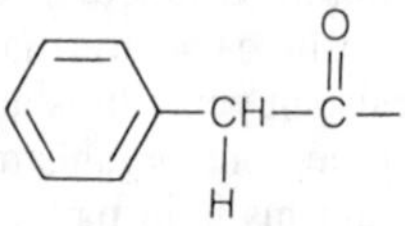

Penicillin G (benzylpenicillin):
High activity against gram-positive bacteria. Low activity against gram-negative bacteria. Acid-labile. Destroyed by β-lactamase. 60% protein-bound.

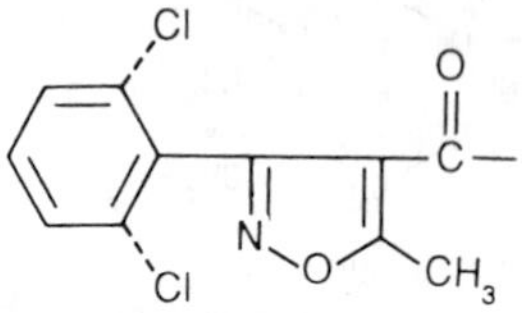

Oxacillin (no Cl atoms); cloxacillin (one Cl in structure) dicloxacillin (2 Cls in structure); flucloxacillin (one Cl and one F in structure) (isoxazolyl penicillins):
Similar to methicillin in β-lactamase resistance, but acid-stable. Can be taken orally. Highly protein-bound (95–98%).

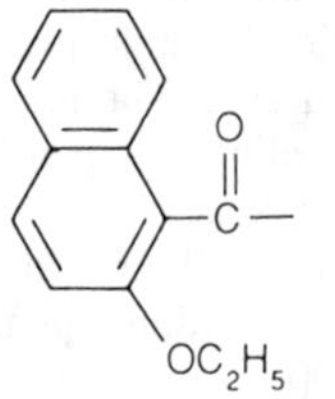

Nafcillin (ethoxynaphthamidopenicillin):
Similar to isoxazolyl penicillins. Less strongly protein-bound (90%). Can be given by mouth or by vein. Resistant to staphylococcal β-lactamase.

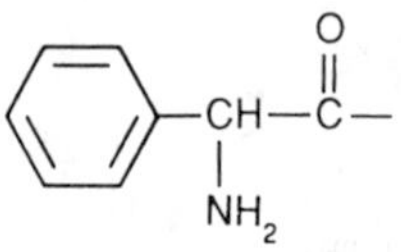

Ampicillin (alpha-aminobenzylpenicillin):
Similar to Penicillin G (destroyed by β-lactamase) but acid-stable and more active against gram-negative bacteria. Cabenicillin has –COONa instead of NH₂ group.

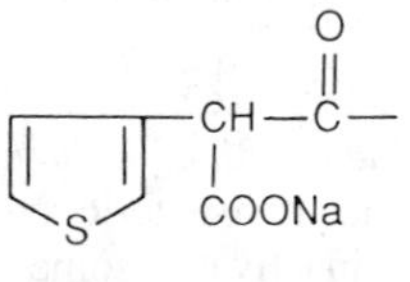

Ticarcillin:
Similar to carbenicillin but gives higher blood levels. Piperacillin, azlocillin, and mezlocillin resemble ticarcillin in action against gram-negative aerobes.

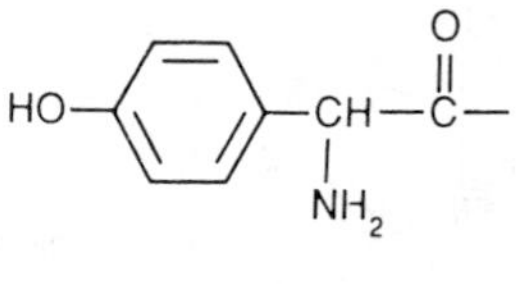

Amoxicillin:
Similar to ampicillin but better absorbed, gives higher blood levels.

Figure 43–2. Structures of some penicillins.

chain. Such penicillins are active against beta-lactamase-producing organisms.

(2) Other bacteria do not produce beta-lactamases but are resistant to the action of penicillins either because they lack specific receptors or because of lack of permeability of outer layers, so that the drug cannot reach the receptors.

(3) Some bacteria may be insusceptible to the killing action of penicillins because the autolytic enzymes in the cell wall are not activated. Such

"tolerant" organisms (eg, certain staphylococci, streptococci, *Listeria*) are inhibited but not killed.

(4) Organisms that lack cell walls (*Mycoplasma*, L forms) or are metabolically inactive are insusceptible to penicillins and other cell wall inhibitors because they do not synthesize peptidoglycans.

(5) Some bacteria (eg, staphylococci) may be resistant to the action of beta-lactamase-resistant penicillins such as methicillin. The mechanism of this resistance appears to depend on a deficiency or inaccessibility of PBP receptors; it is independent of any beta-lactamase production, and its frequency varies greatly with geographic location.

Pharmacokinetics

After parenteral administration, absorption of most penicillins is complete and rapid. Because of the irritation and consequent local pain produced by the intramuscular injection of large doses, administration by the intravenous route (intermittent bolus addition to a continuous drip) is often preferred. After oral administration, absorption differs greatly for different penicillins, depending in part on their acid stability and protein binding. In order to minimize binding to foods, oral penicillins should precede or follow food by at least 1 hour.

After absorption, penicillins are widely distributed in body fluids and tissues. Penicillins are lipid-insoluble and do not enter living cells well. With parenteral doses of 3–6 g (5–10 million units) of penicillin G, injected in divided doses into a continuous infusion or by intramuscular injections, average serum levels of the drug reach 1–10 units (0.6–6 µg)/mL. A relationship of 6 g given parenterally per day yielding serum levels of 1–6 µg/mL also applies to other penicillins. Highly protein-bound penicillins (eg, oxacillin, dicloxacillin) tend to produce lower levels of free drug in serum than less protein-bound penicillins (eg, penicillin G, ampicillin). However, the relevance of protein binding to clinical efficacy of drug is not fully understood.

Special dosage forms of penicillin have been designed for delayed absorption to yield low blood and tissue levels for long periods. The outstanding example is penicillin G benzathine. After a single intramuscular injection of 0.75 g (1.2 million units), serum levels in excess of 0.03 unit/mL are maintained for 10 days and levels in excess of 0.005 unit/mL for 3 weeks. The latter is sufficient to protect against beta-hemolytic streptococcal infection, the former to treat an established infection with these organisms. Procaine penicillin also has delayed absorption, yielding useful levels for 12–24 hours after a single intramuscular injection.

In many tissues, penicillin concentrations are equal to those in serum. Lower levels are found in the eye, the prostate, and the central nervous system. However, with active inflammation of the meninges, as in bacterial meningitis, penicillin levels in the cerebrospinal fluid exceed 0.2 µg/mL with a daily parenteral dose of 12 g. Thus, pneumococcal and meningococcal meningitis may be treated with systemic penicillin, and there is no need for intrathecal injection. It is probable that high levels of penicillins in the cerebrospinal fluid in meningitis are due to (1) increased permeability of meninges, (2) inhibition of the normal active transport of penicillin out of the cerebrospinal fluid, or (3) some binding of penicillin to cerebrospinal fluid proteins. Absorbed penicillins also reach pleural, pericardial, and joint fluids well, so that local injection is rarely warranted.

Most of the absorbed penicillin is rapidly excreted by the kidneys into the urine; small amounts are excreted by other routes. About 10% of renal excretion is by glomerular filtration and 90% by tubular secretion, to a maximum of about 2 g/h in an adult. The normal half-life of penicillin G is ½–1 hour; in renal failure, it may be up to 10 hours. Ampicillin is secreted more slowly than penicillin G. Nafcillin is excreted 80% into the biliary tract and only 20% by tubular secretion; therefore, it is little affected by renal failure. Tubular secretion can be partially blocked by probenecid to achieve higher systemic and cerebrospinal fluid levels. Because renal clearance is less efficient in the newborn, proportionately smaller doses result in higher systemic levels that are maintained longer than in the adult.

Penicillin is also excreted into sputum and milk to levels 3–15% of those present in the serum. This is the case in both humans and cattle. The presence of penicillin in the milk of cows treated for mastitis presents a problem in human allergy.

Clinical Uses

Penicillins are by far the most widely effective and the most extensively used antibiotics. All oral penicillins should be given at other than mealtimes (1 hour before or 1–2 hours after) to reduce binding and acid inactivation. Oxacillin is most strongly bound to food (ie, protein-bound), and dicloxacillin somewhat less so. Blood levels of all penicillins can be raised by simultaneous administration of probenecid, 0.5 g (10 mg/kg in children) every 6 hours orally, which impairs tubular secretion of weak acids.

A. Penicillin G: Penicillin G is the drug of choice for infections caused by pneumococci, streptococci, meningococci, non-beta-lactamase-producing staphylococci and gonococci, *Treponema pallidum* and many other spirochetes, *Bacillus anthracis* and other gram-positive rods, clostridia, *Actinomyces, Listeria,* and *Bacteroides* (except *Bacteroides fragilis*). Most of these infections respond to daily doses of penicillin G, 0.6–10 million units (0.36–6 g). This is generally given by intermittent intravenous injection. Oral administration of **penicillin V** is indicated only in minor infections—eg, of the respiratory tract or its associated structures, especially in children (pharyngitis, otitis, sinusitis)—in a daily dose of 1–4 g. Oral administration is subject to such variable efficacy that it should not be relied upon in seriously ill patients. Many gonococci have developed resistance to penicillin, so that penicillin is no longer a drug of first choice in uncomplicated gonorrhea.

Penicillin G is inhibitory for enterococci, but the simultaneous administration of an aminoglycoside is often necessary for bactericidal effects, eg, in enterococcal endocarditis.

B. Penicillin G Benzathine: This is a salt of

very low water solubility for intramuscular injection that yields low but prolonged drug levels. A single injection of 1.2 million units intramuscularly is satisfactory for treatment of beta-hemolytic streptococcal pharyngitis. A similar injection given intramuscularly once every 3–4 weeks provides satisfactory prophylaxis against reinfection with beta-hemolytic streptococci. Penicillin G benzathine (2.4 million units intramuscularly once a week for 1–3 weeks) is effective in the treatment of early or latent syphilis. This drug should never be given by mouth. Procaine penicillin G (600,000 units intramuscularly twice daily) is used mainly in uncomplicated pneumococcal pneumonia.

C. Ampicillin, Amoxicillin, Carbenicillin, Ticarcillin, Piperacillin, Mezlocillin, Azlocillin: These drugs differ from penicillin G in having greater activity against gram-negative bacteria, but they are inactivated by beta-lactamases.

Ampicillin and amoxicillin have the same spectrum and activity, but amoxicillin is better absorbed from the gut. Thus, a dose of 250–500 mg of amoxicillin 3 times daily is equivalent to the same amount of ampicillin given 4 times daily. These drugs are given orally to treat common urinary tract infections with gram-negative coliform bacteria or mixed secondary bacterial infections of the respiratory tract (sinusitis, otitis, bronchitis). Ampicillin, 300 mg/kg/d intravenously, was a choice for *H influenzae*-caused bacterial meningitis in children. However, because of the frequency of beta-lactamase-producing *H influenzae*, ceftriaxone is now preferred.

Ampicillin is ineffective against *Enterobacter, Pseudomonas,* and indole-positive *Proteus* infections. In invasive *Salmonella* infections (eg, typhoid), ampicillin, 6–12 g/d intravenously, can suppress signs and symptoms and eliminate organisms from some carriers. In typhoid and paratyphoid fevers, ampicillin is an alternative drug. However, it is not beneficial in noninvasive *Salmonella* gastroenteritis and may even prolong carriage and shedding.

Bacampicillin liberates ampicillin after ingestion; it can be given (400–800 mg orally twice daily) for the same indications as ampicillin.

Carbenicillin resembles ampicillin but has more activity against *Pseudomonas* and *Proteus* organisms, though *Klebsiella* species are usually resistant. In susceptible populations of *Pseudomonas,* resistance to carbenicillin may emerge rapidly. Therefore, in *Pseudomonas* sepsis (eg, burns, immunosuppressed patients), carbenicillin, 12–30 g/d intravenously (300–500 mg/kg/d), is usually combined with an aminoglycoside, eg, gentamicin, 5–7 mg/kg/d intramuscularly, to delay emergence of resistance and perhaps to obtain synergistic effects. Carbenicillin contains Na$^+$, 4.7 meq/g. Carbenicillin indanyl sodium is acid-stable and can be given orally in urinary tract infections. Ticarcillin resembles carbenicillin in single and combined activity, but the dose may be lower, eg,

200–300 mg/kg/d intravenously. Piperacillin, mezlocillin, azlocillin, and others resemble ticarcillin and claim special effectiveness against gram-negative aerobic rods, including *Pseudomonas.* However, in serious *Pseudomonas* infections, they should be used in combination with an aminoglycoside.

Ampicillin, amoxicillin, ticarcillin, and others in this group can be protected from destruction by beta-lactamases if they are administered together with beta-lactamase inhibitors such as clavulanic acid, sulbactam, or tazobactam (see below). Such mixtures have been employed against lactamase-producing *H influenzae* or coliform organisms. The possible advantages of such mixtures over appropriate cephalosporins are not fully evident.

D. Penicillins Resistant to Beta-Lactamases: The sole indication for their use is infection by beta-lactamase-producing staphylococci.

Oxacillin, cloxacillin, dicloxacillin, or nafcillin, 0.25–0.5 g orally every 4–6 hours (50–100 mg/kg/d for children), is suitable for treatment of mild localized staphylococcal infections. All of these drugs are relatively acid-stable and reasonably well absorbed from the gut. They are all highly protein-bound (95–98%). Food interferes with absorption, and the drugs must be administered 1 hour before or after meals.

For serious systemic staphylococcal infections, nafcillin, 8–12 g/d, is given by intermittent intravenous infusion of 1–2 g every 2–4 hours (50–100 mg/kg/d for children). Methicillin is more nephrotoxic than nafcillin and is rarely used.

Adverse Reactions

The penicillins undoubtedly possess less direct toxicity than any other antibiotics. Most of the serious adverse effects are due to hypersensitivity.

A. Allergy: All penicillins are cross-sensitizing and cross-reacting. Any preparation containing penicillin, including foods or cosmetics, may induce sensitization. In general, sensitization occurs in direct proportion to the duration and total dose of penicillin received in the past. The responsible antigenic determinants appear to be degradation products of penicillins, particularly penicilloic acid and products of alkaline hydrolysis bound to host protein. Skin tests with penicilloylpolylysine, alkaline hydrolysis products, and undegraded penicillin will identify many hypersensitive individuals. Among positive reactors to skin tests, the incidence of subsequent penicillin reactions is high and is associated with cell-bound IgE antibodies. Although many persons develop IgG antibodies to antigenic determinants of penicillin, the presence of such antibodies does not appear to be correlated with allergic reactivity (except rare hemolytic anemia), and serologic tests have little predictive value. A history of a penicillin reaction is not reliable; about 5–8% of people claim such a history in the USA. However, in such cases, penicillin should be administered with caution or a substitute drug given.

About 10–15% of persons with a history of a penicillin reaction have an allergic reaction when given penicillin again. Less than 1% of persons who previously received penicillin without incident will have an allergic reaction when given penicillin again. The incidence of allergic reactions in small children is negligible.

Allergic reactions may occur as typical anaphylactic shock (very rare—0.05% of recipients); typical serum sickness type reactions (now rare—urticaria, fever, joint swelling, angioneurotic edema, intense pruritus, and respiratory embarrassment occurring 7–12 days after exposure); and a variety of skin rashes, oral lesions, fever, interstitial nephritis (an autoimmune reaction to a penicillin-protein complex), eosinophilia, hemolytic anemia and other hematologic disturbances, and vasculitis.

At times, individuals known to be hypersensitive to penicillin can tolerate the drug during corticosteroid administration. "Desensitization" with gradually increasing doses of penicillin is rarely indicated. Most patients allergic to penicillins can be treated with alternative drugs. Anaphylactic reactions are less common after oral penicillin administration than after parenteral administration.

B. Toxicity: Since the action of penicillin is directed against a unique bacterial structure, the cell wall, it is virtually without effect on most animal cells. However, all penicillins are irritating to the central nervous system and greatly increase the excitability of neurons. For that reason, no more than 20,000 units can be given intrathecally on any one day, but there is little indication for intrathecal administration at present. In rare cases, a patient receiving high doses (eg, > 20 million units of penicillin G daily) has exhibited signs of cerebrocortical irritation as a result of the passage of penicillin into the central nervous system. With doses of this magnitude, direct cation toxicity (Na^+, K^+) can also occur (see Chemistry, above), particularly in patients with renal failure. The local toxic effects of penicillin G are due to the direct irritation caused by intramuscular or intravenous injection of exceedingly high concentrations (eg, 1 g/mL injectate). Such concentrations may cause local pain, induration, thrombophlebitis, or degeneration of an accidentally injected nerve.

Large doses of penicillins given orally may lead to gastrointestinal upset, particularly nausea, vomiting, and diarrhea. This is more pronounced with the broad-spectrum forms (ampicillin, amoxicillin) than with other penicillins. Oral therapy may also be accompanied by luxuriant overgrowth of staphylococci, *Pseudomonas, Proteus,* or yeasts, which may occasionally cause enteritis. Superinfections in other organ systems may occur with penicillins as with any antibiotic therapy. Methicillin, nafcillin, and other penicillins have occasionally caused granulocytopenia, especially in children. Methicillin causes nephritis more commonly than does nafcillin. The tubu-

lar basement membrane protein serves to bind penicillin, and antibody to the carrier-hapten antigen forms a complex, with binding of complement. Carbenicillin can cause hypokalemic alkalosis and transaminase elevation in serum. It can also induce hemostatic defects, leading to a bleeding tendency. Ampicillin frequently causes skin rashes, some of which are not allergic in nature.

Problems Relating to the Use & Misuse of the Penicillins

The penicillins are by far the most widely used antibiotics. Several thousand tons of these drugs have been administered to humans during the past 40 years. Therefore, penicillins have been responsible for some of the most drastic consequences of antibiotic misuse.

A significant proportion (perhaps 1–5%) of the population of many countries has become hypersensitive. In many cases, there is no doubt that sensitization has occurred when penicillin was administered without proper indication. However, hypersensitivity may be temporary.

The saturation of certain environments (eg, hospitals) with penicillin has produced a selection pressure against penicillin-sensitive microorganisms and resulted in greater numbers of penicillin-resistant organisms. In the 1950s, hospitals were an important site for the proliferation and selection of beta-lactamase-producing staphylococci. Now beta-lactamase-producing staphylococci prevail everywhere; they cause about 80% of community-acquired staphylococcal infections.

The suppression of normal flora creates a partial void that is regularly filled with drug-resistant, prevalent organisms. Penicillins are administered to a high proportion of patients in hospitals. These patients are made selectively susceptible to superinfections with microorganisms derived from the hospital environment (*Proteus, Pseudomonas, Enterobacter, Serratia,* staphylococci, yeasts, etc).

Plasmids that control beta-lactamase production are being distributed with increasing frequency among different genera of microorganisms. *Neisseria gonorrhoeae* has acquired such plasmids, probably from *Haemophilus* organisms. In West Africa and in the Philippines, outbreaks of beta-lactamase-producing gonococci are seen. Local endemic foci have also been found in the USA (eg, Los Angeles), presenting problems for their control.

Although pneumococci have long been considered an example of total and regular susceptibility to penicillins, this is no longer entirely true. In New Guinea and South Africa, outbreaks of relatively penicillin-resistant pneumococci have been observed, causing pneumonia and meningitis. Such pneumococci do not produce beta-lactamase, but up to 6 μg/mL of penicillin G may be necessary to kill them. Such concentrations of penicillin cannot be achieved in the central nervous system, and the mortality rate from meningitis has consequently been high. Sporadic cases of similar resistance have been observed in Spain and the USA.

CEPHALOSPORINS

Cephalosporium fungi yielded several antibiotics that resembled penicillins but were resistant to beta-lactamase and were active against both gram-positive and gram-negative bacteria. Methods were eventually developed for the large-scale production of the common nucleus, 7-aminocephalosporanic acid. This made possible the synthesis of a vast array of cephalosporins with varying properties. Cephamycins (fermentation products of *Streptomyces*) and some totally synthetic drugs such as moxalactam resemble cephalosporins.

Chemistry

The nucleus of the cephalosporins, 7-aminocephalosporanic acid, bears a close resemblance to 6-aminopenicillanic acid (Figure 43–1) and also to the nucleus of the cephamycin antibiotics. The intrinsic antimicrobial activity of natural cephalosporins is low, but the attachment of various R_1 and R_2 groups has yielded drugs of good therapeutic activity and low toxicity (Figure 43–3).

The cephalosporins have molecular weights of 400–450. They are soluble in water and relatively stable to pH and temperature changes. They vary in resistance to beta-lactamases. The sodium salt of cephalothin contains 2.4 meq Na^+ per gram.

Antimicrobial Activity

The mechanism of action of cephalosporins is analogous to that of penicillins: (1) binding to specific penicillin-binding proteins (PBPs) that serve as drug receptors on bacteria; (2) inhibition of cell wall synthesis by blocking transpeptidation of peptidoglycan; and (3) activation of autolytic enzymes in the cell wall, which results in lesions that cause bacterial death.

Resistance to cephalosporins can be attributed to (1) poor penetration of bacteria by the drug, (2) lack of PBPs for a specific drug, (3) degradation of drug by beta-lactamases (cephalosporinases; many such enzymes exist), (4) appearance of special beta-lactamases in the course of treatment of certain gram-negative rods (*Enterobacter, Serratia, Pseudomonas* strains), and (5) failure of activation of autolytic enzymes in the cell wall.

Cephalosporins have traditionally been divided into three major groups or "generations," depending mainly on the spectrum of antimicrobial activity. All cephalosporins are inactive against enterococci and methicillin-resistant staphylococci.

FIRST-GENERATION CEPHALOSPORINS

This group includes cefadroxil, cefazolin, cephalexin, cephalothin, cephapirin, and cephradine.

Antimicrobial Activity

These drugs are very active against gram-positive cocci, including pneumococci, viridans streptococci, group A hemolytic streptococci, and *S aureus*. Among gram-negative bacteria, *Escherichia coli, Klebsiella pneumoniae*, and *Proteus mirabilis* are often sensitive, but there is very little activity against *Pseudomonas aeruginosa*, indole-positive *Proteus, Enterobacter, Serratia marcescens, Citrobacter*, and *Acinetobacter*. Anaerobic cocci (eg, *Peptococcus, Peptostreptococcus*) are usually sensitive, but *B fragilis* is not.

Pharmacokinetics & Dosage

A. Oral: Cephalexin, cephradine, and cefadroxil are absorbed from the gut to a variable extent. After oral doses of 500 mg, serum levels are 15–20 μg/mL. Urine concentration is usually very high, but in most tissues levels are variable and generally lower than in serum. Cephalexin and cephradine are given orally in doses of 0.25–0.5 g 4 times daily (15–30 mg/kg/d) and cefadroxil in doses of 0.5–1 g twice daily. Excretion is mainly by glomerular filtration and tubular secretion into the urine. Tubular secretory blocking agents, eg, probenecid, may increase serum levels substantially. In patients with impaired renal function, dosage must be reduced: For creatinine clearance 20–50 mL/min, give half the dose; for creatinine clearance less than 20 mL/min, give one-fourth the normal dose.

B. Intravenous: After an intravenous infusion of 1 g, the peak level of cefazolin is 90–120 μg/mL, while levels of cephalothin or cephapirin are 40–60 μg/mL. The usual intravenous dose of cefazolin for adults is 1–2 g intravenously every 8 hours (50–100 mg/kg/d), and for cephalothin or cephapirin it is 1–2 g every 4–6 hours (50–200 mg/kg/d). Excretion is via the kidney, and with impaired renal function dosage adjustment must be made similar to that suggested for the oral drugs.

C. Intramuscular: This tends to produce local pain, less with cefazolin than with cephapirin, and is therefore rarely employed.

Clinical Uses

Although the first-generation cephalosporins have a broad spectrum of activity and are relatively nontoxic, they are rarely the drug of choice for any infection. Oral drugs may be used for the treatment of urinary tract infections, for minor staphylococcal lesions, or for minor polymicrobial infections such as cellulitis or soft tissue abscess. However, oral cephalosporins should not be relied upon in serious systemic infections.

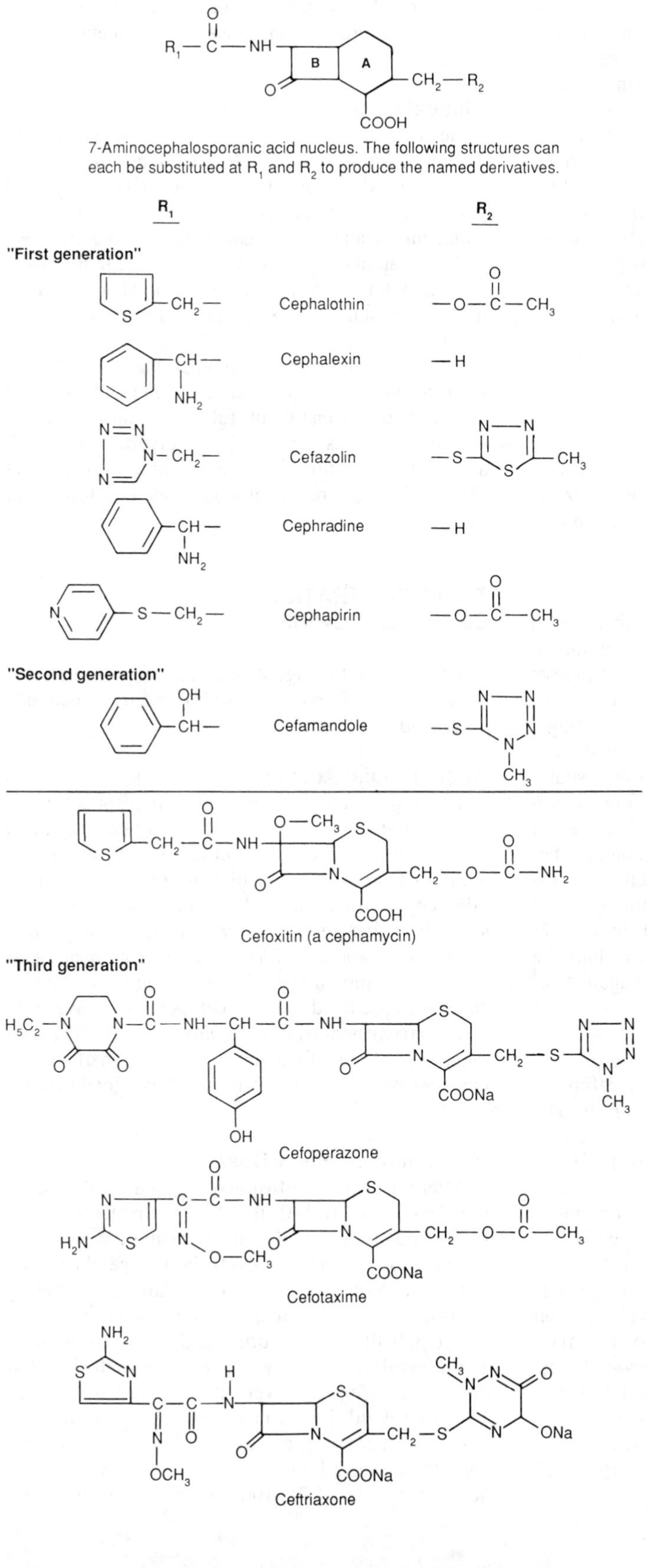

7-Aminocephalosporanic acid nucleus. The following structures can each be substituted at R_1 and R_2 to produce the named derivatives.

R_1   **R_2**

"First generation"

Cephalothin

Cephalexin

Cefazolin

Cephradine

Cephapirin

"Second generation"

Cefamandole

Cefoxitin (a cephamycin)

"Third generation"

Cefoperazone

Cefotaxime

Ceftriaxone

Figure 43–3. Structures of some cephalosporins.

Intravenously injected first-generation cephalosporins penetrate most tissues well and are drugs of choice for surgical prophylaxis, especially cefazolin. Second- and third-generation cephalosporins offer *no* advantage for surgical prophylaxis, are far more expensive, and should not be used for that purpose.

Intravenously injected first-generation cephalosporins may be a choice in infections for which they are the least toxic drugs (eg, *K pneumoniae*) and in persons with a history of a mild penicillin hypersensitivity reaction but not anaphylaxis. First-generation cephalosporins do not penetrate the central nervous system and cannot be used to treat meningitis.

SECOND-GENERATION CEPHALOSPORINS

Members of this group include cefaclor, cefamandole, cefonicid, ceforanide, cefoxitin, cefmetazole, cefotetan, cefuroxime, cefprozil, loracarbef, and cefpodoxime.

Antimicrobial Activity

This is a heterogeneous group of drugs with marked individual differences in activity, pharmacokinetics, and toxicity. In general, they are active against organisms affected by first-generation drugs, but they have an extended gram-negative coverage. *Enterobacter, Klebsiella* (including those resistant to cephalothin), and indole-positive *Proteus* are usually sensitive. Cefamandole, cefuroxime, cefonicid, ceforanide, and cefaclor are active against *H influenzae* but not against *Serratia* or *B fragilis*. In contrast, cefoxitin, cefmetazole, and cefotetan are active against *B fragilis* and some *Serratia* strains but not against *H influenzae*. All second-generation cephalosporins are less active against gram-positive bacteria than the first-generation drugs, and none are active against enterococci or *P aeruginosa*.

Pharmacokinetics & Dosage

A. Oral: Cefaclor, cefuroxime axetil, cefprozil, cefpodoxime, and loracarbef can be given orally. The usual dose for adults is 10–15 mg/kg/d in two to four divided doses; children should be given 20–40 mg/kg/d up to a maximum of 1 g/d.

B. Intravenous Administration: After an intravenous infusion of 1 g, serum levels are usually 75–125 μg/mL, but they reach 200–250 μg/mL for cefonicid. There are marked differences among drugs in half-life, protein binding, and interval between doses. For cefoxitin (50–200 mg/kg/d) or cefamandole (75–200 mg/kg/d), the interval is 4–6 hours. Drugs with longer half-lives are injected less frequently, eg, cefuroxime, 0.75–1.5 g every 8–12 hours; cefotetan, 1–2 g every 8–12 hours; cefonicid or ceforanide, 1–2 g (15–30 mg/kg/d) every 12–24 hours; cefprozil, 500 mg every 24 hours.

In general, intramuscular injection is too painful to be used. In renal failure, dosage adjustments are required.

Clinical Uses

Because of its activity against beta-lactamase-producing *H influenzae* or *Moraxella catarrhalis,* cefaclor is used to treat sinusitis and otitis media in patients who are allergic—or have not responded—to ampicillin or amoxicillin. Cefuroxime is the only second-generation drug that crosses the blood-brain barrier well enough to be considered for the treatment of meningitis. Resistance of *H influenzae* has been encountered.

Because of their activity against anaerobes (including *B fragilis*), cefoxitin and cefotetan (cephamycins) and cefmetazole can be useful in such mixed anaerobic infections as peritonitis or diverticulitis. Cefamandole (or cefuroxime) can be employed to treat community-acquired pneumonia but has few other uses.

THIRD-GENERATION CEPHALOSPORINS

Third-generation agents include cefoperazone, cefotaxime, ceftazidime, ceftizoxime, ceftriaxone, cefixime, and moxalactam.

Antimicrobial Activity

The major feature of these drugs (except cefoperazone) is their expanded gram-negative coverage and their ability to reach the central nervous system. In addition to the gram-negative bacteria inhibited by other cephalosporins, third-generation drugs are consistently active against *Enterobacter, Citrobacter, S marcescens,* and *Providencia* as well as beta-lactamase-producing strains of *Haemophilus* and *Neisseria*. While ceftazidime and cefoperazone have adequate activity against *P aeruginosa*, the other drugs in the group inhibit only a varying proportion of strains. Only ceftizoxime and moxalactam have good activity against *B fragilis.*

Pharmacokinetics & Dosage

After intravenous infusion of 1 g of these drugs, serum levels are 60–140 μg/mL. They penetrate body fluids and tissues well and—with the exception of cefoperazone—achieve levels in the cerebrospinal fluid sufficient to inhibit most pathogens, including gram-negative rods, except perhaps *Pseudomonas.*

The half-life of these drugs and the necessary dosage interval vary greatly: Ceftriaxone (half-life, 7–8 hours) can be injected every 12–24 hours in a dose of 15–30 mg/kg/d, but in meningitis the dose must be 30–50 mg/kg/d injected every 12 hours. Cefoperazone (half-life, 2 hours) can be injected every 8–12 hours in a dose of 25–100 mg/kg/d. The remaining drugs in the group (half-life, 1–1.7 hours) can be injected every 6–8 hours in doses between 2 and 12 g/d, depending on the severity of infection. Cefixime can be given orally (400 mg twice daily) for respiratory or urinary tract infections

The excretion of cefoperazone and ceftriaxone is mainly through the biliary tract; thus, no dosage adjustment is required in renal insufficiency. The others are excreted by the kidney and therefore require dosage adjustment in renal insufficiency.

Clinical Uses

Because of their penetration of the central nervous system, third-generation cephalosporins—except cefoperazone and cefixime—can be used to treat meningitis, including meningitis caused by pneumococci, meningococci, *H influenzae,* and susceptible enteric gram-negative rods. They can usually not be relied on in meningitis caused by *P aeruginosa.* Other potential indications include sepsis of unknown cause in the immunocompetent patient and susceptible infections in which cephalosporins are the least toxic drugs available. In neutropenic, febrile immunocompromised patients, third-generation cephalosporins can be effective if used in combination with an aminoglycoside.

Adverse Effects
of Cephalosporins

A. Allergy: Cephalosporins are sensitizing and may elicit a variety of hypersensitivity reactions, including anaphylaxis, fever, skin rashes, nephritis, granulocytopenia, and hemolytic anemia. The chemical nucleus of cephalosporins is sufficiently different from that of penicillins so that some individuals with a history of penicillin allergy may tolerate cephalosporins. The frequency of cross-allergenicity between the two groups of drugs is uncertain but probably 6–18%. *However, patients with a history of anaphylaxis to penicillins should never receive cephalosporins.*

B. Toxicity: Local irritation can produce severe pain after intramuscular injection and thrombophlebitis after intravenous injection. Renal toxicity, including interstitial nephritis and even tubular necrosis, has been demonstrated and has caused the withdrawal of cephaloridine.

Cephalosporins that contain a methylthiotetrazole group (eg, cefamandole, moxalactam, cefmetazole, cefotetan, cefoperazone) frequently cause hypoprothrombinemia and bleeding disorders. Administration of vitamin K, 10 mg twice weekly, can prevent this. Moxalactam can also interfere with platelet function and has induced severe bleeding. It has been largely abandoned.

Drugs with the methylthiotetrazole ring can also cause severe disulfiram-like reactions; consequently, alcohol and alcohol-containing medications must be avoided.

Superinfection

Many second- and particularly third-generation cephalosporins are ineffective against gram-positive organisms, especially staphylococci and enterococci. During treatment with such drugs, these resistant organisms, as well as fungi, often proliferate and may induce superinfection.

OTHER BETA-LACTAM DRUGS

Monobactams

These are drugs with a monocyclic beta-lactam ring (Figure 43–1). They are resistant to beta-lactamases and active against gram-negative rods (including *Pseudomonas* and *Serratia*), but they have no activity against gram-positive bacteria or anaerobes. The first of such drugs to become available was aztreonam, which resembles aminoglycosides in activity. Aztreonam is given intravenously every 8 hours in a dose of 1–2 g, providing peak serum levels of 100 μg/mL. The half-life is 1–2 hours and is greatly prolonged in renal failure.

Penicillin-allergic patients can apparently tolerate aztreonam without reaction. Occasional skin rashes and elevations of serum transaminase occur during administration of aztreonam, but major toxicity has not yet been reported. Superinfections with staphylococci and enterococci occur. The clinical usefulness of aztreonam has not yet been fully defined.

Beta-Lactamase Inhibitors:
Clavulanic Acid, Sulbactam, Tazobactam

These substances resemble beta-lactam molecules (Figure 43–1) but themselves have very weak antibacterial action. However, they are potent inhibitors of bacterial beta-lactamases and can protect hydrolyzable penicillins from inactivation by these enzymes. Thus, clavulanic acid combined with amoxicillin or ticarcillin can be effective in treating respiratory infections with beta-lactamase-producing *H influenzae.* Sulbactam combined with ampicillin can be effective in various infections caused by beta-lactamase-producing organisms, though it appears to be less effective in intra-abdominal and gynecologic mixed infections than clindamycin plus an aminoglycoside. There appears to be no unequivocal preference for any of these combinations compared with other available drugs.

Carbapenems

The carbapenems are a new class of drugs structurally related to beta-lactam antibiotics (Figure 43–1). The first agent of this class to be extensively studied in humans was imipenem. It has a wide spectrum with good activity against many gram-negative rods, gram-positive organisms, and anaerobes. It is resistant to beta-lactamases but is inactivated by dihydropeptidases in renal tubules, resulting in low urinary concentrations. Consequently, it is administered together with an inhibitor of renal dihydropeptidase, cilastatin, for clinical use.

Imipenem penetrates body tissues and fluids well, including the cerebrospinal fluid. The usual dose is 0.5–1 g given intravenously every 6 hours (half-life, 1 hour). The dose must be reduced in renal insufficiency, and an additional dose must be given after hemodialysis.

The role of imipenem in therapy has not been well defined. It may be indicated for infections caused by susceptible organisms that are resistant to other available drugs. Since *Pseudomonas* may rapidly develop resistance to imipenem, the simultaneous use of an aminoglycoside is required. A combination of imipenem with an aminoglycoside may be effective treatment for febrile neutropenic patients.

The most common adverse effects of imipenem are nausea, vomiting, diarrhea, skin rashes, and reactions at the infusion sites. Excessive levels in patients with renal failure may lead to seizures. Patients allergic to penicillins may be allergic to imipenem as well.

PREPARATIONS AVAILABLE

PENICILLINS

Amoxicillin (generic, Amoxil, others)
Oral: 125, 250 mg chewable tablets; 250, 500 mg capsules; powder to reconstitute for 50 mg/mL solution

Amoxicillin/potassium clavulanate (Augmentin)
Oral: 250, 500 mg tablets; 125, 250 mg chewable tablets; powder to reconstitute for 125, 250 mg/5 mL suspension

Ampicillin (generic, Omnipen, Polycillin, others)
Oral: 250, 500 mg capsules; powder to reconstitute for 100, 125, 250, 500 mg suspensions
Parenteral: powder to reconstitute for injection (125, 250, 500 mg, 1, 2 g per vial; 1, 2 g per IV piggyback unit; 10 g bulk vials)

Ampicillin/sulbactam sodium (Unasyn)
Parenteral: 1, 2 g powder to reconstitute for IV or IM injection

Azlocillin (Azlin)
Parenteral: powder to reconstitute for injection (2, 3, 4 g per vial or IV piggyback unit)

Bacampicillin (Spectrobid)
Oral: 400 mg tablets (equivalent to 280 mg ampicillin); powder to reconstitute for 125 mg/5 mL suspension

Carbenicillin (Geocillin)
Oral: 382 mg tablets
Parenteral: powder for injection (1, 2, 5, 10 g per vial or IV piggyback unit; 10, 20 30 g bulk package)

Cloxacillin (generic, Tegopen)
Oral: 250, 500 mg capsules; powder to reconstitute for 125 mg/5 mL solution

Dicloxacillin (generic, Dynapen, others)
Oral: 125, 250, 500 mg capsules; powder to reconstitute for 62.5 mg/5 mL suspension

Methicillin (Staphcillin)
Parenteral: powder to reconstitute for injection (1, 4, 6 g per vial; 1 g per IV piggyback unit; 10 g bulk package)

Mezlocillin (Mezlin)
Parenteral: powder to reconstitute for injection (in 1, 2, 3, 4 g vials and IV piggyback units, 20 g bulk package)

Nafcillin (generic, Unipen, Nafcil, Nallpen)
Oral: 250 mg capsules; 500 mg tablets; powder to reconstitute for 250 mg/5 mL solution
Parenteral: powder to reconstitute for IV, IM injection (0.5, 1, 2 g per vial); 1, 2 g per IV piggyback units; 10 g bulk package

Oxacillin (Bactocill, Prostaphlin)
Oral: 250, 500 mg capsules; powder to reconstitute for 250 mg/5 mL solution
Parenteral: powder to reconstitute for injection (0.25, 0.5, 1, 2 g per vial; 1, 2, 4 g IV piggyback units; 10 g bulk package)

Penicillin G (generic, Pentids, Pfizerpen)
Oral: 0.2, 0.25, 0.4, 0.5, 0.8 million unit tablets; powder to reconstitute 400,000 units/5mL suspension
Parenteral: powder to reconstitute for injection (0.2, 0.5, 1, 5, 10, 20 million units)

Penicillin G benzathine (Permapen, Bicillin)
Oral: 0.2 million unit tablets
Parenteral: 0.3, 0.6, 1.2, 2.4 million units per dose

Penicillin G procaine (generic)
Parenteral: 0.3, 0.6, 1.2, 2.4 million units for IM injection only

Penicillin V (generic, V-Cillin, Pen-Vee K, others)
Oral: 125, 250, 500 mg tablets; powder to reconstitute for 125, 250 mg/5 mL solution

Piperacillin (Pipracil)
Parenteral: powder to reconstitute for injection (2, 3, 4 g per vial or IV piggyback unit; 40 g bulk package)

Piperacillin and tazobactam sodium (Zosyn)
Parenteral: 2,3,4 g powder to reconstitute for IV injection

Ticarcillin (Ticar)
Parenteral: powder to reconstitute for injection

(1, 3, 6 g per vial; 3 g per IV piggyback unit; 20, 30 g bulk vials)

Ticarcillin and clavulanate potassium (Timentin)

Parenteral: powder to reconstitute for injection (3 g ticarcillin with 0.1 g clavulanic acid per vial or IV piggyback unit)

CEPHALOSPORINS & OTHER BETA-LACTAM DRUGS

Narrow Spectrum (First-Generation) Cephalosporins

Cefadroxil (generic, Duricef, Ultracef)
Oral: 500 mg capsules; 1 g tablets; 125, 250, 500 mg/5 mL suspension

Cefazolin (Ancef, Kefzol)
Parenteral: powder to reconstitute for injection (0.25, 0.5, 1 g per vial or IV piggyback unit; 5, 10, 20 g per bulk vial)

Cephalexin (generic, Keflex, others)
Oral: 250, 500 mg capsules and tablets; 1 g tablets; 125, 250 mg/5 mL suspension; 100 mg/mL pediatric suspension

Cephalothin (generic, Keflin, Seffin)
Parenteral: powder to reconstitute for injection and solution for injection (1, 2 g per vial or infusion pack; 10, 20 g bulk vials)

Cephapirin (generic, Cefadyl)
Parenteral: powder to reconstitute for injection (0.5, 1, 2, 4 g per vial or IV piggyback unit; 20 g bulk package)

Cephradine (generic, Anspor, Velosef)
Oral: 250, 500 mg capsules; 125, 250 mg/5 mL suspension
Parenteral: powder to reconstitute for injection (0.25, 0.5, 1, 2 g per vial)

Intermediate Spectrum (Second-Generation) Cephalosporins

Cefaclor (Ceclor)
Oral: 250, 500 mg capsules; powder to reconstitute for 125, 187, 250, 375 mg/5 mL suspension

Cefamandole (Mandol)
Parenteral: 0.5, 1, 2, 10 g (in vials) for IM, IV injection

Cefmetazole (Zefazone)
Parenteral: 1, 2 g powder for IV injection

Cefonicid (Monocid)
Parenteral: powder to reconstitute for injection (0.5, 1, 10 g per vial)

Ceforanide (Precef)

Parenteral: powder to reconstitute for IM, IV injection (0.5, 1, 10 g per vial)

Cefoxitin (Mefoxin)
Parenteral: powder to reconstitute for injection (1, 2, 10 g per vial)

Cefpodoxime (Vantin)
Oral: 100, 200 mg tablets; 50, 100 mg granules for suspension in 5 mL

Cefprozil (Cefzil)
Oral: 250, 500 mg tablets; powder to reconstitute 125, 250 mg/5mL suspension

Cefuroxime (Ceftin, Kefurox, Zinacef)
Oral: 125, 250, 500 mg tablets
Parenteral: powder to reconstitute for injection (0.75, 1.5, 7.5 g per vial or infusion pack)

Loracarbef (Lorabid)
Oral: 200 mg capsules; powder for 100 mg/5 mL suspension

Broad-Spectrum (Third-Generation) Cephalosporins

Cefixime (Suprax)
Oral: 200, 400 mg tablets; powder for oral suspension, 100 mg/5 mL

Cefoperazone (Cefobid)
Parenteral: powder to reconstitute for injection (1, 2 g per vial)

Cefotaxime (Claforan)
Parenteral: powder to reconstitute for injection (1, 2, 10 g per vial; 10 g bulk package)

Cefotetan (Cefotan)
Parenteral: powder to reconstitute for injection (1, 2, 10 g per vial)

Ceftazidime (Fortaz, Tazidime)
Parenteral: powder to reconstitute for injection (0.5, 1, 2 g per vial; 6 g per bulk package)

Ceftizoxime (Cefizox)
Parenteral: powder to reconstitute for injection and solution for injection (0.5, 1, 2 g per vial)

Ceftriaxone (Rocephin)
Parenteral: powder to reconstitute for injection (0.25, 0.5, 1, 2, 10 g per vial)

Carbapenem

Imipenem/cilastatin (Primaxin)
Parenteral: powder to reconstitute for injection (250, 500 mg imipenem per vial)

Monobactam

Aztreonam (Azactam)
Parenteral: powder to reconstitute for injection (0.5, 1, 2 g)

REFERENCES

Barriere SL, Flaherty JF: Third-generation cephalosporins: A critical evaluation. Clin Pharm 1984;3:351.

Blanca M et al: Cross-reactivity between penicillins and cephalosporins: Clinical and immunologic studies. J Allergy Clin Immunol 1989;83:381.

Brittain DC, Scully BE, Neu HC: Ticarcillin plus clavulanic acid in the treatment of pneumonia and other infections. Am J Med 1985;79(Suppl 5B):81.

Brown NM et al: Cefuroxime resistance in *Haemophilus influenzae*. Lancet 1992;340:552.

Donowitz GR, Mandell GL: Beta lactam antibiotics. (Two parts.) N Engl J Med 1988;318:419, 490.

Eliopoulous GM, Moellering RC Jr: Azlocillin, mezlocillin, and piperacillin: New broad-spectrum penicillins. Ann Intern Med 1982;97:755.

Ellner JJ (editor): Cefixime: A new third generation cephalosporin. Am J Med 1988;85(3A):1.

Erffmeyer JE: Adverse reactions to penicillin. (Two parts.) Ann Allergy 1981;47:288, 294.

EORT Int Antimicrobial Therapy Cooperative Group: Ceftazidime combined with amikacin for empirical therapy of gram negative bacteremia in cancer patients with granulopenia. N Engl J Med 1987;317:1692.

Hackbarth CJ, Chambers HF: Methicillin-resistant staphylococci: Detection methods and treatment of infections. Antimicrob Agents Chemother 1989;33:995.

Handsfiel HH et al: A comparison of single-dose cefixime with ceftriaxone as treatment for uncomplicated gonorrhea. N Engl J Med 1991;325:1337.

Hartman B, Tomasz A: Altered penicillin-binding proteins in methicillin-resistant strains of *Staphylococcus aureus*. Antimicrob Agents Chemother 1981;19:726.

International Rheumatic Fever Study Group: Allergic reactions to long-term benzathine penicillin prophylaxis for rheumatic fever. Lancet 1991;337:1308.

Kass EH, Lode H (editors): Enzyme-mediated resistance to β-lactam antibiotics: Symposium on sulbactam/ampicillin. Rev Infect Dis 1986;8(Suppl 5):S465.

Musher DM: Syphilis, neurosyphilis, penicillin, and AIDS. J Infect Dis 1991;163:1201.

Nelson JD: Emerging role of cephalosporins in bacterial meningitis. Am J Med 1985;79(Suppl 2A):47.

Neu HC: New antibiotics: Areas of appropriate use. J Infect Dis 1987;155:403.

Pakter RL et al: Coagulopathy associated with the use of moxalactam. JAMA 1982;248:1100.

Petz LD: Immunologic cross-reactivity between penicillins and cephalosporins: A review. J Infect Dis 1978;137 (Suppl):S74.

Platt R et al: Serum-sickness-like reactions to amoxicillin, cefaclor, cephalexin, and trimethoprim-sulfamethoxazole. J Infect Dis 1988;158:474.

Platt R, et al: Perioperative antibiotic prophylaxis for herniorrhaphy and breast surgery. N Engl J Med 1990;332:153.

Remington JS (editor): Carbapenems: A new class of antibiotics. (Symposium.) Am J Med 1985;78(Suppl 6A):1.

Rolinson GN: 6-APA and the development of the beta-lactam antibiotics. J Antimicrob Chemother 1979;5:7.

Rolinson GN: β-Lactam antibiotics. J Antimicrob Chemother 1986;17:5.

Rolinson GN: β-Lactamase induction and resistance to lactam antibiotics. J Antimicrob Chemother 1989;23:1.

Rudolph AH, Price EV: Penicillin reactions among patients in venereal disease clinics: A national survey. JAMA 1973;223:499.

Sanders CC: Novel resistance selected by the new expanded-spectrum cephalosporins: A concern. J Infect Dis 1983;147:585.

Schaad UB et al: A comparison of ceftriaxone and cefuroxime for the treatment of bacterial meningitis in children. N Engl J Med 1990;322:141.

Sexually transmitted diseases: Treatment guidelines. MMWR Morb Mortal Wkly Rep 1989;38:S8.

Smith CR et al: Cefotaxime compared with nafcillin plus tobramycin for serious bacterial infections: A randomized, double-blind trial. Ann Intern Med 1984;101:469.

Stone HH et al: Third-generation cephalosporins for polymicrobial surgical sepsis. Arch Surg 1983;118:193.

Swan SK, Bennett WM: Drug dosing guidelines in patients with renal failure. West J Med 1992;156:633.

Sykes RB, Bonner DP: Discovery and development of the monobactams. Rev Infect Dis 1985;7(Suppl 4):S579.

Sykes RB: The classification and terminology of enzymes that hydrolyze beta-lactam antibiotics. J Infect Dis 1982;145:762.

Tipper DJ: Mode of action of beta-lactam antibiotics. Rev Infect Dis 1979;1:39.

Wendel GD et al: Penicillin allergy and desensitization in serious infections during pregnancy. N Engl J Med 1985;312:1229.

White R et al: Halving of mortality of severe melioidosis by ceftazidime. Lancet 1989;2:697.

Chloramphenicol & Tetracyclines

44

Ernest Jawetz, MD, PhD

CHLORAMPHENICOL

Chloramphenicol was first isolated from cultures of *Streptomyces venezuelae* in 1947 and was synthesized in 1949, the first completely synthetic antibiotic of importance to be produced commercially. It is the only available representative of its chemical type.

Chemistry

Crystalline chloramphenicol is a neutral, stable compound with the following structure:

Chloramphenicol

Chloramphenicol consists of colorless crystals with an intensely bitter taste. It is highly soluble in alcohol and poorly soluble in water. Saturated aqueous solutions (0.25%) keep their activity for many months at refrigerator or room temperature if protected from light. Chloramphenicol succinate is highly soluble in water and is hydrolyzed in tissues, with liberation of free chloramphenicol; it is used for parenteral administration.

Antimicrobial Activity

Chloramphenicol is a potent inhibitor of microbial protein synthesis and has little effect on other microbial metabolic functions. Chloramphenicol binds reversibly to a receptor site on the 50S subunit of the bacterial ribosome. There it interferes markedly with the incorporation of amino acids into newly formed peptides by blocking the action of peptidyl transferase (see Chapter 42 and Figures 42–4 and 42–6). Chloramphenicol also inhibits mitochondrial protein synthesis in mammalian bone marrow cells but does not greatly affect other intact cells.

Chloramphenicol is bacteriostatic for many bacteria and for rickettsiae but is clinically ineffective against chlamydiae. Its action is reversible upon removal of the drug. Most gram-positive bacteria are

inhibited by chloramphenicol in concentrations of 1–10 μg/mL, and many gram-negative bacteria are inhibited by concentrations of 0.2–5 μg/mL. *Haemophilus influenzae, Neisseria meningitidis,* and some strains of *Bacteroides* are highly susceptible, and for them chloramphenicol may be bactericidal. Some salmonellae are susceptible, but plasmid-mediated resistance to chloramphenicol has appeared with increasing frequency.

Resistance

In most bacterial species, large populations of chloramphenicol-susceptible cells contain occasional resistant mutants that are less permeable to the drug. These mutants are usually only two to four times more resistant than the parent populations; consequently, they emerge slowly in treated individuals. There is no cross-resistance between chloramphenicol and other drugs, but plasmids may transmit multiple drug resistance (chloramphenicol, tetracycline, streptomycin, etc) from one bacterium to another by conjugation (see Chapter 42). Such plasmid-mediated resistance to chloramphenicol results from the production of chloramphenicol acetyltransferase, a bacterial enzyme that inactivates the drug. Consequently, the resistance of such plasmid-containing microorganisms is of high order.

Pharmacokinetics

After oral administration, crystalline chloramphenicol is rapidly and completely absorbed. With daily doses of 2 g orally, blood levels usually reach 8 μg/mL. Chloramphenicol palmitate, administered to children in doses up to 50 mg/kg/d orally, is hydrolyzed in the intestine to yield free chloramphenicol, but the usual blood levels rarely exceed 10 μg/mL. For parenteral injection, chloramphenicol succinate, 25–50 mg/kg/d intravenously or intramuscularly, yields free chloramphenicol by hydrolysis, giving blood levels somewhat lower than those achieved with the orally administered drug. After absorption, chloramphenicol is widely distributed to virtually all tissues and body fluids, including the central nervous system and cerebrospinal fluid. In fact, the concentration of chloramphenicol in brain tissue may be equal to that in serum—a unique property for the treatment of central nervous system infections. Circulating chloramphenicol is about 30% protein-bound. The drug penetrates cell membranes readily. Most of the drug is inactivated in the body either by conjugation with glucuronic acid (principally in the liver) or by reduction to inactive aryl amines. Excretion of active chloramphenicol (about 10% of the total dose administered) and of inactive degradation products (about 90% of the total) occurs by way of the urine. It may be that the active drug is cleared mainly by glomerular filtration and the inactive products mainly by tubular secretion. Only small amounts of active drug are excreted into bile or feces. The systemic dosage of chloramphenicol need not be altered in renal insufficiency, but it must be reduced markedly in hepatic failure.

Clinical Uses

Because of potential toxicity and the availability of other effective drugs (eg, cephalosporins), chloramphenicol is a possible choice only in the following infections: (1) Symptomatic *Salmonella* infection, eg, typhoid fever. Many strains of *Salmonella* are now resistant, and trimethoprim-sulfamethoxazole is used often. (2) Serious infections with *H influenzae,* eg, meningitis, epiglottitis, or pneumonia. (3) Meningococcal or pneumococcal infections of the central nervous system in patients hypersensitive to beta-lactam drugs. (4) Anaerobic or mixed infections in the central nervous system, eg, brain abscess. (5) Rarely, as an alternative to tetracycline in severe rickettsial infections.

Chloramphenicol is occasionally used topically in the treatment of eye infections because of its wide antibacterial spectrum and its penetration of ocular tissues and the aqueous humor. However, it is not effective in chlamydial infections.

A. Salmonellosis: For *Salmonella* infections (eg, typhoid or paratyphoid fever), adults should receive chloramphenicol, 2–3 g daily orally for 14–21 days, and children 30–50 mg/kg/d orally for 14–21 days. Prolonged treatment tends to reduce the frequency of relapses. A similar program may be followed in severe rickettsial infections (eg, scrub typhus or Rocky Mountain spotted fever).

B. *Haemophilus:* For *H influenzae* meningitis or laryngotracheitis (in small children) or pneumonia (in the elderly), chloramphenicol, 50–100 mg/kg/d orally or intravenously, has been given for 8–14 days, depending upon clinical response and cerebrospinal fluid changes. Since chloramphenicol-resistant *Haemophilus* strains have appeared, ceftriaxone or cefotaxime may now be the drugs of choice.

C. Other Uses: In life-threatening sepsis probably originating in the lower bowel, chloramphenicol, 2 g/d, is sometimes combined with an aminoglycoside (eg, amikacin, 15 mg/kg/d). Because of the ex-

cellent penetration by chloramphenicol of all parts of the central nervous system, it is sometimes used in cerebritis, brain abscess, or meningitis of ill-defined origin. In adult meningitis, the dose of chloramphenicol is 50 mg/kg/d in four divided doses. Sepsis caused by some species of *Bacteroides* and severe melioidosis may respond to chloramphenicol.

Adverse Reactions

A. Gastrointestinal Disturbances: Adults taking chloramphenicol, 1.5–2.5 g daily, occasionally develop nausea, vomiting, and diarrhea in 2–5 days. This is rare in children. After 5–10 days, the results of microbial flora alteration may become apparent, with prominent candidiasis of mucous membranes (especially of the mouth and vagina).

B. Bone Marrow Disturbances: Adults taking chloramphenicol in excess of 50 mg/kg/d regularly exhibit disturbances in red cell maturation after 1–2 weeks of blood levels above 25–30 µg/mL. These are characterized by the appearance of markedly vacuolated nucleated red cells in the marrow, anemia, and reticulocytopenia. These anomalies usually disappear when chloramphenicol is discontinued. The disturbance appears to be a maturation arrest associated with a rise in serum iron concentration and a depression of serum phenylalanine levels and is not related to the rare occurrence of aplastic anemia.

Aplastic anemia is a rare consequence of chloramphenicol administration by any route. It probably represents a specific genetically determined idiosyncrasy of the individual. It is not related to dose or time of intake but is seen more frequently with prolonged use. It tends to be irreversible and fatal. The precise incidence of fatal aplastic anemia as a toxic reaction to chloramphenicol administration is not known, but the disease is estimated to occur 13 times more frequently after the use of the drug than it does spontaneously. Aplastic anemia probably develops in one of every 24,000–40,000 patients who have taken chloramphenicol. Leukemia may follow the development of hypoplastic anemia.

C. Toxicity for Newborn Infants: Newborn infants lack an effective glucuronic acid conjugation mechanism for the degradation and detoxification of chloramphenicol. Consequently, when infants are given doses of 75 mg/kg/d or more, the drug may accumulate, resulting in the **gray baby syndrome,** with vomiting, flaccidity, hypothermia, gray color, shock, and collapse. To avoid this toxic effect, chloramphenicol should be used with caution in infants and the dosage limited to 50 mg/kg/d or less in full-term infants and 30 mg/kg/d or less in prematures.

D. Interaction With Other Drugs: Chloramphenicol may prolong the half-life and raise the blood concentration of phenytoin, tolbutamide, chlorpropamide, and warfarin. This is attributable to inhibition of liver microsomal enzymes by chloramphenicol. It may precipitate a variety of other drugs from solutions. Like other bacteriostatic inhibitors of microbial protein synthesis, chloramphenicol can *antagonize* the bactericidal action of penicillins or aminoglycosides (see Chapter 52).

Medical & Social Implications of Overuse

Because of its "broad spectrum" and its apparent lack of toxicity, chloramphenicol was used indiscriminately between 1948 and 1951 without specific indications. It has been estimated that more than 8 million people received the drug for minor complaints, respiratory (usually viral) illnesses, etc. This inappropriate use was followed by a wave of cases of aplastic anemia, which, in turn, almost resulted in the complete abandonment of an effective drug.

TETRACYCLINES

The tetracyclines are a large group of drugs with a common basic structure and activity. Chlortetracycline, isolated from *Streptomyces aureofaciens,* was introduced in 1948. Oxytetracycline, derived from *Streptomyces rimosus,* was introduced in 1950. Tetracycline, obtained by catalytic dehalogenation of chlortetracycline, has been available since 1953. Demeclocycline was obtained by demethylation of chlortetracycline. More recently developed tetracyclines have emphasized good absorption combined with prolonged blood levels.

Chemistry

All of the tetracyclines have the basic structure shown below.

	R$_7$	R$_6$	R$_5$	Renal Clearance (mL/min)
Chlortetracycline	—Cl	—CH$_3$	—H	35
Oxytetracycline	—H	—CH$_3$	—OH	90
Tetracycline	—H	—CH$_3$	—H	65
Demeclocycline	—Cl	—H	—H	35
Methacycline	—H	=CH$_2$*	—OH	31
Doxycycline	—H	—CH$_3$*	—OH	16
Minocycline	—N(CH$_3$)$_2$	—H	—H	10

*There is no —OH at position 6 on methacycline and doxycycline.

Free tetracyclines are crystalline amphoteric substances of low solubility. They are available as hydrochlorides, which are more soluble. Such solutions are acid and, with the exception of chlortetracycline, fairly stable. Tetracyclines combine firmly with divalent metal ions, and this chelation can interfere with

absorption and activity of the molecule. Tetracyclines fluoresce bright yellow in ultraviolet light of 360 nm wavelength.

Antimicrobial Activity

Tetracyclines are the prototype broad-spectrum antimicrobial drugs. They are bacteriostatic for many gram-positive and gram-negative bacteria, including some anaerobes; for rickettsiae, chlamydiae, mycoplasmas, and L forms; and for some protozoa, eg, amebas. Equal concentrations of tetracyclines in body fluids or tissues have approximately equal antimicrobial activity. Minocycline may have greater lipophilic properties than other congeners. Most differences in activity claimed for individual tetracycline drugs are of small magnitude and limited importance. Differences in clinical efficacy are attributable largely to features of absorption, distribution, and excretion of individual drugs. However, great differences exist in the susceptibility of different strains of a given species of microorganism. Laboratory tests on clinical isolates may therefore be important.

Tetracyclines enter microorganisms in part by passive diffusion and in part by an energy-dependent process of active transport. As a result, susceptible cells concentrate the drug so that the intracellular drug concentration is much higher than the extracellular one. Once inside the cell, tetracyclines bind reversibly to receptors on the 30S subunit of the bacterial ribosome in a position that blocks the binding of the aminoacyl-tRNA to the acceptor site on the mRNA-ribosome complex (see Figure 42–5). This effectively prevents the addition of new amino acids to the growing peptide chain, inhibiting protein synthesis. The selective inhibition of protein synthesis in microorganisms may be explained largely by the failure of mammalian cells to concentrate tetracyclines.

Resistance

Microbial populations containing mostly susceptible organisms also contain small numbers of organisms resistant to tetracyclines. These lack an active transport mechanism across cell membranes and thus do not concentrate tetracycline in their cells. Alternatively, resistant bacteria may lack passive permeability to tetracyclines. The degree of resistance is variable. Among gram-negative bacterial species (especially *Pseudomonas, Proteus,* and coliforms), the selection of highly resistant types has already occurred, and tetracyclines have therefore lost much of their usefulness. Tetracycline resistance is usually transmitted by plasmids. With widespread use, resistance is increasing even among what were at first highly susceptible bacterial species (eg, pneumococci, *Bacteroides*).

Plasmids controlling resistance may be transmitted by transduction or by conjugation. The genes for tetracycline resistance are closely associated with those for other drugs, eg, aminoglycosides, sulfonamides, and chloramphenicol. Plasmids therefore usually transmit resistance to multiple drugs rather than to tetracyclines alone.

Pharmacokinetics

Tetracyclines are absorbed somewhat irregularly from the gastrointestinal tract. A portion of an orally administered dose of tetracycline remains in the gut lumen, modifies intestinal flora, and is excreted in the feces. While only 30% of chlortetracycline and 60–80% of tetracycline, oxytetracycline, and demeclocycline are absorbed in the gut, absorption is 90–100% for doxycycline and minocycline. Absorption occurs mainly in the upper small intestine and is best in the absence of food. It is impaired by chelation with divalent cations (Ca^{2+}, Mg^{2+}, Fe^{2+}) or with Al^{3+}, especially in milk and antacids, and by alkaline pH. Specially buffered tetracycline solutions are formulated for parenteral (usually intravenous) administration in persons unable to take oral medication. The parenteral dosage is generally similar to the oral dosage.

In the blood, 40–80% of various tetracyclines is protein-bound. With oral doses of 500 mg every 6 hours, tetracycline hydrochloride and oxytetracycline reach peak levels of 4–6 µg/mL. With doxycycline and minocycline, the peak levels are somewhat lower (2–4 µg/mL). Intravenously injected tetracyclines give somewhat higher levels only temporarily. The drugs are distributed widely to tissues and body fluids, except for the cerebrospinal fluid, where concentrations are low. Minocycline is unique in reaching very high concentrations in tears and saliva—a feature that permits it to eradicate the meningococcal carrier state. Tetracyclines cross the placenta to reach the fetus and are also excreted in milk. As a result of chelation with calcium, tetracyclines are bound to growing bones and teeth.

Absorbed tetracyclines are excreted mainly in bile and urine. Concentrations in bile are ten times higher than in serum; some of the drug excreted in bile is reabsorbed from the intestine (enterohepatic circulation) and contributes to maintenance of serum levels. Ten to 50 percent of various tetracyclines is excreted into the urine, mainly by glomerular filtration. The renal clearance of tetracyclines ranges from 10 to 90 mL/min. Ten to 40 percent of the drug in the body is excreted in feces.

Doxycycline and minocycline are almost completely absorbed from the gut and are excreted more slowly, leading to persistent serum levels. Doxycycline does not require renal excretion and does not accumulate significantly in renal failure.

Clinical Uses

Tetracyclines were the first broad-spectrum antibiotics. They are effective against a variety of microorganisms and are thus often used indiscriminately.

Tetracyclines are the drugs of choice in infections with *Mycoplasma pneumoniae,* chlamydiae, and rickettsiae and some spirochetes. They are useful in mixed bacterial infections related to the respiratory tract, eg, sinusitis and bronchitis. They may be employed in various gram-positive and gram-negative bacterial infections, including *Vibrio* infections, provided the organism has not become resistant. In cholera, tetracyclines rapidly stop the shedding of vibrios, but tetracycline resistance has appeared during epidemics.

Tetracyclines are effective in most chlamydial infections, including sexually transmitted diseases in which chlamydiae participate. Other uses include treatment of acne, urinary tract infections, exacerbations of bronchitis, Lyme disease, relapsing fever, and leptospirosis. Doxycycline is effective for the prophylaxis of leptospirosis.

In brucellosis, tularemia, and plague, tetracyclines may be given in combination with an aminoglycoside. Tetracyclines are sometimes employed in the treatment of protozoal infections, eg, those due to *Entamoeba histolytica or Plasmodium falciparum.*

While minocycline, 200 mg orally daily for 5 days, can eradicate the meningococcal carrier state, rifampin is generally preferred. Demeclocycline inhibits the action of ADH in the renal tubule and has been used in the treatment of inappropriate secretion of ADH or similar peptides by certain tumors (see Chapter 15).

A. Oral Dosage: The minimal effective oral dose for rapidly excreted tetracyclines, equivalent to tetracycline hydrochloride, is 0.25 g 4 times daily for adults and 20 mg/kg/d for children. For severe systemic infections, a dose two to three times larger for at least 3–5 days is indicated. For chlamydial genital infections, treatment for 10–14 days is advisable.

The minimal effective daily dose is 600 mg for demeclocycline or methacycline, 100 mg for doxycycline, and 200 mg for minocycline. Tetracyclines chelate with metals, as noted above, and thus should not be administered with milk, antacids, or ferrous sulfate. To avoid deposition in growing bones or teeth, tetracyclines are not usually indicated for pregnant women or for children under 8 years of age.

Tetracycline hydrochloride, 250–500 mg daily, is commonly taken for many months to suppress acne, especially in adolescents and young adults. This low dose presumably suppresses lipase activity of propionibacteria (see Chapter 63).

B. Parenteral Dosage: Several tetracyclines are available for intravenous injection in doses of 0.1–0.5 g every 6–12 hours (10–15 mg/kg/d in children). Intramuscular injection is usually unsatisfactory because of pain and inflammatory reactions. There are very few instances (eg, an unconscious patient with rickettsial disease) that warrant parenteral tetracycline administration.

Adverse Reactions

Hypersensitivity reactions (drug fever, skin rashes) to tetracyclines appear to be uncommon. Most adverse effects are due to direct toxicity of the drug or to alteration of microbial flora.

A. Gastrointestinal Adverse Effects: Nausea, vomiting, and diarrhea are the commonest reasons for discontinuing tetracycline medication. During the first few days of administration, they appear to be attributable to direct local irritation of the intestinal tract.

After a few days of oral use, tetracyclines tend to modify the normal flora. Although some coliform organisms are suppressed, *Pseudomonas, Proteus,* staphylococci, resistant coliforms, clostridia, and *Candida* become prominent. This can result in intestinal functional disturbances, anal pruritus, vaginal or oral candidiasis, or even enterocolitis with shock and death.

Nausea, anorexia, and diarrhea can usually be controlled by administering the drug with food or carboxymethylcellulose, reducing drug dosage, or discontinuing the drug. Pseudomembranous enterocolitis associated with *Clostridium difficile* or staphylococci must be recognized promptly and treated with oral vancomycin (see Chapter 50).

B. Bony Structures and Teeth: Tetracyclines are readily bound to calcium deposited in newly formed bone or teeth in young children. When the drug is given during pregnancy, it can be deposited in the fetal teeth, leading to fluorescence, discoloration, and enamel dysplasia; it can also be deposited in bone, where it may cause deformity or growth inhibition. If the drug is given to children under 8 years of age for long periods, similar changes can result.

C. Liver Toxicity: Tetracyclines can probably impair hepatic function, especially during pregnancy, in patients with preexisting hepatic insufficiency, and when high doses are given intravenously. Hepatic necrosis has been reported with daily doses of 4 g intravenously or more.

D. Kidney Toxicity: Renal tubular acidosis and other renal injury resulting in nitrogen retention have been attributed to the administration of outdated tetracycline preparations. Tetracyclines given along with diuretics may produce nitrogen retention. Tetracyclines, except doxycycline, may accumulate to toxic levels in patients with impaired kidney function and may aggravate the condition.

E. Local Tissue Toxicity: Intravenous injection can lead to venous thrombosis. Intramuscular injection produces painful local irritation and should be avoided.

F. Photosensitization: Systemic tetracycline administration, especially of demeclocycline, can induce sensitivity to sunlight or ultraviolet light, particularly in fair-skinned persons.

G. Vestibular Reactions: Dizziness, vertigo, nausea, and vomiting have been particularly noted with minocycline. After doses of 200–400 mg/d of minocycline, 35–70% of patients exhibited such reactions.

Medical & Social Implications of Overuse

The widespread use of tetracyclines for minor illnesses has led to the emergence of resistance even among highly susceptible species, eg, pneumococci and group A streptococci. The large-scale use of these drugs in hospitals has resulted in the emergence of tetracycline-resistant organisms as superinfecting agents. In some measure, the misuse of tetracyclines (among other antibiotics) must be blamed for the rising incidence of mycotic infection in hospitalized severely ill patients.

Tetracyclines have been extensively used in animal feeds to increase the rate of growth. This practice has been widely blamed for the steadily increasing spread of tetracycline resistance among bacteria and of plasmids that promote it. Such use has resulted in tetracycline-resistant infections among farmers, animal handlers, slaughterhouse workers, and perhaps the general public. For this reason, some countries (eg, Great Britain) forbid the use of tetracyclines in animal feeds.

On the other hand, tetracyclines have been of great benefit not only for the control of existing infection but also for the early treatment of acute exacerbations in chronic bronchitis and bronchiectasis, keeping many persons well and at work.

PREPARATIONS AVAILABLE

Chloramphenicol (generic, Chloromycetin)
Oral: 250 mg capsules; 150 mg/5 mL suspension
Parenteral: powder to reconstitute 100 mg/mL solution for injection
Demeclocycline (Declomycin)
Oral: 150, 300 mg tablets; 150 mg capsules
Doxycycline (generic, Vibramycin, others)

Oral: 50, 100 mg tablets and capsules; powder to reconstitute for 25, 50 mg/5 mL suspension; 50 mg/5 mL syrup
Parenteral: powder to reconstitute for injection (100, 200 mg per vial)
Methacycline (Rondomycin)
Oral: 150, 300 mg capsules

Minocycline (Minocin)
Oral: 50, 100 mg tablets and capsules; 50 mg/5 mL suspension
Parenteral: powder to reconstitute for injection (100 mg per vial)
Oxytetracycline (generic, Terramycin)
Oral: 250 mg capsules
Parenteral: 50, 125 mg/mL for IM injection; powder to reconstitute for IV injection (250, 500 mg per vial)
Tetracycline (generic, Achromycin V, others)
Oral: 100, 250, 500 mg capsules; 250 mg tablets; 125 mg/5 mL suspension
Parenteral: powder to reconstitute for IM injection, 100, 250 mg/vial; powder to reconstitute for IV injection, 250, 500 mg/vial.

REFERENCES

Chloramphenicol

Dajani AS, Kauffman RE: The renaissance of chloramphenicol. Pediatr Clin North Am 1981;28:195.

Feder HM Jr, Osier C, Maderazo EG: Chloramphenicol: A review of its use in clinical practice. Rev Infect Dis 1981;3:479.

Hughes WT et al: Guidelines for the use of antimicrobial agents in neutropenic patients with unexplained fever. J Infect Dis 1990;161:381.

Kucers A: Chloramphenicol, erythromycin, vancomycin, tetracyclines. Lancet 1982;2:425.

Nahata MC: Serum concentrations and adverse effects of chloramphenicol in pediatric patients. Chemotherapy 1987;33:322.

O'Brien TF et al: Molecular epidemiology of antibiotic resistance in *Salmonella* from animals and human beings in the United States. N Engl J Med 1982;307:1.

Shann F et al: Absorption of chloramphenicol sodium succinate after intramuscular administration in children. N Engl J Med 1985;313:410.

Snyder MJ et al: Comparative efficacy of chloramphenicol, ampicillin, and co-trimoxazole in the treatment of typhoid fever. Lancet 1976;2:1155.

Wallerstein RO et al: Statewide study of chloramphenicol therapy and fatal aplastic anemia. JAMA 1969; 208: 2045.

West BC et al: Aplastic anemia associated with parenteral chloramphenicol. Possible increased risk with cimetidine. Rev Infect Dis 1988;10:1048.

Tetracyclines

Allen JC: Drugs five years later: Minocycline. Ann Intern Med 1976;85:482.

Chopra I, Hawkey PM, Hinton M: Tetracyclines, molecular and clinical aspects. J Antimicrob Chemother 1992;29: 245.

Chopra I, Howe TGB: Bacterial resistance to tetracyclines. Microbiol Rev 1978;42:707.

Drew TM et al: Minocycline for prophylaxis of infection with *Neisseria meningitidis:* High rate of side effects in recipients. J Infect Dis 1976;133:194.

Holmberg SD et al: Drug-resistant *Salmonella* from animals fed antimicrobials. N Engl J Med 1984;311:617.

Hoshiwara I et al: Doxycycline treatment of chronic trachoma. JAMA 1973;224:220.

Hurwitz S: Acne vulgaris: Current concepts of pathogenesis and treatment. Am J Dis Child 1979;133:536.

Laga M et al: Prophylaxis of gonococcal and chlamydial ophthalmia neonatorum: A comparison of silver nitrate and tetracycline. N Engl J Med 1988;318:653.

Mhalu FS et al: Rapid emergence of El Tor *Vibrio cholerae* resistant to antimicrobials during first six months of fourth cholera epidemic in Tanzania. Lancet 1979;1:345.

Neu HC: Changing mechanisms of bacterial resistance. Am J Med 1984;77(Suppl 1B):11.

Rockhill RC et al: Tetracycline resistance of *Corynebacterium diphtheriae* isolated from diphtheria patients in Indonesia. Antimicrob Agents Chemother 1982; 21:842.

Sack DA et al: Single-dose doxycycline for cholera. Antimicrob Agents Chemother 1978;14:462.

Sauer GC: Safety of long-term tetracycline therapy for acne. Arch Dermatol 1976;112:1603.

Sexually transmitted diseases: Treatment guidelines. MMWR Morb Mortal Wkly Rep 1989;38:S8.

Sigal LH: Current recommendations for the treatment of Lyme disease. Drugs 1992;43:683.

Simpson MB et al: Hemolytic anemia after tetracycline therapy. N Engl J Med 1985;312:840.

Speer BS, Shoemaker MB, Salyers AA: Bacterial resistance to tetracycline: Mechanism, transfer, and clinical significance. Clin Microbiol Rev 1992;5:387.

Aminoglycosides & Polymyxins

45

Ernest Jawetz, MD, PhD

AMINOGLYCOSIDES

Aminoglycosides are a group of bactericidal drugs originally obtained from various *Streptomyces* species and sharing chemical, antimicrobial, pharmacologic, and toxic characteristics. At present, the group includes streptomycin, neomycin, kanamycin, amikacin, gentamicin, tobramycin, sisomicin, netilmicin, and others. All of these agents inhibit protein synthesis in bacteria and suffer the disadvantage of multiple types of resistance.

All aminoglycosides are potentially ototoxic and nephrotoxic. All can accumulate in renal insufficiency, and dosage adjustments must be made in patients with renal impairment.

Aminoglycosides are used most widely against gram-negative enteric bacteria, especially in bacteremia, sepsis, or endocarditis. Streptomycin is the oldest and best-studied of the aminoglycosides. Gentamicin, tobramycin, and amikacin are the most widely employed aminoglycosides at present. Neomycin and kanamycin are now largely limited to topical or oral use.

General Properties of Aminoglycosides

A. Physical and Chemical Properties: Aminoglycosides are water-soluble, stable in solution, and more active at alkaline than at acid pH. They have a hexose nucleus, either streptidine (in streptomycin) or deoxystreptamine (other aminoglycosides), to which amino sugars are attached by glycosidic linkages (Figures 45–1 and 45–2). Each drug is characterized by the number and kind of amino sugars. Aminoglycosides may form complexes with beta-lactam drugs in vitro and may lose some activity.

B. Mechanism of Action: Aminoglycosides are bactericidal for susceptible organisms by virtue of irreversible inhibition of protein synthesis. However, the precise mechanism for this bactericidal activity is not clearly evident. The initial event is penetration through the cell envelope. This is in part an active transport process, in part passive diffusion. The latter can be greatly enhanced by the presence of cell wall-active drugs, eg, penicillins. Since the active transport is an oxygen-dependent process, aminoglycosides are relatively ineffective against strict anaerobes.

Once an aminoglycoside has entered the cell, it binds to receptors on the 30S subunit of the bacterial ribosome. These receptors, some of which have been purified, are proteins under chromosomal control. Ribosomal protein synthesis is inhibited by aminoglycosides in at least three ways: (1) They interfere with the "initiation complex" of peptide formation; (2) they induce misreading of the code on the mRNA template, which causes incorporation of incorrect amino acids into the peptide; and (3) they cause a breakup of polysomes into nonfunctional monosomes.

C. Mechanisms of Resistance: Three principal mechanisms have been established: (1) The microorganism acquires the ability to produce enzymes that inactivate the aminoglycoside by adenylylation, acetylation, or phosphorylation. This is the principal

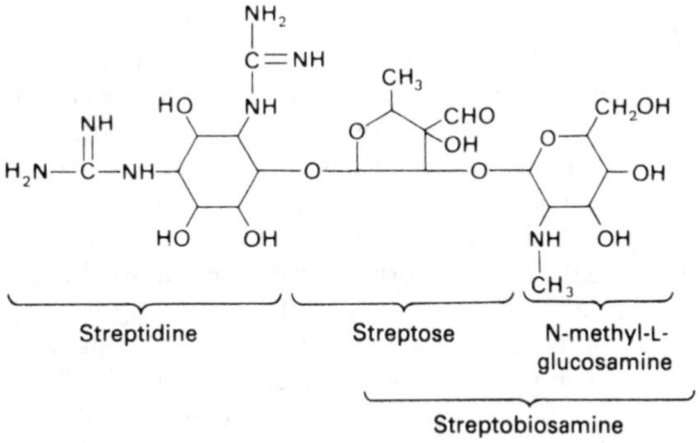

Figure 45–1. Structure of streptomycin.

type of resistance among gram-negative enteric bacteria and is usually plasmid-controlled. This transmissible resistance is of great clinical and epidemiologic concern. (2) Alteration in the cell surface, which interferes with the permeation or transport of aminoglycoside into the cell. This may be chromosomal (eg, enterococci) or plasmid-controlled (eg, gram-negative bacteria). (3) The receptor protein on the 30S ribosomal subunit may be deleted or altered as a result of chromosomal mutation. (4) In addition, facultative organisms growing under anaerobic conditions are usually resistant to aminoglycosides because the oxygen-dependent transport process described above is not functional.

D. Pharmacokinetics: Aminoglycosides are absorbed poorly or not at all from the intact gastrointestinal tract but may be absorbed if ulcerations are present. Virtually the entire oral dose is excreted in feces. After intramuscular injection, aminoglycosides are absorbed well, giving peak concentrations in blood within 30–90 minutes. Only about 10% of the absorbed drugs are bound to plasma proteins. Occasionally, aminoglycosides are injected intravenously.

Being highly polar compounds, aminoglycosides do not enter cells readily and are largely excluded from the central nervous system and the eye. In the presence of active inflammation, cerebrospinal fluid levels reach 20% of plasma levels, and in neonatal meningitis the levels may be higher. Intrathecal or intraventricular injection is required for high levels in cerebrospinal fluid. Even after parenteral injection, concentrations of aminoglycosides are not high in most tissues except the renal cortex. Concentration in most secretions is also modest; in the bile, it may reach 30% of the blood level. Diffusion into pleural or synovial fluid may result in concentrations 50–90% of that of plasma with prolonged therapy. There is no significant metabolic breakdown by host mechanisms. The half-life in serum is 2–3 hours. Excretion is mainly by glomerular filtration and is greatly reduced with impaired renal function. Aminoglycosides are partly and irregularly removed by hemodialysis— eg, 40–60% for gentamicin—and even less effectively by peritoneal dialysis.

In persons with impaired renal function, there is danger of drug accumulation and toxic effects. Therefore, either the dose of drug is kept constant and the interval between doses is increased, or the interval is kept constant and the dose is reduced. Nomograms and formulas have been constructed relating serum creatinine levels to adjustments in treatment regimens. The simplest formula divides the dose (calculated on the basis of normal renal function) by the serum creatinine value (mg/dL). Thus, a 60-kg patient with normal renal function might receive 300 mg/d of gentamicin given as 100 mg every 8 hours. A 60-kg patient with a serum creatinine of 3 mg/dL would receive 100 mg/d as 33 mg every 8 hours. However,

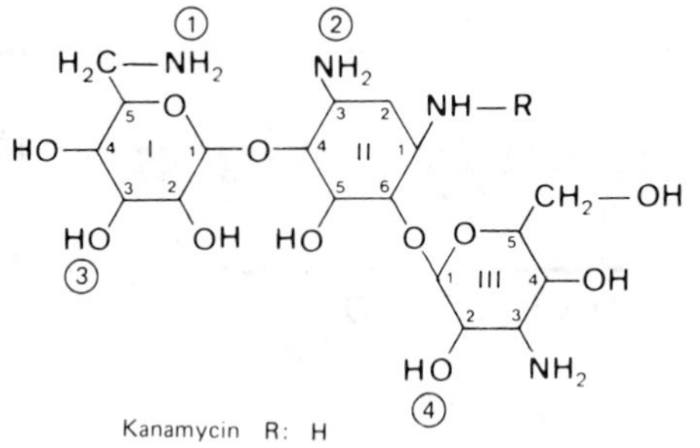

	Ring I			Ring II
	R_1	R_2	C4–C5 bond	R_3
Gentamicin C_1	CH_3	CH_3	Single	H
Gentamicin C_2	CH_3	H	Single	H
Gentamicin C_{1a}	H	H	Single	H
Netilmicin	H	H	Double	C_2H_5

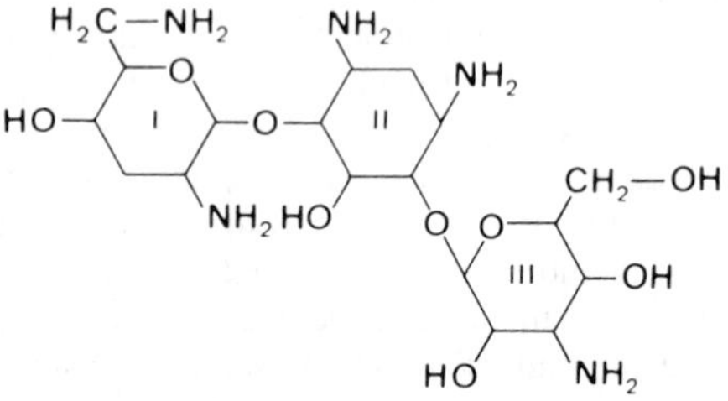

Figure 45–2. Structures of several important aminoglycoside antibiotics. Ring II is 2-deoxystreptamine. The resemblance between kanamycin and amikacin and between gentamicin, netilmicin, and tobramycin can be seen. The circled numerals on the kanamycin molecule indicate points of attack of plasmid-mediated bacterial enzymes that can inactivate this drug. ($\aleph$ and $\mathfrak{Z}$, acetylase; $\mathfrak{R}$, phosphorylase; $\wp$, adenylylase.) Amikacin is resistant to degradation at $\mathfrak{Z}$, $\mathfrak{R}$, and $\wp$

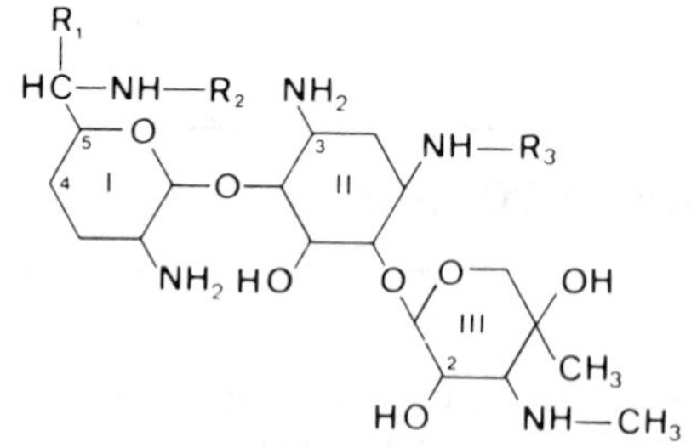

there is considerable variation in aminoglycoside serum levels in different patients with similar serum creatinine values. Therefore, it is highly desirable, especially when using higher dosages, to measure drug levels in blood in order to avoid severe toxicity. Peak levels should be obtained $\frac{1}{2}$–1 hour after infusion; trough levels should be obtained just prior to the next infusion.

E. Adverse Effects: Hypersensitivity occurs infrequently. All aminoglycosides can cause varying degrees of ototoxicity and nephrotoxicity. The ototoxicity can manifest itself either as hearing loss (cochlear damage), noted first with high-frequency tones, or as vestibular damage evident by vertigo, ataxia, and loss of balance. Nephrotoxicity results in rising serum creatinine levels or reduced creatinine clearance. In very high doses, aminoglycosides can produce a curare-like effect with neuromuscular blockade that results in respiratory paralysis. Calcium gluconate (given promptly) or neostigmine can serve as an antidote to this action.

F. Clinical Uses: Aminoglycosides are used most widely against gram-negative enteric bacteria or when there is suspicion of sepsis. In the treatment of bacteremia or endocarditis caused by fecal streptococci or some gram-negative bacteria, the aminoglycoside is given together with a penicillin that enhances permeability and facilitates the entry of the aminoglycoside. Aminoglycosides are selected according to recent susceptibility patterns in a given area or hospital until susceptibility tests become available on a specific isolate. All positively charged aminoglycosides and polymyxins are inhibited in blood cultures by sodium polyanetholsulfonate and other polyanionic detergents.

STREPTOMYCIN

Streptomycin (Figure 45–1) was isolated from a strain of *Streptomyces griseus* by Waksman and his associates in 1944. Dihydrostreptomycin can be produced by catalytic reduction of streptomycin trihydrochloride. Both have similar chemical and identical antimicrobial properties. However, dihydrostreptomycin is more ototoxic than streptomycin and has been abandoned.

The antimicrobial activity of streptomycin is typical of that of other aminoglycosides, as are the mechanisms of resistance. Resistant microorganisms have emerged in most species, severely limiting the current usefulness of streptomycin, with the exceptions listed below. Streptomycin-dependent bacteria require the drug for growth. This results from a mutation in the P 12 receptor protein.

The emergence of resistance in an apparently susceptible isolate tends to be rapid, so that treatment with streptomycin as the sole drug is usually limited to 5 days.

Clinical Uses

A. Mycobacterial Infections: Streptomycin is now rarely chosen for initial therapy of tuberculosis. In advanced tuberculosis, miliary dissemination, meningitis, or serious organ involvement, streptomycin in a dosage of 0.5–1 g (30 mg/kg/d) can be injected intramuscularly in combination with other antimycobacterial drugs. This regimen continues for weeks or months, daily at first and later twice weekly. (See Chapter 46.)

B. Nontuberculous Infections: In plague, tularemia, and sometimes brucellosis, streptomycin, 1 g/d, is injected intramuscularly (15 mg/kg/d for children), while tetracyclines may be given orally.

C. Combined Treatment: In certain infections, simultaneous use of a penicillin plus an aminoglycoside may be bactericidal and may permit eradication of organisms. Examples are infective endocarditis caused by fecal streptococci (enterococci) or viridans streptococci and bacteremia with some gram-negative aerobic bacteria, eg, *Pseudomonas* sp, especially in immunodeficient hosts.

Adverse Reactions

A. Allergy: Fever, skin rashes, and other allergic manifestations may result from hypersensitivity to streptomycin. This occurs most frequently upon prolonged contact with the drug, either in patients who receive a prolonged course of treatment (eg, for tuberculosis) or in medical personnel who handle the drug. (Nurses preparing solutions should wear gloves.) Desensitization is occasionally successful.

B. Toxicity: Pain at the injection site is common but usually not severe. The most serious toxic effect is disturbance of vestibular function—vertigo and loss of balance. The frequency and severity of this disturbance are proportionate to the age of the patient, the blood levels of the drug, and the duration of administration. Vestibular dysfunction may follow a few weeks of unusually high blood levels (eg, in individuals with impaired renal function) or months of relatively low blood levels. After the drug is discontinued, partial recovery frequently occurs.

The concurrent or sequential use of other aminoglycosides with streptomycin should be avoided to reduce the likelihood of ototoxicity. Streptomycin given during pregnancy can cause deafness in the newborn.

General Medical Problems From Overuse

Streptomycin-resistant bacteria have become prevalent as a result of widespread use of the drug, often in unnecessary combination with penicillin. Multiple drug resistance is frequent among bacteria in urinary tract infections, and the hospital transmission of such organisms aggravates treatment problems. Primary infection with streptomycin-resistant tubercle bacilli occurs in up to 15% of cases of pulmonary tuberculosis in children studied in the USA.

GENTAMICIN

Gentamicin is an aminoglycoside complex (Figure 45–2) isolated from *Micromonospora purpurea.* It is effective against both gram-positive and gram-negative organisms, and many of its properties resemble those of other aminoglycosides. Sisomicin is very similar to the C_{1a} component of gentamicin.

Antimicrobial Activity

Gentamicin sulfate, 2–10 µg/mL, inhibits in vitro many strains of staphylococci, coliforms, and other gram-negative bacteria. The simultaneous use of carbenicillin or ticarcillin and gentamicin may result in synergistic enhancement and bactericidal activity against some strains of *Pseudomonas, Proteus, Enterobacter, Klebsiella,* and other gram-negative rods and against viridans and fecal streptococci. However, a penicillin and gentamicin cannot be mixed in vitro.

Resistance

Most streptococci are resistant to gentamicin owing to failure of the drug to reach ribosomes in the cell. However, such streptococci can be killed by the concomitant use of a cell wall-active drug (eg, penicillin) with the aminoglycoside. Among gram-negative bacteria, resistance to gentamicin is increasing in proportion to the amount of drug used in a given hospital environment. This resistance is most commonly attributable to the spread of plasmids that govern gentamicin-inactivating enzymes. Organisms resistant to gentamicin are sometimes resistant to tobramycin but infrequently (as yet) to amikacin.

Clinical Uses

A. Intramuscular or Intravenous: At present, gentamicin and tobramycin are employed mainly in severe infections (eg, sepsis and pneumonia) caused by gram-negative bacteria that are likely to be resistant to other drugs, especially *Pseudomonas, Enterobacter, Serratia, Proteus, Acinetobacter,* and *Klebsiella.* Patients with these infections are often immunocompromised, and the simultaneous action of the aminoglycoside with a cephalosporin or a penicillin may save their lives. In such situations, 5–7 mg/kg/d of gentamicin is given intramuscularly or intravenously in three equal doses. Gentamicin or tobramycin is also used concurrently with penicillin G for bactericidal activity in endocarditis due to viridans streptococci or *Streptococcus faecalis.*

Renal, auditory, and vestibular functions should be monitored, particularly in patients with impaired renal function. Direct enzymatic or radioimmunoassays of gentamicin in serum are available. In renal failure, the dose must be significantly reduced.

B. Topical: Creams, ointments, or solutions containing 0.1–0.3% gentamicin sulfate have been used for the treatment of infected burns, wounds, or skin lesions and the prevention of intravenous catheter infections. Topical gentamicin is partly inactivated by purulent exudates. However, such topical use must be restricted in hospitals to avoid favoring the development of resistant bacteria. Ten milligrams can be injected subconjunctivally for appropriate ocular infections.

C. Intrathecal: Meningitis caused by gram-negative bacteria has been treated by the intrathecal injection of gentamicin sulfate, 1–10 mg/d. In neonates, neither intrathecal nor intraventricular gentamicin was beneficial in meningitis, and intraventricular gentamicin was toxic. Epidural abscess, after aspiration, has been instilled with gentamicin, 20 mg/d for 10 days.

Adverse Reactions

These are analogous to the adverse effects of streptomycin and other aminoglycosides. Nephrotoxicity requires adjustment of regimens, especially in diminished renal function. Whenever possible, measurement of gentamicin serum levels should serve as a guide in difficult clinical situations. Ototoxicity manifests itself mainly as vestibular dysfunction, perhaps due to destruction of hair cells by prolonged elevated drug levels (> 10 µg/mL). Loss of hearing can occur and has occasionally been extensive and irreversible. The incidence of hypersensitivity reactions to gentamicin is poorly documented.

TOBRAMYCIN

This aminoglycoside (Figure 45–2) has an antibacterial spectrum similar to that of gentamicin. While there is some cross-resistance between gentamicin and tobramycin, it is unpredictable in individual strains. Separate laboratory susceptibility tests are therefore necessary.

The pharmacologic properties of tobramycin are virtually identical to those of gentamicin. The daily dose of tobramycin is 5–7 mg/kg/d intramuscularly or intravenously, divided into three equal amounts and given every 8 hours. About 80% of the drug is excreted by glomerular filtration into the urine within 24 hours after administration. In uremia, the drug dosage must be reduced. A formula for such dosage is 1 mg/kg every (6 × serum creatinine [mg/dL] level) hours. Monitoring blood levels in renal insufficiency is desirable and should be used to correct such estimates. Tobramycin can be cleared somewhat during peritoneal dialysis and about 50% during hemodialysis.

Tobramycin has the same antibacterial spectrum as gentamicin. Either tobramycin or gentamicin is the aminoglycoside most often employed in combination with ticarcillin or a cephalosporin against gram-negative bacterial sepsis or in combination with penicillin G against enterococcal endocarditis.

Like other aminoglycosides, tobramycin is ototoxic and nephrotoxic. Nephrotoxicity of tobramycin may be slightly less than that of gentamicin. It should not be used concurrently with other drugs having similar adverse effects or with diuretics, which tend to enhance aminoglycoside tissue concentrations.

AMIKACIN

Amikacin is a semisynthetic derivative of kanamycin that is less toxic (Figure 45–2). It is relatively resistant to several of the enzymes that inactivate gentamicin and tobramycin, and it therefore can be employed against some microorganisms resistant to the latter drugs. However, bacterial resistance due to loss of permeability to amikacin is increasing slowly. Many gram-negative enteric bacteria, including many strains of *Proteus, Pseudomonas, Enterobacter,* and *Serratia,* are inhibited by 1–20 μg/mL amikacin in vitro. After the injection of 500 mg amikacin every 12 hours (15 mg/kg/d) intramuscularly, peak levels in serum are 10–30 μg/mL. Some infections caused by gram-negative bacteria resistant to gentamicin respond to amikacin. Central nervous system infections require intrathecal or intraventricular injection of 3–10 mg daily.

Like all aminoglycosides, amikacin is nephrotoxic and ototoxic (particularly for the auditory portion of the eighth nerve). Its levels should be monitored in patients with renal failure. Concurrent use with loop diuretics (eg, furosemide, ethacrynic acid) should be avoided.

NETILMICIN

This aminoglycoside became available in the USA in 1983. It shares many characteristics with gentamicin and tobramycin. However, the addition of an ethyl group to the 1-amino position of the 2-deoxystreptamine ring (ring II, Figure 45–2) sterically protects the netilmicin molecule from enzymatic degradation at the 3-amino (ring II) and 2-hydroxyl (ring III) positions. Consequently, netilmicin may not be inactivated by many gentamicin-resistant and tobramycin-resistant bacteria.

The dosage (5–7 mg/kg/d) and the routes of administration are the same as for gentamicin. The principal indication for netilmicin may be iatrogenic infections in immunocompromised and severely ill patients at very high risk for gram-negative bacterial sepsis in the hospital setting.

Netilmicin may prove to be less ototoxic and possibly less nephrotoxic than the other aminoglycosides.

KANAMYCIN & NEOMYCIN

These drugs are closely related. Neomycin was isolated by Waksman in 1949 from *Streptomyces fradiae;* kanamycin (Figure 45–2) was isolated by Umezawa in 1957 from *Streptomyces kanamyceticus.* Other members of the group are framycetin and paromomycin. All have similar properties.

Antimicrobial Activity & Resistance

Drugs of the neomycin group are active against gram-positive and gram-negative bacteria and some mycobacteria. *Pseudomonas* and streptococci are generally resistant. Mechanisms of antibacterial action and resistance are the same as with other aminoglycosides. The widespread use of these drugs in bowel preparation for elective surgery has resulted in the selection of resistant organisms and some outbreaks of enterocolitis in hospitals. There is complete cross-resistance between kanamycin and neomycin.

Pharmacokinetics

Drugs of the neomycin group are not significantly absorbed from the gastrointestinal tract. After oral administration, the intestinal flora is suppressed or modified and the drug is excreted in the feces.

Excretion of any absorbed drug is mainly through glomerular filtration into the urine.

Clinical Uses

Because of toxicity, the parenteral administration of kanamycin and neomycin has been abandoned, and they are now limited to topical and oral use.

A. Topical: Solutions containing 1–5 mg/mL are used on infected surfaces or injected into joints, the pleural cavity, tissue spaces, or abscess cavities where infection is present. The total amount of drug given in this fashion must be limited to 15 mg/kg/d because it can be absorbed, giving rise to systemic toxicity. Ointments containing 1–5 mg/g are applied to infected skin lesions or in the nares for suppression of staphylococci. Some ointments contain polymyxin and bacitracin in addition to neomycin.

B. Oral: In preparation for elective bowel surgery, 1 g of neomycin is given orally every 6–8 hours for 1–2 days, often combined with 1 g of erythromycin base. This reduces the aerobic bowel flora with little effect on anaerobes. In hepatic coma, the coliform flora can be suppressed for prolonged periods by giving 1 g every 6–8 hours, together with reduced protein intake, thus reducing ammonia intoxication. Paromomycin, 1 g every 6 hours orally for 2 weeks, has been effective in intestinal amebiasis. Neomycin is occasionally used in the treatment of hyperlipidemia (see Chapter 34).

Adverse Reactions

All members of the neomycin group have nephrotoxic and ototoxic effects. Auditory function is affected more than vestibular. Deafness has occurred especially in adults with impaired renal function and prolonged elevated drug levels.

The sudden absorption of postoperatively instilled kanamycin from the peritoneal cavity (3–5 g) has resulted in curare-like neuromuscular blockade and respiratory arrest. Calcium gluconate and perhaps neostigmine can act as antidotes.

While hypersensitivity is not common, prolonged application of neomycin-containing ointments to skin and eyes has resulted in severe allergic reactions.

SPECTINOMYCIN

Spectinomycin is an aminocyclitol antibiotic (related to aminoglycosides) dispensed as the dihydrochloride pentahydrate for intramuscular injection. While active in vitro against many gram-positive and gram-negative organisms, spectinomycin is proposed only as an alternative treatment for gonorrhea in patients who might be hypersensitive to penicillin or whose gonococci are resistant to penicillin and other drugs. Most gonococci are inhibited by 6 µg/mL of spectinomycin. About 10% of gonococci may be resistant to spectinomycin, but there is no cross-resistance with other drugs used in gonorrhea.

Spectinomycin is rapidly absorbed after intramuscular injection. A single dose of 2 g (40 mg/kg) is given. There is pain at the injection site and occasionally fever and nausea. Nephrotoxicity and anemia have been observed rarely.

POLYMYXINS

The polymyxins are a group of basic polypeptides active against gram-negative bacteria. Because of excessive nephrotoxicity, all but polymyxins B and E have been abandoned.

Chemistry

Polymyxins are cationic, basic polypeptides with molecular weights of about 1400. All contain the fatty acid D-6-methyloctan-1-oic acid and the amino acids L-threonine and L-diaminobutyric acid. The sulfates are water-soluble and very stable. One microgram of pure polymyxin B sulfate equals 10 units.

Antimicrobial Activity & Resistance

Polymyxins are bactericidal for many gram-negative rods, including *Pseudomonas,* in concentrations of 1–5 µg/mL. They attach to cell membranes of bacteria that are rich in phosphatidylethanolamine and disrupt the osmotic properties and transport mechanisms of the membrane. This action is inhibited by cations. Thus, polymyxins act like cationic detergents.

Gram-positive organisms, *Proteus,* and *Neisseria* are highly resistant. This is probably due to the impermeability of the outer membrane to the drug. In susceptible bacterial populations, resistant mutants are rare.

Pharmacokinetics

Polymyxins are not absorbed from the gut. After parenteral injection, blood levels and tissue concentrations are low. Polymyxins are strongly bound by cell debris, acid phospholipids, purulent exudates, and endotoxins of gram-negative bacteria. They do not penetrate into living cells.

Excretion is mainly via the kidneys, and high concentrations may be reached in the urine. Excretion is impaired in renal insufficiency.

Clinical Uses

Polymyxins are rarely considered for systemic administration because of their poor tissue distribution and their substantial nephrotoxicity and neurotoxicity. Other more effective and less toxic drugs are available. Polymyxins are now restricted to topical use.

Solutions containing 1–10 mg/mL of polymyxin B sulfate can be applied to infected surfaces, injected into the pleural cavity and joint spaces, injected subconjunctivally, or inhaled as aerosols. The total dose must not exceed 2.5 mg/kg/d.

Ointments containing polymyxin B, 0.5 mg/g, in mixture with bacitracin or neomycin (or both) are commonly applied to infected superficial skin lesions. Because polymyxins are not absorbed from the gut, the drug has been given orally as a possible prophylactic measure to suppress the aerobic gram-negative members of the intestinal flora in immunosuppressed persons.

Adverse Reactions

Local reactions and hypersensitivity to topical administration are rare. Systemic levels of polymyxins can cause paresthesias, dizziness, and incoordination. These disappear when the drug has been excreted. Very high blood levels (> 30 µg/mL) can cause respiratory paralysis, which can be reversed by calcium gluconate. If polymyxins are absorbed, proteinuria and hematuria occur as signs of tubular injury. In renal insufficiency, nitrogen retention can develop.

PREPARATIONS AVAILABLE

Aminoglycosides
Amikacin (generic, Amikin)
Parenteral: 50, 250 mg (in vials) for IM, IV injection
Gentamicin (generic, Garamycin, Jenamicin)
Parenteral: 60, 80, 100 mg in IV piggyback units; 10, 40 mg/mL vials for IM, IV injection; 2 mg/mL vials for intrathecal use
Kanamycin (generic, Kantrex, Klebcil)
Oral: 500 mg capsules
Parenteral: 500, 1000 mg for IM, IV injection; 75 mg for pediatric injection
Neomycin (generic, Mycifradin, Neobiotic)
Oral: 500 mg tablets; 125 mg/5 mL solution
Parenteral: powder to reconstitute for IM injection (500 mg per vial)
Netilmicin (Netromycin)
Parenteral: 100 mg/mL for IM, IV injection
Paromomycin (Humatin)
Oral: 250 mg capsules
Spectinomycin (Trobicin)

Parenteral: powder to reconstitute for IM injection (2, 4 g per vial)
Streptomycin (generic)
Parenteral: 400 mg for IM injection; also available as powder to reconstitute for injection
Tobramycin (generic, Nebcin)
Parenteral: 10, 40 mg for IM, IV injection; 10, 30, 40 mg powder to reconstitute injection

Polymyxins
Colistimethate (Coly-Mycin M)
Parenteral: powder to reconstitute for IM, IV injection (150 mg per vial)
Colistin [Polymyxin E] (Coly-Mycin S)
Oral: powder to reconstitute for 25 mg/5 mL suspension
Polymyxin B (generic, Aerosporin)
Parenteral: 500,000 units vial; powder to reconstitute for IV, intrathecal injection (500,000 units per vial)

REFERENCES

Appel JB, Neu HC: The nephrotoxicity of antimicrobial agents. (Three parts.) N Engl J Med 1977;296:663, 722, 784.

Bisna AL et al: Antimicrobial treatment of infective endocarditis due to viridans streptococci, enterococci, and staphylococci. JAMA 1989;261:1471.

Blair DC: Inactivation of amikacin and gentamicin by carbenicillin in patients with end-stage renal failure. Antimicrob Agents Chemother 1982;22:376.

Boslego JW et al: Effect of spectinomycin use on the prevalence of spectinomycin-resistant and of penicillinase-producing *Neisseria gonorrhoeae.* N Engl J Med 1987; 317:272.

Brynan LE et al: Mechanism of aminoglycoside antibiotic resistance in anaerobic bacteria. Antimicrob Agents Chemother 1979;15:7.

Chan RA et al: Gentamicin therapy in renal failure: A dosage nomogram. Ann Intern Med 1972;76:773.

Davis SD: Polymyxins, colistin, vancomycin and bacitracin. In: *Antimicrobial Therapy,* 3rd ed. Kagan BM (editor). Saunders, 1980.

Edson RS, Terrell CL: The aminoglycosides: Streptomycin, kanamycin, gentamicin, tobramycin, amikacin, netilmicin, and sisomicin. Mayo Clin Proc 1987;62:916.

Egan EA et al: Prospective controlled trial of oral kanamycin in prevention of neonatal necrotizing enterocolitis. J Pediatr 1976;89:467.

Finitzohieber T et al: Ototoxicity in neonates treated with gentamicin and kanamycin: Results of a 4-year controlled follow-up study. Pediatrics 1979;63:443.

Hughes WT et al: Guidelines for the use of antimicrobial agents in neutropenic patients with unexplained fever. J Infect Dis 1990;161:381.

Krogstad DJ et al: Plasmid-mediated resistance to antibiotic synergism in enterococci. J Clin Invest 1978;61:1645.

Love LJ et al: Randomized trial of empiric antibiotic therapy with ticarcillin in combination with gentamicin, amikacin or netilmicin in febrile patients with granulocytopenia and cancer. Am J Med 1979;66:603.

Maigaard S, Frimodt-Moller N, Madsen PO: Comparison of netilmicin and amikacin in treatment of complicated urinary tract infections. Antimicrob Agents Chemother 1978; 14:554.

McCracken GH et al: Intraventricular gentamicin therapy in gram-negative bacillary meningitis of infancy. Lancet 1980; 1:787.

Meyer RD: Drugs five years later: Amikacin. Ann Intern Med 1981;95:328.

Moellering RC Jr: Have the new beta-lactams rendered the aminoglycosides obsolete for the treatment of serious nosocomial infections? Am J Med 1986;80(Suppl 6B): 44.

Neu HC: New antibiotics: Areas of appropriate use. J Infect Dis 1987;155:403.

Noone M et al: Prospective study of amikacin vs netilmicin in the treatment of severe infections in hospitalized patients. Am J Med 1989;86:809.

Rettig PJ et al: Spectinomycin therapy for gonorrhea in prepubertal children. Am J Dis Child 1980;134:359.

Riff LJ, Jackson GG: Conditions for gentamicin inactivation by carbenicillin. Arch Intern Med 1972;130:887.

Sarubbi FA, Hull JH: Amikacin serum concentrations: Prediction of levels and dosage guidelines. Ann Intern Med 1978;89:612.

Smith CR et al: Double blind comparison of the nephrotoxicity and auditory toxicity of gentamicin and tobramycin. N Engl J Med 1980;302:1106.

Snavely SR, Hodges GR: The neurotoxicity of antibacterial agents. Ann Intern Med 1984;101:92.

Swan SK, Bennett WM: Drug dosing guide lines in patients with renal failure. West J Med 1992;156:633.

Swartz MN: Intraventricular use of aminoglycosides in the treatment of gram-negative bacillary meningitis: Conflicting views. J Infect Dis 1981;143:293.

Tablan OC et al: Renal and auditory toxicity of high-dose, prolonged therapy with gentamicin and tobramycin in *Pseudomonas* endocarditis. J Infect Dis 1984;149:257.

Wolfson JS, Swartz MN: Serum bactericidal activity as a monitor of antibiotic therapy. N Engl J Med 1985; 312:968.

Zaske DE et al: Wide interpatient variations in gentamicin dose requirements for geriatric patients. JAMA 1982; 248:3122.

Antimycobacterial Drugs

46

Ernest Jawetz, MD, PhD

Mycobacterial infections may be symptomatic or asymptomatic but typically are very chronic. Therapy thus presents unusual problems. This chapter describes drugs used for tuberculosis (*Mycobacterium tuberculosis* infections), infections of clinical significance caused by various "atypical" mycobacteria, and leprosy (*Mycobacterium leprae* infections). Following years of diminishing incidence of mycobacterial infections (thanks to effective chemotherapy and public health measures), there has recently evolved a devastating worldwide increase in these diseases in association with the epidemic of AIDS.

DRUGS USED IN TUBERCULOSIS

Streptomycin was the first antimicrobial drug to exhibit striking activity against tubercle bacilli. It remains an important agent in the management of severe tuberculosis, but it is now rarely selected for initial therapy. First-line drugs now are isoniazid, rifampin, ethambutol, and pyrazinamide for initial treatment, with streptomycin as an alternative. Several agents that are drugs of second choice in the treatment of tuberculosis are mentioned here only briefly.

Singular problems exist in the treatment of tuberculosis and related mycobacterial infections. The infections tend to be exceedingly chronic but may also give rise to hyperacute, lethal complications. The organisms are frequently intracellular, exhibit long periods of metabolic inactivity, and tend to develop resistance to any one drug. All these points contribute to the complexity of antituberculosis therapy.

To delay the rapid emergence of resistance in the large mycobacterial populations that occur in clinically active tuberculosis, combinations of first-line drugs are employed. If the organisms are susceptible to these drugs, the patient usually becomes noninfective within 2–3 weeks. While treatment in tubercu-

lous meningitis or miliary tuberculosis is usually continued for 18–24 months, this length of treatment is no longer needed in uncomplicated pulmonary tuberculosis, the most common clinical presentation. With the most effective drug combinations, which include isoniazid and rifampin, "short-course" schedules of 6–9 months of therapy give satisfactory results. The vast majority of patients require little hospitalization.

ISONIAZID (INH)

Isoniazid, introduced in 1952, is the most active drug for the treatment of patients who can tolerate it and whose mycobacteria are susceptible.

Chemistry

Isoniazid is the hydrazide of isonicotinic acid, often called INH. It is a small (MW 137), simple molecule freely soluble in water. The structural similarity to pyridoxine is shown below.

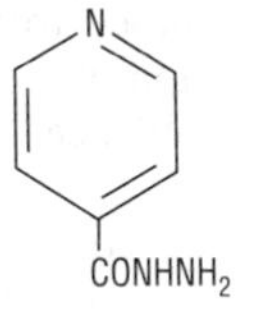

Isoniazid

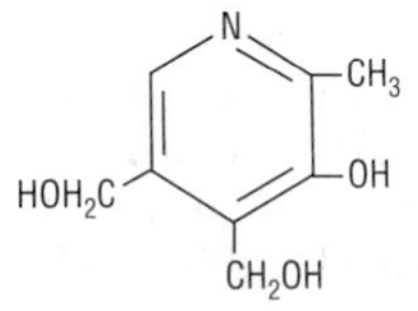

Pyridoxine

Antimycobacterial Activity

In vitro, INH inhibits most tubercle bacilli in a concentration of 0.2 μg/mL or less and is bactericidal for actively growing tubercle bacilli. INH is less effective against many atypical mycobacteria, though *Mycobacterium kansasii* may be susceptible. INH reaches similar concentrations both inside and outside animal cells and thus is able to act on intracellular mycobacteria as well as extracellular ones.

The mechanism of action of INH involves the inhibition of enzymes essential for the synthesis of mycolic acids and mycobacterial cell walls (Quemard, 1991). INH and pyridoxine are structural analogues, and INH exerts competitive antagonism in pyridoxine-catalyzed reactions in *Escherichia coli*. However, this mechanism is not involved in the antituberculous action. The administration of large doses of pyridoxine to patients receiving INH does not interfere with the tuberculostatic action of INH, but it prevents neuritis.

Resistance appears to be associated, at least experimentally, with deletion of a gene (*kat*G) that codes for catalase and peroxidase enzymes in the mycobacteria. Transformation of resistant strains with plasmids containing the *kat*G gene restored sensitivity to INH (Zhang et al, 1992; Zhang, 1993). However, other studies indicate that a large proportion of INH-resistant isolates from patients in New York City carried the gene in question (Stoeckle, 1993), so additional factors may be involved. Resistant mutants occur in susceptible mycobacterial populations with a frequency of about $1:10^7$. Since tuberculous lesions often contain more than 10^8 tubercle bacilli, resistant mutants would be readily selected out if INH were to be given as the sole drug. This has occurred in several countries. There is no cross-resistance between INH, rifampin, and ethambutol. The simultaneous use of any two of these drugs markedly delays the emergence of resistance to any one of them.

Pharmacokinetics

INH is readily absorbed from the gastrointestinal tract. The administration of usual doses (5 mg/kg/d) results in peak plasma concentrations of 3–5 μg/mL within 1–2 hours. INH diffuses readily into all body fluids and tissues. The concentration in the central nervous system and cerebrospinal fluid is about one-fifth of the plasma level. The intracellular and extracellular levels are similar.

The metabolism—particularly the acetylation—of INH is under genetic control (see Chapter 4). The average concentration of active INH in the plasma of rapid inactivators is about one-third to one-half of that in slow inactivators. The average half-life of INH in rapid inactivators is less than $1\frac{1}{2}$ hours, whereas in slow inactivators the half-life is 3 hours. It has been claimed that rapid acetylators are more prone to hepatic toxicity of INH, but this has not been confirmed. The rate of acetylation has little influence in daily dose regimens but may impair antimycobacterial activity in intermittent (1–2 times weekly) administration of INH.

INH is excreted mainly in the urine—partly as unchanged drug, partly as the acetylated form, and partly as other conjugates. The amount of unchanged, free INH in the urine is higher in slow inactivators. In renal failure, normal doses of INH can usually be given, but in severe hepatic insufficiency the dose must be reduced.

Clinical Uses

Isoniazid is probably the most widely useful drug in tuberculosis. In active, clinically manifest disease, it is given in conjunction with ethambutol, rifampin, or streptomycin. The usual dose is 5 mg/kg/d (maximum for adults, 300 mg daily). Twice that dose is sometimes used in severe illness and meningitis, but there is little evidence that the higher dose (10 mg/kg/d) is more effective in adults. Children should receive 10 mg/kg/d, and for maintenance therapy after initial improvement, 15 mg/kg twice weekly is sometimes given. Pyridoxine, 10 mg/100 mg of isoniazid, should be given to prevent neuritis.

Persons converting from negative to positive tuberculin skin tests may be given INH, 5–10 mg/kg/d (maximum 300 mg/d), for 1 year as prophylaxis against the 5–15% risk of meningitis or miliary dissemination. For prophylaxis, INH is given as the sole drug. In addition to skin test converters without active disease, prophylactic INH is also suggested for household and other very close contacts (especially children but also residents of nursing homes) of freshly recognized active cases; and for skin test-positive persons with HIV infections or individuals who undergo immunosuppressive or antineoplastic chemotherapy and have not received adequate antimycobacterial treatment in the past.

INH is usually given by mouth but can be injected parenterally in the same dosage.

In some parts of the world INH has been used as a single drug in the treatment of clinically active tuberculosis, with large mycobacterial populations. Predictably, INH-resistant mutants were selected out. The presence of such resistant mutants in migrants from Southeast Asia is creating major treatment problems. Tuberculosis in such migrants should be started with INH, rifampin, pyrazinamide, and ethambutol until drug susceptibility tests are completed.

Adverse Reactions

The incidence and severity of untoward reactions to INH are related to dosage and duration of administration.

A. Allergic Reactions: Fever, skin rashes, and hepatitis are occasionally seen.

B. Direct Toxicity: The most common toxic effects (10–20%) are on the peripheral and central nervous systems. These have been attributed to a relative pyridoxine deficiency, perhaps resulting from competition of INH with pyridoxal phosphate for the enzyme apotryptophanase. These toxic reactions include peripheral neuritis, insomnia, restlessness, muscle twitching, urinary retention, and even convulsions and psychotic episodes. Most of these complications can be prevented by the administration of pyridoxine, and accidental INH overdose can be treated with pyridoxine in amounts equivalent to the INH ingested.

INH has been associated with hepatotoxicity. Abnormal liver function tests, clinical jaundice, and multilobular necrosis have been observed. In large groups, about 1% of persons develop clinical hepatitis and up to 10% subclinical abnormalities. Some fatalities have occurred. Hepatitis with progressive liver damage is age-dependent. It occurs rarely under age 20, in 1.5% of those between 30 and 50, and in 2.5% of older persons. The risk of hepatitis is greater in alcoholics.

In glucose-6-phosphate dehydrogenase deficiency, INH may cause hemolysis. INH can reduce the metabolism of phenytoin, increasing its blood level and toxicity.

RIFAMPIN

Rifampin is a large (MW 823), complex semisynthetic derivative of rifamycin, an antibiotic produced by *Streptomyces mediterranei*. It is active in vitro against some gram-positive and gram-negative cocci, some enteric bacteria, mycobacteria, chlamydiae, and poxviruses. While many meningococci and mycobacteria are inhibited by less than 1 μg/mL, highly resistant mutants occur in all microbial populations in a frequency of $1:10^7$ or greater. The administration of rifampin as a single drug permits the emergence of these highly resistant organisms. There is no cross-resistance to other antimicrobial drugs. Rifampin resistance may be due to a permeability barrier or to a mutation of the DNA-dependent RNA polymerase.

Antimycobacterial Activity & Pharmacokinetics

Rifampin binds strongly to DNA-dependent RNA polymerase and thus inhibits RNA synthesis in bacteria and chlamydiae. Human RNA polymerase is not affected. Rifampin also blocks a late stage in the assembly of poxviruses, perhaps interfering with envelope formation. When administered together with INH, rifampin is usually bactericidal for mycobacteria and tends to sterilize infected tissues, cavities, or sputum. Rifampin penetrates phagocytic cells well and can kill intracellular mycobacteria and other organisms.

Rifampin is well absorbed after oral administration and excreted mainly through the liver into bile. It then undergoes enterohepatic recirculation, with the bulk excreted in feces and a small amount in the urine. Usual doses result in serum levels of 5–7 μg/mL, and cerebrospinal fluid levels are between 10% and 40% of serum levels. Rifampin is distributed widely in body fluids and tissues.

Clinical Uses

In tuberculosis, rifampin, usually 600 mg/d(10–20 mg/kg) orally, is administered together with INH, ethambutol, or another antituberculosis drug in order to delay the emergence of rifampin-resistant mycobacteria. A similar regimen may apply to atypical mycobacteria. In some short-course therapies, 600 mg of rifampin is given twice weekly. Rifampin is effective in leprosy when used together with a sulfone.

An oral dose of 600 mg twice daily for 2 days can eliminate a majority of meningococci from carriers. Unfortunately, some highly resistant meningococcal strains are selected out by this procedure. Up to 10% of treated meningococcus carriers may exhibit rifampin-resistant organisms. Rifampin, 20 mg/kg/d for 4 days, is used as prophylaxis in contacts of children with *Haemophilus influenzae* type b disease. Rifampin combined with trimethoprim-sulfamethoxazole can sometimes eradicate staphylococcal carriage in the nasopharynx. In urinary tract infections and in chronic bronchitis, the use of rifampin rapidly selects resistant mutants and thus has no place in clinical therapy.

Adverse Reactions

Rifampin imparts a harmless orange color to urine, sweat, tears, and contact lenses. Occasional adverse effects include rashes, thrombocytopenia, nephritis, and impairment of liver function. Rifampin commonly causes light chain proteinuria and may impair antibody response. If administered less often than twice weekly, rifampin causes a "flu syndrome" of uncertain nature and anemia. Rifampin induces microsomal enzymes (eg, cytochrome P450). Thus, it increases the elimination of anticoagulants and contraceptives. Likewise, administration of rifampin with ketoconazole, cyclosporine, or chloramphenicol results in significantly lower serum levels of these drugs. Rifampin increases the urinary excretion of methadone, lowers its plasma concentration, and may result in methadone withdrawal signs.

Caution: The indiscriminate use of rifampin for minor infections may favor the widespread selection of rifampin-resistant mycobacteria and thus deprive the drug of most of its usefulness.

ETHAMBUTOL

Ethambutol is a synthetic, water-soluble, heat-stable compound, the *d* isomer of the structure shown below, dispensed as the dihydrochloride salt.

$$H-\underset{\underset{C_2H_5}{|}}{\overset{\overset{CH_2OH}{|}}{C}}-NH-(CH_2)_2-NH-\underset{\underset{CH_2OH}{|}}{\overset{\overset{C_2H_5}{|}}{C}}-H$$

Ethambutol

Many strains of *M tuberculosis* and other mycobacteria are inhibited in vitro by ethambutol, 1–5 μg/mL. The mechanism of action is not known.

Ethambutol is well absorbed from the gut. Following ingestion of 25 mg/kg, a blood level peak of 2–5 μg/mL is reached in 2–4 hours. About 20% of the drug is excreted in feces and 50% in urine in unchanged form. Excretion is delayed in renal failure. In meningitis, ethambutol appears in the cerebrospinal fluid to the extent of 10–40% of serum levels.

Resistance to ethambutol emerges fairly rapidly among mycobacteria when the drug is used alone. Therefore, ethambutol is always given in combination with other antituberculosis drugs.

Ethambutol hydrochloride, 15 mg/kg, is usually given as a single daily dose in combination with INH or rifampin. As much as 25 mg/kg/d may be used.

Hypersensitivity to ethambutol is rare. The commonest adverse effects are visual disturbances: Reduction in visual acuity, optic neuritis, and perhaps retinal damage occur in some patients given 25 mg/kg/d for several months. Most of these changes apparently regress when ethambutol is discontinued. However, periodic visual acuity testing is desirable during treatment. With doses of 15 mg/kg/d or less, visual disturbances are very rare.

PYRAZINAMIDE

This relative of nicotinamide is stable, slightly soluble in water, and quite inexpensive. At neutral pH, it is inactive in vitro, but at pH 5.0 it strongly inhibits the growth of tubercle bacilli and some other mycobacteria in concentrations of 15 μg/mL. Such concentrations are achieved by daily oral doses of 1.5–2 g (20–30 mg/kg). This can be given once daily or as 0.75 g twice daily. In some cases, 50–70 mg/kg is given 3 times weekly.

Pyrazinamide is well absorbed from the gastrointestinal tract and widely distributed in body tissues. Tubercle bacilli develop resistance to pyrazinamide fairly readily, but there is no cross-resistance with isoniazid or other antimycobacterial drugs.

Major adverse effects of pyrazinamide include hepatotoxicity (in 1–5% of patients), nausea, vomiting, drug fever, and hyperuricemia.

Pyrazinamide (PZA)

STREPTOMYCIN

The pharmacologic features of streptomycin have been discussed in Chapter 45. Most tubercle bacilli are inhibited by streptomycin, 1–10 μg/mL, in vitro. Most "atypical" mycobacteria are resistant to streptomycin in pharmacologic concentrations. All large populations of tubercle bacilli contain some streptomycin-resistant mutants. On the average, $1:10^8$ to $1:10^{10}$ tubercle bacilli can be expected to be resistant to streptomycin at levels of 10–100 μg/mL.

Streptomycin exerts its action mainly on extracellular tubercle bacilli. Only about 10% of the drug penetrates cells that harbor intracellular organisms. Thus, even if the entire microbial population were streptomycin-susceptible, at any one moment a large percentage of the tubercle bacilli would be unaffected by streptomycin. Treatment for many months is therefore required.

Streptomycin sulfate remains an important drug in the treatment of tuberculosis. It is employed principally in individuals with severe, possibly life-threatening forms of tuberculosis, particularly meningitis, miliary dissemination, and severe organ tuberculosis. The usual dosage is 0.5–1 g intramuscularly daily for adults (20–40 mg/kg/d for children) for several weeks, followed by 1 g intramuscularly two or three times weekly for several months. Other drugs are always given simultaneously to delay emergence of resistant strains.

Intrathecal injection of streptomycin in tuberculous meningitis has been largely abandoned, because other drugs such as INH or ethambutol appear in the cerebrospinal fluid. However, the use of streptomycin must still be considered, particularly for INH-resistant mycobacteria.

The eighth nerve toxicity of streptomycin injected intramuscularly for many weeks manifests itself principally as dysfunction of the labyrinth, resulting in inability to maintain equilibrium and in deafness. The latter is often permanent, but some compensation for the former may occur.

ALTERNATIVE SECOND-LINE DRUGS IN TREATMENT OF TUBERCULOSIS

Because of their antimicrobial efficacy and their relative clinical safety, first-line drugs in tuberculosis in 1994 were isoniazid, rifampin, pyrazinamide, and ethambutol. The alternative drugs listed below are usually considered only (1) in the case of resistance to the drugs of first choice (which occurs with increasing frequency); (2) in case of failure of clinical response to conventional therapy; and (3) when expert guidance is available to deal with the toxic effects. For most of the second-line drugs listed below, the dosage, emergence of resistance, and long-term toxicity have not been fully established.

Capreomycin

Capreomycin is a peptide antibiotic obtained from *Streptomyces capreolus.* Daily injection of 1 g intramuscularly results in blood levels of 10 µg/mL or more. Such concentrations in vitro are inhibitory for many mycobacteria. There is some cross-resistance between capreomycin, viomycin, and kanamycin. Capreomycin (20 mg/kg/d) can perhaps take the place of the latter drugs in combined antituberculous therapy. The most serious toxicity is for the kidney, resulting in nitrogen retention, and for the eighth nerve, resulting in deafness and vestibular disturbances. Toxicity is less marked if 1 g is given 2 or 3 times weekly, and such a schedule is sometimes used.

Cycloserine

Cycloserine is an antibiotic analogue of D-alanine. It inhibits alanine racemase. Concentrations of 15–20 µg/mL inhibit many strains of tubercle bacilli. The most serious toxic reactions are various central nervous system dysfunctions and psychotic reactions. Some of these can be controlled by phenytoin, 100 mg/d orally.

The dosage of cycloserine in tuberculosis is 0.5–1 g/d. Cycloserine has been used in urinary tract infections in doses of 15–20 mg/kg/d.

Cycloserine is discussed further in Chapter 50.

Ethionamide

This yellow crystalline substance is stable and almost insoluble in water. It is a close chemical relative of isoniazid and also blocks the synthesis of mycolic acids.

Ethionamide

In spite of this similarity, there is no cross-resistance between isoniazid and ethionamide. Most tubercle bacilli are inhibited in vitro by ethionamide, 2.5 µg/mL or less. Many photochromogenic mycobacteria are also inhibited by ethionamide, 10 µg/mL. Such concentrations in plasma and tissues are achieved by doses of 1 g/d. This dosage is effective in the clinical treatment of tuberculosis, but is poorly tolerated because of the intense gastric irritation and neurologic symptoms it causes. A dose of 0.5 g orally per day is better tolerated but not very effective. Resistance to ethionamide develops rapidly in vitro and in vivo.

Aminosalicylic Acid (PAS)

Among several derivatives of salicylic and benzoic acids, *p*-aminosalicylic acid has the most marked effect on tubercle bacilli. The structural formula of PAS reveals its close similarity to *p*-aminobenzoic aid (PABA) and to the sulfonamides (see Chapter 47).

Aminosalicylic acid (PAS)

PAS is a white crystalline powder only slightly soluble in water and rapidly destroyed by heat. The sodium salt is freely soluble in water and relatively stable at room temperature.

Most bacteria are not affected by PAS. Tubercle bacilli are usually inhibited in vitro by PAS, 1–5 µg/mL, but "atypical" mycobacteria are resistant.

It is likely that PAS and PABA compete for the active center of an enzyme involved in converting PABA to dihydropteroic acid. The receptors of PABA attachment must be quite specific, because PAS is ineffective against most bacteria whereas sulfonamides are ineffective against tubercle bacilli.

PAS is readily absorbed from the gastrointestinal tract. Average daily doses (8–12 g) tend to give blood levels of 10 µg/mL or more. The drug is widely distributed in tissues and body fluids except the cerebrospinal fluid. PAS is rapidly excreted in the urine, in part as active PAS and in part as the acetylated compound and other metabolic products. Very high concentrations of PAS are reached in the urine. To avoid crystalluria, the urine must be kept alkaline.

Aminosalicylic acid was employed in the past together with isoniazid or streptomycin, or both, in the long-term treatment of tuberculosis. It is used infrequently now because other oral drugs are better tolerated. The dosage is 8–12 g/d orally for adults and 300 mg/kg/d for children.

Gastrointestinal symptoms often accompany full doses of PAS. Anorexia, nausea, diarrhea, and epigastric pain and burning may all be diminished by giving PAS with meals and with antacids. Peptic ulceration and hemorrhage may occur. Kidney or liver damage, thyroid gland injury (goiter with or without myxedema), and metabolic acidosis are rare.

Drug fever, joint pains, skin rashes, granulocytopenia, and a variety of neurologic symptoms—all probably due to hypersensitivity—often occur after 3–8 weeks of PAS therapy, making it necessary to stop PAS administration temporarily or permanently.

Viomycin

This antibiotic is produced by certain *Streptomyces* organisms. It is a complex basic polypeptide dispensed as a neutral sulfate that is very soluble in water. Most strains of tubercle bacilli are inhibited in vitro by viomycin, 1–10 µg/mL. Such concentrations can be achieved by the injection of 2 g intramuscularly twice weekly. Tubercle bacilli resistant to viomycin emerge fairly rapidly. There is also some cross-resistance with streptomycin, kanamycin, and capreomycin. The most serious toxic side effects are damage to the kidney and to the eighth nerve, resulting in loss of equilibrium and deafness. Toxic effects are more serious than with streptomycin.

Rifabutin (Ansamycin)

This antibiotic is derived from rifamycin and is related to rifampin. It has significant activity against *M avium-intracellulare* and *M fortuitum* (see below). The dose is 0.15–0.5 g/d orally. Its role in therapy and its toxicity are not well defined.

Other Antimycobacterial Drugs

Amikacin, tetracyclines, and **fluoroquinolones** have been employed in combined therapy of tuberculosis. These drugs can inhibit tubercle bacilli in concentrations that may be achieved in vivo. However, they are much less effective than the drugs of first choice. They are at times useful in treatment of infections due to "atypical" mycobacteria.

SHORT-COURSE CHEMOTHERAPY OF TUBERCULOSIS

Traditional treatment programs have been based on 18–24 months of drug therapy. Schemes of drug combinations for 6–12 months, involving daily or twice-weekly therapy, have achieved good success in inducing complete remissions at least on short-term follow-up.

It must be stressed that these schemes apply only to uncomplicated pulmonary tuberculosis and regimens that contain *both* isoniazid (INH) and rifampin with or without other drugs. Representative protocols for adults consist of INH, 300 mg daily, plus rifampin, 600 mg daily, for a total of 6 months, with pyra-

zinamide, 30 mg/kg daily, added during the first 8 weeks. Alternatively, INH, 300 mg, rifampin, 600 mg, and pyrazinamide, 1.5–2 g, are given daily for 2 weeks; then INH, 15 mg/kg, rifampin, 600 mg, and pyrazinamide, 3 g, are given twice weekly for the next 6 weeks; and for the remainder of the 6-month course the pyrazinamide is omitted. Streptomycin, 1–1.25 g, is sometimes given intramuscularly during the first 2 weeks. Many trials of similar drug regimens have given satisfactory results, with a total length of treatment limited to only 6 months.

DRUGS ACTIVE AGAINST ATYPICAL MYCOBACTERIA

About 10% of mycobacterial infections seen in clinical practice in the USA are not caused by *M tuberculosis* or *M leprae* but by "atypical" mycobacteria. These organisms have distinctive laboratory characteristics, occur in the environment, are generally not communicable from person to person, and are sometimes resistant to several antituberculous drugs. Disease caused by these organisms is often not as severe as tuberculosis and occurs in individuals without contact with tuberculosis yet yielding acid-fast mycobacteria in smears. Chest x-rays may be negative. A few representative pathogens, with the clinical presentation and the drugs to which they are often susceptible, are given in Table 46–1. Some atypical mycobacteria, especially the *M avium* complex, produce serious disseminated disease in AIDS. Such organisms are often multidrug-resistant, and attempts to suppress them employ multidrug treatment. This may include rifampin, ethambutol, clofazimine, amikacin, a fluoroquinolone (eg, ciprofloxacin or ofloxacin), azithromycin or clarithromycin, and rifabutin. The

Table 46–1. Clinical features and treatment of infections due to atypical mycobacteria.

Runyon Group	Pathogen	Frequent Clinical Features	Treatment Possibilities: Often Susceptible to—
I	*M kansasii*	Resembles tuberculous pulmonary disease.	Ethambutol + rifampin (+ INH); erythromycin, ethionamide.
	M marinum	Skin granulomas.	Minocycline, rifampin.
II	*M scrofulaceum*	Cervical adenitis in children.	Amikacin, erythromycin, rifampin, streptomycin. (Surgical excision is treatment of choice.)
III	*M avium-intracellulare*	Occasional pulmonary disease; widespread as asymptomatic infection; serious or fatal dissemination in AIDS patients	Rifampin or rifabutin, ethambutol, clofazimine, ciprofloxacin, amikacin, azithromycin.
IV	*M fortuitum*	Skin ulcers; rarely, lung disease.	Tetracycline, amikacin, ethionamide, capreomycin, rifabutin.
	M ulcerans	Skin ulcers.	Rifampin, streptomycin.

cumulative untoward effects of such drug combinations are difficult to manage.

DRUGS USED IN LEPROSY

Mycobacterium leprae has never been grown in vitro, but animal models, such as growth in injected mouse footpads, have permitted laboratory evaluation of drugs. Only those drugs that have the widest clinical use are presented here. Because of increasing reports of dapsone resistance, treatment of leprosy with combinations of the drugs listed below is now being advocated.

DAPSONE & OTHER SULFONES

Several drugs closely related to the sulfonamides have been used effectively in the long-term treatment of leprosy. Dapsone, the most widely used, is diaminodiphenylsulfone. It probably inhibits folate synthesis. Resistance can emerge in large populations of *M leprae*, eg, in lepromatous leprosy, if very low doses are given. Therefore, the combination of dapsone and rifampin is often recommended for initial therapy. Dapsone may also be used to treat *Pneumocystis* pneumonia in AIDS.

Dapsone

Sulfones are well absorbed from the gut and widely distributed throughout body fluids and tissues. The serum half-life is 1–2 days, and drug tends to be retained in skin, muscle, liver, and kidney. Skin heavily infected with *M leprae* may contain several times as much of the drug as normal skin. Sulfones are excreted into bile and reabsorbed in the intestine. Excretion into urine is variable, and most excreted drug is acetylated. In renal failure, the dose may have to be adjusted.

The usual dosage in leprosy begins with one or two 25-mg tablets of dapsone per week, increasing by one tablet weekly until a full dose of 400–600 mg/wk is reached. For children, the dose is proportionately less.

Untoward reactions to dapsone are common. Many patients develop some hemolysis, particularly if they have glucose-6-phosphate dehydrogenase deficiency. Methemoglobinemia is common. Gastrointestinal intolerance, fever, pruritus, and various rashes occur. During dapsone therapy of lepromatous leprosy, erythema nodosum leprosum develops often. It is sometimes difficult to distinguish reactions to dapsone from manifestations of the underlying illness. Erythema nodosum leprosum may be suppressed by corticosteroids or by thalidomide.

Acedapsone (4,4-diacetamidodiphenylsulfone) is a repository form of dapsone. A single intramuscular injection of 300 mg may maintain inhibitory dapsone levels in tissue for up to 3 months. Several other sulfones related to dapsone have also been used. When intolerance develops, it is to all sulfones.

RIFAMPIN

This drug (see above) in a dose of 600 mg daily can be strikingly effective in lepromatous leprosy. Because of the probable risk of emergence of rifampin-resistant *M leprae*, the drug is usually given in combination with dapsone or another antileprosy drug. A single *monthly* dose of 600 mg may be beneficial in combination therapy. The cost of rifampin is high for use in developing parts of the world, where the need may be greatest.

CLOFAZIMINE

Clofazimine is a phenazine dye that can be used as an alternative to dapsone. Its mechanism of action is unknown but may involve DNA binding. It is relatively expensive.

Absorption of clofazimine from the gut is variable, and a major portion of the drug is excreted in feces. Clofazimine is stored widely in reticuloendothelial tissues and skin, and its crystals can be seen inside phagocytic reticuloendothelial cells. It is slowly released, so that the serum half-life may be 2 months. Only a small proportion of each dose is excreted into urine or bile.

Clofazimine is given for sulfone-resistant leprosy or when patients are intolerant to sulfone. A common dose is 100–300 mg/d orally. In combination therapy, a dose of 50–100 mg/d has been satisfactory. Clofazimine has been used in combination therapy to treat *M avium-intracellulare* infections in patients with

Clofazimine

AIDS. The most prominent untoward effect is skin discoloration ranging from red-brown to nearly black. Gastrointestinal intolerance occurs occasionally.

AMITHIOZONE

Amithiozone is a thiosemicarbazone employed as a substitute for dapsone in intolerant patients. It appears to be more effective in tuberculoid than in lepromatous leprosy. Oral administration of 150 mg daily or 450 mg twice weekly yields serum concentrations inhibitory for mycobacteria, but resistance may develop if the drug is given alone. Gastrointestinal intolerance occurs frequently and hepatic damage has been reported. The drug is currently not available in the USA.

PREPARATIONS AVAILABLE

Drugs Used in Tuberculosis
  Aminosalicylate sodium (Sodium P.A.S.)
    Oral: 0.5 g tablets
  Capreomycin (Capastat Sulfate)
    Parenteral: powder to reconstitute for injection
    (1 g/10 mL vial)
  Cycloserine (Seromycin Pulvules)
    Oral: 250 mg capsules
  Ethambutol (Myambutol)
    Oral: 100, 400 mg tablets
  Ethionamide (Trecator-SC)
    Oral: 250 mg tablets
  Isoniazid (generic)
    Oral: 50, 100, 300 mg tablets; syrup, 50 mg/5 mL
    Parenteral: 100 mg/mL for injection
  Pyrazinamide (generic)

  Oral: 500 mg tablets
  Rifabutin (Mycobutin)
    Oral: 150 mg capsules
  Rifampin (Rifadin, Rimactane)
    Oral: 150, 300 mg capsules
    Parenteral: 600 mg powder for IV infusion
  Streptomycin (generic)
    Parenteral: 400 mg for IM injection; also available as powder to reconstitute for injection

Drugs Used in Leprosy
  Dapsone (generic)
    Oral: 25, 100 mg tablets
  Clofazimine (Lamprene)
    Oral: 50, 100 mg capsules

REFERENCES

Alvarez S, McCabe WR: Extrapulmonary tuberculosis revisited. Medicine (Baltimore) 1984;63:25.

American Thoracic Society: Treatment of tuberculosis and tuberculosis infection in adults and children. Am Rev Respir Dis 1986;134:355.

Byrd RB et al: Toxic effects of isoniazid in tuberculosis chemoprophylaxis. JAMA 1979;241:1239.

Carpenter JL et al: Disseminated disease due to *Mycobacterium chelonei* treated with amikacin and cefoxitin. Arch Intern Med 1984;144:2063.

Citron KM: Ocular toxicity from ethambutol (editorial). Thorax 1986;41:737.

Cohn DL et al: A 62 dose, 6 month therapy for pulmonary and extrapulmonary tuberculosis. Ann Intern Med 1990; 112:407.

Combs DL, et al: USPHS Tuberculosis short course chemotherapy trial 21. Ann Intern Med 1990;112:397.

Cox F et al: Rifampin prophylaxis for contacts of Haemophilus influenzae type b disease. JAMA 1981; 245:1043.

Dutt AK, Moers D, Stead WW: Short-course chemotherapy for extrapulmonary tuberculosis: Nine years' experience. Ann Intern Med 1986:104:7.

Dutt AK, Moers D, Stead WW: Undesirable side effects of

isoniazid and rifampin in largely twice-weekly short-course chemotherapy for tuberculosis. Am Rev Respir Dis 1983;128:419.

Ellard GA: Chemotherapy of leprosy. Br Med Bull 1988; 44:775.

Farr B, Mandell GL: Rifampin. Med Clin North Am 1982; 66:157.

Graber CD et al: Light chain proteinuria and humoral immunoincompetence in tuberculous patients treated with rifampin. Am Rev Respir Dis 1973;107:713.

Horsburgh CR: *Mycobacterium avium* complex in AIDS. N Engl J Med 1991;324:1332.

Iseman MD: Treatment of multidrug-resistant tuberculosis. N Engl J Med 1993;329:784.

Lester TW: Drug-resistant and atypical mycobacterial disease: Bacteriology and treatment. Arch Intern Med 1979; 139:1399.

Maddrey WC, Boitnott JK: Isoniazid hepatitis. Ann Intern Med 1973;79:1.

McKenzie MS et al: Drug treatment of tuberculous meningitis in childhood. Clin Pediatr 1979;18:75.

Mitchison DA: The action of antituberculosis drugs in short-course chemotherapy. Tubercle 1985;66:219.

Mitchison DA, Ellard GA, Grosset J: New antibacterial drugs for the treatment of mycobacterial diseases in man. Br Med Bull 1988;44:757.

Molavi A, LeFrock JL: Tuberculous meningitis. Med Clin North Am 1985;69:315.

Pratt TH: Rifampin induced organic brain syndrome. JAMA 1979;241:2421.

Quemard A, Lacave C, Laneelle G: Isoniazid inhibition of mycolic acid synthesis by cell extracts of sensitive and resistant strains of *Mycobacterium aurum*. Antimicrob Agents Chemother 1991;35:1035.

Snider DE Jr et al: Standard therapy for tuberculosis. Chest 1985;87(Suppl 2):117 S.

Snider DE et al: Drug-resistant tuberculosis. Am Rev Resp Dis 1991;144:732.

Stead WW et al: Tuberculosis as an endemic and nosocomial infection among the elderly in nursing homes. N Engl J Med 1985;312:1483.

Stoeckle MY et al: Catalase-peroxidase gene sequences in isoniazid-sensitive and -resistant strains of *Mycobacterium tuberculosis* from New York City. J Infect Dis 1993;168:1063.

Waters MF et al: Rifampicin for lepromatous leprosy: Nine years' experience. Br Med J 1978;1:133.

Zhang Y et al: The catalase-peroxidase gene and isoniazid resistance of *Mycobacterium tuberculosis*. Nature 1992; 358:591.

Zhang Y, Garbe T, Young D: Transformation with *kat*G restores isoniazid sensitivity in *Mycobacterium tuberculosis* isolates resistant to a range of drug concentrations. Molec Microbiol 1993;8:521.

Sulfonamides & Trimethoprim

47

Ernest Jawetz, MD, PhD

SULFONAMIDES

A red dye, prontosil, was synthesized in Germany by Klarer and Mietzsch in 1932 and tested by the usual (in vitro) screening methods against bacterial cultures. It was found to be ineffective in these tests. However, Domagk reported in 1935 that in vivo it was strikingly active against hemolytic streptococcal and other infections. This was due to the conversion in the body of prontosil to sulfanilamide, the active drug. Since then, the sulfonamide molecule has been chemically altered by the attachment of many different radicals, and there has been a proliferation of active compounds. Perhaps 150 different sulfonamides have been marketed at one time or another, the modifications being designed principally to achieve greater antibacterial potency, a wider antibacterial spectrum, greater solubility in urine, or more prolonged action. In spite of the advent of the antibiotic drugs, the sulfonamides are among the most widely used antibacterial agents in the world today, chiefly because of their low cost and relative efficacy in some common bacterial diseases. The synergistic action of sulfonamide with trimethoprim has brought about an enormous resurgence in sulfonamide use everywhere during the last decade.

Chemistry

The basic formula of the sulfonamides and their relationship to PABA are shown in Figure 47–1.

All have the same nucleus to which various R radicals in the amido group ($-SO_2NH-R$) have been attached or in which various substitutions of the amino group (NH_2) are made. These changes produce compounds with varying physical, chemical, pharmacologic, and antibacterial properties. In general, the sulfonamides are white, odorless, bitter-tasting crystalline weak acids that are much more soluble at alkaline than at acid pH. In a mixture of sulfonamide drugs, each component drug exhibits its own solubility. Therefore, a mixture may be much more soluble, in terms of total sulfonamide present, than one drug

used alone. This is the reason for the use of trisulfapyrimidines, a preparation that permits three times higher dosage than a single drug for comparable solubility in urine.

Most sulfonamides can be prepared as sodium salts that are moderately soluble, and these are used for intravenous administration. Such solutions are highly alkaline and not very stable and may precipitate out of solution with polyionic electrolytes (eg, lactate-chloride-carbonate). Certain sulfonamide molecules were designed for low solubility (eg, phthalylsulfathiazole) so that they would stay in the lumen of the bowel without being absorbed.

Antimicrobial Activity

Different sulfonamides may show quantitative but not necessarily qualitative differences in activity. Sulfonamides can inhibit both gram-positive and gram-negative bacteria, *Nocardia, Chlamydia trachomatis,* and some protozoa. Some enteric bacteria are inhibited but not *Pseudomonas, Serratia, Proteus,* and other multiresistant organisms. Sulfonamides alone are drugs of choice in previously untreated urinary tract infections, nocardiosis, and occasionally other bacterial infections. Many strains of meningococci, pneumococci, streptococci, staphylococci, and gonococci are now resistant. Indications for sulfonamide-trimethoprim mixtures are given below.

Sulfonamides are structural analogues of *p*-aminobenzoic acid (PABA). The action of sulfonamides is bacteriostatic and is reversible by removal of the drug or in the presence of an excess of PABA. The mode of action of the sulfonamides is a good example of **competitive inhibition.** In brief, susceptible microorganisms require extracellular PABA in order to form folic acid (Figure 47–2), an essential step in the production of purines and in the ultimate synthesis of nucleic acids. Sulfonamides can enter into the reaction in place of PABA, compete for the enzyme dihydropteroate synthase, and form nonfunctional analogues of folic acid. As a result, further growth of the microorganisms is prevented. However, growth can

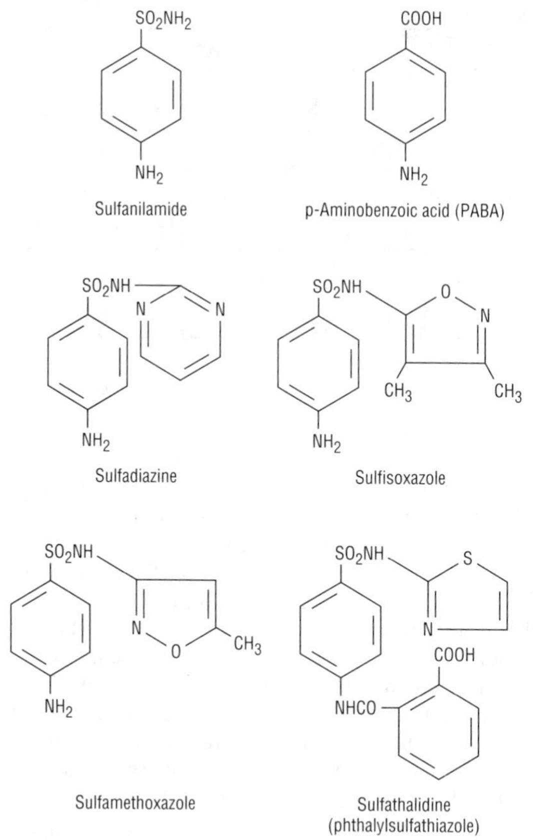

SO₂NH₂

Sulfanilamide

COOH

p-Aminobenzoic acid (PABA)

Sulfadiazine

Sulfisoxazole

Sulfamethoxazole

Sulfathalidine
(phthalylsulfathiazole)

Figure 47–1. Structures of some sulfonamides and para-aminobenzoic acid.

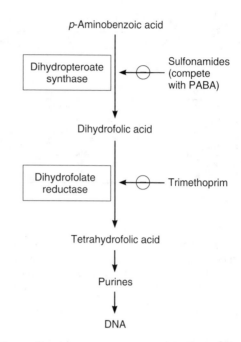

Figure 47–2. Actions of sulfonamides and trimethoprim.

resume when the sulfonamide is displaced by an excess of PABA or when it dissociates from the enzyme.

Resistance

Animal cells (and some bacteria) are unable to synthesize folic acid but depend upon exogenous sources and for this reason are not susceptible to sulfonamide action. Sulfonamide-resistant cells occur in most susceptible bacterial populations and tend to emerge under suitable selection pressure. Sulfonamide resistance may occur as a result of mutation, causing overproduction of PABA, a structural change in the folic acid-synthesizing enzyme with a lowered affinity for sulfonamides, or a loss of permeability. Sulfonamide resistance is most often under the genetic control of a transmissible plasmid that may become rapidly and widely disseminated. Thus, the widespread therapeutic use of sulfonamides against coccal infections (gonococci, meningococci, streptococci) has resulted in the establishment of sulfonamide-resistant strains throughout the world. Other types of

microorganisms—eg, many enteric gram-negative rods—are also commonly resistant. It should be specifically mentioned that rickettsiae not only are not inhibited by sulfonamides but are actually stimulated in their growth.

Pharmacokinetics

Sulfonamides can be divided into three groups on the basis of their half-lives (Table 47–1). Most sulfonamides are given orally. They are rapidly absorbed from the stomach and small intestine and distributed widely to tissues and body fluids (including central nervous system and cerebrospinal fluid), placenta, and fetus. Absorbed sulfonamides become bound to serum proteins to an extent varying from 20% to over 90%. A varying proportion also becomes acetylated or inactivated by other metabolic pathways. Chemical determinations performed on serum may measure free (active) sulfonamide, the acetylated (inactive) sulfonamide, or the total of both. In order to be therapeutically effective after systemic administration, a sulfonamide must generally achieve a concentration of 8–12 mg of free drug per deciliter of blood. Peak blood levels generally occur 2–6 hours after oral intake.

Soluble sulfonamides are excreted mainly by glomerular filtration into the urine. Different compounds exhibit different degrees of reabsorption in the tubules, but the much greater physiologic reabsorption of water results in marked concentration of the drug in the urine. A portion of the drug in the

Table 47–1. Pharmacokinetic properties of some sulfonamides and trimethoprim.

Drug	Half-Life	Oral Absorption
Sulfonamides		
Sulfacytine	No data	Prompt (peak levels in 1–4 hours)
Sulfisoxazole	Short (6 hours)	Prompt
Sulfamethizole	Short (9 hours)	Prompt
Sulfadiazine	Intermediate (10–17 hours)	Slow (peak levels in 4–8 hours)
Sulfamethoxazole	Intermediate (10–12 hours)	Slow
Sulfapyridine	No data	Slow
Sulfadoxine	Long (7–9 days)	Intermediate
Pyrimidines		
Trimethoprim	Intermediate (11 hours)	Prompt

urine is the acetylated metabolite, but enough active drug remains for effective treatment of infections of the urinary tract (usually 10–20 times the concentration present in the blood). In significant renal failure, the dosage of sulfonamide must be reduced.

Sodium salts of sulfonamides are employed for intravenous administration because of their greater solubility. Their distribution and excretion are similar to those of the orally administered drugs.

The "insoluble" sulfonamides (eg, phthalylsulfathiazole) are given orally, are absorbed only slightly in the intestinal tract, and are excreted largely in the feces. Their action is exerted mainly on the aerobic intestinal flora in preparation for bowel surgery.

"Long-acting" sulfonamides, eg, sulfadoxine, sulfamethoxypyridazine, are well absorbed after oral intake and are distributed widely, but urinary excretion—especially of the free form—is very slow. This results in prolonged drug levels in serum. The slow renal excretion is due in part to the high protein binding (more than 85%) and in part to the extensive tubular reabsorption of the free (unacetylated) drug. These drugs are often inadvisable because instances of severe toxicity have resulted from their use. With the exception of sulfadoxine (in Fansidar), they have been withdrawn in the USA but are still available elsewhere. Sulfonamides of "intermediate action," eg, sulfamethoxazole, have no advantage except convenience of dosage, particularly when formulated in a mixture with trimethoprim (80 mg trimethoprim plus 400 mg sulfamethoxazole per tablet).

Bacterial Examinations

When culturing specimens from patients receiving sulfonamides, the incorporation of PABA (5 mg/dL) into the medium overcomes the sulfonamide inhibition of growth of susceptible organisms.

Clinical Uses

A. Topical: In general, the application of sulfonamides to the skin, in wounds, or on mucous membranes is undesirable because of their low activity and high risk of allergic sensitization. One exception may be the application of sodium sulfacetamide solution (30%) or ointment (10%) to the conjunctiva.

A second exception is mafenide acetate (*p*-aminomethylbenzenesulfonamide), a sulfonamide topically applied (as 10% cream) to burned skin surfaces. The drug is absorbed from the vehicle into tissue in 3 hours. It has been effective in reducing burn sepsis but has led to an increase of burn infections by fungi and resistant bacteria. Mafenide causes significant pain on application. Silver sulfadiazine applied to burn wounds causes relatively little pain. The sulfadiazine is released slowly, and only low systemic levels develop. Silver sulfadiazine appears to be effective in controlling infecting flora of most burn wounds, especially if the burns are not too deep.

Oral administration of the "insoluble" sulfonamides, 8–15 g daily, results in a local effect—temporary inhibition of the intestinal aerobic microbial flora—that is of value in preparing the bowel for surgery; it must be timed so that the lowest microbial levels coincide with the time of the operation (fourth to sixth days of administration).

Sulfasalazine (salicylazosulfapyridine) is widely used in ulcerative colitis, enteritis, and other inflammatory bowel disease. This drug appears to be more effective than soluble sulfonamides or other antimicrobials taken orally—all of which may occasionally have a beneficial effect in inflammatory bowel disease. Sulfasalazine is split by intestinal microflora to yield sulfapyridine and 5-aminosalicylate. The latter is released in the colon in high concentration and is responsible for an anti-inflammatory effect, the major source of benefit from this drug. Comparably high concentrations of salicylate cannot be achieved in the colon by oral intake of ordinary formulations of salicylates because of severe gastrointestinal toxicity (see Chapter 64). The sulfapyridine is absorbed and may lead to toxic symptoms if more than 4 g of sulfasalazine is taken per day, particularly in persons who are slow acetylators. Olsalazine, a dimer of salicylic acid, is split by bacteria in the colon and is active in ulcerative colitis. It may be better tolerated than sulfasalazine (see Chapter 64).

B. Oral: The highly soluble and rapidly excreted sulfonamides are most commonly employed for the following clinical indications:

1. First (previously untreated) infections of the urinary tract–In women with uncomplicated, acute symptomatic urinary tract infections who are not pregnant and who have not been treated previously, a single 1-g dose of sulfisoxazole or two tablets twice in 1 day of trimethoprim plus sulfamethoxazole (see below) is effective in 80–90% of patients. Alternatively, sulfisoxazole, 0.5–1 g 4 times daily (30–60 mg/kg), can be given for 3–7 days. Sulfisoxazole, 150 mg/kg/d, is often effective for initial infections in children.

2. Chlamydial infections–*Chlamydia trachomatis* infections of the genital tract, eye, or respiratory tract may be treated with oral sulfonamides, though tetracyclines and erythromycins are drugs of choice. Sulfonamides are not effective in psittacosis.

3. Bacterial infections–In nocardiosis, sulfisoxazole or sulfadiazine, 6–8 g/d, is the treatment of choice. In other bacterial infections, including those caused by beta-hemolytic streptococci, meningococci, and shigellae, sulfonamides were formerly drugs of choice. However, sulfonamide resistance is now widespread among these organisms. In underdeveloped parts of the world, sulfonamides—because of their availability and low cost—are widely used for respiratory tract infections, sinusitis, bronchitis, pneumonitis, otitis media, and bacillary dysentery. Sulfonamide-trimethoprim mixtures are widely employed for these and other bacterial infections everywhere but are much more expensive. Leprosy is treated with sulfones, eg, dapsone (see Chapter 46).

4. Dermatitis herpetiformis– This is not an infectious disorder, but it often responds to sulfapyridine, 2–4 g/d, or dapsone.

C. Intravenous: Sodium salts of sulfonamides in 5% dextrose in water can be given intravenously. This is generally reserved for patients who are comatose or otherwise unable to take medication by mouth.

Adverse Reactions

The sulfonamides can produce a wide variety of untoward effects due partly to allergy and partly to direct toxicity and that must be considered whenever unexplained symptoms or signs occur in a patient who may have received these drugs. Up to 5% of patients exhibit such reactions. *All* sulfonamides are cross-allergenic, including carbonic anhydrase inhibitors, thiazides, furosemide, bumetanide, diazoxide, and the sulfonylurea hypoglycemic agents.

The commonest adverse effects are fever, skin rashes, photosensitivity, urticaria, nausea, vomiting, diarrhea, and difficulties referable to the urinary tract

(see below). Others include stomatitis, conjunctivitis, arthritis, hematopoietic disturbances (see below), hepatitis, exfoliative dermatitis, polyarteritis nodosa, Stevens-Johnson syndrome, psychosis, and many more.

A. Urinary Tract Disturbances: Sulfonamides may precipitate in urine, especially at neutral or acid pH, producing crystalluria, hematuria, or even obstruction. This is best prevented by using the most soluble sulfonamides (sulfisoxazole, trisulfapyrimidines), keeping the urine pH alkaline (5–15 g sodium bicarbonate daily), forcing fluids, and performing urinalysis every week. Sulfonamides must not be given with methenamine compounds, because a precipitate may form.

Sulfonamides have also been implicated in various types of nephrosis and in allergic nephritis. Deterioration of renal function can occur.

In renal insufficiency, the dosage of sulfonamides must be reduced and the interval between doses prolonged.

B. Hematopoietic Disturbances: Sulfonamides can produce anemia (hemolytic or aplastic), granulocytopenia, thrombocytopenia, or leukemoid reactions. These are rare except in certain high-risk patients. Sulfonamides cause hemolytic reactions, especially in patients whose erythrocytes are deficient in glucose-6-phosphate dehydrogenase. Sulfonamides taken near the end of pregnancy increase the risk of kernicterus in newborns.

Medical & Public Health Aspects

Sulfonamides can be made and distributed cheaply and are thus among the principal antimicrobial agents available in many developing areas of the world. They continue to be useful for the treatment of such widespread disorders as urinary tract infections and trachoma, but the emergence of drug resistance has impaired their usefulness in infections with streptococci, gonococci, meningococci, shigellae, and other pathogens. Topical use (skin, eye) on a vast scale has contributed heavily to the sensitization of the population.

TRIMETHOPRIM & TRIMETHOPRIM-SULFAMETHOXAZOLE MIXTURES

Trimethoprim, a trimethoxybenzylpyrimidine, inhibits the dihydrofolic acid reductase of bacteria about 50,000 times more efficiently than the same enzyme of mammalian cells. **Pyrimethamine,** another benzylpyrimidine, inhibits the dihydrofolic acid reductase of protozoa more than that of mammalian cells. Dihydrofolic acid reductases are enzymes that convert dihydrofolic acid to tetrahydrofolic acid, a stage leading to the synthesis of purines and ultimately to DNA. Trimethoprim or pyrimethamine, given together with sulfonamides, produces sequential blocking in this metabolic sequence, resulting in a marked enhancement (synergism) of the activity of both drugs (Figure 47–2).

Microorganisms that lack the step inhibited by trimethoprim (dihydrofolate reductase) can emerge by mutation or by the conjugative transmission of plasmids. Such plasmids inducing trimethoprim resistance exist in coliform bacteria, *Haemophilus,* and other organisms, and this resistance is increasing in frequency.

Trimethoprim

Pyrimethamine

Pharmacokinetics

Trimethoprim is usually given orally, alone or in combination with sulfamethoxazole. This sulfonamide is chosen because it has a similar half-life (Table 47–1). The latter combination can also be given intravenously. Trimethoprim is absorbed well from the gut and distributed widely in body fluids and tissues, including cerebrospinal fluid. Because trimethoprim is more lipid-soluble than sulfamethoxazole, it has a larger volume of distribution than the latter drug. Therefore, when 1 part of trimethoprim is given with 5 parts of sulfamethoxazole (the ratio in the formulation), the peak plasma concentrations are in the ratio of 1:20, which is optimal for the combined effects of these drugs in vitro. About 65–70% of each participant drug is protein-bound, and 30–50% of the sulfonamide and 50–60% of the trimethoprim (or their respective metabolites) are excreted in the urine within 24 hours.

Trimethoprim (a weak base of $pK_a \approx 7.2$) concentrates in prostatic fluid and in vaginal fluid, which are more acid than plasma. Therefore, it has more antibacterial activity in prostatic and vaginal fluids than many other antimicrobial drugs.

Clinical Uses

A. Oral Trimethoprim: Trimethoprim can be given alone (100 mg every 12 hours) in acute urinary tract infections. A majority of community-acquired organisms tend to be susceptible to the high concentrations in urine (200–600 μg/mL).

B. Oral Trimethoprim-Sulfamethoxazole: At present, trimethoprim-sulfamethoxazole mixtures appear to be a treatment of choice for *Pneumocystis carinii* pneumonia, symptomatic *Shigella* enteritis, systemic *Salmonella* infections (caused by ampicillin- or chloramphenicol-resistant organisms), complicated urinary tract infections, prostatitis, and many others.

Two tablets of the regular size (trimethoprim 80 mg + sulfamethoxazole 400 mg) given every 12 hours can be effective in recurrent infections of the lower or upper urinary tract. The same dose may be effective in prostatitis. Two tablets daily may be sufficient for prolonged suppression of chronic urinary tract infections, and one-half of the regular size tablet given 3 times weekly for many months may serve as prophylaxis in recurrent urinary tract infections of some women. Two tablets of the regular size every 12 hours may be effective in some *Shigella, Salmonella,* and other infections. The dose for children treated for shigellosis, urinary tract infection, or otitis media is 8 mg/kg trimethoprim and 40 mg/kg sulfamethoxazole every 12 hours.

Infections with *P carinii* and some other pathogens can be treated with high doses of the combination (trimethoprim, 20 mg/kg, plus sulfamethoxazole, 100 mg/kg, daily) or can be prevented in immunosuppressed patients by two regular tablets twice daily. Some cases of *Serratia* or other resistant bacterial sepsis have responded to trimethoprim-sulfamethoxazole.

C. Intravenous Trimethoprim-Sulfamethoxazole: A solution of the mixture containing 80 mg trimethoprim plus 400 mg sulfamethoxazole per 5 mL diluted in 125 mL of 5% dextrose in water can be administered by intravenous infusion over 60–90 minutes. It may be indicated in severe *P carinii* pneumonia, especially in patients with AIDS; gram-negative bacterial sepsis; shigellosis; or urinary tract infection when patients are unable to take the drug by mouth. Adults may be given 6–12 of these 5 mL ampules in three or four divided doses per day.

D. Oral Pyrimethamine With Sulfonamide: This combination has been used in parasitic infections. In leishmaniasis and toxoplasmosis, full doses of a sulfonamide (6–8 g/d) have been given with pyrimethamine, 50 mg/d. In falciparum malaria, a combination of pyrimethamine with a sulfonamide (Fansidar) or pyrimethamine alone has been occasionally employed (see Chapter 54).

Adverse Effects

Trimethoprim produces the predictable adverse effects of an antifolate drug, especially megaloblastic anemia, leukopenia, and granulocytopenia (see Chapter 56). This can be prevented by the simultaneous administration of folinic acid, 6–8 mg/d. In addition, the combination trimethoprim-sulfamethoxazole may cause all of the untoward reactions associated with sulfonamides. Occasionally, there is also nausea and vomiting, drug fever, vasculitis, renal damage, or central nervous system disturbances. Patients with AIDS and *Pneumocystis* pneumonia have a particularly high frequency of untoward reactions to trimethoprim-sulfamethoxazole, especially fever, rashes, leukopenia, and diarrhea.

PREPARATIONS AVAILABLE

General-Purpose Sulfonamides
Multiple sulfonamides, trisulfapyrimidines (generic)
  Oral: 500 mg (total sulfa) tablets
Sulfacytine (Renoquid)
  Oral: 250 mg tablets
Sulfadiazine (generic)
  Oral: 500 mg tablets
Sulfamethizole (Thiosulfil)
  Oral: 500 mg tablets
Sulfamethoxazole (generic, Gantanol, others)
  Oral: 0.5 g tablets; 500 mg/5 mL suspension
Sulfisoxazole (generic, Gantrisin)
  Oral: 500 mg tablets; 500 mg/5 mL syrup

Sulfonamides for Special Applications
Mafenide (Sulfamylon)
  Topical: 85 mg/g cream
Silver sulfadiazine (generic, Silvadene)
  Topical: 10 mg/g cream
Sulfasalazine (generic, Azaline, Azulfidine)
  Oral: 500 mg tablets and enteric-coated tablets; 250 mg/5 mL suspension

Trimethoprim
Trimethoprim (generic, Proloprim, Trimpex)
  Oral: 100, 200 mg tablets
Trimethoprim-sulfamethoxazole [co-trimoxazole, TMP-SMZ] (generic, Bactrim, Septra, others)
  Oral: 80 mg trimethoprim + 400 mg sulfamethoxazole per single-strength tablet; 160 mg trimethoprim + 800 mg sulfamethoxazole per double-strength tablet; 40 mg trimethoprim + 200 mg sulfamethoxazole per 5 mL suspension
  Parenteral: 80 mg trimethoprim + 400 mg sulfamethoxazole per 5 mL for infusion (in 5 mL ampules and 5, 10, 20, 30, 50 mL vials)

REFERENCES

Ballin JC: Evaluation of a new topical agent for burn therapy: Silver sulfadiazine (Silvadene). JAMA 1974;230:1884.

Bartels RH, van der Spek JA, Oosten HR: Acute pancreatitis due to sulfamethoxazole-trimethoprim. South Med J 1992;85:1006.

Bose W et al: Controlled trial of co-trimoxazole in children with urinary tract infection. Lancet 1974;2:614.

Cockerill FR, Edson RS: Trimethoprim-sulfamethoxazole. Mayo Clin Proc 1987;62:92.

Craig WA, Kunin CM: Trimethoprim-sulfamethoxazole: Effects of urinary pH and impaired renal function. Ann Intern Med 1973;78:491.

Goldman P, Peppercorn MA: Sulfasalazine. N Engl J Med 1975;293:20.

Gordin FM et al: Adverse reactions to trimethoprim-sulfamethoxazole in patients with the acquired immunodeficiency syndrome. Ann Intern Med 1984;100:495.

Hamilton HE, Sheets RF: Sulfisoxazole-induced thrombocytopenic purpura. JAMA 1978;239:2586.

Heikkila E et al: Analysis of localization of the type I trimethoprim resistance gene from Escherichia coli isolated in Finland. Antimicrob Agents Chemother 1991;35:1562.

Heikkila E, Sundstrom L, Huovinen P: Trimethoprim resistance in Escherichia coli isolates from a geriatric unit. Antimicrob Agents Chemother 1990;34:2013.

Huovinen P: Trimethoprim resistance. Antimicrob Agents Chemother 1987;31:1451.

Huovinen P, Wolfson JS, Hooper DC: Synergism of trimethoprinm and ciprofloxacin in vitro against clinical bacterial isolates. Europ J Clin Microbiol Infect Dis 1992;11:255.

Kamada MM, Twarog F, Leung DY: Multiple antibiotic sensitivity in a pediatric population. Allergy Proc 1991;12:347.

Kovacs JA et al: Characterization of de novo folate synthesis in Pneumocystis carinii and Toxoplasma gondii. J Infect Dis 1989;160:312.

Lau WK, Young LS: Trimethoprim-sulfamethoxazole treatment of Pneumocystis carinii pneumonia in adults. N Engl J Med 1976;295:716.

Lee BL et al: Dapsone, trimethoprim-sulfamethoxazole plasma levels during treatment of Pneumocystis pneumonia in patients with AIDS. Ann Intern Med 1989;110:606.

Meares EM Jr: Long-term therapy of chronic bacterial prostatitis with trimethoprim-sulfamethoxazole. Can Med Assoc J 1975;112(13):22.

Modak SM, Fox CL; Sulfadiazine silver-resistant *Pseudomonas* in burns. Arch Surg 1981;116:854.

Murray BE et al: Emergence of high-level trimethoprim resistance in fecal *Escherichia coli* during oral administration of trimethoprim or trimethoprim-sulfamethoxazole. N Engl J Med 1982;306:130.

Pape JW et al: Treatment and prophylaxis of *Isospora belli* infection in patients with AIDS. N Engl J Med 1989;320:1044.

Paradise JL: Antimicrobial prophylaxis for recurrent acute otitis media. Ann Otol Rhinol Laryngol 1992;155 (Suppl):33.

Rubin RH, Swartz MN: Trimethoprim-sulfamethoxazole. N Engl J Med 1980;303:426.

Smego RA Jr, Moeller MB, Gallis HA: Trimethoprim-sulfamethoxazole therapy for *Nocardia* infections. Arch Intern Med 1983;143:711.

Spes CH et al: Sulfadiazine therapy for toxoplasmosis in heart transplant recipients decreases cyclosporine concentration. Clin Invest 1992;70:752.

Stamey TA, Condy M: The diffusion and concentration of trimethoprim in human vaginal fluid. J Infect Dis 1975;131:261.

Then RL, Kohl I, Burdeska A: Frequency and transferability of trimethoprim and sulfonamide resistance in methicillin-resistant *Staphylococcus aureus* and *Staphylococcus epidermidis*. J Chemother 1992;4:67.

Antifungal Agents

48

Ernest Jawetz, MD, PhD

Most fungi are completely resistant to the action of antibacterial drugs. Only a few chemicals have been discovered that inhibit fungi pathogenic for humans, and many of these are relatively toxic. The need for better antifungal drugs has been made more pressing by the greatly increased incidence of local and disseminated fungal infections in immunodeficient patients.

Among the antifungal drugs currently available, amphotericin B is the most difficult to administer and has many adverse effects, but it remains the most effective treatment for severe systemic mycoses. Flucytosine can be used orally for systemic infections, but resistance often develops. The antifungal azoles such as ketoconazole, fluconazole, and some others permit oral therapy of some systemic mycoses. Miconazole, another azole, is effective topically and to a limited degree systemically. Because the azoles inhibit P450 oxidative enzymes in the liver and elsewhere, they may interfere with drug metabolism and synthesis of endogenous compounds. Griseofulvin, taken orally, is effective in dermatophytosis but not in systemic infections. Nystatin, haloprogin, and some others can only be applied topically. Because of the importance of antifungal drugs in dermatology, some are also discussed in Chapter 63.

SYSTEMIC ANTIFUNGAL DRUGS

AMPHOTERICIN B

Amphotericin A and B are antifungal antibiotics produced by *Streptomyces nodosus,* purified in 1956. Amphotericin A is not used in therapy.

Chemistry

Amphotericin B is an amphoteric polyene macrolide (polyene = containing many double bonds; macrolide = containing a large lactone ring of 12 or more atoms). It is almost insoluble in water. It is unstable at 37 °C but stable for weeks at 4 °C. Microcrystalline preparations can be applied topically but are not absorbed to a significant extent. For systemic use by intravenous injection, a colloidal preparation is employed. A liposome preparation is under investigation.

Antifungal Activity

Amphotericin B, 0.1–0.8 μg/mL, inhibits in vitro *Histoplasma capsulatum, Cryptococcus neoformans, Coccidioides immitis, Candida albicans, Blastomyces dermatitidis, Sporothrix schenckii,* and other organisms producing mycotic disease in humans. It has no effect on bacteria, but it can be used with benefit in *Naegleria* meningoencephalitis.

The mode of action of the polyene antibiotics is fairly well understood. These drugs are bound firmly to ergosterol in the fungal cell membrane. The membrane of the fungal cell is altered, perhaps through the formation of amphotericin pores (amphotericin is a "pore-former" in artificial membranes), and cellular macromolecules and ions are lost, producing irreversible damage. Bacteria are not susceptible to polyenes because they lack the ergosterol that is essential for attachment to the cell membrane. Amphotericin resistance may result from a decrease in membrane ergosterol or a modification in its structure so that it combines less well with the drug. Some binding of amphotericin B to cholesterol in animal cell membranes probably accounts in part for its toxicity. Fortunately, this binding is less avid than the binding to ergosterol in fungal cell membranes.

Pharmacokinetics

Amphotericin B is poorly absorbed from the gastrointestinal tract. Orally administered amphotericin B therefore is effective only on fungi within the lumen of the tract and cannot be used for the treatment of systemic disease. The intravenous injection of 0.6 mg/kg/d of amphotericin B results in average blood levels of 0.3–1 μg/mL. Amphotericin B is more than 90% protein-bound and is removed to a very limited extent by hemodialysis. The injected amphotericin B is excreted slowly in the urine over a period of several days. The drug is widely distributed in tissues, but only 2–3% of the blood level is reached in cerebrospinal fluid. Consequently, intrathecal administration is necessary in fungal meningitis.

Amphotericin B can be prepared as liposomal granules with an average diameter of 0.5–3.5 μm. Liposomal amphotericin B in doses up to a cumulative total of 75 mg/kg has been therapeutically effective and has caused little or no renal or neurologic toxicity.

Clinical Uses

For the treatment of systemic fungal infections, amphotericin B is given by slow intravenous infusion over a period of 4–6 hours. The initial dose is 1–5 mg/d, increasing daily by 5 mg increments until a final dosage of 0.4–0.7 mg/kg/d is reached. This is usually continued for 6–12 weeks or longer, with a daily dose rarely exceeding 60 mg. Following an initial response to treatment, doses are given only 2 or 3 times per week, often on an outpatient basis.

In fungal meningitis, intrathecal injection of 0.5 mg amphotericin B may be given 3 times weekly for up to 10 weeks or longer. Continuous infusion with an Ommaya reservoir is sometimes used. Fungal meningitis relapses commonly. Combined treatment with amphotericin B and flucytosine is increasingly used in *Candida* and *Cryptococcus* meningitis and in systemic candidiasis. This delays emergence of resistance to flucytosine and permits use of lower doses of amphotericin B.

In corneal ulcers caused by fungi, a solution (1 mg/mL) dropped onto the conjunctiva every 30 minutes can be curative. Other local routes of administration include injections into joints infected with coccidioidomycosis or sporotrichosis or irrigation of the bladder in *Candida* cystitis.

The clinical use of liposomal amphotericin B in a variety of fungal infections is under investigation.

Adverse Reactions

The intravenous injection of amphotericin B usually produces chills, fever, vomiting, and headache. The severity of adverse reactions may be diminished by reducing the dosage temporarily, administering aspirin, phenothiazines, antihistamines, and corticosteroids, or stopping injections for several days.

Therapeutically active amounts of amphotericin B commonly impair renal and hepatocellular function and produce anemia. There is a fall in glomerular filtration rate and a change in tubular function. These result in a decrease in creatinine clearance and an increase in potassium clearance. Shock-like fall in blood pressure, electrolyte disturbances (especially hypokalemia), and a variety of neurologic symptoms also occur commonly. In impaired kidney function, the dose of amphotericin B must be further reduced.

Liposomal amphotericin B appears to produce less renal and neurologic toxicity.

FLUCYTOSINE

5-Fluorocytosine (flucytosine, 5-FC) is an oral antifungal compound with the structure shown below.

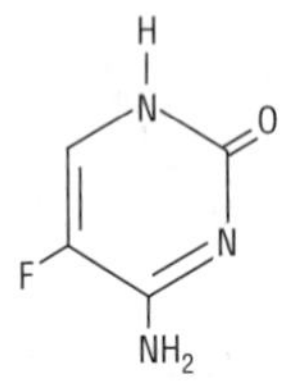

Flucytosine

Flucytosine, 5 μg/mL, inhibits in vitro many strains of *Candida, Cryptococcus,* and *Torulopsis* and some strains of *Aspergillus* and other fungi. Cells are susceptible if they convert flucytosine to fluorouracil, eventually inhibiting thymidylate synthetase and DNA synthesis. Resistant mutants emerge fairly regularly and rapidly and are selected in the presence of the drug, limiting its usefulness. For this reason, combined treatment with flucytosine and amphotericin B is being employed with enhanced antifungal activity in *Candida, Cryptococcus,* and some other infections.

Oral doses of 150 mg/kg/d are well absorbed and widely distributed in tissues—including the cerebrospinal fluid—where the drug concentration may be 60–80% of the serum concentration, which tends to be near 50 μg/mL. About 20% of flucytosine is protein-bound. Flucytosine is largely excreted by the kidneys, and concentrations in the urine reach ten times the concentrations in serum. In the presence of renal failure, the drug may accumulate in serum to toxic levels, but hepatic failure has no effect. Flucytosine is removed by hemodialysis.

Flucytosine appears to be relatively nontoxic for mammalian cells (perhaps because they lack a specific permease). However, prolonged high serum levels often cause depression of bone marrow, loss of hair, and abnormal liver function. Administration of uracil can reduce the hematopoietic toxicity, manifested by bone marrow depression, but seems to have no effect on the antifungal activity of flucytosine. The untoward effects of flucytosine have been attributed to conversion to 5-fluorouracil in the body. Nausea, vomiting, and skin rashes occur occasionally. With daily amounts of 6–12 g administered in divided doses, there have been prolonged remissions of fungemia, sepsis, and meningitis caused by susceptible organisms. The combined use of flucytosine with amphotericin B has been beneficial, particularly in cryptococcal meningitis and in systemic candidiasis, and has permitted a reduction in the amphotericin dose.

ANTIFUNGAL AZOLES: CLOTRIMAZOLE, MICONAZOLE, KETOCONAZOLE, FLUCONAZOLE, & OTHERS

The synthetic antifungal azoles (Figure 48–1) inhibit fungi by blocking the biosynthesis of fungal lipids, especially the ergosterol in cell membranes. This effect has been shown to result from inhibition of P450-dependent 14α-demethylation of lanosterol in fungi. Fortunately, the affinity for mammalian P450 isozymes is less than that for the fungal isozyme; nevertheless, significant depression of several mammalian isozymes has been found.

Clotrimazole as 10 mg troches 5 times daily can suppress oral candidiasis; as 1% cream it is effective topically in dermatophytosis. It is also available as vaginal tablets for candidiasis. It is too toxic for systemic use.

Miconazole has long been used as 2% cream in dermatophytosis and in vaginal candidiasis not responding to topical nystatin. Miconazole has also been given intravenously (30 mg/kg/d) in various disseminated mycoses and has induced some prolonged remissions. However, major adverse effects, including vomiting, hyperlipidemia, hyponatremia, thrombophlebitis, hematologic disturbances, and others, have greatly limited its use.

Ketoconazole, an imidazole, was the first of these drugs that could be given orally and was effective in some systemic mycoses. A single daily dose of 200–400 mg is taken with food. The drug is well absorbed and widely distributed, but concentrations in the cen-

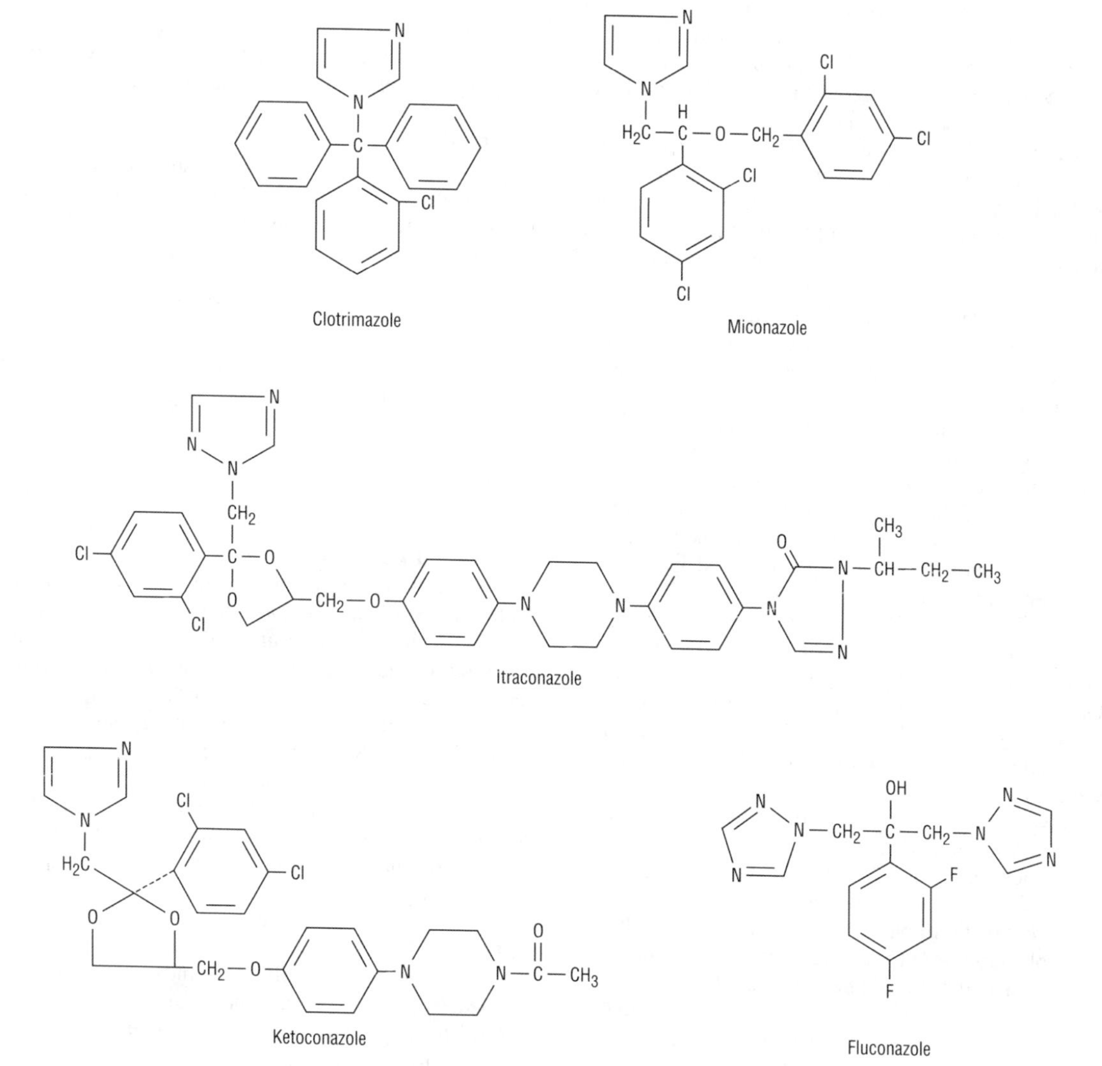

Figure 48–1. Structural formulas of some antifungal azoles.

tral nervous system are low. Daily dosage suppresses *Candida* infections of the mouth or vagina in 1–2 weeks and dermatophytosis in 3–8 weeks. Mucocutaneous candidiasis in immunodeficient children responds in 4–10 months.

Ketoconazole, 200–600 mg/d, effectively suppresses the clinical manifestations of systemic paracoccidioidomycosis and blastomycosis, and sometimes lung, bone, or skin lesions of histoplasmosis and coccidioidomycosis, but not meningitis due to these fungi. In disseminated blastomycosis, ketoconazole appears to be the drug of choice.

With oral doses of 200 mg, peak levels of ketoconazole may be 2–3 μg/mL, persisting for 6 hours or more. The major toxic effects include nausea, vomiting, skin rashes, and elevation of serum transaminase levels. Very rarely, progressive hepatotoxicity has developed with high doses. Ketoconazole inhibits certain mammalian cytochrome P450 isozymes. As a result, it inhibits the synthesis of adrenal steroids and androgens (which requires the action of P450 isozymes; see Chapters 38 and 39) and can cause gynecomastia. Ketoconazole increases levels of cyclosporine, terfenadine, and astemizole (and probably other drugs) by inhibiting P450 (CYP 3A4) in the liver. The effect on antihistamine metabolism has resulted in serious arrhythmias. The emergence of drug resistance is rare. Oral absorption of ketoconazole is impaired by the concomitant administration of antacids, cimetidine, or rifampin.

Fluconazole, a bistriazole (Figure 48–1), is more water-soluble and more readily absorbed from the gastrointestinal tract than ketoconazole. After oral administration of fluconazole, plasma levels are nearly as high as after intravenous administration. Fluconazole is widely distributed in tissues and body fluids, including the cerebrospinal fluid, where levels may be 50–80% of those in serum. The drug is excreted mainly in the urine. The half-life of fluconazole is about 30 hours and is greatly prolonged in patients with renal insufficiency.

Oral fluconazole, 100–200 mg/d, can suppress oral and esophageal candidiasis in immunodeficient patients and may be effective in systemic candidiasis. Oral fluconazole, 400 mg/d, can suppress cryptococcal meningitis in AIDS patients, but relapses are common unless maintenance doses of 200 mg/d are continued for months.

Adverse effects of fluconazole, as of other azoles, include vomiting, diarrhea, rashes, and sometimes impairment of hepatic function. It is probable that all azoles should be discontinued in patients with progressive hepatic impairment. Fluconazole, like ketoconazole, inhibits cytochrome P450 and may increase serum concentrations of phenytoin, cyclosporine, oral hypoglycemic drugs, and anticoagulants. Fluconazole serum levels may be lowered by rifampin and raised by thiazide diuretics.

Itraconazole, another oral azole, has given some promising results in the treatment of invasive aspergillosis, histoplasmosis, coccidioidal and cryptococcal meningitis, and other serious fungal infections. Like the other azoles, it inhibits P450 isozymes and may cause significant elevations of plasma concentrations of drugs such as cyclosporine and terfenadine.

HYDROXYSTILBAMIDINE

Hydroxystilbamidine isethionate is an aromatic diamidine active against *Blastomyces dermatitidis* in vitro and in vivo. It may be severely toxic for liver and kidneys and has been largely replaced by amphotericin B.

GRISEOFULVIN

Griseofulvin is a substance isolated from *Penicillium griseofulvum* in 1939. It was introduced clinically for the treatment of dermatophytoses in 1957.

Chemistry

The structure of griseofulvin is shown below. It is very insoluble in water but quite stable at high temperature, including autoclaving.

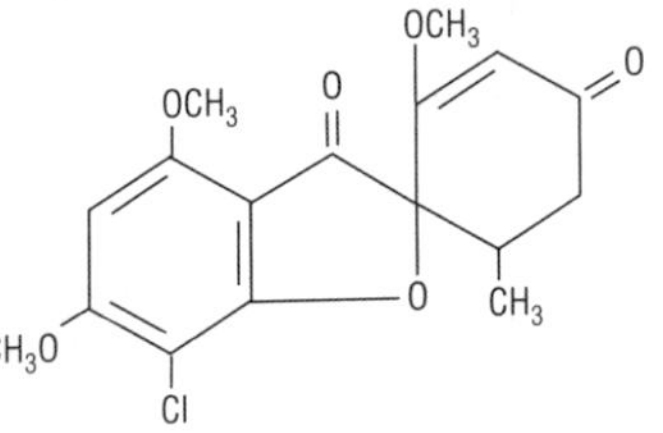

Griseofulvin

Antifungal Activity

Griseofulvin inhibits the growth of dermatophytes, including *Epidermophyton, Microsporum,* and *Trichophyton,* in concentrations of 0.5–3 μg/mL. It has no effect on bacteria, the fungi producing deep mycoses of humans, or certain fungi producing superficial lesions. Resistance can emerge among susceptible dermatophytes. (See Chapter 63.)

The mechanism of action has not been established, but it is probable that griseofulvin interferes with microtubule function or with nucleic acid synthesis and polymerization. The inhibitory effect may be partially reversed by purines.

Pharmacokinetics

Absorption of griseofulvin depends greatly on the physical state of the drug and is aided by high-fat foods. Preparations containing microsize particles of the drug are absorbed twice as well as those with larger particles. Microsize griseofulvin, 1 g daily, gives, in adults, blood levels of 0.5–1.5 μg/mL. Ultramicrosize griseofulvin is absorbed twice as well as the microsize preparation. The absorbed drug has an affinity for diseased skin and is deposited there, bound to keratin. Thus, it makes keratin resistant to fungal growth, and the new growth of hair or nails is freed of infection first. As the keratinized structures are shed, they tend to be replaced by uninfected ones. Little griseofulvin is present in body fluids or tissues. The bulk of ingested griseofulvin is excreted in feces and only a small part in urine.

Clinical Uses

Topical use of griseofulvin has little effect.

An ultramicrosize preparation of griseofulvin is given in an adult dose of 0.3–0.6 g/d orally (7.25 mg/kg/d for children). Treatment must be continued for 3–6 weeks if only hair or skin is involved but for 3–6 months if nails are affected. Griseofulvin is indicated for severe dermatophytosis involving skin, hair, or nails, particularly if caused by *Trichophyton rubrum,* which responds poorly to other measures. Other topical antifungal drugs may have to be used concomitantly.

Griseofulvin may increase the metabolism of warfarin, so that higher doses of the anticoagulant are required. Phenobarbital reduces the bioavailability of griseofulvin.

Adverse Reactions

The overall frequency of side effects is low. However, allergic reactions consisting of fever, skin rashes, leukopenia, and serum sickness-type reactions occur. In addition, direct toxicity consisting of headache, nausea, vomiting, diarrhea, hepatotoxicity, photosensitivity, and mental confusion are reported. Griseofulvin is teratogenic and carcinogenic in laboratory animals.

TOPICAL ANTIFUNGAL DRUGS

NYSTATIN

Chemistry & Mode of Action

This polyene macrolide is stable in dry form but decomposes quickly in the presence of water or plasma. Nystatin has no effect on bacteria or protozoa, but in vitro it inhibits many fungi. In vivo, its action is limited to surfaces where the drug can be in direct contact with the yeast or mold. Resistance to nystatin does not develop in vivo, but drug-resistant strains of *Candida* occur.

The mode of action involves binding of nystatin to fungal membrane sterols, principally ergosterol. There it disturbs membrane permeability and transport, probably by pore formation. This results in loss of cations and macromolecules from the cell. Resistance is due to a decrease in membrane sterols or a change in their structure and binding properties.

Pharmacokinetics

Nystatin is not significantly absorbed from skin, mucous membranes, or the gastrointestinal tract. Virtually all nystatin taken orally is excreted in the feces. There are no significant blood or tissue levels after oral intake, and it is too toxic to administer parenterally.

Clinical Uses

Nystatin can be applied topically to the skin or mucous membranes (buccal, vaginal) in the form of creams, ointments, suppositories, suspensions, or powders for the suppression of local *Candida* infections. Nystatin has been given orally for the partial suppression of *Candida* in the lumen of the bowel. This may be warranted in very small infants or persons with impaired host defenses (diabetes mellitus, leukemia, high doses of steroids), in whom the possibility of disseminated candidiasis exists. However, the addition of nystatin to oral tetracyclines is of dubious merit.

Commercial nystatin preparations often contain antibacterial drugs.

TOLNAFTATE & NAFTIFINE

Tolnaftate is a topical antifungal drug for use in cream, powder, or solution form in the treatment of dermatophytosis. While *Candida* is resistant, many dermatophytes are suppressed, and clinical efficacy is claimed for treatment courses of 1–10 weeks. With topical application, there appears to be no significant systemic absorption. Toxic and allergic reactions appear to be minimal.

Naftifine is an allylamine naphthalene derivative that inhibits the enzyme squalene epoxidase and decreases synthesis of ergosterol. A 1% cream is effective for treatment of tinea cruris and tinea corporis.

CLOTRIMAZOLE & RELATED AZOLES

Clotrimazole and miconazole are effective topical antifungals but are toxic in systemic use. They have been described above. Similar topical azoles include econazole, oxiconazole, and sulconazole. They are used mainly in oral, vaginal, or cutaneous candidiasis in the form of creams or troches. Butoconazole, terconazole, and tioconazole are similar azoles used only in vulvovaginal candidiasis.

NATAMYCIN

This is a polyene antifungal drug active against many different fungi in vitro. Topical application of 5% ophthalmic suspension can be beneficial in the treatment of keratitis caused by *Fusarium, Cephalosporium,* or other fungi. It is approved for such use but must be combined with appropriate ophthalmic surgical measures.

Natamycin may be effective for oral or vaginal candidiasis. Its toxicity via these topical routes appears to be low.

OTHER TOPICAL ANTIFUNGAL DRUGS

Fatty Acids

Fatty acids, particularly undecylenic acid and its salts, are effective topical antifungal drugs (see Chapter 63). They are widely used in tinea pedis and corporis as powders or creams.

Haloprogin

Haloprogin is a topical drug active in vitro against many dermatophytes and in vivo against tinea corporis. It is available as a 1% cream or solution, and 10–20% of the topically applied drug may be absorbed. It occasionally causes local irritation.

PREPARATIONS AVAILABLE

Drugs Used for Systemic or Gastrointestinal Fungal Infections
  Amphotericin B (Fungizone Intravenous)
    Parenteral: 50 mg per vial solution from lyophilized cake
  Fluconazole (Diflucan)
    Oral: 50, 100, 200 mg tablets
    Parenteral: 2 mg/mL in 200 and 400 mL vials
  Flucytosine (Ancobon)
    Oral: 250, 500 mg capsules

  Itraconazole (Sporanox)
    Oral: 100 mg capsules
  Ketoconazole (Nizoral)
    Oral: 200 mg tablets
  Miconazole (Monistat)
    Parenteral: 10 mg/mL for injection

Topical Antifungal Agents & Griseofulvin
See Chapter 63.

REFERENCES

Bennett JE et al: A comparison of amphotericin B alone and combined with flucytosine in the treatment of cryptococcal meningitis. N Engl J Med 1979;301:126.

Bozzette SA et al: A placebo-controlled trial of maintenance therapy with fluconazole after treatment of cryptococcal meningitis in AIDS. N Engl J Med 1991;324:580.

Denning DW et al: Treatment of invasive aspergillosis with itraconazole. Am J Med 1989;86:791.

DeWit S et al: Comparison of fluconazole and ketoconazole for oropharyngeal candidiasis in AIDS. Lancet 1989;1: 746.

Dismukes WE et al: Treatment of cryptococcal meningitis with combination amphotericin B and flucytosine for four as compared with six weeks. N Engl J Med 1987;317: 334.

Drutz DJ, Catanzaro A: Coccidioidomycosis. Am Rev Respir Dis 1978;117:727.

Galgiani JN et al: Fluconazole therapy for coccidioidal meningitis. Ann Intern Med 1993;119:28.

Gallis HA, Drew RH, Pickard WW: Amphotericin B: Thirty years of clinical experience. Rev Infect Dis 1990;12:308.

Goldman L: Griseofulvin. Med Clin North Am 1970;54: 1339.

Hamilton-Miller JMT: Chemistry and biology of polyene antibiotics. Bacteriol Rev 1973;37:166.

Heiberg JK, Svejgaard E: Toxic hepatitis during ketoconazole treatment. Br Med J 1981;283:825.

Hoeprich PD et al: Development of resistance to 5-fluorocytosine in *Candida parapsilosis* during therapy. J Infect Dis 1974;130:112.

Kirkpatrick CH, Alling DW: Treatment of oral candidiasis with clotrimazole troches. N Engl J Med 1978:299:1201.

Koeffler HP, Golde DW: 5-Fluorocytosine: Inhibition of hematopoiesis in vitro and reversal of inhibition by uracil. J Infect Dis 1979;139:438.

Larsen RA et al: Fluconazole compared with amphotericin B plus flucytosine for cryptococcal meningitis in AIDS. Ann Intern Med 1990;113:183.

Lopez-Berestain G et al: Treatment of systemic fungal infections with liposomal amphotericin B. Arch Intern Med 1989;149:2533.

Pont A et al: Ketoconazole blocks adrenal steroid synthesis. Ann Intern Med 1982;97:370.

Restrepo A, Stevens DA, Utz JP (editors): Symposium on ketoconazole. Rev Infect Dis 1980;2:519.

Ross JB et al: Ketoconazole for treatment of chronic pulmonary coccidioidomycosis. Ann Intern Med 1982;96:440.

Smego RA Jr: Combined therapy with amphotericin B and flucytosine for *Candida* meningitis. Rev Infect Dis 1984; 6:791.

Sobel JD: Recurrent vulvovaginal candidiasis: A prospective study of the efficacy of maintenance ketoconazole therapy. N Engl J Med 1986;315:1455.

Sugar AM, Saunders C: Oral fluconazole. Am J Med 1988; 85:481.

Tucker RM et al: Itraconazole therapy for chronic coccidioidal meningitis. Ann Intern Med 1990;112:108.

Woods RA et al: Resistance of polyene antibiotics and correlated sterol changes in isolates of *Candida tropicalis* from a patient with an amphotericin B-resistant funguria. J Infect Dis 1974;129:53.

49

Antiviral Chemotherapy & Prophylaxis

Ernest Jawetz, MD, PhD

Viruses are obligate intracellular parasites whose replication depends primarily on DNA, RNA, and protein synthetic processes of the host cell. Consequently, many chemicals that inhibit virus replication also inhibit some host cell function and cause major toxicity. The search for chemicals that inhibit virus-specific functions is one of the most active areas of pharmacologic investigation.

In many viral infections, replication of the virus reaches a maximum near the time when clinical symptoms first appear or even earlier. Therefore, in order to be clinically effective, chemicals that block virus replication must often be administered before the onset of disease, ie, as chemoprophylaxis. This is the case with amantadine against influenza A and methisazone against poxviruses. In some other infections—particularly those due to herpesviruses—virus replication continues for a time after symptoms and signs have first appeared. In those infections, inhibition of further virus replication may promote healing. This is the case with inhibitors of DNA replication in various herpetic infections.

Virus replication consists of the following steps: (1) adsorption to and penetration of susceptible cells; (2) synthesis of early, nonstructural proteins, eg, nucleic acid polymerases; (3) synthesis of RNA or DNA; (4) synthesis of late, structural proteins; and (5) assembly (maturation) of viral particles and their release from the cell. Antiviral drug action can be considered under these headings (Table 49–1).

INHIBITION OF ADSORPTION & PENETRATION OF SUSCEPTIBLE CELLS

Gamma Globulin

If gamma globulin contains specific antibodies directed against superficial antigens of a given virus, it can interfere with entry of that virus particle into a cell, probably by blocking penetration rather than adsorption. The intramuscular injection of pooled gamma globulin (immune globulin USP), 0.025–0.25

mL/kg of body weight, during the early incubation period can modify infection with the viruses of measles, hepatitis, rabies, poliomyelitis, and perhaps other diseases. The protective effect of a gamma globulin injection lasts 2–3 weeks. For infections that have prolonged incubation periods, injections may have to be given every 3 weeks.

Virus replication is often only partially inhibited, so the development of active immunity may accompany the temporary passive protection conferred by gamma globulin (active-passive immunization).

Specially prepared intravenous immune globulin can be given if intramuscular injection is inadvisable. Special hyperimmune globulins (concentrated from plasma of persons with high antibody levels) are available for rabies, vaccinia, varicella-zoster, hepatitis B, and Rh disease to be administered on specific indications.

Adamantanamines (Amantadine & Rimantadine)

Amantadine and rimantadine are tricyclic symmetric adamantanamines that inhibit the uncoating of certain myxoviruses, eg, influenza A (but not influenza B), rubella, and some tumor viruses after they have entered susceptible cells. They therefore inhibit the replication of these viruses in vitro and in experimental animals. Weak bases such as these amines probably act in part by buffering the pH of endosomes, membrane-bound vacuoles that surround virus particles as they are taken into the cell. Prevention of acidification in these vacuoles blocks the fusion of the virus envelope with the endosome membrane, thereby preventing transfer of the viral genetic material into the cytoplasm of the cell. These drugs may also inhibit virus particle release. In humans, a daily dose of 200 mg of either drug for 2–3 days before and 6–7 days after influenza A infection reduces the incidence and severity of symptoms and the magnitude of the serologic response. There may also be a slight therapeutic effect if the drug is started within 18 hours after the onset of symptoms of influenza.

When given orally, amantadine is almost com-

Table 49–1. Antiviral substances and some of their properties.

Drug	Viral Target	Active Against
Purine and pyrimidine analogues		
Acyclovir	DNA polymerase	Herpes simplex, varicella-zoster
Ganciclovir	DNA polymerase	Cytomegalovirus
Ribavirin[1]	DNA synthesis	Respiratory syncytial virus, influenza A, Lassa fever
Vidarabine	DNA polymerase	Herpes simplex, zoster
Idoxuridine	DNA synthesis	Herpes (corneal)
Trifluridine	DNA synthesis	Herpes (corneal)
Dideoxynucleosides (AZT, ddC, ddI)[2]	Reverse transcriptase, DNA synthesis	HIV
Other drugs		
Amantadine, rimantadine	Adsorption, penetration	Influenza A, rubella
Foscarnet	DNA polymerase, reverse transcriptase	Cytomegalovirus, herpes simplex
Gamma globulin	Adsorption, penetration	Hepatitis B, rabies, polio, others
Interferons	Protein synthesis	Herpes simplex and zoster, hepatitis B, papillomavirus, others
Methisazone	Protein synthesis	Smallpox, other poxviruses
Rifampin	Assembly of mature virus particle	Poxviruses

[1]Ribavirin is not a purine but interferes with guanosine monophosphate.
[2]AZT, zidovudine; ddC, dideoxycytidine; ddI, dideoxyinosine.

pletely absorbed from the gut. The drug is excreted unchanged, mainly by the kidneys. In persons with renal failure, amantadine may accumulate to toxic levels unless dosage is greatly reduced in proportion to the decrease in creatinine clearance. The dose should be reduced in elderly patients. With normal renal function, the half-life is about 12 hours. The pharmacokinetics of rimantadine are similar, but its half-life is longer (about 30 hours) and elimination is dependent on liver function.

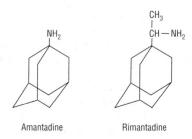

Amantadine   Rimantadine

Chemoprophylaxis with amantadine can be effective in household contacts, in limiting institutional spread of infection, and in protecting adults at high risk during influenza outbreaks. However, drug-resistant influenza A virus mutants can emerge and infect contacts. Rimantadine appears to be equally effective and may require no dosage adjustment in renal insufficiency.

Amantadine has beneficial effects in some cases of Parkinson's disease (see Chapter 27).

The most marked untoward effects of amantadine are insomnia, slurred speech, dizziness, ataxia, and other central nervous system signs. The drug can cause release of stored catecholamines. Experience

with rimantadine in the USA is limited; the frequency of central nervous system adverse effects may be lower than for amantadine.

INHIBITION OF INTRACELLULAR SYNTHESIS

Inhibition of Early Protein Synthesis

Guanidine and hydroxybenzylbenzimidazole are both capable of inhibiting the replication of certain RNA enteroviruses but not of others. Both substances inhibit the formation of RNA polymerases at concentrations that appear to be harmless to host cells in vitro. Mutants resistant to the action of these compounds are common and are rapidly selected out in the presence of the drugs. Therefore, as expected, these compounds do not have significant therapeutic activity in vivo. Trials of biguanidines in RNA virus infections in humans were not encouraging.

Inhibition of Nucleic Acid Synthesis

A. Ribavirin: Ribavirin (ribofuranosyl-triazole-carboxamide; for structure, see below) can inhibit the replication of both RNA and DNA viruses in experimental models. The compound acts by interfering with guanosine monophosphate formation and subsequent nucleic acid synthesis. In experimental animal and human infections with influenza A viruses, doses of 15 mg/kg gave some benefit. When administered as an aerosol, it limits replication of respiratory syncytial virus in infants and reduces the severity and duration of illness. It has also been effective as treatment for influenza A and B infections by accelerating defervescence and shortening symptoms. Ribavirin has been used for respiratory infections and hepatitis in other countries and is approved for respiratory syncytial virus infections in the USA. Health care workers should be protected against extended inhalation exposure.

Ribavirin appears to be the treatment of choice for Lassa fever, provided treatment can be started early in the disease. The drug is not effective in rabies.

B. Pyrimidine and Purine Analogues:

1. Fluorouracil (5-fluorouracil) and **5-bromouracil**—These drugs effectively block the replication of DNA viruses in cell culture systems, but they are relatively ineffective in vivo.

2. Idoxuridine—Idoxuridine (5-iodo-2′-deoxyuridine, IDU, IUDR) inhibits the replication of herpes simplex virus in the cornea and thus aids in the healing of herpetic keratitis in humans. This is a special circumstance, since herpesvirus proliferates in the avascular corneal epithelium and the topically applied drug remains local and is not rapidly removed by the bloodstream. In the vascular conjunctiva, the drug has little therapeutic effect; thus, adenovirus conjunctivitis cannot be controlled by idoxuridine.

For treatment of herpetic keratitis, idoxuridine is applied to the cornea (0.1% solution or 0.5% ointment). This tends to accelerate spontaneous healing. However, DNA synthesis of host cells is also affected, and some toxic effects on corneal cells are occasionally observed if treatment is prolonged. Idoxuridine may induce allergic contact dermatitis. Idoxuridine is too toxic for systemic administration.

Prolonged exposure of herpes viruses to idoxuridine can select drug-resistant mutants.

In deep herpetic stromal keratitis, there is little virus replication in the stroma. Corticosteroids help to reduce the inflammatory response. Idoxuridine is given simultaneously to prevent herpesvirus proliferation in the superficial epithelium.

Topically applied idoxuridine has no effect on skin lesions of herpes simplex or zoster.

3. Cytarabine—Cytarabine (Arabinofuranosylcytosine hydrochloride, cytosine arabinoside, ara-C; see Chapter 56) also inhibits DNA synthesis and interferes with the replication of DNA viruses. By weight it is about ten times more effective than idoxuridine, but it is also ten times more toxic for host cells. Cytarabine, 0.3–2 mg/kg intravenously as a single daily dose for 5 days, was not beneficial in disseminated herpes or varicella.

4. Trifluridine—Trifluridine (5-trifluoromethyl-2-deoxyuridine) inhibits viral DNA synthesis—analogous to the action of idoxuridine. A 1% solution applied to corneas infected with herpes or vaccinia viruses can be curative even with viruses resistant to idoxuridine. It is not given systemically.

5. Vidarabine—Vidarabine (Arabinofuranosyl adenine, ara-A, adenine arabinoside) is the least toxic and most effective of the purine analogues. Its structure is shown below.

Ribavirin   Vidarabine

Vidarabine is phosphorylated in the cell to the triphosphate derivative, which inhibits viral DNA polymerase much more effectively than mammalian DNA polymerase. In vivo, vidarabine is rapidly metabolized to hypoxanthine arabinoside (which is only slightly antiviral) and excreted in urine. Vidarabine monophosphate (Ara-AMP; investigational) is much more water-soluble and readily administered intravenously.

Vidarabine as 3% ointment is effective treatment for herpetic and vaccinial keratitis. Topical vidarabine has no effect on skin or mucous membrane lesions of herpes simplex.

Vidarabine can also be used for systemic administration because of its relatively low toxicity. Toxicity is increased in renal failure. Doses of 10–15 mg/kg/d intravenously over a 12-hour period result in substantial suppression of clinical systemic herpesvirus activity. In herpetic encephalitis proved by biopsy, use of this systemic treatment for 10 days resulted in a significant reduction in the mortality rate. However, only 40% of the treated survivors were able to resume normal life; the rest suffered from severe neurologic sequelae. The most encouraging results were observed in patients with herpetic encephalitis whose treatment was begun before onset of coma.

Systemic vidarabine (15 mg/kg/d) can limit neonatal disseminated herpes simplex, herpes encephalitis, and the dissemination of herpes zoster in immunocompromised patients. However, vidarabine is less effective than acyclovir.

6. Acyclovir—Acyclovir (acycloguanosine) is a guanosine derivative. Its structure is shown below. Herpesvirus contains a thymidine kinase capable of adding a single phosphate to guanosine and deoxyguanosine. It phosphorylates acyclovir 30–100 times faster than does the host cell kinase, in the manner shown in Figure 49–1. The product is then phosphorylated to acycloguanosine triphosphate, which inhibits the herpes DNA polymerase 10–30 times more than it does the host cell polymerase.

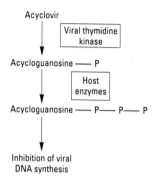

Figure 49–1. Sequence of steps that activate acyclovir in infected cells and result in inhibition of herpesvirus DNA synthesis. Uninfected host cells phosphorylate acyclovir much more slowly because viral thymidine kinase is absent. (P, phosphate groups; host enzymes, cellular GMP kinase and phosphotransferases.)

Given prophylactically before bone marrow transplants to seropositive individuals, acyclovir, 250 mg/m^2 every 8 hours intravenously for 18 days, significantly protected such individuals against severe herpes lesions during posttransplant immunosuppression. Given after heart transplants to prevent dissemination of herpes from existing lesions, it was effective in promoting healing of herpetic lesions but did not prevent subsequent shedding of herpesvirus. In immunocompromised patients with mucocutaneous herpetic lesions, acyclovir promoted healing of lesions and shortened virus shedding. In these trials, acyclovir, 15 mg/kg/d intravenously, produced no noticeable adverse effects in 5–18 days of administration. The same dose of acyclovir also accelerated healing of herpes zoster lesions in immunocompromised patients but had little effect on postherpetic pain. Intravenous acyclovir given early in the course of primary herpes simplex infections—especially of the female genital tract—reduced pain, promoted healing of lesions, and shortened virus shedding. However, such treatment did not prevent the establishment of viral latency in sensory ganglia or the frequency or intensity of recurrences. In herpetic encephalitis and in neonatal herpetic dissemination, acyclovir is more effective than vidarabine.

Oral acyclovir, 200 mg 5 times daily, has the same therapeutic effects as the intravenously administered drug, including benefit in primary genital herpes. However, there is little effect on the lesions of oral or genital recurrences. When taken prophylactically for 4–6 months, it can reduce the frequency and severity of recurrent lesions during this period. Acyclovir can also be effective against varicella.

Topical application of 5% acyclovir ointment can limit mucocutaneous lesions of herpes simplex in immunosuppressed patients but has no effect in patients with normal immunity. Topical acyclovir can also shorten healing time and reduce pain when applied early to lesions in primary genital herpes, but it has no significant effect on recurrent genital lesions. Likewise, the frequency of recurrence is not altered.

Acyclovir-resistant herpesviruses that are thymidine kinase-deficient can emerge during treatment. Such strains are usually not suppressed by acyclovir but may respond clinically to foscarnet (see below).

While latent or subclinical cytomegalovirus infection is very common, reactivation and dissemination of cytomegalovirus occurs in immunocompromised patients, especially in those who receive antineoplastic drugs or organ transplants or who suffer from AIDS. While acyclovir has no beneficial effects—cytomegalovirus does not code for viral thymidine kinase—other guanine derivatives are useful.

7. Ganciclovir–Ganciclovir—9-[(1,3-dihydroxy-2-propoxy)methyl]guanine (DHPG)—enters cells infected with cytomegalovirus and is phosphorylated into a triphosphate that preferentially inhibits cytomegalovirus DNA polymerase. When ganciclovir triphosphate is incorporated into cytomegalovirus DNA, it suppresses chain elongation and inhibits cytomegalovirus replication. When it is given intravenously (5–10 mg/kg/d) for 14 days, virus production is inhibited, and some patients with cytomegalovirus retinitis, pneumonia, or gastrointestinal lesions improve markedly. However, after the drug is stopped, cytomegalovirus replication resumes and clinical relapses follow. With a maintenance dose of 5 mg/kg/d 3–5 times per week, clinical improvement can be maintained longer, and some patients recover entirely. Ganciclovir-resistant strains of cytomegalovirus can emerge during such treatment.

The most important adverse effects of ganciclovir are leukopenia, neutropenia, thrombocytopenia, renal impairment, and seizures. This toxicity has severely limited the dosage and duration of treatment that can be tolerated by many patients. Ganciclovir excretion is reduced—and its toxicity is increased—in renal insufficiency.

8. Zidovudine (AZT) and other dideoxynucleosides–The most dramatic and lethal disease to appear in the last 2 decades is AIDS, caused by human immunodeficiency virus (HIV). This retrovirus can be inhibited by synthetic dideoxynucleosides. These analogues act on the viral DNA polymerase (reverse transcriptase), so that synthesis of viral DNA is inhibited and virus replication markedly decreased. The HIV reverse transcriptase is 20–30 times more susceptible to inhibition by these drugs than the polymerase of mammalian cells. Zidovudine (azidothymidine, AZT) is the most extensively studied and most widely used of these drugs.

AZT is well absorbed from the gut and distributed to most body tissues and fluids, including the cerebrospinal fluid, where drug levels are about 60% of those in serum, The serum half-life is only 1.1 hours, but the intracellular half-life of the active moiety is 3 hours. Fifteen to 20 percent of a dose of AZT is excreted unchanged in the urine, and 75% is metabolized by hepatic glucuronidation before being excreted by the kidneys.

Acyclovir

Zidovudine
(Azidothymidine)

Many controlled clinical trials have documented that treatment of patients with HIV infection—AIDS or ARC (AIDS-related complex)—with AZT can suppress HIV production, prolong life and temporarily reduce morbidity, and reduce the number and severity of opportunistic infections (Table 49–2). CD4+ lymphocyte numbers increase during AZT therapy in both AIDS and ARC, and in ARC this may persist for some time. Neurologic and mental symptoms and signs may be greatly improved. For such therapy, AZT (zidovudine) is administered by mouth in a dosage of 100–200 mg 3–5 times daily. Longer intervals between doses may be possible without reducing efficacy greatly.

AZT has also been given prophylactically to HIV-seropositive but asymptomatic persons with lowered CD4+ cell counts. With oral AZT doses of 500 mg/d, the rate of progression to AIDS and ARC was significantly less than in controls, and the CD4+ counts were better maintained. However, such prophylaxis did not reliably prevent HIV replication even if begun soon after a known infective inoculum. Zidovudine-resistant strains of HIV can be recovered from many AIDS patients who have ingested the drug for 6 months or more.

Less severe adverse effects of AZT include headache, agitation, insomnia, diarrhea, rashes, and fevers. The more severe effects consist of bone marrow suppression with severe anemia (often requiring transfusion), granulocytopenia, and sometimes thrombocytopenia. These tend to limit the dose and duration of drug administration. AZT toxicity may be increased by the concomitant use of drugs that also undergo degradation in the liver, eg, acetaminophen, nonsteroidal anti-inflammatory drugs, and sulfonamides.

Didanosine (dideoxyinosine, ddI) has been studied on a limited scale. Zidovudine-resistant strains of HIV are susceptible to this drug in vitro, and patients infected with such strains appear to benefit from ddI. While the toxicity of ddI may be less than that of AZT, peripheral neuropathy and fatal pancreatitis have been observed with oral doses of 125–300 mg twice daily. It may be that smaller doses would still be effective and better tolerated. The place of ddI in therapy is unknown. The dosage currently recommended is 200 mg twice daily, or 125 mg twice daily for patients weighing less than 60 kg.

Zalcitabine (dideoxycytidine, ddC) has exhibited in vitro and clinical activity, but doses of 0.06 mg/kg/d often result in painful sensory and motor peripheral neuropathy. The recommended dosage is 0.75 mg taken concurrently with 200 mg zidovudine every 8 hours.

Stavudine (3-deoxythymidin-2-ene) appears experimentally to suppress HIV virus and disease.

C. Other Inhibitors of Nucleic Acid Synthesis: Foscarnet is a phosphonoformate drug that does not require phosphorylation for antiviral activity. It inhibits herpesvirus DNA polymerase even in acyclovir-resistant, thymidine kinase-deficient strains. Foscarnet, 50 mg/kg given intravenously 3 times daily, has suppressed such acyclovir-resistant herpetic infections in immunodeficient patients with AIDS and may have some effect on HIV itself.

Table 49–2. Results of azidothymidine (AZT) therapy in AIDS patients during 8–24 weeks of treatment.[1]

	Placebo	AZT
Patients in group	75	85
Patient deaths during study	19	1
Kaposi's sarcoma occurring during study	10	3
Opportunistic infections occuring during study	45	24
Percent requiring transfusions[2]	11	31

[1]Data from Fischl, 1987.
[2]Includes patients with AIDS-related complex (ARC) as well as those with AIDS.

Foscarnet

Phosphonoacetic acid also inhibits herpesvirus DNA polymerase. It is effective as an inhibitor of herpesvirus proliferation in vitro and in some experimental systems. Its clinical potential is unknown.

Interferons

Interferons are a group of endogenous glycoproteins that exert virus-nonspecific antiviral activities, at least in homologous cells, through cellular metabolic processes involving synthesis of both RNA and protein. Interferons were initially found to be produced by cells infected by viruses (type I). It was later discovered that lymphocytes also produced interferons (type II) during the immune response. Interferons express some of their activity as lymphokines and immunomodulators (Chapter 57). Type I interferons, which act mainly as inhibitors of virus replication in cells, do so by inducing host cell ribosomes to produce cellular enzymes that subsequently block viral reproduction by inhibiting the translation of viral messenger RNA into viral proteins.

Interferons are produced in most animal species, but they tend to be active mainly in the species in which they are produced. Among human interferons (IFN), three main substances are described: IFN-α represents human leukocyte interferon (type I); IFN-β represents human fibroblast interferon (type I); and IFN-γ represents human immune interferon (type II). These groupings are tentative at present. Interferons produced by any type of cell may have more than one kind of chemical makeup and more than one type of activity.

Three known enzymes are induced by interferons: (1) a protein kinase that ultimately leads to phosphorylation of elongation factor 2, resulting in inhibition of peptide chain initiation; (2) oligoisoadenylate synthase, which ultimately leads to activation of an RNase and degradation of viral mRNA; and (3) a phosphodiesterase that can degrade the terminal nucleotides of tRNA, inhibiting peptide elongation.

In view of the broad range of viruses that are susceptible to inhibition by interferon, this agent can be considered a potentially valuable antiviral drug. While harmless and potent inducers of endogenous interferon are still being sought, the research emphasis has been to increase production of exogenous human interferon on a large scale. Human interferon was produced from blood leukocytes, fibroblasts, or lymphoblastoid cells in culture. It is now produced by recombinant DNA technology.

Clinical studies with human interferons have shown activity in several viral infections and in neoplasms. If given early, interferon can prevent the dissemination of herpes zoster in cancer patients, reduce cytomegalovirus shedding after renal transplantation, and prevent reactivation of herpes simplex after trigeminal root section. In chronic hepatitis B and C, interferons can suppress clinical and laboratory evidence of disease, at least temporarily. Intralesional injections of interferon into genital warts can speed their regression. If added to pentavalent arsenicals, IFN-γ improves treatment results in severe visceral leishmaniasis.

In several types of cancer, interferon can be used as adjunctive treatment. It is approved in the USA for treatment of hairy cell leukemia, AIDS-related Kaposi's sarcoma, and condyloma acuminatum; its possible role in other tumors is under study.

Dosages of interferon have ranged from 10^6 to 10^9 units daily, given intravenously. Adverse effects include fever, fatigue, headaches, weakness, myalgias, anemia, and gastrointestinal or cardiovascular disturbances. The ultimate potential of interferon treatment in human disease remains to be determined.

Inhibition of Late Protein Synthesis

A number of different amino acid analogues (eg, **fluorophenylalanine**) inhibit the synthesis of structural proteins for the coats of virus particles. The antibiotic **puromycin** has the same effect. However, these inhibitors of protein synthesis show no specificity for the synthesis of virus protein and impair protein synthesis of the host cell to such a degree that they are intensely toxic. Consequently, none of these substances are useful in chemotherapy at present.

In many poxviruses, various **thiosemicarbazones** inhibit virus replication by interfering with the synthesis of a "late" structural protein. As a result, the assembly of normal particles is blocked. **Methisazone** (N-methylisatin-β-thiosemicarbazone) can block replication of smallpox (variola) virus in humans if administered to contacts within 1–2 days after exposure. Methisazone, 2–4 g/d orally (100 mg/kg/d for children) for 3–4 days, provided striking protection against clinical smallpox. The availability of methisazone was an important consideration in abolishing smallpox vaccination. The replication of vaccinia virus can be inhibited by methisazone after symptoms have started, eg, in generalized vaccinia or in progressive vaccinia in immunologically deficient individuals. This is a valid form of antiviral chemotherapy restricted to poxviruses only.

Certain sugar analogues can inhibit the synthesis of virus-specific glycoproteins and glycolipids. Thus, 2-deoxy-D-glucose is incorporated into glycoproteins of herpes simplex virus and appears to block the cellular synthesis of major glycosylated polypeptides of herpesvirus. Clinical benefit has been claimed but has not been confirmed by controlled trials.

INHIBITION OF ASSEMBLY OR RELEASE OF VIRAL PARTICLES

The assembly of intact particles can be inhibited by many agents (eg, **floxuridine [5-fluoro-2'-deoxyuridine]** or **puromycin**) that induce the synthesis of defective viral constituents—whether nucleic acids or structural proteins.

Rifampin (see Chapter 46) inhibits DNA-dependent RNA polymerase in bacteria and mammalian cells. It also inhibits poxviruses but by a different mechanism. Rifampin prevents the assembly of enveloped mature particles. The block apparently occurs during the stage of envelope formation and is reversible upon removal of the drug.

Rifampin has not been used in treatment of human poxvirus infections, but topical application can inhibit human vaccinia lesions.

PREPARATIONS AVAILABLE

Acyclovir (Zovirax)
Oral: 200 mg capsules, 800 mg tablet, 200 mg/5 mL suspension
Parenteral: powder to reconstitute for injection (500, 1000 mg/vial)

Amantadine (generic, Symmetrel)
Oral: 100 mg capsules; 50 mg/5 mL syrup

Cytomegalovirus immune globulin intravenous (human)
Parenteral: Powder to reconstitute for injection, 2500 mg ± 250 mg.

Didanosine (dideoxyinosine, ddI) (Videx)
Oral: 25, 50, 100, 150 mg tablets; 100, 167, 250, 375 mg powder for oral solution; 2, 4 g powder for pediatric solution.

Foscarnet (Foscavir)
Parenteral: 24 mg/mL for IV injection

Ganciclovir (Cytovene)
Parenteral: 500 mg/vial for IV injection

Hepatitis B Immune Globulin (HBIG) (H-BIG, others)
Parenteral: 1, 4, 5 mL vials; 0.5 mL prefilled syringe

Immune globulin intravenous (IGIV) (Gamimune N, others)

Parenteral: 5% in 10, 50, 100 mL vials; 0.5, 1, 2.5, 3, 5, 6 g powder to reconstitute for IV injection

Interferon alfa-2a (Roferon-A)
Parenteral: 3, 6, 36 million IU vials

Interferon alfa-2b (Intron-A)
Parenteral: 3, 5, 10, 18, 25, and 50 million IU vials

Interferon alfa-n3 (Alferon N)
Parenteral: 5 million IU/vial

Ribavirin (Virazole)
Aerosol: powder to reconstitute for 6 g/dL aerosol

Rimantadine (Flumadine)
Oral: 100 mg tablets; 50 mg/5 mL syrup

Varicella-Zoster Immune Globulin (Human)
Parenteral: 125 units globulin in 2.5 mL vial

Vidarabine (Vira-A)
Parenteral: 200 mg/mL suspension for injection

Zalcitabine (dideoxycytidine, ddC) (Hivid)
Oral: 0.375, 0.75 mg tablets

Zidovudine (azidothymidine, AZT) (Retrovir)
Oral: 100 mg capsules, 50 mg/5 mL syrup
Parenteral: 10 mg/mL

REFERENCES

Alderson T: New directions for the anti-retroviral chemotherapy of AIDS—A basis for a pharmacological approach to treatment. Biol Rev 1993;68:265.

Balfour HH et al: A randomized, placebo controlled trial of oral acyclovir for prevention of cytomegalovirus disease in recipients of renal allografts. N Engl J Med 1989;320:1381.

Balfour HH et al: Acyclovir halts progression of herpes zoster in immunocompromised patients. N Engl J Med 1983;308:1448.

Bean B, Aeppli D: Adverse effects of high-dose intravenous acyclovir in ambulatory patients with acute herpes zoster. J Infect Dis 1985;151:362.

Bryson YJ et al: Treatment of first episodes of genital herpes simplex virus infection with oral acyclovir: A randomized double-blind controlled trial in normal subjects. N Engl J Med 1983;308:916.

Buhles WC Jr et al: Ganciclovir treatment of life- or sight-threatening cytomegalovirus infection: experience in 314

immunocompromised patients. Rev Infect Dis 1988;10:S495.

Cheeseman SH et al: Controlled clinical trial of prophylactic human-leukocyte interferon in renal transplantation: Effects on cytomegalovirus and herpes simplex virus infections. N Engl J Med 1979;300:1345.

Deyton LR et al: Reversible cardiac dysfunction associated with interferon alfa therapy in AIDS patients with Kaposi's sarcoma. N Engl J Med 1989;321:1246.

Douglas JM et al: A double-blind study of oral acyclovir for suppression of recurrences of genital herpes simplex virus infection. N Engl J Med 1984;310:1551.

Douglas RG: Prophylaxis and treatment of influenza. N Engl J Med 1990;322:443.

Elion GB: Mechanism of action and selectivity of acyclovir. Am J Med 1982;73:7.

Eron LJ et al: Interferon therapy for condylomata acuminata. N Engl J Med 1986;315:1059.

Fischl MA et al: The efficacy of azidothymidine (AZT) in

the treatment of patients with AIDS and AIDS-related complex: A double-blind, placebo-controlled trial. N Engl J Med 1987;317:185.

Goodrich JM et al: Early treatment with ganciclovir to prevent cytomegalovirus disease after allogenic bone marrow transplantation. N Engl J Med 1991;325:1601.

Hall CB et al: Aerosolized ribavirin treatment of infants with respiratory syncytial viral infection: A randomized double-blind study. N Engl J Med 1983;308:1443.

Hamilton JD et al: A controlled trial of early versus late treatment with zidovudine in symptomatic human immunodeficiency virus infection. N Engl J Med 1992;326:437.

Hay AJ et al: The molecular basis of the specific anti-influenza action of amantadine. EMBO J 1985;4:3021.

Hayden FG et al: Emergence and apparent transmission of rimantadine-resistant influenza A virus in families. N Engl J Med 1989;321:1696.

Hersh EM: Current status of chemotherapy of patients with HIV infection. Int J Immunopharmacol 1991;13:9.

Hirsch MS, Schooley RT: Resistance to antiviral drugs. N Engl J Med 1989;320:313.

Hirsch MS: Chemotherapy of human immunodeficiency virus infections. J Infect Dis 1990;161:845.

Homes GF et al: Lassa fever in the United States. N Engl J Med 1990;323:1120.

Huggins JW et al: Prospective, double blind concurrent placebo-controlled trial of intravenous ribavirin therapy of hemorrhagic fever with renal syndrome. J Infect Dis 1991;164:1119.

Jacobson MA et al: Acyclovir-resistant varicella-zoster virus infection after chronic oral acyclovir therapy in patients with AIDS. Ann Intern Med 1990;112:187.

Keay S, Bissett J, Merigan TC: Ganciclovir treatment of cytomegalovirus infections in iatrogenically immunocompromised patients. J Infect Dis 1987;156:1016.

Lange JMA et al: Failure of zidovudine prophylaxis after accidental exposure to HIV. N Engl J Med 1990;322:1375.

Laskin OL et al: Use of ganciclovir to treat serious cytomegalovirus infections in patients with AIDS. J Infect Dis 1987;155:323.

Leventhal BG et al: Long-term response of recurrent respiratory papillomatosis to treatment with lymphoblastoid interferon alfa-N1. N Engl J Med 1991;325:613.

Matthews T, Boehme R: Antiviral activity and mechanism of action of ganciclovir. Rev Infect Dis 1988;10:S490.

McClung HW et al: Ribavirin aerosol treatment of influenza B virus infection. JAMA 1983;249:2671.

Merigan TC: Interferon: The first quarter century. JAMA 1982;248:2513.

Mertz GJ et al: Double-blind placebo-controlled trial of oral acyclovir in first-episode genital herpes simplex virus infection. JAMA 1984;252:1147.

Mitsuya H et al: Targeted therapy of human immunodeficiency virus-related disease. FASEB J 1991;5:2369.

Nicholson KG: Antiviral agents in clinical practice. (Five parts.) Lancet 1984;2:503, 562, 617, 677, 736.

Reichard O et al: Ribavirin treatment for hepatitis C. Lancet 1991;337:1058.

Reichman RC et al: Treatment of recurrent genital herpes simplex infections with oral acyclovir: A controlled trial. JAMA 1984;251:2103.

Richman DD et al: The toxicity of azidothymidine (AZT) in the treatment of patients with AIDS and AIDS-related complex: A double-blind, placebo-controlled trial. N Engl J Med 1987;317:192.

Richman DD: Antiviral therapy of HIV infection. Annu Rev Med 1991;42:69.

Safrin S et al: Foscarnet therapy for acyclovir-resistant mucocutaneous herpes simplex virus infection in 26 AIDS patients. J Infect Dis 1990;161:1078.

Saral R et al: Acyclovir prophylaxis against herpes simplex infection in patients with leukemia: A randomized, double-blind, placebo-controlled study. Ann Intern Med 1983;99:773.

Seale L et al: Prevention of herpesvirus infections in renal allograft recipients by low-dose oral acyclovir. JAMA 1985;254:3435.

Shepp DH et al: Treatment of varicella-zoster virus infection in severely immunocompromised patients: A randomized comparison of acyclovir and vidarabine. N Engl J Med 1986;314:208.

Spruance SL, Crumpacker CS: Topical 5 percent acyclovir in polyethylene glycol for herpes simplex labialis: Antiviral effect without clinical benefit. Am J Med 1982;73:315.

Straus SE et al: Suppression of frequently recurring genital herpes: A placebo-controlled double-blind trial of oral acyclovir. N Engl J Med 1984;310:1545.

Volberding PA et al: Zidovudine in asymptomatic human immunodeficiency virus infection: A controlled trial in persons with fewer than 500 CD4-positive cells per cubic millimeter. N Engl J Med 1990;322:941.

White DA, Gold JW: Medical management of AIDS patients. Med Clin North Am 1992;76:1.

Whitley RJ et al: Vidarabine versus acyclovir therapy in herpes simplex encephalitis. N Engl J Med 1986;314:144.

Wilson SZ et al: Treatment of influenza A (H1N1) virus infection with ribavirin aerosol. Antimicrob Agents Chemother 1984;26:200.

Yarchoan R et al: Clinical pharmacology of 3'-azido-2',3'-dideoxythymidine (zidovudine) and related dideoxynucleosides. N Engl J Med 1989;321:726. [Erratum appears in N Engl J Med 1990;322:280.]

50 Drugs With Specialized Indications & Urinary Antiseptics

Ernest Jawetz, MD, PhD

CELL WALL INHIBITORS

VANCOMYCIN

Vancomycin is an antibiotic produced by *Streptomyces*. It is active against gram-positive bacteria, particularly staphylococci.

Chemistry

Vancomycin is a glycopeptide of molecular weight 1500. It is soluble in water and quite stable.

Antibacterial Activity

Vancomycin is bactericidal for gram-positive bacteria in concentrations of 0.5–3 μg/mL. Most pathogenic staphylococci, including those producing beta-lactamase and those resistant to nafcillin and methicillin, are killed by 10 μg/mL or less. Resistant mutants are very rare in susceptible populations, and clinical resistance emerges very slowly. There is no cross-resistance with other known antibiotics.

The mechanism of action involves inhibition of cell wall mucopeptide synthesis. Vancomycin inhibits the utilization of disaccharide(-pentapeptide)-P-phospholipid (see Figure 42–3). Apparently the drug binds firmly to the carboxyl terminal D-Ala-D-Ala chain of the growing peptidoglycan and prevents further elongation and cross-linking. The peptidoglycan is thus weakened and the cell becomes susceptible to lysis. Cell membrane function is also damaged.

Vancomycin can be synergistic with aminoglycosides against certain enterococci and other gram-positive bacteria.

Pharmacokinetics
(Table 50–1)

Vancomycin is not absorbed from the intestinal tract and can be given orally only for the treatment of antibiotic-associated enterocolitis. Systemic doses must be administered intravenously. After intravenous injection of 0.5 g, blood levels of 10–20 μg/mL

are maintained for 1–2 hours. The drug is widely distributed in the body. Excretion is mainly through the kidneys into the urine. In the presence of renal insufficiency, striking accumulation may occur. In functionally anephric patients, the half-life of vancomycin is between 6 and 10 days. Vancomycin may also accumulate in the presence of hepatic insufficiency. The drug is not removed by hemodialysis.

Clinical Uses

The main indication for parenteral vancomycin is sepsis or endocarditis caused by staphylococci resistant to other drugs. In such cases, 0.5 g is injected intravenously in 20 minutes every 6–8 hours (20–40 mg/kg/d for children). Rarely, vancomycin is given with an aminoglycoside in enterococcal endocarditis.

Vancomycin penetrates the central nervous system somewhat irregularly, but intravenously administered drug has been used to treat meningitis and shunt infections. Supplemental instillation into the central nervous system site is sometimes necessary.

Oral vancomycin, 0.125–0.5 g every 6 hours, is used to treat antibiotic-associated enterocolitis, especially if caused by *Clostridium difficile*.

Adverse Reactions

Adverse reactions are rare. Vancomycin is irritating to tissue; phlebitis at the site of injection and chills and fever may occur. Ototoxicity and nephrotoxicity are mild with current preparations. Rapid infusion of vancomycin may induce diffuse flushing ("red man syndrome"). It is probably caused by release of histamine and can be largely prevented by pretreatment with antihistamines and a slow infusion rate.

TEICOPLANIN

Teicoplanin is a cell wall inhibitor that is proposed as a "vancomycin substitute" for use in patients who cannot tolerate vancomycin. Like vancomycin, it is not absorbed from the gut; unlike the older drug, it can be given intramuscularly as well as intrave-

Table 50–1. Pharmacokinetic properties of some antimicrobial drugs with special indications.

Drug	Half-life (hours)	Oral Bioavailability	Percent Protein Bound in Plasma	Major Route of Elimination
Cell wall inhibitors				
Vancomycin	5–6	≈0%	<10%	Kidney, liver
Bacitracin	. . .	≈0%	. . .	Kidney
Novobiocin	<6	High	>90%	Liver and bile
Protein synthesis inhibitors: Macrolides				
Erythromycin	1.4	18–45%	72%	Bile
Azithromycin	40–60	40%	50%	Bile
Clarithromycin	5–7	50%	. . .	Bile
Other protein synthesis inhibitors				
Clindamycin	2.7	High	90%	Bile (active metabolite)
DNA synthesis inhibitors: Fluoroquinolones				
Ciprofloxacin	3–4.5	50–80%	15%	Kidney
Enoxacin	3–6	90%	40%	Kidney
Lomefloxacin	8	95%	10%	Kidney
Norfloxacin	3.5–5	30–40%	35%	Kidney
Ofloxacin	5–7	>90%	8%	Kidney
Drugs with other mechanisms				
Metronidazole	6–11	80%	10%	Liver metabolism

nously. Teicoplanin has a long half-life (45–70 hours) and is reported to be free of the histamine-releasing effect that is associated with vancomycin. This drug is investigational.

BACITRACIN

Bacitracin is a cyclic polypeptide mixture first obtained from the Tracy strain of *Bacillus subtilis* in 1943. It is active against gram-positive microorganisms. Because of its marked toxicity when used systemically, it is now generally limited to topical use.

Antibacterial Activity

Bacitracin is most active against gram-positive bacteria, including beta-lactamase-producing staphylococci. There is no cross-resistance between bacitracin and other antimicrobial drugs. Bacitracin inhibits cell wall formation. It interferes with the final dephosphorylation in cycling the isoprenylphosphate carrier that transfers mucopeptide to the growing cell wall (see Figure 42–3).

Pharmacokinetics (Table 50–1)

Bacitracin is little absorbed from gut, skin, wounds, mucous membranes, pleura, or synovia. Topical application thus results in local effects without significant systemic toxicity. Absorbed bacitracin is excreted by glomerular filtration.

Clinical Uses

Because of its systemic toxicity, bacitracin is now used only for topical treatment. Bacitracin, 500 units/g in an ointment base (often combined with polymyxin or neomycin), is useful for the suppression of mixed bacterial flora in surface lesions of the skin, in wounds, or on mucous membranes. Solutions of bacitracin containing 100–200 units/mL in saline can be employed for instillation into joints, wounds, or the pleural cavity—often in conjunction with other drugs given systemically.

Adverse Reactions

Bacitracin is markedly nephrotoxic if absorbed, producing proteinuria, hematuria, and nitrogen retention. Therefore, systemic use has been virtually abandoned. Topical application rarely causes hypersensitivity reactions (eg, skin rashes) or produces significant systemic toxicity.

NOVOBIOCIN

Novobiocin (also called streptonivicin or cardelmycin) is an acidic antibiotic produced by *Streptomyces niveus*. It is a *bacteriostatic* cell wall synthesis inhibitor and is active mainly against gram-positive bacteria.

Until the advent of beta-lactamase-resistant penicillins and cephalosporins, novobiocin was useful in serious staphylococcal infections. To avoid rapid emergence of resistant variants, novobiocin had to be employed in combination with another drug, and the incidence of adverse effects was high. At present, there appears to be no indication for the use of novobiocin.

PROTEIN SYNTHESIS INHIBITORS

ERYTHROMYCINS
(Macrolides)

The erythromycins are a group of closely related macrolide compounds characterized by a macrocyclic lactone ring (usually containing 14 or 16 atoms) to which sugars are attached. The prototype drug, erythromycin, was obtained in 1952 from *Streptomyces erythreus*. Members of the group include carbomycin, oleandomycin, spiramycin, azithromycin, clarithromycin, and many more.

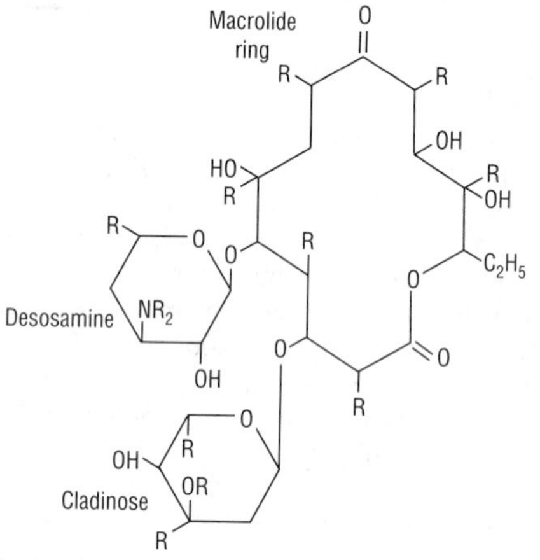

Erythromycin (R = CH₃)

Chemistry

The general structure is shown above with the macrolide ring and the sugars desosamine and cladinose. The molecular weight of erythromycin is 734. It is poorly soluble in water (0.1%) but dissolves readily in organic solvents. Solutions are fairly stable at 4 °C but lose activity rapidly at 20 °C and at acid pH. Erythromycins are usually dispensed as various esters and salts.

Antimicrobial Activity

Erythromycins are effective against gram-positive organisms, especially pneumococci, streptococci, staphylococci, and corynebacteria, in plasma concentrations of 0.02–2 µg/mL. *Mycoplasma, Legionella, Chlamydia trachomatis, Helicobacter,* and certain

mycobacteria *(Mycobacterium kansasii, Mycobacterium scrofulaceum)* are also susceptible.

The antibacterial action of the erythromycins is both inhibitory and bactericidal for susceptible organisms. Activity is enhanced at alkaline pH. Inhibition of protein synthesis occurs by action on the 50S unit of ribosomes. The receptor for erythromycins is a 23S rRNA on the 50S subunit. This receptor is close to the chloramphenicol receptor site. It has been shown experimentally that each drug can interfere with the other's binding, but there is no evidence that this is clinically important. Protein synthesis is inhibited as aminoacyl translocation reactions and the formation of initiation complexes are blocked.

Resistance

In most susceptible microbial populations, organisms occur that are highly resistant to erythromycin (eg, staphylococci). Erythromycin-resistant pneumococci and streptococci are encountered occasionally.

Resistance to erythromycin usually results from methylation of the rRNA-receptor on the 50S unit of the ribosome under control of a plasmid. Inactivation of the drug is not involved. However, among coliform organisms, a transmissible plasmid occurs that specifies an esterase which hydrolyses the lactone ring of macrolides and destroys their activity. Cross-resistance among members of the erythromycin group is virtually complete. Some cross-resistance to lincomycins may occur.

Pharmacokinetics
(Table 50–1)

Erythromycin base is destroyed by stomach acid and must be administered with enteric coating. Stearates and esters are fairly acid-resistant and relatively well absorbed. The lauryl salt of the propionyl ester of erythromycin (erythromycin estolate) is among the best-absorbed oral preparations. Oral doses of 2 g/d result in serum levels of up to 2 µg/mL. Large amounts are lost in feces. Absorbed drug is distributed widely except to the brain and cerebrospinal fluid. It traverses the placenta and reaches the fetus.

Erythromycins are excreted largely in the bile, where levels may be 50 times higher than in the blood. A portion of the drug excreted into bile is reabsorbed from the intestines. Only 5% of the administered dose is excreted in the urine. Some of the newer macrolides (eg, azithromycin, clarithromycin) appear to have better oral activity than the erythromycin esters and, in addition, have longer half-lives than erythromycin.

Clinical Uses

Erythromycins are the drugs of choice in corynebacterial infections (diphtheria, corynebacterial sepsis, erythrasma); in respiratory, neonatal, ocular, or genital chlamydial infections; and in pneumonias caused by *Mycoplasma* and *Legionella.* Clarithromycin and azithromycin have been effective in suppressing disseminated *Mycobacterium avium-intracellulare* infections in AIDS patients. Otherwise, erythromycins are most useful as penicillin substitutes in individuals with streptococcal or pneumococcal infections who are hypersensitive to penicillin. In rheumatic individuals taking penicillin prophylaxis, erythromycin should be given prior to dental procedures as prophylaxis against endocarditis. Although erythromycin estolate is the best-absorbed salt, it imposes the greatest risk of adverse reactions. Therefore, the stearate or succinate salt may be preferred. Erythromycin can enhance gastrointestinal motility in patients with diabetic gastric paresis.

A. Oral Dosage: Give erythromycin base, stearate, or estolate, 0.25–0.5 g every 6 hours (for children, 40 mg/kg/d); or erythromycin ethylsuccinate, 0.4–0.6 g every 6 hours. Oral erythromycin base (1 g) is sometimes combined with oral neomycin or kanamycin for preoperative preparation of the colon. In *M avium-intracellulare* infections, give azithromycin or clarithromycin, 250–500 mg orally twice daily, in combination with another antimycobacterial drug (to avoid rapid development of resistance).

B. Intravenous Dosage: Adults, 0.5 g erythromycin gluceptate or lactobionate every 8–12 hours; children, 40 mg/kg/d.

Adverse Reactions

A. Gastrointestinal Effects: Anorexia, nausea, vomiting, and diarrhea occasionally accompany oral administration.

B. Liver Toxicity: Erythromycins, particularly the estolate, can produce acute cholestatic hepatitis (fever, jaundice, impaired liver function), probably as a hypersensitivity reaction. Most patients recover from this, but hepatitis recurs if the drug is readministered. Other allergic reactions include fever, eosinophilia, and rashes. Erythromycins can inhibit cytochrome P450 and thus increase the effects of oral anticoagulants and oral digoxin. They also increase the concentration of cyclosporine and antihistamines such as terfenadine and astemizole. The resulting high concentrations of these antihistamines may cause serious cardiac arrhythmias.

LINCOMYCIN & CLINDAMYCIN
(Lincosamines)

Lincomycin is an antibiotic elaborated by *Streptomyces lincolnensis.* Clindamycin is a chlorine-substituted derivative of lincomycin.

Lincomycin resembles erythromycin in activity, but there are few valid indications for its use. Clindamycin is more potent and is briefly described here.

Antibacterial Activity

Many gram-positive cocci are inhibited by lincomycins, 0.5–5 μg/mL. Enterococci, *Haemophilus,* neisseriae, and *Mycoplasma* are usually resistant (in contrast to erythromycin). While lincomycins have little or no action against most gram-negative bacteria, *Bacteroides* and other anaerobes are usually susceptible. Lincomycins inhibit protein synthesis by interfering with the formation of initiation complexes and with aminoacyl translocation reactions. The receptor for lincomycins on the 50S subunit of the bacterial ribosome is a 23S rRNA, perhaps identical with the receptor for erythromycins. Thus, these two drug classes may block each other's attachment and may interfere with each other. Resistance to lincomycins appears slowly, perhaps as a result of chromosomal mutation. Plasmid-mediated resistance has not been established with certainty. Resistance to lincomycins is not rare among streptococci, pneumococci, and staphylococci. *C difficile* strains are regularly resistant.

Pharmacokinetics
(Table 50–1)

Oral doses of clindamycin, 0.15–0.3 g every 6 hours (10–20 mg/kg/d for children), yield serum levels of 2–3 μg/mL. When administered intravenously, 600 mg of clindamycin every 8 hours gives levels of 5–15 μg/mL. The drug is widely distributed in the body but does not appear in the central nervous system in significant concentrations. It is about 90% protein-bound. Excretion is mainly through the liver, bile, and urine.

Clinical Uses

Probably the most important indication for clindamycin is the treatment of severe anaerobic infection caused by *Bacteroides* and other anaerobes that often participate in mixed infections. Clindamycin, sometimes in combination with an aminoglycoside or metronidazole, is used to treat penetrating wounds of the abdomen and the gut; infections originating in the female genital tract, eg, septic abortion and pelvic abscesses; or aspiration pneumonia. Lincomycins are *not* effective in meningitis.

Adverse Effects

Common adverse effects are diarrhea, nausea, and skin rashes. Impaired liver function (with or without jaundice) and neutropenia sometimes occur. Severe diarrhea and enterocolitis have followed clindamycin administration and place a serious restraint on its use.

The antibiotic-associated colitis that has followed administration of clindamycin and other drugs is caused by toxigenic *C difficile.* This organism is infrequently part of the normal fecal flora but is selected out during administration of oral antibiotics. It grows to high numbers in the sigmoid colon and secretes a necrotizing toxin that produces pseudomembranous colitis. This potentially fatal complication must be recognized promptly and treated with oral vancomycin, 0.5 g 4–6 times daily (see above) or metronidazole (see below). Variations in the local prevalence of *C difficile* may account for the great differences in incidence of antibiotic-associated colitis.

DNA SYNTHESIS INHIBITORS

QUINOLONES

The important quinolones are synthetic fluorinated analogues of nalidixic acid. They are active against a variety of gram-positive and gram-negative bacteria. Quinolones block bacterial DNA synthesis by inhibiting DNA gyrase, thus preventing the relaxation of supercoiled DNA that is required for normal transcription and duplication (Figure 42–4).

The earlier quinolones (nalidixic acid, oxolinic acid, cinoxacin) did not achieve systemic antibacterial levels and thus were useful only as urinary antiseptics (see below). Newer fluorinated derivatives (norfloxacin, ciprofloxacin, and others; see Figure 50–1 and Table 50–1) have much greater antibacterial activity, achieve bactericidal levels in blood and tissues, and have low toxicity.

Antibacterial Activity

The fluoroquinolones inhibit gram-negative rods including Enterobacteriaceae, *Pseudomonas, Neisse-*

ria, and others in serum concentrations of 1–5 µg/mL. Gram-positive organisms and intracellular pathogens (eg, *Legionella, Chlamydia,* and some mycobacteria) are inhibited by somewhat higher amounts of these drugs, and anaerobes seem to be less susceptible. During fluoroquinolone therapy, resistant organisms emerge with a frequency of about one in 10^9, especially among staphylococci, *Pseudomonas,* and *Serratia.* Resistance is due to a change in the target enzyme, DNA gyrase, or to a change in the permeability of the organism.

Pharmacokinetics (Table 50–1)

After oral administration, the fluoroquinolones are well absorbed and distributed widely in body fluids and tissues, though to different levels. The serum half-life ranges from 3 to 7 hours for different drugs. After ingestion of 400–600 mg, peak serum levels are 1–3 µg/mL for ciprofloxacin, somewhat higher for enoxacin, and 10 µg/mL for ofloxacin. Oral absorption is impaired by divalent cations, eg, antacids. The fluoroquinolones are excreted mainly through the kidney by tubular secretion (which can be blocked by probenecid) and by glomerular filtration. Up to 20% of the dose is metabolized by the liver. In renal insufficiency, some drug accumulation can occur.

Clinical Uses

The fluoroquinolones have significant antimicrobial efficacy, but indications for their use are not clearly defined. Most of these drugs are effective in urinary tract infections even when caused by multidrug-resistant bacteria, eg, *Pseudomonas.* Norfloxacin, 400 mg, or ciprofloxacin, 500 mg, given orally twice daily, is effective for this indication as well as for infectious diarrhea (eg, *Shigella, Salmonella,* toxi-

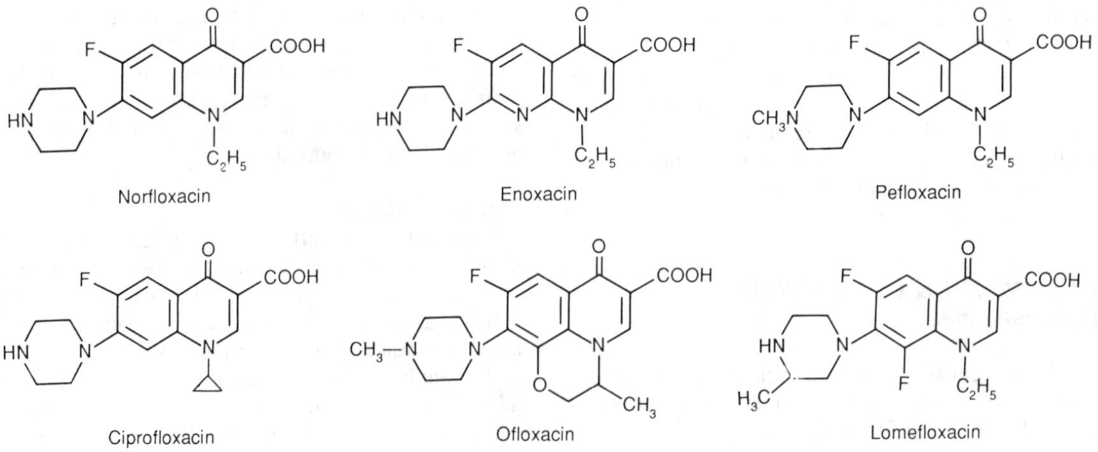

Figure 50–1. Structures of some fluoroquinolones. (Modified and reproduced, with permission, from Brooks GF, Butel JS, Ornston LN: *Jawetz, Melnick, & Adelberg's Medical Microbiology,* 19th ed. Appleton & Lange, 1991.)

genic *E coli, Helicobacter*). The drugs have been employed in infections of soft tissues, bones, and joints, in intra-abdominal and respiratory tract infections, and in sexually transmitted diseases (eg, gonococcal infection, chlamydial infection). They are occasionally given in mycobacterial infections. They may be suitable for eradication of meningococci from carriers or for prophylaxis of infection in neutropenic patients. In addition to the oral fluoroquinolones, ciprofloxacin, ofloxacin, and newer members of the group can be given intravenously.

Adverse Effects

The most prominent effects are nausea, vomiting, and diarrhea. Occasionally, headache, dizziness, insomnia, abnormal liver function tests, or skin rash develops. Concomitant administration of theophylline and quinolones can lead to elevated levels of theophylline with the risk of toxic effects, especially seizures. Fluoroquinolones may damage growing cartilage and should perhaps not be given to patients under 18 years of age. Superinfection with streptococci and *Candida* has been observed.

DRUGS WITH UNKNOWN MECHANISMS

METRONIDAZOLE

This nitroimidazole antiprotozoal drug (Chapter 54) also has striking antibacterial effects against most anaerobes, including *Bacteroides* and clostridia. It is well absorbed after oral administration (Table 50–1), widely distributed in tissues, and reaches serum levels of 4–6 µg/mL after a 250 mg oral dose. It penetrates well into the cerebrospinal fluid, reaching levels similar to those in serum. Metronidazole is metabolized in the liver and may accumulate in hepatic insufficiency, requiring dosage reduction. Metronidazole can also be given intravenously or by rectal suppository.

Metronidazole is considered in the following microbial infections: For anaerobic or mixed infections, 500 mg is given 3 times daily orally or intravenously (30 mg/kg/d). For vaginitis (*Trichomonas, Gardnerella,* mixed), 250 mg is given orally 3 times daily for 7–10 days; some cases of vaginitis respond to a single 2 g dose. In antibiotic-associated enterocolitis, 500 mg is given 3 times daily orally or intravenously as an alternative to vancomycin. Some brain abscesses respond to treatment with metronidazole, often combined with penicillin or cephalosporin. Metronidazole has also been used for preparation of

the colon for surgery. A vaginal gel is available for topical use.

Adverse effects include nausea, diarrhea, stomatitis, and—with prolonged use—peripheral neuropathy. Alcohol ingestion is to be avoided because of metronidazole's disulfiram-like effect. While teratogenic in some animals, metronidazole has not been associated with this effect in humans.

Other properties of metronidazole are discussed in Chapter 54.

URINARY ANTISEPTICS

Many systemic antimicrobial drugs are excreted in high concentration into urine. Doses much below those necessary to achieve systemic effects can therefore be therapeutic in infections of the urinary tract. Short courses or even single doses of drugs such as sulfonamides, certain penicillins (eg, ampicillin, amoxicillin, carbenicillin), aminoglycosides, or fluoroquinolones can sometimes cure acute urinary tract infections.

By contrast, urinary antiseptics are drugs that exert antibacterial activity in the urine but have little or no systemic antibacterial effect. Their usefulness is limited to urinary tract infections. Prolonged suppression of bacteriuria by means of urinary antiseptics may be desirable in chronic urinary tract infections where eradication of infection by short-term systemic therapy has not been possible.

NITROFURANTOIN

Antibacterial Activity

Nitrofurans are bacteriostatic and bactericidal for many gram-positive and gram-negative bacteria. *P aeruginosa* and many strains of *Proteus* are resistant, but in nitrofurantoin-susceptible populations resistant mutants are rare. Clinical drug resistance emerges slowly. There is no cross-resistance between nitrofurans and other antimicrobial agents.

The mechanism of action of the nitrofurans is not known. The activity of nitrofurantoin is greatly enhanced at pH 5.5 or below.

Pharmacokinetics

Nitrofurantoin is well absorbed after ingestion but is metabolized and excreted so rapidly that no systemic antibacterial action is possible. In the kidneys, the drug is excreted in the urine by both glomerular filtration and tubular secretion. With average daily doses, concentrations of 200 µg/mL are reached in urine. In renal failure, urine levels are insufficient for antibacterial action, but high blood levels may cause toxicity.

Clinical Uses

The average daily dose for urinary tract infection in adults is 100 mg orally 4 times daily taken with food or milk. Nitrofurantoin must never be given to patients with severe renal insufficiency. Oral nitrofurantoin can be given for months for the suppression of chronic urinary tract infection. It is desirable to keep urinary pH below 5.5 (see Acidifying Agents, below). A single daily dose of nitrofurantoin, 100 mg, can prevent recurrent urinary tract infections in women.

Another nitrofuran, furazolidone, 400 mg/d orally (5–8 mg/kg/d in children), may reduce diarrhea in cholera and perhaps shorten vibrio excretion. It usually fails in shigellosis.

Adverse Reactions

A. Direct Toxicity: Anorexia, nausea, and vomiting are the principal (and frequent) side effects of nitrofurantoin. Neuropathies and hemolytic anemia occur in glucose-6-phosphate dehydrogenase deficiency. Nitrofurantoin antagonizes the action of nalidixic acid.

B. Allergic Reactions: Various skin rashes, pulmonary infiltration, and other hypersensitivity reactions have been reported.

NALIDIXIC ACID, OXOLINIC ACID, & CINOXACIN

Nalidixic acid, the first antibacterial quinolone, was introduced in 1963. It is not fluorinated and is excreted too rapidly to have systemic antibacterial effects. Oxolinic acid and cinoxacin are similar in structure and function to nalidixic acid.

Antibacterial Activity

Nalidixic acid inhibits many gram-negative bacteria in vitro in concentrations of 1–20 μg/mL. Much higher concentrations are necessary to inhibit gram-positive organisms. Most strains of *E coli* are inhibited, as are some strains of *Enterobacter, Klebsiella,* and *Proteus. Pseudomonas* are usually resistant.

Like all quinolones, nalidixic acid blocks DNA synthesis in bacteria by inhibiting DNA gyrase.

Resistant microorganisms emerge rapidly during therapy, both by selection of drug-resistant mutants in the population and by superinfection with drug-resistant microorganisms of another strain or species. Plasmid-mediated resistance to nalidixic acid has not been demonstrated. There is no cross-resistance with other antimicrobial drugs.

Pharmacokinetics

After oral administration, the drugs are readily absorbed from the gut, rapidly metabolized, and excreted. Thus, there is no significant systemic antibacterial action. About 20% of the absorbed drug is excreted in the urine in the active form and 80% in an inactive form as a glucuronide conjugate. Levels of active drug in the urine reach 50–200 μg/mL.

Clinical Uses

The only indication for these agents is urinary tract infection with coliform organisms. The dose of nalidixic acid for adults is 1 g orally 4 times a day for 1–2 weeks (children, 30–60 mg/kg/d). The dose of oxolinic acid is 0.75 g twice a day and of cinoxacin 1 g/d.

Adverse Reactions

Nalidixic acid excreted in the urine may give rise to false-positive tests for glucose, but true hyperglycemia and glycosuria may also be produced. There are occasional gastrointestinal disturbances, skin rashes, sensitization to sunlight, visual disturbances, and central nervous system stimulation, including seizures. The central nervous system toxicity of oxolinic acid is probably higher.

METHENAMINE MANDELATE & METHENAMINE HIPPURATE

Methenamine mandelate is the salt of mandelic acid and methenamine and possesses to some extent the properties of both of these urinary antiseptics. Methenamine hippurate is the salt of hippuric acid and methenamine. Mandelic acid or hippuric acid taken orally is excreted unchanged in the urine, where these drugs are bactericidal for some gram-negative bacteria if the pH can be kept below 5.5. Methenamine is absorbed readily after oral intake and excreted in the urine. If the urine is strongly acid (pH below 5.5), methenamine releases formaldehyde, which is antibacterial.

Methenamine mandelate, 1 g 4 times daily, or methenamine hippurate, 1 g twice daily by mouth (children, 50 mg/kg/d or 30 mg/kg/d), is used only as a urinary antiseptic. If necessary, acidifying agents (eg, ascorbic acid, 4–12 g/d) may be given to lower urinary pH below 5.5. Sulfonamides cannot be given at the same time because they may form an insoluble compound with the formaldehyde released by methenamine. Persons taking methenamine mandelate may exhibit falsely elevated tests for catecholamine metabolites.

The action of methenamine mandelate or hippurate is nonspecific against many different microorganisms and consists of the simultaneous effects of formaldehyde and acidity. Microorganisms such as *Proteus* that make a strongly alkaline urine through release of ammonia from urea usually are insusceptible.

ACIDIFYING AGENTS

In chronic urinary tract infections, eradication of the organisms often fails. It is then important to suppress bacteria for as long as possible.

Any substance that will produce a urine pH below 5.5 tends to inhibit bacterial growth in urine. Ketogenic diets, ammonium chloride, ascorbic acid, mandelic acid, methionine, and hippuric acid (eg, from ingestion of cranberry juice) all can be employed to that end. It is important to check urinary pH frequently and to ascertain by direct microscopic examination that the bacteriuria is actually suppressed. Prolonged suppression (6–18 months) occasionally permits healing of the infection, probably because it blocks the frequent ascending reinfection of the kidneys from the lower tract.

CYCLOSERINE

Cycloserine is an antibiotic produced by *Streptomyces orchidaceus.*

The substance is water-soluble and very unstable at acid pH. Cycloserine inhibits many microorganisms, including coliforms, *Proteus,* and mycobacteria. Cy-

Cycloserine

closerine inhibits the incorporation of D-alanine into the peptidoglycan of the bacterial cell wall by inhibiting the enzyme alanine racemase. After ingestion of cycloserine, 0.25 g every 6 hours, blood levels reach 20–30 µg/mL—sufficient to inhibit many strains of mycobacteria and gram-negative bacteria. The drug is widely distributed in tissues. Most of the drug is excreted in active form into the urine, where concentrations are sufficiently high to inhibit many organisms causing urinary tract infections. The dose for urinary tract infections is 10–20 mg/kg/d. Cycloserine is occasionally used in treatment of relapsed tuberculosis caused by drug-resistant organisms. The dosage is 0.25 g 2–4 times daily by mouth.

Cycloserine may cause serious central nervous system toxicity with headaches, tremors, acute psychosis, and convulsions. If oral doses are maintained below 0.75 g/d, such effects can usually be avoided.

PREPARATIONS AVAILABLE

Bacitracin (generic)
  Parenteral: powder to reconstitute for 50,000 units for injection
Cinoxacin (Cinobac)
  Oral: 250, 500 mg capsules
Ciprofloxacin (Cipro, Cipro I.V.)
  Oral: 250, 500, 750 mg tablets
  Parenteral: 2, 10 mg/mL
Clindamycin (Cleocin)
  Oral: 75, 150, 300 mg capsules; 75 mg/5 mL granules to reconstitute for solution
  Parenteral: 150 mg/mL in 2, 4, 6, 60 mL vials for injection
Enoxacin (Penetrex)
  Oral: 200, 400 mg tablets
Erythromycin (generic, Ilotycin, Ilosone, E-Mycin, Erythrocin, others)
  Oral (base): 250, 333, 500 mg enteric-coated tablets;
  Oral (base) delayed release: 333, 500 mg tablets, 250 capsules;
  Oral (estolate): 500 mg tablets; 250 mg capsules; 125, 250 mg/5 mL suspension
  Oral (ethylsuccinate): 200, 400 mg film-coated tablets; 200, 400 mg/5 mL suspension
  Oral (stearate): 250, 500 mg film-coated tablets
  Parenteral: lactobionate, powder to reconstitute

for IV injection (0.5, 1 g per vial); glucepate, powder to reconstitute for IV injection (1 g per vial)
Lincomycin (Lincocin)
  Oral: 250, 500 mg capsules
  Parenteral: 300 mg/mL in 2, 10 mL vials for IM or IV injection
Lomefloxacin (Maxaquin)
  Oral: 400 mg tablets
Methenamine hippurate (Hiprex, Urex)
  Oral: 0.5 g tablets
Methenamine mandelate (generic, Mandelamine)
  Oral: 0.5, 1 g tablets; 0.25, 0.5, 1 g enteric-coated tablets; 0.25, 0.5 g/5 mL suspension; 0.5, 1 g granules (packets)
Metronidazole (generic, Flagyl, others)
  Oral: 250, 500 mg tablets
  Parenteral: 500 mg for injection
Nalidixic acid (NegGram)
  Oral: 250, 500, 1000 mg tablets; 250 mg/5 mL suspension
Nitrofurantoin (generic, Furadantin, others)
  Oral: 50, 100 mg capsules and tablets; 25 mg/5 mL suspension; 25, 50, 100 mg macrocrystals (Macrodantin)
  Parenteral: 180 mg powder for reconstitution for IV injection

Norfloxacin (Noroxin)
    Oral: 400 mg tablets
Novobiocin (Albamycin)
    Oral: 250 mg capsules
Ofloxacin (Floxin)
    Oral: 200, 300, 400 mg tablets

Parenteral: 200 mg in 50 mL vial for IV administration
Vancomycin (generic, Vancocin, Vancoled)
    Oral: 125, 250 mg Pulvules; 1, 10 g powder to reconstitute for solution
    Parenteral: 0.5, 1, 5, 10 g powder to reconstitute for IV injection

REFERENCES

Bartlett JG: Anti-anaerobic antibacterial agents. Lancet 1982; 2:478.

Bergan T: Pharmacokinetics of ciprofloxacin with reference to other fluorinated quinolones. J Chemother 1989;1:10.

Counts GM et al: Treatment of cystitis in women with a single dose of trimethoprim-sulfamethoxazole. Rev Infect Dis 1982;4:484.

Cunha BA: Nitrofurantoin—An update. Obstet Gynecol Surv 1989;44:399.

Demotes-Mainard FM, Vincon GA, Albin HC: Pharmacokinetics of a new macrolide, roxithromycin, in infants and children. J Clin Pharmacol 1989;29:752.

Derrick CW Jr, Reilly KM: Erythromycin, lincomycin, and clindamycin. Pediatr Clin North Am 1983;30:63.

Dhawan VK, Thadepalli H: Clindamycin: A review of fifteen years of experience. Rev Infect Dis 1982;4:1133.

Edwards DI: Nitroimidazole drugs—action and resistance mechanisms. (In two parts.) J Antimicrob Chemother 1993;31:9, 201.

Ericsson CD et al: Ciprofloxacin or trimethoprim-sulfamethoxazole as initial therapy for travelers' diarrhea: A placebo-controlled, randomized trial. Ann Intern Med 1987;106:216.

Freeark RJ: Penetrating wounds of the abdomen. N Engl J Med 1974;291:185.

Freeman RB et al: Long-term therapy for chronic bacteriuria in men. Ann Intern Med 1974;83:133.

Gorbach SL, Thadepalli H: Clindamycin in pure and mixed anaerobic infections. Arch Intern Med 1974;134:87.

Hamilton-Miller JM, Brumfitt W: Methenamine and its salts as urinary antiseptics. Invest Urol 1977;14:287.

Hermans PE, Wilhelm MP: Vancomycin. Mayo Clin Proc 1987;62:901.

Hooper DC, Wolfson JS: Fluoroquinolone antimicrobial agents. N Engl J Med 1991;324:384.

Hook EW, Johnson WD: Vancomycin therapy of bacterial endocarditis. Am J Med 1978;65:411.

Johnson AP et al: Resistance to vancomycin and teicoplanin: An emerging clinical problem. Clin Microbiol Rev 1990;3:280.

Kirst HA, Sides GD: New directions of macrolide antibiotics: Pharmacokinetics and clinical efficacy. Antimicrob Agents Chemother 1989;33:1419.

Klainer AS: Clindamycin. Med Clin North Am 1987;71: 1169.

Kucers A: Chloramphenicol, erythromycin, vancomycin, tetracyclines. Lancet 1982;2:425.

Lagast H, Dodion P, Klastersky J: Comparison of pharmacokinetics and bactericidal activity of teicoplanin and vancomycin. J Antimicrob Chemother 1986;18:513.

Lode H: Pharmacokinetics and clinical results of parenter-ally administered new quinolones in humans. Rev Infect Dis 1989;11(Suppl 5):S996.

Martin DH et al: A controlled trial of a single dose of azithromycin for the treatment of chlamydial urethritis and cervicitis. N Engl J Med 1992;327:921.

Mazzei T et al: Chemistry and mode of action of macrolides. J Antimicrob Chemother 1993;31 (Suppl C):1.

McHenry MC, Gavan TL: Vancomycin. Pediatr Clin North Am 1983;30:31.

Moellering RC et al: Vancomycin therapy in patients with impaired renal function: A nomogram for dosage. Ann Intern Med 1981;94:343.

Neu HC (editor): Ciprofloxacin: A major advance in quinolone chemotherapy. (Symposium.) Am J Med 1987; 82(Suppl 4A):1. [Entire issue.]

Peters DH, Clissold SP: Clarithromycin. A review of its antimicrobial activity, pharmacokinetic properties and therapeutic potential. Drugs 1992;44:117.

Radanst JM et al: Interaction of fluoroquinolones with other drugs: Mechanisms, variability, clinical significance, and management. Clin Infect Dis 1992;14:272.

Ronald AR, Harding KM: Urinary infection prophylaxis in women. Ann Intern Med 1981;94:268.

Rosenblatt JE, Edson RS: Metronidazole. Mayo Clin Proc 1987;62:1013.

Sanyal D et al: The emergence of vancomycin resistance in renal dialysis. J Hospit Infect 1993;24:167.

Scully BE: Metronidazole. Med Clin North Am 1988;72: 623.

Sexually transmitted diseases: Treatment guidelines. MMWR Morb Mortal Wkly Rep 1989;38:S8.

Shen L, Baranowski J, Pernet AG: Mechanism of inhibition of DNA gyrase by quinolone antibacterials: specificity and cooperativity of drug binding. Biochemistry 1989;28:3879.

Stamm WE, Hooten TM: Management of urinary tract infections in adults. N Engl J Med 1993;329:1328.

Teasley DG et al: Trial of metronidazole vs. vancomycin for *Clostridium difficile:* Associated diarrhea and colitis. Lancet 1983;2:1043.

Wilson WR, Cockerill FR III: Tetracyclines, chloramphenicol, erythromycin, and clindamycin. Mayo Clin Proc 1987;62:906.

Wolfson JS, Hooper DC: Bacterial resistance to quinolones: Mechanisms and clinical importance. Rev Infect Dis 1989;11 (Suppl 5):S960.

Wolfson JS, Hooper DC: Treatment of genitourinary tract infections with fluoroquinolones: activity in vitro, pharmacokinetics, and clinical efficacy in urinary tract infections and prostatitis. Antimicrob Agents Chemother 1989;33:1655.

Disinfectants & Antiseptics

51

Ernest Jawetz, MD, PhD

The antiseptics and disinfectants differ fundamentally from systemically active chemotherapeutic agents in that they exhibit little or no selective toxicity. Most of these substances are toxic not only for microbial parasites but for host cells as well. Therefore, they may be used to reduce the microbial population in the inanimate environment, but they can usually be applied only topically, not systemically, to humans.

The terms "disinfectants," "antiseptics," and "germicides" have often been used interchangeably, and the definitions overlap greatly in the literature. The term **disinfectant** usually denotes a substance that kills microorganisms in the inanimate environment. The term **antiseptic** often is applied to substances that inhibit bacterial growth both in vitro and in vivo when applied to the surface of living tissue under suitable conditions of contact.

The antibacterial action of antiseptics and disinfectants is largely dependent on concentration, temperature, and time. Very low concentrations may stimulate bacterial growth, higher concentrations may be inhibitory, and still higher concentrations may be bactericidal for certain organisms.

Evaluation of the antiseptics and disinfectants is difficult. Methods of testing are controversial, and results are subject to different interpretations. Ideally, disinfectants should be lethal for microorganisms in high dilution, noninjurious to tissues or inanimate substances, inexpensive, stable, nonstaining, odorless, and rapid-acting even in the presence of foreign proteins, exudates, or fibers. No preparation now available combines these characteristics to a high degree. There is also a need for effective, nontoxic compounds to neutralize disinfectants in vitro.

Many antiseptics and disinfectants were at one time used in medical and surgical practice. Most have now been displaced by chemotherapeutic substances. Mupirocin is a newer antibacterial substance derived from *Pseudomonas* that inhibits staphylococci and streptococci by interfering with bacterial RNA and protein synthesis. While lacking in systemic activity, it can be effective topically in skin infections (see Chapter 63). Most topical antiseptics do not aid wound healing but, on the contrary, often impair healing. In general, cleansing of abrasions and superficial wounds by washing with soap and water is far more effective and less damaging than the application of topical antiseptics. Substances applied topically to skin or mucous membranes are absorbed irregularly and often unpredictably. Occlusive dressings with plastic films often greatly enhance absorption. Penetration of drugs through skin epithelium is also greatly influenced by relative humidity and temperature.

A few chemical classes of disinfectants and antiseptics are briefly characterized in the following paragraphs.

Alcohols

Aliphatic alcohols are antimicrobial in varying degree by denaturing protein. Ethanol (ethyl alcohol) in 70% concentration is bactericidal in 1–2 minutes at 30 °C but less effective at lower and higher concentrations. Ethyl alcohol, 70%, and isopropyl alcohol (isopropanol), 90%, are at present the most satisfactory general antiseptics for skin surfaces. They may be useful for sterilizing instruments but have no effect on spores, and better agents are available for this purpose. Aerosols of 70% alcohol with 1 μm size droplets may be effective disinfectants for mechanical respirators.

Propylene glycol and other glycols have been used as vapors to disinfect air. Precise control of humidity is necessary for good antimicrobial action. Glycol vapors are rarely employed at present.

Aldehydes

Formaldehyde in a concentration of 1–10% effectively kills microorganisms and their spores in 1–6 hours. It acts by combining with and precipitating protein. It is too irritating for use on tissues, but it is widely employed as a disinfectant for instruments. Formaldehyde solution USP contains 37% formaldehyde by weight, with methyl alcohol added to prevent polymerization.

Glutaraldehyde as a 2% alkaline solution in 70% isopropanol (pH 7.5–8.5) serves as a liquid disinfectant for some optical and other instruments and for some prosthetic materials. It kills viable microorganisms in 10 minutes and spores in 3–10 hours, but the solution is unstable, and tissue contact must be avoided.

Methenamine taken orally can release formaldehyde into acid urine. It is employed as a urinary antiseptic (see Chapter 50).

Acids

Several inorganic acids have been used for cauterization of tissue. Although they are effective antimicrobial agents, the tissue destruction they cause precludes their use. Boric acid, 5% in water, or as powder, can be applied to a variety of skin lesions as an antimicrobial agent. However, the toxicity of absorbed boric acid is high, particularly for small children, and its use is not advised. Among the organic acids, benzoic acid, 0.1%, is employed as a food preservative. Esters of benzoic acid (parabens) are used as antimicrobial preservatives of certain other drugs. Acetic acid, 1%, can be used in surgical dressings as a topical antimicrobial agent; 0.25–2% acetic acid is a useful antimicrobial agent in the external ear and for irrigation of the lower urinary tract. It is particularly active against aerobic gram-negative bacteria, eg, *Pseudomonas*. Salicylic and undecylenic and other fatty acids can serve as fungicides on skin. They are employed particularly in dermatophytosis involving intertriginous areas, eg, "athlete's foot" (see Chapter 63).

Mandelic acid is excreted unchanged in the urine after oral intake; 12 g daily taken orally can lower the pH of urine to 5.0, sufficient to be antibacterial. (See Chapter 50.)

Halogens & Halogen-Containing Compounds

A. Iodine: Elemental iodine is an effective germicide. Its mode of action is not definitely known. A 1:20,000 solution of iodine kills bacteria in 1 minute and spores in 15 minutes, and its tissue toxicity is relatively low. Iodine tincture USP contains 2% iodine and 2.4% sodium iodide in alcohol. It is the most effective antiseptic available for intact skin and should be used to disinfect skin when obtaining blood cultures by venipuncture. Its principal disadvantage is the occasional dermatitis that can occur in hypersensitive individuals. This can be avoided by promptly removing the tincture of iodine with alcohol.

Iodine can be complexed with polyvinylpyrrolidone to yield povidone-iodine USP, an iodophore. This is a water-soluble complex that liberates free iodine in solution (eg, 1% free iodine in 10% solution). It is widely employed as a skin antiseptic, particularly for preoperative skin preparation. It is an effective local antibacterial substance, killing not only vegetative forms but also spores. Hypersensitivity reactions are infrequent. Povidone-iodine is available in many

forms: solution, ointment, aerosol, surgical scrub, shampoo, skin cleanser, vaginal gel, vaginal douche, and individual cotton swabs. Povidone-iodine solutions can become contaminated with *Pseudomonas* and other aerobic gram-negative bacteria. Rarely, drops of tincture of iodine are used for the emergency disinfection of small quantities of contaminated drinking water.

B. Chlorine: Chlorine exerts its antimicrobial action in the form of undissociated hypochlorous acid (HOCl), which is formed when chlorine is dissolved in water at neutral or acid pH. Chlorine concentrations of 0.25 ppm are effectively bactericidal for many microorganisms except mycobacteria, which are 500 times more resistant. Organic matter greatly reduces the antimicrobial activity of chlorine. The amount of chlorine bound by organic matter (eg, in water) and thus not available for antimicrobial activity is called the "chlorine demand." The chlorine demand of relatively pure water is low, and the addition of 0.5 ppm chlorine is sufficient for disinfection. The chlorine demand of grossly polluted water may be very high, so that 20 ppm or more of chlorine may have to be added for effective bactericidal action.

Chlorine is used mainly for the disinfection of inanimate objects and particularly for the purification of water. Chlorinated lime forms hypochlorite solution when dissolved. It is a cheap (but unstable) form of chlorine used mainly for disinfection of excreta in the field. Halazone USP is a chloramine employed in tablet form for the sterilization of small quantities of drinking water. The addition of 4–8 mg halazone per liter will sterilize water in 15–60 minutes unless a large quantity of organic material is present. It may not inactivate cysts of *Entamoeba histolytica*.

Sodium hypochlorite solution USP, 0.5% NaOCl (diluted sodium hypochlorite [modified Dakin's]) solution, contains about 0.1 g of available chlorine per deciliter and can be used as an irrigating fluid for the cleansing and disinfecting of contaminated wounds. Household bleaches containing chlorine can serve as disinfectants for inanimate objects.

Oxidizing Agents

Some antiseptics exert an antimicrobial action because they are oxidizing agents. Most are of no practical importance, and only hydrogen peroxide, sodium perborate, and potassium permanganate are occasionally used.

Hydrogen peroxide solution USP contains 3% H_2O_2 in water. Contact with tissues releases molecular oxygen, and there is a brief period of antimicrobial action. There is no penetration of tissues, and the main applications of hydrogen peroxide are as a mouthwash and for the cleansing of wounds. Hydrogen peroxide can be used to disinfect smooth contact lenses that are subsequently applied to the eye. Hydrous benzoyl peroxide USP can be bactericidal to microorganisms. When applied to the skin as a lotion, it is also keratolytic, antiseborrheic, and irritant. It has been used in treating acne and seborrhea, but it bleaches clothing and may produce contact dermatitis.

Potassium permanganate USP consists of purple crystals that dissolve in water to give deep purple solutions that stain tissues and clothing brown. A 1:10,000 dilution of potassium permanganate kills many microorganisms in 1 hour. Higher concentrations are irritating to tissues. The principal use of potassium permanganate solution is in the treatment of weeping skin lesions.

Heavy Metals

A. Mercury: Mercuric ion precipitates protein and inhibits sulfhydryl enzymes. Microorganisms inactivated by mercury can be reactivated by thiols (sulfhydryl compounds). Mercurial antiseptics inhibit the sulfhydryl enzymes of tissue cells as well as those of bacteria. Therefore, most mercury preparations are highly toxic if ingested. Mercury bichloride NF (1:100) can be used as a disinfectant for instruments or unabraded skin.

Ammoniated mercury ointment USP contains 5% of the active insoluble compound ($HgNH_2Cl$). It is a skin antiseptic in impetigo.

Some organic mercury compounds are less toxic than the inorganic salts and somewhat more antibacterial. Nitromersol USP, thimerosal USP (Merthiolate), and phenylmercuric acetate or nitrate are marketed in many different liquid and solid forms as bacteriostatic antiseptics. They are also used as "preservatives" in various biologic products to reduce the chance of accidental contamination. Merbromin (Mercurochrome) is used as a 2% solution that is a feeble antiseptic but stains tissue a brilliant red color. The psychologic effect of this stain has lent support to the otherwise negligible antiseptic properties of this material.

B. Silver: Silver ion precipitates protein and also interferes with essential metabolic activities of microbial cells. Inorganic silver salts in solution are strongly bactericidal. Silver nitrate, 1:1000, destroys most microorganisms rapidly upon contact. Silver nitrate ophthalmic solution USP contains 1% of the salt, to be instilled into the eyes of newborns to prevent gonococcal ophthalmia. It is effective for this purpose but may cause chemical conjunctivitis by being quite acid; therefore, antibiotic ointment has been used instead at times. Other inorganic silver salts are rarely used for their antimicrobial properties because they are strongly irritating to tissues. In burns, compresses of 0.5% silver nitrate can reduce infection of the burn wound, aid rapid eschar formation, and reduce mortality. If silver nitrate is reduced to nitrite by bacteria in the burn, methemoglobinemia may result. Silver sulfadiazine 1% cream slowly releases sulfadiazine and also silver (see Chapter 47) and effectively suppresses microbial flora in burns. It may

have some advantages and causes less pain than mafenide acetate in the treatment of burns, but it has occasionally produced leukopenia.

Colloidal preparations of silver are less injurious to superficial tissues and have significant bacteriostatic properties. Mild silver protein contains about 20% silver and can be applied as an antiseptic to mucous membranes. Prolonged use of any silver preparation may result in argyria.

Other Metals

Other metal salts (eg, zinc sulfate, copper sulfate) have significant antimicrobial properties but are rarely employed in medicine for this purpose.

Soaps

Soaps are anionic surface-active agents, usually sodium or potassium salts of various fatty acids. They vary in composition depending on the specific fats or oils and on the particular alkali from which they are made. Since NaOH and KOH are strong bases, whereas most fatty acids are weak acids, most soaps when dissolved in water are strongly alkaline (pH 8.0–10.0). Thus, they may irritate skin, which has a pH of 5.5–6.5. Special soaps (eg, Neutrogena) use triethanolamine as a base and, when dissolved, are near pH 7.0. While most common soaps are well tolerated, excessive use will dry normal skin. Admixed synthetic fragrances may cause irritation or sensitization of skin.

Most common soaps remove dirt as well as surface secretions, desquamated epithelium, and bacteria contained in them. The physical action of thorough hand washing with plain soaps is quite effective in removing transient bacteria and other contaminating microorganisms from skin surfaces. For additional antibacterial action, certain disinfectant chemicals (hexachlorophene, phenols, carbanilides, etc) have been added to certain soaps. These chemicals may be both beneficial and potentially harmful and are discussed below.

Phenols & Related Compounds

Phenol denatures protein. It was the first antiseptic employed, as a spray, during surgical procedures by Lister in 1867. Concentrations of at least 1–2% are required for antimicrobial activity, whereas a 5% concentration is strongly irritating to tissues. Therefore, phenol is used mainly for the disinfection of inanimate objects and excreta. Substituted phenols are more effective (and more expensive) as environmental disinfectants. Among them are many proprietary preparations containing cresol and other alkyl-substituted phenols. Exaggerated claims have been made for the antibacterial and antiviral properties for some such preparations (eg, Lysol) and their possible health benefits.

Other phenol derivatives such as resorcinol, thymol, and hexylresorcinol have enjoyed some popularity in the past as antiseptics. Several chlorinated phenols are much more active antimicrobial agents.

Hexachlorophene USP is a white crystalline powder that is insoluble in water but soluble in organic solvents, dilute alkalies, and soaps and is an effective bacteriostatic agent. Hexachlorophene liquid soap USP and many proprietary preparations are used widely in surgical scrub routines and as deodorant soaps. Single applications of such preparations are no more effective than plain soaps, but daily use results in a deposit of hexachlorophene on the skin that exerts a prolonged bacteriostatic action. Thus, the number of resident skin bacteria is lower on the surgeon's hands if hexachlorophene soap is used daily and if other soaps, which promptly remove the residual hexachlorophene film, are not employed.

Soaps or detergents containing 3% hexachlorophene are effective in delaying or preventing colonization of the newborn's skin with pathogenic staphylococci in hospital nurseries. However, repeated bathing of newborns (and particularly premature infants) with such preparations may permit sufficient absorption of hexachlorophene to result in toxic effects to the nervous system, especially a spongiform degeneration of the white matter in the brain. For this reason, the "routine prophylactic use" of 3% hexachlorophene preparations was discouraged. Unfortunately, stopping the use of hexachlorophene-containing preparations for bathing of newborns has been accompanied by a resurgence of staphylococcal infections in nursery populations.

Hexachlorophene

Other antiseptics have been added to soaps and detergents, eg, carbanilides or salicylanilides. Trichlorocarbanilide now takes the place of hexachlorophenes in several "antiseptic soaps." Regular use of such antiseptic soaps may reduce body odor by preventing bacterial decomposition of organic material in apocrine sweat. All antiseptic soaps may induce allergic reactions or photosensitization.

Chlorhexidine is a bisdiguanide antiseptic that disrupts the cytoplasmic membrane, especially of gram-positive organisms. It is employed as a skin cleanser, as a constituent of antiseptic soaps, and as a mouthwash for combating plaque-inducing bacteria. A 4% solution of chlorhexidine gluconate can be used to cleanse wounds. When incorporated into soaps, it is used as an antiseptic hand-washing preparation, especially in hospitals, and for surgical scrub and preparation of skin sites for operative procedures. Repeated application of chlorhexidine-containing soap results in persistence of the chemical on the skin to give a cumulative antibacterial effect. Chlorhexidine is somewhat less effective against *Pseudomonas* and *Serratia* strains than against coliform and gram-positive organisms. Several double-blind comparisons have indicated that 0.2% chlorhexidine gluconate can reduce plaque accumulation on teeth and may be of some value in gingivitis. Flushing of the vagina with chlorhexidine solution has been proposed as a prophylaxis for neonatal infections. Chloroxylenol, a chlorine-substituted xylenol, can have similar activity on the skin in concentrations of 0.5–4%.

Cationic Surface-Active Agents

Surface-active compounds are widely used as wetting agents and detergents in industry and in the home. They act by altering the energy relationship at interfaces. Cationic surface-active agents are bactericidal, probably by altering the permeability characteristics of the cell membrane. Cationic agents are antagonized by anionic surface-active agents and thus are incompatible with soaps. Cationic agents are also strongly adsorbed onto porous or fibrous materials, eg, rubber or cotton, and are effectively removed by them from solutions.

A variety of cationic surface-active agents are employed for the disinfection of instruments, mucous membranes, and skin, eg, benzalkonium chloride USP and cetylpyridinium chloride USP. Aqueous solutions of 1:10,000–1:1000 exhibit good antimicrobial activity but have important disadvantages. These quaternary ammonium disinfectants are antagonized by soaps, and soaps should not be used on surfaces where the antibacterial activity of quaternary ammonium disinfectants is desired. They are adsorbed onto cotton and thereby removed from solution. When applied to skin, they form a film under which microorganisms can survive. Because of these properties, these substances have given rise to outbreaks of serious infections due to *Pseudomonas* and other gram-negative bacteria. Therefore, they cannot be employed safely as skin antiseptics and can only rarely be used as disinfectants of instruments.

Nitrofurans

Nitrofurazone USP is used as a topical antimicrobial agent on superficial wounds or skin lesions and as a surgical dressing. The preparations contain about 0.2% of the active drug and do not interfere with wound healing. However, about 2% of patients may become sensitized and may develop reactions, eg, allergic pneumonitis. Nitrofurantoin USP is a urinary antiseptic (see Chapter 50).

PREPARATIONS AVAILABLE

Benzalkonium (generic, Zephiran, others)
Topical: 17% concentrate; 50% solution; 1:750 solution

Chlorhexidine gluconate (Hibiclens, Hibistat, others)
Topical: 2, 4% cleanser, sponge; 0.5% rinse in 70% alcohol (Peridex)
Oral rinse: 0.12%

Hexachlorophene (pHisoHex, Septisol)
Topical: 3% liquid, sponge; 0.25% solution; 0.23% foam

Iodine aqueous (generic, Lugol's Solution)
Topical: 2–5% in water with 2.4% sodium iodide or 10% potassium iodide

Iodine tincture (generic)
Topical: 2% iodine or 2.4% sodium iodide in 47% alcohol, in 15, 30, 120 mL and in larger quantities

Merbromin (Mercurochrome)
Topical: 2% solution

Nitrofurazone (generic, Furacin)
Topical: 0.2% solution, ointment, and cream

Oxychlorosene sodium (Clorpactin)
Topical: 2, 5 g powder for solution for irrigation, instillation, or rinse

Povidone-iodine (generic, Betadine)
Topical: available in many forms, including aerosol, ointment, antiseptic gauze pads, skin cleanser (liquid or foam), solution, and swabsticks

Silver protein (Argyrol S.S. 10%)
Topical: 10% solution

Thimerosal (generic, Merthiolate, Mersol)
Topical: 1:1000 tincture and solution

REFERENCES

Block SS: *Disinfection, Sterilization and Preservation,* 4th ed. Lea & Febiger 1991.

Brecx M et al: Efficacy of Listerine, Meridol and chlorhexidine mouth rinses on plaque, gingivitis and plaque bacteria vitality. J Clin Periodontol 1990;17:292.

Burman LG et al: Prevention of excess neonatal morbidity associated with group B streptococci by vaginal chlorhexidine disinfection during labor. Lancet 1992;340:65.

Craven DE et al: Pseudobacteremia caused by povidone-iodine solution contaminated with *Pseudomonas cepacia.* N Engl J Med 1981;305:621.

Doebbeling BN et al: Comparative efficacy of alternative hand-washing agents in reducing infections in intensive care units. N Engl J Med 1992;327:88.

Donowitz LG: Handwashing technique in a pediatric intensive care unit. Am J Dis Child 1987;141:683.

Fraser GL, Beaulieu JT: Leukopenia secondary to sulfadiazine silver. JAMA 1979;241:1928.

Gezon HM et al: Control of staphylococcal infections in the newborn through the use of hexachlorophene bathing. Pediatrics 1973;51:331.

Kaul F, Jewett JR: Agents and techniques for disinfection of the skin. Surg Gynecol Obstet 1981;152:677.

Kundsin RB, Walter CW: The surgical scrub: Practical considerations. Arch Surg 1973;107:75.

Larson E: Guidelines for use of topical antimicrobial agents. Am J Infect Dis Control 1988;16:233.

Levine AS, Labuza TP, Morley JE: Food technology. N Engl J Med 1985;312:628.

Martin-Bouyer G et al: Outbreak of accidental hexachlorophene poisoning in France. Lancet 1982;1:91.

Peterson AF, Rosenberg A, Alatary SD: Comparative evaluation of surgical scrub preparations. Surg Gynecol Obstet 1978;146:63.

Prince AM et al: Beta-propiolactone/ultraviolet irradiation: A review of its effectiveness for inactivation of viruses in blood derivatives. Rev Infect Dis 1983;5:92.

Russell AD, Hugo WB, Ayliffe GAJ (editors): *Principles and Practice of Disinfection, Preservation and Sterilization.* Blackwell Scientific, 1982.

Taplin D et al: Malathion for treatment of *Pediculus humanus* var capitis infestation. JAMA 1982;247:3103.

Viljanto J: Disinfection of surgical wounds without inhibition of normal wound healing. Arch Surg 1980;115:253.

52

Clinical Use of Antimicrobials

Steven L. Barriere, PharmD, & Richard A. Jacobs, MD

The development of antimicrobial drugs represents one of the most important advances in therapeutics, as effective treatment of serious infections has improved the quality of life and has permitted advances in many other areas of medicine. For example, cancer chemotherapy, organ transplantation, and major surgery (especially involving insertion of prosthetic devices) are almost entirely dependent on the availability of antimicrobials. It is fortunate that most antimicrobials are relatively nontoxic; however, all have adverse effects (eg, allergic reactions, toxic effects, or effects on the normal bacterial flora) that may be troublesome or even life-threatening. Thus, as with all forms of drug therapy, good clinical judgment and overall management are important to optimal patient care.

EMPIRIC ANTIMICROBIAL THERAPY

In many clinical situations in which antimicrobials are used, the pathogen causing the disease is not known at the time therapy is initiated—or, if the pathogen is known, its susceptibility to specific antimicrobials is unknown. This use of antimicrobials constitutes empiric therapy (also called presumptive therapy)—ie, therapy initiated on the presumption of infection based on broad experience with similar clinical situations rather than on specific information about a given patient's disease. The principal justification for empiric therapy is that infections are best treated early. To withhold antimicrobials until the results of cultures and susceptibility testing are available (generally 1–3 days) may expose the patient to risk of serious morbidity or death. There are many clinical circumstances in which this is true—eg, a severely neutropenic patient who develops evidence of infection may die within a few hours if effective therapy is not begun. On the other hand, clinicians must also be cognizant of the many circumstances in which empiric therapy is unnecessary, so that antimicrobials can be withheld pending culture and susceptibility testing. For example, antimicrobial therapy of presumed subacute infective endocarditis should be withheld until several blood cultures have been obtained over a period of 24 hours to improve the likelihood of recovering a pathogen. However, if the patient is hemodynamically unstable or cardiopulmonary function is deteriorating, blood cultures from two sites should be obtained rapidly, antimicrobial therapy instituted promptly, and consideration given to surgery for valve replacement. Empiric therapy has two main disadvantages: (1) If the patient proves not to have an infection, the expense and possible toxicity of antimicrobial drug administration have not been justified; and (2) if proper specimens for diagnosis are not obtained initially, the patient may improve but the diagnosis may be obscured, thus complicating later decisions about definitive therapy.

Initiation of empiric therapy (and, to a certain extent, all antimicrobial therapy) should conform to a well-defined protocol:

(1) Formulate a clinical diagnosis of microbial infection: Using all available data, the clinician should conclude that there is evidence of infection and should then attempt to determine the anatomic site of infection as closely as possible—eg, pneumonia, cellulitis, septicemia.

(2) Obtain specimens for laboratory examination: Examination of specimens by microscopy (Gram's stain or other methods) may provide reliable information within an hour or so about the microbial pathogen. Culture or other specialized examinations (eg, antigen detection by immunofluorescence or other methods) will provide an etiologic diagnosis within 1 or 2 days in most cases. Blood and material from the site of infection (eg, urine from patients with suspected urinary tract infection; sputum from patients with pneumonia) are commonly obtained.

Specimens for microbiologic diagnosis are best collected *before* administration of antimicrobials, because properly selected antimicrobials should eliminate or suppress the causative organisms, thereby making specific diagnosis impossible. Identification of the causative agent permits refining antimicrobial therapy with reduction of toxicity and cost.

(3) Formulate a microbiologic diagnosis:

Based on the history, physical examination, and immediately available laboratory results (eg, Gram-stained smear of sputum), the clinician should formulate as specific a microbiologic diagnosis as possible. In some instances, this may be quite specific and accurate (eg, a patient with lobar pneumonia with organisms resembling pneumococci in a Gram-stained smear of sputum); in other cases, there may be no clues to a specific bacteriologic diagnosis.

(4) Determine the necessity for empiric therapy: This is a clinical decision based partly on experience. Empiric therapy is indicated when there is a significant risk of serious morbidity if the infection is allowed to continue untreated for the time required for the laboratory to identify the causative agent and to determine its antimicrobial susceptibility pattern (usually 1–3 days). Rapid identification and susceptibility testing systems have become available that may significantly reduce this interval.

(5) Institute treatment: Selection of empiric therapy may be based on microbiologic diagnosis, where antimicrobial susceptibility data are lacking (eg, based on a Gram-stained smear or preliminary culture result); on a clinical diagnosis without further microbiologic information (eg, cellulitis, meningitis, pneumonia); or on a combination of the two. If no microbiologic information is available, the antimicrobial spectrum of the drugs chosen must necessarily be broader than if some information about the pathogen is known.

The selection of an antimicrobial agent based on a presumed etiology is not an exact science. Selection from among several potentially active agents is dependent upon host factors, pharmacologic factors, local microbiologic patterns, and prescriber preference. Host factors include prior adverse drug effects, elimination or detoxification capacity (usually dependent upon renal or hepatic function), metabolic or genetic disorders predisposing to drug toxicity (eg, glucose-6-phosphate dehydrogenase deficiency), potential drug interactions resulting from other drug therapy, age of the patient, and pregnancy. Pharmacologic factors include the kinetics of absorption, distribution, and elimination, the route of elimination, ability of the drug to penetrate to the site of infection, and the potential toxicities of the drug. Local microbiologic patterns include knowledge of the organisms and the antimicrobial sensitivities that are prevalent in a given setting (eg, methicillin-resistant *S aureus* or multidrug-resistant gram-negative organisms may be common causes of nosocomial infection). Finally, increasing consideration is being given to the cost of antimicrobial therapy.

Brief guides to empiric therapy based on presumptive microbial diagnosis and site of infection are given in Tables 52–1 and 52–2.

A number of clinical situations may warrant further modification of empiric therapeutic regimens. For example, in the severely leukopenic patient, two drugs (usually an extended-spectrum penicillin with an aminoglycoside) are often used in combination. Serious gram-negative infections in these patients may respond poorly even when two drugs are used; in addition, the variety of pathogens observed is great enough to warrant broad-spectrum coverage.

ANTIMICROBIAL THERAPY OF ESTABLISHED INFECTIONS

INTERPRETATION OF CULTURE RESULTS

Properly obtained and processed specimens for culture frequently yield reliable information about the cause of infection. In some instances, organisms responsible for causing an infection may not be grown in culture. Reasons for this include sampling errors (eg, sending the wrong material for culture); obtaining cultures after antimicrobial agents have been initiated; infections caused by fastidious (eg, nutritionally deficient streptococci), noncultivable (eg, *Treponema pallidum,* rickettsiae) or slow-growing organisms (eg, *Brucella, Cardiobacterium hominis*) where cultures are discarded before they become positive; not requesting that appropriate cultures be done (eg, requesting bacterial cultures when infection is due to mycobacteria or fungi); or not requesting that special media be used (eg, CYE medium to isolate *Legionella*). Similarly, cultures may be positive for organisms that are *not* responsible for infection. This may occur if a specimen is contaminated during collection or during processing in the laboratory but most commonly occurs when specimens from non-sterile sites (eg, sputum, skin) are sent for culture and organisms that normally colonize these sites are grown. Performing semiquantitative cultures may be helpful in this latter instance, because finding large numbers of a pathogen (especially with little of the normal flora) is evidence against the organism being a commensal. Likewise, microscopic examination of stained specimens will be helpful because the presence of leukocytes and a single type of organism favors its role as a pathogen.

GUIDING ANTIMICROBIAL THERAPY OF ESTABLISHED INFECTION

Susceptibility Testing

Testing pathogens for their susceptibility to antimicrobials is a commonplace clinical procedure. Tests measure the concentration of drug required to inhibit growth of the organism (**minimum inhibitory con-**

Table 52–1. Empiric antimicrobial therapy based on microbiologic etiology.

Suspected or Proved Disease or Pathogen	Drug(s) of First Choice	Alternative Drug(s)
Gram-negative cocci (aerobic)		
Gonococcus	Penicillin (parenteral only),[1] ampicillin,[2] ceftriaxone[3]	Cefoxitin,[3] cefotetan,[3] fluoroquinolone
Meningococcus	Penicillin,[1] ampicillin	Chloramphenicol, cefuroxime,[3] cefotaxime[3]
Gram-positive cocci (aerobic)		
Pneumococcus	Penicillin[1]	Erythromycin, cephalosporin[4]
Streptococcus, hemolytic groups A, B, C, G	Penicillin[1]	Erythromycin, cephalosporin[4]
Viridans streptococci	Penicillin[1] (? plus aminoglycoside)	Cephalosporin,[4] vancomycin
Staphylococcus, nonpenicillinase-producing	Pencillin[1]	Cephalosporin,[4] vancomycin
Staphylococcus, penicillinase-producing	Penicillinase-resistant penicillin[5]	Vancomycin, cephalosporin[4]
Staphylococcus, methicillin-resistant	Vancomycin	TMP-SMZ[6] or fluoroquinolone (? plus rifampin)
Enterococcus faecalis	Ampicillin or penicillin plus gentamicin	Vancomycin plus gentamicin
Gram-negative rods (aerobic)		
Coliforms (*E coli, Klebsiella, Proteus*)	Aminoglycoside,[7] third-generation cephalosporin[8]	TMP-SMZ,[6] extended-spectrum penicillin,[9] ciprofloxacin
Enterobacter, Citrobacter, Serratia	Imipenem, fluoroquinolone	TMP-SMZ,[6] extended-spectrum penicillin,[9] aminoglycoside[7]
Shigella	Fluoroquinolones	TMP-SMZ,[6] ampicillin[2]
Salmonella	TMP-SMZ,[6] ciprofloxacin	Chloramphenicol, ampicillin[2]
Haemophilus sp	Cefuroxime,[3] third-generation cephalosporin[8]	TMP-SMZ,[6] ampicillin,[2] chloramphenicol, clarithromycin
Brucella	Tetracycline[10]	Streptomycin plus sulfonamide[11]
Helicobacter sp	Metronidazole	Amoxicillin, tetracycline[10]
Yersinia pestis (plague), *Francisella tularensis* (tularemia)	Tetracycline[10] (? plus streptomycin)	Chloramphenicol, streptomycin, or other aminoglycoside
Vibrio sp	Tetracycline,[10] TMP-SMZ[6]	Ciprofloxacin
Pseudomonas aeruginosa	Aminoglycoside[7] plus extended-spectrum penicillin[9]	Ceftazidime, aztreonam, imipenem ± aminoglycoside; ciprofloxacin ± beta-lactam
Pseudomonas pseudomallei (melioidosis), *Pseudomonas mallei* (glanders)	Tetracycline[10] (? plus streptomycin)	Chloramphenicol
Legionella sp	Erythromycin (? plus rifampin)	TMP-SMZ,[6] fluoroquinolone
Gram-positive rods (aerobic)		
Bacillus sp (eg, anthrax)	Penicillin[1]	Erythromycin, vancomycin
Listeria monocytogenes	Ampicillin[2] (? plus aminoglycoside)	Chloramphenicol, TMP-SMZ[6]
Nocardia	Sulfonamide[11]	Minocycline, TMP-SMZ[6]
Anaerobes		
Gram-positive (peptococci, peptostreptococci, clostridia, etc)	Penicillin[1]	Clindamycin, tetracycline,[10] cephalosporin,[4] cefoxitin
Bacteroides fragilis (some *B bivius* and *B melaninogenicus*)	Metronidazole or clindamycin	Chloramphenicol, imipenem, ampicillin/sulbactam, ticarcillin/clavulanate
Gram-negatives other than *B fragilis* (*Bacteroides, Fusobacterium*)	Penicillin,[1] metronidazole	Clindamycin, tetracycline,[10] cephalosporin,[4] cefoxitin[3]
Mycobacteria		
Mycobacterium tuberculosis	Isoniazid (INH) plus rifampin plus pyrazinamide	Streptomycin, ethambutol, others
Mycobacterium leprae	Dapsone plus rifampin	Clofazimine

(continued)

Table 52–1 (cont'd). Empiric antimicrobial therapy based on microbiologic etiology.

Suspected or Proved Disease or Pathogen	Drug(s) of First Choice	Alternative Drug(s)
Spirochetes		
Borrelia (relapsing fever)	Tetracycline[10]	Penicillin
Borrelia (Lyme disease)	Tetracycline[10] (early), ceftriaxone[3] (neurologic)	Amoxicillin, doxycycline, chloramphenicol
Leptospira	Penicillin[1]	Tetracycline
Treponema (syphilis, yaws)	Penicillin[1]	Erythromycin, tetracycline[10]
Mycoplasma pneumoniae	Tetracycline[10]	Erythromycin, ciprofloxacin
Chlamydia trachomatis, Chlamydia psittaci	Tetracycline[10]	Erythromycin
Rickettsiae	Tetracycline[10]	Chloramphenicol
Fungi		
Candida sp, *Torulopsis*	Amphotericin B	Fluconazole, ketoconazole,[12] flucytosine
Cryptococcus neoformans	Amphotericin B plus flucytosine	Fluconazole
Coccidioidomycosis	Amphotericin B	Fluconazole, itraconazole
Histoplasmosis	Itraconazole	Amphotericin B, ketoconazole[12]
Blastomycosis	Itraconazole	Amphotericin B, ketoconazole[12]
Paracoccidioidomycosis	Ketoconazole[12]	Amphotericin B
Sporotrichosis	Itraconazole	Amphotericin B, ketoconazole[12]
Aspergillosis, mucormycosis	Amphotericin B	Itraconazole

[1]Penicillin G is preferred for parenteral injection; penicillin V for oral administration. Only very susceptible microorganisms should be treated with oral penicillin.

[2]Amoxicillin or ampicillin; ampicillin esters (eg, hetacillin, bacampicillin) and cyclacillin offer no advantages. Amoxicillin is also available with potassium clavulanate as Augmentin.

[3]Effective against beta-lactamase-producing strains.

[4]First-generation cephalosporin; cephalothin, cephapirin, or cefazolin for parenteral administration; cephalexin or cephradine for oral administration.

[5]Parenteral nafcillin, oxacillin, or methicillin. Oral dicloxacillin, cloxacillin, or oxacillin.

[6]Trimethoprim-sulfamethoxazole (TMP-SMZ) is a mixture of 1 part trimethoprim plus 5 parts sulfamethoxazole.

[7]Gentamicin, tobramycin, netilmicin, or amikacin. Kanamycin can be used for some organisms other than *Pseudomonas* sp; streptomycin should be used only for drug-susceptible strains of *M tuberculosis* and streptococci (with penicillin or ampicillin).

[8]Cefotaxime, cefoperazone, ceftizoxime, ceftriaxone, or ceftazidime. Cefoperazone is not effective for meningitis.

[9]Extended-spectrum penicillins: ticarcillin, mezlocillin, piperacillin, or azlocillin.

[10]All tetracyclines have similar activity against microorganisms (with rare exceptions) and comparable therapeutic activity and toxicity. Dosage is determined by the rates of absorption and excretion of different preparations. Doxycycline is generally easier to administer parenterally and is more convenient to give orally (although more expensive).

[11]For oral administration trisulfapyrimidines have the advantage over sulfadiazine of greater solubility in urine; sodium sulfadiazine is suitable for intravenous injection in severely ill persons.

[12]Ketoconazole does not penetrate the central nervous system and is unsatisfactory for meningitis.

centration, MIC) or to kill the organism (**minimum lethal concentration, MLC;** with bacteria, often also called **minimum bactericidal concentration, MBC).** The results of these tests may then be compared with known drug concentrations in various body compartments and with studies correlating clinical outcome with MIC or MLC to determine whether the organism should be considered sensitive or resistant. Only MICs are routinely measured in most laboratories, as this value is adequate basis for treatment of most infections.

Two methods of susceptibility testing in common use are the disk (agar) diffusion or Kirby-Bauer method and the broth dilution method. In the **disk diffusion method,** a disk containing a standardized amount of the test antimicrobial is placed on an agar plate lightly seeded with the test bacteria. The bacteria are then allowed to grow under carefully controlled conditions while the antibiotic diffuses out into the agar. The diameter of the zone of inhibition correlates with MIC, although zone sizes are not comparable from one drug to another. In the **broth dilution method,** the bacteria are inoculated into liquid medium containing graduated concentrations of the test antimicrobial for direct determination of the MIC.

Disk diffusion methods are satisfactory for determining susceptibility of many antimicrobial-organism combinations, and they are all that is required when the susceptibility pattern of the organism is bimodal (ie, very susceptible or very resistant, with few intermediate cases), as is seen with the susceptibility of *S aureus* to penicillin G. However, when there is

Table 52–2. Empiric antimicrobial therapy based on site of infection.

Presumed Site of Infection	Common Pathogens	Drug(s) of First Choice	Alternative Drug(s)
Bacterial endocarditis Acute	Staphylococci, streptococci, aerobic gram-negative rods	PRP[1] plus gentamicin	Vancomycin plus gentamicin
Subacute	Viridans streptococci, enterococci	Penicillin plus gentamicin	Vancomycin plus gentamicin
Hematogenous osteomyelitis	S aureus	PRP[1]	Clindamycin, vancomycin
Septic arthritis Child	H influenzae, S aureus, streptococci	Cefuroxime, third-generation cephalosporin[3]	Ampicillin-sulbactam
Adult	N gonorrhoeae, S aureus, streptococci	Cefuroxime, third-generation cephalosporin[3]	Ampicillin-sulbactam
Cystitis	E coli, P mirabilis, S saprophyticus	Sulfonamide, ampicillin	TMP-SMZ, fluoroquinolone[2]
Pyelonephritis	Coliforms	TMP-SMZ	Third-generation cephalosporin,[3] aminoglycoside,[4] fluoroquinolone[2]
Otitis media and sinusitis	H influenzae, streptococci	Amoxicillin, ampicillin	Erythromycin plus sulfonamide, TMP-SMZ, amoxicillin-clavulanic acid, oral cephalosporin[5]
Bronchitis (bacterial)	H influenzae, pneumococci	Erythromycin or newer macrolide	Ampicillin, TMP-SMZ
Pneumonia (bacterial)[6] Neonate	Group B streptococci, E coli, Listeria	Ampicillin plus aminoglycoside[4]	Chloramphenicol; ampicillin plus third-generation cephalosporin[3]
Child	Pneumococci, S aureus H influenzae	Cefuroxime, cefotaxime	Ampicillin-sulbactam
Adult	Pneumococci, Klebsiella, S aureus	Cephalosporin,[3] cefuroxime	Ampicillin-sulbactam
Cellulitis	Group A streptococci	Penicillin	Cephalosporin
Abscess with cellulitis	Staphylococci	PRP[1] or ampicillin-sulbactam	Clindamycin
Meningitis Neonate	Group B streptococci, E coli, Listeria	Ampicillin plus aminoglycoside[4]	Chloramphenicol; ampicillin plus third-generation cephalosporin[3]
Child	H influenzae, pneumococci, meningococci	Cefotaxime, ceftriaxone	Cefuroxime, chloramphenicol
Adult	Pneumococci, meningococci	Penicillin	Third-generation cephalosporin[3]
Peritonitis due to ruptured viscus	Coliforms, B fragilis, streptococci	Ampicillin-sulbactam, ticarcillin-clavulanate, imipenem	Clindamycin plus third-generation cephalosporin[3]
Septicemia	Any	Third-generation cephalosporin[3] (? plus aminoglycoside[4])	Clindamycin plus aminoglycoside,[4] extended-spectrum penicillin[7]
Septicemia with granulocytopenia	Any (anaerobes are uncommon)	Extended-spectrum penicillin[7] plus aminoglycoside[4] or imipenem	Third-generation cephalosporin[3] plus aminoglycoside[4]

[1]PRP = penicillinase-resistant penicillin, eg, nafcillin, oxacillin.
[2]Ciprofloxacin, ofloxacin, lomefloxacin.
[3]Cefotaxime, cefoperazone, ceftizoxime, ceftriaxone, or ceftazidime. Cefoperazone cannot be used for meningitis.
[4]Gentamicin, tobramycin, netilmicin, or amikacin.
[5]Cefprozil, loracarbef, cefixime, cefpodoxime proxetil, cefuroxime axetil.
[6]Pneumonia may be caused by many different agents, and selection of empiric therapy is complex. Consult more specialized texts for specifics (see References).
[7]Extended-spectrum penicillins: ticarcillin, piperacillin, or mezlocillin.

no sharp dividing line between susceptible and resistant, determination of the MIC may be very helpful for guiding therapy.

The results of laboratory susceptibility testing generally correlate well with clinical response. However, infected patients given antimicrobials shown to be ineffective by in vitro tests may still recover satisfactorily. Host defense mechanisms may be sufficient to permit recovery in many cases, and there is ample evidence that subinhibitory concentrations of antimicrobials may have beneficial effects—eg, enhancing ingestion and killing of bacteria by phagocytes.

Drug Concentrations in Body Fluids

For most antimicrobials, the relationship of dose to resulting body fluid concentrations is well established, and the therapeutic index of most antimicrobials is high enough so that measurement of antimicrobial concentrations in body fluids is rarely necessary. Exceptions are antimicrobials with a low therapeutic index (eg, vancomycin, aminoglycosides), administration of the antimicrobial by an unreliable route for a serious infection (oral therapy), investigation of clinical failure of apparently adequate antimicrobial therapy, and determination of drug concentrations in unusual sites (eg, central nervous system; see Table 52–3).

There are several ways in which antimicrobial concentrations can be determined. The most generally applicable method is bioassay, because it can be modified for use with any antimicrobial drug. In this method, the degree of growth inhibition of a standard organism by the clinical specimen is compared with that produced by several known concentrations of drug, and the concentration in the clinical specimen is determined by interpolation. For antimicrobials such as the aminoglycosides and vancomycin, where drug concentrations are determined frequently, a variety of automated assay methods have been developed that are not different in principle from those used to measure other drugs.

Serum Bactericidal Titers

In many infectious disorders (eg, soft tissue infections, pneumonias, enteritis), host defenses contribute materially to cure. In these conditions, drugs that merely inhibit the growth of the pathogen are often sufficient for successful treatment. In other disorders (infective endocarditis, bacteremia in the immunosuppressed host, bacterial meningitis), host defenses may contribute minimally to cure. Consequently, bactericidal drug concentrations must be achieved in the infected tissue. An assay of the titer of inhibitory as well as bactericidal activity in body fluids may be performed and will establish both susceptibility of the pathogen and adequacy of drug dosage and absorption in one simple test procedure. Serum is obtained from the patient at the appropriate time after the last dose of drug, and serial dilutions of serum are incubated with a standardized amount of the pathogen recovered from the patient. Growth inhibition and killing at a serum dilution (titer) of 1:8 or more is generally considered to be satisfactory, though the data supporting this figure are conflicting. Although

Table 52–3. Penetration of selected antimicrobials into cerebrospinal fluid (CSF).

Antimicrobial	Dosage	Reported concentration in CSF (Inflamed Meninges) (µg/mL)	Plasma Concentration (µg/mL)
Amikacin	15 mg/kg/d	0.8–9.2	5–20
Ampicillin	150–300 mg/kg/d	2–60	16–250
Aztreonam	2 g/d	0.2–8.1	10–107
Cefotaxime	30–150 mg/kg/d	0.3–27	40–100
Ceftazidime	2–3 g/d	3–56	13–100
Ceftriaxone	100 mg/kg/d	0.3–42	30–260
Cefuroxime	200 mg/kg/d	1–17	60–100
Chloramphenicol	25–100 mg/kg/d	3–40	10–128
Ciprofloxacin	400–500 mg/d	0.3–0.4	1.6–2.4
Gentamicin	2–7.5 mg/kg/d	0.5–2	0.7–7
Imipenem	100 mg/kg/d	0.7–10	0.6–27
Nafcillin	150–200 mg/kg/d	2.7–88	36–176
Penicillin G	$2-3 \times 10^5$ units/kg/d	1.7–46	12–740
Sulfamethoxazole	25–50 mg/kg/d	5–40	40–85
Tobramycin	3–4.5 mg/kg/d	0.5–0.9	0.9–6.5
Trimethoprim	5–10 mg/kg/d	0.2–2.4	1.7–3.5
Vancomycin	20–30 mg/kg/d	0.1–8.5	1.4–30

this assay is not fully standardized, it is simple to perform and is useful for confirming choice of antimicrobial and dosage. It is also helpful where *bactericidal* antimicrobials are needed and where antimicrobial combinations are being studied for possible synergism (see below).

Specialized Assay Methods

A. Beta-Lactamase Assay: For some bacteria (eg, gonococci, enterococci, *Haemophilus influenzae*), the susceptibility patterns of all strains are similar except for production of beta-lactamase, which confers resistance to various beta-lactam antimicrobials. In these cases, extensive susceptibility testing may be omitted and a direct test for beta-lactamase done utilizing a chromogenic beta-lactam substrate. This test is sensitive, specific, rapid, and reliable.

B. Synergy Studies: These in vitro tests attempt to measure synergistic, additive, indifferent, or antagonistic drug interactions in vitro. The methods are not standardized and in general have not been correlated with clinical outcome. See section on combination chemotherapy for details.

Selection of Route of Administration

Parenteral therapy is generally preferred for acutely ill patients and when sustained high levels of drug are required for successful therapy (eg, central nervous system syphilis). The choice of intravenous over intramuscular administration is primarily determined by the drug preparations available. A few agents have such reliable oral absorption that parenteral therapy may not be required (eg, chloramphenicol, rifampin, trimethoprim-sulfamethoxazole, metronidazole, fluoroquinolones); however, for other agents, oral therapy is best reserved for mild to moderate infections or for definitive treatment of serious infections in situations where absorption is documented (eg, by drug levels or serum bactericidal titers).

Monitoring Therapeutic Response; Duration of Therapy

The therapeutic response should be monitored both microbiologically and clinically. Cultures of specimens taken from infected sites should show progressively smaller numbers of the pathogen during therapy and should eventually become sterile. Monitoring of cultures is also useful for detecting superinfections or the development of resistance (see below). Clinically, the patient's general manifestations of infection (malaise, fever, leukocytosis, etc) should improve and the specific findings also should abate (eg, clearing of x-ray infiltrates in pneumonia). The speed of clinical response to antimicrobial therapy is generally inversely proportionate to the duration of the illness prior to therapy.

The duration of therapy required for cure depends on the pathogen (bacterial infections are cured with shorter courses of therapy than fungal or mycobacterial infections), the site of infection (endocarditis and osteomyelitis require longer courses of therapy than infections of other organ systems), and host factors (immunocompromised patients are generally treated longer than immunocompetent individuals); precise data on duration of therapy are available for a few infections, eg, streptococcal pharyngitis, cystitis, syphilis, gonorrhea, and tuberculosis. In many other situations, duration of therapy is determined empirically. For serious infections, continuing therapy for 7–10 days after the patient has become afebrile or cultures have become negative is a useful general rule. An important exception is the patient with endocarditis or osteomyelitis, who must receive therapy for a minimum of 6 weeks.

Management of Antimicrobial Drug Toxicity

Because of the large number of antimicrobials available, when drug toxicity occurs it can often be managed by substitution of another drug with equivalent efficacy (Table 52–1). In the rare cases where this is not possible, continuing the drug while simultaneously treating the adverse reaction may be possible, though it is associated with some risk. For example, *Clostridium difficile* colitis induced by antimicrobials may be managed by oral administration of vancomycin, metronidazole, or bacitracin without discontinuing the inducing drug. In addition, some types of drug toxicity (eg, drug fever) may be confused with manifestations of the infection.

Allergic reactions to antimicrobials are common, and management is complex. In the presence of preexisting drug allergy, one should avoid the suspect drug and select a substitute (see Tables 52–1 and 52–2); in virtually every instance, the alternative drugs are of equivalent efficacy. If the patient has a history of a life-threatening reaction to an antimicrobial (eg, anaphylaxis, toxic epidermal necrolysis), all related drugs should probably be avoided. Thus, in the patient with a clear history of anaphylaxis to penicillin, all beta-lactam antimicrobials are best avoided with the possible exception of aztreonam. If there is a commanding need for penicillin treatment of the patient with a history of anaphylactic penicillin reaction, desensitization may be attempted (Wendel, 1985).

Clinical Failure of Antimicrobial Drug Therapy

When the patient has an inadequate clinical or microbiologic response to antimicrobial therapy selected by in vitro susceptibility testing, systematic investigation should be undertaken to determine the cause of the problem (Table 52–4). Errors in susceptibility testing are rare, but the original results should be confirmed by repeated testing. Drug dosing and absorption should be scrutinized and tested directly

Table 52–4. Common causes of failure of antimicrobial therapy.

Drug
  Inappropriate drug.
  Inadequate dose.
  Improper route of administration.
  Malabsorption.
  Accelerated drug excretion or inactivation.
  Poor penetration of drug into a privileged site of infection (eg, brain, eye, prostate).
Host
  Poor host defenses (granulocytopenia, leukopenia, AIDS, etc).
  Undrained pus (eg, abscess).
  Retained infected foreign body.
  Dead tissue (eg, sequestrum).
Pathogen
  Development of drug resistance.
  Superinfection by other pathogens.
  Dual infection initially—only one of the pathogens detected and treated.
Laboratory
  Erroneous report of susceptible pathogen.

with serum drug concentrations or a serum bactericidal titer. However, drug pharmacology problems rarely account for clinical failures.

The clinical data should be reviewed to make certain the patient's host defenses are adequate (adequate numbers of granulocytes, etc) and that there are no abscesses requiring drainage or infected foreign bodies that need to be removed. If the patient has responded well to therapy except for persistence of fever, drug fever should be considered. Lastly, repeat cultures and susceptibility testing should be performed to determine if superinfection has occurred with another organism or if the original pathogen has developed drug resistance.

Adjunctive Measures in the Treatment of Infection

A. Surgery: It is often necessary to drain abscesses, remove foreign bodies, and close persistent sources of contamination (eg, perforated bowel). Although one is often tempted to delay surgery until the patient's systemic symptoms ("toxicity") have abated, in many cases the patient will remain ill until essential surgery is performed. On the other hand, if the patient is improving and particularly if diagnostic tests (eg, ultrasonography, CT scanning) show shrinkage of an abscess, surgery may be postponed. Likewise, some abscesses can be drained by percutaneous needle or catheter under sonographic or CT guidance, thus avoiding an extensive surgical procedure.

B. Management of Fever: Antipyretic drugs should be used to keep the temperature below dangerous levels (40.5 °C [105 °F] in most adults; 39.5 °C [103.2 °F] in children, especially those with a history of febrile seizures) and to make the patient comfortable. If fever is not troublesome and is below danger-

ous levels, antipyretics are not indicated. Do not be concerned about "masking" the infection with antipyretics. In most cases of infection, antipyretic agents will lower the temperature, but some degree of fever will persist as long as the infection is active.

Antipyretics should be administered on a regular basis (usually every 4 hours), *not* given only for an elevated temperature. Intermittent administration produces wide swings in body temperature, making the patient more uncomfortable than if antipyretic drugs were not given.

C. General Supportive Measures: Rest and proper diet will improve the patient's sense of well-being. Aside from correction of obvious malnutrition, however, there is little evidence that such measures are important for recovery from a short illness if adequate antimicrobial therapy has been given.

Correction of host abnormalities associated with infection is an essential component of therapy of infectious diseases. Respiration and circulation must be supported and electrolyte and acid-base disturbances should be corrected. The role of monoclonal antibodies to core glycolipid (endotoxin) in the therapy of gram-negative sepsis and shock remains under investigation. Interleukin-1 receptor antagonist, a protein that prevents interleukin-1 from binding to its receptors, also may prove to be beneficial in the therapy of severe sepsis. Other therapies directed at steps in the inflammatory cascade are also under investigation.

CONDITIONS ALTERING ANTIMICROBIAL PHARMACOLOGY

Diseases of the major excretory organs as well as physiologic states such as infancy or pregnancy alter the disposition of antimicrobials along with other drugs. Some of these changes are shown in Table 52–5. See also Chapter 61. A variety of other clinical states (puerperium, burns, cystic fibrosis) are known to alter antimicrobial pharmacokinetics; thus, measures of adequate dosing (drug concentrations or serum bactericidal titers) are advisable in patients with serious infections and significant underlying disease.

ANTIMICROBIAL DRUG INTERACTIONS

Like other classes of drugs, antimicrobials may interact with other medication being given to the patient, with possible adverse results. Some antimicrobial drug interactions of clinical importance are reviewed in Appendix II. In addition to the interac-

Table 52–5. Antimicrobial pharmacokinetics in renal failure and during dialysis.

Drug	Drug Elimination by Indicated Route (percent)		Approximate Elimination Half-Life (hours)		Dosage Regimen[1]		
					Anuria[2]		
	Renal	Hepatic	Normal	Anuria	Initial Dose	Maintenance	Dialysis[3]
Acyclovir	30–75	...	2–5	Prolonged	5 mg/kg	2.5 mg/kg every 24 h	2.5 mg/kg after HD
Amantadine	90	...	8–18	Prolonged	100 mg	Significant reduction	No change
Amikacin	95–98	...	2.5	60–90	7.5 mg/kg	See footnote 4.	See footnote 5.
Amphotericin B	4–5	5–10	360	Same	No change	No change	No change
Ampicillin	75–90	5–10	0.8–1.5	8–12	3 g	1 g every 6 h	0.5 g after HD
Azithromycin	20	35	120	...	No change	No change	...
Aztreonam	60–70	10–20	1.7	6	1–2 g	0.5–1 g every 6–8 h	0.25–0.5 g after HD
Cefamandole	90–95	5–10	0.8–1	15–24	2 g	1 g every 12 h	0.5 g after HD
Cefazolin	95–98	2–5	1.4	35–56	1 g	0.5 g every 24 h	0.5 g after HD
Cefonicid	95	...	4.5	48–72	2 g	0.25 g twice weekly	No change
Cefoperazone	25	75	2	2	No change	No change	No change
Cefotaxime	40–60	...	0.8–1	3–4	2 g	1 g every 6 h	0.5 g after HD
Cefotetan	50–70	...	3.5	20–35	1–2 g	0.5–1 g every 24 h	0.25 to 0.5 g
Cefoxitin	90	...	0.5–1	8–30	2 g	1 g every 12 h	0.5 g after HD
Ceftazidime	60–90	...	1.9	26–36	1–2 g	1 g every 24 h	0.5 g after HD
Ceftizoxime	95	5–10	1.3	36	1–2 g	1 g every 24 h	0.5 g after HD
Ceftriaxone	40–50	10–60	8	10–12	1 g	No change	No change
Cefuroxime	90–95	...	1.3	15	1.5 g	0.75 g every 12 h	0.75 g after HD
Cephalexin, cephradine	80–95	5–10	0.8–2	20–30	0.5 g	0.5 g every 24 h	0.25 g after HD
Cephalothin, cephapirin	40–60	...	1	3	2 g	1 g every 8 h	0.5 g after HD. Add to PD in desired serum concentration.
Chloramphenicol	5–10	...	2–4	4–6	No change	No change	0.25 g after HD
Ciprofloxacin	50–70	20	4	8	No change	Decrease by 50%	No change
Clarithromycin	30	> 50	3–4	15	500 mg	250 mg	No change
Clindamycin	15	...	2–4	4–6	No change	No change	No change
Doxycycline	20–50	...	15–24	Same	No change	No change	No change
Erythromycin	5–15	...	1.5–3	4–6	No change	No change	No change
Ethambutol	65–80	...	3–4	18–20	15 mg/kg	5 mg/kg every 24 h	5 mg/kg after HD or PD
Fluconazole	80	10	22–31	100	100–400 mg	50–200 mg every 48 h	50–100 mg after HD
Flucytosine	85–90	...	3–6	60–80	30 mg/kg	25 mg/kg every 24 h	15 mg/kg after HD
Foscarnet	>90	...	3–8	...	90–120 mg/kg	Insufficient data	Insufficient data
Ganciclovir	90	10	2.5	28–30	5 mg/kg	2.5 mg/kg every 24 h	2.5 mg/kg after HD
Gentamicin	95–98	...	2.5	60–80	2 mg/kg	See footnote 4.	See footnote 5.
Griseofulvin	<1	...	10–20	Same	No change	No change	No data
Imipenem	70	10–20	0.9	3	0.5–1 g	0.25–0.5 g every 12 h	0.25 g after HD
Isoniazid	5–35	...	1.5	2.5	No change	No change	No change
			5 (slow acetylators)	10 (slow acetylators)			

[1–6]See footnotes at end of table on following page.

(*continued*)

Table 52–5 (cont'd). Antimicrobial pharmacokinetics in renal failure and during dialysis.

Drug	Drug Elimination by Indicated Route (percent)		Approximate Elimination Half-Life (hours)		Dosage Regimen[1]		
					Anuria[2]		
Drug	Renal	Hepatic	Normal	Anuria	Initial Dose	Maintenance	Dialysis[3]
Itraconazole	20	>50	21	25	No change	No change	No change
Ketoconazole	<5	50	4–8	Same	No change	No change	No data
Lomefloxacin	65	. . .	10–12	25	400 mg	200 mg	No change
Metronidazole	30–40	. . .	6–14	8–15	Active metabolite may accumulate: 7.5 mg/kg initially; then 7.5 mg/kg every 12–24 h.		No change
Mezlocillin	40–70	10–20	1	3.5	3 g	2 g every 6 h	2 g after HD
Minocycline	<10	. . .	12–15	14–30	Avoid in renal failure.		No change
Nafcillin	30–50	50–70	0.5	1	No change	No change	No change
Netilmicin	90–95	. . .	2.5	30–40	2.5 mg/kg	See footnote 4.	See footnote 5.
Norfloxacin	30	60	3.5	6	No change	Decrease by 50%	No change
Ofloxacin	75	. . .	6–8	36	400 mg	200 mg	No change
Oxacillin	50	50	0.5	1	No change	No change	No change
Penicillin G	75–90	. . .	0.5	6–20	3 million units	1 million units every 6 h	0.5 million units after HD
Piperacillin	50–90	10–40	1	3–6	3 g	2 g every 8 h	1 g after HD
Rifampin	5–15	80–90	2–3	3–5	No change	No change	No change
Sulfamethoxazole	40–50	. . .	9–11	18–24	See footnote 6.		See footnote 7.
Sulfisoxazole	50	. . .	4.5–7	6–12	15 mg/kg	7.5 mg/kg every 12 h	7.5 mg/kg after HD
Tetracycline	50	20–30	6–12	30–80	Avoid in renal failure.		No change
Ticarcillin	80–90	5–10	1	10–20	3 g	2 g every 12 h	2 g after HD
Tobramycin	95–98	. . .	2.5	60–80	2 mg/kg	See footnote 4.	See footnote 5.
Trimethoprim	65–80	. . .	10–12	24–36	See footnote 6.		See footnote 7.
Vancomycin	95	. . .	4–9	200–240	15 mg/kg	7.5 mg/kg once weekly.[8]	No change
Vidarabine	40–50	. . .	3–4	. . .	Daily dose should be decreased by 25%		5 mg/kg after HD

[1]Dosages shown are for an average adult (70 kg) with a serious infection.
[2]Creatinine clearance less than 5 mL/min.
[3]HD = hemodialysis; PD = peritoneal dialysis.
[4]One-half of initial dose may be given every estimated half-life for maintenance. Serum levels should be monitored.
[5]One-half of initial dose after HD. Add to PD in desired serum concentration.
[6]Daily dose should be decreased to 25% of usual dose.
[7]One-half of daily maintenance doses should be given after HD.
[8]Serum levels should be monitored.

tions listed in Chapter 33, virtually all broad-spectrum antimicrobials (other than rifampin) enhance the effect of coumarin anticoagulants. Likewise, inhibition of bacterial sterol biotransformation by antimicrobial agents may decrease blood levels of contraceptive medication following oral administration, resulting in increased risk of pregnancy in women taking birth control pills.

ANTIMICROBIAL DRUG COMBINATIONS

Possible Indications for Therapy With Multiple Antimicrobials (Table 52–6)

(1) In certain desperately ill patients with suspected infections of unknown origin, it may be desir-

Table 52–6. Some examples of clinically used antimicrobial combinations and their justification.

Indication	Drug Combination	Justification
Empiric therapy of various conditions (see Table 52–2)	Various	Expanded spectrum compared with single agent.
Pseudomonas aeruginosa infections	Beta-lactam plus aminoglycoside	Increased activity (additive or synergistic). Decreased toxicity. Inhibits emergence of resistant strains.
Enterococcal endocarditis	Penicillin or vancomycin plus aminoglycoside	Synergy: converts bacteriostatic drug to bactericidal.
Tuberculosis	Various—especially isoniazid plus rifampin	Inhibits emergence of resistant strains. Accelerated bacterial killing permitting shorter treatment course.
Cryptococcal meningitis	Amphotericin B plus flucytosine	Probably synergy as well as decreased toxicity.
Severely leukopenic patients	Beta-lactam plus aminoglycoside	Increased activity (additive or synergistic). Possibly decreased toxicity.

able to administer more than one antimicrobial drug empirically in an effort to suppress all of the most likely pathogens. Thus, in suspected septicemia, an antistaphylococcal drug (eg, nafcillin) might be combined with a drug having activity against aerobic gram-negative bacilli (gentamicin, tobramycin, or amikacin) until blood cultures yield a specific microorganism (Table 52–2).

(2) In mixed infections, it is possible that two or three drugs may be required to "cover" all of the potential or known pathogens. For example, in peritonitis following perforation of the colon, a drug active against anaerobes and gram-positive bacteria (clindamycin) may be combined with one active against coliforms (an aminoglycoside). However, the availability of beta-lactamase inhibitor combinations (ie, ampicillin/sulbactam, piperacillin/tazobactam, ticarcillin/clavulanate) and imipenem may eliminate the need for such combinations.

(3) In some clinical situations, the rapid emergence of bacteria resistant to one drug may impair the chances for cure. The addition of a second drug may delay or prevent the emergence of resistant strains. This effect has been demonstrated unequivocally in tuberculosis and is the basis for the frequent use of combinations of isoniazid, ethambutol, rifampin, or other drugs in this disease.

(4) The simultaneous use of two drugs may in some situations achieve an effect not obtainable by either drug alone. One drug enhances the antibacterial activity of the second drug against a specific microorganism, eg, the combination of a sulfonamide with trimethoprim. Such an effect can be considered a manifestation of drug synergism. Unfortunately, such synergism is not always predictable: A given combination of drugs must be specifically tailored by laboratory tests to fit a certain strain of a given microorganism. A synopsis of the dynamics of combined antibiotic action is given below. One of the best-established examples of synergism is the cure of infective endocarditis caused by enterococci *(Entero-*

coccus faecalis) by a combination of a penicillin with an aminoglycoside, as compared to the frequent failure of treatment with a penicillin alone.

DYNAMICS OF COMBINED ANTIMICROBIAL DRUG ACTION IN VITRO

Problems in Measuring Antimicrobial Drug Effects

Even when technically feasible, chemical measures of antimicrobial drug concentration may not accurately reflect antibacterial activity. Direct evaluation of bacteriostasis or bactericidal activity is the only useful way of measuring the effects of these drugs. Several methods can be employed, and all may be applicable to the measurement of combined drug action. The results of any one type of examination need not coincide with those of any other type, because the different methods may measure different events in the test system.

A. Bacteriostatic Effect: End points are expressed as the minimum amount of drug necessary to suppress visible growth for a given time.

B. Bactericidal Effect as Shown by Rate of Killing: Results are expressed as the bactericidal rate, ie, the slope of the plot of viable survivors at various time intervals after addition of drug. This is the "time-kill curve" method (Figure 52–1).

C. Bactericidal Effect as Shown by Completeness of Killing: The results are expressed as the smallest concentration of drug resulting in a given number of viable survivors (eg, < 0.1%) in a given time, ie, a bactericidal end point.

D. Curative Effect as Shown in Therapeutic Trials in Vivo: The results are expressed as the smallest drug concentrations measured in patients or experimental animals whose infections are eradicated.

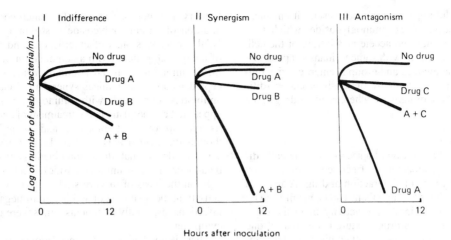

Figure 52–1. Types of combined action of antimicrobial drugs, measuring bactericidal activity by the "time-kill curve" method. *I.* Indifference (A + B = B). *II.* Synergism (A + B > > A or B). *III.* Antagonism (A + C < < A).

OUTCOMES OF COMBINED ANTIMICROBIAL ACTION

The nature of the interaction of two antimicrobial drugs can be judged from the plot of drug activity in Figure 52–1. From the results of measurements (according to any of the methods described in paragraphs A–D, above) with different doses of each drug alone and in combination acting on a given microbial population, it can be determined whether the drugs are additive, synergistic, or antagonistic. These terms can be applied to any specified intensity of bacteriostatic or curative effects as well as to bactericidal effects. Bactericidal action in vitro and in vivo is important, and the three main results that are observed are (1) indifference or additive effect, (2) synergism, and (3) antagonism.

Indifference or Additive Effect

The most common result is indifference. The combined effect of drugs A and B is equal to that of the single more active component of the mixture A + B or is equal to the arithmetic sum of the effects of the individual drugs in their chosen doses. The same total effect could be obtained by the use of a single drug in a dose equivalent to that of the mixture.

Synergism

At times, the simultaneous action of two drugs results in an effect (A + B) far greater than that of either A alone or B alone in much larger dosages and also greater than could be expected from simple addition of individual drug effects.

In at least three types of antimicrobial synergism, the mechanism is fairly well understood (see also Chapter 42):

A. Blocking Successive Steps in a Metabolic Sequence: The best example is the combination of a sulfonamide and trimethoprim. Sulfonamides compete with *p*-aminobenzoic acid, which is required by some bacteria for the synthesis of dihydrofolate. Folate antagonists such as trimethoprim inhibit the enzyme (dihydrofolic acid reductase) that reduces dihydrofolate to tetrahydrofolate. The simultaneous presence of a sulfonamide and trimethoprim results in the simultaneous block of sequential steps leading to the synthesis of purines and nucleic acid and can result in a much more complete inhibition of growth than either component of the mixture alone.

B. One Drug Inhibits an Enzyme That Can Destroy the Second Drug: The best example of this mechanism is the noncompetitive inhibition of beta-lactamase by clavulanic acid or other substances. Organisms that produce beta-lactamase are resistant to the action of penicillin G because the drug is hydrolyzed by the enzyme. However, if the beta-lactamase is inhibited, the penicillin G is protected and can inhibit or kill the microorganism. Combinations of penicillins with clavulanic acid, sulbactam, or tazobactam are available in the USA (see Chapter 43). The combination of imipenem with cilastatin is a special case; cilastatin is necessary to prevent rapid degradation of the active component, imipenem, by dehydropeptidase, an enzyme found in renal tubular cells.

C. One Drug Promotes Entry of a Second Drug Through the Microbial Cell Wall or Cell Membrane: This appears to be a widely applicable mechanism of synergism, with considerable clinical importance. For example, many streptococci exhibit a partial permeability barrier to aminoglycosides. If a cell wall-inhibitory drug is also present, it enhances the penetration of the aminoglycoside, which then acts on ribosomes and accelerates killing of the cell. This effect can occur with some viridans streptococci, group B streptococci, and group D enterococci. Combined therapy permits cure of sepsis or endocarditis caused by these organisms, whereas either drug alone often fails.

Antagonism

At times, the addition of a second drug actually diminishes the antibacterial effectiveness of the first drug, as shown by the interaction of drugs A and C in Figure 52–1. This "antagonism" can be manifested by a decrease in the inhibitory activity or in the early bactericidal rate of a drug mixture below that of one or both of its components. Antagonism can be demonstrated only when the drugs act on organisms capable of multiplication and is most marked when a barely active amount of bacteriostatic drug is added to a minimal bactericidal amount of a second drug. The bacteriostatic drug (tetracycline, chloramphenicol, erythromycin, etc) acts as an inhibitor of bacterial growth; the bactericidal drug (a penicillin, cephalosporin, or aminoglycoside) requires bacterial growth (eg, protein or cell wall synthesis) for killing. In the case of cell wall-active drugs, it has been suggested that the inhibition of protein synthesis by chloramphenicol or tetracycline interferes with the production of some autolytic enzyme system postulated to be an important final step in cell lysis. A recently recognized mechanism of drug antagonism is the combined use of a beta-lactamase-labile antibiotic, even a slowly hydrolyzed one (eg, third-generation cephalosporin), and a beta-lactamase inducer such as imipenem, cefoxitin, ampicillin, or clavulanic acid. These drugs are inducers of Richmond-Sykes type 1 beta-lactamase, which can inactivate even third-generation cephalosporins and produce antagonism, both in vitro and in vivo.

CLINICAL EVIDENCE FOR ANTIMICROBIAL DRUG SYNERGISM OR ANTAGONISM

Although there are multiple in vitro instances of antimicrobial synergism and antagonism, only a few well-substantiated clinical examples are recognized (Table 52–6).

Clinical Evidence for Synergism

The best clinical evidence for antibiotic synergism comes from the treatment of infective endocarditis, a disease that can be cured only if the infecting organisms are eradicated by bactericidal drugs. Endocarditis caused by enterococci (E faecalis) can usually not be cured by penicillin alone, since penicillin is in-

hibitory but not bactericidal for enterococci. The addition of an aminoglycoside is strikingly bactericidal for many strains of enterococci, and the cure of many such patients with a combination of penicillin or ampicillin with an aminoglycoside is an accepted example of clinical synergism. Beta-lactam antibiotics combined with aminoglycosides also appear to be synergistic in the treatment of endocarditis due to other streptococci and staphylococci, though the evidence is weaker. Likewise, there is some evidence that drug combinations (usually a beta-lactam plus an aminoglycoside) selected for synergy on the basis of in vitro studies have synergistic activity in the treatment of aerobic gram-negative rod infections, especially in patients with severe granulocytopenia.

There is good clinical evidence from controlled trials that in cryptococcal meningitis, amphotericin B plus flucytosine is superior to either drug alone. This combination was selected because of in vitro evidence of synergism.

Clinical Evidence for Antagonism

Antagonism is sharply limited by time-dose relationships both in vitro and in vivo. It is readily demonstrated with single-dose treatment of animal infections but only with difficulty in multiple-dose treatment. In clinical practice, it is usual to give a large excess of antimicrobial drug in multiple doses. Consequently, antagonism cannot be expected to be a frequent outcome of clinical antimicrobial therapy, and there are few documented examples. The combination of penicillin and chlortetracycline cured fewer patients with pneumococcal meningitis than did the same dose of penicillin alone. Similarly, the addition of chloramphenicol to ampicillin resulted in more treatment failures in bacterial meningitis than did ampicillin alone.

SELECTION OF ANTIMICROBIAL COMBINATIONS IN CLINICAL PRACTICE

Antimicrobial combinations are used commonly in clinical practice, often with good justification (Tables 52–1 and 52–2). Although the evidence for synergism is not clear in many cases, there is good evidence for clinical benefit for some combinations. On the other hand, the frequent use of antimicrobial combinations that have not been validated by clinical trials—or at least by in vitro or animal testing—should be avoided. The cost and toxicity of antimicrobials increase in direct proportion to the number of drugs used. Whenever drug combinations are employed and a clinical microbial isolate is available, it is desirable to establish the rationale for the choice by in vitro studies. The availability of broad-spectrum antibacterials such as imipenem/cilastatin, third-generation cephalosporins, and the fluoroquinolones may reduce the need for combination therapy.

ANTIMICROBIAL CHEMOPROPHYLAXIS

Anti-infective chemoprophylaxis is the administration of drugs to prevent the acquisition and establishment of pathogenic microorganisms. In a broader sense, it also includes the use of drugs soon after colonization by or inoculation of pathogenic microorganisms but before the development of disease.

Some general principles have emerged from human and animal studies of antimicrobial prophylaxis:

(1) Prophylaxis should be directed against a specific pathogen or defined group of pathogens or used to prevent infection at a specific site. Administration of antimicrobials cannot remove all microorganisms colonizing the host and cannot prevent all types of infections.

(2) The shorter the duration of prophylaxis, the broader the range of infections that may be prevented. Thus, prevention of "all" infections in severely leukopenic patients by broad-spectrum antimicrobial prophylaxis is successful only over the short term (resistance developing with long-term usage), whereas lifetime prophylaxis against group A streptococcal infections is possible.

(3) Prophylaxis is more effective and may be more widely used against pathogens that are poorly able to develop resistance to the drug used. The continued efficacy of penicillin prophylaxis against group A streptococcal infection contrasts with its rapidly dwindling efficacy against gonococcal infection.

(4) Prophylactic administration of antimicrobials generally requires doses equal to those used for therapy. In fact, since the host response to colonization or early infection may be different from that to disease, drugs effective for therapy may be relatively ineffective for prophylaxis and vice versa. For example, penicillin is highly effective treatment for meningococcal disease but is clinically ineffective for prophylaxis, because it does not eliminate colonization of the nasopharynx. Rifampin, highly effective for prophylaxis of meningococcal disease, is not recommended for therapy.

(5) As antimicrobial chemoprophylaxis entails risks (cost, drug toxicity, superinfection, and development of resistant organisms), it should be used only in situations where its efficacy has been documented.

Commonly used prophylactic regimens for nonsurgical infections are shown in Table 52–7. With the exception of the prevention of endocarditis following certain surgical procedures, the efficacy of these measures has been documented by adequate clinical trials. Prevention of endocarditis is now so widely practiced that adequately controlled studies are not possible. Data supporting this practice come from retrospective clinical trials and experiments on animal models of endocarditis. Not dealt with in this table are a multiplicity of clinical situations in which antimicrobial chemoprophylaxis was shown to be *ineffective:* heart failure, viral upper respiratory infections, comatose patients, etc.

In surgery, antimicrobials are given in the perioperative period to prevent postsurgical infectious complications. The general principles outlined above also apply to surgical prophylaxis, though some additional important principles apply to the prevention of postsurgical infections:

(1) The antimicrobial agent must be active against the majority of organisms causing infections after the operation under consideration.

(2) Prophylaxis should be started immediately (not more than 1–2 hours) before surgery and should be continued for not more than 12–48 hours after surgery. Substantial evidence suggests that a single preoperative dose of an antimicrobial offers maximal benefit. Antimicrobial drug activity must be present in the surgical wound at the time of closure.

(3) The antimicrobial should be nontoxic and inexpensive and should not be essential for therapy of serious infections.

(4) Prophylaxis is indicated for surgical procedures in which the wound infection rate (under optimal conditions) is 5% or more except in procedures involving implantation of a foreign body, in which general usage is warranted. Common indications for surgical prophylaxis are shown in Table 52–8.

Many second-and third-generation cephalosporins are promoted for single-dose surgical prophylaxis. There are no data proving that these agents are more effective than a single dose of cefazolin. In particular, third-generation cephalosporins should not be employed for prophylaxis because their use violates several of the principles outlined above, especially number (3).

Table 52–7. Nonsurgical antimicrobial prophylaxis of documented benefit or in common use.[1]

Disease or Infection to Be Prevented	Appropriate Subjects for Prophylaxis	Drugs and Adult Doses	Duration of Prophylaxis	Evidence for Efficacy	Comments
Group A streptococcal infection (post-streptococcal complications of rheumatic fever or glomerulonephritis)	1. Previous rheumatic fever or known rheumatic heart disease. 2 Epidemic of streptococcal impetigo.	1. Benzathine penicillin, 1.2 million units IM monthly. 2. Penicillin G, 125 mg twice a day. 3. Sulfadiazine, 1 g daily.	1. For rheumatic fever, prophylaxis should continue well into adult life. 2. For impetigo, until epidemic has abated.	Excellent (about 95%).	Does not prevent endocarditis.
Meningococcal infection	Close contacts (household, sex partners, day-care center, etc) of index case.	1. Rifampin, 20 mg/kg once a day. 2. Minocycline, 100 mg twice a day. 3. Sulfisoxazole, 1 g twice a day (if organism is susceptible).	Rifampin and sulfonamide: 2 days. Minocycline: 5 days.	Excellent (about 80–90%)	Problems: 1. Rifampin resistance with widespread usage. 2. Vertiginous reactions with minocycline.
Haemophilus influenzae infection	Same as meningococci, but of susceptible age (<5–7 years old).	Rifampin, 20 mg/kg (maximum dose, 600 mg) once a day.	Four days.	Good.	Agreement on clinical use is not uniform. Emergence of resistance has occurred.
Tuberculosis	1. Close contacts of index case (pending tuberculin testing). 2. Tuberculin converters. 3. Positive tuberculin test in high-risk groups (children, etc).	Isoniazid (INH), 300 mg/d.	Six months.	Excellent (about 80%).	Definition of high-risk groups is variable. See American Thoracic Society guidelines for details.
Plague	Close contacts.	Tetracycline, 500 mg twice daily.	One week after exposure has ended.	Good.	
Gonorrhea	1. Contacts of index case. 2. All newborns.	1. As for treatment of gonorrhea. 2. Topical eye drops—silver nitrate or antimicrobial.	One dose. One dose.	Excellent. Excellent.	Required by law in USA.
Syphilis	Contacts of index case.	Benzathine penicillin, 2.4 million units IM.	Once.	Excellent (virtually 100%).	
Toxigenic *E coli* infection	Persons traveling from nonendemic areas to endemic areas.	Many drugs effective. Fluoroquinolones most popular.	Duration of exposure.	Good.	Agreement on clinical use is not uniform. Not effective for antimicrobial-resistant strains.
Rickettsiosis	Exposure in endemic area (eg, scrub typhus).	Tetracycline (or chloramphenicol), 1 g/d.	Duration of exposure.	Good.	Recrudescence may occur when prophylaxis is discontinued.
Malaria	Exposure in endemic area.	Chloroquine phosphate, 500 mg weekly.	Duration of exposure.	Excellent.	1. Not effective for chloroquine-resistant *Plasmodium falciparum*. 2. Recrudescence may occur when prophylaxis is stopped.

[1]Modified, with permission, from Conte JE Jr, Sweet RW: *Infectious Diseases in Clinical Practice*. University of California, San Francisco, 1982. [Course syllabus.]

(continued)

Table 52–7 (cont'd). Nonsurgical antimicrobial prophylaxis of documented benefit or in common use.[1]

Disease or infection to Be Prevented	Appropriate Subjects for Prophylaxis	Drugs and Adult Doses	Duration of Prophylaxis	Evidence for Efficacy	Comments
Influenza A	Exposure in epidemic or to index case with documented infection.	Amantadine, 100 mg twice a day.	Duration of exposure.	Good (about 80%)	Agreement on clinical use is not uniform. Dose of 100 mg daily may be satisfactory.
Mycoplasmal pneumonia	Exposure to index case.	Tetracycline, 500 mg 4 times a day.	One week.	Poor.	Agreement on clinical use is not uniform.
Pneumocystis carinii infection	High-risk individual (high-dose cortico-steroids, AIDS, etc).	Trimethoprim, 5 mg/kg/d (with fixed ratio of sulfamethoxazole).	Uncertain. Probably duration of risk period.	Excellent.	Agreement on indications for use is not uniform. Aerosol pentimidine is an alternative.
African trypano-somiasis	Living in endemic area.	Pentamidine, 3 mg/kg IM every 3–6 months.	Duration of exposure.	Good.	
Endocarditis (endovasculit is)	Individuals with abnormal heart valves (increased susceptibility to endocarditis) or intravascular devices, undergoing a procedure known to cause bacteremia and increased risk of endocarditis (eg, dental extractions).	For dental procedure: amoxicillin, 3 g PO 1 hour before the procedure and 1.5 g 6 hours later; or clindamycin, 300 mg orally 1 hour before the procedure and 150 mg 6 hours later.	Once for each exposure.	None.	For genitourinary or gastrointestinal procedures: ampicillin, 2 g IV, or vancomycin, 1 g IV, plus gentamicin, 1.5 mg/kg 30–60 minutes before the procedure, followed by amoxicillin, 1.5 g 6 hours later.
Otitis media	Individuals with recurrent otitis media.	Ampicillin or sulfonamides or trimethoprim-sulfamethoxazole.	Approximately 1 year.	Good.	
Bite wounds.	Individuals bitten by humans, cats, occasionally other animals (eg, camels, gorillas).	Ampicillin or tetracycline, 0.5 g 4 times daily.	Three to 5 days.	Fair.	Close observation required even with prophylaxis.
Urinary tract infections	Individuals with a history of recurrent UTI.	Trimethoprim-sulfamethoxazole, 1 tablet twice weekly. Nitrofurantoin, 50 mg daily.	1. Continuously for uncertain duration. 2. After coitus (if a clear history of postcoital UTI).	Excellent.	Can substitute prompt, empiric treatment of each recurrence for continuous prophylaxis.
Exacerbations of chronic bronchitis	Individuals with established chronic bronchitis and frequent wintertime exacerbations.	Tetracycline, 0.5 g twice daily.	During the winter.	Good.	Not generally recommended—empiric treatment of each recurrence less toxic, equally efficacious.
Infection in the compromised host	Severely leukopenic patients (circulating granulocytes < 500/μL).	1. Oral, nonabsorbable antimicrobials (various regimens). 2. Trimethoprim-sulfamethoxazole by mouth. 3. Fluoroquinolone by mouth.	Duration of leukopenia.	Variable.	Not generally recommended. Adjunctive measures required: laminar air flow, sterile hospital environment, sterilization of food, etc.

[1]Modified, with permission, from Conte JE Jr, Sweet RW: *Infectious Diseases in Clinical Practice.* University of California, San Francisco, 1982. [Course syllabus.]

Table 52–8. Surgical prophylaxis of documented benefit or in common use.[1]

Disease or Operation	Usual Antimicrobial Employed	Evidence for Efficacy	Comments
Esophagus and stomach	Cephalosporin[2]	Good.	Needed primarily if bacterial flora (normally scanty) is increased by cancer, obstruction, or other disease.
Colon and rectum 　Elective	Oral, poorly absorbed antimicrobials (eg, erythromycin plus neomycin) with mechanical bowel preparation	Good.	Example of short-term "sterilization" of normal flora to prevent infection. Addition of systemic antimicrobials probably not helpful.
Perforation	Cefoxitin alone; clindamycin plus gentamicin (see Table 52–2)	Good	Perhaps should not be considered true prophylaxis, as gross fecal soilage of peritoneum has occurred.
Biliary tract	Cephalosporin[2]	Good.	Indicated.
Hysterectomy 　Vaginal	Cephalosporin[2]	Good.	Indicated.
Routine abdominal	Cephalosporin[2]	Fair.	Use is controversial.
Radical	Various	Fair.	Probably indicated.
Cesarean section	Cephalosporin[2]	Good.	Give after cord has been clamped.
Joint replacement	Cephalosporin[2]	Good.	Benefit greater in group not using laminar flow operating room.
Open fractures	Cephalosporin[2]	Good.	Perhaps should not be considered true prophylaxis as wound is often grossly contaminated.
Cardiac valve replacement	Cephalosporin[2]	Fair to poor.	Has become standard practice—controlled study no longer possible.

[1]Modified, with permission, from Conte JE Jr, Sweet RW: *Infectious Diseases in Clinical Practice.* University of Calfornia, San Francisco, 1982. [Course syllabus.]

[2]First-generation cephalosporins such as cephapirin, cephalothin, cefazolin. Cefazolin is generally preferred. Its long serum half-life and the feasibility of intramuscular administration make this drug generally the least expensive of the group.

REFERENCES

Aoun M, Klastersky J: Drug treatment of pneumonia in the hospital. What are the choices? Drugs 1991;42:962.

Bisno AL et al: Antimicrobial treatment of infective endocarditis due to viridans streptococci, enterococci, and staphylococci. JAMA 1989;261:1471.

Bochner BS, Lichtenstein LM: Anaphylaxis. N Engl J Med 1991;324:1785.

Brown RD, Campbell-Richards DM: Antimicrobial therapy in neonates, infants, and children. Clin Pharmacokinet 1989;17(Suppl 1):105.

Classen DC et al: The timing of prophylactic administration of antibiotics and the risk of surgical-wound infection. N Engl J Med 1992;326:281.

Conte JE, Barriere SL: *Manual of Antibiotics and Infectious Diseases,* 7th ed. Lea & Febiger, 1992.

Eliopoulos GM, Eliopoulos CT: Therapy of enterococcal infections. Eur J Clin Microbiol Infect Dis 1990;9:118.

Eliopoulos GM, Moellering RC Jr: Antibiotic synergism and antimicrobial combinations in clinical infections. Rev Infect Dis 1982;4:282.

Hughes WT et al: Guidelines for the use of antimicrobial agents in neutropenic patients with unexplained fever. J Infect Dis 1990:161:381.

Ludwig KA et al: Prophylactic antibiotics in surgery. Annu Rev Med 1993;44:385.

Mandell GL, Douglas RG Jr, Bennett JE: *Principles and Practice of Infectious Diseases,* 3rd ed. Churchill Livingstone, 1990.

Mosdell DM et al: Antibiotic treatment for surgical peritonitis. Ann Surgery 1991;214:543.

Musher DM: Infections caused by *Streptococcus pneumoniae:* Clinical spectrum, pathogenesis, immunity, and treatment. Clin Infect Dis 1992;14:801.

Raoult D, Drancourt M: Antimicrobial therapy of rickettsial diseases. Antimicrob Agents Chemother 1991;35:2457.

Reves RR et al: A cost-effectiveness comparison of the use of antimicrobial agents for the treatment or prophylaxis of traveler's diarrhea. Arch Intern Med 1988;148:2421.

Sattler FR, Weitekamp MR, Ballard JO: Potential for bleeding with the new beta-lactam antibiotics. Ann Intern Med 1986;105:924.

Snavely SR, Hodges GR: The neurotoxicity of antibacterial agents. Ann Intern Med 1984;101:92.

Wald ER: Sinusitis in children. N Engl J Med 1992;326:319.

Wendel GD Jr et al: Penicillin allergy and desensitization in serious infections during pregnancy. N Engl J Med 1985;312:1229.

Young LS, Glauser MP: Gram-negative septicemia and septic shock. Infect Dis Clin North Am 1991;5:739.

Basic Principles of Antiparasitic Chemotherapy

53

Ching Chung Wang, PhD

In its general scientific sense, the term "parasite" includes all of the known infectious agents such as viruses, bacteria, fungi, protozoa, and helminths. In this and the two following chapters, the term is used in a restricted sense to denote the protozoa and helminths. It has been estimated that 3 billion (3×10^9) humans suffer from parasitic infections, plus a much greater number of domestic and wild animals. Although these diseases constitute the most widespread human health problem in the world today, they have for various reasons also been the most neglected.

In theory, the parasitic infections should be relatively easy to treat because the etiologic agents are known in almost all cases. Furthermore, recent advances in cell culture techniques have made possible in vitro cultivation of many of the important parasites. These advances have not only laid to rest the traditional view that parasites somehow depend on a living host for their existence but have also enabled us to study parasites by methods similar to those employed in investigations of bacteria, including biochemistry, molecular biology, and immunologic pharmacology. However, many problems remain to be solved before effective chemotherapeutic agents will be available for all of the parasitic diseases.

Targets of Chemotherapy

A rational approach to antiparasitic chemotherapy requires comparative biochemical and physiologic investigations of host and parasite to discover differences in essential processes that will permit selective inhibition in the parasite and not in the host. One might expect that the parasite would have many deficiencies in its metabolism associated with its parasitic nature. This is true of many parasites—the oversimplified metabolic pathways are usually indispensable for survival of the parasite and thus represent points of vulnerability. However, oversimplified metabolic pathways are not the only opportunity for attack. Although the parasite lives in a metabolically luxurious environment and may become "lazy," the environment is not entirely friendly and the parasite must have defense mechanisms in order to survive—ie, to defend itself against immunologic attack, proteolytic digestion, etc, by the host. In some instances, necessary nutrients are not supplied to the parasite from the host, though the latter can obtain the same nutrients from the diet. In this situation, the parasite will have acquired the synthetic activity needed for its survival. Finally, the great evolutionary distance between host and parasite has in some cases resulted in sufficient differences among individual enzymes or functional pathways to allow rather selective inhibition of the parasite. Thus, there can be three major types of potential targets for chemotherapy of parasitic diseases: (1) unique enzymes found only in the parasite; (2) enzymes found in both host and parasite but indispensable only for the parasite; and (3) common biochemical functions found in both parasite and host but with different pharmacologic properties. Examples of specific targets and drugs that act on them are summarized in Table 53–1. This chapter discusses antiparasitic mechanisms based upon these examples and provides background information for the drugs described in Chapters 54 and 55.

ENZYMES FOUND ONLY IN PARASITES

These enzymes would appear to be the cleanest targets for chemotherapy. Like inhibition of the enzymes involved in the synthesis of bacterial cell walls (Chapter 42), inhibition of these enzymes should have no effect on the host. Unfortunately, only a few of these enzymes have been discovered among the parasitic protozoa. Furthermore, their usefulness as chemotherapeutic targets is sometimes limited because of the development of drug resistance. Examples of important target enzymes are discussed in the following pages.

Enzymes for Dihydropteroate Synthesis

The intracellular sporozoan parasites such as *Plasmodium*, *Toxoplasma*, and *Eimeria* have long been known to respond to sulfonamides and sulfones. This

Table 53–1. Identified targets for chemotherapy in parasites.

Targets	Parasites	Inhibitors
Unique enzymes		
Enzymes for dihydropteroate synthesis	Sporozoa	Sulfones and sulfonamides
Pyruvate:ferrodoxin oxidoreductase	Anaerobic protozoa	Nitroimidazoles
Nucleoside phosphotransferase	Flagellated protozoa	Allopurinol riboside and formycin B
Trypanothione reductase	Kinetoplastida	Melarsoprol B and nifurtimox
Indispensable enzymes		
Purine phosphoribosyl transferase	Protozoa	Allopurinol
Ornithine decarboxylase	Protozoa	α-Difluoromethylornithine
Glycolytic enzymes	Kinetoplastida	Glycerol plus salicylhydroxamic acid and suramin
Common biochemical functions with different pharmacologic properties		
Thiamine transporter	Coccidia	Amprolium
Mitochondrial electron transporter	Coccidia	4-Hydroxyquinolines
Microtubules	Helminth	Benzimidazoles
Nervous synaptic transmission	Helminth and ectoparasite	Levamisole, piperazine, the milbemycins, and the avermectins.

has led to the assumption that sporozoans must synthesize their own folate in order to survive. The reaction of 2-amino-4-hydroxy-6-hydroxymethyl-dihydropteridine diphosphate with *p*-aminobenzoate to form 7,8-dihydropteroate has been demonstrated in cell-free extracts of the rodent malaria parasite *Plasmodium chabaudi.* 2-Amino-4-hydroxy-6-hydroxymethyl-dihydropteridine pyrophosphokinase and 7,8-dihydropteroate synthase have also been identified, isolated, and purified. Sulfathiazole, sulfaguanidine, and sulfanilamide act as competitive inhibitors of *p*-aminobenzoate in this reaction. It has not been possible to demonstrate dihydrofolate synthase activity in the parasites, which raises the possibility that 7,8-dihydropteroate may have substituted for dihydrofolate in malaria parasites. Similar lack of recognition of folate as substrate was also observed in the dihydrofolate reductase of *Eimeria tenella,* a parasite of chickens.

However, lack of utilization of exogenous folate may not fully explain the apparently indispensable nature of the synthesis of 7,8-dihydropteroate in *Plasmodium, Toxoplasma,* and *Eimeria.* It is known that most of the folate molecules in mammalian cells are linked with polyglutamates in the cytoplasm and are transported across cell membranes with difficulty. This additional factor may compound the problem of obtaining 7,8-dihydropteroate or dihydrofolate for the parasite and makes all of the enzymes involved in their synthesis attractive targets for antisporozoan chemotherapy.

The sulfones and sulfonamides synergize with the inhibitors of dihydrofolate reductase, and combinations have been effective in controlling malaria, toxoplasmosis, and coccidiosis. Although some incidents of drug resistance, especially among coccidia, have been reported, the combinations remain largely effective against malaria and toxoplasmosis. Fansidar, a combination of sulfadoxine and pyrimethamine, has been successful in controlling some strains

of chloroquine-resistant *Plasmodium falciparum* malaria (see Chapter 54).

The pharmacologic properties of parasite 7,8-dihydropteroate synthases may differ from those of the bacterial enzymes. For instance, metachloridine and 2-ethoxy-*p*-aminobenzoate are both ineffective against sulfonamide-sensitive bacteria, but the former has antimalarial activity and the latter is effective against infection by the chicken parasite *Eimeria acervulina;* both activities can be reversed by *p*-aminobenzoate.

Pyruvate:Ferredoxin Oxidoreductase

Certain anaerobic protozoan parasites lack mitochondria and mitochondrial activities for generating ATP. They possess, instead, ferredoxin-like or flavodoxin-like low-redox-potential electron transport proteins to convert pyruvate to acetyl-CoA. In trichomonad flagellates and rumen ciliates, the process takes place in a membrane-limited organelle called the hydrogenosome. By the actions of pyruvate:ferredoxin oxidoreductase and hydrogenase in the hydrogenosome, H_2 is produced by these organisms under anaerobic conditions as the major means of electron disposition. Although *Entamoeba* spp and *Giardia lamblia* have no hydrogenosome, a ferredoxin has been isolated from *Entamoeba histolytica,* and iron-sulfur and flavin centers have been detected by electron paramagnetic resonance studies on *G lamblia.*

Pyruvate:ferredoxin oxidoreductase has no counterpart in the mammalian system. In contrast to the mammalian pyruvate dehydrogenase complex, pyruvate:ferredoxin oxidoreductase is incapable of reducing pyridine nucleotides because of its low redox potential (approximately –400 mV). However, this low potential can also transfer electrons from pyruvate to the nitro groups of metronidazole and other 5-nitroimidazole derivatives to form cytotoxic reduced products that bind to DNA and proteins. This is apparently why anaerobic protozoal species are highly susceptible to drugs such as metronidazole. Despite the recent development of drug resistance in *Trichomonas vaginalis* and the possibility of carcinogenic properties (see Chapter 54), metronidazole remains the drug of choice for controlling anaerobic protozoal parasite infections.

Nucleoside Phosphotransferases

All of the protozoal parasites studied thus far are deficient in de novo synthesis of purine nucleotides. The various purine salvage pathways in these parasites are thus essential for their survival and growth. Among the *Leishmania* species, a unique salvage enzyme has been identified—purine nucleoside phosphotransferase—that can transfer the phosphate group from a variety of monophosphate esters, including *p*-nitrophenylphosphate, to the 5' position of purine nucleosides. This enzyme also phosphorylates purine nucleoside analogues such as allopurinol riboside, formycin B, 9-deazainosine, and thiopurinol riboside, converting them to the corresponding nucleotides. These nucleotides are either further converted to triphosphates and eventually incorporated into nucleic acid of *Leishmania* or become inhibitors of other essential enzymes in purine metabolism. Consequently, allopurinol riboside, formycin B, 9-deazainosine, and thiopurinol riboside all act as potent antileishmanial agents both in vitro and in vivo. Allopurinol riboside is particularly interesting because it is remarkably nontoxic to the mammalian host; it is currently in clinical trials for use in leishmaniasis (Saenz, 1989). The relevant pathways are illustrated in Figure 53–1.

Trichomonad flagellates appear to be deficient in de novo synthesis of both purines and pyrimidines. Pyrimidine as well as purine salvage thus becomes indispensable for these parasites. Among them, *Trichomonas foetus* (the cow parasite), *T vaginalis*, and *G lamblia* also lack dihydrofolate reductase and thymidylate synthase—a deficiency that enables them to grow normally in the presence of methotrexate, the most potent antifolate, in a concentration of 0.5 mmol/L. This metabolic deficiency leads to apparent isolation of the supply route for thymidine 5'-monophosphate (TMP) from the rest of the pyrimidine ribonucleotides; TMP is provided by a single salvage pathway that converts exogenous thymidine to TMP by the action of a thymidine phosphotransferase (Figure 53–2).

The enzyme activity is not affected by thymidine kinase inhibitors such as acyclovir but is inhibitable by guanosine or 5-fluorodeoxyuridine; both compounds also inhibit the in vitro growth of the parasites. This enzyme is an attractive target for chemotherapeutic treatment of the anaerobic protozoal parasites. One could design either a false substrate or an inhibitor of the thymidine phosphotransferase; DNA synthesis in the parasites might be arrested in either case.

Trypanothione Reductase

Certain protozoa (kinetoplastidans) are unusual in that a considerable portion of their intracellular spermidine and glutathione is found as the unique conjugate N^1-N^8-(glutathionyl)spermidine, which has been assigned the name trypanothione. Kinetoplastidans contain neither glutathione reductase nor glutathione peroxidase for maintaining intracellular thiols in the reduced state and removing hydrogen peroxide. Thus, trypanothione plays a central role in kinetoplastida's defense mechanisms against oxidative damage, and trypanothione reductase is among the essential enzymes for the survival of these parasites. Nifurtimox, a nitrofuran derivative effective in treating Chagas' disease (caused by *Trypanosoma cruzi*), has been found to be a potent inhibitor of trypanothione reductase. Other inhibitors are under study (Jockers-Scherubl, 1989). The antitrypanosomal trivalent arsenicals are taken up by the African trypanosome *Trypanosoma brucei* and sequester trypanothione as a product that is also an effective inhibitor of trypanothione reductase.

ENZYMES INDISPENSABLE ONLY IN THE PARASITES

Because of the many metabolic deficiencies among parasites, there are enzymes whose functions may be essential for the survival of parasites, but the same enzymes are not indispensable to the host—ie, the host may be able to achieve the same result through alternative pathways. This discrepancy opens up opportunities for antiparasitic chemotherapy.

Purine Phosphoribosyl Transferases

The absence of de novo purine nucleotide synthesis in protozoal parasites as well as in the trematode *Schistosoma mansoni* is reflected in the relative importance of hypoxanthine-guanine phosphoribosyl transferase in many species. Hypoxanthine is the obligatory base for purine nucleotide synthesis in four species of *Leishmania, Plasmodium berghei, E tenella, T foetus, S mansoni, Crithidia fasciculata,* and perhaps other organisms as well. Unusual substrate specificity of the parasite hypoxanthine-guanine phosphoribosyl transferase (Figure 53–1) has been reported. The enzymes in *Leishmania donovani* and *Trypanosoma cruzi* can recognize allopurinol (see Chapter 35) as the substrate and convert it to allopurinol ribotide, which then accumulates in the parasites and becomes aminated, turned into triphosphate, and finally incorporated into the RNA fraction. This abnormal RNA apparently does not support normal growth (see Figure 53–1). Since allopurinol is an extremely poor substrate for the mammalian hypoxanthine-guanine phosphoribosyl transferase, it has selective antileishmanial and antitrypanosomal effects in vivo. Another enzyme in *L donovani*, xanthine phosphoribosyl trans-

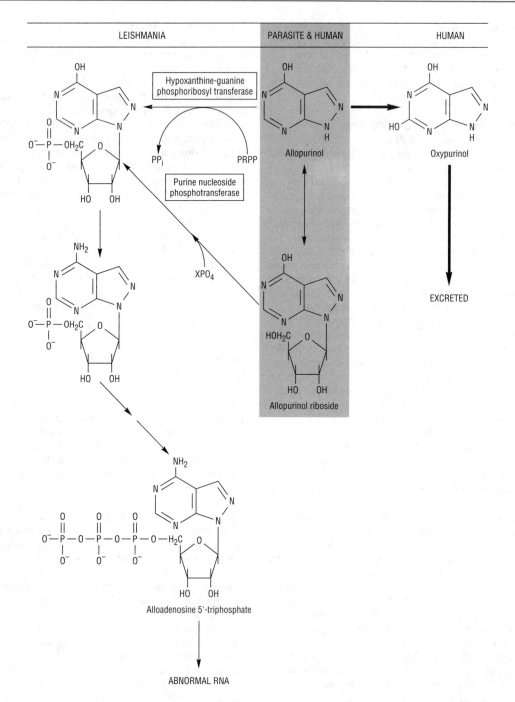

Figure 53–1. Metabolism of allopurinol and allopurinol riboside in *Leishmania* and humans. (PRPP, phosphoribosylpyrophosphate; PP$_i$, inorganic pyrophosphate; XPO$_4$, a phosphate donor.)

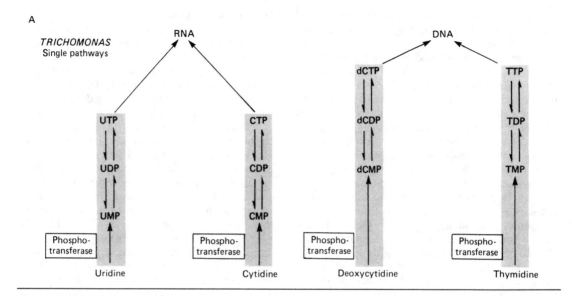

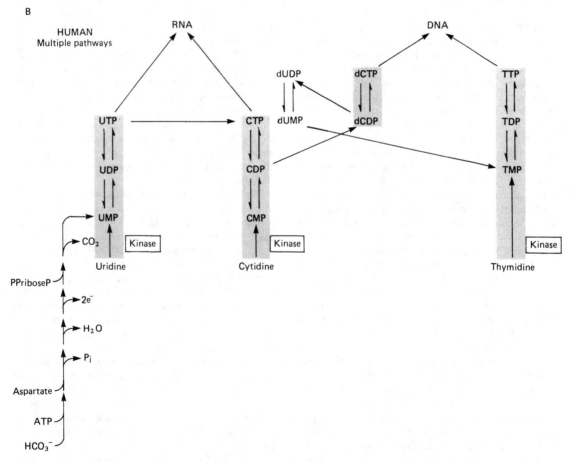

Figure 53–2. Pyrimidine metabolism in *Trichomonas vaginalis* **(A)** and in humans **(B)**. Note that humans have multiple sources for thymidine monophosphate *(TMP)*, an essential precursor for DNA synthesis. The parasite has only one source. (UTP, UDP, UMP, CTP, etc, uridine triphosphate, diphosphate, monophosphate, cytidine triphosphate, etc; PPriboseP, 1-pyrophosphorylribosyl-5-phosphate; P_i, inorganic phosphate.)

ferase, has no counterpart in mammalian systems and thus could be another interesting target for antileishmanial chemotherapy.

G lamblia has an exceedingly simple scheme of purine salvage. It possesses only two pivotal enzymes: the adenine and guanine phosphoribosyl transferases, which convert exogenous adenine and guanine to the corresponding nucleotides. There is no salvage of hypoxanthine, xanthine, or any purine nucleosides and no interconversion between adenine and guanine nucleotides in the parasite. Functions of the two phosphoribosyl transferases are thus both essential for the survival and development of *G lamblia* (Figure 53–3). The guanine phosphoribosyl transferase is an interesting enzyme because it does not recognize hypoxanthine, xanthine, or adenine as substrate. This substrate specificity distinguishes the *Giardia* enzyme from the mammalian enzyme, which uses hypoxanthine, and the bacterial one, which has xanthine as substrate. Design of a highly specific inhibitor of this enzyme is thus possible.

Ornithine Decarboxylase

Polyamines, found in almost all living organisms, are required for cellular proliferation and differentiation. Ornithine decarboxylase, the enzyme that controls the formation of the polyamine putrescine in numerous eukaryotic cells, is an enzyme characterized by its striking inducibility and very short half-life. In many species of trypanosomatids, putrescine and spermidine form the major pool of polyamines, which are synthesized rapidly from ornithine. Alpha-difluoromethylornithine (DFMO), a probable suicide inhibitor of ornithine decarboxylase with known antitumor activities, has been found to possess good activity against African trypanosomes in infected animals. The compound is now available for clinical use and has shown good therapeutic activity against *Trypanosoma brucei gambiense* infections.

DFMO depletes the intracellular polyamine pool of *T brucei*, and its activity is reversible by putrescine, as predicted by an action on ornithine decarboxylase in the parasite. However, since there is little polyamine in mammalian blood—owing to the presence of high levels of polyamine oxidase, the DMFO effect on blood-resident trypanosomes is not reversed in vivo. Since the African trypanosome lives in the blood, DFMO is selectively toxic to it. The physiologic consequence of this action is the transformation of the *long-slender* form of *T brucei* to its nondividing *short-stumpy* form. This nondividing form is apparently incapable of changing its variant surface glycoprotein coat and can eventually be eliminated by the host immune response. In spite of its higher affinity for the mammalian form of ornithine decarboxylase, the drug is less toxic to the host because of more rapid turnover and replacement of the irreversibly inhibited enzyme in the host than in the parasite.

Glycolytic Enzymes

In the bloodstream form of African trypanosomes such as *Trypanosoma brucei brucei,* the single mitochondrion has been reduced to a "peripheral canal" lacking both cytochrome and functional Krebs cycle enzymes. The organism is entirely dependent on glycolysis for its production of ATP. Under aerobic conditions, one glucose molecule can generate only two molecules of ATP, with two pyruvate molecules excreted into the host bloodstream as the end product. This low energy yield makes it necessary to have glycolysis in *T b brucei* proceed at an extremely high rate to enable the trypanosome to divide once every 7 hours. The high glycolytic rate, 50 times that in the mammalian host, is made possible not only by the abundant glucose supply in the host's blood but also by the clustering of most of the glycolytic enzymes of the parasite in membrane-bound microbody organelles, glycosomes (Figure 53–4). Since lactate dehydrogenase is absent from the parasite, the regeneration of NAD from NADH in the glycosome during glycolysis depends on a dihydroxyacetone phosphate:glycerol-3-phosphate shuttle plus a glycerol-3-phosphate oxidase. Thus, under anaerobic conditions, glycerol-3-phosphate cannot be oxidized back to dihydroxyacetone phosphate and accumulates inside the glycosome. This accumulation, together with the accumulation of ADP due to depletion of NAD, eventually drives the reversed glycerol kinase-catalyzed reaction in the glycosome to generate glycerol and ATP. Thus, under anaerobic conditions, *T b brucei* generates only one ATP molecule from each glucose molecule and excretes equimolar pyruvate and glycerol as end products.

This delicate and indispensable glycolytic system appears to be an attractive target for antitrypanosomal chemotherapy. It has been shown that glycerol-3-phosphate oxidase can be inhibited in the parasite with salicylhydroxamic acid (SHAM) to bring *T b brucei* into an anaerobic condition. Glycolysis can then be stopped by inhibiting the reversed glycerol kinase-catalyzed reaction with added glycerol. This SHAM plus glycerol combination can lyse the African trypanosome bloodstream forms in vitro within minutes and is very effective in suppressing parasitemia in infected animals.

The systems involved in glycosome biogenesis may also be targets for antitrypanosomal therapy. The drug suramin contains six negatively charged sulfonyl groups and has a molecular weight of 1429. These sulfonyl groups may facilitate binding of the drug to some of the basic amino acids known to be present in several essential glycosomal enzymes. This would result in binding of the enzymes before transport into the glycosome, with a resultant crippling of glycosomal function.

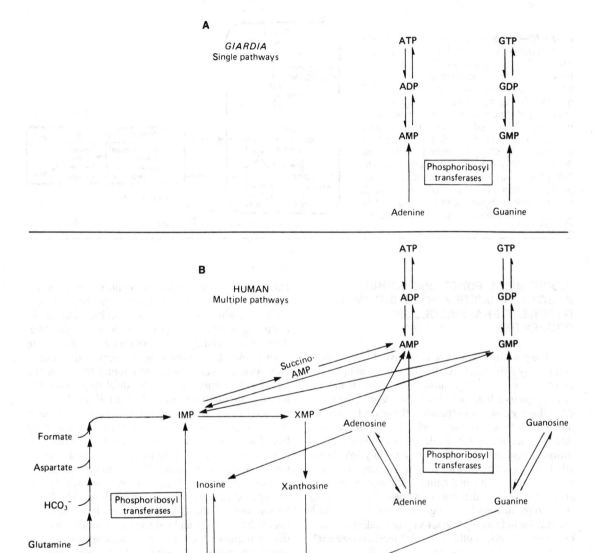

Figure 53–3. Purine metabolism in *Giardia lamblia* **(A)** and in humans **(B)**. *G lamblia* lacks enzymes both for de novo synthesis of essential purine nucleotides and for interconversion of these purine nucleotides. (AMP, GMP, IMP, XMP, etc, adenosine monophosphate, guanosine monophosphate, inosine monophosphate, xanthosine monophosphate, etc.)

Figure 53–4. Glycolytic pathway in long, slender bloodstream forms of *Trypanosoma brucei brucei*. The principal site of inhibition by trypanocidal drugs in vivo is indicated by the bold arrow. (SHAM, salicylhydroxamic acid; G6P, glucose 6-phosphate; F6P, fructose 6-phosphate; FDP, fructose 1,6-diphosphate; GAP, glyceraldehyde 3-phosphate; DHAP, dihydroxyacetone phosphate; GP, *sn*-glycerol 3-phosphate; DPGA, 1,3-diphosphoglycerate; 3PGA and 2PGA, 3- and 2-phosphoglycerate; PEP, phosphoenolpyruvate.) (Modified and reproduced, with permission, from Fairlamb A: Biochemistry of trypanosomiasis and rational approaches to chemotherapy. *Trends Biochem Sci* 1982;7:249.)

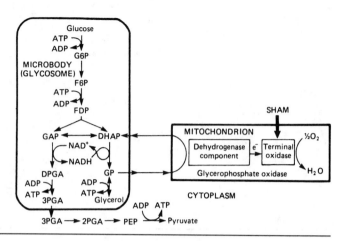

BIOCHEMICAL FUNCTIONS FOUND IN BOTH PARASITE & HOST BUT WITH DIFFERENT PHARMACOLOGIC PROPERTIES

In the parasite, these functions have differentiated sufficiently to become probable targets for antiparasitic chemotherapy, not because of the parasitic nature of the organism but, more likely, because of the long evolutionary distances separating the parasite and the host. It is thus difficult to discover these targets through studying metabolic deficiency or special nutritional requirements of the parasite. They have usually been found by investigating the modes of action of some well-established antiparasitic agents discovered by screening methods in the past. The target of such drugs may not be a single well-defined enzyme but may include transporters, receptors, cellular structural components, or other specific functions essential for the survival of the parasite.

Thiamine Transporter

Carbohydrate metabolism provides the main energy source in coccidia. Diets deficient in thiamine, riboflavin, or nicotinic acid—all cofactors in carbohydrate metabolism—result in suppression of parasitic infestation of chickens by *E tenella* and *E acervulina*. A thiamine analogue, amprolium (1-[(4-amino- 2-propyl-5-pyrimidinyl)methyl]-2-picolinium chloride), has long been used as an effective anticoccidial agent in chickens and cattle with relatively low host toxicity. The antiparasitic activity of amprolium is reversible by thiamine and is now recognized to involve inhibition of thiamine transport in the parasite. Unfortunately, amprolium has a rather narrow spectrum of antiparasitic activity; it has poor activity against toxoplasmosis, a closely related parasitic infection.

Mitochondrial Electron Transporter

Mitochondria of *E tenella* appear to lack cyto-

chrome c and to contain cytochrome o—a cytochrome oxidase commonly found in the bacterial respiratory chain—as the terminal oxidase. Certain 4-hydroxyquinoline derivatives such as buquinolate, decoquinate, and methyl benzoquate that have long been known to be relatively nontoxic and effective anticoccidial agents have been found to act on the parasites by inhibiting mitochondrial respiration. Direct investigation on isolated intact *E tenella* mitochondria indicated that the 4-hydroxyquinolines have no effect on NADH oxidase or succinoxidase activity but that they are extremely potent inhibitors of NADH- or succinate-induced mitochondrial respiration. On the other hand, the ascorbate-induced *E tenella* mitochondrial respiration was totally insusceptible to these 4-hydroxyquinolines. The block by the anticoccidial agents thus may be located between the oxidases and cytochrome b in the electron transport chain. A certain component at this location must be essential for mediating the electron transport and would appear to be highly sensitive to the 4-hydroxyquinolines. This component must be a very specific chemotherapeutic target in *Eimeria* spp, since the 4-hydroxyquinolines have no effect on chicken liver and mammalian mitochondrial respiration and no activity against any parasites other than *Eimeria*.

Microtubules

Microtubules are an important part of the cytoskeleton and the mitotic spindle and consist of α- and β-tubulin subunit proteins. Recent comparisons of α- and β-tubulins from several species of parasitic nematodes indicated the presence of multiple isoforms with varying isoelectric points. This variation is interesting not only in pointing out the evolutionary relations among eukaryotic cells; it is useful also in classifying the tubulins in parasites as potential targets for antiparasitic chemotherapy. A group of benzimidazole derivatives have long been established as highly effective anthelmintics. Mebendazole was among the first such anthelmintics found to act primarily by blocking transport of secretory granules and movement of other subcellular organelles in the parasitic nematode *Ascaris lumbricoides.* This inhibition coincides with the disappearance of cytoplasmic microtubules from the intestinal cells of the worm. The microtubular systems of the host cells are unaffected by the treatment. Mebendazole and fenbendazole, another anthelmintic benzimidazole, have also been shown to compete with colchicine binding to *A lumbricoides* embryonic tubulins with 250–400 times higher potencies than the binding competition to bovine brain tubulins. These differential binding affinities may explain the selective toxicity of the benzimidazoles toward the parasitic nematodes.

Synaptic Transmission

Invertebrate nervous systems in the helminths and the arthropods differ from those of vertebrates in important ways. The motoneurons in invertebrates, for example, are unmyelinated and are thus more susceptible to disturbances of nerve membranes than are the myelinated somatic motor fibers of vertebrates. Muscle fibers in arthropods are innervated by excitatory synapses, in which L-glutamic acid is the neurotransmitter, and by inhibitory nerves, which have γ-aminobutyric acid (GABA) as transmitter. Cholinergic nerves are concentrated in the central nervous system of arthropods. In nematodes, free-living species, eg, *C elegans,* and gastrointestinal parasitic species, eg, *A lumbricoides,* appear to have identical neuronal systems and synaptic transmission. Cholinergic excitatory and GABAergic inhibitory synapses are found at the neuromuscular junctions as well as in the central ventral cords of the worms. The mammalian hosts, on the other hand, have mainly nicotinic receptors at the neuromuscular junctions (see Chapter 6), and the GABA nerves are primarily confined within the central nervous system protected by the blood-brain barrier (Chapter 20).

Neurotoxicant anthelmintics must be administered systemically to mammalian hosts to reach the parasitic nematodes. Therefore, if absorbed, they must be nontoxic to the nervous system of the host. Furthermore, they must penetrate the thick cuticle of the nematodes in order to be effective. It is therefore difficult to find a useful anthelmintic that acts on the nervous system of these parasites. Nevertheless, the majority of presently available anthelmintics do act on the nerves of the nematodes. They can be classified into two groups: (1) those acting as ganglionic nicotinic acetylcholine agonists and (2) those acting directly or indirectly as GABA agonists. The first category includes levamisole, pyrantel pamoate, oxantel pamoate, and bephenium. The acetylcholine receptors at the neuromuscular junctions of nematodes are of the ganglionic nicotinic type; these agonists are quite effective in causing muscular contraction of the worms. Experimentally, the ganglionic nicotinic an-

tagonist mecamylamine can reverse the action of these anthelmintics.

The second category consists of only one drug, piperazine, an older agent that apparently acts as a GABA agonist at the neuromuscular junction and causes flaccid paralysis of the nematode.

An important family of natural compounds, the milbemycins and avermectins, appears to act indirectly to intensify the GABA action on the ventral cord interneuron and on the motoneuron junction to immobilize nematodes—and at the neuromuscular junction of arthropods to cause paralysis. Therefore,

Table 53–2. Some major antiparasitic agents with undefined mechanisms of action.

Antiparasitic Agents	Possibly Relevant Biochemical Activities
Antiamebiasis agents	
Diloxanide furoate	Unknown.
Emetine	Inhibitor of eukaryote protein synthesis.
Halogenated hydroxyquinolines	Unknown.
Paromomycin	Inhibitor of prokaryote protein synthesis.
Antifascioliasis agents	
Bithionol	Oxidative phosphorylation uncoupler.
Rafoxanide	Oxidative phosphorylation uncoupler.
Antifilariasis agents	
Diethylcarbamazine	Inhibitor of lipoxygenase.
Antileishmaniasis agents	
Amphotericin B	Voltage-dependent channel maker in cell membrane.
Pentavalent antimonials	Unknown.
Antimalarials	
Chloroquine	DNA binding, lysosomal neutralization, and hematoporphyrin binding.
Primaquine	Its quinoline quinone metabolite is an oxidant.
Quinacrine	DNA binding and flavoenzyme inhibition.
Quinine	DNA binding and membrane binding.
Antischistosomal agents	
Praziquantel	Opening of Ca^{2+} channels.
Hycanthone	DNA binding.
Metrifonate	Acetylcholinesterase inhibitor.
Niridazole	Metabolites binding to DNA.
Oxamniquine	DNA binding.
Trivalent antimonials	Inhibition of phosphofructokinase.
Antitapeworm agent	
Niclosamide	Oxidative phosphorylation uncoupler.
Antitrypanosomiasis agents	
Melarsen oxide	Inhibitor of trypanothione reductase.
Aromatic diamidines	Transport can be blocked by polyamines; DNA binding.

both the milbemycins and the avermectins are potent anthelmintics, insecticides, and antiectoparasitic agents with no cross-resistance problems with agents acting on the cholinergic systems. Picrotoxin, a specific blocker of the chloride ion channel controlled by postsynaptic GABA binding, can reverse all of the physiologic effects of these drugs (see Chapter 20).

Ivermectin, a simple derivative of the mixture of avermectin B_{1a} and avermectin B_{1b}, is highly effective as an anthelmintic in domestic animals. It is also effective in controlling onchocerciasis by eliminating the microfilariae. It is currently in wide clinical use in West Africa. Avermectins have little effect on the mammalian central nervous system because they do not cross the blood-brain barrier readily. However, when isolated mammalian brain synaptosomes and synaptic membranes are used as models for investigation, specific high-affinity binding sites for the avermectins can be identified in GABAergic nerves. This drug binding stimulates GABA release from the presynaptic end of the GABA nerve and enhances the postsynaptic GABA binding. Avermectins also stimulate benzodiazepine binding to its receptor and enhance diazepam muscle relaxant activity in vivo. There is little doubt that milbemycins and avermectins act on chloride channels associated with GABA receptors and amplify GABA functions. The GABAergic nerves in invertebrates are thus attractive targets for chemotherapy.

Little is known about the nervous systems of cestodes and trematodes except that they probably differ from those of nematodes, since milbemycins and avermectins have no effect on them. However, a highly effective antischistosomal and antitapeworm agent, praziquantel (see Chapter 55), is known to enhance Ca^{2+} influx and induce muscular contraction in those parasites, though it exerts no action on nematodes or insects. Some benzodiazepine derivatives have activities similar to those of praziquantel; these activities are unrelated to the anxiolytic activities in the mammalian central nervous system. The nerves and muscles in schistosomes and tapeworms are thus interesting subjects for future chemotherapeutic studies.

Drugs for Which the Mechanism Has Not Been Identified

In spite of considerable progress in defining the mechanisms of action of the drugs described above, there are still wide gaps in our understanding of a number of other important antiparasitic agents. These include the compounds presented in Table 53–2. From the biochemical activities that have been identified for them, it appears that many are capable of binding DNA, and some can uncouple oxidative phosphorylation in mammals. These types of activity, which are toxic to the host but could also be involved in the antiparasitic action, may have been preferentially detectable in random screens used for antiparasitic agents in the past.

REFERENCES

Aman RA, Wang CC: Identification of two integral glycosomal membrane proteins in *Trypanosoma brucei*. Mol Biochem Parasitol 1987;25:83.

Bacchi CJ et al: In vivo effects of α-DL-difluoromethylornithine on the metabolism and morphology of *Trypanosoma brucei*. Mol Biochem Parasitol 1983;7:209.

Blair KL, Bennett JL, Pax RA: Praziquantel: Physiological evidence for its site(s) of action in magnesium-paralysed *Schistosoma mansoni*. Parasitology 1992;104(Part 1):59.

Borgers M et al: Influence of the anthelmintic mebendazole on microtubules and intracellular organelle movement in nematode intestinal cells. Am J Vet Res 1975;36:1153.

Clarkson AB, Brohn FH: Trypanosomiasis: An approach to chemotherapy by the inhibition of carbohydrate metabolism. Science 1976;194:204.

Craig SP III et al: Analysis of cDNA encoding the hypoxanthine-guanine phosphoribosyltransferase (HGPRTase) of *Schistosoma mansoni;* a putative target for chemotherapy. Nucleic Acids Res 1988;16:7087.

Del Castillo J, de Mello WC, Morales T: Inhibitory action of γ-aminobutyric acid (GABA) on *Ascaris* muscle. Experientia 1964;20:141.

Dovey HF, Parsons M, Wang CC: Biogenesis of glycosomes of *Trypanosoma brucei:* An in vitro model of 3-phosphoglycerate kinase import. Proc Natl Acad Sci USA 1988;85:2598.

Driscoll M et al: Genetic and molecular analysis of a *Caenorhabditis elegans* β-tubulin that conveys benzimidazole sensitivity. J Cell Biol 1989;109:2993.

Fairlamb AH, Henderson GB, Cerami A: Trypanothione is the primary target for arsenical drugs against African trypanosomes. Natl Acad Sci Proc USA 1989;86:2607.

Friedman PA, Platzer EG: Interaction of anthelmintic benzimidazoles with *Ascaris suum* embryonic tubulin. Biochim Biophys Acta 1980;630:271.

Fritz LC, Wang CC, Gorio A: Avermectin B_{1a} irreversibly blocks post-synaptic potentials at the lobster neuromuscular junction by reducing muscle membrane resistance. Proc Natl Acad Sci USA 1979;76:2062.

Hedstrom L, Cheung KS, Wang CC: A novel mechanism of mycophenolic acid resistance in the protozoan parasite *Tritrichomonas foetus*. Biochem Pharmacol 1990;39:151.

Holden-Dye L, Walker RJ: Avermectin and avermectin derivatives are antagonists at the 4-aminobutyric acid (GABA) receptor on the somatic muscle cells of *Ascaris;* is this the site of anthelmintic action? Parasitology, 1990; 101(Part 2):265.

Jockers-Scherubl MC et al: Trypanothione reductase from *Trypanosoma cruzi:* Catalytic properties of the enzyme and inhibition studies with trypanocidal compounds. Eur J Biochem 1989;180:267.

Johnson PJ et al: Molecular analysis of the hydrogenosomal ferredoxin of the anaerobic protist *Trichomonas vaginalis*. Natl Acad Sci Proc USA 1990;87:6097.

Kass IS et al: Avermectin B_{1a}, a paralyzing anthelmintic that affects interneurons and inhibitory motor neurons in *Ascaris*. Proc Natl Acad Sci USA 1980;77:6211.

Kohler P, Davies KP, Zahner H: Activity, mechanism of action and pharmacokinetics of 2-tert-butylbenzothiazole and CGP 6140 (amocarzine) antifilarial drugs. Acta Trop 1992;51:195

Krakow JL, Wang CC: Purification and characterization of glycerol kinase from *Trypanosoma brucei*. Molec Biochem Parasitol 1990;43:17.

Linder E, Thors C: *Schistosoma mansoni:* Praziquantel-induced tegumental lesion exposes actin of surface spines and allows binding of actin depolymerizing factor, gelsolin. Parasitology, 1992;105:71.

Martin RJ, Pennington AJ: A patch-clamp study of effects of dihydroavermectin on *Ascaris* muscle. Br J Pharmacol 1989;98:747.

McCann PP, Pegg AE: Ornithine decarboxylase as an enzyme target for therapy. Pharmacol Ther 1992;54:195.

Müller M: Hydrogenosomes. Symp Soc Gen Microbiol 1980;30:127.

Marr JJ, Berens RL: Pyrazolopyrimidine metabolism in the pathogenic Trypanosomatidae. Mol Biochem Parasitol 1983;7:339.

Osinga KA et al: Topogenesis of microbody enzymes: A sequence comparison of the genes for the glycosomal (microbody) and cytosolic phosphoglycerate kinases of *Trypanosoma brucei*. EMBO J 1985;4:3811.

Pax R, Bennett JL, Fetterer R: A benzodiazepine derivative and praziquantel: Effects on musculature of *Schistosoma mansoni* and *Schistosoma japonicum*. Naunyn Schmiedebergs Arch Pharmacol 1978;304:309.

Phillips MA, Coffino P, Wang CC: Cloning and sequencing of the ornithine decarboxylase gene from *Trypanosoma brucei*. Implications for enzyme turnover and selective difluoromethylornithine inhibition. J Biol Chem 1987;262:8721.

Saenz RE et al: Treatment of American cutaneus leishmaniasis with orally administered allopurinol riboside. J Infect Dis 1989;160:153.

Senft AW et al: Pathways of nucleotide metabolism in *Schistosoma mansoni*. 3. Identification of enzymes in cell-free extracts. Biochem Pharmacol 1973;22:449.

Stretton AOW et al: Structure and physiological activity of the motoneurons of the nematode *Ascaris*. Proc Natl Acad Sci USA 1978;75:3493.

Sweeney TR, Strube RE: Antimalarials. In: *Burger's Medicinal Chemistry,* 4th ed. Wolff ME (editor). Wiley, 1979.

Tang L, Pritchard RK: Characterization of tubulin from *Brugia malayi* and *Brugia pahangi*. Mol Biochem Parasitol 1989;32:145.

Vanden Bossche H: Studies of the mode of action of anthelmintic drugs: Tools to investigate the biochemical peculiarities of helminths. Ann Parasit Hum Comp 1990; 65(Suppl 1):99.

Visser N, Opperdoes FR, Borst P: Subcellular compartmentation of glycolytic intermediates in *Trypanosoma brucei*. Eur J Biochem 1981;118:521.

Wang CC, Aldritt SP: Purine salvage networks in *Giardia lamblia*. J Exp Med 1983;158:1703.

Wang CC, Pong SS: Actions of avermectin B_{1a} on GABA nerves. In: *Membranes and Genetic Disease: Progress in Clinical and Biological Research,* vol 97. Sheppard JR, Anderson VE, Eaton JW (editors). AR Liss, 1982.

Wang CC, Simashkevich PM: Purine metabolism in a protozoan parasite *Eimeria tenella*. Proc Natl Acad Sci USA 1981;78:6618.

Wang CC: A novel suicide inhibitor strategy for antiparasitic drug development. J Cell Biochem 1991;45:49.

Wang CC: Biochemistry and physiology of coccidia. In: *The Biology of the Coccidia*. Long PL (editor). University Park Press, 1982.

Wang CC et al: Pyrimidine metabolism in *Trichomonas foetus*. Proc Natl Acad Sci USA 1983;80:2564.

Yuan L et al: The hypoxanthine-guanine phosphoribosyltransferase of *Schistosoma mansoni*. Further characterization and gene expression in *Escherichia coli*. J Biol Chem 1990;265:13528.

Robert S. Goldsmith, MD, DTM&H

TREATMENT OF MALARIA

Four species of *Plasmodium* are responsible for human malaria: *Plasmodium vivax, Plasmodium malariae, Plasmodium ovale,* and *Plasmodium falciparum.* Although all may cause severe illness, *P falciparum* causes most of the serious complications and deaths. The effectiveness of antimalarial agents varies between parasite species and between stages in their life cycles. In addition, parasite resistance to these drugs is an important therapeutic problem.

PARASITE LIFE CYCLE

The mosquito becomes infected by taking human blood that contains parasites in the sexual form. The sporozoites that develop in the mosquito are then inoculated into humans at its next feeding. In the first stage of development in humans, the **exoerythrocytic stage,** the sporozoites multiply in the liver to form tissue schizonts. Later, the parasites escape from the liver into the bloodstream as **merozoites** to initiate the **erythrocytic stage.** In this stage they invade red blood cells, multiply in them to form **blood schizonts,** and finally rupture the cells, releasing a new crop of merozoites. This cycle may be repeated many times. Meanwhile, the **gametocytes** (the sexual stage) form and are released into the circulation, where they may be taken in by another mosquito.

P falciparum and *P malariae* have only one cycle of liver cell invasion and multiplication, and liver infection ceases spontaneously in less than 4 weeks. Thereafter, multiplication is confined to the red blood cells. Thus, treatment that eliminates these species from the red blood cells 4 or more weeks after inoculation of the sporozoites will cure these infections.

P vivax (and presumably *P ovale*) have, however, a dormant hepatic stage (the **hypnozoite**) that causes subsequent recurrences (**relapses**) of the infection. Therefore, treatment that eradicates parasites from both the red cells and the liver is required to cure these infections.

DRUG CLASSIFICATION

Some major antimalarial drugs are shown by chemical group in Figure 54–1. Others include **antibiotics** (tetracycline, doxycycline), halofantrine, and qinghaosu* and its derivatives. Drug combinations used to treat malaria include Fansidar (pyrimethamine plus sulfadoxine) and Maloprim* (pyrimethamine plus dapsone).

The antimalarial drugs can also be classified by their selective actions on different phases of the parasite's life cycle. Drugs that eliminate developing tissue schizonts or latent hypnozoites in the liver (eg, primaquine) are called **tissue schizonticides.** Those that act on blood schizonts are **blood schizonticides** or **suppressive agents** (eg, chloroquine, amodiaquine, proguanil, pyrimethamine, mefloquine, quinine). **Gametocides** are drugs that prevent infection in mosquitoes by destroying gametocytes in the blood (eg, primaquine for *P falciparum* and chloroquine for *P vivax, P malariae,* and *P ovale.*) **Sporonticidal agents** are drugs that render gametocytes noninfective in the mosquito (eg, pyrimethamine, proguanil).

None of these drugs prevent infection (ie, none are true **causal prophylactic drugs**) except for the antifols (pyrimethamine and proguanil), which prevent maturation of the early *P falciparum* hepatic schizonts. However, blood schizonticides do destroy circulating plasmodia, which prevents attacks and, when used for sufficient time (4 weeks), cures *P falciparum* and *P malariae* malaria. Primaquine destroys the persisting liver hypnozoites of *P vivax* and *P ovale* and, when given with a blood schizonticide, effects radical cure of these infections.

---

*Not available in the USA.

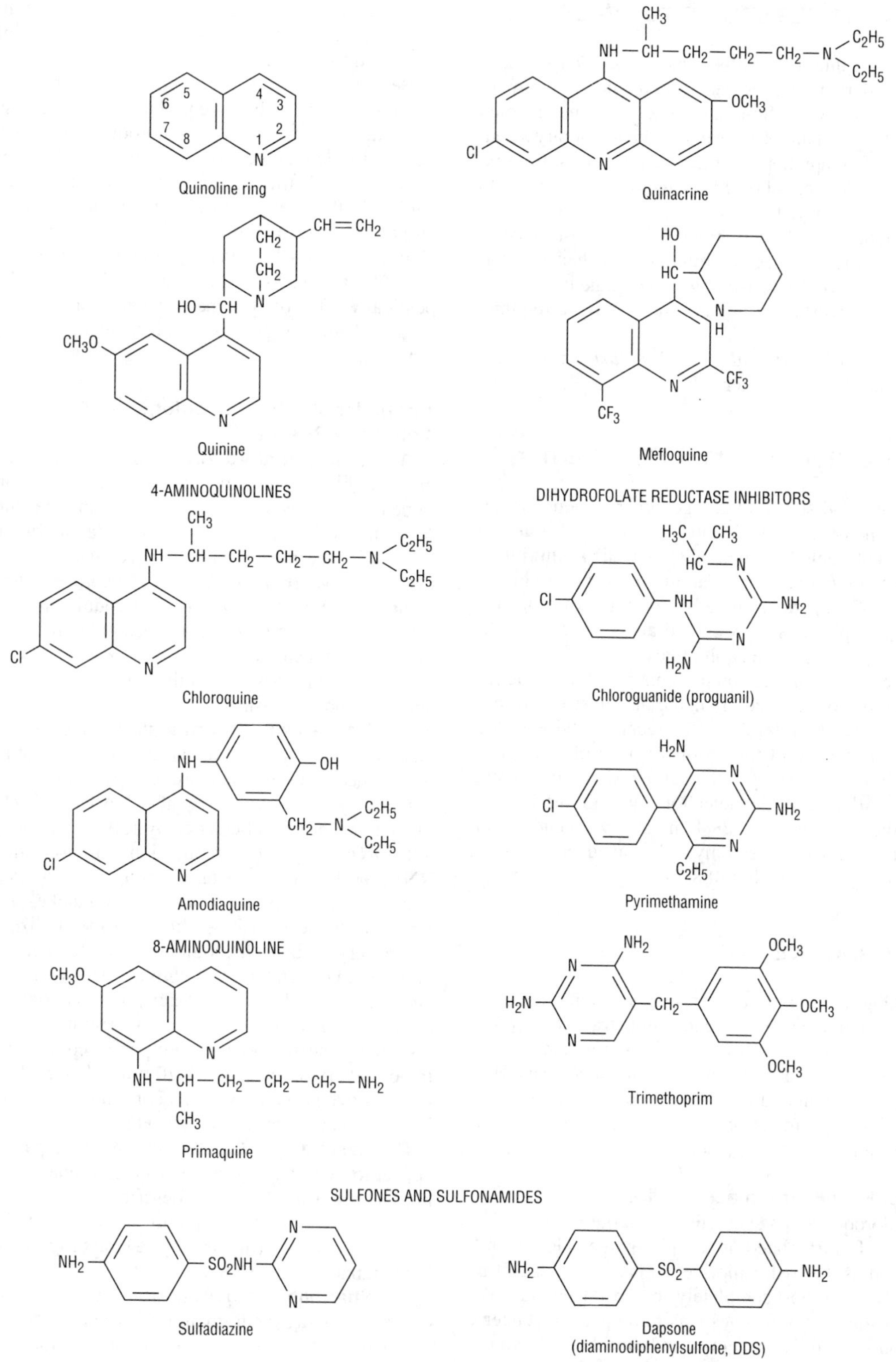

Figure 54–1. Structural formulas of some antimalarial drugs.

PARASITE RESISTANCE TO DRUGS

Chloroquine-resistant strains of *P falciparum* have been reported with increasing frequency in many areas of the world. Sometimes these strains are only partially resistant, manifested by the temporary subsidence of symptoms and a transient decrease in asexual parasitemia, followed by recrudescence of both after several days to weeks.

Instances of *P vivax* blood schizont resistance to chloroquine have been reported. *P vivax* hepatic schizonts are partially resistant to primaquine in some areas of the world, and a larger dose may be required for cure.

Resistance of *P ovale* and *P malariae* to chloroquine has not been observed.

CHEMOPROPHYLAXIS & TREATMENT

Table 54–1 sets forth dosages and regimens for malaria chemoprophylaxis and Table 54–2 outlines treatment, including methods for dealing with infections with *P falciparum* strains resistant to chloroquine. When patients are advised on use of drugs for chemoprophylaxis, they should also be taught methods for preventing mosquito bites.

The rest of this section presents pharmacologic information for selected antimalarial drugs; for further details, see the references. To receive advice in the USA on the use of these drugs—or to obtain quinidine in an emergency—contact the Malarial Branch, CDC, Atlanta, 30333; telephone 404-332-4555 during the day, 404-639-2888 nights, weekends, and holidays (emergencies only). For faxed information on prophylaxis, fax 404-488-7761.

CHLOROQUINE

Chloroquine is used for chemosuppression and treatment of the malarias, except for strains of *P falciparum* that are partially or completely resistant to it. It is also used in the treatment of hepatic amebiasis. Hydroxychloroquine, a derivative of chloroquine, is almost identical in its properties and can be used if chloroquine is not available.

Chemistry & Pharmacokinetics

Chloroquine is a synthetic 4-aminoquinoline (Figure 54–1) formulated as the phosphate salt for oral use and as the hydrochloride for parenteral use. It is rapidly and almost completely absorbed from the gastrointestinal tract, reaches maximum plasma concentrations (50–65% protein-bound) in about 3 hours, and is rapidly distributed to the tissues. Because it is concentrated in the tissues, it has a very large apparent volume of distribution of about 13,000 L. From these sites it is slowly released and metabolized. The drug readily crosses the placenta. It is excreted in the urine with a half-life of 3–5 days. Renal excretion is increased by acidification of the urine.

Because of its very large volume of distribution, a loading dose must be given when an effective schizonticidal plasma level of chloroquine is urgently needed in the treatment of acute attacks. The drug is well absorbed after intramuscular injection, but to avoid life-threatening toxicity, it should be administered in several small doses. Alternatively, parenteral chloroquine may be given by slow intravenous infusion (White: Eur J Clin Pharmacol, 1988). The therapeutically effective plasma concentration appears to be approximately 30 μg/L against sensitive *P falciparum* and 15 μg/L against *P vivax*.

Antimalarial & Pharmacologic Actions & Resistance

A. Antimalarial Action: Chloroquine is a highly effective blood schizonticide and is the 4-aminoquinoline most widely used to prevent or terminate attacks of vivax, ovale, malariae, or sensitive falciparum malaria. It is also moderately effective against gametocytes of *P vivax, P ovale,* and *P malariae* but not against those of *P falciparum.* Chloroquine is not active against the preerythrocytic plasmodium and does not effect radical cures of *P vivax* or *P ovale* infections because it does not eliminate the persisting liver stages of those parasites.

B. Mechanism of Antimalarial Action: The exact mechanism of antimalarial action has not been determined. Chloroquine may act by blocking the enzymatic synthesis of DNA and RNA in both mammalian and protozoal cells or by forming a complex with DNA that prevents replication or transcription to RNA. Within the parasite, the drug concentrates in vacuoles and raises the pH of these organelles, interfering with the parasite's ability to metabolize and utilize erythrocyte hemoglobin. Interference with phospholipid metabolism within the parasite has also been proposed. Selective toxicity for malarial parasites depends on a chloroquine-concentrating mechanism in parasitized cells. Chloroquine's concentration in normal erythrocytes is 10–20 times that in plasma; in parasitized erythrocytes, its concentration is about 25 times that in normal erythrocytes.

C. Resistance: Chloroquine-resistant parasites appear to expel chloroquine via a membrane P-glycoprotein pump similar to that described for multidrug-resistant cancer cells. The pump can be inhibited and resistance reversed (in vitro) by several drugs, including verapamil and desipramine.

D. Pharmacologic Actions: Although chloroquine (and hydroxychloroquine) have anti-inflammatory activity, the mechanism of action in autoimmune disorders is unknown.

Table 54–1. Prevention of malaria in travelers.[1]

TO PREVENT ATTACKS OF ALL FORMS OF MALARIA
AND TO ERADICATE *P FALCIPARUM* AND *P MALARIAE* INFECTIONS[2]

REGIONS WITH CHLOROQUINE-SENSITIVE *P FALCIPARUM* MALARIA: Central America west of the Panama Canal, the Caribbean, North Africa, and parts of the Middle East

Chloroquine[3]

Adult dose: Chloroquine phosphate, 500 mg salt (300 mg base); pediatric dose: 8.3 mg/kg salt (5 mg/kg base) up to the adult dose. Give a single dose of chloroquine weekly starting 2 weeks before entering the endemic area, while there, and for 4 weeks after leaving.

REGIONS WITH CHLOROQUINE-RESISTANT *P FALCIPARUM* MALARIA: All other regions of the world

Mefloquine (preferred method)[4]

Adult dose: one 250-mg tablet salt (228 mg base); pediatric dose: 15–19 kg, ¼ tablet; 20–30 kg, ½ tablet; 31–45 kg, ¾ tablet; >45 kg, one 250-mg tablet. Give a single dose of mefloquine weekly starting 1 week before entering the endemic area, while there, and for 4 weeks after leaving.

Doxycycline (alternative method)[5]

Adult dose: 100 mg daily; pediatric dose is 2 mg/kg (maximum, 100 mg) daily. Give the daily dose for 2 days before departure as a test dose. While in the endemic area, give the daily dose; continue doxycycline daily for 4 weeks after leaving endemic area.

Chloroquine (second alternative method)

Give chloroquine weekly at the above schedule.

    plus

Proguanil[6] (when available)

Adult dose: 200 mg once daily. Pediatric doses: <2 years, 50 mg/d; 2–6 years, 100 mg/d; 7–10 years, 150 mg/d; >10 years, 200 mg/d

    plus

Pyrimethamine-sulfadoxine (Fansidar)[7] (for one-time self-treatment of presumptive infections)

One dose only: Adult dose: 3 tablets; pediatric dose: 5–10 kg, ½ tablet; 11–20 kg, 1 tablet; 21–30 kg, 1½ tablets; 31–45 kg, 2 tablets; >45 kg, 3 tablets.

TO ERADICATE *P VIVAX* OR *P OVALE* INFECTIONS[2]

Primaquine[8]

Primaquine is indicated only for persons who have had a high probability of exposure to *P vivax* or *P ovale*. Start primaquine only after returning home, during the last 2 weeks of chemoprophylaxis. Adult dose: 26.3 mg salt (15 mg base) daily for 14 days; pediatric dose: 0.5 mg salt/kg (0.3 mg base/kg) daily for 14 days.

[1]For additional recommendations for prophylaxis, see the references or call the Centers for Disease Control and Prevention, Atlanta, GA 30333. Telephone (404) 332-4555 during the day for advice; (404) 488-7761 for faxed information.

[2]The blood schizonticides (chloroquine, mefloquine, and doxycycline), when taken for 4 weeks after leaving the endemic area, are curative for sensitive *P falciparum* and *P malariae* infections; primaquine, however, is needed to eradicate the persistent liver stages of *P vivax* and *P ovale*.

[3]Chloroquine can be used by pregnant women and by young children.

[4]Mefloquine is not recommended for use in pregnant women or in children who weigh less than 15 kg, or under certain other conditions (see text). Take with water and after eating.

[5]Doxycycline is contraindicated in pregnant women or in children under 8 years of age. The drug should be taken with the evening meal. Side effects include photosensitivity (preventive measures include the use of sunscreens that absorb ultraviolet radiation and avoidance of exposure to direct sunlight as much as possible), gastrointestinal symptoms, and candidal vaginitis.

[6]Proguanil (Paludrine), when taken in conjunction with chloroquine, is useful in East Africa and possibly in other regions of chloroquine resistance (but not in West Africa). The drug is not available in the USA but can be purchased in other countries.

[7]The drug should not be used for prophylaxis. It is used only for self-treatment of fever when a physician is not immediately available to make the diagnosis; but it is imperative that the patient see a physician promptly. Each tablet of Fansidar contains 25 mg of pyrimethamine and 500 mg of sulfadoxine. The drug is contraindicated in pregnancy at term, in known cases of sulfonamide sensitivity, and in children under 2 months of age. The drug is not effective in Thailand or adjacent countries.

[8]Before taking primaquine, patients should be screened to detect glucose-6-phosphate dehydrogenase deficiency. Primaquine is contraindicated in pregnancy. An alternative regimen in regions where chloroquine can be taken for prophylaxis is chloroquine phosphate, 500 mg (salt), plus primaquine phosphate, 78.9 mg (salt), weekly for 8 weeks.

Table 54–2. Treatment of malaria in nonimmune adult populations.

Treatment[1] of Infection With All Species (Except Chloroquine-Resistant *P falciparum*)	Treatment[1] of Infection With Chloroquine-Resistant *P falciparum* Strains
Oral treatment of *P falciparum*[2] or *P malariae* infection Chloroquine phosphate, 1 g (salt)[3,4] as initial dose, then 0.5 g at 6, 24, and 48 hours. **Oral treatment of *P vivax* or *P ovale* infection** Chloroquine[3,4] as above followed by 0.5 g on days 10 and 17 plus primaquine phosphate, 26.3 mg (salt)[5] daily for 14 days starting about day 4. **Parenteral treatment of severe attacks** Quinine dihydrochloride[6] or quinidine gluconate.[7] Start oral chloroquine therapy as soon as possible; follow with primaquine if the infection is due to *P vivax* or *P ovale*— or Chloroquine hydrochloride IM;[12] repeat every 6 hours. Start oral therapy as soon as possible; follow with primaquine if infection is due to *P vivax* or *P ovale*.	**Oral treatment** Quinine sulfate, 10 mg/kg 3 times daily for 3–7 days,[8] plus one of the following: (1) once only, pyrimethamine, 75 mg, and sulfadoxine, 1500 mg (= 3 tablets of Fansidar); (2) pyrimethamine, 25 mg twice daily for 3 days, and sulfadiazine, 500 mg 4 times daily for 5 days; (3) tetracycline,[9] 250–500 mg 4 times daily for 7 days; (4) doxycycline,[9] 100 mg twice daily for 7 days, or clindamycin,[9] 900 mg 3 times daily for 3 days. or Mefloquine,[10] 15–25 mg/kg (salt) once or in two divided doses 6 hours apart. or Halofantrine[11] **Parenteral treatment of severe attacks** Quinine dihydrochloride[6] or quinidine gluconate.[7] Start oral therapy with quinine sulfate plus a second drug (as above) as soon as possible.

[1] See text for cautions and contraindications for each drug.

[2] In falciparum malaria, if the patient has not shown a clinical response to chloroquine (48–72 hours for mild infections, 24 hours for severe ones), parasite resistance to chloroquine should be considered. Chloroquine should be stopped and oral quinine or mefloquine started.

[3] 500 mg chloroquine phosphate = 300 mg base.

[4] Chloroquine alone is curative for infection with sensitive strains of *P falciparum* and for *P malariae*, but primaquine is needed to eradicate the persistent liver stages of *P vivax* and *P ovale*. Start primaquine after the patient has recovered from the acute illness; continue chloroquine weekly during primaquine therapy. Patients should be screened for glucose-6-phosphate dehydrogenase deficiency before use of primaquine. An alternative mode for primaquine therapy is combined primaquine, 78.9 mg (salt), and chloroquine, 0.5 g (salt), weekly for 8 weeks.

[5] 26.3 mg of primaquine phosphate = 15 mg primaquine base.

[6] Quinine dihydrochloride. Give 10 mg/kg (salt) in 500 mL of normal saline or 5% glucose solution IV slowly over 4 hours; repeat every 8 hours until oral therapy is possible (maximum, 1800 mg/d). Blood pressure and ECG should be monitored constantly to detect arrhythmias or hypotension. A higher initial loading dose of quinine is given (20 mg/kg) to patients who acquired infections in Southeast Asia if it is known with certainty that they have not already taken the medication. Extreme caution is required in treating patients with quinine who previously have been taking mefloquine in prophylaxis. In the USA, quinine dihydrochloride is no longer available from the CDC.

[7] When parenteral quinine is unavailable, quinidine gluconate can be used, administered as a continuous infusion. A loading dose of 10 mg/kg (salt) (maximum, 600 mg) is diluted in 300 mL of normal saline and administered over 1–2 hours, followed by 0.02 mg/kg/min (maximum, 10 mg/kg every 8 hours) until oral quinine therapy is possible. Blood pressure and ECG should be monitored constantly; widening of the QRS interval or lengthening of the QT interval requires discontinuation. Quinidine gluconate is available in the USA from the Centers for Disease Control and Prevention (CDC), Atlanta, GA 30333. Telephone (404) 639-3670 during the day; (404) 639–2888 nights, weekends, and holidays (emergencies only).

[8] Although quinine sulfate is usually given for 3 days, it should be continued for 7 days in patients who acquired infections in Thailand, where diminished sensitivity to quinine has been noted.

[9] Contraindicated in children under the age of 8 years and in pregnant women.

[10] The higher dose is used in Thailand and other areas with increasing resistance and in children, as they metabolize the drug more rapidly than adults. Serious side effects are rare. See text for cautions and contraindications. Mefloquine must not be given with quinine or quinidine.

[11] The adult dosage is 1 tablet (500 mg) every 6 hours for three doses; children under 40 kg, 8 mg/kg (suspension) every 6 hours for three doses.

[12] To avoid potential severe toxicity, give parenteral chloroquine by low-dose intramuscular injection (maximum, 3.5 mg/kg [salt] every 6 hours)

Clinical Uses
(Tables 54–1, 54–2, 54–3)

A. Acute Malaria Attacks: Chloroquine usually terminates the fever (in 24–48 hours) and clears the parasitemia (in 48–72 hours) of acute attacks of *P vivax, P ovale,* and *P malariae* malaria and of malaria due to nonresistant strains of *P falciparum*. To cure malaria caused by *P vivax* and *P ovale,* primaquine must be given concurrently with chloroquine to eradicate the persistent liver stages.

B. Chemoprophylaxis: Chloroquine is the preferred drug for prophylaxis against all forms of malaria except in regions where *P falciparum* is resistant to 4-aminoquinolines.

C. Amebiasis: Chloroquine is used with emetine as an alternative treatment for amebic liver abscess.

D. Autoimmune Disorders: When used daily at high doses for several months, chloroquine (or hydroxychloroquine) has been useful in the treatment of autoimmune disorders (Chapter 35).

Adverse Effects

Patients usually tolerate chloroquine well when it is used for malaria prophylaxis (including prolonged use) or treatment. Gastrointestinal symptoms, mild headache, pruritus (especially in black persons), anorexia, malaise, blurring of vision, and urticaria are uncommon. Taking the drug after meals may reduce some adverse effects. Rare reactions include hemolysis in G6PD-deficient persons, impaired hearing, confusion, psychosis, convulsions, blood dyscrasias, skin reactions, and hypotension.

A total cumulative dosage of 100 g (base) may, theoretically, contribute to the development of irreversible retinopathy, ototoxicity, and myopathy. Baseline and periodic follow-up ophthalmologic and neuromuscular evaluations are recommended if chloroquine is used more than 5 years. The development of retinal or visual field changes or muscular weakness requires stopping the drug. Chloroquine may cause T wave changes and widening of the QRS complex on the ECG.

Large intramuscular injections (10 mg/kg) or rapid intravenous infusions can result in severe hypotension and respiratory and cardiac arrest.

Contraindications & Cautions

Chloroquine is contraindicated in patients with psoriasis or porphyria, in whom it may precipitate acute attacks of these diseases. It should not be combined with other drugs known to cause dermatitis. It should not be used in the presence of retinal or visual field abnormalities unless the benefits outweigh the risks.

Chloroquine should be used with caution in patients with a history of liver damage, alcoholism, or neurologic or hematologic disorders. Certain antacids and antidiarrheal agents (kaolin, calcium carbonate, and magnesium trisilicate) interfere with the absorption of chloroquine and should not be taken within about 4 hours before or after chloroquine administration.

Although the safety of chloroquine in pregnancy has not been completely confirmed, extensive experience with the drug during pregnancy with no reports of teratogenic effects has inclined most workers and WHO authorities to the view that the benefits of the drug outweigh its potential fetal risks. Oral chloroquine can be safely taken by young children. A pediatric solution of chloroquine sulfate (Nivaquine) is widely available outside the USA.

MEFLOQUINE

Mefloquine is used in prophylaxis and treatment of chloroquine-resistant and multidrug-resistant falciparum malaria. It is also effective in prophylaxis against *P vivax* and presumably against *P ovale* and *P malariae*.

Pharmacokinetics

Mefloquine hydrochloride is a synthetic 4-quinoline methanol derivative chemically related to quinine. It can only be given orally, because intense local irritation occurs with parenteral use. It is well absorbed, and peak plasma concentrations are reached in 7–24 hours. A single oral dose of 250 mg of the salt results in a plasma concentration of 290–340 ng/mL, whereas continuation of this dose daily results in mean steady state plasma concentrations of 560–1250 ng/mL. Plasma levels of 200–300 ng/mL may be necessary to achieve chemosuppression in *P falciparum* infections. The drug is highly bound to plasma proteins, concentrated in red blood cells, and extensively distributed to the tissues, including the central nervous system. Mefloquine is cleared in the liver. Its acid metabolites are slowly excreted, mainly in the feces. Its elimination half-life, which varies from 13 days to 33 days, tends to be shortened in patients with acute malaria. The drug can be detected in the blood for months after dosing ceases.

Antimalarial & Pharmacologic Actions

A. Antimalarial Action: Mefloquine has strong blood schizonticidal activity against *P falciparum* and *P vivax* but is not active against *P falciparum* gametocytes or the hepatic stages of *P vivax*. Insufficient information is available to document effectiveness against *P malariae* or *P ovale,* but theoretically the drug should be effective against circulating schizonts of these species. The mechanism of action of mefloquine is unknown.

B. Resistance: Sporadic and low levels of resistance to mefloquine have been reported from Southeast Asia and Africa. Resistance to the drug can emerge rapidly, and resistant strains have been found in areas where the drug has never been used.

B. Pharmacologic Effects: Mefloquine has quinidine-like effects on the heart.

Clinical Uses (Table 54–1)

A. Prophylaxis of Chloroquine-Resistant Strains of *P falciparum:* Mefloquine is effective in prophylaxis against most strains of chloroquine-resistant or pyrimethamine-sulfadoxine-resistant *P falciparum* and is curative when taken weekly for 4 weeks after leaving an endemic area. When used for this purpose, the drug also provides prophylaxis against *P vivax* and probably against *P ovale* and *P malariae.* Eradication of *P vivax* and *P ovale,* however, requires a course of primaquine against their hepatic stages (as used with chloroquine in eradicating *P vivax* infections; see above).

Although the drug is effective against chloroquine-sensitive *P falciparum,* it should be reserved for use in malarious areas in which chloroquine is not effective.

B. Treatment of Chloroquine-Resistant *P falciparum* Infection: The drug is indicated in oral treatment of mild to moderate mefloquine-susceptible *P falciparum* infections. Since mefloquine apparently does not act as quickly as quinine or quinidine and cannot be given parenterally, it should not supplant these drugs in management of severely ill patients. The current dosage recommendation is a single dose of 1250 mg; this recommendation will probably be reduced to either 15 mg/kg or a total of 1000 mg, whichever is lower, in the near future. (***Caution:*** see manufacturer's recommendations before use.)

Adverse Reactions

The frequency and intensity of reactions are dose-related. Most of the symptoms can, however, also occur as a result of malaria itself.

A. Prophylactic Doses: Minor and transient adverse effects include gastrointestinal disturbances (nausea, vomiting, epigastric pain, diarrhea), headache, dizziness, syncope, and extrasystoles, with an incidence not much higher than for placebo or other antimalarials. Transient leukocytosis, thrombocytopenia, and transaminase elevations have been reported. Transient or reversible neuropsychiatric events have also been reported (convulsions, depression, psychoses).

B. Treatment Doses: Particularly with therapeutic doses over 1000 mg, gastrointestinal symptoms and fatigue are more likely and the incidence of neuropsychiatric symptoms (dizziness, headache, visual disturbances, tinnitus, insomnia, restlessness, anxiety, depression, confusion, acute psychosis, or seizures) may be as high as 1%. Reactions may occur 2–3 weeks after the last dose of mefloquine.

C. Animal Toxicity: Ophthalmologic lesions (lens opacity, retinal degeneration) have been reported in animals but not in humans.

D. Mutagenicity, Carcinogenicity, and Teratogenicity: Mutagenicity and carcinogenicity studies have been negative in a variety of assay systems. Adequate controlled studies in human pregnancy are not available.

Contraindications & Cautions

Mefloquine is contraindicated if there is a history of epilepsy or psychiatric disorder. The drug should not be used for children under 15 kg or under 2 years of age; in these groups, the drug appears to be poorly tolerated, and efficacy has not been established. Also contraindicated is concurrent administration of mefloquine with quinine, quinidine, beta-blocking or calcium channel-blocking agents, or any other agent that may prolong or otherwise alter cardiac conduction. If quinine or quinidine precedes the use of mefloquine, 12 hours should elapse before mefloquine is started. Because of the long half-life of mefloquine, extreme caution is required if quinine or quinidine is used to treat malaria after mefloquine has been taken.

The drug should preferably not be used in pregnancy, and women of childbearing potential who take mefloquine for malarial prophylaxis should use reliable precautions against conception.

Mefloquine should not be taken by persons whose work requires fine coordination and spatial discrimination (eg, airline pilots). Patients taking anticonvulsant drugs (particularly valproic acid and divalproex sodium) may have breakthrough seizures; concurrent administration of mefloquine and chloroquine or quinine increases the risk of convulsions.

The safety of mefloquine usage beyond 1 year has not been established. Therefore, if the drug is used for prolonged periods, periodic evaluations, including liver function tests and complete ophthalmologic examinations, are recommended.

PRIMAQUINE

Chemistry & Pharmacokinetics

Primaquine phosphate is a synthetic 8-aminoquinoline derivative (Figure 54–1). After oral administration, the drug is usually well absorbed, reaching peak plasma levels in 1–2 hours, and then is almost completely metabolized and excreted in the urine. Primaquine's plasma half-life is 3–6 hours, and only trace amounts remain at 24 hours. Primaquine is widely distributed to the tissues, but only a small amount is bound there. Its major metabolite is a deaminated derivative that reaches plasma concentrations more than ten times greater than those of the parent compound, is eliminated more slowly, and accumulates with daily dosing. Whether primaquine or one of its metabolites is the active compound has not been determined.

Antimalarial & Pharmacologic Actions

A. Antimalarial Action: Primaquine is active against the late hepatic stages (hypnozoites and schizonts) of *P vivax* and *P ovale* and thus effects radical cure of these infections. Primaquine is also highly active against the primary exoerythrocytic stages of *P falciparum.* When used as a causal prophylactic drug with chloroquine, it effectively protects against *P vivax* and *P ovale* but not against chloroquine-resistant *P falciparum.* Primaquine is highly gametocidal against the four malaria species and occasionally is used to eradicate the gametes of *P falciparum.* At nontoxic doses, primaquine's effect on blood schizonts is too slight to be useful in treatment of acute attacks.

B. Mechanism of Action: The mechanism of primaquine's antimalarial action is not well understood. The quinoline-quinone intermediates derived from primaquine are electron-carrying redox compounds that can act as oxidants. These intermediates probably produce most of the hemolysis and methemoglobinemia associated with primaquine's use.

C. Pharmacologic Effects: At high doses, primaquine may suppress myeloid activity. At standard doses, it may affect erythrocytes in genetically susceptible persons (see below).

Clinical Uses
(Tables 54–1 and 54–2)

A. Terminal Prophylaxis of Vivax and Ovale Malaria: Because of its effect on the persistent liver stages of *P vivax* and *P ovale,* primaquine plus a blood schizonticide, usually chloroquine, are taken together at the end of a period of potential exposure to these parasites to effect radical cure (terminal prophylaxis) (Table 54–1).

B. Radical Cure of Acute Vivax and Ovale Malaria: Primaquine plus chloroquine are used to treat these acute infections (Table 54–2). A 14-day course of primaquine is standard.

C. Causal Prophylaxis of Vivax and Ovale Malaria: The use of combined chloroquine and primaquine taken weekly for suppression and eradication (causal prophylaxis) of the malarias is no longer recommended, because chloroquine alone provides adequate suppression and because extended exposure to primaquine should be avoided.

D. Gametocidal Action: The oral dose of primaquine required to render falciparum gametocytes noninfective is 45 mg (base) once only.

E. *Pneumocystis carinii* Pneumonia: Combined therapy of primaquine with clindamycin is being evaluated in treatment of this pneumonia.

Adverse Effects

Primaquine in recommended doses is generally well tolerated. It infrequently causes nausea, epigastric pain, abdominal cramps, and headache. The more serious adverse effects, leukopenia and agranulocytosis, are rare. Other possible rare reactions are leukocytosis, pruritus, and arrhythmias.

Standard doses of primaquine may cause limited hemolysis, marked hemolysis, or methemoglobinemia (manifested by cyanosis) in persons with some variants of glucose-6-phosphate dehydrogenase deficiency or certain other hereditary erythrocytic pentose phosphate pathway defects. Although primaquine can produce methemoglobinemia in normal persons, the effect is more marked in those with congenital deficiency of nicotinamide adenine dinucleotide methemoglobin reductase.

Contraindications & Cautions

Primaquine should not be prescribed for patients with connective tissue disorders or those with a history of granulocytopenia. It should not be given during the first trimester of pregnancy and preferably not until after delivery. It is never given parenterally, because it may induce marked hypotension.

When feasible, patients should be tested for glucose-6-phosphate dehydrogenase deficiency before primaquine is prescribed. The drug should be stopped if there is any evidence of hemolysis (reddening or darkening of the urine) or anemia. However, sensitive persons can often tolerate and be treated with chloroquine, 0.5 g, plus primaquine, 78.9 mg (45 mg of base), once weekly for 8 weeks.

PYRIMETHAMINE
& PROGUANIL
(Chloroguanide)

Pyrimethamine in fixed combination with sulfadoxine is used in single-dose treatment of susceptible cases of chloroquine-resistant falciparum malaria. Because of the toxicity of the combined drugs, it is no longer used in prophylaxis. Pyrimethamine is also used in the treatment of toxoplasmosis. Proguanil—not available in the USA—is used in some regions of the world for malaria prophylaxis, particularly in combination with chloroquine.

Chemistry & Pharmacokinetics

Pyrimethamine and proguanil are dihydrofolate reductase inhibitors (folic acid antagonists, antifols).

Pyrimethamine is a 2,4-diaminopyrimidine related to trimethoprim, which is used to treat bacterial infections (Chapter 47). Proguanil is a biguanide derivative. Their structures are shown in Figure 54–1.

Both pyrimethamine and proguanil are slowly but adequately absorbed from the gastrointestinal tract. Pyrimethamine reaches peak plasma levels 4–6 hours after an oral dose, is bound to plasma proteins, and has an elimination half-life of about 3.5 days. Proguanil reaches peak plasma levels about 5 hours after an oral dose and has an elimination half-life of about 16 hours. Therefore, in prophylaxis, proguanil must be administered daily, whereas pyrimethamine can be given once a week. Pyrimethamine is extensively metabolized before excretion. Proguanil is a prodrug; only its triazine metabolite, cycloguanil, is active.

Antimalarial & Pharmacologic Actions

A. Antimalarial Action: Pyrimethamine and proguanil are blood schizonticides; however, because they act more slowly than chloroquine or quinine, they can be used alone only in prophylaxis, not in treatment. Proguanil (but not pyrimethamine) has a marked effect on the primary tissue stages of *P falciparum* and therefore may have causal prophylactic action, perhaps effective even when blood schizonts are resistant to the agent. These drugs are neither adequately gametocidal nor effective against the persistent liver stages of *P vivax.*

Pyrimethamine and the triazine metabolite of proguanil have a higher affinity for and more effectively inhibit plasmodial dihydrofolate reductase than the human enzyme; as a result, the reduction of dihydrofolic acid to tetrahydrofolic acid (folinic acid) is selectively inhibited in the parasite.

B. Resistance: Resistant strains of *P falciparum* have appeared worldwide; resistant strains of *P vivax* have appeared less frequently. Therefore, prophylaxis against falciparum malaria with either drug alone is no longer recommended. Although strains of chloroquine-resistant *P falciparum* are usually resistant to pyrimethamine or proguanil as well, they are sometimes susceptible to these drugs in combination with a sulfonamide or sulfone (see below).

C. Pharmacologic Effects: In dosages used for malaria chemoprophylaxis and treatment, the antifols produce no pharmacologic effects in the host. In the higher doses used for toxoplasmosis, macrocytic anemia and other adverse effects may occur.

Clinical Uses

A. Treatment of Chloroquine-Resistant Falciparum Malaria: Pyrimethamine in fixed combination with sulfadoxine (Fansidar; see below) is used to treat known or presumptive acute attacks of chloroquine-resistant falciparum malaria (Table 54–2).

B. Chemoprophylaxis of Chloroquine-Resistant Falciparum Malaria: The use of Fansidar on a continuing schedule for falciparum malaria prophylaxis has been discontinued because of the drug's toxicity.

C. Toxoplasmosis Treatment: The treatment of choice is pyrimethamine, 75 mg/d for 3 days, then 25 mg daily, plus either trisulfapyrimidines (2–6 g/d in four divided doses) or sulfadiazine (100 mg/kg/d [maximum 6 g/d] in four divided doses); continue with this treatment for 3–4 weeks. Leucovorin calcium (folinic acid), 10 mg/d in two to four divided doses, is given to avoid the hematologic effects of pyrimethamine-induced folate deficiency. Platelet and white blood cell counts should be performed at least twice weekly. Patients should be screened for a history of sulfonamide sensitivity.

In the treatment of toxoplasma encephalitis in AIDS, higher doses are used. Primary therapy (for 6 weeks or longer if necessary) is as follows: pyrimethamine, 200 mg as loading dose in two divided doses, then 1–1.5 mg/kg/d; and sulfadiazine or trisulfapyrimidines, 4–6 g/d in four divided doses. Maintenance therapy is as follows: pyrimethamine, 25–50 mg/d; sulfadiazine or trisulfapyrimidines, 2 g/d in two divided doses; and leucovorin calcium, 5–20 g/d in two divided doses. Corticosteroids are often added to reduce increased intracranial pressure.

Adverse Effects

In malaria treatment, most patients tolerate pyrimethamine and proguanil well. Gastrointestinal and allergic reactions are rare.

Cautions & Contraindications

Formerly, pyrimethamine was not recommended in pregnancy because the drug is teratogenic in some animals when administered in large doses. However, pyrimethamine has been widely used in humans for over 20 years, and such effects have not been reported. Proguanil is also now considered safe in pregnancy.

SULFONAMIDES & SULFONES

Sulfonamides and sulfones have blood schizonticidal action against some strains of *P falciparum* by the same mechanism as in bacteria, namely, inhibition of dihydrofolic acid synthesis (Chapter 47). However, the drugs have only weak effects against the blood schizonts of *P vivax,* and they are not active against the gametocytes or liver stages of *P falciparum* or *P vivax.*

When a sulfonamide or sulfone is combined with an antifol, synergistic blockade of folic acid synthesis occurs in susceptible plasmodia (Figure 47–2). Many combinations have been evaluated for prophylaxis and treatment of chloroquine-resistant falciparum; the most useful are sulfadoxine with pyrimethamine (Fansidar) and dapsone with pyrimethamine (Maloprim). However, in many regions of the world, *P falciparum* has also become resistant to these combinations. In addition to drug resistance, major disadvantages of the sulfonamides and sulfones are the slowness of their blood schizonticidal activity and their numerous and sometimes serious adverse effects.

1. FANSIDAR
(Pyrimethamine-Sulfadoxine)

Pharmacokinetics

Fansidar is well absorbed. Its components display peak plasma levels within 2–8 hours and are excreted mainly by the kidneys. Average half-lives are about 170 hours for sulfadoxine and 80–110 hours for pyrimethamine.

Antimalarial Action & Resistance

Fansidar is effective against certain strains of falciparum malaria. However, quinine must be given concurrently in treatment of seriously ill patients, because Fansidar is only slowly active. Fansidar is not effective in vivax malaria, and its usefulness in ovale and malariae malaria has not been adequately studied.

Multidrug resistance (to chloroquine and Fansidar) has occurred in much of southeastern Asia and in areas of the Amazon basin and eastern Africa.

Clinical Uses
(Tables 54–1 and 54–2)

A. Treatment of Chloroquine-Resistant Falciparum Malaria: Fansidar (a slow-acting schizonticide) is used in conjunction with quinine (fast-acting) to treat acute attacks of chloroquine-resistant falciparum malaria (Table 54–2).

B. Presumptive Treatment of Chloroquine-Resistant Falciparum Malaria: Fansidar is used in presumptive self-treatment of malaria—ie, when malaria-like symptoms occur that cannot be immediately diagnosed and managed by a local physician, and the patient decides to self-treat with a single dose (three tablets for an adult). *It is imperative, however, that medical follow-up be sought promptly.* This treatment is not effective for vivax, ovale, or malariae malaria but may be effective for susceptible chloroquine-resistant strains of *P falciparum* if the degree of illness does not require a rapidly acting blood schizonticide such as quinine.

Adverse Effects

Rare adverse effects to single-dose Fansidar are those associated with sulfonamide allergy, including the hematologic, gastrointestinal, central nervous system, dermatologic, and renal systems.

Fansidar is no longer used in continuing prophylaxis because of severe reactions, including erythema multiforme, Stevens-Johnson syndrome, and toxic epidermal necrolysis, that occur with a low but significant frequency.

Contraindications & Cautions

Fansidar is contraindicated in patients who have had adverse reactions to sulfonamides. Fansidar should not be used in pregnancy at term, in nursing women, or in children under 2 months of age. Fansidar should be used with caution in the presence of impaired renal or hepatic function, in patients with glucose-6-phosphate dehydrogenase deficiency (hemolysis occurs in some), and in those with severe allergic disorders, bronchial asthma, or poor nutritional status.

2. MALOPRIM*
(Pyrimethamine-Dapsone)

Because of its potential toxicity (fatal agranulocytosis), this drug is not recommended for routine prophylaxis.

QUININE & QUINIDINE

1. QUININE

Quinine, the principal alkaloid derived from the bark of the cinchona tree, has been used in malaria suppression and treatment for more than 300 years. By 1959, quinine had been superseded by other antimalarials, especially chloroquine. Following the development of widespread resistance to chloroquine, quinine has again become an important antimalarial. It is principally used for the oral treatment of chloroquine-resistant falciparum malaria and where available, for parenteral treatment of severe attacks of falciparum malaria. For parenteral therapy in the USA, The CDC will provide quinidine gluconate on an emergency basis (see Quinidine, below).

Pharmacokinetics

Quinine, a bitter tasting alkaloid, is rapidly ab-

---

*Not available in the USA.

sorbed, reaches peak plasma levels in 1–3 hours, and is widely distributed in body tissues. Approximately 80% of plasma quinine is protein-bound; red blood cell levels are about 20% of the plasma level and cerebrospinal fluid concentrations about 7%. The elimination half-life of quinine is about 10 hours in normal persons but longer in malaria-infected persons in proportion to the severity of the disease. Approximately 80% of the drug is metabolized in the liver and excreted for the most part in the urine. Excretion is accelerated in acid urine.

With constant daily doses, plasma concentrations usually reach a plateau on the third day. In normals or in mild infection, standard oral doses result in plasma levels of about 7 μg/mL; in severe malaria, higher plasma levels are reached. A mean plasma concentration of about 5 μg/mL is necessary to eliminate asexual parasites of vivax malaria and a somewhat higher concentration in falciparum malaria. Concentrations lower than 2 μg/mL have little effect, whereas concentrations over 7 μg/mL are generally accompanied by adverse reactions of "cinchonism." Because of this narrow therapeutic range, adverse reactions are common during falciparum malaria treatment.

Intramuscular use of quinine is now considered safe and effective. Because injections of the concentrated solution (300 mg/mL) are painful and may cause sterile abscess, dilute solutions (50–100 mg/mL) are preferable. Dosage regimens are the same as for intravenous use, and peak plasma levels occur within 4 hours.

Antimalarial & Pharmacologic Actions & Drug Resistance

A. Antimalarial Action: Quinine is a rapidly acting, highly effective blood schizonticide against the four malaria parasites. The drug is gametocidal for *P vivax* and *P ovale* but not very effective against *P falciparum* gametocytes. Quinine has no effect on sporozoites or the liver stages of any of the parasites.

B. Mechanism of Action: The drug's molecular mechanism is unclear. Quinine is known to depress many enzyme systems. It also forms a hydrogen-bonded complex with double-stranded DNA that inhibits strand separation, transcription, and protein synthesis.

C. Pharmacologic Effects: When taken orally, quinine commonly causes gastric irritation. The drug's effect on cardiac muscle is similar to that of its diastereoisomer, quinidine, but less intense. Quinine has a slight oxytocic action on the gravid uterus, especially in the third trimester. In skeletal muscle, quinine has a curare-like effect on the motor endplate; it also appears to lengthen the refractory period of the skeletal muscle membrane. Quinine may diminish tetanic contractions associated with various conditions and has been used to lessen the contractures of myotonia congenita. Obsolete uses include a diagnostic

test for myasthenia gravis, and antipyresis and analgesia. Therapeutic doses sometimes cause hypoglycemia through stimulation of pancreatic B cell release of insulin; this is a particular problem in severe infections and in pregnant patients. Severe or even lethal hypotension can follow too-rapid intravenous injections.

D. Resistance: Resistance of quinine when used alone has been increasing in Southeast Asia. However, there is no unequivocal case of a complete failure to respond to quinine when a second drug is also used.

Clinical Uses
(Tables 54–1 and 54–2)

A. Parenteral Treatment of Severe Falciparum Malaria: Quinine dihydrochloride, if available, is given *slowly* intravenously when parenteral therapy is required for severe *P falciparum* infections, whether sensitive or resistant to chloroquine. Contrary to earlier views, a dilute solution of intramuscular quinine, which is well absorbed, causes little or no local discomfort or tissue necrosis and is an alternative to intravenous administration.

B. Oral Treatment of Falciparum Malaria Resistant to Chloroquine: Quinine sulfate is used with other drugs for the oral treatment of acute attacks of *P falciparum* malaria resistant to chloroquine (Table 54–2). Although quinine effectively reduces parasitemia, combination therapy is necessary because quinine alone fails to completely eliminate the infection. Quinine is less effective than chloroquine and is therefore not used to treat acute attacks of vivax, ovale, or malariae malaria or chloroquine-sensitive falciparum malaria.

C. Prophylaxis: Because of its potential toxicity, quinine is not generally used in prophylaxis. However, in areas where *P falciparum* is resistant to chloroquine and neither mefloquine nor doxycycline is available, quinine prophylaxis can be considered. The dosage is 325 mg daily while in the endemic area and for 4 weeks after leaving. Eradication of *P vivax* or *P ovale* infection requires a course of primaquine, but quinine and primaquine should not be given concurrently.

D. Other Uses: Quinine sulfate, 200–300 mg, sometimes relieves nighttime leg cramps. Quinine is used concurrently with clindamycin in the treatment of severe babesiosis caused by *Babesia microti*.

Adverse Effects

A. Gastrointestinal Effects: Quinine is an irritant to the gastric mucosa and often causes nausea, vomiting, or epigastric pain.

B. Cinchonism: A less common effect is cinchonism, a toxic state that usually develops when plasma levels of quinine exceed 7–10 μg/mL; in some patients, however, symptoms may occur at lower plasma levels. Symptoms of mild to moderate cinchonism include headache, nausea, slight visual disturbances, dizziness, and mild tinnitus. They may abate as treatment continues and usually do not require discontinuance of treatment. If the symptoms become severe, the drug should be discontinued temporarily while plasma quinine levels are determined.

C. Hematologic Effects: Hemolysis directly attributable to quinine occurs in 0.05% of people treated for acute malaria; it may also occur in glucose-6-phosphate dehydrogenase-deficient persons. Leukopenia, agranulocytosis, thrombocytopenic purpura, Henoch-Schönlein purpura, and hypoprothrombinemia are rare.

D. Hypoglycemia: A decrease in blood sugar may occur at therapeutic doses, as noted above. Administration of glucose may evoke greater insulin release followed by further hypoglycemia.

E. Severe Toxicity: Severe toxicity is rare; findings include fever, skin eruptions, deafness, visual abnormalities, central nervous system effects, and quinidine-like effects.

The role of quinine in **blackwater fever** is unclear, but that disorder has been associated with prolonged past use of the drug. In sensitized patients, even a single dose can precipitate the reaction. The syndrome—characterized by massive intravascular hemolysis followed by hemoglobinuria, dark urine, azotemia, intravascular sludging and coagulation, renal failure, and uremia—has a fatality rate of 25–50%.

F. Mutagenicity and Teratogenicity: In humans, large doses of quinine given in failed abortion attempts have resulted in congenital malformations.

G. Other Adverse Effects: Intravenous quinine and quinidine infrequently cause thrombophlebitis. Excessive rate of infusion may result in moderate to marked hypotension, seizures, ventricular fibrillation, and death.

Contraindications & Cautions

Stop the drug immediately if signs of hemolysis appear. Hypersensitivity reactions and other severe reactions require permanent discontinuation of the drug. Quinine should not be given subcutaneously and should not be given in pregnancy or to patients with histories of tinnitus, optic neuritis, or myasthenia gravis. In renal insufficiency, determine plasma quinine levels and reduce dosage appropriately. For patients with cardiac arrhythmias, use the same precautions as with quinidine.

Drug Interactions

Aluminum-containing antacids delay the absorption of quinine. Quinine may delay absorption of digoxin and digitoxin. Concurrent use of digoxin and quinidine may result in increased digoxin serum concentrations. The action of warfarin and other anticoagulants may be enhanced. Quinine may intensify or

reinduce neuromuscular block in patients receiving neuromuscular blockers. Cimetidine slows the elimination of quinine, and acidification of the urine increases quinine clearance.

2. QUINIDINE

Quinidine, the dextrorotatory diastereoisomer of quinine, is formulated as quinidine gluconate for the parenteral treatment of cardiac arrhythmias (see Chapter 14). Quinidine gluconate is also effective in the parenteral treatment of severe malaria and can be used when the parenteral form of quinine, quinine sulfate, is not available. In the USA, quinine sulfate is no longer marketed, but quinidine gluconate, if not locally available, can be obtained from the CDC on an emergency basis (404-639-3670).

ALTERNATIVE DRUGS

The following alternative drugs are particularly useful in regions where *P falciparum* is resistant to both chloroquine and the antifolate-sulfonamide combinations. Some of these drugs are used in prophylaxis. After the patient has left the endemic area, primaquine can be given (in accordance with the guidelines provided above) to provide radical cure for *P vivax* and *P ovale* infections.

1. DOXYCYCLINE

Doxycycline, a tetracycline drug (Chapter 44), is generally effective in prophylaxis against multidrug-resistant *P falciparum* if used in doses of 100 mg/d during residence in the endemic area and for 4 weeks after leaving. In the treatment of acute malaria, it is not used alone but is effective when combined with quinine. Although the drug is appropriate for short-term prophylaxis, its long-term efficacy and safety for this indication have not been evaluated. See Chapter 44 for additional details.

2. HALOFANTRINE*

Halofantrine hydrochloride is a phenanthrene-methanol compound, active against the asexual erythrocytic stages of *P vivax* and chloroquine-sensitive and chloroquine-resistant *P falciparum* but not against the exoerythrocytic stages or against gametocytes. Only limited information is available about its effectiveness in *P ovale* or *P malariae* infections. The

---

*Not available in the USA.

drug is rapidly but incompletely absorbed from the gastrointestinal tract (absorption is improved when the drug is taken with food), widely distributed to the tissues, and reaches peak plasma levels in 3–5 hours. The half-lives of the drug and its principal metabolite, desbutylhalofantrine, are variable: 1–2 days and 3–5 days, respectively. The drug and its metabolite are excreted for the most part in the feces.

The drug is used only in the oral treatment of acute disease, principally falciparum cerebral malaria. Its efficacy in this condition has been estimated as better than 94%. Since no parenteral preparation is available, the drug cannot be used for severely ill persons. The adult oral dosage is 500 mg (for children under 40 kg: 8 mg/kg) given every 6 hours for three doses. For nonimmune persons, the dosage is repeated in 1 week. Currently, the drug is not recommended for prophylaxis.

The drug is embryotoxic in animal studies and is therefore contraindicated in pregnancy unless benefits clearly outweigh the risk. The drug is usually well tolerated.

3. QINGHAOSU*
(Artemisinin)

Qinghaosu is a sesquiterpene lactone endoperoxide, the active principal of a Chinese herbal medicine *(qing hao)* that has been used as an antipyretic in China for over 2000 years.

Because qinghaosu is only sparingly soluble in water and oils, analogues have been synthesized to increase its solubility: water-soluble artesunate (available as tablets for oral use and as an intravenous formulation) and lipid-soluble artemether (available as tablets and as an intramuscular formulation). Arteether, a lipid-soluble derivative similar to artemether, is also under evaluation. Pharmacologic studies have shown that qinghaosu and its analogues are rapidly absorbed (with peak plasma levels occurring in about 1 hour) and undergo rapid hydrolysis to the biologically active metabolite dihydorqinghaosu, following which the parent compound and metabolite are widely distributed in the tissues and eliminated rapidly (with a half-life of about 4 hours).

Qinghaosu and analogues are effective blood schizonticides against all types of malaria, including chloroquine-resistant falciparum malaria. They have no effect on the hepatic stages of the parasites, do not cure the relapsing malarias, and are not causal prophylactics. Their mechanism of action is unknown. They are especially useful in treatment of falciparum

cerebral malaria. The recurrence rate is over 40% when therapy is for 1–3 days but considerably less when treatment is extended to 7 days. Dosage recommendations are as yet largely empirical.

The drugs produce few adverse effects but are said to be embryotoxic in rats and mice. Therefore, they should not be used in pregnancy. Bone marrow depression has been noted in animals, and depression of reticulocyte counts has been reported in humans.

4. QUINACRINE

Quinacrine, a 9-aminoacridine, is a blood schizonticide that can effectively suppress all four types of human malaria and can effect radical cures of *P malariae* and nonresistant strains of *P falciparum.* Until the introduction of chloroquine in 1945, quinacrine was the principal synthetic drug used for antimalarial prophylaxis, but it is now considered obsolete for this purpose. Its disadvantages include occasional drug deposits that turn the skin yellow and rare psychotic reactions.

TREATMENT OF AMEBIASIS

Amebiasis may present as a severe intestinal infection (dysentery), a mild to moderate symptomatic intestinal infection, an asymptomatic intestinal infection, or as an ameboma, liver abscess, or other type of extraintestinal infection.

The choice of drug depends on the clinical presentation and on the desired site of drug action, ie, in the intestinal lumen or in the tissues. Table 54–3 outlines a preferred and an alternative method of treatment for each clinical type of amebiasis. Drug dosages are provided in the table footnotes. No drugs are recommended as safe or effective for chemoprophylaxis.

Drugs Used in Treatment

All of the antiamebic drugs act against *Entamoeba histolytica* trophozoites, but most are not effective against the cyst stage.

A. Tissue Amebicides: These drugs eliminate organisms primarily in the bowel wall, liver, and other extraintestinal tissues. They are not effective against organisms in the bowel lumen.

1. Nitroimidazoles–Metronidazole, tinidazole,* and ornidazole* are highly effective against amebas in the bowel wall and other tissues. They are, however, only partially effective and not adequate as lu-

---

*Not available in the USA.

minal amebicides. For example, metronidazole alone fails to cure up to 50% of intestinal infections.

2. Emetines–Emetine and dehydroemetine† are generally given intramuscularly; in this form, they act on organisms in the bowel wall and other tissues but not on amebas in the bowel lumen.

3. Chloroquine– This drug is active principally against amebas in the liver.

B. Luminal Amebicides: These drugs act primarily in the bowel lumen; they are not effective against organisms in the bowel wall or other tissues.

1. Dichloroacetamides–Diloxanide furoate,† clefamide,* teclozan,* etofamide.*

2. Halogenated hydroxyquinolines–Iodoquinol (diiodohydroxyquin); clioquinol (iodochlorhydroxyquin).*

3. Antibiotics–The oral tetracyclines indirectly affect luminal amebas by inhibiting the bacterial associates of *E histolytica* in the bowel lumen. Paromomycin and erythromycin are directly amebicidal. Except for paromomycin, none of the antibiotics are highly effective against intestinal organisms and therefore should not be used by themselves in treatment. Parenteral antibiotics have little antiamebic activity in any site.

Treatment of Specific Forms of Amebiasis

A. Asymptomatic Intestinal Infection: Persons with asymptomatic infections should be treated, since they may become symptomatic or transmit the infection to others. The drugs of choice, diloxanide furoate and iodoquinol, cure about 80–90% of cases in a single course of treatment. Diloxanide causes fewer adverse effects than iodoquinol. In asymptomatic infection, the additional use of a tissue amebicidal drug is not necessary.

Other alternatives for treatment or re-treatment are paromomycin or metronidazole plus iodoquinol or diloxanide.

B. Mild to Moderate Intestinal Infections: In this stage of intestinal disease, the administration of both a luminal and a tissue amebicidal drug is necessary, since the parasites must be eradicated in the lumen, the intestinal wall, and the liver. The drug combination of choice, metronidazole plus a luminal amebicide (diloxanide furoate or iodoquinol), cures over 90% of cases.

An alternative treatment is to combine a luminal amebicide (iodoquinol or diloxanide furoate) with a tetracycline and then follow with a short course of chloroquine.

C. Severe Intestinal Infection (Dysentery): The amebicidal treatment of severe amebic dysentery is the same as in mild to moderate disease. Fluid and electrolyte therapy and opioids to control bowel motility are necessary adjuncts.

D. Hepatic Abscess: Hospitalization and bed rest are usually necessary. The treatment of choice is metronidazole; if given for 10 days, this drug cures over 95% of uncomplicated cases. However, treatment failures sometimes occur, either during the course of treatment or after its completion. A luminal amebicide such as diloxanide furoate or iodoquinol should also be given to eradicate intestinal infection whether or not organisms are found in the stools. An advantage of metronidazole is its effectiveness against anaerobic bacteria, which are a major cause of bacterial liver abscess.

E. Ameboma or Extraintestinal Forms of Amebiasis: Metronidazole is the drug of choice. Dehydroemetine (or emetine) is an alternative drug; chloroquine cannot be used because it does not reach high enough tissue concentrations to be effective (except in the liver). A simultaneous course of a luminal amebicide should also be given.

CHLOROQUINE

Chloroquine reaches high liver concentrations and is highly effective when given with dehydroemetine (or emetine) in the treatment and prevention of amebic liver abscess. Chloroquine is not used, however, in the treatment of intestinal amebiasis, because the drug is not active against luminal organisms. At the dosage levels used in the treatment of amebiasis, the retinopathy sometimes associated with long-term use of chloroquine does not occur.

EMETINE & DEHYDROEMETINE

Chemistry & Pharmacokinetics

Emetine can be derived from ipecac or synthesized. Racemic 2-dehydroemetine dihydrochloride is a synthetic substance.

Emetine and dehydroemetine are administered parenterally, because oral preparations are absorbed erratically, may induce vomiting, and have low effectiveness. When given parenterally, they are stored primarily in the liver, lungs, spleen, and kidneys. The drugs are cumulative; they are eliminated slowly via the kidneys with trace amounts detectable in the urine 1–2 months after the end of therapy.

Pharmacologic Effects

Emetine and dehydroemetine affect almost all tissues. They irreversibly block the synthesis of protein in eukaryotes by inhibiting the movement of the ribo-

---

†In the USA, available only from the Centers for Disease Control and Prevention, Atlanta 30333; telephone 404-639-3670.
*Not available in the USA.

Table 54–3. Treatment of amebiasis.

	Drug(s) of Choice	Alternative Drug(s)
Asymptomatic intestinal infection	Diloxanide furoate[1,2]	Iodoquinol (diiodohydroxyquin)[3] or paramomycin[4]
Mild to moderate intestinal infection (nondysenteric colitis)	(1) Metronidazole[5] **plus** (2) Diloxanide furoate[2] or iodoquinol[3]	(1) Diloxanide furoate[2] or iodoquinol[3] **plus** (2) A tetracycline[6] **followed by** (3) Chloroquine[7] **or** (1) Paromomycin[4] **followed by** (2) Chloroquine[7]
Sever intestinal infection (dysentery)	(1) Metronidazole[8] **plus** (2) Diloxanide furoate[2] or iodoquinol[3] **If parenteral therapy is needed initially:** (1) Intravenous metronidazole[9] until oral therapy can be started; (2) Then give oral metronidazole[8] plus diloxanide furoate[2] or iodoquinol[3]	(1) A tetracycline[6] **plus** (2) Diloxanide furoate[2] or iodoquinol[3] **followed by** (3) Chloroquine[10] **or** (1) Dehydroemetine[1,11] or emetine[11] **followed by** (2) A tetracycline[6] plus diloxanide furoate[2] or iodoquinol[3] **followed by** (3) Chloroquine[10]
Hepatic abscess	(1) Metronidazole[8,9] **plus** (2) Diloxanide furoate[2] or iodoquinol[3] **followed by** (3) Chloroquine[10]	(1) Dehydroemetine[1,12] or emetine[12] **followed by** (2) Chloroquine[13] **plus** (3) Diloxanide furoate[2] or iodoquinol[3]
Ameboma or extraintestinal infection	As for hepatic abscess, but not including chloroquine	As for hepatic abscess, but not including chloroquine

[1]Available in the USA only from the Parasitic Disease Drug Service, Centers for Disease Control and Prevention, Atlanta 30333. Telephone requests may be made by calling the central number: (404) 639–3670 days; (404)-639–2888 nights, weekends, and holidays (emergencies only).

[2]Diloxanide furoate, 500 mg three times daily with meals for 10 days (for children, 20 mg/kg in three divided doses daily for 10 days).

[3]Iodoquinol (diiodohydroxyquin), 650 mg three times daily for 21 days (for children, 30–40 mg/kg [maximum 2 g] in three divided doses daily for 21 days).

[4]Paromomycin, 25–35 mg/kg (base) (maximum 3 g) in three divided doses after meals daily for 7 days (for children, the same dosage).

[5]Metronidazole, 750 mg three times daily for 10 days (for children, 35 mg/kg in three divided doses daily for 10 days).

[6]A tetracycline, 250 mg four times daily for 10 days; in severe dysentery, give 500 mg 4 times daily for the first 5 days, then 250 mg four times daily for 5 days. Tetracycline should not be used during pregnancy or in children under 8 years of age; in older children, give 20 mg/kg in four divided doses daily for 10 days.

[7]Chloroquine, 500 mg (salt) daily for 7 days (for children, 16 mg/kg [salt] daily for 7 days).

[8]Metronidazole, 750 mg three times daily for 10 days (for children, 35–50 mg/kg in three divided doses daily for 10 days).

[9]An intravenous metronidazole formulation is available; change to oral medication as soon as possible. See manufacturer's recommendation for dosage.

[10]Chloroquine, 500 mg (salt) daily for 14 days (for children, 16 mg/kg [salt] daily for 14 days).

[11]Dehydroemetine or emetine, 1 mg/kg subcutaneously (preferred) or intramuscularly daily for the least number of days necessary to control severe symptoms (usually 3–5 days) (maximum daily dose for dehydroemetine is 90 mg; for emetine, 65 mg). For children, the daily dose is divided into two parts.

[12]Use dosage recommended in footnote 11 for 8–10 days.

[13]Chloroquine, 500 mg (salt) orally twice daily for 2 days and then 500 mg orally daily for 19 days (for children, 16 mg/kg [salt] daily for 21 days).

some along messenger RNA; DNA synthesis is blocked secondarily. In experimental animals, emetine given parenterally in toxic doses causes cellular damage in the liver, kidneys, and skeletal and cardiac muscle. Cardiac conduction and contraction are depressed, which may cause a variety of atrial and ventricular arrhythmias, cardiac dilation, and death. Emetine also has adrenoceptor- and cholinoceptor-blocking actions.

Antiamebic Action

These drugs act only against trophozoites, which they directly eliminate.

Clinical Uses

Emetine and dehydroemetine should not be used to treat asymptomatic or mild intestinal infections. When available, dehydroemetine is the preferred drug, since it is equally effective and may be less toxic than emetine. Dosages are listed in Table 54–3.

A. Severe Intestinal Disease (Amebic Dysentery): Parenterally administered emetine and dehydroemetine rapidly alleviate severe intestinal symptoms but are rarely curative even if a full course is given. For this reason and because of their toxicity, they should be given for the minimum period needed to relieve severe symptoms (usually 3–5 days). Marked toxicity is unlikely when the drugs are used for less than 7 days.

B. Other Parasites: Emetine and dehydroemetine have occasionally been useful in the treatment of infections with *Balantidium coli, Fasciola hepatica,* and *Paragonimus westermani,* but safer drugs should be tried first.

Adverse Effects

Few and (usually) mild adverse effects appear if the drugs are given for 3–5 days; additional mild to severe adverse effects appear if they are given for up to 10 days; serious toxicity is common if they are given for more than 10 days. Therefore, use of these drugs for more than 10 days is contraindicated.

Pain, tenderness, and muscle weakness in the area of the injection are frequent. Occasionally, sterile abscesses develop. Nausea and vomiting, which occur infrequently, are thought to be central in origin. However, diarrhea is induced or exacerbated in many patients, generally beginning several days after the onset of therapy. Minor electrocardiographic changes occur frequently, but severe cardiac toxicity with significant conduction defects is rare. The most serious symptoms and findings are tachycardia and other arrhythmias, precordial pain, and congestive heart failure with dyspnea and hypotension (for details, see Goldsmith and Heyneman, 1989). Generalized muscular weakness—sometimes associated with tenderness, stiffness, aching, or tremors—is reported by many patients. Mild paresthesias are often reported.

Contraindications & Cautions

Hospitalization with careful supervision is essential. Considerable effort should be made to avoid dangerous inadvertent intravenous administration.

Emetine and dehydroemetine should not be used in patients with cardiac or renal disease, in those with a recent history of polyneuritis, or in young children unless alternative drugs have not been effective in controlling severe dysentery or liver abscess. They should not be used during pregnancy.

DILOXANIDE FUROATE

Diloxanide furoate is a dichloroacetamide derivative. The drug is directly amebicidal, but its mechanism of action is not known. It has few pharmacologic effects in vertebrates, but at very high doses it has caused abortion in experimental animals. No teratogenic effects have been reported.

Pharmacokinetics

In the gut, diloxanide furoate is split into diloxanide and furoic acid; about 90% of the diloxanide is rapidly absorbed and then conjugated to form the glucuronide, which is rapidly excreted in the urine. The unabsorbed diloxanide is the active antiamebic substance and is not attacked by gut bacteria.

Clinical Uses
(Table 54–3)

A. Asymptomatic and Mild Intestinal Amebiasis: Diloxanide furoate used alone is the drug of choice for treating asymptomatic infections. For the treatment of mild intestinal disease, it is used with other drugs.

B. Other Forms of Amebiasis: Diloxanide furoate is less effective in moderate to severe intestinal amebiasis. In the treatment of liver abscess, the drug is used to eradicate intestinal infection. It is not effective against extraluminal organisms.

Adverse Effects & Contraindications

Diloxanide furoate does not produce serious adverse effects. Flatulence is common; nausea and abdominal cramps are infrequent. Other toxicities are reported rarely.

The drug should not be used during pregnancy or administered to children under 2 years of age.

IODOQUINOL

Iodoquinol (diiodohydroxyquin) is a halogenated hydroxyquinoline that is effective against organisms in the bowel lumen but not against trophozoites in the intestinal wall or extraintestinal tissues.

Iodoquinol

Chemistry & Pharmacokinetics

Iodoquinol is the nonproprietary name for 8-hydroxy-5,7-diiodoquinoline. Its pharmacokinetics are poorly understood. Metabolic studies in humans indicate it has a half-life of 11–14 hours.

The drug may interfere with certain thyroid function tests by increasing protein-bound serum iodine levels, leading to a decrease in ^{131}I uptake.

Antiamebic Action

The mechanism of action of iodoquinol against trophozoites is unknown.

Clinical Uses

A. Intestinal Amebiasis: Iodoquinol is an alternative drug for the treatment of asymptomatic or mild to moderate intestinal amebiasis. The drug is not effective in the initial treatment of severe intestinal disease but is used in the subsequent eradication of the infection. Although it is not effective against amebomas or extraintestinal forms of the disease, including hepatic amebiasis, it is used to eradicate concurrent intestinal infection.

B. Other Intestinal Parasites: Iodoquinol (650 mg 3 times daily for 10 days) used alone or with a tetracycline (250 mg 4 times daily for 7 days) provides adequate treatment for *Dientamoeba fragilis* infections. Iodoquinol also has been reported to effectively treat some cases of *Giardia lamblia* and *B coli* infection.

Adverse Effects

The halogenated hydroxyquinolines, including iodoquinol, can produce severe neurotoxicity, particularly if they are given at greater than recommended doses and for long periods of time. The principal findings associated with this level of use are optic atrophy, visual loss, and peripheral neuropathy. Although these reactions usually improve when the drug is discontinued, some patients have experienced irreversible neurologic damage. Use of an analogue, clioquinol, is thought to have been responsible for an outbreak of this neurotoxic syndrome, which was given the name **subacute myelo-optic neuropathy (SMON).**

Iodoquinol has not been implicated in the production of neurotoxic effects when used at the standard dosage of 650 mg 3 times daily for 21 days. Mild and infrequent adverse effects that can occur at the standard dosage include diarrhea, which usually stops after several days, nausea and vomiting, gastritis, abdominal discomfort, and slight enlargement of the thyroid gland. Iodoquinol may be more toxic for infants and young children than for adults.

Contraindications & Cautions

Iodoquinol should not be used for the prophylaxis or treatment of travelers' or nonspecific diarrhea. When used to treat amebiasis, it should be taken only for the prescribed period of time at the recommended dosage.

The drug should be discontinued if it produces persistent diarrhea or signs of iodine reactions. It is contraindicated in patients with intolerance to iodine or renal and thyroid disease, and probably in those with severe liver disease not caused by amebiasis.

When the drug is used for young children, careful ophthalmologic assessment should be made before and during the course of therapy.

METRONIDAZOLE

Metronidazole is extremely useful in the treatment of extraluminal amebiasis. It effectively eradicates amebic tissue infections (liver abscess, intestinal wall and extraintestinal infections), but a luminal amebicide must be used with it to achieve satisfactory cure rates for luminal infections. Metronidazole kills trophozoites but does not kill cysts of *E histolytica.*

The chemistry, pharmacokinetics, adverse effects, contraindications, and cautions of this drug are described below (see Treatment of Trichomoniasis & Giardiasis).

OTHER NITROIMIDAZOLES

Other nitroimidazole derivatives include tinidazole, nimorazole, secondizole, and ornidazole. They have similar adverse effects and the same mutagenic action in the *Salmonella* test systems as metronidazole. Because of its short half-life, metronidazole must be administered every 8 hours; the other drugs can be administered at longer intervals. However, with the exception of tinidazole, the other nitroimidazoles have produced poorer results than metronidazole in the treatment of amebiasis.

PAROMOMYCIN SULFATE

Paromomycin sulfate, a broad-spectrum antibiotic, is an alternative drug for the treatment of mild to moderate intestinal amebiasis and is being evaluated in the topical treatment of cutaneous leishmaniasis. This aminoglycoside is derived from *Streptomyces rimosus* and is closely related to neomycin, kanamycin, and streptomycin in properties and structure. Paromomycin is both directly and indirectly amebicidal; the indirect effect is caused by its inhibition of bowel bacteria.

Because paromomycin is not significantly absorbed from the gastrointestinal tract, it can be used only as a luminal amebicide and has no effect in extraintestinal amebic infections. The small amount absorbed is slowly excreted unchanged, mainly by glomerular filtration; some excretion also occurs in the bile. In the presence of ulcerative lesions of the bowel, however, and perhaps with impaired gastrointestinal motility, increased absorption may occur. In renal insufficiency, the drug may accumulate to a toxic level.

Table 54–4. Drugs used in the treatment of other protozoal infections.[1]

Infecting Organism	Drug(s) of Choice	Alternative Drug(s)
Trypanosoma brucei gambiense and T b rhodesiense Hemolymphatic stage	Suramin[2] or eflornithine[3]	Pentamidine isethionate
Late disease with CNS involvement	Melarsoprol[2] or eflornithine[3]	Tryparsamide[4] plus suramin[2]
Trypanosoma cruzi	Nifurtimox[2]	Benznidazole[4]
Babesia species	Clindamycin[5,6] plus quinine[5,6]	None
Balantidium coli	Tetracycline[5]	Iodoquinol[5] or metronidazole[5]
Blastocystis hominis	Iodoquinol[5]	Metronidazole[5]
Cryptosporidium species	None	None
Dientamoeba fragilis	Iodoquinol[5] or paromomycin	Tetracycline[5]
Giardia lamblia	Metronidazole	Furazolidone or quinacrine
Isosospora belli	Trimethoprim-sulfamethoxazole[5]	None
Leishmania braziliensis	Stibogluconate sodium[2]	Amphotericin B[5]
Leishmania mexicana	Stibogluconate sodium[2]	Amphotericin B[5]
Leishmania donovani	Stibogluconate sodium[2]	Pentamidine isethionate
Leishmania tropica	Stibogluconate sodium[2]	Topical drugs
Pneumocystis carinii	Trimethoprim-sulfamethoxazole	Pentamidine isethionate
Toxoplasma gondii	Pyrimethamine plus trisulfapyrimidines	Spiramycin[4]

[1]Modified and reproduced, with permission, from Katzung B (editor): *Drug Therapy*. Appleton & Lange, 1991.
[2]Available in the USA only from the Parastic Disease Drug Service, Centers for Disease Control and Prevention, Atlanta 30333. Telephone 404–639–3670 during the day; 404–639–2888 nights, weekends, and holidays (emergencies only).
[3]Effectiveness in rhodesiense infections is variable.
[4]Not available in the USA; available in some other countries.
[5]Available in the USA but not labeled for this indication.
[6]Effectiveness not established.

OTHER ANTIBIOTICS

Although the tetracyclines have very weak direct amebicidal action, their effects on the gut flora make them (especially oxytetracycline) useful with a luminal amebicide in the eradication of mild to severe intestinal disease. However, because of their potential toxicity, the tetracyclines should not be used to treat pregnant women or children under 8 years of age; erythromycin stearate can be used instead, although it is somewhat less effective.

OTHER PROTOZOAL INFECTIONS

For a list of drugs used in the treatment of other protozoal infections, see Table 54–4.

TREATMENT OF LEISHMANIASIS

Leishmaniasis includes a variety of diseases (visceral [kala-azar], cutaneous, and mucocutaneous) produced by protozoal parasites of the genus *Leishmania*.

Drugs Used

Treatment of leishmaniasis is not satisfactory because of drug toxicity, the long courses required, treatment failures, and the frequent need for hospitalization. The drug of choice is sodium antimony gluconate (sodium stibogluconate). Alternative drugs for some forms of infection, which are generally more toxic, are amphotericin B and pentamidine. Some forms of Old World cutaneous leishmaniasis do not need treatment or can be treated by physical means (cryotherapy, heat therapy, surgery).

A. Sodium Stibogluconate (Sb[5]): Treatment is started with a 200 mg test dose, followed by 20 mg Sb[5]/kg/d. Although the drug can be administered intramuscularly, this route may be locally painful; the intravenous route is preferred when the volume to be injected is high. The drug is given on consecutive days: 20 days for the cutaneous form and 30 days for visceral and mucocutaneous leishmaniasis. Although few adverse effects occur initially, they are more likely to occur with cumulative doses. Most common are gastrointestinal symptoms, fever, and rash; hemolytic anemia and liver, renal, and heart damage are rare. Relapses should be treated at the same dosage levels, for at least twice the previous duration. In the USA, the drug is available only from the CDC Drug Service, Centers for Disease Control and Prevention, Atlanta 30333 (404-639-3670).

B. Pentamidine Isethionate: Pentamidine isethionate, 2–4 mg/kg intramuscularly (preferable) or intravenously, is given daily or on alternate days (up to 15 injections). For some forms of visceral leishmaniasis, a longer duration or repeat of treatment may be necessary. For adverse reactions, see pneumocystosis (below).

C. Amphotericin B: Amphotericin B is injected slowly intravenously over 6 hours on alternate days. The initial dose of 0.25 mg/kg/d is increased to 0.5 mg/kg/d and then to 1 mg/kg/d until a total of about 30 mg/kg has been given. Patients must be closely monitored in hospital, because adverse effects may be severe.

For additional information on the pharmacologic effects, pharmacokinetics, and adverse effects of these drugs, see the references.

TREATMENT OF *PNEUMOCYSTIS CARINII* PNEUMONIA & TRYPANOSOMIASIS

Treatment of Pneumocystosis

The drug of choice for the treatment of pneumocystosis is trimethoprim-sulfamethoxazole (see Chapter 47) in four divided doses for 4 days. Pentamidine isethionate (see below) is an alternative drug in treatment and recently was approved for prophylactic use as an aerosol.

Treatment of Trypanosomiasis

The drug of choice for the treatment of American trypanosomiasis is nifurtimox. Drugs used to treat African trypanosomiasis are suramin, pentamidine, and melarsoprol. Eflornithine has been approved for the meningoencephalitic stage of *T b gambiense* infections in the USA. (See Goldsmith and Heyneman, 1989, for details about these drugs.)

PENTAMIDINE

Chemistry & Pharmacokinetics

Pentamidine is an aromatic diamidine, formulated as isethionate and methanesulfonate salts. Only the isethionate is available in the USA.

Pentamidine is administered parenterally because it is not well absorbed from the gastrointestinal tract. The drug leaves the circulation rapidly and is bound avidly by the tissues, especially the liver, spleen, and kidneys. It is excreted unchanged, mostly in the urine. Pentamidine does not cross the blood-brain barrier but can cross the placenta. Only trace amounts of pentamidine appear in the central nervous system, so other trypanosomicides must be used to treat the central nervous system involvement in late-stage African trypanosomiasis.

Antiparasitic & Pharmacologic Actions

A. Antiparasitic Action: The mechanisms of pentamidine's antiparasitic action are not well understood. In vitro studies indicate that the drug may interfere with the synthesis of DNA, RNA, phospholipids, and proteins.

B. Pharmacologic Effects: Pentamidine causes mast cells to release histamine, which, with peripheral sympathoplegia, is the probable cause of the marked hypotensive reaction that follows intravenous administration. Pentamidine may cause severe hypotension when given by the intravenous route. In addition, pentamidine appears to be selectively toxic to B cells of the pancreatic islets. This initially produces an inappropriate, nonsuppressible insulin release leading to hypoglycemia; up to several months later, this may be replaced by hyperglycemia and diabetes mellitus.

Clinical Uses

A. Leishmaniasis: Pentamidine provides an alternative to sodium stibogluconate for the treatment of several forms of leishmaniasis. The dosage is 2–4 mg/kg/d intramuscularly for up to 15 doses.

B. Trypanosomiasis: Pentamidine provides an alternative to suramin treatment for the early stages of *Trypanosoma brucei gambiense* or *Trypanosoma brucei rhodesiense* infection. Because the drug does not pass the blood-brain barrier, it cannot be used in advanced disease when the central nervous system is involved. (See Goldsmith and Heyneman, 1989, for details on dosage and approach to using the drugs.)

C. Pneumocystosis: Treatment should always be based on a proved diagnosis. Trimethoprim-sulfamethoxazole and pentamidine isethionate are equally effective, but severe adverse reactions can occur in up to 50% of patients receiving either drug. In non-AIDS patients, the former drug is preferred because of its lower incidence of adverse effects. In AIDS patients, however, adverse effects are equivalent, and the choice of agent therefore depends on other factors (oral drug activity, preexisting renal disease, need for fluid loading, history of sulfonamide sensitivity).

For treatment of active pneumocystosis, the drug is administered intravenously or intramuscularly as a single dose of 4 mg (salt)/kg/d for 14–21 days. Some workers recommend 3 mg/kg, which may decrease side effects without reducing efficacy. Aerosolized pentamidine continues under evaluation in treatment trials.

Prophylaxis is recommended by the CDC for all HIV-infected adults who have had an episode of pneumocystosis and for some others. The treatment IND approved for use in the USA for aerosol pentamidine is a 300 mg dose every 4 weeks via jet nebulizer. Further information is available from the manufacturer at 800-727-7003.

D. Blastomycosis: Pentamidine is sometimes used to treat North American blastomycosis.

Adverse Effects

Pain at the injection site is common; infrequently, a sterile abscess develops and ulcerates.

Occasional reactions include rash, neutropenia, abnormal liver function tests, serum folate depression, hyperkalemia, and hypocalcemia. Hypoglycemia (often clinically inapparent), hyperglycemia, hyponatremia, and delayed nephrotoxicity with azotemia may occur.

Because severe hypotension may develop even after a single dose of pentamidine, the patient should be recumbent when the drug is given. Blood pressure should be followed closely during administration and thereafter until stable. Emergency resuscitation equipment should be immediately available.

Rare adverse reactions include megaloblastic anemia, acute pancreatitis, thrombocytopenia, thrombocytopenic purpura, toxic epidermal necrolysis, hyperkalemia, and renal toxicity. Fatalities have occurred from hypotension, hypoglycemia, or arrhythmias.

Contraindications & Cautions

Use pentamidine cautiously in the presence of hypotension, hypertension, latent or clinical diabetes, malnutrition, anemia, thrombocytopenia, or renal or hepatic dysfunction.

ATOVAQUONE

Atovaquone is a new quinone derivative with antiprotozoal activity, especially against *P carinii.* It has been approved by the FDA for treatment of mild to moderate *P carinii* pneumonia. It has not been evaluated, however, in the treatment of severe disease or in prophylaxis. A preliminary study suggests that atovaquone may also be effective in treatment of cerebral toxoplasmosis in patients with AIDS.

The action of atovaquone is not well understood. Its bioavailability is low but is enhanced when taken with meals; its protein binding is greater than 99%, and its half-life in AIDS patients is 2.2–2.9 days. Most of the drug is eliminated unchanged in the feces. The dosage is 750 mg taken with food 3 times daily

for 21 days. Frequent side effects are fever and rash; less frequent are cough, nausea, vomiting, diarrhea, headache, and insomnia.

TREATMENT OF TRICHOMONIASIS & GIARDIASIS

METRONIDAZOLE

Metronidazole is the drug of choice in treatment of urogenital trichomoniasis and an alternative drug in treatment of *Giardia lamblia, Balantidium coli, Blastocystis hominis,* and intestinal and extraintestinal amebiasis infections. Its uses in the treatment of infection with bacterial anaerobes are described in Chapters 50 and 52.

Chemistry & Pharmacokinetics

Oral metronidazole is readily absorbed and permeates all tissues by simple diffusion—including cerebrospinal fluid, breast milk, and alveolar bone. Intracellular concentrations rapidly approach extracellular levels. The half-life of the unchanged drug is 7.5 hours. The drug and its metabolites are excreted in the urine. Plasma clearance of metronidazole is decreased in patients with impaired liver function.

Metronidazole

Mechanism of Action

Within anaerobic bacteria and sensitive protozoal cells, the nitro group of metronidazole is chemically reduced by ferredoxin (or ferredoxin-linked metabolic processes). The reduction products appear to be responsible for killing the organisms by reacting with various intracellular macromolecules. Thus, reduction is responsible for the drug's bactericidal (not bacteriostatic) action against anaerobic bacteria. In vitro, metronidazole is active against most obligate anaerobes, but it does not appear to have significant effect against facultative anaerobes or obligate aerobes.

Metronidazole also has a radiosensitizing effect on tumor cells. As with its antibacterial action, the mechanism of action appears to be dependent on relative hypoxia in the target cells and may involve interaction with free radicals.

In amebiasis, metronidazole kills *Entamoeba histolytica* trophozoites but not cysts.

Clinical Uses

A. Urogenital Trichomoniasis: The treatment of choice is metronidazole, 250 mg orally 3 times a day for 7 days. A single dose of 2 g or 1 g twice in 1 day is also effective. The sexual partner should be treated simultaneously if the organism is found to be present; many workers also treat even if the organism is not found in the partner. In pregnancy, treatment with metronidazole should be delayed until after the first trimester. Metronidazole-resistant strains of *Trichomonas vaginalis* have been described.

B. Giardiasis: The adult dosage of metronidazole is 250 mg orally 3 times a day for 5 days. Children should receive 5 mg/kg 3 times a day for 5 days.

C. Amebiasis: See above.

D. Balantidiasis: If tetracycline is ineffective, give metronidazole, 750 mg 3 times a day for 5 days.

E. *Gardnerella vaginalis:* In refractory infections only, give metronidazole, 500 mg orally twice a day for 5 days.

F. Anaerobic Infections: Metronidazole is used to reduce postoperative anaerobic infections following procedures such as appendectomy, colorectal surgery, and abdominal hysterectomy. Furthermore, serious anaerobic infections involving *Bacteroides fragilis,* clostridia, and other bacteria that are refractory to other agents may respond to metronidazole, in part because of its ability to penetrate abscesses and necrotic tissue.

G. Phagedenic Leg Ulcers, Acute Ulcerative Gingivitis, Cancrum Oris, Decubitus Ulcers, and Other Indolent Lesions: Metronidazole, 250 mg orally 3 times a day, with an appropriate drug for the aerobic infection and appropriate topical treatment, promotes healing and provides relief of pain, inflammatory edema, and purulent discharge.

Adverse Effects & Interactions

Nausea, headache, dry mouth, or a metallic taste in the mouth occur commonly. Urine may be dark or reddish-brown. Infrequent (12%) adverse effects include vomiting, diarrhea, insomnia, weakness, dizziness, stomatitis, rash, urethral burning, vertigo, and paresthesias.

Metronidazole has a disulfiram-like effect, so that nausea and vomiting occur if alcohol is consumed while the drug is still in the body.

Mutagenicity & Carcinogenicity

Metronidazole and its metabolites recovered from the urine of patients taking the drug are mutagenic in certain strains of *Salmonella typhimurium* (Ames test). Chronic oral administration of very large doses to mice has produced a statistically significant increase in the number of lung and liver tumors. This effect has not been found, however, in any nonrodent species. Although the drug has been used in humans for over 20 years, no increase in congenital abnormalities, stillbirths, or low birth weight has been reported. No increase in frequency of chromosomal aberration has been found in patients receiving large doses.

Contraindications & Cautions

Caution should be used in prescribing the drug in multiple courses or over long periods or for patients with a history of blood dyscrasias. Prudence dictates that unless clearly indicated, metronidazole should be avoided in pregnant women (especially in the first trimester), in nursing women, and in young children.

Metronidazole has been reported to potentiate the anticoagulant effect of coumarin-type anticoagulants. Phenytoin and phenobarbital may accelerate elimination of the drug, while cimetidine may decrease plasma clearance. Concurrent usage has resulted in lithium toxicity. Its disulfiram-like effect requires that all patients receiving metronidazole be specifically warned not to use alcohol for 24 hours before starting the drug and for 48 hours after the last dose.

PREPARATIONS AVAILABLE

Chloroquine hydrochloride [80% chloroquine base] (Aralen HCl)
Parenteral: 50 mg/mL for injection

Chloroquine phosphate [60% chloroquine base] (generic, Aralen; outside the USA: Avloclor, Resochin)
Oral: 250, 500 mg tablets

Note: Chloroquine sulfate is available outside the USA as Nivaquine.

Chloroquine phosphate with primaquine phosphate
Oral: Tablets containing 500 mg chloroquine phosphate (300 mg base) plus primaquine phosphate 79 mg (45 mg base).

Dehydroemetine (Mebadin)

Parenteral: solution for injection in 30, 60 mg ampules

Note: Available in the USA only from the Drug Service, Centers for Disease Control and Prevention, Atlanta, 404-639-3670.

Diloxanide furoate (Furamide)

Oral: 500 mg tablets

Note: Available in the USA only from the Drug Service, Centers for Disease Control and Prevention, Atlanta, 404-639-3670.

Doxycycline (generic, Vibramycin, others)

Oral: 50, 100 mg tablets and capsules; 100 mg coated pellets; 25, 50 mg/5 mL suspension from powder; 50 mg/5 mL syrup

Parenteral: powder to reconstitute for injection (100, 200 mg per vial)

Emetine (generic)

Parenteral: 65 mg/mL for injection

Iodoquinol [diiodohydroxyquin] (generic, Yodoxin, Moebequin)

Oral: 210, 650 mg tablets; also available as powder

Note: Iodoquinol is available outside the USA as Embequin, Lanodoxin, Savorquin, Sebaquin.

Mefloquine (Lariam)

Oral: 250 mg tablets (228 mg base).

Metronidazole (generic, Flagyl, others)

Oral: 250, 500 mg tablets

Parenteral: powder to reconstitute for injection (500 mg per vial); ready-to-use for injection (in 500 mg/100 mL vials)

Rectal: suppositories. (*Note:* Not available in the USA.)

Paromomycin (Humatin)

Oral: 250 mg capsules

Pentamidine isethionate

Parenteral (Pentam 300): for injection (300 mg per vial)

Inhaled (NebuPent): 300 mg for nebulization

Primaquine (generic)

Oral: 26.3 mg tablets (equivalent to 15 mg base)

Proguanil [chloroguanide] (generic, Paludrine)

Oral: 100 mg tablets

Note: Not available in the USA.

Pyrimethamine (Daraprim)

Oral: 25 mg tablets

Pyrimethamine/dapsone (Maloprim)

Oral: tablets containing 100 mg dapsone/12.5 mg pyrimethamine

Note: Not available in the USA.

Quinacrine [mepacrine](Atabrine HCl)

Oral: 100 mg tablets

Quinidine gluconate (generic)

Parenteral: 80 mg salt (50 mg base) per mL

Quinine dihydrochloride (generic)

Note: Not available in the USA.

Quinine sulfate [83% quinine base] (generic)

Oral: 130, 195, 200, 300, 325 mg capsules; 260, 325 mg tablets

Stibogluconate [**sodium antimony gluconate**] (Pentostam)

Note: Available in the USA only from the Drug Service, Centers for Disease Control and Prevention, Atlanta, 1-404-639-3670.

Trimethoprim-sulfamethoxazole [co-trimoxazole, TMP-SMZ] (generic, Bactrim, Septra)

Oral: 80 mg TMP/400 mg SMZ single-strength tablets; 160 mg TMP/800 mg SMZ double-strength tablets

Parenteral: 80 mg TMP and 400 mg SMZ per 5 mL for infusion

REFERENCES

General

Goldsmith RS, Heyneman D (editors): *Tropical Medicine and Parasitology.* Appleton & Lange, 1989.

Malaria

Amor D, Richards M: Mefloquine resistant *P vivax* malaria in PNG. Med J Aust 1992;156:883.

Arthur JD et al: A comparative study of gastrointestinal infections in United States soldiers receiving doxycycline or mefloquine for prophylaxis. Am J Trop Med Hyg 1990;43:608.

Bem JL, Kerr L, Stuerchler D: Mefloquine prophylaxis: An overview of spontaneous reports of severe psychiatric reactions and convulsions. J Trop Pediatr 1992; 95:167.

Bruce-Chwatt LJ: Doxycycline prophylaxis in malaria. Lancet 1987;2:1487.

Bryson HM, Goa KL: Halofantrine: A review of its antimalarial activity, pharmacokinetic properties and therapeutic potential. Drugs 1992;43:236.

CDC: Health information for international travel 1992. Atlanta, Georgia: Public Health Service, U.S. Department of Health and Human Services; Publication No. (CDC) 92–8280.

CDC: Recommendations for the prevention of malaria among travelers. MMWR Morb Mortal Wkly Rep 1990;39:1.

CDC: Treatment with quinidine gluconate of persons with severe *Plasmodium falciparum* infection: Discontinuation of parenteral quinine. From CDC Drug Service. MMWR Morb Mortal Wkly Rep 1991;40:21.

Churchill D et al: Chloroquine and proguanil prophylaxis in travellers to Kenya. Lancet 1992;339:63.

Helsby NA et al: The pharmacokinetics and activation of proguanil in man: Consequences of variability in drug metabolism. Br J Clin Pharmacol 1990;30:593.

Hoffman SL: Diagnosis, treatment, and prevention of malaria. Med North Am 1992;76:1327.

Karbwang J et al: Pharmacokinetics and pharmacodynamics of mefloquine in Thai patients with acute falciparum malaria. Bull World Health Organ 1991; 69:207.

Karbwang J et al: Pharmacokinetics of halofantrine in Thai patients with acute uncomplicated falciparum malaria. Br J Clin Pharmacol 1991;31:484.

Keystone JS: Prevention of malaria. Drugs 1990;39:337.

Krogstad DJ, Schlesinger PH, Gluzman IY: The specificity of chloroquine. Parasitology Today 1992;8:183.

Lobel HO et al: Effectiveness and tolerance of long-term malaria prophylaxis with mefloquine. JAMA 1991; 265:361.

Miller KD, Greenberg AE, Campbell CC: Treatment of severe malaria in the United States with a continuous infusion of quinidine gluconate and exchange transfusion. N Engl J Med 1989;321:65.

Peters W: *Chemotherapy and Drug Resistance in Malaria,* 2nd ed. 2 vols. Academic Press, 1987.

Price AH, Fletcher KA: The metabolism and toxicity of primaquine. Prog Clin Biol Res 1986;214:261.

Raccurt CP et al: Failure of falciparum malaria prophylaxis by mefloquine in travelers from West Africa. Am J Trop Med Hyg 1991;45:319.

Rediscovering wormwood: Qinghaosu for malaria. (Editorial.) Lancet 1992;339:649.

Reeve PA et al: Acute intravascular haemolysis in Vanuatu following a single dose of primaquine in individuals with glucose-6-phosphate dehydrogenase deficiency. J Trop Med Hyg 1992;95:349.

Schwartz IK: Prevention of malaria. Infect Dis Clin North Am 1992;6:313.

Slater AFG: Chloroquine: Mechanism of drug action and resistance in *Plasmodium falciparum.* Pharmacol Ther 1993;57:203.

Steffen R, Behrens RH: Travellers' malaria. Parasitology Today 1992;8:61.

Toma E et al: Clindamycin with primaquine for *Pneumocystis carinii* pneumonia. Lancet 1989;1:1046.

Watt G et al: Quinine with tetracycline for the treatment of drug-resistant falciparum malaria in Thailand. Am J Trop Med Hyg 1992;47:108.

Weinke T et al: The efficacy of halofantrine in the treatment of acute malaria in nonimmune travelers. Am J Trop Med Hyg 1992;47:1.

White NJ et al: Comparison of artemether and chloroquine for severe malaria in Gambian children. Lancet 1992;339:317.

White NJ et al: Chloroquine treatment of severe malaria in children. Pharmacokinetics, toxicity, and new dosage recommendations. N Engl J Med 1988;319:1493.

White NJ: Antimalarial pharmacokinetics and treatment regimens. Br J Clin Pharmacol 1992;34:1.

White NJ: Drug treatment and prevention of malaria. Eur J Clin Pharmacol 1988;34:1.

WHO: Development of recommendations for the protection of short-stay travellers to malaria endemic areas: Memorandum from two WHO meetings. Bull WHO 1988;66:177.

WHO: Practical chemotherapy of malaria. Tech Report Series 1990b;No. 805.

WHO: Severe and complicated malaria. Trans R Soc Trop Med Hyg 1990a;84(Suppl 2):1.

Winstanley PA et al: The disposition of oral and intramuscular pyrimethamine/sulfadoxine in Kenyan children with high parasitaemia but clinically non-severe falciparum malaria. Br J Clin Pharmacol 1992;33:143.

Amebiasis, Giardiasis, & Trichomoniasis

Beard CM et al: Cancer after exposure to metronidazole. Mayo Clin Proc 1988;63:147.

Committee on Drugs: Blindness and neuropathy from di-iodohydroxyquin-like drugs. Pediatrics 1974;54:378.

Dombrowski MP et al: Intravenous therapy of metronidazole-resistant *Trichomonas vaginalis*. Obstet Gynecol 1987;69:524.

Dooley CP, O'Morain CAO: Recurrence of hepatic amebiasis after successful treatment with metronidazole. J Clin Gastroenterol 1988;10:339.

El-On J et al: Topical treatment of cutaneous leishmaniasis. J invest Dermatol 1986;87:284.

Friedman GD, Selby JV: Metronidazole and cancer. (Letter.) JAMA 1989;261:866.

Kuntzer T et al: Emetine-induced myopathy and carnitine deficiency. J Neurol 1990;237:495.

McAuley JB, Juranek DD: Luminal agents in the treatment of amebiasis. Clin Infect Dis 1992;14:1161.

McAuley JB et al: Diloxanide furoate for treating asymptomatic *Entamoeba histolytica* cyst passers: 14 years' experience in the United States. Clin Infect Dis 1992; 15:464.

McAuley JB, Juranek DD: Paromomycin in the treatment of mild-to-moderate intestinal amebiasis. Clin Infect Dis 1992;15:551.

Mengel MB et al: The effectiveness of single-dose metronidazole therapy for patients and their partners with bacterial vaginosis. J Family Pract 1989;28:163.

Plaisance KI, Quintilliani R, Nightingale CM: The pharmacokinetics of metronidazole and its metabolites in critically ill patients. J Antimicrob Chemother 1988; 21:195.

Reed S: Amebiasis: An update. Clin Infect Dis 1992; 14:385.

Robertson DH et al: Treatment failure in *Trichomonas vaginalis* infections in females: I. Concentrations of metronidazole in plasma and vaginal content during normal and high dosage. J Antimicrob Chemother 1988;21:373.

Sullam PM et al: Paromomycin therapy of endemic amebiasis in homosexual men. Sex Transm Dis 1986;13: 151.

Wright CW et al: Antiamoebic activity of indole analogues of emetine with in-vitro potency greater than that of emetine J Pharm Pharmacol Suppl 1990;42:1.

Leishmaniasis & Pneumocystosis

Bryceson A: Therapy in man. In: *The Leishmaniases.* Peters W, Killick-Kendrick R (editors). Academic Press, 1987.

CDC: Guidelines for prophylaxis against *Pneumocystis carinii* pneumonia for persons infected with human immunodeficiency syndrome. JAMA 1989;262:335.

Drugs for treatment of systemic fungal infections. Med Lett Drugs Ther 1986;28:41.

Franke ED et al: Efficacy and toxicity of sodium stibogluconate for mucosal leishmaniasis. Ann Intern Med 1990;113:934.

Goa KL, Campoli-Richards DM: Pentamidine isethionate: A review of its antiprotozoal activity, pharmacokinetic properties and therapeutic use in *Pneumocystis carinii* pneumonia. Drugs 1987;33:242.

Herwaldt BL, Berman JD: Recommendations for treating leishmaniasis with sodium stibogluconate (Pentostam) and review of pertinent clinical studies. Am J Trop Med Hyg 1992;46:296.

Hughes WT: A new drug (566C80) for the treatment of *Pneumocystis carinii* pneumonia. Ann Intern Med 1992; 116:953.

Kovacs JA et al: Efficacy of atovaquone in treatment of toxoplasmosis in patients with AIDS. Lancet 1992; 340:637.

Kovacs JA, Masur H: Prophylaxis for *Pneumocystis carinii* pneumonia in patients infected with human immunodeficiency virus. Clin Infect Dis 1992;14:1005.

Martin MA et al: A comparison of the effectiveness of three regimens in the prevention of *Pneumocystis carinii* pneumonia in human immunodeficiency virus infected patients. Arch Intern Med 1992;152:523.

Monk JP, Benfield P: Inhaled pentamidine: An overview of its pharmacological properties and a review of its therapeutic use in *Pneumocystis carinii pneumonia.* Drugs 1990;39:741.

Smaldone GC et al: Deposition of aerosolized pentamidine and failure of pneumocystis prophylaxis. Chest 1992;101:82.

White DA, Zaman MK: Medical management of AIDS patients: Pulmonary disease. Med Clin North Am 1992;76:19.

WHO Expert Committee: Sodium stibogluconate. In: WHO Tech Rep Ser "Control of Leishmaniasis" 793, Chapter 3 1990:50.

55

Clinical Pharmacology of the Anthelmintic Drugs

Robert S. Goldsmith, MD, DTM&H

CHEMOTHERAPY OF HELMINTHIC INFECTIONS

Anthelmintic drugs are used to eradicate or reduce the numbers of helminthic parasites in the intestinal tract or tissues of the body. As noted in Chapter 53, these parasites have many biochemical and physiologic processes in common with their mammalian hosts, yet there are subtle differences that are beginning to yield to pharmacologic investigation. Most of the drugs described below were discovered by traditional screening methods; their mechanisms have been clarified only recently. These mechanisms (where known) are described in Chapter 53.

Table 55–1 lists the major helminthic infections and provides a guide to the drug of choice and alternative drugs for each infection. In the text that follows, these drugs are arranged alphabetically.

Most anthelmintics in use today are active against specific parasites, and some are toxic. Therefore, parasites must be identified before treatment is started, usually by finding the parasite, eggs, or larvae in the feces, urine, blood, sputum, or tissues of the host.

Administration of Anthelmintic Drugs

Unless otherwise indicated, oral drugs should be taken with water during or after meals. In posttreatment follow-up for intestinal nematode infections, stools should be reexamined about 2 weeks after the end of treatment.

Dosages for Children

Dosages for infants and children are on a less secure basis than for adults; when not given in milligrams per kilogram of body weight (or otherwise specified), the dosage may be based on surface area or calculated as a fraction of the adult dose based on Clark's rule or Young's rule (see Chapter 61).

Contraindications

Pregnancy and ulcers of the gastrointestinal tract are contraindications for most of the drugs listed. Specific contraindications are given in the discussions that follow.

ALBENDAZOLE

Albendazole, a broad-spectrum oral anthelmintic, is used for pinworm infection, ascariasis, trichuriasis, strongyloidiasis, and infections with both hookworm species. Albendazole is also the drug of choice in hydatid disease and cysticercosis. Although not available in the USA, the manufacturer (SmithKline Beecham) will make the drug available for compassionate use only (800-366-8900).

Chemistry & Pharmacokinetics

Albendazole is a benzimidazole carbamate.

Albendazole

After oral administration, albendazole is rapidly absorbed and metabolized mainly to albendazole sulfoxide and, to a lesser extent, to other metabolites. About 3 hours after a 400 mg oral dose, the sulfoxide attains a maximum plasma concentration of 250–300 ng/mL; its plasma half-life is 8–9 hours. The metabolites are mainly excreted in the urine; only a small amount is excreted in the feces. Absorption of the drug is about fourfold greater when it is taken with a fatty meal as compared with the fasting state.

Anthelmintic Actions & Pharmacologic Effects

A. Anthelmintic Actions: Albendazole blocks glucose uptake by larval and adult stages of suscepti-

Table 55–1. Drugs for the treatment of helminthic infections.

Infecting Organism	Drug of Choice	Alternative Drugs
Roundworms (nematodes)		
Ascaris lumbricoides (roundworm)	Pyrantel pamoate or mebendazole	Piperazine, albendazole,[1] or levamisol[2]
Trichuris trichiura (whipworm)	Mebendazole	Albendazole[1] or oxantel/pyrantel pamoate[1]
Necator americanus (hookworm); Ancylostoma duodenale (hookworm)	Pyrantel pamoate[2] or mebendazole	Albendazole[1] or levamisole[2]
Combined infection with Ascaris, Trichuris, and hookworm	Mebendazole or albendazole[1]	Oxantel/pyrantel pamoate[1]
Combined infection with Ascaris and hookworm	Mebendazole or pyrantel pamoate[2]	Albendazole[1]
Strongyloides stercoralis (threadworm)	Thiabendazole or ivermectin[3,4]	Albendazole[1] or mebendazole[3]
Enterobius vermicularis (pinworm)	Mebendazole or pyrantel pamoate	Albendazole[1]
Trichinella spiralis (trichinosis)	Mebendazole[2,3] or thiabendazole[3]; add corticosteroids for severe infection	Albendazole[3,5]; add corticosteroids for severe infection
Trichostrongylus species	Pyrantel pamoate[2] or mebendazole[2]	Albendazole[1] or levamisole[2]
Cutaneous larva migrans (creeping eruption)	Albendazole[1]	Thiabendazole
Visceral larva migrans	Thiabendazole[8] or albendazole[1,3]	Mebendazole[2,3,8] or ivermectin[3,4]
Angiostrongylus cantonensis	Levamisole[2,3]	Albendazole[1,5] or mebendazole[2,3]
Wuchereria bancrofti (filariasis); Brugia malayi (filariasis); tropical eosinophilia; Loa loa (loiasis)	Diethylcarbamazine[6]	Ivermectin[3,7]
Onchocerca volvulus (onchocerciasis)	Ivermectin[7]	Diethylcarbamazine[6] plus suramin[7]
Dracunculus medinensis (guinea worm)	Metronidazole[2]	Thiabendazole[2] or mebendazole[2]
Capillaria philippinensis (intestinal capillariasis)	Albendazole[1]	Mebendazole[2] or thiabendazole[2]
Flukes (trematodes)		
Schistosoma haematobium (bilharziasis)	Praziquantel	Metrifonate[1]
Schistosoma mansoni	Praziquantel	Oxamniquine
Schistosoma japonicum	Praziquantel	None
Clonorchis sinensis (liver fluke); Opisthorchis species	Praziquantel[2]	Mebendazole[2,3] or albendazole[1,3]
Paragonimus westermani (lung fluke)	Praziquantel[2]	Bithionol[7]
Fasciola hepatica (sheep liver fluke)	Bithionol[7]	Praziquantel[2,8] or emetine or dehydroemetine[7]
Fasciolopsis buski (large intestinal fluke)	Praziquantel[2] or niclosamide[2]	Tetrachloroethylene[1]
Heterophyes heterophyes; Metagonimus yokogawai (small intestinal flukes)	Praziquantel[2] or niclosamide[2]	Tetrachloroethylene1
Tapeworms (cestodes)		
Taenia saginata (beef tapeworm)	Niclosamide or praziquantel[2]	Mebendazole[2,3]
Diphyllobothrium latum (fish tapeworm)	Niclosamide or praziquantel[2]	
Taenia solum (pork tapeworm)	Niclosamide[2] or praziquantel[2]	
Cysticercosis (pork tapeworm larval stage)	Albendazole[5]	Praziquantel[2]
Hymenolepis nana (dwarf tapeworm)	Praziquantel[2]	Niclosamide
Hymenolepis diminuta (rat tapeworm); Dipylidium caninum	Niclosamide or praziquantel[2]	
Echinococcus granulosus (hydatid disease); Echinococcus multilocularis	Albendazole[5]	Mebendazole[2]

[1]Not available in the USA but available in some other countries.

[2]Available in the USA but not labeled for this indication (see Unlabeled Use, Chapter 66).

[3]Effectiveness not established.

[4]Available in the USA from Merck Sharpe & Dohme. Telephone 215–397–2454.

[5]Available in the USA only from SmithKline Beecham. Telephone 800–366–8900, Ext 5206.

[6]Available in the USA from Lederle Laboratories. Telephone 914–735–5000.

[7]Available in the USA only from the Parasitic Disease Drug Service, Parasitic Diseases Branch, Centers for Disease Control and Prevention, Atlanta 30333. Telephone 404–639–3670 during the day; 404–639–2888 nights, weekends, and holidays (emergencies only).

[8]Effectiveness is low.

ble parasites, depleting their glycogen stores and decreasing formation of ATP. As a result the parasite is immobilized and dies. The drug has larvicidal effects in necatoriasis and ovicidal effects in ascariasis, ancylostomiasis, and trichuriasis. The drug is teratogenic and embryotoxic in some animal species.

B. Pharmacologic Effects: Albendazole does not have pharmacologic effects in humans at therapeutic oral doses (5 mg/kg).

Clinical Uses

Albendazole is probably best administered on an empty stomach when it is used against intraluminal parasites but with a fatty meal when used against tissue parasites.

A. Ascariasis, Trichuriasis, and Hookworm and Pinworm Infections: For pinworm infections, ancylostomiasis, and light ascariasis, necatoriasis, or trichuriasis, the treatment for adults and children over 2 years of age is a single dose of 400 mg orally. In pinworm infection, the dose should be repeated in 2 weeks. This achieves 100% cure rates in pinworm infection and high cure rates for the other infections, or marked reduction in egg counts in those not cured. Although the optimal dosage for achieving high cure rates in heavy ascariasis or satisfactorily reducing worm burden in moderate to heavy necatoriasis and trichuriasis is not established, 400 mg/d for 2–3 days may be tried.

B. Strongyloidiasis: The objective of treatment in strongyloidiasis must be cure. A dosage schedule to accomplish this is not established; 400 mg twice daily for 7–14 days (with meals) may be tried. The drug has been used in mass treatment programs.

C. Hydatid Disease: A current treatment schedule is 800 mg/d with meals for 28 days; this course should be repeated three times, with 2-week intervals between courses. Among 253 patients treated in multiple studies, the results among patients with liver cysts were as follows: 33% cured (disappearance or shrinkage), 44% improved, 21% no change, and 2% worse. In patients with lung cysts, 40% were cured, 37% improved, 22% showed no change, and 1% got worse. In follow-ups extending to 7 years, recurrences have been rare. Bone cysts may prove more refractory to treatment. Pre- and postsurgical use of albendazole to reduce the risk of recurrence due to operative spillage is under evaluation.

D. Neurocysticercosis: Medical treatment—usually preferable to surgery—is most effective for parenchymal cysts, less so for intraventricular, subarachnoid, or racemose cysts, and probably has no effect on cysts that show enhancement or calcification. In short-term (3- to 6-month) follow-up of comparative studies with praziquantel, albendazole appears to be more effective and the drug of choice. Other potential advantages of albendazole over praziquantel are that it is less expensive; that it achieves

better penetration of cerebrospinal fluid; and that when corticosteroids are given concomitantly, the plasma concentration of albendazole increases but that of praziquantel decreases. A suggested approach is to give a course of albendazole plus steroid; if the response is inadequate, follow with a course of praziquantel. For selected patients, some clinicians wait 3 months to see if cysts will spontaneously disappear. Treatment should be conducted in hospital.

The albendazole dosage schedule of 15 mg/kg/d for 8 days is as effective as a 30-day course. Within a few days after the start of treatment, inflammatory reactions around dying parasites may be manifested by headache (analgesics may be sufficient for mild symptoms), vomiting (try antiemetics), hyperthermia, mental changes, and convulsions; decompensation with death is very rare. It remains controversial whether to give a steroid concomitantly to avoid or diminish this reactive inflammation or to use a steroid only if marked symptoms appear or increase. The inflammatory reaction may occur even when steroids are given in advance. One steroid dosage is prednisone, 30 mg/d in two or three divided doses starting 1–2 days before use of the drug and continuing with diminishing doses for about 14 days afterward. The reaction usually subsides in 48–72 hours, but continuing severity may require steroids in higher dosage and mannitol. Following treatment, 50% cure rates (disappearance of cysts and clearing of symptoms) have been reported. Of the remaining patients, many have amelioration of signs and symptoms, including intracranial hypertension and seizures.

E. Other Infections: At a dosage of 200 mg twice daily, albendazole is the drug of choice in treatment of **cutaneous larval migrans** (give daily for 3–5 days) and in **intestinal capillariasis** (10-day course). At a dosage of 400 mg twice daily, it may be useful in **gnathostomiasis** (21-day course) and **trichinosis** (15-day course); for severe symptoms in the latter infection, prednisolone, 40 mg/d, should be given concurrently for about 3 days and then gradually withdrawn. Cure rates were 90% in **clonorchiasis** and 33% in **opisthorchiasis** at a dosage of 400 mg twice daily for 7 days, with a marked reduction in egg counts in those not cured. There have been isolated reports of some effectiveness in treatment of **microsporidiosis** (*Enterocytozoon bieneusi*) and **toxocariasis** and conflicting reports of effectiveness in **taeniasis** and against adult embryogenesis in **onchocerciasis.** In experimental animals, the drug showed promise in **fascioliasis** and **angiostrongyliasis.**

Adverse Reactions

When used for 1–3 days, albendazole seems to be nearly free of significant adverse effects. Mild and transient epigastric distress, diarrhea, headache, nausea, dizziness, lassitude, and insomnia have been attributed to the drug in up to 6% of patients, but in two placebo-controlled studies, the incidence of adverse effects was similar in treatment and control groups.

In 3-month treatment courses for hydatid disease, the following toxicities were observed: reversible low-grade aminotransferase elevations in 17% and jaundice in one patient; gastrointestinal symptoms (nausea, vomiting, abdominal pain) in 4%; alopecia in 2%; rash or pruritus in 1%; and leukopenia to under 2900/μL in 2%. In two patients, pronounced eosinophilia appeared, probably related to cyst fluid leakage. Long-term toxicity studies in animals showed diarrhea, anemia, hypotension, marrow depression, and liver function test abnormalities, varying with different species.

Contraindications & Cautions

The safety of albendazole has not been established in children under 2 years of age. Because the drug is teratogenic and embryotoxic in some animal species, it should not be used in pregnancy. It may be contraindicated in the presence of cirrhosis.

ANTIMONY COMPOUNDS

The trivalent antimony compounds were for many years the principal drugs for the treatment of schistosomiasis (bilharziasis), but because of their toxicity and difficulty of administration, they should no longer be used. Pentavalent stibogluconate is still used in the therapy of leishmaniasis (Chapter 54).

BITHIONOL

Bithionol is the drug of choice for the treatment of fascioliasis (sheep liver fluke), although relatively little is known about its degree of effectiveness. Of the alternative drugs, emetine and dehydroemetine are toxic and praziquantel is usually not effective.

Bithionol is the alternative drug in the treatment of pulmonary paragonimiasis. With one course of treatment, cure rates are over 90%. Several courses may be necessary in acute cerebral paragonimiasis, but the drug is not useful in chronic cerebral paragonimiasis. The mode of action of bithionol against *Paragonimus westermani* has not been established.

Pharmacokinetics

After ingestion, bithionol reaches peak blood levels in 4–8 hours. At a daily dosage of 50 mg/kg orally in three divided doses for 5 days, a serum level of 50–200 μg/mL is maintained. Excretion appears to be mainly via the kidney.

Clinical Uses

For treatment of paragonimiasis and fascioliasis, the dosage of bithionol is 30–50 mg/kg in two or three divided doses, given orally after meals on alternate days for 10–15 doses. For pulmonary paragonimiasis, three negative sputum and stool specimens obtained 3 months after completion of treatment indicate eradication of the parasite. Within 4–6 months, chest film abnormalities will disappear in up to 75% of cases.

Adverse Reactions

Adverse effects, which occur in up to 40% of patients, are generally mild and transient, but occasionally their severity requires interruption of therapy. Diarrhea and abdominal cramps are most common; these may diminish or stop after several days of treatment. Anorexia, nausea, vomiting, dizziness, and headache may also occur. Pruritic, urticarial, or papular skin rashes are less frequent and usually begin after a latent period of 1 week or more of therapy; they are probably allergic in nature, resulting from release of antigens from dying worms. Other infrequent reactions are lassitude, pyrexia, tinnitus, insomnia, proteinuria, and leukopenia. Hypersensitivity reactions to the drug itself are rare.

Contraindications & Cautions

Bithionol should be used with caution in children under 8 years of age because of limited experience in that age group. Treatment should be discontinued if serial liver function and hematologic tests show possible development of toxic hepatitis or leukopenia.

Treatment apparently does not worsen the neurologic condition of patients with cerebral paragonimiasis, but this possibility should be kept in mind and steroid therapy initiated if indicated.

DIETHYLCARBAMAZINE CITRATE

Diethylcarbamazine is a drug of choice in the treatment of filariasis, loiasis, and tropical eosinophilia. It is an alternative drug in the treatment of onchocerciasis.

Chemistry & Pharmacokinetics

Diethylcarbamazine is a synthetic piperazine derivative. It is marketed as a citrate salt, which contains 51% of the active base and is rapidly absorbed from the gastrointestinal tract. The minimum effective blood concentration appears to be 0.8–1 μg/mL. The plasma half-life is 2–3 hours in the presence of acidic urine but about 10 hours if the urine is alkaline. The drug rapidly equilibrates with all tissues except fat. It is excreted, principally in the urine, as unchanged drug and degradation products. Dosage may have to be reduced in patients with persistent urinary alkalosis or renal impairment.

Anthelmintic Actions & Pharmacologic Effects

Diethylcarbamazine immobilizes microfilariae (which results in their displacement in tissues) and alters their surface structure, making them more susceptible to destruction by host defense mechanisms. The mode of action of diethylcarbamazine against adult worms is unknown.

Diethylcarbamazine has shown in vivo and in vitro immunosuppressive actions, the mechanism of which is imperfectly understood. The drug has had no teratogenic effects in experimental animals.

Clinical Uses

The drug should be taken after meals.

A. Wuchereria bancrofti, Brugia malayi, Brugia timori, Loa loa: Diethylcarbamazine is the drug of choice for treatment of infections with these parasites, given its high order of therapeutic efficacy and relative lack of serious toxicity. Microfilariae of all species are rapidly killed; adult parasites are killed more slowly, often requiring several courses of treatment. The drug is highly effective against adult L loa, but the extent to which W bancrofti and B malayi adults are killed is not known. However, if therapy is adequate, microfilariae do not reappear in the majority of patients, which suggests that the adult worms are either killed or permanently sterilized.

These infections are treated with 2 mg/kg 3 times a day for 3 weeks. For W bancrofti infections, to reduce the incidence of allergic reactions to dying microfilariae, a single dose (2 mg/kg) is administered on the first day, two doses on the second day, and three doses on the third day and thereafter. For L loa (with its risk of encephalopathy), or B malayi infection, the same schedule should be used, but individual doses should start at 1 mg/kg once on the first day and gradually increase over 5–6 days.

Antihistamines may be given for the first 4–5 days of diethylcarbamazine therapy to reduce the incidence of allergic reactions. Corticosteroids should be started and doses of diethylcarbamazine temporarily lowered or interrupted if severe reactions occur.

Blood should be checked for microfilariae several weeks after treatment is completed; a course may be repeated after 3–4 weeks. Cure may require several courses of treatment over 1–2 years.

Spaced treatment doses (weekly to monthly) may prove superior as a macrofilaricide to the standard daily dose. The drug may also be used in prophylaxis—300 mg weekly for loiasis and 50 mg monthly for bancroftian and Malayan filariasis.

B. Onchocerca volvulus: Diethylcarbamazine is not effective against the adult worms but does kill the microfilariae. If diethylcarbamazine is used alone, the adult worms survive and the reduction in microfilariae is only temporary; to kill the adult worms, suramin (a toxic drug) must be given. Because of the frequency and severity of reactions when diethylcar-

bamazine is used in the treatment of onchocerciasis, the drug should be administered for this condition only by experts and should preferably be initiated in the hospital. (See Goldsmith and Heyneman, 1989, for details.)

C. Tropical Eosinophilia: Diethylcarbamazine is given orally at a dosage of 2 mg/kg 3 times daily for 7 days.

D. Other Parasites: Diethylcarbamazine is effective in *Mansonella streptocerca* infections, since it kills both adults and microfilariae. Limited information suggests that the drug is not effective, however, against adult *Mansonella ozzardi* or *M perstans* and that it has only a low order of effectiveness or is inactive against microfilariae of these parasites. Diethylcarbamazine is not active against *Dirofilaria immitis*.

In **toxocariasis,** diethylcarbamazine may be tried but its efficacy is not established. The drug has been used in the treatment of *Ascaris* infections and **cutaneous larva migrans,** but other drugs are superior.

E. Mass Therapy: An important application of diethylcarbamazine therapy has been its use for mass treatment of W bancrofti infections to reduce transmission. A common regimen is one dose each week or month for 12 doses. Often, adverse reactions discourage community participation. However, when the drug is administered in low doses in medicated salt, it is stable in cooking, appears to be free of adverse effects, and is active as a microfilaricide and possibly as a macrofilaricide.

Adverse Reactions

A. Drug-Induced Reactions: Reactions to diethylcarbamazine itself are mild and transient and start within 2–4 hours: headache, malaise, anorexia, and weakness are frequent; nausea, vomiting, dizziness, and sleepiness occur less often.

B. Reactions Induced by Dying Parasites: Adverse effects also occur as a result of the release of foreign proteins from dying microfilariae or adult worms in sensitized patients. Eosinophilia and leukocytosis are usually intensified.

1. Reactions in onchocerciasis–In onchocerciasis, adverse reactions affecting the skin and eyes occur in most patients, and systemic reactions may also occur (see Goldsmith and Heyneman, 1989, for details). The reaction may be severe, especially if infection is heavy, or if pruritus is intense, or if microfilariae are near the eyes. Vision can be permanently damaged.

2. Reactions in W bancrofti, B malayi, and L loa infections–Reactions to dying microfilariae are usually mild in W bancrofti (in up to 25% of patients), more intense in B malayi, and occasionally severe in L loa infections. Reactions include fever, malaise, papular rash, headache, gastrointestinal symptoms, cough, chest pains, and muscle or joint pains. Leukocytosis is common; eosinophilia and proteinuria may occur. In W bancrofti and B malayi infections, symptoms are most likely to occur in patients with heavy loads of microfilariae but may also occur even if the patient is apparently amicrofilaremic. In loiasis, severe reactions are more likely to occur if microfilaria counts are greater than 50/μL of blood. Retinal hemorrhages have been described and, rarely, central nervous system involvement that can be life-threatening.

Between the third and twelfth days of treatment, local reactions may occur in the vicinity of dying adult or immature worms. Lymphangitis with localized swellings or nodules and lymph abscesses may occur in *W bancrofti* and *B malayi;* small wheals appear in the skin at the site of dying worms in *L loa;* and flat papules appear in *M streptocerca* infections.

Contraindications & Cautions

There are no absolute contraindications to the use of diethylcarbamazine, but caution is advised in patients with hypertension or renal disease.

Patients suspected of having malaria should be treated before they are given diethylcarbamazine, which may provoke a relapse in asymptomatic malaria infections.

Patients with attacks of lymphangitis due to *W bancrofti* or *B malayi* should be treated during a quiescent period between attacks.

EMETINE HYDROCHLORIDE

Emetine and dehydroemetine are alternative drugs for the treatment of *Fasciola hepatica* infection. Both drugs are sometimes effective in removing the parasite but are more toxic than bithionol (the drug of choice). Dehydroemetine is probably less toxic than emetine; general pharmacologic information, dosage, and precautions in their usage are presented in Chapter 54.

IVERMECTIN

Ivermectin is the drug of choice in onchocerciasis treatment. It is also used in mass treatment, where it is safe and effective in reducing microfilarial loads, and shows promise as a chemotherapeutic control agent. Ivermectin may also prove useful in the treatment of other forms of filariasis, strongyloidiasis, and cutaneous larva migrans.

Chemistry & Pharmacokinetics

Ivermectin, a semisynthetic macrocyclic lactone, is a mixture of avermectin B_{1a} and B_{1b}. It is derived from the soil actinomycete *Streptomyces avermitilis.*

Ivermectin is given only orally in humans. The drug is rapidly absorbed, reaching maximum plasma concentrations (about 50 μg/L) at 4 hours after a 12 mg dose. The drug has a wide tissue distribution and

a volume of distribution of about 50 L. It apparently enters the eye slowly and to a limited extent. Its half-life is about 28 hours. Excretion is almost exclusively in the feces.

Anthelmintic Actions & Pharmacologic Effects

A. Anthelmintic Actions: Ivermectin appears to paralyze nematodes and arthropods (which may lead to their death) by intensifying GABA-mediated transmission of signals in peripheral nerves (see Chapter 53). Ivermectin is an established microfilaricide in onchocerciasis. In addition, recent reports suggest that serial treatments at 6-month or longer intervals result in slow death of some adult worms. In single-dose treatment, the drug acts rapidly against skin microfilariae and slowly (over months) against microfilariae in the anterior chamber of the eye; the drug also affects embryogenesis in female worms (intrauterine microfilariae are damaged and degenerate). Within 2–3 days after a dose, the skin microfilaria counts drop rapidly and remain low for about 12 months. Unsettled is whether adult worms are irreversibly sterilized or killed by repeated doses of ivermectin and whether the drug paralyzes the microfilariae, which might facilitate their removal by the reticuloendothelial system.

B. Pharmacologic Action in Humans: The drug is without known pharmacologic or toxic effects in humans, partly because ivermectin does not readily cross the blood-brain barrier.

In animal studies, ivermectin appears to have a wide margin of safety. However, in mice given high doses, teratogenic effects and occasional unexplained maternal deaths have occurred.

Clinical Uses

A. Onchocerciasis: Treatment is with a single oral dose of 150 μg/kg with water on an empty stomach. Treatment is repeated at 6- to 12-month intervals, based on skin microfilaria levels. A single dose results in marked reduction in skin microfilaria and eosinophil counts and clearance (over months) of microfilariae from the anterior chamber; in some patients, there is improvement of anterior segment eye disease and dermatitis. The long-term effect of repeated treatments on posterior segment disease is unknown.

In comparison studies, ivermectin is as effective as diethylcarbamazine in reducing the numbers of microfilariae—which are responsible for the pathologic features of the disease—in the skin and the anterior chamber, but it does so with significantly fewer systemic and ocular adverse reactions. Furthermore, the reduction in microfilariae persists longer. In comparative studies, ocular changes (punctate keratitis, chorioretinitis, and optic nerve atrophy) were seen in diethylcarbamazine-treated but not in ivermectin-treated patients.

B. Bancroftian Filariasis: In comparisons of ivermectin and diethylcarbamazine, the two drugs appear to be equally efficacious in reducing microfilaria burdens; mild side-effects (myalgia, headache, fever) are similar in some studies but less for ivermectin in others. Although ivermectin has a convenient single-dose or two-dose schedule (under evaluation is a clearing dose of 20 µg/kg followed by 400 µg/kg), it has minimal macrofilaricidal action, and diethylcarbamazine is therefore still needed to kill the adult worms.

C. Other Parasites: Ivermectin has been reported to be useful in *Mansonella ozzardi* but not in *M perstans* infections; a single dose partially cleared *Brugia malayi* microfilariae with minimal side effects. In **loiasis,** the drug may prove useful in patients with high microfilaria loads who might be adversely affected when initially treated with diethylcarbamazine, which is required to eradicate the adult worms. Ivermectin shows promise in **strongyloidiasis;** with a single dose of 200 µg/kg, cure rates may reach over 90%. The drug also appears to be effective in **ascariasis** and possibly in **cutaneous larva migrans.**

Adverse Reactions

The adverse effects of ivermectin are a Mazotti-like reaction, which peaks 2 days after a single oral dose. The reaction is thought to be due to massive killing of microfilariae, not to drug toxicity, and its intensity correlates with skin microfilaria loads. In indigenous adults, the reaction occurs in 5–30% of persons, but it is generally mild, well tolerated, of short duration, and controlled by aspirin and antihistamines. The reaction in expatriate adults—perhaps also in indigenous children—may be more frequent. The Mazotti reaction includes fever (occasionally intermittent for several days), headache, dizziness, somnolence, weakness, rash, increased pruritus, diarrhea, joint and muscle pains, hypotension, tachycardia, lymphadenitis, lymphangitis, and peripheral edema. A more intense Mazotti-like reaction occurs in 1–3% of persons and a severe reaction in 0.3%, including high fever, hypotension, and bronchospasm. Steroids may be necessary for several days. Swellings and abscesses occasionally occur at 1–3 weeks, presumably at sites of adult worms.

Some patients develop punctate corneal opacities several days after treatment. Other uncommon ophthalmologic reactions (all of which can occur with the disease itself) are eyelid edema, anterior uveitis, conjunctivitis, keratitis, optic neuritis, chorioretinitis, and choroiditis. These have rarely been severe or associated with loss of vision and have generally resolved without corticosteroid treatment.

Contraindications & Cautions

Because ivermectin enhances GABA activity, it is best to avoid concomitant use of other drugs with similar effects, eg, barbiturates, benzodiazepines, and valproic acid. Ivermectin should not be used in pregnancy. Safety in children under 5 years has not been established. The proscription against breast feeding by mothers using the drug will probably be reduced to 1 week following the last dose.

The drug should not be administered to patients in whom there may be impairment of the blood-brain barrier, eg, in meningitis and African sleeping sickness.

LEVAMISOLE

Levamisole hydrochloride is a synthetic imidazothiazole derivative and the L isomer of D,L-tetramisole. It is highly effective in eradicating *Ascaris* and *Trichostrongylus* and moderately effective against both species of hookworm. The drug is marketed in the USA but is approved only for its immunomodulating effect as adjunct therapy with fluorouracil for treatment of colon cancer.

MEBENDAZOLE

Mebendazole is a synthetic benzimidazole that has a wide spectrum of anthelmintic activity and a low incidence of adverse effects.

Mebendazole

Chemistry & Pharmacokinetics

Less than 10% of orally administered mebendazole is absorbed. The absorbed drug is protein-bound (> 90%), rapidly metabolized (primarily in the liver to inactive metabolites), and excreted mostly in the urine, either unchanged or as decarboxylated derivatives, within 24–48 hours. In addition, a portion of absorbed drug and its derivatives are excreted in the bile. Absorption is increased if the drug is ingested with a fatty meal.

Anthelmintic Actions
& Pharmacologic Effects

Mebendazole inhibits microtubule synthesis in nematodes, thus irreversibly impairing glucose uptake (see Chapter 53). As a result, intestinal parasites are immobilized or die slowly, and their clearance from the gastrointestinal tract may not be complete until several days after treatment. Efficacy of the drug varies with gastrointestinal transit time, with intensity of infection, with whether or not the drug is chewed, and perhaps with the strain of parasite. The drug kills hookworm, *Ascaris,* and *Trichuris* eggs.

In humans, mebendazole is almost inert. No evidence of carcinogenicity or teratogenicity has been found. However, in pregnant rats the drug has embryotoxic and teratogenic activity at single oral doses as low as 10 mg/kg.

Clinical Uses

In the USA, mebendazole has been approved for use in ascariasis, trichuriasis, and hookworm and pinworm infection. It is investigational for other uses.

The drug can be taken before or after meals; the tablets should be chewed before swallowing. Cure rates decrease in patients who have gastrointestinal hypermotility. In the treatment of trichinosis, hydatid disease, and dracontiasis, the drug should be taken with food containing fat, which enhances absorption.

A. Pinworm Infection: Give 100 mg once and repeat the dose at 2 and 4 weeks. The same dosage is used for children and adults. Cure rates range between 90% and 100%.

B. *Ascaris lumbricoides, Trichuris trichiura,* Hookworm, and *Trichostrongylus:* A dosage of 100 mg twice daily for 3 days is used for adults and for children over 2 years of age. Treatment can be repeated in 2–3 weeks. No pre- or posttreatment purging is necessary. Cure rates are 90–100% for ascariasis and trichuriasis. Although cure rates are lower for hookworm infections of both species (70–95%), a marked reduction in the worm burden occurs in those not cured. Mebendazole is particularly useful in mixed infections with these parasites.

C. Hydatid Disease: Albendazole is the drug of choice. Mebendazole is the alternative and less satisfactory drug, both with regard to cure rates and the high daily doses required to overcome poor absorption. Results of mebendazole therapy have been highly variable. With mebendazole, subjective improvement is reported for most patients and evidence of regression of cysts in some; in other patients, particularly after long-term follow-up, cysts have continued to grow or have proved viable. Unpredictable plasma levels of the drug may contribute to this variability in response. One dosage schedule is 50 mg/kg in three divided doses daily for 3 months. When possible, mebendazole blood levels should be monitored; serum levels in excess of 100 ng/mL 1–3 hours after an oral dose may be necessary for parasite killing.

D. Other Infections: For treatment of **intestinal capillariasis,** mebendazole is an alternative drug at a dosage of 400 mg/d in divided doses for 21 or more days.

In **trichinosis,** limited reports suggest some efficacy against adult worms in the intestinal tract, migrating larvae, and larvae in muscle. The following daily treatment schedule has been recommended for adults: 600 mg initially, increasing stepwise over 3 days to 1200–1500 mg, continuing with the maximum dose for 10 days. Daily doses should be given in three divided portions.

Mebendazole at a dosage of 300 mg twice daily for 3 days has been used in the treatment of **taeniasis** with variable effectiveness. In the treatment of *Taenia solium* infection, mebendazole has a theoretic advantage over niclosamide in that proglottids are expelled intact after therapy with mebendazole.

Cure rates for **strongyloidiasis** using the standard 3-day course of therapy are usually less than 50%; higher doses and longer courses of therapy are being investigated.

In **dracontiasis,** the drug's efficacy has been variable and needs further study. The use of mebendazole or mebendazole plus levamisole in **filariasis, loiasis, onchocerciasis,** and *Mansonella perstans* infection is under study. In the treatment of *Angiostrongylus cantonensis* infection and **visceral larva migrans,** mebendazole can be tried at a dosage of 200–400 mg in divided doses for 5 days; in **gnathostomiasis,** 200 mg every 3 hours for 6 days can be tried.

Adverse Reactions

Low-dose mebendazole for 1–3 days for intestinal nematode therapy has been nearly free of adverse effects even in debilitated patients. Mild nausea, vomiting, diarrhea, and abdominal pain have been reported infrequently, more often in children heavily parasitized by *Ascaris.* Slight headache, dizziness, and hypersensitivity reactions (rash, urticaria) are rare. Oral or nasal passage of ascarids in children under 5 years of age has been reported.

Occasional adverse effects associated with high-dose mebendazole treatment of hydatid disease are pruritus, rash, eosinophilia, reversible neutropenia, musculoskeletal pain, fever, and acute pain in the cyst area. Some of these findings may be due to cyst leakage or rupture with release of antigen. Gastric irritation, cough, transient liver function abnormalities, alopecia, glomerulonephritis, and some cases of drug-induced agranulocytosis (with one death) have been reported.

Contraindications & Cautions

In severe hepatic parenchymal disease, mebendazole is very slowly metabolized and should be used with caution. The drug is contraindicated in the first trimester of pregnancy; alternative drugs are preferred later in pregnancy. Mebendazole should be used with caution in children under 1 year of age because of limited experience and rare reports of convulsions in this age group. Concomitant use of carbamazepine may reduce plasma levels and effectiveness of mebendazole; concomitant use of cimetidine may increase plasma levels.

METRIFONATE

Metrifonate is a safe, low-cost alternative drug for the treatment of *Schistosoma haematobium* infections. It is not active against *S mansoni* or *S japonicum*. The drug is not available in the USA.

Chemistry & Pharmacokinetics

Metrifonate is an organophosphorus compound. It is rapidly absorbed after oral administration. Following a standard oral dose, peak blood levels are reached in 1–2 hours; the half-life is about 1.5 hours. Clearance appears to be through nonenzymatic transformation to dichlorvos, its active metabolite. The amount of dichlorvos in the plasma is about 1% of the metrifonate level. The drug and its derivatives are well distributed to the tissues and are completely eliminated in 24–48 hours.

Anthelmintic Actions & Pharmacologic Effects

Metrifonate acts through its biotransformation to dichlorvos. The mode of action of dichlorvos against both the mature and immature stages of *S haematobium* is not established but is thought to be in part related to its function as a cholinesterase inhibitor. The cholinesterase inhibition temporarily paralyzes the adult worms, resulting in their shift from the bladder venous plexus to small arterioles of the lungs, where they are trapped, encased, and die. The drug is not effective against *S haematobium* eggs, and live eggs will therefore continue to pass in the urine for several months after all adult worms have been killed.

Therapeutic dosages of metrifonate in humans produce no untoward physiologic or chemical abnormalities except for cholinesterase inhibition. Following oral ingestion of 7.5–12.5 mg/kg of metrifonate by infected persons, there is an almost complete inhibition of plasma butyrylcholinesterase and a marked reduction (about 50%) of erythrocytic acetylcholinesterase. Recovery of plasma cholinesterase is usually 70% (or more) by 2 weeks and is complete by 4 weeks, but erythrocyte enzyme recovery may take up to 15 weeks.

Metrifonate or perhaps impurities associated with its manufacture show weak mutagenicity in the *Salmonella typhimurium* direct test system. It induces mutations in *Escherichia coli* but causes no chromosomal abnormalities in animals or humans. Reproduction toxicity studies showed negative results except for suggestions of impaired spermatogenesis.

Clinical Uses

In the treatment of *S haematobium,* a single dose of 7.5–10 mg/kg is given orally 3 times at 14-day intervals. Cure rates on this schedule range from 44% to 93%, with marked reductions in egg counts in those not cured.

Metrifonate was also effective as a prophylactic when given monthly to children in a highly endemic area. The drug is used in mass treatment programs. In mixed infections with *S haematobium* and *S mansoni,* metrifonate has been successfully combined with oxamniquine.

Adverse Reactions

Some studies report no adverse effects; others note mild and transient cholinergic symptoms, including nausea and vomiting, diarrhea, abdominal pain, bronchospasm, headache, sweating, fatigue, weakness, dizziness, and vertigo. These symptoms may begin within 30 minutes and persist up to 12 hours. The drug is well tolerated by patients in the advanced hepatosplenic stage of the disease.

One case of typical organophosphate poisoning following a standard dose has been reported; the patient responded well to the use of atropine.

Contraindications & Cautions

Metrifonate should not be used after recent exposure to insecticides or drugs that might potentiate cholinesterase inhibition. The use of muscle relaxants should be avoided for 48 hours after administration of the drug. Metrifonate is contraindicated in pregnancy.

NICLOSAMIDE

Niclosamide is a drug of choice for the treatment of most tapeworm infections.

Chemistry & Pharmacokinetics

Niclosamide is a salicylamide derivative. It appears to be minimally absorbed from the gastrointestinal tract: neither the drug nor its metabolites have been recovered from the blood or urine.

Anthelmintic Actions & Pharmacologic Effects

Following oral administration in animals and humans, no hematologic, renal, or hepatic abnormalities have been noted.

The scoleces and segments of cestodes–but not the ova–are rapidly killed on contact with niclosamide. This may be due to the drug's inhibition of oxidative phosphorylation or to its ATPase-stimulating property. With the death of the parasite, the scolex is released from the intestinal wall and digestion of segments begins.

The drug has not been fully evaluated for carcinogenic and mutagenic potential. Human peripheral lymphocytes show a dose-related increase in clastogenicity and an increase in chromosome aberrations. Urine from mice fed niclosamide shows mutagenicity in the Ames test.

Clinical Uses

The adult dosage is 2 g (four tablets, 500 mg each).

Children weighing more than 34 kg are given three tablets; 11–34 kg, two tablets; and under 11 kg, one tablet. Niclosamide should be given in the morning on an empty stomach. The tablets *must be chewed thoroughly* and are then swallowed with water. For small children, pulverize the tablets and then mix with water. The patient may eat 2 hours later. Posttreatment purges to expel the worm are not necessary except for an occasional patient with chronic constipation. Even if a purge is used to determine cure by finding the scolex, the scolex and proglottids may be partially digested and difficult to identify. In treating infections with large tapeworms, segments may continue to pass for several days with normal peristalsis.

A. *T saginata* **(Beef Tapeworm),** *T solium* **(Pork Tapeworm), and** *Diphyllobothrium latum* **(Fish Tapeworm):** A single dose of niclosamide results in cure rates of over 85% for *D latum* and about 95% for *T saginata.* It is probably equally effective against *T solium,* but 2 hours after treatment an effective purge (such as 15–30 g of magnesium sulfate) should be given to eliminate all mature segments before ova can be released. The patient should be monitored to ensure that prompt evacuation occurs. Cysticercosis is theoretically possible after treatment of *T solium* infections, since viable ova are released into the gut lumen following digestion of segments. However, after more than 2 decades of use, no cases of cysticercosis have been reported. In taeniasis, if the scolex is not found or is not searched for after treatment, cure can be presumed only if regenerated segments have not reappeared after 3–5 months.

B. *Hymenolepis nana* **(Dwarf Tapeworm):** Praziquantel is the drug of choice. Although niclosamide is effective against the adult parasites in the lumen of the intestine, it is not effective against cysticercoids embedded in the villi. For the drug to be successful, therefore, it must be given until all of the cysticercoids have emerged (about 4 days). Thus, the minimum course of treatment must be 7 days; some workers repeat the course 5 days later. The overall cure rate with niclosamide is about 75%.

C. Other Tapeworms: Results have been promising in patients treated for *Hymenolepis diminuta* and *Dipylidium caninum* infections. Most patients are cured with a 7-day course of treatment; a few require a second course. Niclosamide is not effective against cysticercosis or hydatid disease.

D. Intestinal Fluke Infections: Niclosamide can be used as an alternative drug for the treatment of *Fasciolopsis buski, Heterophyes heterophyes,* and *Metagonimus yokogawai* infections. The standard dose is given every other day for three doses.

Adverse Reactions

Adverse effects are infrequent, mild, and transitory. Nausea, vomiting, diarrhea, and abdominal discomfort occur in less than 4% of patients. Rarely described are headache, skin rash, urticaria, pruritus ani, and vertigo, some of which may be related to release of antigenic material from disintegrating parasites.

Contraindications & Cautions

The consumption of alcohol should be avoided on the day of treatment and for 1 day afterward.

There are no contraindications to the use of niclosamide. In children under 2 years of age, the safety of the drug has not been established. Reproductive studies in animals were negative, but there are no adequate studies in pregnant women.

OXAMNIQUINE

Oxamniquine is a drug of choice for the treatment of *S mansoni* infections. It has also been used extensively for mass treatment. It is not effective against *S haematobium* or *S japonicum.*

Pharmacokinetics

Oxamniquine is a semisynthetic tetrahydroquinoline. It is readily absorbed orally and is not given intramuscularly, because it causes intense and prolonged local pain by this route. After therapeutic doses, its plasma half-life is about 2.5 hours. The drug is extensively metabolized to inactive metabolites and excreted, primarily in the urine.

Intersubject variations in serum concentration have been noted, which could explain some treatment failures. Although the drug is taken with food to decrease adverse effects, food does delay its absorption.

Anthelmintic Actions & Pharmacologic Effects

Oxamniquine is active against both mature and immature stages of *S mansoni* but does not appear to be cercaricidal. Although the exact mechanism is not known, the drug may act by DNA binding. Contraction and paralysis of the worms results in detachment from terminal venules in the mesentery and a shift to the liver, where many die; surviving females cease to lay eggs. The drug has no immunoregulating effect on perioval granuloma formation.

Strains of *S mansoni* in different parts of the world vary in susceptibility by dosage. Although *S mansoni* resistance to oxamniquine can be induced experimentally in mice, resistance following treatment in humans has not been established.

Clinical Uses

Oxamniquine, effective only against *S mansoni,* is safe and effective in all stages of the disease, including advanced hepatosplenomegaly. In the acute (Katayama) syndrome, treatment results in disappearance of acute symptoms and subsequent failure to develop infection.

The drug is generally less effective in children, who require higher doses than adults. It is better tolerated if given with food. When divided doses are given in a single day, they should be separated by 6–8 hours.

Optimal dosage schedules vary for different regions of the world. In the Western Hemisphere and western Africa, the adult dose is 12–15 mg/kg given once (children under 30 kg, 10 mg/kg twice in 1 day). In northern and southern Africa, give 15 mg/kg twice daily for 2 days (children under 30 kg, twice daily for 2-3 days). In eastern Africa and the Arabian peninsula, give 15–20 mg/kg twice in 1 day (children under 30 kg, twice daily for 1 day). Cure rates are 70–95%, with marked reduction in egg excretion in those not cured.

In mixed infections with *S mansoni* and *S haematobium,* oxamniquine has been successfully used in combination with metrifonate. Oxamniquine's potential for suppressive prophylaxis as shown in animals needs further study in humans.

Adverse Reactions

Experience with the drug in millions of persons has shown it to be nearly free of significant toxicity. However, mild symptoms—starting about 3 hours after a dose, and lasting for several hours—do occur in more than one-third of patients. Central nervous system symptoms (dizziness, headache, drowsiness) are most common; nausea and vomiting, diarrhea, colic, pruritus, and urticaria also occur. Infrequent adverse effects are low-grade fever, an orange to red discoloration of the urine, proteinuria, microscopic hematuria, and a transient decrease in leukocytes and lymphocytes. Seizures are rare and generally occur within hours after ingestion, most often in persons with a history of seizures. Insomnia, amnesia, behavioral changes, and hallucinations are rare.

Liver enzyme elevations, eosinophilia, transient pulmonary infiltrates (sometimes associated with cough and rhonchi), urticaria, and fever (especially in Egypt) that occur from several days to 1 month after treatment have been ascribed to the death of parasites and release of antigens rather than to a direct toxic effect of the drug.

Oxamniquine has shown low mutagenicity in the *S typhimurium* test system and when assayed in mice, but chromosomal abnormalities were not found in other animals or humans. Oxamniquine has also been shown to have an embryocidal effect in rabbits and mice when given in doses ten times the equivalent human dose.

Contraindications & Cautions

It appears prudent to observe patients for about 3 hours after ingestion of the drug for signs of central nervous system disturbances. Patients with a history of epilepsy should be hospitalized for treatment, or an alternative drug used. Since the drug makes many patients dizzy or drowsy, it should be used with caution

(eg, no driving for 24 hours) in patients whose work or activity requires mental alertness.

Oxamniquine is contraindicated in pregnancy.

OXANTEL PAMOATE & OXANTEL/PYRANTEL PAMOATE

Oxantel pamoate, a tetrahydroxypyrimidine and metaoxyphenol analogue of pyrantel pamoate, is effective only in the treatment of trichuriasis infections. Since trichuriasis commonly occurs as a multiple infection with the other soil-transmitted helminths, oxantel is now being marketed in combination with pyrantel pamoate because the latter is active against *Ascaris* and hookworm infections. Neither oxantel nor oxantel/pyrantel is effective in strongyloidiasis. These drugs are not available in the USA.

PIPERAZINE

The piperazine salts are alternative drugs in the treatment of ascariasis. Cure rates are over 90% when patients are treated for 2 days. Piperazine is not useful for treatment of hookworm infection, trichuriasis, or strongyloidiasis. The drug is no longer recommended in this text in the treatment of pinworm infection, because a 7-day course of treatment is required.

Chemistry & Pharmacokinetics

Piperazine is available as the hexahydrate (which contains about 44% of the base) and as a variety of salts: citrate, phosphate, adipate, tartrate, and others.

Piperazine is readily absorbed from the gastrointestinal tract, and maximum plasma levels are reached in 2–4 hours. Most of the drug is excreted unchanged in the urine in 2–6 hours, and excretion is complete within 24 hours.

Anthelmintic Actions & Pharmacologic Effects

Orally administered piperazine in therapeutic dosage is almost free of pharmacologic action in the host.

The formation of a potentially carcinogenic nitrosamine metabolite, N-mononitrosopiperazine, has been reported in gastric contents and urine of volunteers given therapeutic doses of piperazine; the significance of this finding remains to be determined.

Piperazine causes a paralysis of *Ascaris* by blocking acetylcholine at the myoneural junction. Piperazine has a similar (but much weaker) myoneural blocking action on mammalian skeletal muscle. When the drug is used in humans, the paralyzed roundworms are unable to maintain their position in the host and are expelled live by normal peristalsis.

Clinical Uses

For ascariasis, the dosage of piperazine (as the

hexahydrate) is 75 mg/kg orally (maximum dose, 3.5 g) for 2 days in succession, before or after breakfast. For heavy infections, treatment should be continued for 3–4 days or be repeated after 1 week. No pre- or posttreatment cathartics are used. In the nonsurgical management of intestinal obstruction caused by heavy *Ascaris* infection, piperazine syrup is administered via an intestinal drainage tube.

Adverse Reactions

There is a wide range between the therapeutic and toxic doses of piperazine. Mild adverse effects occur occasionally, including nausea, vomiting, diarrhea, abdominal pain, and headache. At high dosage, neurotoxic adverse effects (somnolence, dizziness, ataxia, seizures, chorea, and others) occur but are rare. Patients with epilepsy may have an exacerbation of seizures. Piperazine is potentially allergenic. Serum sickness-like syndromes (urticaria, purpura, fever, eczematous skin reactions, bronchospasm) have rarely been reported 2–4 days after an initial dose of piperazine.

Contraindications & Cautions

Piperazine compounds should not be given to patients with impaired renal or hepatic function or with a history of epilepsy or chronic neurologic disease. Piperazine and phenothiazines should not be given together. Caution should be exercised in patients with severe malnutrition or anemia. In view of its partial conversion to a nitrosamine (see above), the drug should be given to pregnant women only if clearly indicated and if alternative drugs are not available.

PRAZIQUANTEL

Praziquantel is effective in the treatment of schistosome infections of all species and most other trematode and cestode infections, including cysticercosis. The drug's safety and effectiveness as a single oral dose have also made it useful in mass treatment of several of the infections. Praziquantel is not effective against *Fasciola hepatica* or in hydatid disease. In the USA, although the drug is only labeled for schistosomiasis treatment, it is the drug of choice (as an investigational drug) for many other cestode and trematode infections.

Chemistry & Pharmacokinetics

Praziquantel is a synthetic isoquinoline-pyrazine derivative. The drug should be stored below 30 °C. It is rapidly absorbed, with a bioavailability of about 80% after oral administration. Peak serum concentrations of 0.2–2 µg/mL of the unchanged drug are reached 1–3 hours after a therapeutic dose. About 80% of the drug is bound to plasma proteins. Cerebrospinal fluid concentrations of praziquantel reach 14–20% of the drug's plasma concentration; esti-

mates for bile, breast milk, and feces are 10–20% of plasma levels. Most of the drug is rapidly metabolized to inactive mono- and polyhydroxylated products after a first pass in the liver; the half-life of the drug is 0.8–1.5 hours, while that of its metabolites is 4–6 hours. Excretion is mainly via the kidneys (60–80%) and bile (15–35%).

Pharmacologic Effects

In humans, no major alterations in biochemical or hematologic tests have been described. Transient elevations in liver function tests and, rarely, minor electrocardiographic changes may occur, but no significant damage to vital organs has been reported. In severe liver dysfunction, plasma levels rise.

In experimental animals, no effects are seen until doses approximately 100 times the therapeutic range are reached; signs of central nervous system toxicity are then noted.

A wide variety of mutagenicity, carcinogenicity, embryotoxicity, and teratogenicity studies have been negative. One laboratory (not confirmed by others) reported that praziquantel and a urinary metabolite acted as a mutagen or comutagen in *S typhimurium* and mammalian cell test systems. On balance, the present evidence indicates that praziquantel probably does not present a genotoxic risk.

Anthelmintic Actions

The threshold serum concentration of praziquantel for therapeutic effect is about 0.3 µg/mL. In spite of its short half-life, praziquantel is the active agent; its metabolites are inactive. However, in vivo evidence suggests that host antibody to the parasite is also essential to eliminate tissue parasites.

Praziquantel's in vitro action on all platyhelminths appears to be the same—the drug increases cell membrane permeability to calcium, resulting in marked contraction, followed by paralysis of worm musculature. Vacuolization and disintegration of the tegmen occur, and parasite death follows. Although *F hepatica* does absorb the drug, no reaction occurs and the infection is not cleared.

In schistosome infections of experimental animals, praziquantel is effective against adult worms and immature stages; adult worms are rapidly immobilized and then passively shift to the liver. In addition, when a single high dose of praziquantel is given concurrently with an infecting dose of cercariae, all immature forms are killed; thus, praziquantel has a prophylactic effect.

Clinical Uses

Praziquantel tablets are taken with liquid after a meal; they should be swallowed immediately without chewing because their bitter taste can induce retching and vomiting. If the drug is taken more than once on the same day, the interval between doses should be no less than 4 hours and no more than 8 hours.

A. Schistosomiasis: Praziquantel is a drug of choice for all forms of schistosomiasis. The dosage is 20 mg/kg at intervals of 4–6 hours for a total of three doses. Other schedules, some with lower total doses, have been effective in some regions: 40 mg/kg once for *S haematobium* and 40 mg/kg in two divided doses for *S mansoni*. High cure rates are achieved when patients are evaluated at 3–6 months; there is marked reduction in egg counts in those not cured. The drug is effective in adults and children and is generally well tolerated by patients in the hepatosplenic stage of advanced disease. It is not clear, however, whether the drug can be safely used during the acute stage of the disease (Katayama fever) because release of antigens from dying immature worms may exacerbate symptoms. Use of the drug prophylactically has not been established. Schistosomes apparently do not develop resistance to praziquantel.

B. Clonorchiasis and Opisthorchiasis: The dosage of 25 mg/kg 3 times daily for 1 day for *Opisthorchis* and 2 days for *Clonorchis* infections results in nearly 100% cure rates.

C. Paragonimiasis: When treated with 25 mg/kg 3 times daily for 2 days, cure rates for pulmonary paragonimiasis are 89–100%.

D. Taeniasis and Diphyllobothriasis: A single dose of praziquantel, 10 mg/kg, results in cure rates of 97–100% for *T saginata* and *T solium*. In cysticercosis-endemic areas, it may be safer but equally effective to use 2.5 mg/kg. A single dose of 25 mg/kg results in similar cure rates for *D latum* infections. Within 24–48 hours after treatment, a disintegrating worm is usually passed by normal peristalsis. Pre- and posttreatment purges are not necessary. If the scolex is searched for but not found or is not searched for, cure can be presumed only if regenerated segments have not reappeared 3–5 months after treatment. For *T solium*, the recommendation continues that an effective purge (eg, magnesium sulfate, 15–30 g) be given 2 hours after treatment to eliminate all mature segments before eggs can be released from disintegrating segments. Since praziquantel does not kill the eggs, it is theoretically possible that larvae released from eggs in the large bowel could penetrate the intestinal wall and give rise to cysticercosis. However, as with the use of niclosamide, this hazard is probably minimal.

E. Neurocysticercosis: Neurocysticercosis should be treated in hospital by a physician with neurologic expertise. The indications, cautions, use of concomitant corticosteroids, and outcome for praziquantel treatment are similar to those for albendazole use. However, in comparable studies, albendazole (see above) appears to be the preferred drug. The praziquantel dosage is 50 mg/kg/d in three divided doses for 14 days. If appropriate services are available, blood levels should be monitored. Therapy may result in apparent cure, with clearance of symptoms, changes in cysts by cerebral tomograms (disappear-

ance, reduction in size, or calcification), and clearing of abnormal cerebrospinal fluid findings. In other patients, there may be remarkable improvement, including reduction in cerebral hypertension and amelioration of seizures. Still other patients, however, show no change or continued progression of the disease.

F. H nana: Praziquantel is the drug of choice for *H nana* infections and the first drug to be highly effective. A single dose of 25 mg/kg is used. Re-treatment may be required.

G. Other Parasites: Limited trials at a dosage of 25 mg/kg 3 times a day for 1–2 days indicate a high order of effectiveness of praziquantel against **fasciolopsiasis, metagonimiasis,** and other forms of **heterophyiasis.** In **fascioliasis,** however, praziquantel had only a low effectiveness at dosages as high as 25 mg/kg 3 times daily for 3–7 days. In **hydatid disease,** praziquantel adversely affects protoscoleces of *Echinococcus granulosus* in vitro, though it does not affect the germinal membrane in vivo. The drug is being evaluated as an adjunct during surgery to protect against cyst spillage.

Adverse Reactions

Mild and transient adverse effects directly attributable to the drug are common. They begin within several hours after ingestion and may persist for hours to 1 day. Most frequent are headache, dizziness, drowsiness, and lassitude; others include nausea, vomiting, abdominal pain, loose stools, pruritus, urticaria, arthralgia, myalgia, and low-grade fever. Minimal elevations of liver enzymes have occasionally been reported. Low-grade fever, pruritus, and skin rashes (macular and urticarial), sometimes associated with augmented eosinophilia, may also appear several days after starting the medication and are more likely to be due to the release of foreign proteins from dying worms than to a direct action of the drug.

Praziquantel appears to be better tolerated in children than in adults. Adverse effects may be more frequent in heavily infected patients, especially in *S mansoni* infections. The intensity and frequency of adverse effects also increase with dosage: They are mild and infrequent at dosages of 10 mg/kg given once but occur in up to 50% of patients who receive 25 mg/kg 3 times in 1 day.

Two types of adverse reactions in treatment of neurocysticercosis are (1) those characteristic of praziquantel usage at high dosage (described above) and (2) new neurologic reactions or exacerbations of existing ones due to inflammatory reactions around dying parasites. Common findings in up to 90% of patients who do not receive corticosteroids are headache, meningismus, nausea, vomiting, mental changes, and seizures (often accompanied by increased cerebrospinal fluid pleocytosis). These occur during or shortly after completion of therapy, last 48–72 hours, and usually are sufficiently mild that they can be ameliorated with analgesics, antiemetics, diuretics, or anticonvulsants. However, arachnoiditis, hyperthermia, and intracranial hypertension may also occur. Many workers give dexamethasone concurrently to decrease the inflammatory reaction; this is controversial, especially with the recent recognition that steroids reduce the plasma level of praziquantel. It is not established, however, that the steroidal reduction in plasma levels also reduces the effectiveness of praziquantel.

Drug interactions

In the treatment of cysticercosis, concomitant use of dexamethasone reduces plasma levels of praziquantel about 50%; the bioavailability of praziquantel is also reduced by phenytoin and carbamazepine and is increased by cimetidine. A digitalis-antagonistic effect has been seen in animal studies.

Contraindications & Cautions

The only specific contraindication is ocular cysticercosis; parasite destruction in the eye may cause irreparable damage. Some workers also caution against use of the drug in spinal neurocysticercosis. In cysticercosis-endemic areas, patients treated with praziquantel for conditions other than cysticercosis should be observed carefully in hospital for about 48 hours after completion of treatment. The drug can be used in the presence of liver impairment, but a reduction in dose may be necessary. Although safety of the drug in children under age 4 years is not established, no pediatric-specific problems have been documented.

Because the drug induces dizziness and drowsiness, patients should not drive and should be warned if their work requires physical coordination or alertness.

The drug should preferably not be taken during pregnancy; an increase in abortion rate was found in rats treated with three times the human dose. In lactating women, although praziquantel appears in milk at about one-fourth of the plasma levels, the drug may be given to the mother provided the infant is not nursed on the day of treatment and for 3 subsequent days.

Patients should be cautioned against chewing the bitter-tasting drug; the retching that results can become a special problem in treatment of *T solium* infection because regurgitation of segments might result, which could be hazardous.

PYRANTEL PAMOATE

Pyrantel pamoate is a broad-spectrum anthelmintic highly effective for the treatment of pinworm, *Ascaris,* and *Trichostrongylus orientalis* infections. It is moderately effective against both species of hookworm but less so against *N americanus*. It is not ef-

fective in trichuriasis or strongyloidiasis. Oxantel pamoate, an analogue of pyrantel, has been used successfully in the treatment of trichuriasis.

Chemistry & Pharmacokinetics

Pyrantel pamoate is a tetrahydropyrimidine derivative. Because it is poorly absorbed from the gastrointestinal tract, it is active mainly against luminal organisms. Peak plasma levels of 50–130 ng/mL are reached in 1–3 hours. Over half the administered dose is recovered unchanged in the feces; about 7% is excreted in the urine as unchanged drug and metabolites.

Anthelmintic Actions & Pharmacologic Effects

Pyrantel is effective against mature and immature forms of susceptible helminths within the intestinal tract but not against migratory stages in the tissues. The drug is a depolarizing neuromuscular blocking agent that causes release of acetylcholine, inhibits cholinesterase, and stimulates ganglionic receptors. Although pyrantel is not vermicidal (or ovicidal), the paralyzed worm is expelled from the host's intestinal tract.

Clinical Uses

The standard dose is 11 mg (base)/kg (maximum, 1 g), given with or without food.

A. Enterobius vermicularis: Pyrantel is given as a single dose and repeated in 2 and 4 weeks. Cure rates are greater than 95%.

B. A lumbricoides: Pyrantel is given as a single dose. Cure rates are 85–100%. Treatment should be repeated if eggs are still found 2 weeks later.

C. Hookworm and T orientalis: A single dose produces cures in over 90% of *Ancylostoma duodenale* and *T orientalis* infections and a marked reduction in the worm burden in the remainder. However, for *N americanus* infections, the cure rate depends on the intensity of infection. A single dose may give a satisfactory cure rate in light infections, but for moderate or heavy infections (> 2000 ova per gram of feces), a 3-day course is necessary to reach 90% cure rates. Hookworm burdens should be markedly reduced, but it is not always possible or essential to eradicate the infection. If iron deficiency accompanies the infection, it should be treated with iron medication and a high-protein diet. A course of treatment can be repeated in 2 weeks.

Adverse Reactions; Contraindications & Cautions

Adverse effects, which occur in 4–20% of patients, are infrequent, mild, and transient. They include nausea, vomiting, diarrhea, abdominal cramps, dizziness, drowsiness, headache, insomnia, rash, fever, and weakness. No important effects on hematologic, renal, or hepatic function have been recorded.

There are no contraindications to pyrantel, but it should be used with caution in patients with liver dysfunction, since low, transient transaminase elevations have been noted in a small number of patients. Experience with the drug in children under age 2 years is limited. Although teratogenic studies in animals have been negative, adequate studies in pregnant women have not been done.

QUINACRINE HYDROCHLORIDE

Quinacrine was formerly an alternative drug for the treatment of tapeworm infections. Because of its toxicity, it should no longer be used unless niclosamide or alternative drugs (praziquantel, mebendazole, or dichlorophen) are not available.

SURAMIN

Suramin is an alternative drug for the eradication of adult parasites of *Onchocerca volvulus* and the drug of choice in the treatment of the hemolymphatic stage of African trypanosomiasis due to *Trypanosoma brucei gambiense* and *Trypanosoma brucei rhodesiense* The drug is being evaluated as an anticancer agent, including prostate and breast cancer.

Suramin is a nonspecific inhibitor of many enzymes. Toxic reactions are frequent and sometimes severe, including nausea, vomiting, urticaria, fever, nephrotoxicity, peripheral neuritis, anemia, jaundice, and exfoliative dermatitis. Some deaths have occurred. The drug should be given only under expert guidance.

TETRACHLOROETHYLENE

Tetrachloroethylene was introduced in 1925 for the treatment of hookworm infections due to *Necator americanus* or *Ancylostoma duodenale*. Other drugs with fewer adverse effects are now preferred, but tetrachloroethylene remains an effective, inexpensive alternative drug, with mild adverse reactions. It is not available in the USA.

THIABENDAZOLE

Thiabendazole is the drug of choice for the treatment of strongyloidiasis and an alternative drug for cutaneous larva migrans. It may also be tried in trichinosis and visceral larva migrans, given the absence of other effective drugs. It is no longer recommended for the treatment of pinworm, ascarid, trichurid, or hookworm infection unless the safer drugs of choice are not available.

Chemistry

Thiabendazole is a benzimidazole compound. It is tasteless and nearly insoluble in water. Although it is a chelating agent that forms stable complexes with a number of metals, including iron, it does not bind calcium.

Pharmacokinetics

Thiabendazole is rapidly absorbed after ingestion. With a standard dose, drug concentrations in plasma peak within 1–2 hours (5 µg/mL) and are barely detectable after 8 hours; the half-life is 1.2 hours. The drug is almost completely metabolized in the liver to the 5-hydroxy form, which appears in the urine largely as the glucuronide or sulfonate conjugate. Ninety percent of the drug is excreted in the urine. Thiabendazole can also be absorbed from the skin. In some clinical situations, it may be useful to monitor serum drug concentrations.

Anthelmintic Actions & Pharmacologic Effects

Thiabendazole has anti-inflammatory properties, which may be an important factor in its ability to relieve symptoms in some parasitic diseases, particularly dracontiasis. It also has immunomodulating effects on T cell function—it appears to be an immunorestorative agent, demonstrating maximum immunopotentiation in the immunosuppressed host. Thiabendazole also has antipyretic and mild antifungal and scabicidal actions. The drug appears to be free of carcinogenic and mutagenic effects. Most studies for teratogenicity were negative, but one study that used high doses in rats and mice was positive.

Thiabendazole's vermicidal action may be a result of interference with microtubule aggregation (see Chapter 53) acting through inhibition of the enzyme fumarate reductase. The drug has ovicidal effects for some parasites.

Clinical Uses

The standard dose is 25 mg/kg (maximum, 1.5 g). The drug should be given after meals, and the tablet formulation should be chewed well. Pre- and posttreatment purges are not necessary.

A. Strongyloides stercoralis: The standard dose is given twice daily for 2 days. Cure rates are 93%. A course can be repeated in 1 week if indicated. In patients with hyperinfection syndrome, the standard dose is continued twice daily for 5–7 days.

B. Cutaneous Larva Migrans (Creeping Eruption): Thiabendazole is highly effective in the treatment of cutaneous larva migrans. The standard dose is given twice daily for 2 days. If active lesions are still present 2 days after completion of therapy, a second course should be given. Excellent results have also followed daily application, for 5 days, of a cream containing 15% thiabendazole in a hygroscopic base or of a 2% solution in dimethyl sulfoxide.

C. Other Infections: For the treatment of **trichinosis,** the standard dosage is given twice daily for 2–4 days; for **visceral larva migrans,** twice daily for up to 7 days, depending upon the response of the patient. Information on the effectiveness of the drug for both conditions is limited. During the first 24 hours after ingestion of trichinous pork, the drug may have an effect on adult worms, resulting in a decrease of larvae released. During the invasive stage, thiabendazole provides some symptomatic relief, and biopsy evidence suggests that the drug destroys some (though not all) larvae in muscle. Corticosteroids and ACTH are effective in reducing inflammatory reactions to the larvae and may be lifesaving in severe infections.

Intestinal capillariasis has been successfully treated with thiabendazole at a dosage of 12 mg/kg given twice daily for 30 days.

For the treatment of **dracontiasis,** the drug is often effective at a dosage of 50–75 mg/kg/d in two divided doses for 1–3 days. Local inflammation subsides rapidly, and many worms are then spontaneously extruded or can be extracted manually. Re-treatment is occasionally needed.

Several reports have indicated the usefulness of topical thiabendazole for the treatment of **scabies** and **tinea nigra palmaris.**

Adverse Reactions

At the standard dosage of 25 mg/kg twice daily for 2 days, adverse effects occur in 7–50% of patients, generally 3–4 hours after ingestion of the drug, and last 2–8 hours. Higher doses or treatment beyond 2 days increases the frequency and intensity of symptoms. Although toleration may occasionally be improved by reducing the dosage to 25 mg/kg once daily, effectiveness is likely to decrease.

Adverse effects are generally mild and transient but can be severe; the most common are dizziness, anorexia, nausea, and vomiting. Less frequent are epigastric pain, abdominal cramps, diarrhea, pruritus, headache, drowsiness, giddiness, and other neuropsychiatric symptoms. Rarely reported are perianal rashes, tinnitus, paresthesias, bradycardia, hypotension, hyperglycemia, convulsions, transient leukopenia, hematuria, crystalluria, visual disturbances, intrahepatic cholestasis, and parenchymal liver damage; jaundice and liver function abnormalities may result. In some patients, a medically insignificant asparagine odor is imparted to the urine.

Rare hypersensitivity reactions include fever, chills, skin rashes, pruritus, conjunctival edema, angioedema, lymphadenopathy, toxic epidermal necrolysis, anaphylaxis, and erythema multiforme. Fatal Stevens-Johnson syndrome has occurred in children.

Contraindications & Cautions

Experience with thiabendazole is limited in children weighing less than 15 kg. The drug should not be used in pregnancy, except for life-threatening strongyloidiasis. It may be best to use alternative drugs in patients with hepatic or renal dysfunction. The drug should be used with caution where drug-induced vomiting may be dangerous or in patients with severe malnutrition or anemia. There are a few reports of ascarids becoming hypermotile after treatment and appearing at the nose or mouth.

Since the drug makes some patients dizzy or drowsy, it should not be used during the day for patients whose work or activity requires mental alertness.

Thiabendazole may compete with theophylline for sites of metabolism in the liver. Discontinue the drug immediately if hypersensitivity symptoms appear.

PREPARATIONS AVAILABLE

Albendazole (Zental)
Oral: 200 mg tablets; 100 mg/5 mL suspension
Note: Albendazole is not approved in the USA but can be obtained from the manufacturer (SmithKline Beecham, 800-366-8900) for compassionate use.

Bithionol (Bitin)
Oral: 200 mg tablets
Note: Bithionol is not marketed in the USA but can be obtained from the Parasitic Disease Drug Service, Centers for Disease Control and Prevention, Atlanta, Georgia; 404-639-3670.

Diethylcarbamazine (Hetrazan)
Oral: 50, 200, 400 mg tablets
Note: Diethylcarbamazine is no longer marketed in the USA but is available upon request from Lederle Laboratories; 914-732-5000.

Ivermectin (Mectizan)
Oral: 6 mg tablets
Note: Ivermectin is not commercially available but will be provided on a compassionate basis by the manufacturer, Merck Sharp and Dohme 215-397-2454.

Levamisole (Decaris, Ethnor, Ketrax, Solaskil)
Oral: 50, 150 mg tablets and syrup.

Mebendazole (Vermox)
Oral: 100 mg chewable tablets; outside the USA, 100 mg/5 mL suspension

Metrifonate (Bilarcil)
Oral: 100 mg tablets
Note: Metrifonate is not available in the USA.

Niclosamide (Niclocide)
Oral: 500 mg chewable tablets
Oxamniquine (Vansil, Mansil)
Oral: 250 mg capsules; outside the USA, 50 mg/mL syrup
Oxantel pamoate (Quantrel); **oxantel/pyrantel pamoate** (Telopar)
Oral: tablets containing 100 mg (base) of each drug; suspensions containing 20 or 50 mg (base) per mL
Note: Oxantel pamoate and oxantel/pyrantel pamoate are not available in the USA.
Piperazine (generic, Vermizine)
Oral: piperazine citrate tablets equivalent to 250 mg of the hexahydrate; piperazine citrate syrup equivalent to 500 mg of the hexahydrate per 5 mL
Praziquantel (Biltricide; others outside the USA)

Oral: 600 mg tablets (other strengths outside the USA)
Pyrantel pamoate (Antiminth, Combantrin)
Oral: 50 mg (base)/mL suspension; 125 mg tablets are available in Canada and some other countries but not in the USA.
Suramin (Bayer 205, others)
Parenteral: ampules containing 0.5 or 1 g powder to be reconstituted as a 10% solution and used immediately
Note: Suramin is not marketed in the USA but can be obtained from the Parasitic Disease Drug Service, Centers for Disease Control, Atlanta, GA, 404-639-3670.
Thiabendazole (Mintezol)
Oral: 500 mg chewable tablets; suspension, 500 mg/mL.

REFERENCES

General References

Cook GC: Anthelmintic agents: Some recent developments and their clinical application. Postgrad Med J 1991;67:16.

Drugs for parasitic infections. Med Lett Drugs Ther 1993;35:111.

Edwards E, Breckenridge AM: Clinical pharmacokinetics of anthelmintic drugs. Clin Pharmacokinet 1988;15:67.

Goldsmith R, Heyneman D (editors): *Tropical Medicine & Parasitology.* Appleton & Lange, 1989.

MacLeod C: *Parasitic Infections in Pregnancy and the Newborn.* Oxford Medical Publications, 1988.

Singh SK, Sharma S: Current status of medicinal research in helminth diseases. Med Res Rev 1991;11:581.

WHO: *WHO Model Prescribing Drugs: Drugs Used in Parasitic Diseases.* WHO, 1990.

Albendazole

Blanshard C et al: Treatment of intestinal microsporidiosis with albendazole in patients with AIDS. AIDS 1992;6:3.

Chanthavanich P et al: Repeated doses of albendazole against strongyloidiasis in Thai children. Southeast Asian J Trop Med Public Health 1989;20:221.

Firth M (editor): Symposium on albendazole in helminthiasis. *Royal Society of Medicine International Congress and Symposium Series,* No. 57. The Royal Society of Medicine, Academic Press, and Grune & Stratton, 1983.

Horton RJ: Chemotherapy of *Echinococcus* infection in man with albendazole. Trans R Soc Trop Med Hyg 1989;83:97.

Jung H et al: Dexamethasone increases plasma levels of albendazole. J Neurol 1990;237:279.

Kraivichian P et al: Albendazole in the treatment of human gnathostomiasis. Trans R Soc Trop Med Hyg 1992;86:418

Rossignol JF, Maisonneuve H: Albendazole: Placebo-controlled study in 870 patients with intestinal helminthiasis. Trans R Soc Trop Med Hyg 1983;77:707.

Sanguigini S et al: Albendazole in the therapy of cutaneous larva migrans. Trans R Soc Trop Med Hyg 1990;84:831.

Sotelo J et al: Comparison of therapeutic regimen of anticysticercal drugs for parenchymal brain cysticercosis. J Neurol 1990;237:69.

Sturchler D et al: Thiabendazole vs. albendazole in treatment against toxocariasis: A clinical trial. Ann Trop Med Parasitol 1989;83:473.

Takayanagui OM, Jardim E: Therapy for neurocysticercosis: Comparison between albendazole and praziquantel. Arch Neurol 1992;49:290.

Todorov T et al: Chemotherapy of human cystic echinococcosis: Comparative efficacy of mebendazole and albendazole. Ann Trop Med Parasitol 1992;86:59.

Bithionol

Bassiouny HK et al: Human fascioliasis in Egypt: Effect of infection and efficacy of bithionol treatment. J Trop Med Hyg 1991;94:333.

Coleman DL, Barry M: Relapse of *Paragonimus westermani* lung infection after bithionol therapy. Am J Trop Med Hyg 1982;31:71.

Diethylcarbamazine

Carme B et al: Five cases of encephalitis during treatment of loiasis with diethylcarbamazine. Am J Trop Med Hyg 1991;44:684.

Eberhard ML et al: Evidence of nonsusceptibility to diethylcarbamazine in *Wuchereria bancrofti.* J Infect Dis 1991;163:1157.

Mackenzie CD, Kron MA: Diethylcarbamazine: A review of its action in onchocerciasis, lymphatic filariasis and inflammation. Trop Dis Bull 1985;82:R1.

Ottesen EA: Efficacy of diethylcarbamazine in eradicating infection with lymphatic-dwelling filariae in humans. Rev Infect Dis 1985;7:341.

Vijayan VK et al: Tropical eosinophilia: clinical and physiological response to diethylcarbamazine. Respir Med 1991;85:17.

Ivermectin

Campbell WC: Ivermectin as an antiparasitic agent for use in humans. Annu Rev Microbiol 1991;45:445.

Chippaux JP et al: Ivermectin treatment of loiasis. Trans R Soc Trop Med Hyg 1992;86:289.

Duke BOL et al: Effects of three-month doses of ivermectin on adult *Onchocerca volvulus*. Am J Trop Med Hyg 1992;46:189.

Goa KL, McTavish D, Clissold SP: Ivermectin. A review of its antifilarial activity, pharmacokinetic properties and clinical efficacy in onchocerciasis. Drugs 1991;42:640.

Sabry M et al: A placebo-controlled double-blind trial for the treatment of Bancroftian filariasis with ivermectin or diethylcarbamazine. Trans R Soc Trop Med Hyg 1991;85:640.

Whitworth J: Treatment of onchocerciasis with ivermectin in Sierra Leone. Parasitol Today 1992;8:138.

Wijesundera MS, Sanmuganathan PS: Ivermectin therapy in chronic strongyloidiasis. Trans R Soc Trop Med Hyg 1992;86:291.

Mebendazole

Bartoloni C et al: The efficacy of chemotherapy with mebendazole in human cystic echinococcosis: Long-term follow-up of 52 patients. Ann Trop Med Parasitol 1992;86:249.

Chippaux JP: Mebendazole treatment of dracunculiasis. Trans Roy Soc Trop Med Hyg 1991;85:280.

Sebastian VJ, Bhattacharya S, Ray S: Mebendazole retention enema for severe *Trichuris trichiura* (whipworm) infection: A CAE report. J Trop Med Hyg 1989;92:39.

Shikiya K et al: Treatment of strongyloidiasis with mebendazole: Long term eradication and new trials. J Japan Assoc Infect Dis 1991;65:433.

Todorov T et al: Chemotherapy of human cystic echinococcosis: Comparative efficacy of mebendazole and albendazole. Ann Trop Med Parasitol 1992;86:59.

Metrifonate

Abdi Y, Gustafsson LL: Field trial of the efficacy of a simplified and standard metrifonate treatment of *Schistosoma haematobium*. Eur J Clin Pharmacol 1989;37:371.

Aden-Abdi Y et al: Metrifonate in healthy volunteers: Interrelationship between pharmacokinetic properties, cholinesterase inhibition and side- effects. Bull World Health Organ 1990;68:731.

Nhachi CFB et al: Effect of single oral dose of metrifonate on human plasma cholinesterase levels. Bull Environ Contam Toxicol 1991;47:641.

Niclosamide

Jones WE: Niclosamide as a treatment for *Hymenolepis*

diminuta and *Dipylidium caninum* infection in man. Am J Trop Med Hyg 1979;28:300.

Pearson RD, Hewlett EL: Niclosamide therapy for tapeworm infections. Ann Intern Med 1985;102:550.

Oxamniquine

Coles GC et al: Tolerance of Kenyan *Schistosoma mansoni* to oxamniquine. Trans R Soc Trop Med Hyg 1987;81:782.

El-Masry NA et al: Oxamniquine treatment for schistosomal polyposis: A 1–2 year follow-up study. J Trop Med Hyg 1986;89:19.

Foster R: A review of clinical experience with oxamniquine. Trans R Soc Trop Med Hyg 1987;81:55.

Sleigh AC et al: Manson's schistosomiasis in Brazil: 11-year evaluation of successful disease control with oxamniquine. Lancet 1986:1:635.

Piperazine

Bellander BTD, Hagmar LE, Osterdahl BG: Nitrosation of piperazine in the stomach. Lancet 1981;2:372.

Fletcher KA et al: Urinary piperazine excretion in healthy Caucasians. Ann Trop Med Parasitol 1982; 76:77.

Ukadgaonkar NG, Bjagwat RB, Kulkarni MU: Transient cerebellar syndrome due to piperazine citrate. Clinician 1982;46:461.

Praziquantel

Bittencourt PRM et al: Phenytoin and carbamazepine decrease oral bioavailability of praziquantel. Neurology 1992;42:492

Doehring E et al: Ultrasonographical investigation of periportal fibrosis in children with *Schistosoma mansoni* infection: Reversibility of morbidity twenty-three months after treatment with praziquantel. Am J Trop Med Hyg 1992;46:409.

Farid Z, Kamal M, Mansour N: Praziquantel and *Fasciola hepatica* infection. Trans R Soc Trop Med Hyg 1989:83.

King CH, Mahmoud AAF: Drugs five years later: Praziquantel. Ann Intern Med 1989;110:290.

Ohmae H et al: Improvement of ultrasonographic and serologic changes in *Schistosoma japonicum*-infected patients after treatment with praziquantel. Am J Trop Med Hyg 1992;46:99.

Pawlowski ZS: Efficacy of low doses of praziquantel in taeniasis. Acta Tropica 1991;48:83.

Takayanagui OM, Jardim E: Therapy for neurocysticercosis: Comparison between albendazole and praziquantel. Arch Neurol 1992;49:290.

Vanijanonta S et al: The treatment of neurocysticercosis with praziquantel. Southeast Asian J Trop Med Public Health 1991;22(Suppl):275.

Pyrantel Pamoate

Davis A: *Drug Treatment in Intestinal Helminthiases.* World Health Organization, 1973.

Kale OO: Controlled comparative study of the efficacy of pyrantel pamoate and a combined regimen of piperazine citrate and bephenium hydroxynaphthoate in the treatment of intestinal nemathelminthiasis. Afr J Med Sci 1981;10:63.

Sinniah B, Sinniah D: The anthelmintic effects of pyrantel pamoate, oxantel-pyrantel pamoate, levamisole and mebendazole in the treatment of intestinal nematodes. Ann Trop Med Parasitol 1981;75:315.

Suramin

Duke BO: Suramin and the time it takes to kill *Onchocerca volvulus*. Trop Med Parasitol 1991;42:346.

Thiabendazole

Grove DI: Treatment of strongyloidiasis with thiabendazole: An analysis of toxicity and effectiveness. Trans R Soc Trop Med Hyg 1982;76:114.

Kale OO, Elemile T, Enahoro F: Controlled comparative trial of thiabendazole in the treatment of dracontiasis. Ann Trop Med Parasitol 1983;77:151.

Lew G et al: Theophylline-thiabendazole drug interaction. Clin Pharm 1989;8:225.

Roy MA et al: Micronodular cirrhosis after thiabendazole. Dig Dis Sci 1989;34:938.

Winter PAD, Fripp PJ: Treatment of cutaneous larva migrans (sandworm disease). S Afr Med J 1978;54:556.

Cancer Chemotherapy

56

Sydney E. Salmon, MD, & Alan C. Sartorelli, PhD

The incidence, geographic distribution, and behavior of specific types of cancer are related to multiple factors including sex, age, race, genetic predisposition, and exposure to environmental carcinogens. Of these factors, the last is probably most important. Chemical carcinogens (particularly those in tobacco smoke) as well as agents such as azo dyes, aflatoxins, and benzene have been clearly implicated in cancer induction in humans and animals. Identification of potential carcinogens in the environment has been greatly simplified by the widespread use of the "Ames test" for mutagenic agents. Ninety percent of carcinogens can be shown to be mutagenic on the basis of this assay. Ultimate identification of potential human carcinogens requires, however, testing in at least two animal species.

Certain herpes and papilloma group DNA viruses and type C RNA viruses have also been implicated as causative agents in animal cancers and might be responsible for some human cancers as well. Oncogenic RNA viruses all appear to contain a "reverse transcriptase" enzyme that permits translation of the RNA message of the tumor virus into the DNA code of the infected cell. Thus, the information governing transformation can become a stable part of the genome of the host cell. Expression of virus-induced neoplasia probably also depends on additional host and environmental factors that modulate the transformation process. A specific human T cell leukemia virus (HTLV-I) has been identified as causative of this specific type of leukemia. The virus (HIV-1) that causes AIDS is closely related. Cellular genes are known that are homologous to the transforming genes of the retroviruses, a family of RNA viruses, and induce oncogenic transformation. These mammalian cellular genes, known as **oncogenes,** have been shown to code for specific growth factors and their receptors and may be amplified (increased number of gene copies) or modified by a single nucleotide in malignant cells.

Another class of genes, **tumor suppressor genes,** may be deleted or damaged, with resulting neoplastic change. A single gene in this class, the p53 gene, has been shown to have mutated from a tumor suppressor gene to an oncogene in a high percentage of cases of several human tumors, including liver, breast, colon, lung, cervix, bladder, prostate, and skin. The normal "wild" form of this gene appears to play an important role in suppressing neoplastic transformation; mutation places the cell at high risk of transformation (Harris, 1993).

CANCER AS A DISEASE OF CELLS

Whatever the cause, cancer is basically a disease of cells characterized by a shift in the control mechanisms that govern cell proliferation and differentiation. Cells that have undergone neoplastic transformation usually express cell surface antigens that appear to be of normal fetal type and have other signs of apparent "immaturity" and may exhibit qualitative or quantitative chromosomal abnormalities, including various translocations and the appearance of amplified gene sequences. Such cells proliferate excessively and form local tumors that can compress or invade adjacent normal structures. A small subpopulation of cells within the tumor can be described as **tumor stem cells.** They retain the ability to undergo repeated cycles of proliferation as well as to migrate to distant sites in the body to colonize various organs in the process called **metastasis.** Such tumor stem cells thus can express **clonogenic** or colony-forming capability. Tumor stem cells often have chromosome abnormalities reflecting their genetic instability, which leads to progressive selection of subclones that can survive more readily in the multicellular environment of the host. Quantitative abnormalities in various metabolic pathways and cellular components accompany this neoplastic progression. The invasive and metastatic processes as well as a series of metabolic abnormalities resulting from the cancer cause illness and eventual death of the patient unless the neoplasm can be eradicated with treatment.

CANCER THERAPEUTIC MODALITIES

Next to heart disease, cancer is the major cause of death in the USA, causing over 500,000 fatalities annually. With present methods of treatment, one-third of patients are cured with local measures (surgery or radiation therapy), which are quite effective when the tumor has not metastasized by the time of treatment. Earlier diagnosis might lead to increased cure of patients with such local treatment; however, in the remaining cases, early micrometastasis is a characteristic feature of the neoplasm, indicating that a systemic approach such as can be attained with chemotherapy will be required (often along with surgery or radiation) for effective cancer management. At present, about 50% of patients with cancer can be cured, with chemotherapy contributing to cure in about 17% of patients.

Cancer chemotherapy as currently employed can be curative in certain disseminated neoplasms that have undergone either gross or microscopic spread by the time of diagnosis. These include testicular cancer, diffuse large cell lymphoma, Hodgkin's disease, and choriocarcinoma as well as childhood tumors such as acute lymphoblastic leukemia, Burkitt's lymphoma, Wilms' tumor, and embryonal rhabdomyosarcoma. Of major importance are recent demonstrations that use of chemotherapy along with initial surgery can increase the cure rate in relatively early-stage breast cancer and osteogenic sarcoma. Common carcinomas of the lung and colon are generally refractory to currently available treatment and have usually disseminated by the time of diagnosis.

At present, chemotherapy provides palliative rather than curative therapy for many other forms of disseminated cancer. Effective palliation results in temporary clearing of the symptoms and signs of cancer and prolongation of useful life. In the past decade, advances in cancer chemotherapy have also begun to provide evidence that chemical control of neoplasia may become a reality for many forms of cancer. This will probably be achieved first through combined therapy in which optimal combinations of surgery, radiotherapy, and chemotherapy are used to eradicate both the primary neoplasm and its occult micrometastases before gross spread can be detected on physical or x-ray examination. Use of endocrine agents to modulate tumor growth is playing an increasing role in hormone-responsive tumors thanks to the development of hormone antagonists and partial agonists. Several recombinant biologic agents have recently been identified as being active for cancer therapy. These include interferon and interleukin-2. Gene therapy is the latest investigational approach to cancer treatment and is now in the earliest stages of clinical investigation. It is too soon to make a judgment about whether it will be useful.

ANTICANCER DRUG DEVELOPMENT

A major effort to develop anticancer drugs through both empirical screening and rational design of new compounds has now been under way for 3 decades. Recent advances in this field have included the synthesis of peptides and proteins with recombinant DNA techniques and monoclonal antibodies. The drug development program has employed testing in a few well-characterized transplantable animal tumor systems. The development of a simple in vitro colony assay for measuring drug sensitivity of human tumor stem cells may augment and shorten the testing program in the future. After new drugs with potential anticancer activity are identified, they are subjected to preclinical toxicologic and limited pharmacologic studies in animals as described in Chapter 5. Promising agents that do not have excessive toxicity are then advanced to phase I clinical trials wherein their pharmacologic and toxic effects are tested in patients with advanced cancer rather than in healthy volunteers. The remainder of clinical testing is similar to that for other drugs but may be accelerated.

Ideal anticancer drugs would eradicate cancer cells without harming normal tissues. Unfortunately, no currently available agents meet this criterion and clinical use of these drugs involves a weighing of benefits against toxicity in a search for a favorable therapeutic index.

Classes of drugs that have recently entered development include inducers of differentiation, intended to force neoplastic cells past a maturation block to form end-stage cells with little or no proliferative potential; antimetastatic drugs, designed to perturb surface properties of malignant cells and thus alter their invasive and metastatic potential; hypoxic tumor stem cell-specific agents, designed to exploit the greater capacity for reductive reactions in these therapeutically resistant cells created by oxygen deficiency within solid tumors; tumor radiosensitizing and normal tissue radioprotecting drugs, aimed at increased therapeutic effectiveness of radiation therapy; and "biologic response modifiers," which alter tumor-host metabolic and immunologic relationships.

IMPORTANCE OF NEOPLASTIC CELL BURDEN

Patients with widespread cancer (eg, acute leukemia) may have 10^{12} tumor cells throughout the body at the time of diagnosis (Figure 56–1). If tolerable dosing of an effective drug is capable of killing 99.9% of clonogenic tumor cells, this would induce a clinical remission of the neoplasm associated with symptomatic improvement. However there would still be nine "logs" of tumor cells (10^9) remaining in the body, including some that may be inherently re-

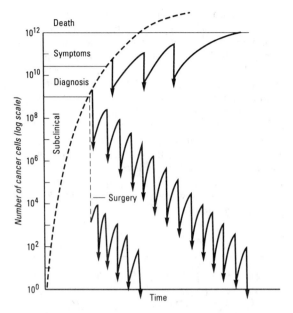

Figure 56–1. The "log-kill hypothesis." Relationship of tumor cell number to time of diagnosis, symptoms, treatment, and survival. Three alternative approaches to drug treatment are shown for comparison with the course of tumor growth when no treatment is given *(dashed line)*. In the protocol diagrammed at top, treatment (indicated by the arrows) is given infrequently and the result is manifested as prolongation of survival but with recurrence of symptoms between courses of treatment and eventual death of the patient. The combination chemotherapy treatment diagrammed in the middle section is begun earlier and is more intensive. Tumor cell kill exceeds regrowth, drug resistance does not develop, and "cure" results. In this example, treatment has been continued long after all clinical evidence of cancer has disappeared (1–3 years). This approach has been established as effective in the treatment of childhood acute leukemia, testicular cancers, and Hodgkin's disease. In the treatment diagrammed near the bottom of the graph, early surgery has been employed to remove the primary tumor and intensive adjuvant chemotherapy has been administered long enough (up to 1 year) to eradicate the remaining tumor cells that comprise the occult micrometastases.

sistant to the drug because of heterogeneity, and others that might reside in pharmacologic sanctuaries (eg, the central nervous system, testes) where effective drug concentrations may be difficult to achieve. When cell cycle-specific (CCS) drugs are used, the tumor stem cells must also be in the sensitive phase of the cell cycle (not in G_0), so scheduling of these agents is particularly important. In common bacterial infections, a three-log reduction in microorganisms might be curative because host resistance factors can eliminate residual bacteria through immunologic and

microbicidal mechanisms; however, host mechanisms for eliminating moderate numbers of cancer cells appear to be generally ineffective.

Combinations of agents with differing toxicities and mechanisms of action are often employed to overcome the limited "log kill" of individual anticancer drugs. If the drugs do not have too much overlap in toxicity, they can be used at almost full dosage and at least additive cytotoxic effects can be achieved with combination chemotherapy; furthermore, subclones resistant to only one of the agents can potentially be eradicated. Some combinations of anticancer drugs also appear to exert true synergism wherein the effect of the two drugs is greater than additive. The efficacy of combination chemotherapy has now been validated in many forms of human cancer, and the scientific rationale appears to be sound. As a result, combination chemotherapy is now the standard approach to curative treatment of testicular cancer and lymphomas and improved palliative treatment of many other tumor types. This important therapeutic approach was first formulated by Skipper and Schabel and described as the "log-kill hypothesis" (Figure 56–1).

IMPORTANCE OF CELL CYCLE KINETICS

Information on cell and population kinetics of cancer cells in part explains the limited effectiveness of most available anticancer drugs. A schematic summary of cell cycle kinetics is presented in Figure 56–2. This information is relevant to the mode of action, indications, and scheduling of cell cycle-specific (CCS) and cell cycle-nonspecific (CCNS) drugs. Agents falling in these two major classes are summarized in Table 56–1.

In general, CCS drugs have proved most effective in hematologic malignancies and other tumors in which a relatively large proportion of the cells are proliferating or are in the **growth fraction.** CCNS drugs (many of which bind to DNA and damage these macromolecules) are useful in low-growth-fraction "solid tumors" as well as in high-growth-fraction tumors. In all instances, effective agents sterilize or inactivate tumor stem cells, which are often only a small fraction of the cells within a tumor. Non-stem cells (eg, those that have irreversibly differentiated) are considered sterile by definition and are not a significant component of the cancer problem.

Resistance to Cytotoxic Drugs

A major problem in cancer chemotherapy is **drug resistance.** Some tumor types, eg, non-small cell lung cancer and colon cancer, exhibit *primary* resistance, ie, absence of response on the first exposure, to currently available standard agents. *Acquired resis-*

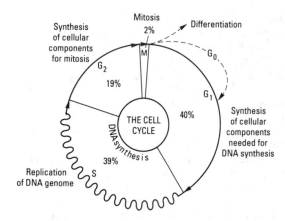

Figure 56–2. The cell cycle and cancer. A conceptual depiction of the cell cycle phases that all cells—normal and neoplastic—must traverse before and during cell division. The percentages given represent the approximate percentage of time spent in each phase by a typical malignant cell; the duration of G_1, however, can vary markedly. Many of the effective anticancer drugs exert their action on cells traversing the cell cycle and are called cell cycle-specific (CCS) drugs (Table 56–1). A second group of agents called cell cycle-nonspecific (CCNS) drugs can sterilize tumor cells whether they are cycling or resting in the G_0 compartment. CCNS drugs can kill both G_0 and cycling cells (although cycling cells are more sensitive).

tance develops in a number of drug-sensitive tumor types. Experimentally, drug resistance can be highly specific to a single drug and usually is based on a change in the tumor cells' genetic apparatus with *amplification* or increased expression of one or more specific genes. In other instances, a multidrug-resistant phenotype occurs—resistance to a variety of natural product anticancer drugs of differing structures developing after exposure to a single agent. This form of multidrug resistance is often associated with increased expression of a normal gene (the *MDR1* gene) for a cell surface glycoprotein (P-glycoprotein)

Table 56–1. Cell cycle relationships of major classes of drugs.

Cell Cycle-Specific (CCS) Agents	Cell Cycle-Nonspecific (CCNS) Agents
Antimetabolites (azacitidine, cytarabine, fluorouracil, mercaptopurine, methotrexate, thioguanine)	Alkylating agents (busulfan, cyclophosphamide, mechlorethamine, melphalan, thiotepa)
Bleomycin peptide antibiotics	Antibiotics (dactinomycin, daunorubicin, doxorubicin, plicamycin, mitomycin)
Podophyllin alkaloids (etoposide, VP-16; teniposide, VM-26)	
Plant alkaloids (vincristine, vinblastine, paclitaxel)	Cisplatin
	Nitrosoureas (BCNU, CCNU, methyl-CCNU)

involved in drug efflux. This transport molecule (Figure 56–3) uses the energy of ATP to expel a variety of foreign molecules (not limited to antitumor drugs) from the cell. It occurs constitutively in normal tissues such as epithelial cells of the kidney, large intestine, and adrenal gland as well as in a variety of tumors. Multidrug resistance can be reversed experimentally by calcium channel blockers, such as verapamil, and a variety of other drugs, which inhibit the transporter. Preliminary clinical results suggest that reversal of resistance by these drugs may be possible in patients. A second mechanism of multiple drug resistance involves qualitative or quantitative changes in topoisomerase II, which repairs the lesions created in DNA by antitumor drugs.

I. BASIC PHARMACOLOGY OF CANCER CHEMOTHERAPEUTIC DRUGS

POLYFUNCTIONAL ALKYLATING AGENTS

The major clinically useful alkylating agents (Figure 56–4) have a structure containing a bis(chloroethyl)amine, ethylenimine, or nitrosourea moiety. Among the bis(chloroethyl)amines, cyclophosphamide, mechlorethamine, melphalan, and chlorambucil are the most useful. Ifosfamide is closely related to cyclophosphamide but has a somewhat different spectrum of activity and toxicity. Thiotepa and busulfan are used for specialized purposes for ovarian cancer and chronic myeloid leukemia, respectively. The major nitrosoureas are BCNU (carmustine), CCNU (lomustine), and methyl-CCNU (semustine). A variety of investigational alkylating agents have been synthesized that link various carrier molecules such as amino acids, nucleic acid bases, hormones, or sugar moieties to a group capable of alkylation; however, successful "site-directed" alkylation has not to date been achieved.

As a class, the alkylating agents act by exerting cytotoxic effects via transfer of their alkyl groups to various cellular constituents. Alkylations of DNA within the nucleus probably represent the major interactions that lead to cell death. However, these drugs react chemically with sulfhydryl, amino, hydroxyl, carboxyl, and phosphate groups of other cellular nucleophiles as well. The general mechanism of action of these drugs involves intramolecular cyclization to form an **ethyleneimonium ion** that may directly or

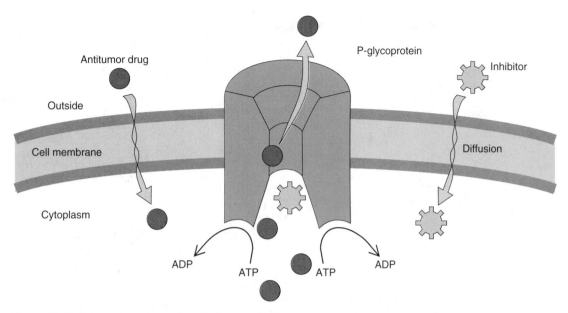

Figure 56–3. Schematic concept of the P-glycoprotein drug transport molecule responsible for multidrug resistance in cancer cells. ATP is used to drive the efflux process. The protein consists of 12 transmembrane domains with two ATP binding sites, only one of which must be occupied for drug transport to occur. Verapamil, quinidine, cyclosporine, and certain other drugs are able to inhibit transport at concentrations as low as 3 μmol/L, probably by acting as competitive substrates.

through formation of a **carbonium ion** transfer an alkyl group to a cellular constituent. In addition to alkylation, a secondary mechanism that occurs with nitrosoureas involves carbamoylation of lysine residues of proteins through formation of isocyanates.

The major site of alkylation within DNA is the N7 position of guanine (Figure 56–5); however, other bases are also alkylated to lesser degrees, including N1 and N3 of adenine, N3 of cytosine, and O6 of guanine, as well as phosphate atoms and proteins associated with DNA. These interactions can occur on a single strand or both strands of DNA through cross-linking, as most major alkylating agents are bifunctional, with two reactive groups. Alkylation of guanine can result in miscoding through abnormal base pairing with thymine or in depurination by excision of guanine residues. The latter effect leads to DNA strand breakage through scission of the sugar-phosphate backbone of DNA. Cross-linking of DNA appears to be of major importance to the cytotoxic action of alkylating agents, and replicating cells are most susceptible to these drugs. Thus, although alkylating agents are not cell cycle-specific, cells are most susceptible to alkylation in late G_1 and S phases of the cell cycle and express block in G_2.

Drug Resistance

The mechanism of acquired resistance to alkylating agents may involve increased capability to repair DNA lesions, decreased permeability of the cell to the alkylating drug, and increased production of glutathione, which inactivates the alkylating agent through conjugation in a reaction catalyzed by glutathione S-transferase.

Pharmacologic Effects

Active alkylating agents have direct vesicant effects and can damage tissues at the site of injection as well as produce systemic toxicity. Toxicities are generally dose-related and occur particularly in rapidly growing tissues such as bone marrow, gastrointestinal tract, and gonads. After intravenous injection, nausea and vomiting usually occur within 30–60 minutes with mechlorethamine, cyclophosphamide, or BCNU. The emetic effects are of central nervous system origin and can be reduced by pretreatment with phenothiazines or cannabinoids (tetrahydrocannabinol, nabilone). Subcutaneous injection of mechlorethamine or BCNU leads to tissue necrosis and sloughing. Cyclophosphamide does not have direct vesicant effects and must be activated to cytotoxic forms by microsomal enzymes (Figure 56–6).

The liver microsomal cytochrome P450 mixed-function oxidase system converts cyclophosphamide to 4-hydroxycyclophosphamide, which is in equilibrium with aldophosphamide. These active metabolites are believed to be carried by the bloodstream to tumor and normal tissue, where nonenzymatic cleavage of aldophosphamide to the cytotoxic forms—phosphoramide mustard and acrolein—occurs. The

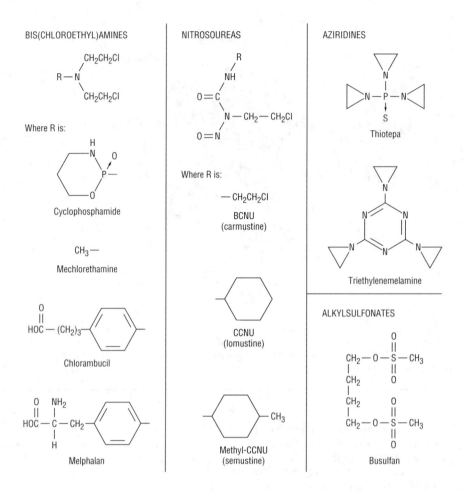

BIS(CHLOROETHYL)AMINES
R—N(CH2CH2Cl)2
Where R is:
Cyclophosphamide
CH3—
Mechlorethamine
Chlorambucil
Melphalan
NITROSOUREAS
Where R is:
—CH2CH2Cl
BCNU
(carmustine)
CCNU
(lomustine)
Methyl-CCNU
(semustine)
AZIRIDINES
Thiotepa
Triethylenemelamine
ALKYLSULFONATES
Busulfan

Figure 56–4. Structures of major classes of alkylating agents.

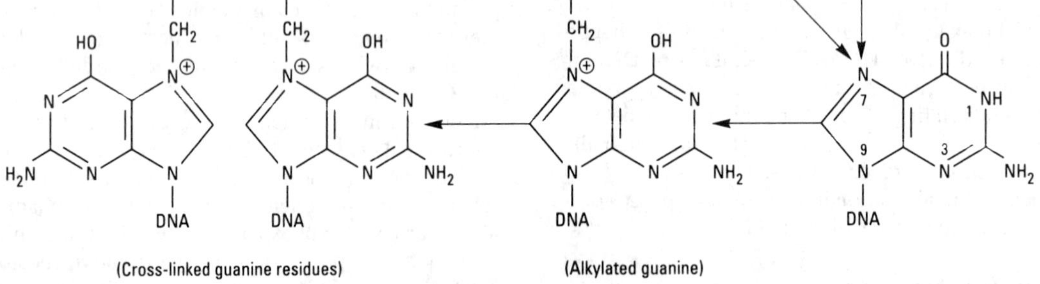

Cl⁻
DNA
(Cross-linked guanine residues)
(Alkylated guanine)

Figure 56–5. Mechanism of alkylation of DNA guanine. A bis(chloroethyl)amine forms an ethyleneimonium ion and a carbonium ion that react with a base such as N7 of guanine in DNA, producing an alkylated purine. Alkylation of a second guanine residue, through the illustrated mechanism, results in cross-linking of DNA strands.

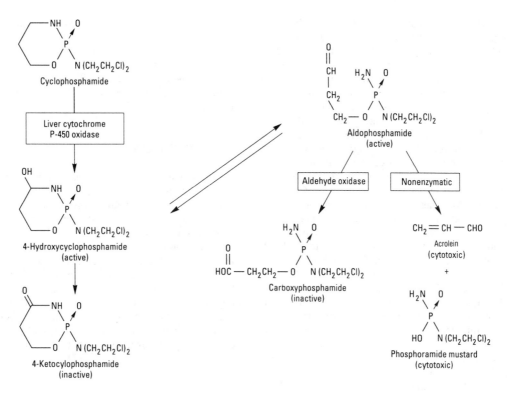

Figure 56–6. Cyclophosphamide metabolism.

liver appears to be protected through the enzymatic formation of the inactive metabolites 4-ketocyclophosphamide and carboxyphosphamide. The major toxicity of alkylating agents is on the bone marrow and results in dose-related suppression of myelopoiesis. The white blood count and absolute granulocyte count reach their low point 10–12 days after injection of mechlorethamine or cyclophosphamide, with subsequent recovery within 21 (cyclophosphamide) to 42 (mechlorethamine) days. The white count nadir with nitrosoureas is delayed to 28 days, with recovery by 42 days. Effects on megakaryocytes and platelets parallel those on granulocytes. Because of the long life span of the erythrocyte, effects on erythropoiesis are minor and the red cell count is usually only mildly reduced. Adverse effects on the bone marrow may be more severe when an alkylating agent is given along with other myelosuppressive drugs or radiation therapy, and dose reductions are often required in such circumstances to avoid excessive toxicity.

Following hematopoietic recovery, these agents may be given again on an intermittent dosage schedule at sufficient intervals to permit blood count recovery. Ovarian or testicular failure is a common late sequela of alkylating agent therapy, while acute leukemia is a relatively rare complication of use of these mutagenic agents (Boice, 1983).

Oral dosage forms of alkylating agents have been of great value and have been developed using relatively less reactive alkylating drugs. Oral administration of cyclophosphamide, melphalan, chlorambucil, busulfan, and CCNU represents the most common route of administration of these agents and produces effects similar to those observed with parenteral administration. In general, if a tumor is resistant to one alkylating agent, it will be relatively resistant to other agents of this class (although not necessarily to nitrosoureas); however, there are distinct exceptions to this rule for specific tumor types. Overall, cyclophosphamide is the most useful alkylating agent currently available. The oral drug busulfan has a major degree of specificity for the granulocyte series and therefore is of particular value in therapy of chronic myelogenous leukemia. With all oral alkylating agents, some degree of leukopenia is necessary to provide evidence that the drug has been absorbed adequately. Repeated blood counts are essential during administration of these agents, because the development of severe leukopenia or thrombocytopenia necessitates interruption of therapy.

NITROSOUREAS

Carmustine (BCNU), lomustine (CCNU), and semustine (methyl-CCNU) appear to be non-cross-reactive (as regards tumor resistance) with other alkylating agents; all appear to require biotransformation, which occurs by nonenzymatic decomposition, to derivatives with both alkylating and carbamoylating activities. The nitrosoureas are highly lipid-soluble and cross the blood-brain barrier, making them useful in the treatment of brain tumors. The nitrosoureas appear to function by cross-linking through alkylation of DNA. The drugs may be more effective against plateau phase cells than exponentially growing cells, although within a cycling cell population the drugs appear to slow cell progression through the DNA synthetic phase. After oral administration of CCNU or methyl-CCNU, plasma metabolites account for virtually all the administered drug, with peak plasma levels of metabolites appearing within 1–4 hours and prompt central nervous system appearance of 30–40% of the activity present in the plasma. While the initial plasma half-life is in the range of 6 hours, a second half-life is in the range of 1–2 days. Urinary excretion appears to be the major route of elimination from the body. One naturally occurring sugar-containing nitrosourea, streptozocin, is interesting because it has minimal bone marrow toxicity but is frequently effective in the treatment of insulin-secreting islet cell carcinoma of the pancreas and occasionally in non-Hodgkin lymphomas.

RELATED DRUGS PROBABLY ACTING AS ALKYLATING AGENTS

A variety of other compounds have mechanisms of action that involve alkylation. These include procarbazine, dacarbazine, altretamine (hexamethylmelamine), and cisplatin.

1. PROCARBAZINE

The oral agent procarbazine is a methylhydrazine derivative with chemotherapeutic activity (particularly in Hodgkin's disease). The drug is also leukemogenic and has teratogenic and mutagenic properties.

The mechanism of action of procarbazine is uncertain; however, the drug inhibits the synthesis of DNA, RNA, and protein; prolongs interphase; and produces chromosome breaks. Oxidative metabolism of this drug by microsomal enzymes generates azoprocarbazine and H_2O_2, which may be responsible for DNA strand scission. A variety of other metabolites of the drug are formed that may be cytotoxic. One metabolite is a monoamine oxidase (MAO) inhibitor, and adverse side effects can occur when procarbazine is given with other MAO inhibitors. In addition to predictable nausea, vomiting, and myelosuppression, hemolytic anemia, pulmonary reactions, and adverse responses with alcohol (disulfiram-like) have also

been reported, as have skin rashes when procarbazine is given with phenytoin.

Procarbazine is often used in combination chemotherapy of Hodgkin's disease; however, its leukemogenic properties may eventually lead to its replacement with drugs that have lesser carcinogenic potential.

2. DACARBAZINE

Dacarbazine is a synthetic compound that functions as an alkylating agent following metabolic activation by liver microsomal enzymes by oxidative N-demethylation to the monomethyl derivative that spontaneously decomposes to 5-aminoimidazole-4-carboxamide, which is excreted in the urine, and diazomethane. The diazomethane generates a methyl carbonium ion that is believed to be the likely cytotoxic species. Dacarbazine is administered parenterally and is not schedule-dependent. It produces marked nausea, vomiting, and myelosuppression. Its major applications are in melanoma, Hodgkin's disease, and some soft tissue sarcomas. In the latter two tumors, its activity is potentiated by doxorubicin.

3. ALTRETAMINE (Hexamethylmelamine)

Altretamine is structurally similar to triethylenemelamine. It is relatively insoluble and available only in oral form. A related compound, pentamethylmelamine, which is a major metabolite of hexamethylmelamine, is more soluble and is now in clinical trial in an intravenous form. Both agents are rapidly biotransformed by demethylation, presumably to active intermediates. These agents cause nausea, vomiting, and central and peripheral nervous system neuropathies but relatively mild myelosuppression. Altretamine is useful in alkylating agent-resistant ovarian carcinoma.

4. CISPLATIN

Cisplatin (*cis*-diamminedichloroplatinum [II]) is an inorganic metal complex discovered by Rosenberg and his colleagues, who made the serendipitous observation that neutral platinum complexes inhibit division and induce filamentous growth of *Escherichia coli*. Many platinum analogues of this very important drug have been synthesized. While the precise mechanism of action of cisplatin is still undefined, it is thought to act analogously to alkylating agents. It kills cells in all stages of the cell cycle, inhibits DNA biosynthesis, and binds DNA through the formation of interstrand cross-links. The primary binding site is the N7 of guanine, but covalent interaction with adenine and cytosine also occurs. The platinum complexes appear to synergize with certain other anticancer drugs. After intravenous administration, the major acute toxicity is nausea and vomiting. Cisplatin has relatively little effect on the bone marrow, but it can induce significant renal dysfunction and occasional acoustic nerve dysfunction. Hydration with saline infusion alone or with mannitol or other diuretics appears to minimize nephrotoxicity.

Cisplatin

Cisplatin has major antitumor activity in genitourinary cancers, particularly testicular, ovarian, and bladder cancer. Its use along with vinblastine and bleomycin has been a major advance in the development of curative therapy for nonseminomatous testicular cancers. A platinum analogue (carboplatin) with significantly less gastrointestinal and renal toxicity but with myelosuppressive toxicity provides a useful alternative to cisplatin.

Dosage & Toxicity of the Alkylating Agents

The alkylating agents are used in the treatment of a wide variety of hematologic and solid cancers, generally as components of combination chemotherapy. These are discussed under various specific tumors. Dosages and major toxicities are listed in Table 56–2.

Nausea and vomiting are almost universally reported with intravenously administered mechlorethamine, cyclophosphamide, and carmustine and occur with moderate frequency with oral cyclophosphamide.

The important toxic effect of therapeutic doses of virtually all the alkylating drugs is depression of bone marrow and subsequent leukopenia and thrombocytopenia. Severe infections and septicemia may result, with granulocytopenia below 600 PMNs/μL. Platelet depression below 40,000/μL may be accompanied by induced hemorrhagic phenomena. Cyclophosphamide may produce slight to severe alopecia in up to 30% of patients. It may also cause hemorrhagic cystitis. The cystitis can often be averted with adequate hydration.

The hematopoietic effects of toxic doses of alkylating drugs are treated by discontinuing the agent. Red cell and platelet transfusions and antibiotics to con-

Table 56–2. Polyfunctional alkylating agents and probable alkylating agents: Dosages and toxicity.

Alkylating Agent	Single-Agent Dosage	Acute Toxicity	Delayed Toxicity
Nitrogen mustard (HN2, mechlorethamine, Mustargen)	0.4 mg/kg IV in single or divided doses	Nausea and vomiting	Moderate depression of peripheral blood count. Excessive doses produce severe bone marrow depression with leukopenia, thrombocytopenia, and bleeding. Alopecia and hemorrhagic cystitis occasionally occur with cyclophosphamide. Cystitis can be prevented with adequate hydration. Busulfan is associated with skin pigmentation, pulmonary fibrosis, and adrenal insufficiency.
Chlorambucil (Leukeran)	0.1–0.2 mg/kg/d orally; 6–12 mg/d	None	
Cyclophosphamide (Cytoxan)	3.5–5 mg/kg/d orally for 10 days; 1 g/m² IV as single dose	Nausea and vomiting	
Melphalan (Alkeran)	0.25 mg/kg/d orally for 4 days every 4–6 weeks	None	
Thiotepa (triethylenethiophosphoramide)	0.2 mg/kg IV for 5 days	None	
Busulfan (Myleran)	2–8 mg/d orally; 150–250 mg/course	None	
Carmustine (BCNU)	200 mg/m² IV every 6 weeks	Nausea and vomiting	Leukopenia and thrombocytopenia. Rarely hepatitis.
Lomustine (CCNU)	150 mg/m² orally every 6 weeks	Nausea and vomiting	
Semustine (methyl-CCNU)	150 mg/m² orally every 6 weeks	Nausea and vomiting	
Altretamine (hexamethylmelamine)	10 mg/kg/d for 21 days	Nausea and vomiting	Leukopenia, thrombocytopenia, and peripheral neuropathy.
Procarbazine (Matulane)	50–200 mg/d orally	Nausea and vomiting	Bone marrow depression, central nervous system depression.
Dacarbazine	300 mg/m² daily IV for 5 days	Nausea and vomiting	Bone marrow depression.
Cisplatin (Platinol)	20 mg/m²/d IV for 5 days or 50–70 mg/m² as single dose every 3 weeks	Nausea and vomiting	Renal dysfunction. Acoustic nerve dysfunction.
Carboplatin (Paraplatin)	360 mg/m² IV every 4 weeks	Nausea and vomiting	Leukopenia and thrombocytopenia. Rarely neuropathy or hepatic dysfunction.

trol infections are employed as needed until the marrow has regenerated.

ANTIMETABOLITES
(Structural Analogues)

The development of drugs with actions on intermediary metabolism of proliferating cells has been important both clinically and conceptually. While biochemical properties unique to all cancer cells have yet to be discovered, neoplastic cells do have a number of quantitative differences in metabolism from normal cells that render them more susceptible to a number of antimetabolites or structural analogues. Many of these agents have been rationally designed and synthesized, based on knowledge of cellular processes, although a few have been discovered as antibiotics.

Mechanisms of Action

The biochemical pathways that have thus far proved to be most exploitable with antimetabolites have been those relating to nucleotide and nucleic acid synthesis. In a number of instances, when an enzyme is known to have a major effect on pathways leading to cell replication, inhibitors of the reaction it catalyzes have proved to be useful anticancer drugs.

These drugs and their doses and toxicities are shown in Table 56–3. The principal drugs are discussed below.

METHOTREXATE

Methotrexate (MTX) is a folic acid antagonist that binds to the active catalytic site of dihydrofolate reductase (DHFR), interfering with the synthesis of the reduced form that accepts one-carbon units. Lack of this cofactor interrupts the synthesis of thymidylate, purine nucleotides, and the amino acids serine and methionine, thereby interfering with the formation of DNA, RNA, and protein. The enzyme binds methotrexate extremely tightly, and at pH 6.0 virtually no dissociation of the enzyme-inhibitor complex occurs (inhibition constant about 1 nmol/L). At physiologic pH, reversible competitive kinetics occur (inhibition constant about 1 μmol/L). Intracellular formation of polyglutamate derivatives appears to be important in the therapeutic action of methotrexate (Jolivet, 1983). The polyglutamates of methotrexate are retained by cells longer than methotrexate and have increased inhibitory effects on enzymes involved in folate metabolism, making them important determinants in the duration of action of methotrexate.

Drug Resistance

Tumor cell resistance to methotrexate has been attributed to (1) decreased drug transport, (2) altered DHFR with lower affinity for methotrexate, (3) decreased polyglutamate formation, and (4) synthesis of

Table 56–3. Structural analogues: Dosages and toxicity.

Chemotherapeutic Agent	Single-Agent Dosage	Delayed Toxicity[1]
Azacitidine[2]	200 mg/m^2/d IV for 5 days	Nausea and vomiting, diarrhea, fever, hypotension, prolonged marrow hypoplasia.
Cladribine (Leustatin)	0.09 mg/kg/d for 9 days by IV infusion	Severe myelosuppression for about 2 weeks after therapy.
Cytarabine (ara-C, Cytosar-U)	100 mg/m^2/d for 5–10 days, either by continuous IV infusion or SC every 8 hours	Nausea and vomiting, bone marrow depression, megaloblastosis, leukopenia, thrombocytopenia.
Fludarabine (Fludara)	25 mg/m^2/d for 5 days every 28 days (administer IV over 30 minutes)	Myelosuppression. *Note:* High doses can cause serious neurotoxicity.
Fluorouracil (5-FU, Adrucil)	15 mg/kg/d IV for 5 days by 24-hour infusion; 15 mg/kg weekly IV	Nausea, oral and gastrointestinal ulceration, bone marrow depression.
Mercaptopurine (6-MP, Purinethol)	2.5 mg/kg/d orally	Usually well tolerated. Larger dosages may cause bone marrow depression.
Methotrexate (amethopterin, MTX)	2.5–5 mg/d orally (Rheumatrex); 10 mg intrathecally (Folex) once or twice weekly	Oral and gastrointestinal tract ulceration, bone marrow depression, leukopenia, thrombocytopenia.
Thioguanine (6-TG)	2 mg/kg/d orally	Usually well tolerated. Larger dosages may cause bone marrow depression.
Supportive agent with all drugs Allopurinol (Zyloprim)	300–800 mg/d orally for prevention or relief of hyperuricemia	Usually none. Enhances effects and toxicity of mercaptopurine when used in combination.

[1]These drugs do not cause acute toxicity.
[2]For use only in approved treatment protocols.

increased levels of DHFR. This occurs through gene amplification and results in a marked increase in DHFR messenger RNA. It remains to be established whether this genetic resistance mechanism is relevant for other drugs or for resistant tumors in patients receiving methotrexate.

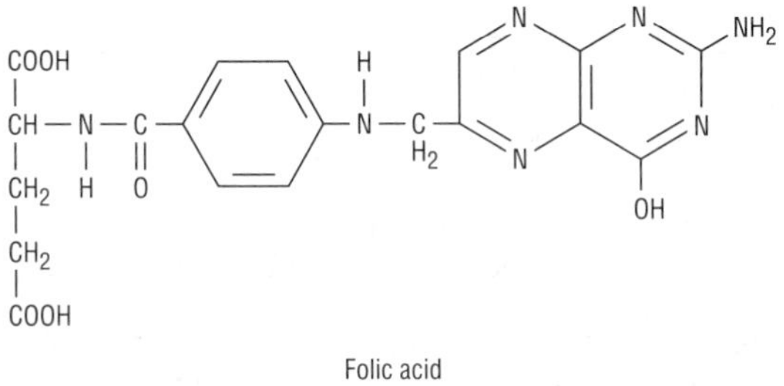

Folic acid

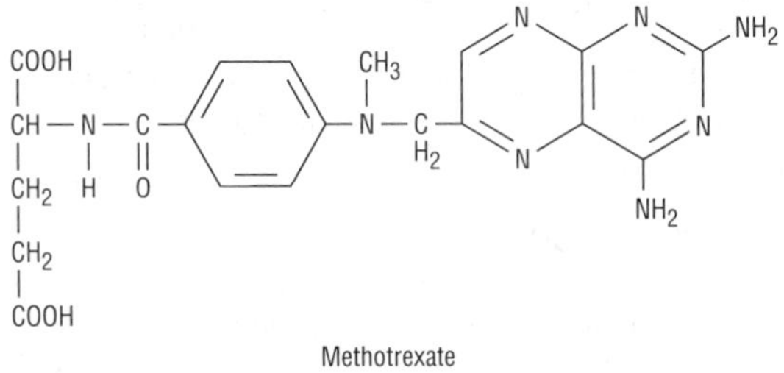

Methotrexate

Dosage & Toxicity

Methotrexate is administered by the intravenous or oral route (Table 56–3). Up to 90% of an oral dose is excreted in the urine within 12 hours. The drug is not subject to metabolism, and serum levels are therefore proportionate to dose as long as renal function and hydration status are adequate. Toxic effects to proliferating tissues are usually observed on the bone marrow and to a lesser extent on the skin and gastrointestinal mucosa. The effects of methotrexate can be reversed by administration of leucovorin (citrovorum factor). Leucovorin "rescue" has been used with accidental overdose or experimentally along with high-dose methotrexate therapy in a protocol intended to rescue normal cells while still leaving the tumor cells subject to its cytotoxic action.

Other Applications

Methotrexate also has important applications in the treatment of rheumatoid arthritis (Chapter 35) and psoriasis. It is in clinical trials for the treatment of asthma (Chapter 19) and (with a prostaglandin) as an abortifacient.

PURINE ANTAGONISTS

1. 6-THIOPURINES

Mercaptopurine (6-MP) was the first of the thiopurine series found useful as an anticancer drug.

Like other thiopurines, it must be metabolized by hypoxanthine-guanine phosphoribosyl transferase (HGPRT) to the nucleotide form (6-thioinosinic acid), which in turn inhibits a number of the enzymes of purine interconversion. Significant amounts of thioguanylic acid and 6-methylmercaptopurine ribotide (MMPR) also are formed from 6-MP. These metabolites may also contribute to the action of the mercaptopurine. 6-MP is used primarily in the treatment of childhood acute leukemia, and a closely related analogue, azathioprine, is used as an immunosuppressive agent (see Chapter 57).

Thioguanine (6-TG) inhibits several enzymes in the purine nucleotide pathway. A variety of metabolic lesions are associated with the cytotoxic action of the purinethiols. These include inhibition of purine nucleotide interconversion; decrease in intracellular levels of guanine nucleotides, which leads to inhibition of glycoprotein synthesis; interference with the formation of DNA and RNA; and incorporation of purinethiols into both DNA and RNA. 6-TG has a synergistic action when used together with cytarabine in the treatment of adult acute leukemia.

Drug Resistance

Resistance to both 6-MP and 6-TG occurs most commonly by decrease in HGPRT activity; an alternative mechanism in acute leukemia involves elevation of levels of alkaline phosphatase, which results in dephosphorylation of thiopurine nucleotide and cellular loss of the resulting ribonucleoside.

Dosage & Toxicity

Mercaptopurine and thioguanine are both given orally (Table 56–3) and excreted mainly in the urine. However, 6-MP is converted to an inactive metabolite (6-thiouric acid) by an oxidation catalyzed by xanthine oxidase, whereas 6-TG requires deamination before it is metabolized by this enzyme. This factor is important because the purine analogue allopurinol, a potent xanthine oxidase inhibitor, is frequently used with chemotherapy in hematologic cancers to

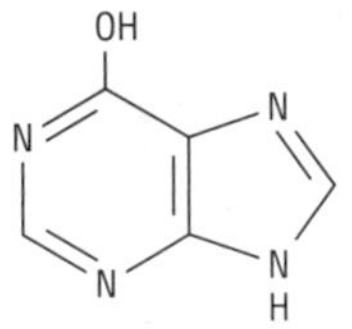

Hypoxanthine

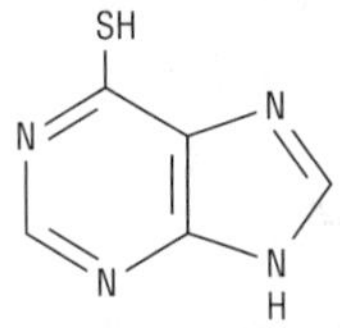

6-Mercaptopurine

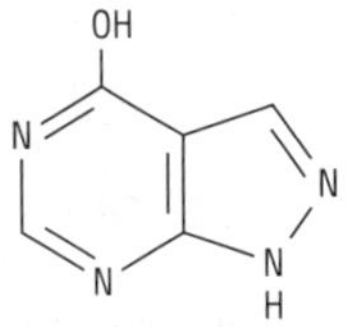

Allopurinol

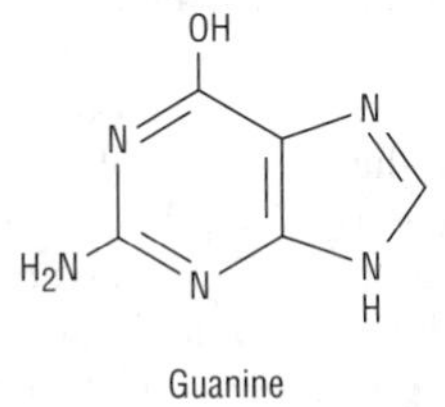

Guanine

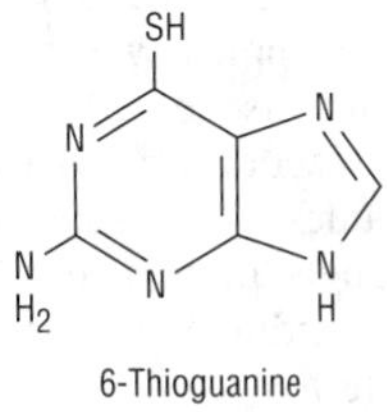

6-Thioguanine

prevent hyperuricemia after tumor cell lysis. It prevents this by blocking purine breakdown, allowing excretion of cellular purines that are relatively more soluble than uric acid. Nephrotoxicity and acute gout produced by excessive uric acid are thereby prevented. Simultaneous therapy with allopurinol and 6-MP results in excessive mercaptopurine toxicity unless the dose of mercaptopurine is reduced to 25–30% of the usual level. This effect does not occur with 6-TG, which can be used in full doses with allopurinol.

2. FLUDARABINE PHOSPHATE

Fludarabine phosphate (2-fluoro-arabinofuranosyl-adenine monophosphate) is rapidly dephosphorylated in vivo to 2-fluoro-arabinofuranosyladenine and then phosphorylated intracellularly by deoxycytidine kinase to the triphosphate. This product interferes with DNA synthesis through inhibition of DNA polymerase and ribonucleotide reductase. Fludarabine phosphate is used chiefly in the treatment of lymphoproliferative diseases. Fludarabine phosphate is given parentally and is excreted primarily in the urine; its dose-limiting toxicity is myelosuppression.

3. CLADRIBINE

Cladribine (2-chlorodeoxyadenosine) achieves high intracellular concentrations because of its resistance to adenosine deaminase; it is phosphorylated by deoxycytidine kinase and is incorporated into DNA. Cladribine causes DNA strand breaks (presumably through interference with DNA repair) and loss of NAD (through activation of poly[ADP-ribose]synthase). Cladribine has been recommended for the treatment of hairy cell leukemia. It is given as a single continuous 7-day infusion; under these conditions its toxicity, which consists of transient marrow suppression, is low.

PYRIMIDINE ANTAGONISTS

1. FLUOROURACIL

Fluorouracil (5-FU) undergoes biotransformation to ribosyl and deoxyribosyl nucleotide metabolites. One of these metabolites, 5-fluoro-2'-deoxyuridine 5'-phosphate (FdUMP), forms a covalently bound ternary complex with the enzyme thymidylate synthase and its cofactor $N^{5,10}$-methylenetetrahydrofolate, a reaction critical for the synthesis of thymine nucleotides. This results in inhibition of DNA synthesis through "thymineless death." 5-FU is converted to 5-fluorouridine triphosphate, incorporated into RNA, and interferes with RNA processing and function.

Cytotoxicity of 5-FU is thus due to its effects on both DNA and RNA.

Uracil   5-FU

5-FU is normally given intravenously (Table 56–3) and has a short metabolic half-life. Although it is active when given orally, its bioavailability is erratic by that route of administration. Floxuridine (5-fluorodeoxyuridine, FUDR) has an action similar to that of 5-FU and is used for hepatic artery infusions. A cream incorporating 5-FU is used topically for treating skin cancers. Fluorouracil is used systemically in the treatment of a variety of adenocarcinomas. Its major toxicities are myelosuppression and mucositis.

2. CYTARABINE

Cytarabine (cytosine arabinoside, ara-C) is an S phase-specific antimetabolite that is converted by deoxycytidine kinase to the 5'-mononucleotide (AraCMP). AraCMP is further metabolized to the triphosphate (AraCTP), which competitively inhibits DNA polymerase. This results in blockade of DNA synthesis while RNA and protein formation continues and leads to unbalanced growth. Cytarabine is also incorporated into RNA and DNA. Incorporation into DNA leads to interference with chain elongation and defective ligation of fragments of newly synthesized DNA. The cellular retention time for AraCTP appears to correlate with its lethality to malignant cells.

Cytosine   Cytosine
deoxyriboside   arabinoside
                  (Cytarabine)

After intravenous administration (Table 56–3), the drug is cleared rapidly, with most of it being deaminated to an inactive form. The ratio of the anabolic enzyme deoxycytidine kinase to the inactivating catalyst cytidine deaminase is important to the cytotoxicity of cytarabine.

In view of cytarabine's S phase specificity, the drug is highly schedule-dependent and must be given either by continuous infusion or every 8–12 hours for 5–7 days. Its activity is limited almost entirely to treatment of acute myelogenous leukemia, for which it is a major drug. Adverse effects include nausea, severe myelosuppression, and varying degrees of stomatitis or alopecia.

3. AZACITIDINE

Azacitidine (5-azacytidine) produces multiple effects associated with its cytotoxicity. It is phosphorylated to the mononucleotide form by uridine-cytidine kinase. Azacytidine 5'-phosphate then inhibits orotidylate decarboxylase, which reduces production of pyrimidine nucleotides. Further metabolism results in incorporation of azacitidine into DNA and RNA and inhibition of DNA, RNA, and protein synthesis.

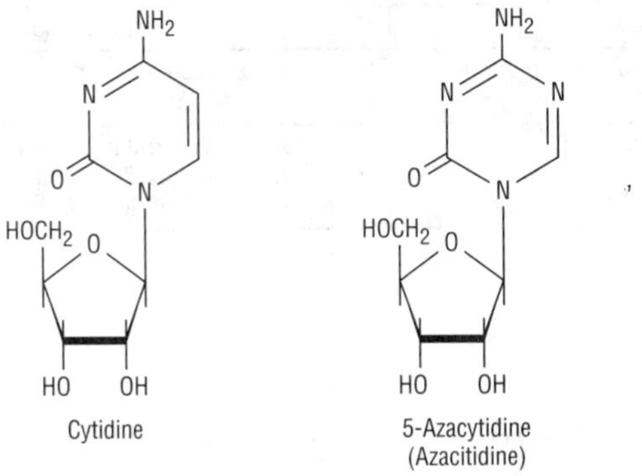

Cytidine

5-Azacytidine
(Azacitidine)

Azacitidine is administered intravenously (Table 56–3) and must be shielded from light and kept at slightly acid pH, because it is unstable and can undergo ring opening. Nausea and fever are observed during drug administration. The half-life is 3–6 hours, with most of the drug excreted either unchanged or in deaminated form.

Azacitidine is currently an investigational agent in the USA, but it is a recognized "second-line agent" in the treatment of acute leukemia. Optimal dosage schedules have yet to be developed. The drug can produce profound myelosuppressive toxicity of long duration.

PLANT ALKALOIDS

VINBLASTINE

Vinblastine is an alkaloid derived from *Vinca rosea*, the periwinkle plant. Its mechanism of action involves depolymerization of microtubules, which are an important part of the cytoskeleton and the mitotic spindle. The drug binds specifically to the microtubular protein tubulin in dimeric form; the drug-tubulin complex adds to the forming end of the microtubules to terminate assembly, and depolymerization of the microtubules then occurs. This results in mitotic arrest at metaphase, dissolution of the mitotic spindle, and interference with chromosome segregation. It produces nausea and vomiting and marrow depression as well as alopecia. It has value in the treatment of systemic Hodgkin's disease and other lymphomas. See clinical section below and Table 56–4. Several related agents, including desacetylvinblastine (vindesine) and vinzolidine, are currently in clinical trial as investigational drugs.

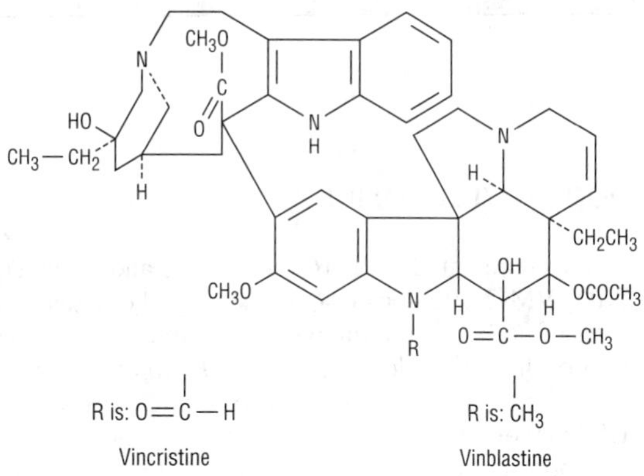

Vincristine

Vinblastine

VINCRISTINE

Vincristine, also an alkaloid derivative of *V. rosea*, is closely related in structure to vinblastine. Its mechanism of action is considered to be identical to that of vinblastine, and it also appears to be a "spindle poison" and to cause arrest of the mitotic cycle. Despite these similarities to vinblastine, vincristine has a strikingly different spectrum of clinical activity and qualitatively different toxicities.

Vincristine has been used with considerable success in combination with prednisone for remission induction in acute leukemia in children. It is also useful in certain other rapidly proliferating neoplasms. It causes a significant incidence of neurotoxicity (Table 56–4), which limits its use to short courses. It occasionally produces bone marrow depression.

Table 56–4. Natural product cancer chemotherapy drugs: Dosages and toxicity.

Drug	Single-Agent Dosage	Acute Toxicity	Delayed Toxicity
Bleomycin (Blenoxane)	Up to 15 mg/m^2 twice weekly to a total dose of 200 mg/m^2	Allergic reactions, fever, hypotension	Edema of hands, pulmonary fibrosis, stomatitis, alopecia.
Dactinomycin (actinomycin D, Cosmegen)	0.04 mg/kg IV weekly	Nausea and vomiting	Stomatitis, gastrointestinal tract upset, alopecia, bone marrow depression.
Daunorubicin (daunomycin, Cerubidine)	30–60 mg/m^2 daily IV for 3 days, or 30–60 mg/m^2 IV weekly	Nausea, fever, red urine (not hematuria)	Cardiotoxicity, bone marrow depression, alopecia.
Doxorubicin (Adriamycin)	60 mg/m^2 IV every 3 weeks to a maximum total dose of 550 mg/m^2	Nausea, red urine (not hematuria)	Cardiotoxicity, alopecia, bone marrow depression, stomatitis.
Etoposide (VePesid, VP-16)	50–100 mg/m^2 daily for 5 days	Nausea, vomiting, hypotension	Alopecia, bone marrow depression.
Idarubicin (Idamycin)	12 mg/m^2 IV daily for 3 days (with cytarabine)	Nausea and vomiting	Bone marrow suppression, mucositis, cardiotoxicity.
Paclitaxel (Taxol)	130–170 mg/m^2 IV over 3 or 24 hrs every 3–4 weeks	Nausea, vomiting, hypotension, arrhythmias	Bone marrow suppression.
Plicamycin (mithramycin, Mithracin)	25–50 µg/kg IV every other day for up to 8 doses	Nausea and vomiting	Thrombocytopenia, hepatotoxicity.
Mitomycin (Mutamycin)	20 mg/m^2 every 6 weeks	Nausea	Thrombocytopenia, leukopenia.
Vinblastine (Velban)	0.1–0.2 mg/kg IV weekly	Nausea and vomiting	Alopecia, loss of reflexes, bone marrow depression.
Vincristine (Oncovin)	1.5 mg/m^2 IV (maximum: 2 mg weekly)	None	Areflexia, muscle weakness, peripheral neuritis, paralytic ileus, mild bone marrow depression, alopecia.

PODOPHYLLOTOXINS

Two compounds, VP-16 (etoposide) and a related drug, VM-26 (teniposide), are semisynthetic derivatives of podophyllotoxin, which is extracted from the root of the mayapple or mandrake *(Podophyllum peltatum)*. Etoposide is approved for clinical use in the USA; an oral formulation is still investigational.

Etoposide and teniposide are quite similar in chemical structure, in their block of cells in the late S-G$_2$ phase of the cell cycle, and clinically. The mode of action involves inhibition of topoisomerase II, which results in DNA damage through strand breakage induced by the formation of a ternary complex of drug, DNA, and enzyme. The drugs are water-insoluble and require a solubilizing vehicle for clinical formulation. After intravenous administration (Table 56–4), they are protein-bound and distributed throughout the body, except for the brain. Excretion is predominantly in the urine, with a lesser amount excreted in bile. In addition to nausea, vomiting, and alopecia, significant toxicity occurs to the hematopoietic and lymphoid systems. Thus far, etoposide has shown activity in monocytic leukemia, testicular cancer, and oat cell carcinoma of the lung; teniposide has activity in various lymphomas.

PACLITAXEL

Paclitaxel is an alkaloid ester derived from the Western yew *(Taxus brevifolia)* and the European yew *(Taxus baccata)*. The drug functions as a mitotic spindle poison through the enhancement of tubulin polymerization. This promotion of microtubule assembly by paclitaxel occurs in the absence of microtubule-associated proteins (MAPs) and guanosine triphosphate.

Paclitaxel has significant activity in ovarian and advanced breast cancer. Neutropenia, thrombocytopenia and peripheral neuropathy are its primary dose-limiting toxicities. A related drug, taxotere, is currently in clinical trial.

ANTIBIOTICS

Screening of microbial products has led to the discovery of a number of growth inhibitors that have proved to be clinically useful in cancer chemotherapy. Many of these antibiotics bind to DNA through intercalation between specific bases and block the synthesis of new RNA or DNA (or both), cause DNA strand scission, and interfere with cell replication. All of the clinically useful antibiotics now available are products of various strains of the soil fungus *Streptomyces*. These include the anthracyclines, actinomycin, bleomycin, mitomycin, and plicamycin.

ANTHRACYCLINES

The anthracycline antibiotics, isolated from *Streptomyces peucetius* var *caesius,* are among the most useful cytotoxic anticancer drugs. Two congeners doxorubicin and daunorubicin are FDA-approved and in general use. Their structures are shown below.

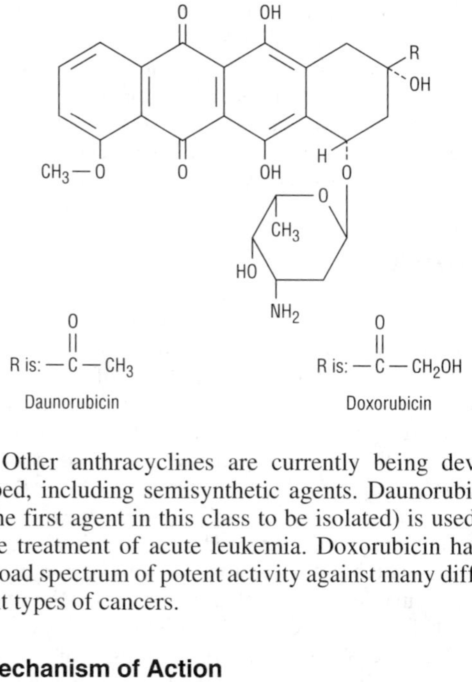

Daunorubicin   Doxorubicin

Other anthracyclines are currently being developed, including semisynthetic agents. Daunorubicin (the first agent in this class to be isolated) is used in the treatment of acute leukemia. Doxorubicin has a broad spectrum of potent activity against many different types of cancers.

Mechanism of Action

Three major actions have been documented for the organ and tumor toxicities of the anthracyclines. These include (1) high-affinity binding to DNA through intercalation with consequent blockade of the synthesis of DNA and RNA, and DNA strand scission through effects on topoisomerase II; (2) binding to membranes to alter fluidity and ion transport; and (3) generation of the semiquinone free radical and oxygen radicals through an enzyme-mediated reductive process. This latter action may be responsible for cardiac toxicity through oxygen radical-mediated damage to membranes.

Pharmacokinetics

In clinical use, anthracyclines are administered by the intravenous route (Table 56–4). Peak blood concentration decreases by 50% within the first 30 minutes after injection, but significant levels persist for up to 20 hours. The anthracyclines are metabolized by the liver, with reduction and hydrolysis of the ring substituents. An alcohol form is an active metabolite, whereas the aglycone is inactive. Most of the drug and its metabolites are excreted in bile, and about one-sixth is excreted in urine. Some metabolites retain antitumor activity. The biliary route of excretion includes enterohepatic recirculation of cytotoxic moieties. In patients with significant elevations of serum bilirubin (> 2.5 mg/dL), the initial dose of anthracyclines must be reduced by 75%.

Clinical Uses

Doxorubicin is one of the most important anticancer drugs, with major clinical application in carcinomas of the breast, endometrium, ovary, testicle, thyroid, and lung and in treatment of many sarcomas, including neuroblastoma, Ewing's sarcoma, osteosarcoma, and rhabdomyosarcoma. It is useful also in hematologic cancers, including acute leukemia, multiple myeloma, Hodgkin's disease, and the diffuse non-Hodgkin lymphomas. It is used in adjuvant therapy in osteogenic sarcoma and breast cancer. It is generally used in combination with other agents (eg, cyclophosphamide, cisplatin, and nitrosoureas), with which it often synergizes, yielding longer remissions than are observed when it is used as a single agent. This approach can also minimize some of the toxicities that would otherwise be associated with use of higher dosages of doxorubicin.

The major use of daunorubicin is in acute leukemia, and for this purpose the drug may have slightly greater activity than doxorubicin. However, daunorubicin appears to have a far narrower spectrum of utility; its efficacy in solid tumors appears to be limited.

A new anthracycline analogue, idarubicin, has completed clinical trials and now is approved for use in acute myeloid leukemia. When combined with cytarabine, idarubicin appears to be somewhat more active than daunorubicin in producing complete remissions in patients with AML. There is also some improvement in survival duration with idarubicin plus cytarabine as compared with daunorubicin plus cytarabine.

Adverse Reactions

In common with many other cytotoxic drugs, the anthracyclines cause bone marrow depression, which is of short duration with rapid recovery. Toxicities more pronounced with anthracyclines (doxorubicin and daunorubicin) than with other agents include a potentially irreversible, cumulative dose-related cardiac toxicity. The mechanism of cardiac toxicity is still under study but appears to involve excessive intracellular production of free radicals within the myocardium by doxorubicin. This is rarely seen at doxorubicin dosages below 500 mg/m^2. Use of lower weekly doses or continuous infusions of doxorubicin that avoid high peak plasma concentrations appear to reduce the frequency of cardiac toxicity as compared to intermittent (every 3–4 weeks) higher dosage schedules.

A second toxicity of doxorubicin and daunorubicin is the almost universal occurrence of severe or total alopecia at standard dosages.

DACTINOMYCIN

Dactinomycin is an antitumor antibiotic isolated from a *Streptomyces*.

Mechanism of Action & Pharmacokinetics

Dactinomycin binds tightly to double-stranded DNA through intercalation between adjacent guanine-cytosine base pairs. Dactinomycin inhibits all forms of DNA-dependent RNA synthesis, with ribosomal RNA formation being most sensitive to drug action. DNA replication is much less reduced, but protein synthesis is blocked in affected cells. The degree of responsiveness to dactinomycin appears to be dependent on the cellular capability for accumulation and retention of the antibiotic.

Approximately half of the intravenous dose of dactinomycin (Table 56–4) remains unmetabolized and is excreted in the bile; a small amount is lost by urinary excretion. The plasma half-life is short. Because the drug is irritating to tissues, it is usually administered with caution to avoid extravasation and with "flushing" with normal saline to wash out the vein.

Clinical Uses

Dactinomycin is used in combination with surgery and vincristine (with or without radiotherapy) in the adjuvant treatment of Wilms' tumor. It is also used along with methotrexate to provide potentially curative treatment for patients with localized or disseminated gestational choriocarcinoma.

Adverse Reactions

Bone marrow depression, the major dose-limiting toxicity of this agent, is usually evident within 7–10 days. All blood elements are affected, but platelets and leukocytes are affected most profoundly and severe thrombocytopenia sometimes occurs. Nausea and vomiting, diarrhea, oral ulcers, and skin eruptions may also be noted. The agent is also immunosuppressive, and patients receiving this drug should not receive live virus vaccines. Alopecia and various skin abnormalities occur occasionally. As with anthracyclines, dactinomycin can interact with radiation, producing a "radiation recall" skin abnormality associated with inflammation at sites of prior radiation therapy.

PLICAMYCIN

Plicamycin (formerly mithramycin) is one of the chromomycin antibiotics isolated from *Streptomyces plicatus*. Plicamycin's mechanism of action appears to involve its binding to DNA, possibly through an antibiotic-Mg^{2+} complex; this interaction interrupts DNA-directed RNA synthesis. In addition, the drug causes plasma calcium levels to decrease, apparently through an action on osteoclasts that is independent of its action on tumor cells (useful in hypercalcemia; see Chapter 41). The drug has some usefulness in testicular cancers refractory to standard treatment, but it is of more use in reversing severe hypercalcemia associated with malignant disease.

Toxic effects of plicamycin include nausea and vomiting, thrombocytopenia, leukopenia, hypocalcemia, bleeding disorders, and liver toxicity. Aside from its use in management of hypercalcemia, plicamycin currently has few other indications.

MITOMYCIN

Mitomycin (mitomycin C) is an antibiotic isolated from *Streptomyces caespitosus*. It contains quinone, carbamate, and aziridine groups, all of which may contribute to its activity. The drug is a "bioreductive" alkylating agent that undergoes metabolic reductive activation through an enzyme-mediated reduction to generate an alkylating agent that cross-links DNA. Hypoxic tumor stem cells of solid tumors exist in an environment conducive to reductive reactions and are more sensitive to the cytotoxic actions of mitomycin than normal and oxygenated tumor cells. Mitomycin is thought to be a CCNS alkylating agent. While this agent is one of the more toxic drugs available for clinical use, it is the best available drug for use as an adjuvant to x-irradiation to attack hypoxic tumor cells. It is being used increasingly in combination chemotherapy (with bleomycin and vincristine) for squamous cell carcinoma of the cervix and for adenocarcinomas of the stomach, pancreas, and lung (along with doxorubicin and fluorouracil). The drug also has some usefulness as a second-line agent for metastatic colon cancer. A special application of mitomycin has been in topical intravesical treatment of small bladder papillomas. Instillations of the agent in distilled water are usually held in the bladder for 3 hours, and the procedure is repeated over a course of weeks. Very little of the agent is absorbed systemically, and it can be quite effective at reducing the frequency of such bladder tumors.

Mitomycin

When mitomycin is administered intravenously, it is cleared rapidly from the vascular compartment; it appears to be eliminated primarily by liver metabolism. Mitomycin causes severe myelosuppression with relatively late toxicity against all three formed elements from the bone marrow. Increasingly profound toxicity occurs after repeated doses. This late form of toxicity suggests an action on hematopoietic stem cells as opposed to later progenitors. Nausea, vomiting, and anorexia commonly occur shortly after injection, and occasional instances of renal toxicity and interstitial pneumonitis have also been reported.

BLEOMYCIN

The bleomycins are a series of antineoplastic antibiotics produced by *Streptomyces verticillus.* A mixture (Blenoxane) of 11 different glycopeptides is used in therapy with the major components being bleomycin A_2 and bleomycin B_2. Bleomycin appears to act through binding to DNA, which results in single- and double-strand breaks following free radical formation, and inhibition of DNA biosynthesis. The fragmentation of DNA seems to be due to oxidation of a DNA-bleomycin-Fe(II) complex and leads to chromosomal aberrations. Bleomycin is a CCS drug that causes accumulation of cells in G_2. It appears to be schedule-dependent, and chronic low-dose administration by repeated injection or continuous infusion seems to be the most effective schedule. The drug synergizes with other drugs such as vinblastine and cisplatin in curative treatment for testicular cancers. It is also used in squamous cell carcinomas of the head and neck, cervix, skin, penis, and rectum, and in combination chemotherapy for the lymphomas. A special use has been for intracavitary therapy of malignant effusions in ovarian and breast cancer. The drug can be given subcutaneously, intramuscularly, or intravenously as well as by the intracavitary route (Table 56–4). Peak blood levels of bleomycin after intramuscular injection appear within 30–60 minutes. Intravenous injection of similar dosages yields higher peak concentrations and a terminal half-life of about 2.5 hours.

Adverse effects include lethal anaphylactoid reactions and a high incidence of fever, with or without chills, particularly in patients with lymphoma. Fever may result in dehydration and hypotension in susceptible patients, and small test doses of the drug are commonly used to anticipate this potentially serious toxicity. More common toxic effects include anorexia and blistering and hyperkeratosis of the palms. A form of pulmonary fibrosis is an uncommon but sometimes fatal adverse effect seen particularly in older patients. The drug does not have significant myelosuppressive effects, which means that it may be incorporated into a number of different combination chemotherapy programs with no significant addition to bone marrow toxicity.

HORMONAL AGENTS

STEROID HORMONES & ANTISTEROID DRUGS

The relationship between hormones and hormone-dependent tumors was initially demonstrated in 1896 when Beatson showed that oophorectomy produced improvement in women with advanced breast cancer. Sex hormones and adrenocortical hormones are now employed in the management of several types of neoplastic disease. Since the sex hormones are concerned with the stimulation and control of proliferation and function of certain tissues, including the mammary and prostate glands, cancer arising from these tissues may be inhibited or stimulated by appropriate changes in hormone balance. Cancer of the breast and cancer of the prostate can be palliated with sex hormone therapy or ablation of appropriate endocrine organs.

The adrenal corticosteroids (particularly the glucocorticoid analogues) have been useful in the treatment of acute leukemia, lymphomas, myeloma, and other hematologic cancers as well as in advanced breast cancer and as supportive therapy in the management of hypercalcemia resulting from many types of cancer. These steroids cause dissolution of lymphocytes, regression of lymph nodes, and inhibition of growth of certain mesenchymal tissues.

The most useful steroid hormones in cancer therapy are listed in Table 56–5.

Pharmacologic Effects

The mechanisms of action of steroid hormones on lymphoid, mammary, or prostatic cancer have been partially clarified. Steroid hormones bind to receptor proteins in cancer cells, and high levels of receptor proteins are predictive for responsiveness of endocrine therapy. Highly specific receptor proteins have been identified for estrogens, progesterone, cortico-

Table 56–5. Hormonally active agents: Dosages and toxicity.

	Usual Adult Dosage	Acute Toxicity	Delayed Toxicity
Androgens Testosterone propionate	100 mg IM 3 times weekly	None	Fluid retention, masculinization
Fluoxymesterone (Halotestin)	10–20 mg/d orally	None	Cholestatic jaundice in some patients receiving fluoxymesterone
Antiandrogen Flutamide (Eulexin)	500 mg/d orally	None	None
Estrogens Diethylstilbestrol	1–5 mg orally 3 times daily	Occasional nausea and vomiting	Fluid retention, feminization, uterine bleeding
Ethinyl estradiol (Estinyl)	3 mg/d orally		
Antiestrogen Tamoxifen (Nolvadex)	20 mg/d orally	None	None
Progestins Hydroxyprogesterone caproate	1 g IM twice weekly	None	None
Medroxyprogesterone (Provera)	100–200 mg/d orally; 200–600 mg orally twice weekly	None	None
Megestrol acetate (Megace)	40 mg orally 4 times daily	None	Fluid retention
Adrenocorticosteroids Hydrocortisone	40–200 mg/d orally	None	Fluid retention, hypertension, diabetes, increased susceptibility to infection, "moon facies"
Prednisone	20–100 mg/d orally	None	
Gonadotropin-releasing hormone agonists Goserelin acetate (Zoladex)	3.6 mg SC monthly	Transient flare of symptoms	None
Leuprolide (Lupron)	7.5 mg SC monthly	Hot flashes	None
Aromatase inhibitor Aminoglutethimide (Cytadren)	250 mg orally twice daily, with hydrocortisone, 20 mg twice daily	Dizziness, rash	None
Peptide hormone inhibitor Octreotide (Sandostatin)	100–600 µg/d SC in 2–4 divided doses	Nausea and vomiting	None

steroids, and androgens in certain neoplastic cells. As in normal cells, steroid hormones form a mobile steroid-receptor complex that ultimately binds directly to nuclear nonhistone protein of DNA to activate transcription of associated clusters of genes.

Most steroid-sensitive cancers have specific receptors. Prednisone-sensitive lymphomas and estrogen-sensitive breast and prostatic cancers contain, respectively, specific receptors for corticosteroids, estrogens, and androgens. It is now possible to assay biopsy specimens for steroid receptor content and to predict from the results which individual patients are likely to benefit from steroid therapy. Measurement of the estrogen receptor (ER) and progesterone receptor (PR) proteins in breast cancer tissue is now a standard clinical test. ER- or PR-positive results predict responsiveness to endocrine ablation or additive therapy, whereas patients whose tumors are ER-negative generally fail to respond to such treatment.

Clinical Uses

The sex hormones are employed in cancer of the female and male breast, cancer of the prostate, and cancer of the endometrium of the uterus (Table 56–7). Extensive studies with the androgenic, estrogenic, and progestational sex hormones have demonstrated their value in advanced inoperable mammary cancer, cancer of the prostate, and cancer of the endometrium (see Clinical Pharmacology, below). In replacement doses, estrogen can stimulate breast and endometrial cancer growth. Surprisingly, high dose estrogen is useful therapeutically in metastatic breast cancer, but has largely been replaced by antiestrogens. In prostate cancer, androgens stimulate growth and estrogen administration results in suppression of androgen production. Drugs that block androgen receptors or the reduction of testosterone to dihydrotestosterone (the active androgen in the prostate) are also valuable in prostate cancer.

Adverse Reactions

Androgens, estrogens, and adrenocortical hormones all can produce fluid retention through their sodium-retaining effect. Prolonged use of androgens and estrogens will cause masculinization and feminization, respectively. Extended use of the adrenocortical steroids may result in hypertension, diabetes, increased susceptibility to infection, and the development of cushingoid appearance ("moon facies"; see Chapter 38 and Table 56–5).

ESTROGEN & ANDROGEN INHIBITORS

The estrogen inhibitor tamoxifen has proved to be extremely useful for the treatment of breast cancer. It also has activity against progesterone-resistant endometrial cancer. Tamoxifen is also currently undergoing clinical trial as a chemopreventive agent in women at high risk for breast cancer. Tamoxifen functions as a competitive partial agonist-inhibitor of estrogen and binds to the estrogen receptors of estrogen-sensitive tissues and tumors. However, tamoxifen has a tenfold lower affinity constant for ER than does estradiol, indicating the importance of ablation of endogenous estrogen for optimal antiestrogen effect.

Excellent plasma levels of tamoxifen are obtained after oral administration, and the agent has a much longer biologic half-life than estradiol. The usual dosage is 10 mg twice daily (Table 56–5), although doses up to 100 mg/m^2 have been administered without major toxicity. Because it may take several weeks to achieve a steady-state level of the active metabolite (monohydroxytamoxifen) with the dosage of 20 mg/d, it is advisable to give an 80 mg "loading course" on the first day to achieve good blood levels rapidly.

Adverse effects in the usual dose range are quite mild. Hot flashes are the most frequent effect. Nausea is observed occasionally, as is fluid retention. Occasional "flares" of breast cancer are observed that usually subside with continued therapy.

Tamoxifen

In advanced breast cancer, clinical improvement is observed in 40–50% of patients who receive tamoxifen. Patients who show objective benefit with treatment are largely those who (1) lack endogenous estrogens (oophorectomy or postmenopausal state) and (2) have breast cancers in which the cytoplasmic ER or PR protein is demonstrable. Tamoxifen has also been effective at prolonging survival when used as surgical adjuvant therapy for postmenopausal women with ER-positive breast cancer. In addition to its direct antiestrogen effects on tumor cells, tamoxifen also suppresses serum levels of insulin-like growth factor-1 and up-regulates local production of transforming growth factor-beta (TGFβ). These endocrine effects of tamoxifen may account for some of its antitumor actions in other tumor types such as ovarian cancer and melanoma.

An antiandrogen, flutamide, has been approved by the FDA for use in the treatment of prostate cancer. It is used to antagonize residual androgenic effects after orchiectomy or with leuprolide (see below). Finasteride, a nonsteroidal inhibitor of 5α-testosterone reductase (Chapter 39), the enzyme that converts testosterone to dihydrotestosterone, is investigational in the treatment of cancer. It is promising because it may prevent androgen effects in prostatic tumor tissue without suppressing androgen production or effects in other tissues.

GONADOTROPIN-RELEASING HORMONE AGONISTS

Leuprolide acetate and goserelin are synthetic peptide analogues of naturally occurring gonadotropin-releasing hormone (GnRH, LHRH). They are described in Chapters 36 and 39. These analogues are more potent than the natural hormone and function as GnRH agonists, with paradoxic results, when given continuously (or as a depot preparation), on the pituitary—initial stimulation followed by inhibition of the release of follicle-stimulating hormone and luteinizing hormone. This results in reduced testicular androgen synthesis. The latter effect underlies the efficacy of these agents in the treatment of metastatic carcinoma of the prostate.

Leuprolide has been directly compared with standard endocrine therapy of prostatic cancer with diethylstilbestrol (DES). Suppression of androgen synthesis and reductions in serum prostatic acid phosphatase (a marker of metastatic tumor burden) are comparable with both leuprolide and DES. However, painful gynecomastia, nausea, vomiting, edema, and thromboembolism occur significantly less frequently with leuprolide than with DES. Leuprolide and goserelin are more expensive than DES, but that is more than offset by the overall cost of complications of DES or the surgical and hospitalization costs associated with surgical orchiectomy. Long-acting depot formulations of both leuprolide and goserelin are administered once monthly. The endocrine effects of these agents may also prove useful in the management of hormone receptor-positive breast cancer, but this application remains to be established.

AROMATASE INHIBITORS

Aminoglutethimide is an inhibitor of adrenal steroid synthesis at the first step (conversion of cholesterol to pregnenolone; see Chapter 38). Aminoglutethimide also inhibits the extra-adrenal synthesis of estrone and estradiol. Aside from its direct effects on adrenal steroidogenesis, aminoglutethimide is an inhibitor of an aromatase enzyme that converts the adrenal androgen androstenedione to estrone. This aromatization of an androgenic precursor into an estrogen can occur in body fat. Since estrogens promote the growth of breast cancer, estrogen synthesis in extragonadal adipose tissue can be important in breast cancer growth in postmenopausal women.

Aminoglutethimide is effective in the treatment of metastatic breast cancer in women whose tumors contain significant levels of estrogen or progesterone receptors. Aminoglutethimide is normally administered with adrenal replacement doses of hydrocortisone to avoid symptoms of adrenal insufficiency. Hydrocortisone is preferable to dexamethasone, because the latter agent accelerates the rate of catabolism of aminoglutethimide. Adverse effects of aminoglutethimide include occasional dizziness, lethargy, visual blurring, and rash.

Aminoglutethimide plus hydrocortisone is normally used as second-line therapy for women who have been treated with tamoxifen, largely because aminoglutethimide causes somewhat more adverse effects than tamoxifen. However, it can be used as primary endocrine therapy also. Other purportedly more potent and selective aromatase inhibitors are under investigation.

MISCELLANEOUS ANTICANCER DRUGS
(See Table 56–6.)

AMSACRINE

Amsacrine is a 9-anilinoacridine derivative that causes chromosome breakage. This drug intercalates between base pairs in DNA, distorts the double helix, and produces single- and double-strand breaks in DNA and DNA-protein cross-links. DNA strand breaks appear to be mediated by formation of topoisomerase II-DNA complexes trapped by amsacrine in the breaking-sealing action of the enzyme.

Amsacrine is predominantly metabolized by the liver with a half-life of 8–9 hours; thus, liver impairment causes considerable prolongation of plasma concentrations. Amsacrine has significant activity against anthracycline- and cytarabine-refractory

Table 56–6. Miscellaneous anticancer drugs: Dosages and toxicity.

Drug	Usual Dosage	Acute Toxicity	Delayed Toxicity
Amsacrine	90 mg/m^2 IV for 5 days (leukemia)	Nausea	Bone marrow depression.
Asparaginase (Elspar)	20,000 IU/m^2 daily IV for 5–10 days	Nausea and fever, allergic reactions	Hepatotoxicity, mental depression, pancreatitis.
Hydroxyurea (Hydrea)	300 mg/m^2 orally for 5 days	Nausea and vomiting	Bone marrow depression.
Mitotane (Lysodren)	6–15 g/d orally	Nausea and vomiting	Dermatitis, diarrhea, mental depression.
Mitoxantrone (Novantrone)	10–12 mg/m^2 IV every 3–4 weeks	Nausea	Bone marrow depression, occasional cardiac toxicity, mild alopecia.
Quinacrine	100–300 mg/d by intracavitary injection for 5 days	Local pain and fever	None.

acute myelogenous leukemia, advanced ovarian carcinomas, and lymphomas. Hematologic toxicity is dose-limiting, and cardiac arrest has been reported during amsacrine infusions.

ASPARAGINASE

Asparaginase (L-asparagine amidohydrolase) is an enzyme that is isolated for clinical use from various bacteria. The drug is used to treat childhood acute leukemia. Asparaginase acts indirectly by catabolic depletion of serum asparagine to aspartic acid and ammonia. Blood glutamine levels are also reduced. This results in inhibition of protein synthesis in neoplastic cells requiring an external source of asparagine because of low or deficient levels of asparagine synthase, and cell proliferation is blocked. Most normal cells can synthesize asparagine and thus are less susceptible to the action of asparaginase.

HYDROXYUREA

Hydroxyurea ($H_2NCONHOH$) is an analogue of urea whose mechanism of action involves the inhibition of DNA synthesis. It exerts its lethal effect on cells in S phase by inhibiting the enzyme ribonucleotide reductase, resulting in the depletion of deoxynucleoside triphosphate pools. The drug is administered orally. Its major uses are in melanoma and chronic myelogenous leukemia; however, it plays a secondary role in both these circumstances. The major adverse effect of this agent is bone marrow depression. At high dosages (> 40 mg/kg/d), megaloblastosis unresponsive to vitamin B_{12} or folic acid may appear. Gastrointestinal symptoms, including nausea, vomiting, and diarrhea, are common in patients receiving high doses of this drug.

MITOXANTRONE

Mitoxantrone (dihydroxyanthracenedione, DHAD) is an anthracene compound whose structure resembles the anthracycline ring. It binds to DNA to produce strand breakage and inhibits both DNA and RNA synthesis. It was recently approved for treatment of refractory acute leukemia. The plasma half-life of mitoxantrone in patients is approximately 32 hours; it is predominantly excreted in the feces. Mitoxantrone is active in both pediatric and adult acute myelogenous leukemia, non-Hodgkin lymphomas, and breast cancer. Leukopenia is the dose-limiting toxicity, and mild nausea and vomiting, stomatitis, and alopecia also occur. The drug also produces some cardiac toxicity, usually manifested as arrhythmias.

MITOTANE

This drug (Figure 38–4) is a DDT congener that was first found to be adrenolytic in dogs. Subsequently it was found to be useful in the treatment of adrenal carcinoma. The drug produces tumor regression and relief of the excessive adrenal steroid secretion that often occurs with this malignancy. Toxicities include skin eruptions, diarrhea, and mental depression. The drug also causes anorexia, nausea, somnolence, and dermatitis.

The utility of mitotane appears to be limited to adrenal carcinoma, and it is labeled for that one indication.

RETINOIC ACID DERIVATIVES

all-*trans*-Retinoic acid (etretinate) produces remissions in patients with acute promyelocytic leukemia (APL) through the induction of terminal differentiation, in which the leukemic promyelocytes lose their ability to proliferate. APL is associated with a t(15;17) chromosomal translocation, which disrupts the gene for the nuclear receptor-α for retinoic acid and fuses it to a gene called PML. This chimeric gene, which expresses aberrant forms of the retinoic acid receptor-α, is present in virtually all PML patients and appears to be responsible for sensitivity to all-*trans*-retinoic acid.

13-*cis*-Retinoic acid (isotretinoin) has achieved a significant objective response rate as a chemopreven-tive adjuvant to prevent second primary tumors in patients with head and neck squamous cell carcinoma.

The most frequent toxicities of the retinoids include mucocutaneous, skeletal, liver, and teratogenic effects.

BONE MARROW GROWTH FACTORS

Use of bone marrow stimulating factors with chemotherapy can reduce the frequency and severity of neutropenic sepsis and other complications. Two bone marrow growth factors that stimulate neutrophil growth were recently approved: granulocyte colony stimulating factor (G-CSF) and granulocyte-macrophage stimulating factor (Chapter 32). Their specific indications are still being developed, but it is clear that they can shorten hospitalization after bone marrow transplantation and reduce the incidence of infection associated with severe neutropenia.

INVESTIGATIONAL AGENTS

Several of the drugs mentioned in the text remain in investigational status in the USA until their efficacy and safety for cancer chemotherapy can be established. In specific instances where treatment with one of these agents seems warranted, it usually can be arranged through a university hospital or cancer center or by contacting the Division of Cancer Treatment of the National Cancer Institute, which can provide further information and identify investigators who are authorized to administer these drugs.

This status applies to gencytabine, amonafide, azacitidine, and amsacrine, agents useful in acute leukemias. Other products still in the investigational phase include suramin, taxotere, tenizolamide, and 9-amino-20(S)-camptothecin. All of these drugs have substantial toxicities. Until their pharmacology is more completely understood and their net effects have proved to be beneficial, their use will be restricted to clinical research.

II. CLINICAL PHARMACOLOGY OF CANCER CHEMOTHERAPEUTIC DRUGS (Table 56–7)

Knowledge of the kinetics of tumor cell proliferation as well as information on the pharmacology and mechanism of action of cancer chemotherapeutic agents has become important in designing optimal chemotherapeutic regimens for patients with cancer. The strategy for developing drug regimens requires a knowledge of the particular characteristics of specific tumors—eg, Is there a high growth fraction? Is there a high spontaneous cell death rate? Are most of the cells in G_0? Is a significant fraction of the tumor composed of hypoxic stem cells? Are their normal counterparts under hormonal control? Similarly, knowledge of the pharmacology of specific drugs is equally important—eg, Does the drug have a particular affinity for uptake by the tumor cells (streptozocin)? Are the tumor cells sensitive to the drug? Is the drug cell cycle-specific?

Drugs that affect cycling cells can often be used most effectively after treatment with a cell cycle-nonspecific agent (eg, alkylating agents); this principle has been tested in a few human tumors with increasing success. Similarly, recognition of true drug synergism (tumor cell kill by the drug combination greater than the additive effects of the individual drugs) or antagonism is important in the design of combination chemotherapeutic programs. The combination of cytarabine with an anthracycline in acute myelogenous leukemia and the use of vinblastine or etoposide along with cisplatin and bleomycin in testicular tumors are good examples of true drug synergism against cancer cells but not against normal tissues.

In general, it is preferable to use cytotoxic chemotherapeutic agents in intensive "pulse" courses every 3–4 weeks rather than to use continuous daily dosage schedules. This allows for maximum effects against neoplastic cell populations with complete hematologic and immunologic recovery between courses rather than leaving the patient continuously suppressed with cytotoxic therapy. This approach reduces adverse effects but does not reduce therapeutic efficacy.

The application of these principles is well illustrated in the current approach to the treatment of acute leukemia, lymphomas, Wilms' tumor, and testicular neoplasms.

Adjuvant Chemotherapy for Micrometastases: Multimodality Therapy

The most important role for effective cancer chemotherapy is undoubtedly as an adjuvant to initial or "primary field" treatment with other methods such as surgery or radiation therapy. Failures with primary field therapy are due principally to occult micrometastases outside the primary field. With the currently available treatment modalities, this form of multimodality therapy appears to offer the greatest chance of curing patients with solid tumors.

Distant micrometastases are usually present in patients with one or more positive lymph nodes at the time of surgery (eg, in breast cancer) and in patients with tumors having a known propensity for early hematogenous spread (eg, osteogenic sarcoma, Wilms' tumor). The risk of recurrent or metastatic disease in such patients can be extremely high (80%). Only systemic therapy can adequately attack micrometastases. Chemotherapy regimens that are at least moderately effective against advanced cancer may have curative potential (at the right dosage and schedule) when combined with primary therapy such as surgery. Several studies show that adjuvant chemotherapy prolongs both disease-free and overall survival in patients with osteogenic sarcoma, rhabdomyosarcoma, or breast cancer. Similar comments apply to the use of three cycles of combination chemotherapy (eg, "MOPP") prior to total nodal radiation in stage IIB Hodgkin's disease.

In breast cancer, premenopausal women with positive lymph nodes at the time of mastectomy have benefited from combination chemotherapy. It has been established that several programs of cytotoxic chemotherapy achieve prolonged disease-free and overall survival times; this method of treatment has increased the cure rate in high-risk primary breast cancer. Active regimens have included, in various combinations, the agents cyclophosphamide, methotrexate, fluorouracil, doxorubicin, and vincristine. In general, regimens with at least three active drugs have been useful. The results produced by combination chemotherapy are superior to the results produced by single agents, because combination chemotherapy copes better with tumor cell heterogeneity and produces a greater tumor cell log kill. Full protocol doses of cytotoxic agents are required to maximize the likelihood of efficacy. Clinical trials have proved tamoxifen to be an effective adjuvant in postmenopausal women with positive estrogen receptor tests on the primary tumor. Because it is cytostatic rather than cytocidal, adjuvant therapy with tamoxifen will probably need to be continued for many years. Tamoxifen adjuvant chemotherapy is now standard in node-positive postmenopausal women with positive ER or PR tests on tumor specimens. Tamoxifen appears to exert an effect on ER-negative

Table 56–7. Malignancies responsive to chemotherapy.

Diagnosis	Current Treatment of Choice	Other Valuable Agents
Acute lymphocytic leukemia	Induction: vincristine plus prednisone. Remission maintenance: mercaptopurine, methotrexate, and cyclophosphamide in various combinations	Asparaginase, daunorubicin, carmustine, doxorubicin, cytarabine, allopurinol,[1] craniospinal radiotherapy
Acute myelocytic and myelomonocytic leukemia	Combination chemotherapy: cytarabine and mitoxantrone or daunorubicin or idarubicin	Methotrexate, thioguanine, mercaptopurine, allopurinol,[1] mitoxantrone, asacitidine,[2] amsacrine,[2] etoposide
Chronic lymphocytic leukemia	Chlorambucil and prednisone (if indicated)	Vincristine, androgens,[1] allopurinol,[1] doxorubicin, fludarabine[2]
Chronic myelogenous leukemia	Busulfan or interferon	Vincristine, mercaptopurine, hydroxyurea, melphalan, interferon, allopurinol[1]
Hodgkin's disease (stages III and IV)	Combination chemotherapy: mechlorethamine, vincristine, procarbazine, prednisone (MOPP)	Vinblastine, doxorubicin, lomustine, dacarbazine, etoposide, ifosfamide, bleomycin, interferon
Non-Hodgkin lymphomas	Combination chemotherapy: cyclophosphamide, doxorubicin, vincristine, prednisone	Bleomycin, lomustine, carmustine, etoposide, interferon, mitoxantrone, ifosfamide
Multiple myeloma	Melphalan plus prednisone or multiagent combination chemotherapy	Cyclophosphamide, vincristine, carmustine, interferon, doxorubicin, androgens[1]
Macroglobulinemia	Chlorambucil	Fludarabine,[2] prednisone
Polycythemia vera	Busulfan, chlorambucil, or cyclophosphamide	Radioactive phosphorus 32
Carcinoma of lung	Etoposide plus cisplatin	Methotrexate, vincristine, vinblastine, doxorubicin, mitomycin C
Carcinomas of head and neck	Fluorouracil plus cisplatin	Methotrexate, bleomycin, hydroxyurea, doxorubicin, vincristine
Carcinoma of endometrium	Progestins or tamoxifen	Doxorubicin, cisplatin, carboplatin
Carcinoma of ovary	Cyclophosphamide and cisplatin or carboplatin	Doxorubicin, melphalan, fluorouracil, vincristine, altretamine (hexamethylmelamine), bleomycin, taxol
Carcinoma of cervix	Cisplatin, carboplatin	Lomustine, cyclophosphamide, doxorubicin, methotrexate, mitomycin, bleomycin, vincristine, interferon, 13-*cis*-retinoic acid
Breast carcinoma	(1) Adjuvant chemotherapy or tamoxifen after primary breast surgery. (2) Combination chemotherapy or hormonal manipulation for late recurrence	Cyclophosphamide, doxorubicin, vincristine, methotrexate, fluorouracil, taxol, mitoxantrone, prednisone,[1] megestrol, androgens,[1] aminoglutethimide
Choriocarcinoma (trophoblastic neoplasms)	Methotrexate alone or etoposide and cisplatin	Vinblastine, mercaptopurine, chlorambucil, doxorubicin
Carcinoma of testis	Combination chemotherapy: cisplatin, bleomycin, and etoposide	Methotrexate, dactinomycin, plicamycin, vinblastine, doxorubicin, cyclophosphamide, etoposide, ifosfamide plus mesna[1]
Carcinoma of prostate	Estrogens or GnRH agonist plus flutamide	Aminoglutethimide, doxorubicin, cisplatin, prednisone,[1] estramustine, fluorouracil, progestins, suramin
Wilms' tumor	Vincristine plus dactinomycin after surgery and radiotherapy	Methotrexate, cyclophosphamide, doxorubicin
Neuroblastoma	Cyclophosphamide plus doxorubicin and vincristine	Dactinomycin, daunorubicin, cisplatin
Carcinoma of thyroid	Radioiodine (^{131}I), doxorubicin, cisplatin	Bleomycin, fluorouracil, melphalan
Carcinoma of adrenal	Mitotane	Suramin[2]
Carcinoma of stomach or pancreas	Fluorouracil plus doxorubicin and mitomycin	Hydroxyurea, lomustine, cisplatin
Carcinoma of colon	Fluorouracil plus leucovorin or interferon (or both)	Cyclophosphamide, mitomycin, nitrosoureas
Carcinoid	Doxorubicin plus cyclophosphamide	Interferon, dactinomycin, methysergide,[1] streptozocin, octreotide

(continued)

Table 56–7 (cont'd). Malignancies responsive to chemotherapy.

Diagnosis	Current Treatment of Choice	Other Valuable Agents
Insulinoma	Streptozocin, interferon	Doxorubicin, fluorouracil, mitomycin, streptozocin
Osteogenic sarcoma	Doxorubicin, or methotrexate with citrovorum rescue initiated after surgery	Cyclophosphamide, dacarbazine, interferon
Miscellaneous sarcomas	Doxorubicin plus dacarbazine	Methotrexate, dactinomycin, ifosfamide plus mesna,[1] vincristine, vinblastine
Melanoma	Dacarbazine, cisplatin	Lomustine, hydroxyurea, mitomycin, dactinomycin, interferon, tamoxifen

[1]Supportive agent, not oncolytic.
[2]Investigational agent. Treatment available through qualified investigators and centers authorized by National Cancer Institute and Cooperative Oncology Groups.

tumors as well, perhaps via mechanisms other than the estrogen receptor. For example, tamoxifen administration reduces serum concentrations of insulin-like growth factor-1 and increases concentrations of the growth-suppressing factor TGFβ in stromal cells within a tumor.

Other applications of adjuvant chemotherapy include colorectal (fluorouracil plus levamisole or leucovorin), testicular (vinblastine, bleomycin, and cisplatin), head and neck, and gynecologic neoplasms (various drugs). Thus, adjuvant chemotherapy (with curative intent) should now be considered for patients who undergo primary surgical staging and therapy and are found to have a stage and histologic type of cancer with a high risk of micrometastasis. This policy is germane to those tumor types for which palliative chemotherapy has already been developed and has been shown to induce complete remissions in advanced stages of the disease. In each instance, the benefit:risk ratio must be closely examined.

Primary chemotherapy (prior to local surgery) is now extensively used in patients with osteogenic sarcoma and has facilitated limb-sparing procedures. Primary chemotherapy is now also being evaluated in breast cancer to "downstage" patients prior to surgery.

THE LEUKEMIAS

1. ACUTE LEUKEMIA

Childhood Leukemia

Acute lymphoblastic leukemia (ALL) is the predominant form of leukemia in childhood and the most common form of cancer in children. Children with this disease now have a relatively good prognosis. A subset of patients with neoplastic lymphocytes expressing surface antigenic features of T lymphocytes have a poor prognosis (see Chapter 57). A cytoplasmic enzyme expressed by normal thymocytes, terminal deoxycytidyl transferase (terminal transferase), is also expressed in many cases of ALL. T cell ALLs also express high levels of the enzyme adenosine

deaminase (ADA). (This led to interest in the use of ADA inhibitor pentostatin [deoxycoformycin] for treatment of such T cell cases.) Until 1948, the median length of survival in ALL was 3 months. With the advent of the folic acid antagonists, the length of survival was greatly increased. Subsequently, corticosteroids, mercaptopurine, cyclophosphamide, vincristine, daunorubicin, and asparaginase were all found to act against this disease. A combination of vincristine and prednisone plus other agents is currently used to initially induce remission. Over 90% of children enter complete remission with this therapy, with only minimal toxicity. However, circulating tumor stem cells often lodge in the brain, and such cells are not killed by these drugs because they do not cross the blood-brain barrier. The value of "prophylactic" intrathecal methotrexate therapy for prevention of central nervous system leukemia (a major mechanism of relapse) has been clearly demonstrated. Intrathecal therapy with methotrexate should therefore be considered as a standard component of the induction regimen for children with ALL. Alternative approaches for prevention of central nervous system leukemia that also appear to be efficacious are intrathecal cytarabine and craniospinal irradiation. However, radiation therapy to the neuraxis can cause skeletal growth retardation. Once a complete remission has been induced (> three log cell kill), "maintenance" or "consolidation" therapy is always indicated. This usually consists of a combination of oral methotrexate, mercaptopurine, and cyclophosphamide administered either in pulses, simultaneously, or in various sequences. This "total therapy" approach should be considered the standard form of treatment, because it has produced a substantial increase in the cure rate of children with acute leukemia. Although many of the clinical trials are still under way, such therapy appears to offer the best hope of cure for an increasing percentage of patients. The median length of survival in childhood acute leukemia is now approaching 4 years. Many centers discontinue intensive chemotherapy in patients who have shown no sign of relapse after 3 years of intensive chemotherapy. Children who survive for 5 years in complete remission have a greater than 60% chance of having a permanent remission or cure (Rivera, 1993).

If leukemia does recur in a patient in remission, the same drugs are used again to try to reinduce the remission. If resistance is observed, reinduction is attempted with different agents (daunorubicin, vincristine, asparaginase, methotrexate, etc) in various combinations. The possibility of curing this fatal childhood disease has fueled current investigations into intensive combination chemotherapy with proved agents plus asparaginase, daunorubicin, and other experimental agents and has led to increased interest in combination chemotherapy for other kinds of neoplastic diseases.

Adult Leukemia

Acute leukemia in adults is predominantly myelocytic, although some cases of lymphoblastic leukemia are also seen. Unlike ALL, induction therapy in acute myelogenous leukemia (AML) requires the use of drugs toxic to normal bone marrow cells. The single most active agent for AML is cytarabine; however, it is best used in combination. Recent trials with combinations of anthracyclines with cytarabine have induced complete remissions in about 70% of patients.

The patient often requires intensive supportive care during the toxic period of induction chemotherapy before remission is achieved. Such care includes platelet transfusions to prevent bleeding, G-CSF to shorten periods of neutropenia, and bactericidal antibiotics plus granulocyte transfusions to combat infections. Younger patients (eg, < age 55) who are in complete remission and have an HLA-compatible donor are candidates for allogeneic bone marrow transplantation. The transplant procedure is preceded by high-dose chemotherapy and total body irradiation and followed by immunosuppression. This procedure may cure 40% of eligible acute leukemia patients. Patients over age 60 respond less well to chemotherapy, primarily because their resistance to infection is lower. Remission maintenance is usually with thioguanine and cytarabine courses. Mitoxantrone, azacitidine, and amsacrine are used as secondary agents for patients who develop resistance to standard therapy. The median life expectancy of patients with AML who enter complete remission is now in excess of 1 year, and some patients are in remission for over 3 years. About 20% of adult patients who achieve complete remission with current standard chemotherapy appear to remain free of recurrent leukemia and are probably cured.

2. CHRONIC MYELOGENOUS LEUKEMIA

Chronic myelogenous leukemia (CML) arises from a chromosomally abnormal hematopoietic stem cell. An abnormal chromosome 22 with deletion of a short arm or translocation to the long arm of chromosome 9 is present in 90% of cases. It is called the Philadelphia chromosome (Ph[1]). The clinical symptoms and course are related to the leukocyte level and its rate of increase. Most patients with leukocyte counts over 50,000/μL should be treated. The goals of treatment are to reduce the granulocytes to normal levels, to raise the hemoglobin concentration to normal, and to relieve metabolic symptoms. The most useful forms of systemic treatment to induce remission are with alpha interferon or busulfan, with other oral alkylating agents, or with hydroxyurea. Local splenic x-ray therapy is occasionally used. In the early stages of the disease, treatment produces a prompt decrease in spleen size, a decrease in the leukocyte count, and an increase in subjective well-being. Recent results obtained with alpha interferon indicate that this agent can reduce or eliminate the expression of the Ph[1] chromosome in bone marrow myeloid progenitors, whereas this rarely occurs with cytotoxic agents. Prolonged chemotherapy relieves symptoms and signs of CML but does not prolong survival. A major advance in the treatment of younger patients with CML has been in the application of allogeneic bone marrow transplantation performed when the patient is in remission and preferably within the first year after the diagnosis has been made. Bone marrow transplantation can be curative in up to 50% of such CML patients.

Patients who are not eligible for bone marrow transplantation (eg, those over age 55 and those who lack an HLA-compatible donor) and those who are not cured by the procedure develop an accelerated or acute leukemic phase 3–5 years after diagnosis. At this point, agents such as hydroxyurea or mercaptopurine may provide partial temporary improvement. Combination chemotherapy, including cytarabine, asparaginase, and vincristine or hydroxyurea with or without prednisone, may have transient benefit in a subset of patients, but the prognosis for patients with CML in blastic transformation remains grim.

3. CHRONIC LYMPHOCYTIC LEUKEMIA

Treatment of chronic lymphocytic leukemia (CLL) is markedly different from that of CML. Whereas CML is a proliferative neoplasm requiring systemic treatment for symptomatic control, CLL appears to result from a gradual accumulation of monoclonal B lymphocytes rather than from rapid neoplastic cell proliferation. CLL is often detected accidentally long before the development of symptoms. Although the average life expectancy after diagnosis is only 3 years, the disease occurs frequently in elderly patients, which skews the survival data. Many asymptomatic patients may survive for long periods (ie, 5–15 years) without any therapy. In patients whose disease is restricted to lymphocytosis in the peripheral blood, it is reasonable to withhold treatment unless the lymphocyte count is well above 150,000/μL. When anemia or thrombocytopenia, immunodeficiency, weight loss, fever, or generalized organ involvement does occur, treatment is indicated.

The therapeutic methods used to treat CLL include corticosteroids, alkylating agent chemotherapy, or use of fludarabine. Prednisone is often quite effective, and after an initial course of 80 mg/d for several weeks the dose can be gradually decreased or switched to an intermittent (every other day) schedule, which virtually eliminates adverse effects. Hemolytic anemia may respond dramatically to prednisone, although thrombocytopenia is often more refractory.

Chlorambucil is probably the most easily administered oral alkylating agent and has the fewest adverse effects. The dose is usually 0.1 mg/kg/d, with monitoring of blood counts at weekly intervals. Alternatively, cyclophosphamide can be given in "pulse courses" of 1 g/m^2 orally over 4 days every 4–6 weeks. Fludarabine is rapidly becoming the treatment of choice in CLL. The goal of therapy is to eliminate the systemic manifestations of the disease; complete normalization of the lymphocyte count is not necessary. Therapy can be discontinued once the patient's condition has stabilized, but maintenance therapy should be considered if symptoms reappear quickly. Local x-ray therapy is useful for shrinking symptomatic enlarged lymph nodes but is only occasionally indicated. It is important not to overtreat these usually elderly patients because of their poor host resistance.

4. HAIRY CELL LEUKEMIA

This rare form of leukemia originates in a specific subset of B cells and has symptoms and signs similar to those of CLL; however, it responds poorly to conventional chemotherapy. Alpha interferon, which is currently the preferred treatment for hairy cell leukemia (HCL), is approved by the FDA for this indication. Approximately 90% of patients with HCL achieve hematologic improvement with alpha interferon. The adenosine deaminase inhibitors cladribine and pentostatin are very active in HCL and can induce complete remissions (indicated by negative biopsies) even in patients who relapse from interferon.

THE LYMPHOMAS

1. HODGKIN'S DISEASE

Although remarkably little is known about the cause of Hodgkin's disease, its therapy has undergone revolutionary improvement. Hodgkin's disease is a lymphoma with certain unique characteristics in its natural history: (1) its apparent tendency to progress from a single involved node to anatomically adjacent nodes in a somewhat "orderly" fashion, and (2) its tendency to appear confined to the lymphoid system for a long period of time. Extranodal involvement may also occur, and involvement of the liver, bone marrow, lungs, or other sites is taken as evidence of more "malignant" behavior of the tumor. To effectively treat this disorder, the extent of disease must be adequately staged in order to prepare a rational treatment plan. Widespread involvement is manifested by symptoms such as sweats, fever, anorexia, and weight loss and by infiltration of other organs, including the lungs, liver, and bone marrow.

Intensive x-ray therapy with supervoltage equipment is curative in most cases of early Hodgkin's disease confined to one lymph node area or several adjacent areas above the diaphragm (stages I and II). Radiation therapy is also of some use in asymptomatic patients with stage III Hodgkin's disease, although its use is decreasing. As can be seen in Table 56–7, a variety of chemotherapeutic agents are active in Hodgkin's disease; however, it is now clear that combination chemotherapy produces the best results.

Combination chemotherapy is now indicated in patients presenting with stage III or IV Hodgkin's disease. Results in stage IIIA Hodgkin's disease with three cycles of chemotherapy (see below) followed by total nodal radiotherapy are clearly superior to those achieved with radiotherapy alone. Standard chemotherapy is with a four-drug combination known as MOPP, consisting of mechlorethamine, Oncovin (vincristine), procarbazine, and prednisone. This form of treatment is given repeatedly for at least 6 months and sometimes for as long as 1 year. Over 80% of previously untreated patients with advanced Hodgkin's disease (stages III and IV) go into complete remission, including the disappearance of all symptoms and objective evidence of tumors.

A "non-cross-resistant" alternative to the MOPP regimen developed by Bonadonna consists of doxorubicin (Adriamycin), bleomycin, vinblastine, and dacarbazine (ABVD). The ABVD program appears to be similar in efficacy to MOPP and, more importantly, has been of value in treatment of MOPP failures. Complex treatment regimens such as these should be under the direction of a medical oncologist who is familiar with the individual and the synergistic toxicities and contraindications for the drugs involved. After remission induction with at least six courses of MOPP or ABVD, approximately 50% of patients will remain free of all signs of Hodgkin's disease for over 2 years. The ABVD combination has not been associated with the late development of acute leukemia, perhaps because it lacks alkylating agents and procarbazine.

About half of patients who have achieved complete remission with MOPP or ABVD are cured of Hodgkin's disease.

Nitrosoureas such as lomustine are also effective in Hodgkin's disease and have been used with other drugs to reinduce remission in patients who relapse from the standard regimens. New agents observed to be active in Hodgkin's disease include mitoxantrone and isotopically labeled ferritin antibody.

2. NON-HODGKIN LYMPHOMAS

The clinical characteristics of non-Hodgkin lymphomas (NHL) are related to major histopathologic features and the immunologic origin of the neoplastic cells. The simplest useful pathologic classification is one based on cell type plus the presence or absence of nodularity in the lymphomatous tissues. In general, the nodular lymphomas have a far better prognosis (median survival up to 7 years) than do the diffuse ones (median survival about 1–2 years).

Liver and bone marrow, gastrointestinal, and localized extralymphatic involvement are all observed more commonly in NHL than in Hodgkin's disease, and a higher fraction of patients (about one-third) have stage IV disease at presentation—in contrast to 15% of patients with Hodgkin's disease.

Combination chemotherapy is clearly preferred to single-agent therapy for diffuse but not for nodular lymphomas. The nodular lymphomas are "low-grade" indolent tumors and respond much better to palliative treatment with single agents than do the diffuse lymphomas. Some of the diffuse lymphomas are curable with available drugs, whereas nodular lymphomas are not. In fact, there is no evidence that combination chemotherapy is any better than single agent chlorambucil in the treatment of low-grade nodular lymphomas.

Doxorubicin has been found to be extremely active in the treatment of non-Hodgkin lymphomas. While a number of aggressive drug combinations—including doxorubicin, vincristine, cyclophosphamide, prednisone, cytarabine, bleomycin, methotrexate, and etoposide—have been evaluated, none appear to yield superior results than a four-drug combination of cyclophosphamide, doxorubicin, vincristine and prednisone ("CHOP"). Current data suggest that one-third to one-half of patients with diffuse large cell lymphomas are cured with intensive combination chemotherapy. The new agents mitoxantrone and paclitaxel are also active in non-Hodgkin lymphomas. Alpha interferon has been observed to cause tumor regression in some nodular lymphomas; this finding will undoubtedly be investigated further. Alpha interferon is also useful in peripheral T cell lymphomas. Monoclonal antibodies directed against T or B cell antigens have recently been tested in a few patients with leukemias or lymphomas, and some antitumor effects have been observed.

MULTIPLE MYELOMA

This plasma cell tumor is now one of the "models" of neoplastic disease in humans because the tumor arises from a single tumor stem cell, and the tumor cells produce a marker protein (myeloma immunoglobulin) that allows the total body burden of tumor cells to be quantified. The tumor grows principally in the bone marrow and the surrounding bone, causing anemia, bone pain, lytic lesions, bone fractures, and anemia as well as increased susceptibility to infection. Treatment with oral alkylating agents such as melphalan or cyclophosphamide and intermittent high doses of prednisone is effective in most patients with myeloma. Relatively simple combination chemotherapy was therefore developed by combining melphalan and prednisone. Somewhat better results have been obtained in advanced disease with the use of more intensive regimens containing alkylating agents, doxorubicin, a nitrosourea, and a *Vinca* alkaloid. About 75% of myeloma patients improve with this treatment, experiencing significant relief of symptoms and prolonged survival. Resistance to chemotherapy usually develops after 2–3 years of treatment in most responding cases. Allogeneic bone marrow transplants are a possibility for patients under age 55.

An alternative strategy has been developed that may prolong remission. With this approach, patients who achieve remission with 6–12 months of induction chemotherapy are switched to long-term remission maintenance therapy with alpha interferon. Interferon maintenance may prolong remissions, but has not prolonged survival. Given its cost and toxicity, its role in myeloma remains uncertain. For patients who relapse after an initial response to chemotherapy, the combination of vincristine and doxorubicin by 4-day infusion with high-dose dexamethasone induces second remissions in about 70% of patients. Patients relapsing again after this program may be "chemosensitized" by the addition of verapamil or cyclosporine to the regimen. High-dose glucocorticoids alone are also useful in some patients.

CARCINOMA OF THE BREAST

1. STAGE I & STAGE II NEOPLASMS

The management of primary carcinoma of the breast is undergoing remarkable change as a result of major efforts at early diagnosis (through encouragement of self-examination as well as through the use of cancer detection centers) and the implementation of multimodality clinical trials incorporating systemic chemotherapy as an adjuvant to surgery. Women with stage I lateral lesions at the time of breast surgery (small primaries and negative axillary lymph node dissections) are currently treated with surgery, and have an 80% chance of cure. The current trend is toward more conservative surgery. While the standard surgical procedure is now the modified radical mastectomy, segmental mastectomy (lumpectomy) plus an axillary lymph node sampling is equally effective in treating primary tumors less than 4 cm in diameter.

Women with one or more positive lymph nodes have a very high risk of systemic recurrence and death from breast cancer. Thus, lymph node status directly indicates the risk of occult distant micrometastasis. In this situation, postoperative use of systemic cytotoxic chemotherapy in six monthly cycles of cyclophosphamide-methotrexate-fluorouracil (CMF) reduces the relapse rate and prolongs survival. Other drug combinations such as fluorouracil-doxorubicin (Adriamycin)-cyclophosphamide (FAC) are also useful. All these chemotherapy regimens have been of most benefit in women with stage II breast cancer with one to three involved lymph nodes. Women with four or more involved nodes have had limited benefit thus far from adjuvant chemotherapy. High-dose chemotherapy with autologous stem cell rescue and growth factor support is now being evaluated in women with ten or more involved nodes. Long-term analysis has clearly shown improved survival rates in node-positive premenopausal women who have been treated aggressively with multiagent combination chemotherapy. Tamoxifen is useful in postmenopausal women when used alone or with cytotoxic chemotherapy. Results from a number of randomized trials of chemotherapy for breast cancer have established that adjuvant chemotherapy for premenopausal women and adjuvant tamoxifen for postmenopausal women are of benefit to women with stage I (node-negative) breast cancer. While this group of patients has the lowest overall risk of recurrence after surgery alone (about 35–50% over 15 years), this risk can be further reduced with adjuvant therapy. The major benefit of radiotherapy appears to be that it replaces radical surgery, thus allowing the far better cosmetic results obtained with limited breast surgery.

2. STAGE III & STAGE IV NEOPLASMS

Until such multimodality programs as those discussed above are fully effective in the population at risk, the treatment of women with advanced breast cancer remains a major problem. Indeed, some women still present with inoperable "local" lesions with suspected metastases (stage III) or overt distant metastases (stage IV). Currently, most women with local or distant recurrence have had prior breast cancer surgery, or surgery plus radiotherapy.

Current treatment of advanced breast cancer is only palliative. Combination chemotherapy or endocrine therapy (or both) modestly prolongs the survival of most patients as well as relieving their symptoms. Biochemically differentiated breast cancers (as deter-

mined by the presence of receptors for estrogen or progesterone) retain many of the intrinsic hormonal sensitivities of the normal breast—including the growth stimulatory response to ovarian, adrenal, and pituitary hormones. Oophorectomy alone or with tamoxifen is reasonable in premenopausal women with ER- or PR-positive tumors who have skin, lymph node, pleural, or bone metastases. Patients who show improvement with ablative procedures also respond to the addition of tamoxifen. Patients with moderate to severe lung, liver, brain, or visceral involvement rarely benefit from hormonal maneuvers, and initial systemic chemotherapy is indicated in such cases. Irrespective of sites of involvement, if the estrogen receptor is absent, the likelihood of observing a response to hormonal therapy is less than 5%. Males with breast cancer show similar therapeutic responses to castration at almost any age.

Use of Antiestrogens

While both androgens and estrogens are useful in some patients with hormone receptor-positive breast cancer, tamoxifen has proved to be a virtually nontoxic alternative to conventional endocrine therapy of breast cancer. It has already supplanted other agents in many settings and can be considered the drug of choice for hormone receptor-positive breast cancer. "Flare" of disease is observed occasionally with tamoxifen and can herald the subsequent achievement of an excellent remission, but meticulous supportive care (eg, for bone pain or hypercalcemia) is required. Tamoxifen is effective in both pre- and postmenopausal women whose tumors are ER- or PR-positive. Tamoxifen slightly increases risk of developing uterine cancer in a frequency similar to that occuring with estrogens.

Use of Aromatase Inhibitors

Aminoglutethimide plus hydrocortisone is effective against hormone receptor-positive breast cancers. It is often used in women who have previously responded to tamoxifen or who have ER- or PR-positive breast cancers.

Systemic Chemotherapy

The use of cytotoxic drugs and hormones has become a highly specialized and increasingly effective means of treating cancer. Combination chemotherapy has improved considerably for patients with visceral involvement from advanced breast cancer. Doxorubicin is the most active single agent, with an average response rate of 40%. Combination chemotherapy has been found to induce much more durable remissions in 50–80% of patients. Combination regimens not based on doxorubicin have generally employed cyclophosphamide plus methotrexate and fluorouracil (CMF) alone or plus vincristine and prednisone (CMFVP). Doxorubicin-based combinations have generally included cyclophosphamide with either vincristine or fluorouracil. In most combination chemotherapy regimens, partial remissions have a median duration of about 10 months and complete remissions a duration of about 15 months. Unfortunately, only 10–20% of patients achieve complete remissions with any of these regimens, and complete remissions are usually not very long-lasting in metastatic breast cancer. The addition of tamoxifen to such programs yields only modest additional improvement. When doxorubicin is used in such combinations, it is generally discontinued before the patient reaches cardiotoxic limits. At that point, other drugs are generally substituted. Paclitaxel has recently been found to be active in previously treated women with metastatic breast cancer, with up to 50% of patients responding.

CHORIOCARCINOMA OF THE UTERUS

This rare tumor that arises from fetal trophoblastic tissue was the first metastatic cancer cured with chemotherapy. Massive doses of methotrexate—25 mg/d for 4 or 5 days—will produce a high percentage of cures associated with complete regression of metastatic lesions and disappearance of chorionic gonadotropic hormones in the urine. Therapy should be given repeatedly until some months after all evidence of the disease has disappeared. An alternative regimen with a high cure rate (including cures of methotrexate treatment failures) combines etoposide with cisplatin.

CARCINOMA OF THE OVARY

This neoplasm often remains occult until it has metastasized to the peritoneal cavity; it may present with malignant ascites. It is important to stage such neoplasms accurately using laparoscopy, ultrasound, or CT scanning. Patients with stage I tumors appear to benefit from pelvic radiotherapy and might receive additional benefit from combination chemotherapy. Combination chemotherapy is now the standard approach to stage III and stage IV disease. The most useful combinations include cyclophosphamide and cisplatin or carboplatin, which produce remission in 70–80% of patients and complete remission in approximately 40%. Paclitaxel was recently approved by the FDA for use in women with refractory ovarian cancer and induces remissions in up to one-third of such patients. It is currently being studied in combination with cisplatin. Radiotherapy (including whole-abdomen radiotherapy) does not improve the survival rates of patients with higher stages of involvement and is generally not indicated. Multimodality therapy utilizing surgery, radiotherapy, and adjuvant combination chemotherapy in patients with stage I and stage II neoplasms has shown promising signs of effi-

cacy in current clinical trials. Assays of tumor stem cells are being increasingly used to tailor treatment regimens for individual patients with ovarian cancer.

TESTICULAR NEOPLASMS

Single-agent chemotherapy has produced impressive tumor regressions in some advanced nonseminomatous testicular neoplasms but few complete responses lasting longer than 1 year. The introduction of combination chemotherapy with cisplatin, vinblastine, and bleomycin (PVB) has made an impressive change in these statistics. Ninety-five percent of patients respond to chemotherapy, with approximately 90% entering complete remission. It now seems likely that over half of patients achieving complete remission are cured with chemotherapy. Substitution of etoposide for vinblastine yields similar remission and cure rates with significantly less hematologic toxicity. In advanced disease (patients who have positive lymph nodes), adjuvant use of this treatment is generally not indicated because over half of patients do not relapse after primary surgery that includes retroperitoneal lymphadenectomy and because the salvage rate with chemotherapy in recurrent disease is quite good.

CARCINOMA OF THE PROSTATE

Carcinoma of the prostate was one of the first forms of cancer shown to be responsive to hormonal manipulation. Orchiectomy or low-dose estrogen therapy (or both) has resulted in prolonged improvement in patients with bone lesions. Similar results have also been obtained with the gonadotropin-releasing hormone agonists. These agents appear to be less toxic than estrogens but are much more expensive. Use of the antiandrogen flutamide after orchiectomy or with leuprolide is also of palliative value. Hormonal treatment reduces symptoms in 70–80% of patients and produces a significant degree of regression of established metastases. Subjective relief of bone pain, objective evidence of normalization of involved bones, and reduction of prostate-specific antigen and prostatic alkaline phosphatase are common criteria of response to therapy for this disorder. The antifungal agent ketoconazole inhibits androgenic steroid synthesis and may find increasing application in the treatment of prostate cancer in the future. The growth factor antagonist (and antiparasitic drug) suramin has recently been reported to have anticancer activity in patients with metastatic prostate cancer. It is assumed to act via an endocrine mechanism. However, chemotherapy is still of minimal curative value for this disease.

CARCINOMA OF THE THYROID

Until recently, only radioactive iodine (^{131}I) had therapeutic activity in metabolic thyroid cancer, and its effects were limited to well-differentiated tumors that could concentrate iodine. It is now clear that doxorubicin and cisplatin have significant activity against a variety of histologic types of thyroid cancer (particularly anaplastic lesions), induce excellent regressions of tumor, and prolong survival. The use of combination chemotherapy with ^{131}I therapy in thyroid cancer appears promising for high-risk patients who have anaplastic cell characteristics on histologic examination or vascular invasion of the thyroid gland.

GASTROINTESTINAL CARCINOMAS

This group of neoplasms has only limited sensitivity to available chemotherapeutic agents. All these lesions release carcinoembryonic antigen (CEA), and radioimmunoassay can be used to detect recurrence after surgery as well as response to (or relapse from) systemic chemotherapy. Colorectal adenocarcinoma is the most common type, and only 43% of cases are curable with surgery. Patients with micrometastases to regional lymph nodes are candidates for adjuvant chemotherapy with fluorouracil plus levamisole. This combination has been reported to reduce the recurrence rate after surgery by 35% in these patients and clearly improves survival as compared with surgery alone. Fluorouracil is the most active single agent for patients with metastatic disease, but it induces only a 21% remission rate with virtually no complete remissions. The effects of fluorouracil can be enhanced in patients with metastatic colorectal cancer by coadministration of leucovorin or interferon (or both). Lomustine, mitomycin, and cyclophosphamide all have definite but lesser degrees of activity. Mitomycin or carmustine also acts against these carcinomas when used with fluorouracil. All of these regimens induce substantial hematologic toxicity. Because these combinations do not induce complete remission, do not prolong survival, and are rather toxic, their use should be limited to patients with symptomatic metastatic disease. Recently, hepatic artery catheterization and repeated arterial infusion of fluorouracil or FUDR have proved useful for treating patients with colorectal cancer that has metastasized only to the liver. Fluorouracil alone has been extensively tried as a surgical adjuvant and has produced a minor reduction in the relapse rate observed with surgery alone.

Gastric carcinoma and pancreatic carcinoma are less common but far more aggressive lesions that usually cannot be completely resected surgically and are generally grossly metastatic at the time of surgery. The combination of fluorouracil, doxorubicin, and mitomycin relieves symptoms in some patients.

"Neoadjuvant" chemotherapy with aggressive use of 5-FU prior to surgery appears to have some promise.

Islet cell carcinoma of the pancreas arising from B cells and secreting insulin has been found to be exquisitely sensitive to the antibiotic streptozocin. The results have been good in this rare tumor, and this therapy may be curative in some patients. Streptozocin is often used with several other agents, eg, fluorouracil, doxorubicin, and mitomycin.

BRONCHOGENIC CARCINOMA

The management of epidermoid cancers, large cell cancers, and adenocarcinomas of the lung is very unsatisfactory, and prevention (primarily through avoidance of cigarette smoking) remains the most important means of control. The average life expectancy after diagnosis has been 8 months. The tumor can rarely be cured by surgery, and x-ray therapy is used primarily for palliation of pain, obstruction, or bleeding. However, in most cases of lung cancer, distant metastases have occurred by the time of diagnosis and chemotherapy therefore appears to be the most feasible approach.

Although lung cancer had been notoriously resistant to all conventional forms of cancer chemotherapy, several novel approaches now show promise. Histologic examination of tumor tissue has been found to be important in identifying subgroups of patients who will respond to chemotherapy. Patients with small cell (oat cell) lung cancer (the most rapidly growing type) show the best responses to combination chemotherapy with agents such as cisplatin, etoposide, doxorubicin, cyclophosphamide, methotrexate, and nitrosoureas. Patients with limited small cell carcinomas respond best to such regimens. They may also require whole brain irradiation to sterilize occult central nervous system metastases, which are often present. However, the role of prophylactic whole brain irradiation remains uncertain because of the significant impairment of brain function that eventually develops in such patients. For non-small cell lung cancer, combinations of etoposide and cisplatin have some limited benefit.

MALIGNANT MELANOMA & MISCELLANEOUS SARCOMAS

Metastatic melanoma is one of the most difficult neoplasms to treat. Most chemotherapeutic agents are reported to induce regression in at least 10% of melanoma patients; however, spontaneous regressions also occur, especially in skin metastases, so regression of cutaneous lesions does not necessarily imply sensitivity to chemotherapy. Immunologic reactivity to the tumor by host lymphocytes may partially explain the evanescent changes in skin lesions, but "spontaneous regression" of visceral disease is rare and metastases occur in virtually every organ in the body. Dacarbazine and cisplatin are the most active cytotoxic agents. Biologic agents, including human leukocyte interferon (natural or recombinant), may have a similar order of activity. Interleukin-2 may also be of occasional benefit. Tamoxifen may potentiate the effects of multidrug combinations that include cisplatin.

Osteogenic sarcoma and Ewing's sarcoma respond to doxorubicin, and a combination of doxorubicin and dacarbazine may induce substantial regressions in about 40% of cases of rhabdomyosarcoma, fibrosarcoma, osteogenic sarcoma, and related tumors. The use of adjuvant therapy that includes doxorubicin after primary surgery for osteosarcoma has already lengthened the median survival time. This therapy appears likely to increase the long-term salvage rate for this otherwise almost uniformly fatal neoplasm. Similar results have recently been reported for patients with soft tissue sarcomas of the extremities for whom adjuvant chemotherapy has clearly prolonged disease-free survival. When this approach has been applied together with limb-salvage surgery, it has reduced the need for amputation as part of initial surgery. For grossly metastatic soft-tissue sarcomas, first-line therapy uses doxorubicin-based combinations. Patients in relapse from these regimens sometimes benefit from therapy with ifosfamide.

BRAIN TUMORS

Stage III and stage IV astrocytomas (predominantly glioblastoma multiforme) are the most common primary brain tumors, and they have been extraordinarily refractory to surgical therapy. Although advances in diagnostic methods such as computerized tomography (CT) scanning have better delineated the site of primary involvement for surgical therapy, the median survival time with surgery alone is still about 20 weeks. The addition of whole brain radiotherapy (approximately 5500 cGy) or carmustine alone (220 mg/m^2 every 6–8 weeks) increases the median survival time to 36 weeks, whereas the use of multimodality therapy (surgery plus radiotherapy plus carmustine) increases it to 50 weeks, with approximately 25% of patients still alive at 18 months. This multimodality approach, although still limited in efficacy, can be recommended as palliation for patients with such tumors until more effective regimens are developed. The experimental agent tenizolamide appears to be active in brain tumor therapy and is currently in early clinical trials.

CONTROL OF MALIGNANT EFFUSIONS & ASCITES

The direct injection of mechlorethamine or other anticancer drugs into the involved cavity will eliminate or suppress ascites and effusions caused by carcinoma in about two-thirds of patients. The method is useful irrespective of the type of primary tumor.

The procedure involves withdrawing most of the pleural or ascitic fluid and then injecting the drug into the cavity. The dose of mechlorethamine employed intrapleurally is 0.4 mg/kg, or a total dose of 20–30 mg in the average patient. The solution is prepared immediately before administration so as to avoid loss of potency through hydrolysis. A free flow of fluid from the cavity must be established before the drug is injected to avoid injection into the tissues. Pleural or peritoneal effusions caused by ovarian or breast carcinoma are frequently responsive to an intracavitary dose of 60 mg/m^2 of bleomycin. After the drug is injected, the patient is placed in a variety of positions in order to distribute the drug throughout the pleural cavity. On the following day, the remaining fluid is withdrawn.

Pain, nausea, and vomiting sometimes occur following injection of mechlorethamine into the pleural cavity. Nausea and vomiting can often be controlled by giving an intramuscular dose of a phenothiazine immediately before the procedure and at intervals following the injection. Bone marrow depression is mild with this method of administration, except in patients who have received extensive radiation therapy. Agents such as bleomycin or thiotepa are preferable to mechlorethamine for intraperitoneal use, since they cause significantly less peritoneal irritation and pain.

Tetracycline has been employed intrapleurally with similar therapeutic benefit. Local pain and fever are commonly noted, but there is no systemic hematopoietic depression.

EVALUATION OF TUMOR RESPONSE

Since cancer chemotherapy can induce clinical improvement, significant toxicity, or both, it is extremely important to critically assess the effects of treatment to determine that the net effect is beneficial. Preliminary evidence regarding the use of the tumor stem cell assay to determine the appropriate form of chemotherapy is quite encouraging, particularly with respect to rejecting drugs that would probably cause toxicity without compensating clinical benefit. The assay also appears to be relatively accurate (70%) in identifying drugs that will prove useful in the patient. The following paragraphs discuss the most valuable signs to follow to determine the benefits of current chemotherapy.

Shrinkage in tumor size can be demonstrated by physical examination, chest film or other x-ray, or special scanning procedures such as bone scanning (breast, prostate cancer), CT scan, MRI, or ultrasonography.

Another sign of therapeutic response is a significant decrease in the quantity of a tumor product or marker substance that reflects the amount of tumor in the body. Examples of such markers include paraproteins in the serum or urine in multiple myeloma and macroglobulinemia, chorionic gonadotropin in choriocarcinoma and testicular tumors, urinary steroids in adrenal carcinoma and paraneoplastic Cushing's syndrome, 5-hydroxyindoleacetic acid in carcinoid syndrome, and prostate-specific antigen in prostatic carcinoma. Secreted tumor antigens such as alpha-fetoprotein can be found in hepatoma, in teratoembryonal carcinoma, and in occasional cases of gastric carcinoma; the carcinoembryonic antigen can be found in carcinomas of the colon, lung, and breast. The tumor antigen CA 125 is very useful in following the response to treatment in women with ovarian cancer.

Normalization of function of organs that were previously impaired by the presence of a tumor is a useful indicator of drug effectiveness. Examples of such improvement include the normalization of liver function (eg, increased serum albumin) in patients known to have liver metastases and improvement in neurologic findings in patients with cerebral metastases. Disappearance of the signs and symptoms of the paraneoplastic syndromes often falls in this general category and can be taken as an indication of tumor response.

A valuable sign of clinical improvement is the general well-being of the patient. Although this finding is a combination of subjective and objective factors and may be subject to placebo effects, it nonetheless serves as an obvious and useful sign of clinical improvement and can be used to reassess some of the objective observations listed above. Factors to be considered in determining general well-being include improved appetite, weight gain, and improved "performance status" (eg, ambulatory versus bedridden).

Evaluation of factors such as activity status has the advantage of summarizing beneficial and toxic effects of chemotherapy and enables the physician to judge whether the net effect of chemotherapy is worthwhile palliation. Standardized scales are available (Karnovsky Scale, Eastern Cooperative Oncology Group Scale).

SECOND MALIGNANCIES & CANCER CHEMOTHERAPY

Second malignancy is a late complication of some types of cancer chemotherapy. The most frequent second malignancy is acute myelogenous leukemia (AML). Aside from AML, other second malignancies are sporadic. AML has been observed in up to 15% of patients with Hodgkin's disease who have received radiotherapy plus MOPP and in patients with multiple myeloma, ovarian, or breast carcinoma treated with melphalan. Several alkylating agents (as well as ionizing radiation) are considered to be leukemogenic. Additionally, procarbazine (a component of the MOPP combination) is known to be mutagenic to bacteria and carcinogenic in animals. The mechanisms of carcinogenesis with these other agents remain poorly understood. While the risk of AML is relatively small, the benefit of complete remission or cure of Hodgkin's disease or remission of other neoplasms is considerable. As further advances are made in chemical control and cure of cancer, the problem of the second malignant tumor assumes greater importance. There are already hints that certain alkylating agents (eg, cyclophosphamide) may be less carcinogenic than others. Systematic testing of the carcinogenicity of anticancer drugs in several animal species allows less toxic agents to be identified and substituted for other more carcinogenic ones in chemotherapy regimens. In this fashion, the risk of second tumors should be reduced without sacrificing therapeutic benefit.

PREPARATIONS AVAILABLE

The reader is referred to the manufacturers' literature for the most recent information.

REFERENCES

General
Bonadonna G, Valagussa P: Adjuvant systemic therapy for resectable breast cancer. J Clin Oncol 1985;3:259.

Chabner BA, Collins JM (editors): *Cancer Chemotherapy: Principles and Practice.* Lippincott, 1990.

Cheng KK et al: Pickled vegetables in the aetiology of oesophageal cancer in Hong Kong Chinese. Lancet 1992;339:1314.

DeVita VT Jr, Hellman S, Rosenberg SA (editors): *Cancer: Principles and Practice of Oncology,* 4th ed. Lippincott, 1993.

Druker BJ et al: Oncogenes, growth factors, and signal transduction. N Engl J Med 1989;321:1383.

Endicott JA, Ling V: The biochemistry of P-glycoprotein-mediated multidrug resistance. Annu Rev Biochem 1989;58:137.

Giovanella BC et al: DNA topoisomerase I-targeted chemotherapy of human colon cancer in xenografts. Science 1989;246:1046.

Gottesman MM, Pastan I: Biochemistry of multidrug resistance mediated by the multidrug transporter. Annu Rev Biochem 1993;62:385.

Harris CC, Hollstein M: Clinical implications of the p53 tumor-suppressor gene. N Engl J Med 1993;329:1318.

Kaiser HE (editor): *Cancer Growth and Progression.* Kluwer, 1989.

Koutsky LA et al: A cohort study of the risk of cervical intraepithelial neoplasia grade 2 or 3 in relation to papillomavirus infection. N Engl J Med 1992;27:1272.

McManaway ME et al: Tumour-specific inhibition of lymphoma growth by an antisense oligodeoxynucleotide. Lancet 1990;335:808.

Moertel CG: Chemotherapy for colorectal cancer. N Engl J Med 1994;330:1136.

Munzarova M, Kovarik J: Is cancer a macrophage-mediated autoaggressive disease? Lancet 1987;1:952.

Reiss M et al: Induction of tumor cell differentiation as a therapeutic approach: Preclinical models for hematopoietic and solid neoplasms. Cancer Treat Rep 1986;70: 201.

Rinsky RA et al: Benzene and leukemia: An epidemiologic risk assessment. N Engl J Med 1987;316:1044.

Rosenberg SA The low grade non-Hodgkin's lymphomas: Challenges and opportunities. J Clin Oncol 1985;3:299.

Salmon SE (editor): *Adjuvant Therapy of Cancer VII.* Lippincott, 1993.

Salmon SE: Malignant disorders. In: *Current Medical Diagnosis & Treatment 1991.* Schroeder SA et al (editors). Appleton & Lange, 1991.

Sartorelli AC: Therapeutic attack of hypoxic cells of solid tumors: Presidential address. Cancer Res 1988; 48:775.

Someveld P et al: Modulation of multidrug-resistant multiple myeloma by cyclosporin. Lancet 1992;340:255.

Toguchida J et al: Prevalence and spectrum of germline mutations of the p53 gene among patients with sarcoma. N Engl J Med 1992;326:1301.

Vähäkangas KH et al: Mutations of p53 and *ras* genes in radon-associated lung cancer from uranium miners. Lancet 1992;339:576.

Vokes EE et al: Head and neck cancer. N Engl J Med 1993;328:184.

Williams SD et al. Immediate adjuvant chemotherapy versus observation with treatment at relapse in pathological stage II testicular cancer. N Engl J Med 1987; 317:1433.

Withers HR: Biological basis of radiation therapy for cancer. Lancet 1992;339:156.

Yandell DW et al: Oncogenic point mutations in the human retinoblastoma gene: Their applications to genetic counseling. N Engl J Med 1989;321:1689.

Alkylating Agents
Boice JD Jr et al: Leukemia and preleukemia after adjuvant treatment of gastrointestinal cancer with semustine (methyl-CCNU). N Engl J Med 1983;309:1079.

Curtis RE et al: Risk of leukemia after chemotherapy and radiation treatment for breast cancer. N Engl J Med 1992; 326:1745.

Antimetabolites
Jolivet J et al: The pharmacology and clinical use of methotrexate. N Engl J Med 1983;309:1094.

Juliusson G, Elmhorn-Rosenborg A, Liliemark J: Response to 2-chlorodeoxyadenosine in patients with B-cell chronic lymphocytic leukemia resistant to flu-darabine. N Engl J Med 1992;327:1056.

Koren G et al: Systemic exposure to mercaptopurine as a prognostic factor in acute lymphocytic leukemia in children. N Engl J Med 1990;323:17.

Piro LD et al: Lasting remissions in hairy-cell leukemia induced by a single infusion of 2-chlorodeoxyadenosine. N Engl J Med 1990;322:1117.

Antibiotics & Other Agents
Weissberg JB: Randomized clinical trial of mitomycin C as an adjunct to radiotherapy in head and neck cancer. Int J Rad Oncol Biol Phys 1989;17:3.

Winick NJ et al: Secondary acute myeloid leukemia in children with acute lymphoblastic leukemia treated with etoposide. J Clin Oncol 1993;11:209.

Young RC et al: The anthracycline antineoplastic drugs. N Engl J Med 1981;305:139.

Hormonally Active Agents
Ahmann FR et al: Zoladex: A sustained-release, monthly luteinizing hormone-releasing hormone analogue for the treatment of advanced prostate cancer. J Clin Oncol 1987;5:912.

Butturini A et al: Use of recombinant granulocyte-macrophage colony-stimulating factor in the Brazil radiation accident. Lancet 1988;2:471.

Fisher B et al: A randomized clinical trial evaluating tamoxifen in the treatment of patients with node-negative breast cancer who have estrogen receptor-positive tumors. N Engl J Med 1989;320:479.

Leuprolide Study Group: Leuprolide versus diethylstilbestrol for metastatic prostate cancer. N Engl J Med 1984;311:1281.

Love RR et al: Effects of tamoxifen on bone mineral density in postmenopausal women with breast cancer. N Engl J Med 1992;326:852.

Biologic Response Modifiers
& Immunologic Agents

Bar MH et al: Metastatic malignant melanoma treated with combined bolus and continuous infusion of interleukin-2 and lymphokine-activated killer cells. J Clin Oncol 1990;8:1138.

Dianzani F, Antonelli G, Capobianchi MR: *The Interferon System.* Serono Symposium Publications. Raven Press, 1989.

Grander D et al: Interferon-induced enhancement of 2′,5′-oligoadenylate synthetase in mid-gut carcinoid tumors. Lancet 1990;336:337.

Groopman JE, Molina JM, Scadden DT: Hematopoietic growth factors: Biology and clinical applications. N Engl J Med 1989;321:1449.

Hong WK et al: Prevention of second primary tumors with isotretinoin in squamous cell carcinoma of the head and neck. N Engl J Med 1990;323:795.

Krown SE et al: Preliminary observations on the effect of recombinant leukocyte A interferon in homosexual men with Kaposi's sarcoma. N Engl J Med 1983; 308:1071.

Kwak LW et al: Induction of immune responses in patients with B-cell lymphoma against the surface-immunoglobulin idiotype expressed by their tumors. N Engl J Med 1992;327:1209.

Mandelli F et al: Maintenance treatment with recombinant interferon alfa-2b in patients with multiple myeloma responding to conventional induction chemotherapy. N Engl J Med 1990;322:1430.

Ohno R et al: Effect of granulocyte colony-stimulating factor after intensive induction therapy in relapsed or refractory acute leukemia. N Engl J Med 1990;323: 871.

Rosenberg SA et al: A progress report on the treatment of 157 patients with advanced cancer using lymphokine-activated killer cells and interleukin-2 or high-dose interleukin-2 alone. N Engl J Med 1987;316:889.

Rosenberg SA et al: Gene transfer into humans: Immunotherapy of patients with advanced melanoma, using tumor-infiltrating lymphocytes modified by retroviral gene transduction. N Engl J Med 1990;323:570.

Socinski MA et al: Granulocyte-macrophage colony stimulating factor expands the circulating haemopoietic progenitor cell compartment in man. Lancet 1988; 1:1194.

Vadhan-Raj S et al: Effects of recombinant human granulocyte-macrophage colony-stimulating factor in patients with myelodysplastic syndromes. N Engl J Med 1987;317:1545.

Combined Modality or Drug Combinations

Al-Sarraf M: Head and neck cancer: Chemotherapy concepts. Semin Oncol 1988;15:70.

Baum M: Controlled trial of tamoxifen as adjuvant agent in management of early breast cancer (for Nolvadex Adjuvant Trial Organization). Lancet 1983;1:257.

Bell DR et al: Detection of P-glycoprotein in ovarian cancer: A molecular marker associated with multidrug resistance. J Clin Oncol 1985;3:311.

Bunn PA et al: Clinical course of retrovirus-associated adult T-cell lymphoma in the United States. N Engl J Med 1983;309:257.

Canellos GP et al: Chemotherapy of advanced Hodgkin's disease with MOPP, ABVD, or MOPP alternating with ABVD. N Engl J Med 1992;327:1478.

Champlin R, Gale RP: Acute myelogenous leukemia: Recent advances in therapy. Blood 1987;69:1551.

Coates A et al: Improving the quality of life during chemotherapy for advanced breast cancer: A comparison of intermittent and continuous treatment strategies. N Engl J Med 1987;317:1490.

Cocconi G et al: Treatment of metastatic malignant melanoma with dacarbazine plus tamoxifen. N Engl J Med 1992;327:516.

Early Breast Cancer Trialists' Collaborative Group: Effects of adjuvant tamoxifen and of cytotoxic therapy on mortality in early breast cancer: An overview of 61 randomized trials among 28,896 women. N Engl J Med 1988;319:1681.

Early Breast Cancer Trialists' Collaborative Group: Systemic treatment of early breast cancer by hormonal, cytotoxic, or immune therapy. Lancet 1992;339:1.

Fisher RI et al: Comparison of a standard regimen (CHOP) with three intensive chemotherapy regimens for advanced non-Hodgkin's lymphoma. N Engl J Med 1993;328:1002.

Friedman EL et al: Therapeutic guidelines and results in advanced seminoma. J Clin Oncol 1985;3:1325.

Harris JR et al: Breast cancer. (Three parts.) N Engl J Med 1992;327:319, 390, 473.

Herskovic A et al: Combined chemotherapy and radiotherapy compared with radiotherapy alone in patients with cancer of the esophagus. N Engl J Med 1992; 326:1593.

Jaakkimainen L et al: Counting the costs of chemotherapy in a National Cancer Institute of Canada randomized trial in non-small cell lung cancer. J Clin Oncol 1990;8:1301.

Kaldor JM et al: Leukemia following chemotherapy for ovarian cancer. N Engl J Med 1990;322:1.

Kaldor JM et al: Leukemia following Hodgkin's disease. N Engl J Med 1990;322:7.

Kaye FJ et al: A randomized trial comparing electron-beam radiation and chemotherapy with topical therapy in the initial treatment of mycosis fungoides. N Engl J Med 1989;321:1784.

Kaye SB et al: Randomised study of two doses of cisplatin with cyclophosphamide in epithelial ovarian cancer. Lancet 1992;340:329.

Link MP et al: Results of treatment of childhood localized non-Hodgkin's lymphoma with combination chemotherapy with or without radiotherapy. N Engl J Med 1990;322:1169.

Merlano M et al: Treatment of advanced squamous-cell carcinoma of the head and neck with alternating chemotherapy and radiotherapy. N Engl J Med 1992; 327:1115.

Miller TP, Jones SE: Initial chemotherapy for clinically localized lymphomas of unfavorable histology. Blood 1983;62:413.

Moertel CG et al: Levamisole and fluorouracil for adjuvant therapy of resected colon carcinoma. N Engl J Med 1990;322:352.

Pedersen-Bjergaard J: Carcinoma of the urinary bladder after treatment with cyclophosphamide for non-Hodgkin's lymphoma. N Engl J Med 1988;318:1028.

Rivera GK et al: Treatment of acute lymphoblastic leukemia: 30 years' experience at St. Jude Children's Research Hospital. N Engl J Med 1993;329:1289.

Rosenberg SA et al: Prospective randomized evaluation of adjuvant chemotherapy in adults with soft tissue sarcomas of the extremities. Cancer 1983;52:424.

Salmon SE et al: Alternating combination chemotherapy improves survival in multiple myeloma: A southwest oncology study. J Clin Oncol 1983;1:453.

Santoro A et al: Alternating drug combinations in the treatment of advanced Hodgkin's disease. N Engl J Med 1982;306:770.

Williams SD et al: Treatment of disseminated germ-cell tumors with cisplatin, bleomycin, and either vinblastine or etoposide. N Engl J Med 1987;316:1435.

Young RC et al: Adjuvant therapy in stage I and stage II epithelial ovarian cancer. N Engl J Med 1990;322:1021

Miscellaneous

Byrne TN: Spinal cord compression from epidural metastases. N Engl J Med 1992;327:614.

Chan HSL et al: Immunohistochemical detection of P-glycoprotein: Prognostic correlation in soft tissue sarcoma of childhood. J Clin Oncol 1990;8:689.

Clarkson B: Retinoic acid in acute promyelocytic leukemia: The promise and the paradox. Cancer Cells 1991; 3:211.

Cubeddu LX et al: Efficacy of ondansetron (GR 38032F) and the role of serotonin in cisplatin-induced nausea and vomiting. N Engl J Med 1990;322:810.

Gabert J et al: Detection of residual bcr/abl translocation by polymerase chain reaction in chronic myeloid leukaemia patients after bone marrow transplantation. Lancet 1989;2:1125.

Harris AL et al: Comparison of short-term and continuous chemotherapy (mitoxantrone) for advanced breast cancer. Lancet 1990;335:186.

Hong WK et al: Prevention of second primary tumors with isotretinoin in squamous cell carcinoma of the head and neck. N Engl J Med 1990;323:795

Luton JP et al: Clinical features of adrenocortical carcinoma, prognostic factors, and the effect of mitotane therapy. N Engl J Med 1990;322:1195.

Patt YZ et al: Imaging with Indium[111]-labeled anticarcinoembryonic antigen monoclonal antibody ZCE-025 of recurrent colorectal or carcinoembryonic antigen-producing cancer in patients with rising serum carcinoembryonic antigen levels and occult metastases. J Clin Oncol 1990;8:1246.

Ralston SH et al: Comparison of three intravenous bisphosphonates in cancer-associated hypercalcaemia. Lancet 1989;2:1180.

Rifkin MD et al: Comparison of magnetic resonance imaging and ultrasonography in staging early prostate cancer. N Engl J Med 1990;323:621.

Tavorian T et al: Prolonged disease-free survival after autologous bone marrow transplantation in patients with non-Hodgkin's lymphoma with a poor prognosis. N Engl J Med 1987;316:1499.

57

Immunopharmacology

Jose Alexandre M. Barbuto, MD, PhD, Evan M. Hersh, MD, & Sydney E. Salmon, MD

THE IMMUNE MECHANISM

Agents that suppress the immune response now play an important role in tissue transplantation procedures and in certain diseases associated with disorders of immunity. Although some of the details of the overall immune mechanism are still uncertain, a general scheme of the steps involved in the genesis of specific immunity can be sketched (Figures 57–1 and 57–2) as a means of placing the effects and toxicities of immunosuppressive agents in perspective.

Specific immunity appears to result from the interaction of antigens (substances the host normally recognizes as foreign) with mononuclear cells that circulate in the blood, lymph, and tissues. The nature of self-recognition, or "tolerance," is complex, but it appears to be defined in utero, during the development of the lymphoid tissues. Mechanisms that have been implicated in tolerance include clonal deletion, blockade of antigen receptor by antigen-antibody complex, antibody to cell surface immunoglobulin, and active T cell-mediated suppression. Although lymphoid cells derived embryologically from the thymus and bone marrow play the major role in the development of specific immunity, a critical initial "antigen-processing" step occurs in **antigen-presenting cells (APCs),** which include the dendritic cell (thought to be derived from the blood monocyte or the tissue macrophage), Langerhans cells, macrophages, and B lymphocytes. Macrophages or supernatants from macrophage cultures also can stimulate or inhibit proliferative reactions among immune cells. These reactions are mediated by peptide growth factors. Interleukins have also been identified that promote or inhibit proliferation of B cells, T cells, or both. Monocytes and macrophages also secrete prostaglandin E_2, which has been found to inhibit proliferation of B and T cell precursors. The ability of lymphoid cells to interact with specific antigens appears to be genetically determined, with different lymphoid clones having individual specificities for different antigenic determinants. Part of the genetic regulation of proliferation of cells of the immune system also appears to reside in the antigen-presenting cell that expresses major

ACRONYMS USED IN THIS CHAPTER	
ALG	Antilymphocyte globulin
APC	Antigen-presenting cell
ATG	Antithymocyte globulin
CD	Cluster of differentiation
CSF	Colony-stimulating factor
CTLC	Cytotoxic T lymphocyte
FKBP	FK-binding protein
HAMA	Human anti-mouse antibody
HLA	Human leukocyte antigen
IFN	Interferon
IgE, IgG, IgM, etc	Immunoglobulin E, G, M, etc
IL	Interleukin
MHC	Major histocompatibility complex
NK	Natural killer
PAF	Platelet-activating factor
TNF	Tumor necrosis factor

histocompatibility antigens which present the foreign antigen to T lymphocytes.

Individual cell types involved in the immune response can be recognized by means of monoclonal antibodies to specific cell surface constituents designated as **clusters of differentiation (CDs)** and identified by number. While some CDs are identified only as membrane antigens and have unknown functions, others are now recognized to be specific receptors or enzymes. An important set of molecules on the surface of antigen-presenting cells is the **major histocompatibility complex** (MHC) class II antigens (also known as Ia antigens). The MHC class II antigens bind antigen fragments, and the resulting complex is recognized by helper T cells. The interaction of T cells with antigen bound to class II antigens greatly potentiates immune responses, including the B cell and antibody response.

A basic dualism governs the function of the lym-

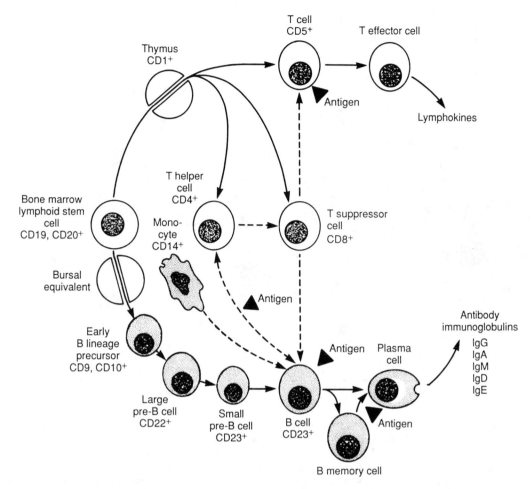

Figure 57–1. Genesis and interactions of the immune system. Solid arrows denote stimulation or development. Dashed arrows indicate inhibition. Cell surface antigen markers *(CDs)* are shown at the earliest point in their appearance. They generally persist at later stages of differentiation in a given cell lineage.

phoid system. Two different types of lymphoid cells—**T** and **B cells**—mediate cellular immunity and serologic immunity, respectively (Figure 57–3). Both types of cells are found in the blood and in various tissues of the body as well as in peripheral lymphoid tissues (including lymph nodes, spleen, and bone marrow). Long-lived clones of small lymphoid cells derived from the thymus (T cells) appear to recognize the antigen in the context of MHC antigens. The CD3a+7+ T cell appears to arise from a bone marrow progenitor under the influence of thymic hormones, which are produced by the epithelioid component of the thymus. The earliest-developing T cells in the immune system are the CD1+ thymocytes. The proliferation of clones of antigen-specific T cells, which occurs after contact with antigen fragments, is responsible for the development of "cellular immunity," which can be demonstrated in delayed hypersensitivity reactions and is important in tissue

graft rejection as well as resistance to viral, fungal, and mycobacterial infections.

Specific T cell receptors for antigen on the cell surface account for their immunologic specificity. Specific subsets of T cells also influence or modulate antibody synthesis by B cells. These include both CD4+ "helper" and CD8+ "suppressor" T cells. The T cell subsets can be assayed functionally and with monoclonal antibodies directed against specific cell surface antigens that differ on the T helper and suppressor cells. T helper and suppressor cells interact with different classes of MHC molecules. T suppressor cells interact with the antigens bound to MHC class I, whereas T helper cells interact with MHC class II (Ia) antigens. Another important T cell subtype is the cytotoxic T lymphocyte (CTLC), normally a CD8+ cell, involved in transplant rejection. T cells appear to exert their effects by direct cytotoxic interaction (eg, with tumor cells or transplants) and by release of ef-

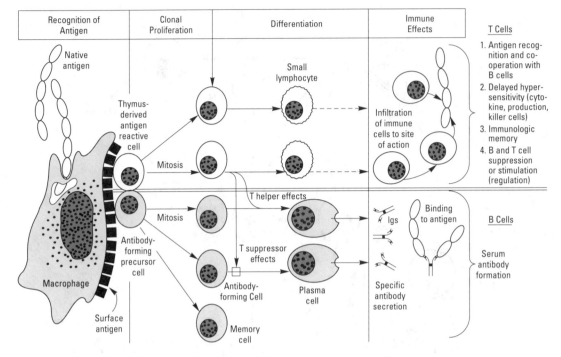

Figure 57–2. A simplified scheme of cellular and humoral immunity.

fector substances called **cytokines** (Table 57–1). Other cells in the lymphoreticular apparatus also produce cytokines.

The genesis of specific antibody **immunoglobulins** resides in the progeny of a second type of lymphoid cell, the B cell, derived from the bone marrow. The first identifiable cell committed to this series is the pro-B cell, which has unrearranged immunoglobulin genes and expresses HLA class II antigens, CD19, CD37, CD38, and CD40. B cells can be identified by the presence of intact monoclonal immunoglobulins on their surfaces that serve as antigen receptors. B cells also have receptors for complement components and immune complexes and present cell surface MHC (Ia) antigen. Prior to contact with antigen, lymphocyte surface immunoglobulin is predominantly of the IgD and IgM classes.

By the time of birth, lymph node and splenic architecture includes parafollicular cuffs of thymus-derived lymphocytes and follicular nests of immunoglobulin-synthesizing cells that form germinal centers. Intimate interactions between antigen-presenting cells, bearing the antigen in an immunogenic form on the cell surface and complementary clones of T cells, are thought to be required before the clonal proliferation of T cells can result in the development of cellular immunity. Antigen-specific activated T cells interact with B cells and induce their differentiation into antibody-forming cells (Figures 57–1 and 57–2). The primary immunoproliferative response is

augmented or inhibited by T cells with helper or suppressor function.

Natural killer (NK) cells (CD16,56,57+) may play an important role in tumor rejection and viral immunity. NK cells are large granular lymphocytes (with azurophilic cytoplasmic granules) that are surface immunoglobulin-negative and Fc receptor-positive, with low affinity for sheep red blood cells. Studies with monoclonal antisera suggest that NK cells may be of T cell or monocytic origin, but they may represent an entirely separate lineage of lymphoid cells. NK cells have reactivity against tumor and normal cells and may play an important role in host defense. However, their in vivo relevance remains uncertain.

Antibody-forming cells can increase their synthetic capacity by further differentiation into plasma cells, clones of which specifically secrete large amounts of antibody of one of the immunoglobulin classes— **IgG, IgA, IgM, IgD, or IgE.** During the course of this differentiation, individual clones may "switch" their immunoglobulin type from IgD to IgM, IgG, IgA, or IgE, even though the active site of the secreted antibody retains the identical structure after this "switch." Finally, specific antibody binds to the foreign antigen, leading to its precipitation, inactivation (eg, virus), lysis (eg, red cells), or opsonization followed by phagocytosis (eg, bacteria). In some of these circumstances, complement is bound to the antigen-antibody complex and facilitates the destruction or phagocytosis of the antigen. Once an antibody re-

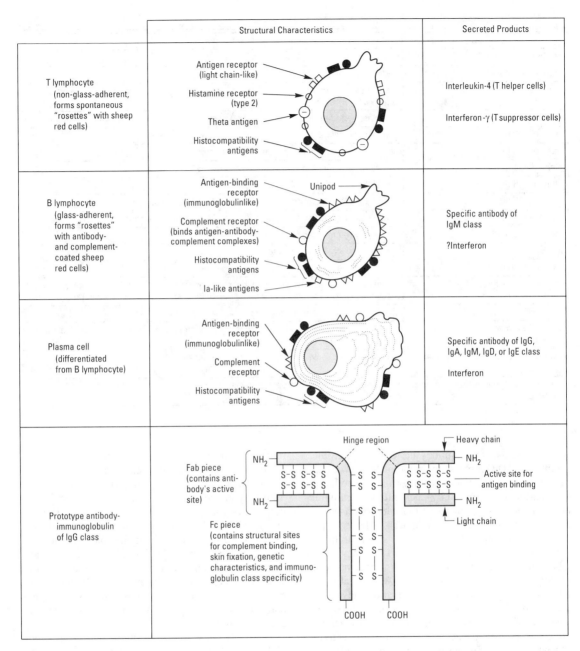

	Structural Characteristics	Secreted Products
T lymphocyte (non-glass-adherent, forms spontaneous "rosettes" with sheep red cells)	Antigen receptor (light chain-like) Histamine receptor (type 2) Theta antigen Histocompatibility antigens	Interleukin-4 (T helper cells) Interferon-γ (T suppressor cells)
B lymphocyte (glass-adherent, forms "rosettes" with antibody- and complement-coated sheep red cells)	Antigen-binding receptor (immunoglobulinlike) Unipod Complement receptor (binds antigen-antibody-complement complexes) Histocompatibility antigens Ia-like antigens	Specific antibody of IgM class ?Interferon
Plasma cell (differentiated from B lymphocyte)	Antigen-binding receptor (immunoglobulinlike) Complement receptor Histocompatibility antigens	Specific antibody of IgG, IgA, IgM, IgD, or IgE class Interferon
Prototype antibody-immunoglobulin of IgG class	Hinge region — Heavy chain Fab piece (contains antibody's active site) Fc piece (contains structural sites for complement binding, skin fixation, genetic characteristics, and immunoglobulin class specificity) NH₂ — Active site for antigen binding — Light chain — COOH COOH	

Figure 57–3. Effectors in the immune response. Specific cell types, including T lymphocytes, B lymphocytes, and plasma cells—as well as secreted antibody-immunoglobulin—have binding sites for specific antigen as well as differential genetic and functional characteristics. Membrane features as well as secreted products can thus be seen to have important functions in the immune response.

sponse is established, reexposure to antigen leads to an immediate chemical combination of antigen and antibody and also serves to provide a "booster" for a rapid secondary wave of cell proliferation and antibody synthesis.

The dual nature of immunity is underscored by certain "experiments of nature," or **genetic diseases.** For

example, DiGeorge's syndrome, resulting from absence of the third branchial cleft, is associated with absent thymic development and impaired delayed hypersensitivity but normal antibody formation. In contrast, delayed hypersensitivity is usually normal in another congenital immunodeficiency disease, namely, X-linked congenital agammaglobulinemia,

Table 57–1. The cytokines.

Cytokine	Properties
Interferon-α (IFN-α)	Generates antiviral and antiproliferative actions.
Interferon-β (IFN-β)	Generates antiviral and antiproliferative actions.
Interferon-γ (IFN-γ)	Generates immunomodulatory action; up-regulates cytokine production and microbial activity of leukocytes.
Interleukin-1 (IL-1)	Stimulates endogenous pyrogen and bone marrow growth; inflammation mediator.
Interleukin-2 (IL-2)	Stimulates proliferation of T cells and their activation to "killer cells."
Interleukin-3 (IL-3)	Stimulates early bone marrow progenitors; "multi-CSF."
Interleukin-4 (IL-4)	Stimulates proliferation of antigen-primed B and T cells.
Interleukin-5 (IL-5)	Stimulates eosinophil proliferation.
Interleukin-6 (IL-6)	Stimulates plasma cell and early bone marrow progenitors.
Interleukin-7 (IL-7)	Stimulates proliferation and differentiation of early cell progenitors.
Interleukin-8 (IL-8)	Neutrophil chemotactic factor.
Interleukin-9 (IL-9)	Mast cell growth-enhancing factor.
Interleukin-10 (IL-10)	Suppresses immune response.
Tumor necrosis factor-β (TNFβ)	Generates antiparasitic action (malaria, trypanosomiasis); mediates inflammatory reactions in endotoxic shock and antitumor actions; stimulates B cell proliferation.
Tumor necrosis factor (TNF)	Mobilizes calcium from bone; generates other actions similar to those of TNFβ.
Granulocyte-macrophage colony-stimulating factor (GM-CSF)	Stimulates granulocyte, neutrophil monocyte-macrophage, and eosinophil proliferation and differentiation.
Granulocyte colony-stimulating factor (G-CSF)	Stimulates granulocyte proliferation and differentiation.
Macrophage colony-stimulating factor (M-CSF)	Stimulates monocyte-macrophage proliferation.

which presents as an antibody deficiency syndrome. Infants with DiGeorge's syndrome or those with severe combined immunodeficiency (missing both cellular and humoral immunity) lack circulating thymic hormone activity. A number of children with severe combined immunodeficiency appear to have a specific deficiency in the enzyme adenosine deaminase, which plays a critical role in normal lymphocyte metabolism and prevents the intracellular accumulation of toxic products such as deoxy-ATP. Stabilized adenosine deaminase enzyme preparations have been used to treat such children. More recently, the use of gene transfection has been initiated to provide sustained restitution of adenosine deaminase activity ("gene therapy"). Studies of circulating T and B cells in the blood have shown that patients with DiGeorge's syndrome lack T cells, whereas those with congenital agammaglobulinemia lack B cells.

AIDS has also underscored the profound defect that can occur in host immunity to both infection and cancer that occurs when CD4+ T helper cells are depleted. In this illness, as CD4+ T cells are progressively depleted, there is a progressive increase in the frequency of opportunistic infections and malignancies.

The complexity of the immune system appears to provide a sufficient number of control points to render the emergence of a "forbidden clone," which is reactive against the host's own constituents, a relatively rare event. Normally, most components of the lymphoid system remain in a highly "repressed" state until they are selectively activated for a specific immune response. The numerous steps of the process also imply that immunosuppressive agents can be directed at various steps along this pathway (Figure 57–4), including the induction of specific tolerance. Because the immune system provides a major barrier against invading microorganisms, including oncogenic viruses, as well as toxins and foreign cells, generalized immunosuppression can potentially be very dangerous to the host.

With only one notable exception—Rh$_o$(D) immune globulin—the clinically useful immunosuppressive agents that are now available may have general immunosuppressive properties and must be used with caution. Generalized immunosuppression increases the risk of infection and may also increase the risk of development of lymphoreticular and other forms of cancer. In general, it is easier to prevent or attenuate a primary immune response with immunosuppressive drugs than to suppress an established immune response. Even with these limitations and cautions, immunosuppression is of proved usefulness in a number of acquired immune disorders as well as in organ transplantation. While there is no simple definition for autoimmunity, it is associated with activation and

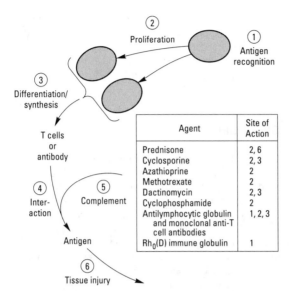

Figure 57–4. The sites of action of immunosuppression agents on the immune response.

Agent	Site of Action
Prednisone	2, 6
Cyclosporine	2, 3
Azathioprine	2
Methotrexate	2
Dactinomycin	2, 3
Cyclophosphamide	2
Antilymphocytic globulin and monoclonal anti-T cell antibodies	1, 2, 3
$Rh_0(D)$ immune globulin	1

proliferation of T cells and the production of antibodies against host-tissue constituents. Even though such autoimmune reactions may be due to eclipsed viruses (eg, retroviruses), the symptoms and signs of disease can often be reduced with immunosuppressive therapy.

TESTS OF IMMUNOCOMPETENCE

A wide variety of techniques have been used to test immunologic competence and its drug-induced alteration. The simplest tests that can be used to detect the effects of immunosuppressive or immunostimulating agents include the following:

(1) Delayed hypersensitivity testing with skin test antigens to detect the ability to respond to recall antigens. These are antigens, usually microbial, to which the individual has had prior exposure. Common examples include mumps, streptokinase-streptodornase, *Candida albicans,* tetanus, diphtheria, and *Pseudomonas* antigen as well as tuberculin. Other antigens would include sensitizing chemicals such as dinitrochlorobenzene.

(2) Measurement of serum immunoglobulins, serum complement, and specific antibodies to various natural and acquired antigens.

(3) Serial measurements of antibody response after primary immunization or a secondary booster injection (Figure 57–4).

(4) Absolute circulating lymphocyte counts.

(5) Measurement of the percentages of B cells, T cells, and subsets (eg, with monoclonal antibodies) that comprise the circulating blood lymphocyte count.

(6) In vitro lymphocyte proliferative responses to mitogens such as phytohemagglutinin, concanavalin A, and pokeweed mitogen.

(7) Mixed-lymphocyte reaction, in which the lymphocytes of one individual are mixed with and proliferate in response to allogeneic lymphocytes of another individual.

(8) NK cell cytotoxicity to target tumor cells.

RELATIONSHIP BETWEEN IMMUNOSUPPRESSIVE THERAPY & CANCER CHEMOTHERAPY

Although there is definite overlap between the drugs used for immunosuppression (Figure 57–4) and those used in cancer chemotherapy (see Chapter 56), different principles govern their use in these two disease categories. The character and kinetics of cancer cell proliferation are not identical to immune cell proliferation and allow different features to be exploited in immunosuppression. For example, whereas cancer cell proliferation appears to be "unstimulated," immune cell proliferation usually occurs in response to the presence of a specific antigen. While division of individual malignant cells within a large cancer cell population appears to occur randomly in an apparently unsynchronized way, immune cell proliferation appears to be partially "synchronized" in a burst of mitotic division that occurs after introduction of the antigen, with a large fraction of the responding cells going through the generation cycle in order to produce specific immunity. Thus, when cytotoxic drugs are used at the time of initial exposure to foreign antigen (eg, a kidney transplant), a very high percentage of an initially small number of precursor cells can be destroyed, because the antigen stimulates selected relevant clones to proliferate rather than all clones of immune cells. Therefore, a greater degree of selective toxicity can be initially obtained against the unwanted immune clone, whereas this objective is harder to achieve in cancer chemotherapy. Additionally, when cytotoxic drugs are used for immunosuppression, they are generally administered in a low-dosage daily schedule to block immunoproliferation continuously. In contrast, when these same drugs (eg, cyclophosphamide) are used for cancer chemotherapy, they are administered intermittently in high-dosage "pulse" courses every 3–6 weeks. Such "pulse" administration permits rapid immune rebound between treatments, which is desirable for augmentation of tumor immunity but undesirable in immunosuppressive therapy.

IMMUNOSUPPRESSIVE AGENTS

CORTICOSTEROIDS

Corticosteroids were the first class of hormonal agents recognized to have lympholytic properties. Administration of a glucocorticoid (eg, prednisone, dexamethasone) reduces the size and lymphoid content of the lymph nodes and spleen, though it has essentially no toxic effect on proliferating myeloid or erythroid stem cells in the bone marrow. Glucocorticoids are thought to interfere with the cell cycle of activated lymphoid cells. The mechanism of their action is described in Chapters 38 and 56. Glucocorticoids are quite cytotoxic to certain subsets of T cells, but their immunologic effects are probably due to their ability to modify cellular functions rather than direct cytotoxicity. Glucocorticoids inhibit the production of inflammatory mediators, including platelet-activating factor, leukotrienes, prostaglandins, histamine, and bradykinin. In monocytes and neutrophils, glucocorticoids cause diminished chemotaxis and impaired bactericidal and fungicidal activities but do not alter their phagocytic ability. Leukocyte distribution is also changed by corticosteroids, which can cause lymphopenia (probably due to lymphoid tissue sequestration) and neutrophilia (due to demargination and impaired extravasation of neutrophils). By inhibiting IL-1 production by monocytes, glucocorticoids also cause a decrease in IL-2 and γ-interferon production. Although cellular immunity is more affected than humoral immunity, the primary antibody response can be diminished, and, with continued use, previously established antibody responses are also decreased. Furthermore, continuous administration of prednisone increases the fractional catabolic rate of IgG, the major class of antibody immunoglobulins, thus lowering the effective concentration of specific antibodies. Cutaneous delayed hypersensitivity is usually abrogated by corticosteroid therapy.

Glucocorticoids are used in a wide variety of clinical circumstances where it is thought that their immunosuppressive and anti-inflammatory properties account for their beneficial effects. Indications include autoimmune disorders such as autoimmune hemolytic anemia, idiopathic thrombocytopenic purpura, inflammatory bowel disease, lupus erythematosus, and some cases of Hashimoto's thyroiditis. Corticosteroids also modulate allergic reactions and are used in bronchial asthma, as will be discussed later in this chapter. Corticosteroids are also used liberally in the management of organ transplant recipients and are of particular value during rejection crises because the dosage can be increased without fear of bone marrow toxicity. The usual dosage range for prednisone

as an immunosuppressive agent is 10–100 mg orally daily. The potential adverse effects of corticosteroids, including adrenal suppression and serious viral, bacterial, and fungal infections, are also relevant when these agents are used chronically for immunosuppression.

CYCLOSPORINE

Cyclosporine (Figure 57–5) is an immunosuppressive agent that has shown impressive efficacy in human organ transplantation, in the treatment of graft-versus-host syndrome after bone marrow transplantation, and in the treatment of selected autoimmune disorders. Patients in whom it is used as the only immunosuppressant or combined with prednisone have similar graft survival frequency and a lower incidence of rejection and infectious complications than patients treated with combinations of drugs such as azathioprine, prednisone, and antilymphocyte antibodies. Substantial investigation in animals has also shown excellent results. The drug is a fat-soluble peptide antibiotic that appears to act at an early stage in the antigen receptor-induced differentiation of T cells and blocks their activation. Recent in vitro studies have indicated that cyclosporine inhibits the gene transcription of IL-2, IL-3, IFN-γ, and other factors produced by antigen-stimulated T cells, but it does not block the effect of such factors on primed T cells nor does it block interaction with antigen.

Cyclosporine has been given orally on a daily basis in a dosage of 7.5–25 mg/kg. Toxicities include nephrotoxicity, hyperglycemia and hyperlipidemia, some increase in hair growth, and transient liver dysfunction. Regular monitoring of blood levels can help in avoiding these effects. There is very little bone marrow toxicity. While a slightly increased incidence of lymphoma has been seen in transplant recipients receiving cyclosporine, there is also an increased incidence of lymphoma in other transplant recipients who have received other immunosuppressive agents.

A number of reports indicate that cyclosporine is of sufficient potency and efficacy to obviate the need for simultaneous use of corticosteroids, azathioprine, cyclophosphamide, or other immunosuppressive drugs in some patients, whereas in other patients it must be combined with other immunosuppressive drugs. It has been used with apparent success as the sole im-

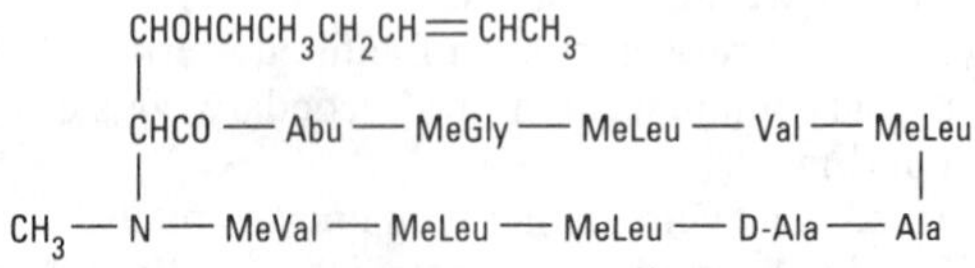

Figure 57–5. Cyclosporine. (Abu, L-2-aminobutyryl.)

munosuppressant for cadaveric transplants of the kidney, pancreas, and liver, and it has proved extremely useful in cardiac transplants as well. Cyclosporine (7.5 mg/kg/d or less) has also proved useful in a variety of autoimmune disorders, including uveitis, rheumatoid arthritis, and the early treatment of type I diabetes. About two-thirds of children with early symptoms of diabetes can discontinue or reduce insulin therapy within 6 weeks after starting cyclosporine therapy. This indicates that nontoxic doses of cyclosporine may be useful in abrogating the anti-islet cell autoimmune process responsible for the genesis of type I diabetes.

Cyclosporine is slowly and incompletely absorbed (20–50%) after oral administration. It has an elimination half-life of 24 hours. An administered dose is almost totally metabolized and excreted in the bile.

Cyclosporine appears to be a major step in the direction of a more specific and selective agent effective against a subpopulation of lymphocytes, but its adverse effects are still considerable–though perhaps less than those of corticosteroids and other cytotoxic agents used for immunosuppression.

TACROLIMUS (FK 506)

FK 506 is an immunosuppressant macrolide antibiotic produced by *Streptomyces tsukubaensis*. It is not chemically related to cyclosporine, but their mechanisms of action seem to be very similar. Both drugs bind to cytoplasmic peptidyl-prolyl-isomerases that are abundant in all tissues. Cyclosporine binds to cyclophilin and FK 506 binds to FK-binding protein (FKBP). Both complexes inhibit the same cytoplasmic phosphatase, calcineurin, which seems to be necessary to the activation of a T cell-specific transcription factor. This transcription factor, NF-AT, is involved in the synthesis of interleukins by activated T cells.

On a weight basis, FK 506 is 10–100 times more potent that cyclosporine in inhibiting immune responses. FK 506 is currently undergoing clinical trials in liver, heart, kidney, and pancreas transplantation. In kidney transplantation, results with FK 506 are similar to those obtained with cyclosporine. For liver transplantation, FK 506 appears to be more effective—in terms of graft and patient survival—when compared to historical controls treated with cyclosporine. Furthermore, it has proved to be effective as rejection rescue therapy after failure of standard rejection therapy, including anti-T cell antibodies.

The drug can be administered orally or intravenously. After oral intake, peak concentrations are reached after 1–4 hours. The half-life of the intravenous form is approximately 9–12 hours, and the drug is metabolized primarily by P450 enzymes in the liver. Its toxic effects are similar to those of cyclosporine, including nephrotoxicity, neurotoxicity, hyperglycemia (requiring insulin therapy), and gastrointestinal dysfunction.

NEW IMMUNOSUPPRESSIVE AGENTS

New immunosuppressive agents are being investigated in an attempt to obtain less toxic and more specific drugs. **Mycophenolate mofetil** (RS-61443) is a semisynthetic derivative of mycophenolic acid, isolated from the mold *Penicillium glaucum*. In vitro, it inhibits a series of lymphocyte responses, including mitogen and mixed lymphocyte responses. Its action depends on its ability to inhibit the de novo pathway of purine synthesis. Recently, it has been tested in kidney and liver transplantation patients, with promising results in rescue therapy for refractory rejections or, in combination with prednisone, as an alternative to cyclosporine or FK 506 in patients who did not tolerate these drugs. A closely related drug, **mizoribine**, which inhibits the same nucleotide synthesis pathway, is also known to be effective in kidney transplantation. In Japan, it is used as an alternative to the more toxic azathioprine. Another drug in this group is **brequinar sodium**. It is an inhibitor of the de novo pathway of pyrimidine synthesis. It has been used in the treatment of cancer, and clinical trials for its use in transplantation were begun in 1992. In animal models, it has shown a very potent immunosuppressive effect and synergism with cyclosporine.

15-Deoxyspergualin was isolated from *Bacillus laterosporus*. It has potent antimonocytic effects, including decreased MHC antigen expression and inhibition of free radical generation. It also has antilymphocytic effects, inhibiting antibody production after immunization, as well as cytotoxic cell generation during mixed lymphocyte reactions. It apparently acts late in the response of T and B cells to activation and is able to suppress even secondary antibody responses. It has been successful in the treatment of acute rejection in renal transplantation. Experiments are currently being conducted to see whether this agent can prevent the development of human antimouse antibody (HAMA) after mouse monoclonal antibody therapy.

Rapamycin[*] is a macrolide antibiotic isolated from *Streptomyces hygroscopicus* that shows structural similarity to FK 506. Accordingly, it has been shown (like FK 506) to bind to FKBP. However, it does not block interleukin production by activated T cells but blocks the response of T cells to cytokines. In vitro, it inhibits T cell responses to FK 506 but seems to be synergistic with cyclosporine. In animal studies, alone or in combination with other immunosuppressants, it has been effective preventing kidney and heart allograft rejection.

---

[*] New name: sirolimus.

CYTOTOXIC AGENTS

Azathioprine

Azathioprine is an imidazolyl derivative of mercaptopurine (6-mercaptopurine, 6-MP) and functions as a structural analogue or antimetabolite (see Chapter 56). Although its action is presumably mediated by mercaptopurine as the active form, it has received more widespread use than mercaptopurine for immunosuppression in humans. These agents represent prototypes of the structural analogue or cytotoxic types of immunosuppressive drugs, and many other agents that kill proliferative cells seem to work at a similar level in the immune response.

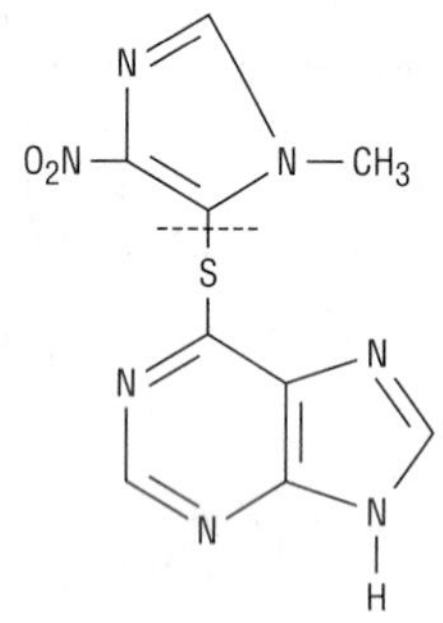

Azathioprine

Azathioprine is well absorbed from the gastrointestinal tract and is metabolized primarily to mercaptopurine (portion below the dashed line in the above figure). Xanthine oxidase splits much of the active material to 6-thiouric acid prior to excretion in the urine. After administration of azathioprine, small amounts of unchanged drug and mercaptopurine are also excreted by the kidney, and as much as a twofold increase in toxicity may occur in anephric or anuric patients. Since much of the drug's inactivation depends on xanthine oxidase, patients who are also receiving allopurinol (see Chapter 56) for control of hyperuricemia should have the dose of azathioprine reduced to one-fourth to one-third the usual dose to prevent excessive toxicity.

Immunosuppression with azathioprine or mercaptopurine therapy seems to result from interference with nucleic acid metabolism at steps that are required for the wave of cell proliferation that follows antigenic stimulation. The purine analogues are thus cytotoxic agents that destroy stimulated lymphoid cells. Although continued messenger RNA synthesis is necessary for sustained antibody synthesis by plasma cells, these analogues appear to have less effect on this process than on nucleic acid synthesis in proliferating cells. Cellular immunity as well as primary and secondary serum antibody responses can be blocked by these cytotoxic agents.

Azathioprine and mercaptopurine appear to be of definite benefit in maintaining renal allografts and may also be of value in transplantation of other tissues. These analogues have also been used with some success in the management of acute glomerulonephritis and in the renal component of systemic lupus erythematosus.

As with mercaptopurine, the chief toxicity of azathioprine is bone marrow depression, usually manifest as leukopenia, though anemia, thrombocytopenia, and bleeding may also occur. Skin rashes, drug fever, nausea and vomiting, and sometimes diarrhea occur, with the gastrointestinal symptoms seen mainly at higher dosages. Hepatic dysfunction, manifested by very high serum alkaline phosphatase levels and mild jaundice, occurs occasionally.

Although these agents are potentially toxic to bone marrow elements, including the megakaryocytes and red cell precursors, the favorable effects often outweigh the toxic effects. The drugs have been of occasional use in prednisone-resistant antibody-mediated idiopathic thrombocytopenic purpura and autoimmune hemolytic anemias.

Cyclophosphamide

The alkylating agent cyclophosphamide has recently been the focus of considerable interest as an immunosuppressive agent in animals and humans. It is perhaps the most potent immunosuppressive drug that has been synthesized. Cyclophosphamide destroys proliferating lymphoid cells but also appears to alkylate some resting cells. It has been observed that very large doses (eg, > 120 mg/kg intravenously over several days) may induce an apparent specific tolerance to a new antigen if the drug is administered simultaneously with—or shortly after—the antigen. In smaller doses, it has been very effective in autoimmune disorders (including systemic lupus erythematosus), in patients with acquired factor XIII antibodies and bleeding syndromes, in autoimmune hemolytic anemia, in antibody-induced pure red cell aplasia, and in patients with Wegener's granulomatosis.

Although treatment with large doses of cyclophosphamide carries considerable risk of pancytopenia and hemorrhagic cystitis, the drug has aided in "takes" of bone marrow transplants and may have value in other types of organ transplantation also. Although cyclophosphamide appears to induce tolerance for marrow or immune cell grafting, its use does not prevent the subsequent graft-versus-host syndrome, which may be serious or lethal if the donor is a poor histocompatibility match. Specialized medical care and supportive facilities are mandatory for patient survival during the period of intensive therapy.

Other Cytotoxic Agents

Other cytotoxic agents, including vincristine, methotrexate, and cytarabine (see Chapter 56), also have immunosuppressive properties. Methotrexate has recently been used extensively in rheumatoid arthritis (Chapter 35). Although the other agents can be used for immunosuppression, they have not received as widespread use as the purine antagonists, and their indications for immunosuppression are less certain. The use of methotrexate (which can be given orally) appears reasonable in patients with idiosyncratic reactions to purine antagonists. The antibiotic dactinomycin has also been used with some success at the time of impending renal transplant rejection. Vincristine appears to be quite useful in idiopathic thrombocytopenic purpura refractory to prednisone. The related *Vinca* alkaloid vinblastine has been shown to prevent mast cell degranulation in vitro by binding to microtubule units within the cell and to prevent release of histamine and other vasoactive compounds.

ANTIBODIES AS IMMUNOSUPPRESSIVE AGENTS

Until recently, development of specific antibodies required immunization and collection of antisera with subsequent purification of the gamma globulin fraction. The development of "hybridoma" technology by Milstein and Köhler has revolutionized this field and radically increased the purity and specificity of antibodies used for immunosuppression and other applications. Hybridomas consist of antibody-forming cells fused to plasmacytoma cells. Hybrid cells that are stable and produce the required antibody can be cloned for mass culture for antibody production. Fermentation facilities are now being used for this purpose in the pharmaceutical industry.

Antilymphocyte & Antithymocyte Antibodies

Antisera directed against lymphocytes have been prepared sporadically since Metchnikoff's first observations just before the turn of the century. With the era of human organ homotransplantation, heterologous antilymphocytic globulin (ALG) suddenly took on new importance. ALG and antithymocyte globulin (ATG) and monoclonal anti-T cell antibodies are now in clinical use in many medical centers that have organ transplantation programs. The antiserum is usually obtained by immunization of large animals with human lymphoid cells or by the hybridoma technique for monoclonal antibody generation.

Antilymphocytic antibody acts primarily on the small, long-lived peripheral lymphocytes that circulate between the blood and lymph. With continued administration, the "thymus-dependent" lymphocytes from the cuffs of lymphoid follicles are also depleted, as they normally participate in the recirculating pool. Antilymphocytic antibody binds to the surface of these T cells (Figure 57–2) and induce immunosuppression by a variety of mechanisms. Opsonization and phagocytosis of antibody-bound cells takes place in the liver and spleen. Cytotoxic destruction of the cells, mediated by serum complement, may occur with some polyclonal antibody preparations (but not with murine monoclonal antibodies, since these do not activate human complement). Antibody-dependent cell-mediated cytotoxicity is another possible mechanism. Besides cell lysis, an antibody preparation may block immune function by modulating the surface expression of molecules involved in lymphocyte function. This is more readily demonstrated with monoclonal antibodies, mainly those directed against the CD3-TCR complex. As a result of destruction or inactivation of the T cells, a rather specific impairment of delayed hypersensitivity and cellular immunity occurs while humoral antibody formation remains relatively intact. Furthermore, antibodies, both polyclonal and monoclonal, are the most selective means of affecting the immune response and thus play a definite role in the management of organ transplantation. The use of monoclonal antibodies directed against specific subsets of immune cells further improves the selectivity of the therapy and provides the possibility of use of this approach also for the treatment of autoimmune disorders.

In the management of transplants, ALG and monoclonal antibodies can be used in the induction of immunosuppression, in the treatment of initial rejections, or in the treatment of steroid-resistant rejections. Since such antibodies have not been adequately standardized, only generalizations about dosage and treatment can be given. After transplantation of an organ such as the kidney, ALG is often administered (by intramuscular injection) first on a daily basis and subsequently less often. Because ALG is usually administered along with azathioprine and prednisone, it has not been possible to assess the effect of ALG alone in human kidney transplants. Since cyclosporine has shown increased nephrotoxicity when used shortly after kidney transplantation, ALG and monoclonal antibodies have been used frequently in protocols that avoid the initial use of cyclosporine. Investigators who treat their renal transplant recipients with ALG believe that it reduces the dosage requirements for the other immunosuppressive drugs and improves survival in patients who receive kidneys from unrelated or cadaver donors. There has been some success in the use of ALG for recipient preparation for bone marrow transplantation. In this procedure, the recipient is treated with ALG in large doses for 7–10 days prior to transplantation of bone marrow cells from the donor. Residual ALG appears to destroy the T cells in the donor marrow graft, and the probability of severe graft-versus-host syndrome is reduced.

The adverse effects of ALG are mostly those of the injection of a foreign protein obtained from heterologous serum. Local pain and erythema often occur at the injection site. Since the humoral antibody mechanism remains active, skin-reactive and precipitating antibodies can be formed against the foreign IgG. Similar reactions occur with monoclonal antibodies of murine origin, but reactions thought to be caused by the release of cytokines by the T cells and monocytes have also been described. With the use of monoclonal antibodies, another undesirable effect is the development of human anti-mouse antibody responses that cause rapid clearance of the mouse antibodies and preclude their continuous use. For this reason, development of human-to-human hybridomas is a major current research objective, since it should eliminate most heterologous protein reactions. Another approach that has received much effort recently is the "humanization" of murine antibodies using molecular biology techniques, where antigen-binding portions of the murine monoclonal antibody are inserted into a human immunoglobulin framework. These chimeric or hybrid antibodies are less immunogenic than murine monoclonal antibodies.

Anaphylactic and serum sickness reactions have been observed and usually require cessation of ALG or monoclonal antibody therapy. In addition, complexes of host antibodies with horse ALG may precipitate and localize in the glomerulus of the transplanted kidney. Even more disturbing has been the development of histiocytic lymphoma in the buttock at the site of ALG injection. The incidence of lymphoma as well as other forms of cancer is increased in kidney transplant patients, and it may be as high as 2% in long-term survivors. It appears likely that part of the increased risk of cancer is related to the suppression of a normally potent defense system against oncogenic viruses or transformed cells. It is felt that the preponderance of lymphoma in these cancer cases is related to the concurrence of chronic immune suppression with chronic low-level lymphocyte proliferation.

Standardization of antilymphocytic antibody with antithymocyte globulin (ATG) of monoclonal origin offers considerable promise, because some of these antisera are selective for T cell subsets and are potentially available in unlimited quantities with very well defined specificity. Monoclonal antibodies currently in use or under investigation include mouse and rat antibodies directed against the CD3-TCR complex of T cells, the IL-2 receptor (expressed only on activated T cells), the CD4 molecule, and against lymphokines.

Clinical studies have shown that the murine monoclonal antibody (**muromonab-CD3; OKT3**) directed against the CD3 molecule on the surface of human thymocytes and mature T cells can also be useful in the treatment of renal transplant rejection. In vitro, OKT3 blocks both killing by cytotoxic human T cells and the generation of other T cell functions. In a prospective randomized multicenter trial with cadaveric renal transplants, use of OKT3 (along with lower doses of steroids or other immunosuppressive drugs) proved more effective at reversing acute rejection than did conventional steroid treatment. This was associated also with a better 1-year survival rate (62% with OKT3) as compared to steroid therapy (45%). Accordingly,

OKT3 is now marketed (as muromonab-CD3) for the treatment of renal allograft rejection crises.

A ricin-conjugated murine monoclonal antibody (xomen H-65) is currently in clinical trials and appears to be quite potent in reversing the graft-versus-host syndrome after allogeneic bone marrow transplantation.

$Rh_o(D)$ Immune Globulin

One of the major advances in immunopharmacology was the development of a technique for preventing Rh hemolytic disease of the newborn. The technique is based on the observation that a primary antibody response to a foreign antigen can be blocked if specific antibody to that antigen is administered passively at the time of exposure to antigen. $Rh_o(D)$ immune globulin is a concentrated (15%) solution of human IgG globulin containing a higher titer of antibodies against the $Rh_o(D)$ antigen of the red cell.

Sensitization of Rh-negative mothers to the D antigen occurs usually at the time of birth of an $Rh_o(D)$-positive or D^u-positive infant, when fetal red cells may leak into the mother's bloodstream. Sensitization might also occur occasionally with miscarriages or ectopic pregnancies. With subsequent pregnancies, maternal antibody against Rh-positive cells is transferred to the fetus during the third trimester, leading to the development of erythroblastosis fetalis or hemolytic disease of the newborn.

If an injection of $Rh_o(D)$ antibody is administered to the mother within 72 hours after the birth of an Rh-positive baby, the mother's own antibody response to the foreign $Rh_o(D)$-positive cells is suppressed. When the mother has been treated in this fashion, Rh hemolytic disease of the newborn has not been observed in the subsequent pregnancy. For this prophylactic treatment to be successful, the mother must be $Rh_o(D)$-negative and D^u-negative and must not already be immunized to the $Rh_o(D)$ factor. Treatment is also often advised for Rh-negative mothers who have had miscarriages, ectopic pregnancies, or abortions when the blood type of the fetus is unknown.

Note: $Rh_o(D)$ immune globulin is administered to the mother and must not be given to the infant.

The usual dose of $Rh_o(D)$ immune globulin is 2 mL intramuscularly. Adverse reactions are infrequent and consist of local discomfort at the injection site or, rarely, a slight temperature elevation.

The mechanism of suppression of the immune response by passive administration of specific antibody may consist of prompt elimination of the foreign antigen after combination with the antibody or may be a type of "feedback immunosuppression" in which a change in the antigen results from its combination with antibody, so that it is no longer recognized as foreign. If antibody produces feedback immunosuppression, it presumably acts on the macrophage, the T lymphocyte, or the B lymphocyte (Figures 57–1 to 57–3).

CLINICAL USES OF IMMUNOSUPPRESSIVE DRUGS

Immunosuppressive agents are currently used in three clinical circumstances: (1) organ transplantation, (2) autoimmune disorders, and (3) isoimmune disorders (Rh hemolytic disease of the newborn). The agents used differ somewhat for the specific disorders treated (see specific agents and Table 57–2), as do administration schedules. Optimal treatment schedules have yet to be established in many clinical situations in which these drugs are used.

Organ Transplantation

In organ transplantation, tissue typing, based on donor and recipient histocompatibility matching with the human leukocyte antigen (HLA) haplotype system and in vitro mixed lymphocyte culture (MLC), is of definite value. Close histocompatibility matching reduces the likelihood of graft rejection and may also reduce the requirements for intensive immunosuppressive therapy. Response to transplantation and immunosuppressive drugs in renal disease may be dependent on the nature of the primary renal lesions in patients undergoing transplant.

Primary renal disease itself is frequently immunologic in nature. Two major types of glomerular injury, the renal component of systemic lupus erythematosus and acute glomerulonephritis, are mediated by immune mechanisms. Although immunosuppressive therapy may be of benefit in both of these circumstances, the data are incomplete. Since patients with severe glomerulonephritis are often candidates for kidney transplantation, pathologic factors that might persist and also damage the transplanted kidney are of great importance. It has been observed that patients with anti-basement membrane antibody may experience an acute graft rejection when they receive a kidney transplant. Patients with anti-basement membrane antibodies are likely to need immunosuppressive therapy for 6–8 weeks after bilateral nephrectomy, being maintained on a dialysis program, before transplantation of a donor kidney can be considered. Similarly, patients with a disease such as systemic lupus erythematosus are poor candidates for renal transplant until the systemic cause of the renal injury is under control.

Even with all these immunologic obstacles, the response to renal transplantation has become increasingly gratifying, including transplants with unmatched kidneys from cadaver donors. Patients who have received prior blood transfusions have a higher success rate with cadaveric renal grafts. The introduction of cyclosporine in the management of transplants has improved graft survival but, more importantly, has decreased the morbidity rate and increased overall patient survival. At present, over 80% of carefully selected but nonrelated transplanted kidneys may survive beyond 2 years after the transplant, and 5-year survival is not an unrealistic hope. As discussed above, use of the monoclonal anti-T cell antibody muromonab-CD3 has reduced acute graft rejection significantly.

Recently, increasing success has been achieved with bone marrow transplantation in patients with aplastic anemia, refractory acute leukemia, or severe combined immunodeficiency disease (congenital) who have an HLA- and MLC-matched donor. Pa-

Table 57–2. Clinical uses of immunosuppressive agents.

Disease	Immunosuppressive Agents Used	Response
Autoimmune Idiopathic thrombocytopenic purpura	Prednisone,[1] vincristine, occasionally mercaptopurine or azathioprine, high-dose gamma-globulin	Usually good
Autoimmune hemolytic anemia	Predisone,[1] cyclophosphamide, chlorambucil, mercaptopurine, azathioprine	Usually good
Acute glomerulonephritis	Prednisone,[1] mercaptopurine, cyclophosphamide	Usually good
Acquired factor XIII antibodies	Cyclophosphamide plus factor XIII	Usually good
Miscellaneous "autoreactive" disorders[2]	Prednisone, cyclophosphamide, azathioprine, cyclosporine	Often good
Isoimmune Hemolytic anemia of the newborn	Rh$_o$ (D) immune globulin[1]	Excellent
Organ transplantation Renal	Cyclosporine, azathioprine, prednisone, ALG, OKT3 monoclonal antibody, dactinomycin, cyclophosphamide	Very good
Heart		Good
Liver	Cyclosporine, prednisone	Fair
Bone marrow (HLA-matched)	Cyclosporine, cyclophosphamide, prednisone, methotrexate, ALG, total body irradiation, donor marrow purging with monoclonal anti-T cell antibodies, immunotoxins	Very good

[1]Drug of choice.
[2]Systemic lupus erythematosus, rheumatoid arthritis, Wegener's granulomatosis, chronic active hepatitis, lipoid nephrosis, inflammatory bowel disease.

tients with aplastic anemia or leukemia require intensive immunosuppression prior to transplantation. Monoclonal antibodies to leukemia-, lymphoma-, and neuroblastoma-associated antigens have been used to "clean up" patients' bone marrow for autologous bone marrow storage and reinfusion after high-dose chemotherapy. Use of monoclonal antibody-immunotoxin conjugates appears particularly promising in this regard and may markedly broaden the use of autologous bone marrow transplantation. Patients who do not receive autologous bone marrow or a graft from an identical twin require postengraftment immunosuppression to minimize the graft-versus-host syndrome attributable to donor immunocytes in the marrow graft. Recent investigations indicate that anti-T cell antiserum or cyclosporine can modify or reverse established graft-versus-host syndrome in a significant proportion of cases.

Cyclosporine has proved to be an effective immunosuppressive drug for use in renal, cardiac, hepatic, and bone marrow transplantation. Together with newer drugs, it is now being evaluated as an alternative to other more complex immunosuppressive regimens.

Autoimmune Disorders

The effectiveness of immunosuppressive drugs in autoimmune disorders varies widely. Nonetheless, with immunosuppressive therapy, remissions can be obtained in many instances of autoimmune hemolytic anemia, idiopathic thrombocytopenic purpura, type 1 diabetes mellitus, Hashimoto's thyroiditis, and temporal arteritis. Apparent improvement is also often seen in patients with systemic lupus erythematosus, acute glomerulonephritis, acquired factor VIII inhibitors (antibodies), and certain other autoimmune states. Some cases of idiopathic aplastic anemia also appear to have an autoimmune basis. In some instances, it appears to be the result of increased activity of CD8+ T suppressor cells. In such instances, γ-interferon produced by T suppressor cells may be the humoral mediator of hematopoietic suppression. A recent series of aplastic anemia patients showed significant clinical improvement and prolonged survival with ATG alone. Some prior cases treated with bone marrow transplantation after conditioning with cyclophosphamide, cyclosporine, or ALG have also shown prolonged improvement in blood counts even though there was evidence of graft rejection and recovery of recipient marrow function, again supporting an autoimmune basis for some cases of aplastic anemia. Recently, the use of high doses of normal gamma globulin (administered intravenously) has been found useful in therapy of refractory idiopathic thrombocytopenic purpura. Furthermore, high-dose intravenous immunoglobulin (2 g/kg) therapy has been shown to be safe and effective in the management of Kawasaki syndrome, reducing systemic inflammation and preventing coronary artery aneurysms. Possible mechanisms of action of intravenous immunoglobulin include diminution of helper T cells, increase in suppressor T cells, decrease in spontaneous immunoglobulin production, and idiotypic-anti-idiotypic interactions with "pathologic antibodies."

Another new approach to the control of this condition is plasma immunoabsorption using protein A columns. This presumably removes the immunoreactive antibody, particularly in the form of immune complexes. This approach is currently FDA-approved for AIDS-related idiopathic thrombocytic purpura.

In most instances it is only assumed that it is the immunosuppressive properties of drugs such as prednisone, cyclosporine, cyclophosphamide, mercaptopurine, or ALG that produce these improvements. Anti-inflammatory effects of some of these drugs may also contribute to their efficacy.

IMMUNOMODULATING AGENTS

A new frontier in pharmacology—still in the stage of exploration and debate—is the development of agents that modulate the immune response rather than suppress it. The rationale underlying all research contributing to the development of these agents is that they can be used to increase the immunoresponsiveness of patients who have either selective or generalized immunodeficiency. The major potential uses are in immunodeficiency disorders, chronic infectious disease, and cancer. At present, all but two of the immunostimulating or immunomodulating agents (BCG and levamisole) are classed as investigational drugs. The AIDS epidemic has greatly increased interest in developing more effective immunomodulatory drugs. The HIV organism resides in and destroys CD4+ helper cells, leading to progressive immunologic paralysis.

Thymosin & Other Thymic Peptides

Thymosin is composed of a group of protein hormones synthesized by the epithelioid component of the thymus. They have been isolated and purified from bovine and human thymus glands. Thymosin, which has a molecular weight of approximately 10,000, appears to convey T cell specificity to uncommitted lymphoid stem cells. Lower-molecular-weight fractions may also have thymic hormone-like activity. Thymosin levels are high through normal childhood and early adulthood, begin to fall in the third to fourth decades, and are low in elderly people. Serum levels are also low in DiGeorge's syndrome of T cell deficiency. In vitro treatment of lymphocytes with thymosin increases the number of cells that manifest T cell surface markers and function.

Mechanistically, thymosin is considered to induce the maturation of pre-T cells. The effects of fetal thymus transplantation in DiGeorge's syndrome are probably attributable to the action of thymosin. The purified hormone therefore has potential therapeutic applications in DiGeorge's syndrome and other T cell deficiency states. A recombinant peptide derived from this hormone, **thymosin α-1**, induces enhanced production of IL-2 and increases the expression of IL-2 receptors on T lymphocytes. This peptide is undergoing clinical trials for the treatment of cancer and chronic active hepatitis with encouraging preliminary results.

Two other thymus-related peptides, **thymopentin** and **thymic humoral factor,** also have T cell-stimulating properties and are under investigation for the treatment of AIDS as well as cancer and hepatitis.

Cytokines

The cytokines are a large heterogeneous group of proteins with diverse functions. Some are immunoregulatory proteins synthesized within lymphoreticular cells and play numerous interacting roles in the function of the immune system and in the control of hematopoiesis. Cytokines that have been clearly identified are summarized in Table 57–1. In most instances, cytokines mediate their effects via cell surface receptors in relevant target cells and appear to act in a manner similar to that of hormones. In other instances, cytokines may have antiproliferative or antimicrobial effects.

The first group of cytokines discovered were the interferons (also discussed in Chapter 49), followed by the colony-stimulating factors (CSFs, also discussed in Chapter 32). The latter regulate the proliferation and differentiation of bone marrow progenitor cells. Most of the more recently discovered cytokines have been classified as interleukins and numbered in the order of their discovery. The identification of most interleukins and the production of highly purified cytokines of all types have been greatly facilitated by the development and biopharmaceutical application of gene cloning techniques.

Now that they have become available through genetic engineering, the cytokines are playing an increasingly important role in immunopharmacology and will probably find a variety of applications in the treatment of infectious, inflammatory, autoimmune, and neoplastic disorders. At present, IFN-α has been approved by the Food and Drug Administration for clinical use in various neoplasms, including hairy cell leukemia and Kaposi's sarcoma. IFN-α has also shown activity as an anticancer agent in malignant melanoma, renal cell carcinoma, carcinoid syndrome, and T cell leukemia. Interferon beta-1b has been approved by the FDA for use in relapsing-type multiple sclerosis. This cytokine appears to reduce the number of moderate to severe exacerbations of the disease over a period of 2 years, though it did not change the total disability scores of the patients. IFN-γ has been approved for the treatment of chronic granulomatous disease and IL-2 for the treatment of metastatic renal cell carcinoma. IFN-α is also useful in the treatment of hepatitis. Numerous clinical investigations of the other cytokines, including IL-1, IL-3, IL-4, and IL-6, are now in progress. Tumor necrosis factor-α (TNF) has been extensively tested in the therapy of various malignancies with disappointing results. Even at highly toxic doses, TNF induced almost no positive results. One exception is the use of intra-arterial high-dose TNF for malignant melanoma of the extremities.

Cytokines as adjuvants to vaccines have been under clinical investigation recently. Interferons and IL-2 have shown some positive effects in the response of human subjects to hepatitis B vaccine. However, recombinant cytokines are expensive drugs and may never reach wide use as vaccine adjuvants.

One of the most promising new areas of investigation has been the attempt to reverse leukopenia and inadequate granulocyte reserve resulting from disease states or cancer therapy by application of granulocyte-macrophage colony stimulating factor (GM-CSF) and granulocyte colony-stimulating factor (G-CSF). Both GM-CSF (as sargramostim) and G-CSF (as filgrastim) have been approved for clinical use in the control of neutropenia associated with chemotherapy. Therapy starting 1 day after the end of chemotherapy, with daily injections of cytokine, shortens the period and lessens the severity of neutropenia significantly. The CSFs may also prove useful in the supportive care of burn patients or patients with a variety of infectious disorders. CSFs probably will be administered with antibiotics to patients who have poor leukocyte responses to infection. It is important to emphasize that in normal immunophysiology, cytokine interaction with target cells often occurs with a cascade of different cytokines exerting their effects sequentially or simultaneously. For example, prior IFN-γ exposure increases the number of cell surface receptors on target cells for TNF.

A more recent approach to immunomodulation involves the use of cytokine inhibitors for the treatment of inflammatory diseases and septic shock, conditions where cytokines such as IL-1 and TNF are involved in the pathogenetic mechanisms. Anticytokine monoclonal antibodies, soluble cytokine receptors (both soluble IL-1 receptors and soluble TNF receptors occur naturally in humans), and the IL-1 receptor antagonist IL-1Ra (also a naturally occurring molecule that binds to IL-1 receptors but does not induce biologic responses) are under investigation. In various animal models, these molecules have shown efficacy in the treatment of a series of conditions, including septic shock, experimental arthritis, immune complex-mediated colitis, and diabetes. Phase I clinical studies demonstrated the safety of the use of monoclonal antibodies anti-TNF and of IL-1Ra in human volunteers. Preliminary data from phase III studies with monoclonal anti-TNF antibodies suggest that these antibodies may be effective in the treatment of septic shock when bacteremia is present. Furthermore, results from a phase III study of IL-1Ra with 893 patients indicated that among high-risk patients (595 patients with a mortality risk ≥ 24%), treatment with IL-1Ra improved survival significantly (P < .03). Other clinical trials using IL-1Ra for the treatment of ulcerative colitis, rheumatoid arthritis, and myelogenous leukemia are also being conducted.

Synthetic Agents

Several synthetic chemical agents have been discovered to have immunomodulating properties. The chemical agent levamisole was first synthesized for the treatment of parasitic infections. Later studies suggested that it increases the magnitude of delayed hypersensitivity or T cell-mediated immunity in humans. In immunodeficiency associated with Hodgkin's disease, levamisole has been noted to increase the number of T cells in vitro and to enhance skin test reactivity in vivo. Levamisole has also been widely tested in rheumatoid arthritis and found to have some efficacy. However, it has induced severe agranulocytosis (mainly in HLA-B27-positive patients), which caused discontinuation of its use for that condition. The drug also potentiates the action of fluorouracil in adjuvant therapy of colorectal cancer, and in this combination it has been approved by the FDA for clinical use in the treatment of Dukes class C colorectal cancer after surgery. Its use in these cases markedly reduces recurrences, and the mechanism probably relates to macrophage activation and the killing of residual tumor cells by activated macrophages. Inosiplex (isoprinosine) has been found to have immunomodulating activities also, and in various preclinical and clinical settings this agent has increased natural killer cell cytotoxicity as well as T cell and monocyte functional activities. It has been tested in AIDS, with some (slight) benefit observed. Other synthetic drugs, including cyanoaziridine compounds (azimexon, ciamexon, and imexon) and methyl-inosine monophosphate, are currently under investigation for the treatment of AIDS and neoplasia.

BCG (Bacille Calmette-Guérin) & Other Adjuvants

BCG is a viable strain of *Mycobacterium bovis* that has been used for immunization against tuberculosis. It has also been employed as a nonspecific adjuvant or immunostimulant in cancer therapy but has been successful only in intravesical therapy for superficial bladder cancer. BCG appears to act at least in part via activation of macrophages to make them more effective killer cells in concert with lymphoid cells in the efferent limb of the immune response. Lipid extracts of BCG (eg, methanol-extractable residue) as well as nonviable preparations of *Corynebacterium parvum*

may have similar nonspecific immunostimulant properties. A chemically defined derivative of the BCG cell wall, [Lys^{18}] muramyl dipeptide, has been licensed in Japan to induce bone marrow recovery after cancer chemotherapy. These agents prepare macrophages for the release of various cytokines, including IL-1, colony-stimulating factors, and TNF. TNF is released into the serum of BCG-treated animals after endotoxin challenge. TNF is also considered an important mediator of the hypotensive reaction observed in patients with endotoxic shock associated with gram-negative bacteremia.

IMMUNOLOGIC REACTIONS TO DRUGS & DRUG ALLERGY

The basic immune mechanism and the ways in which it can be suppressed or stimulated by drugs are discussed in the foregoing sections of this chapter. Drugs also *activate* the immune system in undesirable ways that appear as adverse drug reactions. These reactions are generally lumped in a broad classification as "drug allergy." Indeed, many drug reactions such as those to penicillin, iodides, phenytoin, and sulfonamides are allergic in nature. These drug reactions are manifested as skin eruptions, edema, anaphylactoid reactions, fever, and eosinophilia. The underlying mechanism of the allergic sensitization to drugs was clarified by the discovery of the IgE class of immunoglobulins and by a better understanding of the process of sensitization and activation of blood basophils and tissue mast cells.

Drug reactions mediated by immune processes may have different mechanisms. Thus, any one of the four major types of hypersensitivity can be associated with a drug allergy reaction:

Type I: IgE-mediated acute allergic reactions to stings, pollens, and drugs, including anaphylaxis, urticaria, and angioedema. IgE is fixed to tissue mast cells and blood basophils.

Type II: Allergic reactions that are complement-dependent and therefore involve IgG or IgM antibodies in which the antibody is fixed to a circulating blood cell subject to complement-dependent lysis.

Type III: Drug reactions that are exemplified by serum sickness, which involves immune complexes containing IgG and is a multisystem complement-dependent vasculitis.

Type IV: Cell-mediated allergy that is the mechanism involved in allergic contact dermatitis from topically applied drugs.

In a number of drug reactions, several of these hypersensitivity reactions may present simultaneously.

Some adverse reactions to drugs may be mistakenly classified as allergic or immune when they are in reality genetic deficiency states or are idiosyncratic and not mediated by immune mechanisms (eg, hemolysis due to primaquine in glucose-6-phosphate dehydrogenase deficiency, or aplastic anemia due to chloramphenicol).

IMMEDIATE (TYPE I) DRUG ALLERGY

The mechanisms of immune activation that are operative in drug allergy are similar to the normal humoral antibody responses to foreign macromolecules. These mechanisms can now be placed in a theoretical construct that includes an afferent limb of the immune response (Figure 57–6) as well as an efferent limb that includes the pharmacologic mediators of allergy (Figure 57–7). Landsteiner and his associates first demonstrated that animals could be sensitized to simple chemicals such as picric acid (a hapten) if the chemical was linked to a carrier protein. This linkage can occur in the body with a normal tissue or serum protein serving as the carrier. The subsequent immune response will be specific for the hapten even though linkage to a carrier is necessary for immune recognition. Surprisingly, carrier recognition is genetically determined even though the host does not produce antibodies against the carrier protein. When drugs serve as haptens, the antibody-forming precursor cells that respond are often the precursors of cells that produce antibodies of the IgE class. IgE class-specific antibody responses are very dependent on helper T cells, which secrete IL-4 and promote the differentiation of B cells to IgE-forming cells. Suppressor T cells secrete IFN-γ, which can block B cell differentiation to IgE production and inhibit the IgE response. In nonallergic individuals, IgE globulin levels are the lowest of any immunoglobulin (< 1 μg/mL), whereas in allergy they may be increased tenfold or more. IgE antibodies have the interesting property of fixing to blood basophils and tissue mast cells and are skin-sensitizing or reaginic antibodies.

Fixation of the IgE antibody to high-affinity Fc receptors (Fc$_\varepsilon$R) on blood basophils or their tissue equivalent (mast cells) sets the stage for an acute allergic reaction. Among the sites for mast cell distribution and IgE sensitization, the skin, lung, and gastrointestinal tract are most important. When the offending drug is reintroduced into the body, IgE antibody molecules attached to Fc$_\varepsilon$R on the surface of sensitized basophilic leukocytes and mast cells bind to the antigenic form of the drug (Figure 57–7). Sensitized tissue mast cells or blood basophils are stimulated to release mediators (eg, histamine, leukotrienes; Chapters 16 and 18) from granules when IgE molecules on two adjacent Fc$_\varepsilon$R are bridged by binding specific antigen. Mediator release is associated with a fall in intracellular cAMP within the mast cell. Many of the drugs that block mediator release appear to act through the cAMP mechanism (eg, catecholamines, corticosteroids, theophylline), with different loci of action in the pathway of cAMP synthesis or degradation. Other vasoactive substances such as kinins may also be generated during histamine release.

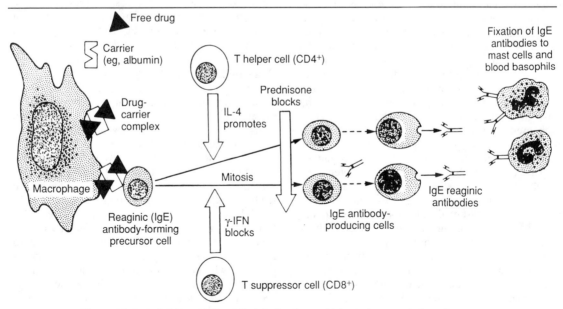

Figure 57–6. Induction of IgE-mediated allergic sensitivity to drugs and other allergens.

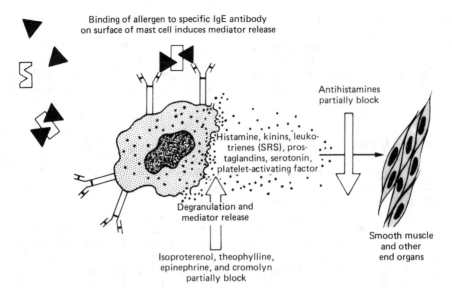

Figure 57–7. Response of IgE-sensitized cells to subsequent exposure to allergens.

These mediators cause immediate skin and smooth muscle responses and thus initiate tissue injury and the inflammatory response. Mediator-induced reactions can be devastating or lethal to the patient, especially when they produce laryngospasm, bronchospasm, or hypotension.

Drug Treatment of Immediate Allergy

One can test an individual for possible sensitivity to a drug by a simple scratch test, ie, by applying an extremely dilute solution of the drug to the skin and making a scratch with the tip of a needle. If allergy is present, an immediate wheal and flare will often occur. However, in many instances the skin test may be negative in spite of marked hypersensitivity to a hapten or to a metabolic product of the drug, or at times when the antibody may be of a class other than IgE.

Drugs that modify allergic responses act at several links in this chain of events. Prednisone, which is often used in severe allergic reactions, is immunosuppressive and probably blocks proliferation of the IgE-producing clones and inhibits IL-4 production by helper T cells in the IgE response. In the efferent limb of the allergic response, isoproterenol, epinephrine, and theophylline reduce the release of mediators from mast cells and basophils and produce bronchodilation, whereas antihistamines competitively inhibit histamine, which would otherwise produce bronchoconstriction and increased capillary permeability in the end organ. Corticosteroids may also act to reduce tissue injury and edema in the inflamed tissue as well as by "unblocking" beta-blocked cells, thereby facilitating the actions of catecholamines in cells that may

have become refractory to epinephrine or isoproterenol. Several agents directed toward the inhibition of leukotriene synthesis are currently in clinical trial, with the view that they may be useful in acute allergic and inflammatory disorders. Cromolyn sodium, a drug that is useful for treatment of allergic asthma, appears to inhibit the liberation of the mediators of anaphylaxis that are released after antibody-antigen interaction (see Chapter 19). However, its complete mechanism of action is still obscure. Ketotifen, an antihistaminic drug that has been used in the prophylaxis of diverse allergic diseases, can prevent allergic reactions by similar mechanisms that are independent of its antihistaminic properties and probably related to its effects on eosinophils.

Desensitization To Drugs

When reasonable alternatives are not available, certain drugs (eg, penicillin) must be used for life-threatening illnesses even in the presence of known allergic sensitivity. In such cases, desensitization can sometimes be accomplished by starting with minute dosages of the drug and gradually increasing over a period of hours or days to the full therapeutic range. This practice is hazardous, and one must always be ready to manage an episode of acute anaphylactic shock before desensitization has been achieved. This form of desensitization differs from immunosuppression in that the immune mechanism often appears to be stimulated and reactivity is only predictably diminished while the treatment is continued. With the advent of cephalosporins and other antibiotics, the need for such desensitization procedures to administer penicillin has been essentially eliminated.

The exact mechanism of desensitization to drugs is complex and incompletely understood. It may be due to controlled anaphylaxis (with gradual depletion of mast cells and basophils) while symptoms are suppressed, or it may be due to antigen excess, which can under certain circumstances block mediator release. In some instances, allergic desensitization appears to be accomplished by the stimulation of competing clones of cells that produce "blocking" antibodies, often of the IgG or IgA immunoglobulin class. Additionally, desensitization with antigen could induce the generation of specific suppressor T cells.

AUTOIMMUNE (TYPE II) REACTIONS TO DRUGS

Certain autoimmune syndromes can be induced by drugs. Examples of this phenomenon include systemic lupus erythematosus following hydralazine or procainamide therapy, "lupoid hepatitis" due to cathartic sensitivity, autoimmune hemolytic anemia resulting from methyldopa administration, thrombocytopenic purpura due to quinidine, and agranulocytosis due to a variety of drugs. In these drug-induced autoimmune states, antibodies to tissue constituents or to the drug can be demonstrated. Immune mechanisms also appear to be involved in many additional cases of so-called idiopathic thrombocytopenic purpura, but it is more difficult to demonstrate the specific antibodies. The blood platelet or granulocyte is sometimes an innocent bystander to an immunologic reaction to a drug but manages to be damaged or activated by antigen-antibody complexes or destroyed by the reticuloendothelial system, leading to the development of "idiopathic" thrombocytopenic purpura or agranulocytosis.

Fortunately, autoimmune reactions to drugs usually subside within several months after the offending drug is withdrawn. Immunosuppressive therapy is warranted only when the autoimmune response is unusually severe.

SERUM SICKNESS & VASCULITIC (TYPE III) REACTIONS

Serum sickness reactions to drugs are more common than immediate anaphylactic responses. The clinical features of serum sickness include urticarial skin eruptions, arthralgia or arthritis, lymphadenopathy, and fever. The reactions generally last 6–12 days and usually subside once the offending drug is eliminated. Although IgE antibodies may play some role, complement-fixing antibodies of the IgM or IgG class are usually involved. Corticosteroids are useful in attenuating severe serum sickness reactions to drugs.

Immune vasculitis can also be induced by drugs. The sulfonamides, penicillin, thiouracil, anticonvulsants, and iodides have all been implicated in the initiation of hypersensitivity angiitis. Erythema multiforme is a relatively mild vasculitic skin disorder that may be secondary to drug hypersensitivity. Stevens-Johnson syndrome is probably a more severe form of this hypersensitivity reaction and includes erythema multiforme, arthritis, nephritis, central nervous system abnormalities, and myocarditis. It has frequently been associated with sulfonamide therapy.

CLINICAL IDENTIFICATION OF IMMUNOLOGIC REACTIONS TO DRUGS

In view of the multiplicity of drugs administered to hospitalized patients, it is not always easy to determine which drug has initiated an allergic or immune syndrome of drug sensitivity. Careful questioning about the history of prior drug sensitivities is an important part of every patient's medical record, and errors of omission can be dangerous. In almost all instances, once an offending drug is identified, its use is discontinued. If an alternative drug is to be used (eg, an antibiotic), it is important to select one from a different class of agents to avoid cross-sensitivity reactions. Since certain commonly used drugs such as the penicillins are among the more common offenders, direct questions about penicillin sensitivity should always be included in the patient's history. Skin testing may be very useful in confirming drug allergy when the history is equivocal and the proper antigens are available. Skin testing is considerably less hazardous than a therapeutic trial and is usually indicated where there is an equivocal allergic history and a strong clinical indication for treatment with the drug. An alternative to skin testing that is increasingly available is the radioallergosorbent test (RAST), a form of radioimmunoassay procedure.

Warnings of known sensitivities should be prominently displayed in the patient's record or hospital chart. When drug intolerance is suspected, an assessment of the patient's anaphylactic potential should be made, since delayed rashes carry a different prognosis from that of urticaria and angioedema. Once a drug allergy is defined, this information should always be conveyed to the patient in clear language to prevent repeated challenges with the same agent in the future, when the reaction may be much more severe. In the case of known severe sensitivity to common drugs, the patient should be advised to carry a clearly written notice of the sensitivity to lessen the chance of being given the agent during incapacitation, as after an accident.

PREPARATIONS AVAILABLE[*]

Azathioprine (Imuran)
Oral: 50 mg tablets
Parenteral: 100 mg/mL for injection (in 20 mL vials)

Cyclophosphamide (Cytoxan, Neosar)
Oral: 25, 50 mg tablets
Parenteral: powder to reconstitute for injection (in 100, 200, 500 mg and 1, 2 g vials)

Cyclosporine (Sandimmune)
Oral: 25, 50 mg capsules; 100 mg/mL solution
Parenteral: 50 mg/mL for IV administration

Interferon beta-1b (Betaseron)

Parenteral: 0.3 mg vial for SC injection

Lymphocyte immune globulin (Atgam)
Parenteral: 50 mg/mL for injection (in 5 mL ampules)

Muromonab-CD3 [OKT3] (Orthoclone OKT3)
Parenteral: 5 mg/5 mL ampule for injection

Rh$_o$(D) immune globulin micro-dose (HypRho-D Mini-Dose, MICRhoGAM, Mini-Gamulin Rh)
Parenteral: in single-dose and micro-dose vials

Tacrolimus [FK 506] (Prograf)
Oral: 1,5 mg capsules
Parenteral: 5 mg/mL for injection

REFERENCES

Current Concepts in Immunology

Adams DH et al: Soluble interleukin-2 receptors in serum and bile of liver transplant recipients. Lancet 1989;1:469.

Ahonen P et al: Clinical variation of autoimmune poly- endocrinopathy-candidiasis-ectodermal dystrophy (APECED) in a series of 68 patients. N Engl J Med 1990;322:1829.

Akira S et al: Biology of multifunctional cytokines: IL 6 and related molecules (IL 1 and TNF). FASEB J 1990;4:2860.

Banchereau J, Rousset F: Human B lymphocytes: Phenotype, proliferation and differentiation. Adv Immunol 1992;52:125.

Blaese RM: Development of gene therapy for immunodeficiency: Adenosine deaminase deficiency. Pediatr Res 1993;33(Suppl):S49.

Chatila T et al: An immunodeficiency characterized by defective signal transduction in T lymphocytes. N Engl J Med 1989;320:696.

Ferrara JLM, Deeg HJ: Graft-versus-host disease. N Engl J Med 1991;324:667.

Hall BM et al: Comparison of three immunosuppressive regimens in cadaver renal transplantation: Long-term cyclosporine, short-term cyclosporine followed by azathioprine and prednisolone, and azathioprine and prednisolone without cyclosporine. N Engl J Med 1988;318:1499.

Johnston RB Jr: Current concepts in immunology: Monocytes and macrophages. N Engl J Med 1988; 318:747.

Jones RJ et al: Induction of graft-versus-host disease after autologous bone marrow transplantation. Lancet 1989;2:754.

Krensky AM et al: T-lymphocyte-antigen interactions in transplant rejection. N Engl J Med 1990;322:510.

Ledbetter J et al: Evolutionary conservation of surface molecules that distinguish T lymphocyte helper/inducer and cytotoxic suppressor subpopulation in mouse and man. J Exp Med 1981;153:310.

Lipsky PE: The control of antibody production by immunomodulatory molecules. Arthritis Rheum 1989;32: 1989.

Miyajima A et al: Coordinate regulation of immune and inflammatory responses by T cell-derived lymphokines. FASEB J 1988;2:2462.

Nossal GJV: Immunologic tolerance: Collaboration between antigen and lymphokines. Science 1989;245: 147.

Ortaldo JR et al: Determination of surface antigens on highly purified human NK cells by flow cytometry with monoclonal antibodies. J Immunol 1981;127: 2401.

Paul W (editor): *Fundamental Immunology,* 3rd ed. Raven Press, 1993.

Rock B et al: The pathogenic effect of IgE4 antibodies in endemic pemphigus foliaceus (fogo selvagem). N Engl J Med 1989;320:1463.

Roitt I, Brostoff J, Male D (editors): *Immunology.* Mosby, 1985.

Stites DP, Terr AI (editors): *Basic & Clinical Immunology,* 7th ed. Appleton & Lange, 1991.

Vogelsang G et al: An in vitro predictive test for graft versus host disease in patients with genotypic HLA-identical bone marrow transplants. N Engl J Med 1985;313:645.

Weinberg K, Parkman R: Severe combined immunodeficiency due to a specific defect in the production of interleukin-2. N Engl J Med 1990;322:1718.

Wilkin TJ: Receptor autoimmunity in endocrine disorders. N Engl J Med 1990;323:1318.

Wirt DP et al: Novel T-lymphocyte population in combined immunodeficiency with features of graft-versus-host disease. N Engl J Med 1989;321:370.

Immunosuppressive Agents

Armitage JM et al: A clinical trial of FK 506 as primary and rescue immunosuppression in cardiac transplantation. Transplant Proc 1991;23:1149.

Ash RC et al: Successful allogeneic transplantation of T-

---

[*]Several interleukin products and other monoclonal antibodies are available as orphan drugs. Other drugs discussed in this chapter and not listed here will be found in other chapters (see Index).

cell-depleted bone marrow from closely HLA-matched unrelated donors. N Engl J Med 1990; 322:485.

Atkinson K et al: Cyclosporin A associated nephrotoxicity in the first 100 days after allogeneic bone marrow transplantation. Br J Haematol 1983;54:59.

Bougneres PF et al: Factors associated with early remission of type I diabetes in children treated with cyclosporine. N Engl J Med 1988;318:663.

Brynskov J et al: A placebo-controlled, double-blind, randomized trial of cyclosporine therapy in active chronic Crohn's disease. N Engl J Med 1989;321:845.

Bumgardner GL, Roberts JP: New immunosuppressive agents. Gastroenterol Clin North Am 1993;22:421.

Eisen D et al: Effect of topical cyclosporine rinse on oral lichen planus. N Engl J Med 1990;323:290.

European Multicentre Trial Group: Cyclosporine in cadaveric renal transplantation. Lancet 1983;2:986.

Fehr J, Hofmann V, Kappeler CM: Transient reversal of thrombocytopenia in idiopathic thrombocytopenia purpura by high-dose intravenous gamma globulin. N Engl J Med 1982;306:1254.

First MR et al: Concomitant administration of cyclosporine and ketoconazole in renal transplant recipients. Lancet 1989;2:1198.

Freda VJ et al: Prevention of Rh hemolytic disease: Ten years' experience with Rh immune globulin. N Engl J Med 1975;292:1014.

Fung J et al: A randomized trial of primary liver transplantation under immunosuppression with FK 506 vs cyclosporine. Transplant Proc 1991;23:2977.

Fung J et al: Randomized trial in primary liver transplantation under immunosuppression with FK 506 or cyclosporine. Transplant Proc 1993;25(1 Pt 2): 1130.

Gernsheimer T et al: Mechanisms of response to treatment in autoimmune thrombocytopenic purpura. N Engl J Med 1989;320:974.

Hayes JM: The immunobiology and clinical use of current immunosuppressive therapy for renal transplantation. J Urol 1993;149:437.

Hoffman GS: Immunosuppressive therapy for autoimmune diseases. Ann Allergy 1993;70:263.

Imbach P et al: Intravenous immunoglobulin versus oral corticosteroids in acute immune thrombocytopenic purpura in childhood. Lancet 1985;2:464.

Jenkins MK, Schwartz RH, Pardoll DM: Effects of cyclosporine A on T cell development and clonal deletion. Science 1988;241:1655.

Kahan BD: Cyclosporine. N Engl J Med 1989;321:1725.

Larick JW: Potential of monoclonal antibodies as pharmacological agents. Pharmacol Rev 1989;41:539.

Lichtiger S, Present DH: Preliminary report: Cyclosporine in treatment of severe active ulcerative colitis. Lancet 1990;336:16.

Liu J: FK 506 and cyclosporin, molecular probes for studying intracellular signal transduction. Immunol Today 1993;14:290.

Mathieson PW et al: Monoclonal antibody therapy in systemic vasculitis. N Engl J Med 1990;323:250.

Moran M et al: Prevention of acute graft rejection by the prostaglandin E$_1$ analogue misoprostol in renal-transplant recipients treated with cyclosporine and prednisone. N Engl J Med 1990;322:1183.

Morris RE: Immunopharmacology of new xenobiotic immunosuppressive molecules. Semin Nephrol 1992;12:304.

Ortho Multicenter Transplant Study Group: Randomized trial of OKT3 monoclonal antibody for acute rejection of cadaveric renal transplants. N Engl J Med 1985; 313:337.

Prummel MF et al: Prednisone and cyclosporine in the treatment of severe Graves' ophthalmopathy. N Engl J Med 1989;321:1353.

Schindler R (editor): Cyclosporin in Autoimmune Diseases. Springer Verlag, 1985.

Showstack J et al: The effect of cyclosporine on the use of hospital resources for kidney transplantation. N Engl J Med 1989;321:1086.

Schreiber SL, Crabtree GR: The mechanism of action of cyclosporin A and FK 506. Immunol Today 1992; 13:136.

Sigal NH, Dumont FJ: Cyclosporin A, FK-506, and rapamycin: Pharmacologic probes of lymphocyte signal transduction. Annu Rev Immunol 1992;10:519.

Snyder HW Jr et al: Experience with protein A-immunoadsorption in treatment-resistant adult immune thrombocytopenic purpura. Blood 1992;79:2237.

Soulillou J-P et al: Randomized controlled trial of monoclonal antibody against the interleukin-2 receptor (33B3.1) as compared with rabbit antithymocyte globulin for prophylaxis against rejection of renal allografts. N Engl J Med 1990;322:1175.

Starzl TE et al: Liver transplantation with the use of cyclosporin A and prednisone. N Engl J Med 1981; 305:266.

Tugwell P et al: Low-dose cyclosporine versus placebo in patients with rheumatoid arthritis. Lancet 1990; 335:1051.

Venkataramanan R et al: Pharmacokinetics of FK 506. Transplant Proc 1991;23:2736.

Yee GC et al: Serum cyclosporine concentration and risk of acute graft-versus-host disease after allogeneic marrow transplantation. N Engl J Med 1988;319:65.

Immunomodulating Agents

Atkinson MA et al: 64000 M$_r$ autoantibodies as predictors of insulin-dependent diabetes. Lancet 1990;335: 1357.

Audibert FM, Lise LD: Adjuvants: current status, clinical perspectives and future prospects. Immunol Today 1993;14:281.

Dinarello CA: Modalities for reducing interleukin 1 activity in disease. Immunol Today 1993;14:260.

Dinarello CA, Gelfand JA, Wolff SM: Anticytokine strategies in the treatment of systemic inflammatory response syndrome. JAMA 1993;14:1829.

Ezekowitz AR et al: Partial correction of the phagocyte defect in patients with X-linked chronic granulomatous disease by subcutaneous interferon gamma. N Engl J Med 1988;319:146.

Foon KA: Biological response modifiers: The new immunotherapy. Cancer Res 1989;49:1621.

Gresser I (editor): Interferon. Academic Press, 1981.

Hadden JW: Immunostimulants. Immunol Today 1993; 14:275.

Lee B, Ciardelli TL: Clinical applications of cytokines

for immunostimulation and immunosuppression. Prog Drug Res 1992;39:167.

Lewis V: Circulating thymic-hormone activity in congenital immunodeficiency. Lancet 1977;2:471.

Norman DJ: Antilymphocyte antibodies in the treatment of allograft rejection: Targets, mechanisms of action, monitoring and efficacy. Semin Nephrol 1992;12:315.

Starzl TE et al: FK 506 for liver, kidney, and pancreas transplantation. Lancet 1989;2:1000.

Starzl TE, Makowka L, Todo S (editors): FK 506: A potential breakthrough in immunosuppression. Transplant Proc 1987;19(Suppl 6):3.

St Georgiev V: New synthetic immunomodulating agents. Trends Pharmacol Sci 1988;9:446.

Vilcek J, Gresser I, Merigan TC (editors): Regulatory functions of interferons. Ann NY Acad Sci 1980; 350:1.

Vitetta ES, Thorpe PE, Uhr JW: Immunotoxins: Magic bullets or misguided missiles? Immunol Today 1993; 14:252.

Winter G, Harris WJ: Humanized antibodies. Immunol Today 1993;14:243.

Wybran J: Immunomodulatory properties of isoprinosine in man: In vitro and in vivo data. Int J Immunopharmacol 1980;2:197.

Immunologic Reactions to Drugs & Allergy

Anderson JA, Adkinson NF Jr: Allergic reactions to drugs and biologic agents. JAMA 1987;258:2891.

Askenase PW: Effector and regulatory mechanisms in delayed type hypersensitivity. In: *Allergy Principles and Practice,* 2nd ed. Middleton E Jr, Reed C, Ellis EF (editors). Mosby, 1983.

Morley J: Immunopharmacology of asthma. Immunol Today 1993;14:317.

Nabe M et al: The effect of ketotifen on eosinophils as measured at LTC4 release and by chemotaxis. Allergy Proc 1991;12:267.

Rieder MJ: Immunopharmacology and adverse drug reactions. J Clin Pharmacol 1993;33:316.

Samuelsson B et al: Leukotrienes and slow reacting substance of anaphylaxis (SRS-A). Allergy 1980;35:375.

Section IX.
Toxicology

Introduction to Toxicology: Occupational & Environmental Toxicology

58

Gabriel L. Plaa, PhD

Humans live in a chemical environment. Estimates indicate that more than 60,000 chemicals are in common use and about 500 new chemicals are said to enter the commercial market annually. Pollution has paralleled technologic advances. Industrialization and the creation of large urban centers have led to the contamination of air, water, and soil. The principal causes of pollution are related to the production and use of energy, the production and use of industrial chemicals, and increased agricultural activity.

TOXICOLOGY & ITS SUBDIVISIONS

Toxicology is concerned with the deleterious effects of chemical and physical agents on all living systems. In the biomedical area, however, the toxicologist is primarily concerned with adverse effects in humans resulting from exposure to drugs and other chemicals as well as the demonstration of safety or hazard associated with their use.

Occupational Toxicology
Occupational toxicology deals with the chemicals found in the workplace. Industrial workers may be exposed to these agents during the synthesis, manufacturing, or packaging of these substances or through their use in an occupational setting. Agricultural workers, for example, may be exposed to harmful amounts of pesticides during their application in the field. The major emphasis of occupational toxicology is to identify the agents of concern, define the conditions leading to their safe use, and prevent absorption of harmful amounts. Guidelines have been elaborated to establish safe ambient air concentrations for many chemicals found in the workplace. The American Conference of Governmental Industrial Hygienists periodically prepares lists of recommended **threshold limit values (TLV)** for about 600

such chemicals (Lu, 1991). Three different categories of air concentrations (expressed in parts per million [ppm] or milligrams per cubic meter [mg/m^3]) have been elaborated to cover various exposure conditions: (1) threshold limit value-time-weighted average (TLV-TWA) is the concentration for a normal 8-hour workday or 40-hour workweek to which workers may be repeatedly exposed without adverse effect; (2) threshold limit value-short-term exposure limit (TLV-STEL) is the maximum concentration (a value greater than the TLV-TWA) that should not be exceeded at any time during a 15-minute exposure period; and (3) threshold limit value-ceiling (TLV-C) is the concentration that should not be exceeded even instantaneously. These guidelines are reevaluated as new information becomes available.

Environmental Toxicology
Environmental toxicology deals with the potentially deleterious impact of chemicals, present as pollutants of the environment, to living organisms. The term "environment" includes all the surroundings of an individual organism, but particularly the air, soil, and water. A "pollutant" is a substance that occurs in the environment, at least in part as a result of human activity, and which has a deleterious effect on living organisms. While humans are considered a target species of particular interest, other terrestrial and aquatic species are of considerable importance as potential biologic targets.

Air pollution is a product of industrialization, technologic development, and increased urbanization. Humans may also be exposed to chemicals used in the agricultural environment as pesticides or in food processing that may persist as residues or ingredients in food products. The Food and Agriculture Organization and the World Health Organization (FAO/WHO) Joint Expert Commission on Food Additives adopted the term **acceptable daily intake (ADI)** to denote "the daily intake of a chemical which, during an entire lifetime, appears to be without appreciable risk on the basis of all the known facts at the time" (Lu, 1991). After evaluation of the pertinent scientific data, the FAO/WHO periodically lists ADI values (expressed in milligrams per kilogram of body weight per day) for many pesticides and food additives that may enter the human food chain. These guidelines are reevaluated as new information becomes available.

Ecotoxicology

Ecotoxicology has evolved relatively recently as an extension of environmental toxicology. It is concerned with the toxic effects of chemical and physical agents on living organisms, especially in populations and communities within defined ecosystems; it includes the transfer pathways of those agents and their interactions with the environment. Traditional toxicology is concerned with toxic effects on individual organisms; ecotoxicology is concerned with the impact on populations of living organisms or on ecosystems (Truhaut, 1977). It is possible that an environmental event, exerting severe effects on *individual* organisms, has no important impact on populations or an ecosystem. Thus, the terms "environmental toxicology" and "ecotoxicology" are not interchangeable.

TOXICOLOGIC TERMS & DEFINITIONS

Toxicity, Hazard, & Risk

Toxicity is *the ability of a chemical agent to cause injury.* It is a qualitative term. Whether or not these injuries occur depends on the amount of chemical absorbed (severity of the exposure, dose). Hazard, on the other hand, is *the likelihood that injury will occur in a given situation or setting;* the conditions of use and exposure are primary considerations. To assess hazard, one needs to have knowledge about both the inherent toxicity of the substance (qualitative aspect) and the amounts to which individuals are liable to be exposed (quantitative aspect). Humans can safely use potentially toxic substances when the necessary conditions minimizing absorption are established and respected. The presence of a potentially toxic substance in the workplace or in the environment does not necessarily mean that a hazardous situation exists.

Risk is defined as the *expected frequency of the occurrence of an undesirable effect* arising from exposure to a chemical or physical agent. Estimation of risk makes use of dose-response data and extrapolation from the observed relationships to the expected responses at doses occurring in actual exposure situations. The quality and suitability of the biologic data used in such estimates are major limiting factors. A number of mathematical models have been devised and are often used for calculating risk of carcinogene-

sis (Ecobichon, 1992); they may also be used to assess the risk involved with other forms of toxicity.

Routes of Exposure

The route of entry for chemicals into the body differs in different exposure situations. In the industrial setting, inhalation is the major route of entry. The transdermal route is also quite important, but oral ingestion is a relatively minor route. Consequently, preventive measures are largely designed to eliminate absorption by inhalation or by topical contact. Atmospheric pollutants gain entry by inhalation, whereas for pollutants of water and soil, oral ingestion is the principal route of exposure for humans.

Duration of Exposure

Toxic reactions may differ qualitatively depending on the duration of the exposure. A single exposure—or multiple exposures occurring over 1 or 2 days—represents **acute exposure.** Multiple exposures continuing over a longer period of time represent a **chronic exposure.** In the occupational setting, both acute (eg, accidental discharge) and chronic (eg, repetitive handling of a chemical) exposures may occur, whereas with chemicals found in the environment (eg, pollutants in ground water), chronic exposure is more likely. Society is also concerned with the possible harmful effects of contact with small concentrations of chemicals over long periods of time; this type of chronic situation is called **low-level, long-term exposure.** The appearance of the toxic effect after acute exposure may appear rapidly or after a variable interval; the latter is called **delayed toxicity.** With chronic exposures, the toxic effect may not be discernible until after several months of repetitive exposure. The harmful effect resulting from either acute or chronic exposure may be reversible or irreversible. The relative reversibility of the toxic effect depends on the recuperative properties of the affected organ.

Presence of Mixtures

Humans normally come in contact with several (or many) different chemicals concurrently or sequentially. This complicates the assessment of potentially hazardous situations encountered in the workplace or in the environment. The resulting biologic effect of combined exposure to several agents can be characterized as **additive, supra-additive (synergistic),** or **infra-additive (antagonistic).** Another type of interaction, **potentiation** (a special form of synergism), may be observed. In cases of potentiation, one of two agents exerts no effect upon exposure; but when exposure to both together occurs, the effect of the active agent is increased. All these types of interactions have been observed in humans. In the absence of contrary evidence, one usually assumes that the toxic effects of mixtures of chemicals are likely to be additive.

ENVIRONMENTAL CONSIDERATIONS

Certain chemical and physical characteristics are known to be important for estimating the potential hazard involved for environmental toxicants. In addition to information regarding effects on different organisms, knowledge about the following properties is essential to predict the environmental impact: The **degradability** of the substance; its **mobility** through air, water, and soil; whether or not **bioaccumulation** occurs; and its transport and **biomagnification** through food chains. Chemicals that are poorly degraded (by abiotic or biotic pathways) exhibit *environmental persistence* and thus can accumulate. Lipophilic substances tend to bioaccumulate in body fat, resulting in tissue residues. When the toxicant is incorporated into the food chain, biomagnification occurs as one species feeds upon others and concentrates the chemical. The pollutants that have the widest environmental impact are poorly degradable; are relatively mobile in air, water, and soil; exhibit bioaccumulation; and also exhibit biomagnification. Attempts have been made to estimate for humans the bioaccumulation potential of organic chemicals found in the environment (Geyer, 1986).

In ecotoxicology there are three interacting components; the toxicant, the environment, and the organisms (community, population, or ecosystem). Ecotoxicologic studies are designed to determine emission and entry of the toxicant in the abiotic environment, including distribution and fate; entry and fate of the toxicant in the biosphere; and the qualitative and quantitative toxic consequences to the ecosystem.

SPECIFIC CHEMICALS

AIR POLLUTANTS

The five major substances that account for about 98% of air pollution are carbon monoxide (about 52%), sulfur oxides (about 18%), hydrocarbons (about 12%), particulate matter (about 10%), and nitrogen oxides (about 6%) (Amdur, 1991). The sources of these chemicals include transportation, industry, generation of electric power, space heating, and refuse disposal. Considerable progress has been made in our understanding of the chemistry of urban air pollution (Seinfeld, 1989). The "reducing type" of pollution (sulfur dioxide and smoke resulting from incomplete combustion of coal) has been associated with acute adverse effects, particularly among the elderly and individuals with preexisting cardiac or respiratory disease. The association of acute adverse

effects, other than severe irritation of the eyes, is less striking with the "oxidizing or photochemical type" of pollution (hydrocarbons, nitrogen oxides, and photochemical oxidants). Ambient air pollution has been implicated as a contributing factor in bronchitis, obstructive ventilatory disease, pulmonary emphysema, bronchial asthma, and lung cancer (Sarnet, 1991).

1. CARBON MONOXIDE

Carbon monoxide (CO) is a colorless, tasteless, odorless, and nonirritating gas, a by-product of incomplete combustion. The average concentration of CO in the atmosphere is about 0.1 ppm; in heavy traffic, the concentration may exceed 100 ppm. The recommended threshold limit values (TLV-TWA and TLV-STEL) are shown in Table 58–1.

Mechanism of Action

CO combines reversibly with the oxygen-binding sites of hemoglobin and has an affinity for hemoglobin which is about 220 times that of oxygen. The product formed, carboxyhemoglobin, cannot transport oxygen. Furthermore, the presence of carboxyhemoglobin interferes with the dissociation of oxygen from the remaining oxyhemoglobin, thus reducing the transfer of oxygen to tissues. The brain and the heart are the organs most affected. Normal nonsmoking adults have carboxyhemoglobin levels of less than 1% saturation (1% of total hemoglobin is in the form of carboxyhemoglobin); this level has been attributed to the endogenous formation of CO from heme catabolism. Smokers may exhibit 5–10% saturation, depending on their smoking habits. An individual breathing air containing 0.1% CO (1000 ppm) would have a carboxyhemoglobin level of about 50%.

Clinical Effects

The principal signs of CO intoxication are those of

Table 58–1. Threshold limit values (TLV) of some common air pollutants and solvents. (NA = none assigned.)

Compound	TLV (ppm) TWA[1]	TLV (ppm) STEL[1]
Benzene	10	NA
Carbon monoxide	25	NA
Carbon tetrachloride	5	NA
Chloroform	10	NA
Nitrogen dioxide	3	5
Ozone	0.1	NA
Sulfur dioxide	2	5
Tetrachloroethylene	50	200
Toluene	50	NA
1,1,1-Trichloroethane	350	450
Trichloroethylene	50	200

[1]See text for definitions.

hypoxia and progress in the following sequence: (1) psychomotor impairment; (2) headache and tightness in the temporal area; (3) confusion and loss of visual acuity; (3) tachycardia, tachypnea, syncope, and coma; and (4) deep coma, convulsions, shock, and respiratory failure. Individual variability in response to a given carboxyhemoglobin concentration is quite high. Carboxyhemoglobin levels below 15% rarely produce symptoms; collapse and syncope may appear around 40%; above 60%, death may ensue. Prolonged hypoxia and posthypoxic unconsciousness can result in residual irreversible damage to the brain and the myocardium. The clinical effects may be aggravated by heavy labor, high altitudes, and high ambient temperatures. The presence of cardiovascular disease is considered to increase the risks associated with CO exposure (Folinsbee, 1992).

While CO intoxication is usually thought of as a form of acute toxicity, there is some evidence that chronic exposure to low levels may lead to undesirable effects, including the development of atherosclerotic coronary disease in cigarette smokers. However, convincing experimental evidence is lacking (Penney, 1991). The fetus may be quite susceptible to the effects of CO exposure.

Treatment

In cases of acute intoxication, removal of the individual from the exposure source and maintenance of respiration is essential, followed by administration of oxygen—the specific antagonist to CO—within the limits of oxygen toxicity. With room air at 1 atm, the elimination half-time of CO is about 320 minutes; with 100% oxygen, the half-time is about 80 minutes; and with hyperbaric oxygen (2–3 atm), the half-time can be reduced to about 20 minutes. The role of hyperbaric oxygen in the treatment of CO intoxication remains controversial (Ellenhorn, 1988).

2. SULFUR DIOXIDE

Sulfur dioxide (SO_2) is a colorless, irritant gas generated primarily by the combustion of sulfur-containing fossil fuels. The TLV-TWA and TLV-STEL are given in Table 58–1.

Mechanism of Action

On contact with moist membranes, SO_2 forms sulfurous acid, which is responsible for its severe irritant effects on the eyes, mucous membranes, and skin. It is estimated that approximately 90% of inhaled SO_2 is absorbed in the upper respiratory tract, the site of its principal effect. The inhalation of SO_2 causes bronchial constriction; altered smooth muscle tone and parasympathetic reflexes appear to be involved in this reaction (Chapter 19). Exposure to 5 ppm for 10 minutes leads to increased resistance to air flow in most humans. Exposures to 5–10 ppm are reported to cause severe bronchospasm; 10–20% of the healthy young adult population is estimated to be reactive to even lower concentrations. The phenomenon of adaptation to irritating concentrations is a recognized occurrence in workers. Asthmatic individuals are especially sensitive to SO_2 (Amdur, 1991; Folinsbee, 1992).

Clinical Effects & Treatment

The signs and symptoms of intoxication include irritation of the eyes, nose, and throat and reflex bronchoconstriction. If severe exposure has occurred, delayed onset pulmonary edema may be observed. Cumulative effects from chronic low-level exposure to SO_2 are not striking, particularly in humans. Chronic exposure, however, has been associated with aggravation of chronic cardiopulmonary disease (Ellenhorn, 1988). Treatment is not specific for SO_2 but depends on therapeutic maneuvers utilized in the treatment of irritation of the respiratory tract.

3. NITROGEN OXIDES

Nitrogen dioxide (NO_2) is a brownish irritant gas sometimes associated with fires. It is formed also from fresh silage; exposure of farmers to NO_2 in the confines of a silo can lead to "silo-filler's disease." The 1993 TLV-TWA and TLV-STEL values are shown in Table 58–1.

Mechanism of Action

NO_2 is a deep lung irritant capable of producing pulmonary edema. The type I cells of the alveoli appear to be the cells chiefly affected on acute exposure. Exposure to 25 ppm is irritating to some individuals; 50 ppm is moderately irritating to the eyes and nose. Exposure for 1 hour to 50 ppm can cause pulmonary edema and perhaps subacute or chronic pulmonary lesions; 100 ppm can cause pulmonary edema and death.

Clinical Effects & Treatment

The signs and symptoms of acute exposure to NO_2 include irritation of the eyes and nose, cough, mucoid or frothy sputum production, dyspnea, and chest pain. Pulmonary edema may appear within 1–2 hours. In some individuals, the clinical signs may subside in about 2 weeks; the patient may then pass into a second stage of abruptly increasing severity, including recurring pulmonary edema and fibrotic destruction of terminal bronchioles (bronchiolitis obliterans). Chronic exposure of laboratory animals to 10–25 ppm NO_2 has resulted in emphysematous changes; thus, chronic effects in humans are of concern. There is no specific treatment for acute intoxication by NO_2; therapeutic measures for the management of deep lung irritation and noncardiogenic pulmonary edema are employed. These measures include maintenance of gas exchange with adequate oxygenation and alveolar ventilation. Drug therapy may include bronchodilators, sedatives, and antibiotics; the use of corticosteroids is controversial (Ellenhorn, 1988).

4. OZONE

Ozone (O_3) is a bluish irritant gas that occurs normally in the earth's atmosphere, where it is an important absorbent of ultraviolet light. In the workplace, it can occur around high-voltage electrical equipment and around ozone-producing devices used for air and water purification. It is also an important oxidant found in polluted urban air. See Table 58–1 for TLV-TWA and TLV-STEL values.

Clinical Effects & Treatment

O_3 is an irritant of mucous membranes. Mild exposure produces upper respiratory tract irritation. Severe exposure can cause deep lung irritation, with pulmonary edema, when inhaled at sufficient concentrations. Some of the effects of O_3 resemble those seen with radiation, suggesting that O_3 toxicity may result from the formation of reactive free radicals. The gas causes shallow, rapid breathing and a decrease in pulmonary compliance. Enhanced sensitivity of the lung to bronchoconstrictors is also observed. Exposures around 0.1 ppm for 10–30 minutes causes irritation and dryness of the throat; above 0.1 ppm, one finds changes in visual acuity, substernal pain, and dyspnea. Pulmonary function is impaired at concentrations exceeding 0.8 ppm. Airway hyperresponsiveness and airway inflammation have been observed in humans (Folinsbee, 1992). Animal studies indicate that the response of the lung to O_3 is a dynamic one. The morphologic and biochemical changes are the result of both direct injury and secondary responses to the initial damage (Wright, 1990). Long-term exposure in animals results in morphologic and functional pulmonary changes. Chronic bronchitis, bronchiolitis, fibrosis, and emphysematous changes have been reported in a variety of species exposed to concentrations above 1 ppm. There is no specific treatment for acute O_3 intoxication. Management depends on therapeutic measures utilized for deep lung irritation and noncardiogenic pulmonary edema. (See Nitrogen Oxides, above.)

SOLVENTS

1. HALOGENATED ALIPHATIC HYDROCARBONS

These agents find wide use as industrial solvents, degreasing agents, and cleaning agents. The substances include carbon tetrachloride, chloroform, trichloroethylene, tetrachloroethylene (perchloroethylene), and 1,1,1-trichloroethane (methyl chloro-

form). See Table 58–1 for recommended threshold limit values.

Mechanism of Action & Clinical Effects

In laboratory animals, the halogenated hydrocarbons cause central nervous system depression, liver injury, kidney injury, and some degree of cardiotoxicity. These substances are depressants of the central nervous system in humans, although their relative potencies vary considerably; chloroform is the most potent and was widely used as an anesthetic agent. Chronic exposure to tetrachloroethylene can cause impaired memory and peripheral neuropathy. Hepatotoxicity is also a common toxic effect that can occur in humans after acute or chronic exposures, the severity of the lesion being dependent on the amount absorbed. Carbon tetrachloride is the most potent of the series in this regard. Nephrotoxicity can occur in humans exposed to carbon tetrachloride, chloroform, and trichloroethylene. With chloroform, carbon tetrachloride, trichloroethylene, and tetrachloroethylene, carcinogenicity has been observed in lifetime exposure studies performed in rats or mice. The potential effects of low-level, long-term exposures to humans, however, are yet to be determined.

Treatment

There is no specific treatment for acute intoxication resulting from exposure to halogenated hydrocarbons. Management depends upon the organ system involved (Arena, 1979).

2. AROMATIC HYDROCARBONS

Benzene is widely used for its solvent properties and as an intermediate in the synthesis of other chemicals. The 1993 recommended TLV-TWA and TLV-STEL values are given in Table 58–1. The acute toxic effect of benzene is depression of the central nervous system. Exposure to 7500 ppm for 30 minutes can be fatal. Exposure to concentrations larger than 3000 ppm may cause euphoria, nausea, locomotor problems, and coma; vertigo, drowsiness, headache, and nausea may occur at concentrations ranging from 250 to 500 ppm. No specific treatment exists for the acute toxic effect of benzene.

Chronic exposure to benzene can result in very serious toxic effects, the most significant being an insidious and unpredictable injury to the bone marrow; aplastic anemia, leukopenia, pancytopenia, or thrombocytopenia may occur. Bone marrow cells in early stages of development appear to be most sensitive to benzene. The early symptoms of chronic benzene intoxication may be rather vague (headache, fatigue, and loss of appetite). Epidemiologic data suggest an association between chronic benzene exposure and an increased incidence of leukemia in workers; such effects have yet to be produced in laboratory animals (Yardley-Jones, 1991).

Toluene (methylbenzene) does not possess the myelotoxic properties of benzene, nor has it been associated with leukemia. It is, however, a central nervous system depressant. See Table 58–1 for the TLV-TWA and TLV-STEL values. Exposure to 800 ppm can lead to severe fatigue and ataxia; 10,000 ppm can produce rapid loss of consciousness. Chronic effects of long-term toluene exposure are unclear because human studies indicating behavioral effects usually concern exposures to several solvents, not toluene alone (Ellenhorn, 1988).

INSECTICIDES

1. CHLORINATED HYDROCARBON INSECTICIDES

These agents are usually classified in four groups: DDT (chlorophenothane) and its analogues, benzene hexachlorides, cyclodienes, and toxaphenes (Table 58–2). They are aryl, carbocyclic, or heterocyclic compounds containing chlorine substituents. The individual compounds differ widely in their biotransformation and capacity for storage; toxicity and storage are not always correlated. They can be absorbed through the skin as well as by inhalation or oral ingestion. There are, however, important quantitative differences between the various derivatives; DDT in solution is poorly absorbed by the skin, whereas dieldrin absorption from the skin is very efficient.

Table 58–2. Chlorinated hydrocarbon insecticides.

Chemical Class	Compounds	Toxicity Rating[1]	ADI[2]
DDT and analogues	Dichlorodiphenyl-trichloroethane (DDT)	4	0.005
	Methoxychlor	3	0.1
	Tetrachlorodiphenyl-ethane (TDE)	3	—
Benzene hexachlorides	Benzene hexachloride (BHC; hexachlorocyclohexane)	4	—
	Lindane	4	0.01
Cyclodienes	Aldrin	5	0.0001
	Chlordane	4	0.001
	Dieldrin	5	0.0001
	Heptachlor	4	0.0005
Toxaphenes	Toxaphene (camphechlor)	4	—

[1]Toxicity rating: Probable human oral lethal dosage for class 3 = 500–5000 mg/kg, class 4 = 50–500 mg/kg, and class 5 = 5–50 mg/kg. (See Gosselin reference.)
[2]ADI = acceptable daily intake (mg/kg body weight/d).

Human Toxicology

The acute toxic properties of the chlorinated hydrocarbon insecticides in humans are qualitatively similar. These agents interfere with inactivation of the sodium channel in excitable membranes and cause rapid repetitive firing in most neurons. Calcium ion transport is also inhibited. These events affect repolarization and enhance the excitability of neurons. The major effect is central nervous stimulation. With DDT, tremor may be the first manifestation, possibly continuing on to convulsions, whereas with the other compounds convulsions often appear as the first sign of intoxication. There is no specific treatment for the acute intoxicated state, management being symptomatic. Chronic administration of some of these agents to laboratory animals over long periods has resulted in enhanced tumorigenicity; there is no agreement regarding the potential carcinogenic properties of these substances, and extrapolation of these observations to humans is controversial (Ames, 1987, 1992). Evidence of carcinogenic effects in humans has not been established.

Environmental Toxicology

The chlorinated hydrocarbon insecticides are considered "persistent" chemicals. Degradation is quite slow when compared to other insecticides, and bioaccumulation, particularly in aquatic ecosystems, is well documented. Their mobility in soil depends on the composition of the soil; the presence of organic matter favors the adsorption of these chemicals onto the soil, whereas adsorption is poor in sandy soils. Once adsorbed, they do not readily desorb.

Because of their environmental impact, use of the chlorinated hydrocarbon insecticides has been largely curtailed in North America and Europe. Some of them are still used, however, in tropical countries.

2. ORGANOPHOSPHORUS INSECTICIDES

These agents, some of which are listed in Table 58–3, are utilized to combat a large variety of pests. They are useful pesticides when in direct contact with insects or when used as "plant systemics," where the agent is translocated within the plant and exerts its effects on insects that feed on the plant. Some of these agents are used in human and veterinary medicine as local or systemic antiparasitics or in circumstances in which prolonged inhibition of cholinesterase is indicated (Chapter 7). The compounds are absorbed by the skin as well as by the respiratory and gastrointestinal tracts. Biotransformation is rapid, particularly when compared to the rates observed with the chlorinated hydrocarbon insecticides.

Table 58–3. Organophosphorus insecticides.

Compound	Toxicity Rating[1]	ADI[2]
Azinphos-methyl	5	0.0025
Chlorfenvinphos	—	0.002
Diazinon	4	0.002
Dichlorvos	—	0.004
Dimethoate	4	0.02
Fenitrothion	—	0.005
Leptophos	—	—
Malathion	4	0.02
Parathion	6	0.005
Parathion-methyl	5	—
Trichlorfon	4	0.01

[1]Toxicity rating: Probable human oral lethal dosage for class 4 = 50–500 mg/kg, class 5 = 5–50 mg/kg, and class 6 = <5 mg/kg. (See Gosselin reference.)
[2]ADI = acceptable daily intake (mg/kg body weight/d).

Human Toxicology

In mammals as well as insects, the major effect of these agents is inhibition of acetylcholinesterase, because of phosphorylation of the esteratic site. The signs and symptoms that characterize acute intoxication are due to inhibition of this enzyme, resulting in the accumulation of acetylcholine; some of the agents also possess direct cholinergic activity. These effects and their treatment are described in Chapter 7.

In addition to—and independent of—inhibition of acetylcholinesterase, some of these agents are capable of phosphorylating another enzyme present in neural tissue, the so-called neuropathy target esterase (Johnson MK, 1990; Lotti, 1992). This results in development of a delayed neurotoxicity characterized by polyneuropathy, associated with paralysis and axonal degeneration (organophosphorus ester-induced delayed polyneuropathy; OPIDP); hens are particularly sensitive to these properties and have proved very useful for studying the pathogenesis of the lesion and for identifying potentially neurotoxic organophosphorus derivatives. In humans, neurotoxicity has been observed with triorthocresyl phosphate (TOCP), a noninsecticidal organophosphorus compound, and is thought to occur with the insecticides dichlorvos, trichlorfon, leptophos, methamidophos, mipafox, and trichloronat (Lotti, 1992). The polyneuropathy usually begins with burning and tingling sensations, particularly in the feet, with motor weakness following a few days later. Sensory and motor difficulties may extend to the legs and hands. Gait is affected, and ataxia may be present. There is no specific treatment for this form of delayed neurotoxicity.

Environmental Toxicology

Organophosphorus insecticides are not considered to be "persistent" pesticides. As a class they are considered to have a small impact on the environment in spite of their acute effects on organisms.

3. CARBAMATE INSECTICIDES

These compounds (Table 58–4) inhibit acetylcholinesterase by carbamoylation of the esteratic site. Thus, they possess the toxic properties associated with inhibition of this enzyme as described for the organophosphorus insecticides. The effects and treatment are described in Chapter 7. Generally speaking, the clinical effects due to carbamates are of shorter duration than those observed with organophosphorus compounds. The range between the doses that cause minor intoxication and those which result in lethality is larger with carbamates than that observed with the organophosphorus agents. Spontaneous reactivation of cholinesterase is more rapid after inhibition by the carbamates.

The carbamate insecticides are considered to be "nonpersistent" pesticides in the environment, and they are thought to exert a small impact on the environment.

4. BOTANICAL INSECTICIDES

Insecticides derived from natural sources include **nicotine, rotenone,** and **pyrethrum.** Nicotine is obtained from the dried leaves of *Nicotiana tabacum* and *Nicotiana rustica.* It is rapidly absorbed from mucosal surfaces; the free alkaloid, but not the salt, is readily absorbed from the skin. Nicotine reacts with the acetylcholine receptor of the postsynaptic membrane (sympathetic and parasympathetic ganglia, neuromuscular junction), resulting in depolarization of the membrane. Toxic doses cause stimulation rapidly followed by blockade of transmission. These actions are described in Chapter 7. Treatment is directed toward maintenance of vital signs and suppression of convulsions.

Rotenone (Figure 58–1) is obtained from *Derris el-*

Table 58–4. Carbamate insecticides.

Compound	Toxicity Rating[1]	ADI[2]
Aldicarb	6	0.005
Aminocarb	5	—
Carbaryl	4	0.01
Carbofuran	5	0.01
Dimetan	4	—
Dimetilan	4	—
Isolan	5	—
Methomyl	5	—
Propoxur	4	0.02
Pyramat	4	—
Pyrolan	5	—
Zectran	5	—

[1]Toxicity rating: Probable human oral lethal dosage for class 4 = 50–500 mg/kg, class 5 = 5–50 mg/kg, and class 6 = <5 mg/kg. (See Gosselin reference.)
[2]ADI = acceptable daily intake (mg/kg body weight/d).

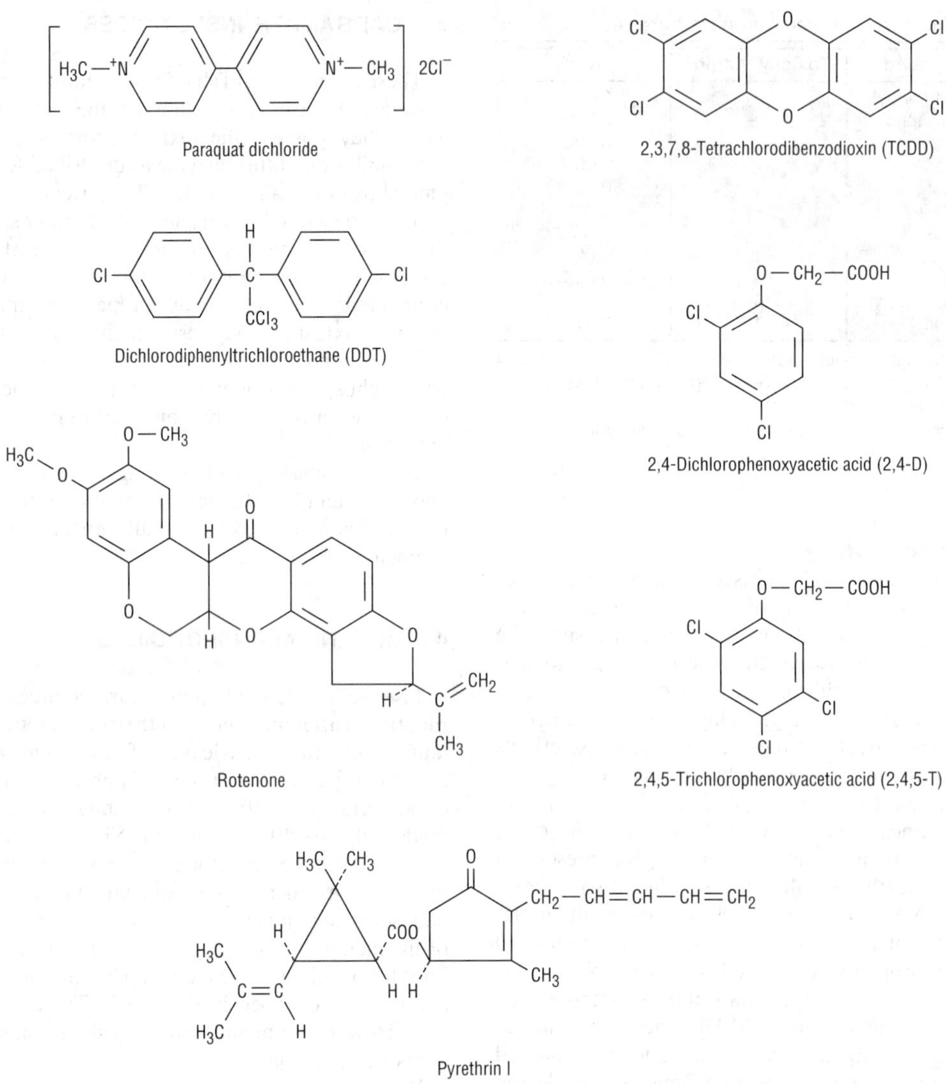

Figure 58–1. Chemical structures of selected agents.

liptica, Derris mallaccensis, Lonchocarpus utilis, and *Lonchocarpus urucu.* The oral ingestion of rotenone produces gastrointestinal irritation. Conjunctivitis, dermatitis, pharyngitis, and rhinitis can also occur. Treatment is symptomatic.

Pyrethrum consists of six known insecticidal esters: pyrethrin I (Figure 58–1), pyrethrin II, cinerin I, cinerin II, jasmolin I, and jasmolin II. Synthetic pyrethroids account for about 30% of worldwide insecticide usage (Ecobichon, 1991). Pyrethrum may be absorbed after inhalation or ingestion; absorption from the skin is not significant. The esters are extensively biotransformed. Pyrethrum insecticides are not highly toxic to mammals. When absorbed in sufficient quantities, the major site of toxic action is the central nervous system; excitation, convulsions, and tetanic paralysis can occur by a sodium channel mechanism resembling that of DDT. Treatment is with anticonvulsants. The most frequent injury reported in humans results from the allergenic properties of the substance, especially contact dermatitis. Cutaneous paresthesias have been observed in workers spraying synthetic pyrethroids. Severe occupational exposures to synthetic pyrethroids in China resulted in marked effects on the central nervous system, including convulsions (Ecobichon, 1991).

HERBICIDES

1. CHLOROPHENOXY HERBICIDES

2,4-Dichlorophenoxyacetic acid (2,4-D), 2,4,5-trichlorophenoxyacetic acid (2,4,5-T), and their salts and esters are the major compounds of interest as herbicides used for the destruction of weeds (Figure 58–1). They have been assigned toxicity ratings of 4 or 3, respectively, which place the probable human lethal dosages at 50–500 or 500–5000 mg/kg, respectively (Gosselin, 1984).

In humans, 2,4-D in large doses can cause coma and generalized muscle hypotonia. Rarely, muscle weakness and marked myotonia may persist for several weeks. With 2,4,5-T, coma may occur, but the muscular dysfunction is less evident. In laboratory animals, signs of liver and kidney dysfunction have also been reported. There is limited evidence that occupational exposure to phenoxy herbicides is associated with an increased risk of non-Hodgkin's lymphoma; the evidence for soft-tissue sarcoma, however, is considered equivocal (Morrison, 1992).

The toxicologic profile for these agents, particularly with 2,4,5-T, has been confusing because of the presence of chemical contaminants (dioxins) produced during the manufacturing process. The presence of 2,3,7,8-tetrachlorodibenzo-*p*-dioxin (TCDD) is believed to be largely responsible for the teratogenic effects detected in some animal species as well as the contact dermatitis and chloracne observed in workers involved in the manufacture of 2,4,5-T. In spite of exhaustive studies, it has been very difficult to document long-term toxic effects of TCDD in humans (Bertai, 1989).

TCDD as a contaminant in herbicides has stimulated interest in its possible carcinogenic properties in humans. Soft tissue sarcomas and malignant lymphomas have received considerable attention. A causal role for TCDD in malignant melanoma, however, appears unlikely, and the evidence for soft tissue sarcoma is considered unconvincing; a role for TCDD in the etiology of other cancers remains to be evaluated (Johnson ES, 1992, 1993).

2. BIPYRIDYL HERBICIDES

Paraquat is the most important agent of this class (Figure 58–1). It has been given a toxicity rating of 4, which places the probable human lethal dosage at 50–500 mg/kg. A number of lethal human intoxications (accidental or suicidal) have been reported.

In humans, the first signs and symptoms after oral exposure are attributable to gastrointestinal irritation (hematemesis and bloody stools). Within a few days, however, respiratory distress may appear (delayed toxicity) with the development of congestive hemorrhagic pulmonary edema accompanied by widespread cellular proliferation. Evidence of hepatic, renal, or myocardial involvement may also be present. The interval between ingestion and death may be several weeks. Because of the delayed pulmonary toxicity, prompt removal of paraquat from the digestive tract is important. Gastric lavage, the use of cathartics, and the use of adsorbents to prevent further absorption have all been advocated; after absorption, treatment is successful in fewer than 50% of cases. Oxygen should be used cautiously to combat dyspnea or cyanosis, as it may aggravate the pulmonary lesions (Arena, 1979). Patients require prolonged observation, because the proliferative phase begins 1–2 weeks after ingestion (Ellenhorn, 1988).

ENVIRONMENTAL POLLUTANTS

The **polychlorinated biphenyls (PCBs)** have been used in a large variety of applications as dielectric and heat transfer fluids, plasticizers, wax extenders, and flame retardants. Their industrial use and manufacture in the USA was terminated by 1977. Unfortunately, they persist in the environment. The products used commercially were actually mixtures of PCB isomers and homologues containing 12–68% chlorine. These chemicals are highly stable and highly lipophilic, poorly metabolized, and very resistant to environmental degradation; they bioaccumulate in food chains. Food is the major source of PCB residues in humans.

A serious exposure to PCBs, lasting several months, occurred in Japan in 1968 as a result of cooking oil contamination with PCB-containing transfer medium (Yusho disease). Possible effects on the fetus and the development of offspring of poisoned women were reported (Yen, 1989). It is now known that the contaminated cooking oil contained not only PCBs but also polychlorinated dibenzofurans (PCDFs) and polychlorinated quaterphenyls (PCQs). Consequently, the effects that were initially attributed to the presence of PCBs are now thought to have been largely caused by the other contaminants. Workers occupationally exposed to PCBs have exhibited the following clinical signs: dermatologic problems (chloracne, folliculitis, erythema, dryness, rash, hyperkeratosis, hyperpigmentation), some hepatic involvement, and elevated plasma triglycerides. Effects of PCBs alone on reproduction and development, as well as carcinogenic effects, have yet to be established in humans, even though some subjects have been exposed to very high levels of PCBs. The bulk of the evidence from human studies indicates that PCBs pose little hazard to human health except in situations where food is contaminated with high concentrations of these congeners.

REFERENCES

General

Ecobichon DJ: *The Basis of Toxicity Testing.* CRC Press 1992.

Lu FC: *Basic Toxicology: Fundamentals, Target Organs, and Risk Assessment,* 2nd ed. Hemisphere, 1991.

National Research Council: *Complex Mixtures.* National Academy Press, 1988

Air Pollution

Amdur MO: Air pollutants. In: *Casarett and Doull's Toxicology,* 4th ed. Amdur MO, Doull J, Klaassen CD (editors). Pergamon, 1991.

Folinsbee LJ: Human health effects of air pollution. Environ Health Perspect 1992;100:45.

Penney DG, Howley, JW: Is there a connection between carbon monoxide exposure and hypertension? Environ Health Perspect 1991;95:191.

Sarnet JM, Utell MJ: The environment and the lung. JAMA 1991;266:670.

Seinfeld JH: Urban air pollution: State of the science. Science 1989;243:745.

Wright ES, Dziedzic D, Wheeler CS: Cellular, biochemical, and functional effects of ozone: New research and perspectives on ozone health effects. Toxicol Lett 1990;51: 125.

Occupational Toxicology

Cullen MR, Cherniak MG, Rosenstock L: Occupational medicine. (Two parts.) N Engl J Med 1990;322:594, 675.

Proctor NH, Hughes JP: *Chemical Hazards of the Workplace,* 3rd ed. Lippincott, 1991.

Yardley-Jones A, Anderson D, Parke DV: The toxicity of benzene and its metabolism and molecular pathology in human risk assessment. Brit J Indust Med 1991;48:437.

Environmental Toxicology & Ecotoxicology

Ames BN: Pollution, pesticides, and cancer. J AOAC Int 1992;75:1.

Ames BN, Magaw R, Gold LS: Ranking possible carcinogenic hazards. Science 1987;236:271.

Bertai PA et al: Ten-year mortality study of the population involved in the Seveso incident in 1976. Am J Epidemiol 1989;129:1187.

Geyer H, Scheunert I, Korte F: Bioconcentration potential of organic environmental chemicals in humans. Regul Toxicol Pharmacol 1986;6:313.

Johnson ES: Human exposure to 2,3,7,8-TCDD and risk of cancer. CRC Crit Rev Toxicol 1992;21:451.

Johnson ES: Important aspects of the evidence for TCDD carcinogenicity in man. Environ Health Perspect 1993; 99:383.

Moriarty F: *Ecotoxicology.* Academic Press, 1983.

Reggiani G, Bruppacher R: Symptoms, signs and findings in humans exposed to PCBs and their derivatives. Environ Health Perspect 1985;60:225.

Silberhorn EM, Glauert HP, Robertson LW: Carcinogenicity of polyhalogenated biphenyls: PCBs and PBBs. CRC Crit Rev Toxicol 1990;20:440.

Truhaut R: Ecotoxicology: Objectives, principles and perspectives. Ecotoxicol Environ Safety 1977;1:151.

Yen YY et al: Follow-up study of reproductive hazards of multiparous women consuming PCBs-contaminated rice oil in Taiwan. Bull Environ Contam Toxicol 1989;43: 647.

Pesticides & Herbicides

Ecobichon DJ: Toxic effects of pesticides. In: *Casarett and Doull's Toxicology,* 4th ed. Amdur MO, Doull J, Klaassen CD (editors). Pergamon, 1991.

Johnson MK: Organophosphates and delayed neuropathy: Is NTE alive and well? Toxicol Appl Toxicol 1990;102: 385.

Lotti M: The pathogenesis of organophosphate polyneuropathy. CRC Crit Rev Toxicol 1992;213:465.

Morrison HI et al: Herbicides and cancer. J Natl Cancer Inst 1992;84:1866

Clinical Toxicology

Arena JM: *Poisoning,* 4th ed. Thomas, 1979.

Ellenhorn MJ, Barceloux DG: *Medical Toxicology.* Elsevier, 1988.

Gosselin RE, Smith RP, Hodge HC: *Clinical Toxicology of Commercial Products,* 5th ed. Williams & Wilkins, 1984.

Chelators & Heavy Metal Intoxication

59

Maria Almira Correia, PhD, & Charles E. Becker, MD

Some metals such as iron are essential for life, while others such as lead are present in all organisms but serve no useful biologic purpose. However, heavy metals in the environment pose a hazard to biologic organisms. Some of the oldest diseases of humans can be traced to heavy metal poisoning associated with the development of metal mining, refining, and use. Even with the present recognition of the hazards of heavy metals, the incidence of intoxication remains significant and the need for effective therapy remains high.

PHARMACOLOGY OF CHELATORS

Chelating agents are the most versatile and effective antidotes for metal intoxication. These compounds are usually flexible molecules with two or more electronegative groups that form stable coordinate-covalent bonds with the cationic metal atom. The complexes thus formed are then excreted by the body. The action of these drugs provides an excellent application of the principle of chemical antagonism. Edetate (ethylenediamine-tetraacetate, Figure 59–1) is an important example.

The efficiency of the chelator is partly determined by the number of ligands available for metal binding. The greater the number of these ligands, the more stable the metal-chelator complex. Depending on the number of metal-ligand bonds, the complex may be referred to as mono-, bi-, or polydentate. The chelating ligands include functional groups such as –OH, –SH, and –NH, which can donate electrons for coordination with the metal. Such bonding effectively prevents interaction of the metal with similar functional groups of enzymes, coenzymes, cellular nucleophiles, and membranes. Unfortunately, chelators are nonspecific and may chelate essential metals such as Ca^{2+} and Zn^{2+}, which are vital for body function. Such interactions are determined by the relative affinities of the toxic metal and the essential metal for the chelator. Thus, the toxicity associated with administration of some chelators may be caused by chelation of essential metals. This problem may be circumvented by judicious administration of the essential metal along with the chelating agent.

The relative efficacy of various chelators in facilitating excretion of metals from the body is also determined in part by the pharmacokinetics of the chelator. For any significant metal sequestration to occur, the affinity of the metal for the chelator must be greater than its affinity for endogenous ligands, and the relative rate of exchange of the metal between the endogenous ligands and the chelator must be faster than the rate of elimination of the chelator. If a chelator is eliminated more rapidly than the dissociation of the metal-endogenous ligand complex, it may not be present in sufficient concentrations for effective competition with the endogenous binding sites. This would be particularly critical if sequestration occurred via a ternary complex (endogenous ligand–metal–exogenous chelator). The above considerations also dictate that efficient mobilization can be accomplished only when the physiologic distribution of the chelator includes the body compartment containing the metal. For example, lead may be stored in bone and not be available for chelation. Following absorption, the tissue distribution profile of the metal may change markedly with time. For example, lead is first distributed to soft tissue such as bone marrow, brain, kidneys, and testes. Distribution to bone occurs subsequently. Therefore, the choice of chelator may also be determined on the basis of its distribution to primary and secondary tissue sites. Combination therapy with two or more chelating agents, each capable of permeating different target tissue compartments, may prove useful. Specific agents are presented below.

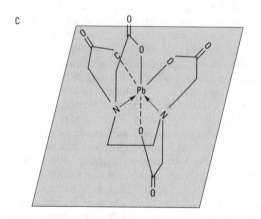

Figure 59–1. Salt and chelate formation with ethyl-enediamine-tetraacetate (EDTA). *A:* In a solution of the disodium salt of EDTA, the sodium and hydrogen ions are chemically and biologically available. *B:* In solutions of calcium disodium edetate, calcium is bound by coordinate-covalent bonds with nitrogens as well as by the usual ionic bonds. Calcium ions are effectively removed from solution. *C:* In the lead-edetate chelate, lead is incorporated into five heterocyclic rings. (Modified and reproduced, with permission, from Meyers FH, Jawetz E, Goldfien A: *Review of Medical Pharmacology,* 7th ed. Lange, 1980.)

BIDENTATE

1. DIMERCAPROL
(2,3-Dimercaptopropanol)

Dimercaprol (BAL) (Figure 59–2) is a colorless oily liquid with an offensive odor of rotten eggs. It is soluble in water, but aqueous solutions are unstable and oxidize readily. Dimercaprol is therefore dispensed in 10% solution in peanut oil and must be administered by a painful intramuscular injection. It interacts directly with metals in blood and tissue fluids and reactivates cellular sulfhydryl-containing enzymes. However, it is most efficient if administered immediately following exposure to the metals. This indicates that its salutary effects may be due primarily to *prevention* of metal binding to cellular constituents rather than *removal* of metal already bound.

Indications & Toxicity

Dimercaprol is thought to be a useful antidote in arsenic, mercury, and perhaps childhood lead poisoning. It has also been used in cadmium poisoning. Given intramuscularly, it is readily absorbed, metabolized, and excreted by the kidney within 4 hours. It produces a variety of adverse effects of which the cardiovascular (hypertension and tachycardia) are most significant. It also causes headache, nausea, vomiting, lacrimation, salivation, paresthesias, and pain at the injection site.

Because of the high incidence of adverse effects with dimercaprol, several congeners have been intensively investigated. Two of the most promising were succimer (2,3-dimercaptosuccinic acid, DMSA, dimercaprol succimer) and 2,3-dimercaptopropane-1-sulfonate (DMPS). These agents are more polar than dimercaprol, appear to be relatively confined to the extracellular space, and thus have less cellular toxicity. In comparative studies in mice, both agents were found to be more effective and less toxic than dimercaprol (Aposhian, 1990). Preliminary clinical evidence suggests that they are effective in mercury and arsenic poisoning as well as lead intoxication (Graziano, 1988). Succimer is now approved for use in lead poisoning in children with blood lead levels > 45 mg/dL and is investigational in several other types of heavy metal intoxication, with good results reported for treating poisoning with arsenic and mercury. It is also investigational for use in prevention of kidney stones in patients with homozygous cystinuria who are prone to stone development. Succimer may cause small changes in liver function and white blood count.

2. PENICILLAMINE
(D-β,β-Dimethylcysteine)

Penicillamine (Figure 59–2) is a white crystalline, water-soluble degradation product of penicillin. The D isomer is relatively nontoxic compared to the L form and consequently is the preferred form of the antidote. Penicillamine is readily absorbed from the gut and is resistant to metabolic degradation. Even greater resistance to metabolic degradation has been achieved by N-acetylation, as in N-acetylpenicillamine.

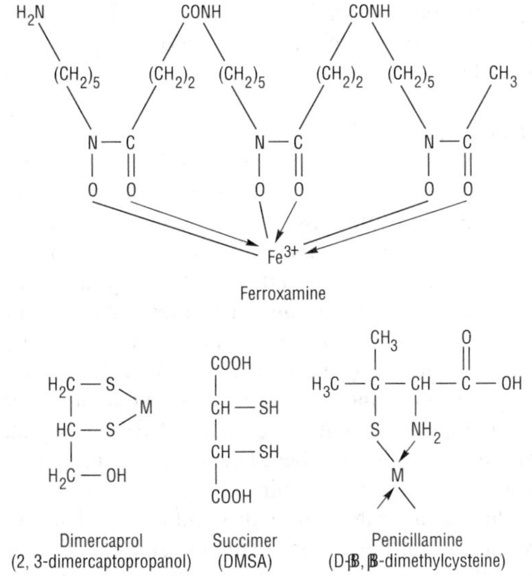

Figure 59–2. Chemical structures of several metal chelates. Ferroxamine without the chelated iron is deferoxamine. It is represented here to show the functional groups; the iron is actually held in a caged system. Dimercaprol incorporates the metal into a stable heterocyclic ring by covalent bonding. Succimer is closely related to dimercaprol. A single molecule of copper or other metal may be held by two molecules of penicillamine. (M = metal molecules.) (Modified and reproduced, with permission, from Meyers FH, Jawetz E, Goldfien A: *Review of Medical Pharmacology,* 7th ed. Lange, 1980.)

Indications & Toxicity

Penicillamine is used chiefly for poisoning with copper or to prevent copper accumulation, as in Wilson's disease. It is also used occasionally as adjunctive therapy in the treatment of lead, mercury, and arsenic poisoning and in the treatment of severe rheumatoid arthritis (Chapter 35). Pyridoxine deficiency is a frequent toxic effect of other forms of the drug but is rarely seen with the D form. Acute allergic reactions, especially in patients allergic to penicillin, may preclude the continued use of the drug. Nephrotoxicity with proteinuria has also been reported and with protracted use of the drug may result in renal insufficiency. Bone marrow toxicity resulting in aplastic anemia has been associated with prolonged drug intake. Autoimmune diseases, including lupus erythematosus and hemolytic anemia, have been reported also.

POLYDENTATE

1. EDETATE CALCIUM DISODIUM

Ethylenediamine-tetraacetic acid (EDTA) (Figure 59–1) is an efficient chelator of many divalent and trivalent metals in vitro. However, chelation of essential calcium in vivo—due to this very property—limits its clinical use. This limitation is partially circumvented by administration of its calcium disodium salt.

EDTA penetrates cell membranes relatively poorly and therefore chelates extracellular metal ions much more effectively than intracellular ions.

The highly polar ionic character of EDTA precludes significant oral absorption, and consequently the chelator (calcium disodium salt) is administered either by slow intravenous infusion or intramuscularly. It is excreted by glomerular filtration in 24 hours if kidney function is normal. Its effects (including renal toxicity; see below) may be prolonged in patients in renal failure.

Indications & Toxicity

Metals such as lead and a few other heavy metals capable of binding EDTA and displacing Ca^{2+} are effectively chelated. EDTA-induced mobilization of mercury, in contrast to that of lead, is unsuccessful, perhaps owing to the relatively poor distribution of the chelator into tissue compartments where mercury is found as well as to the less successful competition of mercury with the chelated calcium. EDTA is *not* useful in the treatment of atherosclerotic cardiovascular disease.

In high doses, EDTA is toxic to the kidney, and the renal tubules appear relatively sensitive to its toxic effects, which include hydropic degeneration of the proximal tubules, progressing to total destruction. Mild effects disappear with cessation of therapy. Other (rare) toxic effects include chills, fever, nausea, vomiting, myalgia, allergic reactions, and glycosuria.

2. TRIENTINE

Trientine (triethylenetetramine HCl) is a polydentate chelating agent that has affinity for copper and is useful in the treatment of Wilson's disease (hepatolenticular degeneration). It is available for this use in the USA. Early reports suggested that it may be less toxic than penicillamine in this application. It also has some effect in nickel poisoning. However, it was found to be teratogenic in long-term studies of rats. Another agent, tetrathiomolybdate, an effective

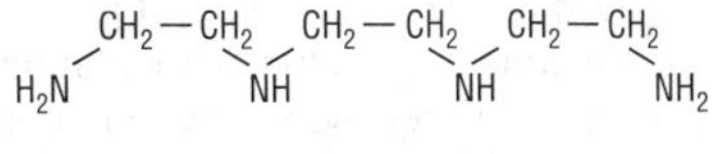

Trientine

and apparently less toxic copper chelator in sheep, is being explored as a potential replacement.

3. DEFEROXAMINE

Deferoxamine mesylate is isolated from *Streptomyces pilosus.* It binds iron avidly but essential trace metals poorly. Furthermore, while competing for loosely bound iron in iron-carrying proteins (hemosiderin and ferritin), it fails to compete with biologically chelated iron, as in microsomal and mitochondrial cytochromes and hemoproteins. Consequently, it is the chelator of choice for iron poisoning. It may also be useful in the treatment of aluminum toxicity in renal failure (Jones, 1991).

Deferoxamine is poorly absorbed when administered orally. To be effective, it must be administered intramuscularly or intravenously. It is believed to be metabolized, but the pathways are unknown. The products are excreted almost completely in the urine, turning the urine dark red if free iron exceeds the iron binding capacity. Intravenous administration may result in hypotensive shock owing to histamine release, especially if given rapidly. Neurotoxicity has been described with long-term therapy for iron overload.

Adverse idiosyncratic responses such as flushing, blotchy erythema, intestinal irritation, and urticaria have also been observed. Additional complications of deferoxamine therapy include severe coagulopathies, hepatic failure, renal failure, and intestinal infarction.

Use of deferoxamine in iron poisoning is described in Chapter 32.

TOXICOLOGY OF HEAVY METALS

LEAD

The toxic effects of lead probably constitute the oldest occupational disease in the world. Lead is now widely distributed in air, food, and water, so that a completely lead-free environment would be difficult or impossible to achieve. With a greater understanding of the kinetics and toxicology of lead and more childhood lead screening programs, acute lead poisoning is fortunately much less frequent than in the past. Hazardous working conditions have been improved, exposure of children to flaking lead-base paints has been reduced, and adult exposure to illicit whiskey and battery casings is less frequent (Schneitzer, 1990). However, important public health questions remain concerning environmental pollution and the hazard to renal, reproductive, hematopoietic, and neurologic function imposed by chronic low-level lead exposure (Landrigan, 1989). Lead serves no useful purpose in the human body. No safe threshold for the effects of lead on these organ systems has been demonstrated.

Pharmacokinetics

Metallic lead is slowly but consistently absorbed by inhalation and gastrointestinal absorption. *Inorganic* lead is poorly absorbed through the skin but *organic* lead compounds are well absorbed by this route. Absorption of lead dust via the respiratory tract is the most common cause of industrial poisoning. The intestinal tract is the primary route of entry in nonindustrial exposure (Table 59–1). Absorption via the gastrointestinal tract varies with the nature of the lead compound, but in general, about 10% of ingested inorganic lead is absorbed. Dietary calcium, iron, and phosphorus alter gastrointestinal lead absorption. Studies in laboratory animals demonstrate that a diet low in calcium and iron increases lead retention and that there are associated biochemical and morphologic manifestations of enhanced lead toxicity.

Once absorbed from the respiratory or gastrointestinal tract, lead is bound to erythrocytes and widely distributed initially to soft tissues such as bone marrow, brain, kidney, and testes. Its half-life in these tissues is about 30 days. Lead also crosses the placenta and poses a potential hazard to the fetus. Most lead entering the body is eventually bound in the skeleton; the half-life of elimination from bone is in excess of 20 years. The bony reservoir may provide a source of lead if bone breakdown occurs (eg, renal failure). The lead burden in bone has been quantitated using x-ray fluorescence techniques (Kosnett, 1994). Lead is also bound in hair and nails, which could theoretically be a useful method of estimating the body burden. However, external contamination creates special problems in interpreting these levels. Ingested lead is excreted in the stool (over 90%) and urine. Most of the absorbed lead is excreted via renal elimination. Small amounts of lead are also eliminated through sweat and in mother's milk.

Pharmacodynamics

Lead is capable of forming complex ligands with many compounds. It interferes with the activity of enzymes and affects a variety of organ systems.

A. Blood: Hypochromic microcytic anemia is common, but not all patients with lead poisoning are anemic. Lead induces critical derangements in heme biosynthesis, leading to excretion of porphyrins and their precursors in urine. The enzymes most sensitive to lead inhibition are delta-aminolevulinic acid dehydratase and ferrochelatase. Inhibition of the first enzyme blocks conversion of delta-aminolevulinic acid to porphobilinogen. Delta-aminolevulinic acid is excreted in the urine, and its urine concentration can be used as a diagnostic test. Inhibition of ferrochelatase results in decreased production of heme and accumu-

Table 59–1. Toxicology of arsenic, lead, and mercury.

	Form Entering Body	Route of Absorption	Distribution	Target Organs for Toxicity	Metabolism	Elimination
Arsenic	Inorganic arsenic salts.	Gastrointestinal, skin, respiratory (all mucous surfaces).	Red cells (95–99% bound to globin) (24 hours); then to liver, lung, kidney, wall of gastrointestinal tract, spleen, muscle, nerve tissue (2 weeks); then to skin, hair, and bone (years).	Increased vascular permeability leading to vasodilation and vascular collapse. Uncoupling of oxidative phosphorylation resulting in impaired cellular metabolism.	Binds avidly to cellular sulfhydryl groups of various critical enzymes to form stable cyclic thioarsenicals. Substitutes for inorganic phosphorus in synthesis of high-energy phosphates.	Principally renal. Sweat and feces minor.
Lead	Inorganic lead oxides and salts.	Gastrointestinal, respiratory, skin (minor).	Bone (90%), teeth, hair, blood (erythrocytes), liver, kidney.	Hematopoietic tissues and liver, CNS, kidney, neuromuscular junction.	Dissociation and binding of lead to critical tissue sulfhydryl groups.	Urine and feces (major); sweat (minor).
	Organic (tetraethyl lead).	Skin (major), gastrointestinal.	Liver.	CNS.	Hepatic dealkylation (fast)→trialkymetabolites (slow)→ dissociation to lead.	Urine and feces (major); sweat (minor).
Mercury	Elemental mercury.	Respiratory tract.	CNS (where it is trapped as Hg^{2+}), kidney (following conversion of elemental Hg to Hg^{2+}).	CNS (neuropsychiatric due to elemental Hg and its Hg^{2+} metabolite), kidney (substantial due to conversion of elemental Hg to Hg^{2+}).	Elemental Hg converted to Hg^{2+}.	Urine (major; feces (minor).
	Inorganic: Hg^+ (less toxic); Hg^{2+} (more toxic).	Gastrointestinal, skin (minor).	Kidney (predominant), blood, brain (minor).	Kidney, gastrointestinal.	Hg^{2+} plus R–SH converted to Hg^+–S–R, $Hg(S–R)_2$.	Urine.
	Organic: alkyl, aryl, alkoxylkyl.	Gastrointestinal, skin (substantial).	Kidney, brain, blood.	CNS.	R–Hg^+ converted to Hg^{2+} plus R (slow).	Urine.

lation of its precursor, protoporphyrin IX. In addition, the shortened life span of erythrocytes contributes to lead-induced anemia.

B. Nervous System: Lead affects the peripheral and central nervous systems. The lowest concentration of lead associated with neurologic damage is still uncertain (Needleman, 1990). Even at very high blood levels and marked alterations of hematopoietic function, some individuals may have no apparent neurologic manifestations. The most common sign of peripheral neuropathy is painless weakness of the extensor muscles of the hand (wristdrop). The lower limb is less often involved. Sensory function is usually not affected. Lead-induced neuropathy usually develops after months of chronic exposure but may occur subacutely in 2–3 weeks.

Lead encephalopathy is an important acute disorder usually seen in children who have eaten lead-base paints. It is rare in adults. Encephalopathy most often begins with convulsions and is associated with increased intracranial pressure and brain edema. The mortality rate is high, and urgent chelation therapy is required. Cognitive abnormalities have been docu-

mented in association with chronic heavy exposure in lead workers (Stollery, 1989).

C. Kidneys: Lead may cause interstitial kidney damage and hypertension. In acute intoxication, lead may affect uric acid metabolism and cause both acute gout and gouty nephropathy. Lead nephropathy itself develops only after years of prolonged lead exposure. Recent studies suggest that renal damage, hypertension, or both in adults may result from childhood lead exposure. Environmental exposures to lead from gasoline and cigarettes may contribute to hypertension in adults, especially black males (Osterloh, 1989).

D. Reproductive Organs: Lead also affects reproductive function. It has long been known that lead poisoning is associated with decreased fertility in women and an increased incidence of stillbirths. Little is known about the effects of lead on male reproductive function, though sterility and testicular atrophy have been noted in severe cases, and asymptomatic lead exposure has been associated with dose-related alteration of sperm.

E. Gastrointestinal Tract: Lead poisoning may cause loss of appetite, epigastric distress, abdominal colicky pains, and constipation. The mechanism of lead colic is unclear but involves contraction of smooth muscles of the intestinal wall. The gastrointestinal symptoms are reversible with chelation therapy.

Major Forms of Lead Intoxication
A. Inorganic Lead Poisoning:
1. Acute–Acute inorganic lead poisoning is uncommon today. It usually results from industrial inhalation of large quantities of lead oxide or, in small children, from ingestion of a large oral dose of lead in lead-based paints. Acute intoxication is associated with severe gastrointestinal distress that progresses to marked central nervous system abnormalities. If absorption of lead is slower, abdominal colic and encephalopathy may develop over days. The diagnosis of acute inorganic lead poisoning may be difficult. Disorders that simulate lead poisoning include appendicitis, peptic ulcer, and pancreatitis.

2. Chronic–The most common manifestations of chronic inorganic lead poisoning are weakness, anorexia, nervousness, tremor, weight loss, headache, and gastrointestinal symptoms. The association of recurrent abdominal pain and extensor muscle weakness without sensory disturbances suggests the possibility of lead poisoning. The most characteristic neurologic finding in chronic lead poisoning is wristdrop.

The diagnosis is confirmed by measuring lead in the blood and identifying abnormalities of porphyrin metabolism. The zinc erythrocyte protoporphyrin test is valuable to diagnose chronic lead poisoning if iron deficiency anemia can be ruled out. Peripheral blood smears may show basophilic stippling. Lead deposits in long bones are uncommon, as are lead lines on the gums. In difficult cases an EDTA chelation test or K x-ray fluorescence bone tests are used to confirm a suspected diagnosis of lead poisoning.

B. Organic Lead Poisoning:
Organic lead poisoning is usually caused by tetraethyl or tetramethyl lead, which is used as an "antiknock" agent in gasoline. Organic lead is highly volatile and lipid-soluble. Thus, it can be readily absorbed through the skin and respiratory tract. Severe poisoning has resulted from deliberate "sniffing" of gasoline. Acute central nervous system disorders result. These can progress rapidly, causing hallucinations, insomnia, headache, and irritability (similar to severe alcohol withdrawal). Organic lead causes relatively few hematologic abnormalities. Tetraethyl and tetramethyl lead are metabolized by the liver to trialkyl lead and inorganic lead. Trialkyl lead is thought to be responsible for the acute poisoning syndrome. Chronic poisoning with organic lead is fortunately uncommon. Most organic lead exposures occur in the course of cleaning gasoline storage tanks or from sniffing leaded gasoline. With massive organic lead exposure, seizures may terminate in coma and death. Blood and urine lead levels are relatively unreliable in organic lead poisoning but may be elevated.

Treatment
A. Inorganic Lead Poisoning: Treatment of symptomatic inorganic lead poisoning involves immediate termination of exposure and use of chelation therapy. For severe intoxication, use an intravenous infusion of calcium disodium EDTA in a dose of approximately 8 mg/kg; dimercaprol, 2.5 mg/kg/dose intramuscularly, is suggested by some for lead-poisoned children. Oral succimer is approved specifically for lead poisoning in children. Blood and urine levels of lead should be monitored as a guide to therapy. Availability of succimer makes the use of penicillamine unnecessary. Treating asymptomatic patients with chelating agents is not recommended. Prophylactic use of chelating agents in workers exposed to lead is contraindicated because it may increase absorption of the metal from the gastrointestinal tract. After chelation therapy is discontinued, blood lead and porphyrin function should be assessed by serial analysis in order to identify a rebound increase in lead as lead is mobilized from bone.

B. Organic Lead Poisoning: Initial treatment consists of decontaminating the skin and preventing further exposure. Treatment of seizures requires judicious use of anticonvulsants.

ARSENIC

Elemental arsenic and arsenic compounds are widely distributed in nature. Arsenic is a common contaminant of coal and of many metal ores, especially copper, lead, and zinc. The two largest sources of industrial arsenic are coal-burning power plants and smelters. Approximately 1.5 million employees in the USA are potentially exposed to arsenic compounds.

The chemical forms of arsenic of toxicologic importance are elemental arsenic, inorganic arsenic, organic arsenicals, and arsine gas (AsH_3). The important toxic forms of the metal are trivalent arsenic and arsine gas.

Arsenic was used as both a therapeutic agent and poison in ancient Greek and Roman times. More recently (until the advent of penicillin), arsenic was used in the treatment of syphilis and as a tonic in Fowler's solution. Its only therapeutic use today is in the treatment of trypanosomiasis involving the central nervous system. The most common nonmedical uses of arsenic compounds are as insecticides, herbicides, fungicides, algicides, and wood preservatives. Arsenic is also used for doping semiconductor chips, for alloying, and in glassmaking.

Pharmacokinetics

Environmental and dietary exposure to arsenic and its compounds is possible, since arsenic is present in ocean water, especially near the mouths of estuaries draining industrial areas. Alcoholic beverages when improperly prepared occasionally contain large amounts of arsenic. Many types of seafood contain nontoxic forms of arsenic. These environmental contaminants may account for elevated urinary arsenic levels, as the usual urine arsenic test does not distinguish the form of arsenic. The average daily intake of arsenic from environmental sources is less than 1 mg. The total body burden of arsenic in adults is about 20 mg, mostly in bone and to a lesser extent in hair and skin. Inorganic arsenic can be absorbed from the lungs, the gut, and rarely through intact skin (Table 59–1).

Gastrointestinal absorption of arsenic compounds is a function of their water solubility. Trivalent arsenites are poorly soluble and pentavalent arsenates more soluble. Organic arsenicals are usually poorly absorbed from the gastrointestinal tract. Arsenic can cross the placenta and may cause fetal damage. The trivalent form of arsenic is excreted slowly, chiefly by the fecal route, whereas the pentavalent form is more rapidly excreted in urine in a methylated form. Absorption of arsenic through the skin is a function of lipid solubility, with the trivalent form being more lipid-soluble than the pentavalent form. Trivalent inorganic arsenicals are partially oxidized in the body to the pentavalent form, and some are methylated.

Pharmacodynamics

All of the major toxicologic effects of inorganic arsenical compounds are attributable to the trivalent form of arsenic. Trivalent arsenic inhibits sulfhydryl enzymes and is corrosive to epithelium lining the respiratory and gastrointestinal tracts, to skin, and to other tissues. The primary target organs for trivalent arsenic are the nervous system, bone marrow, liver, skin, and respiratory tract. Arsenic is now a recognized carcinogen in humans (Bates, 1992).

Major Forms of Arsenic Intoxication

A. Acute and Subacute Inorganic Arsenic Poisoning: Acute and subacute forms of inorganic arsenic poisoning may produce acute violent nausea, vomiting, abdominal pain, skin irritation, laryngitis, and bronchitis. The gastroenteritis may be so severe as to be hemorrhagic. A sweet metallic garlicky odor is imparted to breath and feces. Vomiting may be severe, and diarrhea may be characterized as "rice water stool." The trivalent form of arsenic also damages capillaries, causing increased permeability, dehydration, shock, and death. If patients survive the acute episodes, bone marrow depression, encephalo-

pathy, and a crippling sensory neuropathy may follow.

Treatment of acute arsenic poisoning includes induction of emesis or gastric lavage, correction of dehydration and electrolyte imbalance, and supportive care for liver and other tissue injury. In severe cases, immediate chelation therapy with dimercaprol, 3–5 mg/kg intramuscularly every 4 hours for 48 hours, is indicated. Dimercaprol is continued every 12 hours for 10 days while monitoring urinary excretion of arsenic. Some studies suggest that succimer is more effective than dimercaprol (Jones, 1991).

B. Chronic Inorganic Arsenic Poisoning: Chronic inorganic arsenic poisoning may present as perforation of the nasal septum, irritation of the skin, sensory neuropathy, hair loss, bone marrow depression, fatty infiltration of the liver, or renal damage. The skin manifestations include cutaneous vasodilation and pallor (from anemia), resulting in a characteristic "milk and roses" complexion. Prolonged arsenic exposure may lead to hyperkeratosis of the palms and soles, increased skin pigmentation, hair loss, and white lines over the nails. Patients may become cachectic owing to chronic nausea and gastrointestinal complaints. Conjunctivitis and irritation of the mucous membranes, larynx, and respiratory passages are common.

Laboratory diagnosis of inorganic arsenic poisoning may be difficult. Urinary arsenic measurements and hair and nail analyses are indications of prior exposure but not intoxication. Urinary arsenic levels are influenced by intake of seafood. Most unexposed persons taking an average amount of seafood in the diet will excrete less than 100 μg of arsenic per 24 hours in the urine. Laboratory evidence of bone marrow suppression, abnormal liver function tests, proteinuria, and hematuria may also be diagnostically useful.

C. Organic Arsenic Poisoning: Organic arsenical poisoning is rare. Organic arsenicals are absorbed to a varying extent depending on their valences and are usually rapidly excreted. Benzene arsenicals are not converted to inorganic arsenic compounds under most circumstances. The mechanism of organic arsenical toxicity involves inhibition of sulfhydryl enzymes, especially in the central nervous system. Cerebral lesions are occasionally observed in both gray and white matter.

D. Arsine Gas Poisoning: Arsine gas (AsH_3) is one of the most powerful hemolytic agents known. It is absorbed primarily through inhalation. Arsine combines with hemoglobin and is oxidized to a hemolytic compound. Destruction of red blood cells leads to hemoglobinuria, causing acute renal failure. Extensive renal tubular damage occurs, along with thickening of glomerular basement membranes. Initial symptoms are dark urine, jaundice, and severe abdominal pain. Severe arsine exposure will lead to high arsenic levels in the urine. Laboratory findings consist of hemolysis and severe anemia. Chelation therapy is not useful to prevent red cell destruction. Supportive care, including exchange transfusion and hemodialysis for renal failure, determines the outcome with acute arsine poisoning.

E. Other Manifestations of Arsenic Poisoning: Increased incidence of skin cancer is recognized in patients undergoing prolonged treatment for psoriasis and other skin disease with inorganic arsenicals, especially Fowler's solution. A study of smelter workers in the USA suggests an increased risk of respiratory system cancer that is probably dose-related. Since smelter workers have multiple exposures and confounding variables for enhanced risk of respiratory cancer, further studies are required to define the risk. Attempts to demonstrate the carcinogenic potential of arsenic compounds in animals have generally been unrewarding. Mutagenic testing, especially with the Ames test, has failed to show any mutagenic effects of arsenic compounds, though chromosomal abnormalities have been reported. Despite these laboratory uncertainties, arsenic is now considered a human carcinogen for the skin and lung. It is "suspected" in cancers of the liver, gastrointestinal tract, hematopoietic system, kidney, and bladder (Bates, 1992).

MERCURY

Metallic mercury as "quicksilver"—the only metal that is liquid under ordinary conditions—has attracted scholarly and scientific interest from earliest times. It was quickly recognized that the mining of mercury was hazardous to health. As industrial uses of mercury became common during the past 200 years, new forms of toxicity were recognized that were found to be associated with inorganic compounds of the element or with the metal itself. In 1953, a mysterious epidemic occurred in the Japanese fishing village of Minamata. The village is located near the effluent of a large factory in which vinyl plastic is manufactured. The epidemic of poisoning was traced to the consumption of fish contaminated by the effluent discharged by the factory. The causative agent was methylmercury, formed in ocean water by bacterial action on inorganic mercury from the effluent.

The main sources of inorganic mercury as a toxic hazard include materials used in dental laboratories, wood preservatives, herbicides, insecticides, spermicidal jellies, fireworks, batteries, thermometers, barometers, gauges, and preparations of chlorine and sodium hydroxide. Organic mercury compounds are used as seed dressings, as fungicides, and in preventing mold.

Pharmacokinetics

The absorption of mercury varies considerably depending on the chemical form of the metal. Elemental mercury is quite volatile and can be absorbed from the lungs (Table 59–1). It is poorly absorbed from the gastrointestinal tract. Inhaled mercury is the primary source of occupational exposure. Organic short-chain alkyl mercury compounds are volatile and potentially harmful by the same route. After absorption, mercury is distributed to the tissues in a few hours, with the highest concentration occurring in the proximal renal tubules. Mercury is readily bound to sulfhydryl groups. Excretion of mercury is primarily through the urine, although some is removed through the gastrointestinal tract and the sweat glands. Most inorganic mercury gaining entrance into the body is excreted over a 1-week period, but the kidney and the brain retain mercury for longer periods.

The acute and chronic poisoning syndromes with mercury depend on the form of the metal. Oral metallic mercury has little effect. Oral mercurous chloride has relatively low toxicity. Mercuric chloride is very toxic and causes acute kidney damage. Organic mercurials, especially methyl mercury, are more completely absorbed from the gastrointestinal tract. The short-chain organic mercury compounds are usually distributed to the central nervous system and are devoid of renal toxicity. There is no solid evidence that mercury amalgam in dental fillings poses a risk to patients.

Major Forms of Mercury Intoxication

A. Acute: Acute mercury poisoning most frequently occurs from inhalation of high concentrations of mercury vapor. Symptoms include chest pain and shortness of breath, metallic taste, and nausea and vomiting. Acute damage to the kidney occurs next. If the patient survives, severe gingivitis and gastroenteritis occur on the third to fourth days. In the most severe cases, severe muscle tremor and psychopathology develop.

B. Chronic: Chronic mercury poisoning may be difficult to diagnose. Complaints of mouth and gastrointestinal disorders may be reported, and signs of renal insufficiency may be present. Gingivitis, discolored gums, and loosening of the teeth are common. The salivary glands may be enlarged. Tremor involving the fingers, arms, and legs is often present. Chronic mercury poisoning may simulate drug intoxication, cerebellar dysfunction, or Wilson's disease. An alteration of handwriting is frequently observed. Ocular changes, including deposition of mercury in the lens, are reported. Personality changes with unusual fearfulness, inability to concentrate, and irritability have been described. This psychologic disorder is known as erethism.

Diagnosis of chronic mercury poisoning depends primarily on a history of exposure. Concentrations of mercury in the body vary widely, apparently owing to pharmacokinetic factors. Hair analysis may be useful in diagnosing mercury poisoning.

Treatment

A. Acute: Treatment of acute mercury poisoning consists of removal from exposure and chelation treatment with dimercaprol, usually in a dosage of 3–5 mg/kg intramuscularly every 4 hours for 48 hours and then every 12 hours for 10 days. Succimer has

been reported to be more effective and less toxic (Jones, 1991). If renal damage occurs, hemodialysis will be required. Oral charcoal therapy is not useful in binding mercury in the gastrointestinal tract.

B. Chronic: Succimer may prove to be of value. Urinary mercury levels should be monitored to observe enhanced removal. Treatment of organic mercury poisoning has been poorly studied. Administration of chelating agents requires further study.

PREPARATIONS AVAILABLE

Deferoxamine (Desferal Mesylate)
  Parenteral: powder to reconstitute for injection (500 mg per vial)
Dimercaprol, BAL (in oil)
  Parenteral: 100 mg/mL for injection (in 3 mL ampules)
Edetate calcium [calcium EDTA](Calcium Disodium Versenate)

  Parenteral: 200 mg/mL for injection
Penicillamine (Cuprimine, Depen)
  Oral: 125, 250 mg capsules; 250 mg tablets
Succimer (Chemet)
  Oral: 100 mg capsules
Trientine (Syprine)
  Oral: 250 mg capsules

REFERENCES

Chelating Agents

Aposhian HV, Aposhian MM: *meso*-2,3-Dimercaptosuccinic acid: chemical, pharmacological and toxicological properties of an orally effective metal chelating agent. Annu Rev Pharmacol Toxicol 1990;30:279.

Graziano JH: Role of 2,3-dimercaptosuccinic acid in the treatment of heavy metal poisoning. Med Toxicol 1986;1:155.

Graziano JH, Lolacono NJ, Meyer P: Dose-response study of oral 2,3-dimercaptosuccinic acid in children with elevated lead concentrations. J Pediatr 1988;113:751.

Jones MM: New developments in therapeutic chelating agents as antidotes for metal poisoning. Crit Rev Toxicol 1991;21:209.

Mann KV, Travers JD: Succimer, an oral lead chelator. Clin pharmacy 1991;10:914.

Netter P et al: Clinical pharmacokinetics of D-penicillamine. Clin Pharmacokinet 1987;13:317.

Walshe JM: Treatment of Wilson's disease with trientine (triethylene tetramine) dihydrochloride. Lancet 1982;1:643.

Weinberger HL et al: An analysis of 248 initial mobilization tests performed on an ambulatory basis. Am J Dis Child 1987;141:1266.

Heavy Metals

Friberg L, Nordberg GF, Vouk V (editors): *Handbook on the Toxicology of Metals,* 2nd ed. Elsevier, 1986.

Greenhouse AH, Glaeske CS: Heavy metal intoxication. In: *Textbook of Clinical Neurotoxicology and Therapeutics,* 2nd ed. Klawans HL et al (editors). Raven Press, 1992.

Landrigan PJ: Occupational and community exposures to toxic metals: Lead, cadmium, mercury and arsenic. West J Med 1982;137:531.

Lead

Baghurst PA et al: Environmental exposure to lead and children's intelligence at the age of seven years. The Port Pirie cohort study. N Engl J Med 1992;327:1279.

Brangstrup-Hanse JP: Chelatable lead burden by calcium disodium EDTA and blood lead concentration in man. J Occup Med 1981;93:39.

Bushnell PJ, Jaeger RJ: Hazards from environmental lead exposure: A review of recent literature. Vet Hum Toxicol 1986;28:255.

Chisolm JJ: The continuing hazard of lead exposure and its effects in children. Neurotoxicology 1985;5:23.

Cory-Slechta DA, Weiss B, Cox C: Mobilization and redistribution of lead over the course of calcium disodium ethylenediamine tetraacetate chelation therapy. J Pharmacol Exp Ther 1987;243:804.

Cory-Slechta DA, Weiss B: Efficacy of the chelating agent CaEDTA in reversing lead-induced changes in behavior. Neurotoxicology 1990;10:685.

Craswell PW et al: Chronic renal failure with gout: A marker of chronic lead poisoning. Kidney Int 1984;26:319.

Hemberg SL: Lead in occupational medicine. In: *Principles and Practical Approach of Occupational Medicine,* 2nd ed. Zenz C (editor). Year Book, 1988.

Ibels LS, Pollock CA: Lead intoxication. Med Toxicol 1986;1:387.

Kosnett MJ et al: Factors influencing bone lead concentration in a suburban community assessed by noninvasive K x-ray fluorescence. JAMA 1994;271:197.

Landrigan PJ: Toxicity of lead at low dose. Br J Ind Med 1989;46:593.

Markowitz ME et al: Effects of calcium disodium versenate (CaNa$_2$EDTA) chelation in moderate childhood lead poisoning. Pediatrics 1993;92:265.

Nadig RJ: Treatment of lead poisoning. JAMA 1990; 263:2181.

Needleman HL et al: The long-term effects of exposure to low doses of lead in childhood: An 11-year follow-up report. N Engl J Med 1990;322:83.

Nriagu JO: *Lead and Lead Poisoning in Antiquity.* Wiley, 1983.

O'Connor ME: CaEDTA vs CaEDTA plus BAL to treat children with elevated blood levels. Clin Pediatrics 1992;31:386.

Oheme FW: Mechanism of heavy metal toxicity. J Clin Toxicol 1972;5:151.

Osterloh JD et al: Body burdens of lead in hypertensive nephropathy. Arch Environ Health 1989;44:304.

Pagliuca A et al: Lead poisoning: clinical, biochemical, and haematological aspects of a recent outbreak. J Clin Pathol 1990;43:277.

Pirkle JL et al: The relationship between blood lead levels and blood pressure and its cardiovascular risk implication. Am J Epidemiol 1985;121:246.

Rempel D: The lead-exposed worker. JAMA 1989;262: 532.

Schneitzer L et al: Lead poisoning in adults from renovation of an older home. Ann Emerg Med 1990;19:415.

Schwartz J: Lead, blood pressure, and cardiovascular disease in men and women. Environ Health Perspect 1991;91:71.

Settle DM: Lead in albacore: Guide to lead pollution in America. Science 1980;207:1167.

Sharp DS, Becker CE, Smith AH: Chronic low-level lead exposure: Its role in the pathogenesis of hypertension. Med Toxicol 1987;2:210.

Staessen JA et al: Impairment of renal function with increasing blood lead concentrations in the general population. N Engl J Med 1992;327:151.

Stollery BT et al: Cognitive functioning in lead workers. Br J Ind Med 1989;46:698.

Arsenic

Bates MN, Smith AH, Hopenhayn-Rich C: Arsenic ingestion and internal cancers: A review. Am J Epidemiol 1992;135:462.

Martin DW Jr, Woeber KA: Arsenic poisoning. Calif Med (March) 1973;118:13.

Mathieu D et al: Massive arsenic poisoning: Effect of hemodialysis and dimercaprol on arsenic kinetics. Intensive Care Med 1992;18:47.

National Institute of Safety and Health: *Occupational Exposure to Inorganic Arsenic: New Criteria.* US Department of Health, Education, and Welfare Publication No. 75–140, 1975.

Peterson RG, Rumack BH: D-Penicillamine therapy of acute arsenic poisoning. J Pediatr 1977;91:661.

Mercury

Agocs MM et al: Mercury exposure from interior latex paint. N Engl J Med 1990;323:1096.

Done AK: The toxic emergency: The many faces of mercurialism. Emerg Med (Jan) 1980;12:137.

Jung RC, Aaronson J: Death following inhalation of mercury vapor at home. West J Med 1980;132:539.

Kahn A, Denis R, Blum D: Accidental ingestion of mercuric sulphate in a 4-year-old child. Clin Pediatr 1977; 16:956.

Krohn IT et al: Subcutaneous injection of metallic mercury. JAMA 1980;243:548.

Roels H et al: Surveillance of workers exposed to mercury vapor: Validation of previously proposed biological threshold limit value for mercury concentration in the urine. Am J Ind Med 1985;7:45.

Snodgrass W et al: Mercury poisoning from home gold ore processing. JAMA 1981;246:1929.

Management of the Poisoned Patient

60

Charles E. Becker, MD, & Kent R. Olson, MD

Over a million cases of acute poisoning occur each year. Most of the deaths are due to intentional suicidal overdose with a drug or toxic substance. Childhood deaths due to accidental ingestion of a toxic product have been markedly reduced in the past 20 years as a result of safety packaging and effective poisoning prevention education.

In spite of the relatively large number of poisonings that occur every year, poisoning is rarely fatal if the victim receives medical attention promptly and good supportive care is given. Careful management of airway obstruction, respiratory failure, hypotension, seizures, and thermoregulatory disturbances has resulted in improved survival of overdosed patients who reach the hospital alive.

This chapter reviews the basic principles of poisoning, the pathophysiology of lethal poisoning, initial management of the overdose, diagnosis of toxic syndromes, and specialized treatment of poisoning including methods of increasing the elimination of drugs and toxins.

TOXICOKINETICS & TOXICODYNAMICS

Toxicologic problems are best viewed in a classic pharmacologic model. This model is based on the pharmacologic properties of chemical agents and the effects of "normal" doses on "normal" people. Toxicology extends this information to excessive doses.

The term "toxicokinetics" denotes the absorption, distribution, excretion, and metabolism of toxins, toxic doses of therapeutic agents, and their metabolites. The term "toxicodynamics" is used to denote the injurious effects of these substances on vital function. Although there are many similarities between the pharmacokinetics and toxicokinetics of most substances, there are also important differences. The same caution applies to pharmacodynamics and toxicodynamics.

SPECIAL ASPECTS OF TOXICOKINETICS

Volume of Distribution

The volume of distribution (V_d) is defined as the apparent volume into which a substance is distributed. It is calculated from the dose given and the resulting plasma concentration: V_d = dose/concentration, as described in Chapter 3. If a chemical is highly tissue-bound or otherwise sequestered outside the plasma, then the plasma concentration will be low and the V_d very large. A large V_d implies that the drug is not readily accessible to measures aimed at purifying the blood, such as hemodialysis. Drugs with large volumes of distribution (> 5–10 L/kg) include antidepressants, phenothiazines, lindane, and phencyclidine (PCP). Drugs with relatively small volumes of distribution (< 1 L/kg) include theophylline, salicylate, phenobarbital, lithium, and phenytoin (Table 3–1).

Clearance

Clearance is a measure of the volume of plasma that is cleared of drug per unit time. For most drugs, the total amount of drug removed per unit time is dependent on the plasma drug concentration as well as the clearance. The body has intrinsic mechanisms for clearing drugs, and the total clearance is the sum of clearances by excretion by the kidneys, metabolism by the liver, and elimination in sweat, feces, and expired air (see Chapter 3). In planning detoxification strategy, it is important to know the contribution of each organ to total clearance. For example, if a drug is 95% cleared by liver metabolism and only 5% cleared by renal excretion (eg, phencyclidine, PCP), then even a dramatic increase in urinary output would have little effect on overall elimination.

Overdosage of a drug can alter the usual pharmacokinetic processes, and this must be considered when applying kinetics to poisoned patients. For example, dissolution of tablets or gastric emptying time may be altered so that peak effects of the toxin are delayed. Drugs may injure the gastrointestinal tract and thereby alter absorption. If the capacity of the liver to metabolize a drug is exceeded, then more drug will be delivered to the circulation. With a dramatic increase in the concentration of drug in the blood, tissue-binding and protein-binding capacity may be exceeded, resulting in an increased fraction of free drug and greater toxicologic effect. At normal dosage, most drugs are eliminated at a rate proportionate to the plasma concentration (first-order kinetics). If the plasma concentration is very high and normal metabolism is saturated, the rate of elimination may become fixed (zero-order kinetics). This change in kinetics may markedly prolong the apparent serum half-life and increase toxicity.

SPECIAL ASPECTS OF TOXICODYNAMICS

Knowledge of basic pharmacology may also help the physician anticipate important toxicodynamic problems in the diagnosis and management of the intoxicated patient. The general dose-response principles described in Chapter 2 are of crucial importance in determining the severity of the intoxication. When considering **quantal dose-response** data, both the therapeutic index and the overlap of therapeutic and toxic response curves must be considered. The safety margin, if known, takes the latter factor into account. For instance, as shown in Figure 60–1, drugs A and B have the same therapeutic index. However, drug B is much more likely to cause inadvertent intoxication, because its toxic response curve overlaps the therapeutic dose range much more than in the case of drug A. For some drugs, eg, sedative-hypnotics, the major toxic effect is a direct extension of the therapeutic action, as shown by their **graded dose-response curve** (Figure 60–2). In the case of a drug with a flat dose-response curve (drug A), lethal effects may require

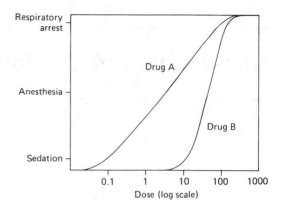

Figure 60–2. Graded dose-response comparison of two sedative-hypnotic drugs. A much larger multiple of the normal prescription dose of drug A is required to cause respiratory arrest, ie, it is safer than drug B.

100 times the normal therapeutic dose. In contrast, a drug with a steeper curve (drug B) may be lethal at 10 times the normal dose.

For many drugs, at least part of the toxic effect may be distinct from the therapeutic action yet interact with it. For example, intoxication with drugs that have atropine-like effects (eg, tricyclic antidepressants) will reduce sweating, making it more difficult to dissipate heat. In tricyclic antidepressant intoxication, there may also be increased muscular activity or seizures; the body's production of heat is thus enhanced, and lethal hyperpyrexia may result. Overdoses of drugs that depress the cardiovascular system, eg, beta-adrenoceptor-blocking agents or barbiturates, can profoundly alter not only target organ function but all functions that are dependent on blood flow. These include renal and hepatic elimination of the toxin and any other drugs that may be given.

Conversely, lack of tissue perfusion with falling blood pressure may lead to a transient decrease in target organ drug levels. When blood pressure is restored to adequate levels, enhanced delivery of the toxin can lead to an apparent increase in the degree of intoxication. The result may be a confusing waxing and waning of the signs and symptoms. Thus, an appreciation of the toxicodynamics of an agent will allow for better understanding of changes in the clinical course of intoxicated patients.

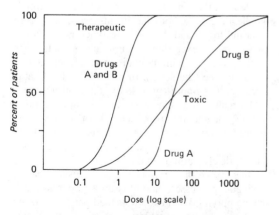

Figure 60–1. Quantal dose-response comparison of two drugs with differing safety margins. Both drugs have the same therapeutic index (TD50/ED50). However, at the dose required for therapeutic effects in 90% of patients, less than 1% of patients receiving drug A have toxicity, but 20% of those taking drug B have toxicity.

APPROACH TO THE POISONED PATIENT

HOW DOES THE POISONED PATIENT DIE?

In the majority of cases of poisoning, supportive measures are the mainstay of treatment. An understanding of common mechanisms of death due to poisoning can help prepare the physician to treat patients effectively.

Many toxins depress the central nervous system, resulting in obtundation or coma. Comatose patients frequently lose their airway protection and their respiratory drive. Thus, they are likely to die as a result of airway obstruction by the flaccid tongue, aspiration of gastric contents into the tracheobronchial tree, or respiratory arrest. These are the most common causes of death due to overdoses of narcotics, barbiturates, alcohol, and other sedative-hypnotic drugs.

Cardiovascular toxicity is also frequently encountered in poisoning. Hypotension may be due to direct depression of cardiac contractility; hypovolemia, due to fluid sequestration or fluid or blood loss; peripheral vascular collapse, due to blockade of alpha-adrenoceptor-mediated vascular tone; and brady- and tachyarrhythmias, due to direct cardiac effects. Hypotension is common with overdoses of tricyclic antidepressants, phenothiazines, beta-adrenoceptor blockers, calcium channel blockers, theophylline, and phenobarbital and other sedative-hypnotic drugs. Hypothermia due to exposure as well as the temperature-dysregulating effects of many drugs can also produce hypotension. Hypothermia may be worsened by rapid infusion of intravenous fluids at room temperature (24 °C). Lethal arrhythmias such as ventricular tachycardia and fibrillation can occur with overdoses of many cardioactive drugs such as amphetamines, cocaine, tricyclic antidepressants, digitalis, and theophylline.

Cellular hypoxia may occur in spite of adequate ventilation and oxygen administration when poisoning is due to cyanide, hydrogen sulfide, carbon monoxide, and other poisons that interfere with transport or utilization of oxygen. In such patients, cellular hypoxia is evident by the development of tachycardia, hypotension, severe lactic acidosis, and signs of ischemia on the ECG.

Seizures, muscular hyperactivity, and rigidity may result in death. Seizures may lead to pulmonary aspiration and hypoxia and lactic acidosis. Hyperthermia may result from sustained muscular hyperactivity and can lead to muscle breakdown and myoglobinuria, renal failure, lactic acidosis, hyperkalemia, and brain damage, features typical of heat stroke. Drugs and toxins that may induce seizures are tricyclic antidepressants, theophylline, isoniazid (INH), phenothiazines, cocaine, lithium, strychnine, and chlorinated hydrocarbons such as camphor and lindane.

Other organ system damage may be delayed after poisoning. Paraquat characteristically attacks lung tissue, resulting in pulmonary fibrosis several days after ingestion. Massive hepatic necrosis due to poisoning by acetaminophen or certain mushrooms results in hepatic encephalopathy and death 24–48 hours after ingestion.

Finally, some patients may die before hospitalization because the behavioral effects of the ingested drug may result in traumatic injury. Intoxication with alcohol and other sedative-hypnotic drugs is a frequent contributing factor to vehicle accidents. Patients under the influence of hallucinogens such as phencyclidine may die in gun battles or in falls from high places.

INITIAL MANAGEMENT OF THE POISONED PATIENT

The initial management of a patient with coma, seizures, or otherwise altered mental status should follow the same approach regardless of the poison involved. Attempting to make a specific toxicologic diagnosis only delays the application of supportive measures that form the basis ("ABCDs") of poisoning treatment.

First, the **airway** (A) should be cleared of vomitus or any other obstruction and an oral airway or endotracheal tube inserted if needed. For many patients, simple positioning in the lateral decubitus position is sufficient to move the flaccid tongue out of the airway. Adequacy of **breathing** (B) should be assessed by observation and by measuring arterial blood gases. Patients with respiratory insufficiency should be intubated and mechanically ventilated. Adequacy of the **circulation** (C) should be assessed by measurement of pulse rate, blood pressure, urinary output, and evaluation of peripheral perfusion. An intravenous line should be placed and blood drawn for serum glucose and other routine determinations.

At this point, every patient with altered mental status should receive a challenge with concentrated **dextrose** (D). Adults are given 25 g (50 mL of 50% dextrose) intravenously. This should be routine, because patients comatose from hypoglycemia are rapidly and irreversibly losing brain cells. Hypoglycemic patients may appear to be intoxicated, and there is no rapid and reliable way to distinguish them from poisoned patients. It is not generally harmful to give glucose while awaiting the blood sugar determination.

Alcoholic or malnourished patients should also receive 100 mg of thiamine intramuscularly at this time to prevent Wernicke's syndrome.

The narcotic antagonist naloxone (Narcan) may be given in a dose of 0.4–2 mg intravenously. Naloxone will reverse respiratory and central nervous system depression due to all varieties of narcotic drugs. It is useful to remember that these drugs cause death primarily by respiratory depression; therefore, if airway and breathing assistance have already been instituted, naloxone may not be necessary. The benzodiazepine antagonist flumazenil (Chapter 21) is of value in patients with suspected benzodiazepine overdose, but it should not be used if there is a history of seizures or of tricyclic antidepressant overdose, and it should not be used as a substitute for careful airway management.

Management of poisoning requires a thorough knowledge of how to treat hypoventilation, coma, shock, seizures, and psychosis. Sophisticated toxicokinetic considerations are of little value if vital functions are not maintained. Hypoventilation and coma require particular attention to airway management. Arterial blood gases must be checked frequently, and aspiration of gastric contents must be prevented. Fluid and electrolyte management may be complex. Monitoring body weight, central venous pressure, pulmonary capillary wedge pressure, and arterial blood gases is necessary to ensure adequate but not excessive administration of fluid. With appropriate support for coma, shock, seizures, and agitation, most patients will survive the poisoning.

History & Physical Examination

Once these essential initial interventions have been carried out, one can begin a more detailed evaluation to make a specific diagnosis. This includes gathering any available history and performing a toxicologically oriented brief physical examination. Other causes of coma or seizures such as head trauma, meningitis, or metabolic abnormalities should be looked for and treated.

A. History: Oral statements about the amount and even the type of drug ingested in toxic emergencies may be unreliable. Even so, family members, police, and fire department or paramedical personnel should be asked to describe the environment in which the toxic emergency occurred and should bring to the emergency room all syringes, empty bottles, household products, or over-the-counter medications in the immediate vicinity of the possibly poisoned patient.

B. Physical Examination: A brief examination should be performed emphasizing those areas most likely to give clues to the toxicologic diagnosis. These include vital signs, eyes and mouth, skin, abdomen, and nervous system.

1. Vital signs—Careful evaluation of vital signs (blood pressure, pulse, respirations, and temperature) is essential in all toxicologic emergencies. Hypertension and tachycardia are typical with amphetamines, cocaine, phencyclidine, nicotine, and anti-muscarinic drugs. Hypotension and bradycardia are characteristic features of overdose with narcotics, clonidine, sedative-hypnotics, and beta blockers. Tachycardia and hypotension are common with tricyclic antidepressants, phenothiazines, and theophylline. Rapid respirations are typical of amphetamines and other sympathomimetics, salicylates, carbon monoxide, and other toxins that produce metabolic acidosis. Hyperthermia may be due to sympathomimetics, antimuscarinics, salicylates, and drugs producing seizures or muscular rigidity. Hypothermia can be caused by severe overdoses of the narcotics, phenothiazines, and sedative drugs, especially when accompanied by exposure to a cold environment or room temperature intravenous infusions.

2. Eyes—The eyes are a valuable source of toxicologic information. Constriction of the pupils (miosis) is typical of narcotics, clonidine, phenothiazines, organophosphate insecticides and other cholinesterase inhibitors, and deep coma due to sedative drugs. Dilation of the pupils (mydriasis) is common with amphetamines, cocaine, LSD, and atropine and other antimuscarinic drugs. Horizontal nystagmus is characteristic of intoxication with phenytoin, alcohol, barbiturates, and other sedative drugs. The presence of both vertical and horizontal nystagmus is strongly suggestive of phencyclidine poisoning. Ptosis and ophthalmoplegia are characteristic features of botulism.

3. Mouth—The mouth may show signs of burns due to corrosive substances, or soot from smoke inhalation. Typical odors of alcohol, hydrocarbon solvents, paraldehyde, or ammonia may be noted. Poisoning due to cyanide can be recognized by some examiners as an odor like bitter almonds. Arsenic and organophosphates have been reported to produce a garlicky odor.

4. Skin—The skin often appears flushed, hot, and dry in poisoning with atropine and other antimuscarinics. Excessive sweating occurs with organophosphates, nicotine, and sympathomimetic drugs. Cyanosis may be caused by hypoxemia or by methemoglobinemia. Icterus may suggest hepatic necrosis due to acetaminophen or *Amanita phalloides* mushroom poisoning.

5. Abdomen—Abdominal examination may reveal ileus, which is typical of poisoning with antimuscarinic, narcotic, and sedative drugs. Hyperactive bowel sounds, abdominal cramping, and diarrhea are common in poisoning with organophosphates, iron, arsenic, theophylline, and *A phalloides*.

6. Nervous system—A careful neurologic examination is essential. Focal seizures or motor deficits suggest a structural lesion (such as intracranial hemorrhage due to trauma) rather than toxic or metabolic encephalopathy. Nystagmus, dysarthria, and ataxia are typical of phenytoin, alcohol, barbiturate, and other sedative intoxication. Rigidity and muscular hyperactivity are common with methaqualone, haloperidol, phencyclidine (PCP), and sympathomimetic drugs. Seizures are often caused by overdose with tricyclic antidepressants, theophylline, isoniazid, and phenothiazines. Flaccid coma with absent reflexes and even an isoelectric EEG may be seen with deep coma due to narcotic and sedative-hypnotic drugs and may mimic brain death.

Toxic Syndromes

Based on the initial physical examination, a tenta-tive diagnosis of the type of poisoning may be possible. Table 60–1 lists the characteristics of some important toxic syndromes.

Laboratory & X-Ray Procedures

Routine laboratory tests that are valuable in toxicologic diagnosis include the following:

A. Arterial Blood Gases: Hypoventilation will result in an elevated PCO_2 (hypercapnia). The PO_2 may be low with aspiration pneumonia or drug-induced pulmonary edema. Poor tissue oxygenation

Table 60–1. Common toxic syndromes associated with major drug groups.

Drug Group	Clinical features	Key Interventions
Antidepressants (eg, amitriptyline, doxepin, maprotiline, others)	Anticholinergic features common: dilated pupils, tachycardia, hot dry skin, decreased bowel sounds. The "three Cs"—coma, convulsions, and cardiac problems—are the most common causes of death. A major diagnostic feature is widening of the QRS complex greater than 0.1 s on ECG (not seen with amoxapine). Hypotension and ventricular arrhythmias are common.	Control seizures, correct acidosis and cardiotoxicity with ventilation and HCO_3. Do not use physostigmine or flumazenil. Watch for hyperthermia.
Antimuscarinic drugs (eg, atropine, scopolamine, antihistamines, tricyclic antidepressants, jimsonweed, *Amanita muscaria* mushrooms)	Hallucinations, delirium, coma. Seizures may occur with tricyclic antidepressants, antihistamines. Tachycardia, hypertension. Hyperthermia with hot, dry skin. Mydriasis. Decreased bowel sounds, urinary retention. Delayed gastric emptying is expected.	Control hyperthermia. Physostigmine is of potential value but should not be given for cyclic antidepressants.
Cholinomimetic drugs (eg, organophosphate and carbamate insecticides)	Anxiety, agitation, seizures, coma. May see brady-cardia(muscarinic effect) or tachycardia (nicotinic effect). Pinpoint pupils. Excessive salivation, sweating. Bowel sounds hyperactive, with abdominal cramping, diarrhea. Muscle fasciculations and twitching followed by flaccid paralysis. Death due to respiratory muscle paralysis.	Respiratory support, atropine, pralidoxime (2-PAM). Remove clothes, wash skin.
Opioid drugs (eg, morphine, heroin, meperidine, codeine, methadone)	Sleepiness, lethargy, or coma, depending on dose. Blood pressure and heart rate usually decreased. Hypoventilation or apnea. Pinpoint pupils. Skin cool; may show signs of intravenous drug abuse with associated infectious disease complications. Bowel sounds decreased. Muscle tone flaccid; occasionally see twitching, rigidity. Clonidine overdose may present with identical syndrome.	Airway support. Frequent supplements of naloxone may be necessary because of its short half-life.
Salicylates	Confusion, lethargy, coma, seizures. Hyperventilation, hyperthermia. Anion gap metabolic acidosis. Dehydration, potassium loss. Acute overdose: 6-hour level over 100 mg/dL (1000 mg/L) very serious. Chronic or accidental overdose: level not reliable; more severe toxicity; often mistakenly diagnosed as upper respiratory infection or gastroenteritis.	Correct acidosis and fluid and electrolyte abnormalities; alkalinize the urine; hemodialysis if pH or CNS symptoms cannot be controlled.
Sedative-hypnotics (eg, benzodiazepines, barbiturates, ethanol)	Highly variable depending on stage of intoxication; initially disinhibition and rowdiness, later lethargy, stupor, coma. With deep coma: hypotension, small pupils. Nystagmus common with moderate intoxication. Bowel sounds decreased in deep coma. Muscle tone usually flaccid. May be associated with hypothermia.	Airway and respiratory support. Avoid fluid overload. Flumazenil may reverse benzodiazepine-induced coma.
Stimulant drugs (eg, amphetamines, cocaine, PCP)	Agitation, psychosis, seizures. Hypertension, tachycardia, arrhythmias. Mydriasis (usually). Vertical and horizontal nystagmus are common with PCP poisoning. Skin warm and sweaty. Muscle tone increased; muscle necrosis is possible. Hyperthermia may be major complication.	Control seizures, blood pressure, and hyperthermia.

due to hypoxia, hypotension, or cyanide poisoning will result in metabolic acidosis. The PO_2 measures only oxygen dissolved in the plasma and not total blood oxygen content and therefore may appear normal despite significant oxyhemoglobin deficiency in carbon monoxide poisoning.

B. Electrolytes: Sodium, potassium, chloride, and bicarbonate should be measured. The anion gap is then calculated by subtracting the measured anions from cations:

$$\text{Anion gap} = (Na^+ + K^+) - (HCO_3^- + Cl^-)$$

It is normally no greater than 12–16 meq/L. A larger-than-expected anion gap is caused by the presence of unmeasured anions accompanying metabolic acidosis. This is caused by, for example, diabetic ketoacidosis, renal failure, or shock-induced lactic acidosis. Drugs that may induce an elevated anion gap metabolic acidosis (Table 60–2) include aspirin, methanol, ethylene glycol, isoniazid, and iron.

Alterations in serum potassium level are hazardous because they may result in cardiac arrhythmias. Drugs that may cause hyperkalemia despite normal renal function include potassium itself, beta-adrenoceptor blockers, digitalis glycosides, fluoride, and lithium. Drugs associated with hypokalemia include barium, beta-adrenoceptor agonists, caffeine, theophylline, diuretics, and toluene.

C. Renal Function Tests: Some toxins have direct nephrotoxic effects; in other cases, renal failure is due to shock, disseminated intravascular coagulation (DIC), or myoglobinuria. Blood urea nitrogen and creatinine levels should be measured and urinalysis performed. Elevated serum creatine phosphokinase (CPK) and myoglobin in the urine suggest muscle necrosis due to seizures or muscular rigidity. Oxalate crystals in the urine suggest ethylene glycol poisoning.

D. Serum Osmolality: The calculated serum osmolality is dependent mainly on the serum sodium and glucose and the blood urea nitrogen and can be estimated from the following formula:

$$2 \times Na^+ \, (meq/L) + \frac{\text{Glucose (mg/dL)}}{18} + \frac{BUN \, (mg/dL)}{3}$$

This calculated value is normally 280–290 mosm/kg. Ethanol and other alcohols may contribute significantly to the measured serum osmolality but, since they are not included in the calculation, cause an osmolar gap:

$$\text{Osmolar gap} = \\ \text{Measured osmolality} - \text{Calculated osmolality}$$

In the absence of significant levels of an osmotically active intoxicant molecule, the osmolar gap is zero. Table 60–3 lists the concentration and expected contribution to the serum osmolality in ethanol, methanol, ethylene glycol, and isopropanol poisonings.

E. Electrocardiogram: Widening of the QRS complex duration to greater than 0.1 s is typical of tricyclic antidepressant and quinidine overdoses (Figure 60–3). The QT interval may be prolonged in quinidine, phenothiazine, and tricyclic antidepressant poisoning. Variable atrioventricular block and multiple ventricular arrhythmias are common with digitalis poisoning. The ECG may show typical abnormalities when hypothermia and electrolyte abnormalities accompany overdose. Hypoxemia due to carbon monoxide poisoning may result in ischemic changes on the ECG.

F. X-Ray Findings: A plain film of the abdomen may be useful, since some tablets, particularly iron and potassium, may be radiopaque. Chest x-ray may reveal aspiration pneumonia, hydrocarbon pneumonia, or pulmonary edema. When head trauma is suspected, a CT scan is recommended.

Screening Tests

It is a common misconception that a "stat" toxicology "screen" is the best way to diagnose and manage an acute poisoning. The "screen" is time-consuming, expensive, and often unreliable; some drugs are not sought for. The clinical examination of the patient and selected routine laboratory tests are usually sufficient to generate a tentative diagnosis and an appropriate treatment plan. When a specific antidote or invasive therapy such as hemodialysis is under consideration, in-depth laboratory testing may be in-

Table 60–2. Drug-induced anion gap acidosis.

Type of Elevation of the Anion Gap	Agents
Metabolic acidosis	Methanol, ethylene glycol, salicylates.
Lactic acidosis	Any drug-induced seizures, iron, phenformin, hypoxia.
Ketoacidosis	Ethanol.

Note: The normal anion gap calculated from $(Na^+ + K^+) - (HCO_3^- + Cl^-)$ is 12–16 meq/L; calculated from $(Na^+) - (HCO_3^- + Cl^-)$, it is 8–12 meq/L.

Table 60–3. Substances that cause osmolar gap.

	Potentially Lethal Level (mg/dL)	Corresponding Osmolar Gap (mosm/kg)
Ethanol	350	75
Methanol	80	25
Ethylene glycol	200	35
Isopropanol	350	60

Note: Most laboratories use the freezing point method of determining osmolality. However, if the vaporization point method is used, the alcohols may be driven off and their contribution to osmolality will be lost.

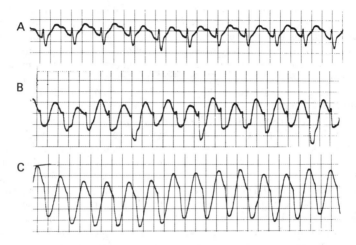

Figure 60–3. Changes in the ECG in tricyclic antidepressant overdosage. **A:** Slowed intraventricular conduction results in prolonged QRS interval (0.18 s; normal, 0.08 s). **B** and **C:** Supraventricular tachycardia with progressive widening of QRS complexes mimics ventricular tachycardia. (Reproduced, with permission, from Benowitz NL, Goldschlager N: Cardiac disturbances in the toxicologic patient. In: *Clinical Management of Poisoning and Drug Overdose.* Haddad LM, Winchester JF [editors]. Saunders, 1983.)

dicated. For example, quantitative determination of acetaminophen is useful in determining antidotal therapy with N-acetylcysteine. Serum levels of theophylline, lithium, salicylates, and other drugs may indicate the need for hemodialysis or hemoperfusion (Table 60–4).

Time of Ingestion of Poison

To estimate the severity of poisoning, it is important to consider the time since ingestion and compare it with the plasma level, if available. The importance of time in evaluating plasma levels has been particularly well demonstrated for aspirin poisoning. An aspirin concentration of 50 mg/dL 4–6 hours after ingestion is associated with only mild intoxication; the same level obtained 36 hours after ingestion is associated with very severe poisoning. The basis for this relationship lies in the fact that the clinical manifestation of toxic effects in some target organs such as the brain may lag significantly behind the peak levels in the blood.

Blood Levels of Toxins

Note: Supportive treatment should not be delayed while waiting for laboratory reports.

There are relatively few acute toxic emergencies in which measurement of blood levels is necessary to

Table 60–4. Indications for hemodialysis (HD) and hemoperfusion (HP).

	Toxin	Procedure
Indicated immediately if significant intoxication has occurred	Ethylene glycol	HD
	Methanol	HD
	Salicylate	HD
	Theophylline	HP or HD
	Procainamide	HD or HP
Indicated if supportive measures fail or if prolonged coma is expected	Meprobamate	HP
	Ethchlorvynol	HP
	Phenobarbital	HP
	Lithium	HD
	Carbamazepine	HP
Not indicated	Amphetamines, PCP, cocaine	
	Benzodiazepines	
	Chlorpromazine, other antipsychotics	
	Digoxin	
	Glutethimide	
	Narcotics	
	Quinidine	
	Tricyclic antidepressants	

evaluate severity and guide management. Examples include acetaminophen, aspirin, lithium, carbon monoxide, digoxin, carbamazepine, and theophylline poisoning. Poisoning with ethanol, methanol, and ethylene glycol can usually be diagnosed on clinical grounds but must be confirmed by the toxicology laboratory. Quantitative analysis of blood and urine for sedative-hypnotic drugs is only important when simple supportive procedures do not appear adequate and especially when dialysis is being considered, eg, in phenobarbital poisoning. Quantitative comprehensive screening should also be performed in cases of suspected brain death. Table 60–5 lists common sedative-hypnotic drugs, their kinetic parameters, and treatment methods.

Decontamination

Decontamination procedures should be undertaken after initial diagnostic assessment and laboratory evaluation. Decontamination involves removing toxins from the skin or gastrointestinal tract.

A. Skin: Contaminated clothing should be completely removed and saved for analysis. Percutaneous penetration by toxins has been poorly studied but should be anticipated. Vigorous washing with copious amounts of water and soap should be carried out.

B. Gastrointestinal Tract: There is considerable controversy regarding the efficacy of gut decontamination, especially when treatment is initiated more than 1 hour after ingestion. Some authorities recommend simple administration of activated charcoal without prior gut emptying in selected patients.

Caution: It is essential to protect the airway. All necessary emergency equipment such as suction must be readily available. Seizures, absence of the gag reflex, and ulcerated oral mucous membranes are contraindications to emesis. Gastric lavage is contraindicated if the airway is at risk (eg, unconscious patient with no gag reflex). Acid and alkaline corrosives should be diluted but not neutralized. Therapists should not put their fingers in the patient's throat and should not use salt water or mustard as emetic agents.

1. Emesis–Induce emesis by oral administration of **ipecac syrup**, 30 mL for adults or 10–15 mL for children, repeated once after 15 minutes if necessary. (Ipecac *fluid extract* should be avoided because of its high concentration of emetic and cardiotoxic alkaloids.) Home use of ipecac has been documented to be safe and effective and should be part of the home treatment of children in poisoning emergencies. Ipecac is effective even when antiemetic medications have been taken in overdose. Ipecac should *not* be used if the suspected intoxicant is a convulsant (eg, tricyclic antidepressant), since seizures may occur abruptly and aspiration is extremely likely if vomiting occurs during a seizure. Apomorphine is much more toxic than ipecac, especially in children, because of its persistent emetic effects and the central nervous system depression it causes. Apomorphine should not be used.

2. Gastric lavage–If the patient is awake or if the airway is protected by an endotracheal tube, gastric lavage may be performed (Figure 60–4). As large a tube as possible should be used. Lavage solutions (usually 0.9% saline) should be at body temperature to prevent hypothermia.

Table 60–5. Toxicologic features of some sedative-hypnotic overdoses.

Drug	V_d (L/kg)	Normal Doses $t_{1/2}$ (hours)	Overdoses $t_{1/2}$ (hours)	Maximum Therapeutic Level (mg/L)	Treatment	Comments
Phenobarbital	0.75	60–100	70–120	20	Supportive. Repeat-dose charcoal by gastric tube and urinary alkalinization may enhance elimination.	Avoid fluid overload. Hemoperfusion may be required if serum level >250 mg/L or if intractable hypotension develops.
Pentobarbital	1–2	20–30	50	50	Supportive.	Short-acting.
Chloral hydrate	0.6	4–8	19–20	15	Supportive.	Gastritis, arrhythmias. Radiopaque pills.
Glutethimide (Doriden)	20–25	8–12	34–40	0.5	Supportive.	Cyclic variation in coma; mydriasis.
Ethchlorvynol (Placidyl)	3–4	10–20	20–100	100	Supportive.	Pink or green aspirate with pungent odor. Prolonged coma with overdose.
Diazepam (Valium)	1–2	30–70	50–140	5	Supportive.	Severe overdose uncommon unless combined with other drugs. Flumazenil is a benzodiazepine antagonist.

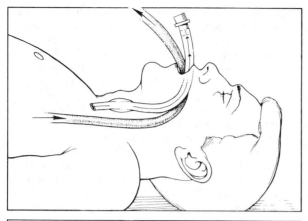

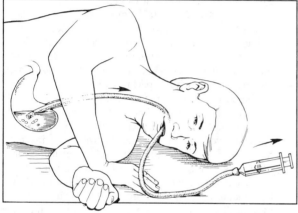

Figure 60–4. Positioning of lavage tube and patient for gastric decontamination ("pumping the stomach"). Upper panel shows the relative positions of the endotracheal tube (clear) with cuff in the trachea and the lavage tube (stippled). Lower panel shows the left-lateral position that is optimal for the removal of stomach contents. (Reproduced, with permission, from Olson KR [editor]: *Poisoning & Drug Overdose.* Appleton & Lange, 1990.)

3. Catharsis–Administration of a cathartic agent should hasten removal of toxins from the gastrointestinal tract and reduce absorption, though no controlled studies have been done. Pediatricians have reported finding whole tablets—especially enteric-coated ones—in stools after administration of cathartic agents. If charcoal is also administered, this procedure marks the stool with charcoal, so that total gastrointestinal transit time can be estimated. Sorbitol (70%) is the preferred cathartic agent. Magnesium sulfate may also be used if renal function is unimpaired. Cathartic agents with an oil base are of no value and are potentially harmful. Table 60–6 lists some common cathartics.

4. Activated charcoal–Administration of activated charcoal is a valuable decontamination procedure if given in sufficient quantity because it binds many toxins. It is best to give it in a ratio of at least 10:1 of charcoal to estimated dose of toxin. Charcoal does not bind iron, lithium, or potassium, and it binds alcohols and cyanide only poorly. It does not appear to be useful in poisoning due to corrosive alkaline or acidic substances, boric acid, ethanol or other alcohols, iron, lithium, methylcarbamate, or tolbutamide.

Generally, charcoal is underutilized and given in

Table 60–6. Usual doses of cathartics in decontamination.[1]

Magnesium citrate (10%) (magnesium = 1.6 meq/mL)	Adult: 100–150 mL Child: 1 mL/kg
Magnesium sulfate (10%) magnesium = 0.8 meq/mL	Adult: 150–250 mL Child: 1–2 mL/kg
Sodium sulfate (10%) (sodium = 1.4 meq/mL)	Adult: 150–250 mL Child: 1–2 mL/kg
Sorbitol (70%) (contains no sodium or magnesium)	Adult: 50–100 mL Child: 1 mL/kg

[1]Modified and reproduced, with permission, from Riegel JM, Becker CE: Use of cathartics in toxic ingestions. *Ann Emerg Med* 1981;**10**:254.

Note:
1. Avoid magnesium cathartics in renal disease and cases of nephrotoxin ingestion.
2. Avoid sodium cathartics in congestive heart failure and hypertension.
3. *Never* use oil-based cathartics.

insufficient doses. In most studies in humans, charcoal was administered after normal therapeutic doses of drug; controlled studies of the use of charcoal after overdose are few. However, recent studies suggest that activated charcoal given without prior gastric emptying may be just as effective as traditional emptying followed by charcoal. Other studies suggest that repeated doses of charcoal every 4 hours may be of value in poisoning due to carbamazepine, chlordecone, dapsone, digitoxin, nadolol, phenobarbital, and theophylline.

Specific Antidotes

There is a popular misconception that there is an antidote for every poison. The opposite is true—relatively selective antidotes are available for only a few classes of toxins. The major antidotes and their characteristics are listed in Table 60–7. These drugs are supplemented by immunologic agents such as snake antivenin (see below) and digoxin antibodies.

Methods of Enhancing Elimination of Toxins

After appropriate diagnostic and decontamination procedures and administration of antidotes, it is important to consider measures for enhancing elimination, such as forced diuresis, dialysis, or exchange procedures. If a patient is able to eliminate a toxin rapidly, the period of coma will be shortened, metabolites removed, and organ damage reduced. It is thus important to have knowledge of the toxicokinetics of the poison.

In cases of massive overdose, elimination pathways with limited capacities are often saturated. Drugs that have been demonstrated to exhibit concentration-dependent toxicokinetics in the overdose setting are ethanol, salicylate, phenytoin, chloral hydrate, etchlorvynol, some barbiturates, theophylline, and acetaminophen. In cases of toxic ingestion of these drugs, methods of enhancing elimination that contribute to total body clearance may significantly improve the clinical outcome.

A. Techniques Available:

1. Dialysis procedures, including peritoneal dialysis, hemodialysis, and hemoperfusion, are theoretically appealing as a means of removing toxins that are eliminated through metabolic mechanisms that cannot be enhanced.

2. Renal elimination of a few toxins is enhanced by alteration of urinary pH. Urinary alkalinization is useful in cases of salicylate or phenobarbital overdose. Forced diuresis with excessive fluid volumes enhances the risk of fluid and electrolyte imbalance and of worsening pulmonary function.

B. Dialysis (Table 60–4):

1. Peritoneal dialysis–This is a relatively simple and available technique but is inefficient in removing most drugs.

2. Hemodialysis–Hemodialysis is more efficient than peritoneal dialysis and has been well studied. It assists in correction of fluid and electrolyte imbalance and may also enhance removal of toxic metabolites, eg, formate in cases of methanol poisoning. The efficiency of both peritoneal dialysis and hemodialysis is a function of the molecular weight, water solubility, protein binding, endogenous clearance, and distribution in the body of the specific toxin. Removal of drug with these procedures can be enhanced by increasing the time on dialysis or by altering the dialysis medium to bind the toxin. However, the complications of these procedures also increase with the length of time of dialysis. Hemodialysis is especially useful in overdose cases in which fluid and electrolyte imbalances are present or when toxic by-products are removable.

C. Hemoperfusion: Hemoperfusion for treatment of drug intoxication has been used increasingly in the past 5 years. Blood is pumped from the patient via a venous catheter through a column of adsorbent material and then recirculated to the patient. Systemic anticoagulation with heparin is required to prevent the blood from clotting in the cartridge. Hemoperfusion does not improve fluid and electrolyte balance and does not remove all toxic products. However, it does remove many high-molecular-weight toxins that have poor water solubility, because the perfusion cartridge has a large surface area for adsorption that is directly perfused with the blood and is not impeded by a membrane. The rate-limiting factors in removal of toxins by hemoperfusion are the affinity of the adsorbent resin for the drug, the rate of blood flow through the cartridge, and the rate of equilibration of the drug from the peripheral tissues to the blood. Many different hemoperfusion cartridges are now being studied for use in various toxic circumstances.

Although relatively few toxins have been studied, there is evidence that hemoperfusion may enhance whole body clearance of salicylate, phenytoin, ethchlorvynol, phenobarbital, theophylline, and carbamazepine. Complications such as embolization of adsorbed particles, depletion of blood cells, and removal of proteins, solutes, and steroids have been minimized with increasing clinical experience.

D. Selection of Technique to Be Used: Drugs or toxins with extremely large volumes of distribution such as tricyclic antidepressants and digoxin are poorly removed by hemodialysis or hemoperfusion. Therefore, critical review of kinetic parameters and dialysis capability is required before undertaking dialysis procedures. Table 60–4 lists intoxications requiring immediate dialysis, those in which it is used only if supportive measures fail, and those for which dialysis is not indicated. The toxicology laboratory should monitor methanol, ethylene glycol, salicylate, theophylline, phenobarbital, paraquat, and lithium blood levels during dialysis.

The problems of enhancing elimination are well illustrated in PCP intoxication. Studies in laboratory

Table 60–7. Specific antidotes.

Antidote	Poison(s)	Comments
Acetylcysteine (Mucomyst)	Acetaminophen	Best results if given within 8–10 hours of overdose. Follow liver function tests and acetaminophen blood levels. Little recognized toxicity. Dose: 140 mg/kg orally as loading dose, then 70 mg/kg orally every 4 hours for 17 doses or until serum acetaminophen level is zero. Intravenous acetylcysteine has been used successfully in Europe and is currently under trial in the USA.
Atropine	Anticholinesterases: organophosphates, carbamates	A test dose of 1–2 mg (for children, 0.05 mg/kg) is given IV until symptoms of atropinism appear (tachycardia, dilated pupils, ileus). Dose may be repeated every 10–15 minutes, with decrease of secretions as therapeutic end point.
Bicarbonate, sodium	Membrane depressant cardiotoxic drugs (tricyclic antidepressants, quinidine, etc)	1–2 meq/kg IV bolus usually reverses cardiotoxic effects (wide QRS, hypotension). Give cautiously in heart failure (avoid sodium overload).
Deferoxamine (Desferal)	Iron salts	If poisoning is severe, give 15 mg/kg/h IV. Urine may become pink. 100 mg of deferoxamine binds 8.5 mg of iron.
Digoxin-specific FAB antibodies	Digoxin and related cardiac glycosides	One vial binds 0.6 mg digoxin; indications include serious arrhythmias, hyperkalemia.
Esmolol	Theophylline, caffeine, metaproterenol	Short-acting beta blocker reverses $beta_1$-induced tachycardia and $beta_2$-induced vasodilation. Infuse 25–50 µg/kg/min IV.
Ethanol	Methanol, ethylene glycol	Ethanol therapy can be started before laboratory diagnosis is confirmed. A loading dose is calculated so as to give a blood level of at least 100 mg/dL (42 g/70 kg in adults.).
Flumazenil	Benzodiazepines	Adult dose is 0.2 mg IV, repeated as necessary to a maximum of 3 mg. Do not give to patients with seizures, benzodiazepine dependence, or tricyclic overdose.
Glucagon	Beta-adrenoceptor blockers	5–10 mg IV bolus may reverse hypotension and bradycardia that was resistant to beta agonist drugs. May cause vomiting
Metal chelators Calcium disodium ethyl- enediamine-tetraacetate (CaEDTA)	Lead	Give 50–75 mg/kg/d IM or IV in 3–6 divided doses for up to 5 days in cases of lead encephalopathy. Modify dose in renal failure. Toxicity: zinc depletion and vitamin B_6 deficiency. Avoid oral therapy.
Dimercaprol (BAL)	Arsenic, lead, mercury	Give 3–5 mg/kg every 4 hours IM for 2 days, then 2.5–3 mg/kg every 6 hours for 7 days. Not effective for arsine gas. Try to keep urine pH alkaline. Monitor for hypertension. No proved efficacy if delayed for 24 hours.
Penicillamine	Lead, gold, arsenic	Give 1 g orally daily in 4 divided doses before meals.
Naloxone (Narcan)	Narcotic drugs, other opioid derivatives	A specific antagonist of opioids; 1–2 mg initially by IV, IM, or subcutaneous injection. Larger doses may be needed to reverse the effects of overdose with propoxyphene, codeine, or fentanyl derivatives. Duration of action (2–3 h) may be significantly shorter than that of the opioid being antagonized.
Oxygen	Carbon monoxide.	Give 100% by high-flow nonrebreathing mask; use of hyperbaric chamber controversial.
Physostigmine salicylate	"Suggested" for antimuscarinic anticholinergic agents; not for tricyclic antidepressants	Adult dose is 0.5–1 mg IV slowly. The effects are transient (30–60 minutes), and the lowest effective dose may be repeated when symptoms return. May cause bradycardia, increased bronchial secretions, seizures. Have atropine ready to reverse excess effects. *Do not use for tricyclic antidepressant overdose.*
Pralidoxime (2-PAM)	Organophosphate cholinesterases	Adult dose is 1 g IV, which may be repeated every 3–4 hours as needed or preferably as a constant infusion 250–400 mg/h. Pediatric dose is approximately 250 mg. No proven benefit in carbamate poisoning.
Hydroxocobalamin	Cyanide	Orphan drug. Available at Selected Poison Control Centers.

animals suggest that there is limited renal clearance and little effect of blood pH changes on the distribution of the drug. However, urinary acidification has been demonstrated to increase the renal clearance of phencyclidine. Gastric suction increases the diffusion of phencyclidine into gastric contents. Based on these preliminary data, large numbers of patients have been treated by acidification of the urine and gastric suction but with little documentation of the effectiveness of these techniques. Because intoxication with PCP has a waxing and waning clinical pattern, it has been difficult to evaluate improvement in the clinical status. Because phencyclidine poisoning is associated with muscle destruction and excretion of myoglobin in the urine, inappropriate acidification of the urine may increase the likelihood of precipitation of myoglobin in the renal tubules, thereby increasing the likelihood of renal failure.

Treatment of Snake, Spider, & Scorpion Envenomation

The venoms of several snakes and scorpions and (in very small children) that of black widow spiders are important toxicologic emergencies. In the USA, rattlesnake bite is by far the most important because of the amount of venom that may be injected, its intrinsic toxicity, and the fact that victims may be far from medical help when the bite occurs.

A. Rattlesnake Envenomation: Evidence of rattlesnake envenomation includes local bleeding, severe pain, superficial edema of rapid onset and progression, hemorrhagic bleb formation, lymphadenitis, and obvious fang marks. Many studies have shown that emergency field remedies such as incision and suction, tourniquets, and ice packs are far more damaging than useful. Avoidance of unnecessary motion, on the other hand, does help to limit the spread of the venom. Definitive therapy relies on antivenins and should be started as soon as possible.

Blood should be typed and cross-matched before antivenin is administered. Clotting and bleeding times should be monitored. Dose of the antivenin should be adjusted according to the presence and rate of progression of signs of systemic intoxication, including nausea, vomiting, paresthesias, bleeding disorder, shock, arrhythmias, renal failure, and pulmonary edema. For significant rattlesnake bite, at least five vials of mixed crotalid antivenin should be administered; if envenomation is severe, 10–20 vials

may be required. After large doses of antivenin, signs of serum sickness often develop 10–12 days after treatment. Skin testing is usually done to determine horse serum sensitivity, but a negative test does not rule out anaphylaxis. Steroids are useful only for severe serum sickness.

Common Errors in Management of Poisoning

"Universal antidote" (burnt toast, magnesium oxide, tannic acid) is of no value and may be harmful. If ipecac syrup is to be used, it should be given at once and not postponed until arrival at the hospital or during the evaluation procedure in the emergency room. Clinical experience, especially in pediatrics, suggests that ipecac can be administered by a lay person, especially when instructed by the physician over the telephone.

In the past, ingested acid and alkaline substances were neutralized; this liberates heat and increases tissue destruction. Dilution of caustics or acid substances is preferred. Copious amounts of milk or water (up to 15 mL/kg) may be used. Inducing emesis by placing a finger in the throat or with copper salts or hypertonic salt solution is hazardous to the mouth and esophagus. Use of oil-based cathartic agents may cause lipid pneumonia. Lavage fluids containing large quantities of sodium and phosphate may cause severe electrolyte imbalances. Excessive hydration may worsen pulmonary function. Large amounts of glucose may lower phosphate and potassium. Respiratory stimulants and analeptic agents are of no value and are harmful in toxic emergencies.

Monitoring of renal and hepatic function is essential. Muscle destruction (rhabdomyolysis) may result in acute renal failure. Inadvertent acidification of the urine may increase the likelihood of renal insufficiency resulting from myoglobin destruction and excretion. Catheters in veins and arteries or in the bladder may become sources of infection. Large amounts of fluid at room temperature or dialysis procedures may lower body temperature and worsen cardiovascular function. Appropriate supportive treatment may on occasion result in physiologic survival of a neurologically impaired patient. One must be extremely cautious in diagnosing brain death, however, especially in cases of sedative hypnotic drug overdose, such patients may awaken after several days of absent EEG activity.

REFERENCES

Basic Texts and Indexes

Berg GL (editor): *Farm Chemicals Handbook 1989.* Meister, 1989.

Ellenhorn MJ, Barcelou DG: Medical Toxicology. *Diag-*

nosis and Treatment of Human Poisoning. Elsevier, 1988.

Goldfrank LR et al (editors): *Toxicologic Emergencies,* 5th ed. Appleton & Lange, 1993

Gosselin RE et al: *Clinical Toxicology of Commercial Products,* 6th ed. Williams & Wilkins, 1988.

Haddad LM, Winchester JF (editors): *Clinical Management of Poisoning and Drug Overdose,* 2nd ed. Saunders, 1990.

Hathaway GL et al: *Proctor and Hughes' Chemical Hazards of the Workplace,* 2nd ed. Van Nostrand, Reinhold, 1991.

Klaassen CD, Amdur MO, Doull J (editors): *Casarett and Doull's Toxicology: The Basic Science of Poisons,* 4th ed. Macmillan, 1991.

Olson KR et al (editors): *Poisoning & Drug Overdose.* (2nd ed) Appleton & Lange, 1994.

Olson KR, Becker CE: Poisoning. In *Current Emergency Diagnosis & Treatment,* 4th ed. Saunders CE, Ho MT (editors). Appleton & Lange, 1992.

Rumack BH (editor): *Poisindex.* Micromedex, Inc., 1994. [National Center for Poison Information, Denver 80204.] Revised quarterly.

Other Sources

Alldredge BK, Lowenstein DH, Simon RP: Seizures associated with recreational drug abuse. Neurology 1989;39:1037.

Baud FJ et al: Elevated cyanide concentrations in victims of smoke inhalation. N Engl J Med 1991;325:1761.

CDC: Unintentional poisoning mortality: United States, 1980–1986. MMWR 1989;10:153.

Curtis RA, Barone J, Giacona N: Efficacy of ipecac and activated charcoal/cathartic. Prevention of salicylate absorption in a simulated overdose. Arch Int Med 1984;144:48.

Dawson AH, Whyte IM: The assessment and treatment of theophylline poisoning. Med J Aust 1989;151:689.

Eastaugh J, Shepherd S: Infectious and toxic syndromes from fish and shellfish consumption. A review. Arch Intern Med 1989;149:1736.

Fine JS, Goldfrank LR: Update in medical toxicology. Pediatr Clin North Am 1992;39:1031.

Frommer D et al: Tricyclic antidepressant overdose: A review. JAMA 1987;257:521.

Hepler B, Sutheimer C, Sunshine I: Role of the toxicology laboratory in suspected ingestions. Pediatr Clin North Am 1986;33:245.

Hursting MJ, Raisys VA, Opheim KE: Drug-specific Fab therapy in drug overdose. Arch Path Lab Med 1987;111:693.

Jackson JE: Phencyclidine pharmacokinetics after a massive overdose. Ann Intern Med 1989;111:613.

Kirschenbaum LA et al: Whole-bowel irrigation versus activated charcoal in sorbitol for the ingestion of modified-release pharmaceuticals. Clin Pharmacol Ther 1989;46:264.

Kulig K: Initial management of ingestions of toxic substances. N Engl J Med 1992;326:1677.

Mortensen ML: Management of acute childhood poisonings caused by selected insecticides and herbicides. Pediatr Clin North Am 1986;33:421.

Olson KR, Pentel PR, Kelley MT: Physical assessment and differential diagnosis of the poisoned patient. Med Toxicol 1987;2:52.

Pellinen TJ et al: Electrocardiographic and clinical features of tricyclic antidepressant intoxication: A survey of 88 cases and outlines of therapy. Ann Clin Res 1987;19:12.

Pentel PR et al: Effect of hypertonic sodium bicarbonate in encainide overdose. Am J Cardiol 1986;57:878.

Pentel PR, Benowitz NL: Tricyclic antidepressant poisoning: Management of arrhythmias. Med Toxicol 1986;1:101.

Rich J et al: Isopropyl alcohol intoxication. Arch Neurol 1990;47:322.

Shelling JR et al: Increased osmolal gap in alcoholic ketoacidosis and lactic acidosis. Ann Intern Med 1990; 113:580.

Smilkstein MJ et al: Efficacy of oral N-acetylcysteine in the treatment of acetaminophen overdose: Analysis of the National Multicenter Study (1976 to 1985). N Engl J Med 1988;319:1557.

Su Y-J, Shannon M: Pharmacokinetics of drugs in overdose. Clin Pharmacokinet 1992;23:93.

Wiley JF II: Difficult diagnoses in toxicology. Poisons not detected in the comprehensive drug screen. Pediatr Clin North Am 1991;38:725.

Special Aspects of Perinatal & Pediatric Pharmacology

61

Gideon Koren, MD, & Martin S. Cohen, MD

The effects of drugs on the fetus and newborn infant are based on the general principles set forth in Chapters 1–4 of this book. However, the physiologic contexts in which these pharmacologic laws operate are different in pregnant women and in rapidly maturing infants. At present, the special pharmacokinetic factors operative in these patients are beginning to be understood, whereas information regarding pharmacodynamic differences (eg, receptor characteristics and response) is still quite preliminary. This chapter presents basic principles of pharmacology in the special context of perinatal and pediatric therapeutics.

DRUG THERAPY IN PREGNANCY

Pharmacokinetics

Most drugs taken by pregnant women can cross the placenta and expose the developing embryo and fetus to their pharmacologic and teratogenic effects. Critical factors affecting placental drug transfer and drug effects on the fetus include the following: (1) The physicochemical properties of the drug. (2) The rate at which the drug crosses the placenta and the amount of drug reaching the fetus. (3) The duration of exposure to the drug. (4) Distribution characteristics in different fetal tissues. (5) The stage of placental and fetal development at the time of exposure to the drug. (6) The effects of drugs used in combination.

A. Lipid Solubility: As is true also of other biologic membranes, drug passage across the placenta is dependent on lipid solubility and the degree of drug ionization. Lipophilic drugs tend to diffuse readily across the placenta and enter the fetal circulation. For example, thiopental, a drug commonly used for cesarean sections, crosses the placenta almost immediately and can produce sedation or apnea in the newborn infant. Highly ionized drugs such as succinylcholine and tubocurarine, also used for cesarean sections, cross the placenta slowly and achieve very low concentrations in the fetus. Impermeability of the

placenta to polar compounds is relative rather than absolute. If high enough maternal-fetal concentration gradients are achieved, polar compounds cross the placenta in measurable amounts. Salicylate, which is almost completely ionized at physiologic pH, crosses the placenta rapidly. This occurs because the small amount of salicylate that is not ionized is highly lipid-soluble.

B. Molecular Size: The molecular weight of the drug also influences the rate of transfer and the amount of drug transferred across the placenta. Drugs with molecular weights of 250–500 can cross the placenta easily, depending upon their lipid solubility and degree of ionization; those with molecular weights of 500–1000 cross the placenta with more difficulty; and those with molecular weights greater than 1000 cross very poorly. An important clinical application of this property is the choice of heparin as an anticoagulant in pregnant women. Because it is a very large (and polar) molecule, heparin is unable to cross the placenta. Unlike warfarin, which is teratogenic and should be avoided during the first trimester, heparin may be safely given to pregnant women who need anticoagulation. Apparent exceptions to the "size rule" are maternal antibody globulins and certain polypeptides that cross the placenta by some selective mechanism that has not yet been identified.

C. Protein Binding: The degree to which a drug is bound to plasma proteins (particularly albumin) may also affect the rate of transfer and the amount transferred. However, if a compound is very lipid-soluble (eg, some anesthetic gases), it will not be affected greatly by protein binding. Transfer of these more lipid-soluble drugs and their overall rates of equilibration are more dependent on (and proportionate to) placental blood flow. This is because very lipid-soluble drugs diffuse across placental membranes so rapidly that their overall rates of equilibration do not depend on the free drug concentrations becoming equal on both sides. If a drug is poorly lipid-soluble and is ionized, its transfer is slow and will probably be impeded by its binding to maternal plasma proteins. Differential protein binding is also important, since some drugs exhibit greater protein binding in maternal plasma than in fetal plasma because of a lowered binding affinity of fetal proteins. This has been shown for sulfonamides, barbiturates, phenytoin, and local anesthetic agents.

D. Placental and Fetal Drug Metabolism:
Two mechanisms help to protect the fetus from drugs in the maternal circulation: (1) The placenta itself plays a role both as a semipermeable barrier and as a site of metabolism of some drugs passing through it. Several different types of aromatic oxidation reactions (eg, hydroxylation, N-dealkylation, demethylation) have been shown to occur in placental tissue. Ethanol and pentobarbital are oxidized in this way. Conversely, it is possible that the metabolic capacity of the placenta may lead to creation of toxic metabolites, and the placenta may therefore augment toxicity (eg, ethanol, benzpyrenes). (2) Drugs that have crossed the placenta enter the fetal circulation via the umbilical vein. About 40–60% of umbilical venous blood flow enters the fetal liver; the remainder bypasses the liver and enters the general fetal circulation. A drug that enters the liver may be partly metabolized there before it enters the fetal circulation. In addition, a large proportion of drug present in the umbilical artery (returning to the placenta) may be shunted through the placenta back to the umbilical vein and into the liver again. It should be noted that metabolites of some drugs may be more active than the parent compound and may affect the fetus adversely.

Pharmacodynamics

A. Maternal Drug Actions: The effects of drugs on the reproductive tissues (breast, uterus, etc) of the pregnant woman are sometimes altered by the endocrine environment appropriate for the stage of pregnancy. Drug effects on other maternal tissues (heart, lungs, kidneys, central nervous system, etc) are not changed significantly by pregnancy, though the physiologic context (cardiac output, renal blood flow, etc) may be altered and may require the use of drugs that are not needed in the same woman when she is not pregnant. For example, cardiac glycosides and diuretics may be needed for congestive heart failure precipitated by the increased cardiac workload of pregnancy, or insulin may be required for control of blood glucose in pregnancy-induced diabetes.

B. Therapeutic Drug Actions in the Fetus:
Fetal therapeutics is an emerging area in perinatal pharmacology. This involves drug administration to the pregnant woman with the fetus as the target of the drug. At present, corticosteroids are used to stimulate fetal lung maturation when premature birth is expected. Phenobarbital, when given to pregnant women near term, can induce fetal hepatic enzymes responsible for the glucuronidation of bilirubin, and the incidence of jaundice is lower in newborns when mothers are given phenobarbital than when phenobarbital is not used. Recently, administration of phenobarbital to the mother has been shown to decrease the risk of intracranial bleeding in preterm infants. Antiarrhythmic drugs have also been given to mothers for treatment of fetal cardiac arrhythmias.

C. Predictable Toxic Drug Actions in the Fetus: Chronic use of opioids by the mother may produce dependence in the fetus and newborn. This dependence may be manifested after delivery as a neonatal withdrawal syndrome. A less well understood fetal drug toxicity is caused by the use of angiotensin-converting enzyme inhibitors during pregnancy. These drugs can result in significant and irreversible renal damage in the fetus and are therefore contraindicated in pregnant women. Adverse effects may also be delayed, as in the case of female fetuses exposed to diethylstilbestrol (DES), who may be at increased risk for adenocarcinoma of the vagina after puberty.

D. Teratogenic Drug Actions: A single intrauterine exposure to a drug can affect the fetal structures undergoing rapid development at the time of exposure. Thalidomide is an example of a drug that may profoundly affect the development of the limbs after only brief exposure. This exposure, however, must be at a critical time in the development of the limbs. The thalidomide phocomelia risk occurs during the fourth through the seventh weeks of gestation because it is during this time that the arms and legs develop (Figure 61–1).

The mechanisms by which different drugs produce teratogenic effects are poorly understood and are probably multifactorial. For example, drugs may have a direct effect on maternal tissues with secondary or indirect effects on fetal tissues. Drugs may interfere with the passage of oxygen or nutrients through the placenta and therefore have effects on the most rapidly metabolizing tissues of the fetus. Finally, drugs may have important direct actions on the processes of differentiation in developing tissues. For example, vitamin A (retinol) has been shown to have important differentiation-directing actions in normal tissues. Several vitamin A analogues (isotretinoin, etretinate) are powerful teratogens, suggesting that they alter the normal processes of differentiation. Finally, deficiency of a critical substance appears to play a role in some types of abnormalities. For example, folic acid supplementation during pregnancy appears to reduce the incidence of neural tube defects, eg, spina bifida.

Continued exposure to a teratogen may produce cumulative effects or may affect several organs going through varying stages of development. Chronic consumption of high doses of ethanol during pregnancy, particularly during the first and second trimesters, may result in the fetal alcohol syndrome (Chapter 22). In this syndrome, the central nervous system, growth, and facial development may be affected.

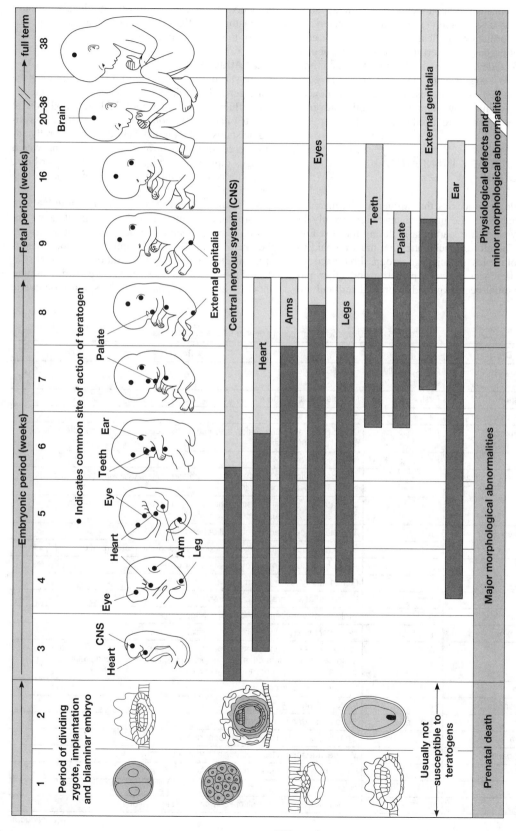

Figure 61–1. Schematic diagram of critical periods of human development. (Reproduced, with permission, from Moore KL: *The Developing Human, Clinically Oriented Embryology*, 4th ed. Saunders, 1988.

To be considered teratogenic, a candidate substance or process should (1) result in a characteristic set of malformations, indicating a selectivity for certain target organs; (2) exert its effects at a particular stage of fetal development, ie, during the limited time period of organogenesis of the target organs (Figure 61–1); and (3) show a dose-dependent incidence. Some drugs with known teratogenic or other adverse effects in pregnancy are listed in Table 61–1.

DRUG THERAPY IN INFANTS & CHILDREN

Physiologic processes that influence pharmacokinetic variables in the infant change significantly in the first year of life, particularly during the first few months. Therefore, special attention must be paid to pharmacokinetics in this age group. Pharmacodynamic differences between pediatric and other patients have not been explored in great detail and are probably small except for those specific target tissues that mature at birth or immediately thereafter, eg, closure of the ductus arteriosus.

Drug Absorption

Drug absorption in infants and children follows the same general principles as in adults. Unique factors that influence drug absorption include blood flow at the site of administration, as determined by the physiologic status of the infant or child; and, for orally administered drugs, gastrointestinal function, which changes rapidly during the first few days after birth. Age after birth also influences the regulation of drug absorption.

A. Blood Flow at the Site of Administration: Absorption after intramuscular or subcutaneous injection depends mainly, in neonates as in adults, on the rate of blood flow to the muscle or subcutaneous area injected. Physiologic conditions that might reduce blood flow to these areas are cardiovascular shock, vasoconstriction due to sympathomimetic

Drug	Trimester	Effect
ACE inhibitors	All, especially second and third	Renal damage.
Aminopterin	First	Multiple gross anomalies.
Aminoglycosides	All	Eighth nerve toxicity.
Amphetamines	All	Cystic cerebral cortical lesions, abnormal developmental patterns, decreased school performance.
Androgens	Second and third	Masculinization of female fetus.
Antidepressants, tricyclic	First	Anecdotal evidence for congenital anomalies associated with use of imipramine, amitriptyline, and nortriptyline.
	Third	Neonatal withdrawal symptoms have been reported with clomipramine, desipramine, and imipramine.
Barbiturates	All	Chronic use can lead to neonatal dependence.
	First	Some evidence for increased incidence of congenital malformations.
Busulfan	All	Various congenital malformations; low birth weight.
Chlorambucil	All	Genitourinary tract malformations.
Chloramphenicol	Third	Increased risk of gray baby syndrome.
Chlorpropamide	All	Prolonged symptomatic neonatal hypoglycemia.
Clomipramine	Third	Neonatal lethargy, hypotonia, cyanosis, hypothermia.
Cocaine	All	Increased risk of spontaneous abortion, abruptio placentae, and premature labor; neonatal cerebral infarction, cystic cortical lesions, abnormal development, and decreased school performance.
Cortisone	First	Increased risk of cleft palate.
Cyclophosphamide	First	Various congenital malformations.
Cytarabine	First, second	Various congenital malformations.
Diazepam	All	Chronic use leads to neonatal dependence.
Diethylstilbestrol	All	Vaginal adenosis, clear cell vaginal adenocarcinoma.
Disulfiram	First	Malformations of lower extremity, "VACTERL" syndrome.[1]
Ethanol	All	High risk of fetal alcohol syndrome.
Etretinate	All	Extremely high risk of multiple congenital malformations.

Table 61–1. Drugs with significant adverse effects on the fetus.

(continued)

Table 61–1 (cont'd). Drugs with significant adverse effects on the fetus.

Drug	Trimester	Effect
Heroin	All	Chronic use leads to neonatal dependence.
Hydroflumethiazide	First	Some evidence for increased risk of congenital malformations.
Iodide	All	Congenital goiter, hypothyroidism.
Isotretinoin	All	Extremely high risk of congenital anomalies.
Lithium	First	Cardiovascular defects.
Methadone	All	Chronic use leads to neonatal dependence.
Methotrexate	First	Multiple congenital malformations.
Methylthiouracil	All	Hypothyroidism.
Metronidazole	First	May be mutagenic (from animal studies; there is no evidence for mutagenic or teratogenic effects in humans).
Penicillamine	First	Cutis laxa, other congenital malformations.
Phencyclidine	All	Abnormal neurologic examination, poor suck reflex and feeding.
Phenytoin	All	Cleft lip and palate.
Progestins	All	Ambiguous genitalia, cardiovascular defects.
Propylthiouracil	All	Congenital goiter.
Tamoxifen	All	Increased risk of spontaneous abortion or fetal damage.
Tetracycline	All	Discoloration and defects of teeth and altered bone growth.
Thalidomide	First	Phocomelia (shortened or absent long bones of the limbs.)
Trimethadione	All	Multiple congenital anomalies.
Vaccines, live virus	All	Risk of fetal infection with attenuated viruses.
Valproic acid	All	Various congenital anomalies, especially spina bifida.
Warfarin	First	Hypoplastic nasal bridge, chondrodysplasia.
	Third	Risk of bleeding. Discontinue use 1 month before delivery.

[1]VACTERL = Vertebral anomalies, Anal atresia, Cardiovascular anomalies, Tracheo-Esophageal fistula, Renal anomalies, Limb defects.

agents, and heart failure. However, sick premature infants requiring intramuscular injections may have very little muscle mass. This is further complicated by diminished peripheral perfusion to these areas. In such cases, absorption becomes irregular and difficult to predict, because the drug may remain in the muscle and be absorbed more slowly than expected. If perfusion suddenly improves, there can be a sudden and unpredictable increase in the amount of drug entering the circulation, resulting in high and potentially toxic concentrations of drug. Examples of drugs especially hazardous in such situations are cardiac glycosides, aminoglycoside antibiotics, and anticonvulsants.

B. Gastrointestinal Function: Significant biochemical and physiologic changes occur in the neonatal gastrointestinal tract shortly after birth. In full-term infants, gastric acid secretion begins soon after birth and increases gradually over several hours. In premature infants, the secretion of gastric acid occurs more slowly, with the highest concentration appearing on the fourth day of life. Therefore, drugs that are partially or totally inactivated by the low pH of gastric contents should not be administered orally.

Gastric emptying time is prolonged (up to 6 or 8 hours) in the first day or so of life. Therefore, drugs that are absorbed primarily in the stomach may be ab-

sorbed more completely than anticipated. In the case of drugs absorbed in the small intestine, therapeutic effect may be delayed. Peristalsis in the neonate is irregular and may be slow. The amount of drug absorbed in the small intestine may therefore be unpredictable; more than the usual amount of drug may be absorbed if peristalsis is slowed, and this could result in potential toxicity from an otherwise standard dose. Table 61–2 summarizes data on oral bioavailability of various drugs in neonates as opposed to older children and adults. An increase in peristalsis, as in diarrheal conditions, tends to decrease the extent of absorption, since contact time with the large absorptive surface of the intestine is decreased.

Gastrointestinal enzyme activities tend to be lower in the newborn than in the adult. Activities of α-amylase and other pancreatic enzymes in the duodenum are low in infants up to 4 months of age. Neonates also have low concentrations of bile acids and lipase, which may decrease the absorption of lipid-soluble drugs.

Drug Distribution

As body composition changes with development, the distribution volumes of drugs are also changed. The neonate has a higher percentage of its body

Table 61–2. Oral drug absorption (bioavailability) of various drugs in the neonate compared with older children and adults.

Drug	Oral Absorption
Acetaminophen	Decreased
Ampicillin	Increased
Diazepam	Normal
Digoxin	Normal
Penicillin G	Increased
Phenobarbital	Decreased
Phenytoin	Decreased
Sulfonamides	Normal

weight in the form of water (70–75%) than does the adult (50–60%). Differences can also be observed between the full-term neonate (70% of body weight as water) and the small premature neonate (85% of body weight as water). Similarly, extracellular water is 40% of body weight in the neonate, compared with 20% in the adult. Most neonates will experience diuresis in the first 24–48 hours of life. Since many drugs are distributed throughout the extracellular water space, the size (volume) of the extracellular water compartment may be important in determining the concentration of drug at receptor sites. This is especially important for water-soluble drugs (such as aminoglycosides) and less crucial for lipid-soluble agents.

Premature infants have much less fat than full-term infants. Total body fat in premature infants is about 1% of total body weight, compared with 15% in full-term neonates. Therefore, organs that generally accumulate high concentrations of lipid-soluble drugs in adults and older children may accumulate smaller amounts of these agents in more immature infants.

Another major factor determining drug distribution is drug binding to plasma proteins. Albumin is the plasma protein with the greatest binding capacity. In general, protein binding of drugs is reduced in the neonate. This has been seen with local anesthetic drugs, diazepam, phenytoin, ampicillin, and phenobarbital. Therefore, the concentration of free (unbound) drug in plasma is increased. Because the free drug exerts the pharmacologic effect, this can result in greater drug effect or toxicity despite a normal or even low plasma concentration of total drug (bound plus unbound). As a practical example, consider a therapeutic dose of a drug, eg, diazepam, given to a patient. The concentration of total drug in the plasma is 300 µg/L. If the drug is 98% protein-bound in an older child or adult, then 6 µg/L is the concentration of free drug. Assume that this concentration of free drug produces the desired effect in the patient without producing toxicity. However, if this drug is given to a premature infant in a dosage adjusted for body weight and it produces a total drug concentration of 300

µg/L—and protein binding is only 90%—then the free drug concentration will be 30 µg/L, or five times higher! Although the higher free concentration may result in faster elimination (Chapter 3), this concentration may be quite toxic initially.

Some drugs compete with serum bilirubin for binding to albumin. Drugs given to a neonate with jaundice can displace bilirubin from albumin. Because of the greater permeability of the neonatal blood-brain barrier, substantial amounts of bilirubin may enter the brain and cause kernicterus. This was in fact observed when sulfonamide antibiotics were given to premature neonates as prophylaxis against sepsis. Conversely, as the serum bilirubin rises for physiologic reasons or because of a blood group incompatibility, bilirubin can displace a drug from albumin and substantially raise the free drug concentration. This may occur without altering the total drug concentration and would result in greater therapeutic effect or toxicity at normal concentrations. This has been shown to happen with phenytoin.

Drug Metabolism

The metabolism of most drugs occurs in the liver (Chapter 4). The drug-metabolizing activities of the cytochrome P450-dependent mixed-function oxidases and the conjugating enzymes are substantially lower (50–70% of adult values) in early neonatal life than later. The point in development at which enzymatic activity is maximal depends upon the specific enzyme system in question. Glucuronide formation reaches adult values (per kilogram body weight) between the third and fourth years of life. Because of the neonate's decreased ability to metabolize drugs, many drugs have slow clearance rates and prolonged elimination half-lives. If drug doses and dosing schedules are not altered appropriately, this immaturity predisposes the neonate to adverse effects from drugs that are metabolized by the liver. Table 61–3 demonstrates how neonatal and adult drug elimina-

Table 61–3. Approximate half-lives of various drugs in neonates and adults.

Drug	Neonatal Age	Neonates $t_{1/2}$ (hours)	Adults $t_{1/2}$ (hours)
Acetaminophen		2.2–5	1.9–2.2
Diazepam		25–100	40–50
Digoxin		60–70	30–60
Phenobarbital	0–5 days	200	64–140
	5–15 days	100	
	1–30 months	50	
Phenytoin	0–2 days	80	12–18
	3–14 days	18	
	14–50 days	6	
Salicylate		4.5–11	10–15
Theophylline	Neonate	13–26	5–10
	Child	3–4	

tion half-lives can differ and how the half-lives of phenobarbital and phenytoin decrease as the neonate grows older. The process of maturation must be considered when administering drugs to this age group, especially if the drug or drugs are administered over long periods.

Another consideration for the neonate is whether or not the mother was receiving drugs (such as phenobarbital) that can induce early maturation of fetal hepatic enzymes. In this case, the ability of the neonate to metabolize certain drugs will be greater than expected, and one may see less therapeutic effect and lower plasma drug concentrations when the usual neonatal dose is given.

Drug Excretion

The glomerular filtration rate is much lower in newborns than in older infants, children, or adults, and this limitation persists during the first few days of life. Calculated on the basis of surface area, glomerular filtration in the neonate is only 30–40% of the adult value. The glomerular filtration rate is even lower in neonates born before 34 weeks of gestation. Function improves substantially during the first week of life. At that time, the glomerular filtration rate and renal plasma flow have increased 50% from the first day. By the end of the third week, glomerular filtration is 50–60% of the adult value; by 6–12 months, it reaches adult values (per unit surface area). Therefore, drugs that depend on renal function for elimination are cleared from the body very slowly in the first weeks of life.

Penicillins, for example, are cleared by premature infants at 17% of the adult rate based on comparable surface area and 34% of the adult rate when adjusted for body weight. The dosage of ampicillin for a neonate less than 7 days old is 50–100 mg/kg/d in two doses at 12-hour intervals. The dosage for a neonate over 7 days old is 100–200 mg/kg/d in three doses at 8-hour intervals. A decreased rate of renal elimination in the neonate has also been observed with aminoglycoside antibiotics (kanamycin, gentamicin, neomycin, streptomycin). The dosage of gentamicin for a neonate less than 7 days old is 5 mg/kg/d in two doses at 12-hour intervals. The dosage for a neonate over 7 days old is 7.5 mg/kg/d in three doses at 8-hour intervals. Total body clearance of digoxin is directly dependent upon adequate renal function, and accumulation of digoxin can occur when glomerular filtration is decreased. Since renal function in a sick infant may not improve at the predicted rate during the first weeks and months of life, appropriate adjustments in dosage and dosing schedules may be very difficult. In this situation, adjustments are best made on the basis of plasma drug concentrations determined at intervals throughout the course of therapy.

Special Pharmacodynamics Features in the Neonate

The appropriate use of drugs has made possible the survival of neonates with severe abnormalities who would otherwise die within days or weeks after birth. For example, administration of indomethacin (Chapter 35) causes the rapid closure of a patent ductus arteriosus, which would otherwise require surgical closure in an infant with a normal heart. Infusion of prostaglandin E_1, on the other hand, causes the ductus to remain open, which can be life-saving in an infant with transposition of the great vessels or tetralogy of Fallot (Chapter 18). An unexpected effect of such PGE_1 infusion has recently been described. The drug caused antral hyperplasia with gastric outlet obstruction as a clinical manifestation in 6 of 74 infants who received it (Peled et al, 1992). This phenomenon appears to be dose-dependent.

PEDIATRIC DOSAGE FORMS & COMPLIANCE

The form in which a drug is manufactured and the way in which the parent dispenses the drug to the child determine the actual dose administered. Many drugs prepared for children are in the form of elixirs or suspensions. Elixirs are alcoholic solutions in which the drug molecules are dissolved and evenly distributed. No shaking is required, and unless some of the vehicle has evaporated, the first dose from the bottle and the last dose should contain equivalent amounts of drug.

Suspensions contain undissolved particles of drug that must be distributed throughout the vehicle by shaking. If shaking is not thorough each time a dose is given, the first doses from the bottle may contain less drug than the last doses, with the result that less than the expected plasma concentration or effect of the drug may be achieved early in the course of therapy. Conversely, toxicity may occur late in the course of therapy, when it is not expected. This uneven distribution is a potential cause of inefficacy or toxicity in children taking phenytoin suspensions. It is thus essential that the prescriber know the form in which the drug will be dispensed and provide proper instructions to the pharmacist and patient or parent.

Compliance may be more difficult to achieve in pediatric practice than otherwise, since it involves not only the parent's conscientious effort to follow directions but also such practical matters as measuring errors, spilling, and spitting out. For example, the measured volume of "teaspoons" ranges from 2.5 to 7.8 mL. The parents should obtain a calibrated medicine spoon or syringe from the pharmacy. These devices improve the accuracy of dose measurements and simplify administration of drugs to children.

When evaluating compliance, it is often helpful to ask if an attempt has been made to give a further dose after the child has spilled half of what was offered. The parents may not always be able to say with confidence how much of a dose the child actually received. The parents must be told whether or not to wake the baby for its every-6-hour dose day or night. These matters should be discussed and made clear, and no assumptions should be made about what the parents may or may not do. Noncompliance frequently occurs when antibiotics are prescribed to treat otitis media or urinary tract infections and the child feels well after 4 or 5 days of therapy. The parents may not feel there is any reason to continue giving the medicine even though it was prescribed for 10 or 14 days. This common situation should be anticipated so the parents can be told why it is important to continue the medicine for the prescribed period even if the child seems to be "cured."

Practical and convenient dosage forms and dosing schedules should be chosen to the extent possible. The easier it is to administer and take the medicine and the easier the dosing schedule is to follow, the more likely it is that compliance will be achieved.

Consistent with their ability to comprehend and cooperate, children should also be given some responsibility for their own health care and for taking medications. This should be discussed in appropriate terms both with the child and the parents. Possible adverse effects and drug interactions with over-the-counter medicines or foods should also be discussed. Whenever a drug does not achieve its therapeutic effect, the possibility of noncompliance should be considered. There is ample evidence that in such cases parents' or children's reports may be grossly inaccurate. Random measurement of serum concentrations and pill count may help disclose noncompliance. Recently, the use of computerized pill containers, which record each lid opening, has been shown to be very effective in measuring compliance.

DRUG USE DURING LACTATION
(Table 61–4)

Drugs should be used conservatively during lactation, and the physician must know which drugs are potentially dangerous to nursing infants (Table 61–4). Most drugs administered to lactating women are detectable in breast milk. Fortunately, the concentration of drugs achieved in breast milk is usually low. Therefore, the total amount the infant would receive in a day is substantially less than what would be considered a "therapeutic dose." If the nursing mother must take medications and the drug is a relatively safe one, she should optimally take it 30–60 minutes after nursing and 3–4 hours before the next feeding. This allows time for many drugs to be cleared from the mother's blood, and the concentrations in breast milk will be relatively low. Drugs for which no data are available on safety during lactation should be avoided or breast feeding discontinued while they are being given.

Most antibiotics taken by nursing mothers can be detected in breast milk. Tetracycline concentrations in breast milk are approximately 70% of maternal serum concentrations and present a risk of permanent tooth staining in the infant. Chloramphenicol concentrations in breast milk are not sufficient to cause the gray baby syndrome, but there is a remote possibility of causing bone marrow suppression, and chloramphenicol should be avoided during lactation. Isoniazid reaches a rapid equilibrium between breast milk and maternal blood. The concentrations achieved in breast milk are high enough so that pyridoxine deficiency may occur in the infant if the mother is not given pyridoxine supplements.

Most sedatives and hypnotics achieve concentrations in breast milk sufficient to produce a pharmacologic effect in some infants. Barbiturates taken in hypnotic doses by the mother can produce lethargy, sedation, and poor suck reflexes in the infant. Chloral hydrate can produce sedation if the infant is fed at peak milk concentrations. Diazepam can have a sedative effect on the nursing infant, but most importantly, its long half-life can result in significant drug accumulation.

Opioids such as heroin, methadone, and morphine enter breast milk in quantities potentially sufficient to prolong the state of neonatal narcotic dependence if the drug was taken chronically by the mother during pregnancy. If conditions are well controlled and there is a good relationship between the mother and the physician, an infant could be breast-fed while the mother is taking methadone. She should not, however, stop taking the drug abruptly; the infant can be tapered off the methadone as the mother's dose is tapered. The infant should be watched for signs of narcotic withdrawal.

Minimal use of alcohol by the mother has not been reported to harm nursing infants. Excessive amounts of alcohol, however, can produce alcohol effects in the infant. Nicotine concentrations in the breast milk of smoking mothers are low and do not produce effects in the infant. Very small amounts of caffeine are excreted in the breast milk of coffee-drinking mothers.

Lithium enters breast milk in concentrations equal to those in maternal serum. Clearance of this drug is almost completely dependent upon renal elimination, and women who are receiving lithium may expose the baby to relatively large amounts of the drug.

Drugs such as propylthiouracil and tolbutamide enter breast milk in quantities sufficient to affect endocrine function in the infant. They should be avoided if possible or breast feeding discontinued.

Radioactive substances such as iodinated ^{125}I albumin and radioiodine can cause thyroid suppression in

Table 61–4. Drugs often used during lactation and possible effects on the nursing infant.

Drug	Effect on Infant	Comments
Ampicillin	Minimal	No significant adverse effects; possible occurrence of diarrhea or allergic sensitization.
Aspirin	Minimal	Occasional doses probably safe; high doses may produce significant concentration in breast milk.
Caffeine	Minimal	Caffeine intake in moderation is safe; concentration in breast milk is about 1% of total dose taken by mother.
Chloral hydrate	Significant	May cause drowsiness if fed at peak concentration in milk.
Chloramphenicol	Significant	Concentrations too low to cause gray baby syndrome; possibility of bone marrow suppression does exist; recommend not taking chloramphenicol while breast feeding.
Chlorothiazide	Minimal	No adverse effects reported.
Chlorpromazine	Minimal	Appears insignificant.
Codeine	Minimal	No adverse effects reported.
Diazepam	Significant	Will cause sedation in breast-fed infants; accumulation can occur in newborns.
Dicumarol	Minimal	No adverse side effects reported; may wish to follow infant's prothrombin time.
Digoxin	Minimal	Insignificant quantities enter breast milk.
Ethanol	Moderate	Moderate ingestion by mother unlikely to produce effects in infant; large amounts consumed by mother can produce alcohol effects in infant.
Heroin	Significant	Enters breast milk and can prolong neonatal narcotic dependence.
Iodine (radioactive)	Significant	Enters milk in quantities sufficient to cause thyroid suppression in infant.
Isoniazid (INH)	Minimal	Milk concentrations equal maternal plasma concentrations. Possibility of pyridoxine deficiency developing in the infant.
Kanamycin	Minimal	No adverse effects reported.
Lithium	Significant	Avoid breast feeding.
Methadone	Significant	(See heroin.) Under close physician supervision, breast-feeding can be continued. Signs of opiate withdrawal in the infant may occur if mother stops taking methadone or stops breast feeding abruptly.
Oral contraceptives	Minimal	Will suppress lactation in high doses.
Penicillin	Minimal	Very low concentrations in breast milk.
Phenobarbital	Moderate	Hypnotic doses can cause sedation in the infant.
Phenytoin	Moderate	Amounts entering breast milk may be sufficient to cause adverse effects in infant.
Prednisone	Moderate	Low maternal doses (5 mg/d) probably safe. Doses 2 or more times physiologic amounts (> 15 mg/d) should probably be avoided.
Propranolol	Minimal	Very small amounts enter breast milk.
Propylthiouracil	Significant	Can suppress thyroid function in infant.
Spironolactone	Minimal	Very small amounts enter breast milk.
Tetracycline	Moderate	Possibility of permanent staining of developing teeth in the infants. Should be avoided during lactation.
Theophylline	Moderate	Can enter breast milk in moderate quantities but not likely to produce significant effects.
Thyroxine	Minimal	No adverse effects in therapeutic doses.
Tolbutamide	Minimal	Low concentrations in breast milk.
Warfarin	Minimal	Very small quantities found in breast milk.

infants and may increase the risk of subsequent thyroid cancer as much as tenfold. Breast feeding is contraindicated after large doses and should be withheld for days to weeks after small doses. Similarly, breast feeding should be avoided in mothers receiving cancer chemotherapy or being treated with similar agents for collagen diseases such as lupus erythematosus or post transplant.

PEDIATRIC DRUG DOSAGE

Because of differences in pharmacokinetics in infants and children, simple proportionate reduction in the adult dose may not be adequate to determine a safe and effective pediatric dose. The most reliable pediatric dose information is usually that provided by the manufacturer in the package insert. If such information is not available for a given product, an approximation can be made by any of several methods based on age, weight, or surface area. These rules are not precise and should not be used if the manufacturer provides a pediatric dose. Most drugs approved for use in children have recommended pediatric doses, generally stated as milligrams per kilogram or per pound. When pediatric doses are calculated (either from one of the methods set forth below or from a manufacturer's dose), the pediatric dose should never exceed the adult dose.

Surface Area

Calculations of dosage based on age or weight (see below) are conservative and tend to underestimate the required dose. Doses based on surface area (Table 61–5) are more likely to be adequate.

Age (Young's rule):

$$\text{Dose} = \text{Adult dose} \times \frac{\text{Age (years)}}{\text{Age} + 12}$$

Weight (Somewhat more precise is Clark's rule):

Table 61–5. Determination of drug dosage from surface area.[1,2]

Weight		Approximate Age	Surface Area (m²)	Percent of Adult Dose
(kg)	(lb)			
3	6.6	Newborn	0.2	12
6	13.2	3 months	0.3	18
10	22	1 year	0.45	28
20	44	5.5 years	0.8	48
30	66	9 years	1	60
40	88	12 years	1.3	78
50	110	14 years	1.5	90
60	132	Adult	1.7	102
70	154	Adult	1.76	103

[1]Reproduced, with permission, from Silver HK, Kempe CH, Bruyn HB: *Handbook of Pediatrics,* 14th ed. Lange, 1983.
[2]For example, if adult dose is 1 mg/kg, dose for 3-month-old infant would be 2 mg/kg (18% of 70 mg/6 kg).

$$\text{Dose} = \text{Adult dose} \times \frac{\text{Weight (kg)}}{70}$$

or

$$\text{Dose} = \text{Adult dose} \times \frac{\text{Weight (lb)}}{150}$$

REFERENCES

American Academy of Pediatrics, Committee on Drugs: Emergency drug doses for infants and children. Pediatrics 1988;81:462.

Benitz WE, Tatro DS: *The Pediatric Drug Handbook,* 2nd ed. Year Book, 1988.

Besunder JB, Reed MD, Blumer JL: Principles of drug biodisposition in the neonate: A critical evaluation of the pharmacokinetic-pharmacodynamic interface. (Two parts.) Clin Pharmacokinet 1988;14:189, 261.

Briggs GG, Freeman RK, Yaffe SJ: *Drugs in Pregnancy and Lactation.* Williams & Wilkins, 1990.

Drug toxicity in the newborn. (Symposium.) Fed Proc 1985; 44:2301.

Gilman JT: Therapeutic drug monitoring in the neonate and paediatric age group: Problems and clinical pharmacokinetic implications. Clin Pharmacokinet 1990;19:1.

Hansten PD: *Drug Interactions.* Applied Therapeutics, Lea & Febiger, 1993. [Quarterly.]

Heymann MA: Non-narcotic analgesics: Use in pregnancy and fetal and perinatal effects. Drugs 1986;32(Suppl 4): 164.

Koren G: *Maternal-Fetal Toxicology; A Clinician's Guide.* Dekker, 1990.

Koren G, Prober C, Gold R: *Antimicrobial Therapy in Infants and Children.* Dekker, 1987.

Morselli PL: Clinical pharmacology of the perinatal period and early infancy. Clin Pharmacokinet 1989;17(Suppl 1): 13.

Nau H: Clinical pharmacokinetics in pregnancy and perinatology: 2. Penicillins. Dev Pharmacol Ther 1987;10:174.

Nottarianni LJ: Plasma protein binding of drugs in pregnancy and in neonates. Clin Pharmacokinet 1990;18:20.

Paap CM, Nahata MC: Clinical pharmacokinetics of antibacterial drugs in neonates. Clin Pharmacokinet 1990; 19:280.

Peled N et al: Gastric-outlet obstruction induced by prostaglandin therapy in neonates. N Engl J Med 1992;327: 505.

Roberts RJ: *Drug Therapy in Infants: Pharmacologic Principles and Clinical Experience.* Saunders, 1984.

Rousseaux CG, Blakely PM: Fetus. In *Handbook of Toxicologic Pathology.* Haschek WM, Rousseaux CG (editors). Academic Press, 1991.

Safety of antimicrobial drugs in pregnancy. Med Lett Drugs Ther 1987;29:61.

Stewart CF, Hampton EM: Effect of maturation on drug disposition in pediatric patients. Clin Pharm 1987;6:548.

Valdes-Dapena M: Iatrogenic disease in the perinatal period. Pediatr Clin North Am 1989;36:67.

Wilson JT (editor): *Drugs in Breast Milk.* ADIS Press, 1981.

Special Aspects of Geriatric Pharmacology

62

Bertram G. Katzung, MD, PhD

Society often classifies everyone over 65 as "elderly," but most authorities consider the field of geriatrics to apply to persons over 75—even though this too is an arbitrary definition. Furthermore, chronologic age is only one determinant of the changes pertinent to drug therapy that occur in older adults. Important changes in responses to some drugs occur with increasing age in most individuals. Drug usage patterns also change as a result of the increasing incidence of disease with age and the tendency to prescribe heavily for patients in nursing homes. General changes in the lives of older people have significant effects on the way drugs are used. Among these changes are the increased incidence with advancing age of multiple diseases, nutritional problems, reduced financial resources, and—in some patients—decreased dosing compliance for a variety of reasons.

The health practitioner thus should be aware of the changes in pharmacologic responses that may occur in older people and how to deal with these changes.

PHARMACOLOGIC CHANGES ASSOCIATED WITH AGING

Measurements of functional capacity of most of the major organ systems show a decline beginning in young adulthood and continuing throughout life. As shown in Figure 62–1, there is no "middle-age plateau" but rather a linear decrease beginning no later than age 45. However, these data reflect the mean and do not apply to every person above a certain age; approximately one-third of healthy subjects have no age-related decrease in, eg, creatinine clearance. Thus, the elderly do not lose specific functions at an accelerated rate compared to young and middle-aged adults but rather accumulate more deficiencies with the passage of time. Some of these changes result in altered pharmacokinetics. For the pharmacologist and the clinician, the most important of these is the decrease in renal function. Other changes and concurrent diseases may alter the pharmacodynamic characteristics of the patient.

Pharmacokinetic Changes

A. Absorption: There is little evidence that there is any major alteration in drug absorption with age. However, conditions associated with age may alter the rate at which some drugs are absorbed. Such conditions include altered nutritional habits, greater consumption of nonprescription drugs (eg, antacids, laxatives), and changes in gastric emptying, which is often slower in older persons.

B. Distribution: As noted in Chapters 1 and 3, the distribution of a drug is a function of the chemical characteristics of the drug molecule and the size and composition of the compartments of the body. The elderly have reduced lean body mass, reduced total and percentage body water, and an increase in fat as a percentage of body mass. Some of these changes are shown in Table 62–1. There is usually a decrease in serum albumin, which binds many drugs, especially weak acids. There may be a concurrent increase in serum orosomucoid (α-acid glycoprotein), a protein that binds many basic drugs. Thus, the ratio of bound to free drug may be significantly altered. As explained in Chapter 3, these changes may alter the appropriate loading dose of a drug. However, since both the clearance and the effects of drugs are related to the free concentration, the steady-state effects of a maintenance dosage regimen should not be altered by these factors alone. For example, the loading dose of digoxin in an elderly patient with congestive heart failure should be reduced because of the decreased apparent volume of distribution. The maintenance dose may have to be reduced because of reduced clearance of the drug.

C. Metabolism: The capacity of the liver to metabolize drugs does not appear to decline consistently with age for all drugs. Animal studies and some clinical studies have suggested that certain drugs are metabolized more slowly; some of these drugs are listed in Table 62–2. It would appear that the greatest changes are in phase I reactions, ie, those carried out by the microsomal mixed function oxidase system; there are much smaller changes in the ability of the liver to carry out conjugation (phase II) reactions

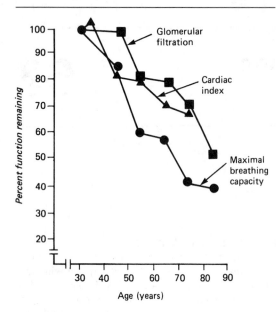

Figure 62–1. Effect of age on some physiologic functions. (Modified and reproduced, with permission, from Kohn RR: *Principles of Mammalian Aging.* Prentice-Hall, 1978.)

Table 62–2. Effects of age on hepatic clearance of some drugs. (1) Phase I metabolism by hepatic mixed function oxidase system; (2) phase II metabolism (conjugation) or phase I metabolism by nonmicrosomal systems.

Age-Related Decrease in Hepatic Clearance Found	No Age Difference Found
Alprazolam (1)	Ethanol (2)
Barbiturates (1)	Isoniazid (2)
Carbenoxolone (1)	Lidocaine (1)
Chlordiazepoxide (1)	Lorazepam (2)
Chlormethiazole (1)	Nitrazepam (2)
Clobazam (1)	Oxazepam (2)
Desmethyldiazepam (1)	Prazosin (1)
Diazepam (1)	Salicylate (2)
Flurazepam (1)	Warfarin (1)
Imipramine (1)	
Meperidine (1)	
Nortriptyline (1)	
Phenylbutazone (1)	
Propranolol (1)	
Quinidine, quinine (1)	
Theophylline (1)	
Tolbutamide (1)	

(Chapter 4). Some of these changes may be caused by decreased liver blood flow (Table 62–1), an important variable in the clearance of drugs that have a high hepatic extraction ratio. In addition, there is a decline with age of the liver's ability to recover from injury, eg, that caused by alcohol or viral hepatitis. Therefore, a history of recent liver disease in an older person should lead to caution in dosing with drugs that are cleared primarily by the liver, even after apparently complete recovery from the hepatic insult. Finally, diseases that affect hepatic function, eg, congestive heart failure, are more common in the elderly. Congestive heart failure may dramatically alter the ability of the liver to metabolize drugs and may also reduce hepatic blood flow. Similarly, severe nutritional deficiencies, which occur more often in old age, may impair hepatic function.

D. Elimination: Because the kidney is the major organ for clearance of drugs from the body, the "natural" decline of renal functional capacity referred to above is very important. As shown in Table 62–3, there is an age-related decline in creatinine clearance; this occurs in about two-thirds of the population. It is important to note that this decline is not reflected in an equivalent rise in serum creatinine because the production of creatinine is also reduced as muscle mass declines with age. The practical result of this change is marked prolongation of the half-life of many drugs (Figure 62–2) and the possibility of accumulation to toxic levels if dosage is not reduced in size or frequency. Dosing recommendations for the elderly often include an allowance for reduced renal

Table 62–1. Some changes related to aging that affect pharmacokinetics of drugs.[1]

Variable	Young Adults (20–30 years)	Geriatric Adults (60–80 years)
Body water (% of body weight)	61	53
Lean body mass (% of body weight)	19	12
Body fat (% of body weight)	26–33 (women) 18–20 (men)	38–45 (women) 36–38 (men)
Serum albumin (g/dL)	4.7	3.8
Kidney weight (% of young adult)	100	80
Hepatic blood flow (% of young adult)	100	55–60

[1]Compiled from various sources.

Table 62–3. Effects of age on creatinine clearance, serum concentration, and total body creatinine production.[1]

Age (years)	Creatinine Clearance (mL/min)[2]	Serum Creatinine Concentration (mg/dL)	Creatinine Production (mg/24 h)
17–24	140	0.81	1790
25–34	140	0.81	1862
35–44	133	0.81	1746
45–54	127	0.83	1689
55–64	120	0.84	1580
65–74	110	0.83	1409
75–84	97	0.84	1259

[1]Modified and reproduced, with permission, from Rowe JW et al: *J Gerontol* 1976;311:155.
[2]Normalized to 1.73 m^2 body surface area.

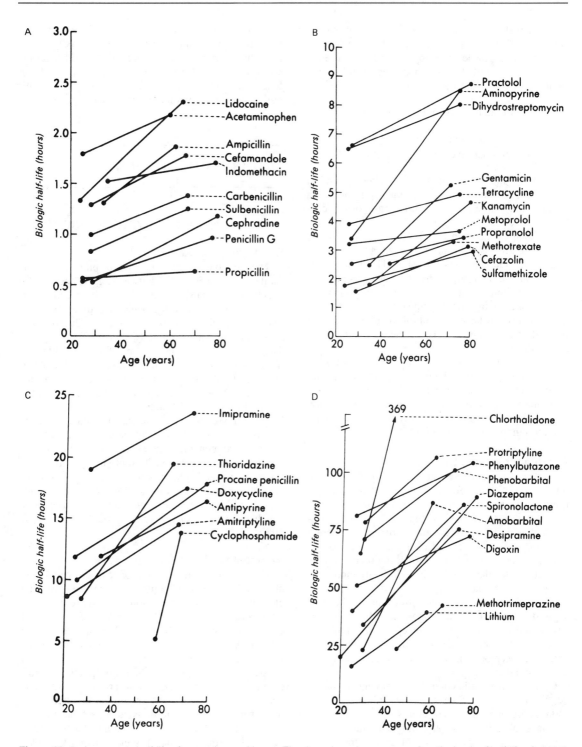

Figure 62–2. Increase in half-life of some drugs with age. The drugs have been grouped on the basis of half-life. **A:** 0.5–3 hours; **B:** 1–10 hours; **C:** 5–25 hours; **D:** 20–370 hours. Note that the lines merely connect the end points of the age range; they do not imply a linear relationship between age and half-life. (Modified and reproduced, with permission, from Ritschel WA: Pharmacokinetics in the aged. In: *Pharmacologic Aspects of Aging.* Pagliaro LA, Pagliaro AM [editors]. Mosby, 1983.)

clearance. If only the young adult dosage is known for a drug that requires renal clearance, a rough correction can be made by using the Cockcroft-Gault formula (Cockcroft, 1976), which is applicable to patients from age 40 through age 80:

Creatinine clearance (mL/min) =

$$\frac{(140 - age) \times (weight~in~kg)}{72 \times serum~creatinine~in~mg/dL}$$

For women, the result should be multiplied by 0.85. If the patient has normal renal function (up to one-third of patients), a dose corrected on the basis of this estimate will be too low—but a low dose is initially desirable if one is uncertain of the renal function in any patient. If a precise measure is needed, a standard 12- or 24-hour creatinine clearance should be done. As indicated above, nutritional changes alter pharmacokinetic parameters. A patient who is severely dehydrated (not uncommon in patients with stroke or other motor impairment) may have an additional marked reduction in renal drug clearance that is completely reversible by rehydration.

The lungs are important for the excretion of volatile drugs. As a result of reduced respiratory capacity (Figure 62–1) and the increased incidence of active pulmonary disease in the elderly, the use of inhalation anesthesia is less common and parenteral agents more common in this age group. (See Chapter 24.)

Pharmacodynamic Changes

It was long believed that geriatric patients were much more "sensitive" to the action of many drugs, implying a change in the pharmacodynamic interaction of the drugs with their receptors. It is now recognized that many—perhaps most—of these apparent changes result from altered pharmacokinetics or diminished homeostatic responses. Clinical studies have supported the idea that the elderly are more sensitive to *some* sedative-hypnotics and analgesics. In addition, there are some data from animal studies that suggest actual changes with age in the characteristics or numbers of certain types of receptors. The most extensive studies show a decrease in responsiveness to beta-adrenoceptor stimulants and blockers. Other examples are discussed below.

Certain homeostatic control mechanisms appear to be blunted in the elderly. Since homeostatic responses are often important components of the total response to a drug, these physiologic alterations may change the pattern or intensity of drug response. In the cardiovascular system, the cardiac output increment required by mild or moderate exercise is successfully provided to at least age 75 (in individuals without obvious cardiac disease), but the increase is the result primarily of increased stroke volume in the elderly and not tachycardia, as in young adults. Average blood pressure goes up with age (in most Western

countries), but the incidence of symptomatic orthostatic hypotension also increases markedly. Similarly, the average 2-hour postprandial blood sugar increases by about 1 mg/dL for each year of age above 50. Temperature regulation is also impaired, and hypothermia is poorly tolerated in the elderly.

MAJOR DRUG GROUPS

CENTRAL NERVOUS SYSTEM DRUGS

Sedative-Hypnotics

The half-lives of many benzodiazepines and barbiturates increase 50–150% between age 30 and age 70. Much of this change occurs during the decade from 60 to 70. For many of the benzodiazepines, both the parent molecule and its metabolites (produced in the liver) are pharmacologically active (Chapter 21). The age-related decline in renal function and liver disease, if present, both contribute to the reduction in elimination of these compounds. In addition, an increased volume of distribution has been reported for some of these drugs. Lorazepam and oxazepam may be less affected by these changes than the other benzodiazepines. In addition to these pharmacokinetic factors, it is generally believed that the elderly are more variable in their sensitivity to the sedative-hypnotic drugs on a pharmacodynamic basis as well. Among the toxicities of these drugs, ataxia and other aspects of motor impairment should be particularly watched for in order to avoid accidents (Ray, 1987, 1992).

Analgesics

The opioids (narcotic analgesics) show variable changes in pharmacokinetics with age. However, the elderly are often markedly more sensitive to the respiratory effects of these agents because of age-related changes in respiratory function. Therefore, this group of drugs should be used with caution until the sensitivity of the particular patient has been evaluated, and the patient should then be dosed appropriately for full effect. Studies show that opioids are consistently *underutilized* in patients who require strong analgesics for chronic painful conditions such as cancer (Portenoy, 1992). There is no justification for underutilization of these drugs, especially in the care of the elderly, and good pain management plans are readily available (Ashburn, 1993; Schug, 1992).

Antipsychotic & Antidepressant Drugs

The antipsychotic agents (phenothiazines and haloperidol) have been very heavily used (and probably misused) in the management of a variety of psychiatric diseases in the elderly. There is no doubt that they are useful in the management of schizophrenia in old age, and they are probably useful also in the treatment of symptoms associated with delirium or dementia, agitation and combativeness, and a paranoid syndrome that appears in some geriatric patients. However, they are not fully satisfactory in these geriatric conditions, and dosage should not be increased on the assumption that full control is possible. There is no evidence that these drugs have any beneficial effects in Alzheimer's dementia, and on theoretical grounds the antimuscarinic effects of the phenothiazines might be expected to worsen memory impairment and intellectual dysfunction (see below). Much of the apparent improvement in agitated and combative patients may simply reflect the sedative effects of the drugs. When a sedative antipsychotic is desired, a phenothiazine such as thioridazine is appropriate. If sedation is to be avoided, haloperidol is more appropriate. The latter drug has increased extrapyramidal toxicity, however, and should be avoided in patients with preexisting extrapyramidal disease. The phenothiazines, especially older drugs such as chlorpromazine, often induce orthostatic hypotension in young adults because of their alpha-adrenoceptor-blocking effects. They are even more prone to do so in the elderly. (See also Chapter 28.)

Because of increased responsiveness to all these drugs, dosage should usually be started at a fraction of that used in young adults. The half-lives of some phenothiazines are increased in the geriatric population (Figure 62–2). Thioridazine's half-life, for example, is more than doubled. Plasma protein binding of fluphenazine is reduced, which results in an increase of the free drug:total drug ratio.

Lithium is often used in the treatment of mania in the aged. Because it is cleared by the kidneys, doses must be adjusted appropriately. Concurrent use of thiazide diuretics reduces the clearance of lithium and should be accompanied by further reduction in dosage and more frequent measurement of lithium blood levels.

Psychiatric depression is thought to be underdiagnosed and undertreated in the elderly. The suicide rate in the over-65 age group (twice the national average) supports this view. Unfortunately, the apathy, flat affect, and social withdrawal of major depression may be mistaken for senile dementia. Limited evidence suggests that the elderly are as responsive to the antidepressants (both tricyclic agents and MAO inhibitors) as younger patients but are more sensitive to their toxic effects (Preskorn, 1993). This factor along with the reduced clearance of some of these drugs underlines the importance of careful dosing and strict attention to the appearance of toxic effects. If a tricyclic antidepressant is to be used, a drug with reduced antimuscarinic effects should be selected, eg, nortriptyline or desipramine (Table 29–2).

Drugs Used in Alzheimer's Disease

Alzheimer's disease is characterized by progressive impairment of memory and cognitive functions and may lead to a completely vegetative state. The biochemical defects responsible for these changes have not been identified, but there is much evidence for a marked decrease in choline acetyltransferase and other markers of cholinergic neuron activity and for decreases in brain dopamine, norepinephrine, serotonin, and somatostatin activity. Eventually, cholinergic and possibly other neurons die or are destroyed. Patients with Alzheimer's disease are often exquisitely sensitive to the central nervous system toxicities of drugs with antimuscarinic effects. Many methods of treatment of Alzheimer's disease have been explored (Gottlieb, 1993). Most attention has been focused on the cholinomimetic drugs because of the evidence for loss of cholinergic neurons noted above. MAO type B inhibition with selegiline (L-deprenyl) has been suggested to have some beneficial effects (Tariot, 1987). So-called cerebral vasodilators are ineffective (Thompson, 1990).

Tacrine (tetrahydroaminoacridine, THA), a long-acting cholinesterase inhibitor and muscarinic modulator, has been extensively studied (Freeman, 1991; Schneider, 1993). Tacrine is an orally active amine that enters the central nervous system readily and has a duration of effect of 6–8 hours. (In contrast, physostigmine has a duration of action of 1–2 hours.) Tacrine blocks both acetylcholinesterase and butyrylcholinesterase and has complex inhibitory effects on M_1 and M_2 cholinoceptors. It is also a weak nicotinic blocker. The drug apparently increases the release of acetylcholine from cholinergic nerve endings as well. Finally, tacrine may inhibit MAO, decrease the release of GABA, and increase the release of norepinephrine, dopamine, and serotonin from nerve endings. Other receptors (NMDA, adenosine) and potassium channels may also be affected at higher concentrations of tacrine. In spite of its extremely broad range of effects, attention has focused on tacrine's cholinergic actions and cholinomimetic analogues (eg, velnacrine) are currently under investigation. Tacrine causes cholinomimetic adverse effects, including nausea and vomiting, and significant hepatic toxicity. The latter is manifested by a reversible increase in serum AST or ALT levels of sufficient magnitude to require dose reduction or withdrawal in 40–50% of patients. Hepatocellular necrosis with jaundice has been reported (Schneider, 1993).

Although tacrine appeared to be effective in a very small initial double-blind clinical trial, it was no better than placebo in several subsequent larger double-blind trials. The largest double-blind trial to date showed a modest positive effect (Davis, 1992). Nevertheless, since better drugs are lacking, tacrine has been approved for use in the USA.

CARDIOVASCULAR DRUGS

Antihypertensive Drugs

As noted previously, blood pressure, especially systolic pressure, increases with age in Western countries and in most cultures in which salt intake is high. The increase is especially marked after age 50 in women. The high frequency and sometimes benign course of this form of late-onset systolic hypertension encourage a conservative approach to its treatment. On the other hand, diastolic hypertension and significant elevation of the systolic pressure above the age-corrected norm should be vigorously treated since they are associated with a marked increase in the incidence of stroke, congestive heart failure, and renal failure (Gifford, 1987), and because effective treatment has been clearly shown to reduce the incidence of these sequelae.

The basic principles of therapy are not different in the geriatric age group from those described in Chapter 11, but the usual cautions regarding altered pharmacokinetics and sensitivity apply. Because of its safety, nondrug therapy (weight reduction in the obese and salt restriction) should be encouraged. Thiazides are a reasonable first step in drug therapy. The hypokalemia, hyperglycemia, and hyperuricemia toxicities of these agents are more relevant in the elderly because of the higher incidence of arrhythmias, non-insulin-dependent diabetes, and gout in these patients. Thus, use of low antihypertensive doses, rather than maximum diuretic doses, is important. Calcium channel blockers are effective and safe if titrated to the appropriate response. They are especially useful if the patient also has atherosclerotic angina (Chapter 12). Beta-blockers are potentially hazardous in patients with obstructive airway disease and are considered less useful than calcium channel blockers in the older patient. For more severe hypertension, methyldopa and hydralazine have proved effective and safe. The most powerful drugs, such as guanethidine and minoxidil, are rarely needed.

Positive Inotropic Agents

Congestive heart failure is a common and particularly lethal disease in the elderly. Fear of this condition may be one reason why physicians overuse cardiac glycosides in this age group. In one study, 90% of a group of elderly patients who were withdrawn from digoxin therapy had no recurrence of symptoms or signs of failure, ie, the drug was being used unnecessarily. The toxic effects of this drug group are particularly dangerous in the geriatric population, since the elderly are more susceptible to arrhythmias. The clearance of digoxin appears to be decreased in the older age group, and while the volume of distribution is often decreased as well, the half-life of this drug may be increased by 50% or more. Because the drug is cleared by the kidneys, renal function must be considered in designing a dosage regimen. There is no

evidence that there is any increase in pharmacodynamic sensitivity to the therapeutic effects of the cardiac glycosides; in fact, animal studies suggest a possible decrease in therapeutic sensitivity. On the other hand, as noted above, there is probably an increase in sensitivity to the toxic arrhythmogenic actions. Hypokalemia, hypomagnesemia, hypoxemia (from pulmonary disease), and coronary atherosclerosis all contribute to the high incidence of digitalis-induced arrhythmias in geriatric patients. The less common toxicities of digitalis such as delirium, visual changes, and endocrine abnormalities (Chapter 13) also occur more often in the elderly than in younger patients.

Antiarrhythmic Agents

The treatment of arrhythmias in the elderly is particularly challenging because of the lack of good hemodynamic reserve, the frequency of electrolyte disturbances, and the high incidence of severe coronary disease. The clearances of quinidine and procainamide decrease and their half-lives increase with age. Disopyramide should probably be avoided in the geriatric population, because its major toxicities—antimuscarinic action, leading to voiding problems in men; and negative inotropic cardiac effects, leading to congestive heart failure—are particularly undesirable in these patients. The clearance of lidocaine appears to be little changed, but the half-life is increased in the elderly. Although this observation implies an increase in the volume of distribution, it has been recommended that the loading dose of this drug be reduced in geriatric patients because of their greater sensitivity to its toxic effects.

ANTIMICROBIAL DRUGS

Several age-related changes contribute to the high incidence of infections in geriatric patients. There appears to be a reduction in host defenses in the elderly; this is manifested in the increase in both serious infections and cancer. This may reflect an alteration in T lymphocyte function. In the case of the lungs, a major age- and tobacco-dependent decrease in mucociliary clearance significantly increases susceptibility to infection. In the urinary tract, the incidence of serious infection is greatly increased by urinary retention and catheterization in men. Since 1940, the antimicrobial drugs have contributed more to the prolongation of life than any other drug group, because they can compensate to some extent for this deterioration in natural defenses.

The basic principles of therapy of the elderly with these agents are no different from those applicable in younger patients and have been presented in Chapter 52. The major pharmacokinetic changes relate to decreased renal function; because most of the beta-lactam, aminoglycoside, and fluoroquinolone antibiotics are excreted by this route, important changes in half-life may be expected. This is particularly important in the case of the aminoglycosides, because they cause concentration-dependent toxicity in the kidney and in other organs. For gentamicin, kanamycin, and netilmicin, the half-lives are more than doubled. According to one study, the increase may not be so marked for tobramycin.

ANTI-INFLAMMATORY DRUGS

Osteoarthritis is a very common disease of the elderly. Rheumatoid arthritis is less exclusively a geriatric problem, but the same drug therapy is usually applicable. The basic principles laid down in Chapter 35 and the properties of the anti-inflammatory drugs described there apply fully here.

The nonsteroidal anti-inflammatory agents must be used with special care in the geriatric patient because they cause toxicities to which the elderly are very susceptible. In the case of aspirin, the most important of these is gastrointestinal irritation and bleeding. In the case of the newer NSAIDs, the most important is renal damage, which may be irreversible. Because they are cleared primarily by the kidneys, these drugs will accumulate more rapidly in the geriatric patient and especially in the patient whose renal function is already compromised beyond the average range for his or her age. A vicious cycle is easily set up in which cumulation of the NSAID causes more renal damage, which causes more cumulation, and so on. Benoxaprofen, a very efficacious NSAID, was withdrawn shortly after it was released because several elderly patients died in renal failure as a result of improper dosing. Elderly patients receiving high doses of any NSAID should be carefully monitored for changes in renal function.

Corticosteroids are extremely useful in elderly patients who cannot tolerate full doses of NSAIDs. However, they consistently cause a dose- and duration-related osteoporosis, an especially hazardous toxic effect in the elderly. It is not certain whether this drug-induced effect can be reduced by increased calcium and vitamin D intake, but it would seem prudent to use these agents and to encourage frequent exercise in any patient taking corticosteroids.

ADVERSE DRUG REACTIONS IN THE ELDERLY

The positive relationship between number of drugs taken and the incidence of adverse reactions to them has been well documented. In long-term care facilities, which have a high population of the elderly, the average number of prescriptions per patient varies between 6.6 and 7.7. Studies have shown that the percentage of patients with adverse reactions increases from about 10% when a single drug is being taken to nearly 100% when ten drugs are taken. Thus, it may be expected that about half of patients in long-term care facilities will have recognized or unrecognized reactions at some time. The overall incidence of drug reactions in geriatric patients is estimated to be at least twice that in the younger population. Reasons for this high incidence undoubtedly include errors in prescribing on the part of the practitioner and errors in drug usage by the patient.

Practitioner errors sometimes occur because the physician does not appreciate the importance of changes in pharmacokinetics with age and age-related diseases. Some errors occur because the practitioner is unaware of incompatible drugs prescribed by other practitioners for the same patient. For example, cimetidine, a drug heavily prescribed to the elderly, has a much higher incidence of untoward effects (eg, confusion, slurred speech) in the geriatric population than in younger patients. It also inhibits the hepatic metabolism of many drugs, including phenytoin, warfarin, beta-blockers, and other agents. A patient who has been taking one of the latter agents without ill effect may develop markedly elevated blood levels and severe toxicity if cimetidine is added to the regimen without adjustment of dosage of the other drugs. Additional examples of drugs that inhibit liver microsomal enzymes and lead to adverse reactions are described in Appendix II.

Patient errors may result from noncompliance for reasons described below. In addition, they often result from use of nonprescription drugs that are taken without the knowledge of the physician. As noted in Chapter 65, many OTC agents contain "hidden ingredients" with potent pharmacologic effects. For example, many antihistamines have significant sedative effects and are inherently more hazardous in patients with impaired cognitive function. Similarly, their antimuscarinic action may precipitate urinary retention in the geriatric male or glaucoma in a patient with a narrow anterior chamber. If the patient is also taking a metabolism inhibitor such as cimetidine, the probability of an adverse reaction is greatly increased.

PRACTICAL ASPECTS OF GERIATRIC PHARMACOLOGY

The quality of life in elderly patients can be greatly improved and life can be prolonged by the intelligent use of drugs. However, there are several practical obstacles to compliance that the prescriber must recognize.

The expense of drugs can be a major disincentive in patients receiving marginal retirement incomes who are not covered by health insurance. The prescriber must be aware of the cost of the prescription and of cheaper alternative therapies. For example, the monthly cost of arthritis therapy with newer NSAIDs exceeds $75, while that for generic aspirin is about $2 and for ibuprofen, an older NSAID, about $15.

Noncompliance may result from forgetfulness or confusion, especially if the patient has several prescriptions and different dosing intervals. Surveys show that in 1986 the population over 65 years of age accounted for 25% of physician visits and 32% of drugs prescribed in the USA although they represented only 11–12% of the population (Food and Drug Administration, 1989). Since the prescriptions are often written by several different practitioners, there is usually no attempt to design "integrated" regimens that use drugs with similar dosing intervals for the conditions being treated. Patients may forget instructions regarding the need to complete a fixed duration of therapy when a course of treatment is being given, eg, for an infection. The disappearance of symptoms is often regarded as the best reason to halt drug taking, especially if the prescription was expensive.

Noncompliance may also be deliberate. A decision not to take a drug may be based on prior experience with it. There may be excellent reasons for such "intelligent" noncompliance, and the practitioner should try to elicit them. Such efforts may also improve compliance with alternative drugs, because enlisting the patient as a participant in therapeutic decisions tends to increase motivation to succeed.

Some errors in drug taking are caused by physical disabilities. Arthritis, tremor, and visual problems may all contribute. Liquid medications that are to be measured out "by the spoonful" are especially inappropriate for patients with any type of tremor or motor disability. "Childproof" containers are often "patient-proof" if the patient has arthritis. Cataracts and macular degeneration occur in a large number of patients over 70; therefore, labels on prescription bottles should be large enough for the patient with diminished vision to read, or color-coded if the patient can see but can no longer read.

Drug therapy has considerable potential for both helpful and harmful effects in the geriatric patient. The balance may be tipped in the right direction by adherence to a few principles:

(1) Take a careful drug history. The disease to be treated may be drug-induced, or drugs being taken may lead to interactions with drugs to be prescribed.

(2) Prescribe only for a specific and rational indication. Do not prescribe cimetidine for "dyspepsia."

(3) Define the goal of drug therapy. Then start with small doses and titrate to the response desired. Wait at least three geriatric half-lives before increasing the dose. If the expected response does not occur at the normal adult dosage, check blood levels. If the expected response does not occur at the appropriate blood level, one should switch to a different drug.

(4) Maintain a high index of suspicion regarding drug reactions and interactions. Know what other drugs the patient is taking.

(5) Simplify the regimen as much as possible. When multiple drugs are prescribed, try to use drugs that can be taken at the same time of day. Whenever possible, reduce the number of drugs being taken.

REFERENCES

Abrams WB: Cardiovascular drugs in the elderly. Chest 1990;98:980.

Ashburn MA, Lipman AG: Management of pain in the cancer patient. Anesth Analg 1993;76:402.

Avorn J et al: Use of psychoactive medication and the quality of care in rest homes: Findings and policy implications of a statewide study. N Engl J Med 1989;320:227.

Avorn J et al: A randomized trial of a program to reduce the use of psychoactive drugs in nursing homes. N Engl J Med 1992;327:168.

Bellamy N: Treatment considerations in the elderly rheumatic patient. Gerontology 1988;34(Suppl 1):16.

Birnbaum LS: Pharmacokinetic basis of age-related changes in sensitivity to toxicants. Annu Rev Pharmacol Toxicol 1991;31:101.

Blazer D: Depression in the elderly. N Engl J Med 1989; 320:164.

Carlsson A: Brain neurotransmitters in aging and dementia: Similar changes across diagnostic dementia groups. Gerontology 1987;33:159.

CDC: Hospitalizations for the leading causes of death among the elderly: United States, 1987. MMWR 1990; 39:777.

Chatellier G, Lacomblez L, Groupe Français d'Étude de la Tetrahydroaminoacridine: Tacrine (tetrahydroaminoacridine; THA) and lecithin in senile dementia of the Alzheimer type: A multicentre trial. Br Med J 1990;300:495.

Cockcroft DW, Gault MH: Prediction of creatinine clearance from serum creatinine. Nephron 1976;16:31.

Cody RJ: Physiologic changes due to age: Implications for drug therapy of congestive heart failure. Drugs Aging 1993;3:320.

Davis KL et al: A double-blind, placebo-controlled multicenter study of tacrine for Alzheimer's disease. N Engl J Med 1992;327:1253.

Dean BS, Krenzelok EP: Poisoning in the elderly: An increasing problem for health care providers. J Toxicol Clin Toxicol 1987;25:411.

Eisen SA et al: The effect of prescribed daily dose frequency on patient medication compliance. Arch Intern Med 1990:150:1881.

Food and Drug Administration: *Drug Utilization in the United States 1988: Tenth Annual Review.* Office of Epidemiology and Biostatistics, 1989.

Freeman SE, Dawson RM: Tacrine: A pharmacological review. Prog Neurobiol 1991;36:257.

Gauthier S et al: Tetrahydroaminoacridine-lecithin combination treatment in patients with intermediate-stage Alzheimer's disease. N Engl J Med 1990;322:1272.

Gifford RW Jr: Myths about hypertension in the elderly. Med Clin North Am 1987;71:1003.

Gottlieb GL, Kumar A: Conventional pharmacologic treatment for patients with Alzheimer's disease. Neurology 1993;43(Suppl 4):S56.

Greenblatt DJ: Disposition of cardiovascular drugs in the elderly. Med Clin North Am 1989;73:487.

Greenblatt DJ, Shader RI, Harmatz JS: Implications of altered drug disposition in the elderly: Studies of benzodiazepines. J Clin Pharmacol 1989;29:866.

Gurwitz JH, Avorn J: The ambiguous relationship between aging and adverse drug reactions. Ann Intern Med 1991; 114:956.

Hayflick L: Theories of biological aging. Exp Gerontol 1985;20:145.

Hyams DE: The elderly patient: A special case for diuretic therapy. Drugs 1986;31(Suppl 4):138.

Katzman R: Alzheimer's disease. N Engl J Med 1986; 314:964.

Kohn RR: *Principles of Mammalian Aging.* Prentice-Hall, 1978.

Lebel M, Bergeron MG: Pharmacokinetics in the elderly. Studies on ciprofloxacin. Am J Med 1987;82(Suppl 4A): 108.

Lindeman RD, Tobin J, Shock NW: Longitudinal studies on the rate of decline in renal function with age. J Am Geriatr Soc 1985;33:278.

Lipowski ZJ: Delirium in the elderly patient. N Engl J Med 1989;320:578.

Loi CM, Vestal RE: Drug metabolism in the elderly. Pharmacol Ther 1988;36:131.

Massoro EJ: Biology of aging: Facts, thoughts, and experimental approaches. Lab Invest 1991;65:500.

Materson BJ et al: Treatment of hypertension in the elderly: I. Blood pressure and clinical changes. Results of a Department of Veterans Affairs Cooperative Study. Hypertension 1990;15:348.

Meyers BR, Wilkinson P: Clinical pharmacology of antibacterial drugs in the elderly. Implications for selection and dosage. Clin Pharmacokinet 1989;17:385.

Montamat SC, Cusack BJ, Vestal RE: Management of drug therapy in the elderly. N Engl J Med 1989;321:303.

Pan HY et al: Decline in beta-adrenergic receptor-mediated vascular relaxation with aging in man. J Pharmacol Exp Ther 1986;239:802.

Portenoy RK et al: Pain in ambulatory patients with lung or colon cancer: Prevalence, characteristics and impact. Cancer 1992;70:1616.

Preskorn SH: Recent advances in antidepressant therapy for the elderly. Am J Med 1993;95(Suppl 5):2S.

Prinz PN et al: Geriatrics: Sleep disorders and aging. N Engl J Med 1990;323:520.

Ray WA et al: Psychotropic drug use and the risk of hip fracture. N Engl J Med 1987;316:363.

Ray WA: Psychotropic drugs and injuries among the elderly: A review. J Clin Psychopharmacol 1992;12:386.

Roberts J, Tumer N: Age and diet effects on drug action. Pharmacol Ther 1988;37:111.

Rowe JW: Health care of the elderly. N Engl J Med 1985; 312:827.

Rowe JW, Besdine RW: Approach to the elderly patient: Physiologic and clinical considerations. In: *Drug Treatment in the Elderly.* Vestal RE (editor). ADIS Health Science Press, 1984.

Salzman C: Geriatric psychopharmacology. Annu Rev Med 1985;36:217.

Schmucker DL: Aging and drug disposition: An update. Pharmacol Rev 1985;37:133.

Schneider LS: Clinical pharmacology of aminoacrines in Alzheimer's disease. Neurology 1993;43(Suppl 4):S64.

Schug SA, Dunlap R, Zech D: Pharmacologic management of cancer pain. Drugs 1992;43:44.

Schwartz JB, Abernethy DR: Cardiac drugs: Adjusting their use in aging patients. Geriatrics 1987;42:31.

Sunderland T et al: Anticholinergic sensitivity in patients with dementia of the Alzheimer type and age-matched controls: A dose-response study. Arch Gen Psychiat 1987;44:418.

Tariot PN et al: L-Deprenyl in Alzheimer's disease. Arch Gen Psychiatry 1987;44:427.

Thompson TL II, Moran MG, Nies AS: Psychotropic drug use in the elderly. (2 parts.) N Engl J Med 1983;308:134, 194.

Thompson TL II et al: Lack of efficacy of hydergine in patients with Alzheimer's disease. N Engl J Med 1990;323: 445.

Tonkin A, Wing L: Aging and susceptibility to drug-induced orthostatic hypotension. Clin Pharmacol Ther 1992;52:277.

Tsujimoto G, Hashimoto K, Hoffman BB: Pharmacokinetic and pharmacodynamic principles of drug therapy in old age. (Two parts.) Int J Clin Pharmacol Therap Toxicol 1989;27:13, 102.

Tumer N, Scarpace PJ, Lowenthal DT: Geriatric pharmacology: Basic and clinical considerations. Annu Rev Pharmacol Toxicol 1992;32:271.

Vestal RE (editor): *Drug Treatment in the Elderly.* ADIS Health Science Press, 1984.

Vestal RE: Wood AJJ, Shand DG: Reduced β-adrenoceptor sensitivity in the elderly. Clin Pharmacol Ther 1979;26: 181.

Whalley LJ: Drug treatments of dementia. Br J Psychiatry 1989;155:595.

63

Dermatologic Pharmacology*

Dirk B. Robertson, MD, & Howard I. Maibach, MD

The skin offers a number of special problems and opportunities to the therapist. Topical therapy is especially appropriate for diseases of the skin, although some dermatologic diseases respond as well or better to drugs administered systemically.

The general pharmacokinetic principles governing the use of drugs applied to the skin are the same as those involved in other routes of drug administration (Chapters 1 and 3). However, human skin, though often depicted as a simple three-layered structure, is a complex series of diffusion barriers. Quantitation of the flux of drugs and drug vehicles through these barriers is the basis of pharmacokinetic analysis of dermatologic therapy; techniques for making such measurements are rapidly increasing in number and sensitivity.

Major variables that determine pharmacologic response to drugs applied to the skin include the following:

(1) Regional variation in drug penetration: For example, the scrotum, face, axilla, and scalp are far more permeable than the forearm and may require less drug for equivalent effect.

(2) Concentration gradient: Increasing the concentration gradient increases the mass of drug transferred per unit time, just as in the case of diffusion across other barriers (Chapter 1). Thus, resistance to topical corticosteroids can sometimes be overcome by use of higher concentrations of drug.

(3) Dosing schedule: Because of its physical properties, the skin acts as a reservoir for many drugs. As a result, the "local half-life" may be long enough to permit once-daily application of drugs with short systemic half-lives. For example, once-daily application of corticosteroids appears to be just as effective as multiple applications in many conditions.

(4) Vehicles and occlusion: An appropriate vehicle maximizes the ability of the drug to penetrate the outer layers of the skin. In addition, through their physical properties (moistening or drying effects), vehicles may themselves have important therapeutic effects.

Occlusion (application of a plastic wrap to hold the drug and its vehicle in close contact with the skin) is extremely effective in maximizing absorption of many drugs.

DERMATOLOGIC VEHICLES

Topical medications usually consist of active ingredients incorporated in a vehicle that facilitates cutaneous application. Important considerations in selection of a vehicle include the solubility of the active agent in the vehicle; the rate of release of the agent from the vehicle; the ability of the vehicle to hydrate the stratum corneum, thus enhancing penetration; the stability of the therapeutic agent in the vehicle; and interactions, chemical and physical, of the vehicle, stratum corneum, and active agent. Vehicles have traditionally been considered pharmacologically inert; however, owing to their unique physical properties, many are therapeutically beneficial themselves.

Depending upon the vehicle, dermatologic formulations may be classified as tinctures, wet dressings, lotions, gels, aerosols, powders, pastes, creams, and ointments. The ability of the vehicle to retard evaporation from the surface of the skin increases in this series, being least in tinctures and wet dressings and greatest in ointments. In general, acute inflammation with oozing, vesiculation, and crusting is best treated with drying preparations such as tinctures, wet dressings, and lotions, while chronic inflammation with xerosis, scaling, and lichenification is best treated with more lubricating preparations such as creams and ointments. Tinctures, lotions, gels, and aerosols are convenient for application to the scalp and hairy

---

*Because of the large number and great diversity of dermatologic preparations, the most important formulations are described throughout this chapter rather than in a separate preparations section.

areas. Emulsified vanishing type creams may be used in intertriginous areas without causing maceration.

Emulsifying agents are used to provide homogeneous, stable preparations when mixtures of immiscible liquids such as oil-in-water creams are compounded. Some patients develop irritation from these agents. Substituting a preparation that does not contain them or using one containing a lower concentration may resolve the problem.

ANTIBACTERIAL AGENTS

TOPICAL ANTIBACTERIAL PREPARATIONS

Topical antibacterial agents may be useful in preventing infections in clean wounds, in the early treatment of infected dermatoses and wounds, in reducing colonization of the nares by staphylococci, in axillary deodorization, and in the management of acne vulgaris. The efficacy of antibiotics in these topical applications is not uniform. The general pharmacology of the antimicrobial drugs is discussed in Chapters 42–52.

Numerous topical anti-infectives contain corticosteroids in addition to antibiotics. There is no convincing evidence that topical corticosteroids inhibit the antibacterial effect of antibiotics when the two are incorporated in the same preparation. In the treatment of secondarily infected dermatoses, which are usually colonized with streptococci, staphylococci, or both, combination therapy may prove superior to corticosteroid therapy alone. Antibiotic-corticosteroid combinations may be useful in treating diaper dermatitis, otitis externa, and impetiginized eczema.

The selection of a particular antibiotic depends of course upon the diagnosis and, whenever possible, in vitro culture and sensitivity studies of clinical samples. The pathogens isolated from most infected dermatoses are group A beta-hemolytic streptococci, *Staphylococcus aureus,* or both. The pathogens present in surgical wounds will be those resident in the environment. Information about regional epidemiologic data and the prevailing patterns of drug resistance is therefore important in selecting a therapeutic agent. Prepackaged topical antibacterial preparations that contain multiple antibiotics are available in fixed dosages well above the therapeutic threshold. These formulations offer the advantages of efficacy in mixed infections, broader coverage for infections due to undetermined pathogens, and delayed microbial resistance to any single component antibiotic.

1. BACITRACIN & GRAMICIDIN

Bacitracin and gramicidin are polypeptide antibiotics, active against gram-positive organisms such as streptococci, pneumococci, and staphylococci. In addition, most anaerobic cocci, neisseria, tetanus bacilli, and diphtheria bacilli are sensitive. Bacitracin is compounded in an ointment base alone or in combination with neomycin, polymyxin B, or both. The use of bacitracin in the anterior nares temporarily decreases colonization by pathogenic staphylococci. Microbial resistance may develop following prolonged use. Bacitracin-induced contact urticaria syndrome occurs rarely. Allergic contact dermatitis occurs more frequently. Bacitracin is poorly absorbed through the skin, so systemic toxicity is rare.

Gramicidin is available only for topical use, in combination with other antibiotics such as neomycin, polymyxin, bacitracin, and nystatin. Systemic toxicity limits this drug to topical use. The incidence of sensitization following topical application is exceedingly low in therapeutic concentrations.

2. MUPIROCIN

Mupirocin (pseudomonic acid A) is structurally unrelated to other currently available topical antibacterial agents. Most gram-positive aerobic bacteria, including methicillin-resistant *S aureus,* are sensitive to mupirocin. It has been demonstrated to be effective in the treatment of impetigo caused by *S aureus* and group A beta-hemolytic streptococci. Intranasal use for temporarily eliminating nasal carriage of *S aureus* may be associated with irritation of mucous membranes caused by the polyethylene glycol vehicle. Mupirocin is not appreciably absorbed systemically after topical application to intact skin.

3. POLYMYXIN B SULFATE

Polymyxin B is a polypeptide antibiotic effective against gram-negative organisms, including *Pseudomonas aeruginosa, Escherichia coli, Enterobacter,* and *Klebsiella.* Most strains of *Proteus* and *Serratia* are resistant, as are all gram-positive organisms. Topical preparations may be compounded in either a solution or ointment base. Numerous prepackaged antibiotic combinations containing polymyxin B are available. Detectable serum concentrations are difficult to achieve from topical application, but the total daily dose applied to denuded skin or open wounds should not exceed 200 mg in order to reduce the likelihood of neurotoxicity and nephrotoxicity. Hypersensitivity to topically applied polymyxin B sulfate is uncommon.

4. NEOMYCIN & GENTAMICIN

Neomycin and gentamicin are aminoglycoside antibiotics active against gram-negative organisms, including *E coli, Proteus, Klebsiella,* and *Enterobacter.* Gentamicin generally shows greater activity against *P aeruginosa* than neomycin. Gentamicin is also more active against staphylococci and group A beta-hemolytic streptococci. Widespread topical use of gentamicin, especially in a hospital environment, should be avoided to slow the appearance of gentamicin-resistant organisms.

Neomycin is available in numerous topical formulations, both alone and in combination with polymyxin, bacitracin, and other antibiotics. It is also available as a sterile powder for topical use. Gentamicin is available as an ointment or cream.

Topical application of neomycin rarely results in detectable serum concentrations. However, in the case of gentamicin, serum concentrations of 1–18 μg/mL are possible if the drug is applied in a water-miscible preparation to large areas of denuded skin, as in burned patients. Both drugs are water-soluble and are excreted primarily in the urine. Renal failure may permit the accumulation of these antibiotics, with possible nephrotoxicity, neurotoxicity, and ototoxicity.

Neomycin frequently causes sensitization, particularly if applied to eczematous dermatoses or if compounded in an ointment vehicle. When sensitization occurs, cross-sensitivity to streptomycin, kanamycin, paromomycin, and gentamicin is possible.

5. TOPICAL ANTIBIOTICS IN ACNE

Several parenteral antibiotics that have traditionally been used in the treatment of acne vulgaris have been shown to be effective when applied topically. Currently, four antibiotics are so utilized: clindamycin phosphate, erythromycin base, metronidazole, and tetracycline hydrochloride. The effectiveness of topical therapy is less than that achieved by systemic administration of the same antibiotic. Therefore, topical therapy is generally suitable in mild to moderate cases of inflammatory acne.

Clindamycin

Clindamycin has in vitro activity against *Propionibacterium (Corynebacterium) acnes:* this has been postulated as the mechanism of its beneficial effect in acne therapy. Approximately 10% of an applied dose is absorbed, and rare cases of bloody diarrhea and pseudomembranous colitis have been reported following topical application. The hydroalcoholic vehicle may cause drying and irritation of the skin, with complaints of burning and stinging. The water-based gel vehicle is well tolerated and less likely to cause dehydration and irritation. Allergic contact dermatitis is uncommon.

Erythromycin

In topical preparations, the base of erythromycin rather than a salt is used to facilitate penetration. Although the mechanism of action of topical erythromycin in inflammatory acne vulgaris is unknown, it is presumed to be due to its inhibitory effects on *P acnes.* One of the possible complications of topical therapy is the development of antibiotic-resistant strains of organisms, including staphylococci. If this occurs in association with a clinical infection, topical erythromycin should be discontinued and appropriate systemic antibiotic therapy started. Adverse local reactions may include a burning sensation at the time of application and drying and irritation of the skin. Allergic hypersensitivity appears to be uncommon. Erythromycin is also available in a fixed combination preparation with benzoyl peroxide (Benzamycin) for topical treatment of acne vulgaris.

Metronidazole

Topical metronidazole gel is effective in the treatment of acne rosacea. The mechanism of action is unknown, but it may relate to the inhibitory effects of metronidazole on *Demodex brevis.* Oral metronidazole had been shown to be a carcinogen in susceptible rodent species, and topical use during pregnancy and by nursing mothers and children is therefore not recommended. Adverse local effects include dryness, burning, and stinging.

Tetracycline

Two topical tetracycline antibiotics are currently available for topical treatment of acne vulgaris: (1) tetracycline hydrochloride in a hydroalcoholic base containing *n*-decyl methyl sulfoxide and (2) meclocycline sulfosalicylate in a cream base. Serum levels of tetracycline obtained from continued twice-daily topical use of hydroalcoholic preparations are 0.1 μg/mL or less, and no demonstrable absorption has been reported following extensive twice-daily topical application of the meclocycline sulfosalicylate preparation over 4 weeks.

The beneficial effect of these preparations on acne vulgaris has been attributed to their inhibitory action on *P acnes.* Their use is associated with temporary yellow staining of the skin, which is most noticeable in fair-skinned individuals. Although photosensitivity has not been a problem, this hazard should be considered when using these potentially phototoxic antibiotics. As with all tetracycline derivatives, these agents should not be used in patients who are pregnant or have a history of significant renal or hepatic dysfunction.

ANTIFUNGAL AGENTS

The treatment of superficial fungal infections caused by dermatophytic fungi may be accomplished (1) with topical antifungal agents, eg, clotrimazole, miconazole, econazole, ketoconazole, naftifine, tolnaftate, and haloprogin; or (2) with orally administered agents, eg, griseofulvin and ketoconazole. Superficial infections caused by *Candida* sp may be treated with topical applications of clotrimazole, miconazole, econazole, ketoconazole, nystatin, or amphotericin B. Chronic generalized mucocutaneous candidiasis is responsive to long-term therapy with oral ketoconazole.

TOPICAL ANTIFUNGAL PREPARATIONS

1. TOPICAL AZOLE DERIVATIVES

The imidazoles, which currently include clotrimazole, econazole, ketoconazole, miconazole, oxiconazole, and sulconazole, have a wide range of activity against dermatophytes (*Epidermophyton, Microsporum,* and *Trichophyton*) and yeasts, including *Candida albicans* and *Pityrosporum orbiculare,* the cause of tinea versicolor.

Miconazole (Monistat, Micatin) is available for topical application as a cream or lotion and as vaginal cream or suppositories for use in vulvovaginal candidiasis. Clotrimazole (Lotrimin, Mycelex) is available for topical application to the skin as a cream or lotion and as vaginal cream and tablets for use in vulvovaginal candidiasis. Econazole (Spectazole) is available as a cream for topical application. Oxiconazole (Oxistat) is available as a cream and lotion for topical use. Ketoconazole (Nizoral) is available as a cream for topical treatment of dermatophytosis and candidiasis and as a shampoo for the treatment of seborrheic dermatitis. Sulconazole (Exelderm) is available as a solution. Topical antifungal-corticosteroid fixed combinations have recently been introduced on the basis of providing more rapid symptomatic improvement than an antifungal agent alone. Clotrimazole-betamethasone dipropionate cream (Lotrisone) is one such example.

Once- or twice-daily application to the affected area will generally result in clearing of superficial dermatophyte infections in 2–3 weeks, although the medication should be continued until eradication of the organism is confirmed. Paronychial and intertriginous candidiasis can be treated effectively by any of these agents when applied three or four times daily. Seborrheic dermatitis should be treated with twice-daily applications of ketoconazole until clinical clearing is obtained.

Adverse local reactions to the imidazoles may include stinging, pruritus, erythema, and local irritation. Allergic contact dermatitis appears to be uncommon.

2. CICLOPIROX OLAMINE

Ciclopirox olamine is a synthetic broad-spectrum antimycotic agent with inhibitory activity against dermatophytes, *Candida* species, and *P orbiculare.* This agent appears to inhibit the uptake of precursors of macromolecular synthesis; the site of action is probably the cell membrane.

Pharmacokinetic studies indicate that 1–2% of the dose is absorbed when applied as a solution on the back under an occlusive dressing. Ciclopirox olamine is available as a 1% cream (Loprox) for the topical treatment of dermatomycosis, candidiasis, and tinea versicolor. The incidence of adverse reactions has been low. Pruritus and worsening of clinical disease have been reported. The potential for delayed allergic contact hypersensitivity appears small.

3. NAFTIFINE

Naftifine hydrochloride is an allylamine that is highly active against dermatophytes but less active against yeasts. The antifungal activity derives from selective inhibition of squalene epoxidase, a key enzyme for the synthesis of ergosterol.

Naftifine (Naftin) is available as a 1% cream for the topical treatment of dermatophytosis, to be applied on a twice-daily dosing schedule. Adverse reactions include local irritation, burning sensation, and erythema. Contact with mucous membranes should be avoided.

4. TERBINAFINE

Terbinafine (Lasmisil) is an *n*-allylamine with activity similar to that of naftifine hydrochloride. It will be available as a 1% cream for the topical treatment of dermatophyte infections. Reported adverse reactions include local irritation with erythema, dryness, and stinging. Contact with eyes and mucous membranes should be avoided.

5. TOLNAFTATE

Tolnaftate is a synthetic antifungal compound that is effective topically against dermatophyte infections caused by *Epidermophyton, Microsporum,* and

Trichophyton. It is also active against *P orbiculare* but not against *Candida.*

Tolnaftate (Aftate, Tinactin) is available as a cream, solution, powder, or powder aerosol for application twice daily to infected areas. Recurrences following cessation of therapy are common, and infections of the palms, soles, and nails are usually unresponsive to tolnaftate alone. The powder or powder aerosol may be used chronically following initial treatment in patients susceptible to tinea infections. Tolnaftate is generally well tolerated and rarely causes irritation or allergic contact sensitization.

6. HALOPROGIN

Haloprogin is a synthetic halogenated phenolic ether, active against *Epidermophyton, Microsporum,* and *Trichophyton* as well as *P orbiculare.* Although this compound does exhibit in vitro activity against *Candida,* its use is generally restricted to the treatment of dermatophyte infections and tinea versicolor.

Haloprogin (Halotex) is available as cream or solution. There is only slight penetration of intact skin, and systemic toxicity following topical application has not been observed. The small amounts of drug that are absorbed are converted to trichlorophenol, which is excreted predominantly in the urine. Twice-daily application to the affected area usually results in clearing in 2–3 weeks. Infections of the palms, soles, and nails are generally resistant to topical therapy. Adverse reactions include local irritation, burning sensations, vesiculation, increased maceration, and exacerbation of the preexisting lesion. Contact with the eyes must be avoided. Allergic contact hypersensitivity is uncommon.

7. NYSTATIN & AMPHOTERICIN B

Nystatin and amphotericin B are useful in the topical therapy of *C albicans* infections but ineffective against dermatophytes. Nystatin is limited to topical treatment of cutaneous and mucosal *Candida* infections because of its narrow spectrum and negligible absorption from the gastrointestinal tract following oral administration. Amphotericin B has a broader antifungal spectrum and is used intravenously in the treatment of many systemic mycoses (Chapter 48) and to a lesser extent in the treatment of cutaneous *Candida* infections.

The recommended dosage for topical preparations of nystatin in treating paronychial and intertriginous candidiasis is application two or three times a day. Oral candidiasis (thrush) is treated by holding 5 mL (infants, 2 mL) of nystatin oral suspension in the mouth for several minutes four times daily before swallowing. An alternative therapy for thrush is to retain a vaginal tablet in the mouth until dissolved four times daily. Recurrent or recalcitrant perianal, vaginal, vulvar, and diaper area candidiasis may respond to oral nystatin, 0.5–1 million units in adults (100,000 units in children) four times daily in addition to local therapy. Vulvovaginal candidiasis may be treated by insertion of 1 vaginal tablet twice daily for 14 days, then nightly for an additional 14–21 days.

Amphotericin B (Fungizone) is available for topical use in cream, ointment, and lotion form. The recommended dosage in the treatment of paronychial and intertriginous candidiasis is application two to four times daily to the affected area.

Adverse effects associated with oral administration of nystatin include mild nausea, diarrhea, and occasional vomiting. Topical application is nonirritating, and allergic contact hypersensitivity is exceedingly uncommon. Topical amphotericin B is well tolerated and only occasionally locally irritating. Hypersensitivity is exceedingly rare. The drug may cause a temporary yellow staining of the skin, especially when the cream vehicle is used.

ORAL ANTIFUNGAL AGENTS

1. GRISEOFULVIN

Griseofulvin is effective orally against dermatophyte infections caused by *Epidermophyton, Microsporum,* and *Trichophyton.* It is ineffective against *Candida* and *P orbiculare.*

Griseofulvin's antifungal activity has been attributed to inhibition of hyphal cell wall synthesis, effects on nucleic acid synthesis, and inhibition of mitosis. Griseofulvin interferes with microtubules of the mitotic spindle and with cytoplasmic microtubules. The destruction of cytoplasmic microtubules may result in impaired processing of newly synthesized cell wall constituents at the growing tips of hyphae. Griseofulvin is active only against growing cells.

Following the oral administration of 1 g of micronized griseofulvin, peak serum levels of 1.5–2 µg/mL are obtained in 4–8 hours. The drug can be detected in the stratum corneum 4–8 hours following oral administration, with the highest concentration in the outermost layers and the lowest in the base. Reducing the particle size of the medication greatly increases absorption of the drug. Formulations which contain the smallest particle size are labeled "ultramicronized." Ultramicronized griseofulvin achieves bioequivalent plasma levels with half the dose of micronized drug. In addition, solubilizing griseofulvin in polyethylene glycol enhances absorption even further. Micronized griseofulvin is available as 250 mg and 500 mg tablets, and ultramicronized drug is available as 125 mg, 165 mg, and 330 mg tablets and as 250 mg capsules.

The usual adult dose of the micronized ("microsize") form of the drug is 500 mg daily in single or divided doses with meals; occasionally, 1 g/d is indicated in the treatment of recalcitrant infections. The pediatric dose is 10 mg/kg of body weight daily in single or divided doses with meals. An oral suspension is available for use in children.

Griseofulvin is most effective in treating tinea infections of the scalp and glabrous (nonhairy) skin. In general, infections of the scalp respond to treatment in 4–6 weeks, and infections of glabrous skin will respond in 3–4 weeks. Dermatophyte infections of the nails respond only to prolonged administration of griseofulvin. Fingernails may respond to 6 months of therapy, whereas toenails are quite recalcitrant to treatment and may require 8–18 months of therapy; relapse almost invariably occurs.

Adverse effects seen with griseofulvin therapy include headaches, nausea, vomiting, diarrhea, photosensitivity, peripheral neuritis, and occasionally mental confusion. Griseofulvin is derived from a *Penicillium* mold, and cross-sensitivity with penicillin may occur. It is contraindicated in patients with porphyria or hepatic failure or those who have had hypersensitivity reactions to it in the past. Its safety in pregnant patients has not been established. Leukopenia and proteinuria have occasionally been reported. Therefore, in patients undergoing prolonged therapy, routine evaluation of the hepatic, renal, and hematopoietic systems is advisable. Coumarin anticoagulant activity may be altered by griseofulvin, and anticoagulant dosage may require adjustment.

2. ORAL AZOLE DERIVATIVES

Azole derivatives currently available for oral treatment of systemic mycosis include fluconazole (Diflucan), itraconazole (Sporanox), and ketoconazole (Nizoral). As discussed in Chapter 48, imidazole derivatives act by affecting the permeability of the cell membrane of sensitive cells through alterations of the biosynthesis of lipids, especially sterols, in the fungal cell.

Ketoconazole was the first imidazole derivative used for oral treatment of systemic mycoses. Patients with chronic mucocutaneous candidiasis respond well to a once-daily dose of 200 mg of ketoconazole, with a median clearing time of 16 weeks. Most patients require long-term maintenance therapy. Variable results have been reported in treatment of chromomycosis.

Ketoconazole has been shown to be quite effective in the therapy of cutaneous infections caused by *Epidermophyton, Microsporum,* and *Trichophyton* species. Infections of the glabrous skin often respond within 2–3 weeks to a once-daily oral dose of 200 mg. Palmar-plantar skin is slower to respond, often taking 4–6 weeks at a dosage of 200 mg twice daily. Infections of the hair and nails may take even longer before resolving with low cure rates noted for tinea

capitis. Tinea versicolor is very responsive to short courses of a once-daily dose of 200 mg.

Nausea or pruritus has been noted in approximately 3% of patients taking ketoconazole. More significant side effects include gynecomastia, elevations of hepatic enzyme levels, and hepatitis. Caution is advised when using ketoconazole in patients with a history of hepatitis. Routine evaluation of hepatic function is advisable for patients on prolonged therapy.

The newer azole derivatives for oral therapy include fluconazole and itraconazole. Fluconazole is well absorbed following oral administration with a prolonged plasma half-life of 30 hours. In light of this, daily dosing of 100 mg is sufficient to treat mucocutaneous candidiasis; alternate day dosing is sufficient for dermatophyte infections. The plasma half-life of itraconazole is similar to fluconazole, with detectable therapeutic concentrations remaining in the stratum corneum for up to 28 days following end of therapy. Recommended dosage of itraconazole is 200 mg daily taken with food to ensure maximum absorption.

Coadministration of oral azoles with terfenadine or astemizole may increase the plasma concentration of terfenadine and astemizole by inhibiting their metabolism. This may result in severe cardiac dysrhythmias including ventricular tachycardia and death. *Therefore, coadministration of the oral azoles with either terfenadine or astemizole is absolutely contraindicated.*

ANTIVIRAL AGENTS

ACYCLOVIR

Acyclovir is a synthetic guanine analogue with inhibitory activity against members of the herpesvirus family, including herpes simplex types 1 and 2. As explained in Chapter 49, acyclovir is phosphorylated preferentially by herpes simplex virus-coded thymidine kinase and, following further phosphorylation, the resultant acyclovir triphosphate interferes with herpesvirus DNA polymerase and viral DNA replication. Indications and usage of oral and parenteral acyclovir in the treatment of cutaneous infections are discussed in Chapter 49.

Topical acyclovir (Zovirax) is available as a 5% ointment for application to primary cutaneous herpes simplex infections and to limited mucocutaneous herpes simplex virus infections in immunocompromised patients. In primary infections, the use of topical acyclovir shortens the duration of viral shedding and may decrease healing time. In localized, limited mucocutaneous infections in immunocompromised patients, its use may be associated with a decrease in the duration of viral shedding. There is no evidence that the topical use of acyclovir is of any benefit in the treatment of recurrent disease in nonimmunocompromised patients. Indiscriminate use of acyclovir may result in the selection of resistant strains of herpes simplex virus, which are deficient in viral-coded thymidine kinase. This should be considered when contemplating the use of topical acyclovir in other than nonimmunocompromised patients with primary herpes simplex infection.

Adverse local reactions to acyclovir may include pruritus and mild pain with transient stinging or burning.

ECTOPARASITICIDES

LINDANE
(Hexachlorocyclohexane)

The gamma isomer of hexachlorocyclohexane was commonly called gamma benzene hexachloride, which was a misnomer, since no benzene ring is present in this compound. Lindane is an effective pediculicide and scabicide.

Percutaneous absorption studies using a solution of lindane in acetone have shown that almost 10% of a dose applied to the forearm is absorbed, to be subsequently excreted in the urine over a 5-day period. Serum levels following the application of a commercial lindane lotion reach maximum at 6 hours and decline thereafter with a half-life of 24 hours. After absorption, lindane is concentrated in fatty tissues, including the brain.

Lindane (Kwell, Scabene) is available as a shampoo, lotion, or cream. For pediculosis capitis or pubis, one application of 30 mL of shampoo is worked into a lather and left on the scalp or genital area for 5 minutes and then rinsed off. No additional application is indicated unless living lice are present 1 week after treatment. Then reapplication may be required. Recent concerns about the toxicity of lindane have altered treatment guidelines for its use in scabies; the current recommendation calls for a single application to the entire body from the neck down, left on for 8–12 hours, and then washed off. Patients should be retreated only if active mites can be demonstrated, and never within 1 week of initial treatment.

Much controversy exists about the possible systemic toxicities of topically applied lindane used for medical purposes. Concerns about neurotoxicity and hematotoxicity have resulted in warnings that lindane should be used with caution in infants, children, and pregnant women. The current USA package insert recommends that it not be used as a scabicide in premature infants and in patients with known seizure disorders. The risk of adverse systemic reactions to lindane appears to be minimal when it is used properly and according to directions in adult patients. However, local irritation may occur, and contact with the eyes and mucous membranes should be avoided.

CROTAMITON

Crotamiton, N-ethyl-*o*-crotonotoluidide, is a scabicide with some antipruritic properties. Its mechanism of action is not known, and studies on percutaneous absorption have not been performed.

Crotamiton (Eurax) is available as cream or lotion. Suggested guidelines for scabies treatment call for two applications to the entire body from the chin down at 24-hour intervals, with a cleansing bath 48 hours after the last application. Crotamiton is an effective agent that can be used as an alternative to lindane. Allergic contact hypersensitivity and primary irritation may occur, necessitating discontinuance of therapy. Application to acutely inflamed skin or to the eyes or mucous membranes should be avoided.

BENZYL BENZOATE

Benzyl benzoate is effective as a pediculicide and scabicide. It has generally been supplanted by lindane. The mechanism of action of benzyl benzoate is unknown. Although it appears to be relatively nontoxic after topical application, there are no studies of its toxic potential in the treatment of scabies.

SULFUR

Sulfur has a long history of use as a scabicide. Although it is nonirritating, it has an unpleasant odor, is staining, and is disagreeable to use. It has been replaced by more esthetic and effective scabicides in recent years, but it remains a possible alternative drug for use in infants and pregnant women. The usual formulation is 5% precipitated sulfur in petrolatum.

MALATHION

Malathion is an organophosphate cholinesterase inhibitor (Chapter 7) which is an effective pediculicide and is indicated for the treatment of pediculosis capitis. In vitro studies have shown malathion to be both lousicidal and ovicidal at a concentration of 0.5%.

Malathion (Prioderm) is available as an alcohol-based 0.5% lotion. For pediculosis capitis, one application of 30 mL is applied to dry hair and scalp and allowed to remain for 8–12 hours before shampooing. Patients should be re-treated only if active lice can be demonstrated 7–10 days after initial treatment. Approximately 8% of an applied dose in an acetone vehicle is percutaneously absorbed. Although animal studies have not shown malathion to be carcinogenic, mutagenicity has not been determined, and caution is therefore advised with use in pregnant women, nursing mothers, and infants. This formulation is a weak primary irritant and is unlikely to cause allergic contact hypersensitivity.

PERMETHRIN

Permethrin is neurotoxic to *Pediculus humanus, Pthirus pubis,* and *Sarcoptes scabiei.* Less than 2% of an applied dose is absorbed percutaneously. Residual drug persists up to 10 days following application.

It is recommended that permethrin 1% cream rinse (Nix) be applied undiluted to affected areas of pediculosis for 10 minutes and then rinsed off with warm water. For the treatment of scabies, a single application of 5% cream (Elimite) is applied to the body from the neck down, left on for 8–12 hours, and then washed off. Adverse reactions to permethrin include transient burning, stinging, and pruritus. Cross-sensitization to pyrethrins or chrysanthemums may occur.

AGENTS AFFECTING PIGMENTATION

HYDROQUINONE & MONOBENZONE

Hydroquinone and monobenzone, the monobenzyl ether of hydroquinone, are used to *reduce hyperpigmentation* of the skin. Topical hydroquinone usually results in temporary lightening, whereas monobenzone causes irreversible depigmentation.

The mechanism of action of these compounds appears to involve inhibition of the enzyme tyrosinase, thus interfering with the biosynthesis of melanin. In addition, monobenzone may be toxic to melanocytes, resulting in permanent depigmentation. Some percutaneous absorption of these compounds takes place, because monobenzone may cause hypopigmentation at sites distant from the area of application. Both hydroquinone and monobenzone may cause local irritation. Allergic sensitization to these compounds does occur, and it is advisable to do a patch test on a small area of the body prior to use on the face.

TRIOXSALEN & METHOXSALEN

Trioxsalen and methoxsalen are psoralens used for the *repigmentation* of depigmented macules of vitiligo. With the recent development of high-intensity long-wave ultraviolet fluorescent lamps, photochemotherapy with oral methoxsalen for psoriasis and with oral trioxsalen for vitiligo has been under intensive investigation.

Psoralens must be photoactivated by long-wavelength ultraviolet light in the range of 320–400 nm (UVA) to produce a beneficial effect. Psoralens intercalate with DNA and, with subsequent UVA irradiation, cyclobutane adducts are formed with pyrimidine bases. Both monofunctional and bifunctional adducts may be formed, the latter causing interstrand crosslinks. These DNA photoproducts may inhibit DNA synthesis. The major long-term risks of psoralen photochemotherapy are cataracts and skin cancer.

SUNSCREENS

Topical medications useful in protecting against sunlight contain either chemical compounds that absorb ultraviolet light, called **sunscreens;** or opaque materials such as titanium dioxide that reflect light, called **sunshades.** The three classes of chemical compounds most commonly used in sunscreens are *p*-aminobenzoic acid (PABA) and its esters, the benzophenones, and the dibenzoylmethanes.

Most sunscreen preparations are designed to absorb ultraviolet light in B ultraviolet wavelength range from 280 to 320 nm, which is the range responsible for most of the erythema and tanning associated with sun exposure. Chronic exposure to light in this range induces aging of the skin and photocarcinogenesis. Para-aminobenzoic acid and its esters are the most effective available absorbers in the B region.

The benzophenones include oxybenzone, dioxybenzone, and sulisobenzone. These compounds provide a broader spectrum of absorption from 250 to 360 nm, but their effectiveness in the UVB erythema range is less than that of *p*-aminobenzoic acid. The dibenzoylmethanes include Parasol and Eusolex. These compounds absorb wavelengths throughout the longer ultraviolet A range, 320 nm to 400 nm, with maximum absorption at 360 nm. Patients particularly sensitive to ultraviolet A wavelengths include individuals with polymorphous light eruption, cutaneous lupus erythematosus, and drug-induced photosensitivity. In these patients, butyl-methoxydibenzoylmethane-containing sunscreen (UVA Guard) may provide superior photoprotection.

The protection factor (PF) of a given sunscreen is a measure of its effectiveness in absorbing erythrogenic ultraviolet light. It is determined by measuring the minimal erythema dose (MED) with and without the sunscreen in a group of normal people. The ratio of the minimal erythema dose with sunscreen to the minimal erythema dose without sunscreen is the protection factor. Fair-skinned individuals who sunburn easily are advised to use a product with a high protection factor of 15 or greater; those with darker skins may use a sunscreen with a lower protection factor of 10–15.

ACNE PREPARATIONS

RETINOIC ACID

Retinoic acid, also known as tretinoin or all-*trans*-retinoic acid, is the acid form of vitamin A. It is an effective topical treatment for acne vulgaris. Several analogues of vitamin A, eg, 13-*cis*-retinoic acid (isotretinoin), have been shown to be effective in various dermatologic diseases when given *orally*. Vitamin A alcohol is the physiologic form of vitamin A. The topical therapeutic agent, retinoic acid, is formed by the oxidation of the alcohol group, with all four double bonds in the side chain in the *trans* configuration as shown.

Retinoic acid

Retinoic acid is insoluble in water but soluble in many organic solvents. It is susceptible to oxidation and ester formation, particularly when exposed to light. Topically applied retinoic acid remains chiefly in the epidermis, with less than 10% absorption into the circulation. The small quantities of retinoic acid absorbed following topical application are metabolized by the liver and excreted in bile and urine.

Retinoic acid has several effects on epithelial tissues. It stabilizes lysosomes, increases ribonucleic acid polymerase activity, increases prostaglandin E_2, cAMP, and cGMP levels, and increases the incorporation of thymidine into DNA. Its action in acne has been attributed to decreased cohesion between epidermal cells and increased epidermal cell turnover. This is thought to result in the expulsion of open comedones and the transformation of closed comedones into open ones.

Topical retinoic acid (Retin-A) is applied initially in a concentration sufficient to induce slight erythema with mild peeling. The concentration or frequency of application may be decreased if too much irritation is produced. Topical retinoic acid should be applied to dry skin only, and care should be taken to avoid contact with the corners of the nose, eyes, mouth, and mucous membranes. During the first 4–6 weeks of therapy, comedones not previously evident may appear and give the impression that the acne has been aggravated by the retinoic acid. However, with continued therapy, the lesions will clear, and in 8–12 weeks optimal clinical improvement should occur.

The most common adverse effects of topical retinoic acid are the erythema and dryness that occur in the first few weeks of use, but these can be expected to resolve with continued therapy. Animal studies suggest that tretinoin may increase the tumorigenic potential of ultraviolet radiation. In light of this, patients using retinoic acid should be advised to avoid or minimize sun exposure and use a protective sunscreen. Allergic contact dermatitis to topical retinoic acid is rare.

ISOTRETINOIN

Isotretinoin (Accutane) is a synthetic retinoid currently restricted to the treatment of severe cystic acne that is recalcitrant to standard therapies. The precise mechanism of action of isotretinoin in cystic acne is not known, although it appears to act by inhibiting sebaceous gland size and function. The drug is well absorbed, extensively bound to plasma albumin, and has an elimination half-life of 10–20 hours.

Isotretinoin

Most cystic acne patients respond to 1–2 mg/kg, given in two divided doses daily for 4–5 months. If severe cystic acne persists following this initial treatment, after a period of 2 months, a second course of therapy may be initiated. Common adverse effects resemble hypervitaminosis A and include dryness and itching of the skin and mucous membranes. Less common side effects are headache, corneal opacities, pseudotumor cerebri, inflammatory bowel disease, anorexia, alopecia, and muscle and joint pains. These effects are all reversible on discontinuance of therapy. Skeletal hyperostosis has been observed in patients receiving isotretinoin with premature closure of epiphyses noted in children treated with this medication. Lipid abnormalities (triglycerides, HDL) are frequent; their clinical relevance is unknown at present.

Teratogenicity is a significant risk in patients taking isotretinoin; therefore, women of childbearing potential *must* use an effective form of contraception for at least 1 month before, throughout isotretinoin therapy, and for one or more menstrual cycles following discontinuance of treatment. A serum pregnancy test *must* be obtained within 2 weeks before starting therapy in these patients, and therapy should be initiated only on the second or third day of the next normal menstrual period.

ETRETINATE

Etretinate (Tigason) is an aromatic retinoid that is quite effective in the treatment of psoriasis, especially pustular forms. It is given orally at a dosage of 1–5 mg/kg/d, starting with 0.5 mg/kg/d in patients with erythrodermic psoriasis. Chronic dosing studies reveal a slow terminal elimination phase of several months' duration. Adverse effects attributable to etretinate therapy are similar to those seen with isotretinoin and resemble hypervitaminosis A. Lipid abnormalities are not frequently seen with etretinate; however, transient liver enzyme elevations have been reported. Etretinate is more teratogenic than isotretinoin in the animal species studied to date, which is of special concern in view of its prolonged elimination time after chronic administration. The drug should not be taken by women with childbearing potential.

BENZOYL PEROXIDE

Benzoyl peroxide is an effective topical agent in the treatment of acne vulgaris. It penetrates the stratum corneum or follicular openings unchanged and is converted metabolically to benzoic acid within the epidermis and dermis. Less than 5% of an applied dose is absorbed from the skin in an 8-hour period.

It has been postulated that the mechanism of action of benzoyl peroxide in acne is related to its antimicrobial activity against *P acnes* and to its peeling and comedolytic effects.

To decrease the possibility of irritation, application should be limited to a low concentration (2.5%) once daily for the first week of therapy and increased in frequency and strength if the preparation is well tolerated. Recently, a fixed combination formulation of 5% benzoyl peroxide with 3% erythromycin base (Benzamycin) has become available.

Benzoyl peroxide is a potent contact sensitizer in experimental studies, and this adverse effect may occur in up to 1% of acne patients. Care should be taken to avoid contact with the eyes and mucous membranes. Benzoyl peroxide is an oxidant and may rarely cause bleaching of the hair or colored fabrics.

ANTI-INFLAMMATORY AGENTS

TOPICAL CORTICOSTEROIDS

The remarkable efficacy of topical corticosteroids in the treatment of inflammatory dermatoses was noted soon after the introduction of hydrocortisone in 1952. Subsequently, numerous analogues have been developed that offer extensive choices of potencies, concentrations, and vehicles. The therapeutic effectiveness of topical corticosteroids is based primarily on their anti-inflammatory activity. Definitive explanations of the effects of corticosteroids on endogenous mediators of inflammation such as histamine, kinins, lysosomal enzymes, prostaglandins, and leukotrienes await further experimental clarification. The antimitotic effects of corticosteroids on human epidermis may account for an additional mechanism of action in psoriasis and other dermatologic diseases associated with increased cell turnover. The general pharmacology of these endocrine agents is discussed in Chapter 38.

The original topical glucocorticosteroid was hydrocortisone, the natural glucocorticosteroid of the adrenal cortex. Prednisolone and methylprednisolone are as active topically as hydrocortisone. The 9α-fluoro derivatives of hydrocortisone were active topically, but their salt-retaining properties made them undesirable even for topical use. The 9α-fluorinated steroids dexamethasone and betamethasone subsequently developed did not have any advantage over hydrocortisone. However, triamcinolone and fluocinolone, the acetonide derivatives of the fluorinated steroids, have a distinct advantage in topical therapy. Similarly, betamethasone is not very active topically, but attaching a 5-carbon valerate chain to the 17-hydroxyl position results in a compound over 300 times as active as hydrocortisone for topical use. Fluocinonide is the 21-acetate derivative of fluo- cinolone acetonide; the addition of the 21-acetate enhances the topical activity about fivefold. Fluorination of the steroid is not required for high potency; hydrocortisone valerate and butyrate have activity similar to that of triamcinolone acetonide.

Corticosteroids are only minimally absorbed following application to normal skin, eg, approximately 1% of a dose of hydrocortisone solution applied to the ventral forearm is absorbed. Occlusion with an impermeable film, such as plastic wrap, is an effective method of enhancing penetration, yielding a tenfold increase in absorption. There is a marked regional anatomic variation in corticosteroid penetration. Compared to the absorption from the forearm, hydrocortisone is absorbed 0.14 times as well through the plantar foot arch, 0.83 times as well through the palm, 3.5 times as well through the scalp, 6 times as well through the forehead, 9 times as well through vulvar skin, and 42 times as well through scrotal skin. Penetration is increased severalfold in the inflamed skin of atopic dermatitis; and in severe exfoliative diseases, such as erythrodermic psoriasis, there appears to be little barrier to penetration.

Experimental studies on the percutaneous absorption of hydrocortisone fail to reveal a significant increase in absorption when applied on a repetitive basis compared to a single dose, and a single daily application may be effective in most conditions. Ointment bases tend to give better activity to the corticosteroid than do cream or lotion vehicles. Increasing the concentration of a corticosteroid increases the penetration but not to the same degree. For example, approximately 1% of a 0.25% hydrocortisone solution is absorbed from the forearm. A tenfold increase in concentration only causes a fourfold increase in absorption. Solubility of the corticosteroid in the vehicle is a significant determinant of the percutaneous absorption of a topical steroid. Marked increases in efficacy are noted when optimized vehicles are used, as demonstrated by newer formulations of betamethasone dipropionate and diflorasone diacetate.

Table 63–1 groups topical corticosteroid formulation according to approximate relative efficacy. Table 63–2 lists major dermatologic diseases in order of their responsiveness to these drugs. In the first group of diseases, low-to medium-efficacy corticosteroid preparations often produce clinical remission. In the second group, it is often necessary to use high-efficacy preparations, occlusion therapy, or both. Once a remission has been achieved, every effort should be made to maintain the patient with a low-efficacy corticosteroid.

The limited penetration of topical corticosteroids can be overcome in certain clinical circumstances by the intralesional injection of relatively insoluble corticosteroids, eg, triamcinolone acetonide, triamcinolone diacetate, triamcinolone hexacetonide, and betamethasone acetate-phosphate. When these agents are injected into the lesion, measurable amounts remain in place and are gradually released for 3–4 weeks. This form of therapy is often effective for the lesions listed in Table 63–2 that are generally unresponsive to topical corticosteroids. The dosage of the triamcinolone salts should be limited to 1 mg per treatment site, ie, 0.1 mL of 10 mg/mL suspension, to decrease the incidence of local atrophy (see below).

Adverse Effects

All absorbable topical corticosteroids possess the potential to suppress the pituitary-adrenal axis (Chapter 38). Although most patients with pituitary-adrenal axis suppression demonstrate only a laboratory test abnormality, cases of severely impaired stress response can occur. Iatrogenic Cushing's syndrome

Table 63–1. Relative efficacy of some topical corticosteroids in various formulations.

Lowest efficacy	
0.25–2.5%	Hydrocortisone
0.25%	Methylprednisolone acetate (Medrol)
0.04%	Dexamethasone[1] (Hexadrol)
0.1%	Dexamethasone[1] (Decaderm)
1.0%	Methylprednisolone acetate (Medrol)
0.5%	Prednisolone (Meti-Derm)
0.2%	Betamethasone[1] (Celestone)
Low efficacy	
0.01%	Fluocinolone acetonide[1] (Fluonid, Synalar)
0.01%	Betamethasone valerate[1] (Valisone)
0.025%	Fluorometholone[1] (Oxylone)
0.05%	Aclometasone dipropionate (Aclovate)
0.025%	Triamcinolone acetonide[1] (Aristocort, Kenalog, Triacet)
0.1%	Clocortolone pivalate[1] (Cloderm)
0.03%	Flumethasone pivalate[1] (Locorten)
Intermediate efficacy	
0.2%	Hydrocortisone valerate (Westcort)
0.1%	Mometasone furoate (Elocon)
0.1%	Hydrocortisone butyrate (Locoid)
0.025%	Betamethasone benzoate[1] (Benisone, Flurobate, Uticort)
0.025%	Flurandrenolide[1] (Cordran)
0.1%	Betamethasone valerate[1] (Valisone)
0.05%	Fluticasone propionate (Cutivate)
0.05%	Desonide (Tridesilon, Desowen)
0.025%	Halcinonide[1] (Halog)
0.05%	Desoximetasone[1] (Topicort L.P.)
0.05%	Flurandrenolide[1] (Cordran)
0.1%	Triamcinolone acetonide[1]
0.025%	Fluocinolone acetonide[1]
High efficacy	
0.05%	Betamethasone dipropionate[1] (Diprosone)
0.1%	Amcinonide[1] (Cyclocort)
0.25%	Desoximetasone[1] (Topicort)
0.5%	Triamcinolone acetonide[1]
0.2%	Fluocinolone acetonide[1] (Synalar-HP)
0.05%	Diflorasone diacetate[1] (Florone, Maxiflor)
0.1%	Halcinonide[1] (Halog)
Highest efficacy	
0.05%	Betamethasone dipropionate[1] in optimized vehicle (Diprolene)
0.05%	Diflorasone diacetate[1] in optimized vehicle (Psorcon)
0.05%	Halobetasol propionate[1] (Ultravate)
0.05%	Clobetasol propionate[1] (Temovate)

[1]Fluorinated steroids.

Table 63–2. Dermatologic disorders responsive to topical corticosteroids ranked in order of sensitivity.

Very responsive
 Atopic dermatitis
 Seborrheic dermatitis
 Lichen simplex chronicus
 Pruritus ani
 Later phase of allergic contact dermatitis
 Later phase of irritant dermatitis
 Nummular eczematous dermatitis
 Stasis dermatitis
 Psoriasis, especially of genitalia and face
Less responsive
 Discoid lupus erythematosus
 Psoriasis of palms and soles
 Necrobiosis lipoidica diabeticorum
 Sarcoidosis
 Lichen striatus
 Pemphigus
 Familial benign pemphigus
 Vitiligo
 Granuloma annulare
Least responsive: intralesional injection required
 Keloids
 Hypertrophic scars
 Hypertrophic lichen planus
 Alopecia areata
 Acne cysts
 Prurigo nodularis
 Chondrodermatitis nodularis helicus

may occur as a result of protracted use of topical corticosteroids in large quantities. Applying potent corticosteroids to extensive areas of the body for prolonged periods, with or without occlusion, increases the likelihood of systemic side effects. Fewer of these factors are required to produce adverse systemic effects in children, and growth retardation is of particular concern in the pediatric age group.

Adverse local effects of topical corticosteroids include the following: atrophy, which may present as depressed, shiny, often wrinkled "cigarette paper"-appearing skin with prominent telangiectases and a tendency to develop purpura and ecchymosis; steroid rosacea, with persistent erythema, telangiectatic vessels, pustules, and papules in central facial distribution; perioral dermatitis, steroid acne, alterations of cutaneous infections, hypopigmentation, hypertrichosis, and increased intraocular pressure; and allergic contact dermatitis, which may be confirmed by patch testing with high concentrations of corticosteroids, ie, 1% in petrolatum, because topical corticosteroids are not irritating. Topical corticosteroids are contraindicated in individuals who demonstrate hypersensitivity to them.

TAR COMPOUNDS

Coal tar is the principal by-product of the destructive distillation of bituminous coal and an exceedingly complex mixture, containing about 10,000 compounds. These include naphthalene, phenanthrene, fluoranthrene, benzene, xylene, toluene, phenol, creosols, other aromatic compounds, pyridine bases, ammonia, and peroxides. Coal tar is available in many over-the-counter preparations in the form of bath additives, shampoos, and hydroalcoholic base gels. Coal tar may also be compounded in accordance with *United States Pharmacopeia, National Formulary,* or other formulations in concentrations ranging from 2% to 10%.

Liquor carbonis detergens (LCD) is a coal tar solution prepared by extracting coal tar with alcohol and an emulsifying agent, such as polysorbate 80. This solution contains 20 g of coal tar per 100 mL and may be compounded in concentrations of 2–10% in creams, ointments, or shampoos.

Tar preparations are used mainly in the treatment of psoriasis, dermatitis, and lichen simplex chronicus. The phenolic constituents endow these compounds with antipruritic properties, making them particularly valuable in the treatment of chronic lichenified dermatitis. Acute dermatitis with vesiculation and oozing may be irritated by even weak tar preparations, which should be avoided. However, in the subacute and chronic stages of dermatitis and psoriasis, these preparations are quite useful and offer an alternative to the use of topical corticosteroids.

The most common adverse reaction to coal tar compounds is an irritant folliculitis, necessitating discontinuance of therapy to the affected areas for a period of 3–5 days. Phototoxicity and allergic contact dermatitis may also occur. Tar preparations should be avoided in patients who have previously exhibited sensitivity to them. Care should be exercised when using tar compounds in patients with erythrodermal or generalized pustular psoriasis, because of the risk of total body exfoliation.

KERATOLYTIC & DESTRUCTIVE AGENTS

SALICYLIC ACID

Salicylic acid was chemically synthesized in 1860 and has been extensively used in dermatologic therapy as a keratolytic agent. It is a white powder quite soluble in alcohol but only slightly soluble in water.

Salicylic acid

Salicylic acid is absorbed percutaneously and distributed in the extracellular space, with maximum plasma levels occurring 6–12 hours after application. Since 50–80% of salicylate is bound to albumin, transiently increased serum levels of free salicylates are found in patients with hypoalbuminemia. The urinary metabolites of topically applied salicylic acid include salicyluric acid and acyl and phenolic glucuronides of salicylic acid; only 6% of the total recovered is unchanged salicylic acid. About 95% of a single dose of salicylate is excreted in the urine within 24 hours after its absorption.

The mechanism by which salicylic acid produces its keratolytic and other therapeutic effects is poorly understood. The drug may solubilize cell surface proteins that keep the stratum corneum intact, thereby resulting in desquamation of keratotic debris. Salicylic acid is keratolytic in concentrations of 3–6%. In concentrations greater than 6%, it can be destructive to tissues.

Salicylism and death have occurred following topical application. In an adult, 1 g of a topically applied 6% salicylic acid preparation will raise the serum salicylate level not more than 0.5 mg/dL of plasma; the threshold for toxicity is 30–50 mg/dL. Higher serum levels are possible in children, who are therefore at a greater risk to develop salicylism. In cases of severe intoxication, hemodialysis is the treatment of choice (see Chapter 60). It is advisable to limit both the total amount of salicylic acid applied and the frequency of application. Urticarial, anaphylactic, and erythema multiforme reactions may occur in patients allergic to salicylates. Topical use may be associated with local irritation, acute inflammation, and even ulceration with the use of high concentrations of salicylic acid. Particular care must be exercised when using the drug on the extremities of diabetics or patients with peripheral vascular disease.

PROPYLENE GLYCOL

Propylene glycol is extensively used in topical preparations because it is an excellent vehicle for organic compounds. Propylene glycol has recently been used alone as a keratolytic agent in 40–70% concentrations, with plastic occlusion, or in gel with 6% salicylic acid.

Only minimal amounts of a topically applied dose are absorbed through normal stratum corneum. Percutaneously absorbed propylene glycol is oxidized by the liver to lactic acid and pyruvic acid, with subsequent utilization in general body metabolism. Approximately 12–45% of the absorbed agent is excreted unchanged in the urine.

Propylene glycol is an effective keratolytic agent for the removal of hyperkeratotic debris. Propylene glycol is also an effective humectant and increases the water content of the stratum corneum. The hygro-

scopic characteristics of the agent may help it to develop an osmotic gradient through the stratum corneum, thereby increasing hydration of the outer-most layers by drawing water out from the inner layers of the skin.

Propylene glycol is used under polyethylene occlusion or with 6% salicylic acid for the treatment of ichthyosis, palmar and plantar keratodermas, psoriasis, pityriasis rubra pilaris, keratosis pilaris, and hypertrophic lichen planus.

In concentrations greater than 10%, propylene glycol may act as an irritant in some patients; those with eczematous dermatitis may be more sensitive. Allergic contact dermatitis occurs with propylene glycol, and at present a 4% aqueous propylene glycol solution is recommended for the purpose of patch testing.

UREA

Urea in a compatible cream vehicle or ointment base has a softening and moisturizing effect on the stratum corneum. It has the ability to make creams and lotions feel less greasy, and this has been utilized in dermatologic preparations to decrease the oily feel of a preparation that otherwise might feel unpleasant. It is a white crystalline powder with a slight ammonia odor when moist.

Urea is absorbed percutaneously, although the precise amount absorbed is not well documented. It is distributed predominantly in the extracellular space and excreted in urine. Urea is a natural product of metabolism, and systemic toxicities with topical application do not occur.

Urea allegedly increases the water content of the stratum corneum, presumably as a result of the hygroscopic characteristics of this naturally occurring molecule. Urea is also keratolytic. The mechanism of action appears to involve alterations in prekeratin and keratin, leading to increased solubilization. In addition, urea may break hydrogen bonds that keep the stratum corneum intact.

As a humectant, urea is used in concentrations of 2–20% in creams and lotions. As a keratolytic agent, it is used in 20% concentration in diseases such as ichthyosis vulgaris, hyperkeratosis of palms and soles, xerosis, and keratosis pilaris. Concentrations of 30–50% in ointment base applied to the nail plate under occlusion have been useful in softening the nail prior to avulsion. Concentrations of 10–20% applied to the diaper area, groin, or areas of eczematous dermatitis may be associated with an unpleasant stinging sensation that may necessitate discontinuance of use of the preparation.

PODOPHYLLUM RESIN & PODOFILOX

Podophyllum resin, an alcoholic extract of *Podophyllum peltatum,* commonly known as mandrake root or May apple, is used in the treatment of condyloma acuminatum and other verrucae. It is a mixture of podophyllotoxin, alpha and beta peltatin, desoxypodophyllotoxin, dehydropodophyllotoxin, and other compounds. It is soluble in alcohol, ether, chloroform, and compound tincture of benzoin.

Percutaneous absorption of podophyllum resin occurs, particularly in intertriginous areas and from applications to large moist condylomas. It is soluble in lipids and therefore is distributed widely throughout the body, including the central nervous system.

The major use of podophyllum resin is in the treatment of condyloma acuminatum. Podophyllotoxin and its derivatives are active cytotoxic agents with specific affinity for the microtubule protein of the mitotic spindle. Normal assembly of the spindle is prevented, and epidermal mitoses are arrested in metaphase. A 25% concentration of podophyllum resin in compound tincture of benzoin is recommended for the treatment of condyloma acuminatum. Application should be restricted to wart tissue only, to limit the total amount of medication used and to prevent severe erosive changes in adjacent tissue. In treating cases of large extensive condylomas, it is advisable to limit application to sections of the affected area to minimize systemic absorption. The patient is instructed to wash off the preparation 2–3 hours after the initial application, since the irritant reaction is variable. Depending on the individual patient's reaction, this period can be extended to 6–8 hours on subsequent applications. If three to five applications have not resulted in significant resolution, other methods of treatment should be considered.

Toxic symptoms associated with excessively large applications include nausea, vomiting, alterations in sensorium, muscle weakness, neuropathy with diminished tendon reflexes, coma, and even death. Local irritation is common, and inadvertent contact with the eye may cause severe conjunctivitis. Use during pregnancy is contraindicated in view of possible cytotoxic effects on the fetus.

Recent clinical trials utilizing pure podophyllotoxin (podofilox) resulted in the approval of a 0.5% podophyllotoxin preparation (Condylox) for application by the patient in the treatment of genital condylomas. The low concentration of podofilox significantly reduces the potential for systemic toxicity. Most men with penile warts may be treated with less than 70 μL per application. At this dose, podofilox is not routinely detected in the serum. Treatment is self-administered in treatment cycles of twice-daily application for 3 consecutive days followed by a 4-day drug-free period. Local adverse effects include inflammation, erosions, burning pain, and itching.

CANTHARIDIN

Cantharidin is the active irritant isolated from cantharides, or dried blister beetles (*Lytta [Cantharis] vesicatoria,* also known as Russian fly or Spanish fly). The ability of insects of the *Cantharis* type to produce vesicles and bullae on human skin led to the investigation of possible therapeutic uses of the vesicant cantharidin in dermatology. The major clinical use is in the treatment of molluscum contagiosum and verruca vulgaris, particularly periungual warts.

The amount of cantharidin absorbed following cutaneous application is unknown. It is excreted by the kidney, and in cases of oral ingestion of significant amounts, marked irritation of the entire urinary tract has resulted, with pain, urinary urgency, and priapism.

Cantharidin acts on mitochondrial oxidative enzymes, resulting in decreased ATP levels. This leads to changes in the epidermal cell membranes, acantholysis, and blister formation. This effect is entirely intraepidermal, and no scarring ensues.

The main use of cantharidin is in the treatment of verruca vulgaris. Periungual warts are treated by applying cantharidin to the wart surface, allowing it to dry, and occluding it with a nonporous plastic tape. A blister will form that will resolve in 7–14 days, at which time the area is debrided and any remaining wart is re-treated. Several applications may be required to effect a cure. Plantar warts are treated by paring and then applying several layers of cantharidin. An occlusive plastic tape is then applied. The resulting blister is removed in 10–14 days, and any residual wart is re-treated. Molluscum contagiosum will often respond to a single application without occlusion. Painless application and lack of residual scarring make cantharidin ideally suited for treatment of children.

A ring of warts may develop at the periphery of a cantharidin-treated wart as a result of intraepidermal inoculation. These may be re-treated with cantharidin or by an alternative method. Systemic toxic effects have not been observed with topical therapy, although ingestion of as little as 10 mg has resulted in abdominal pain, nausea, vomiting, and shock.

FLUOROURACIL

Fluorouracil is a fluorinated pyrimidine antimetabolite that resembles uracil, with a fluorine atom substituted for the 5-methyl group. Its systemic pharmacology is described in Chapter 56. Fluorouracil is used topically for the treatment of multiple actinic keratoses and intralesionally for keratoacanthomas.

The pharmacokinetics of intralesional therapy have not been determined. Approximately 6% of a topically applied dose is absorbed—an amount insufficient to produce adverse systemic effects. Most of the

Table 63–3. Antiseborrhea agents.

Chloroxine shampoo (Capitrol)
Coal tar shampoo (Ionil-T, Pentrax, Theraplex-T, T-Gel)
Ketoconazole shampoo (Nizoral)
Selenium sulfide shampoo (Selsun, Exsel)
Zinc pyrithione shampoo (DHS-Zinc, Theraplex-Z)

Table 63–4. Miscellaneous oral medications and the dermatologic conditions in which they are used.

Drug or Group	Conditions	
Antihistamines	Pruritus (any cause)	See also Chapter 16.
Antimalarials	Lupus erythematosus, photosensitization	See also Chapter 35.
Antimetabolites	Psoriasis, pemphigus, pemphigoid	See also Chapter 56.
Dapsone	Dermatitis herpetiformis, erythema elevatum diutinum, pemphigus, pemphigoid, bullous lupus erythematosus	See also Chapter 46.
Corticosteroids	Pemphigus, pemphigoid, lupus erythematosus, allergic contact dermatoses, and certain other dermatoses	See also Chapter 38.

absorbed drug is metabolized and excreted as carbon dioxide, urea, and α-fluoro-β-alanine. A small percentage is eliminated unchanged in the urine. Fluorouracil inhibits thymidylate synthetase activity, interfering with the synthesis of deoxyribonucleic acid and to a lesser extent ribonucleic acid. These effects are most marked in atypical, rapidly proliferating cells.

The response to treatment begins with erythema and progresses through vesiculation, erosion, superficial ulceration, necrosis, and finally reepithelialization. Fluorouracil should be continued until the inflammatory reaction reaches the ulceration and necrosis stage, usually in 3–4 weeks, at which time treatment should be terminated. The healing process may continue for 1–2 months after therapy is discontinued. Local adverse reactions may include pain, pruritus, a burning sensation, tenderness, and residual postinflammatory hyperpigmentation. Excessive exposure to sunlight during treatment may increase the intensity of the reaction and should be avoided. Allergic contact dermatitis to fluorouracil has been reported, and its use is contraindicated in patients with known hypersensitivity. Intralesional injections of keratoacanthomas with a 5% aqueous solution of fluorouracil have recently been advocated. Weekly injections of 25–50 mg are given until 70–80% involution of the lesion is noted. If the lesion does not involute after five injections, excisional surgery is performed. Local reactions include erythema, inflammation, and subsequent necrosis of the tumor. Systemic adverse effects have not been observed and are not anticipated in view of the comparatively small amounts of fluorouracil administered on a weekly basis. Recent trials demonstrated similar effectiveness of 10% masoprocol cream (Actinex).

MINOXIDIL

Topical minoxidil is effective in reversing the progressive miniaturization of terminal scalp hairs associated with androgenic alopecia. Vertex balding is more responsive to therapy than frontal balding. The mechanism of action of minoxidil on hair follicles is unknown. Chronic dosing studies have demonstrated that the effect of minoxidil is not permanent, and cessation of treatment will lead to hair loss in 4–6 months. Percutaneous absorption of minoxidil in normal scalp is minimal, but possible systemic effects on blood pressure (Chapter 11) should be monitored in patients with cardiac disease.

ANTISEBORRHEA AGENTS

Table 63–3 lists topical formulations for the treatment of seborrheic dermatitis. These are of variable efficacy and may necessitate concomitant treatment with topical corticosteroids for severe cases.

MISCELLANEOUS ORAL MEDICATIONS

A number of drugs used primarily for other conditions also find use as oral therapeutic agents for dermatologic conditions. A few such preparations are listed in Table 63–4.

REFERENCES

General

Braun-Falco O, Korting H, Maibach HI: *Liposome Dermatics.* Springer, 1992.

Bronaugh R, Maibach HI: *Percutaneous Penetration: Principles and Practices,* 2nd ed. Dekker, 1991.

Guy RH et al: Kinetics of drug absorption across human skin in vivo. Developments in methodology. Pharmacol Skin 1987;1:70.

Lorette G, Vaillant L: Pruritus: Current concepts in pathogenesis and treatment. Drugs 1990;39:218.

Orkin M, Maibach HI, Dahl MV (editors): *Dermatology.* Appleton & Lange, 1991.

Phillips TJ, Dover JS: Recent advances in dermatology. N Engl J Med 1992;326:167.

Steigleder G, Maibach HI: *Pocket Atlas of Dermatology.* Thieme, 1993.

Antibacterial Drugs

Eady EA, Holland KT, Cunliffe WJ: Topical antibiotics in acne therapy. J Am Acad Dermatol 1981;5:455.

Hirschmann JV: Topical antibiotics in dermatology. Arch Dermatol 1988;124:1691.

Leyden JJ et al: Topical antibiotics and topical antimicrobial agents in acne therapy. Acta Derm Venereol (Stockh) 1980;89(Suppl):75.

Milstone EM, McDonald AJ, Scholhamer CF: Pseudomembranous colitis after topical application of clindamycin. Arch Dermatol 1981;117:154.

Rasmussen JE: Topical antibiotics. J Dermatol Surg 1976;2:69.

Wachs GN, Maibach HI: Cooperative double blind trial of an antibiotic corticoid combination in impetiginized atopic dermatitis. Br J Dermatol 1976;95:323.

Antifungal Drugs

Borgers M: Mechanism of action of antifungal drugs with special reference to the imidazole derivatives. Rev Infect Dis 1980;2:250.

Graybill JR et al: Ketoconazole treatment of chronic mucocutaneous candidiasis. Arch Dermatol 1980;116:1137.

Heel RC et al: Econazole: A review of its antifungal activity and therapeutic efficacy. Drugs 1978;16:177.

Jones HE: Ketoconazole. Arch Dermatol 1982;118:217.

Jones HE, Simpson JG, Artis WW: Oral ketoconazole: An effective and safe treatment for dermatophytosis. Arch Dermatol 1981;117:129.

Katz R, Cahn B: Haloprogin therapy for dermatophyte infections. Arch Dermatol 1972;106:837.

Knight AG: The activity of various griseofulvin preparations and the appearance of oral griseofulvin in the stratum corneum. Br J Dermatol 1974;91:49.

Sakurai K et al: Mode of action of 6-cyclohexyl-1-hydroxy-4-methyl-2(1H)-pyridone ethanolamine salt (ciclopirox olamine). Chemotherapy 1978;25:68.

Urcuyo FG, Zaias N: The successful treatment of pityriasis versicolor by systemic ketoconazole. J Am Acad Dermatol 1982;6:24.

Weber K, Wehland J, Herzog W: Griseofulvin interacts with microtubules both in vivo and in vitro. J Mol Biol 1976;102:817.

Antiviral Agents

Corey L et al: A trial of topical acyclovir in genital herpes simplex virus infection. N Engl J Med 1982;306:1313.

Douglas JM et al: A double-blind study of oral acyclovir for suppression of recurrences of genital herpes simplex virus infection. N Engl J Med 1984;310:1551.

Mertz GJ et al: Double-blind placebo-controlled trial of oral acyclovir in first episode genital herpes simplex virus infection. JAMA 1984;252:1147.

Pagano JS: Acyclovir comes of age. J Am Acad Dermatol 1982;6:396.

Ectoparasiticides

Cubela V, Yawalkar SJ: Clinical experience with crotamiton cream and lotion in the treatment of infants with scabies. Br J Clin Pract 1978;32:229.

Konstantinou D, Stanoeva L, Yawalkar SJ: Crotamiton cream and lotion in the treatment of infants and young children with scabies. J Int Med Res 1979;7:443.

Orkin M et al (editors): *Scabies and Pediculosis.* CRC Press, 1990.

Rasmussen JE: The problem of lindane. J Am Acad Dermatol 1981;5:507.

Schacter B: Treatment of scabies and pediculosis with lindane preparation: An evaluation. J Am Acad Dermatol 1981;5:517.

Agents Affecting Pigmentation

Engasser PG, Maibach HI: Cosmetics and dermatology: Bleaching creams. J Am Acad Dermatol 1981;5:143.

Epstein JH et al: Current status of oral PUVA therapy for psoriasis. J Am Acad Dermatol 1979;1:106.

Kaidbey KH, Kligman AM: An appraisal of the efficacy and substantivity of the new high-potency sunscreens. J Am Acad Dermatol 1981;4:566.

Mosher DB, Parrish JA, Fitzpatrick TB: Monobenzylether of hydroquinone: A retrospective study of treatment of 18 vitiligo patients and a review of the literature. Br J Dermatol 1977;97:669.

Pathak MA, Kramer DM, Fitzpatrick TB: Photobiology and photochemistry of furocoumarins (psoralens). In: *Sunlight and Man: Normal and Abnormal Photobiologic Responses.* Tokyo Univ Press, 1974.

Sayre RM et al: Performance of six sunscreen formulations on human skin. Arch Dermatol 1979;115:46.

Stolk LML, Siddiqui AH: Biopharmaceutics, pharmacokinetics, and pharmacology of psoralens. Gen Pharmacol 1988;19:649.

Thompson SC et al: Reduction of solar keratoses by regular sunscreen use. N Engl J Med 1993;329:1147.

Retinoids & Other Acne Preparations

Allen JG, Bloxham DP: The pharmacology and pharmacokinetics of the retinoids. Pharmacol Ther 1989;40:1.

Bigby M, Stern RS: Adverse reactions to isotretinoin. J Am Acad Dermatol 1988;18:543.

Ehmann CW, Voorhees JJ: International studies of the efficacy of etretinate in the treatment of psoriasis. J Am Acad Dermatol 1982;6:692.

Ellis CN et al: Etretinate therapy reduces inpatient treatment of psoriasis. J Am Acad Dermatol 1987;17:787.

Lammer EJ et al: Retinoic acid embryopathy. N Engl J Med 1985;313:837.

Larsen FG et al: Pharmacokinetics and therapeutic efficacy of retinoids in skin diseases. Clin Pharmacokinetic 1992;23:42.

Lever L, Marks R: Current views on the aetiology, pathogenesis, and treatment of acne vulgaris. Drugs 1990;39: 681.

Lippman SM, Meyskens FL Jr: Results of the use of vitamin A and retinoids in cutaneous malignancies. Pharmacol Ther 1989;40:107.

Nacht S et al: Benzoyl peroxide: Percutaneous penetration and metabolic disposition. J Am Acad Dermatol 1981; 4:31.

Orfanos CE, Ehlert R, Gollnick H: The retinoids: A review of their clinical pharmacology and therapeutic use. Drugs 1987;34:459.

Weinstein GD et al: Topical tretinoin for treatment of photodamaged skin. Arch Dermatol 1991;127:659.

Weiss JS et al: Topical tretinoin improves photoaged skin: A double-blind vehicle-controlled study. JAMA 1988; 259:527.

Anti-inflammatory Agents

Grupper C: The chemistry, pharmacology and use of tar in the treatment of psoriasis. In: *Psoriasis: Proceedings of the International Symposium, Stanford University.* Farber E, Cos AJ (editors). Stanford Univ Press, 1971.

Jackson DB et al: Bioequivalence (bioavailability) of generic topical corticosteroids. J Am Acad Dermatol 1989; 20:791.

Maibach HI, Stoughton RB: Topical corticosteroids. In: *Steroid Therapy.* Arzanoff DL (editor). Saunders, 1975.

Miller JA, Munro DD: Topical corticosteroids: Clinical pharmacology and therapeutic use. Drugs 1980;19: 119.

Robertson DB, Maibach HI: Topical corticosteroids: A review. Int J Dermatol 1982;21:59.

Keratolytic & Destructive Agents

Ashton H, Frenk E, Stevenson CJ: Urea as a topical agent. Br J Dermatol 1971;84:194.

Chamberlain MJ, Reynolds AL, Yeoman WB: Toxic effects of podophyllum applications in pregnancy. Br Med J 1972;3:391.

Epstein WL, Kligman AM: Treatment of warts with cantharidin. Arch Dermatol 1958;77:508.

Fine JD, Arndt KA: *Propylene Glycol: A Review.* Excerpta Medica, 1980.

Geotte DK: Topical chemotherapy with 5-fluorouracil. J Am Acad Dermatol 1981;4:633.

Geotte DK, Odom RB: Successful treatment of keratoacanthoma with intralesional fluorouracil. J Am Acad Dermatol 1980;2:212.

Roenigk H, Maibach HI (editors): *Psoriasis.* Marcel Dekker, 1985.

Taylor JR, Halprin KM: Percutaneous absorption of salicylic acid. Arch Dermatol 1975;111:740.

Dermatotoxicology

Menne T, Maibach HI: *Exogenous Dermatoses: Environmental Dermatitis.* CRC Press, 1991.

Marzelli F, Maibach H (editors): *Dermatotoxicology,* 2nd ed. Hemisphere Press, 1985.

Rougier A, Goldberg A, Maibach H: *In Vitro Skin Toxicology.* M. Liebert, 1994.

Wang R, Knaak J, Maibach HI: Dermal Inhalation, Exposure, & Absorption of Toxicants. CRC Press, 1993

Drugs Used in Gastrointestinal Diseases

64

David F. Altman, MD

Many drugs discussed elsewhere in this book have applications in the treatment of gastrointestinal diseases. Antimuscarinic drugs inhibit the food-stimulated secretion of gastric acid and also affect intestinal smooth muscle; these drugs are useful in some forms of functional bowel disease. Muscarinic agonists stimulate smooth muscle and are used to promote gastrointestinal motility. Nicotine from tobacco smoke is one of the strongest risk factors for ulcer recurrence; conversely, nicotine (from nicotine chewing gum or a transdermal patch) may have beneficial effects in ulcerative colitis. Some phenothiazines have excellent antiemetic properties, and narcotic analgesics and some of their derivatives are useful antidiarrheal medications by virtue of their ability to inhibit intestinal motility. Several other groups of medications are used almost exclusively in gastrointestinal disease; these are grouped and discussed below according to their therapeutic uses.

DRUGS USED IN ACID-PEPTIC DISEASE

Acid-peptic disease includes peptic ulcer (gastric and duodenal), gastroesophageal reflux, and pathologic hypersecretory states such as Zollinger-Ellison syndrome. The pathogenesis of peptic ulcer is not completely understood. It is clear that gastric acid and pepsin secretion are necessary for the development of a peptic ulcer. However, factors relating to mucosal resistance to acid, particularly the production of gastroduodenal mucus and secretion of bicarbonate by epithelial cells, may be equally important. A role for the bacterium *Helicobacter pylori* in ulcer pathogenesis is widely accepted. Salicylates and other nonsteroidal anti-inflammatory drugs may not only cause dyspepsia but can also cause or exacerbate peptic ulcers and their complications. Currently, drugs are available that may neutralize gastric acid, reduce gastric acid secretion, or enhance mucosal defenses through "cytoprotective" or possibly antimicrobial activities. Most clinicians treat patients with recurrent ulcers with antimicrobial drugs to eradicate *H pylori* colonization.

ANTACIDS

Gastric antacids are weak bases that react with gastric hydrochloric acid to form a salt and water. Their usefulness in peptic ulcer disease appears to lie in their ability to reduce gastric acidity and, since pepsin is inactive in solutions above pH 4.0, to reduce peptic activity. However, recent trials demonstrating ulcer healing with the administration of relatively low daily doses of antacid suggest that this may not be the only reason for their effectiveness. Animal studies have demonstrated mucosal protection by antacids, either through the stimulation of prostaglandin production or the binding of an unidentified injurious substance. The roles played by these various mechanisms remain to be determined.

Most antacids in current use have as their principal constituent either magnesium or aluminum hydroxide, alone or in combination, and occasionally in combination with sodium bicarbonate or a calcium salt. The chemical activities, neutralizing capacity, solubility, and side effects of some of these ingredients are summarized in Table 64–1. The net buffering capacity of any compound is determined by its ability to neutralize gastric acid and the duration of the medication's residence in the stomach. Thus, the combinations available for administration (Table 64–2) have been developed in an effort to maximize effectiveness and minimize inconvenience. Antacids also vary significantly in palatability and price.

Clinical Use of Antacids

After a meal, gastric acid is produced at a rate of about 45 meq/h. A single dose of 156 meq of antacid given 1 hour after a meal effectively neutralizes gastric acid for 2 hours. A second dose given 3 hours after eating maintains the effect for over 4 hours after

Table 64–1. Major constituents of antacids.

Constituent	Neutralizing Capacity	Salt Formed in Stomach	Solubility of Salt	Adverse Effects
$NaHCO_3$	High	NaCl	High	Systemic alkalosis, fluid retention
$CaCO_3$	Moderate	$CaCl_2$	Moderate	Hypercalcemia, nephrolithiasis, milk-alkali syndrome
$Al(OH)_3$	High	$AlCl_3$	Low	Constipation, hypophosphatemia; drug adsorption reduces bioavailability
$Mg(OH)_2$	High	$MgCl_2$	Low	Diarrhea, hypermagnesemia (in patients with renal insufficiency)

the meal. The dose-response relationship of antacids is variable, depending on the gastric secretory capacity (some individuals are "hypersecretors," some "hyposecretors") and the rate at which the antacid is emptied from the stomach. In addition, as implied by the discussion of the individual antacid compounds, antacids vary widely in their potency. The relative amounts of the various compounds and their reactivity will not be clear on the product label. However, commercially available antacids vary as much as sevenfold in in vitro acid-neutralizing capacity. Antacids can be effective in promoting healing of duodenal ulcers. Their benefit in gastric ulcers is less clear. In the best controlled trial of duodenal ulcer therapy, 140 meq of antacid given 1 and 3 hours after each meal and at bedtime accelerated the healing of duodenal ulcers, although pain relief was not much better than that seen with placebo. Different doses of antacid are required to achieve this degree of neutralizing capability, depending on the commercial product used (Table 64–2). Tablet antacids are generally weak in their neutralizing capability, and a large number of tablets would be required for this high-dose regimen. They are not recommended for the treatment of active peptic ulcer. Thus, an optimum antacid regimen for active peptic ulcer disease—one that would maxi-

mally neutralize gastric acid throughout a 24-hour period—would use 140 meq of a liquid antacid given 1 and 3 hours after meals and at bedtime. The actual volume of antacid given should be adjusted to provide 140 meq of acid-neutralizing effect. A final important variable, as noted above, is palatability. Patients will often state a strong preference for one antacid over another.

As noted earlier, some studies suggest that accelerated healing may also occur with tablet or liquid antacids at doses far lower than those necessary to neutralize gastric acid. It is possible that the beneficial effects of antacids reflect something other than simple neutralization of gastric acid. Aluminum compounds may act via a direct cytoprotective action or by binding injurious substances.

Adverse reactions to antacids often include a change in bowel habits. As indicated in Table 64–1, magnesium salts often have a cathartic effect, and aluminum hydroxide may be constipating. These problems can be managed by either combining or alternating compounds with these effects. Other potential problems with antacids relate to cation absorption (sodium, magnesium, aluminum, calcium) and systemic alkalosis. Fortunately, these become clinical problems only in patients with renal impairment. In

Table 64–2. Representative liquid antacids.

Proprietary Preparation	Ingredients	Acid-Neutralizing Capability (meq/mL)	Volume Required to Neutralize 140 meq (mL)	Sodium Content (mg/dose)	Cost of High-Dose Regimen[1]
Alternagel	Aluminum hydroxide	3.2	44	17	$148
Amphojel	Aluminum hydroxide	1.3	107	150	$301
Gelusil	Aluminum hydroxide, magnesium hydroxide, simethicone	4.8	29	7.5	$ 98
Maalox	Aluminum hydroxide, magnesium hydroxide	2.7	52	14	$132
Maalox HRF	Aluminum hydroxide, magnesium hydroxide	5.7	25	4.0	$107
Mylanta-DS	Aluminum hydroxide, magnesium hydroxide, simethicone	5.1	27	6.2	$ 90

[1]Cost to the pharmacist of 1 month's treatment with high-dose regimen (see text) based on manufacturers' listings in *Drug Topics Red Book 1994*.

large doses, the sodium content of some antacids may become an important factor in patients with congestive heart failure. Antacids have long been a mainstay of therapy for gastroesophageal reflux. However, they appear to have little impact on the natural history of the disease. Antacid in combination with alginic acid (Gaviscon) does lead to reduced acid reflux and symptomatic improvement. Antacids have been used for pain relief from esophagitis, gastric ulcer, and duodenal ulcer. However, placebo-controlled trials have shown no effect of a single "effective" antacid dose for pain relief in any of these conditions.

GASTRIC ANTISECRETORY DRUGS

Gastric acid secretion is under the control of three principal agonists: histamine, acetylcholine, and gastrin (Figure 64–1). The final common pathway is through the proton pump H^+/K^+ ATPase. Inhibitors of the activities of the first two secretagogues and of the proton pump have been developed.

H_2-Receptor Antagonists

Since their introduction in the mid 1970s, these compounds have gained wide acceptance. The four drugs in use in the USA are **cimetidine, ranitidine, famotidine,** and **nizatidine** (see Chapter 16). These agents are capable of over 90% reduction in basal, food-stimulated, and nocturnal secretion of gastric

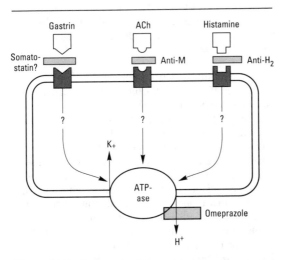

Figure 64–1. Schematic diagram of hormonal and pharmacologic control of hydrogen ion secretion by the gastric parietal cell.(Anti-M, antimuscarinic agents; anti-H_2, histamine H_2-blocking drugs.) The intracellular events are not completely understood (question marks). Some recent evidence places the histamine receptor, and possibly the cholinoceptor, on nearby tissue cells rather than on the parietal cell itself.

acid after a single dose. Many trials have demonstrated their effectiveness in promoting the healing of duodenal and gastric ulcers and preventing their recurrence. It is also apparent that these medications are essentially equally effective in treating these conditions. In addition, they are important in the medical management of Zollinger-Ellison syndrome and gastric hypersecretory states seen in systemic mastocytosis.

A. Dosage: Suppression of nocturnal acid secretion appears to be the most important determinant of the rate of healing of duodenal ulcers. Whereas previous recommendations were to administer these agents at least twice a day, a single bedtime dose may be just as effective and may elicit better compliance. For active ulcer, cimetidine can be given in doses of 400–600 mg twice daily or 800 mg at bedtime; ranitidine and nizatidine can be given in a dosage of 150 mg twice daily or 300 mg at bedtime; and famotidine can be given at 20 mg twice daily or 40 mg at bedtime. To prevent recurrence, half of the above bedtime doses can be given daily at bedtime.

B. Toxicity: All of the H_2-receptor antagonists have been generally well tolerated with few side effects reported. The longest clinical experience has been with cimetidine; there have been reports relating this drug to confusional states, particularly in elderly patients. Cimetidine therapy, particularly when prolonged and at high doses, may cause reversible gynecomastia. This has been reported only rarely with ranitidine and famotidine. Cimetidine is known to cause a dose-dependent elevation in serum prolactin and may alter estrogen metabolism in men. Headache occurs in 34% of people taking famotidine or ranitidine. Reversible hematologic abnormalities have been a rare occurrence with all members of this class of drugs. Cimetidine also slows hepatic microsomal metabolism of some drugs, such as warfarin, theophylline, diazepam, and phenytoin. Ranitidine appears to have less effect and famotidine and nizatidine no effect on hepatic drug metabolism.

C. Combination Therapy: Although combinations of H_2-receptor antagonists and antacids are widely prescribed, there is little rationale for this potentially expensive practice. Although higher 24-hour intragastric pH has been reported in patients receiving this combination, no benefit with respect to either accelerated healing or the promotion of pain relief has been demonstrated.

D. Refractory Disease: Intractability (lack of response to H_2 blockers or antacids) of peptic ulcers remains a problem, especially among older people and cigarette smokers, and as many as 20% of ulcers will fail to heal with 4 weeks of conventional therapy. Alternative pharmacologic approaches to failure of a course of an H_2-blocker include using a higher dose or prolonged course of the initial agent, switching to another H_2-receptor antagonist, or switching to a "cytoprotective" agent. All have been shown to be effective in small trials. In patients who are demonstrated to have *H pylori* infection, intractability warrants a trial of the combination of antibiotics and bismuth (see below). Patients with Zollinger-Ellison syndrome often require higher doses of an H_2-blocker, eg, up to 2400 mg/d of cimetidine.

Antimuscarinic Agents

Cholinoceptor antagonists (discussed in greater detail in Chapter 8) are now most useful as adjuncts to H_2-receptor antagonists, especially in those patients refractory to treatment with the latter or those with nocturnal pain. **Pirenzepine,** an antimuscarinic agent with activity relatively selective for gastric M_1 muscarinic receptors, is under investigation and may prove more useful in ulcer therapy. **Tricyclic antidepressants** (discussed in Chapter 29) also may promote the healing of peptic ulcers, but their precise mechanism of action (H_2-receptor blockade, antimuscarinic, or both) is not clear, and careful clinical trials have not been done (Ries, 1984).

Proton Pump Inhibitors

Omeprazole is a substituted benzimidazole that irreversibly inhibits the gastric parietal cell proton pump (H^+/K^+ ATPase; Figure 64–1). The drug requires activation in the acid environment of the secretory canaliculus of the parietal cell, ie, it is a prodrug and probably acts from the external side of the membrane. A single daily dose can inhibit essentially 100% of gastric acid secretion. Omeprazole is now approved for the treatment of severe gastroesophageal reflux disease or disease that is unresponsive to other treatment and for short-term treatment of active duodenal ulcers. It is also used for pathologic hypersecretory syndromes such as Zollinger-Ellison syndrome, multiple endocrine neoplasias, and systemic mastocytosis. The initial dose is 60 mg once daily. Omeprazole given 3 days per week has been shown to prevent recurrence of duodenal ulcers. Duodenal ulcer prevention and prophylaxis for reflux disease are not yet approved indications for this drug, however. Safety concerns with omeprazole relate to the effects of prolonged complete suppression of acid secretion on bacterial colonization of the stomach and on hypergastrinemia. In rats, chronic administration of large doses of omeprazole causes development of gastric carcinoid tumors. This has not been reported in humans, and omeprazole appears to be safe in trials to date. A second drug of this class, **lansoprazole,** is under investigation.

Octreotide

Octreotide is a long-acting synthetic somatostatin analogue. It has been found to significantly inhibit the secretion of several circulating peptide hormones and to inhibit gastric and pancreatic secretion. Although no controlled prospective trials have been reported, several patients with Zollinger-Ellison syndrome have been treated with octreotide, with some reporting symptomatic improvement and others reporting decreased size of metastases or slowed tumor growth. There is also evidence that in patients with portal hypertension due to chronic liver disease, octreotide can lower portal pressures and reduce the risk of variceal hemorrhage—though renal function may be impaired in some individuals. Because the drug requires parenteral administration, its use for these indications will be limited. However, its apparent effectiveness will further stimulate the search for orally active somatostatin analogues.

MUCOSAL PROTECTIVE AGENTS

Sucralfate

Sucralfate, or aluminum sucrose sulfate, is a sulfated disaccharide developed for use in peptic ulcer disease. Its mechanism of action is thought to involve selective binding to necrotic ulcer tissue, where it may act as a barrier to acid, pepsin, and bile. In addition, sucralfate may directly absorb bile salts. Finally, the drug may stimulate endogenous prostaglandin synthesis. Whatever the mechanism, sucralfate has been shown to be effective in the healing of duodenal ulcers. It is poorly absorbed systemically (though rising blood levels have been documented in patients with renal failure), and few adverse effects have been reported. The dosage is 1 g 4 times daily on an empty stomach (at least 1 hour before meals). It also requires an acid pH to be activated and so should not be administered simultaneously with antacids or an H_2-receptor antagonist.

Colloidal Bismuth Compounds

Like sucralfate, bismuth compounds also appear to work by selective binding to an ulcer, coating it and protecting it from acid and pepsin. Other postulated mechanisms of action include inhibition of pepsin activity, stimulation of mucous production, and increased prostaglandin synthesis. They may also have some antimicrobial activity against *H pylori* although this has been disputed. When combined with antibiotics such as metronidazole and tetracycline, ulcer healing rates of up to 98% have been seen. The cost and potential toxicity of this regimen may limit its use to serious ulcers or patients subject to frequent relapses. **Bismuth subsalicylate** (Pepto-Bismol[R]) has been used in these trials in the USA. **Tripotassium dicitrato bismuthate** has been extensively tested in Europe and shown to be superior to placebo in the healing of both duodenal and gastric ulcers. Adverse effects have been minimal, and the encephalopathy reported with long-term use of other bismuth compounds has not been noted.

Carbenoxolone

Carbenoxolone is a synthetic derivative of glycyrrhizic acid (an agent extracted from licorice) and has been shown to be effective in healing both gastric and duodenal ulcers. The mechanism of action of carbenoxolone is not clear but is thought to involve an increase in the production, secretion, and viscosity of intestinal mucus. Although its ulcer-healing properties are evident, the drug has a major aldosterone-like side effect, so that hypertension, fluid retention, and hypokalemia have limited its clinical usefulness. The concurrent administration of spironolactone controls the fluid retention but also abolishes the ulcer-healing effect; thiazides prevent sodium retention without abolishing the beneficial effect in peptic disease. Carbenoxolone, though widely used in Europe, is investigational in the USA.

Prostaglandins

These derivatives of arachidonic acid are discussed in detail in Chapter 18. Misoprostol, a methyl analogue of prostaglandin E_1, is now approved for the prevention of ulcers induced by the administration of nonsteroidal anti-inflammatory drugs (NSAIDs). Although prostaglandins are produced by the gastric mucosa and are thought to have a cytoprotective effect, at the doses needed in experimental animals to prevent or heal ulcers, the principal mechanism of action of prostaglandins appears to be inhibition of gastric secretion. This effect may be mediated through inhibition of histamine-stimulated cAMP production. Cyclic AMP is thought to be the major second messenger for histamine-induced acid secretion. Misoprostol causes a dose-dependent diarrhea, and its stimulant effect on the uterus makes it contraindicated in women of childbearing potential. The optimal role of misoprostol in ulcer treatment is difficult to define. Routine clinical prophylaxis of NSAID-induced ulcers may not be justified except in patients

with recent or current ulcers in whom NSAID use cannot be discontinued.

DRUGS PROMOTING GASTROINTESTINAL MOTILITY

Cholinergic mechanisms are responsible for modulating motor phenomena in the gut; thus it is not surprising that cholinomimetic agents such as **bethanechol** are effective in promoting gastrointestinal motility.

Metoclopramide and **cisapride** are promoted as more selective motility stimulants (prokinetic agents). In addition to its cholinomimetic properties, metoclopramide is a potent dopamine antagonist. Both drugs apparently release acetylcholine from cholinergic neurons in the enteric nervous system's myenteric plexus. They may also sensitize intestinal smooth muscle cells to the action of acetylcholine. They do not increase gastric or pancreatic secretion. These drugs hasten esophageal clearance, raise lower esophageal sphincter pressure, accelerate gastric emptying, and shorten small bowel transit time. Metoclopramide's central dopamine antagonist effect is thought to be responsible for its significant antiemetic properties, an action that cisapride appears to lack.

Clinical applications follow these effects. Metoclopramide is useful for facilitating small bowel intubation. In addition, in patients with gastric motor failure—particularly diabetic gastroparesis but possibly also after vagotomy and in other disorders of gastric emptying–metoclopramide and cisapride can produce significant symptomatic relief (Drenth, 1992). In patients with chronic gastroesophageal reflux disease,

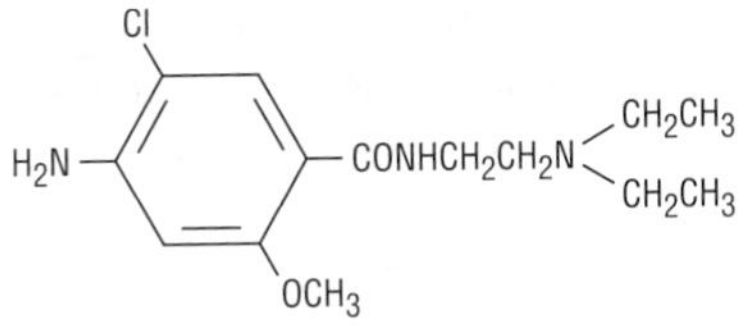

Metoclopramide

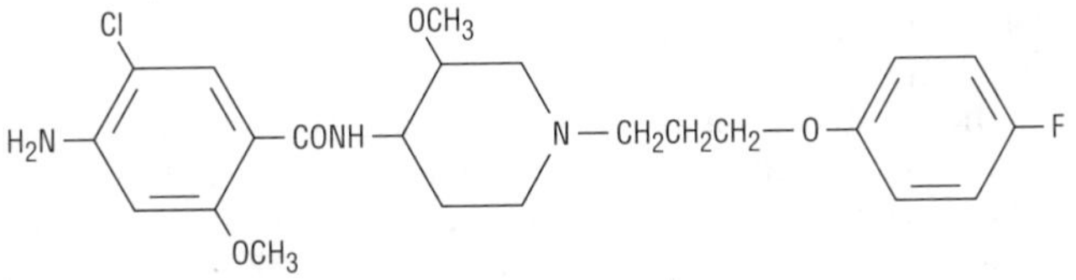

Cisapride

both agents are effective in decreasing the incidence of heartburn, though long-term effects are uncertain. Finally, metoclopramide is an effective antiemetic, particularly useful in association with cancer chemotherapy and in emergency surgery or labor and delivery to prevent aspiration of gastric contents. Both drugs are rapidly absorbed, with peak concentrations after a single oral dose seen in 40–120 minutes. Their plasma half-lives are 2–4 hours.

The usual dose of metoclopramide is 10 mg 4 times daily with meals and at bedtime. Larger doses (up to 1–2 mg/kg) have been used in conjunction with cancer chemotherapy. A dose of 20 mg given by slow intravenous infusion is used for small bowel intubation. The most common side effects of metoclopramide are somnolence, nervousness, and dystonic reactions. Parkinsonism and tardive dyskinesia have also been reported. The drug also causes increased pituitary prolactin release, and galactorrhea and menstrual disorders have been reported. Cisapride is currently labeled only for use in gastroesophageal reflux ("heartburn"), and the recommended dosage is 10 mg 4 times a day. In clinical trials in patients with diabetic gastroparesis, 5–10 mg of cisapride appeared to improve gastric emptying significantly.

Erythromycin, a macrolide antibiotic described elsewhere, has prokinetic activity in the stomach as a motilin agonist. It appears to be clinically effective in conditions such as diabetic gastroparesis and intestinal pseudo-obstruction.

ANTIEMETIC DRUGS

Nausea and vomiting may be manifestations of a wide variety of conditions, including pregnancy, motion sickness, gastrointestinal obstruction, peptic ulcer, drug toxicity, myocardial infarction, renal failure, and hepatitis. In cancer chemotherapy, drug-induced nausea and vomiting may occur so regularly that anticipatory vomiting occurs when patients return for treatment—before the chemotherapeutic agent is given. If not controlled, the discomfort associated with drug-induced emesis may cause a patient to refuse further chemotherapy.

The physiologic mechanisms responsible for nausea and vomiting are not fully understood. Coordination of the complex motor activity of the stomach and abdominal musculature takes place in the "vomiting center," which is located in the reticular formation in the medulla. The vomiting center receives input from the chemoreceptor trigger zone located on the floor of the fourth ventricle, the vestibular apparatus, and other areas. The trigger zone responds to chemical stimuli such as cancer chemotherapeutic agents, apparently through activation of dopamine or serotonin receptors.

The major categories of antiemetic agents include H_1 antihistamines, phenothiazines, metoclopramide, and ondansetron.

The antihistamines with good antiemetic activity (eg, diphenhydramine, hydroxyzine) possess significant antimuscarinic and sedative effects (see Chapter 16). It appears probable that both of these actions and the H_1-blocking effect contribute to the antiemetic efficacy. They are particularly effective for the nausea and vomiting associated with motion sickness, perhaps because of specific depression of conduction in the vestibulocerebellar pathway. Anticholinergic agents, especially scopolamine, are also used to prevent motion sickness (Chapter 8).

The phenothiazines block dopamine receptors in the chemoreceptor trigger zone as well as other areas of the brain (see Chapter 28). Prochlorperazine and promethazine are often used as antiemetics. Although nearly all phenothiazines possess some antiemetic activity, their use is limited by the degree of sedation associated with the antiemetic action. Extrapyramidal symptoms, especially dystonias, can be severe when large doses are used to combat the nausea and vomiting associated with chemotherapy. The dystonias can usually be reversed by intravenous administration of 50 mg of diphenhydramine.

Metoclopramide also acts as a dopamine antagonist (see above) and has been used in the prevention and treatment of nausea and vomiting. **Ondansetron**, a 5-HT$_3$ inhibitor, is also approved for use in the prevention of chemotherapy-induced and postoperative nausea and vomiting (see Chapter 16). Marijuana derivatives, including tetrahydrocannabinol (THC, dronabinol) itself are effective antiemetics in some patients, including some in whom other antiemetics are ineffective. Dronabinol is approved for this indication. The mechanism of action of this drug is not known but appears to involve receptors in the chemoreceptor trigger zone. Corticosteroids are antiemetics, but their mechanism is unknown. Finally, sedative-hypnotics such as the benzodiazepines are often used to control anticipatory nausea and vomiting.

PANCREATIC ENZYME REPLACEMENT PRODUCTS

Steatorrhea occurs in pancreatic insufficiency when lipase output is reduced below 10% of normal. It is estimated that in the postprandial period, approximately 100,000 units of lipase are delivered to the intestinal lumen per hour. Thus, the goal of pancreatic enzyme replacement should be to deliver at least 10,000 units per hour. However, because of inactivation of the enzyme below pH 4.0, only about 8% of the ingested lipase activity reaches the distal duodenum. Different pancreatic enzyme preparations vary markedly in enzyme activity. Manufacturers' listings of enzyme content may not always match a well-standardized in vitro laboratory assay. Two major types of preparation in use are pancreatin, an alcoholic extract of hog pancreas, and pancrelipase, a lipase-enriched hog pancreas preparation. The enzyme content of several pancreatic enzyme preparations as measured by in vitro assay is given in Table 64–3. As indicated in the table, variation in enzyme content can be partly compensated for by increases in dosage; the in vivo response–measured as reduction in stool fat and nitrogen—can be appreciable. Various dosage schedules have been recommended for pancreatic enzyme replacement, but there appears to be little difference between giving the medication with meals and giving it every 2 hours through the day. Because individual dosage requirements vary, it is essential that the result of therapy—the daily stool fat excretion—be monitored and the number of capsules or tablets increased until a therapeutic effect is seen. Supplementing the regimen with cimetidine enhances the effectiveness of the enzymes, presumably by decreasing the destruction of enzyme activity by gastric acid. Because the enzyme preparations have a high purine content, uric acid renal stones may be seen as a side effect. Also, the lactose in the pills may be sufficient to cause symptoms in lactose-intolerant patients. Finally, pancreatic enzyme replacement is expensive, costing up to $1500 per year for adequate therapy. Ineffectiveness of generic brands of enzyme preparations has been reported; bioequivalence studies are not required of these products (Hendeles, 1990).

LAXATIVES

Laxatives of various types are widely prescribed and more widely purchased without prescription, indicating a cultural preoccupation with "regularity." These drugs are generally classified by simplified mechanism of action as irritants or stimulants, bulking agents, and stool softeners. However, laxatives work through more complex actions such as the interaction of osmotic effects with epithelial transport, changes in the enteric nervous system, and the release of extracellular regulators such as prostaglandins.

IRRITANT OR STIMULANT LAXATIVES

Castor oil is hydrolyzed in the upper small intestine to ricinoleic acid, a local irritant that increases intestinal motility. The onset of action is prompt and continues until the compound is excreted via the colon. **Cascara, senna,** and **aloes** contain emodin alkaloids that are liberated after absorption from the intestine and are excreted into the colon, where peristalsis is stimulated. Thus, their onset of activity is delayed for 6–8 hours. Chronic stimulation of the colon is thought to lead to chronic colonic distention and perpetuation of the perceived need for laxatives. **Phenolphthalein** and **bisacodyl,** which are chemically similar, are also potent colonic stimulants. Their action may be prolonged by an enterohepatic circulation.

BULK LAXATIVES

Hydrophilic colloids, prepared from the indigestible parts of fruits, vegetables, and seeds, form gels within the large intestine, distending the intestine and thereby stimulating its peristaltic activity. Agar, psyllium seed, and methylcellulose all act in this manner as well. Bran and other forms of vegetable fiber have the same effect. **Saline cathartics** such as magnesium citrate and magnesium hydroxide also distend the bowel and stimulate its contractions. These nonabsorbable salts hold water in the intestine by osmotic force and cause distention. Isosmotic electrolyte solutions containing polyethylene glycol serve as colonic lavage solutions, chiefly in preparation for radiologic or endoscopic procedures and for removal of ingested toxins. **Lactulose** is a synthetic disaccharide (galac-

Table 64–3. Enzyme activities in some pancreatic enzyme replacement products. (nd = data not available.)

Proprietary Preparation	Amount (Units per Tablet or Capsule)			Number of Tablets or Capsules per Meal	Percentage Reduction in Feces	
	Lipase	Trypsin	Amylase		Fat	Nitrogen
Ilozyme[1]	3600	3444	329,600	3	48	nd
Cotazyme[1]	2014	1797	499,200	5	nd	35
Pancrease[1]	2005	nd	nd	3	73	40
Viokase[1]	1636	1828	277,333	6	49	40

[1]Generic pancrelipase.

tose-fructose) that is not absorbed, thus acting as an osmotic laxative when given in doses of 10–20 g up to 4 times daily.

STOOL SOFTENERS

Agents that become emulsified with stool serve to soften it and make passage easier. Examples are **mineral oil, glycerin suppositories,** and detergents such as **dioctyl sodium sulfosuccinate (docusate).**

ANTIDIARRHEAL DRUGS

The two most widely used prescription drugs for diarrhea are **diphenoxylate** (with atropine), a weak analogue of meperidine, and **loperamide,** which is chemically related to haloperidol. Loperamide is also available without prescription. **Difenoxin** is the active metabolite of diphenoxylate and is available as a prescription medication. Their mechanism of action on the gut is similar to that of the opioids (see Chapter 30) and involves inhibition of acetylcholine release through presynaptic opioid receptors in the enteric nervous system. Loperamide may not cross the blood-brain barrier and thus may cause less sedation and be less addicting than diphenoxylate. None of these drugs should be used in patients with severe ulcerative colitis, since toxic megacolon may be precipitated. It has been suggested that these drugs may prolong the duration of diarrhea in patients with *Shigella* or *Salmonella* infection. On the other hand, in patients with irritable bowel syndrome with predominant diarrhea, loperamide in doses of 2–4 mg 4 times a day may lead to substantial clinical improvement, especially when combined with increased dietary fiber, use of anticholinergic agents as antispasmodics, and supportive counseling. Adsorbents such as **kaolin** and **pectin** are also widely used. Their action is through their ability to adsorb compounds from solution, presumably binding potential intestinal toxins. Overall, however, they are much less effective than the drugs mentioned above, and they may also interfere with the absorption of other medications. Experimental and clinical observations indicate that α_2-adrenoceptor agonists such as clonidine can reduce electrolyte secretion by the bowel in conditions like diabetic diarrhea (Fedorak, 1985). Similar α_2-selective drugs with reduced transport into the central nervous system are being investigated for this purpose.

DRUGS USED FOR THE DISSOLUTION OF GALLSTONES

Cholesterol is solubilized in aqueous bile by the combined effect of bile acids and lecithin, which, together with cholesterol, form the mixed micelle. When cholesterol is secreted in bile in relative excess to lecithin and bile acids, cholesterol crystals precipitate and may coalesce into cholesterol gallstones. Patients with these stones may have impaired bile salt secretion, excess cholesterol secretion, or some combination of both.

Oral Therapy

Chenodiol, a primary bile acid in man, and **ursodiol,** the 7β epimer of chenodiol, are both effective in dissolving cholesterol stones in some patients. Both compounds expand the total bile salt pool, but their principal effect appears to be more complicated. Chenodiol inhibits the rate-limiting enzyme of the conversion of bile salts to cholesterol, HMG-CoA reductase, thus causing an increase in bile salt excretion and a decrease in cholesterol secretion. Ursodiol causes the transport of cholesterol in a liquid crystal form, and it appears also to stabilize the canalicular membrane of hepatocytes. In addition, as 7β epimers do not appear to exert suppression of 7α-hydroxylase, the rate-limiting enzyme for bile acid synthesis, the addition of ursodiol to the bile acid pool does not cause hepatic bile acid synthesis to be down-regulated. These physicochemical differences between the two compounds probably account for some of the differences in their toxicities.

The use of chenodiol is limited by adverse effects. A dose-related diarrhea is seen in up to 30% of patients, and a similar percentage will have increased serum transaminase or cholesterol levels. Ursodiol appears to have substantially fewer adverse effects, but it is more expensive. Studies are now in progress to determine whether a combination of ursodiol with chenodiol can be effective at reduced cost and toxicity.

These agents are most effective in dissolving small (< 5 mm) floating stones in a functioning gallbladder. They cannot dissolve stones that are more than 4% calcium by weight; unfortunately, stones with lower calcium concentrations are not often radiopaque and will not be discovered. Thus, many patients will be poor candidates or will not respond with complete dissolution of their stones even with 2 years of therapy. In addition, the recurrence rate after therapy is stopped is sufficiently high that lifelong therapy may be considered for patients who respond well to an initial course of treatment. An alternative to pharmacologic treatment—shock wave lithotripsy—may have its benefits enhanced by the concurrent administration of chenodiol or ursodiol. This combination is under investigation.

Other conditions in which these agents have been tried include cholestatic disorders of the liver and biliary tree. Recent studies have indicated that ursodiol is effective in primary biliary cirrhosis and sclerosing cholangitis. The exact mechanism is unknown, but it is postulated that by modifying the endogenous bile acid pool, ursodiol reverses the intracellular accumulation of toxic bile acids. Therapeutic trials show an improvement in both hepatic enzyme levels and histopathology.

Other Drugs

Methyl *tert*-butyl ether can dissolve cholesterol stones in the gallbladder and bile ducts when it is infused via a catheter directly into the gallbladder or bile duct lumen. The ether has a boiling point of 52.2 °C and thus remains liquid at body temperature. Ethers are excellent solvents for lipids, and dissolution of stones can usually be accomplished within hours. The exact therapeutic role of methyl *tert*-butyl ether remains to be defined, and it is likely that for now it will be reserved for selected patients who are not surgical candidates. **Monoctanoin** (glyceryl-1-monooctanoate) is another agent that is infused into the common bile duct through a catheter or T tube to dissolve retained bile duct stones. Stones may be completely dissolved or sufficiently reduced in size to facilitate their subsequent removal.

DRUGS USED IN THE TREATMENT OF CHRONIC INFLAMMATORY BOWEL DISEASE

The principal drugs used in the treatment of chronic inflammatory bowel disease (ulcerative colitis, Crohn's disease) are corticosteroids and other immunosuppressive agents and salicylate derivatives.

Salicylates

Most evidence suggests that nonabsorbed 5-aminosalicylic acid (5-ASA) is an active anti-inflammatory agent in inflammatory bowel disease. 5-Aminosalicylic acid (mesalamine) can affect multiple sites in the arachidonic acid pathway critical in the pathogenesis of inflammation. Although its interruption of the cyclooxygenase pathway would inhibit prostaglandin production, recent studies suggest that leukotriene formation is also inhibited and may be more important. The drug may also act as a free-radi-

cal scavenger. Further studies are needed to answer these questions.

Unfortunately, 5-ASA itself cannot be taken orally in sufficient dosage to produce a useful effect in the colon without excessive upper gastrointestinal tract irritation and systemic toxicity. **Sulfasalazine** combines sulfapyridine with 5-aminosalicylic acid linked by an azo bond. The drug is poorly absorbed from the intestine, and the azo linkage is broken down by the bacterial flora in the distal ileum and colon to release 5-ASA. Sulfasalazine was first introduced in the 1940s for the treatment of rheumatoid arthritis. It was subsequently shown to be effective in mildly to moderately active ulcerative colitis and Crohn's colitis but less so in Crohn's disease of the small intestine. In ulcerative colitis, it is more effective in maintaining than in achieving clinical remission.

The usual therapeutic dose of sulfasalazine is 3–4 g/d in divided doses. Smaller doses, usually 2 g/d, are needed to maintain remission in ulcerative colitis. Dose-related side effects such as malaise, nausea, abdominal discomfort, or headache occur in up to 20% of patients given 4 g/d. Some of these effects may be avoided by beginning at a lower dose and slowly increasing to the desired dosage level or by using enteric-coated or liquid suspension preparations. The inhibition of folic acid absorption by sulfasalazine has been reported, so supplemental folate should be administered. Finally, as with other sulfonamides, serum sickness-like reactions and severe bone marrow suppression have occasionally been seen.

Three other oral forms of 5-aminosalicylate have been developed that can deliver the active moiety to the distal bowel while avoiding the toxicity of sulfapyridine as well as excessive systemic absorption of 5-ASA. **Olsalazine** links two 5-ASA molecules via a diazo bond that is broken down by bacterial action in the colon, releasing the active agent. **Balsalazide** (investigational) links 5-ASA to an inert carrier via a diazo bond, which can be similarly broken down in the colon. 5-ASA itself is available (as **mesalamine**) in two forms: as an enema (see below) and in slow-release microspheres for oral administration. Controlled trials have shown encouraging results in mild and moderate ulcerative colitis and Crohn's disease. Currently, mesalamine is approved only for treatment of active colitis, and olsalazine is approved only for maintenance of remission. These drugs all appear to be well tolerated. The most frequent adverse effect is watery diarrhea, which occurs in 15–35% of patients receiving olsalazine and is thought to be caused by the drug's secretagogue properties. In addition, 5-ASA appears to be responsible for the rarely observed exacerbation of ulcerative colitis associated with sulfasalazine. All of these newer preparations are more expensive than sulfasalazine, and their clinical advantages in patients tolerant of this drug remain to be demonstrated. Topical 5-ASA, delivered in a retention enema or as a suppository, has proved effective in the treatment of active distal colitis and is approved for use. A full response may require months, however, and enemas will reach, at best, only to the splenic flexure. Fortunately, topical therapy has also proved effective as prophylaxis against recurrence in patients who have achieved remission.

Immunosuppressive agents

Immunosuppressive agents applied in inflammatory bowel disease include the corticosteroids, which have been used for many years to control acute episodes, and cytotoxic drugs. Both ACTH and standard corticosteroids such as hydrocortisone and prednisone have been used with comparable clinical efficacy. Topical corticosteroids given in enema form are effective for patients with distal colitis, but over the long term their use may be associated with the same side effects as are seen with systemic corticosteroids. Studies of newer topical preparations with the same anti-inflammatory effects but no systemic effects, such as tixocortol pivalate, have been promising. However, none of these compounds are yet available in the USA. Cytotoxic agents, particularly azathioprine and mercaptopurine, are being used more often in the treatment of inflammatory bowel disease. Their steroid-sparing properties can be beneficial to patients with Crohn's disease and ulcerative colitis, and they seem to be particularly helpful in the treatment of fistulas complicating Crohn's disease. Both drugs appear to be more effective than corticosteroids as prophylaxis in patients with Crohn's disease. The doses used are relatively low, beginning at 50 mg/d and not exceeding 1.5 mg/kg daily. At these dose levels, hematologic complications are minimized al-

though careful monitoring is still essential. In addition, the long-term risk of drug-induced malignancy would seem to be minimal at these doses. Cyclosporine may also be of value in these conditions, but its toxicity may limit its application in chronic therapy.

DRUGS USED IN THERAPY OF PORTAL-SYSTEMIC ENCEPHALOPATHY

The broad-spectrum, nonabsorbable antibiotic neomycin (see Chapter 45) has been combined with dietary restriction of protein for the treatment of portal-systemic encephalopathy. **Lactulose** is also effective in this condition. The mechanism of action of lactulose is unclear. It is apparently degraded by intestinal bacteria to lactic acid, acetic acid, and other organic acids. It is thought that this may facilitate the "trapping" of ammonium ion or other putative central nervous system toxins in the intestinal tract. Modification of the normal intestinal flora by lactulose has been suggested as another mechanism of action, but this has not been demonstrated with certainty. Lactulose is available as a syrup and is given in doses of 15–30 mL 4 times daily or until the patient has four or five soft bowel movements daily. The drug is well tolerated and may be given in combination with neomycin, although this combination has no clear advantage over lactulose alone. Lactulose may also be administered as an enema.

PREPARATIONS AVAILABLE
(See Table 64–2 for antacid preparations.)

H₂ Histamine Receptor Blockers
Cimetidine (Tagamet)
Oral: 200, 300, 400, 800 mg tablets; 300 mg/5 mL liquid
Parenteral: 300 mg/2 mL aqueous injection; 300 mg/50 mL (0.9% sodium chloride)
Famotidine (Pepcid)
Oral: 20, 40 mg tablets; 400 mg powder to reconstitute for 40 mg/5 mL suspension
Parenteral: 10 mg/mL for injection
Nizatidine (Axid)
Oral: 150, 300 mg capsules
Ranitidine (Zantac)
Oral: 150, 300 mg tablets; syrup, 15 mg/mL
Parenteral: 0.5, 25 mg/mL for injection

Anticholinergic Drugs
Anisotropine (generic, Valpin)
Oral: 50 mg tablets
Atropine (generic)
Oral: 0.4, 0.6 mg tablets
Parenteral: 0.05, 0.1, 0.3, 0.4, 0.5, 0.8, 1 mg/mL for injection
Clidinium (Quarzan)
Oral: 2.5, 5 mg capsules
Dicyclomine (generic, Bentyl, others)
Oral: 10, 20 mg capsules; 10 mg/5 mL syrup
Parenteral: 10 mg/mL for injection
Glycopyrrolate (generic, Robinul)
Oral: 1, 2 mg tablets
Parenteral: 0.2 mg/mL for injection

Isopropamide (Darbid)
Oral: 5 mg tablets
Mepenzolate (Cantil)
Oral: 25 mg tablets
Methantheline (Banthine)
Oral: 50 mg tablets
Methscopolamine (Pamine)
Oral: 2.5 mg tablets
Oxyphencyclimine (Daricon)
Oral: 10 mg tablets
Propantheline (generic, Pro-Banthine, others)
Oral: 7.5, 15 mg tablets
Tridihexethyl (Pathilon)
Oral: 25 mg tablets

Proton Pump Inhibitor
Omeprazole (Prilosec)
Oral (sustained-release): 20 mg capsules

Mucosal Protective Agents
Misoprostol (Cytotec)
Oral: 100, 200 μg tablets
Sucralfate (Carafate)
Oral: 1 g tablets

Drugs For Motility Disorders & Selected Antiemetics
Cisapride (Propulsid)
Oral: 10 mg tablets
Dronabinol (Marinol)
Oral: 2.5, 5, 10 mg tablets
Metoclopramide (generic, Reglan, others)
Oral: 5, 10 mg tablets; 5 mg/5 mL syrup
Parenteral: 5 mg/mL for injection
Ondansetron (Zofran)
Oral: 4, 8 mg tablets
Parenteral: 2 mg/mL for IV injection
Prochlorperazine (Compazine)
Oral: 5, 10, 25 mg tablets; 10, 15, 30 mg capsules; 1 mg/mL solution
Rectal: 2.5, 5, 25 mg suppositories
Parenteral: 5 mg/mL for injection

Selected Anti-inflammatory Drugs Used in Gastrointestinal Disease
Hydrocortisone (Cortenema, Cortifoam)
Rectal: 100 mg/60 mL unit retention enema; 90 mg/applicatorful intrarectal foam
Mesalamine (Asacol, Rowasa)
Oral: 400 mg tablets
Rectal: 4 g/60 mL suspension; 500 mg suppositories
Methylprednisolone (Medrol Enpack)
Rectal: 40 mg/bottle retention enema
Olsalazine (Dipentum)
Oral: 250 mg capsules
Sulfasalazine (generic, Azulfidine, others)

Oral: 500 mg tablets and enteric-coated tablets; 250 mg/5 mL suspension

Selected Antidiarrheal Drugs
Bismuth subsalicylate (Pepto-Bismol, others)
Oral: 262 mg chewable tablets and suspension; 524 mg/15 mL suspension
Difenoxin (Motofen)
Oral: 1 mg (with 0.025 mg atropine sulfate) tablets
Diphenoxylate (generic, Lomotil, others)
Oral: 2.5 mg (with 0.025 mg atropine sulfate) tablets and liquid
Kaolin/pectin (generic, Kaopectate, others)
Oral: 5.85 g kaolin and 130 mg pectin per 30 mL suspension
Loperamide (Imodium)
Oral: 2 mg capsules; 1 mg/5 mL liquid
Paregoric (generic)
Oral: 2 mg morphine (equivalent) per 5 mL liquid

Selected Laxative Drugs
Bisacodyl (generic, Dulcolax, others)
Oral: 5 mg tablets
Rectal: 5, 10 mg suppositories
Cascara sagrada (generic)
Oral: 325 mg tablets; 5 mL per dose fluid extract (approximately 18% alcohol)
Castor oil (generic, others)
Oral: liquid or liquid emulsion
Docusate (generic, Colace, others)
Oral: 50, 100, 240, 250 mg capsules; 100 mg tablets; 50, 60, 150 mg/15 mL syrup; 50 mg/mL solution
Glycerin suppository (generic, Sani-Supp, Fleet Babylax)
Lactulose (Chronulac, Cephulac)
Oral: 10 g/15 mL syrup
Magnesium hydroxide [milk of magnesia, Epsom Salt] (generic)
Oral: 7–8.5% aqueous suspension
Methylcellulose
Oral: 450 mg/5 mL liquid
Mineral oil (generic, others)
Oral: liquid, jelly, or emulsion
Phenolphthalein (generic, Ex-Lax, others)
Oral: 60, 90 mg tablets
Polycarbophil (Equalactin, Mitrolan, FiberCon, Fiber-Lax)
Oral: 500, 625 mg tablets; 500, 1250 mg tablets and chewable tablets
Polyethylene glycol electrolyte solution (CoLyte, GoLYTELY, others)
Oral: Powder for oral solution, makes one gallon (approx 4 L)
Psyllium (generic, Serutan, Metamucil, others)

Oral: 3.4, 3.5, 4.94 g psyllium powder per packet; 50%, 100% psyllium also available
Senna (Senokot, others)
Oral: 187, 217 mg tablets; 600 mg senna (eq) tablets; 326, 326.1 mg granules; 1.65 g senna (eq) per ½ tsp granules; 218 mg/5 mL syrup; 6.5, 7% liquid
Rectal: 652 mg suppositories

Drugs That Dissolve Gallstones
Chenodiol (Chenix)
Oral: 250 mg tablets
Monoctanoin (Moctanin)
Parenteral: 120 mL infusion bottle
Ursodiol (Actigall)
Oral: 300 mg capsules

REFERENCES

Pharmacokinetics

Lauritsen K, Laursen LS, Rask-Madsen J: Clinical pharmacokinetics of drugs used in the treatment of gastrointestinal diseases. (Two parts.) Clin Pharmacokinet 1990;19:11, 94.

Acid-Peptic Disease

Blum AL: Treatment of acid-related disorders with gastric acid inhibitors: The state of the art. Digestion 1990;47(Suppl 1):3.

Burgess E, Muruve D: Aluminum absorption and excretion following sucralfate therapy in chronic renal insufficiency. Am J Med 1992;92:471.

Chamberlain CE, Peura DA: *Campylobacter (Helicobacter) pylori:* Is peptic disease a bacterial infection? Arch Intern Med 1990;150:951.

Farup PG et al: Low-dose antacids versus 400 mg cimetidine twice daily for reflux oesophagitis: A comparative, placebo-controlled, multicentre study. Scand J Gastroenterol 1990;25:315.

Galmiche JP et al: Double-blind comparison of cisapride and cimetidine in treatment of reflux esophagitis. Dig Dis Sci 1990;35:649.

Graham DY et al: Effect of treatment of *Helicobacter pylori* infection on the long-term recurrence of gastric or duodenal ulcer: A randomized, controlled study. Ann Intern Med 1992;116:705.

Gugler R, Allgayer H: Effects of antacids on the clinical pharmacokinetics of drugs: An update. Clin Pharmacokinet 1990;18:210.

Hentschel E et al: Effect of ranitidine and amoxicillin plus metronidazole on the eradication of *Helicobacter pylori* and the recurrence of duodenal ulcer. N Engl J Med 1993;328:308.

Hetzel DJ: Controlled clinical trials of omeprazole in the long-term management of reflux disease. Digestion 1992;5(Suppl 1):35.

Hixson LJ et al: Current trends in the pharmacotherapy for gastroesophageal reflux disease. Arch Intern Med 1992;152:717.

Maton PN: Omeprazole. N Engl J Med 1991; 324:965.

Maton PN, Gardner JD, Jensen RT: Use of long-acting somatostatin analog SMS 201-995 in patients with pancreatic islet cell tumors. Dig Dis Sci 1989;34 (Suppl):28S.

Maton PN et al: The effect of Zollinger-Ellison syndrome and omeprazole therapy on gastric oxyntic endocrine cells. Gastroenterology 1990;99:943.

McCarthy DM: Sucralfate. N Engl J Med 1991;325: 1017.

Ramirez B, Richter JE: Review article: promotility drugs in the treatment of gastro-esophageal reflux disease. Aliment Pharmacol Ther 1993;7:5.

Ries RK, Gilbert DA, Katon W: Tricyclic antidepressant therapy for peptic ulcer disease. Arch Intern Med 1984;144:566.

Soll AH: Pathogenesis of peptic ulcer and implications for therapy. N Engl J Med 1990;322:909.

Soll AH (moderator): Nonsteroidal anti-inflammatory drugs and peptic ulcer disease. Ann Intern Med 1991; 114:307.

Sontag S et al: Cimetidine, cigarette smoking, and recurrence of duodenal ulcer. N Engl J Med 1984;311:689.

Walt RP: Misoprostol for the treatment of peptic ulcer and anti-inflammatory-drug-induced gastroduodenal ulceration. N Engl J Med 1992;327:1575.

Walt RP, Langman MJS: Antacids and ulcer healing. Drugs 1991;42:205.

Wilson DE: Prostaglandins in peptic ulcer disease: Their postulated role in the pathogenesis and treatment. Postgrad Med 1987;81:309.

Wolfe MM, Soll AH: The physiology of gastric acid secretion. N Engl J Med 1988;319:1707.

Motility Disorders

Binder HJ, Donowitz M: A new look at laxative action. Gastroenterology 1975;69:1001.

Drenth JPH, Engels LGJB: Diabetic gastroparesis: A critical appraisal of new treatment strategies. Drugs 1992;44:537.

Drossman DA, Thompson WG: The irritable bowel syndrome: Review and a graduated multicomponent treatment approach. Ann Intern Med 1992;116:1009.

Fedorak RN, Field M, Chang EB: Treatment of diabetic diarrhea with clonidine. Ann Intern Med 1985;102: 197.

Lynn RB, Friedman LS: Irritable bowel syndrome. N Engl J Med 1993;329:1940.

Tack J et al: Effect of erythromycin on gastric motility in controls and in diabetic gastroparesis. Gastroenterology 1992;103:72.

Gallstone Therapy

Hoffman AF: Nonsurgical treatment of gallstone disease. Annu Rev Med 1990;41:401.

Johnston DE, Kaplan MM: Pathogenesis and treatment of gallstones. N Engl J Med 1993;328:412.

Poupon RE et al: A multicenter, controlled trial of ursodiol for the treatment of primary biliary cirrhosis. N Engl J Med 1991;324:1548.

Inflammatory Bowel Disease

Klotz U et al: Therapeutic efficacy of sulfasalazine and its metabolites in patients with ulcerative colitis and Crohn's disease. N Engl J Med 1980;303:1499.

Kozarek RA: Review article: immunosuppressive therapy for inflammatory bowel disease. Aliment Pharmacol Ther 1993;7:117.

Lashner BA et al: Testing nicotine gum for ulcerative colitis patients. Dig Dis Sci 1990;35:827.

Peppercorn MA: Advances in drug therapy for inflammatory bowel disease. Ann Intern Med 1990:112:50.

Schroeder KW, Tremaine WJ, Ilstrup DM: Coated oral 5-aminosalicylic acid therapy for mildly to moderately active ulcerative colitis: A randomized study. N Engl J Med 1987;317:1625.

Shanahan F, Targan S: Medical treatment of inflammatory bowel disease. Annu Rev Med 1992;43:125.

Watkinson G: Sulphasalazine: A review of 40 years' experience. Drugs 1986;32(Suppl 1):1.

Antiemetics

Aapro MS et al: Antiemetic efficacy of droperidol or me-toclopramide combined with dexamethasone and diphenhydramine: Randomized open parallel study. Oncology 1991;48:116.

Herrstedt J et al: Ondansetron plus metopimazine compared with ondansetron alone in patients receiving moderately emetogenic chemotherapy. N Engl J Med 1993;328:1076.

Lane M et al: Dronabinol and prochlorperazine alone and in combination as antiemetic agents for cancer chemotherapy. Am J Clin Oncol 1990;13:480.

Marin J, Ibanez MC, Arribas S: Therapeutic management of nausea and vomiting. Gen Pharmacol 1990; 21:1.

Mitchelson F: Pharmacological agents affecting emesis. A review. (Two parts) Drugs 1992;43:295,443.

Stewart DJ: Cancer therapy, vomiting, and antiemetics. Can J Physiol Pharmacol 1990;68:304.

Tortorice PV, O'Connell MB: Management of chemotherapy-induced nausea and vomiting. Pharmacotherapy 1990;10:129.

Miscellaneous

Hendeles L et al: Treatment failure after substitution of generic pancrelipase capsules: Correlation with in vitro lipase activity. JAMA 1990;263:2459.

65

Therapeutic & Toxic Potential of Over-the-Counter Agents

Mary Anne Koda-Kimble, PharmD

In the USA, drugs are divided by law into two classes: those restricted to sale by prescription only and those for which directions for safe use by the public can be written. The latter category constitutes the nonprescription or over-the-counter (OTC) drugs. In 1992, the American public spent approximately $12 billion on an estimated 300,000 OTC products to medicate themselves for self-diagnosed ailments ranging from acne to warts. These 300,000 products represent about 700 active ingredients in various forms and combinations. It is thus apparent that many are no more than "me too" products advertised to the public in ways that suggest that there are significant differences between them. For example, there are over 100 different systemic analgesic products almost all of which contain aspirin, acetaminophen, salicylamide, phenacetin, ibuprofen, or a combination of these agents as primary ingredients. They are made different from one another by the addition of questionable ingredients such as caffeine or antihistamines; by brand names chosen to suggest a specific use or strength ("feminine pain," "arthritis," "maximum," "extra"); or by their special dosage form (enteric-coated tablets, liquids, sustained-release products, powders, seltzers). There is a price attached to all of these gimmicks, and in most cases a less expensive generic product can be equally effective. It is probably safe to assume that the public is generally overwhelmed and confused by the wide array of products presented and will probably use those that are most heavily advertised.

Since 1972, the Food and Drug Administration has been engaged in a methodical review of OTC ingredients for both safety and efficacy. There have been two major outcomes of this review: (1) ingredients designated as ineffective or unsafe for their claimed therapeutic use are being eliminated from OTC product formulations (eg, antimuscarinic agents have been eliminated from OTC sleep aids); and (2) agents previously available by prescription only have been made available for OTC use because they were judged by the review panel to be generally safe and effective for consumer use without medical supervision (eg, topical hydrocortisone 0.5 and 1%, diphen-

hydramine, ibuprofen, clotrimazole). Some OTC ingredients previously available in low doses only are now available in higher concentrations. Table 65–1 lists some prescription drugs that have been recommended for OTC use. Although few final regulations have been issued on these recommendations, the FDA's position has been to allow manufacturers to incorporate these ingredients into their OTC formulations upon publication of the review panel's preliminary report unless it (the FDA) finds compelling reason to dissent. Examples of other prescription drugs currently under consideration for OTC sales include H_2 antagonists, sucralfate, nonsedating antihistamines, other nonsteroidal anti-inflammatory drugs, oral contraceptives, nicotine chewing gum, albuterol, and cromolyn.

There are three reasons why it is important for the clinician to be familiar with this class of products. First, many of the ingredients contained in these products are effective in treating common ailments, and it is important to be able to help the patient select a safe, effective product. (See Table 65–2.) Second, many of the active ingredients contained in OTC drugs may worsen existing medical conditions or interact with prescription medications. (See Appendix II, Drug Interactions.) Finally, the misuse or abuse of OTC products may actually produce significant medical complications. Phenylpropanolamine, for example, a sympathomimetic included in many cold, allergy, and weight control products, has been abused by adolescents and is often sold in the illicit market as a cocaine or amphetamine substitute. In only two to three times the therapeutic dose, this drug can cause severe hypertension, seizures, and intracranial hemorrhage. A general awareness of these products and their formulation will enable clinicians to more fully appreciate the potential for OTC drug-related problems in their patients.

Table 65–2 lists examples of OTC products that may be used effectively to treat medical problems commonly encountered in ambulatory patients. The selection of one ingredient over another may be important in patients with certain medical problems or in patients taking certain prescription medications.

Table 65–1. Ingredients that have been recommended by over-the-counter (OTC) review panel to be switched from prescription to OTC status.

Ingredient and Dosage	Indication	Single-Ingredient Product Examples
Systemic		
Brompheniramine 4 mg every 4–6 hours	Antihistamine	Dimetane Extentabs
Chlorpheniramine 4 mg every 4–6 hours	Antihistamine	Chlor-Trimeton, Teldrin
Diphenhydramine hydrochloride 25–50 mg every 4–6 hours	Antihistamine Antitussive Sleep aid	Benadryl Benylin Syrup Sominex 2, Sleep-Eze 3
Doxylamine 7.5–12.5 mg every 4–6 hours	Antihistamine	None
Dyclonine hydrochloride 0.05–0.10%	Oral local anesthetic, analgesic	Sucret's maximum strength sprays
Fluoride (various salts) Sodium 0.05% rinse Stannous 0.1% rinse Acidulated phosphate 0.02% rinse	Dental caries prophylactic	None
Methoxyphenamine hydrochloride 100 mg every 4–6 hours	Bronchodilator[1]	None
Promethazine hydrochloride 6.25–12.5 mg every 8–12 hours	Antihistamine[1]	None
Pseudoephedrine hydrochloride and sulfate 60 mg every 4–6 hours	Nasal decongestant	D-Feda, Sudafed
Pyrantel pamoate 11 mg/kg as single dose	Anthelmintic (pinworms)	Reese's Pinworm Medicine
Topical		
Ephedrine sulfate 2–25%	Hemorrhoidal vasoconstrictor	None
Epinephrine hydrochloride 100–200 μg aqueous solution 4 times daily	Hemorrhoidal vasoconstrictor	None
Haloprogin 1%	Antifungal (anticandidal[1])	None
Hydrocortisone (base and various salts) 0.5–1%	Anti-inflammatory (antifungal[1]) Dandruff (seborrheic dermatitis) Antipruritic, anti-inflammatory	None Aeroseb-HC CaldeCort, Cortaid, Lanacort
Miconazole nitrate 2%	Antifungal Anticandidal	Micatin cream, spray, powder, liquid Monistat vaginal cream, suppositories
Nystatin 100,000 units/g	Anticandidal[1]	None
Oxymetazoline hydrochloride 0.1%	Nasal decongestant	Afrin, Duration, Neo-Synephrine 12 Hour
Phenylephrine hydrochloride 0.5 mg aqueous solution 4 times daily	Hemorrhoidal vasoconstrictor	None
Xylometazoline 0.1%	Nasal decongestant	Dristan Long Lasting Nasal Mist, Neo-Synephrine II Long Acting, Sine-Off Once-A-Day, Sinex Long-Acting Decongestant Nasal Spray

[1]Despite review panel recommendation, the FDA has dissented from OTC use for this application at this time.

These are discussed in detail in other chapters. The recommendations listed in Table 65–2 are based upon the efficacy of the ingredients and on the principles set forth in the following paragraphs:

(1) Select the product that is simplest in formulation with regard to ingredients and dosage form. In general, single-ingredient products are preferred. Although some combination products contain effective doses of all ingredients, others contain therapeutic doses of some ingredients and subtherapeutic doses of others. Furthermore, there may be differing durations of action among the ingredients, and there is always a possibility that the clinician or patient will be unaware of the presence of certain active ingredients in the product. Aspirin, for example, is present in many cough and cold preparations; a patient unaware

Table 65–2. Ingredients of known efficacy for selected over-the-counter (OTC) classes.

OTC Category	Ingredient and Dosage	Product Examples	Comments
Acne preparations	Benzoyl peroxide, 2.5, 5, 10%	Generic, Benoxyl, Clearasil, Oxy-5, Oxy-10	One of the most effective acne preparations. Apply sparingly once or twice daily. Decrease dose if excessive skin irritation occurs.
Allergy preparations	Chlorpheniramine, 4 mg every 4–6 hours; 12 mg every 12 hours	Generic, Chlor-Trimeton (4 mg/tab or 10 mL syrup), Long Acting Chlor-Trimeton[1] (8 mg/tab), Teldrin Time-Release Capsules[1] (8 mg and 12 mg/cap).	Antihistamines alone relieve most symptoms associated with allergic rhinitis or hay fever. Chlorpheniramine, brompheniramine, and clemastine cause less drowsiness than diphenhydramine, methapyriline, pyrilamine, doxylamine, and phentoloxamine. Occasionally, symptoms unrelieved by the antihistamine respond to the addition of a sympathomimetic.
	Brompheniramine, 4 mg every 4–6 hours; 12 mg every 12 hours	Symptom 3 (4 mg/10 mL), Dimetane Extentab[1] (12 mg).	
	Clemastine fumarate, 1.34 mg every 12 hours	Tavist-1 (1.34 mg/tab)	
	Diphenhydramine,[1] 25–50 mg every 4–6 hours	Benadryl (25 mg/cap; 12.5 mg/5 mL elixir).	
	Chlorpheniramine (4 mg) with pseudoephedrine (60 mg)	Novahistine, elixir and tabs (per 10 mL or 2 tabs); Triaminicin Allergy (per tab).	
	Clemastine fumarate (1.34 mg) with phenylpropanolamine (75 mg) every 12 hours	Tavist-D	
	Triprolidine HCl (2.5 mg) with pseudoephedrine (60 mg)	Actifed	
Analgesics and antipyretics	Aspirin, 300–600 mg every 4–6 hours	Generic, Bayer Aspirin (325 mg/tab)	There are numerous product modifications, including the addition of antacid, caffeine, and methapyriline; enteric-coated tabs and seltzers; long-acting or extra-strength formulations; and various mixtures of analgesics. None have any substantial advantage over a single-ingredient product. Acetaminophen lacks anti-inflammatory activity but is available as a liquid; this dosage form is used primarily for infants and children who cannot chew or swallow tablets. Aspirin should be used cautiously in certain individuals (see text). Avoid products that contain phenacetin, eg, A.S.A. compound, Bromo-Seltzer, A.P.C. Capsules. Extra-strength formulations contain 400–600 mg of active ingredient.
	Acetaminophen, 300–600 mg every 4–6 hours	Generic, Datril, Tylenol (325 mg/tab various strengths available).	
	Ibuprofen,[1] 200–400 mg every 4–6 hours	Generic, Advil, Nuprin, Mediprin (200 mg/tab)	
	Naproxen, 200 mg every 8–10 hours	Aleve (200 mg/tab)	
Antacids	Magnesium hydroxide and aluminum hydroxide combinations	Gelusil, Gelusil II, Maalox No.1, Maalox No. 2, Mylanta, Mylanta II, Wingel, others.	Combinations of magnesium and aluminum hydroxide are less likely to cause constipation or diarrhea and offer high neutralizing capacity. The "II" formulations are approximately twice as potent on a meq/mL basis. The products listed are liquid products with a low sodium content.
Antidiarrheal agents	Bismuth subsalicylate, 600 mg 4 times daily to prevent traveler's diarrhea	Pepto-Bismol (262 mg/tab or 524 mg/30 mL suspension).	Can turn tongue and stools black. Salicylates are absorbed and can cause tinnitus.
	Loperamide, 4 mg initially, then 2 mg after each loose stool, not to exceed 16 mg/d	Imodium (2 mg/cap or 1 mg/5 mL liquid).	A synthetic opioid that does not penetrate the CNS. Not considered a controlled substance. Avoid in febrile patients.
	Opium, powdered, 15–20 mg 1–4 times daily, not to exceed 2 days (≈ 1.5–2 mg morphine)	Diabismal suspension (0.47 mg/mL), Donnagel-PG (0.8) mg/mL), Infantol Pink (0.5 mg/mL).	A schedule V substance when combined with other antidiarrheal substances. Not available OTC in some states. Avoid use in febrile patients and those predisposed to toxic megacolon. CNS depression possible.

(continued)

OTC Category	Ingredient and Dosage	Product Examples	Comments
Antidiarrheal agents (continued)	Tincture of opium (paregoric), 4–5 mL 1–4 times daily, not to exceed 2 days. (1 mL paregoric contains 4 mg opium.)	Kaodene with Paregoric (0.125 mg/mL), Parepectolin (0.12 mg/mL).	See previous page
Antifungal topical preparations	Tolnaftate, 1% solution, cream, or powder	Generic, Aftate, Tinactin	Fungicidal. Effective for the treatment of tinea pedis, tinea cruris, and tinea corporis.
	Clotrimazole, 1% cream or 100 mg vaginal inserts[1]	Fem-Care, Gyne-Lotrimin, Mycelex 7	Clotrimazole and miconazole also effective against *Candida albicans* vaginitis. Insert one applicatorful or one insert at bedtime for 7 days.
	Miconazole nitrate, 2% cream or 100 mg vaginal tablet[1]	Monistat-7	
Anti-inflammatory topical preparations	Hydrocortisone, 0.5%	Generic, Cortaid (cream, lotion, ointment), Dermolate, Lanacort	Used to temporarily relieve itching and inflammation associated with minor rashes due to contact or allergic dermatitides, insect bites, and hemorrhoids. Apply small amounts and thoroughly rub into skin 3–4 times daily.
	Hydrocortisone, 1% cream or spray.[1]	Generic, Caldecort, Cortizone 10, Lanacort 10, Maximum Strength Cortaid	
Antiseborrheal agents	Selenium sufide, 1–2%	Selsun Blue	Both are cytostatic agents that decrease epidermal turnover rates. Work into clean scalp for 5–10 minutes 2 or 3 times weekly. Selenium sulfide can be irritating to the eyes and skin.
	Zinc pyrithione, 1–2%	Many. Breck One, Head and Shoulders	
Antitussives	Codeine, 10–20 mg every 4–6 hours (with guaifenesin)	Cheracol, Robitussin A–C (both contain 2 mg/mL).	In doses required for cough suppression, the addictive liability associated with codeine is low. Codeine is a schedule V narcotic, and its OTC sale is restricted in some states. The efficacy of expectorants, which are included in almost all antitussives, is questionable. Guaifenesin has the least potential for toxicity. Watch for hidden ingredients in these products.
	Dextromethorphan, 10–20 mg every 4 hours or 30 mg every 6 hours (with guaifenesin)	Cheracol D (2 mg/mL), 2/G-DM (3 mg/mL), Novahistine Cough Formula (5 mg/mL, Pertussin 8-Hour Cough Formula (1.5 mg/mL), Robitussin-DM (3 mg/mL).	
Decongestants	Topical Oxymetazoline	Afrin	Topical sympathomimetics are effective in the acute management of rhinorrhea associated with common colds and allergies. Long-acting agents (oxymetazoline and xylometazoline) are generally preferred, although phenylephrine is equally effective. Oral decongestants have a prolonged duration of action but may cause more systemic effects. Pseudoephedrine has the least CNS stimulatory effect. Phenylpropanolamine is also effective. Oral phenylephrine is unpredictably absorbed.
	Xylometazoline	Dristan Long Lasting Nasal Mist, Neo-Synephrine II, Sinex-L.A., Sinutab Nasal Spray	
	Phenylephrine	Allerest, Coricidin Nasal Spray, Neo-Synephrine, NTZ	
	Oral Pseudoephedrine 60 mg every 4 hours or 120 mg every 12 hours	Novafed (30 mg/5 mL), Sudafed (30 mg/tab or 5 mL),	
	Phenylpropanolamine 25 mg every 4 hours	Sudafed SA (120 mg/cap) No single-ingredient product available.	
Expectorants	Guaifenesin (20 mg/mL): age >12, 200–400 mg every 4 hours; age 6–12, 100–200 mg every 4 hours; age 2–6, 50–100 mg every 4 hours	1/G, Nortussin, Robitussin Syrups	The only expectorant ingredient listed by FDA panel as having scientific evidence of safety and efficacy.
Laxatives	Bulk formers	Metamucil, Serutan	The safest laxatives for chronic use include the bulk formers and stool softeners. Saline laxatives and stimulants may be used acutely but not chronically (see text).
	Stool softeners-docusate sodium	Generic, Colace, Coloctyl, Doxinate	
	Saline laxatives	Philips' Milk of Magnesia	

(*continued*)

Table 65–2 (cont'd). Ingredients of known efficacy for selected over-the-counter (OTC) classes.

OTC Category	Ingredient and Dosage	Product Examples	Comments
Pediculicides	Permethrin 1%	NIX Cream Rinse	Effective. Apply to dry hair and scalp, wetting entire area. Leave on for 10 minutes. Lather with water and rinse. Avoid contact with eyes. Repeat once if reinfestation occurs. comb out nits.
	Pyrethrums combined with piperonyl butoride	A-200 Pediculicide Shampoo and Gel; RID Lice Killing Shampoo	
Sleep aids	Diphenhydramine,[1] 25–50 mg at bedtime	Sominex 2, Sleep-Eze 3 (25 mg/tab or cap); Sleepinal (50 mg).	Diphenydramine, an antihistamine with well-documented CNS depressant effects, is now available over the counter for sedative use.

[1]Previously available by prescription only. Now available over the counter.

Table 65–3. Hidden ingredients in over-the-counter (OTC) products.

Hidden Drug or Drug Class	OTC Class Containing Drug	Product Examples
Alcohol (percent ethanol)	Cough syrups/cold preparations.	Breacol (10%), Cotussis (20%), Formula 44D (20%), Halls (22%), Novahistine DMX (10%), NyQuil Nighttime Cold Medicine (25%), Pertussin 8-Hour Cough Formula (9.5%), Prunicodeine (25%), Romilar III (20%), Romilar CF (20%), Tussar SF (12%)
	Mouthwashes.	Astring-O-Sol (65%), Cepacol Mouthwash/Gargle (14%), Listerine Antiseptic (75%), Scope (19%).
Antihistamines	Analgesics.	Allerest Headache Strength Tablets, Excedrin PM, Percogesic, Sinarest Tablets.
	Asthma products.	Bronitin, Primatene M.
	Cold/allergy products.	Many. Alka-Seltzer Plus, Allerest, Benylin Cough Syrup, Chlor-Trimeton, Contac, Coricidin, Co-Tylenol, Dristan, Novahistine, Ny-Quil, Sinarest, Sine-Off, Sinutab, Super Anahist, Triminic, Triaminicin, 4-Way Cold Tablets.
	Dermatologic preparations.	Pyribenzamine Cream or Ointment.
	Menstrual products.	Cardui, Pamprin, Sunril.
	Motion sickness products, antiemetics.	Bonine, Dramamine, Marezine.
	Sleep aids.	Compoz Tablets, Nervine, Nyutol, Sleep-Eze, Sominex.
	Topical decongestants.	Dristan, Sinex.
Antimuscarinic agents	Antidiarrheals.	Donnagel, Donnagel-PG.
	Coug/ cold/allergy preparations.	Sinulin Tablets.
	Hemorrhoidal products.	Wyanoids Hemorrhoidal Suppositories.
Aspirin and other salicylates	Analgesics.	Many. Alka-Seltzer, Anacin, Aspergum, Cope, Ecotrin, Excedrin, Fizrin Powder, Measurin, Persistin, Stanback Tablets and Powder, Vanquish.
	Antidiarrheals.	Pepto-Bismol (bismuth subsalicylate).
	Cold/alergy preparations.	Alka-Seltzer Plus, Congespirin, Coricidin, Dristan Tablets, Sine-Off, Triaminicin, 4-Way Cold Tablets.
	Menstrual products.	Diurex (potassium salicylate), Midol.
	Sleep aids.	Quiet World Tablets, Tranquil Capsules (sodium salicylate)

(continued)

Table 65–3 (cont'd). Hidden ingredients in over-the-counter (OTC) products.

Hidden Drug or Drug Class	OTC Class Containing Drug	Product Examples
Caffeine	Analgesics.	Anacin, Bromo-Seltzer, Cope, Excedrin, Stanback Tablets and Powder, Vanquish.
	Cold/allergy products.	Coryban D, Dristan, Super Anahist, Triaminicin.
	Menstrual/diuretic products.	Aqua-Ban, Midol, Tri-Aqua.
	Stimulants.	Awake, NoDoz, Vivarin.
	Weight control products.	Anorexin Capsules, Dexatrim
Estrogens	Hair creams.	Le Kair.
Local anesthetics (usually benzocaine)	Antitussives.	Formula 44 Cough Disc, Silexin Cough Tablets. Vicks Cough Silencer Tablets.
	Dermatologic preparations.	Americaine First Aid Spray or Ointment. Dermoplast, Nupercainal Cream or Ointment, Medi-Quick, Solarcaine, Unguentine Spray. Unguentine Plus.
	Hemorrhoidal products.	Americaine, Anusol Ointment, Lanacane Medicated Creme, Nupercainal Cream or Ointment, Tronolane Anesthetic Hemorrhoidal Cream.
	Lozenges.	Cepacol Troches, Hold, Spec-T Sore Throat Products, Trokettes, Vicks Throat Lozenges.
	Toothache, cold sore, and teething products.	Baby Orajel, Benzodent, Numzident, Orabase B with Benzocaine, Orajel teething lotion, toothache drops.
	Weight loss products.	Diet Trim Tablets, Slim Line Candy and Gum, Spantrol.
Sodium (mg/tablet or mg/ 5 mL or as stated)	Analgesics.	Alka-Seltzer Effervescent Pain Reliever and Antacid (567), Bromo-Seltzer (761), Fizrin Powder (673), sodium salicylate (50 mg, 300 mg).
	Antacids.	Alka-Seltzer Effervescent Antacid (276), Amphojel Liquid (7), A.M.T. (7), BisoDol (157), Rolaids (53), Soda Mint (89).
	Cough syrups.	Coryban D (31), Cerose (38), Dristan (59), Pertussin 8-Hour Cough Formula (24), Formula 44 (68) Vicks Cough Syrup (54)
	Laxatives.	Instant Mix Metamucil (250 mg/packet), Fleets Enema (500 mg, of which 250–300 mg is absorbed), Phospho-Soda (55), Sal Hepatica (1000).
Sympathomimetics	Analgesics.	Allerest Headache Strength Tablets, Sinarest Tablets, Sine-Aid Sinus Headache Tablets.
	Asthma products.	Bronkaid, Bronkotabs, Primatene, Tedral.
	Cold/allergy preparations.	Many. Alka-Seltzer Plus, Allerest, Chlor-trimeton Decongestant, Contac, Coricidin 'D' Decongestant Tablets, Co-Tylenol, Dristan, Novafed, Novahistine Sinus Tablets, NyQuil, Sinarest, Sine-Aid, Sine-Off, Sinutab, Sudafed, Super Anahist, Triaminicin, 4-Way Cold Tablets.
	Cough syrups.	Cerose DM, Formula 44D, Robitussin-PE, Triaminic Expectorant, Triaminicol, and many others.
	Hemorrhoidal products.	A-Caine, Epinephricaine Rectal Ointment, HTO Stainless Manzan Hemorrhoidal Tissue Ointment, Pazo Hemorrhoid Ointment, Wyanoids Ointment.
	Lozenges.	Spec-T Sore Throat/Decongestant, Sucrets Cold Decongestant Formula.
	Menstrual products.	Femcaps, Fluidex-Plus with Diadax.
	Topical decongestants.	Many. Afrin, Benzedrex, Neo-Synephrine Hydrochloride, NTZ, Privine Sinex, Vicks Inhaler.
	Weight control products.	Appedrine Tablets, Dexatrim Capsules, Prolamine Capsules.

of this may take separate doses of analgesic in addition to that contained in the cold preparation.

(2) Select a product that contains a therapeutically effective dose.

(3) Select a product that lists its ingredients and their amounts. The label of a product should always be read carefully, since ingredients may be changed without public notification or change of brand name.

(4) Recommend a generic product if one is available.

(5) Be wary of "gimmicks" or advertising claims that claim specific superiority over similar products.

(6) For children, the dose, dosage form, and palatability of the product will be prime considerations.

Certain ingredients in OTC products should be avoided or used with caution in selected patients because they may exacerbate existing medical problems or interact with prescription medications the patient is taking. Many of the more potent OTC ingredients are "hidden" in products where their presence would not ordinarily be expected (Table 65–3). This lack of awareness of the ingredients present in OTC products and the belief by many physicians that OTC products are "ineffective and harmless" may cause diagnostic confusion and perhaps interfere with therapy.

For example, innumerable OTC products, including cough and cold preparations, decongestants, and appetite control products, contain sympathomimetics. These agents should be avoided or used cautiously in insulin-dependent diabetics and patients with hypertension, angina, or hyperthyroidism. Aspirin should be avoided by individuals with active peptic ulcer disease, certain platelet disorders, or patients taking oral anticoagulants.

Finally, overuse or misuse of OTC products may induce significant medical problems. A prime example is rebound congestion from the regular use of nasal sprays for more than 3 or 4 days. The improper and chronic use of some antacids (eg, aluminum hydroxide) may cause constipation and even impaction in elderly people as well as hypophosphatemia. Laxative abuse (chiefly by older people) can result in abdominal cramping and fluid and electrolyte disturbances. Insomnia, nervousness, and restlessness can result from the use of sympathomimetics or caffeine hidden in many OTC products (Table 65–3). The chronic systemic use of some analgesics containing large amounts of caffeine may produce rebound headaches, and long-term use of analgesics, especially those containing phenacetin, has been associated with interstitial nephritis. Acute ingestion of large amounts of aspirin or acetaminophen by adults or children causes serious toxicity. Antihistamines may cause sedation or drowsiness, especially when taken concurrently with sedative-hypnotics, tranquilizers, alcohol, or other central nervous system depressants. Finally, antihistamines, local anesthetics, antibiotics, antibacterial agents, counterirritants, p-aminobenzoic acid (PABA), preservatives, and deodorants contained in a myriad of OTC topical and vaginal products may induce allergic reactions.

There are three major drug information sources for OTC products. *Handbook of Nonprescription Drugs* is the most comprehensive resource for OTC medications; it evaluates ingredients contained in major OTC drug classes and lists the ingredients included in many OTC products. *Physicians' Desk Reference for Nonprescription Drugs,* a compendium of manufacturers' information regarding OTC products, is somewhat incomplete with regard to the number of products included and the consistency of information provided. *The New Medicine Show,* a consumer guide to the use of OTC products, critically evaluates these products and discusses their rational use. It is well written and factually correct. Any clinician who seeks more specific information regarding OTC products should find these references useful.

REFERENCES

Derby LE, Jick H. Renal parenchymal disease related to over-the-counter analgesic use. Pharmacotherapy 1991; 11:467–471.

Estrogens in cosmetics. Med Lett Drugs Ther (June 21) 1985;27:54.

Editors of Consumers Reports: *The New Medicine Show: Consumer's Union Practical Guide to Some Everyday Health Problems.* Consumer's Union of The United States, Inc, 1989.

Fredd SB. The OTC drug approval process. Am J Gastroenterol 1990;85:12–14.

Gossel TA. Implications of the reclassification of drugs from prescription-only to over-the-counter status. Clinical Therapeutics 1991;13:201–215.

Handbook of Nonprescription Drugs, 10th ed. American Pharmaceutical Association, 1993.

Kofoed LL. OTC drug overuse in the elderly: What to watch for. Geriatrics 1985;40:55–59.

Oster G et al. The risks and benefits of an Rx-to-OTC switch: The case of over-the-counter H2-blockers. Medical Care 1990;28:834–852.

Palmer HA. New OTCs: A selected review. Am Pharm 1992;NS32:26–38.

Pentel P. Toxicity of over-the-counter stimulants. JAMA. 1984;252:1898–1903.

Physicians' Desk Reference for Nonprescription Drugs, 14th ed. Medical Economics, 1994.

Smith MBH, Feldman W. Over-the-counter cold medications. A critical review of clinical trials between 1950 and 1991. JAMA 1993;269:2258–2263.

Rational Prescribing & Prescription Writing

66

Paul W. Lofholm, PharmD, & Bertram G. Katzung, MD, PhD

A practitioner's decision to treat a patient assumes that the patient has been evaluated and diagnosed. The practitioner then can select from a variety of therapeutic approaches. Medication, surgery, psychiatric treatment, radiation, physical therapy, health education, counseling, further consultation, or no therapy are some of the options available. Of these options, drug therapy is by far the most commonly chosen. In most cases this requires the writing of a prescription. A prescription is the prescriber's order to prepare or dispense a specific treatment—usually medication—for a specific patient. When a patient comes for an office visit, the physician or other authorized health professional will prescribe medications 67% of the time, and an average of one prescription per office visit is written because more than one prescription may be written at a single visit.

In this chapter, a plan for prescribing is presented. The physical form of the prescription, common prescribing errors, and legal requirements that govern various features of the prescribing process are then discussed. Finally, some of the social and economic factors involved in prescribing and drug use are described.

RATIONAL PRESCRIBING

Like any other process in medicine, writing a prescription should be based on a series of rational steps. These operations can be described as follows.

(1) Make a specific diagnosis. Prescriptions based merely on a desire to satisfy the patient's psychologic need for some type of therapy are often unsatisfactory and may result in adverse effects. A specific diagnosis, even if it is "presumptive," is required to move to the next step. In a 35-year-old woman with symmetric joint stiffness, pain, and inflammation that are worse in the morning and not associated with a history of infection, the diagnosis of rheumatoid arthritis would be considered. This diagnosis and the reasoning underlying it should be shared with the patient.

(2) Consider the pathophysiology of the diagnosis selected. If the pathology is well understood, the prescriber is in a much better position to select effective therapy. For example, increasing knowledge about the mediators of inflammation makes possible more effective use of NSAIDs and other agents used in rheumatoid arthritis. The patient should be provided with the appropriate level and amount of information about the pathophysiology. Many disease-oriented public and private agencies (eg, American Heart Association, American Cancer Society, Arthritis Foundation) provide information sheets suitable for patients.

(3) Select a specific therapeutic objective. A therapeutic objective should be chosen for each of the pathophysiologic processes defined in the preceding step. In a patient with rheumatoid arthritis, relief of pain by reduction of the inflammatory process is one of the major therapeutic goals that defines the drug groups which will be considered. Arresting the course of the disease process in rheumatoid arthritis is a different therapeutic goal that might give rise to consideration of other drug groups and prescriptions.

(4) Select a drug of choice. One or more drug groups will be suggested by each of the therapeutic goals specified in the preceding step. Selection of a drug of choice from among these groups will follow from a consideration of the specific characteristics of the patient and the clinical presentation. For certain drugs, characteristics such as age, race, other diseases, and other drugs being taken are extremely important in determining the most suitable drug for management of the present complaint. In the example of the patient with probable rheumatoid arthritis, it would be important to know whether she has a history of aspirin intolerance or ulcer disease, whether the cost of medication is an especially important factor, and whether there is a need for once-daily dosing. Based on this information, a drug would probably be selected from the nonsteroidal anti-inflammatory group. If the patient is intolerant of aspirin and does not have ulcer disease but does have a need for low-cost treatment, ibuprofen would be a rational choice.

(5) Determine the appropriate dosing regimen. The dosing regimen is determined primarily by the pharmacokinetics of the drug in that patient. If the patient is known to have disease of the major organs required for elimination of the drug selected, adjustment of the "average" regimen will be needed. For a drug such as ibuprofen, which is eliminated mainly by the kidney, renal function should be assessed. If renal function is normal, the half-life of ibuprofen (about 2 hours) requires administration 3 or 4 times daily. The dose suggested in drug handbooks and the manufacturer's literature is 400–800 mg 4 times daily.

(6) Devise a plan for monitoring the drug's action and determine an end point for the therapy. The prescriber should be able to describe to the patient the kinds of drug effects that will be monitored and in what way, including laboratory tests (if necessary) and signs and symptoms that the patient should report. For conditions that call for a limited course of therapy (eg, most infections), the duration of therapy should be made clear so that the patient will not stop taking the drug prematurely and will understand why the prescription probably need not be renewed. For the patient with rheumatoid arthritis, the need for prolonged—perhaps indefinite—therapy should be explained. The prescriber should also specify any changes in the patient's condition that would call for changes in therapy. For example, in the patient with rheumatoid arthritis, development of gastrointestinal bleeding would require an immediate change in drug therapy and a prompt workup of the bleeding. Major toxicities that require immediate attention should be explained clearly to the patient.

(7) Plan a program of patient education. The prescriber and other members of the health team should be prepared to repeat, extend, and reinforce the information transmitted to the patient as often as necessary. The more toxic the drug prescribed, the greater the importance of this educational program. The importance of informing and involving the patient in each of the above steps must be recognized, as shown by experience with teratogenic drugs (Shulman, 1989).

THE PRESCRIPTION

While a prescription can be written on any piece of paper (as long as all of the legal elements are present), it usually takes a specific form. A typical printed prescription form for outpatients is shown in Figure 66–1.

In the hospital setting, drugs are prescribed on a particular page of the patient's hospital chart called the physician's order sheet (POS) or a **chart order.** The contents of that prescription are specified in the medical staff rules by the hospital's Pharmacy and

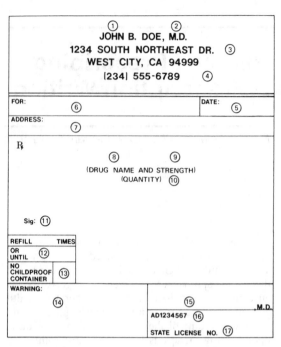

Figure 66–1. Common form of outpatient prescription. Circled numbers are explained in the text.

Therapeutics Committee. The patient's name is typed or written on the form; therefore, the orders consist of the name and strength of the medication, the dose, the route and frequency of administration, the date, other pertinent information, and the signature of the prescriber. Often the duration of therapy or the number of doses is not specified; therefore, medications are continued until the prescriber discontinues the order or until it is terminated as a matter of policy routine, eg, a stop order policy.

A typical chart order might be as follows:

6/14/94 (1) Ampicillin 500 mg IV q6h × 5 days
(2) ASA 0.6 g per rectum q6h prn temp over 101

[Signed] Janet B. Doe, M.D.

Thus, the elements of the hospital chart order are equivalent to the central elements (8–11) of the outpatient prescription.

Whether in the hospital or in an office practice setting, the implications of each element of the prescription should be understood.

Elements of the Prescription

The first four elements of the outpatient prescription establish the identity of the prescriber: name, license classification (ie, professional degree), address, and office telephone number. Before dispensing a prescription, the pharmacist must establish the prescriber's bona fides and should be able to contact the prescriber by telephone should any question arise. Element ° is the date the prescription was written. It should be near the top of the prescription form or at the beginning (left margin) of the order. Since the order has legal significance and usually has some temporal relationship to the date of the patient-prescriber interview, a pharmacist should refuse to fill a prescription without verification by telephone if too much time has elapsed since its writing.

Elements ± and " identify the patient by name and address. The patient's name and full address should be clearly spelled out.

The body of the prescription contains the elements ≥ to ⑩ that specify the medication, the quantity to be dispensed, the dose, and complete directions for use. When writing the drug name (element ≥), either the brand name (proprietary name) or generic name (nonproprietary name) may be used. Reasons for using one or the other are discussed below. The strength of the medication (element ×) should be written in metric units. However, the prescriber should be familiar with both systems now in use: apothecary and metric. For practical purposes, the following approximate conversions are useful:

> 1 grain (gr) = 0.065 grams (g), often rounded to 60 milligrams (mg)
> 15 gr = 1 g
> 1 ounce (oz) = 30 milliliters (mL)
> 1 teaspoonful (tsp) = 5 mL
> 1 tablespoonful (tbsp) = 15 mL
> 1 quart (qt) = 1000 mL
> 20 drops (gtt) = 1 mL
> 2.2 pounds (lb) = 1 kilogram (kg)
> 1 minim = 1 drop

The strength of a solution is usually expressed as the quantity of solute in sufficient solvent to make 100 mL; for instance, 20% potassium chloride solution is 20 grams per deciliter (g/dL). Both the concentration and the volume should be explicitly written out.

The quantity of medication prescribed should reflect the anticipated length of therapy, the cost, the need for continued contact with the clinic or physician, the potential for abuse, and the potential for toxicity or overdose. Consideration should be given also to the standard sizes in which the product is available and whether this is the initial prescription of the drug or a repeat prescription or refill. If 10 days of therapy are required to effectively cure a streptococcal infection, an appropriate quantity for the full course should be prescribed. Birth control pills are often prescribed for 1 year or until the next examination is due; however, some patients may not be able to afford a year's supply at one time; therefore, a 3-month supply might

be ordered, with refill instructions to renew three times or for 1 year (element 12). Finally, when first prescribing medications that are to be used for the treatment of a chronic disease, the initial quantity should be small, with refills for larger quantities. The purpose of beginning treatment with a small quantity of drug is to reduce the cost if the patient cannot tolerate the drug. Once it is determined that intolerance is not a problem, a larger quantity purchased less frequently is usually less expensive.

The directions for use (element ⑪) must be drug-specific and patient-specific. The simpler the directions, the better; and the fewer the number of doses (and drugs) per day, the better. Patient noncompliance (failure to adhere to the drug regimen) is a major cause of treatment failure. To help patients remember to take their medications, prescribers often give an instruction that medications be taken at or around mealtimes and at bedtime. However, it is important to inquire about the patient's eating habits and other life-style patterns, since many patients do not eat three regularly spaced meals a day, especially if they are sick or dieting.

The instructions on how and when to take medications, the duration of therapy, and the purpose of the medication must be explained to each patient by the physician and by the pharmacist. (Neither should assume that the other will do it.) Furthermore, the drug name, the purpose for which it is given, and the duration of therapy should be written on each label so that the drug may be identified easily in case of overdose. An instruction to "take as directed" may save the time it takes to write the orders out but often leads to noncompliance, patient confusion, and medication error. The directions for use must be clear and concise to avoid toxicity and to obtain the greatest benefits from therapy.

Patient education has been of concern to the FDA and professional groups and has resulted in several programs. The United States Pharmacopeial Convention (USP) annually publishes a three-volume work entitled *USP DI* ("Drug Information"). The first volume contains information for the professional (prescriber) and the second consists of short informational notes prepared for patients' use in understanding the drugs they are given. Over 1000 medications are covered in the 1994 edition. A program sponsored by the American Medical Association has the potential for similar usefulness to patients. Patient medication instruction (PMI) sheets in lay language for about 100 drugs have been prepared that provide patient information about individual drugs or classes of drugs. The content of the PMI sheet is similar to that of the *USP DI* note for the same drug. Information about *USP DI* and PMI sheets may be obtained from the USP Drug Information Division, 12601 Twinbrook Parkway, Rockville, MD 20852–1790.

Although directions for use are no longer written in

Latin, many Latin apothecary abbreviations (and some others included below) are still in use. Knowledge of these abbreviations is essential for the dispensing pharmacist and often useful for the prescriber. Some of the abbreviations still used are listed in Table 66–1.

Elements ⑫ to ⑭ of the prescription include refill information, waiver of the requirement for childproof containers, and additional labeling instructions (eg, name of drug on label, "may cause drowsiness," "do not drink alcohol"). Most pharmacists now put the name of the medication on the label unless directed otherwise by the prescriber, and some medications have the name of the drug stamped or imprinted on the tablet or capsule. Pharmacists also place the expiration date for the drug on the label. If the patient or prescriber does not request waiver of childproof containers, the pharmacist or dispenser must place the medication in such a container. Pharmacists may not refill a pre-

scription medication without authorization from the prescriber. Prescribers may grant authorization to renew prescriptions at the time of writing the prescription or over the telephone. Finally, the prescriber may request that special warning notices be placed on the label by the pharmacist. Elements ⑮ to ⑰ are the prescriber's signature and other identification data.

PRESCRIBING ERRORS

All prescription orders should be legible, unambiguous, dated (and timed in the case of a chart order), and signed clearly for optimal communication between prescriber, pharmacist, and nurse. Furthermore, a good prescription or chart order should contain sufficient information to permit the pharmacist or nurse to discover possible errors before the drug is dispensed or administered.

Table 66–1. Abbreviations used in prescriptions and chart orders. Note that several abbreviations have more than one meaning. It is always safer to write out the direction without abbreviating.

Abbreviation	Explanation	Abbreviation	Explanation
ā	before	p̄	after
ac	before meals	pc	after meals
AD	right ear	PO	by mouth
AS	left ear	PR	per rectum
AU	both ears	prn	when needed
agit	shake, stir	q	every
Aq	water	qam, om	every morning
Aq dest	distilled water	qd	every day
bid	twice a day	qh, q1h	every hour
c̄	with	q2h, q3h, etc	every 2 hours, every 3 hours, etc
cap	capsule		
D5W, D₅W	dextrose 5% in water	qhs	every night at bedtime
dil	dissolve, dilute	qid	four times a day
disp, dis	dispense	qod	every other day
dL	deciliter	qs	sufficient quantity
elix	elixir	rept, repet	may be repeated
ext	extract	Rx	take
g	gram	s̄	without
gr	grain	SC, SQ	subcutaneous
gtt	drops	Sig, S	label
h	hour	sos	if needed
hs	at bedtime	ss, s̄s̄	one-half
IA	intra-arterial	stat	at once
IM	intramuscular	sup, supp	suppository
IV	intravenous	susp	suspension
IVPB	IV piggyback	tab	tablet
kg	kilogram	tbsp, T	tablespoon (always write out "15 mL")
L, l	liter		
mEq, meq	milliequivalent	tid	three times a day
mg	milligram	tr, tinct	tincture
mL	milliliter	tsp	teaspoon (always write out "5 mL")
mcg, µg	microgram (always write out "microgram")	U (do not use this abbreviation)	units (always write out "units")
no	number		
non rep	do not repeat	vag	vaginal
OD	right eye	i, ii, iii, iv, etc	one, two, three, four, etc
OS, OL	left eye	ʒ	dram (in fluid measure, 3.7 mL)
OTC	over-the-counter		
OU	both eyes		

Several types of prescribing errors are particularly common. These include errors involving omission of needed information; poor writing perhaps leading to errors of drug dose or timing; and prescription of drugs that are inappropriate for the specific situation.

Omission Of Information

Errors of omission are common in hospital orders and may include instructions to "resume pre-op meds," which assumes that a full and accurate record of the "pre-op meds" is available; "continue present IV fluids," which fails to state exactly what fluids are to be given, in what volume, and over what time period; or "continue eye drops," which omits mention of which eye is to be treated as well as the drug, concentration, and frequency of administration. Chart orders may also fail to discontinue a prior medication when a new one is begun; may fail to state whether a regular or long-acting form is to be used; may fail to specify a strength or notation for long-acting forms; or may authorize "as-needed" (prn) use that fails to state what conditions will justify the need.

Poor Prescription Writing

Poor prescription writing is traditionally exemplified by illegible handwriting. However, other types of poor writing are common and often more dangerous. One of the most important is the misplaced or ambiguous decimal point. Thus ".1" is easily misread as "1," a tenfold overdose, if the decimal point is not unmistakably clear. This danger is easily avoided by always preceding the decimal point with a zero. On the other hand, appending an unnecessary zero after a decimal point increases the risk of a tenfold overdose, because "1.0 mg" is easily misread as "10 mg," whereas "1 mg" is not. The slash or virgule ("/") was traditionally used as a substitute for a decimal point. This should be abandoned because it is too easily misread as the numeral "1." Similarly, the abbreviation "U" for units should never be used because "10U" is easily misread as "100"; the word "units" should *always* be written out. Doses in micrograms should *always* have this unit written out because the abbreviated form ("μg") is very easily misread as "mg," a 1000-fold overdose! Orders for drugs specifying only the number of dosage units and not the total dose required should not be filled if more than one size dosage unit exists for that drug. For example, ordering "one ampule of furosemide" is unacceptable because furosemide is available in ampules that contain 20, 40, or 100 mg of the drug. Unclear handwriting can be lethal when drugs with similar names but very different effects are available, eg, acetazolamide and acetohexamide, methotrexate and metolazone (Huseby, 1991). In this situation, errors are best avoided by noting the indication for the drug in the body of the prescription, eg, "acetazolamide, for glaucoma."

Inappropriate Drug Prescriptions

Prescribing an inappropriate drug for a particular patient results from failure to recognize contraindications imposed by other diseases the patient may have, failure to obtain information about other drugs the patient is taking (including over-the-counter drugs), or failure to recognize possible physicochemical incompatibilities between drugs that may react with each other. Contraindications to drugs in the presence of other diseases or pharmacokinetic characteristics are listed in the discussions of the drugs described in this book. The manufacturer's package insert usually contains similar information. Some of the important drug interactions are listed in Appendix II of this book as well as in package inserts.

Physicochemical incompatibilities are of particular concern when parenteral administration is planned. For example, when calcium and phosphate ion concentrations are excessively high in a total parenteral nutrition (TPN) solution, precipitation will occur. Similarly, the simultaneous administration of antacids or products high in metal content may compromise the absorption of many drugs in the intestine, eg, tetracyclines. The package insert and the *Handbook of Injectable Drugs* are good sources for this information.

COMPLIANCE

Compliance is the extent to which patients follow instructions. There are four types of noncompliance leading to medication errors:

(1) The patient fails to obtain the medication. Some studies suggest that one-third of patients never have their prescriptions filled. Some patients leave the hospital without discharge medications, while others leave the hospital without having their prehospitalization medications resumed. Some patients cannot afford the medications prescribed.

(2) The patient fails to take the medication as prescribed. Examples include wrong dosage, wrong frequency of administration, improper timing or sequencing of administration, wrong route or technique of administration, or taking medication for the wrong purpose.

(3) The patient prematurely discontinues the medication. This can occur, for instance, if the patient incorrectly assumes that the medication is no longer needed because the bottle is empty or symptomatic improvement has occurred.

(4) The patient (or another person) takes medication inappropriately. For example, the patient may share a medication with others for any of several reasons.

Several factors encourage noncompliance. Some diseases cause no symptoms (eg, hypertension); patients with these diseases therefore have no symptoms to remind them to take their medications. Patients with very painful conditions, such as arthritis, may continually change medications in hope of finding a better one. Characteristics of the therapy itself can limit the degree of compliance; patients taking a drug once a day are much more likely to be compliant than those taking a drug four times a day. Various patient factors also play a role in compliance. Men living alone are much less likely to be compliant than married men of the same age. Packaging may also be a deterrent to compliance—elderly arthritic patients often have difficulty opening their medication containers. Lack of transportation as well as various social or personal beliefs about the use of medications are likewise barriers to compliance.

Strategies for improving compliance include enhanced communication between the patient and health care team members; assessment of personal, social, and economic conditions reflected in the patient's lifestyle; development of a routine for taking medications (eg, at mealtimes if the patient has regular meals); and provision of systems to assist taking medications (ie, devices that separate drug doses by day of the week, or medication alarm clocks that remind patients to take their medications); and mailing of refill reminders by the pharmacist to patients taking drugs chronically. The patient who is likely to discontinue a medication because of a perceived drug-related problem should receive instruction and education about how to monitor and understand the effects of the medication. Compliance can often be improved by enlisting the patient's active participation in the treatment.

LEGAL FACTORS (USA)

The United States government recognizes two classes of drugs: (1) over-the-counter (OTC) drugs and (2) those that require a prescription from a licensed prescriber (legend drugs). OTC drugs are those that can be safely self-administered by the layman for self-limiting conditions and for which appropriate labels can be written for lay comprehension. Half of all drug doses consumed by the American public are OTC drugs.

Physicians, dentists, podiatrists, and veterinarians—and, in some states, specialized pharmacists, nurses, physician's assistants, and optometrists—are granted authority to prescribe dangerous drugs (those bearing the federal legend statement, "Federal law prohibits dispensing without a prescription") on the basis of their training in diagnosis and treatment. Pharmacists are authorized to dispense prescriptions pursuant to a prescriber's order, provided that the medication order is appropriate and rational for the patient. Nurses are authorized to administer medications to patients subject to a prescriber's order.

Prescription drugs are controlled by the United States Food and Drug Administration. The federal legend statement as well as the package insert are part of the packaging requirements for all prescription drugs. The package insert is the official brochure setting forth the indications, contraindications, warnings, and dosing for the drug.

The prescriber, by writing and signing a prescription order, controls who may obtain prescription drugs. The pharmacist may purchase these drugs, but they may be dispensed only on the order of a legally qualified prescriber. Thus a "prescription" is actually three things: the physician's order in the patient's chart, the written order to which the pharmacist refers when dispensing, and the patient's medication vial with a label affixed.

While the federal government controls the drugs and their labeling and distribution, the state legislatures control who may prescribe drugs through their licensing boards, eg, the Board of Medical Examiners. Prescribers must pass examinations, pay fees, and—in the case of some states and some professions—meet other requirements for relicensure such as continuing education. If these requirements are met, the prescriber is licensed to order dispensing of drugs.

The federal government and the states further impose special restrictions on drugs with a potential for abuse. Drugs with abuse potential include opioids, hallucinogens, stimulants, and depressants (Chapter 31). Special requirements must be met when these drugs are to be prescribed. The Controlled Drug Act requires prescribers and dispensers to register with the Drug Enforcement Agency (DEA), pay a fee, receive a personal registration number, and keep records of all controlled drugs prescribed or dispensed. Every time a controlled drug is prescribed, a valid DEA number must appear on the prescription blank.

Table 66–2. Classification of controlled substances. (See inside front cover for examples.)

	Potential for Abuse	Other Comments
Class I	High	No accepted medical use; lack of accepted safety as drug.
Class II	High	Current accepted medical use. Abuse may lead to psychologic or physical dependence.
Class III	Less than I or II	Current accepted medical use. Moderate or low potential for physical dependence and high potential for psychologic dependence.
Class IV	Less than III	Current accepted medical use. Limited potential for dependence.
Class V	Less than IV	Current accepted medical use. Limited dependence possible.

Controlled drugs are classified according to their potential for abuse as shown in Table 66–2.

Prescriptions for substances with a high potential for abuse (class II) cannot be refilled. Prescriptions for class III, IV, and V drugs can be refilled, but there is a five-refill maximum, and in no case may the prescription be refilled after 6 months from the date of writing. Class II drug prescriptions may not be transmitted over the telephone, and some states require a special state-issued prescription blank. These restrictive prescribing laws are intended to limit the amount of drugs of abuse that are made available to the public.

Labeled & Unlabeled Uses of Drugs

In the USA, the FDA approves a drug only for the specific uses proposed and documented by the manufacturer in its New Drug Application (NDA; see Chapter 5). These approved (labeled) uses or indications are set forth in the package insert that accompanies the drug. For a variety of reasons, these labeled indications may not include all the conditions in which the drug might be useful. Therefore, a clinician may wish to prescribe the agent for some other, unapproved (unlabeled) clinical condition, often on the basis of adequate or even compelling scientific evidence. Federal laws governing FDA regulations and drug use place no restrictions on such unapproved use.* Even if the patient suffers injury from the drug, its use for an unlabeled purpose does not in itself constitute "malpractice." However, the courts may consider the package insert labeling as a complete listing of the indications for which the drug is considered safe unless the clinician can show (from the literature, etc) that his or her use of the agent is considered reasonable by his or her peers.

SOCIOECONOMIC FACTORS

Generic Prescribing

Prescribing by generic name offers the pharmacist flexibility in selecting the particular drug product to fill the order and the patient a potential savings if there is price competition. The brand name of a popular sedative is, for example, Valium by Roche. The generic (public nonproprietary) name of the same chemical substance adopted by United States Adopted Names (USAN) and approved by the Food

---

*"Once a product has been approved for marketing, a physician may prescribe it for uses or in treatment regimens or patient populations that are not included in the approved labeling. Such 'unapproved' or, more precisely, 'unlabeled' uses may be appropriate and rational in certain circumstances, and may, in fact, reflect approaches to drug therapy that have been extensively reported in medical literature."—FDA Drug Bull 1982;12:4.

and Drug Administration (FDA) is diazepam. All diazepam drug products in the USA meet the pharmaceutical standards expressed in *United States Pharmacopeia (USP)*. However, there are several manufacturers, and prices vary many fold. For other drugs, the difference in cost between the trade name product and generic products varies from less than twofold to more than 100 fold.

In some states and in many hospitals, pharmacists have the option of supplying a generically equivalent drug product even if a proprietary name has been specified in the order. If the physician wants a particular brand of drug product dispensed, handwritten instruction to "dispense as written" or words of similar meaning are required. Some government-subsidized health care programs require that pharmacists dispense the cheapest generically equivalent product in the inventory. However, the principles of drug product selection by pharmacists do not permit substituting one therapeutic agent for another; ie, dispensing trichlormethiazide for hydrochlorothiazide would not be permitted without the prescriber's permission even though these two diuretics may be considered pharmacodynamically equivalent.

It should not be assumed that all generic drug products are as satisfactory as trade name products, though most generics are satisfactory. Bioavailability—the effective absorption of the drug product—varies between manufacturers and sometimes between different lots of a drug produced by the same manufacturer. In the case of a very small number of drugs, which usually have a low therapeutic index, poor solubility, or a high ratio of inert ingredients to active drug content, a specific manufacturer's product may give more consistent results. In the case of life-threatening diseases, the advantages of generic substitution are probably outweighed by the clinical urgency so that the prescription should be filled as written.

In an effort to codify bioequivalence information, the FDA publishes *Approved Drug Products With Therapeutic Equivalence Evaluations,* with monthly supplements, commonly called "the Orange Book." The book contains listings of multisource products in one of two categories: Products coded "A" are considered bioequivalent to all other versions of that product with a similar "A" coding. Products not considered bioequivalent are coded "B." Of the approximately 8000 products listed, 90% are coded "A." This information is also published in volume 3 of *USP DI.*

Mandatory drug product selection on the basis of price is rapidly becoming common practice in the USA as third-party payers (insurance companies, etc) enforce money-saving regulations. The prescriber can usually override these controls by writing "dispense as written" on a prescription that calls for a brand-named product. However, in such cases, the patient may have to pay the difference between the dispensed product and the cheaper one.

Other Cost Factors

The private pharmacist bases his or her charges on the cost of the drug plus a fee for providing a professional service. Each time a prescription is dispensed, there is a fee. The prescriber controls the frequency of filling prescriptions by authorizing refills and specifying the quantity to be dispensed. Thus, the prescriber can save the patient money by prescribing standard sizes (so that drugs do not have to be repackaged) and, when chronic treatment is involved, by ordering the largest quantity consistent with safety and expense. Thus, optimal prescribing often involves consultation between the prescriber and the pharmacist.

REFERENCES

Bloom BS, Wierz DJ, Pauly MV: Cost and price of comparable branded and generic pharmaceuticals. JAMA 1986; 256:2523.

California Business and Professions Code, Chapter 9, Division 2, Pharmacy Law. Department of Consumer Affairs, Sacramento, Calif, 1985.

Do we pay too much for prescriptions? Consumer Reports 1993;58:668.

Final Report: *Task Force on Prescription Drugs.* Department of Health, Education, and Welfare, 1969.

Frazier LM et al: Can physician education lower the cost of prescription drugs? Ann Intern Med 1991;115:116.

Friedman D et al: Physician attitudes toward and knowledge about generic drug substitution. N Y State J Med 1987; 87:539.

Gennaro AR (editor): *Remington's Pharmaceutical Sciences,* 18th ed. Mack, 1990.

Huseby JS, Anderson P: Confusion about drug names. (Letter.) N Engl J Med 1991;325:588.

Jerome JB, Sagan P: The USAN nomenclature system. JAMA 1975;232:294.

King RE (editor): *Dispensing of Medication. A Practical Manual on the Formulation and Dispensing of Pharmaceutical Products,* 9th ed. Mack, 1984.

Krawelski JE, Pitt L, Dowd B: The effects of competition on prescription-drug product substitution. N Engl J Med 1983;309:213.

Kuehm SL, Doyle MJ: Medication errors: 1977 to 1988. Experience in medical malpractice claims. N J Med 1990; 87:27.

Lindley CM et al: Inappropriate medication is a major cause of adverse drug reactions in elderly patients. Age Aging 1992;21:294.

Shulman SR: The broader message of Accutane. Am J Public Health 1989;79:1565.

Strom BL: Generic drug substitution revisited. N Engl J Med 1987;316:1456.

United States Pharmacopeial Convention: *1994 USP DI.* Vol 1: *Advice for the Health Care Professional;* Vol 2: *Advice for the Patient;* Vol 3: *Approved Drug Products and Legal Requirements,* 14th ed. United States Pharmacopeial Convention, Inc., 1994.

Use of approved drugs for unlabeled indications. FDA Drug Bull 1982;12:4.

Vagelos PR: Are prescription prices high? Science 1991; 252:1080.

WHO Drug Action Committee: *Model Guide to Good Prescribing.* WHO, 1994.

Wu AW et al: Do house officers learn from their mistakes? JAMA 1991;265:2089.

Appendix I: Vaccines, Immune Globulins, & Other Complex Biologic Products

I

Steven L. Barriere, PharmD

Vaccines and related biologic products constitute an important group of agents that bridge the disciplines of microbiology, infectious disease, immunology, and immunopharmacology. While a complete discussion of these agents is beyond the scope of this book, a listing of the most important preparations is provided here. The reader who requires more complete information is referred to the sources listed at the end of this appendix.

ACTIVE IMMUNIZATION

Active immunization means the administration of antigens to the host to induce formation of antibodies and cell-mediated immunity. Immunization is practiced to induce protection against many infectious agents and may utilize either inactivated (killed) material or live attenuated agents (Table I–1). Desirable features of the ideal immunogen include complete prevention of disease, prevention of the carrier state, production of prolonged immunity with a minimum of immunizations, absence of toxicity, and suitability for mass immunization (ie, cheap and easy to administer). Active immunization is generally preferable to passive immunization, because host resistance is better (higher levels of antibody present at the time of exposure; coexisting cellular immunity in some cases) and the procedure need not be repeated as frequently. However, active immunization is associated with complications that do not occur with passive immunization, largely related to administering foreign proteins (eg, allergy, nonspecific toxic reactions).

Current recommendations for routine active immunization are given in Table I–2.

PASSIVE IMMUNIZATION

Passive immunization means transfer of immunity to a host using preformed immunologic effectors. From a practical standpoint, only immunoglobulins have been utilized for passive immunization, since passive administration of immune effector cells is technically difficult and has been associated with graft-versus-host reactions. Note, however, that nonimmune effector cells (eg, granulocytes) have been administered to humans with success, and cellular immunity has been transferred or augmented by other means (interferon, transfer factor).

Passive immunization with antibodies may be accomplished with either animal or human immunoglobulins in varying degrees of purity. These may contain relatively high titers of antibodies directed against a specific antigen or, as is true for pooled immune globulin, may simply contain antibodies found in most of the population.

Passive immunization is useful (1) for individuals unable to form antibodies (eg, congenital agammaglobulinemia); (2) for prevention of disease when time does not permit active immunization (eg, postexposure); (3) for treatment of certain diseases normally prevented by immunization (eg, tetanus); and (4) for treatment of conditions for which active immunization is unavailable or impractical (eg, snakebite).

Complications from administration of human immunoglobulins are rare. The injections may be moderately painful, and, rarely, sterile abscesses occur. Individuals with certain immunoglobulin deficiency states (IgA deficiency, etc) may occasionally develop hypersensitivity reactions to immune globulin that may limit therapy. Conventional immune globulin contains aggregates of IgG; it will cause severe reactions if given intravenously.

However, if the passively administered antibodies

Table I–1. Materials commonly used for active immunization. (DTP = diphtheria and tetanus toxoids and pertussis vaccine; DT = diphtheria and tetanus toxoids; Td = tetanus and diphtheria toxoids, adult type; and T = tetanus toxoid.)[1]

Pathogen or Disease	Product (Source)	Type of Agent	Route of Administration	Primary Immunization	Duration of Effect	Comments
Cholera	Cholera vaccine.	Killed bacteria	Subcut, IM	Two doses 1 week to 1 month apart.	6 months[2]	Fifty percent protective. Booster doses should be given every 6 months.
Diphtheria	DTP, DT (adsorbed) for child under 6; Td (adsorbed) for all others. Also available as diphtheria-toxoid alone.	Toxoid	IM	Three doses 4 weeks or more apart, with an additional dose 1 year later for a child under 6. (Can be given at the same time as polio vaccine if doses at least 8 weeks apart.)	10 years[3]	Use DT if convulsions follow use of DTP. Give schoolchildren and adults third dose 6–12 months after second.
Haemophilus influenzae infection	Purified type b polysaccharide (polyribosylribitol phosphate) and polysaccharide-protein (diphtheria toxoid) conjugate.	Polysaccharide ± protein	IM	One dose to children age 18–24 months.	Uncertain	Efficacy best when given above age 2 years, but recommended for high-risk infants at age 18 months. Conjugate vaccine is the preferred product.
Hepatitis B	Hepatitis B virus and surface antigen, inactivated (human plasma from carriers; recombinant protein).	Purified and inactivated virus coat protein	IM	Three doses: one initially, one at 1 month, and one at 6 months. Double dosage recommended for immunocompromised patients. One-tenth of standard dose (0.1 mL) given intradermally may be equally effective.	Years	Greater than 90% protective. Give preexposure to individuals who are not immune (ie, lack HBs antibody) and who are at high risk of acquiring disease (medical personnel, spouses of carriers, etc).
Influenza	Influenza virus vaccine, monovalent, bivalent, or trivalent (chick embryo). Composition of the vaccine is changed depending upon types of viruses causing disease.	Killed whole or split virus; types A and B	IM	One dose. (Two doses 4 weeks or more apart are preferable when a major new antigenic component is first incorporated into the vaccine. Two doses of the split virus products should be used in persons under age 13 years because of a lower incidence of adverse effects.)	1–3 years	Give immunization by November. Recommended annually for patients with cardiorespiratory disease, diabetes, other chronic diseases, and the elderly. Patients receiving chemotherapy for malignant disease are likely to respond better if immunized between or before courses of treatment.
Measles	Measles virus vaccine, live attenuated (chick embryo).	Live virus	Subcut	One dose at age 15 months. Give earlier if risk of measles is high (eg, an epidemic).	Permanent	Reimmunize if given before 15 months of age; may prevent natural disease if given less than 48 hours after exposure.
Meningococcal meningitis	Meningococcal polysaccharide vaccine, group A, group C, or both. A tetravalent preparation is also available containing serotypes A, C, W-135, and Y.	Polysaccharide	Subcut	One dose. Since primary antibody response requires at least 5 days, antibiotic prophylaxis with rifampin (600 mg or 10 mg/kg every 12 hours for 4 doses) should be given to household contacts.	?Permanent	Recommended in epidemic situations, for use by the military to prevent outbreaks in recruits, and possibly as an adjunct to antibiotic prophylaxis in preventing secondary cases in family contacts. Not reliably effective in children less than 2 years old.

Mumps	Mumps virus vaccine, live, Jeryl Lynn strain (chick embryo).	Live virus	Subcut	One dose.	Permanent	Reimmunize if given before 1 year of age.
Pertussis	DTP; also pertussis vaccine alone.	Killed bacteria	IM	As for DTP.	See[3]	Not generally recommended after age 6.
Pneumococci	Pneumococcal polysaccharide vaccine, polyvalent (23 of the most common serotypes).	Polysaccharide	Subcut, IM	0.5 mL.	Uncertain; probably at least 5 years	Recommended for individuals at high risk of serious pneumococcal disease: asplenia, sickling hemoglobinopathies, chronic cardiorespiratory ailments, etc. Variable efficacy in children; not recommended for those less than 2 years old.
Poliomyelitis	Poliovirus vaccine, live, oral, trivalent (monkey kidney, human diploid). Monovalent vaccines also available.)	Live virus types I, II, and III	Oral	Two doses 6–8 weeks or more apart, followed by a third dose 12 months later. (Can be given at the same time as primary DTP immunization.) A fourth dose before entering school is recommended for children immunized in the first 1–2 years of life.	Permanent	Recommended for adults only if at increased risk by travel to epidemic or highly endemic areas or occupational contact. (Inactivated vaccine may be preferable in this circumstance.) Individuals who have completed a primary series may take a single booster dose if the risk of exposure is high.
	Poliomyelitis vaccine. (Use the enhanced potency vaccine where possible.)	Killed virus types I, II, and III	IM	Three doses 1–2 months apart, followed by a fourth dose 6–12 months later and a fifth dose before entering school.[3]	2–5 years, perhaps longer	Killed virus vaccines are licensed but not readily available and are no longer recommended except for immunologically deficient patients or possibly for unimmunized adults who are at risk of exposure to poliomyelitis by reason of travel or immunization of their children.
Rabies	Rabies vaccine (human diploid cell–derived). Duck embryo or mouse brain–derived vaccines may still be available outside the USA but are generally more toxic than the human diploid cell-derived vaccine.	Killed virus	IM	**Preexposure:** Two doses 1 week apart, followed by third dose 2–3 weeks later. **Postexposure:** Five doses on days 0, 3, 7, 14, and 28. Always give rabies immune globulin as well (see Table II–3).	Unknown; probably > 2 years	Preexposure immunization only for occupational or avocational risk or residence in hyperendemic area. Antibody responses should be measured 3–4 weeks after last injection to ensure successful immunization, and repeat injection should be given if no response. Wounds should be copiously swabbed and flushed with soap and water. (See Table II–3 regarding use of hyperimmune serum or immune globulin.) For animal bite, consider antitetanus measures as well.

(continued)

Table I–1 (cont'd). Materials commonly used for active immunization. (DTP = diphtheria and tetanus toxoids and pertussis vaccine; DT = diphtheria and tetanus toxoids; Td = tetanus and diphtheria toxoids, adult type; and T = tetanus toxoid.)[1]

Pathogen or Disease	Product (Source)	Type of Agent	Route of Adminis- tration	Primary Immunization	Duration of Effect	Comments
Rubella	Rubella virus vaccine, live (human diploid).	Live virus	Subcut	One dose.	Permanent	Give after 15 months of age. Do not give during pregnancy. Women must prevent pregnancy for 3 months after immunization. Prevents disease but not infection.
Smallpox	Small pox vaccine (calf lymph, chick embryo).	Live vaccinia virus	Intrader- mal	One dose.	3 years	The only groups for whom smallpox vaccine is indicated at the present time are (1) military personnel and (2) laboratory personnel working with poxviruses. No longer required for international travel, as smallpox has been eradicated. Production for civilian use discontinued in May, 1983.
Tetanus	DTP, DT (adsorbed) for children under age 6; Td or T (adsorbed) for all others.	Toxoid	IM	Two doses 4 weeks or more apart; third dose 6–12 months after second dose.	10 years[3,4]	Give schoolchildren and adults a fourth dose 6–12 months after initial series of injections.
Tuberculosis	BCG vaccine (bacille Calmette-Guérin). Only the Danish substrain is available in the USA.	Live attenuated *Mycobacterium bovis*	Intrader- mal or subcut (per manu- facturer's recom- menda- tion)	One dose (0.1 mL intradermally).	?Permanent[5]	Not recommended for use in USA. Has shown highly variable efficacy.
Typhoid	Typhoid vaccine.	Killed bacteria	Subcut or intrader- mal	Two doses 4 weeks or more apart or 3 doses 1 week apart (less desirable).	3 years[3]	Seventy percent protective. Recommended only for exposure from travel, epidemic, or household carrier and not, eg, because of floods.
Yellow fever	Yellow fever vaccine (chick embryo) (17-D strain).	Live virus	Subcut	One dose.	10 years[2]	Recommended for residence in or travel to endemic areas of Africa and South America.

[1]Dosages for the specific product, including variations for age, are best obtained from the manufacturer's package insert. Immunizations should be given by the route suggested for the product.

[2]Revaccination interval required by international regulations.

[3]A single dose is a sufficent booster at any time after the effective duration of primary immunization has passed.

[4]For contaminated or severe wounds, give booster if more than 5 years has elapsed since full immunization or last booster.

[5]Test for PPD conversion 2 months later and reimmunize if there is no conversion.

Table I–2. Recommended schedule for active immunization and skin testing of children.[1]

Age	Product Administered	Test Recommended
Birth–4 days	HBV[2]	
2 months	DTP[3], HBV Oral poliovaccine,[4] trivalent	
4 months	DTP Oral poliovaccine, trivalent	
6 months	DTP, HBV Oral poliovaccine, trivalent (optional)	
15–19 months (15 months preferred)	DTP Measles vaccine[5] Mumps vaccine[6] Rubella vaccine[8] Oral poliovaccine, trivalent	
18–24 months	*Haemophilus influenzae* vaccine[4]	
4–6 years	DTP Oral poliovaccine, trivalent	Tuberculin test[7]
14–16 years	Rubella vaccine[8] Td[10]	Tuberculin test[7]

[1]Adapted from *MMWR* 1986;**35:**577.

[2]HBV: Hepatitis B vaccine.

[3]DTP: Toxoids of diphtheria and tetanus, alum-precipitated or aluminum hydroxide adsorbed, combined with pertussis bacterial antigen. Suitable for young children. Three doses of 0.5 mL intramuscularly at intervals of 4–8 weeks. Fourth injection of 0.5 mL intramuscularly given about 1 year later.

[4]Oral live poliomyelitis virus vaccine: Trivalent (types 1, 2, and 3 combined) given 3 times at intervals of 6–8 weeks and then as a booster 1 year later. Monovalent vaccine is rarely used now; it can be given at 6-week intervals, followed by a booster of trivalent vaccine 1 year later. Inactive (Salk type) trivalent vaccine is available but not recommended. *Note:* One sequence of monovalent vaccines (type 2, then 1, then 3) is in accordance with the recommendations of the US Public Health Service Advisory Committee on Immunization Practices. The American Academy of Pediatrics recommends the sequence 1, 3, 2.

[5]Live measles virus vaccine, 0.5 mL intramuscularly. When using attenuated (Edmonston) strain, give human gamma globulin, 0.01 mL/lb, injected into the opposite arm at the same time, to lessen the reaction to the vaccine. This is not advised with "further attenuated" (Schwarz) strain vaccine. Inactivated measles vaccine should not be used.

[6]Live mumps virus vaccine (attenuated), 0.5 mL intramuscularly.

[7]The frequency with which tuberculin tests are administered depends on the risk of exposure, ie, the prevalence of tuberculosis in the population group. The intervals indicated are the recommended minimum.

[8]Rubella live virus vaccine (attenuated) can be given between age 1 and puberty. Some physicians recommend rubella vaccine only for prepubertal girls. The entire contents of a single-dose vaccine vial, reconstituted from the lyophilized state, are injected subcutaneously. The vaccine must *not* be given to women who are pregnant or are liable to become pregnant within 3 months of vaccination. Women must be warned that there is a possibility of developing arthralgias or arthritis after vaccination. The cell culture-grown RA 27/3 rubella virus vaccine was licensed in the USA in 1979. No live vaccine should be given to immunodeficient patients, other than children with human immunodeficiency virus infection.

[9]*H influenzae* polysaccharide or polysaccharide-protein conjugate vaccine (preferred).

[10]Tetanus toxoid and diphtheria toxoid, purified, suitable for adults, given every 7–10 years.

are derived from animal sera, hypersensitivity reactions ranging from anaphylaxis to serum sickness may occur. Highly purified immunoglobulins, especially from rodents or lagomorphs, are the least likely to cause reactions. To avoid anaphylactic reactions, tests for hypersensitivity to the animal serum must be performed. If the tests give evidence of hypersensitivity, it is best to avoid that specific type of foreign protein (eg, horse serum) and obtain antibodies made in another animal (eg, human, goat, rabbit). If an alternative preparation is not available and administration of the specific antibody is deemed essential, desensitization can be carried out. Tests for hypersensitivity and desensitization protocols for antibody-containing proteins are described in Stites (1994).

Antibodies derived from human serum not only avoid the risk of hypersensitivity reactions but also have a much longer half-life in humans (about 23 days for IgG antibodies) than those from animal sources (5–7 days or less). Consequently, much smaller doses of human antibody can be administered to provide therapeutic concentrations for several weeks. These advantages point to the desirability of using human antibodies for passive protection whenever possible. Materials available for passive immunization are summarized in Table I–3.

LEGAL LIABILITY FOR UNTOWARD REACTIONS

It is the physician's responsibility to inform the patient of the risk of immunization and to employ vaccines and antisera in an appropriate manner. This may require skin testing to assess the risk of an untoward reaction. Some of the risks described above are, however, currently unavoidable; on balance, the patient and society are clearly better off for accepting the risks for routinely administered immunogens (eg, poliomyelitis and tetanus vaccines).

Manufacturers should be held legally accountable for failure to adhere to existing standards for production of biologicals. However, in the present litigious atmosphere in the USA, the filing of large liability claims by the statistically inevitable victims of good public health practice has caused manufacturers to abandon efforts to develop and produce low-profit but medically valuable therapeutic agents such as vaccines. Since the use and sale of these products are subject to careful review and approval by government bodies such as the Surgeon General's Advisory Committee on Immunization Practices and the Food and Drug Administration, "strict product liability" (liability without fault) may be an inappropriate legal standard to apply when rare reactions to biologicals, produced and administered according to government guidelines, are involved.

RECOMMENDED IMMUNIZATION OF ADULTS FOR TRAVEL

Every adult, whether traveling or not, must be immunized with tetanus toxoid and should also be fully immunized against poliomyelitis and diphtheria. In addition, every traveler must fulfill the immunization requirements of the health authorities of the countries to be visited. These are listed in *Health Information for International Travel,* available from the Superintendent of Documents, US Government Printing Office, Washington, DC 20402. *The Medical Letter on Drugs and Therapeutics* also offers periodically updated recommendations for international travelers (eg, see issue of April 6, 1990). Immunizations received in preparation for travel should be recorded on the International Certificate of Immunization. *Note:* Smallpox immunization is not recommended or required for travel anywhere.

Table I–3. Materials available for passive immunization.

Indication	Product	Dosage	Comments
Black widow spider bite	Black widow spider antivenin, equine.	One vial (6000 units) IM or IV	Use should be limited to children <15 kg, the only group with significant morbidity or mortality. Available from Merck Sharp & Dohme.
Botulism	ABE polyvalent anti-toxin, equine, (Hexavalent ABCDEF, bivalent AB, and monovalent E antitoxins are also available.)	One vial IV and 1 vial IM; repeat after 2–4 hours if symptoms worsen, and after 12–24 hours.	For treatment of botulism. Available from CDC.[1] Twenty percent incidence of serum reactions. Only type E antitoxin has been shown to affect outcome of illness. Prophylaxis is not routinely recommended but may be given to asymptomatic persons with unequivocal exposure.
Diphtheria	Diphtheria antitoxin, equine.	20,000 (1 vial)–120,000 units IM depending on severity and duration of illness. Same dose for children and adults.	For treatment of diphtheria. Active immunization and (perhaps) erythromycin prophylaxis rather than antitoxin prophylaxis should be given to nonimmune contacts of active cases. Contacts should be observed for signs of illness so that antitoxin may be administered if needed. Available from CDC.[1]
Hepatitis A ("infectious")	Immune globulin (ISG).	For postexposure prophylaxis, 0.02 mL/kg IM as soon as possible after exposure up to 2 weeks.	Modifies but does not prevent infection. Recommended for household contacts and other contacts of similar intensity. Also recommended prior to travel to endemic areas. Not recommended for office or school contacts unless an epidemic appears to be in progress.
		For chronic exposure, a dose of 0.06 mL/kg is recommended every 6 months. (0.02 mL/kg is effective for 2–3 months.)	Personnel of mental institutions, facilities for retarded children, and prisons appear to be at chronic risk of acquiring hepatitis A, as are those who work with nonhuman primates.
Hepatitis B ("serum")	Hepatitis B immune globulin (HBIG). Regular immune globulin may be effective as well.	0.06 mL/kg IM as soon as possible after exposure, preferably within 7 days. A second injection should be given 25–30 days after exposure, unless hepatitis B vaccine was given with first dose of HBIG.	Administer to nonimmune individuals as postexposure prophylaxis following either parenteral exposure to or direct mucous membrane contact with HBsAg-positive materials. Should not be given to persons already demonstrating anti-HBsAg antibody. Give a single dose of 0.13 mL/kg to newborns of mothers who develop hepatitis B in the third trimester and who have HBs antigenemia at time of delivery.
Hepatitis non-A, non-B	Immune globulin (ISG).	0.06 mL/kg IM as soon as possible after exposure.	Give to individuals with parenteral exposure to sera from patients with hepatitis, or other close contacts. Efficacy uncertain.
Hypogamma-globulinemia	Immune globulin (ISG).	0.6 mL/kg IM every 3–4 weeks; or 2–4 mL/kg IV every 4 weeks (it is the only globulin modified for IV use).	Give double dose at onset of therapy. Immune globulin is of no value in prevention of frequent infections in the absence of demonstrable hypogammaglobuinemia.
Measles	Immune globulin (ISG). (Measles immune globulin no longer available.)	0.25 mL/kg IM as soon as possible after exposure. This dose may be ineffective in immunoincompetent patients, who should receive 20–30 mL.	Live measles vaccine will usually prevent natural infection if given within 48 hours following exposure. If immunoglobulin is administered, delay immunization with live virus for 3 months.
Organ transplant	Antilymphocyte or antithymocyte immune serum or globulin, equine	Variable. See manufacturer's guidelines.	Used as adjunctive immuosuppressive agent in patients undergoing organ transplantation.
Pertussis	Pertussis immune globulin.	1.25 mL IM (child).	Efficacy doubtful, for treatment as well as for prophylaxis. Available from Cutter Laboratories.
Poliomyelitis	Immune globulin (ISG).	0.15 mL/kg IM.	Indicated only for exposed, unimmunized subject. Immunize with live or inactivated vaccine after 2–3 months, with subsequent boosters.

(continued)

Table I–3 (cont'd). Materials available for passive immunization.

Indication	Product	Dosage	Comments
Rabies	Rabies immune globulin. (equine antirabies serum is available but is much less desirable and requires a higher dose of about 500 units/20 kg of body weight.)	20 IU/kg, up to half of which is infiltrated locally at the wound site, and the remainder given IM.	Give as soon as possible after exposure. Recommended for all bite or scratch exposure to carnivores, especially bat, skunk, fox, coyote, or raccoon, despite animal's apparent health, if the brain cannot be immediately examined and found rabies-free. Not recommended for individuals with demonstrated antibody response from preexposure prophylaxis. Must be combined with rabies immunization. Available through CDC.[1]
Rh isoimmunization (from fetal-maternal transfusion)	Rh_0 (D) immune globulin.	In an Rh(D)-negative woman, one dose IM within 72 hours of abortion, amniocentesis, obstetric delivery of an Rh-positive infant, or transfusion of Rh-positive blood.	For nonimmune females only. May be effective at much greater postexposure interval; therefore, give even if more than 72 hours have elapsed. One vial contains 300 µg antibody and can reliably inhibit the immune response to a fetal-maternal bleed of up to 30 mL as estimated by the Betke-Kleihauer smear technique.
Rubella	Immune globulin (ISG).	20–40 mL IM at time of exposure.	Prevents disease in recipient but *not* in fetus of exposed mother—hence *not recommended*.
Snakebite	Coral snake antivenin, equine. Crotalid (pit viper) anti-venin, polyvalent, equine.	At least 3–5 vials IV (preferred) or IM.	Dose should be sufficient to reverse symptoms of envenomation. Consider antitetanus measures as well. Available from Wyeth Laboratories ([215] 688–4400) or CDC.[1]
Tetanus	Tetanus immune globulin. (Bovine and equine antitoxins are available but are not recommended. They are used at 10 times the dose of tetanus immune globulin.)	Prophylaxis: 250–500 units IM. Therapy: 3000–6000 units IM.	Give in separate syringe at different site from that of simultaneously adminstered toxoid. Recommended only for major or contaminated wounds in individuals who have had fewer than 2 doses of toxoid at any time in the past (fewer than 3 doses if wound is more than 24 hours old or otherwise highly tetanus-prone).
Vaccinia	Vaccinia immune globulin.	Prophylaxis: 0.3 mL/kg IM. Therapy: 0.6 mL/kg IM. May be repeated as necessary for treatment and at intervals of 1 week for prophylaxis.	May be useful in treatment of vaccinia of the eye, eczema vaccinatum, generalized vaccinia, and vaccinia necrosum and in the prevention of such complications in exposed patients with skin disorders. Available from CDC.[1]
Varicella	Varicella-zoster immune globulin or zoster immune globulin. (Regular immune globulin may be effective if this is unavailable.)	Give 125 units/10 kg (patients ≤ 50 kg), up to maximum of 625 units (patients > 50 kg). Give IM within 96 hours of exposure.	For immunosuppressed or immunoincompetent children under 15 years of age, known to be nonimmune (by laboratory test if possible), and with household, hospital (same 2- or 4-bed room or adjacent beds in large ward), or playmate (> 1 hour play indoors) contact with a known case of varicella-zoster; and for neonates whose mothers have developed varicella within 4 days before or 48 hours after delivery. The products modify natural disease but may not prevent the development of immunity. Expensive (about $400 to treat one adult).

[1]Centers for Disease Control, central number (404) 639–3670 during the day; (404) 639–2888 nights, weekends, and holidays (emergencies only).

Note: Passive immunotherapy or immunoprophylaxis should always be administered as soon as possible after exposure to the offending agent

Immune antisera and globulin are always given intramuscularly unless otherwise noted. Always question carefully and test for hypersensitivity before administering animal sera (see text).

In general, administration of live virus vaccines should be delayed at least 2 months after passive immunization with pooled human gamma globulin preparations.

REFERENCES

Brooks GF, Butel JS, Ornston LN: *Jawetz, Melnick, & Adelberg's Medical Microbiology,* 19th ed. Appleton & Lange, 1991.

*Centers for Disease Control: Diphtheria, tetanus, and pertussis: Guidelines for vaccine prophylaxis and other preventive measures. MMWR 1985;34:405.

*Centers for Disease Control: General recommendations on immunization. MMWR 1994;43:1.

*Centers for Disease Control: Health Information for International Travelers. [Updated annually with supplemental information in *Morbidity and Mortality Weekly Reports* as needed.]

*Centers for Disease Control: *Immunobiologic Agents and Drugs Available From the Centers for Disease Control: Descriptions, Recommendations and Adverse Reactions,* 3rd ed. 1982.

*Centers for Disease Control: Update: Prevention of *Haemophilus influenzae* type b disease. MMWR 1988;37:13.

*Centers for Disease Control: Recommendations for protection against viral hepatitis. MMWR 1985;34:313.

*Centers for Disease Control: Rubella prevention. MMWR 1984;33:301.

Committee on Immunization, American College of Physicians: *Guide for Adult Immunization.* American College of Physicians, 1985.

Conte JE, Barriere S: *Manual of Antibiotics and Infectious Diseases.* Lea & Febiger, 1992.

Cremer KJ et al: Vaccinia virus recombinant expressing herpes simplex virus type 1 glycoprotein D prevents latent herpes in mice. Science 1985;228:737.

Dreesman GR, Bronson JG, Kennedy RC (editors): *High Technology Route to Virus Vaccines.* American Society for Microbiology, 1985.

Germanier R (editor): *Bacterial Vaccines.* Beecham, 1984.

Grossman M, Cohen SN: Immunization. In: *Basic & Clinical Immunology,* 7th ed. Stites DP, Terr AI (editors). Appleton & Lange, 1991.

Health and Public Policy Committee, American College of Physicians: Compensation for vaccine-related injuries. Ann Intern Med 1984;101:559.

Iglehart JK: Compensating children with vaccine-related injuries. N Engl J Med 1987;316:1283.

Plotkin SA, Mortimer EA: *Vaccines.* Saunders, 1988.

Robbins JB, Hill JC, Sadoff JC: *Bacterial Vaccines.* Thieme-Stratton, 1982.

Sato Y, Kimura M, Fukumi H: Development of a pertussis component vaccine in Japan. Lancet 1984;1:122.

Schoenbaum SC: A perspective on the benefits, costs and risks of immunization. Chapter 9 in: *Seminars in Infectious Diseases.* Vol 3. Wernstein L, Fields BN (editors). Thieme- Stratton, 1980.

Scolnick EM et al: Clinical evaluation in healthy adults of a hepatitis B vaccine made by recombinant DNA. JAMA 1984;251:2812.

Simonsen O, Kjeldsen K, Heron I: Immunity against tetanus and effect of revaccination 25–30 years after primary vaccination. Lancet 1984;2:1240.

Stiehm ER: Standard and special human immune serum globulins as therapeutic agents. Pediatrics 1979;63:301.

Stites DP, Terr AI, Parslow TG (editors): *Basic & Clinical Immunology,* 8th ed. Appleton & Lange, 1994.

*May be obtained from the CDC, Building 1, Room SB 253, Atlanta 30333.

Appendix II: Important Drug Interactions

Philip D. Hansten, PharmD

MECHANISMS OF DRUG INTERACTIONS

One of the factors that can alter the response to drugs is the concurrent administration of other drugs. There are several mechanisms by which drugs may interact, but most can be categorized as pharmacokinetic (absorption, distribution, metabolism, excretion), pharmacodynamic, or combined toxicity. Knowledge of the mechanism by which a given drug interaction occurs is often clinically useful, since the mechanism may influence both the time course and the methods of circumventing the interaction. Some important drug interactions occur as a result of two or more mechanisms.

Pharmacokinetic Mechanisms

The gastrointestinal **absorption** of drugs may be affected by concurrent use of other agents that (1) have a large surface area upon which the drug can be adsorbed, (2) bind or chelate, (3) alter gastric pH, or (4) alter gastrointestinal motility. One must distinguish between effects on absorption *rate* and effects on *extent* of absorption. A reduction in only the absorption rate of a drug is seldom clinically important, whereas a reduction in the extent of absorption will be clinically important if it results in subtherapeutic serum levels of the drug.

The mechanisms by which drug interactions alter drug **distribution** include (1) competition for plasma protein binding and (2) displacement from tissue binding sites. Although competition for plasma protein binding can increase the free concentration (and thus the effect) of the displaced drug in plasma, the increase tends to be temporary owing to a compensatory increase in drug disposition. The clinical importance of protein binding displacement has probably been overemphasized; current evidence suggests that

such interactions are unlikely to result in adverse effects. Displacement from tissue binding sites would tend to increase the blood concentration of the displaced drug. Such a mechanism may contribute to the elevation of serum digoxin concentration by concurrent quinidine therapy.

The **metabolism** of drugs can be stimulated or inhibited by concurrent therapy. Induction (stimulation) of hepatic microsomal drug-metabolizing enzymes can be produced by drugs such as barbiturates, carbamazepine, glutethimide, phenytoin, primidone, rifampin, and rifabutin. Enzyme induction does not take place quickly; maximal effects usually occur after 7–10 days and require an equal or longer time to dissipate after the enzyme inducer is stopped. Inhibition of metabolism generally takes place more quickly than enzyme induction and may begin as soon as sufficient hepatic concentration of the inhibitor in achieved. However, if the half-life of the affected drug is long, it may take a week or more to reach a new steady-state serum level. Drugs that may inhibit hepatic microsomal metabolism of other drugs include allopurinol, chloramphenicol, cimetidine, ciprofloxacin, clarithromycin, diltiazem, disulfiram, enoxacin, erythromycin, fluconazole, isoniazid, itraconazole, ketoconazole, metronidazole, miconazole, omeprazole, phenylbutazone, propoxyphene, sulfonamides, and verapamil.

The renal **excretion** of active drug can also be affected by concurrent drug therapy. The renal excretion of certain drugs that are weak acids or weak bases may be influenced by other drugs that affect urinary pH. This is due to changes in ionization of the drug, thus altering its lipid solubility and therefore its ability to be absorbed back into the blood from the kidney tubule. For some drugs, active secretion into the renal tubules is an important elimination pathway. This process may be affected by concurrent drug therapy, thus altering serum drug levels and pharmacologic response.

Pharmacodynamic Mechanisms

When drugs with similar pharmacologic effects are administered concurrently, an additive or synergistic response is usually seen. The two drugs may or may not act on the same receptor to produce such effects. Conversely, drugs with opposing pharmacologic effects may reduce the response to one or both drugs. Pharmacodynamic drug interactions are relatively common in clinical practice, but adverse effects can be minimized if the interactions are anticipated and appropriate countermeasures taken.

Combined Toxicity

The combined use of two or more drugs, each of which has toxic effects on the same organ, can greatly increase the likelihood of organ damage. For example, concurrent administration of two nephrotoxic drugs can produce kidney damage even though the dose of either drug alone may have been insufficient to produce toxicity. Furthermore, some drugs can enhance the organ toxicity of another drug even though the enhancing drug has no intrinsic toxic effect on that organ.

PREDICTABILITY OF DRUG INTERACTIONS

The designations listed below (Table II–1) will be used here to *estimate* the predictability of the drug interactions. These estimates are intended to indicate simply whether or not the interaction will occur and do not always mean that the interaction is likely to produce an adverse effect. Whether the interaction occurs and produces an adverse effect or not depends upon (1) the presence or absence of factors that predispose to the adverse effects of the drug interaction (diseases, organ function, dose of drugs, etc) and (2) awareness on the part of the prescriber, so that appropriate monitoring can be ordered or preventive measures taken.

Table II–1. Important drug interactions.

HP = Highly predictable. Interaction occurs in almost all patients receiving the interacting combination.
P = Predictable. Interaction occurs in most patients receiving the combination.
NP = Not predictable. Interaction occurs only in some patients receiving the combination.
NE = Not established. Insufficient data available on which to base estimate of predictability.

Drug or Drug Group	Properties Promoting Drug Interaction	Clinically Documented Interactions

Alcohol	Chronic alcoholism results in enzyme induction. Acute alcoholic intoxication tends to inhibit drug metabolism (whether person is alcoholic or not). Severe alcohol-induced hepatic dysfunction may inhibit ability to metabolize drugs. Disulfiram-like reaction in the presence of certain drugs. Additive central nervous system depression with other central nervous system depressants.	**Acetaminophen:** [NE] Increased formation of hepatotoxic acetaminophen metabolites (in chronic alcoholics).
		Anticoagulants, oral: [NE] Increased hypoprothrombinemic effect with acute alcohol intoxication.
		Central nervous system depressants: [HP] Additive or synergistic central nervous system depression.
		Insulin: [NE] Acute alcohol intake may increase hypoglycemic effect of insulin (especially in fasting patients).
		Drugs that may produce a disulfiram-like reaction:
		  Cephalosporins: [NP] Disulfiram-like reactions noted with cefamandole, cefoperazone, cefotetan, and moxalactam.
		  Chloral hydrate: [NP] Mechanism not established.
		  Disulfiram: [HP] Inhibits aldehyde dehydrogenase.
		  Metronidazole: [NP] Mechanism not established.
		  Sulfonylureas: [NE] Chlorpropamide is most likely to produce a disulfiram-like reaction; acute alcohol intake may increase hypoglycemic effect (especially in fasting patients).

Allopurinol	Inhibits hepatic drug-metabolizing enzymes.	**Anticoagulants, oral:** [NP] Increased hypoprothrombinemic effect. **Azathioprine:** [P] Decreased azathioprine detoxification resulting in increased azathioprine toxicity. **Mercaptopurine:** [P] Decreased mercaptopurine metabolism resulting in increased mercaptopurine toxicity.
Antacids	Antacids may adsorb drugs in gastrointestinal tract, thus reducing absorption. Antacids tend to speed gastric emptying, thus delivering drugs to absorbing sites in the intestine more quickly. Some antacids (eg, magnesium hydroxide + aluminum hydroxide) alkalinize the urine somewhat, thus altering excretion of drugs sensitive to urinary pH.	**Digoxin:** [NP] Decreased gastrointestinal absorption of digoxin. **Iron:** [P] Decreased gastrointestinal absorption of iron with some antacids. **Ketoconazole:** [P] Reduced gastrointestinal absorption of ketoconazole due to increased pH (ketoconazole requires acid for absorption). **Quinolones:** [HP] Decreased gastrointestinal absorption of ciprofloxacin, norfloxacin, enoxacin (and probably other quinolones). **Salicylates:** [P] Increased renal clearance of salicylates due to increased urine pH; occurs only with large doses of salicylates. **Sodium polystyrene sulfonate:** [NE] Binds antacid cation in gut, resulting in metabolic alkalosis. **Tetracyclines:** [HP] Decreased gastrointestinal absorption of tetracyclines.
Anticholinergics	*See* Antimuscarinics.	*See* Antimuscarinics.

Anticoagulants, oral	Metabolism inducible. Susceptible to inhibition of metabolism. Highly bound to plasma proteins. Anticoagulation response altered by drugs that affect clotting factor synthesis or catabolism.	*Drugs that may increase anticoagulant effect:*
		  Amiodarone: [P] Inhibits anticoagulant metabolism.
		  Anabolic steroids: [P] Alter clotting factor disposition?
		  Chloramphenicol: [NE] Decreased dicumarol metabolism (possibly also warfarin).
		  Cimetidine: [HP] Decreased anticoagulant metabolism.
		  Ciprofloxacin: [NE] Probably inhibits anticoagulant metabolism.
		  Clofibrate: [P] Mechanism not established.
		  Danazol: [NE] Impaired synthesis of clotting factors?
		  Dextrothyroxine: [P] Enhances clotting factor catabolism?
		  Disulfiram: [P] Decreased anticoagulant metabolism.
		  Erythromycin: [NE] Probably inhibits anticoagulant metabolism.
		  Fluconazole: [NE] Decreased warfarin metabolism.
		  Metronidazole: [P] Decreased anticoagulant metabolism.
		  Miconazole: [NE] Mechanism not established.
		  Nonsteroidal anti-inflammatory drugs: [P] Inhibition of platelet function, gastric erosions; some agents increase hypoprothrombinemic response (unlikely with ibuprofen or naproxen).
		  Phenylbutazone: [HP] Inhibits anticoagulant metabolism.
		  Quinidine: [NP] Additive hypoprothrombinemia.
		  Salicylates: [HP] Platelet inhibition with aspirin but not with other salicylates; [P] large doses have hypoprothrombinemic effect.
		  Sulfinpyrazone: [NE] Mechanism not established.
		  Sulfonamides: [NE] Inhibit anticoagulant metabolism; displace protein binding.
		  Thyroid hormones: [P] Enhance clotting factor catabolism.

Table II–1 (cont'd.). Important drug interactions.

HP = Highly predictable. Interaction occurs in almost all patients receiving the interacting combination.
P = Predictable. Interaction occurs in most patients receiving the combination.
NP = Not predictable. Interaction occurs only in some patients receiving the combination.
NE = Not established. Insufficient data available on which to base estimate of predictability.

Drug or Drug Group	Properties Promoting Drug Interaction	Clinically Documented Interactions

Anticoagulants oral (*cont'd.*)	(see preceding page)	**Trimethoprim-sulfamethoxazole:** [P] Inhibits anticoagulant metabolism; displaces from protein binding.
		See also Alcohol; Allopurinol.
		Drugs that may decrease anticoagulant effect:
		  Aminoglutethimide: [P] Enzyme induction.
		  Barbiturates: [P] Enzyme induction.
		  Carbamazepine: [P] Enzyme induction.
		  Cholestyramine: [P] Reduces absorption of anticoagulant.
		  Glutethimide: [P] Enzyme induction.
		  Nafcillin: [NE] Mechanism not established.
		  Primidone: [P] Enzyme induction.
		  Rifampin: [P] Enzyme induction.
		Effects of anticoagulants on other drugs:
		  Hypoglycemics, oral: [P] Dicumarol inhibits hepatic metabolism of tolbutamide and chlorpropamide.
		  Phenytoin: [P] Dicumarol inhibits metabolism of phenytoin.

Antidepressants, tricyclic and second generation	Inhibition of amine uptake into postganglionic adrenergic neuron. Antimuscarinic effects may be additive with other antimuscarinic drugs. Metabolism inducible.	**Barbiturates:** [P] Increased antidepressant metabolism. **Carbamazepine:** [NE] Enhanced metabolism of antidepressants. **Cimetidine:** [P] Decreased antidepressant metabolism. **Clonidine:** [P] Decreased clonidine antihypertensive effect. **Fluoxetine:** [NE] Inhibits antidepressant metabolism. **Guanadrel:** [P] Decreased uptake of guanadrel into sites of action. **Guanethidine:** [P] Decreased uptake of guanethidine into sites of action. **Monoamine oxidase inhibitors:** [NP] Some cases of excitation, hyperpyrexia, mania, and convulsions, but many patients have received combination without ill effects. **Quinidine:** [NE] Inhibits antidepressant metabolism. **Sympathomimetics:** [P] Increased pressor response to norepinephrine, epinephrine, and phenylephrine.
Antihistamines, nonsedating (terfenadine, astemizole)	Susceptible to inhibition of hepatic metabolism.	**Erythromycin:** [NP] Reduced antihistamine metabolism; possible cardiac arrhythmias. Clarithromycin may produce similar effects. **Ketoconazole:** [P] Reduced antihistamine metabolism, increased serum levels, possible cardiac arrhythmia.
Antimuscarinics	Decreased gastrointestinal motility. This may increase bioavailability of poorly soluble drugs and reduce bioavailability of drugs degraded in gut. Combined use of more than one antimuscarinic or combination of an antimuscarinic with another drug with "hidden" antimuscarinic actions (especially OTC antihistamines) increases likelihood of antimuscarinic adverse effects.	**Combined antimuscarinics:** [P] Antimuscarinic adverse effects (eg, paralytic ileus, urinary retention, blurred vision). **Levodopa:** [P] Increased degradation of levodopa in gut; serum levodopa levels lowered.
Barbiturates	Induction of hepatic microsomal drug-metabolizing enzymes. Additive central nervous system depression with other central nervous system depressants.	**Beta-adrenoceptor blockers:** [P] Increased beta-blocker metabolism. **Calcium channel blockers:** [P] Increased calcium channel blocker metabolism. **Central nervous system depressants:** [HP] Additive central nervous system depression. **Corticosteroids:** [P] Increased corticosteroid metabolism. **Cyclosporine:** [NE] Increased cyclosporine metabolism. **Doxycycline:** [P] Increased doxycycline metabolism. **Estrogens:** [P] Increased estrogen metabolism. **Phenothiazines:** [P] Increased phenothiazine metabolism. **Quinidine:** [P] Increased quinidine metabolism. **Theophylline:** [NE] Increased theophylline metabolism; reduced theophylline effect. **Valproic acid:** [P] Decreased phenobarbital metabolism. *See also* Anticoagulants, oral; Antidepressants, tricyclic.

(*continued*)

Table II–1 (cont'd.). Important drug interactions.

HP = Highly predictable. Interaction occurs in almost all patients receiving the interacting combination.
P = Predictable. Interaction occurs in most patients receiving the combination.
NP = Not predictable. Interaction occurs only in some patients receiving the combination.
NE = Not established. Insufficient data available on which to base estimate of predictability.

Drug or Drug Group	Properties Promoting Drug Interaction	Clinically Documented Interactions
Beta-adrenoceptor blockers	Beta blockade (especially with nonselective agents such as propranolol) alters response to sympathomimetics with beta-agonist activity (eg, epinephrine). Beta-blockers that undergo extensive first-pass metabolism may be affected by drugs capable of altering this process. Beta blockers may reduce hepatic blood flow.	*Drugs that may increase beta-blocker effect:* **Chlorpromazine:** [P] Decreased metabolism of propranolol. **Cimetidine:** [P] Decreased metabolism of beta blockers that are cleared primarily by the liver, eg, propranolol. Less effect (if any) on those cleared by the kidneys, eg, atenolol, nadolol. **Furosemide:** [P] Decreased metabolism of propranolol. **Hydralazine:** [P] Decreased metabolism of propranolol. *Drugs that may decrease beta-blocker effect:* **Enzyme inducers:** [P] Barbiturates, phenytoin, and rifampin may enhance beta-blocker metabolism; other enzyme inducers may produce similar effects. **Nonsteroidal anti-inflammatory drugs:** [P] Indomethacin reduces antihypertensive response; other prostaglandin inhibitors probably also interact. *Effects of beta-blockers on other drugs:* **Clonidine:** [NE] Hypertensive reaction if clonidine is withdrawn while patient is taking propranolol. **Insulin:** [P] Inhibition of glucose recovery from hypoglycemia; inhibition of symptoms of hypoglycemia (except sweating); increased blood pressure during hypoglycemia. **Lidocaine:** [NE] Decreased clearance of intravenous lidocaine; increased plasma lidocaine levels. **Prazosin:** [P] Increased hypotensive response to first dose of prazosin. **Sympathomimetics:** [P] Increased pressor response to epinephrine (and possibly other sympathomimetics); this is more likely to occur with nonspecific beta-blockers.
Bile acid-binding resins	Resins may bind with orally adminstered drugs in gastrointestinal tract. Resins may bind in gastrointestinal tract with drugs that undergo enterohepatic circulation, even if the latter are given parenterally.	**Acetaminophen:** [NE] Decreased gastrointestinal absorption of acetaminophen. **Digitalis glycosides:** [NE] Decreased gastrointestinal absorption of digitoxin (possibly also digoxin). **Methotrexate:** [NE] Reduced gastrointestinal absorption of methotrexate. **Thiazide diuretics:** [P] Reduced gastrointestinal absorption of thiazides. **Thyroid hormones:** [P] Reduced thyroid absorption. *See also* Anticoagulants, oral.
Calcium channel blockers	Verapamil, diltiazem, and possibly nicardipine (but not nifedipine) inhibit hepatic drug-metabolizing enzymes. Metabolism of diltiazem, nifedipine, verapamil, and possibly other calcium channel blockers is inducible.	**Carbamazepine:** [P] Decreased carbamazepine metabolism with diltiazem and verapamil; possible increase in calcium channel blocker metabolism. **Cimetidine:** [NP] Decreased metabolism of calcium channel blockers. **Cyclosporine:** [P] Decreased cyclosporine metabolism with diltiazem, nicardipine, verapamil. **Rifampin:** [P] Increased metabolism of calcium channel blockers. *See also* Barbiturates, Theophylline.
Carbamazepine	Induction of hepatic microsomal drug-metabolizing enzymes. Susceptible to inhibition of metabolism.	**Cimetidine:** [P] Decreased carbamazepine metabolism. **Corticosteroids:** [P] Increased corticosteroid metabolism. **Danazol:** [P] Decreased carbamazepine metabolism. **Diltiazem:** [P] Decreased carbamazepine metabolism. **Doxycycline:** [P] Increased doxycycline metabolism. **Erythromycin:** [NE] Decreased carbamazepine metabolism. **Estrogens:** [P] Increased estrogen metabolism. **Fluoxetine:** [NE] Decreased carbamazepine metabolism. **Haloperidol:** [P] Increased haloperidol metabolism. **Isoniazid:** [P] Decreased carbamazepine metabolism. **Propoxyphene:** [HP] Decreased carbamazepine metabolism. **Theophylline:** [NE] Increased theophylline metabolism. **Troleandomycin:** [P] Decreased carbamazepine metabolism. **Verapamil:** [P] Decreased carbamazepine metabolism. *See also* Anticoagulants, oral; Antidepressants, tricyclic; Calcium channel blockers.
Chloramphenicol	Inhibits hepatic drug-metabolizing enzymes.	**Phenytoin:** [P] Decreased phenytoin metabolism. **Sulfonylurea hypoglycemics:** [P] Decreased sulfonylurea metabolism. *See also* Anticoagulants, oral.

Table II–1 (cont'd.). Important drug interactions.

HP = Highly predictable. Interaction occurs in almost all patients receiving the interacting combination.
P = Predictable. Interaction occurs in most patients receiving the combination.
NP = Not predictable. Interaction occurs only in some patients receiving the combination.
NE = Not established. Insufficient data available on which to base estimate of predictability.

Drug or Drug Group	Properties Promoting Drug Interaction	Clinically Documented Interactions
Cimetidine	Inhibits hepatic microsomal drug-metabolizing enzymes. (Ranitidine and newer H_2 blockers do not appear to do so.) May inhibit the renal tubular secretion of weak bases. Purportedly reduces hepatic blood flow, thus reducing first-pass metabolism of highly extracted drugs. (However, the ability of cimetidine to affect hepatic blood flow has been disputed.)	**Benzodiazepines:** [P] Decreased metabolism of alprazolam, chlordiazepoxide, diazepam, halazepam, prazepam, and clorazepate but not oxazepam, lorazepam, or temazepam. **Carmustine:** [NE] Increased bone marrow suppression. **Ketoconazole:** [NE] Decreased gastrointestinal absorption of ketoconazole due to increased pH in gut; other H_2 blockers would be expected to have the same effect. **Lidocaine:** [P] Decreased metabolism of lidocaine; increased serum lidocaine. **Phenytoin:** [NE] Decreased phenytoin metabolism; increased serum phenytoin. **Procainamide:** [P] Decreased renal excretion of procainamide; increased serum procainamide levels. Similar effect with ranitidine but smaller. **Quinidine:** [P] Decreased metabolism of quinidine; increased serum quinidine levels. **Theophylline:** [P] Decreased theophylline metabolism; increased plasma theophylline. *See also* Anticoagulants, oral; Antidepressants, tricyclic; Beta-adrenoceptor blockers; Calcium channel blockers, Carbamazepine.
Cyclosporine	Metabolism inducible. Susceptible to inhibition of metabolism.	**Aminoglycosides:** [NE] Possible additive nephrotoxicity. **Amphotericin B:** [NE] Possible additive nephrotoxicity. **Androgens:** [NE] Increased serum cyclosporine. **Diltiazem:** [NE] Decreased cyclosporine metabolism; increased cyclosporine effect. **Erythromycin:** [NE] Decreased cyclosporine metabolism; increased cyclosporine effect. **Fluconazole:** [NE] Decreased cyclosporine metabolism; increased cyclosporine effect. **Ketoconazole:** [NE] Increased serum cyclosporine with nephrotoxicity; due to decreased cyclosporine metabolism. **Lovastatin:** [NE] Myopathy and rhabdomyolysis noted in patients taking both drugs. **Phenytoin:** [NE] Increased cyclosporine metabolism; reduced cyclosporine effect. **Rifampin:** [P] Increased cyclosporine metabolism; reduced cyclosporine effect. **Verapamil:** [NE] Decreased cyclosporine metabolism; increased cyclosporine effect. *See also* Barbiturates; Calcium channel blockers
Digitalis glycosides	Digoxin susceptible to inhibition of gastrointestinal absorption. Digitalis toxicity may be increased by drug-induced electrolyte imbalance (eg, hypokalemia). Digitoxin metabolism inducible. Renal excretion of digoxin susceptible to inhibition.	*Drugs that may increase digitalis effect:* **Amiodarone:** [P] Reduced renal digoxin excretion leads to increased plasma digoxin concentrations. **Diltiazem:** [P] Increased plasma digoxin (usually 20–30 %) due to reduced renal and nonrenal clearance. **Erythromycin:** [NP] Increased gastrointestinal absorption of digoxin in certain patients; probably due to decreased inactivation of digoxin by intestinal flora. **Potassium-depleting drugs:** [P] Increased likelihood of digitalis toxicity. **Quinidine:** [HP] Reduced digoxin excretion; displacement of digoxin from tissue binding sites; digitoxin may also be affected. **Spironolactone:** [NE] Decreased renal digoxin excretion and interference with some serum digoxin assays. **Verapamil:** [P] Increased plasma digoxin levels. *Drugs that may decrease digitalis effect:* **Kaolin-pectin:** [P] Decreased gastrointestinal digoxin absorption. **Penicillamine:** [NE] Decreased plasma digoxin. **Rifampin:** [NE] Increased metabolism of digitoxin and possibly digoxin. **Sulfasalazine:** [NE] Decreased gastrointestinal digoxin absorption. *See also* Antacids; Bile acid-binding resins.

(continued)

Table II–1 (cont'd.). Important drug interactions.		

HP = Highly predictable. Interaction occurs in almost all patients receiving the interacting combination.
P = Predictable. Interaction occurs in most patients receiving the combination.
NP = Not predictable. Interaction occurs only in some patients receiving the combination.
NE = Not established. Insufficient data available on which to base estimate of predictability.

Drug or Drug Group	Properties Promoting Drug Interaction	Clinically Documented Interactions
Disulfiram	Inhibits hepatic microsomal drug-metabolizing enzymes. Inhibits aldehyde dehydrogenase.	**Benzodiazepines:** [P] Decreased metabolism of chlordiazepoxide and diazepam but not lorazepam and oxazepam. **Metronidazole:** [NE] Confusion and psychoses reported in patients receiving this combination; mechanisms unknown. **Phenytoin:** [P] Decreased phenytoin metabolism. *See also* Alcohol; Anticoagulants, oral.
Estrogens	Metabolism inducible. Entero-hepatic circulation of estrogen may be interrupted by alteration in bowel flora (eg, due to antibiotics).	**Ampicillin:** [NP] Interruption of enterohepatic circulation of estrogen; possible reduction in oral contraceptive efficacy. **Croticosteroids:** [P] Decreased metabolism of corticosteroids leading to increased corticosteroid effect. **Diazepam:** [NE] Decreased diazepam metabolism. **Griseofulvin:** [NE] Possible inhibition of oral contraceptive efficacy; mechanism unknown. **Phenytoin:** [NP] Increased estrogen metabolism; possible reduction in oral contraceptive efficacy. **Rifampin:** [NP] Increased estrogen metabolism; possible reduction in oral contraceptive efficacy. *See also* Barbiturates; Carbamazepine.
Iron	Binds with drugs in gastrointestinal tract, reducing absorption.	**Methyldopa:** [NE] Decreased methyldopa absorption. **Quinolones:** [P] Decreased absorption of ciprofloxacin, norfloxacin, and probably other quinolones. **Tetracyclines:** [P] Decreased absorption of tetracyclines; decreased efficacy of iron. *See also* Antacids.
Levodopa	Levodopa degraded in gut prior to reaching sites of absorption. Agents that alter gastrointestinal motility may alter degree of intraluminal degradation. Antiparkinsonism effect of levodopa susceptible to inhibition by other drugs.	**Clonidine:** [NE] Inhibits antiparkinsonism effect. **Monoamine oxidase inhibitors:** [P] Hypertensive reaction (carbidopa prevents the interaction). **Papaverine:** [NE] Inhibits antiparkinsonism effect. **Phenothiazines:** [P] Inhibits antiparkinsonism effect. **Phenytoin:** [NE] Inhibits antiparkinsonism effect. **Pyridoxine:** [P] Inhibits antiparkinsonism effect (carbidopa prevents the interaction). *See also* Antimuscarinics.
Lithium	Renal lithium excretion sensitive to changes in sodium balance. (Sodium depletion tends to cause lithium retention.) Susceptible to drugs enhancing central nervous system lithium toxicity.	**ACE inhibitors:** [NE] Probable reduced renal clearance of lithium; increased lithium effect. **Diuretics (especially thiazides):** [P] Decreased excretion of lithium; furosemide may be less likely to produce this effect than thiazide diuretics. **Haloperidol:** [NP] Occasional cases of neurotoxicity in manic patients, especially with large doses of one or both drugs. **Methyldopa:** [NE] Increased likelihood of central nervous system lithium toxicity. **Nonsteroidal anti-inflammatory drugs:** [NE] Reduced renal lithium excretion (except sulindac). **Theophylline:** [P] Increased renal excretion of lithium; reduced lithium effect.
Monoamine oxidase inhibitors	Increased norepinephrine stored in adrenergic neuron. Displacement of these stores by other drugs may produce acute hypertensive response. MAOIs have intrinsic hypoglycemic activity.	**Antidiabetic agents:** [P] Additive hypoglycemic effect. **Dextromethorphan:** [NE] Severe reactions (hyperpyrexia, coma, death) have been reported. **Fluoxetine:** [NE] Fatalities have been reported in patients taking this combination; more studies are needed. **Guanethidine:** [P] Reversal of the hypotensive action of guanethidine. **Narcotic analgesics:** [NP] Some patients develop hypertension, rigidity, excitation; meperidine may be more likely to interact than morphine. **Phenylephrine:** [P] Hypertensive episode, since phenylephrine is metabolized by monoamine oxidase. **Sympathomimetics (indirect-acting):** [HP] Hypertensive episode due to release of stored norepinephrine. *See also* Levodopa.

Table II–1 (cont'd.). Important drug interactions.

HP = Highly predictable. Interaction occurs in almost all patients receiving the interacting combination.
P = Predictable. Interaction occurs in most patients receiving the combination.
NP = Not predictable. Interaction occurs only in some patients receiving the combination.
NE = Not established. Insufficient data available on which to base estimate of predictability.

Drug or Drug Group	Properties Promoting Drug Interaction	Clinically Documented Interactions
Nonsteroidal anti-inflammatory drugs	Prostaglandin inhibition may result in reduced renal sodium excretion, impaired resistance to hypertensive stimuli, and reduced renal lithium excretion. Most NSAIDs inhibit platelet function; may increase likelihood of bleeding due to other drugs that impair hemostasis. Most NSAIDs are highly bound to plasma proteins. Phenylbutazone may inhibit hepatic microsomal drug metabolism (also seems to act as enzyme inducer in some cases). Phenybutazone may alter renal excretion of some drugs.	**ACE inhibitors:** [P] Decreased antihypertensive response. **Furosemide:** [P] Decreased diuretic, natriuretic, and antihypertensive response to furosemide. **Hydralazine:** [NE] Decreased antihypertensive response to hydralazine. **Methotrexate:** [NE] Possible increase in methotrexate toxicity (especially with anticancer doses of methotrexate). **Phenytoin:** [P] Decreased hepatic phenytoin metabolism. **Triamterene:** [NE] Decreased renal function noted with triamterene plus indomethacin in both healthy subjects and patients. *See also* Anticoagulants, oral; Beta-adrenoceptor blockers; Lithium.
Phenytoin	Induces hepatic microsomal drug metabolism. Susceptible to inhibition of metabolism.	*Drugs whose metabolism is stimulated by phenytoin:* **Corticosteroids:** [P] Decreased serum corticosteroid levels. **Doxycycline:** [P] Decreased serum doxycycline levels. **Methadone:** [P] Decreased serum methadone levels; withdrawal symptoms. **Mexiletine:** [NE] Decreased serum mexiletine levels. **Quinidine:** [P] Decreased serum quinidine levels. **Theophylline:** [NE] Decreased serum theophylline levels. **Verapamil:** [NE] Decreased serum verapamil levels. *See also* Cyclosporine, Estrogens. *Drugs that inhibit phenytoin metabolism:* **Amiodarone:** [P] Increased serum phenytoin; possible reduction in serum amiodarone. **Chloramphenicol:** [P] Increased serum phenytoin. **Felbamate:** [P] Increased serum phenytoin. **Fluconazole:** [P] Increased serum phenytoin. **Fluoxetine:** [P] Increased serum phenytoin. **Isoniazid:** [NP] Increased serum phenytoin; problem primarily with slow acetylators of isoniazid. *See also* Cimetidine; Disulfiram; Phenylbutazone. *Drugs that enhance phenytoin metabolism:* **Rifampin:** [P] Decreased serum phenytoin levels.
Potassium-sparing diuretics (amiloride, spironolactone, triamterene)	Additive effects with other agents increasing serum potassium concentration. May alter renal excretion of substances other than potassium (eg, digoxin, hydrogen ions).	**ACE inhibitors:** [NE] Additive hyperkalemic effect. **Potassium supplements:** [P] Additive hyperkalemic effect; especially a problem in presence of renal impairment. *See also* Digitalis glycosides; Nonsteroidal anti-inflammatory drugs.
Probenecid	Interference with renal excretion of drugs that undergo active tubular secretion, especially weak acids. Inhibition of glucuronide conjugation of other drugs.	**Clofibrate:** [P] Reduced glucuronide conjugation of clofibric acid. **Methotrexate:** [P] Decreased renal methotrexate excretion; possible methotrexate toxicity. **Penicillin:** [P] Decreased renal penicillin excretion. **Salicylates:** [P] Decreased uricosuric effect of probenecid (interaction unlikely with less than 1.5 g of salicylate daily).
Quinidine	Metabolism inducible. Inhibits cytochrome P450 2D6. Renal excretion susceptible to changes in urine pH.	**Acetazolamide:** [P] Decreased renal quinidine excretion due to increased urinary pH; elevated serum quinidine. **Amiodarone:** [NE] Increased serum quinidine levels; mechanism not established. **Kaolin-pectin:** [NE] Decreased gastrointestinal absorption of quinidine. **Rifampin:** [P] Increased hepatic quinidine metabolism. *See also* Anticoagulants, oral; Antidepressants, tricyclic; Barbiturates; Cimetidine; Digitalis glycosides; Phenytoin.

(continued)

Table II–1 (cont'd.). Important drug interactions.

HP = Highly predictable. Interaction occurs in almost all patients receiving the interacting combination.
P = Predictable. Interaction occurs in most patients receiving the combination.
NP = Not predictable. Interaction occurs only in some patients receiving the combination.
NE = Not established. Insufficient data available on which to base estimate of predictability.

Drug or Drug Group	Properties Promoting Drug Interaction	Clinically Documented Interactions
Quinolone antibiotics	Susceptible to inhibition of gastrointestinal absorption. Some quinolones inhibit hepatic microsomal drug metabolizing enzymes.	**Caffeine:** [P] Ciprofloxacin, enoxacin, pipedemic acid, and to a lesser extent, norfloxacin, inhibit caffeine metabolism. **Sucralfate:** [HP] Reduced gastrointestinal absorption of ciprofloxacin, norfloxacin, and probably other quinolones. **Theophylline:** [P] Ciprofloxacin, enoxacin, and to a lesser extent norfloxacin inhibit theophylline metabolism; lomefloxacin and ofloxacin appear to have little effect. *See also* Antacids; Anticoagulants, oral.
Rifampin	Induction of hepatic microsomal drug-metabolizing enzymes.	**Corticosteroids:** [P] Increased corticosteroid hepatic metabolism; reduced corticosteroid effect. **Ketoconazole:** [NE] Increased ketoconazole metabolism; reduced ketoconazole effect. **Mexiletine:** [NE] Increased mexiletine metabolism; reduced mexiletine effect. **Sulfonylurea hypoglycemics:** [P] Increased hepatic metabolism of tolbutamide and probably other sulfonylureas metabolized by the liver (including chlorpropamide). **Theophylline:** [P] Increased theophylline metabolism; reduced theophylline effect. *See also* Anticoagulants, oral; Beta-adrenoceptor blockers; Calcium channel blockers; Cyclosporine; Digitalis glycosides; Estrogens.
Salicylates	Interference with renal excretion of drugs that undergo active tubular secretion. Salicylate renal excretion dependent on urinary pH when large doses of salicylate used. Aspirin (but not other salicylates) interferes with platelet function. Large doses of salicylates have intrinsic hypoglycemic activity. Salicylates may displace drugs from plasma protein binding sites.	**Carbonic anhydrase inhibitors:** [NE] Increased acetazolamide serum concentrations; increased salicylate toxicity due to decreased blood pH. **Corticosteroids:** [P] Increased salicylate elimination; possible additive toxic effect on gastric mucosa. **Heparin:** [NE] Increased bleeding tendency with aspirin, but probably not with other salicylates. **Methotrexate:** [P] Decreased renal methotrexate clearance; increased methotrexate toxicity. **Sulfinpyrazone:** [HP] Decreased uricosuric effect of sulfinpyrazone (interaction unlikely with less than 1.5 g of salicylate daily). *See also* Antacids; Anticoagulants, oral; Probenecid.
Theophylline	Susceptible to inhibition of hepatic metabolism. Metabolism inducible.	**Benzodiazepines:** [NE] Inhibition of benzodiazepine sedation. **Diltiazem:** [P] Decreased theophylline metabolism; increased theophylline effect. **Clarithromycin:** [NE] Decreased theophylline metabolism; increased theophylline effect. **Erythromycin:** [P] Decreased theophylline metabolism; increased theophylline effect. **Smoking:** [HP] Increased theophylline metabolism; decreased theophylline effect. **Tacrine:** [P] Decreased theophylline metabolism; increased theophylline effect. **Troleandomycin:** [P] Decreased theophylline metabolism; increased theophylline effect. **Verapamil:** [P] Decreased theophylline metabolism; increased theophylline effect. *See also* Barbiturates; Carbamazepine, Cimetidine; Lithium, Phenytoin; Quinolones, Rifampin.

REFERENCES

Cluff LE, Petrie JC: *Clinical Effects of Interaction Between Drugs.* Excerpta Medica, 1974.

Hansten PD, Horn JR: *Drug Interactions.* Applied Therapeutics, Lea & Febiger. [Quarterly.]

Jankel CA, Speedie SM: Detecting drug interactions. A review of the literature. Ann Pharmacother 1990;24:982.

Lam YWF, Shepherd AMM: Drug interactions in hypertensive patients. Pharmacokinetic, pharmacodynamic and genetic considerations. Clin Pharmacokinet 1990; 18: 295.

Rizack MA (editor): *The Medical Letter Handbook of Adverse Interactions.* The Medical Letter, 1993.

Sands BF, Ciraulo DA: Cocaine drug-drug interactions. J Clin Psychopharmacol 1992;12:49.

Smith NT, Miller RD, Corbascio AN: *Drug Interactions in Anesthesia.* Lea & Febiger, 1981.

Tatro DS (editor): *Drug Interaction Facts.* Lippincott. [Quarterly.]

Index

NOTE: A *t* following a page number indicates tabular material and an *f* following a page number indicates a figure. Most drugs are listed under their generic names. Insofar as possible, when a drug trade name is listed, page references are for preparations available. For further detail refer to the generic name provided.